MOSBY'S POCKET DICTIONARY
of Medicine, Nursing, & Allied Health

Second Edition

Kenneth N. Anderson

Lois E. Anderson

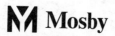 Mosby

St. Louis Baltimore Berlin Boston Carlsbad Chicago London Madrid

Naples New York Philadelphia Sydney Tokyo Toronto

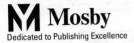
Mosby
Dedicated to Publishing Excellence

Executive Editor: N. Darlene Como
Senior Developmental Editor: Laurie Sparks
Project Manager: Karen A. Edwards
Senior Production Editor: Amy Adams Squire Strongheart
Manufacturing Supervisor: Theresa Fuchs

SECOND EDITION

Printed in the United States of America
Composition by Clarinda Company
Printing/binding by R.R. Donnelley & Sons Company

Mosby–Year Book, Inc.
11830 Westline Industrial Drive
St. Louis, Missouri 63146

Library of Congress Cataloging in Publication Data

Mosby's pocket dictionary of medicine, nursing, & allied health /
[edited by] Kenneth N. Anderson, Lois E. Anderson. — 2nd ed.
  p. cm.
 Abridgement of: Mosby's medical, nursing, and allied health
dictionary. 4th ed. 1993.
 ISBN 0-8016-7226-0
  1. Medicine—Dictionaries. 2. Nursing—Dictionaries.
I. Anderson, Kenneth II. Anderson, Lois E. III. Mosby's
medical, nursing, and allied health dictionary. IV. Title: Pocket
dictionary of medicine, nursing, & allied health.
 [DNLM: 1. Dictionaries, Medical. 2. Nursing—dictionaries. W 13
M8942 1994]
R121.M892 1994
610'.3—dc20
DNLM/DLC
for Library of Congress   94-4392
                 CIP

94 95 96 97 98 9 8 7 6 5 4 3 2 1

Contents

Consultants

The following individuals assisted in the development of this dictionary by acting as consultants to *Mosby's Medical, Nursing, and Allied Health Dictionary*, ed. 4, from which this dictionary is derived:

Betty J. Ackley, MSN, EdS, RN
Beth Arnold
Emilie J. Aubert, MA, PT
Addison Ault, PhD
Miriam G. Austrin, RN, BA
Edward S. Bennett, OD, MS, MEd
Diane M. Billings, EdD, RN, FAAN
Jackie Birmingham, RN, BSN, MS
Joseph Bittengle, MEd, RT(R) (ARRT)
Christine Bolwell, RN, MSN
Edward T. Bope, MD
Violet Breckbill, PhD, RN
Frances R. Brown, RN, PhD
Lynda Burroughs, BSN, MAN
Katharine G. Butler, PhD
Mary Butts, RN, CSN, MEd
Deborah Cameron, RN, BAAN, MEd (pending)
Gayle Kathleen Campbell, RN, BSN, BHSA
Toni Cascio, RN, MN, CCRN
Carol J. Chancey, RN, MS
Jane C. Clark, MN, RN, OCN
Jacqueline J. Clibourn, RN, HP (ASCP)
Charlene D. Coco, RN, MN
Jeffrey A. Cokely, PhD
Bruce Colbert, MS, RRT
Mary Boudreau Conover, RN, BS
Patricia Dardis, MS, RNC, CNS, FNP
Mardell Davis, RN, MSN, CETN
Hetty L. DeVroom, RN, BSN, CNRN
Clarice L. Dietrich, RDH, MA
Marcelline Eachus, RN, BSN
Jody A. Eckler, RN, BSN
Janet E. Edens, MSN, RN
Irene Eskildsen, RN, BSN
Ann Fagerness, RN, BSN, CNRN, CCRN, RNC
Neil B. Ford, PhD
Stephanie Fox-Young
Kerry E. George
Patty Hale, RN, MSN
M.A. Gray, MEd, BA, DipNEd
Mark Hamelink, CRNA, MSN

Wendy B. Hamilton, RN, BA, MEd
Mildred L. Hamner, RNC, EdD
Mary Barb Haq, PhD, RN, CS
Janice Hausauer, RN, MS, CCRN
E. Charles Healey, PhD
Susan R. Herman, MSN, RN
Marcia J. Hill, RN, MSN
Shirley P. Hoeman, PhD, RN
Michael S. Hudecki, PhD, DSc
Terry Karapas, RN, MS
Larita Norris Kaspar, MSN, RN
Jerry H. Kennedy, MN, RNCS
Patricia T. Ketcham, MSN, RN
Marjorie Knox, MPA, MA, RN
Kathy Kozak, RN, BA, BScN
Thomas Kraker, MEd, RT(R)
Joan M. Kulpa, EdD, MSN, RN
Mavis Kyle, RN, BScN, MHSA
Gail B. Ladwig, MSN, RN
Diane Langevin, CDA, RDH, MA
Linda Armstrong Lazure, RN, MSN
Elaine Lee
Donna M. Lewis-Stevens, RN, CMNP
Maxine E. Loomis, RNCS, PhD, FAAN
Carolyn Loop, BSRT, RT
Ruth Ludwick, RNC, PhD
Lois Irby Mack, MS, RN, CMAC
Jannetta MacPhail, PhD, MSN, FAAN, LLD(Hon)
Ann Marriner-Tomey, RN, BS, MS, PhD, FAAN
Lori Martell, BS, PhD
Sheryl A. Martz, RN, MSN
Edwina A. McConnell, RN, PhD
Linda McLeod, RegN, BSN, MContEd
Bozena B. Michniak, BSc, PhD, MRPharmSoc
Christina M. Mumma, CRRN, PhD
Helen K. Mussallem CC, BN, MA, EdD, LLD, DSc, DStJ, FRCN, MRSH
Dennis R. Myers, BA, RT(R)
Kim A. Neudorf, RN, BSN
Susan Jenkinson Neuman, RN, AS, BA
Donna Ortega, RN, MSN

Martin Owen
Kathleen Deska Pagana, PhD, RN
Michael A. Pagliarulo, EdD, PT
Glenda Paisley, BA, RN, BScN
Emma Ree Pelham, RN
Cindy A. Peternelj-Taylor, RN, BScN, MSc
Olga Carol Petrozella, RN, BSN, MSEd, MSN
Timothy Philipp, RN, PhD
Victoria Poole, RN, DSN
Joyce Powers, RN, MSN, CS
Joanne Profetto-McGrath, RN, BAPsych, BScN, MEd
Dale Rajacich, MS, CN, RN
William G. Rector Jr, MD
Diana Reding, RN, BS, MS
Kathlyn L. Reed, PhD, OTR, MLIS
Malvin E. Ring, DDS, MLS, FACD
Janet T. Robuck, MS, RD
Elizabeth A. Schenk, MSN, CRRN, RNCS
Sister Mary Arthur Schramm, CRNA, PhD
Charlotte Searle, RN, RM, BA, MA, LLD, DCur, DLitt et Phil
Kay See-Lasley, MS, RPh
Brenda K. Shelton, MS, RN, CCRN, OCN
Kim Sherer, RN, MN
Dan Shock, MA, RT(T)
Sandra L. Siehl, RN, BA, BSN, MSN
Nancy Simmons, RN, MS, CNA
Kathleen Simpson, RNC, MSN
Candace Skrapek, RegN, BN
Ida L. Slusher, MSN

Donna Phillips Smith, MS, RN
Robert R. Smith, BS, MS, PhD
Joanne Spaide, PhD, RD, LD
Sandra Mason Spengler, RN, MSN
Annette Smith Stacy, MSN, RN, CS, OCN
Kaye L. Stanek, PhD, RD, CN
Ruth Anderson Stephens, RN, PhD
Bernice D. Stiansen, RN, BScN
Stephen P. Storfer, MD
Michael Strysick
Patricia Greb Sullivan, RN, MS
Dorothy Thomas, RN, MSN
June D. Thompson, RN, MS
Catherine A. Trombly, ScD OTR/L, FAOTA
Mary L. Turgeon, EdD
Jean Urick, RN, MN
Margaret Uyeda
Louis Verardo, MD
Carole J. Petrosky Vozel, RN, C, PhD
Patricia Wells, AB
Pamela Becker Weilitz, MSN(R), RN
OT Wendel, PhD
Thomas Wenzka
John R. White Jr, PharmD
Jo Wiggens, RN, BSN, CEN
P. Sharon Wilson, RN, MEd, MN
William Wojciechowski, MS, RRT
Gale Woolley, EdD, ARNP
Caroline M. Wright, RN, CM, DipTeach(Nurs), MA(Hon), PhD
Bonnie Young, RN, BSN
Katherine E. Yutzy, RN, MSN
Hana Zemplenyi, MSc

Foreword

The complexity and continuing evolution of health science vocabularies require that students and professionals alike have an affordable, compact, yet thorough, quick reference to the language of their fields. *Mosby's Pocket Dictionary of Medicine, Nursing, and Allied Health* provides students and practitioners of the health sciences with a succinct and portable abridgement of *Mosby's Medical, Nursing, and Allied Health Dictionary,* which has been used by hundreds of thousands of nurses, allied health professionals, and physicians in their education and practice. The first edition of *Mosby's Pocket Dictionary of Medicine, Nursing, and Allied Health* was the first pocket dictionary to address the broad spectrum of health science terminology in the medical, nursing, and allied health professions.

To reflect new developments in many facets of health care, nearly 6,000 new entries have been added to this edition, and several hundred obsolete entries have been deleted. In addition, all new and former entries were reviewed by experts and updated, as needed, to reflect current knowledge and practice. To increase the durability of this portable reference, a hard yet flexible cover has been used for the second edition. We have also printed tabs on the edge of each page to designate the letter of the alphabet covered by that page. This will assist in quickly locating definitions.

The extensive vocabulary of the larger dictionary has been retained by restructuring and condensing its many encyclopedic entries while retaining the essential content of the definitions. An example can be seen in a comparison of the entries for drugs. The pocket edition defines the drug and relates the indications for its use, while the parent volume includes further information on contraindications and adverse effects.

In our pocket dictionary, the user will continue to find many of the valuable features of our larger dictionary, including clear pronunciations and etymologies for thousands of terms.

Development of this second edition of our pocket dictionary has taken the effort of many people. We gratefully acknowledge and appreciate the work of all who participated. The valuable contributions by all who were involved in the parent work, in particular, the authors whose works were consulted and the writers and editors, are also gratefully acknowledged.

The extremely positive response to the first edition leads us to believe that *Mosby's Pocket Dictionary of Medicine, Nursing, and Allied Health* will remain an eminently useful and usable resource. We welcome your comments and suggestions for improving future editions.

Guide to the Dictionary

A. Alphabetic order

The entries are alphabetized in dictionary style, that is, letter by letter, disregarding spaces or hyphens between words:

analgesic	**artificial lung**
anal	**artificially acquired**
membrane	**immunity**
analog	**artificial pacemaker**

The alphabetization is alphanumeric: words and numbers form a single list with numbers positioned as though they were spelled-out numerals: Nilstat / 90-90 traction / ninth nerve. (An example of the few exceptions to this rule is the sequence 17-hydroxycorticosteroid / 11-hydroxyetiocholanolone / 5-hydroxyindoleacetic acid, which can be found between the entries hydroxochloroquine sulfate and hydroxyl, not, as may be expected, 17-. . . in letter "S," 11-. . . in letter "E," and 5-. . . in letter "F.")

Small subscript and superscript numbers are disregarded in alphabetizing: No / N_2O / nobelium.

Compound headwords are given in their natural word order: abdominal surgery, not surgery, abdominal; achondroplastic dwarf, not dwarf, achondroplastic. There are few exceptions to this natural word order; nearly all of these concern formal classifications, for example: "comfort, alteration in: pain, a NANDA-accepted nursing diagnosis . . ."

(NOTE: In this guide, the term "headword" is used to refer to any alphabetized and nonindented definiendum, be it a single-word term or a compound term).

In some cases, there may be one or more terms that are synonymous with a headword or derived from a headword. If the synonym or derivation would immediately precede or follow the definition, it is not included as a separate entry. Therefore, if a term is not listed at the expected place, the reader might find it among the boldface terms of the immediately preceding or immediately following entry.

B. Etymology

ETYMOLOGY is shown for principal entries and in other instances where it contributes immediately to a better understanding of the meaning: "lysergide, . . . Also called LSD (an abbreviation of the original German name, *Lyserg-Säure-Diäthylamid), lysergic acid diethylamide, (slang) acid." "hangnail, . . . painful . . . (Hang is not related to the verb but is an old English word for pain.) . . ."

C. Pronunciation

All sounds, both English and non-English, are represented by letters or combinations of letters of the alphabet with few adaptations, and with the schwa (/ə/), the neutral vowel. Pronunciations are shown between slants. The following pronunciation key shows the symbols used:

Vowels

SYMBOLS	KEY WORDS
/a/	hat
/ä/	father
/ā/	fate
/e/	flesh
/ē/	she
/er/	air, ferry
/i/	sit
/ī/	eye
/ir/	ear
/o/	proper
/ō/	nose
/ô/	saw
/oi/	boy
/o͞o/	move
/o͝o/	book
/ou/	out
/u/	cup, love
/ur/	fur, first
/ə/	(the neutral vowel, always unstressed, as in) ago, focus
/ər/	teacher, doctor
/œ/	as in (French) feu /fœ/; (German) schön /shœn/
/Y/	as in (French) tu /tY/; (German) grün /grYn/

/N/	This symbol does not represent a sound but indicates that the preceding vowel is a nasal, as in French bon /bôN/, or international /aNternäsyōnäl'/.

Consonants

SYMBOLS	KEY WORDS
/b/	book
/ch/	chew
/d/	day
/f/	fast
/g/	good
/h/	happy
/j/	gem
/k/	keep
/l/	late
/m/	make
/n/	no
/ng/	sing, drink
/ng·g/	finger
/p/	pair
/r/	ring
/s/	set
/sh/	shoe, lotion
/t/	tone
/th/	thin
/th/	than
/v/	very
/w/	work
/y/	yes
/z/	zeal
/zh/	azure, vision

/kh/	as in (Scottish) loch /lokh/; (German) Rorschach /rôr′shokh/
/kh/	as in (German) ich /ikh/ (or, approximated, as in English fish: /ish/, /rīsh/)
/nyə/	Occurring at the end of French words, this symbol is not truly a separate syllable but an /n/ with a slight /y/ (similar to the sound in "onion") plus a near-silent /ə/, as in Bois de Boulogne /bo͞olō′nyə/

ACCENTS: Pronunciation is shown with primary and secondary accents. A raised dot shows that two vowels (or occasionally, two consonants) are pronounced separately.

Many of the numerous *Latin* terms in this dictionary are not given with pronunciation, mainly because there are different ways (all of them understood) in which Latin is pronounced by the English speaker and may be pronounced by speakers elsewhere. However, guidance is given in many cases, often to reflect common usage.

LATIN AND GREEK PLURALS: The spelling of Latin and Greek plurals is shown in most instances. However, when the plural formation is regular according to Latin and Greek rules, the pronunciation is usually not included.

NOTE: Notwithstanding the listing of Latin and Greek plurals in this dictionary, and the rules of Latin and Greek pluralization, in most instances it is acceptable or even preferable to pluralize Latin and Greek words according to the rules of English words. (For certain kinds of entries, both the English and the foreign plurals are given in this dictionary, usually showing the English form first, as, for example, in nearly all -oma nouns: hematoma, *pl.* hematomas, hematoma.)

A

a, symbol for **arterial blood.**

A, 1. abbreviation for **accommodation.** 2. symbol for **alveolar gas.** 3. abbreviation for **ampere.** 4. abbreviation for **anterior.** 5. abbreviation for **atomic weight.** 6. abbreviation for **axial.** 7. symbol for **mass number.**

A68, symbol for a protein found in the brain tissue of Alzheimer's disease patients. It is also found in the developing normal brains of fetuses and infants but begins to disappear by the age of 2 years.

Å, symbol for **angstrom.**

AA, 1. abbreviation for **achievement age.** 2. abbreviation for **Alcoholics Anonymous.** 3. abbreviation for **amplitude of accommodation.**

āa, āā, ĀĀ, (in prescriptions) abbreviation for *ana,* indicating an equal amount of each ingredient to be compounded.

AAAI, abbreviation for **American Academy of Allergy and Immunology.**

AACN, 1. abbreviation for **American Association of Colleges of Nursing.** 2. abbreviation for **American Association of Critical Care Nurses.**

AAFP, abbreviation for *American Academy of Family Practice.*

AAGP, abbreviation for *American Academy of General Practice.* Now called *American Academy of Family Practice.*

AAIN, abbreviation for **American Association of Industrial Nurses.**

AAMC, abbreviation for **American Association of Medical Colleges.**

AAMI, abbreviation for **Association for the Advancement of Medical Instrumentation.**

AAN, abbreviation for **American Academy of Nursing.**

AANA, abbreviation for **American Association of Nurse Anesthetists.**

AANN, 1. abbreviation for **American Association of Neuroscience Nurses.** 2. abbreviation for **American Association of Neurosurgical Nurses.**

AANNT, abbreviation for **American Association of Nephrology Nurses and Technicians.**

AAOHN, abbreviation for *American Association of Occupational Health Nurses.*

AAOMS, abbreviation for *American Association of Oral and Maxillofacial Surgeons.*

AAPA, abbreviation for **American Academy of Physicians' Assistants.**

AAPB, abbreviation for **American Association of Pathologists and Bacteriologists.**

AAPMR, abbreviation for **American Academy of Physical Medicine and Rehabilitation.**

AARP, abbreviation for **American Association of Retired Persons.**

AART, abbreviation for *American Association for Respiratory Therapy.*

AAUP, abbreviation for **American Association of University Professors.**

AAV, abbreviation for **adenoassociated virus.**

Ab, abbreviation for **antibody.**

abacterial /ab'aktir'ē·əl/, any atmosphere or condition free of bacteria; literally, without bacteria.

abaissement /ä'bäsmäN'/ [Fr, a lowering], a falling or depressing; in ophthalmology, the displacement of a lens.

abalienation /abāl'yənā'shən/ 1. a state of physical deterioration or mental decay. 2. a state of insanity. **–abalienate,** *v.,* **abalienated,** *adj.*

A band, the area between two I bands of a sarcomere, marked by partial overlapping of actin and myosin filaments.

abandonment of care, (in law) wrongful cessation of the provision of care to a patient, usually by a physician.

abarticular /ab'ärtik'yŏŏlər/ 1. of or pertaining to a condition that does not affect a joint. 2. of or pertaining to a site or structure remote from a joint.

abarticulation /ab'ärtik'yəlā'shən/, 1. dislocation of a joint. 2. a synovial joint.

abasia /əbā'zhə/ [Gk *a, basis* not step], the inability to walk, as in paralytic abasia that paralyzes the leg muscles. **–abasic, abatic,** *adj.*

abasia-astasia, See astasia-abasia.

abate /əbāt'/, [ME *abaten,* to beat down], to decrease or reduce in severity or degree.

abaxial /abak'sē·əl/ [L *ab, axis* from axle], 1. of or pertaining to a position outside the axis of a body or structure. 2. of or pertaining to a position at the opposite extremity of a structure.

Abbé-Estlander operation /ab'ē-est'-/ [Robert Abbé, American surgeon, b. 1851; Jakob A. Estlander, Finnish surgeon, b. 1831], a surgical procedure that transfers a full-thickness section of one oral lip to the other lip.

Abbé-Zeiss apparatus, /äbā'tsīs'/ [Abbé; Carl Zeiss, German optician, b. 1816], an apparatus for calculating the number of blood cells in a measured amount of blood.

Abbott pump /ab'ət/, a small portable pump that can be adjusted and finely calibrated to deliver precise amounts of medication in solution through an intravenous infusion set.

ABC, abbreviation for **aspiration biopsy cytology.**

abdomen /ab'dəmən, abdō'mən/ [L, belly], the portion of the body between the thorax and the pelvis. The abdominal cavity contains the lower portion of the esophagus, the stomach, the intestines, the liver, the spleen, the pancreas, and other visceral organs. The abdominal cavity is lined with two layers of peritoneum, a serous membrane. **–abdominal** /abdom'-/, adj.

abdominal actinomycosis. See **actinomycosis.**

abdominal adhesion, the binding together of tissue surfaces of abdominal organs, usually involving the intestines and causing obstruction. The condition may be the result of trauma or inflammation and may form after abdoninal surgery. The patient experiences pain, nausea, vomiting, and increased pulse rate. Surgery may be required.

abdominal aorta, the portion of the descending aorta that passes from the aortic hiatus of the diaphragm into the abdomen. It supplies many different parts of the body, such as the testes, ovaries, kidneys, and stomach. Its branches are the celiac, superior mesenteric, inferior mesenteric, middle suprarenal, renal, testicular, ovarian, inferior phrenic, lumbar, middle sacral, and common iliac arteries.

abdominal aortography, the process of producing a radiograph of the abdominal aorta using a radiopaque contrast medium.

abdominal aponeurosis, the conjoined tendons of the oblique and transverse muscles of the abdomen.

abdominal bandage, a broad supportive bandage commonly used after abdominal surgery.

abdominal binder, a bandage or elasticized wrap that is applied around the lower part of the torso to support the abdomen, sometimes applied after abdominal surgery to decrease discomfort. One kind of

abdominal binder is the **Scultetus binder.**

abdominal breathing, breathing in which the majority of respiratory work is done by the diaphragm and abdominal muscles.

abdominal cavity, the space within the abdominal walls between the diaphragm and the pelvic area, containing the liver, stomach, intestines, spleen, kidneys, and associated tissues and vessels.

abdominal delivery, the delivery of a child through a surgical incision in the abdomen. The procedure performed may be any of the several kinds of cesarean section.

abdominal fistula, an abnormal passage from an abdominal organ to the surface of the body. In a colostomy, a passage from the bowel to an opening on the surface of the abdomen is created surgically.

abdominal gestation, the implantation of a fertilized ovum outside the uterus but within the peritoneal cavity.

abdominalgia, /abdom'ənal'jə/ [L, abdomen, belly; Gk, algos, pain], a pain in the abdomen.

abdominal girth, the circumference of the abdomen, usually measured at the umbilicus.

abdominal hernia, a hernia in which a loop of bowel protrudes through the abdominal musculature, often through the site of an old surgical scar.

abdominal hysterectomy, the excision of the uterus through the abdominal wall.

abdominal nephrectomy, [L, abdominis, belly; Gk, nrphros, kidney, ektome, cutting out], the surgical removal of a kidney through an incision into the abdomen.

abdominal pain, acute or chronic localized or diffuse pain in the abdominal cavity. Abdominal pain is a significant symptom because its cause may require immediate surgical or medical intervention. The most common causes of severe abdominal pain are inflammation, perforation of an intraabdominal structure, circulatory obstruction, intestinal or ureteral obstruction, or rupture of an organ located within the abdomen. Specific conditions include appendicitis, perforated gastric ulcer, strangulated hernia, superior mesenteric arterial thrombosis, and small and large bowel obstruction. Conditions producing acute abdominal pain that may require surgery include appendicitis, acute or severe and chronic diverticulitis, acute and chronic cholecystitis, cholelithiasis, acute pancreatitis, perforation of a peptic ulcer, various intestinal obstructions, abdominal aortic aneurysms, and trauma affecting any of the abdominal organs. Gynecologic causes of acute abdominal pain that may require surgery include acute pelvic inflammatory disease, ruptured ovarian cyst, and ectopic pregnancy. Abdominal pain associated with pregnancy may be caused by the weight of the enlarged uterus; rotation, stretching, or compression of the round ligament; or squeezing or displacement of the bowel. Chronic abdominal pain may be functional or the result of overeating or aerophagia. Organic sources of abdominal pain include peptic ulcer, hiatus hernia, gastritis, chronic cholecystitis and cholelithiasis, chronic pancreatitis, pancreatic carcinoma, chronic diverticulitis, intermittent low-grade intestinal obstruction, and functional indigestion.

abdominal paracentesis, [L, *abdominis,* belly; Gk, *para,* near, *kentesis,* puncturing], the surgical puncturing of the abdominal cavity in order to remove fluid for diagnosis or treatment.

abdominal pregnancy, an extrauterine pregnancy in which the conceptus develops in the abdominal cavity after being extruded from the fimbriated end of the fallopian tube or through a defect in the tube or uterus. The placenta may implant on the abdominal or visceral peritoneum. Abdominal pregnancy may be suspected when the abdomen has enlarged but the uterus has remained small for the length of gestation. Abdominal pregnancies constitute approximately 2% of ectopic pregnancies and approximately 0.01% of all pregnancies. The condition results in perinatal death of the fetus in approximately 90% of cases, maternal death in approximately 6%. Because of its rarity, the condition may be unsuspected, and diagnosis is often delayed. Surgical removal of the placenta, sac, and embryo or fetus is necessary.

abdominal pulse, the pulse of the abdominal aorta.

abdominal quadrant, any of four topographic areas of the abdomen divided by two imaginary vertical and horizontal lines intersecting at the umbilicus. The divisions are the left upper quadrant (LUQ), the left lower quadrant (LLQ), the right upper quadrant (RUQ), and the right lower quadrant (RLQ).

abdominal reflex, a superficial neurologic reflex obtained by firmly stroking the skin of the abdomen, normally resulting in a brisk contraction of abdominal muscles in which the umbilicus moves toward the site of the stimulus. This reflex is lost in diseases of the pyramidal tract.

abdominal regions, the nine topographic subdivisions of the abdomen, determined by four imaginary lines, in a tic-tac-toe pattern, imposed over the anterior surface.

The upper horizontal line passes along the level of the cartilages of the nine ribs; the lower along the iliac crests. The two vertical lines extend on each side of the body from the cartilage of the eighth rib to the center of the inguinal ligament. The lines divide the abdomen into three upper, three middle, and three lower zones: right hypochondriac, epigastric, and left hypochondriac regions (upper zones); right lateral, umbilical, and left lateral regions (middle zones); right inguinal, pubic, and left inguinal regions (lower zones).

abdominal splinting, a rigid contraction of the muscles of the abdominal wall. It may result in hypoventilation and respiratory complications.

abdominal sponge, [L, *abdommen,* belly; Gk, *spoggia,* sponge], a thin, flat surgical sponge used as packing, absorbent, and covering for the viscera.

abdominal surgery, any operation that involves an incision into the abdomen, usually performed under general anesthesia. Some kinds of abdominal surgery are **appendectomy, cholecystectomy, colostomy, gastrectomy, herniorrhaphy,** and **laparotomy.**

abdominal tenaculum. See **tenaculum.**

abdominocentesis. See **paracentesis.**

abdominocyesis /abdom′inōsī·ē′sis/, an abdominal pregnancy.

abdominohysterectomy. See **abdominal hysterectomy.**

abdominohysterotomy, hysterotomy through an abdominal incision.

abdominopelvic cavity, the space between the diaphragm and the groin. There is no structurally distinct separation between the abdomen and pelvic regions.

abdominoperineal, pertaining to the abdomen and the perineum, including the pelvic area, female vulva and anus, and the male anus and scrotum.

abdominoplasty /abdom′ənōplas′tē/ plastic surgery involving the abdominal tissues.

abdominoscopy /abdom′inos′kəpē/ [L *abdomen;* Gk *skopein* to view], a procedure for examining the contents of the peritoneum in which an electrically illuminated tubular device is passed through a trocar into the abdominal cavity.

abducens, [L, drawing away], pertaining to a movement away from the median line of the body.

abducens muscle, the extraocular lateral rectus muscle that moves the eyeball outward.

abducens nerve /abd͞oo′sənz/ [L *abducere* to take away], the sixth cranial nerve. It controls the external rectus muscle, turn-

4

ing the eye outward. Also called *abducent nerve.*

abduct /abdukt'/, to move away from the median plane of the body.

abduction /abduk'shən/ [L *abducere* to take away], movement of a limb away from the body.

abduction boots, a pair of orthopedic casts for the lower extremities, available in both short-leg and long-leg configurations, with a bar incorporated at ankle level to provide hip abduction.

abductor /abduk'tər/ [L *abducere*], a muscle that draws a body part away from the midline, or one part from another.

Abernethy's sarcoma /ab'ərnē'thēz/, a malignant neoplasm of fat cells, usually occurring on the trunk.

aberrancy. See **aberrant ventricular conduction.**

aberrant /aber'ənt/ [L *aberrare* to wander] **1.** of or pertaining to a wandering from the usual or expected course, such as various ducts, nerves, and vessels in the body. **2.** (in botany and zoology) of or pertaining to an abnormal individual, such as certain atypical members of a species.

aberrant goiter, an enlargement of a supernumerary or ectopic thyroid gland.

aberrant ventricular conduction (AVC), the temporary abnormal intraventricular conduction of a supraventricular impulse, usually associated with a change in cycle length.

aberration /ab'ərā'shən/ [L *aberrare* to wander], **1.** any departure from the usual course or normal condition. **2.** abnormal growth or development. **3.** (in psychology) an illogical and unreasonable thought or belief, often leading to an unsound mental state. **4.** (in genetics) any change in the number or structure of the chromosomes. **5.** (in optics) any imperfect image formation caused by unequal refraction or focalization of light rays through a lens.

abetalipoproteinemia /əbā'təlip'ōprō'tinē'mē·ə/ [Gk *a, beta* not beta, *lipos* fat, *proteios* first rank, *haima* blood], a rare inherited disorder of fat metabolism, characterized by acanthocytosis, low or absent serum betalipoproteins, and hypocholesterolemia.

ABG, abbreviation for **arterial blood gas.**

abient /ab'ē·ənt/ [L *abire* to go away], characterized by a tendency to move away from stimuli. **−abience,** *n.*

ability, the capacity to act in a specified way because of the possession of appropriate skills and mental or physical fitness.

abiogenesis /ab'ē·ōjen'əsis/ [Gk *a, bios* not life, *genein* to produce], spontaneous

generation; the theory that organic life can originate from inanimate matter. **−abiogenetic,** *adj.*

abiosis /ab'ē·ō'sis/ [Gk *a, bios* not life], a nonviable condition or a situation that is incompatible with life. **−abiotic,** *adj.*

abiotrophy /ab'ē·ot'rəfē/ [Gk *a, bios* + *trophe* nutrition], a premature depletion of vitality or the deterioration of certain cells and tissues, especially those involved in genetic degenerative diseases. **−abiotrophic** /ab'ē·ətrō'fik/, *adj.*

ablate /ablāt'/, [L, *ab, latus,* carried away], to cut away or remove.

ablation /ablā'shən/ [L *ab, latus,* carried away], an amputation, an excision of any part of the body, or a removal of a growth or harmful substance.

ablatio placentae. See **abruptio placentae.**

ablepsia /əblep'sē·ə/ [Gk *a, blepein* not to see], the condition of being blind.

ABMS, abbreviation for *American Board of Medical Specialties.*

abnerval current [L *ab* from; Gk *neuron* nerve], an electric current that passes from a nerve to and through muscle.

abnormal behavior [L *ab, norma* away from rule], maladaptive acts or activities detrimental to the individual and to society.

abnormality /ab'nôrmal'itē/, [L *ab* away from; *norma* the rule], a condition that differs from the usual physical or mental state.

abnormal psychology, the study of mental disorders and maladaptive behavior, including neuroses and psychoses, and of normal phenomena that are not completely understood, such as dreams and altered states of consciousness.

ABO blood groups, the most important of several systems for classifying human blood based on the antigenic components of the red blood cell. The ABO blood group is identified by the presence or absence of two different antigens, A or B, on the surface of the erythrocyte. The four blood types in this grouping, A, B, AB, and O, are determined by and named for these antigens. Type AB indicates the presence of both antigens; type O the absence of both.

aboiement /ä'bô·ämäN'/, an involuntary making of abnormal, animal-like sounds, such as barking. Aboiement may be a clinical sign of Gilles de la Tourette's syndrome.

abort /abôrt'/ [L *ab* away from, *oriri* to be born] **1.** to deliver a nonviable fetus; to miscarry. **2.** to terminate a pregnancy before the fetus has developed enough to live ex utero. **3.** to terminate in the early stages or to discontinue before completion, as to arrest the usual course of a disease, to stop growth and development, or to halt a project.

aborted systole, a contraction of the heart that is usually weak and is not associated with a radial pulse.

abortifacient /əbôr′tifā′shənt/, **1.** producing abortion. **2.** an agent that causes abortion.

abortion [L ab + oriri], the spontaneous or induced termination of pregnancy before the fetus has developed enough to be expected to live if born. Kinds of abortion include **habitual abortion, infected abortion, septic abortion, threatened abortion,** and **voluntary abortion.**

abortion on demand, a concept promoted by pro-choice health advocates that it is the right of a pregnant woman to have an abortion performed at her request.

abortive infection, an infection in which some or all viral components have been synthesized, but no infective virus is produced.

abortus /əbôr′təs/, any incompletely developed fetus that results from an abortion, particularly one that weighs less than 500 g.

abortus fever, a form of brucellosis, the only one endemic to North America. It is caused by *Brucella abortus,* an organism so named because it causes abortion in cows. Infection in humans results from contact with cows infected with *B. abortus.*

abouchement /ä′bŏŏshmäN′/ [Fr, a tube connection], the junction of a small blood vessel with a large blood vessel.

aboulia. See **abulia.**

ABP, abbreviation for **arterial blood pressure.**

ABPM, abbreviation for **ambulatory blood pressure monitoring.**

abrachia /əbrā′kē·ə/ [Gk a, brachion not arm], the absence of arms. **–abrachial,** adj.

abrade, /əbrād′/ to remove the epidermis or other skin layers, usually by scraping or rubbing.

abrasion /əbrā′zhən/ [L abradere to scrape off], a scraping, or rubbing away of a surface by friction. Abrasion may be the result of trauma, such as a skinned knee; of therapy, as in dermabrasion of the skin for removal of scar tissue; or of normal function, such as the wearing down of a tooth by mastication. **–abrade,** v., **abrasive,** adj.

abreaction /ab′rē·ak′shən/ [L ab from, re again, agere to act], an emotional release resulting from mentally reliving or from bringing into consciousness, through the process of catharsis, a long-repressed, painful experience.

abrosia /əbrō′zhə/ [Gk, fasting], a condition caused by fasting or abstaining from food.

abruptio placentae [L ab away from, rumpere to rupture], separation of the placenta implanted in normal position in a pregnancy of 20 weeks or more or during labor before delivery of the fetus. It occurs approximately once in 200 births, and, because it often results in severe hemorrhage, it is a significant cause of maternal and fetal mortality. In severe cases, shock and death can occur in minutes. Cesarean section must be performed immediately and rapidly. If the pregnancy is near term, labor may be permitted or induced by means of amniotomy.

abscess /ab′səs/ [L abscedere to go away], a cavity containing pus and surrounded by inflamed tissue, formed as a result of suppuration in a localized infection (characteristically, a staphylococcal infection). Healing usually occurs when an abscess drains or is incised.

abscess of liver [L abscedere; AS lifer], an abscess in the liver cells, usually caused by an amebic infection, bacterial infections, or trauma, characterized by sweats and chills, pain, nausea, and vomiting.

abscissa /absis′ə/ [L ab away; scindere to cut], a point on a horizontal Cartesian coordinate plane measured from the y-axis running perpendicular to the plane.

absence seizure, an epileptic seizure characterized by a sudden, momentary loss of consciousness occasionally accompanied by minor myoclonus of the neck or upper extremities, slight symmetric twitching of the face, or a loss of muscle tone. The seizures usually occur many times a day without a warning aura and are most frequent in children and adolescents, especially at the time of puberty. The patient experiencing a typical seizure has a vacant facial expression and ceases all voluntary motor activity; with the rapid return of consciousness, the patient may resume conversation at the point of interruption without realizing what occurred. During and between seizures, the patient's electroencephalogram shows three cycle-per-second spike and wave discharges. Anticonvulsant drugs used to prevent absence seizures include ethosuximide and valproic acid.

absenteeism, (for health or related reasons) absence from work. The most common causes of absenteeism include influenza and occupationally related skin diseases.

absentia epileptica [L, *absens,* not present; Gk, *epilepsia,* seizure], a brief loss of consciousness. It usually occurs without convulsions but may be accompanied by minor involuntary muscle contractions. Formerly called **petit mal seizures.**

absent without leave (AWOL) /ā'wôl/ [L *absentia*], describing a patient who leaves a psychiatric facility without authorization.

absolute agraphia [L, *absolutus,* set loose; Gk, *a,* not, *graphein,* to write], a complete inability to write due to a central nervous system lesion. The person is unable to write even the letters of the alphabet.

absolute alcohol. See **dehydrated alcohol.**

absolute cephalopelvic disproportion. See **cephalopelvic disproportion.**

absolute discharge [L *absolutus* set free], a final and complete termination of the patient's relationship with a hospital.

absolute growth, the total increase in size of an organism or a particular organ or part, such as the limbs, head, or trunk.

absolute humidity, the actual weight or content of water in a measured volume of air. It is usually expressed in grams per cubic meter or pounds per cubic foot or cubic yard.

absolute refractory period. See **refractory period.**

absolute temperature, temperature that is measured from a base of absolute zero on either the Kelvin scale or the Rankine scale.

absolute threshold, [L *absolutus* set loose; AS *therscold*], the lowest point at which a stimulus can be perceived.

absolute zero, the temperature at which all molecular activity ceases. On the Kelvin scale, absolute zero is estimated to be equal to $-273°$ C.

absolutum glaucoma [L *abolutus;* Gk *cataract*], complete blindness in which vision is permanently lost and intraocular pressure is increased. The optic disc is white and deeply excavated and the pupil is usually widely dilated and immobile.

absorb /əbsôrb', əbzôrb'/ [L *absorbere* to swallow], 1. the act of taking up various substances; for example, the tissues of the intestines absorb fluids. 2. the energy transferred to tissues by radiation, such as an absorbed dose of radioactivity.

absorbable gauze, a gauzelike material, produced from oxidized cellulose, that can be absorbed. It is applied directly to bleeding tissue for hemostasis.

absorbable surgical suture, [L *absorbere;* Gk *cheirourgos,* surgery; L *sutura*], sutures made from material that can be completely removed by the body's phagocytes.

absorbance /əbsôr'bəns/, the degree of absorption of light or other radiant energy by a medium through which the radiant energy passes.

absorbed dose, (in radiotherapy) the energy imparted by ionizing radiation per unit mass of irradiated material at the place of interest. The SI unit of absorbed dose is the gray, which is 1 joule/kg and equals 100 rad.

absorbent /absôr'bənt/ [L *absorbere*], 1. capable of attracting and absorbing substances into itself. 2. a product or substance that can absorb liquids or gases.

absorbent dressing, a dressing of any material applied to a wound or incision to absorb secretions.

absorbent gauze, a gauze for absorbing fluids. The form, weight, and use vary. Gauze may be a fine fabric in rolled single layers for spiral bandages, or it may be a thick, many-layered pad for a sterile pressure dressing.

absorbifacient /absôr'bifā'shənt/ [L *absorbere* + *facere* to make], 1. any agent that promotes or enhances absorption. 2. causing or enhancing absorption.

absorption /absôrp'shən/ [L *absorbere*], 1. the incorporation of matter by other matter through chemical, molecular, or physical action, as the dissolving of a gas in a liquid or the taking up of a liquid by a porous solid. 2. (in physiology) the passage of substances across and into tissues, such as the passage of digested food molecules into intestinal cells or the passage of liquids into kidney tubules. Kinds of absorption are **agglutinin, cutaneous, external, interstitial, intestinal, parenteral,** and **pathologic absorption.** 3. (in radiology) the process of absorbing radiant energy by living or nonliving matter with which the radiation reacts.

absorption coefficient, (in radiology) the fractional loss in intensity of radioactive energy as it interacts with an absorbing material. It is usually expressed per unit of thickness or per unit mass.

absorption rate constant, a value describing how much drug is absorbed per unit of time.

absorption spectrum, the range of electromagnetic energy that is used for spectroanalysis, including both visible light and ultraviolet radiation; also, a graph of spectrum for a specific compound.

absorptivity /ab'sôrptiv'itē/, absorbance divided by the product of the concentration of a substance and the sample path length.

abstinence /ab'stinəns/, voluntary avoidance of any substance or the performance

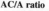

of any act for which the person has an appetite.

abstinence syndrome [L *abstinere* to hold back; Gk *syn* together, *dromos* course], the withdrawal symptoms experienced by a chemically dependent person who is suddenly deprived of a regular intake of alcohol or other drugs.

abstract /ab′strakt, abstrakt′/, a condensed summary of a scientific article, literary piece, or address.

abstraction /abstrak′shən/ [L *abstrahere* to drag away], a condition in which the teeth or other maxillary and mandibular structures are below their normal position or away from the occlusal plane.

abstract thinking, the final stage in the development of the cognitive thought processes in the child. During this phase, thought is characterized by adaptability, flexibility, and the use of concepts and generalizations.

abulia /əbōō′lyə/ [Gk *a, boule* not will], a loss of the ability or a reduced capacity to function voluntarily or to make decisions. Also spelled **aboulia.**

abuse /abyōōz/ [L *abuti* to waste], **1.** improper use of equipment, a substance, or a service, such as a drug or program, either intentionally or unintentionally. **2.** to attack or injure. A kind of abuse is **child abuse.**

abuse of the elderly, physical, psychologic, or material abuse, as well as violation of the rights of safety, security, and adequate health care of older adults. The victim of such abuse is generally an older woman with physical or mental impairment who lives with an adult child or another relative.

abutment [Fr *abouter* to place end to end], a tooth, root, or implant for the support and retention of a fixed or movable prosthesis.

abutment tooth, a tooth selected to support a prosthesis.

ABVD, an anticancer drug combination of doxorubicin, bleomycin, vinblastine, and dacarbazine.

Ac, symbol for the element **actinium.**

a.c., (in prescriptions) abbreviation for *ante cibum,* a Latin phrase meaning "before meals." The times of administration are commonly 7 AM, 11 AM, and 5 PM.

A-C, abbreviation for *alveolar-capillary.*

acacia gum, a dried, gummy exudate of the acacia tree *(Acacia senegal)* used as a suspending or emulsifying agent in medicines.

academic ladder [Gk *akademeia* school], the hierarchy of faculty appointments in a university through which a faculty member must advance from instructor to assis-

tant professor, to associate professor, and, finally, to professor.

acalculia /a′kalkōō′lyə/ [Gk *a* not; L *calculare* to reckon], a type of aphasia characterized by the inability to solve simple mathematic calculations.

acampsia /əkamp′sē·ə/ [Gk *a, kampsein* not to bend], a condition in which a joint becomes rigid.

acantha /əkan′thə/ [Gk *akantha* thorn], a spine or a spinous projection. **–acanthoid,** *adj.*

acanthiomeatal line /əkan′thē·ō′mē·ā′təl/ a hypothetical line extending from the external auditory meatus to the acanthion. In dentistry, a full maxillary denture is constructed so that its occlusal plane is parallel with this line.

acanthion, a point at the center of the base of the anterior nasal spine.

Acanthocheilonema perstans, /akan′-thōkī′lənē′mə/ a threadworm usually found in Africa. It commonly infects wild and domestic animals and occasionally invades the bloodstream of humans, causing a skin rash, muscle and joint pains, and various neurologic disorders.

acanthocyte /əkan′thəsīt′/ [Gk *akantha* + *kytos* cell], an abnormal red blood cell with spurlike projections giving it a thorny appearance.

acanthocytosis /akan′thōsītō′sis/ [Gk *akantha, kytos* + *osis* condition], the abnormal presence of acanthocytes in the circulating blood system.

acanthoid. See **acantha.**

acanthoma /ak′anthō′mə/ [Gk *akantha* + *oma* tumor], any benign or malignant tumor arising from the prickle-cell layer of the epidermis.

acanthoma adenoides cysticum. See **trichoepithelioma.**

acanthoma verrucosa seborrheica. See **seborrheic keratosis.**

acanthosis /ak′ənthō′sis/ [Gk *akantha* + *osis* condition], an abnormal thickening of the prickle-cell layer of the skin, as in eczema and psoriasis. **–acanthotic,** *adj.*

acanthosis nigricans /nē′grikanz′/, a skin disease characterized by hyperpigmented, warty lesions of the axillae and perianal body folds.

acapnia, /akap′nē·ə/ a deficiency of carbon dioxide in the blood. The condition is usually the result of hyperventilation.

AC/A ratio, in ophthalmology, the proportion between accommodative convergence (AC) and accommodation (A), or the amount of convergence automatically resulting from the dioptric focusing of the eyes at a specified distance. The ratio of accommodative convergence to accommodation is usually expressed as the quotient of accommodative convergence in prism diopters divided by the accommodative response in diopters.

acarbia /akär′bē·ə/ [Gk *a* not; L *carbo*, coal], **1.** a decrease in the bicarbonate level in the blood. **2.** any condition that lowers the bicarbonate level in the blood.

acardia /akär′dē·ə/ [Gk *a, kardia* not heart], a rare congenital anomaly in which the heart is absent. It is sometimes seen in a conjoined twin whose survival until birth depended on the circulatory system of its twin. **–acardiac,** *adj.*

acardius acephalus, an acardiac fetus that lacks a head and most of the upper part of the body.

acardius acormus, an acardiac fetus that has a grossly defective trunk.

acardius amorphus, an acardiac fetus with a rudimentary body that does not resemble the normal form.

acariasis /ak′ərī′əsis/ [Gk *akari* mite, *osis* condition], any disease caused by an acarid, such as scrub typhus, which is transmitted by trombiculid mites.

acarid /ak′ərid/, one of the many mites that are members of the order Acarina, which includes a great number of parasitic and free-living organisms. Important as vectors of scrub typhus and other rickettsial agents are the six-legged larvae of trombiculid mites, which are parasitic of humans, many other mammals, and birds.

acc, Acc, abbreviation for **accommodation.**

accelerated hypertension. See **malignant hypertension.**

accelerated idiojunctional rhythm /id′ē·ō-/, an automatic junctional rhythm at a rate exceeding the normal firing rate of the junction but slower than 100 per minute (60 to 100 per minute) and without retrograde conduction to the atria.

accelerated idioventricular rhythm (AIVR), an automatic ectopic ventricular rhythm, faster than the normal rate of the His-Purkinje system but slower than 100 per minute (50 to 100 per minute) and without retrograde conduction to the atria.

accelerated junctional rhythm, an ectopic junctional heart rhythm with a rate that exceeds the normal firing rate of junctional tissue, with or without retrograde atrial conduction.

acceleration [L *accelerare* to quicken], an increase in the speed or velocity of an object or reaction. **–accelerator,** *n.*

acceleration phase, (in obstetrics) the first period of active labor, characterized by an increased rate of dilatation of the cervical os as charted on a Friedman curve.

accelerator urinae. See **bulbocavernosus.**

accentuation, [L *accentus* accent], an increase in distinctness or loudness, as in heart sounds.

acceptable daily intake (ADI), the maximum amount of any substance that can be safely ingested by a human. Ingestion in excess of this amount may cause toxic effects.

acceptance of individuality, (in psychiatry) an index of family health by which diff erentiation or individuation is a valued goal.

acceptance of separation, an indicator of mental well-being in a family by which a loss is mourned and the family moves on to growth issues.

acceptor [L *accipere* to receive], **1.** an organism that receives from another person or organism living tissue, such as transfused blood or a transplanted organ. **2.** a substance or compound that combines with a part of another substance or compound.

access cavity [L *accedere* to approach], a coronal opening in a tooth, required for effective cleaning, shaping, and filling of the pulp space.

accessory /akses′ərē/ [L *accessonis* appendage], **1.** a supplement used chiefly for convenience or for safety, such as the electric elevator mechanisms for hospital beds. **2.** a structure that serves one of the main anatomic systems, such as the accessory organs of the skin, the hair, the nails, and the skin glands.

accessory chromosome, an unpaired X or Y sex chromosome.

accessory diaphragm, a congenital defect in which a second diaphragm or portion of a diaphragm develops in the chest. It may be separated from the true diaphragm by a lobe of a lung.

accessory ligament, [L *accessionis* a thing added, *ligare* to bind], a ligament that helps to strengthen a union between two bones, although it is not part of a joint capsule.

accessory movements, joint movements that are necessary for a full range of motion, but that are not under direct voluntary control of the individual. Examples include rotation and gliding motions.

accessory muscle, a relatively rare anatomic duplication of a muscle that may appear anywhere in the muscular system.

accessory muscles of respiration [L, *supplementary*], additional or reinforcing muscles, such as muscles of the neck, back, and abdomen, that may play a more prominent role in respiration during a breathing disorder or during exercise.

accessory nasal sinuses [L *accessus* extra + *nasus* nose + *sinus* hollow], the paranasal sinuses that occur as hollows within the skull but open into the nasal cavity and are lined with a mucous membrane that is continuous with the nasal mucous membrane.

accessory nerve, either of a pair of cranial nerves essential for speech, swallowing, and certain movements of the head and shoulders. Each nerve has a cranial and a spinal portion, communicates with certain cervical nerves, and connects to the nucleus ambiguus of the brain.

accessory pancreas [L *accessus;* Gk *pan* all, *kreas* flesh], small clusters of pancreas cells detached from the pancreas and sometimes found in the wall of the stomach or intestines.

accessory pancreatic duct, a small duct opening into the pancreatic duct or duodenum near the mouth of the common bile duct.

accessory pathway, an extramuscular tract between atrium and ventricle.

accessory phrenic nerve, the nerve that joins the phrenic nerve at the root of the neck or in the thorax, forming a loop around the subclavian vein.

accessory placenta [L *accessus* + *placenta* flat cake], a small placenta that may develop attached to the main placenta by umbilical blood vessels.

accessory root canal, a lateral branching of the pulp canal in a tooth, usually occurring in the apical third of the root.

accessory sinus of the nose. See **paranasal sinus.**

accessory spleen [L *accessus;* Gk *splen*], small nodules of spleen tissue that may occur in the gastrosplenic ligament, greater omentum, or other visceral sites.

accessory thymus [L, *accessus,* extra; Gk, *thymos,* thymelike], a nodule of thymus tissue that is isolated from the gland.

accessory tooth, a supernumerary tooth that does not resemble a normal tooth in size, shape, or position.

ACCH, abbreviation for **Association for the Care of Children's Health.**

accident /ak'sidənt/ [L *accidere* to happen], any unexpected or unplanned event that may result in death, injury, property damage, or a combination of serious effects.

accidental hemorrhage. See **abruptio placentae.**

acclimate /əklī'mit, ak'limāt/ [L *ad* toward; Gk *klima* region], to adjust physiologically to a different climate, especially to changes in altitude and temperature. Also **acclimatize** /əklī'mətīz'/. –**acclimation, acclimatization,** *n.*

accommodation (A, acc, Acc) /əkom'-ədā'shən/ [L *acommodatio* adjustment], **1.** the state or process of adapting or adjusting one thing or set of things to another. **2.** the continuous process or effort of the individual to adapt or adjust to his or her surroundings to maintain a state of homeostasis, both physiologically and psychologically. **3.** the adjustment of the eye to variations in distance. **4.** (in sociology) the reciprocal reconciliation of conflicts between individuals or groups concerning habits and customs, usually through a process of compromise, arbitration, or negotiation.

accommodation reflex, an adjustment of the eyes for near vision, consisting of pupillary constriction, convergence of the eyes, and increased convexity of the lens.

accommodative strabismus [L, *accommodatio,* adjustment; Gk, *strabismos,* squint], **1.** strabismus resulting from abnormal demand on accommodation, such as convergent strabismus, due to uncorrected hypermetropia or divergent strabismus due to uncorrected myopia. **2.** strabismus resulting from the act of accommodating in association with a high AC/A ratio.

accomplishment quotient, a numerical evaluation of a person's achievement age compared with mental age, expressed as a ratio multiplied by 100.

accountability /əkoun'təbil'itē/, being accountable or responsible for the moral and legal requirements of proper patient care.

accreditation, /əkred'itā'shən/ a process whereby a professional association or nongovernmental agency grants recognition to a school or institution for demonstrated ability in a special area of practice or training.

accrementition /ak'rəmentish'ən/, growth or increase of size by the addition of similar tissue or material, as in cellular division, simple fission, budding, or gemmation.

accretio cordis /əkrē'shē·ō/ [L *accrescere* to increase; *cordis* heart], an abnormal condition in which there is an adhesion of the pericardium to a structure around the heart.

accretion /əkrē'shən/ [L *accrescere* to increase], **1.** growth or increase by the addition of material of the same nature that is already present. **2.** the adherence or growing together of parts that are normally separated. **3.** the accumulation of foreign material, especially within a cavity. –**accrete,** *v.,* –**accretive,** *adj.*

acculturation, /əkul'chərā'shən/ the process of adopting the cultural traits or social patterns of another population group.

accumulated dose equivalent, an estimated lifetime maximum permissible dose (MPD) of radiation for persons working with radioactive materials or x-rays. It is based on the formula $(n-18) \times 5$ rems, where n represents one's age in years.

accuracy, the extent to which a measurement is close to the true value.

accurate empathy, a communication technique used by a nurse to convey an understanding of the patient's feelings and experiences.

ACE, abbreviation for **angiotensin-converting enzyme.**

Ace bandage, trademark for a woven elastic bandage.

acebutolol /as'əbōō'təlol/, a beta-adrenergic blocking agent prescribed for the treatment of hypertension, angina pectoris, cardiac arrhythmias, and other cardiovascular disorders.

acedia /əsē'dē·ə/ [Gk *akedia* apathy], a condition of listlessness and a form of melancholy, marked by indifference and sluggish mental processes.

acelius /āsē'lē·əs/, an individual without a body cavity.

acentric /āsen'trik/ [Gk *a, kentron* not center], **1.** having no center. **2.** (in genetics) describing a chromosome fragment that has no centromere.

acephalobrachia /asef'əlōbrā'kē·ə/ [Gk *a, kephale* + *brachion* arm], a congenital anomaly in which a fetus lacks both arms and a head.

acephaly /əsef'əlē/ [Gk *a, kephale* not head], a congenital defect in which the head is absent or not properly developed. **–acephalic,** *adj.*

acet, abbreviation for an acetate carboxylate anion.

acetabulum /as'ətab'yələm/, *pl.* **acetabula** [L, vinegar cup], the large, cup-shaped, articular cavity at the juncture of the ilium, the ischium, and the pubis, containing the ball-shaped head of the femur. **–acetabular,** *adj.*

acetaldehyde, /əs'ətəlde'hīd/ a colorless, volatile liquid with a pungent odor produced by the oxidation of ethyl alcohol. In the human body, acetaldehyde is produced in the liver by the action of alcohol dehydrogenase and other enzymes.

acetaminophen /əset'əmin'əfin/, an analgesic and antipyretic drug prescribed for mild to moderate pain and fever.

acetaminophen poisoning, a toxic reaction to the ingestion of excessive doses of acetaminophen. In adults dosages exceeding 10 to 15 g can produce liver failure, and doses greater than 25 g can be fatal. Large amounts of acetaminophen metabolites can overwhelm the glutathione-detoxifying mechanism of the liver, result-ing in progressive necrosis of the liver within 5 days. The onset of symptoms may be marked by nausea and vomiting, profuse sweating, pallor, and oliguria.

acetanilide /as'ətan'ilīd/, an analgesic drug with antipyretic and antirheumatic properties, derived from aniline.

acetate /as'itāt/, a salt of acetic acid.

acetate kinase, an enzyme that catalyzes the transfer of a phosphate group from adenosine triphosphate to acetate.

acetazolamide /as'ətəzō'ləmīd/, a carbonic anhydrase inhibitor prescribed for edema, glaucoma, and epilepsy (primarily petit mal).

acetic [L *acetum* vinegar], pertaining to substances having the sour properties of vinegar or acetic acid; also, chemical compounds possessing the radical, $CH_3CO—$.

acetic acid /əsē'tik, əset'ik/[L *acetum* vinegar], a clear, colorless, pungent liquid that is miscible with water, alcohol, glycerin, and ether and that constitutes 3% to 5% of vinegar.

acetic acid test. See **albumin test.**

acetic fermentation, the production of acetic acid or vinegar from a weak alcoholic solution.

acetoacetic acid /as'ətō·əsē'tik, əsē'tō-/, a colorless, oily keto acid produced by the metabolism of lipids and pyruvates. It is excreted in trace amounts in normal urine and in elevated levels in diabetes mellitus.

acetohexamide /-hek'səmīd/, a sulfonyl-urea oral antidiabetic prescribed in the treatment of non-insulin-dependent diabetes mellitus.

acetokinase. See **acetate kinase.**

acetol kinase, an enzyme that catalyzes the transfer of a phosphate group from adenosine triphosphate to hydroxyacetone.

acetone /as'ətōn/, a colorless, aromatic, volatile liquid ketone body found in small amounts in normal urine and in larger quantities in the urine of diabetics.

acetone bodies. See **ketone bodies.**

acetone carboxylic acid. See **acetoacetic acid.**

acetone in urine test, a test for the presence of dimethylketone in the urine of patients, used as a laboratory indication of ketosis and the severity of diabetes. The test consists of exposing chemically treated test paper strips or sticks to urine. If acetone is present in the urine as the result of incomplete breakdown of fatty and amino acids in the body, the test strips change color. A similar test utilizes a compound added directly to a urine sample.

acetonide grouping, an acetone-like chemical combination commonly present in some corticosteroid drugs, such as flucinolone acetonide.

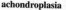

acetonuria /as′ətōn ŏŏr′ē·ə/, the presence of acetone and diacetic bodies in the urine.

acetophenetidin. See **phenacetin.**

acetpyrogall /as′ətpī′rəgal/, a topical irritant used as a caustic and keratolytic agent.

acetylacetic acid. See **acetoacetic acid.**

acetylcholine (ACh) /as′ətilkō′lēn, əsē′til-/, a neurotransmitter substance widely distributed in body tissues, with a primary function of mediating synaptic activity of the nervous system. Its active phase is transient because it is rapidly destroyed by acetylcholinesterase. Acetylcholine activity also can be blocked by atropine at junctions of nerve fibers with glands and smooth muscle tissue.

acetylcholinesterase (AChe), an enzyme that inactivates the neurotransmitter acetylcholine by hydrolyzing the substance to choline and acetate. The action reduces or prevents excessive firing of neurons at neuromuscular junctions.

acetylcoenzyme A /əsē′tilkō·en′zīm, as′ətil-/, a molecule that is formed in the course of several important metabolic processes. The formation of acetylcoenzyme A is the critical intermediate step between anaerobic glycolysis and the Krebs′ citric acid cycle.

acetylcysteine /-sis′tēn/, a mucolytic prescribed in the treatment of chronic pulmonary disease, acute bronchopulmonary disease, and atelectasis resulting from mucus obstruction.

acetylsalicylic acid. See **aspirin.**

acetylsalicylic acid poisoning, the toxic effects of overdose of the commonly used antipyretic and analgesic drug, aspirin. Early symptoms of overdose include dizziness, ringing in the ears, changes in body temperature, gastrointestinal discomfort, and hyperventilation. Severe poisoning is marked by respiratory alkalosis, which may lead to metabolic acidosis. Children are particularly vulnerable to the potential toxic effects of salicylates.

acetyltransferase /-trans′fərās′/, any of several enzymes that transfer acetyl groups from one compound to another.

ACG, abbreviation for *apexcardiography.*

ACh, abbreviation for **acetylcholine.**

ACH, abbreviation for **adrenocortical hormone.**

achalasia /ak′əlā′zhə/ [Gk *a, chalasis* not relaxation], an abnormal condition characterized by the inability of a muscle to relax, particularly the cardiac sphincter of the stomach.

Achard-Thiers syndrome /ash′ärtērz′/ [Émile C. Achard, French physician, b. 1860; Joseph Thiers, French physician, b. 1873], a hormonal disorder seen in postmenopausal women with diabetes, charac-

terized by growth of body hair in a masculine distribution.

ache /āk/ [OE *acan* to hurt], **1.** a pain characterized by persistence, dullness, and, usually, moderate intensity. An ache may be localized, as a stomach ache, headache, or bone ache, or general, as the myalgia that accompanies a viral infection or a persistent fever. **2.** to suffer from a dull, persistent pain of moderate intensity.

AChE, abbreviation for **acetylcholinesterase.**

achievement age, the level of a person′s educational development as measured by an achievement test and compared with the normal score for chronologic age.

achievement quotient (AQ), a numeric expression of a person′s achievement age, determined by various achievement tests, divided by the chronologic age and expressed as a multiple of 100.

achievement test, a standardized test for the measurement and comparison of knowledge or proficiency in various fields of vocational or academic study.

Achilles tendon /əkil′ēz/ [Achilles, Greek mythologic hero], the common tendon of the soleus and gastrocnemius muscles. It is the thickest and strongest tendon in the body and begins near the middle of the posterior part of the leg.

Achilles tendon reflex, a deep tendon reflex consisting of plantar flexion of the foot when a sharp tap is given directly to the tendon of the gastrocnemius muscle at the back of the ankle. This reflex is often absent in diabetics and people with peripheral neuropathies.

achlorhydria /ā′klôrhī′drē·ə/ [Gk *a, chloros* not green, *hydor* water], an abnormal condition characterized by the absence of hydrochloric acid in the gastric juice. Achlorhydria in a patient with symptoms of gastric ulcer almost always indicates that the lesion is malignant. **–achlorhydric,** *adj.*

acholia /akō′lē·ə/ [Gk *a, chole* not bile], **1.** the absence or decrease of bile secretion. **2.** any condition that suppresses the flow of bile into the small intestine. **–acholic,** *adj.*

acholuria [Gk *a, chole* + *ouron* urine], the absence or lack of pigments in the urine.

achondrogenesis /əkon′drōjen′əsis/, a form of dwarfism characterized by gross limb shortening and hydropic head and trunk.

achondroplasia /ākon′drōplā′zhə/ [Gk *a, chondros* not cartilage, *plassein* to form], a disorder of the growth of cartilage in the epiphyses of the long bones and skull that results in premature ossification, permanent limitation of skeletal development, and dwarfism typified by protruding forehead, and short, thick arms and legs on a normal trunk.

achondroplastic dwarf, the most common type of dwarf, characterized by disproportionately short limbs, a normal-sized trunk, large head with a depressed nasal bridge and small face, stubby trident hands, and lordosis.

achromatic lens, [Gk *a* without, *chroma* color; L *lentil*], a lens in which the focal lengths for red and blue colors of the spectrum are the same, refracting light without decomposing it into its component colors.

achromatic vision. See color blindness.

achromia /akrō'mē·ə/ [Gk *a, chroma* not color], the absence or loss of normal skin pigment. The condition may be congenital, as in albinism, or the result of a disease, such as psoriasis.

achromocyte /ākrō'məsīt/, a sickle-shaped, hypochromic erythrocyte, perhaps the result of a ruptured red blood cell that lost hemoglobin.

achylia /ākī'lē·ə/ [Gk *a, chylos* not juice], an absence or severe deficiency of hydrochloric acid and pepsinogen in the stomach. This condition may also occur in the pancreas, when the exocrine portion of that gland fails to produce digestive enzymes.

achylous /əkī'ləs/, 1. of or pertaining to a lack of gastric juice or other digestive secretions. 2. of or pertaining to a lack of chyle.

acicular /əsik'yələr/ [L *aciculus* little needle], needle-shaped, such as certain leaves and crystals.

acid /as'id/ [L *acidus* sour], 1. a compound that yields hydrogen ions when dissociated in solution. Acids turn blue litmus red, have a sour taste, and react with bases to form salts. Acids have chemical properties essentially opposite to those of bases. 2. *slang.* lysergic acid diethylamide (LSD).

acid-base balance, a condition existing when the net rate at which the body produces acids or bases equals the net rate at which acids or bases are excreted. The result of acid-base balance is a stable concentration of hydrogen ions in body fluids.

acid-base metabolism, the metabolic processes that maintain the balance of acids and bases essential in regulating the composition of body fluids. Metabolic buffer systems within the body maintain this ratio, and, when it is upset, either acidosis or alkalosis results.

acid bath, a bath taken in water containing a mineral acid to help reduce excessive sweating.

acid burn, damage to tissue caused by exposure to a strong acid. The severity of the burn is determined by the kind of acid and the duration and extent of exposure. Emergency treatment includes washing the affected area with large amounts of water.

acid dust, an accumulation of highly acidic particles of dust in the atmosphere.

acid-fast bacillus (AFB), a type of bacillus that resists decoloring by acid after accepting a stain. Examples include *Mycobacterium tuberculosis* and *M. leprae.*

acid-fast stain, a method of staining used in bacteriology in which a smear on a slide is treated with carbol-fuchsin stain, decolorized with acid alcohol, and counterstained with methylene blue to identify acid-fast bacteria.

acid flush, a runoff of precipitation with a high acid content, as may occur during thaws.

acidify /asid'əfī/, 1. to make a substance acid, as through the addition of an acid. 2. to become acid.

acidity /asid'itē/ [L *acidus* sour], the degree of sourness, sharpness of taste, or ability of a chemical to yield hydrogen ions in an aqueous solution.

acidity of the stomach, the degree of gastric acid in the stomach. Acidity varies during any 24-hour period but averages in the range of pH 0.9 to 1.5. The main source of stomach acidity is hydrochloric acid secreted by gastric glands of the stomach.

acid mist, mist containing a high concentration of acid or particles of any toxic chemical, such as carbon tetrachloride or silicon tetrachloride.

acid mucopolysaccharide, a major chemical constituent of ground substance in the dermis.

acidophil /as'idōfil, əsid'əfil/ [L *acidus* + Gk *philein* to love], 1. a cell or cell constituent with an affinity for acid dyes. 2. an organism that thrives in an acid medium. –**acidophilic,** *adj.*

acidophilic adenoma, a tumor of the pituitary gland characterized by cells that can be stained red with an acid dye. Gigantism and acromegaly are caused by an acidophilic adenoma.

acidophilus milk /as'idof'ələs/, milk inoculated with cultures of *Lactobacillus acidophilus,* used in various enteric disorders to change the bacterial flora of the GI tract.

acidosis /as'idō'sis/ [L *acidus* + Gk *osis* condition], an abnormal increase in hydrogen ion concentration in the body resulting from an accumulation of an acid or the loss of a base. The various forms of acidosis are named for the cause of the condition; for example, respiratory acidosis results from respiratory retention of CO_2. Treatment depends on diagnosis of the underlying pathology and correction of the acid-base imbalance. **–acidosic, acidotic** *adj.*

acidosis dialysis, a type of metabolic acidosis that may develop when contaminating bacteria alter the pH of the dialysis bath. The condition is most likely to occur after prolonged hemodialysis.

acid-perfusion test, a test to demonstrate sensitivity of the esophagus to acid, a condition suggestive of reflux esophagitis. A weak hydrochloric acid solution and normal saline are dripped alternately into the esophagus via a nasal-esophageal tube without telling the patient which solution is being infused. A positive response is pain with acid but not with saline.

acid phosphatase, an enzyme found in the kidneys, serum, semen, and prostate gland. It is elevated in serum in cancers of the prostate and in trauma.

acid poisoning, a toxic condition caused by the ingestion of a toxic acid agent such as hydrochloric, nitric, phosphoric, or sulfuric acids, some of which are ingredients in cleaning compounds. Emergency treatment includes giving copious amounts of water, milk, or beaten eggs to dilute the acid. Vomiting is not induced, and mild solutions of alkali are not given.

acid rain, the precipitation of moisture, as rain, with high acidity caused by release into the atmosphere of pollutants from industry, motor vehicle exhausts, and other sources.

acid rebound, a condition of hypersecretion of gastric acid that may occur after the initial buffering effect of an antacid.

acid salt, a salt that is formed from only partial replacement of hydrogen ions from the related acid, leaving some degree of acidity in the salt. An example is sodium bicarbonate.

acid therapy, a method for removing warts that uses plaster patches impregnated with acid.

acidulous /əsid′yələs/, slightly acidic or sour.

aciduria [L *acidus* + Gk *ouron* urine], the presence of acid in the urine. The condition may be caused by a diet rich in meat proteins or certain fruits, the introduction of a medication for the treatment of a urinary tract disorder, an inborn error of metabolism, or ketoacidosis.

acinar adenocarcinoma. See **acinic cell adenocarcinoma.**

acinar cell /as′inər/ [L *acinus* grape], a cell of the tiny lobules of a compound gland or similar saclike structure such as an alveolus.

Acinetobacter /as′inē′təbak′tər/, a genus of nonmotile, aerobic bacteria of the family Neisseriaceae that often occurs in clinical specimens.

acinic cell adenocarcinoma /asin′ik/ [L *acinus* grape], an uncommon, low-grade malignant neoplasm that develops in the secreting cells of racemose glands, especially the salivary glands.

acinitis /as′inī′tis/, any inflammation of the tiny, grape-shaped portions of certain glands.

acinous adenocarcinoma. See **acinic cell adenocarcinoma.**

acinus /as′inəs/, *pl.* **acini** [L, grape] **1.** any small saclike structure, particularly one found in a gland. **2.** a subdivision of the lung consisting of the tissue distal to a terminal bronchiole.

AC joint, abbreviation for *acromioclavicular joint.*

ACLS, abbreviation for **advanced cardiac life support.**

ACMC, abbreviation for **Association of Canadian Medical Colleges.**

acme, the peak or highest point, such as the peak of intensity of a uterine contraction during labor.

acne /ak′nē/ [Gk *akme* point], an inflammatory, papulopustular skin eruption occurring usually in or near the sebaceous glands on the face, neck, shoulders, and upper back. Its cause is unknown but involves bacterial breakdown of sebum into fatty acids irritating to surrounding subcutaneous tissue. Kinds of acne include **acne conglobata, acne vulgaris, chloracne,** and **rosacea.**

acne artificialis, an eruption in the skin caused by an external irritant, such as tar, or ingestion of halogen compounds.

acne cachecticorum, an eruption or irritation of the skin that may occur in patients who are very weak and debilitated. It is characterized by soft, mildly infiltrated pustular lesions.

acne conglobata /kong′glōbā′tə/, a severe form of acne with abscess, cyst, scar, and keloid formation.

acneform /ak′nifôrm/, resembling acne. Also **acneiform** /aknē′əfôrm/.

acneform drug eruption, any one of various skin reactions to a drug, characterized by papules and pustules erupting in acne, with or without comedones.

acnegenic /ak′nijen′ik/ [Gk *akme* + *genein* to produce], causing or producing acne.

acne indurata, a pathologic skin condition characterized by extensive papular lesions that often produce severe scars.

acne keloid, [Gk *akme* point, *kelis* spot, *eidos* form], a cellular overgrowth at the site of an acne lesion.

acne keratosa, a skin condition characterized by hard conic plugs that usually appear at the corners of the mouth and inflame surrounding tissue.

acne necrotica miliaris, a rare, chronic type of folliculitis of the scalp, occurring mostly in adults and characterized by tiny pustules.

acne neonatorum, a skin condition of infants caused by sebaceous gland hyperplasia and characterized by the formation of comedones, nodules, and cysts on the nose, cheeks, and forehead.

acne papulosa, a common pathologic skin condition that develops small papular lesions that usually do not become inflamed. It is considered a papular form of acne vulgaris.

acne rosacea. See rosacea.

acne vulgaris, a common form of acne seen predominantly in adolescents and young adults. Acne vulgaris is probably an effect of androgenic hormones and *Propionibacterium acnes* in the hair follicle.

ACNM, abbreviation for *American College of Nurse-Midwives.*

ACOG, abbreviation for **American College of Obstetricians and Gynecologists.**

acognosia /ak′og·nō′zhə/, a knowledge of remedies.

acoria /akôr′ē·ə/ [Gk *a, koros* not satiety], a condition characterized by constant hunger, even when the appetite is small.

acorn-tipped catheter, a flexible catheter with an acorn-shaped tip used in various diagnostic procedures, especially in urology.

acousma /əkooz′mə/, *pl.* **acousmas, acousmata** [Gk *akousma* something heard], a hallucinatory impression of strange sounds.

acoustic, acoustical [Gk *akouein* to hear], of or pertaining to sound or hearing.

acoustic cavitation, a potential biologic effect of ultrasonography, marked by large-amplitude oscillations of microscopic gas bubbles.

acoustic center, the portion of the brain in the temporal lobe of the cerebrum in which the sense of hearing is located.

acoustic impedance, resistance to the passage of sound waves, such as that generated by ultrasound equipment, by objects in the path of the sound wave. Testing of middle ear impedance is part of audiologic test batteries to detect middle ear problems.

acoustic meatus [Gk *akoustikos* hearing; L *meatus,* a passage], either the external or internal canal of the ear.

acoustic microscope, a microscope in which the object being viewed is scanned with sound waves and its image reconstructed with light waves.

acoustic nerve, either of a pair of cranial nerves composed of fibers from the cochlear nerve and the vestibular nerve in the inner ear, conveying impulses of both the sense of hearing and the sense of balance. Also called **eighth cranial nerve.**

acoustic neuroma, a benign tumor that develops from the eighth cranial (auditory) nerve and grows within the auditory canal. Tinnitus, increasing deafness, headache, facial numbness, papilledema, dizziness, and an unsteady gait may result. It may be unilateral or bilateral.

acoustic reflex, contraction of the stapedius muscle in the middle ear in response to a loud noise. The **acoustic reflex threshold** is the lowest level of sound that will elicit an acoustic reflex and is in the range of 85 to 90 dB HL in individuals with normal hearing.

acoustics /əkoōs′tiks/ [Gk *akoustikos* hearing], the perception of sound.

acoustic shadow, an ultrasound image produced by the presence of dense material, such as calculi, in a scan of soft tissue.

acoustic trauma, a gradual loss of hearing caused by exposure to loud noise over an extended time or a sudden loss of hearing, partial or complete, caused by an explosion, a severe blow to the head, or other accident. Hearing loss may be temporary or permanent.

acoustooptics /əkoōs′tō·op′tiks/, a field of physics that studies the generation of light waves by ultrahigh-frequency sound waves.

ACP, 1. abbreviation for *American College of Pathologists.* 2. abbreviation for **American College of Physicians.** 3. abbreviation for **American College of Prosthodontists.**

acquired [L *acquiere* to obtain], of or pertaining to a characteristic, condition, or disease originating after birth and caused not by hereditary or developmental factors but by a reaction to environmental influences outside the organism.

acquired hypogammaglobulinemia [L *acquirere* to obtain; Gk *hypo* a deficiency, *gamma* third letter of Greek alphabet; L *globulus* small globe; Gk *haima* blood], an acquired deficiency of the gamma globulin blood fraction.

acquired immunodeficiency syndrome (AIDS) /ādz/, a disease involving a defect in cell-mediated immunity. The disorder is found primarily in homosexual men, intravenous drug users, female sex partners of infected men, and children of those with the disease. The causative agent is a retrovirus, identified as HTLV-3 (Human T-cell Lymphotropic Virus) usually transmitted through sexual contact or exposure to contaminated blood or sharing of hypodermic needles. Initial symptoms include extreme fatigue, intermittent fever, night sweats, chills, lymphadenopathy, enlarged spleen, anorexia and consequent weight loss, severe diarrhea, apathy, and depression. As the disease progresses, there is a general failure to thrive, anergy, and any number and kind of recurring infections, such as *Pneumocystis carinii* pneumonia. Most patients with the disorder are susceptible to malignant neoplasms, especially Kaposi's sarcoma, Burkitt's lymphoma, and non-Hodgkin's lymphoma. The fatality rate is 90% in those diagnosed more than 2 years.

acquired immunity, any form of immunity that is not innate and is obtained during life. It may be natural or artificial and actively or passively induced. **Naturally acquired immunity** is obtained by the development of antibodies resulting from an attack of infectious disease or by the transmission of antibodies from the mother through the placenta to the fetus or to the infant through the colostrum. **Artificially acquired immunity** is obtained by vaccination or by the injection of antiserum.

acquired reflex. See **conditioned reflex.**

acquired sterility [L *acquiere + sterilis,* barren], the failure to conceive after once bearing a child.

acquired trait [L *acquiere + trahere,* to draw], a physical characteristic that is not inherited, but which may be an effect of the environment or a mutation.

ACR, abbreviation for **American College of Radiology.**

acrid /ak'rid/, sharp or pungent, bitter and unpleasant to the smell or taste.

acridine /ak'rīdēn/, a dibenzopyridine compound used in the synthesis of dyes and drugs.

acrimony /ak'rəmō'nē/ [L *acrimonia* pungency], a quality of bitterness, harshness, or sharpness.

acrocentric /ak'rōsen'trik/ [Gk *akron* extremity, *kentron* center], pertaining to a chromosome in which the centromere is located near one of the ends so that the arms of the chromatids are extremely uneven.

acrocephalosyndactylism. See **Apert's syndrome.**

acrocephaly. See **oxycephaly.**

acrochordon /ak'rōkôr'don/, a benign, pedunculated skin tag commonly occurring on the eyelids or neck or in the axilla or groin.

acrocyanosis /ak'rōsī'ənō'sis/ [Gk *akron + kyanos* blue], a condition characterized by cyanotic discoloration, coldness, and sweating of the extremities, especially the hands, caused by arterial spasm that is usually precipitated by cold or by emotional stress. A kind of acrocyanosis is **peripheral acrocyanosis of the newborn.**

acrodermatitis /-dur'mətī'tis/ [Gk *akron + derma* skin, *itis* inflammation], any eruption of the skin of the hands and feet caused by a parasitic mite, which is a member of the order Acarina.

acrodermatitis enteropathica /en'tərōpath'ikə/, a rare, chronic disease of infants characterized by vesicles and bullae of the skin and mucous membranes, alopecia, diarrhea, and failure to thrive.

acrodynia /ak'rōdin'ē·ə/ [Gk *akron + odyne* pain], a disease that occurs in infants and young children. Symptoms include edema, pruritus, generalized skin rash, with pink coloration of the extremities and scarlet coloration of the cheeks and nose, profuse sweating, digestive disturbances, photophobia, polyneuritis, extreme irritability alternating with periods of listlessness and apathy, and failure to thrive.

acrokeratosis verruciformis /ak'rōker'ətō'sis/, an inherited skin disorder characterized by the appearance of wartlike lesions on the dorsum of the hands and feet and occasionally on the wrists, forearms, and knees.

acrokinesis /-kīnē'sis/ [Gk *akron* extremity, *kinesis* motion], a state in which there is an abnormally wide range of motion of the limbs.

acromegalic eunuchoidism, a rare disorder characterized by genital atrophy and the development of female secondary sex characteristics, occurring in men with advanced acromegaly caused by a chromophobe adenoma in the anterior pituitary gland.

acromegaly /ak'rəmeg'əlē/ [Gk *akron + megas* great], a chronic metabolic condition characterized by a gradual, marked enlargement and elongation of the bones of the face, jaw, and extremities. The condition is caused by the overproduction of growth hormone. **–acromegalic** /-məgal'-ik/, *adj.*

acromial process [Gk *akron + omos* shoulder], a flat triangular plate at the end of the scapula.

acromicria /ak'rəmik'rē·ə/, an anomaly characterized by abnormally small hands and feet.

acromioclavicular articulation, the gliding joint between the acromial end of the clavicle and the medial margin of the acromion of the scapula.

acromiocoracoid /-kôr'əkoid/, pertaining to the acromion and coracoid process.

acromiohumeral, pertaining to the acromion and the humerus.

acromion /əkrō'mē·ən/ [Gk akron + omos shoulder], the lateral extension of the spine of the scapula, forming the highest point of the shoulder and connecting with the clavicle at a small oval surface in the middle of the spine. It gives attachment to the deltoideus and trapezius. −**acromial,** adj.

acromioscapular, pertaining to the acromion process and the scapula.

acroosteolysis, an occupational disease that mainly affects people who work with polyvinylchloride (PVC) plastic materials. It is characterized by Raynaud's phenomenon, loss of bone tissue in the hands, and sensitivity to cold temperatures.

acroparesthesia /ak'rōpar'isthē'zhə/ [Gk akron + para near, aisthesis feeling] **1.** an extreme sensitivity at the tips of the extremities of the body, caused by compression of the nerves in the affected area or by polyneuritis. **2.** a disease characterized by tingling, numbness, and stiffness in the extremities, especially in the fingers, hands, and forearms.

acrophobia [Gk akron + phobos fear], a pathologic fear or dread of high places that results in extreme anxiety.

acrosomal cap, acrosomal head cap. See **acrosome.**

acrosomal reaction, the pattern of various chemical changes that occur in the anterior of the head of the spermatozoon in response to contact with the ovum and that lead to the penetration by the sperm and fertilization of the ovum.

acrosome /ak'rəsōm'/ [Gk akron + soma body], the caplike structure surrounding the anterior end of the nucleus of a spermatozoon. −**acrosomal,** adj.

acrotic /əkrot'ik/ [Gk a, krotos not beating], **1.** of or pertaining to the surface or to the skin glands. **2.** of or pertaining to the absence or the weakness of a pulse.

acrylic resin base, (in dentistry) a denture base made of acrylic resin.

acrylic resin dental cement, a dental cement for restoring or repairing damaged teeth.

ACS, 1. abbreviation for American Cancer Society. **2.** abbreviation for American Chemical Society. **3.** abbreviation for **American College of Surgeons. 4.** abbreviation for **anodal closing sound.**

ACSM, abbreviation for American College of Sports Medicine.

ACTH, abbreviation for **adrenocorticotropic hormone.**

actigraph /ak'tigraf'/, any instrument that records changes in the activity of a substance or an organism and produces a graphic record of the process, such as an electrocardiograph machine, which produces a record of cardiac activity.

actin, a protein found in muscle fibers that acts with myosin to bring about contraction and relaxation.

acting out, the expression of intrapsychic conflict or painful emotion through overt behavior that is usually neurotic, defensive, and unconscious and that may be destructive or dangerous.

actinic /aktin'ik/ [Gk aktis ray], of or pertaining to radiation, such as sunlight or x-rays.

actinic conjunctivitis [Gk actis ray; L conjunctivus connecting, + Gk, itis, inflammation], an eye inflammation caused by exposure to the ultraviolet radiation of sunlight or other UV sources, such as acetylene torches, therapeutic lamps (sun lamps), and kleig lights.

actinic dermatitis, a skin inflammation or rash resulting from exposure to sunlight, x-ray, or atomic particle radiation. Chronic or recurrent actinic dermatitis can predispose to skin cancer.

actinic keratosis, a slowly developing, localized thickening of the outer layers of the skin as a result of chronic, excessive exposure to the sun. Treatment of this potentially malignant lesion includes surgical excision, cryotherapy, and topical chemotherapy.

actinium (Ac), a rare, radioactive metallic element. Its atomic number is 89; its atomic weight is 227. It occurs in some ores of uranium.

Actinomyces /ak'tinōmī'sēz/ [Gk aktis ray, mykes fungus], a genus of anaerobic, gram-positive bacteria. Several species that may cause disease in humans, such as *Actinomyces israelii,* are normally present in the mouth and throat.

actinomycin A, the first of a group of chromopeptide antibiotic agents derived from soil bacteria. Most are derivatives of phenoxazine and contain actinocin. They are generally active against gram-positive bacteria, fungi, and neoplasms.

actinomycin B, an antibiotic agent derived from *Actinomyces antibioticus.*

actinomycin D. See **dactinomycin.**

actinomycosis /ak'tinōmīkō'sis/, a chronic, systemic disease characterized by deep, lumpy abscesses that extrude a thin, granular pus through multiple sinuses. The various species of *Actinomyces* are species specific. The causative organism in humans is *A. israelii*, a normal inhabitant of the bowel and mouth. Disease occurs after tissue damage, usually in the presence of another infectious organism. **Cervicofacial actinomycosis** occurs with the spread of the bacterium into the subcutaneous tissues of the mouth, throat, and neck, as a result of dental or tonsillar infection. **Thoracic actinomycosis** may represent proliferation of the organism from cervicofacial abscesses into the esophagus, bronchi, lungs, pleura, or mediastinum. Fever, cough, draining sinuses, weight loss, night sweats, and, rarely, pleural effusion are characteristic of this form of the disease. **Abdominal actinomycosis** usually follows an acute inflammatory process in the stomach or intestines, such as appendicitis, diverticulum of the large bowel, or a perforation of the stomach. Generalized actinomycosis may involve the skin, brain, liver, and urogenital system. A pelvic form of abdominal actinomycosis occurs after insertion of an intrauterine contraceptive device.

action current. See **action potential.**

action level, the level of concentration at which an undesirable or toxic component of a food is considered dangerous enough to public health to warrant government prohibition of the sale of that food. The United States Food and Drug Administration tests foods for action levels.

action potential, an electric impulse consisting of a self-propagating series of polarizations and depolarizations, transmitted across the cell membranes of a nerve fiber during the transmission of a nerve impulse and across the cell membranes of a muscle cell during contraction or other activity of the cell.

action tremor, [L *agere* to do, *tremor* shaking], a tremor that occurs or is evident during voluntary movements.

activate, [L, *activus*, active], to induce or prolong an activity or render optimal action

activated charcoal, a general-purpose antidote and a powerful pharmaceutical adsorbent prescribed in the treatment of acute poisoning and to control flatulence.

activated 7-dehydrocholesterol. See **vitamin D₃.**

activated partial thromboplastin time (APTT), a timed blood test that determines the efficacy of various clotting factors used in the diagnosis of coagulation disorders. The normal value in venous blood is 32 to 51 seconds.

activating enzyme, an enzyme that promotes or sustains an activity, as an enzyme

that catalyzes the combining of amino acids to form peptides or proteins.

activation energy [L *activus* active], the energy required to convert reactants to activated or transition-state species that will spontaneously proceed to products.

activation factor. See **factor XII.**

activator, **1.** a substance, force, or device that stimulates activity in another substance or structure, especially a substance that activates an enzyme. **2.** a substance that stimulates the development of an anatomic structure in the embryo. **3.** an internal secretion of the pancreas. **4.** an apparatus for making substances radioactive, such as a cyclotron or neutron generator. **5.** (in dentistry) a removable orthodontic appliance that functions as a passive transmitter and stimulator of the perioral muscles.

active algognia. See **sadism.**

active anaphylaxis [Gk, *ana*, up, *phylaxis, protection*], a condition of hypersensitivity caused by the reaction of the body's immune system to injection of a foreign protein.

active assisted exercise [L *activus*], the movement of the body or any of its parts primarily through the individual's own efforts but accompanied by the aid of a therapist or some device, such as an exercise machine.

active carrier [OFr, *carier*], a person without signs or symptoms of an infectious disease who carries the causal microorganisms.

active electrode [Gk *elektron* amber, *hodos* way], an electrode that is applied at a specific point to produce stimulation in a concentrated area in electrotherapy.

active euthanasia. See **euthanasia.**

active exercise, repetitive movement of a part of the body as a result of voluntary contraction and relaxation of the controlling muscles.

active expiration [L *expirare* to breathe out], forced exhalation, utilizing the muscles of the abdominal wall and rib cage, in addition to the diaphragm and recoil of elastic tissues.

active hyperemia [L *activus*; Gk *hyper* excessive, *haima* blood], the increased flow of blood into a particular body part.

active immunity, a form of long-term acquired immunity that protects the body against a new infection, as the result of antibodies that develop naturally after an initial infection or artificially after a vaccination.

active labor [L *activus, labor* work], the normal progress of the birth process, including uterine contractions, dilatation of the cervix, and descent of the fetus into the birth canal.

active listening, an attitude of alert hearing and of showing an interest in what a person has to say.

active movement, muscular action at a joint as a result of voluntary effort without outside help.

active-passive, (in psychiatry) a concept that characterizes persons as either actively involved in shaping events or passively reacting to events.

active play, any activity from which one derives amusement, entertainment, enjoyment, or satisfaction by taking a participatory rather than a passive role.

active range of motion (AROM), the range of movement through which a joint can be moved without assistance.

active resistance exercise, the movement or exertion of the body or any of its parts performed totally through the individual's own efforts against a resisting force.

active resistance training (ART), a conditioning or rehabilitation program designed to enhance a patient's muscular strength, power, and endurance through progressive resistance exercises and muscle overloading.

active sensitization [L *agere* to do + *sentire* to feel], the condition that results when a specific antigen is injected into a person known to be susceptible.

active site, the place on the surface of an enzyme where its catalytic action occurs.

active specific immunotherapy, a therapy in which a cancer patient is injected with irradiated tumor cells. The injected cells stimulate the production of antibodies that resist the tumor cells.

active transport, the movement of materials across the membrane of a cell by means of chemical activity that allows the cell to admit larger molecules than would otherwise be able to enter. Expediting active transport are carrier molecules within the cell that bind themselves to incoming molecules, rotate around them, and disconnect, setting the incoming molecule free inside the cell wall. Certain enzymes play a role in active transport, providing a chemical "pump" that helps move substances through the cell membrane.

activities of daily living (ADL), the activities usually performed in the course of a normal day in the person's life, such as eating, dressing, washing, or brushing the teeth. The ability to perform ADL may be compromised by a variety of causes, including chronic illnesses and accidents. An ADL checklist is often used before discharge from a hospital. If any activities cannot be adequately performed, arrange-

ments are made with an outside agency, such as a visiting nurse service, to provide the necessary assistance.

activity, the action of an enzyme on an amount of substrate that is converted to product per unit time under defined conditions.

activity coefficient, a proportionality constant, γ, relating activity, α, to concentration, expressed in the equation, $\alpha = \gamma c$.

activity intolerance, a NANDA-accepted nursing diagnosis of insufficient physiologic or psychologic energy to endure or complete required or desired daily activities. Defining characteristics include verbal report of fatigue or weakness, abnormal heart rate or blood pressure response to activity, exertional discomfort or dyspnea, and electrocardiographic changes reflecting arrhythmias or ischemia.

activity intolerance, high risk for, a NANDA-accepted nursing diagnosis of the risk of experiencing insufficient physiologic or psychologic energy to endure or complete required or desired daily activities. Risk factors include a history of previous intolerance, deconditioned status, presence of circulatory or respiratory problems, and inexperience with activity.

activity theory, a concept proposed by Robert J. Havighurst, an American gerontologist, that activity promotes well-being and satisfaction in aging.

activity tolerance, the type and amount of exercise a patient may be able to perform without undue exertion or possible injury.

actual cautery [L *actus* act], the application of heat, rather than a chemical substance, in the destruction of tissue.

actual charge, the amount actually charged or billed by a medical practitioner for a service. The actual charge may not be the same as that paid for the service by an insurance plan.

actual damages. See **damages.**

actualize, the act of fulfilling a potential, as by a person who may develop capabilities through experience and education.

acuity /əkyōō′itē/, the clearness or sharpness of perception, such as visual acuity.

acuminate wart, See **condyloma acuminatum.**

acupressure /ak′yəpresh′ər/ [L *acus* needle, *pressura* pressure], a therapeutic technique of applying digital pressure in a specified way on designated points on the body to relieve pain, produce anesthesia, or regulate a body function.

acupuncture /ak′yəpunk′tshər/ [L *acus* + *punctura* puncture], a method of producing analgesia or altering the function of a system of the body by inserting fine, wire-thin needles into the skin at specific sites on the body along a series of lines or channels called meridians. The needles are twirled or energized electrically or warmed. Acupuncture originated in the Far East and has gained increasing attention in the West since the early 1970s. **–acupuncturist,** *n.*

acupuncture point, one of many discrete points on the skin along the several meridians or chains of points of the body. Stimulation of any of the various points may induce an increase or decrease in function or sensation in an area or system of the body.

acute /əkyōōt'/ [L *acutus* sharp], **1.** (of a disease or disease symptoms) beginning abruptly with marked intensity or sharpness, then subsiding after a relatively short time. **2.** sharp or severe.

acute abdomen, an abnormal condition characterized by the acute onset of severe pain within the abdominal cavity. An acute abdomen requires immediate evaluation and diagnosis, because it may indicate a condition that calls for surgical intervention. Information about the onset, duration, character, location, and symptoms associated with the pain is critical in making an accurate diagnosis.

acute abscess, [L *acutus* sharp, *abscedere* to go away], a collection of pus in a body cavity accompanied by localized inflammation, pain, pyrexia, and swelling.

acute air trapping, a condition of bronchiolar collapse that may occur without warning. The patient's respiratory system becomes immobilized in a position of partial exhalation, unable to either inhale or exhale.

acute alcoholism, drunkenness or intoxication resulting from excessive consumption of alcoholic beverages. The syndrome is temporary and is characterized by depression of the higher nerve centers causing impaired motor control, stupor, lack of coordination, and often nausea, dehydration, headache, and other physical symptoms.

acute angle, [L *acutus* + *angulus*], any angle of less than 90 degrees.

acute anicteric hepatitis [Gk *a* without, *ikteros* jaundice, *hepar* liver, *itis* inflammation], acute hepatitis that is not accompanied by jaundice.

acute articular rheumatism [L *articulare* to divide into joints; Gk *rheumatismos* that which flows], a common form of adult rheumatism, possibly associated with a pyogenic infection in the joints. Symptoms include fever and arthritis.

acute ascending myelitis [L *ascendere* to go up; Gk *myelos* marrow, *itis*], an in-

flammation of the spinal cord that extends progressively upward with corresponding interference in nerve functions.

acute ascending spinal paralysis, progressive spinal paralysis that spreads upward toward the brain.

acute atrophic paralysis [Gk *a* without, *trophe* nourishment, *paralyein* to have palsy], acute poliomyelitis involving the anterior horns of the spinal cord and resulting in flaccid paralysis of involved muscle groups and later by atrophy.

acute bacterial arthritis. See **septic arthritis.**

acute care, a pattern of health care in which a patient is treated for an acute episode of illness, for the sequelae of an accident or other trauma, or during recovery from surgery. Acute care is usually given in a hospital by specialized personnel using complex and sophisticated technical equipment and materials, and it may involve intensive care.

acute catarrhal sinusitis [Gk, *kata* + *rhoia,* flow; L, *sinus,* hollow], an inflammation that involves both the nose and the sinuses.

acute cervicitis. See **cervicitis.**

acute childhood leukemia, a progressive, malignant disease of the blood-forming tissues that is characterized by the uncontrolled proliferation of immature leukocytes and their precursors, particularly in the bone marrow, spleen, and lymph nodes. It is the most frequent cancer in children, with a peak onset occurring between 2 and 5 years of age. Acute leukemia is classified according to cell type: **acute lymphoid leukemia (ALL)** includes lymphatic, lymphocytic, lymphoblastic, and lymphoblastoid types; **acute nonlymphoid leukemia (ANLL)** includes granulocytic, myelocytic, monocytic, myelogenous, monoblastic, and monomyeloblastic types (the myelocytic and monocytic series are abbreviated **AML**). ALL is predominantly a disease of childhood, whereas AML occurs in all age groups. The exact cause of the disease is unknown, although various factors are implicated, including genetic defects, immune deficiency, viruses, and carcinogenic environmental factors, primarily ionizing radiation.

acute cholecystitis. See **cholecystitis.**

acute circulatory failure, a drop in heart output resulting from either cardiac or noncardiac causes and leading to tissue hypoxia. If not controlled immediately, the condition usually progresses to one of shock syndrome.

acute circumscribed edema [L *circum* around, *scribere* to draw; Gk *oidema* swelling], localized edema, often associated with an inflammatory lesion or process.

acute confusional state, a form of central nervous system dysfunction caused by interference with the metabolic or other biochemical processes essential for normal brain functioning. Symptoms may include disturbances in cognition, levels of awareness, memory, and orientation.

acute decubitus [L, *decumbere,* to lie down], an ulceration that may develop secondary to increased pressure.

acute delirium, an episode of delirium that is sudden, severe, and transient.

acute diarrhea [Gk *dia, rhein* to flow], a sudden severe attack of diarrhea.

acute diffuse peritonitis [L *diffundere* to pour out; Gk *peri* near, *tenein* to stretch, *itis*], an acute widespread attack of peritonitis affecting most of the peritoneum and usually caused by a perforation of the stomach or appendix.

acute disease, a disease characterized by a relatively short duration of symptoms that are usually severe. An episode of acute disease results in recovery to a state comparable to the patient's state of health and activity before the disease, in passage into a chronic phase, or in death.

acute endarteritis [Gk *endon* within, *arteria* windpipe, *itis*], an inflamed condition of the cells lining an artery. It may be caused by an infection or the proliferation of fibrous tissue inside the wall of a large artery.

acute epiglottitis, a severe, rapidly progressing bacterial infection of the upper respiratory tract that occurs in young children, primarily between 2 and 7 years of age. It is characterized by sore throat, croupy stridor, and an inflamed epiglottis, which may cause sudden respiratory obstruction and be quickly fatal. The infection is generally caused by *Haemophilus influenzae,* type B, although streptococci may occasionally be the causative agent. Transmission occurs by infection with airborne particles or contact with infected secretions.

acute febrile polyneuritis. See **Guillain-Barré syndrome.**

acute fibrinous pericarditis [L *fibra* fibrous; Gk *peri* near, *kardia* heart, *itis*], an acute inflammation of the pericardium with fibers extending into the pericardial sac. The endothelial cells of the pericardium become inflamed.

acute glomerulonephritis. See **postinfectious glomerulonephritis.**

acute goiter, [L *guttur* throat], a condition of sudden enlargement of the thyroid gland.

acute hallucinatory paranoia, a form of paranoia in which hallucinations are combined with the systematized delusions.

acute hallucinosis. See **alcoholic hallucinosis.**

acute hemorrhagic conjunctivitis, a highly contagious eye disease usually caused by enterovirus type 70 and found primarily in densely populated humid areas, particularly the developing countries or places with a high immigration or refugee population. Clinical features include sudden onset of ocular pain, itching, redness, photophobia, edema of the eyelid, and profuse watery discharge.

acute hemorrhagic leukoencephalitis. See **acute necrotizing hemorrhagic encephalopathy.**

acute hemorrhagic pancreatitis [Gk *haima* blood, *rhegnynei* to gush, *pan* all, *kreas* flesh], a potentially fatal inflammation of the pancreas characterized by bleeding, tissue necrosis, and digestive tract paralysis.

acute hydrocele [Gk *hydor* water, *kele* hernia], a benign fluid accumulation within the tunica vaginalis that causes swelling of the scrotum. It is a frequent, minor disorder in infant boys and adults. Surgery eliminates the condition.

acute hypoxia, a sudden or rapid depletion in available oxygen, as may result from asphyxia, airway obstruction, acute hemorrhage, or abrupt cardiorespiratory failure. Clinical signs may include either hypoventilation or hyperventilation to the point of air hunger, and neurologic deficits ranging from headache to loss of consciousness.

acute idiopathic polyneuritis. See **Guillain-Barré syndrome.**

acute illness, any illness characterized by signs and symptoms that are of a short duration, are usually severe, and impair the normal functioning of the patient.

acute infectious paralysis [L *inficere* to stain; Gk *paralyein* to be palsied], **1.** an alternative term for acute anterior poliomyelitis. **2.** infectious polyneuritis.

acute intermittent porphyria (AIP), a genetically transmitted metabolic disorder characterized by acute attacks of neurologic dysfunction that can be started by either environmental or endogenous factors. Women are affected more frequently than men, and attacks often are precipitated by female sex hormones. Other precipitating factors include starvation or crash dieting, bacterial or viral infections, and a wide range of pharmaceutical products. Any part of the nervous system can be affected, and a common effect is mild to severe abdominal pain associated with autonomic neuropathy.

acute laryngotracheobronchitis. See croup.

acute lymphoblastic leukemia. See acute lymphocytic leukemia.

acute lymphocytic leukemia (ALL), a progressive, malignant disease characterized by large numbers of immature cells, closely resembling lymphoblasts in the bone marrow, the circulating blood, the lymph nodes, the spleen, the liver, and other organs. The number of normal blood cells is reduced. About 80% of the 2,250 cases a year in the United States occur in children, with the greatest number diagnosed between 2 and 5 years of age.

acute mountain sickness. See altitude sickness.

acute myelitis, a sudden, severe inflammation of the spinal cord.

acute myelocytic leukemia (AML), a malignant neoplasm of blood-forming tissues characterized by the uncontrolled proliferation of immature granular leukocytes that usually have azurophilic Auer rods in their cytoplasm. The typical symptoms, appearing abruptly or, more often, gradually, are spongy bleeding gums, anemia, fatigue, fever, dyspnea, moderate splenomegaly, joint and bone pains, and repeated infections. Chloromas (greenish granulocytic sarcomas) may develop in bone or soft tissue. AML may occur at any age, but it most frequently affects adolescents and young adults.

acute myocardial infarction (AMI) [L acutus + Gk mys muscle, kardia heart; L infarcire to stuff], the early critical stage of myocardial infarction, characterized by elevated ST segments in the reflecting leads.

acute necrotizing hemorrhagic encephalopathy, a degenerative, often fatal disease of the brain, characterized by marked edema, numerous minute hemorrhages, necrosis of blood vessel walls, especially those of small veins, demyelination of nerve fibers, and infiltration of the meninges with neutrophils, lymphocytes, and histiocytes. Typical signs are severe headache, fever, and vomiting; convulsions may occur, and the patient may rapidly lose consciousness.

acute necrotizing ulcerative gingivitis (ANUG), a fusospirochetal infection characterized by necrotic, foul-smelling ulcers of the gums and throat, fever, and enlarged lymph nodes in the neck. It is usually associated with poor oral hygiene and is most common in conditions in which there is crowding and malnutrition.

acute nephritis, a sudden inflammation of the kidney, characterized by albuminuria and hematuria, but without edema or urine retention. It affects children most commonly and usually involves only a few glomeruli.

acute nicotine poisoning [L Nicotiana, potio drink], toxic effect produced by nicotine, usually in the insecticide form. Characteristics include burning sensation in the mouth, nausea and vomiting, diarrhea, palpitations, pulmonary edema, and convulsions that may lead to death.

acute nongonorrheal vulvitis [L non not; Gk gone seed + rhoia flow; L vulva wrapper; Gk itis], an inflammation of the vulva that is due to chafing, accumulation of sebaceous material, or other causes that are nonvenereal.

acute nonlymphocytic leukemia. See acute myelocytic leukemia.

acute nonspecific pericarditis [Gk peri around, kardia heart, itis], an inflammation of the pericardium, with or without effusion. It often is associated with myocarditis but usually resolves without complications.

acute pain, severe pain, as may follow surgery or trauma or accompany myocardial infarction or other conditions and diseases. Acute pain occurring in the first 24 to 48 hours after surgery is often difficult to relieve, even with drugs. Acute pain in individuals with orthopedic problems originates from the periosteum, the joint surfaces, and the arterial walls. Muscle pain associated with bone surgery results from muscle ischemia rather than muscle tension. Acute abdominal pain often causes the individual involved to lie on one side and draw up the legs in the fetal position.

acute pancreatitis [Gk pan all, kreas flesh, itis], a sudden inflammation of the pancreas marked by symptoms of acute abdomen and escape of pancreatic enzymes into the pancreas tissues. The condition is associated with biliary disease or alcoholism.

acute paranoid disorder, a psychopathologic condition characterized by a persecutory delusional system of rapid onset, quick development, and short duration, usually lasting less than 6 months. The disorder, which rarely becomes chronic, is most commonly seen in persons who have experienced drastic changes in their environment, such as immigrants, refugees, prisoners, military inductees, and, in a less severe form, those leaving home for the first time.

acute pharyngitis, a sudden, severe inflammation of the pharynx.

acute pleurisy, an inflammation of the pleura, often secondary to a disease of the lung. It is characterized by irritation without recognizable effusion and is localized.

acute primary myocarditis, 1. an inflammation of the heart muscle caused by a bacterial infection initiated locally or carried through the bloodstream. **2.** a severe inflammation of the heart muscle associated with degeneration in the muscle fibers with the release of leukocytes into the interstitial tissues.

acute promyelocytic leukemia, a malignancy of the blood-forming tissues, characterized by severe bleeding, scattered bruises, a low fibrinogen level and platelet count, and the proliferation in bone marrow of promyelocytes and blast cells with distinctive Auer rods.

acute prostatitis [L *acutus* sharp, Gk *prostates* one standing before, *itis*], a sudden, severe inflammation of the prostate gland.

acute psychosis, one of a group of disorders in which the ability to process information is diminished and disordered. The cause of the particular disorder may be a known physiologic abnormality. In other cases the physiologic abnormality may not be recognized, but the defect in function is clearly present. Delirium and acute brain syndrome are associated with known pathophysiology in the brain and are characterized by disorientation, disturbance of memory, and lapses in consciousness. Acute functional psychosis is associated with unknown pathophysiology and varying signs and symptoms that progress from insomnia and agitation to paranoid or grandiose delusions, mania, emotional lability, and hallucinations.

acute pyogenic arthritis, an acute bacterial infection affecting one or more joints, caused by trauma or a penetrating wound and occurring most frequently in children. Typical signs are pain, redness, and swelling in the affected joint, muscular spasms in the area, chills, fever, diaphoresis, and leukocytosis.

acute radial nerve palsy, a type of mononeuropathy characterized by damage to the radial nerve and consequent weakening of the muscles of the forearm. It may be caused by excessive compression of the radial nerve against a hard surface in individuals insensitized by the intake of alcohol or sedatives.

acute radiation exposure, exposure of short duration to intense ionizing radiation, usually occurring as the result of an accident in an industrial installation, a nuclear power plant, or a vehicle transporting radioactive material or from proximity to a detonated atom bomb. Exposure of the whole body to approximately 10,000 rad (100 gray) causes neurologic and car-

diovascular breakdown and is fatal within 24 hours. A dose between 500 and 1,200 rad (5 and 12 gray) destroys GI mucosa, produces bloody diarrhea, and may cause death in several days. Death may occur weeks after exposure to a dose of 200 to 500 rad (2 to 5 gray) because of the destructive effect on blood-forming organs, but 600 rad (6 gray) is generally considered the fatal dose.

acute rejection [L *rejicere* to throw back], the rapid reaction against allograph or xenograph tissue that is incompatible after about a week's delay while the immune response increases in intensity.

acute respiratory distress syndrome. See adult respiratory distress syndrome.

acute respiratory failure (ARF) [L *acutus* + *respirare* respiratory, *fallere* to deceive], a sudden inability of the lungs to maintain normal respiratory function. It may be caused by an obstruction in the airways or failure of the lungs to exchange gases in the alveoli.

acute rheumatic arthritis, arthritis that occurs during the acute phase of rheumatic fever.

acute schizophrenia, a form of schizophrenia that is characterized by the sudden onset of personality disorganization with symptoms that include confusion, emotional turmoil, fear, depression, dreamlike dissociation, and bizarre behavior. Episodes appear suddenly in persons whose previous behavior has been relatively normal and are usually of short duration.

acute secondary myocarditis, a sudden severe inflammation of the heart muscle secondary to a disease of the endocardium or the pericardium, or a generalized infection.

acute septic myocarditis [Gk *septikos* putrid, *mys* muscle, *kardia* heart, *itis*], a severe inflammation of the myocardium associated with pus formation, necrosis, and abscess formation.

acute suppurative sinusitis [L *acutus* + *suppurare* to form pus + *sinus* hollow; Gk *itis* inflammation], a purulent infection of the sinuses. Symptoms are pain over the inflamed area, headache, chills, and fever.

acute tonsillitis, [L *acutus* + *tonsilla;* Gk *itis* inflammation], an inflammation of one or both tonsils associated with either a catarrhal exudate over the tonsil or the discharge of caseous or suppurative material from the tonsil crypts.

acute toxicity, the harmful effect of a toxic agent that manifests itself in seconds, minutes, hours, or days after entering the patient.

acute transverse myelitis, an inflammation of the entire thickness of the spinal cord, affecting both the sensory and the motor nerves. It is the most destructive form of myelitis and can develop rapidly, accompanied by necrosis and neurologic disorder that commonly persist after recovery. Patients who develop spastic reflexes soon after the onset of this disease are more likely to recover. This disorder may develop from a variety of causes, such as acute multiple sclerosis, measles, pneumonia, and the ingestion of certain toxic agents, such as carbon monoxide, lead, and arsenic. Such poisonous substances can destroy the entire circumference of the spinal cord, including the myelin sheaths, the axis cylinders, and the neurons, and can also cause hemorrhage and necrosis.

acute tubular necrosis (ATN) [L *tubulus* tubule; Gk *nekros* dead, *osis* condition], sudden failure of the kidney tubules. The condition is commonly caused by an interruption of the blood supply to the tubules, resulting in ischemia.

acute urethral syndrome [Gk *ourethra* urethra, *syn* together, *dromos* course], a group of pelvic area symptoms experienced by women, including dysuria, urinary frequency, urinary tenesmus, lower back pain, and suprapubic aching and cramping. However, clinical evidence of a pathogen or other factor to account for the symptoms is usually absent.

acyanotic /ā′sī-ənot′ik/ [Gk *a* not, *kyanos* blue], pertaining to the absence of the blue appearance of the skin and mucous membranes.

acyanotic congenital defect /āsī′ənot′ik/ [Gk *a, kyanos* not blue], a congenital heart defect that does not produce cyanosis under normal circumstances.

acyclovir /əsī′klōvir/, an antiviral (acycloguanosine) prescribed topically in an ointment for the treatment of herpes simplex keratitis and both topically and systemically in other types of herpes infections, including genital herpes. Acyclovir appears to act selectively by inhibiting the functions of herpesvirus DNA molecules.

acyesis /ā′sī-ē′sis/, **1.** the absence of pregnancy. **2.** a condition of sterility in women.

acylation /as′ilā′shən/, the incorporation into a molecule of an organic compound of an acyl group.

a.d., abbreviation for the Latin phrase, *auris dextra,* right ear.

ADA, 1. abbreviation for *American Dental Association.* **2.** abbreviation for *American Diabetes Association.* **3.** abbreviation for *American Dietetic Association.* **4.** abbreviation for **adenosine deaminase.**

adactyly /ādak′tilē/ [Gk *a, daktylos* not fin-

ger or toe], a congenital defect in which one or more digits of the hand or foot are missing.

adamantinoma,   adamantoblastoma. See **ameloblastoma.**

ADAMHA, abbreviation for United States **Alcohol, Drug Abuse, and Mental Health Administration.**

Adam's apple, *informal.* the bulge at the front of the neck produced by the thyroid cartilage of the larynx.

Adams-Stokes syndrome [Robert Adams, Dublin surgeon, b. 1791; William Stokes, Dublin physician, b. 1804], a condition characterized by sudden recurrent episodes of loss of consciousness because of incomplete heart block. Seizures may accompany the episodes.

adaptation [L *adaptatio* act of adapting], a change or response to stress of any kind, such as inflammation of the nasal mucosa in infectious rhinitis or an increase in crying in a frightened child. Adaptation may be normal, self-protective, and developmental, such as a child learning to talk; it may be all encompassing, creating further stress, such as polycythemia, naturally occurring at high altitudes, which provides more oxygen-carrying red blood cells but which may also lead to thrombosis, venous congestion, or edema.

adaptation model, (in nursing) a conceptual framework that focuses on the patient as an adaptive system, one in which nursing intervention is required when a deficit develops in the patient's ability to cope with the internal and external demands of the environment. These demands are classified in four groups: physiologic needs, the need for a positive self-concept, the need to perform social roles, and the need to balance dependence and independence. Nursing care is planned to promote adaptive responses to cope successfully with the current stress on the patient's wellbeing.

adaptation syndrome. See **general adaptation syndrome.**

adapted clothing, clothing that has been modified to permit disabled persons to dress themselves with a minimum of difficulty.

adaptive device [L *adaptatio* process of adapting; OFr *devise*], any structure, design, instrument, contrivance, or equipment that enables a person with a disability to function independently.

adaptive hypertrophy [L *adaptatio*; Gk *hyper* excessive, *trophe* nourishment], an increase in amount of tissue that compensates for a loss of the same or similar tissue so that function is not impaired.

adaptive response, an appropriate reaction to an environmental demand.

adaptor RNA. See **transfer RNA.**

ADC, abbreviation for **AIDS-dementia complex.**

Addams, Jane (1860–1935), an American social reformer. In 1889 she founded Hull House in Chicago, one of the first social settlements in the United States, where volunteers from many disciplines, including nursing, lived and continued working in their professions. She was co-recipient of the Nobel peace prize in 1931.

addict /ad'ikt/ [L *addicere* to devote], a person who has become physiologically or psychologically dependent on a chemical, such as alcohol or other drugs, so that normal social, occupational, and other responsible life functions are disrupted.

addiction [L *addictere* to devote], compulsive, uncontrollable dependence on a substance, habit, or practice to such a degree that cessation causes severe emotional, mental, or physiologic reactions.

addictive personality, a personality marked by traits of compulsive and habitual use of a substance or practice to cope with psychic pain engendered by conflict and anxiety.

Addis count, a method for counting red blood cells, white blood cells, epithelial cells, casts, and protein content in a sedimented 12-hour urine sample. Results are expressed as the number of each formed element excreted per 24 hours. The count is useful for diagnosing and managing kidney disease.

addisonian anemia. See **pernicious anemia.**

addisonian crisis, Addison's crisis. See **adrenal crisis.**

addisonism, [Thomas Addison, London physician, b. 1793], a condition characterized by the physical signs of Addison's disease, although loss of adrenocortical functions is not involved. The signs include increased pigmentation of the skin and mucous membranes, general debility, and a tendency to develop tubercular infections.

Addison's disease [Thomas Addison], a life-threatening condition caused by partial or complete failure of adrenocortical function, often resulting from autoimmune processes, infection (especially tubercular or fungal), neoplasm, or hemorrhage in the gland. All three general functions of the adrenal cortex are lost: glucocorticoid, mineralocorticoid, and androgenic.

Addison's keloid. See **morphea.**

Addison's syndrome. See **Addison's disease.**

addition [L *additio* something added], a chemical reaction in which two complete molecules combine to form a new product, usually by attachment to carbon atoms at a double or triple bond of one of the molecules.

additive effect [L *additio* + *effectus*], the combined effect of drugs, which when used in combination produce an enhanced effect that is no greater than the sum of their separately measured individual effects.

adduct /ədukt'/ [L *adducere* to bring to], to move toward the median line or axis of the body.

adduction /əduk'shən/ [L *adducere*], movement of a limb toward the axis of the body.

adductor /əduk'tər/, a muscle that acts to draw a part toward the axis or midline of the body.

adductor brevis, a somewhat triangular muscle in the thigh and one of the five medial femoral muscles. Arising from the inferior ramus of the pubis between the gracilis and the obturator externus, it passes downward, backward, and to the side to insert into the line leading from the lesser trochanter to the linea aspera of the femur. It acts to adduct and rotate the thigh medially and to flex the leg.

adductor canal, a triangular channel beneath the sartorius muscle and between the adductor longus and vastus medialis through which the femoral vessels and the saphenous nerve pass.

adductor longus, the most superficial of the three adductor muscles of the thigh and one of five medial femoral muscles. A triangular muscle that arises from the anterior surface of the pubis, it spreads to form a broad fleshy belly, passing downward, backward, and to the side to insert into the linea aspera of the femur, between the vastus medialis and the adductor magnus. It functions to adduct and flex the thigh.

adductor magnus, the long, heavy triangular muscle of the medial aspect of the thigh. It arises from the inferior rami of the ischium and pubis and the inferior margin of the ischial tuberosity. The fibers of the muscle insert into the rough surface of the greater trochanter, into the linea aspera via a broad aponeurosis, and into the distal third of the femur via a rounded, thick tendon. The adductor magnus acts to adduct the thigh. The proximal portion acts to rotate the thigh medially and to flex it on the hip; the distal portion acts to extend the thigh and rotate it laterally.

adenalgia /ad'ənal'jə/ [Gk *aden* gland, *algos* pain], a condition characterized by pain in any of the glands.

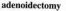
adenectomy /ad′ənek′təmē/ [Gk *aden* + *ektome* excision], the surgical removal of any gland.

Aden fever. See **dengue fever.**

adenine /ad′ənin/, a purine-base component of the nucleic acids, DNA and RNA, and a constituent of cyclic AMP and the adenosine portion of AMP, ADP, and ATP.

adenine arabinoside. See **vidarabine.**

adenine-D-ribose. See **adenosine.**

adenitis /ad′ənī′tis/, an inflammatory condition of a lymph node or gland. Acute adenitis of the cervical lymph nodes manifests itself as a sore throat and stiff neck. Inflammation of the lymph nodes of the mesenteric portion of the peritoneum often produces pain and other symptoms similar to those of appendicitis. Generalized adenitis is a secondary symptom of syphilis. Therapy requires treatment of the primary infection by the administration of antimicrobial agents, application of warm compresses, and, in rare cases, incision and drainage.

adenoacanthoma /ad′ənō·ak′anthō′mə/ [Gk *aden* + *akantha* thorn, *oma* tumor], a neoplasm that may be malignant or benign, derived from glandular tissue with squamous differentiation shown by some of the cells.

adenoameloblastoma /ad′ən·amel′ōblastō′mə/, *pl.* **adenoameloblastomas, adenoameloblastomata,** a benign tumor of the maxilla composed of ducts lined with columnar or cuboidal epithelial cells. It develops in tissue that normally gives rise to the teeth, and it is most often seen in young people.

adenoassociated virus (AAV) /ad′ənō-/, a defective virus that can reproduce only in the presence of adenoviruses. It is not yet known what role, if any, these organisms have in causing disease.

adenocarcinoma /ad′ənōkärsinō′mə/, *pl.* **adenocarcinomas, adenocarcinomata** [Gk *aden* + *karkinos* crab, *oma*], any one of a large group of malignant, epithelial cell tumors of the glands. Specific tumors are diagnosed and named by cytologic identification of the tissue affected; for example, an adenocarcinoma of the uterine cervix is characterized by tumor cells resembling the glandular epithelium of the cervix. **–adenocarcinomatous,** *adj.*

adenocarcinoma in situ, a localized growth of abnormal glandular tissue that may become malignant. It is most common in the endometrium and in the large intestine.

adenocarcinoma of the kidney. See **renal cell carcinoma.**

adenocele /ad′ənōsēl′/, a cystic, glandular tumor.

adenochondroma /ad′ənōkondrō′mə/, *pl.* **adenochondromas, adenochondromata** [Gk *aden* + *chondros* cartilage, *oma*], a neoplasm of cells derived from glandular and cartilaginous tissues, as a mixed tumor of the salivary glands.

adenocyst /ad′ənōsist′/ [Gk *aden* + *kytis* bag], a benign epithelial tumor in which the cells form glandular structures and cysts. A kind of adenocyst is **papillary adenocystoma lymphomatosum.**

adenocystic carcinoma, a malignant neoplasm composed of cords of uniform small epithelial cells arranged in a sievelike pattern around cystic spaces that often contain mucus. The tumor occurs most frequently in the salivary glands, breast, mucus glands of the upper and lower respiratory tract, and, occasionally, in vestibular glands of the vulva.

adenodynia. See **adenalgia.**

adenoepithelioma /ad′ənō·ep′ithē′lē·ō′mə/, *pl.* **adenoepitheliomas, adenoepitheliomata** [Gk *aden* + *epi* on, *thele* nipple, *oma*], a neoplasm consisting of glandular and epithelial components.

adenofibroma /ad′ənōfībrō′mə/, *pl.* **adenofibromas, adenofibromata**[Gk *aden* + L *fibra* fiber, *oma*], a tumor of the connective tissues that contains glandular elements.

adenofibroma edematodes, a neoplasm consisting of glandular elements and connective tissue in which there is marked edema, as in a nasal polyp.

adenohypophysis /ad′ənōhīpof′isis/ [Gk *aden* + *hypo* beneath, *phyein* to grow], the anterior lobe of the pituitary gland. It secretes growth hormone, thyrotropin, adrenocorticotropic hormone, melanocyte stimulating hormone, follicle stimulating hormone, luteinizing hormone, prolactin, beta lipotropin molecules, and endorphins. Releasing hormones from the hypothalamus regulate secretion by the anterior pituitary. Adenohypophyseal hormones control activities of the thyroid, gonads, adrenal cortex, breast, and other endocrine glands.

adenoid /ad′ənoid/ [Gk *aden* + *eidos* form] **1.** having a glandular appearance, particularly lymphoid. **2.** adenoids, hypertrophy of the pharyngeal tonsil. **–adenoidal,** *adj.*

adenoidal speech, an abnormal manner of speaking caused by hypertrophy of the adenoidal tissue that normally exists in the nasopharynx of children. It is often characterized by a muted, nasal quality.

adenoid cystic carcinoma. See **adenocystic carcinoma.**

adenoidectomy /ad′ənoidek′təmē/ [Gk *aden* + *eidos* form, *ektome* excision], removal of the lymphoid tissue in the nasopharynx. The surgical procedure may be performed because the adenoids are enlarged, causing obstruction, or chronically infected, and normal adenoids may be excised as a prophylactic measure during tonsillectomy.

adenoid hyperplasia, a condition in which enlarged adenoid glands cause partial respiratory obstruction, especially in children. Enlarged adenoids, often in association with enlarged tonsils, are a frequent cause of recurrent otitis media, sinusitis, and conduction deafness.

adenoid hypertrophy [Gk *aden* + *eidos* + *hyper* excessive, *trophe* nourishment], an enlargement of the pharyngeal tonsil.

adenoids, small masses of lymphoid tissue forming the pharyngeal tonsils on the posterior wall of the nasopharynx.

adenoid tissue, the lymphoid tissue that forms the pharyngeal tonsils.

adenoleiomyofibroma /ad′ənōlī′ōmī′ō-fībrō′mə/, *pl.* **adenoleiomyofibromas, adenoleiomyofibromata** [Gk *aden* + *leios* smooth, *mys* muscle; L *fibra* fiber; Gk *oma*], a glandular tumor with smooth muscle, connective tissue, and epithelial elements.

adenolipoma /ad′ənōlipō′mə/, *pl.* **adenolipomas, adenolipomata** [Gk *aden* + *lipos,* fat, *oma*], a neoplasm consisting of elements of glandular and fatty tissue.

adenolipomatosis /ad′ənōlipōmətō′sis/, a condition characterized by the growth of numerous adenolipomas in the groin, axilla, and neck.

adenolymphoma. See **papillary adenocystoma lymphomatosum.**

adenoma /ad′ənō′mə/, *pl.* **adenomas, adenomata** [Gk *aden* + *oma*], a tumor of glandular epithelium in which the cells of the tumor are arranged in a recognizable glandular structure. Kinds of adenomas include **acidophilic adenoma, basophilic adenoma, fibroadenoma,** and **insulinoma.** –**adenomatous,** *adj.*

adenoma sebaceum /sebā′sē·əm/, an abnormal skin condition consisting of multiple, wartlike, yellowish red, waxy papules on the face, composed chiefly of fibrovascular tissue. The lesions are not true adenomas but fibromas and part of the complex known as tuberous sclerosis.

adenomatoid /ad′ənō′mətoid/ [Gk *aden, oma* + *eidos* form], resembling a glandular tumor.

adenomatosis /ad′ənōmətō′sis/, an abnormal condition in which hyperplasia or tumor development affects two or more glands, usually the thyroid, adrenals, or pituitary.

adenomatous goiter /ad′ənō′mətəs/, an enlargement of the thyroid gland because of an adenoma or numerous colloid nodules.

adenomatous polyp [Gk *aden, oma* + *polys* many, *pous* foot], a tumor that develops in glandular tissue.

adenomatous polyposis coli (APC), a gene associated with **familial adenomatous polyposis,** an inherited disorder characterized by the development of myriad polyps in the colon beginning in late adolescence or early adulthood. Untreated, the condition may lead to colon cancer.

adenomyoepithelioma. See **adenocystic carcinoma.**

adenomyofibroma /ad′ənōmī′ōfībrō′mə/, *pl.* **adenomyofibromas, adenomyofibromata** [Gk *aden* + *mys* muscle; L *fibra* fiber; Gk *oma*], a fibrous tumor that contains glandular and muscular components.

adenomyoma /ad′ənōmī·ō′mə/, *pl.* **adenomyomas, adenomyomata,** a tumor of the endometrium of the uterus characterized by a mass of smooth muscle containing endometrial tissue and glands. It usually causes dysmenorrhea.

adenomyomatosis /ad′ənōmī′ōmətō′sis/, an abnormal condition characterized by the formation of benign nodules resembling adenomyomas, found in the uterus or in parauterine tissue.

adenomyosarcoma /ad′ənōmī′ōsärkō′mə/, *pl.* **adenomyosarcomas, adenomyosarcomata,** a malignant tumor of soft tissue containing glandular elements and striated muscle. A kind of adenomyosarcoma is **Wilms' tumor.**

adenomyosis /ad′ənōmī·ō′sis/, **1.** a benign neoplastic condition characterized by tumors composed of glandular tissue and smooth muscle cells. **2.** a malignant neoplastic condition characterized by the invasive growth of uterine mucosa in the wall of the uterus or the oviducts.

adenopathy /ad′ənop′əthē/ [Gk *aden* + *pathos* suffering], an enlargement of any gland, especially a lymphatic gland. –**adenopathic,** *adj.*

adenosarcoma /ad′ənōsärkō′mə/, *pl.* **adenosarcomas, adenosarcomata** [Gk *aden* + *sarx* flesh, *oma*], a malignant glandular tumor of the soft tissues of the body.

adenosarcorhabdomyoma /ad′ənōsär′kōrab′dōmī′ō′mə/, *pl.* **adenosarcorhabdomyomas, adenosarcorhabdomyomata,** a tumor composed of glandular and connective tissue and striated muscle elements.

adenosine /əden′əsin, -sēn/, a compound derived from nucleic acid, composed of adenine and a sugar, D-ribose. Adenosine is the major molecular component of nucleotides and of the nucleic acids.

adenosine deaminase /dē·am′inās,/ an enzyme that catalyzes the conversion of adenosine to the nucleoside inosine through the removal of an amino group.

adenosine diphosphate, a product of the hydrolysis of adenosine triphosphate.

adenosine hydrolase, an enzyme that catalyzes the conversion of adenosine into adenine and ribose.

adenosine kinase, an enzyme in the liver and kidney that catalyzes the transfer of a phosphate group from adenosine triphosphate to produce adenosine phosphate.

adenosine monophosphate (AMP), an ester, composed of adenine, D-ribose, and phosphoric acid, that affects energy release in work done by a muscle.

adenosine phosphate, a compound consisting of the nucleotide adenosine attached through its ribose group to one, two, or three phosphoric acid molecules. Kinds of adenosine phosphate, all of which are interconvertible, are **adenosine diphosphate, adenosine monophosphate,** and **adenosine triphosphate.**

adenosine 3′:5′-cyclic phosphate. See **cyclic adenosine monophosphate.**

adenosine triphosphatase (ATPase), an enzyme in skeletal muscle that catalyzes the hydrolysis of adenosine triphosphate to adenosine diphosphate and inorganic phosphate. Mitochondrial ATPase is involved in obtaining energy for cellular metabolism, and myosin ATPase is involved in muscle contraction.

adenosine triphosphate (ATP), a compound consisting of the nucleotide adenosine attached through its ribose group to three phosphoric acid molecules. It stores energy in muscles, which is released when it is hydrolized to adenosine diphosphate.

adenosis /ad′ənō′sis/, **1.** a disease in any gland, especially a lymphatic gland. **2.** an abnormal development or enlargement of glandular tissue.

adenovirus /ad′ənōvī′rəs/ [Gk *aden* + L *virus* poison], any one of the 33 medium-sized viruses of the Adenoviridae family, pathogenic to humans, that cause conjunctivitis, upper respiratory infection, or GI infection. –**adenoviral,** *adj.*

adenylate /əden′ilāt/, a salt or ester of adenylic acid.

adenylate cyclase, an enzyme that initiates the conversion of adenosine triphosphate (ATP) to cyclic adenosine monophosphate (cAMP), a mediator of many physiologic activities.

adenylate kinase, an enzyme in skeletal muscle that makes possible the reaction ATP + AMP = 2ADP.

adenylic acid. See **adenosine monophosphate.**

adequate and well-controlled studies, clinical and laboratory studies that the sponsors of a new drug are required by law to conduct to demonstrate the truth of the claims made for its effectiveness.

adermia /ədur′mē·ə/ [Gk *a, derma* not skin], a congenital or acquired skin defect or the absence of skin.

ADH, abbreviation for **antidiuretic hormone.**

ADHA, abbreviation for the **American Dental Hygienists' Association.**

adhere /adhir′/, to stick together or become fastened together, as two surfaces.

adherence, 1. the quality of clinging or being closely attached. **2.** the process in which a person follows rules, guidelines, or standards, especially as a patient follows prescription and recommendations for a regimen of care.

adherent, [L *adhaerens* sticking to], the tendency of one substance to cling to the surface of another substance.

adherent placenta, a placenta that remains attached to the uterine wall beyond the normal time after delivery of the fetus.

adhesion /adhē′zhən/ [L *adhesio* clinging to], a band of scar tissue that binds together two anatomic surfaces that are normally separate from each other. Adhesions are most commonly found in the abdomen where they form after abdominal surgery, inflammation, or injury.

adhesiotomy /adhē′sē·ot′əmē/ [L *adhesio* + Gk *temnein* to cut], the surgical dividing or separating of adhesions, usually performed to relieve an intestinal obstruction.

adhesive /adhē′siv/ [L *adhesio*], a quality of a substance that enables it to become attached to another substance.

adhesive absorbent dressing, an absorbent dressing on an adhesive backing.

adhesive pericarditis, a condition characterized by adhesions between the visceral and the parietal layers of the pericardium or by adhesions between the pericardium and the mediastinum, diaphragm, or chest wall.

adhesive peritonitis, an inflammation of the peritoneum, characterized by adhesions between adjacent serous surfaces.

adhesive plaster, See **adhesive tape.**

adhesive pleurisy, inflammation of the pleura with exudation, causing obliteration of the pleural space through the fusion of the visceral pleural layer covering the lungs and the parietal layer lining the walls of the thoracic cavity.

adhesive skin traction, one of two kinds of skin traction in which the therapeutic pull of traction weights is applied with adhesive straps that stick to the skin over the body structure involved, especially a fractured bone. Adhesive skin traction is used only when continuous traction is desired and skin care for the affected area presents no serious problem.

adhesive tape, a strong fabric material covered on one side with an adhesive. Often water-repellent, it may be used to hold bandages and dressings in place, to immobilize a part, or to exert pressure. Also called **adhesive plaster.**

ADI, abbreviation for **acceptable daily intake.**

adiadochokinesia /ā'dē·ad'əkōkinē'sis, ədī'ədō'kō-/, an inability to perform rapidly alternating movements, such as pronation and supination, or elbow flexion and extension.

adiastole /ā'dī·as'təlē/ [Gk *a* not, *dia* across, *stellein* to set], absence or imperceptibility of the diastolic stage of the cardiac cycle.

adiathermance /a'dī·əthur'məns/ [Gk *a, dia* not through, *therme* heat], the quality of being unaffected by radiated heat.

adient /ad'ē·ənt/ [L *adire* moving toward], characterized by a tendency to move toward rather than away from stimuli. –**adience,** *n.*

Adie's pupil /ā'dēz/ [William J. Adie, London physician, b. 1816], an abnormal condition of the eyes marked by one pupil that reacts much more slowly to light changes or accommodation or convergence than the pupil of the other eye.

Adie's syndrome, the condition of Adie's pupil accompanied by depressed or absent tendon reflexes, particularly the ankle and knee-jerk reflexes.

adipectomy. See **lipectomy.**

adiphenine hydrochloride /ədif'ənin/, an anticholinergic with smooth muscle relaxant properties that has been used for spastic disorders of the GI and genitourinary tract.

adipic /ədip'ik/ [L *adeps* fat], of or pertaining to fatty tissue.

adipocele /ad'ipōsēl'/ [L *adeps* + Gk *kele* hernia], a hernia containing fat or fatty tissue.

adipocyte /ad'ipōsīt'/, a fat cell.

adipofibroma /ad'ipōfībrō'mə/, *pl.* **adipofibromas, adipofibromata** [L *adeps* + *fibra* fiber; Gk *oma*], a fibrous neoplasm of the connective tissue in which there are fatty components.

adipokinesis /ad'ipō'kinē'sis/, the mobilization of fat or fatty acids in lipid metabolism.

adiponecrosis /ad'ipōnikrō'sis/ [L *adeps* + Gk *nekros* dead, *osis* condition], a necrosis of fatty tissue in the body. –**adiponecrotic,** *adj.*

adiponecrosis subcutanea neonatorum, a dermatologic condition of the newborn characterized by patchy areas of hardened subcutaneous fatty tissue and a bluish red discoloration of the overlying skin.

adipose /ad'ipōs/, fatty. Adipose tissue is composed of fat cells arranged in lobules.

adipose tissue [L *adeps* fat; OFr *tissu*], a collection of fat cells.

adipose tumor. See **lipoma.**

adiposogenital dystrophy /ad'ipō'sōjen'itəl/ [L *adeps* + *genitalis* generation], a disorder occurring in adolescent boys, characterized by genital hypoplasia and feminine secondary sex characteristics, including female distribution of fat. It is caused by hypothalamic malfunction or by a tumor in the anterior pituitary gland.

adipsia /ādip'sē·ə/ [Gk *a, dipsa* not thirst], absence of thirst.

aditus /ad'itəs/ [L, going to], an approach or an entry.

adjunct [L *adjungere* to join], (in health care) an additional substance, treatment, or procedure used for increasing the efficacy or safety of the primary substance, treatment, or procedure or to facilitate its performance. –**adjunctive,** *adj.*

adjunctive group, a group with specific activities and focuses, such as socialization, sensory stimulation, or reality orientation.

adjunctive psychotherapy, a form of psychotherapy that concentrates on improving a person's general mental and physical outlook without trying to resolve basic emotional problems. Some kinds of adjunctive psychotherapy are **music therapy, occupational therapy, physical therapy,** and **recreational therapy.**

adjunct to anesthesia, one of a number of drugs of five different classes. Each class of drug has a use in anesthetic procedures, as well as a therapeutic indication in other aspects of health care. Adjuncts to anesthesia are used as premedications, as intravenous supplements to hypnotic or analgesic medications, and as neuromuscular blocking agents, analeptics, and therapeutic gases.

adjustable orthodontic band, a thin metal ring, usually made of stainless steel, equipped with an adjusting screw to allow alteration in size, fitted to a tooth and serving for the attachment of orthodontic appliances.

adjusted death rate. See **standardized death rate.**

adjustment. See **accommodation.**

adjustment, impaired, a NANDA-accepted nursing diagnosis of an individual's inability to modify his or her life-style behavior in a manner consistent with a change in health status. Defining characteristics include verbalization of nonacceptance of health status change, nonexistent or unsuccessful ability to be involved in problem solving or goal setting, lack of movement toward independence, lack of future-oriented thinking, and extended period of shock, disbelief, or anger regarding health status change.

adjustment reaction [L adjuxtare to bring together], a temporary disorder of varying severity that occurs as an acute reaction to overwhelming stress in persons of any age who have no apparent underlying mental disorders. Symptoms include anxiety, withdrawal, depression, brooding, temper outbursts, crying spells, attention-getting behavior, enuresis, loss of appetite, aches, pains, and muscle spasms. Symptoms usually recede and eventually disappear as stress diminishes.

adjuvant [L, ad, juvare, to help], 1. a substance, especially a drug, added to a prescription to assist in the action of the main ingredient. 2. in immunology, a substance added to an antigen that enhances or modifies the antibody response to the antigen.

adjuvant chemotherapy /ad′jəvənt/, the use of anticancer drugs in the absence of any detectable residual cancer, as after surgical removal of a cancer. The method is used when there is a significant risk that undetectable cancer cells may still be present.

adjuvant therapy, the treatment of a disease with substances that enhance the action of drugs, especially drugs that promote the production of antibodies.

ADL, abbreviation for **activities of daily living.**

ad lib, an abbreviation of the Latin phrase ad libitum, meaning to be taken as desired and sometimes used in pharmaceutical prescriptions.

administration of parenteral fluids, the intravenous infusion of various solutions to maintain adequate hydration, restore blood volume, reestablish lost electrolytes, or provide partial nutrition.

Administration On Aging (AOA), the principal agency designated to carry out the provisions of the Older Americans Act of 1965. The AOA advises the Secretary of the Department of Health and Human Services and other Federal Departments and agencies on the characteristics and needs of older people and develops programs designed to promote their welfare.

ADN, abbreviation for **Associate Degree in Nursing.**

ad nauseam [L ad, to; Gk nausia seasickness], a situation or condition that induces nausea and vomiting.

adnexa /adnek′sə/, sing. **adnexus** [L adnectere to tie together], tissue or structures in the body that are next to or near another, related structure. The ovaries and the uterine tubes are adnexa of the uterus. **–adnexal,** adj.

adnexitis /ad′neksī′tis/, an inflammation of the adnexal organs of the uterus, such as the ovaries or the fallopian tubes.

adolescence [L adolescere to grow up], 1. the period in development between the onset of puberty and adulthood. It usually begins between 11 and 13 years of age, with the appearance of secondary sex characteristics, and spans the teen years, terminating at 18 to 20 years of age with the acquisition of completely developed adult form. During this period the individual undergoes extensive physical, psychologic, emotional, and personality changes. 2. the state or quality of being adolescent or youthful.

adolescent, 1. of, pertaining to, or characteristic of adolescence. 2. one in the state or process of adolescence; a teenager.

adolescent vertebral epiphysitis. See **Scheuermann's disease.**

adoption [L adoptere to choose], to select and bring into a previously established relationship.

ADP, abbreviation for **adenosine diphosphate.**

adrenal /adrē′nəl/ [L ad to, ren kidney], pertaining to the adrenal or suprarenal glands that are located atop the kidneys.

adrenal cortex [L ad, ren to kidney], the greater portion of the adrenal or suprarenal gland, fused with the gland's medulla and producing mineralocorticoids, androgens, and glucocorticoids, hormones essential to homeostasis. The outer cortex is normally a deep yellow; the inner part, dark red or brown.

adrenal cortical carcinoma, a malignant neoplasm of the adrenal cortex that may cause adrenogenital syndrome or Cushing's syndrome. Such tumors vary in size, occur at any age, and are more common in females than in males.

adrenal crisis, an acute, life-threatening state of profound adrenocortical insufficiency in which immediate therapy is required. It is characterized by glucocorticoid deficiency, a drop in extracellular fluid volume, and hyperkalemia.

adrenalectomy /ədrē′nalek′təmē/ [L ad, ren + Gk ektome excision], the surgical removal of one or both adrenal glands or the resection of a portion of one or both glands, performed to reduce the excessive secretion of adrenal hormones when an adrenal tumor or a malignancy of the breast or prostate is present. If both glands are removed, maintenance dosage of steroids continues for life. Stress and fatigue must be avoided.

adrenal gland, either of two secretory organs perched atop the kidneys. Each consists of two parts having independent functions: the cortex and the medulla. The adrenal cortex, in response to adrenocorticotropic hormone secreted by the anterior pituitary, secretes cortisol and androgens. Adrenal androgens are precursors that are converted by the liver to testosterone and estrogens. Renin from the kidney controls adrenal cortical production of aldosterone. The adrenal medulla manufactures the catecholamines epinephrine and norepinephrine.

adrenaline. See **epinephrine.**

adrenal insufficiency [L *ad, ren* kidney, *in* not, *sufficere* to suffice], a condition in which the adrenal gland is unable to function adequately.

adrenalize /ədrē′nəlīz/, to stimulate or excite.

adrenal medulla, the inner portion of the adrenal gland. Adrenal medulla cells secrete epinephrine and norepinephrine.

adrenal virilism, a condition characterized by hypersecretion of adrenocortical androgens, resulting in somatic masculinization. Excessive production of the hormone may be caused by a virilizing adrenal tumor, congenital adrenal hyperplasia, or an inborn deficiency of enzymes required to transform endogenous androgenic steroids to glucocorticoids. Girls born with adrenogenitalism may be pseudohermaphroditic with clitoral enlargement and labial fusion in infancy and later hirsutism, low vocal pitch, acne, amenorrhea, and masculine distribution of hair and development of muscles. Boys with congenital adrenogenitalism show precocious development of the penis and prostate and of pubic and axillary hair, but their testes remain small and immature because negative feedback from the high level of adrenal androgens prevents the normal pubertal increase in pituitary gonadotropin.

adrenarche /ad′rinär′kē/ [L *ad, ren* + Gk *arche* beginning], the intensified activity in the adrenal cortex that occurs at about 8 years of age and increases the elaboration of various hormones, especially androgens.

adrenergic /ad′rinur′jik/ [L *ad, ren* + Gk *ergon* work], of or pertaining to sympa-

thetic nerve fibers of the autonomic nervous system that use as neurotransmitters epinephrine or epinephrine-like substances.

adrenergic blocking agent. See **antiadrenergic.**

adrenergic bronchodilator, a drug that acts on the sympathetic nervous system receptors to cause relaxation of the bronchial smooth muscle cells. Examples include drugs that contain epinephrine, ephedrine, isoproterenol, or albuterol.

adrenergic drug. See **sympathomimetic.**

adrenergic fibers, nerve fibers of the autonomic nervous system that release the neurotransmitter norepinephrine and, in some areas, dopamine. Most postganglionic sympathetic fibers are of this type.

adrenergic nerve [L *ad, ren;* Gk *ergon* work; L *nervus*], a nerve of the autonomic system that controls the release of norepinephrine at its synapses.

adrenergic receptor, a site in a sympathetic effector cell that reacts to adrenergic stimulation. Two types of adrenergic receptors are recognized: alpha-adrenergic receptors and beta-adrenergic receptors. In general, stimulation of alpha receptors is excitatory of the function of the host organ or tissue, and stimulation of the beta-receptors is inhibitory.

adrenocortical /-kôr′tikəl/ [L *ad,ren* + *cortex* bark], pertaining to the outer or superficial portion of the adrenal gland.

adrenocortical hormone (ACH) [L *ad, ren, cortex;* Gk *hormaein* to set in motion], any of the hormones secreted by the cortex of the adrenal gland, including the glucocorticoids, mineral corticoids, and sex hormones.

adrenocorticotropic /ədrē′nōkôr′tikōtrop′-ik/ [L *ad, ren* + *cortex* rind; Gk *trope* a turning], of or pertaining to stimulation of the adrenal cortex. Also **adrenocorticotrophic** /-trof′ik/.

adrenocorticotropic hormone (ACTH), a hormone of the anterior pituitary gland that stimulates the growth of the adrenal gland cortex and the secretion of corticosteroids. ACTH secretion, regulated by corticotropin releasing factor (CRF) from the hypothalamus, increases in response to a low level of circulating cortisol and to stress, fever, acute hypoglycemia, and major surgery.

adrenocorticotropin, the adrenocorticotropic hormone (**ACTH**), secreted by the anterior pituitary gland that stimulates secretion of other hormones by the adrenal cortex.

adrenodoxin /ədrē′nōdok′sin/, a protein produced by the adrenal glands that participates in the transfer of electrons within animal cells.

adrenogenital syndrome. See **adrenal virilism.**

adrenoleukodystrophy (ALD), a rare, hereditary childhood metabolic disease that is transmitted as a recessive sex-linked trait and that affects only boys. It is characterized by adrenal atrophy and widespread cerebral demyelination, producing progressive mental deterioration, aphasia, apraxia, and eventual blindness.

adrenomegaly /-meg'əlē/ [L *ad,ren;* Gk *megaly* large], an abnormal enlargement of one or both adrenal glands.

adromia /ədrō'mē·ə/ [Gk *a, dromos* not course], the absence of the conductive capacity of any nerve that normally innervates a muscle.

ADRV, abbreviation for **adult rotavirus.**

adsorbent, a substance that takes up another by the process of adsorption, as by the attachment of one substance to the surface of the other.

adsorption [L *ad, sorbere* to suck in], a natural process whereby molecules of a gas or liquid adhere to the surface of a solid. The phenomenon depends on an assortment of factors such as surface tension and electrical charges. Many biologic reactions involve adsorption. In chemistry, adsorption is the principle on which chromatography is based and allows for the separation of a mixture into component fractions for qualitative analysis.

ADT, abbreviation for *Accepted Dental Therapeutics,* a journal published by the Council on Dental Therapeutics of the American Dental Association.

adult [L *adultus* grown up], **1.** one who is fully developed and matured and who has attained the intellectual capacity and the emotional and psychologic stability characteristic of a mature person. **2.** a person who has reached full legal age.

adult celiac disease. See **celiac disease.**

adult day-care center, a facility for the supervised care of older adults, providing activities such as meals and socialization during specified day hours, with the participants returning to their homes each evening.

adult ego state, (in psychiatry) a part of the self that analyzes and solves problems using information received from the parent ego and child ego states.

adulteration /ədul'tərā'shən/ [L *adulterare* to defile], the debasement or dilution of the purity of any substance, process, or activity by the addition of extraneous material.

adult hemoglobin. See **hemoglobin A.**

adulthood, the phase of development characterized by physical and mental maturity.

adult nurse practitioner, a registered nurse who has received additional education and training in the primary health care of adults. The additional education may be obtained through a master's degree program or a nondegree continuing education certificate program.

adult-onset diabetes. See **non-insulin-dependent diabetes.**

adult polycystic disease. See **polycystic kidney disease.**

adult respiratory distress syndrome (ARDS), a respiratory emergency characterized by respiratory insufficiency and failure usually after aspiration of a foreign body, cardiopulmonary bypass surgery, gram-negative sepsis, multiple blood transfusions, oxygen toxicity, trauma, pneumonia, or other respiratory infection. The symptoms and signs of ARDS include shortness of breath, rapid breathing, inadequate oxygenation of the arterial blood, and decreased lung compliance.

adult rickets, a disease affecting adults that resembles rickets.

adult rotavirus (ADRV), a form of rotavirus that causes severe diarrhea in adults.

advance [Fr *avancer* to move forward], a surgical technique in which a muscle or tendon is brought forward.

advanced cardiac life support (ACLS), emergency medical procedures in which basic life support efforts of cardiopulmonary resuscitation are augmented by establishment of an intravenous fluid line, drug administration, control of cardiac arrhythmias, and ventilation equipment. The procedures usually require direct or indirect supervision by a physician.

advance declaration. See **advance directive, living will.**

advance directive [Fr *avancer;* L *dirigere* to direct], **1.** an advance declaration by a patient adjudged to be hopelessly and terminally ill that the person does not want to be connected to life-support equipment. The document, signed and witnessed, may generally serve as a "Living Will," depending on current state laws. **2.** a Durable Power of Attorney for Health Care, in which a terminally ill person assigns to someone else the power to make health care decisions if the patient is no longer able to make such decisions. The document directs the surrogate person to function as "attorney-in-fact" and make the final decision regarding cessation of treatment.

advanced life support. See **Emergency Medical Technician-Advanced Life Support.**

adventitia [L *adventitius* coming from abroad], the outermost layer, composed of connective tissue with elastic and collagenous fibers, of an artery or other structure.

adventitious /ad'ventish'əs/ [L *adventitius*], of or pertaining to an accidental condition or an arbitrary action.

adventitious bursa, an abnormal bursa that develops as a response to friction or pressure.

adventitious crisis, an accidental, uncommon tragedy that may affect an entire community or population, such as an earthquake, flood, or airplane crash.

adventitious sounds, breath sounds that are not normally heard, such as crackles and rhonchi.

adverse drug effect, a harmful, unintended reaction to a drug administered at normal dosage.

adverse reaction, any harmful or unintended effect of a medication, diagnostic test, or therapeutic intervention.

advocacy, 1. a process whereby a nurse provides a patient with the information to make certain decisions. 2. a method by which groups can work together to develop programs that ensure the availability of high-quality health care for a community.

adynamia /ad'inā'mē·ə/ [Gk *a, dynamis* not strength], lack of physical and emotional drive because of a pathologic condition. **–adynamic,** *adj.*

adynamia episodica hereditaria, a condition seen in infancy, characterized by muscle weakness and episodes of flaccid paralysis. It is inherited as an autosomal dominant trait.

adynamic fever, an elevated temperature with a feeble pulse, nervous depression, and a cool, moist skin.

adynamic ileus. See **ileus.**

AE amputation, the amputation of the arm above the elbow.

Aedes /ā·ē'dēz/ [Gk *aedes* unpleasant], a genus of mosquito, prevalent in tropical and subtropical regions. Several species are capable of transmitting pathogenic organisms to humans, including dengue, equine encephalitis, St. Louis encephalitis, tularemia, and yellow fever.

aerate /er'āt/ [Gk *aer* air], to charge a substance or a structure with air, carbon dioxide, or oxygen.

aeration [Gk, *aer,* air], 1. exchange of carbon dioxide for oxygen by blood in the lungs. 2. a process of exposing a tissue or fluid to the air, or artificially charging it with oxygen or another gas, such as carbon dioxide.

Aerobacter aerogenes. See *Enterobacter cloacae.*

aerobe /er'ōb/ [Gk *aer* + *bios* life], a microorganism that lives and grows in the presence of free oxygen. Kinds of aerobe are **facultative aerobe** and **obligate aerobe.**

aerobic /erō'bik/, 1. of or pertaining to the presence of air or oxygen. 2. able to live and function in the presence of free oxygen. 3. requiring oxygen for the maintenance of life. 4. of or pertaining to aerobic exercise.

aerobic exercise, any physical exercise that requires additional effort by the heart and lungs to meet the increased demand by the skeletal muscles for oxygen. The exercise generally requires heavier breathing than passive muscular activity and results in increased heart and lung efficiency with a minimum of wasted energy.

aerobic glycolysis. See **glycolysis.**

aerobics. See **aerobic exercise.**

aerobic training, physical exercises designed to require an increased intake and distribution of oxygen. Such exercises involve depletion of the body's normal tissue stores of oxygen by comparatively strenuous exertion and replacement of the oxygen through deep breathing. This training can be accomplished by biking, walking, jogging, or other similar activities for at least 20 minutes, three times per week.

aerodontalgia /er'ōdontal'jə/ [Gk *aer* + *odous* tooth, *algos* pain], a painful sensation in the teeth because of decreased atmospheric pressure, as may occur at high altitudes.

aeroembolism. See **embolism.**

aerophagy /erof'əjē/ [Gk *aer* + *phagein* to eat], the swallowing of air, usually followed by belching, gastric distress, and flatulence.

aerosinusitis /er'ōsī'nəsī'tis/ [Gk *aer* + L *sinus* curve; Gk *itis*], inflammation, edema, or hemorrhage of the frontal sinuses caused by expansion of air within the sinuses when barometric pressure is decreased, as in aircraft at high altitudes.

aerosol /er'əsol'/ [Gk *aer* + *hydor* water; L *solutus* dissolved], 1. nebulized particles suspended in a gas or air. 2. a pressurized gas containing a finely nebulized medication for inhalation therapy. 3. a pressurized gas containing a nebulized chemical agent for sterilizing the air of a room.

aerosol bronchodilator therapy, the use of drugs that provide relaxation of the respiratory tract smooth muscle tissue when administered as a mist to be inhaled.

aerospace medicine, a branch of medicine concerned with the physiologic and

psychologic effects of living and working in an artificial environment beyond the atmospheric and gravitational forces of the earth. The stress of extraterrestrial travel requiring long periods of weightlessness is a major concern.

aerotitis /er′əti′tis/ [Gk *aer* + *otikos* ear, *itis*], an inflammation of the ear caused by changes in atmospheric pressure.

aerotitis media, inflammation or bleeding in the middle ear caused by a difference between the air pressure in the middle ear and that of the atmosphere, as occurs in sudden changes in altitude, in diving, or in hyperbaric chambers. Symptoms are pain, tinnitus, diminished hearing, and vertigo.

Æsculapius /es′kyŏŏlā′pē·əs/, the ancient Greek god of medicine. Serpents were regarded as sacred by Æsculapius, and he is symbolized in modern medicine by a staff with a serpent entwined about it.

AF, abbreviation for **atrial fibrillation.**

AFB, abbreviation for **acid-fast bacillus.**

afebrile /āfē′bril, āfeb′ril/ [Gk *a, febris* not fever], without fever.

affect /əfekt′/ [L *affectus* influence], an outward manifestation of a person's feelings or emotions. –**affective,** *adj.*

affection [L *affectare* to be influenced], **1.** an emotional state expressed by a warm or caring feeling toward another individual. **2.** a morbid process affecting all or a part of the human body.

affective [L *affectus*], pertaining to emotion, mood, or feeling.

affective disorder. See **major affective disorder.**

affective intimacy, a measure of well-being in a family group in which members feel close to one another but do not lose their individuality.

affective learning, the acquisition of behaviors involved in expressing feelings in attitudes, appreciations, and values.

affective psychosis, a psychotic reaction in which the primary clinical feature is a severe disorder of mood or emotions.

affect memory, a particular emotional feeling that recurs whenever a significant experience is recalled.

afferent /af′ərənt/ [L *ad, ferre* to carry], proceeding toward a center, as applied to arteries, veins, lymphatics, and nerves.

afferent nerves [L *ad, ferre* + *nervus*], nerve fibers that transmit impulses from the periphery toward the central nervous system.

afferent pathway [L *ad, ferre;* AS *paeth, weg*], the course or route taken, usually by a linkage of neurons, from the periphery of the body toward the center.

afferent tract [L *ad, ferre* + *tractus*], a pathway for nerve impulses traveling inward, or toward the brain, the center of an organ or other body structure.

affidavit /af′idā′vit/ [L *affidare* under oath], a written statement that is sworn to before a notary public or an officer of the court.

affiliated hospital [L *ad, filius* to son], a hospital that is associated to some degree with a medical school or health program.

affinity [L *affinis* related], the measure of the binding strength of the antibody-antigen reaction.

affirmative defense [L *affirmare* to make firm], (in law) a denial of guilt or wrongdoing based on new evidence rather than on simple denial of a charge, as a plea of immunity according to a good samaritan law. The defendant bears the burden of proof in an affirmative defense.

afibrinogenemia /afi′brinōjenē′mē·ə/ [Gk *a* not; L *fibra* fiber; Gk *genein* to produce, *haima* blood], a rare, hematologic disorder characterized by a relative lack or absence of fibrinogen in the blood.

aflatoxins /af′lätok′sins/ [Gk *a* not; L *flavus* yellow; Gk *toxikon* poison], a group of carcinogenic and toxic factors produced by *Aspergillus flavus* food molds. The mucotoxins have been found to cause liver cancer in laboratory animals.

AFO, abbreviation for **ankle-foot orthosis.**

AFP, abbreviation for **alpha fetoprotein.**

African lymphoma. See **Burkitt's lymphoma.**

African sleeping sickness. See **African trypanosomiasis.**

African tick fever. See **relapsing fever.**

African tick typhus, a rickettsial infection transmitted by ixodid ticks and characterized by fever, maculopapular rash, and swollen lymph nodes.

African trypanosomiasis, a disease caused by the parasites *Trypanosoma brucei gambiense* or *Trypanosoma brucei rhodesiense,* transmitted to humans by the bite of the tsetse fly. The disease is fatal unless treated. Kinds of African trypanosomiasis are **Gambian trypanosomiasis** and **Rhodesian trypanosomiasis.**

afterbirth [AS *aefter;* ME *burth*], the placenta, the amnion and the chorion, and some amniotic fluid, blood, and blood clots expelled from the uterus after childbirth.

aftercare [AS *aefter, caru*], health care offered a patient after discharge from a hospital or other medical facility.

afterdepolarization, a slow channel depolarization that follows in the wake of an action potential. It is thought to be responsible for atrial and ventricular ectopic beats, especially in the setting of digitalis toxicity.

afterload [AS *aefter;* ME *lod*], the load, or resistance, against which the left ventricle must eject its volume of blood during contraction.

afterloading, (in radiotherapy) a technique in which an unloaded applicator or needle is placed within the patient at the time of an operative procedure and subsequently loaded with the radioactive source under controlled conditions in which health care personnel are protected against exposure to radiation. A kind of afterloading is **remote afterloading.**

aftermovement, an involuntary muscle contraction that causes a continued movement of a limb after a strong exertion against resistance has stopped.

afterpains [AS *aefter;* Gk *poine* penalty], contractions of the uterus common during the first days postpartum. They tend to be strongest in nursing mothers and multiparas, resolve spontaneously, and may require analgesia.

afterpotential wave, either of two smaller waves, positive or negative, that follows the main spike potential wave of a nerve impulse, as recorded on an oscillograph tracing.

Ag, symbol for the element **silver.**

AGA, abbreviation for **appropriate for gestational age.**

against medical advice (ama), pertaining to a client's decision to discontinue a therapy despite the advice of medical professionals.

agalactia /ā′gəlak′shə/ [Gk *a, gala* not milk], the failure of the mother to secrete enough milk to breast-feed an infant after childbirth.

agamete /āgam′ēt/ [Gk *a, gamos* not marriage] **1.** any of the unicellular organisms that reproduce asexually by multiple fission, such as bacteria and protozoa. **2.** any asexual reproductive cell, such as a spore or merozoite, that forms a new organism without fusion with another cell.

agametic /āgəmē′tik/, asexual; without recognizable sex organs or gametes. Also **agamous** /ag′əməs/.

agamic /āgam′ik/, reproducing asexually, without the union of gametes; asexual.

agammaglobulinemia /agam′əglob′yŏŏlinē′mē·ə/ [Gk *a, gamma* not gamma (third letter of Greek alphabet); L *globulus* small sphere; Gk *haima* blood], a rare disorder characterized by the absence of the serum immunoglobulin, gamma globulin, associated with an increased susceptibility to infection. The condition may be transient, congenital, or acquired.

agamogenesis /əgam′ōjen′əsis/ [Gk *a, gamos* not marriage, *genein* to produce], asexual reproduction, as by budding or simple fission of cells; parthenogenesis. –**agamocytogenic, agamogenetic, agamogenic, agamogonic** *adj.*

agamont. See **schizont.**

agamous. See **agametic.**

aganglionic megacolon. See **Hirschsprung's disease.**

agar-agar /a′gärä′gär/ [Malay], a dried hydrophilic, colloidal product obtained from certain species of red algae. It is widely used as the basic ingredient in solid culture media in bacteriology.

agarose /ag′ərōs/, an essentially neutral fraction of agar used as a medium in electrophoresis, particularly for separation of serum proteins, hemoglobin variants, and lipoprotein fractions.

agastric [Gk *a* not, *gaster* stomach], a condition of lacking a stomach or digestive tract.

age [L *aetus*], a stage of development at which the body has arrived, as compared by physical and laboratory examinations to what is normal for a man or woman of the same chronologic span of life.

aged, a state of having grown older or more mature than others of the population group.

ageism /ā′jizəm/ [L *aetas* lifetime], an attitude that discriminates, separates, stigmatizes, or otherwise disadvantages older adults on the basis of chronologic age.

agency [L *agere* to do], (in law) a relationship between two parties in which one authorizes the other to act in his or her behalf as an agent.

agenesia corticalis [Gk *a, genein* not to produce; L, cortex], the failure of the cortical cells of the brain, especially the pyramidal cells, to develop in the embryo, resulting in infantile cerebral paralysis and severe mental retardation.

agenesis /ājen′əsis/ [Gk *a, genein* not to produce] **1.** congenital absence of an organ or part, usually caused by a lack of primordial tissue and failure of development in the embryo. **2.** impotence or sterility. –**agenic,** *adj.*

agenetic fracture, a spontaneous fracture caused by an imperfect osteogenesis.

ageniocephaly /ājen′ē·ōsef′əlē/ [Gk *a, genein* not to produce; *kephale* head], a form of otocephaly in which the brain, cranial vault, and sense organs are intact but the lower jaw is malformed. –**ageniocephalic, ageniocephalous,** *adj.*

agenitalism /ājen′itəliz′əm/, a condition caused by the lack of sex hormones and the absence or malfunction of the ovaries or testes.

agenosomia /əjen′əsō′mē·ə/, a congenital malformation characterized by the absence or defective formation of the genitals and protrusion of the intestines through an incompletely developed abdominal wall.

agenosomus /əjen′əsō′məs/ [Gk *a, genein* not to produce, *soma* body], a fetus with agenosomia.

agent [L *agere* to do], (in law) a party authorized to act on behalf of another and to give the other an account of such actions.

Agent Orange, a U.S. military code name for a mixture of two herbicides, 2,4-D and 2,4,5-T, used as a defoliant in Southeast Asia during the 1960s war in Vietnam. The herbicides were unintentionally contaminated with the highly toxic chemical dioxin, a cause of cancer and birth defects in animals and of chloracne and porphyria cutanea tarda in humans.

age of majority, the age at which a person is considered to be an adult in the eyes of the law.

age 30 transition, in psychiatry, a period between the ages of 28 and 33 when an individual may reevaluate the choices made in his or her twenties.

ageusia /əgyōō′sē·ə/ [Gk *a* not, *geusis* taste], a loss or impairment of the sense of taste. The degree and cause may vary.

agglutinant [L *agglutinare* to glue], something that causes adhesion, such as an antibody produced in the blood that is stimulated by the presence of an antigen to adhere to it.

agglutination /əglōō′tinā′shən/ [L *agglutinare* to glue], the aggregation or clumping together of cells as a result of their interaction with specific antibodies called agglutinins, commonly used in blood typing and in identifying or estimating the strength of immunoglobulins or immune sera.

agglutination-inhibition test, a serologic technique useful in testing for certain unknown soluble antigens.

agglutinin /əglōō′tinin/, a specific kind of antibody whose interaction with antigens is manifested by agglutination.

agglutinin absorption, the removal from immune serum of antibody by treatment with homologous antigen, followed by centrifugation and separation of the antigen-antibody complex.

agglutinogen /ag′lōōtin′əjin/ [L *agglutinare* + Gk *genein* to produce], any antigenic substance that causes agglutination by the production of agglutinin.

aggregate /ag′rəgāt/ [L *ad, gregare* to gather together], the total of a group of substances or components making up a mass or complex.

aggregate anaphylaxis, an exaggerated reaction of hypersensitivity rapidly induced by the injection of an antigen that forms a soluble antigen-antibody complex.

aggregation [L *ad, gregare* to form a flock], an accumulation of substances, objects, or individuals, as in the clumping of blood cells or the clustering of clients with the same disorder.

aggression [L *aggressio* to attack], a forceful, self-assertive action or attitude that is expressed physically, verbally, or symbolically. Kinds of aggression are **constructive aggression, destructive aggression,** and **inward aggression.**

aggressive personality, a personality with behavior patterns characterized by irritability, tantrums, destructiveness, or violence in response to frustration.

aggressive-radical therapy, (in psychiatry) a form of therapy that introduces the political and social viewpoints of the therapist into the therapeutic process.

aging [L *aetas* lifetime], the process of growing old, resulting in part from a failure of body cells to function normally or to produce new body cells to replace those that are dead or malfunctioning.

agitated [L *agitare* to shake], describing a condition of psychomotor excitement characterized by purposeless, restless activity. Pacing, crying, and laughing without apparent cause are often seen and may release nervous tension associated with anxiety, fear, or other mental stress. **–agitate,** *v.,* **agitation,** *n.*

agitated depression, a form of depression characterized by severe anxiety accompanied by continuous physical restlessness.

agitation, a state of chronic restlessness, generally observed as a psychomotor expression of emotional tension.

agitographia /aj′itōgraf′ē·ə/ [L *agitare* + Gk *graphein* to write], a condition characterized by abnormally rapid writing in which words or parts of words are unconsciously omitted.

agitophasia /aj′itōfā′zhə/ [L *agitare* + Gk *phasis* speech], a condition characterized by abnormally rapid speech in which words, sounds, or syllables are unconsciously omitted, slurred, or distorted. The condition is commonly associated with agitographia.

aglycemia /ā′glīsē′mē·ə/ [Gk *a, glykis* not sweet, *haima* blood], an absence of blood sugar.

agnathia /ag·nath′ē·ə/ [Gk *a, gnathos* not jaw], a developmental defect characterized by total or partial absence of the lower jaw. **–agnathous,** *adj.*

agnathocephalus /ag·nath′əsef′ələs/, a fetus with agnathocephaly.

agnathocephaly /ag·nath'əsef'əlē/ [Gk *a, gnathos* + *kephale* head], a congenital malformation characterized by the absence of the lower jaw, defective formation of the mouth, and placement of the eyes low on the face with fusion or approximation of the zygomas and the ears. **–agnathocephalic, agnathocephalous,** *adj.*

agnathus /ag·nath'əs/ [Gk *a, gnathos* not jaw], a fetus with agnathia.

agnathy. See **agnathia.**

agnogenic myeloid metaplasia. See **myeloid metaplasia.**

agnosia /ag·nō'zhə/ [Gk *a, gnosis* not knowledge], total or partial loss of the ability to recognize familiar objects or persons through sensory stimuli as a result of organic brain damage.

agonal [Gk *agon* struggle], pertaining to death and dying.

agonal respiration /ag'ənəl/ [Gk *agon* struggle], a type of breathing that usually follows a pattern of gasping succeeded by apnea. It generally indicates the onset of respiratory arrest.

agonal thrombus, an aggregation of blood platelets, fibrin, clotting factors, and cellular elements that forms in the heart in the process of dying.

agonist /ag'ənist/ [Gk *agon* struggle], **1.** a contracting muscle whose contraction is opposed by another muscle (an antagonist). **2.** a drug or other substance having a specific cellular affinity that produces a predictable response.

agony [Gk *agon*], severe physical or emotional anguish or distress, as in pain.

agoraphobia /ag'ərə-/ [Gk *agora* marketplace, *phobos* fear], an anxiety disorder characterized by a fear of being in an open, crowded, or public place, such as a field, tunnel, bridge, congested street, or busy department store, where escape may be difficult or help not available in case of sudden incapacitation.

agranular endoplasmic reticulum. See **endoplasmic reticulum.**

agranulocyte /āgran'yoŏlōsīt'/ [Gk *a* not; L *granulum* small grain; Gk *kytos* cell], any leukocyte that does not contain cytoplasmic granules, such as a monocyte or lymphocyte. **–agranulocytic,** *adj.*

agranulocytic /-sī'tik/ [Gk *a, granule* + *kytos* cell], pertaining to a leukocyte or white blood cell, which upon being stained, shows no granules in the cytoplasm.

agranulocytosis /āgran'yoŏlōsītō'sis/, an abnormal condition of the blood, characterized by a severe reduction in the number of granulocytes (basophils, eosinophils, and neutrophils), resulting in fever,

prostration, and bleeding ulcers of the rectum, mouth, and vagina.

agraphia /āgraf'ē-ə/ [Gk *a, graphein* not to write], an abnormal neurologic condition characterized by loss of the ability to write, resulting from injury to the language center in the cerebral cortex. **–agraphic,** *adj.*

A:G ratio, the ratio of protein albumin to globulin in the blood serum. On the basis of differential solubility, with neutral salt solution the normal values are 3.5 to 5 g/dl for albumin and 2.5 to 4 g/dl for globulin.

agrypnia. See **insomnia.**

agrypnocoma /agrip'nōkō'mə/ [Gk *agrypnos* sleepless], a coma in which there is some degree of wakefulness.

agrypnotic /ag'ripnot'ik/, **1.** insomniac. **2.** a drug or other substance that prevents sleep.

agyria /əjī'rē-ə/, **1.** an abnormal condition caused by excessive absorption and tissue deposition of silver salts. It is marked by a slate-gray coloration of the skin and mucous membranes. **2.** a cerebral cortex abnormality in which the gyri are poorly developed.

AHA, abbreviation for **American Hospital Association.**

"aha" reaction /ähä'/, (in psychology) a sudden realization or inspiration, experienced especially during creative thinking.

AHF, abbreviation for **antihemophilic factor.**

AHH, abbreviation for **aryl hydrocarbon hydroxylase.**

Ahumada-del Castillo syndrome, /ä'hōōmä'dädel'kästē'yō/ a form of secondary amenorrhea that may be associated with a pituitary gland tumor.

AI, 1. abbreviation for **artificial insemination. 2.** abbreviation for **artificial intelligence.**

aid, assistance given a person who is ill, injured, or otherwise unable to cope with normal demands of life.

AID, abbreviation for **artificial insemination-donor.**

AIDS /ādz/, abbreviation for **acquired immunodeficiency syndrome.**

AIDS-dementia complex (ADC), a neurologic effect of encephalitis or brain inflammation experienced by nearly one third of all AIDS patients. The condition is characterized by memory loss and other forms of dementia. A suggested cause is that the AIDS virus may destroy neurons without actually entering the brain cells. Autopsies indicate the neuron density in AIDS patients may be 40% lower than in the brains of persons who have not experienced AIDS.

AIDS-wasting syndrome, a category of acquired immunodeficiency syndrome (AIDS). Signs and symptoms may include weight loss, fever, malaise, lethargy, oral thrush, and immunologic abnormalities characteristic of AIDS.

AIH, abbreviation for **artificial insemination-husband.**

ailment [OE *eglan*], any disease or physical disorder or complaint, generally of a chronic, acute, or mild nature.

ainhum. See **autoamputation.**

air [Gk aer], the colorless, odorless gaseous mixture constituting the earth's atmosphere. It consists of 78% nitrogen; 21% oxygen; almost 1% argon; small amounts of carbon dioxide, hydrogen, and ozone; traces of helium, krypton, neon, and xenon; and varying amounts of water vapor.

air bath, the exposure of the naked body to warm air for therapeutic purposes.

airborne contaminants, materials in the atmosphere that can affect the health of persons in the same or nearby environments. Particularly vulnerable are tissues of the upper respiratory tract and lungs.

air compressor, a contrivance that compresses air for storage and use in handpieces and other air-driven medical and dental tools.

air embolism, the abnormal presence of air in the cardiovascular system, resulting in obstruction of the flow of blood through the vessel. Air may be inadvertently introduced by injection, during intravenous therapy or surgery, or traumatically, as by a puncture wound.

air encephalography. See **encephalography.**

air entrainment, the movement of room air into the chamber of a jet nebulizer used to treat respiratory diseases. It increases the rate of nebulization and the amount of liquid administered per unit of time.

airflow pattern, the pattern of movement of respiratory gases through the respiratory tract. The pattern is affected by factors such as gas density and viscosity.

air fluidization, the process of blowing warm air through a collection of microspheres to create a fluidlike environment.

air-fluidized bed, a bed with body support provided by thousands of tiny sodalime glass beads suspended by pressurized warm air.

air hunger, a form of respiratory distress characterized by gasping, labored breathing, or dyspnea.

airplane splint, a splint used for immobilizing a fractured humerus during healing. The splint holds the arm in an abducted position at shoulder level, with the elbow bent.

air pump, a pump that forces air in or out of a cavity or chamber.

air sickness. See **motion sickness.**

air spaces, the alveolar ducts, alveolar sacs, and alveoli of the respiratory system.

air splint, a device for temporarily immobilizing fractured or otherwise injured extremities. It consists of an inflatable cylinder that can be closed at both ends and become rigid when filled with air under pressure.

air thermometer, a thermometer using air as its expansible medium.

airway [Gk *aer* + AS *weg* way], any tubular passage for the movement of air into and out of the lungs, such as the trachea and bronchi, a respiratory anesthesia device, or an oropharyngeal tube used for mouth-to-mouth resuscitation. An airway with a diameter greater than 2 mm is defined as a large, or central, airway; one smaller than 2 mm is called a small, or peripheral, airway.

airway clearance, ineffective, a NANDA-accepted nursing diagnosis of an individual's inability to clear secretions or obstructions from the respiratory tract to maintain airway patency. Defining characteristics include abnormal breath sounds, change in the rate or depth of respiration, tachypnea, cough, cyanosis, and dyspnea.

airway conductance, the instantaneous volumetric gas flow rate in the airway per unit of pressure difference between the mouth, nose, or other airway opening and the alveoli. It is also the reciprocal of airway resistance. It is indicated by the symbol G_{aw}.

airway division, one of the 18 segments of the bronchopulmonary system. The segments are usually numbered from 1 to 10 for both the right and left lungs.

airway obstruction, an abnormal condition of the respiratory system characterized by a mechanical impediment to the delivery or to the absorption of oxygen in the lungs, as in bronchospasm, choking, croup, laryngospasm, chronic obstructive lung disease, goiter, tumor, or pneumothorax.

airway resistance, the ratio of pressure difference between the mouth, nose, or other airway opening and the alveoli to the simultaneously measured resulting volumetric gas flow rate. It is indicated by the symbol R_{aw}.

AK, abbreviation for *above the knee,* a term referring to amputations, amputees, prostheses, and orthoses.

akathisia /ak'athē'zhə/ [Gk *a, kathizein* not to sit], an abnormal condition characterized by restlessness and agitation, as seen in tardive dyskinesia. **–akathisiac,** *adj.*

akinesia /ā′kinē′zhə, ā′kīnē′zhə/ [Gk *a, kinesis* not movement], an abnormal state of motor and psychic hypoactivity or muscular paralysis. **–akinetic** /ā′kinet′ik/, *adj.*

akinetic apraxia, the inability to perform a spontaneous movement.

akinetic mutism, a state in which a person is unable or refuses to move or to make sounds, resulting from neurologic or psychologic disturbance.

akinetic seizure, a type of seizure disorder observed in children. It is a brief, generalized seizure in which the child suddenly falls to the ground.

Al, symbol for the element **aluminum.**

ala /ā′lə/, *pl.* **alae** [L, wing], **1.** any winglike structure. **2.** the axilla.

Ala, abbreviation for **alanine.**

ALA, abbreviation for **aminolevulinic acid.**

ala auris, the auricle of the ear.

ala cerebelli /ser′əbel′ī/, the ala of the central lobule of the cerebellum.

ala cinerea /sinir′ē·ə/, the triangular area on the floor of the fourth ventricle of the brain from which the autonomic fibers of the vagus nerve arise.

alactasia. See **lactase deficiency.**

ala nasi /nā′sī/, the outer flaring cartilaginous wall of each nostril.

alanine (Ala) /al′ənin/, a nonessential amino acid found in many proteins in the body. It is degraded in the liver to produce pyruvate and glutamate.

alanine aminotransferase (ALT), an enzyme normally present in the serum and tissues of the body, especially the tissues of the liver. This enzyme catalyzes the transfer of an amino group from l-alanine to alpha-ketoglutarate, forming pyruvate and l-glutamate.

Al-Anon, an international organization that offers guidance and counseling for the relatives, friends, and associates of alcoholics.

ala of the ethmoid, a small projection on each side of the crista galli of the ethmoid bone. Each ala fits into a corresponding depression of the frontal bone.

ala of the ilium, the upper flaring portion of the iliac bone.

ala of the sacrum, the flat extension of bone on each side of the sacrum.

alar /ā′lär/ [L *ala* wing], pertaining to a winglike structure, such as the shoulder.

alar lamina [L *ala* + *lamina* thin plate], the posterolateral area of the embryonic neural tube through which sensory nerves enter.

alar ligament, one of a pair of ligaments that connects the axis to the occipital bone and limits rotation of the cranium.

alar process [L *ala* + *processus*], a projection of the cribriform plate of the ethmoid bone articulating with the frontal bone.

alarm reaction, the first stage of the general adaptation syndrome, characterized by the mobilization of the various defense mechanisms of the body or the mind to cope with a stressful situation of a physical or emotional nature.

alastrim /al′əstrim/ [Port *alastrar* to spread], a mild form of smallpox, thought to be caused by a weak strain of *Poxvirus variolae.*

Alateen, an international organization that offers counseling and counseling for the children of alcoholics.

ala vomeris /vō′məris/, an extension of bone on each side of the upper border of the vomer.

alba /al′bə/, literally, "white," as in *linea alba.*

Albers-Schönberg disease [Heinrich E. Albers-Schönberg, Hamburg radiologist, b. 1865], a form of osteopetrosis characterized by marblelike calcification of bones.

Albert's disease, an inflammation of the bursa that lies between the Achilles tendon and the calcaneus. It is most frequently caused by injury. If treatment is delayed, the inflammation may cause erosion of the calcaneus.

albicans /al′bikənz/ [L *albus* white], pertaining to the whitish yellow scar tissue of the **corpus albicans** of the ovary. The scar tissue forms following rupture of the ovarian follicle after ovulation. The scar decreases in size and eventually disappears over time.

albinism /al′biniz′əm/, an abnormal congenital condition characterized by partial or total lack of melanin pigment in the body. Total albinos have pale skin that does not tan, white hair, pink eyes, nystagmus, astigmatism, and photophobia.

albino /albī′nō/, [L *albus*], an individual with a marked deficiency of pigment in the eyes, hair, and skin. Because of a lack of eye pigment, the choroid is vulnerable to adverse effects of sunlight frequently resulting in photophobia, astigmatism, and other visual disorders. Lack of skin pigment predisposes the individual to skin cancer.

Albright's syndrome /ôl′brīts/ [Fuller Albright, Boston physician, b. 1900], a disorder characterized by fibrous dysplasia of bone, isolated brown macules on the skin, and endocrine dysfunction. It causes precocious puberty in girls but not in boys.

albumin /alby͞oo′min/ [L *albus* white], a water-soluble, heat-coagulable protein containing carbon, hydrogen, oxygen, nitrogen, and sulfur. Various albumins are found in practically all animal tissues and in many plant tissues.

albumin A, a blood serum constituent that gathers in cancer cells but is deficient in circulation in cancer patients.

albumin (human), a plasma-volume expander prescribed in the treatment of hypoproteinemia, hyperbilirubinemia, and hypovolemic shock.

albumin test [L *albus*], any of several tests for the presence of albumin, a class of simple proteins, in the urine, a common sign of renal or functional disorders. One type of albumin test depends on the change in color of a chemically treated strip of paper in the presence of albumin. The **Heller's test** involves the addition of a thin layer of urine on a small amount of concentrated nitric acid and is regarded as positive if an opaque line forms at the junction of the two fluids. In an **acetic acid test,** a test tube of urine is heated until a cloudiness develops. The test is considered positive if the cloudiness increases when three drops of acetic acid are added.

albuminuria. See proteinuria.

albuterol, an adrenergic used as a bronchodilator. It is prescribed in the treatment of bronchospasm in patients with reversible obstructive airway disease.

alcalase /ˈalkəlās/, a protein enzyme contained in concentrations of about 60 ppm in certain laundry detergents. It is a cause of enzymatic detergent asthma.

alclometasone dipropionate, a topical corticosteroid prescribed for the relief of symptoms of inflammation and pruritus of corticosteroid-responsive dermatoses.

Alcock's canal [Joseph Alcock, English surgeon, b. 1784], a canal formed by the obturator internus muscle and the obturator fascia through which the pudendal nerve and vessels pass.

alcohol [Ar *alkohl* subtle essence], **1.** (USP) a preparation containing at least 92.3% and not more than 93.8% by weight of ethyl alcohol, used as a topical antiseptic and solvent. **2.** a clear, colorless, volatile liquid that is miscible with water, chloroform, or ether, obtained by the fermentation of carbohydrates with yeast. **3.** a compound derived from a hydrocarbon by replacing one or more hydrogen atoms with an equal number of hydroxyl (OH) groups. Depending on the number of hydroxyl radicals, alcohols are classified as monohydric, dihydric, or trihydric. Some kinds of alcohol are **rubbing alcohol, sugar alcohol,** and **unsaturated alcohol.**

alcohol bath, a procedure for decreasing an elevated body temperature. A tepid solution of 25% to 50% alcohol in water is sponged lightly on each limb, then on the trunk. As the alcohol evaporates quickly, the bed is less likely to get wet, the patient does not need to be dried, and, for an equal result, the solution does not need to be as cold as a plain bath with cold water.

Alcohol, Drug Abuse, and Mental Health Administration (ADAMHA), an agency of the U.S. Department of Health and Human Services with three components—the National Institute on Alcohol Abuse and Alcoholism, the National Institute on Drug Abuse, and the National Institute of Mental Health. It conducts and supports research on the biologic, psychologic, epidemiologic, and behavioral aspects of alcoholism, drug abuse, and mental health and illness.

alcoholic ataxia [Ar *alkohl* essence; Gk *ataxia* disorder], a loss of control of voluntary movements associated with peripheral neuritis secondary to alcoholism. A similar form of ataxia may occur with neuritis due to other toxic agents.

alcoholic cardiomyopathy [Ar *alkohl*; Gk *kardia* heart, *mys* muscle, *pathos* disease], cardiac disease associated with alcohol abuse. It is characterized by an enlarged heart and low cardiac output.

alcoholic coma [Ar *alkohl*; Gk *koma* deep sleep], a state of unconsciousness that results from severe alcoholic intoxication.

alcoholic dementia [Ar *alkohl*; L *de* away, *mens* mind], a deterioration of normal cognitive and intellectual functions associated with long-term alcohol abuse.

alcoholic fermentation, the conversion of carbohydrates to ethyl alcohol.

alcoholic hallucinosis, a form of alcoholic psychosis characterized primarily by auditory hallucinations, abject fear, and delusions of persecution. The condition develops in acute alcoholism as withdrawal symptoms shortly after stopping or reducing the intake of alcohol.

alcoholic hepatitis, acute toxic liver injury associated with excess ethanol consumption. This is characterized by necrosis, polymorphonuclear inflammation, and in many instances Mallory bodies.

alcoholic ketoacidosis, the fall in blood pH (acidosis) sometimes seen in alcoholics and associated with a rise in serum ketone bodies (acetone, beta-hydroxybutyric acid, and acetoacetic acid).

alcoholic-nutritional cerebellar degeneration, a sudden, severe incoordination in the lower extremity, characteristic of poorly nourished alcoholics. The patient walks, if at all, with an ataxic or wide-based gait.

alcoholic paralysis [Ar *alkohl;* Gk *paralyein* to be palsied], paralysis affecting the peripheral nerves as a result of alcohol consumption.

alcoholic psychosis, any of a group of severe mental disorders, such as pathologic intoxication, delirium tremens, Korsakoff's psychosis, and acute hallucinosis, characterized by brain damage or dysfunction that results from the excessive use of alcohol.

Alcoholics Anonymous (AA), an international nonprofit organization, founded in 1935, consisting of abstinent alcoholics whose purpose is to help other alcoholics stop drinking and maintain sobriety through group support, shared experiences, and faith in a power greater than themselves.

alcoholic trance, a state of automatism resulting from ethanol intoxication.

alcoholism, the extreme dependence on excessive amounts of alcohol, associated with a cumulative pattern of deviant behaviors. Alcoholism is a chronic illness with frequent medical consequences of central nervous system depression and cirrhosis of the liver. The severity of each of these is increased in the absence of food intake. The severe form of alcohol withdrawal is called delirium tremens.

alcohol poisoning, poisoning caused by the ingestion of any of several alcohols, of which ethyl, isopropyl, and methyl are the most common. Ethyl alcohol (grain alcohol) is found in whiskies, brandy, gin, and other beverages. Isopropyl alcohol is more toxic: Ingestion of 8 ounces may result in respiratory or circulatory failure. Methyl alcohol (wood alcohol) is extremely poisonous: In addition to nausea, vomiting, and abdominal pain, it may cause blindness, and death may follow the consumption of only 2 ounces.

alcohol withdrawal syndrome, the clinical symptoms associated with cessation of alcohol consumption. These may include tremor, hallucinations, autonomic nervous system dysfunction, and seizures.

ALD, abbreviation for **adrenoleukodystrophy.**

aldehyde /al'dəhīd'/ [Ar *alkohl* + L *dehydrogenatum* dehydrogenated], any of a large category of organic compounds derived from a corresponding alcohol by the removal of two hydrogen atoms, as in the conversion of ethyl alcohol to acetaldehyde. Each aldehyde is characterized by a carbonyl (-CHO) group in its empiric formula and can be converted into a corresponding acid by the addition of one oxygen atom, as in the conversion of acetaldehyde to acetic acid.

aldolase /al'dəlās/, an enzyme found in muscle tissue that catalyzes the step in anaerobic glycolysis involving the breakdown of fructose 1,6-diphosphate to glyceraldehyde 3-phosphate.

aldose /al'dōs/, the chemical form of monosaccharides in which the carbonyl group is an aldehyde.

aldosterone /al'dōstərōn', aldos'tərōn/, a steroid hormone produced by the adrenal cortex to regulate sodium and potassium balance in the blood.

aldosteronism /al'dōstərō'nizəm, aldos'-/, a condition characterized by hypersecretion of aldosterone, occurring as a primary disease of the adrenal cortex or, more often, as a secondary disorder in response to various extra-adrenal pathologic processes. Primary aldosteronism may be caused by adrenal hyperplasia or by an aldosterone-secreting tumor. Secondary aldosteronism is associated with increased plasma renin activity and may be induced by the nephrotic syndrome, hepatic cirrhosis, idiopathic edema, congestive heart failure, trauma, burns, or other kinds of stress.

aldosteronoma /al'dōstir'ənō'mə/, *pl.* **aldosteronomas, aldosteronomata,** an aldosterone-secreting adenoma of the adrenal cortex that is usually small and occurs more frequently in the left than the right adrenal gland, causing hyperaldosteronism with salt retention, expansion of the extracellular fluid volume, and increased blood pressure.

Aleppo boil. See **oriental sore.**

alertness [Fr *alerte*], a condition of being quick, active, and keenly aware of the environment.

aleukemic leukemia /ā'lookē'mik/, a type of leukemia in which the total leukocyte count remains within normal limits and few abnormal forms appear in the peripheral blood.

aleukemic myelosis. See **myeloid metaplasia.**

aleukia /āloo'kē-ə/ [Gk *a, leukos* not white], a marked reduction in or the complete absence of white blood cells or blood platelets.

aleukocythemic leukemia. See **aleukemic leukemia.**

Alexander technique, a body-focused mental health therapy introduced by Frederick Alexander. It focuses on individual variations in body musculature, posture, and the breathing process and the correction of defects.

alexia /əlek'sē-ə/ [Gk *a, lexis* not speech], an abnormal neurologic condition characterized by an inability to comprehend written words. **–alexic,** *adj.*

alexithymia /əlek′sithī′mē·ə, -thim′ē·ə/, an inability to consciously experience and communicate feelings.

alfa. See **alpha.**

alga /al′gə/, *pl.* **algae** /al′jī, al′jē/ [L, seaweed], any of a large group of nonmotile, or motile, marine plants containing chlorophyll. Many genera and species of algae are found worldwide in fresh water, in salt water, and on land. All belong to the phylum Thallophyta. **–algal,** *adj.*

algid malaria [L *algere* to be cold], a form of malaria caused by the protozoan *Plasmodium falciparum,* characterized by coldness of the skin, profound weakness, and severe diarrhea.

algodystrophy /al′gōdis′trəfē/, a painful wasting of the muscles of the hands, often accompanied by tenderness and a loss of bone calcium.

algolagnia /al′gōlag′nē·ə/ [Gk *algos* pain, *lagneia* lust], a form of sexual perversion characterized by sadism or masochism.

algologist /algol′əjist/, **1.** a person who specializes in the study of or the treatment of pain. **2.** also called **phycologist.** a person who specializes in the study of algae.

algology, 1. the branch of medicine that is concerned with the study of pain. **2.** also called **phycology.** the branch of science that is concerned with algae.

algophobia [Gk *algos,* pain, *phobos* fear], an anxiety disorder characterized by an abnormal, pervasive fear of experiencing pain or of witnessing pain in others.

algorithm /al′gərith′əm/, **1.** a step-by-step procedure for the solution of a problem by computer, using specific mathematic or logical operations. **2.** an explicit protocol with well-defined rules to be followed in solving a health care problem.

algor mortis, the reduction in body temperature and accompanying loss of skin elasticity that occur after death.

alien [L *alienare* to estrange], something or someone strange, unusual, or foreign.

alienate [L *alienare*], to cause a withdrawal or transference of affection, or detachment.

alienation [L *alienare*], the act or state of being estranged or isolated.

alignment, 1. the arrangement of a group of points or objects along a line. **2.** the placing or maintaining of body structures in their proper anatomic positions, such as repairing a fractured bone.

alimentary /al′əmen′tərē/ [L *alimentum* nourishment], pertaining to food or nourishment and to the digestive organs.

alimentary bolus. See **bolus.**

alimentary canal. See **digestive tract.**

alimentary system [L *alimentum;* Gk *systema*], the digestive system.

alimentation. nourishment.

aliphatic /al′ifat′ik/ [Gk *aleiphar* oil], pertaining to fat or oil, specifically to those hydrocarbon compounds that are open chains of carbon atoms, such as the fatty acids, rather than ring structures.

aliphatic acid, an acid of a nonaromatic hydrocarbon.

aliphatic alcohol, an alcohol that contains an open chain or fatty series of hydrocarbons. Examples include ethyl alcohol and isopropyl alcohol.

alkalemia [Ar *al, qalīy* wood ash; Gk *haima* blood], a condition of increased pH of the blood.

alkali /al′kəlī/ [Ar *al, qalīy* wood ash], a compound with the chemical characteristics of a base. Alkalis combine with fatty acids to form soaps, turn red litmus blue, and enter into reactions that form water-soluble carbonates. **–alkaline,** *adj.* **alkalinity,** *n.*

alkali burn, tissue damage caused by exposure to an alkaline compound like lye. The victim should be immediately taken to a medical facility if the tissue damage is more than slight and superficial.

alkaline-ash, residue in the urine having a pH of higher than 7.

alkaline-ash producing foods, foods that may be ingested in order to produce an alkaline pH in the urine, thereby reducing the incidence of acidic urinary calculi, or that may be avoided in order to reduce the incidence of alkaline calculi. Some of the foods that result in alkaline ash are milk, cream, fruit (except prunes, plums, and cranberries), vegetables (except corn and lentils), almonds, chestnuts, coconuts, and olives.

alkaline bath, a bath taken in water containing sodium bicarbonate, used especially for skin disorders.

alkaline phosphatase, an enzyme present in bone, the kidneys, the intestine, plasma, and teeth. It may be elevated in the serum in some diseases of the bone and liver and in some other illnesses.

alkaline reserve, an additional amount of sodium bicarbonate the body produces to maintain an arterial blood pH of 7.40 when the carbon dioxide level increases as a result of hypoventilation.

alkalinity /al′kəlin′itē/, pertaining to the acid-base relationship of any solution that has fewer hydrogen ions or more hydroxyl ions than pure water, which is an arbitrarily neutral standard with a pH of 7.00.

alkalinize /al′kəliniz′/, **1.** to make a substance alkaline, as through the addition of a base. **2.** to become alkaline.

alkali poisoning, a toxic condition caused by the ingestion of an alkaline agent like liquid ammonia, lye, and some detergent powders. Emergency treatment includes giving copious amounts of water or milk to dilute the alkali. Vomiting is not induced, and mild acids are not administered.

alkali reserves [Ar *al-qalīy* wood ashes; L *reservare* to save], the volume of carbon dioxide or carbonates at standard temperature and pressure held by 100 ml of blood plasma to be neutralized by lactic or other acids. The principal buffer in blood is bicarbonate, which essentially represents the alkali reserve. Hemoglobin phosphates and additional bases also act as buffers. If the alkali reserve is low, a state of acidosis exists; if the alkali reserve is high, alkalosis exists.

alkaloid /al'kəloid/ [Ar *al, qalīy* + Gk *eidos* form], any of a large group of organic compounds produced by plants, including many pharmacologically active substances, such as atropine, caffeine, cocaine, morphine, nicotine, and quinine.

alkalosis /al'kəlō'sis/ [Ar *al, qalīy* + Gk *osis* condition], an abnormal condition of body fluids, characterized by a tendency toward a pH level greater than 7.44, as from an excess of alkaline bicarbonate or a deficiency of acid. Respiratory alkalosis may be caused by hyperventilation, resulting in an excess loss of carbon dioxide and a carbonic acid deficit. Metabolic acidosis may result from an excess intake or retention of bicarbonate, loss of gastric acid in vomiting, potassium depletion, or any stimulus that increases the rate of sodium-hydrogen exchange.

alkaptonuria /alkap'tōnŏŏr'ē·ə/ [Ar *al, qalīy* + Gk *haptein* to possess, *ouron* urine], a rare inherited disorder resulting from the incomplete metabolism of tyrosine, an amino acid, in which abnormal amounts of glycosuric acid are excreted, staining the urine dark. **–alkaptonuric,** *adj.*

alkene /a'kēn/, an unsaturated aliphatic hydrocarbon containing one double bond in the carbon chain, such as ethylene.

alkyl /al'kil/, a hydrocarbon molecule from which one of the hydrogen atoms has been removed, producing an alkyl radical.

alkylamine /al'kiləmīn'/, an amine in which an alkyl group replaces one to three of the hydrogen atoms that are attached to the nitrogen atom, such as methylamine.

alkylating agent /al'kilā'ting/, any substance that contains an alkyl radical and is therefore capable of replacing a free hydrogen atom in an organic compound. Because this type of chemical reaction results

in interference with mitosis and cell division, such agents are particularly useful in the treatment of cancer.

alkylation, a chemical reaction in which a hydrogen atom in an organic compound is replaced by an alkyl radical from an alkylating agent.

ALL, abbreviation for **acute lymphocytic leukemia.**

allantoidoangiopagus /al'əntoidō·an'jē-op'əgəs/ [Gk *allantoeides* sausagelike, *aggeion* vessel, *pagos* fixed], conjoined monozygotic twin fetuses of unequal size that are united by the vessels of the umbilical cord. **–allantoidoangiopagous,** *adj.*

allantoin /əlan'tō·in/, a chemical compound (5-ureidohydantoin), $C_4H_6N_4O_3$, that occurs as a white crystallizable substance found in many plants and in the allantoic and amniotic fluids and fetal urine of primates.

allantois /əlan'tois/ [Gk *allas* sausage, *eidos* form], a tubular extension of the yolk sac endoderm that extends with the allantoic vessels into the body stalk of the embryo. In human embryos, allantoic vessels become the umbilical vessels, and the chorionic villi. **–allantoic** /al'əntō'ik/, *adj.*

allele /əlēl'/, **1.** one of two or more alternative forms of a gene that occupy corresponding loci on homologous chromosomes. **2.** also called **allelomorph** /əlēl'əmôrf'/. one of two or more contrasting characteristics transmitted by alternative genes.

allelomorph. See **allele.**

Allen correction, multichromatic analysis of reaction to correct for background absorbance.

Allen-Doisy test [Edgar Allen, American anatomist, b. 1892; Edward Doisy, American physiologist, b. 1893], a bioassay test for estrogen and gonadotropins by injecting ovariectomized mice with an estrogenic substance. The appearance of cornified cells on vaginal smears is regarded as positive.

Allen test, a test for the patency of the radial artery after insertion of an indwelling monitoring catheter.

allergen /al'ərjin/ [Gk *allos* other, *ergein* to work, *genein* to produce], a substance that can produce a hypersensitive reaction in the body but is not necessarily intrinsically harmful. Some common allergens are pollen, animal dander, house dust, feathers, and various foods. The body normally protects itself against allergens or antigens by the complex chemical reactions of the humoral immune and the cell-mediated immune systems. **–allergenic,** *adj.*

allergenic extract, an extract of the protein of a substance to which a person may be sensitive. The extract, which may be prepared from a wide variety of substances from food to fungi, can be used for diagnosis or for desensitization therapy.

allergic, 1. of or pertaining to allergy. 2. having an allergy.

allergic alveolitis. See **diffuse hypersensitivity pneumonia.**

allergic asthma, a form of asthma caused by the exposure of the bronchial mucosa to an inhaled airborne antigen. This allergen causes the production of antibodies that bind to mast cells in the bronchial tree. The mast cells then release histamine, which stimulates contraction of bronchial smooth muscle and causes mucosal edema. Psychologic factors may provoke asthma attacks in bronchi already sensitized by allergens.

allergic bronchopulmonary aspergillosis, a form of aspergillosis that occurs in asthmatics when the fungus *Aspergillus fumigatus,* growing within the bronchial lumen, causes a hypersensitivity reaction. The characteristics of the condition are similar to those of asthma, including dyspnea and wheezing.

allergic conjunctivitis, an abnormal condition characterized by hyperemia of the conjunctiva caused by an allergy. Common allergens that cause this condition are pollen, grass, topical medications, air pollutants, occupational irritants, and smoke. It is bilateral and usually starts before puberty and lasts about 10 years, commonly recurring in a seasonal pattern.

allergic coryza, acute rhinitis caused by exposure to any allergen to which the person is hypersensitive.

allergic dermatitis [Ger *Allergie* reaction; Gk *derma,* skin, *itis* inflammation], an acute inflammatory condition of the skin following exposure of a body area to an allergen to which the patient is hypersensitive.

allergic interstitial pneumonitis. See **diffuse hypersensitivity pneumonia.**

allergic purpura [Gk *allos* other, *ergein* to work; L *purpura* purple], a chronic disorder of the skin associated with urticaria, erythema, asthma, and rheumatic joint swellings. Unlike in other forms of purpura, platelet count, bleeding time, and blood coagulation are normal.

allergic reaction, a hypersensitive response to an allergen to which an organism has previously been exposed and to which the organism has developed antibodies. Subsequent exposure causes the release of histamine and a variety of symptoms including urticaria, eczema, dyspnea,

bronchospasm, diarrhea, rhinitis, sinusitis, laryngospasm, and anaphylaxis.

allergic rhinitis, inflammation of the nasal passages, usually associated with watery nasal discharge and itching of the nose and eyes because of a localized sensitivity reaction to house dust, animal dander, or an antigen, commonly pollen. The condition may be seasonal, as in hay fever, or perennial, as in allergy to dust or animals.

allergic vasculitis, an inflammatory condition of the blood vessels that is induced by an allergen. Allergic cutaneous vasculitis is characterized by itching, malaise, and a slight fever and by the presence of papules, vesicles, urticarial wheals, or small ulcers on the skin.

allergist, a physician who specializes in the diagnosis and treatment of allergic disorders.

allergy [Gk *allos* other, *ergein* to work], a hypersensitive reaction to intrinsically harmless antigens, most of which are environmental. Allergies are classified according to types I, II, III, and IV hypersensitivity. Types I, II, and III involve different immunoglobulin antibodies and their interaction with different antigens. Type IV allergy is associated with contact dermatitis and T cells, which react directly with the antigen and cause local inflammation. Allergies are divided into those that produce immediate or antibody-mediated reactions and those that produce delayed or cell-mediated reactions. Immediate allergic reactions involve types I, II, and III hypersensitivity and antigen-antibody reactions that activate certain enzymes, creating an imbalance between these enzymes and their inhibitors. Some common symptoms of allergy are bronchial congestion, conjunctivitis, edema, fever, urticaria, and vomiting. Severe allergic reactions, such as anaphylaxis, can cause systemic shock and death. When allergic reactions are life threatening, steroids may be administered intravenously. For milder diseases, such as serum sickness and hay fever, antihistamines are usually administered.

allergy testing, any one of the various procedures used in identifying the specific allergens that afflict the patients involved. Such tests are helpful in prescribing treatment to prevent allergic reactions or to reduce their severity. The most common kinds of allergy testing include the intradermal, scratch, patch, conjunctival, and use tests.

all fours position, the sixth stage in the Rood system of ontogenetic motor patterns. The lower trunk and lower extremities are brought into a cocontraction pattern while stretching of the trunk and limb girdles develops cocontractions of the trunk flexors and extensors.

allied health personnel. See **paramedical personnel.**

alligator forceps, 1. a forceps with heavy teeth and a double clamp used in orthopedic surgery. 2. a forceps with long, thin, angular handles and interlocking teeth.

allodiploid /al'ōdip'loid/ [Gk *allos* other, *diploos* double, *eidos* form], 1. also **allodiploidic.** of or pertaining to an individual, organism, strain, or cell that has two genetically distinct sets of chromosomes derived from different ancestral species, as occurs in hybridization. 2. such an individual, organism, strain, or cell.

allodiploidy /al'ōdip'loidē/, the state or condition of having two genetically distinct sets of chromosomes derived from different ancestral species.

alloeroticism, alloerotism. See **heteroeroticism.**

alloesthesia /al'ō·esthē'zhə/, a referred pain or other sensation that may be perceived on the same or opposite side of the body but not at the site stimulated.

allogamy. See **cross fertilization.**

allogenic /al'ōjen'ik/ [Gk *allos* + *genein* to produce] 1. (in genetics) denoting an individual or cell type that is from the same species but genetically distinct. 2. (in transplantation biology) denoting tissues that are from the same species but antigenically distinct; homologous.

allograft /al'əgraft/ [Gk *allos* + *graphion* stylus], the transfer of tissue between two genetically dissimilar individuals of the same species, such as a tissue transplant between two humans who are not identical twins.

allohexaploid, allohexaploidic. See **allopolyploid.**

allometric growth, the increase in size of different organs or parts of an organism at various rates.

allometron /əlom'itron/, a quantitative change in the proportional relationship of the parts of an organism as a result of the evolutionary process.

allometry /əlom'itrē/ [Gk *allos* + *metron* measure], the measurement and study of the changes in proportions of the various parts of an organism in relation to the growth of the whole or within a series of related organisms. –**allometric,** *adj.*

allomorphism, [Gk *allos* + *morphe* form], 1. a change in crystalline form without a change in chemical composition. 2. a change in the shape of a group of cells due to pressure or other physical factors.

allopathic physician /al'ōpath'ik/, a physician who treats disease and injury with active interventions, such as medical and surgical treatment, intended to bring about effects opposite from those produced by the disease or injury.

allopathy /əlop'əthē/ [Gk *allos* + *pathos* suffering], a system of medical therapy in which a disease or an abnormal condition is treated by creating an environment that is antagonistic to the disease or condition; for example, an antibiotic toxic to a pathogenic organism is given in an infection, or an iron supplement may be given to increase the synthesis of hemoglobin in iron deficiency anemia.

allopentaploid, allopentaploidic. See **allopolyploid.**

alloplastic maneuver [Gk *allos* + *plassein* to form], (in psychology) a process that is part of adaptation, involving an adjustment or change in the external environment.

alloploid, alloploidic. See **allodiploid, allopolyploid.**

alloploidy. See **allodiploidy, allopolyploidy.**

allopolyploid /al'əpol'iploid/ [Gk *allos* + *polyplous* many times, *eidos* form], 1. also **allopolyploidic.** of or pertaining to an individual, organism, strain, or cell that has more than two genetically distinct sets of chromosomes derived from two or more different ancestral species, as occurs in hybridization. They are referred to as allotriploid, allotetraploid, and so on, depending on the number of multiples of haploid sets of chromosomes they contain. 2. such an individual, organism, strain, or cell.

allopolyploidy /al'əpol'iploi'dē/, the state or condition of having more than two genetically distinct sets of chromosomes from two or more ancestral species.

allopurinol /al'əpyŏŏr'ənôl/, a xanthine oxidase inhibitor prescribed in the treatment of gout and other hyperuricemic conditions.

all-or-none law, 1. the principle in neurophysiology that if a stimulus is strong enough to trigger a nerve impulse, the entire impulse is discharged. A weak stimulus will not produce a weak reaction. 2. the principle that the heart muscle, under any stimulus above a threshold level, will respond either with a maximum strength contraction or not at all.

allosteric sites [Gk *allos* + *stereos* solid], the sites, other than the active site or sites, of an enzyme that bind regulatory molecules.

allotetraploid, allotetraploidic. See **allopolyploid.**

allotriploid, allotriploidic. See **allopolyploid.**

allowable charge, the maximum amount

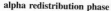

allowable costs that a third party, usually an insurance company, will pay to reimburse a provider for a specific service.

allowable costs, components of an institution's costs that are reimbursable as determined by a payment formula. In general, costs of services not considered to be reasonable or necessary to the proper provision of health services are excluded from allowable costs.

allowable dose. See **maximum permissible dose.**

allowable error, the amount of error that can be tolerated without invalidating the medical usefulness of the analytic result. Allowable error is defined as having a 95% limit of analytic error; only one sample in 20 can have an error greater than this limit.

alloxan /əlok′san/, an oxidation product of uric acid that is found in the human intestine in diarrhea. Because it can destroy the insulin-secreting islet cells of the pancreas, alloxan may cause diabetes.

alloy /al′oi/ [Fr *aloyer* to combine metals], a mixture of two or more metals or of substances with metallic properties. Most alloys are formed by mixing molten metals that dissolve in each other.

aloe /al′ō/ [Gk], the inspissated juice of various species of *Aloe* plants, formerly used as a cathartic but generally discontinued because it often causes severe intestinal cramps.

alopecia /al′əpē′shə/ [Gk *alopex* fox (mange)], partial or complete lack of hair resulting from normal aging, endocrine disorder, drug reaction, anticancer medication, or skin disease. Kinds of alopecia include **alopecia areata, alopecia totalis,** and **alopecia universalis.**

alopecia areata /er′ē·ā′tə/, a disease of unknown cause in which there are well-defined bald patches, usually round or oval, on the head and other hairy parts of the body. The condition is usually self-limited and clears completely within 6 to 12 months without treatment.

alopecia totalis, an uncommon condition characterized by the loss of all the hair on the scalp. The cause is unknown, and the baldness is usually permanent. No treatment is known.

alopecia universalis, a total loss of hair on all parts of the body, occasionally an extension of alopecia areata.

alpha (α), the first letter of the Greek alphabet, often used in chemical nomenclature to distinguish one variation in a chemical compound from others. Also **alfa.**

alpha₁-antitrypsin [Gk *anti* against + trypsin], a plasma protein produced in the liver that inhibits the action of proteolytic enzymes such as trypsin. Deficiencies are associated with hepatitis in children and panacinar emphysema in adults. The latter is an inherited condition.

alpha-adrenergic blocking agent. See **antiadrenergic.**

alpha-adrenergic receptor. See **alpha receptor.**

alpha alcoholism, a mild form of alcoholism in which the dependence is psychologic rather than physical.

alpha-aminoisovalerianic acid. See **valine.**

alpha cells, [Gk *alpha* + L *cella* storeroom], cells located in the anterior lobe of the pituitary gland or in the pancreatic islets. In the pancreas, they produce glucagon.

alpha fetoprotein (AFP), a protein normally synthesized by the liver, yolk sac, and GI tract of a human fetus, but which may be found elevated in the sera of adults having certain malignancies.

alpha-galactosidase, a form of the enzyme that catalyzes the conversion of alpha-D-galactoside to D-galactose.

alpha hemolysis, the development of a greenish zone around a bacterial colony growing on blood-agar medium, characteristic of pneumococci and certain streptococci and caused by the partial decomposition of hemoglobin.

alpha-hydroxypropionic acid. See **lactic acid.**

alpha₂-interferon /in′tərfir′on/, a protein molecule that has been found effective in controlling the spread of common colds caused by rhinoviruses. It is administered as a nasal spray.

alpha-methyldopa. See **methyldopa.**

alphanumeric, pertaining to a system of characters in which information is coded in combinations of letters and numerals. The characters, which also may include punctuation, are used commonly in computer programming to code signals or data.

alpha particle, a particle emitted from an atom during one kind of radioactive decay. It consists of two protons and two neutrons, the equivalent of a helium nucleus.

alpha receptor, any one of the postulated adrenergic components of receptor tissues that responds to norepinephrine and to various blocking agents. The activation of the alpha receptors causes such physiologic responses as increased peripheral vascular resistance, dilatation of the pupils, and contraction of pilomotor muscles.

alpha redistribution phase, a period following intravenous administration of a drug when the blood level begins to fall from its peak.

alpha rhythm. See **alpha wave.**

alpha state, a condition of relaxed, peaceful wakefulness devoid of concentration and sensory stimulation. It is characterized by the alpha rhythm of brain wave activity and is accompanied by feelings of tranquillity and a lack of tension and anxiety.

Alpha Tau Delta /al'fə tou' del'tə/, a national fraternity for professional nurses.

alpha-tocopherol. See **vitamin E.**

alphavirus /al'fəvī'rəs/, any of a group of very small togaviruses consisting of a single molecule of single-stranded DNA within a lipoprotein capsule.

alpha wave, one of the four types of brain waves, characterized by a relatively high voltage or amplitude and a frequency of 8 to 13 Hz. Alpha waves are the "relaxed waves" of the brain.

Alport's syndrome, a form of hereditary nephritis with symptoms of glomerulonephritis, hematuria, progressive sensorineural hearing loss, and occasional ocular disorders.

alprazolam /al'praz'ələm/, an antianxiety agent prescribed for the treatment of anxiety disorders or the short-term relief of the symptoms of anxiety.

alprostadil, a proprietary form of prostaglandin E_1 used to maintain the patency of ductus arteriosus in certain neonates. It is recommended as a palliative therapy for neonates awaiting surgery to correct congenital heart defects, such as tetralogy of Fallot and tricuspid atresia.

ALS, **1.** abbreviation for **advanced life support. 2.** abbreviation for **amyotrophic lateral sclerosis. 3.** abbreviation for **antilymphocyte serum.**

Alstrom syndrome, an inherited disease characterized by multiple end organ resistance to hormones. Clinical features include retinal degeneration leading to childhood blindness, vasopressin-resistant diabetes insipidus, and hypogonadism.

ALT, abbreviation for **alanine aminotransferase.**

altered state of consciousness (ASC) [Gk *alterare* to change], any state of awareness that differs from the normal awareness of a conscious person. Altered states of consciousness have been achieved, especially in Eastern cultures, by many individuals using various techniques, such as long fasting, deep breathing, whirling, and chanting.

alternans /ôl'tərnənz/ [L *alternare* to alternate], a regular rhythm of the heart where the pulse alternates between strong beats and weak beats (pulsus alternans).

alternate generation [L *alter* other of two], a type of reproduction in which a sexual generation alternates with one or more asexual generations, as in many plants and lower animals.

alternating current (AC), an electric current that reverses direction, according to a consistent sinusoidal pattern.

alternating mydriasis, a visual disorder in which there is abnormal dilatation of the pupils of the eyes that affects the left and right eyes alternately.

alternating pulse, See **pulsus alternans.**

alternation of generations. See **alternate generation.**

alternation rules, (in psychology) the sociolinguistic rules that establish options available to a person when he or she is speaking to someone else.

alternative inheritance, the acquisition of all genetic traits and conditions from one parent, as in self-pollinating plants and self-fertilizing animals.

alternative pathway of complement activation, a process of antibody formation in which activation of the C3 step occurs without prior activation of C1, C4, and C2.

alternobaric vertigo, a condition of dysequilibrium caused by unequalized pressure differences in the middle ear, as may be experienced by divers during ascent.

alt.h., abbreviation for the Latin prescription term *alternis horis,* meaning "every other hour."

altitude [L *altitudo* height], pertaining to any location on earth with reference to a fixed surface point, which is usually sea level. Several types of health effects are associated with altitude extremes, including a greater intensity of ultraviolet radiation that results from a thinner atmosphere.

altitude anoxia [L *altus* high; Gk *a* without, *oxys* sharp, *genein* to produce], oxygen deprivation in a high altitude atmosphere.

altitude sickness, a syndrome associated with the relatively low concentrations of oxygen in the atmosphere at altitudes encountered during mountain climbing or travel in unpressurized aircraft. The acute symptoms may include dizziness, headache, irritability, breathlessness, and euphoria.

altruism /al'trōō·iz'əm/, a sense of concern for the welfare of others. It may be expressed at the level of the individual or the larger social system.

alum /al'əm/ [L *alumen*], a topical astringent, used primarily in lotions and douches. Common potassium is applied topically as a 0.5% to 5% solution.

alum bath, a bath taken in water containing alum, used primarily for skin disorders.

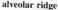

aluminum (Al) [L *alumen* alum], a widely used metallic element and the third most abundant of all the elements. Its atomic number is 13; its atomic weight is 26.97. It is a component of many antacids, antiseptics, astringents, and styptics. Aluminum hydroxychloride is the most commonly used agent in antiperspirants and is also effective as a deodorant.

aluminum acetate solution. See **Burow's solution.**

aluminum attenuator, an aluminum filter used to control the hardness of an x-ray beam. The attenuator removes low-energy x-ray photons before they can reach the patient and be absorbed.

aluminum hydroxide gel [L *alumen*; Gk *hydor* water, *oxys* sharp; L *gelare* to congeal], an antacid that works by chemical neutralization and also by adsorption of hydrochloric acid, gases, and toxins.

Alu sequences, a family of repeated sequences in the human genome.

alveobronchitis [L *alveolus* little hollow; Gk *brogchos* windpipe, *itis* inflammation], inflammation of the alveoli and bronchioles.

alveolar adenocarcinoma /alvē′ələr/ [L *alveolus* small hollow], a neoplasm in which the tumor cells form alveoli.

alveolar air, the respiratory gases in an alveolus, or air sac, of the lung.

alveolar air equation, a method of calculating the approximate alveolar oxygen tension from the arterial partial pressure of carbon dioxide, fractional inspired oxygen, and the ratio of carbon dioxide production to oxygen consumption.

alveolar-arterial end-capillary gas pressure difference, the gas pressure difference that exists between alveolar gas and pulmonary capillary blood as the latter leaves the alveolus. It is measured in torr units or mm Hg.

alveolar-arterial gas pressure difference, the difference between the measured or calculated mean partial pressure of a gas, such as CO_2, in the alveoli and the simultaneously measured partial pressure of that gas in systemic arterial blood. It is measured in torr units.

alveolar bone. See **alveolar process.**

alveolar canal, any of the canals of the maxilla through which the posterior superior alveolar blood vessels and the nerves to the upper teeth pass.

alveolar-capillary membrane, a lung tissue structure through which diffusion of oxygen and carbon dioxide molecules occurs during the respiration process.

alveolar cell carcinoma, a malignant pulmonary neoplasm that arises in a bronchiole and spreads along alveolar surfaces.

This form of lung cancer is characterized clinically by a severe cough and copious sputum.

alveolar cleft, a form of cleft palate in which the fusion failure extends forward to include the alveolar ridge.

alveolar dead space. See **dead space.**

alveolar distending pressure, the pressure difference between the alveolus and the intrapleural space.

alveolar duct, any of the air passages in the lung that branch out from the respiratory bronchioles. From the ducts arise the alveolar sacs.

alveolar edema, an accumulation of fluid within the alveoli.

alveolar fiber, any one of the many white collagenous fibers of the peridontal ligament that extend from the alveolar bone to the intermediate plexus where their terminations mix with those of the cemental fibers.

alveolar fistula. See **dental fistula.**

alveolar gas, the gas mixture within the gas-exchange regions of the lungs, reflecting the combined effects of alveolar ventilation and respiratory gas exchange, or the expired gas that has come from the alveoli and gas exchange regions.

alveolar gas volume, the aggregate volume of gas in the lung regions within which respiratory gas exchange occurs. It is indicated by the symbol V_A.

alveolar gingiva, gingiva that covers the alveolar bone and process in the maxilla and mandible. It is firmly attached to the bone and to the cementum of the teeth.

alveolar macrophages, defense cells within the lungs that act by engulfing and digesting foreign substances that may be inhaled into the alveoli.

alveolar microlithiasis, a disease characterized by the presence of calcium phosphate deposits in the alveolar sacs and ducts. It is familial in about half of cases.

alveolar periosteum [L *alveolus*; Gk *peri* near, *osteon* bone], a dense layer of connective tissue that lines the alveolar cavities of the upper and lower jaws, joining the bones to the cementum of the teeth.

alveolar pressure (P_A), the pressure in the alveoli of the lungs.

alveolar process, the portion of the maxilla or the mandible that forms the dental arch and serves as a bony investment for the teeth.

alveolar proteinosis, a disorder marked by the accumulation of plasma proteins, lipoproteins, and other blood components in the alveoli of the lungs.

alveolar ridge, the bony ridge of the maxilla or the mandible that contains the alveoli of the teeth.

alveolar sac [L *alveolus;* Gk *sakkos*], an air sac at one of the terminal cavities of lung tissue.

alveolar socket [L *alveolus;* OFr *soket*], a cavity in the alveolar bone of the maxilla and mandible that accommodates a tooth.

alveolar soft part sarcoma, a tumor in subcutaneous or fibromuscular tissue, consisting of numerous large round or polygonal cells in a netlike matrix of connective tissue.

alveolar ventilation, the volume of air that ventilates all the perfused alveoli, measured as minute volume in liters. The figure is also the difference between total ventilation and dead space ventilation. The normal average is between 4 and 5 liters per minute.

alveolectomy /al'vē·əlek'təmē/ [L *alveolus* + Gk *ektome* excision], the excision of a portion of the alveolar process for aiding the extraction of a tooth or teeth, the modification of the alveolar contour after tooth extraction, or the preparation of the mouth for dentures.

alveoli /alvē'əlī/, small outpouchings of walls of alveolar space through which gas exchange takes place between alveolar air and pulmonary capillary blood.

alveolitis /al'vē·əlī'tis/, an allergic pulmonary reaction to the inhalation of antigenic substances characterized by acute episodes of dyspnea, cough, sweating, fever, weakness, and pain in the joints and muscles. Kinds of alveolitis include **bagassosis, farmer's lung,** and **pigeon breeder's disease.**

alveolus /alvē'ələs/, *pl.* **alveoli** [L, small hollow], a small saclike structure. Often used interchangeably with **acinus.** –**alveolar,** *adj.*

alymphocytosis /alim'fōsītō'sis/ [Gk *a* not; L *lympha* water; Gk *kytos* cell, *osis* condition], an abnormal reduction in the total number of lymphocytes circulating in the blood.

Alzheimer's disease /älts'hīmərz/ [Alois Alzheimer, German neurologist, b. 1864], presenile dementia, characterized by confusion, memory failure, disorientation, restlessness, agnosia, speech disturbances, inability to carry out purposeful movements, and hallucinosis. The disease usually begins in later middle life with slight defects in memory and behavior and occurs with equal frequency in men and women.

Alzheimer's sclerosis [Alois Alzheimer; Gk *sklerosis* hardening], the degeneration of small cerebral blood vessels resulting in mental changes.

am, abbreviation for an ammonium cation.

Am, symbol for the element **americium.**

ama, abbreviation for **against medical advice.**

AMA, abbreviation for **American Medical Association.**

amalgam /amal'gəm/ [Gk *malagma* soft mass] **1.** a mixture or combination. **2.** an alloy of mercury and another metal or metals.

amalgam carrier, (in dentistry) an instrument for carrying plastic amalgam for inserting into a prepared tooth cavity or mold.

amalgam carver, a dental instrument for shaping plastic amalgams used in some tooth cavity fillings.

amalgam condenser, (in dentistry) an instrument used for compacting plastic amalgam in filling teeth.

amalgam core, a rigid base for the retention of a cast crown restoration, used in the replacement of a damaged tooth crown.

amalgam tattoo, a discoloration of the gingiva or buccal membrane caused by particles of silver amalgam filling material that became embedded under the surface.

Amanita [Gk *amanitai* fungus], a genus of mushrooms. Some species, as *Amanita phalloides,* are poisonous, causing hallucinations, GI upset, and pain that may be followed by liver, kidney, and central nervous system damage.

amantadine hydrochloride /əman'tədēn/, an antiviral and antiparkinsonian drug prescribed in the prophylaxis and early treatment of influenza virus A₂, and for symptomatic treatment of parkinsonian symptoms.

amastia /əmas'tē·ə/ [Gk *a, mastos* not breast], absence of the breasts in women caused by a congenital defect, an endocrine disorder resulting in faulty development, lack of development of secondary sex characteristics, or a bilateral mastectomy.

amaurosis /am'ôrō'sis/ [Gk *amauroein* to darken], blindness, especially lack of vision resulting from an extraocular cause, such as disease of the optic nerve or brain, diabetes, renal disease, or systemic poisoning produced by excessive use of alcohol or tobacco, rather than from damage to the eye itself. –**amaurotic,** *adj.*

amaurosis fugax /fōō'gaks/, transient episodic blindness.

amaurosis partialis fugax, transitory partial blindness, usually caused by vascular insufficiency of the retina or optic nerve as a result of carotid artery disease.

amaurotic familial idiocy. See **Tay-Sachs disease.**

amazia. See **amastia.**

amber mutation [Ar *anbar* ambergris], (in molecular genetics) a genetic alteration in which a polypeptide chain terminates prematurely because an erroneous nucleotide code signals the end of the chain.

ambidextrous [L, *ambo*, both, *dexter*, right], pertaining to an ability to use use either the left or right hand to perform a task.

ambient [L *ambire* on both sides], pertaining to the surrounding area or atmosphere.

ambient air standard, the maximum tolerable concentration of any air pollutant, such as lead, nitrogen dioxide, sodium hydroxide, or sulfuric dioxide.

ambient noise, the total noise in a specific environment.

ambient pressure, the atmospheric pressure, or pressure in the environment or surrounding area. It is given a reference value of zero (0) cm H_2O.

ambient temperature, the temperature of the environment.

ambiguous genitalia [L *ambigere* to go around], external genitalia that are not normal and morphologically typical of either sex, as occurs in pseudohermaphroditism.

ambilhar. See **niridazole.**

ambiopia. See **diplopia.**

ambivalence /ambiv′ələns/ [L *ambo* both, *valentia* strength], **1.** a state in which a person experiences conflicting feelings, attitudes, drives, desires, or emotions, such as love and hate, tenderness and cruelty, pleasure and pain. **2.** uncertainty and fluctuation caused by an inability to make a choice between opposites. **3.** a continuous oscillation or fluctuation. **–ambivalent,** *adj.*

ambivalent [L *ambo* + *valentia* strength], **1.** having equal power on both sides. **2.** in psychology, having equally strong but opposing emotions, as love and hate for the same person.

ambivert /am′bivurt′/ [L *ambo* both, *vertere* to turn], a person who possesses some of the characteristics of both introversion and extroversion.

amblyopia /am′blē·ō′pē·ə/ [Gk *amblys* dull, *ops* eye], reduced vision in an eye that appears to be structurally normal when examined with an ophthalmoscope. Kinds of amblyopia are **alcoholic amblyopia, suppression amblyopia, tobacco amblyopia,** and **toxic amblyopia.**

ambulance, an emergency vehicle usually used for the transport of patients to a medical facility in cases of accident, trauma, or sudden, severe illness.

ambulatory [L *ambulare* to walk about], able to walk, hence describing a patient who is not confined to bed, or designating a health service for people who are not hospitalized.

ambulatory automatism, aimless wandering or moving about or performance of mechanical acts without conscious awareness of the behavior.

ambulatory blood pressure monitoring (ABPM), a device that permits recording of a patient's blood pressure under normal living and working conditions.

ambulatory care, health services provided on an outpatient basis to those who visit a hospital or other health care facility and depart after treatment on the same day.

ambulatory schizophrenia, a mild form of schizophrenia, characterized by a tendency to respond to questions with vague and irrelevant answers. The person also may seem somewhat eccentric and wander aimlessly.

ambulatory surgery center, a medical facility designed and equipped to handle relatively minor surgery cases, such as cataracts, herniorrhaphy, and meniscectomy, which do not require overnight hospitalization.

AM care, routine hygiene care that is given patients before breakfast or early in the morning.

amcinonide, a topical corticosteroid used as an antiinflammatory agent.

amdinocillin /am′dinōsil′in/, a penicillin derivative that is used as a parenteral antibiotic. It is prescribed for the treatment of urinary infections caused by susceptible strains of *Escherichia coli* and various species of *Klebsiella* and *Enterobacter.*

ameba /əmē′bə/ [Gk *amoibe* change], a microscopic, single-celled, parasitic organism. Several species may be parasitic in humans, including *Entamoeba coli* and *E. histolytica.* Also spelled **amoeba.** **–amebic,** *adj.*

amebiasis /am′ēbī′əsis/, an infection of the intestine or liver by species of pathogenic amebas, particularly *Entamoeba histolytica,* acquired by ingesting food or water contaminated with infected feces. Mild amebiasis may be asymptomatic; severe infection may cause profuse diarrhea, acute abdominal pain, jaundice, anorexia, and weight loss.

amebic abscess, a collection of pus formed by disintegrated tissue in a cavity, usually in the liver, caused by the protozoan parasite *Entamoeba histolytica.*

amebic carrier state, a condition in which a patient may be a carrier of amebic organisms without showing signs or symptoms of an amebic infection. A **precocious carrier** may appear healthy but subsequently develop the amebic infection.

amebic dysentery, an inflammation of the intestine caused by infestation with *Entamoeba histolytica* and characterized by frequent, loose stools flecked with blood and mucus.

amebicide, a drug or other agent that is destructive to amebas.

ameboid movement [Gk *amoibe* + *eidos*, form; L *movere* to move], the ameba-like movement of certain types of body cells that can migrate through tissues. The movement generally consists of extension of a portion of the cell wall through a small opening between other tissue cells, which allows the cytoplasmic contents to follow.

amelanic melanoma /am'ilan'ik/, a melanoma that lacks melanin.

amelanotic /am'ilənot'ik/ [Gk *a, melas* not black], of or pertaining to tissue that is unpigmented because it lacks melanin.

amelia /əmē'lyə/ [Gk *a, melos* not limb] **1.** a birth defect, marked by the absence of one or more limbs. The term may be modified to indicate the number of legs or arms missing at birth, such as **tetramelia** for the absence of all four limbs. **2.** a psychologic trait of apathy or indifference associated with certain forms of psychosis.

amelification /əmel'ifikā'shən/ [OFr *amel* enamel; L *facere* to make], the differentiation of ameloblasts, or enamel cells, into the enamel of the teeth.

amelioration [L *ad* to, *melior* better], an improvement in conditions.

ameloblast /am'ilōblast'/ [OFr *amel* + Gk *blastos* germ], an epithelial cell from which tooth enamel is formed. **–ameloblastic** /-blas'tik/, *adj.*

ameloblastic fibroma, an odontogenic neoplasm in which there is a simultaneous proliferation of mesenchymal and epithelial tissues but no development of dentin or enamel.

ameloblastic hemangioma, a highly vascular tumor of cells covering the dental papilla.

ameloblastic odontoma, an odontogenic tumor characterized by an ameloblastoma within an odontoma.

ameloblastic sarcoma, a malignant odontogenic tumor, characterized by the proliferation of epithelial and mesenchymal tissue without the formation of dentin or enamel.

ameloblastoma /am'əlōblastō'mə/ [OFr *amel* + Gk *blastos* germ, *oma*], a highly destructive, malignant, rapidly growing tumor of the jaw.

amelodentinal /am'əlōden'tinəl/ [OFr *amel*

+ L *dens* tooth], pertaining to both the enamel and dentin of the teeth.

amelogenesis /am'əlōjen'əsis/ [OFr *amel* + Gk *genein* to produce], the formation of the enamel of the teeth. **–amelogenic,** *adj.*

amelogenesis imperfecta, a hereditary dental defect characterized by a brown coloration of the teeth and resulting from either severe hypocalcification or hypoplasia of the enamel.

amenorrhea /ā'menərē'ə/ [Gk *a, men* not month, *rhoia* to flow], the absence of menstruation. Amenorrhea is normal before sexual maturity, during pregnancy, after menopause, and during the intermenstrual phase of the monthly hormonal cycle but is otherwise caused by dysfunction of the hypothalamus, pituitary gland, ovary, or uterus, by the congenital absence or surgical removal of both ovaries or the uterus, or by medication. **Primary amenorrhea** is the failure of menstrual cycles to begin. **Secondary amenorrhea** is the cessation of menstrual cycles once established. **–amenorrheic.** *adj.*

American Academy of Allergy and Immunology (AAAI), a national organization of physicians specializing in the diagnosis and treatment of allergies and immune system disorders.

American Academy of Nursing (AAN), the honorary organization of the American Nurses' Association, created to recognize superior achievement in nursing in order to promote advances and excellence in nursing practice and education. A person who is elected to membership is given the title of Fellow of the American Academy of Nursing and may use the abbreviation FAAN as an honorific.

American Academy of Physical Medicine and Rehabilitation (AAPMR), a national association of professional health care workers concerned with the diagnosis of physical impairment and the development of therapies and devices to improve physical function.

American Academy of Physicians' Assistants (AAPA), a national organization of physicians' assistants or associates.

American Association for Respiratory Therapy (AART), a national organization of nurses and other health workers in the field of respiratory therapy.

American Association of Colleges of Nursing (AACN), an organization of baccalaureate and graduate schools of nursing that was established to deal with various issues of nursing education.

American Association of Critical Care Nurses (AACN), a national organization of nurses who work in critical care units.

American Association of Industrial Nurses (AAIN), a national professional association of nurses working in industry and concerned with issues in occupational health.

American Association of Medical Colleges (AAMC), a national organization of faculty members and deans of medical schools.

American Association of Nephrology Nurses and Technicians (AANNT), an organization of nurses and technicians working in the fields of dialysis and renal diseases.

American Association of Neuroscience Nurses (AANN), a national organization of nurses working with neurologically impaired patients. The organization is affiliated with the American Association of Neurological Surgeons.

American Association of Nurse Anesthetists (AANA), a professional association of certified registered nurse anesthetists. The AANA is the accrediting agency for schools of nurse anesthetists.

American Association of Pathologists and Bacteriologists (AAPB), a national professional organization of specialists in pathology and bacteriology.

American Association of Retired Persons (AARP), a voluntary U.S. organization of older persons, who may or may not be retired, with the goal of improving the welfare of persons over the age of 50. The AARP claims a membership of 30,000,000 and advises members of congress and state legislatures regarding legislation affecting older individuals.

American Association of University Professors (AAUP), a national organization of faculty members of institutions of higher learning.

American College of Obstetricians and Gynecologists (ACOG), the national organization of obstetricians and gynecologists.

American College of Physicians (ACP), a national professional organization of physicians.

American College of Prosthodontists, an organization of dentists who specialize in restoration of dental or oral structures, such as dentures, crowns, and bridges, and in the diagnosis and treatment of temporomandibular joint and maxillofacial disorders.

American College of Radiology (ACR), a national professional organization of physicians who specialize in radiology.

American College of Surgeons (ACS), a national professional organization of physicians who specialize in surgery.

American Dental Hygienists' Association, a national organization, a tripartite group, composed of constituent or state, local (city), and regional associations. National headquarters are in Chicago, Illinois.

American Hospital Association (AHA), a national organization of individuals, institutions, and organizations that works to promote the improvement of health services for all people.

American Journal of Nursing, the professional journal of the American Nurses' Association (ANA). It contains articles of general and specialized clinical interest to nurses and is the principal resource regarding the profession in the United States.

American leishmaniasis, a group of mucocutaneous infections caused by various species of *Leishmania,* characterized by disfiguring ulcerative lesions of the nose, mouth, and throat. Kinds of American leishmaniasis are **chiclero's ulcer, espundia, forest yaws,** and **uta.**

American Medical Association (AMA), a professional association whose membership is made up of licensed physicians in the United States, including practitioners in all recognized medical specialties, as well as general primary care physicians. The AMA maintains directories of all qualified physicians (including nonmembers) in the United States, including graduates of foreign medical colleges, advises congressional and state legislators regarding proposed health care laws, and publishes a variety of journals.

American mountain fever. See **Colorado tick fever.**

American National Standards Institute, a private, nonprofit organization that coordinates voluntary developments of standards for medical and other devices in the United States and represents the United States in areas of international standardization.

American Nurses' Association (ANA), the national professional association of registered nurses in the United States. It was founded in 1896 to improve standards of health and the availability of health care given in order to foster high standards for nursing, to promote the professional development of nurses, and to advance the economic and general welfare of nurses. The ANA is made up of 53 constituent associations from 50 states, the District of Columbia, Guam, and the Virgin Islands. Members may join one or more of the five Divisions on Nursing Practice: Community Health, Gerontological, Maternal and Child Health, Medical-Surgical, and Psychiatric and Mental Health Nursing. These

Divisions are coordinated by the Congress for Nursing Practice. The Congress evaluates changes in the scope of practice, monitors scientific and educational developments, encourages research, and develops statements that describe ANA policies regarding legislation affecting nursing practice. In addition, the ANA is politically active on the federal level in all issues relevant to nursing. The publications of the ANA include the *American Nurse,* a newspaper, the *Publications List,* and *The American Journal of Nursing,* the professional journal of the Association.

American Psychiatric Association (APA), a national professional psychiatric society concerned with the development of standards for psychiatric facilities, the formulation of mental health programs, the dissemination of data, and the promotion of psychiatric education and research. It publishes the *Diagnostic and Statistical Manual of Mental Disorders.*

American Red Cross, a national organization that seeks to reduce human suffering through various health, safety, and disaster relief programs in affiliation with the International Committee of the Red Cross. The Committee and all Red Cross organizations evolved from the Geneva Convention of 1864, following the example and urging of Swiss humanitarian Jean Henri Dunant, who aided wounded French and Austrian soldiers at the Battle of Solferino in 1859. The American Red Cross has more than 130 million members in about 3,100 chapters throughout the United States. Volunteers comprise the entire staffs of about 1,700 chapters. The organization annually collects about 4 million blood donations and gives blood to more than 4,000 hospitals. American Red Cross nursing and health programs include courses in the home on parenthood, prenatal and postnatal care, hygiene, and venereal disease. The symbol of the American Red Cross is a red cross on a field of white.

American Registry of Radiologic Technologists (ARRT), a national professional organization of technicians specializing in radiology.

American Society of Parenteral and Enteral Nutrition, an organization that provides education, support, and accreditation to persons who specialize in nutrition that is provided through intravenous, enteral, or related types of feeding.

American Speech, Language, and Hearing Association (ASHA), the professional association that certifies audiologists and speech-language pathologists.

American trypanosomiasis. See **Chagas' disease.**

American Type Culture Collection (ATCC), a nonprofit, nongovernmental organization that is concerned with the preservation of specimens of cellular and microbiologic cultures and with the distribution of the cultures to research centers and laboratories in the academic, scientific, and medical communities.

americium (Am), a synthetic radioactive element of the actinide group. Its atomic number is 95; its atomic weight is 243.

Ameslan /am′islan/, abbreviation for *American Sign Language,* a method of communication with the deaf that relies primarily on the position, shape, and motion of the hands and fingers for the transmission of concepts and messages.

Ames test, a method for testing substances for possible carcinogenicity by exposing a strain of *Salmonella* bacteria to a sample of the substance.

amethocaine hydrochloride. See **tetracaine hydrochloride.**

amethopterin. See **methotrexate.**

ametropia /am′itrō′pē·ə/ [Gk *ametros* irregular, *opsis* sight], a condition characterized by an optic defect involving an error of refraction, such as astigmatism, hyperopia, or myopia. **–ametropic,** *adj.*

AMI, 1. abbreviation for *anterior myocardial infarction.* **2.** abbreviation for **acute myocardial infarction.**

amide-compound local anesthetic, any of more than two dozen compounds that are safe, versatile, and effective local anesthetics. Some kinds of amide-compound local anesthetics are **bupivacaine, dibucaine, etiodocaine, lidocaine, mepivacaine,** and **prilocaine.**

amidobenzene. See **aniline.**

amikacin sulfate /am′ikā′sin/, an aminoglycoside antibiotic prescribed in the treatment of various severe infections that are resistant to other antibiotics.

amiloride hydrochloride /am′ilôr′īd/, a diuretic and hypertensive agent prescribed as adjunctive therapy in the treatment of congestive heart failure or hypertension. It is often given with a thiazide medication.

amine /am′in, əmēn′/ [L *ammonia*], (in chemistry) any organic compound that contains nitrogen.

amine pump, *informal.* an active transport system in the presynaptic nerve endings that takes up released amine neurotransmitters.

aminoacetic acid. See **glycine.**

amino acid, an organic chemical compound composed of one or more basic amino groups and one or more acidic carboxyl groups. Twenty of the more than

100 amino acids that occur in nature are the building blocks of peptides, polypeptides, and proteins. The eight essential amino acids are isoleucine, leucine, lysine, methionine, phenylalanine, threonine, tryptophan, and valine. Arginine and histidine are essential in infants. Cysteine and tyrosine are quasiessential because they may be synthesized from methionine and phenylalanine, respectively. The main nonessential amino acids are alanine, asparagine, aspartic acid, glutamine, glutamic acid, glycine, proline, and serine.

amino acid group, a category of organic chemicals containing the monovalent amine radical NH_2, an acid or COOH, and a group idiosyncratic to that particular amino acid group.

aminoaciduria /əmē′nō·as′id͝oōr′ē·ə/, the abnormal presence of amino acids in the urine that usually indicates an inborn metabolic defect, as in cystinuria.

aminobenzene. See **aniline.**

aminobenzoic acid /-benzō′ik/, a metabolic product of the catabolism of the amino acid tryptophan.

aminocaproic acid /əmē′nōkəprō′ik, am′inō-/, a hemostatic prescribed to stop excessive bleeding that results from hyperfibrinolysis.

aminoglycoside antibiotic. See **antibiotic.**

aminolevulinic acid (ALA) /am′inōlev′-oōlin′ik/, the aliphatic precursor of heme. It may be detected in the urine of some patients with porphyria, liver disease, and lead poisoning.

aminophylline /am′ənōfil′in, əmē′nō-/, a bronchodilator prescribed in the treatment of bronchial asthma, emphysema, and bronchitis.

aminosalicylic acid. See **paraaminosalicylic acid.**

aminosuccinic acid. See **aspartic acid.**

aminotransferase /-trans′fərās/, an enzyme that catalyzes the transfer of an amino group from an alpha-amino acid to an alpha-keto acid, with pyridoxal phosphate and pyridoxamine phosphate acting as coenzymes. Aspartate amino transferase (AST), normally present in serum and various tissues, is released by damaged cells, and, as a result, a high serum level of AST may be diagnostic in myocardial infarction or hepatic disease. Alanine aminotransferase (ALT), a normal constituent of serum and various tissues, may be present in high concentrations in the sera of patients with acute liver disease.

amiodarone hydrochloride, an oral antiarrhythmic drug prescribed for the treatment of life-threatening, recurrent ventricular fibrillation and recurrent, hemody-namically unstable ventricular tachycardia refractory to other drugs.

amitosis /am′ətō′sis/ [Gk *a, mitos* not thread], direct cell division in which there is simple fission of the nucleus and cytoplasm. It does not involve the complex stages of chromatin separation of the chromosomes that occur in mitosis. –**amitotic,** *adj.*

amitriptyline /am′itrip′tilin/, a tricyclic antidepressant prescribed in the treatment of depression.

AML, abbreviation for **acute myelocytic leukemia.**

ammonia [Gk *ammoniakos* salt of Ammon, Egyptian god], a colorless aromatic gas consisting of nitrogen and hydrogen, produced by the decomposition of nitrogenous organic matter. Some of its many uses are as an aromatic stimulant, a detergent, and an emulsifier.

ammoniacal fermentation, the production of ammonia and carbon dioxide from urea by the enzyme urease.

ammonium ion, an NH_4^+ ion formed by the reaction of ammonia (NH_3) with a hydrogen ion (H^+).

Ammon's horn. See **hippocampus major.**

amnesia [Gk *a, mnemonic* not memory], a loss of memory caused by brain damage or by severe emotional trauma. Kinds of amnesia are **anterograde, hysteric, posttraumatic,** and **retrograde amnesia.** –**amnesic,** *adj.*

amnesic aphasia [Gk *amnesia* + *a, phasis* without speech], an inability to remember spoken words, or to use words for names of objects, circumstances, or characteristics.

amnestic apraxia, the inability to carry out a movement in response to a request because of a lack of ability to remember the request rather than to a loss of motor function.

amniocentesis /am′nē·ōsentē′sis/ [Gk *amnos* lamb's caul, *kentesis* pricking], an obstetric procedure in which a small amount of amniotic fluid is removed for laboratory analysis. It is usually performed between the sixteenth and twentieth weeks of gestation to aid in the diagnosis of fetal abnormalities.

amniography /am′nē·og′rəfē/, a procedure used to detect placement of the placenta by x-ray examination.

amnion /am′nē·on/ [Gk *amnos* lamb's caul], a membrane, continuous with and covering the fetal side of the placenta, that forms the outer surface of the umbilical cord and becomes the outermost layer of the skin of the developing fetus.

amnionitis /am'nē·ōnī'tis/, an inflammation of the amnion. The condition may develop after early rupture of the fetal membranes.

amnioscopy /am'nē·os'kəpē/, direct visual examination of the fetus and amniotic fluid with an endoscope that is inserted into the amniotic cavity through the uterine cervix or an incision in the abdominal wall.

amniotic /am'nē·ot'ik/, pertaining to the amnion.

amniotic band syndrome, an abnormal condition of fetal development characterized by the development of fibrous bands within the uterus that entangle the fetus, leading to deformities in structure and function.

amniotic cavity, [Gk *amnion*; L *cavum*], the fluid-filled cavity of the amniotic sac surrounding the fetus.

amniotic fluid, a liquid produced by the fetal membranes and the fetus. It surrounds the fetus throughout pregnancy, usually totaling about 1,000 ml at term. In addition to providing the fetus with physical protection, the amniotic fluid is a medium of active chemical exchange. Amniotic fluid itself is clear, though desquamated fetal cells and lipids give it a cloudy appearance.

amniotic fluid embolism [Gk *amnion*; L *fluere* to flow; Gk *embolos* plug], an embolism resulting from amniotic fluid entering the maternal blood system during labor and/or delivery. It is usually fatal for the mother if it is a pulmonary embolism.

amniotic sac, a thin-walled bag that contains the fetus and amniotic fluid during pregnancy, having a capacity of 4 to 5 L at term. The wall of the sac extends from the margin of the placenta. The amnion, chorion, and decidua that make up the wall are each a few cell layers thick. The intact sac and its fluid provide for the equilibration of hydrostatic pressure within the uterus and, during labor, effect the uniform transmission of the force of uterine contractions to the cervix for dilatation.

amniotomy /am'nē·ot'əmē/ the artificial rupture of the fetal membranes (ARM). It is usually performed to stimulate the onset of labor.

amobarbital /am'ōbär'bətal/, a barbiturate sedative-hypnotic prescribed for the relief of anxiety and insomnia and as an anticonvulsant.

A-mode, the amplitude modulation display in diagnostic ultrasonography. It represents the time taken for the ultrasound beam to strike a tissue interface and return its signal to the transducer.

A-mode ultrasound [L *ultra* beyond + *so-*

nus sound], a display of ultrasonic echoes in which the horizontal axis of the cathode ray tube display represents the time required for the return of the echo and the vertical oscilloscope trace represents the strength of the echo. The mode is used in echoencephalography.

amoeba. See ameba.

amoebiasis. See amebiasis.

amoebic dysentery. See amebic dysentery.

amok [Malay *amoq* furious], a psychotic frenzy with a desire to kill anybody encountered. The murderous episodes may follow periods of severe depression.

amorph /ā'môrf, əmôrf'/ [Gk *a, morphe* not shape], **1.** inactive gene; a mutant allele that has little or no effect on the expression of a trait. **2.** abbreviation for **amorphous,** such as amorph IZS (amorphous insulin zinc suspension).

amorphic, (in genetics) of or pertaining to a gene that is inactive or nearly inactive so that it has no determinable effect.

amorphous crystals, shapeless, ill-defined crystals, usually phosphates.

amoxapine /əmôk'sepin/, an antidepressant similar to the tricyclics. It is prescribed in the treatment of mental depression.

amoxicillin /əmok'səsil'in/, a semisynthetic oral penicillin antibiotic similar to ampicillin. It is prescribed in the treatment of several infections that are caused by a susceptible gram-negative or gram-positive organism.

AMP, abbreviation for **adenosine monophosphate.**

ampere (A) /am'pēr/ [André M. Ampère, French physicist, b. 1775], a unit of measurement of the amount of electric current. An ampere, according to the meter-kilogram-second (MKS) system, is the amount of current passed through a resistance of 1 ohm by an electrical potential of 1 volt.

amperometry /am'pərom'ətrē/, the measurement of current at a single applied potential.

amphetamines, a group of nervous system stimulants, including amphetamine and its chemical congeners dextroamphetamine and methamphetamine, that are subject to abuse because of their ability to produce wakefulness and euphoria. Abuse leads to compulsive behavior, paranoia, hallucinations, and suicidal tendencies.

amphetamine poisoning, toxic effects of overdosage of amphetamines. Symptoms usually include excitement, tremors, tachycardia, hallucinations, delirium, convulsions, and circulatory collapse. Emergency first aid requires gastric lavage with tap water and charcoal or induced emesis.

amphiarthrosis. See **cartilaginous joint.**

amphigenesis. See **amphigony.**

amphigenetic /am'fijənet'ik/ [Gk *amphi* both sides, *genein* to produce], **1.** produced by the union of gametes from both sexes. **2.** bisexual; having both testicular and ovarian tissue.

amphigenous inheritance /amfij'ənəs/, the acquisition of genetic traits and conditions from both parents.

amphigonadism /am'figō'nədiz'əm/, true hermaphroditism; having both testicular and ovarian tissue. **–amphigonadic,** *adj.*

amphigony /amfig'ənē/ [Gk *amphi* + *gonos* generation], sexual reproduction. **–amphigonic** /am'figon'ik/, *adj.*

amphikaryon /am'fiker'ē·on/ [Gk *amphi* + *karyon* nucleus], a nucleus containing the diploid number of chromosomes. **–amphikaryotic,** *adj.*

amphimixis /am'fimik'sis/ [Gk *amphi* + *mixis* mingling] **1.** the union of germ cells in reproduction so that both maternal and paternal hereditary characteristics are derived; interbreeding. **2.** (in psychoanalysis) the union and integration of oral, anal, and genital libidinal impulses in the development of heterosexuality.

amphipathic [Gk *amphi* + *pathos* suffering], pertaining to a molecule having two sides with characteristically different properties, such as a detergent, which has both a polar (hydrophilic) end and a nonpolar (hydrophobic) end but is long enough so that each end demonstrates its own solubility characteristics.

amphoric breath sound [Gk *amphoreus* jug], an abnormal, resonant, hollow blowing sound heard with a stethoscope. It indicates a cavity opening into the bronchus, or a pneumothorax.

amphoteric /am'fōter'ik/ [Gk *amphoteros* pertaining to both], a substance that can have a positive, zero, or negative charge, depending on conditions.

amphotericin B /am'fəter'əsin/, an antifungal medication prescribed for topical or systemic use in the treatment of fungal infections.

amphotericin methyl ester (AME), an antiviral drug used in experimental treatment of HIV infections.

amphoterism [Gk *amphoteros*], a quality of a chemical compound that permits it to act as either an acid or a base.

ampicillin /am'pəsil'in/, a semisynthetic penicillin prescribed in the treatment of a variety of infections caused by a broad spectrum of sensitive gram-negative and gram-positive organisms.

amplification [L *amplificare* to make wider], **1.** (in molecular genetics) a process in which the amount of plasmid DNA is increased in proportion to the amount of bacterial DNA by treatment with certain substances, including chloramphenicol. **2.** the replication in bulk of an entire gene library. **–amplify,** *v.*

amplitude [L *amplus* wide], width or breadth of range or extent, such as amplitude of accommodation or amplitude of convergence.

amplitude of accommodation (AA), the total accommodative power of the eye, determined by the difference between the refractive power for farthest vision and that for nearest vision.

amplitude of convergence, the difference in the power needed to turn the eyes from their far point to their near point of convergence.

ampule /am'pyool/ [Fr *ampoule* phial], a small, sterile glass or plastic container that usually contains a single dose of a solution to be administered parenterally. Also spelled **ampoule.**

ampulla /ampool'ə/ [L, flasklike bottle], a rounded, saclike dilatation of a duct, canal, or any tubular structure, such as the lacrimal duct, semicircular canal, uterine tube, rectum, or vas deferens.

ampulla of Vater. See **hepatopancreatic ampulla.**

ampullary aneurysm. See **saccular aneurysm.**

ampullary tubal pregnancy /ampool'ərē, am'pəler'ē/, a kind of tubal pregnancy in which implantation occurs in the ampulla of one of the fallopian tubes.

amputation [L *amputare* to excise], the surgical removal of a part of the body or a limb or part of a limb, performed to treat recurrent infections or gangrene in peripheral vascular disease, to remove malignant tumors, and in severe trauma. With the patient under general anesthesia, the part is removed and a shaped flap is cut from muscular and cutaneous tissue to cover the end of the bone, with a section left open for drainage if infection is present. Kinds of amputation include **closed, congenital, open, primary,** and **secondary amputation.**

amputation neuroma, a form of traumatic neuroma that may develop near the stump after the amputation of an extremity.

amputee, a person who has had one or more extremities traumatically, congenitally, or surgically removed.

AMRA, abbreviation for *American Medical Records Association.*

amrinone lactate /am'rinōn/, an intravenous cardiac inotropic drug prescribed in the short-term management of congestive heart failure in patients who do not respond to therapy with digitalis, diuretics, and vasodilators.

Amsler grid [Marc Amsler, Swiss ophthalmologist, b. 1891], a checkerboard grid of intersecting dark horizontal and vertical lines with one dark spot in the middle. To discover a visual field defect, the person simply covers or closes one eye and looks at the spot with the other.

AMT, abbreviation for *American Medical Technologists.*

amu, abbreviation for **atomic mass unit.**

amusia /əmyoō′sē·ə/, a form of agnosia characterized by a loss of the ability to recognize melodies.

amyelinic neuroma [Gk *a, myelos* not marrow, *neuron* nerve, *oma*], a tumor that contains only nonmyelinated nerve fibers.

amygdala /əmig′dələ/ [Gk *amygdale* almond], an almond-shaped mass of gray matter in the front portion of the temporal lobe of the brain.

amygdalin /əmig′dəlin/ [Gk *amygdale* almond], a naturally occurring cyanogenic glycoside obtained from bitter almonds and apricot pits. It has been promoted as a potential cancer remedy under the trademark of Laetrile.

amygdaloid fossa, a space in the wall of the oropharynx, between the pillars of the fauces, that is occupied by the palatine tonsil.

amygdaloid nucleus [Gk *amygdale* + *eidos*; L *nucleus* nut], one of the basal nuclei found in the inferior horn of the lateral ventricle.

amyl alcohol [Gk *amylon* starch], a colorless, oily liquid that is only slightly soluble in water but can be mixed with ethyl alcohol, chloroform, or ether.

amyl alcohol tertiary. See **amylene hydrate.**

amylase /am′iləs/ [Gk *amylon* starch], an enzyme that catalyzes the hydrolysis of starch into smaller carbohydrate molecules. Alpha-amylase, found in saliva, pancreatic juice, malt, certain bacteria, and molds, catalyzes the hydrolysis of starches to dextrins, maltose, and maltotriose. Beta-amylase, found in grains, vegetables, and malt, is involved in the hydrolysis of starch to maltose.

amylene hydrate, a clear, colorless liquid with a camphorlike odor, miscible with alcohol, chloroform, ether, or glycerin and used as a solvent and a hypnotic.

amylic fermentation /əmil′ik/, the formation of amyl alcohol from sugar.

amyl nitrite, a vasodilator prescribed to relieve the vasospasm of angina pectoris.

amylobarbitone. See **amobarbital.**

amyloid /am′iloid/ [Gk *amylon* + *eidos* form], **1.** pertaining to or resembling starch. **2.** a starchlike protein-carbohydrate complex that is deposited abnormally in some tissues during certain chronic disease states, such as amyloidosis, rheumatoid arthritis, and tuberculosis.

amyloid disease. See **amyloidosis.**

amyloid liver [Gk *amylon* + *eidos*; AS, *lifer*], liver in which the cells have been infiltrated with amyloid deposits.

amyloidosis /am′iloid′sis/ [Gk *amylon* + *eidos* form, *osis* condition], a disease in which a waxy, starchlike glycoprotein (amyloid) accumulates in tissues and organs, impairing their function. There are two major forms of the condition. **Primary amyloidosis** usually occurs with multiple myeloma. Patients with **secondary amyloidosis** usually suffer from another chronic infectious or inflammatory disease, as tuberculosis, osteomyelitis, rheumatoid arthritis, or Crohn's disease. The cause of both types of amyloidosis is unknown. Almost all organs are affected, most often the heart, lungs, tongue, and intestines in primary amyloidosis, and the kidneys, liver, and spleen in the secondary type.

amylopectinosis. See **Andersen's disease.**

amyoplasia congenita. See **arthrogryposis multiplex congenita.**

amyotonia /ā′mī·ōtō′nē·ə/ [Gk *a, mys* not muscle, *tonos* tone], an abnormal condition of skeletal muscle, characterized by a lack of tone, weakness, and wasting, usually the result of motor neuron disease. –**amyotonic,** *adj.*

amyotrophic lateral sclerosis (ALS) /ā′mī·ōtrof′ik/ [Gk *a, mys* + *trophe* nourishment], a degenerative disease of the motor neurons, characterized by atrophy of the muscles of the hands, forearms, and legs spreading to involve most of the body. It results from degeneration of the motor neurons, beginning in middle age.

ana (**āa, āā, AA**), (in prescriptions) "so much of each," indication of the amount of each ingredient to be compounded. Usually written as an abbreviation.

ANA, 1. abbreviation for **American Nurses' Association. 2.** abbreviation for **antinuclear antibody.**

anabolic steroid [Gk *anaballein* to build up], any one of several compounds derived from testosterone or prepared synthetically to promote general body growth, to oppose the effects of endogenous estrogen, or to promote masculinizing effects. All such compounds cause a mixed androgenic-anabolic effect. Anabolic steroids are prescribed in the treatment of aplastic anemia, red-cell aplasia, and he-

anabolism /ənab'əliz'əm/ [Gk *anaballein* to build up], constructive metabolism characterized by the conversion of simple substances into the more complex compounds of living matter. **–anabolic** /an'əbol'ik/, *adj.*

anacatadidymus /an'əkat'ədid'iməs/ [Gk *ana* up, again *kata* down, *didymos* twin], conjoined twins that are fused in the middle but separated above and below.

anaclisis /ən'əkli'sis/ [Gk *ana* + *klisis* leaning] **1.** a condition, normal in childhood but pathologic in adulthood, in which a person is emotionally dependent on other people. **2.** a condition in which a person consciously or unconsciously chooses a love object because of a resemblance to the mother, father, or other person who was an important source of comfort and protection in infancy. **–anaclitic** /an'əklit'ik/, *adj.*

anaclitic depression, a syndrome occurring in infants, usually after sudden separation from the mothering person. Symptoms include apprehension, withdrawal, incessant crying, refusal to eat, sleep disturbances, leading to impairment of the infant's physical, social, and intellectual development.

anacrotic pulse /an'əkrot'ik/ [Gk *ana* + *krotos* stroke], (on a sphygmographic tracing) a pulse characterized by one transient drop in amplitude on the curve of the primary elevation. It is seen in valvular aortic stenosis.

anacusis /an'əkoo'sis/ [Gk *a, akouein* not to hear], a total loss of hearing.

anadicrotic pulse /an'ədīkrot'ik/ [Gk *ana* + *dis* twice, *krotos* stroke], (on a sphygmographic tracing) a pulse characterized by two transient drops in amplitude on the curve of primary elevation.

anadidymus /an'ədid'iməs/ [Gk *ana* + *dydymos* twin], conjoined twins that are united at the pelvis and lower extremities but are separated in the upper half.

anadipsia /an'ədip'sē·ə/ [Gk *ana* + *dipsa* thirst], extreme thirst, often occurring in the manic phase of manic-depressive psychosis. The condition is the result of dehydration caused by the excessive perspiration, continuous urination, and relentless physical activity produced by the intense excitement characteristic of the manic phase.

anaerobe /aner'ōb/ [Gk *a, aer* not air, *bios* life], a microorganism that grows and lives in the complete or almost complete absence of oxygen. An example is *Clostridium botulinum.* Some kinds of anaer-

molytic anemia and in anemias associated with renal failure, myeloid metaplasia, and leukemia.

obes are **facultative anaerobe** and **obligate anaerobe.**

anaerobic /an'ərō'bik/, **1.** pertaining to the absence of air or oxygen. **2.** able to grow and function without air or oxygen.

anaerobic catabolism, the breakdown of complex chemical substances into simpler compounds, with the release of energy, in the absence of oxygen.

anaerobic exercise, muscular exertion sufficient to result in metabolic acidosis because of accumulation of lactic acid as a product of muscle metabolism.

anaerobic glycolysis. See **glycolysis.**

anaerobic infection, an infection caused by an anaerobic organism, usually occurring in deep puncture wounds that exclude air or in tissue that has diminished oxygen-reduction potential as a result of trauma, necrosis, or overgrowth of bacteria. Kinds of anaerobic infection are **gangrene** and **tetanus.**

anaerobic myositis. See **gas gangrene.**

anal /ā'nəl/ [L *anus*], of or pertaining to the anus.

anal agenesis. See **imperforate anus.**

anal canal, the final portion of the alimentary tract, about 4 cm long, between the rectal ampulla and the anus.

anal character, (in psychoanalysis) a kind of personality exhibiting patterns of behavior originating in the anal phase of infancy, characterized by extreme orderliness, obstinacy, perfectionism, cleanliness, punctuality, and miserliness, or their extreme opposites.

anal crypt, the depression between rectal columns that encloses networks of veins that, when inflamed and swollen, are called hemorrhoids.

analeptic. See **central nervous system stimulant.**

anal eroticism, (in psychoanalysis) libidinal fixation at or regression to the anal stage of psychosexual development, often reflected in such personality traits as miserliness, stubbornness, and overscrupulousness.

anal fissure, a linear ulceration or laceration of the skin of the anus.

anal fistula, an abnormal opening on the cutaneous surface near the anus, usually resulting from a local crypt abscess and also common in Crohn's disease. A perianal fistula may or may not communicate with the rectum.

analgesia /an'əljē'zē·ə/ [Gk *a, algos* not pain], a lack of pain without loss of consciousness.

analgesia algera. See **anesthesia dolorosa.**

analgesic /an'əljē'zik/, **1.** relieving pain. **2.** a drug that relieves pain. The narcotic analgesics act on the central nervous system and alter the patient's perception; they are more often used for severe pain. The nonnarcotic analgesics act at the site of the pain, do not produce tolerance or dependence, and do not alter the patient's perception; they are used for mild to moderate pain.

analgesic nephropathy [Gk *a* without, *algos* pain + *nephros* kidney, *pathos* disease], a condition of kidney damage resulting from consuming excessive amounts of aspirin or similar analgesic pills.

analgia [Gk *a* without, *algos* pain], an absence of pain.

anal incontinence [L *anus, incontinentia* an inability to retain], the lack of voluntary control over fecal discharge.

anal membrane. See **cloacal membrane.**

anal membrane atresia. See **imperforate anus.**

analog /an'əlog/ [Gk *analogos* proportionate] 1. a substance, tissue, or organ that is similar in appearance or function to another but differing in origin or development, such as the eye of a fly and the eye of a human. 2. a drug or other chemical compound that resembles another in structure or constituents but has different effects.

analogous [Gk *analogos*], pertaining to objects that are similar in function but different in origin or structure, as wings of birds and flies.

analog signal, a continuous electric signal representing a specific condition, such as temperature or ECG waveforms.

analogy [Gk *analogos*], a resemblance between two things that are similar to a degree in function or form, but differ structurally or in origin.

anal reflex, a superficial neurologic reflex obtained by stroking the skin or mucosa of the region around the anus, which normally results in a contraction of the external anal sphincter.

anal sadism, (in psychoanalysis) a sadistic form of anal eroticism, manifested by behavior such as aggressiveness and selfishness.

anal stage, (in psychoanalysis) the pregenital period in psychosexual development, occurring between 1 and 3 years of age, when preoccupation with the function of the bowel and the sensations associated with the anus are the predominant source of pleasurable stimulation.

anal stenosis. See **imperforate anus.**

anal verge [L *anus* + *vergere* to bend], the area between the anal canal and the perianal skin.

analysand /ənal'isand'/, a person undergoing psychoanalysis.

analysis [Gk *ana* + *lyein* to loosen], the separation of substances into their constituent parts and the determination of the nature, properties, and composition of compounds. In chemistry, **qualitative analysis** is the determination of the elements present in a substance; **quantitative analysis** is the determination of how much of each element is present in a substance. Analysis is also an informal term for **psychoanalysis.** –**analytic,** *adj.* **analyze,** *v.*

analysis of variance (ANOVA), a series of statistic procedures for determining the differences, attributable to chance alone, among two or more groups of scores.

analyst, 1. a psychoanalyst. 2. a person who analyzes the chemical, physical, or other properties of a substance or product.

analyte, any substance that is measured. The term is usually applied to a component of a biologic section.

analytic psychology, 1. the system in which phenomena, such as sensations and feelings, are analyzed and classified by introspective rather than by experimental methods. 2. also called **Jungian psychology.** a system of analyzing the psyche according to the concepts developed by Carl Gustav Jung. It differs from the psychoanalysis of Sigmund Freud in stressing a "racial" or collective unconscious and a mystic, religious factor in the development of the personal unconscious and in minimizing the importance of sexual influence on early emotional and psychologic development.

analyzing, (in five-step nursing process) a category of nursing behavior in which the health care needs of the client are identified and the goals of care are selected. The nurse interprets data; identifies problems involving the client, the client's family, and significant others; establishes priorities among goals; integrates the information; and projects the expected outcomes of nursing activities.

anamnesis /an'amnē'sis/ [Gk *anamimneskein* to recall] 1. remembrance of the past. 2. the accumulated data concerning a medical or psychiatric patient and the patient's background, including family, previous environment, experiences, and, particularly, recollections, for use in analyzing his or her condition.

anaphase /an'əfāz/ [Gk *ana* + *phainein* to appear], the third of four stages of nuclear division in mitosis and in each of the two divisions of meiosis. In mitosis and the second meiotic division, the centromeres divide, and the two chromatids, which are arranged along the equatorial plane of the spindle, separate and move to the opposite poles of the cell, forming daughter chromosomes. In the first meiotic division, the pairs of homologous chromosomes separate from each other and move intact to the opposite poles of the spindle.

anaphia /ənā'fē·ə/, the loss of the ability to perceive tactile stimuli.

anaphylactic hypersensitivity /an'əfilak'-tik/, an IgE- or IgG-dependent, immediate-acting humoral hypersensitivity response to an exogenous antigen. Histamine, kinins, and other substances are released from mast cells, causing vasodilatation and muscle contraction. Systemic anaphylaxis, atopic allergies, hayfever, and insect-sting reactions are all anaphylactic hypersensitivity reactions.

anaphylactic reactions [Gk ana, phylaxis protection; L re, agere to act], a hypersensitive condition induced by contact with certain antigens. The second contact with the same antigen may result in dyspnea, severe convulsions, shock, and, in some cases, death. The reaction is particularly severe if the antigen contact is by injection.

anaphylactic shock, a severe and sometimes fatal systemic hypersensitivity reaction to a sensitizing substance, such as a drug, vaccine, certain food, serum, allergen extract, insect venom, or chemical. This condition may occur within seconds from the time of exposure to the sensitizing factor and is commonly marked by respiratory distress and vascular collapse. The more quickly any systemic atopic reaction occurs in the individual after exposure, the more severe the associated shock is likely to be. The involved allergen enters the systemic circulation and triggers an incomplete humoral response that allows the allergen to combine with IgE and cause the release of histamine. Also entering into the reaction are IgG and IgM, which cause the release of complement fractions, further stimulating histamine action.

anaphylactoid purpura. See **Henoch-Schönlein purpura.**

anaphylatoxin /an'əfī'lətok'sin/, a polypeptide derived from complement. It mediates changes in mast cells leading to the release of histamine and other pharmacologically active substances.

anaphylaxis /an'əfilak'sis/ [Gk ana + phylaxis protection], an exaggerated hypersensitivity reaction to a previously encountered antigen. The response, which is mediated by antibodies of the IgE class of immunoglobulins, causes the release of histamine, kinin, and substances that affect smooth muscle. The reaction may be a lo-

calized wheal and flare of generalized itching, hyperemia, angioneurotic edema, and in severe cases vascular collapse, bronchospasm, and shock. The severity of symptoms depends on the original sensitizing dose of the antigen, the amount and distribution of antibodies, and the route of entry and size of the dose of antigen producing anaphylaxis. Penicillin injection is the most common cause of anaphylactic shock. Kinds of anaphylaxis are **aggregate, antiserum, cutaneous, cytotoxic, indirect,** and **inverse.** –**anaphylactic,** adj.

anaplasia /an'əplā'zhə/ [Gk ana + plassein to shape], a change in the structure of cells and in their orientation to each other characterized by a loss of differentiation and reversion to a more primitive form. Anaplasia is characteristic of malignancy. –**anaplastic,** adj.

anaplastic astrocytoma. See **glioblastoma multiforme.**

anarthria /anär'thrē·ə/ [Gk a, arthron not joint], a loss of control of the muscles of speech, resulting in the inability to utter words. The condition is usually caused by damage to a central or peripheral motor nerve.

anasarca /an'əsär'kə/ [Gk ana + sarx flesh], generalized, massive edema. Anasarca is often observed in edema associated with renal disease when fluid retention continues for an extended period of time. –**anasarcous,** adj.

anastomose /ənas'təmōs/, [Gk anastomoein to provide a mouth], to open a channel or passage between two vessels or cavities that are normally separate.

anastomosis /ənas'tōmō'sis/, pl. **anastomoses** [Gk anastomoien to provide a mouth], a surgical joining of two ducts or blood vessels to allow flow from one to the other. It may be performed to bypass an aneurysm or a vascular or arterial occlusion. Kinds of anastomoses are **end-to-end anastomosis, side-to-side anastomosis.** –**anastomotic,** adj.

anastomosis at elbow joint, a convergence of blood vessels at the elbow joint consisting of various veins and portions of the brachial and deep brachial arteries and their branches.

anatomic age, the estimated age of an individual based on the stage of development or deterioration of the body as compared with other persons of the same chronologic age.

anatomic neck of the humerus [Gk ana up, temnein to cut; AS hnecca; L humerus shoulder], the portion of the humerus where there is a slight constriction adjoining the head.

anatomic topography [Gk *ana, temnein* + *topos* place + *graphein* to write], a system of identification of a body part in terms of the region in which it is located and its nearby structures.

anatomic crown, the portion of the dentin of a tooth, covered by dental enamel.

anatomic curve, the curvature of the different segments of the vertebral column. In the lateral contour of the back, the cervical curve appears concave, the thoracic curve appears convex, and the lumbar curve appears concave.

anatomic dead space. See **dead space.**

anatomic height of contour, a line that encircles and designates the greatest convexity of a tooth.

anatomic impotence. See **impotence.**

anatomic pathology [Gk *ana, temnein* + *pathos* disease, *logos* science], the study of the effects of disease on the structure of the body.

anatomic position, a position of the body in which a person stands erect, facing directly forward, feet pointed forward slightly apart, arms hanging down at the sides with palms facing forward.

anatomic snuffbox, a small, cuplike depression on the back of the hand near the wrist formed by the tendons reaching toward the thumb and index finger as the thumb is abducted, the wrist flexed, and the digits extended.

anatomic zero joint position, the beginning point of a joint range of motion.

anatomy [Gk *ana* + *temnein* to cut], **1.** the study, classification, and description of structures and organs of the body. Kinds of anatomy are **applied, comparative, descriptive, gross, microscopic,** and **surface. 2.** the structure of an organism. **3.** a text on anatomy. **-anatomic,** *adj.*

ANC, abbreviation for **Army Nurse Corps.**

ancillary /an'səler'ē/, pertaining to something that is subordinate, auxiliary, or supplementary.

anconeus /angkō'nē·əs/ [Gk *agkon* elbow], one of seven superficial muscles of the posterior forearm. A small triangular muscle, it originates on the dorsal surface of the lateral condyle and inserts in the olecranon process of the ulna. It functions to extend the forearm.

ancrod /ang'krod/, the venom of the Malayan pit viper, used to remove fibrinogen from the circulation, thus preventing clotting of the blood.

Ancylostoma /ang'kilos'təmə/ [Gk *agkylos* crooked, *stoma* mouth], a genus of nematode that is an intestinal parasite and causes hookworm disease.

ancylostomiasis /an'sələs'təmī'əsis/, hookworm disease, more specifically that caused by *Ancylostoma duodenale, A. braziliense,* or *A. cannium.* Infection by *A. duodenale* is generally more harmful and less responsive to treatment than that by *Necator americanus,* which is the hookworm most often found in the southern United States.

Andersen's disease [Dorothy H. Andersen, American pediatrician, b. 1901], a rare glycogen storage disease characterized by a genetic deficiency of branching enzyme (amylo-1:4, 1:6 transglucosidase), causing the deposition in tissues of abnormal glycogen with long inner and outer chains.

andreioma, andreoblastoma. See **arrhenoblastoma.**

androgamone /an'drōgam'ōn/ [Gk *andros* man, *gamos* marriage], a gamone secreted by the male gamete.

androgen /an'drəjin/ [Gk *andros* + *genein* to produce], any steroid hormone that increases male characteristics. Natural hormones, such as testosterone and its esters and analogs, are primarily used as substitutional therapy during the male climacteric. Androgens may be administered orally or parenterally. **-androgenic,** *adj.*

androgynous /androj'inəs/, **1.** (of a man or woman) having some characteristics of both sexes. Social role, behavior, personality, and appearance are reflections of individuality and are not determined by gender. **2.** hermaphroditic. **-androgyny,** *n.*

android [Gk *andros* + *eidos* form], pertaining to something that is typically masculine, or manlike, such as an android pelvis.

android pelvis, a type of pelvis in which the structure is characteristic of the male. The bones are thick and heavy, and the inlet is heart-shaped.

androma. See **arrhenoblastoma.**

andropause /an'drəpôs/, a change of life for men that may be expressed in terms of a reordering of life. It is associated with a decline in androgen levels that occurs in men during their late forties or early fifties.

androsterone /andros'tərōn/ [Gk *andros* + *stereos* solid], a male sex hormone. The greater potency of several other male sex hormones has relegated androsterone largely to historic biochemical interest.

anecdotal [Gk *anekdotos* unpublished], pertaining to medical knowledge based on isolated observations and not yet verified by controlled scientific studies.

anechoic /an'ekō'ik/, (in ulrasonography) free of echoes or without echoes.

anemia [Gk *a, haima* not blood], a disorder characterized by a decrease in hemoglobin in the blood to levels below the normal range, decreased red cell production or increased red cell destruction, or blood loss. A separate and distinct morphologic classification system describes anemia by the hemoglobin content of the red cells (normochromic or hypochromic) and by differences in red cell size (macrocytic, normocytic, or microcytic). **–anemic** *adj.*

anemia of pregnancy, a condition of pregnancy characterized by a reduction in the concentration of hemoglobin in the blood. It may be physiologic or pathologic. In physiologic anemia of pregnancy, the reduction in concentration results from dilution because the plasma volume expands more than the red blood cell volume. In pathologic anemia of pregnancy, the oxygen-carrying capacity of the blood is deficient because of disordered erythrocyte production or excessive loss of erythrocytes through destruction or bleeding.

anemic anoxia, a condition characterized by a deficiency of oxygen in body tissues, resulting from a decrease in the number of erythrocytes in the blood or in the amount of hemoglobin.

anencephaly /an′ensef′əlē/ [Gk *a, egkephalos* not brain], congenital absence of the brain and spinal cord in which the cranium does not close and the vertebral canal remains a groove. Transmitted genetically, anencephaly is not compatible with life.

anephrogenesis /anef′rōjen′əsis/ [Gk *a* without, *nephros* kidney, *genein* to produce], to be born without kidneys.

anergic stupor, a kind of dementia characterized by quietness, listlessness, and nonresistance.

anergy [Gk *a, ergon* not work], **1.** lack of activity. **2.** an immunodeficient condition characterized by a lack of or diminished reaction to an antigen or group of antigens. This state may be seen in advanced tuberculosis and other serious infections, acquired immunodeficiency syndrome, and some malignancies. **–anergic,** *adj.*

aneroid /an′əroid/, not containing a liquid, used especially to describe a device that does contain liquid, such as aneroid sphygmomanometer, which does not contain a column of liquid mercury.

aneroid barometer, a device consisting of a flexible spring in a sealed, evacuated metal box that is used to measure atmospheric pressure.

anesthesia [Gk *anaisthesia* lack of feeling], the absence of normal sensation, especially sensitivity to pain, as induced by an anesthetic substance or by hypnosis or as occurs with traumatic or pathophysiologic damage to nerve tissue. Anesthesia induced for medical or surgical purposes may be topical, local, regional, or general and is named for the anesthetic agent used, the method or procedure followed, the area or organ anesthetized, or the age or class of patient served.

anesthesia dolorosa, a severe tactile or spontaneous, paradoxical pain in an anesthetized area.

anesthesia machine, an apparatus for administering inhalant anesthetic agents.

anesthesia paralysis [Gk *anaisthesia + paralyein* to be palsied], paralysis that may develop following administration of a general anesthetic.

anesthesia patients, classification of, the system by which the American Society of Anesthesiologists classifies anesthesia patients in five categories by anesthetic risk factors. Class I includes patients who are generally healthy; without serious organic, physiologic, biochemical, or psychiatric problems; and for whom anesthesia is required only for a local condition, such as an inguinal hernia or fibroid uterus. Class II includes patients who have mild to moderate systemic problems, whether involving or extraneous to the condition requiring anesthesia, such as anemia, mild diabetes, essential hypertension, extreme obesity, or chronic bronchitis. Class III includes patients who have severe systemic disturbances or disease, whether or not related to the procedure requiring surgical anesthesia. Class IV includes patients who are suffering from a life-threatening, but not necessarily terminal, condition that may or may not be related to the intended surgical procedure. Class V includes the moribund patient who has little chance of survival, such as a person in shock with a burst abdominal aneurysm or a massive pulmonary embolus. The letter *E* is added to the Roman numeral to indicate an emergency procedure, such as a patient scheduled for an elective herniorrhaphy who becomes an emergency case when his hernia becomes an obstruction.

anesthesia screen, a metal inverted U-shaped frame that attaches to the sides of an operating table, 12 to 18 inches above a patient's upper chest. It is covered with a sheet to prevent contamination of an operative site on the chest or abdomen by airborne infection from the patient or the anesthetist and to provide a wide sterile field for the surgeon.

anesthesia shock, [Gk *anaisthesia;* Fr *choc*], a condition of shock produced by an overdose of anesthetic.

anesthesiologist /an'əsthē'zē·ol'əjist/, a physician trained in the administration of anesthetics and in the provision of respiratory and cardiovascular support during anesthetic procedures.

anesthesiologist's assistant (AA), an allied health professional who assists the anesthesiologist in performing various preoperative tasks, in administering supportive therapy, in providing anesthesia monitoring services, and in other functions and tasks.

anesthesiology, the branch of medicine concerned with the relief of pain and the administration of medication to relieve pain during surgery.

anesthetic, a drug or agent that is capable of producing a complete or partial loss of feeling (anesthesia).

anesthetist /ənes'thətist/, **1.** a person who administers anesthesia. **2.** an anesthesiologist.

anesthetize, to induce a state of anesthesia.

anetoderma /an'ətōdur'mə/ [Gk *anetos* relaxed, *derma* skin], an idiopathic, patchy atrophy and looseness of skin for which there is no known effective treatment.

aneuploid /an'yōōploid/ [Gk *a, eu* not good, *ploos* fold, *eidos* form], **1.** of or pertaining to an individual, organism, strain, or cell that has a chromosome number that is not an exact multiple of the normal, basic haploid number characteristic of the species. **2.** such an individual, organism, strain, or cell.

aneuploidy /an'yōōploi'dē/, any variation in chromosome number that involves individual chromosomes rather than entire sets. There may be fewer chromosomes, as in Turner's syndrome, or more chromosomes, as in Down syndrome.

aneurysm /an'yōōriz'əm/ [Gk *aneurysma* widening], a localized dilatation of the wall of a blood vessel, usually caused by atherosclerosis and hypertension, or, less frequently, by trauma, infection, or a congenital weakness in the vessel wall. Aneurysms are common in the aorta but also occur in peripheral vessels and are fairly common in the lower extremities of older people, especially in the popliteal arteries. A sign of an arterial aneurysm is a pulsating swelling that produces a blowing murmur on auscultation. An aneurysm may rupture, causing hemorrhage, or thrombi may form in the dilated pouch and give rise to emboli that may obstruct smaller vessels. Kinds of aneurysms include **aortic, bacterial, berry, cerebral, compound, dissecting, fusiform, mycotic, racemose, Rasmussen's, saccular, vari-**cose and **ventricular aneurysm.** **–aneurysmal** /an'yōōriz'məl/, *adj.*

aneurysmal bone cyst, a cystic bone lesion that tends to develop in the metaphyseal region of long bones but may occur in any bone, including the vertebrae. It produces pain and swelling.

aneurysmal varix [Gk *aneurysma* a widening; L *varix* a dilated vein], a varicose vein in which the enlargement is of aneurysmal proportions.

aneurysm needle, a needle equipped with a handle, used to ligate aneurysms.

aneurysmoid varix. See **aneurysmal varix.**

ANF, abbreviation for *American Nurses Foundation; Australian Nursing Federation.*

angel dust. See **phencyclidine hydrochloride (PCP).**

anger [L *angere* to hurt], an emotional reaction characterized by extreme displeasure, rage, indignation, or hostility. It is considered to be of pathologic origin when such a response does not realistically reflect a person's actual circumstances.

angiitis /anjē·ī'tis/ [Gk *aggeion* vessel, *itis*], an inflammatory condition of a vessel, chiefly a blood or lymph vessel. A kind of angiitis is **consecutive angiitis.**

angina /anji'nə, an'jinə/ [L *angor* quinsy (strangling)], **1.** a spasmodic, cramplike choking feeling. **2.** a term now used primarily to denote angina pectoris, the paroxysmal chest pain caused by anoxia of the myocardium. **3.** a descriptive feature of various diseases characterized by a feeling of choking, suffocation, or crushing pressure and pain. Kinds of angina are **intestinal, Ludwig's, Prinzmetal's, stable, unstable,** and **streptococcal angina.** **–anginal,** *adj.*

angina decubitus, a condition characterized by periodic attacks of angina pectoris that occur when the person is lying down.

angina pectoris, a paroxysmal thoracic pain caused most often by myocardial anoxia as a result of atherosclerosis of the coronary arteries. The pain usually radiates down the inner aspect of the left arm and is frequently accompanied by a feeling of suffocation and impending death. Attacks of angina pectoris are often related to exertion, emotional stress, and exposure to intense cold.

angina sine dolore /sē'nə dolôr'ə, sī'nē/, a painless episode of coronary insufficiency.

angina trachealis. See **croup.**

angioblastic meningioma /an'jē-ōblas'tik/, a tumor of the blood vessels of the meninges covering the spinal cord or the brain.

angioblastoma /an'jē-ōblastō'mə/, *pl.* **an-**

gioblastomas, angioblastomata [Gk *aggeion* vessel, *blastos* germ, *oma*], a tumor of blood vessels in the brain. Kinds of angioblastomas are **angioblastic meningioma** and **cerebellar angioblastoma.**

angiocardiography /an'jē-ōkär'dē-ōgram'/ [Gk *aggeion* + *kardia* heart, *graphein* to record], the process of producing a radiograph of the heart and great vessels of the heart. A radiopaque contrast medium is injected directly into the heart by means of a catheter introduced through the antecubital veins.

angiocardiopathy [Gk *aggeion* + *kardia* heart, *pathos* disease], a disease of the blood vessels of the heart.

angiocatheter /an'jē-ōkath'ətər/, a hollow, flexible tube inserted into a blood vessel to withdraw or instill fluids.

angiochondroma /an'jē-ōkondrō'mə/, pl. **angiochondromas, angiochondromata** [Gk *aggeion* + *chondros* cartilage, *oma*], a cartilaginous tumor characterized by an excessive formation of blood vessels.

angioedema. See **angioneurotic edema.**

angioendothelioma. See **hemangioendothelioma.**

angiofibroma /an'jē-ōfībrō'mə/, pl. **angiofibromas, angiofibromata** [Gk *aggeion* + L *fibra* fiber; Gk *oma*], an angioma containing fibrous tissue.

angiogenesis /an'jē-ōjen'əsis/ [Gk *aggeion* + *genesis* origin], the ability to evoke blood vessel formation, a common property of malignant tissue.

angiogenin /an'jē-ōjen'in/, a protein that mediates the formation of blood vessels. It is used experimentally to stimulate the development of new blood vessels in wound healing, stroke, or coronary heart disease.

angioglioma /an'jē-ōglē-ō'mə/, pl. **angiogliomas, angiogliomata** [Gk *aggeion* + *glia* glue, *oma*], a highly vascular tumor composed of neuroglia.

angiogram /an'jē-ogram/ [Gk *aggeion* + *gramma* writing], a radiographic image of a blood vessel after the injection of a contrast medium.

angiograph, [Gk *aggeion* + *graphein* to record], a sphygmographic device that records the patterns of pulse waves.

angiography /an'jē-og'rəfē/ [Gk *aggeion* + *graphein* to record], the radiographic visualization of the internal anatomy of the heart and blood vessels after the intravascular introduction of radiopaque contrast medium. —**angiographic,** *adj.*

angiohemophilia. See **von Willebrand's disease.**

angiokeratoma /an'jē-ōker'ətō'mə/, pl. **angiokeratomas, angiokeratomata** [Gk

aggeion + *keras* horn, *oma*], a vascular, horny neoplasm on the skin, characterized by clumps of dilated blood vessels, clusters of warts, and thickening of the epidermis, especially the scrotum and the dorsal aspect of the fingers and toes.

angiokeratoma circumscriptum, a rare skin disorder characterized by discrete papules and nodules in small patches on the legs or on the trunk.

angiokeratoma corporis diffusum, an uncommon familial disease in which phospholipids are stored in many parts of the body, especially the blood vessels, causing vasomotor, urinary, and cutaneous disorders and, in some cases, muscular abnormalities.

angiolipoma /an'jē-ōlipō'mə/, pl. **angiolipomas, angiolipomata** [Gk *aggeion* + *lipos* fat, *oma*], a benign neoplasm containing blood vessels and tissue.

angioma /an'jē-ō'mə/, pl. **angiomas, angiomata** [Gk *aggeion* vessel, *oma* tumor], any benign tumor with blood vessels (hemangioma) or lymph vessels (lymphangioma). Most angiomas are congenital; some, like cavernous hemangiomas, may disappear spontaneously.

angioma arteriale racemosum /ärtir'ē-ā'lē ras'əmō'səm/ [Gk *aggeion*, *oma* + L *arteria* airpipe, *racemus* grape], a vascular neoplasm characterized by the intertwining of many small, newly formed, dilated blood vessels.

angioma cavernosum. See **cavernous hemangioma.**

angioma cutis, a nevus composed of a network of dilated blood vessels.

angioma lymphaticum. See **lymphangioma.**

angioma serpiginosum/ [Gk *aggeion*, *oma* + L *serpere* to creep], a cutaneous disease characterized by rings of tiny vascular points appearing as red dots.

angiomatosis /an'jē-ōmətō'sis/, a condition characterized by the presence of numerous vascular tumors.

angiomyoma, pl. **angiomyomas, angiomyomata** [Gk *aggeion* + *mys* muscle, *oma*], a tumor composed of vascular and muscular tissue elements.

angiomyoneuroma. See **glomangioma.**

angiomyosarcoma /an'jē-ōmī'ōsärkō'mə/, pl. **angiomyosarcomas, angiomyosarcomata** [Gk *aggeion* + *mys* muscle, *sarx* flesh, *oma*], a tumor containing vascular, muscular, and connective tissue elements.

angioneuroma. See **glomangioma.**

angioneurotic anuria [Gk *aggeion* + *neuron* nerve; *a, ouron* not urine], an abnormal condition characterized by an almost complete absence of urination caused by destruction of tissue in the renal cortex.

angioneurotic edema [Gk *aggeion* + *neuron* nerve; *oidema* swelling], an acute, painless, dermal, subcutaneous or submucosal swelling of short duration involving the face, neck, lips, larynx, hands, feet, genitalia, or viscera. It may result from food or drug allergy, infection, or emotional stress, or it may be hereditary.

angioneurotic gangrene, the death and putrefaction of tissue due to an interruption of the blood supply resulting from thrombotic arteries or veins.

angiopathy [Gk *aggeion* + *pathos* disease], a disease of the blood vessels.

angioplasty /an'jē-ōplas'tē/ [Gk *aggeion* + *plassein* to mold], the reconstruction of blood vessels damaged by disease or injury.

angiorraphy /an'jē-ôr'əfē/ [Gk *aggeion* + *rhaphe* suture], the repair by suture of any blood vessel.

angiosarcoma /an'jē-ōsärkō'mə/, a rare, malignant tumor consisting of endothelial and fibroblastic tissue that proliferates and eventually surrounds vascular channels.

angiosclerosis [Gk *aggeion* + *skleros* hard + *osis* condition], a thickening and hardening of the walls of the blood vessels.

angiospasm, a sudden, transient constriction of a blood vessel.

angiotensin /an'jē-ōten'sin/ [Gk *aggeion* + L *tendere* to stretch], a polypeptide occurring in the blood causing vasoconstriction, increased blood pressure, and the release of aldosterone from the adrenal cortex. Angiotensin is formed by the action of renin on angiotensinogen, an alpha-2-globulin that is produced in the liver and constantly circulates in the blood.

angiotensin-converting enzyme (ACE), a protein (dipeptidyl carboxypeptidase) that catalyzes the conversion of angiotensin I to angiotensin II by splitting two terminal amino acids.

angiotensinogen, a serum globulin produced in the liver that is the precursor of angiotensin.

angiotensin sensitivity test (AST), a test for sensitivity to angiotensin II by infusion of angiotensin-II-amide into the right cubital vein.

angle [L *angulus*], 1. the space or the shape formed at the intersection of two lines, planes, or borders. The divergence of the lines, planes, or borders may be measured in degrees of a circle. 2. (in anatomy and physiology) the geometric relationships between the surfaces of body structures and the positions affected by movement.

angle board, (in dentistry) a device used for facilitating the establishment of reproducible angular relationships between a patient's head, the x-ray beam, and the x-ray film.

angle-closure glaucoma. See **glaucoma.**

angle former, (in dentistry) one of a series of paired cutting instruments having cutting edges at an angle other than a right angle in relation to the axis of the blade.

angle of incidence, the angle at which an ultrasound beam hits the interface between two different types of tissues, such as the facing surfaces of bone and muscle.

angle of Louis, the sternal angle between the manubrium and the body of the sternum.

angle of mandible, the angular relationship between the body and the ramus of the mandible.

angle of refraction [L *angulus* + *refringere* to break apart], the angle between a refracted ray and the normal to the surface of the refracting medium.

angle of Treitz /trīts/, a sharp curve or flexure at the junction of the duodenum and jejunum.

Angle's Classification of Malocclusion, a classification of the various types of malocclusion, established by Edward Hartley Angle, American orthodontist (1855–1930). This system has since been modified. Classification is based on the relation of different teeth in the upper and lower jaws, such as the maxillary and the mandibular molars.

angstrom (Å) /ang'strəm/ [Anders J. Angström, Swedish physicist, b. 1814], a unit of measure of length equal to 0.1 millimicron (1/10,000,000 meter), or 10^{-10} meter.

angstrom unit (AU). See **angstrom (Å).**

angular gyrus [L *angulus* + Gk *gyros*], a folded convolution in the inferior parietal lobe where it unites with the temporal lobe of the cerebral cortex.

angular movement [L *angularis* sharply bent], one of the four basic kinds of movement allowed by the various joints of the skeleton in which the angle between two adjoining bones is decreased, as in flexion, or increased, as in extension.

angular spinal curvature [L *angulus* + *spina* backbone + *curvatura* bend], a sharp bending or sloping of the vertebral column.

angular stomatitis, inflammation at the corner of the mouth.

angular vein, one of a pair of veins of the face, formed by the junction of the frontal and the supraorbital veins.

angulated fracture, a fracture in which the fragments of bone are at angles.

angulation [L *angulatus* bent], **1.** an angular shape or formation. **2.** the discipline of precisely measuring angles, as in mechanical drafting and surveying. **3.** (in radiography) the direction of the primary beam of radiation in relation to the object being radiographed and the film used to record its image.

anhedonia /an'hēdō'nē·ə/ [Gk *a, hedone* not pleasure], the inability to feel pleasure or happiness from experiences that are ordinarily pleasurable. **–anhedonic,** *adj.*

anhidrosis /an'hidrō'sis, an'hī-/ [Gk *a, hidros* not sweat], an abnormal condition characterized by inadequate perspiration.

anhidrotic /an'hidrot'ik, an'hī-/, **1.** of or pertaining to anhidrosis. **2.** an agent that reduces or suppresses sweating.

anhydrase /anhī'drās/ [Gk *a* not, *hydor* water], an enzyme that catalyzes the elimination of water molecules from certain compounds, as carbonic anhydrase dehydrates carbonic acid, thereby controlling the amount of carbon dioxide in the blood and lungs.

anhydride [Gk *a, hydor* not water], a chemical compound, especially an acid, derived by the removal of water from a substance. **–anhydrous,** *adj.*

anicteric /an'ikter'ik/ [Gk *a, icterus* not jaundice], pertaining to the absence of jaundice.

anicteric hepatitis, a mild form of hepatitis in which there is no jaundice (icterus). Symptoms include anorexia, GI disturbances, and slight fever. AST and ALT are elevated. The infection may be mistaken for flu or go unnoticed.

anidean /anid'ē·ən/ [Gk *a, eidos* not form], formless; shapeless; denoting an undifferentiated mass, such as an anideus.

anideus /anid'ē·əs/, an anomalous, rudimentary embryo consisting of a simple rounded mass with little indication of the body parts. A kind of anideus is **embryonic anideus.**

aniline /an'ilēn/ [Ar *alnil* indigo], an oily, colorless, poisonous liquid with a strong odor and burning taste, formerly extracted from the indigo plant and now made synthetically using nitrobenzene in the manufacture of aniline dyes.

anilism, [Ar *alnil* indigo + Gk *ismos* state], a condition of poisoning from exposure to aniline compounds. Symptoms generally include cyanosis, weakness, cold sweats, irregular pulse, breathing difficulty, coma, convulsions, and possible sudden heart failure.

anilinparasulfonic acid. See **sulfanilic acid.**

anima /an'imə/ [L, soul], **1.** the soul or life. **2.** the active ingredient in a drug. **3.** (in Jungian psychology) a person's true, inner, unconscious being or personality, as distinguished from overt personality, or persona. **4.** (in analytic psychology) the female component of the male personality.

animal pole [L *anima*], the active, formative part of the ovum protoplasm that contains the nucleus and bulk of the cytoplasm and where the polar bodies form. In mammals it is also the site where the inner cell mass gives rise to the ectoderm.

animal starch. See **glycogen.**

animus /an'iməs/ [L, spirit], **1.** the active or rational soul; the animating principle of life. **2.** the male component of the female personality. **3.** (in psychiatry) a deepseated antagonism that is usually controlled but may erupt with virulence under stress.

anion /an'ī·ən/ [Gk *ana, ion,* backward going], **1.** a negatively charged ion that is attracted to the positive electrode (anode) in electrolysis. **2.** a negatively charged atom, molecule, or radical.

anion exchange resin, any one of the simple organic polymers with high molecular weights that exchange anions with other ions in solution. Anion exchange resins are used as antacids in treating ulcers.

anion gap, the difference between the concentrations of serum cations and anions, determined by measuring the concentrations of sodium cations and chloride and bicarbonate anions. It is helpful in the diagnosis and treatment of acidosis.

anionic /an'ī·on'ik/ [Gk *ana* not, *ion* going], pertaining to an anion.

anise /an'is/, the fruit of the *Pimpinella anisum* plant. Extract of anise is used in the preparation of carminatives and expectorants.

aniseikonia /an'īsīkō'nē·ə/ [Gk *anisos* unequal, *eikon* image], an abnormal ocular condition in which each eye perceives the same image as being of a different form and size.

anisocytosis /anī'sōsītō'sis/ [Gk *anisos* + *kytos* cell], an abnormal condition of the blood characterized by red blood cells of variable and abnormal size.

anisogamete [Gk *anisos* + *gamos* marriage], a gamete that differs considerably in size and structure from the one with which it unites, as the macrogamete and microgamete of certain sporozoa. **–anisogametic,** *adj.*

anisogamy /an'īsog'əmē/, sexual conjugation of gametes that are of unequal size and structure, as in certain thallophytes and sporozoa. **–anisogamous,** *adj.*

anisognathic, /an'īsōnath'ik/ [Gk *anisos* + *gnathos* jaw], of or pertaining to an abnormal condition in which the maxillary and the mandibular arches or jaws are of significantly different sizes in the same individual.

anisokaryosis /anĭ'sōker'ē·ō'sis/, significant variation in the size of the nucleus of cells of the same general type. **–anisokaryotic,** adj.

anisomastia /anĭ'sōmas'tē·ə/, a condition in which one female breast is much larger than the other.

anisometropia /anĭ'sōmetrō'pē·ə/ [Gk anisos + metron measure, ops eye], an abnormal ocular condition characterized by a difference in the refractive powers of the eyes.

anisopia /an'isō'pē·ə/, a condition in which the visual power of one eye is greater than that of the other.

anisotropine methylbromide, an anticholinergic drug prescribed as adjunctive therapy in the treatment of peptic ulcer.

ankle [AS ancleow], **1.** the joint of the tibia, the talus, and the fibula. **2.** the part of the leg where this joint is located.

ankle bandage, a figure-of-eight bandage looped under the sole of the foot and around the ankle. The heel may be covered or left exposed, although covering is preferable because it prevents "window edema."

ankle bone. See **talus.**

ankle clonus, an involuntary tendon reflex that causes repeated flexion and extension of the foot.

ankle-foot orthosis (AFO), any of a variety of protective external devices that can be applied to the ankle area to prevent injury in a high-risk athletic activity, to protect a previous injury such as a sprain, and to compensate for chronic joint instability.

ankle joint [AS ancleow; L jungere to join], a synovial hinge joint at the lower end of the tibia. The rounded malleous prominences on either side of the joint form a mortise for the upper surface of the talus.

ankle reflex. See **Achilles tendon reflex.**

ankyloglossia [Gk agkylos crooked, glossa tongue], an oral defect, characterized by an abnormally short lingual frenum that limits tongue movement and impairs the speech. It may be surgically corrected by a frenotomy.

ankylosed, pertaining to the immobility of a joint resulting from pathologic changes in the joint or in adjacent tissues.

ankylosing spondylitis /ang'kilō'sing/, a chronic inflammatory disease of unknown origin, first affecting the spine and adjacent structures, and commonly progressing to eventual fusion (ankylosis) of the involved joints. In extreme cases the patient develops a forward flexion of the spine called a "poker spine" or "bamboo spine."

ankylosis /ang'kilō'sis/ [Gk agkylosis bent condition], **1.** fixation of a joint, often in an abnormal position, usually resulting from destruction of articular cartilage and subchondral bone, as occurs in rheumatoid arthritis. **2.** also called **arthrodesis, fusion.** surgically induced fixation of a joint to relieve pain or provide support.

anlage /on'lägə/ [Ger Anlage, disposition, aptitude], (in embryology) the undifferentiated layer of cells from which a particular organ, tissue, or structure develops; primordium rudiment.

ANLL, abbreviation for **acute nonlymphocytic leukemia.**

annihilation, the total transformation of matter into energy.

annular. See **anular.**

annular ligament. See **anular ligament.**

annulus /an'yələs/ [L, a ring], any ring-shaped structure, such as the outer edge of an intervertebral disc.

anodic stripping voltammetry /anod'ik/, a process of electroanalytic chemistry used to detect trace metals.

anodontia /an'ōdon'tē·ə/ [Gk a, not odous tooth], a congenital defect in which some or all of the teeth are missing.

anodyne /an'ədīn/ [Gk a, odyne not pain], a drug that relieves or lessens pain.

anomaly /ənom'əlē/ [Gk anomalos irregular], **1.** deviation from what is regarded as normal. **2.** congenital malformation, such as the absence of a limb or the presence of an extra finger. **–anomalous,** adj.

anomia /ənō'mē·ə/ [Gk a, onoma not name], a form of aphasia characterized by the inability to name objects, caused by a lesion in the temporal lobe of the brain.

anomie /an'əmē/, a state of apathy, alienation, anxiety, personal disorientation, and distress resulting from the loss of social norms and goals previously valued. Also spelled **anomy.**

anoopsia /an'ō·op'sē·ə/ [Gk ana up, ops eye], a strabismus in which one or both eyes are deviated upward.

Anopheles /ənof'əlēz/ [Gk anopheles harmful], a genus of mosquito, many species of which transmit malaria-causing parasites to humans.

anopia /anō'pē·ə/ [Gk a, ops not eye], blindness resulting from a defect in or the absence of one or both eyes.

anoplasty [L anus; Gk plassein to shape], a restorative operation on the anus.

anorchia /anôr'kē·ə/ [Gk a, orchis not testis], congenital absence of one or both testes.

anorectal /an′ōrek′təl/, ā′nō- [L *anus* + *rectus* straight], of or pertaining to the anal and rectal portions of the large intestine.

anorectal abscess [L *anus* + *rectus* straight, *abscedere* to go away], an abscess in the area of the anus and rectum.

anorectal stricture [L *anus, rectus* + *strictura* compression], a narrowing of the anorectal canal, sometimes congenital but also the result of surgery to correct a fissure or to remove hemorrhoids.

anorectic /an′ōrek′tik/, **1.** of or pertaining to anorexia. **2.** lacking appetite. **3.** causing a loss of appetite, as anorexiant drug.

anorexia /an′ōrek′sē·ə/ [Gk *a, orexis* not appetite], lack or loss of appetite, resulting in the inability to eat. –**anorexic, anorectic,** *adj.*

anorexia nervosa, a disorder characterized by a prolonged refusal to eat, resulting in emaciation, amenorrhea, emotional disturbance concerning body image, and an abnormal fear of becoming obese.

anorexiant, a drug or other agent that suppresses the appetite, such as amphetamine.

anorthopia /an′ôrthō′pē·ə/, a visual distortion in which straight lines appear to be curved or angular.

anosigmoidoscopy /an′ōsig′moidos′kəpē/, a procedure in which an endoscope is used for direct examination of the lining of the anus, rectum, and colon.

anosmia /anoz′mē·ə/ [Gk *a, osme* not smell], loss or impairment of the sense of smell, usually occurring as a temporary condition resulting from a head cold or respiratory infection or when intranasal swelling or other obstruction prevents odors from reaching the olfactory region. It becomes a permanent condition when the olfactory neuroepithelium or any part of the olfactory nerve is destroyed. Kinds of anosmia are **anosmia gustatoria** and **preferential anosmia.** –**anosmatic, anosmic,** *adj.*

anosmia gustatoria, the inability to smell foods.

anosmic [Gk *a* without, *osme* smell], pertaining to a loss of the sense of smell.

anosognosia /an′əsog·nō′zhə/ [Gk *a, nosos* not disease, *gnosis* knowing], an abnormal condition characterized by a real or feigned inability to perceive a defect, especially paralysis, on one side of the body, possibly attributable to a lesion in the right parietal lobe of the brain.

anosphrasia, anosphresia. See **anosmia.**

anotia /anō′tē·ə/ [Gk *a* without, *ous* ear], a congenital absence of one or both ears.

ANOVA, abbreviation for **analysis of variance.**

anovaginal [L *anus* + *vagina* sheath], pertaining to the perineal region of the anus and vagina.

anovesical [L *anus* + *vesicula* small bladder], pertaining to the anus and bladder.

anovular /anov′yələr/ [Gk *a* not, *ovulum*], pertaining to a menstrual discharge not associated with the production or release of an ovum.

anovular menstruation [Gk *a, ovulum* not egg], menstrual bleeding that occurs even though ovulation has not taken place.

anovulation /an′ovy ōōlā′shən/, failure of the ovaries to produce, mature, or release eggs as a result of ovarian immaturity or postmaturity; of altered ovarian function, as in pregnancy and lactation; of primary ovarian dysfunction, as in ovarian dysgenesis; or of disturbance of the interaction of the hypothalamus, pituitary gland, and ovary caused by stress or disease. –**anovulatory** /anov′y ōōlətôr′ē/, *adj.*

anoxemia /an′oksē′mē·ə/, a deficiency of oxygen in the blood.

anoxia /anok′sē·ə/ [Gk *a, oxys* not sharp, *genein* to produce], an abnormal condition characterized by a lack of oxygen. Anoxia may be local or systemic and may be the result of an inadequate supply of oxygen to the respiratory system or of an inability of the blood to carry oxygen to the tissues or of the tissues to absorb the oxygen from the circulation, as in histotoxic anoxia. Kinds of anoxia include **cerebral anoxia** and **stagnant anoxia.** –**anoxic,** *adj.*

ansa /an′sə/, *pl.* **ansae** [L, handle], (in anatomy) a looplike structure resembling a curved handle of a vase.

ansa cervicalis, one of three loops of nerves in the cervical plexus, branches of which innervate the infrahyoid muscles.

ANSI, abbreviation for **American National Standards Institute.**

antacid /antas′id/ [Gk *anti* against, *acidus* sour], **1.** opposing acidity. **2.** a drug or dietary substance that buffers, neutralizes, or absorbs hydrochloric acid in the stomach.

antagonism [Gk *antagonisma* struggle], an inhibiting action between physiologic processes, such as muscle actions, opposing actions of drugs. Also,

antagonist /antagə′nist/, [Gk *antagonisma* struggle], **1.** one who contends with or is opposed to another. **2.** (in physiology) any agent, such as a drug or muscle, that exerts an opposite action to that of another or competes for the same receptor sites. Kinds of antagonists include **antimetabolite, associated, direct,** and **narcotic. 3.** (in dentistry) a tooth in the upper jaw that articulates during mastication or occlusion with a tooth in the lower jaw. **–antago-nistic,** *adj.,* **antagonize,** *v.*

antagonistic reflexes [Gk *antagonisma;* L *reflectere* to bend back], two or more re-flexes initiated at the same time that pro-duce opposite effects. The most adaptive or persistent response occurs.

antecardium. See **epigastric region.**

antecubital [L *ante* before, *cubitum* elbow], in front of the elbow; at the bend of the elbow.

antecubital fossa [L *ante* before, *cubitum* elbow, *fossa* ditch], a depression at the bend of the elbow.

anteflexion /-flek′shən/ [L *ante* + *flectare* bend], an abnormal position of an organ in which the organ is tilted acutely for-ward, folded over on itself.

antegonial notch [L *ante* + *gonia* angle], a depression or concavity commonly present at the junction of the ramus and the mandible, near the attachment of the anterior margin of the masseter.

antegrade [L *ante* + *gredi* to go], mov-ing forward or proceeding toward the front.

ante mortem [L *ante* + *mors* death], be-fore death.

antenatal. See **prenatal.**

antenatal diagnosis. See **prenatal diag-nosis.**

antepartal [L *ante* + *parturire* to have la-bor pains], pertaining to the period span-ning conception and labor.

antepartal care, care of a pregnant woman during the time in the maternity cycle that begins with conception and ends with the onset of labor.

antepartum hemorrhage [Gk *ante;* L, *par-turire* to have labor pains; Gk *haima* blood, *rhegnynei* to gush], bleeding from the uterus during a pregancy in which the placenta appears to be normally situated, particularly after the 28th week.

antepyretic [L *ante* + Gk *pyretos* fever], before the onset of fever.

anterior (A) [L *ante, prior* foremost], **1.** the front of a structure. **2.** of or pertaining to a surface or part situated toward the front or facing forward.

anterior Achilles bursitis. See **Albert's disease.**

anterior asynclitism. See **asynclitism.**

anterior atlantoaxial ligament, one of five ligaments connecting the atlas to the axis. It is fixed to the inferior border of the anterior arch of the atlas and to the ventral surface of the body of the axis.

anterior atlantooccipital membrane, one of two broad, densely woven fibrous sheets that form part of the atlantooccipi-tal joint between the atlas and the occipi-tal bone.

anterior cardiac vein, one of several small vessels that return deoxygenated blood from the ventral portion of the myo-cardium of the right ventricle to the right atrium.

anterior cerebral commissure [L *ante, prior* + *cerebrum* brain, *commissura* ajoining], a bundle of fibers in the ante-rior wall of the forebrain connecting the olfactory bulb and cortex on one side with the similar structures on the other side.

anterior chamber, the part of the anterior cavity of the eye in front of the iris. It con-tains the aqueous humor.

anterior common ligament. See **ante-rior longitudinal ligament.**

anterior crural nerve. See **femoral nerve.**

anterior cutaneous nerve, one of a pair of cutaneous branches of the cervical plexus. It arises from the second and the third cervical nerves, bends around the middle of the sternocleidomastoideus, crosses the muscle obliquely, passes be-neath the platysma, and divides into the as-cending and descending branches.

anterior determinants of cusp, (in den-tistry) the characteristics of the anterior teeth that determine the cusp elevations and the fossa depressions in restoration of the postcanine teeth.

anterior fontanel, a diamond-shaped area between the frontal and two parietal bones just above the baby's forehead at the junction of the coronal and sagittal sutures.

anterior guide, (in dentistry) the portion of an articulator that is contacted by the incisal guide pin to maintain the selected separation of the upper and lower mem-bers of the articulator.

anterior horn cell, a large nerve cell, as seen in cross-section, of the anterior col-umn of the spinal cord. It is the axon of a somatic efferent nerve.

anterior horn of the spinal cord, one of the hornlike projections of gray matter into the white matter of the spinal cord. The an-terior, or ventral horn, contains efferent fi-bers innervating muscle tissue.

anterior longitudinal ligament, the broad, strong ligament attached to the ven-tral surfaces of the vertebral bodies. It ex-tends from the occipital bone and the an-terior tubercle of the atlas to the sacrum.

anterior mediastinal node, a node in one of the three groups of thoracic visceral nodes of the lymphatic system that drains lymph from the nodes of the thymus, the pericardium, and the sternum.

anterior mediastinum, a caudal portion of the mediastinum in the middle of the thorax, bounded ventrally by the body of the sternum and parts of the fourth through the seventh ribs and dorsally by the parietal pericardium, extending downward as far as the diaphragm.

anterior nares, the ends of the nostrils that open anteriorly into the nasal cavity and allow the inhalation and the exhalation of air. The anterior nares connect with the nasal fossae.

anterior neuropore, the opening of the embryonic neural tube in the anterior portion of the forebrain.

anterior pituitary. See **adenohypophysis.**

anterior rhizotomy [L *ante, prior;* Gk *rhiza* root + *temnein* to cut], the surgical cutting of the ventral root of a spinal nerve, usually to relieve persistent spasm or involuntary movement.

anterior tibial artery, one of the two divisions of the popliteal artery, arising in back of the knee, dividing into six branches, and supplying various muscles of the leg and foot.

anterior tibial node, one of the small lymph glands of the lower limb, lying on the interosseous membrane near the proximal portion of the anterior tibial vessels.

anterior tooth, any one of the incisors or canine teeth.

anterocclusion /an′tərōkloo′shən/ [L *ante* + *occludere* to shut], (in dentistry) a malocclusion in which the mandibular teeth are anterior to their normal position relative to the teeth in the maxillary arch.

anterograde amnesia [L *ante, prior* foremost, *gredi* to go], the inability to recall events of long ago with normal recall of recent events.

anterograde memory, the ability to recall events of long ago but not those of recent occurrence.

anterolateral, pertaining to a position that is in front and on either side of another structure or object.

anterolateral thoracotomy /an′tərōlat-′ərəl/, a chest surgery technique in which entry to the chest is made with an incision below the breast but above the costal margins.

anteroposterior (AP) /an′tərōpostir′ē·ər/ [L *ante, prior* foremost, *posterus* coming after], from the front to the back of the body, commonly associated with the direction of the x-ray beam.

anteroposterior vaginal repair, a surgical procedure in which the upper and lower walls of the vagina are reconstructed to correct relaxed tissue.

anteversion [L *ante* + *versio* turning], **1.** an abnormal position of an organ in which the organ is tilted forward on its axis, away from the midline. **2.** (in dentistry) the tipping or the tilting of teeth or other man-

dibular structures more anteriorly than normal. **3.** the angulation created in the transverse plane between the neck and shaft of the femur. **–anteverted,** *adj.*

anthelmintic /ant′helmin′tik/ [Gk *anti, helmins* against worms], **1.** of or pertaining to a substance that destroys or prevents the development of parasitic worms, such as filariae, flukes, hookworms, pinworms, roundworms, schistosomes, tapeworms, trichinae, and whipworms. **2.** an anthelmintic drug. An anthelmintic may interfere with the parasites' carbohydrate metabolism, inhibit their respiratory enzymes, block their neuromuscular action, or render them susceptible to destruction by the host's macrophages.

anthracosis /an′thrəkō′sis/ [Gk *anthrax* coal, *osis* condition], a chronic lung disease occurring in coal miners, characterized by the deposit of coal dust in the lungs and the formation of black nodules on the bronchioles, and resulting in focal emphysema.

anthracosis linguae. See **parasitic glossitis.**

anthralin /an′thrəlin/, a topical antipsoriatic prescribed in the treatment of psoriasis and chronic dermatitis.

anthranilic acid. See **aminobenzoic acid.**

anthrax /an′thraks/ [Gk, coal, carbuncle], a disease affecting primarily farm animals (cattle, goats, pigs, sheep, and horses), caused by the bacterium *Bacillus anthracis.* Anthrax in animals is usually fatal. Humans most often acquire it when a break in the skin comes into direct contact with infected animals and their hides, or by inhaling the spores of the bacterium.

anthropoid, [Gk *anthropos* human, *eidos* form], a term generally applied to humanlike apes or other primates. Also a term used to describe a certain kind of pelvis in gynecology and obstetrics.

anthropoid pelvis [Gk *anthropos* human, *eidos* form], a type of pelvis in which the inlet is oval; the anteroposterior diameter is much greater than the transverse, and, because of the posterior inclination of the sacrum, the posterior portion of the space in the true pelvis is much greater than the anterior portion.

anthropology [Gk *anthropos* + *logos* science], the science of human beings, from animal-like characteristics to social and environmental aspects.

anthropometry /an′thrəpom′ətrē/ [Gk *anthropos* + *metron* measure], the science of measuring the human body as to height, weight, and size of component parts, including measurement of skinfolds, to study and compare the relative proportions under normal and abnormal conditions. **–anthropometric,** adj.

antiadrenergic /an'ti·ad'rənur'jik/ [Gk anti + L ad, ren to kidney], **1.** of or pertaining to the blocking of the effects of impulses transmitted by the adrenergic postganglionic fibers of the sympathetic nervous system. **2.** an antiadrenergic agent. Drugs that block the response to norepinephrine by alpha-adrenergic receptors reduce the tone of smooth muscle in peripheral blood vessels, causing increased peripheral circulation and decreased blood pressure.

antiagglutinin [Gk anti + L agglutinare to glue], a specific antibody that counteracts the effects of an agglutinin.

antianabolic, pertaining to drugs or other agents that inhibit or retard anabolic processes, such as cell division or the creation of new tissue by protein synthesis.

antianaphylaxis /-an'əfilak'sis/ [Gk anti, ana back, phylaxis protection], a procedure to prevent anaphylactic reactions by injecting a patient with small desensitizing doses of the antigen.

antianemic [Gk anti + a, haima without blood], **1.** of or pertaining to a substance or procedure that counteracts or prevents a deficiency of erythrocytes. **2.** an agent used to treat or to prevent anemia.

antianginal drug, any medication that has the effect of dilating the coronary arteries, thereby improving the blood flow to the myocardium to prevent symptoms of angina pectoris.

antiantibody [Gk anti, anti + AS bodig], an immunoglobulin formed as the result of the administration of an antibody that acts as an immunogen. The antiantibody then interacts with the antibody.

antiantitoxin [Gk anti + anti + toxikon poison], an antiantibody that may form in the body during immunization that inhibits or counteracts the effect of the antitoxin administered.

antianxiety agent. See **sedative-hypnotic.**

antiarrhythmic [Gk anti + rhythmos rhythm], **1.** of or pertaining to a procedure or substance that prevents, alleviates, or corrects an abnormal cardiac rhythm. **2.** an agent used to treat a cardiac arrhythmia. A defibrillator that delivers a precordial electric shock is often used to restore a normal rhythm to rapid, irregular atrial or ventricular contractions. A pacemaker may be implanted in a patient with an extremely slow heart rate or other arrhythmia. The beta-adrenergic blocking agent propranolol may be used in treating arrhythmias. Verapamil and other calcium antagonists control arrhythmias by inhibiting calcium ion influx across the cell membrane of cardiac muscle, thus slowing atrioventricular conduction and prolonging the effective refractory period within the atrioventricular node.

antiarthritic /-ärthrit'ik/ [Gk anti + arthron joint, itis inflammation], pertaining to a therapy that relieves symptoms of arthritis.

antibacterial [Gk anti + bakterion small staff], **1.** of or pertaining to a substance that kills bacteria or inhibits their growth or replication. **2.** an antibacterial agent. Antibiotics synthesized chemically or derived from various microorganisms exert their bactericidal or bacteriostatic effect by interfering with the production of the bacterial cell wall, by interfering with protein synthesis, nucleic acid synthesis, or cell membrane integrity, or by inhibiting critical biosynthetic pathways in the bacteria.

antiberiberi factor. See **thiamine.**

antibiotic [Gk anti + bios life], **1.** of or pertaining to the ability to destroy or interfere with the development of a living organism. **2.** an antimicrobial agent, derived from cultures of a microorganism or produced semisynthetically, used to treat infections. The penicillins exert their action by inhibiting mucopeptide synthesis in bacterial cell walls during multiplication of the organisms. Aminoglycoside antibiotics interfere with the synthesis of bacterial proteins and are used primarily for the treatment of infections caused by gram-negative organisms. Macrolide antibiotics interfere in protein synthesis of susceptible bacteria during multiplication without affecting nucleic acid synthesis. Antifungals apparently bind to sterols in fungus cell membranes and change their permeability. The tetracyclines are primarily bacteriostatic and are thought to exert their effect by inhibiting protein synthesis in the organisms. Tetracycline therapy may cause GI irritation, photosensitivity, renal toxicity, and hepatic toxicity, and administration of a drug of this group during the last half of pregnancy, during infancy, or before 8 years of age may result in permanent discoloration of the teeth. The cephalosporins inhibit bacterial cell wall synthesis. Chloramphenicol, a broad-spectrum antibiotic initially derived from *Streptomyces venezuelae,* inhibits protein synthesis in bacteria by interfering with the transfer of activated amino acids from soluble RNA to ribosomes.

antibiotic anticancer agents, drugs that may have both antibiotic and anticancer activity. Examples include bleomycin, dactinomycin, daunorubicin, and mitomycin.

antibiotic sensitivity tests, a laboratory method for determining the susceptibility of bacterial infections to therapy with antibiotics. After the infecting organism has been recovered from a clinical specimen, it is cultured and tested against several antibiotic drugs. If the growth of the organism is inhibited by the action of the drug, it is reported as sensitive to that antibiotic.

antibody (Ab) [Gk *anti* + AS *bodig*], an immunoglobulin, essential to the immune system, produced by lymphoid tissue in response to bacteria, viruses, or other antigenic substances. An antibody is specific to an antigen. Each class of antibody is named for its action. Among the many antibodies are agglutinins, bacteriolysins, opsonins, precipitin.

antibody absorption, the process of removing or tying up undesired antibodies in an antiserum reagent by allowing it to react with undesired antigens.

antibody instructive theory, a theory that each antigenic contact in the life of an individual develops a new antibody, as when an immunoglobulin-covered B cell comes in contact with an antigen and subsequently produces plasma cells and memory cells.

antibody specific theory, (in immunology) a theory of antibody formation proposed by F.M. Burnet, stating that preprogramed, or precommitted, clones of lymphoid cells that are produced in the fetus are capable of interacting with a limited number of antigenic determinants with which the host may come in contact. The theory holds that the body contains an enormous number of diverse clones of cells, each genetically programed to synthesize a different antibody.

antibromic. See **deodorant.**

anticancer diet, a diet, based on recommendations of the American Cancer Society (ACS), National Cancer Institute (NCI), and National Academy of Sciences, to reduce risk factors associated with eating habits. It includes a fat intake of not more that 30% of total calories and a daily intake of high-fiber foods.

anticarcinogenic /-kär′sinəjen′ik/ [Gk *anti* + *karkinos* crab, *oma* tumor, *genein* to produce], pertaining to a substance or device that neutralizes the effects of a carcinogen.

anticholinergic /-kōlənur′jik/ [Gk *anti* + *chole* bile, *ergein* to work] **1.** of or pertaining to a blockade of acetylcholine receptors that results in the inhibition of the transmission of parasympathetic nerve impulses. **2.** an anticholinergic agent that functions by competing with the neurotransmitter acetylcholine for its receptor sites at synaptic junctions. Anticholinergic drugs reduce spasms of smooth muscle in the bladder, bronchi, and intestine; relax the iris sphincter; decrease gastric, bronchial, and salivary secretions; decrease perspiration; and accelerate impulse conduction through the myocardium by blocking vagal impulses.

anticholinergic agent. See **anticholinergic.**

anticholinesterase /an′tikol′ənes′tərās/, a drug that inhibits or inactivates the action of acetylcholinesterase. Drugs of this class cause acetylcholine to accumulate at the junctions of various cholinergic nerve fibers and their effector sites or organs, allowing potentially continuous stimulation of cholinergic fibers throughout the central and peripheral nervous systems.

anticipatory adaptation /antis′əpətôr′ē/ [L *anticipare* to receive before], the act of adapting to a potentially distressing situation before actually confronting the problem, as when a person tries to relax before learning the results of a medical examination.

anticipatory grief, feelings of grief that develop before, rather than after, the loss of a loved one.

anticipatory guidance, the psychologic preparation of a patient to help relieve fear and anxiety of an event expected to be stressful, such as the preparation of a child for surgery by explaining what will happen.

anticoagulant /-kō·ag′yələnt/ [Gk *anti* + *coagulare* curdle], **1.** of or pertaining to a substance that prevents or delays coagulation of the blood. **2.** an anticoagulant drug. Heparin, obtained from the liver and lungs of domestic animals, is a potent anticoagulant that interferes with the formation of thromboplastin, with the conversion of prothrombin to thrombin and with the formation of fibrin from fibrinogen.

anticoagulant therapy [Gk *anti;* L *coagulare* to curdle; Gk *therapeia*], the administration of drugs that reduce the tendency of blood to coagulate, thereby reducing the risk of thrombosis.

anticodon /an′tikō′don/ [Gk *anti* + *caudex* book], (in genetics) a sequence of three nucleotides in transfer RNA that pairs complementarily with a specific codon of messenger RNA during protein synthesis to specify a particular amino acid in the polypeptide chain.

anticonvulsant [Gk *anti* + L *convellere* to shake], **1.** of or pertaining to a substance or procedure that prevents or reduces the severity of epileptic or other convulsive seizures. **2.** an anticonvulsant drug. Hydantoin derivatives, especially phenytoin, apparently exert their anticonvulsant effect by stabilizing the cell membrane and decreasing intracellular sodium, with the result that the excitability of the epileptogenic focus is reduced. Phenacemide and primidone are also used in treating grand mal epilepsy, and succinic acid derivatives, valproic acid, paramethadione, and various barbiturates are among the drugs prescribed to limit or prevent petit mal seizures.

antideformity positioning and splinting, the use of splints, braces, or similar devices to prevent or control contractures or other musculoskeletal deformities that may result from disuse, burns, or other injuries.

antidepressant, 1. of or pertaining to a substance or a measure that prevents or relieves depression. 2. an antidepressant agent. Tricyclic antidepressant agents block re-uptake of amine neurotransmitters, but the exact mechanism of the antidepressant action of these drugs is unknown. Monoamine oxidase (MAO) inhibitors increase the concentration of epinephrine, norepinephrine, and serotonin in storage sites in the nervous system.

antidiarrheal, a drug or other agent that relieves the symptoms of diarrhea. Antidiarrheals work by absorbing water from the digestive tract, by altering intestinal motility, by altering electrolyte transport, or by adsorption of toxins or microorganisms.

antidiuretic [Gk *anti* + *dia* through, *ourein* to urinate] 1. of or pertaining to the suppression of urine formation. 2. an antidiuretic agent. Antidiuretic hormone (vasopressin), produced in hypothalamic nuclei and stored in the posterior lobe of the pituitary gland, suppresses urine formation by stimulating the resorption of water in distal tubules and collecting ducts in the kidneys. –antidiuresis, *n.*

antidiuretic hormone (ADH), a hormone that decreases the production of urine by increasing the reabsorption of water by the renal tubules. ADH is secreted by cells of the hypothalamus and stored in the posterior lobe of the pituitary gland. It is released in response to a decrease in blood volume or an increased concentration of sodium or other substances in plasma, or by pain, stress, or the action of certain drugs.

antidotal [Gk *anti* + *dotos*, that which is given] a substance that renders a poison or drug ineffective.

antidote /an'tidōt/ [Gk *anti* + *dotos* that which is given], a drug or other substance that opposes the action of a poison. An antidote may coat the stomach and pre-

vent absorption, make the toxin inert, or oppose the action of the poison.

antidromic conduction /an'tidrom'ik/ [Gk *anti* + *dromos* course], the conduction of a neural impulse backward from a receptor in the midportion of an axon. It is an unnatural phenomenon and may be produced experimentally.

antiembolism hose [Gk *anti* + *embolos* plug], elasticized stockings worn to prevent the formation of emboli and thrombi, especially in patients after surgery or those restricted to bed. Return flow of the venous circulation is promoted, preventing venous stasis and dilatation of the veins, conditions that predispose to varicosities and thromboembolic disorders.

antiemetic /-imet'ik/ [Gk *anti* + *emesis* vomiting], 1. of or pertaining to a substance or procedure that prevents or alleviates nausea and vomiting. 2. an antiemetic drug or agent. Belladonna derivatives, bromides, barbiturates and other sedatives, and substances that protect the stomach lining, such as lime water or mild gastric astringents, have weak antiemetic properties. Chlorpromazine and other phenothiazines are the most effective antiemetic agents. In motion sickness scopolamine and antihistamines provide relief.

antiepileptic. See **anticonvulsant.**

antiestrogen drug, any of a group of hormone-based products used predominantly in cancer chemotherapy.

antifebrile. See **antipyretic.**

antifungal, 1. of or pertaining to a substance that kills fungi or inhibits their growth or reproduction. 2. an antifungal, antibiotic drug. Amphotericin B and ketoconazole, both effective against a broad spectrum of fungi, probably act by binding to sterols in the fungal cell membrane and changing the membrane's permeability. Griseofulvin, another broad-spectrum antifungal agent, binds to the host's new keratin and renders it resistant to further fungal invasion. Miconazole inhibits the growth of common dermatophytes, including yeastlike *Candida albicans,* and nystatin is effective against yeast and yeast-like fungi.

antigalactic, pertaining to a drug or other agent that prevents or reduces milk secretion in some mothers of newborns.

anti-GBM disease, an immunologically mediated kidney disorder involving the glomerular basement membrane (GBM), which is damaged in the antigen-antibody reaction. The kidney itself may serve as the antigenic target in the reaction.

antigen /an'tijən/ [Gk *anti* + *genein* to produce], a substance, usually a protein, that causes the formation of an antibody and reacts specifically with that antibody.

antigen-antibody reaction, a process of the immune system in which immuno-globulin-coated B cells recognize an intruder or antigen and stimulate antibody production to protect the body against infection. The T cells of the body assist in the antigen-antibody reaction, but the B cells play the key role. Antigen-antibody reactions activate the complement system of the body, amplifying the humoral immunity response of the B cells and causing lysis of the antigenic cells. Antigen-antibody reactions involve the binding of antigens to antibodies to form antigen-antibody complexes that may render the toxic antigen harmless, agglutinize antigens on the surface of microorganisms, or activate the complement system by exposing the complement-binding sites on the antibody molecule. Antigen-antibody reactions normally produce immunity, but they can also produce allergy, autoimmunity, and fetomaternal hematologic incompatibility. In immediate allergic reactions, antigens provoke the production of specific antibodies that may circulate freely in the serum or may become attached to specific cells. Autoimmunity makes it impossible for the immune system to distinguish between self and a foreign substance.

antigen determinant, a small area on the surface of an antigen molecule that fits a combining site of an antibody molecule and binds the antigen in the formation of an antigen-antibody complex. Antigen determinants commonly consist of a sequence of amino acids that decrees the shape of these reactive areas.

antigenic drift [Gk *anti, genein* to produce; AS *drifan* drift], the tendency of a virus or other microorganism to alter its genetic makeup periodically resulting in a mutant antigen, requiring new antibodies and vaccines to combat its effects.

antigenicity /an'tijənis'ətē/, the quality of causing the production of antibodies. The degree of antigenicity depends on the kind and amount of the particular substance, the condition of the host, and the degree to which the host is sensitive to the antigen and able to produce antibodies.

antigerminal pole. See **vegetal pole.**

antiglobulin /an'tiglob'y ōōlin/ [Gk *anti* + L *globulus* small globe], an antibody against human globulin, occurring naturally or prepared in laboratory animals. Specific antiglobulins are used in the detection of specific antibodies, as in blood typing.

antiglobulin test, a test for the presence of antibodies that coat and damage red blood cells as a result of any of several diseases or conditions. The test can detect Rh antibodies in maternal blood and is used to anticipate hemolytic disease of the newborn.

antigravity muscles, the muscle groups involved with stabilization of joints or other body parts by opposing the effects of gravity on the body.

antihemophilic C factor. See **factor XI.**

antihemophilic factor (AHF), blood factor VIII, a systemic hemostatic. It is prescribed in the treatment of hemophilia A, a deficiency of factor VIII.

antihemophilic factor plasma, blood plasma that contains the antihemophilic Factor VIII.

antihemorrhagic, any drug or agent used to prevent or control bleeding, such as thromboplastin or thrombin, either of which mediates the blood clotting process.

antihidrotic /-hidrot'ik/ [Gk *anti* + *hidros* sweat], an agent that inhibits or prevents the production of sweat.

antihistamine [Gk *anti* + *histos* tissue, amine (ammonia compound)], any substance capable of reducing the physiologic and pharmacologic effects of histamine, including a wide variety of drugs that block histamine receptors. Many such drugs are readily available as nonprescriptive medicines for the management of allergies. These substances do not stop the release of histamine, and the ways in which they act on the central nervous system (CNS) are not completely understood. The antihistamines are divided into H_1 and H_2 blockers, depending on the responses to histamine they prevent. –**antihistaminic,** *adj.*

antihypercholesterolemic, a drug that prevents or controls an increase of cholesterol in the blood. Examples include clofibrate and colestipol.

antihypertensive, **1.** of or pertaining to a substance or procedure that reduces high blood pressure. **2.** an antihypertensive agent. Various drugs achieve their antihypertensive effect by depleting tissue stores of catecholamines in peripheral sites by stimulating pressor receptors in the carotid sinus and heart, by blocking autonomic nerve impulses that constrict blood vessels, by stimulating central inhibitory alpha-adrenergic receptors, or by direct vasodilatation. Thiazides and other diuretic agents reduce blood pressure by decreasing blood volume.

antiimmune [Gk *anti* + L *immunis* free from], pertaining to the prevention or inhibition of immunity.

antiinfection vitamin. See **vitamin A.**

antiinfectious [Gk *anti* + L *inficere* to

stain], pertaining to an agent that prevents or treats infection.

antiinflammatory [Gk *anti* + L *inflammare* to set afire] **1.** of or pertaining to a substance or procedure that counteracts or reduces inflammation. **2.** an antiinflammatory drug or agent. The basis of the antiinflammatory effect of salicylates and nonsteroidal antiinflammatory agents, such as phenylbutazone and indomethacin, appears to involve inhibition of prostaglandin biosynthesis.

antiinitiator, a substance that is a potential co-carcinogen but that may protect cells against cancer development if given before exposure to an initiator.

antileprotic, a drug or other agent that is effective in treating leprosy.

antilipidemic /an'tilip'idē'mik/ [Gk *anti* + *lipos* fat, *haima* blood], **1.** of or pertaining to a regimen, diet, or agent that reduces the amount of lipids in the serum. **2.** a drug used to reduce the amount of lipids in the serum.

antilymphocyte serum (ALS), a serum prescribed as an immunosuppressive agent for the reduction of rejection reactions in organ transplant and as an adjunct in chemotherapy for malignant neoplasms.

antimalarial, **1.** of or pertaining to a substance that destroys or suppresses the development of malaria plasmodia or to a procedure that exterminates the mosquito vectors of the disease, such as spraying insecticides or draining swamps. **2.** an antimalarial drug that destroys or prevents the development of plasmodia in human hosts.

antimessage, a strand of RNA that cannot act as mRNA because of its negative coding sequence. It must be converted to a positive-strand sequence by a viral transcriptase before it can function as a messenger.

antimetabolite [Gk *anti* + *metabole* change], a drug or other substance that is an antagonist or that resembles a normal human metabolite and interferes with its function in the body, usually by competing for the metabolite's receptors or enzymes.

antimicrobial [Gk *anti* + *mikros* small, *bios* life], **1.** of or pertaining to a substance that kills microorganisms or inhibits their growth or replication. **2.** an agent that kills or inhibits the growth or replication of microorganisms.

antimicrobial drugs [Gk *anti* + *mikros* small, *bios* life; Fr *drogue*], drugs that destroy or inhibit the growth of microorganisms.

antimitochondrial antibody, an antibody that acts specifically against mitochondria. These antibodies are not normally present in the blood of healthy people. A laboratory test for the presence of the antibodies in the blood is a valuable diagnostic aid in liver disease.

antimitotic /-mītot'ik/, pertaining to the inhibition of cell division.

antimony /an'təmō'nē/ [L *antimonium*], a bluish, crystalline metallic element occurring in nature, both free and as salts. Various antimony compounds are used in the treatment of filariasis, leishmaniasis, lymphogranuloma, schistosomiasis, and trypanosomiasis and as an emetic.

antimony poisoning, poisoning caused by the ingestion or inhalation of antimony or antimony compounds, characterized by vomiting, sweating, diarrhea, and a metallic taste in the mouth. Irritation of the skin or mucous membrane may result from external exposure. Severe poisoning resembles arsenic poisoning.

antimorph /an'təmôrf/ [Gk *anti* + *morphe* form], a mutant gene that inhibits or antagonizes the normal influence of its allele in the expression of a trait.

antimuscarinic [Gk *anti* + L *musca* fly], inhibiting the stimulation of the postganglionic parasympathetic receptor.

antimutagen /an'timy oo'təjən/ [Gk *anti* + L *mutare* to change; Gk *genein* to produce], **1.** any substance that reduces the rate of spontaneous mutations or counteracts or reverses the action of a mutagen. **2.** any technique that protects cells against the effects of mutagenic agents. –**antimutagenic,** *adj.*

antimycotic. See **antifungal.**

antineoplastic [Gk *anti* + *neos* new, *plasma* something formed] **1.** of or pertaining to a substance, procedure, or measure that prevents the proliferation of malignant cells. **2.** a chemotherapeutic agent that controls or kills cancer cells. Drugs used in the treatment of cancer are cytotoxic but are generally more damaging to dividing cells than to resting cells. Cycle-specific antineoplastic agents are more effective in killing proliferating cells than in killing resting cells, and phase-specific agents are most active during a specific phase of the cell cycle. Most anticancer drugs prevent the proliferation of cells by inhibiting the synthesis of DNA by various mechanisms.

antineoplastic antibiotic, a chemical substance derived from a microorganism or a synthetic analog of the substance used in cancer chemotherapy.

antineoplastic hormone, a chemical substance produced by an endocrine gland or a synthetic analog of the naturally occurring compound used to control certain disseminated cancers. Hormonal therapy is

antineuritic vitamin. See **thiamine.**

antinuclear antibody (ANA), an autoantibody that reacts with nuclear material. Antinuclear antibodies are found in the blood serum of patients with rheumatoid arthritis, systemic lupus erythematosus, Sjögren's syndrome, polymyositis, and a number of nonrheumatic disorders.

antioxidant /-ok'sidənt/, a chemical or other agent that inhibits or retards oxidation of a substance to which it is added. Examples include butylated hydroxyanisole (BHA) and butylated hydroxytoluene (BHT), which are added to foods containing fats or oils to prevent oxygen from combining with the fatty molecules, thereby causing them to become rancid.

antiparallel [Gk *anti* + *parallelos* side-by-side], (in molecular genetics) the condition in which molecules, such as strands of DNA, are parallel but point in opposite directions.

antiparasitic /-pər'əsit'ik/ [Gk *anti* + *parasitos* guest], **1.** of or pertaining to a substance or procedure that kills parasites or inhibits their growth or reproduction. **2.** an antiparasitic drug including amebicides, anthelmintics, antimalarials, schistosomicides, trichomonacides, and trypanosomicides.

antiparkinsonian, of or pertaining to a substance or procedure used to treat parkinsonism. Drugs for this neurologic disorder are of two kinds: those that compensate for the lack of dopamine in the corpus striatum of parkinsonism patients and anticholinergic agents that counteract the activity of the abundant acetylcholine in the striatum.

antipathy [Gk *anti* + *pathos* suffering], a strong feeling of aversion or antagonism to particular objects, individuals, or substances.

antiperistaltic [Gk *anti* + *peristellein* to wrap around] **1.** of or pertaining to a substance that inhibits or diminishes peristalsis. **2.** an antiperistaltic agent. Narcotics, such as paregoric, diphenoxylate, and loperamide hydrochloride, are antiperistaltic agents used to provide symptomatic relief in diarrhea. Anticholinergic (parasympatholytic) drugs reduce spasms of intestinal smooth muscle and are frequently prescribed to decrease excessive GI motility.

antipernicious anemia factor. See **cyanocobalamin.**

antiprotoplasmatic, pertaining to agents that damage the protoplasm of cells.

antipruritic /-prŏŏrit'ik/ [Gk *anti* + L *prurire* to itch], **1.** of or pertaining to a substance or procedure that tends to relieve or prevent itching. **2.** an antipruritic drug. Topical anesthetics, corticosteroids, and antihistamines are used as antipruritic agents.

antipsoriatic /an'tisôr'ē·at'ik/ [Gk *anti* + *psora* itch], pertaining to an agent that relieves the symptoms of psoriasis.

antipsychotic [Gk *anti* + *psyche* mind, *osis* condition] **1.** of or pertaining to a substance or procedure that counteracts or diminishes symptoms of a psychosis. **2.** an antipsychotic drug. Phenothiazine derivatives are the most frequently prescribed antipsychotics for use in the treatment of schizophrenia and other major affective disorders.

antipyresis /-pīrē'sis/ [Gk *anti* + *pyretos* fever], treatment to reduce and ameliorate fever.

antipyretic /-pīret'ik/ [Gk *anti* + *pyretos* fever], **1.** of or pertaining to a substance or procedure that reduces fever. **2.** an antipyretic agent. Such drugs usually lower the thermodetection set point of the hypothalamic heat regulatory center, with resulting vasodilatation and sweating. A tepid alcohol sponge bath or lukewarm tub bath may decrease an elevated temperature, and hypothermia produced by a cooling blanket is sometimes used for patients with a prolonged, high fever.

antipyretic bath, a bath in which tepid water is used to reduce the temperature of the body.

antipyrotic /-pīrot'ik/ [Gk *anti* + *pyr* fire], pertaining to the treatment of burns or scalds.

antirachitic, pertaining to an agent used to treat rickets.

antirheumatic [Gk *anti* + *rheumatismos* that which flows], pertaining to the relief of symptoms of any painful or immobilizing disorder of the musculoskeletal system.

antiscorbutic vitamin. See **ascorbic acid.**

antiseborrheic, pertaining to a drug or agent that is applied to the skin to control seborrhea or seborrheic dermatitis.

antisense, (molecular genetics) an Rna molecule that is complementary to the mRNA (sense) molecule produced by transcription of a given gene. The antisense strands of many genes have been synthesized in the laboratory and are useful because they hybridize with the mRNA sense strand and block their translation into amino acids and proteins.

antisepsis [Gk *anti* + *sepein* putrefaction], destruction of microorganisms to prevent infection.

antiseptic, 1. tending to inhibit the

---

designed to counteract the effect of an endogenous hormone required for the growth of the tumor.

growth and reproduction of microorganisms. **2.** a substance that tends to inhibit the growth and reproduction of microorganisms.

antiseptic dressing, a dressing treated with an antiseptic, germicide, or bacteriostat and applied to a wound or an incision to prevent or treat infection.

antiseptic gauze, gauze permeated with an antiseptic solution, sometimes packaged in individual, sealed packets.

antiserum, *pl.* **antisera, antiserums** [Gk *anti* + L, whey], serum of an animal or human containing antibodies against a specific disease used to confer passive immunity to that disease. Antisera do not provoke the production of antibodies. There are two types of antiserum. Antitoxin is an antiserum that neutralizes the toxin produced by specific bacteria, but it does not kill the bacteria. Antimicrobial serum destroys bacteria by making them more susceptible to the leukocytic action.

antiserum anaphylaxis, an exaggerated reaction of hypersensitivity in a normal person caused by the injection of serum from a sensitized individual.

antisialogogue, a drug that reduces saliva secretion.

antisocial personality [Gk *anti* + L *socius* companion], a person who exhibits attitudes and overt behavior contrary to the customs, standards, and moral principles accepted by society.

antisocial personality disorder, a condition characterized by repetitive behavioral patterns that lack moral and ethical standards and bring a person into continuous conflict with society. Symptoms include aggressiveness, callousness, impulsiveness, irresponsibility, hostility, a low frustration level, marked emotional immaturity, and poor judgment.

antisocial reaction. See **antisocial personality disorder.**

antispasmodic, a drug or other agent that prevents smooth muscle spasms, as in the uterus, digestive system, or urinary tract.

antistreptolysin-O test (ASOT, ASLT) /an′tistrep′təli′sinō′/, a streptococcal antibody test for finding and measuring serum antibodies to streptolysin-O, an exotoxin produced by most group A and some group C and G streptococci. The test is often used as an aid in the diagnosis of rheumatic fever.

antithermic. See **antipyretic.**

antithymocyte globulin (ATG) /an′tithī′məsīt/, a gamma globulin fraction that has been rendered immune to T lymphocytes.

antithyroid drug, any one of several preparations that can inhibit the synthesis of thyroid hormones and are commonly used in the treatment of hyperthyroidism. In the body such substances interfere with the incorporation of iodine into the tyrosyl residues of thyroglobulin required for the production of the hormones thyroxine and triiodothyronine.

antitoxin /-tok′sin/ [Gk *anti* + *toxikon* poison], a subgroup of antisera usually prepared from the serum of horses immunized against a particular toxin-producing organism, such as botulism antitoxin given therapeutically in botulism and tetanus and diphtheria antitoxin given prophylactically to prevent those infections.

antitrust, (in law) against the operation, establishment, or maintenance of a monopoly in the manufacture, production, or sale of a commodity, providing of a service, or practice of a profession.

antitrypsin, a protein produced in the liver that blocks the action of trypsin and other proteolytic enzymes.

antitubercular, any agent or any of a group of drugs used to treat tuberculosis. At least two drugs, and usually three, are required in various combinations in pulmonary tuberculosis therapy.

antitussive /an′titus′iv/ [Gk *anti* + L *tussive* cough] **1.** against a cough. **2.** any of a large group of narcotic and nonnarcotic drugs that act on the central and peripheral nervous systems to suppress the cough reflex. Because the cough reflex is necessary for clearing the upper respiratory tract of obstructive secretions, antitussives should not be used with a productive cough.

antivenin /an′tiven′in/ [Gk *anti* + L *venenum* poison], a suspension of venom-neutralizing antibodies prepared from the serum of immunized horses. Antivenin confers passive immunity and is given as a part of emergency first aid for various snake and insect bites.

antiviral, destructive to viruses.

antivitamin [Gk *anti* + L *vita* life, amine], a substance that inactivates a vitamin.

antixerophthalmic vitamin. /-zir′əfthal′-mik/ See **vitamin A.**

Anton's syndrome, a form of anosognosia in which a person with partial or total blindness denies being visually impaired, despite medical evidence to the contrary.

antral gastritis [Gk *antron* cave], an abnormal narrowing of the antrum, or distal portion of the stomach. The narrowing is not a true gastritis, but a radiographic finding that may represent gastric ulcer or tumor.

antrum cardiacum, a constricted passage from the esophagus to the stomach, lying just inside the opening formed by the cardiac sphincter.

antrum of Highmore. See **maxillary sinus.**

ANUG, abbreviation for **acute necrotizing ulcerative gingivitis.**

anular [L *annulus* ring], describing a ring-shaped lesion surrounding a clear, normal, unaffected disk of skin.

anular ligament, a ligament that encircles the head of the radius and holds it in the radial notch of the ulna. Distal to the notch, the anular ligament forms a complete fibrous ring.

anulus, a ring of circular tissue, such as the whitish tympanic anulus around the perimeter of the tympanic membrane.

anuresis. See **anuria.**

anuria /ənō̄or′ē-ə/ [Gk *a, ouron* not urine], the inability to urinate, the cessation of urine production, or a urinary output of less than 100 to 250 ml per day. Anuria may be caused by kidney failure or dysfunction, a decline in blood pressure below that required to maintain filtration pressure in the kidney, or an obstruction in the urinary passages. Although patients can live up to 2 weeks with anuria, death may occur within 24 hours of the total loss of urinary function. Kinds of anuria include **angioneurotic, calculus, obstructive, postrenal, prerenal,** and **renal.** –**anuric, anuretic,** *adj.*

anus /ā′nəs/, the opening at the terminal end of the anal canal.

anxietas /angzī′ətas/ [L, anxiety], a state of anxiety, nervous restlessness, or apprehension, often accompanied by a feeling of oppression in the epigastrium. Kinds of anxietas are **anxietas presenilis** and **restless legs syndrome.**

anxietas presenilis [L *anxietas; prae* before, *senex* aged], a state of extreme anxiety associated with the climacteric period of life.

anxietas tibiarum. See **restless legs syndrome.**

anxiety [L *anxietas*], a NANDA-accepted nursing diagnosis of a feeling of apprehension, uneasiness, agitation, uncertainty, and fear resulting from the anticipation of some threat or danger, usually of intrapsychic rather than external origin, whose source is generally unknown or unrecognized. Defining characteristics may be subjective or objective. The subjective characteristics include feelings of increased tension, helplessness, inadequacy, fear, overexcitedness, distress, and worry. Objective characteristics include cardiovascular excitation, superficial vasoconstriction, pupil dilatation, restlessness, insomnia, poor eye contact, trembling, facial tension, quivering voice, continuous focus on the self, increased perspiration, and expressed concern regarding change in life events. Kinds of anxiety include **castration, free-floating, separation,** and **situational.**

anxiety attack, an acute, psychobiologic reaction manifested by intense anxiety and panic. Symptoms vary according to the individual and the intensity of the attack but typically include palpitations, shortness of breath, dizziness, faintness, profuse sweating, pallor of the face and extremities, GI discomfort, and a vague feeling of imminent death.

anxiety complex. See **castration anxiety.**

anxiety disorders, disorders characterized by persistent worry. The symptoms range from mild, chronic tenseness, with feelings of timidity, fatigue, apprehension, and indecisiveness, to more intense states of restlessness and irritability that may lead to aggressive acts or indecisiveness. In extreme cases, the overwhelming emotional discomfort is accompanied by physical reactions, including tremor, sustained muscle tension, tachycardia, dyspnea, hypertension, increased respiration, and profuse perspiration.

anxiety dream, a dream that occurs during rapid-eye-movement (REM) sleep and is accompanied by restlessness and a gradual increase in pulse rate.

anxiety hysteria [L *anxietas;* Gk *hystera* womb], a disorder characterized by symptoms of both anxiety and hysteria.

anxiety reaction [L *anxietas + re, agere* to act], any of a group of disorders in which anxiety is the predominant characteristic or is experienced by a person facing a dreaded siuation to the extent that the individual's functioning is impaired. The reaction may be expressed as a panic disorder, a phobia, or a compulsion.

anxiety state [L *anxietas + state*], a mental reaction characterized by apprehension, uncertainty, and fear. Anxiety states may be accompanied by physiologic changes as sweating and tremors.

anxiolytic /angk′sē-ōlit′ik/, a sedative or minor tranquilizer used primarily to treat episodes of anxiety. Kinds of anxiolytics include barbiturates, benzodiazepines, chlormezanone, hydroxyzine, meprobamate, and tybamate.

AOA, abbreviation for **Administration on Aging.**

AORN, abbreviation for **Association of Operating Room Nurses.**

aorta /ā-ôr′tə/ [Gk *aerein* to raise], the main trunk of the systemic arterial circulation, comprising four parts: the ascending aorta, the arch of the aorta, the thoracic portion of the descending aorta, and the abdominal portion of the descending aorta. It starts at the aortic opening of the left ventricle, where it has a diameter of about 3 cm, rises a short distance toward the neck, bends to the left and dorsally over the root of the left lung, descends within the thorax on the left side of the vertebral column, and passes through the aortic hiatus of the diaphragm into the abdominal cavity. –aortic, adj.

aortic aneurysm, a localized dilatation of the wall of the aorta caused by atherosclerosis, hypertension, or, less frequently, syphilis. The lesion may be a saccular distention, a fusiform or cylindroid swelling of a length of the vessel, or a longitudinal dissection between the outer and middle layers of the vessel wall.

aortic arch syndrome, any of a group of occlusive conditions of the aortic arch producing a variety of symptoms related to obstruction of the large branch arteries, including the innominate, left common carotid, or left subclavian. Such conditions as atherosclerosis, Takayasu's arteritis, and syphilis may cause aortic arch syndrome.

aortic atresia [Gk aerein + a, tresis a boring], a congenital anomaly in which the left side of the heart is defective and there is an imperforation of the aortic valve.

aortic balloon pump. See **intraaortic balloon pump.**

aortic body. See **carotid body.**

aortic body reflex, See **carotid body reflex.**

aortic notch [Gk aerein to raise; OFr enochier], the dicrotic notch on the descending limb of an arterial pulse sphygmogram. It marks the closure of the aortic valve and immediately precedes a dicrotic wave.

aortic regurgitant murmur [Gk aerein + L re again, gurgitare to flow + murmur, humming], a heart murmur that is a sign of aortic incompetence. A failure of the aortic valves to close completely during ventricular diastole allows some blood to flow back into the left ventricle.

aortic regurgitation, the flow of blood from the aorta back into the left ventricle.

aortic sinus [Gk, aerein + L sinus little hollow], any of three dilatations, one anterior and two posterior, between the aortic wall and the semi-lunar cusps of the aortic valve.

aortic stenosis (AS), a cardiac anomaly characterized by a narrowing or stricture of the aortic valve because of congenital malformation or of fusion of the cusps, as may result from rheumatic fever. Aortic stenosis obstructs the flow of blood from the left ventricle into the aorta, causing decreased cardiac output and pulmonary vascular congestion.

aortic thrill [Gk aerein + AS thyrlian], a palpable chest vibration caused by stenosis of the aortic valve or by an aortic aneurysm. It is usually felt or palpated in the second intercostal space to the right of the sternum in systole using the flat of the hand or the fingertips.

aortic valve, a valve in the heart between the left ventricle and the aorta. It is composed of three semilunar cusps that close in diastole to prevent blood from flowing back into the left ventricle from the aorta.

aortitis /ā′ôrtī′tis/, an inflammatory condition of the aorta, occurring most frequently in tertiary syphilis and occasionally in rheumatic fever. Kinds of aortitis are **rheumatic aortitis** and **syphilitic aortitis.**

aortocoronary [Gk aerein + L corona crown], pertaining to the aorta and coronary arteries.

aortocoronary bypass [AS bi alongside; Fr passer], a surgical procedure in which a saphenous vein, mammary artery, or other blood vessel is used to build a shunt from the aorta to one of the coronary arteries in order to bypass a circulatory obstruction.

aortogram /ā·ôr′təgram/ [Gk aerein + gramma record], a radiographic image of the aorta made after the injection of a radiopaque medium in the blood.

aortography /ā·ôrtog′rəfē/ [Gk aerein + graphein to record], a radiographic process in which the aorta and its branches are injected with any of various contrast media for visualization. –aortographic, adj.

aortopulmonary fenestration [Gk aerein + L pulmoneus lung; fenestra window], a congenital anomaly characterized by an abnormal fenestration in the ascending aorta and the pulmonary artery cephalad to the semilunar valve, allowing oxygenated and unoxygenated blood to mix.

aosmic. See **anosmia.**

AOTA, abbreviation for American Occupational Therapy Association.

AOTF, abbreviation for American Occupational Therapy Foundation.

AP, abbreviation for **anteroposterior.**

APA, 1. abbreviation for **American Psychiatric Association.** 2. abbreviation for American Psychological Association.

apareunia /ā′pərōō′nē·ə/, an inability to perform sexual intercourse because of a physical or psychologic sexual dysfunction.

apathetic hyperthyroidism, a form of

thyrotoxicosis that tends to affect mainly older adults who have stereotyped "senile" physical features and are apathetic and inactive rather than hyperkinetic.

apathy /ap'əthē/ [Gk *a, pathos* not suffering], an absence or suppression of emotion, feeling, concern, or passion; an indifference to things found generally to be exciting or moving. **–apathetic,** *adj.*

apatite /ap'ətīt/ [Gk *apate* deceit], an inorganic mineral composed of calcium and phosphate that is found in the bones and teeth.

APC, 1. abbreviation for **aspirin, phenacetin, caffeine. 2.** abbreviation for *atrial premature contraction.* **3.** abbreviation for **adenomatous polyposis coli.**

APD, abbreviation for **adult polycystic disease.** See **polycystic kidney disease.**

apepsia /āpep'sē-ə/ [Gk *a* without, *pepsis* digestion], a condition of a failure of the digestive functions.

aperient /əpir'ē-ənt/ [L *aperire* to open], a mild laxative.

aperistalsis /āper'istal'sis/ [Gk *a* without, *peristellein* to clasp], a failure of the normal waves of contraction and relaxation which move contents through the digestive tract.

aperitive /əper'itiv/ [L *aperere* to open], a stimulant of the appetite.

Apert's syndrome /operz'/ [Eugene Apert, French pediatrician, b. 1868], a rare condition characterized by an abnormal craniofacial appearance in combination with partial or complete syndactyly of the hands and feet.

aperture /ap'ərchər/ [L *apertura* an opening], an opening or hole in an object or anatomic structure. See specific apertures.

aperture of frontal sinus, an external opening of the frontal sinus into the nasal cavity.

aperture of glottis, an opening between the true vocal cords and the arytenoid cartilages.

aperture of larynx, an opening between the pharynx and larynx.

aperture of sphenoid sinus, a round opening between the sphenoid sinus and nasal cavity, situated just above the superior nasal concha.

apex /ā'peks/, *pl.* **apices** /ā'pisēz/ [L, tip], the top, the end, or the tip of a structure, such as the apex of the heart or the apices of the teeth.

apex beat, a pulsation of the left ventricle of the heart, palpable and sometimes visible at the fifth intercostal space.

apexcardiogram, a graphic representation of the pulsations of the chest over the heart in the region of the cardiac apex.

apex cordis [L *apex + cordis* of the heart], the pointed lower border of the heart. It is directed downward, forward, to the left, and usually located at the level of the fifth intercostal space.

apexification /-if'ikāshən/ [L *apex + facere* to make], (in dentistry) the process of induced tooth root development, or apical closure of the root by the deposit of hard tissue.

apexigraph /āpek'sigraf'/, (in dentistry) a device used for determining the position of the apex of a tooth root.

apex murmur [L *apex + murmur* humming], a murmur heard best at the apex of the heart. Also called **apical murmur.**

apex pneumonia [L *apex;* Gk *pnemon* lung], pneumonia in which consolidation is limited to the upper lobe of one lung.

apex pulmonis /polmō'nis/ [L *apex + pulmoneus* lung], the rounded upper border of each lung, projecting above the clavicle into the root of the neck.

Apgar score /ap'gär/ [Virginia Apgar, American anesthesiologist, b. 1909], the evaluation of an infant's physical condition, usually performed 1 minute, and, again, 5 minutes after birth, based on a rating of five factors that reflect the infant's ability to adjust to extrauterine life. The infant's heart rate, respiratory effort, muscle tone, reflex irritability, and color are scored from a low value of 0 to a normal value of 2. The five scores are combined, and the totals at 1 minute and 5 minutes are noted; for example, Apgar 9/10 is a score of 9 at 1 minute and 10 at 5 minutes.

APHA, abbreviation for *American Public Health Association.*

aphagia /əfā'jē-ə/ [Gk *a, phagein* not to eat], a condition characterized by the loss of the ability to swallow as a result of organic or psychologic causes. A kind of aphagia is **aphagia algera.**

aphagia algera, a condition characterized by the refusal to eat or swallow because doing so causes pain.

aphakia /əfā'kē-ə/ [Gk *a, phakos* not lens], (in ophthalmology) a condition in which part or all of the crystalline lens of the eye is absent, usually because it has been surgically removed, as in the treatment of cataracts. **–aphakic, aphacic,** *adj.*

aphasia /əfā'zhə/ [Gk *a, phasis* not speech], an abnormal neurologic condition in which language function is defective or absent because of an injury to certain areas of the cerebral cortex. The deficiency may be sensory or receptive, in which language is not understood, or expressive or motor, in which words cannot be formed or expressed. **–aphasic,** *adj.*

aphemia /əfē′mē·ə/, a loss of the ability to speak applied to emotional disorders as well as neurologic causes.

apheresis /əfer′əsis, af′ərē′sis/,[Gk *aphairesis* removal], a procedure in which blood is temporarily withdrawn, one or more components are selectively removed, and the remainder of the blood is reinfused into the donor. The process is used in treating various disease conditions in the donor and for obtaining blood elements for treating other patients or for research purposes.

aphonia /āfō′nē·ə/ [Gk *a, phone* not voice], a condition characterized by loss of the ability to produce normal speech sounds because of overuse of the vocal cords, organic disease, or psychologic causes, such as hysteria. Kinds of aphonia include **aphonia paralytica, aphonia paranoica,** and **spastic aphonia. –aphonic, aphonous,** adj.

aphonia paralytica /par′əlit′ikə/, a condition characterized by a loss of the voice because of paralysis or disease of the laryngeal nerves.

aphonia paranoica, an inability to speak that lacks an organic basis and that is characteristic of some forms of mental illness.

aphonic speech /āfon′ik/, abnormal speech in which vocalizations are whispered.

aphoria /əfôr′ē·ə/, a condition in which physical weakness is not improved as a result of exercise.

aphrasia /əfā′zhə/, a form of aphasia in which a person may be able to speak or understand single words but is not able to communicate with words that are arranged in meaningful phrases or sentences.

aphronia /əfrō′nē·ə/ [Gk *a, phronein* not to understand], (in psychiatry) a condition characterized by an impaired ability to make common-sense decisions. **–aphronic,** n., adj.

aphthae /af′thē/, [Gk *aphtha* eruption], a condition of shallow, painful ulcerations that usually affect the oral mucosa. Aphthae occasionally may affect other body tissues, including the GI tract and the external genitalia. **–aphthous,** adj.

aphthous fever. See **foot-and-mouth disease.**

aphthous stomatitis /af′thəs/ [Gk *aptha* eruption; *stoma* mouth, *itis* inflammation], a recurring condition characterized by the eruption of painful ulcers (commonly called canker sores) on the mucous membranes of the mouth.

APIC, abbreviation for **Association for Practitioners of Infection Control.**

apical /ap′ikəl, ā′pi-/ [L *apex* tip], **1.** of or pertaining to the summit or apex. **2.** of or pertaining to the end of a tooth root.

apical curettage [L *apex;* Fr, scraping], (in dentistry) debridement of the apical surface of a tooth and removal of diseased soft tissues in the surrounding bony crypt.

apical fiber, any one of the many fibers of the periodontal ligament that radiate apically from tooth to bone.

apical lordotic view, a radiograph made by positioning the patient leaning backward at an angle of approximately 45 degrees.

apical odontoid ligament, a ligament connecting the axis to the occipital bone. It extends from the process of the axis to the anterior margin of the foramen magnum.

apical periodontitis [L *apex;* Gk *peri* near, *odous* tooth, *itis* inflammation], an inflammation around the apex of the root of a tooth.

apical pneumonia. See **apex pneumonia.**

apical pulse, the heartbeat as taken with the bell or disk of a stethoscope placed on the apex, or pointed extremity, of the heart.

apicectomy /ap′isek′təmē/ [L *apex* + Gk *ektome* excision], the surgical removal of the apex or the apical portion of a tooth root, usually in conjunction with apical curettage or root canal therapy.

apituitarism, [Gk *a* without + L *pituita* phlegm + Gk *ismos* a state], an absence or loss of function of the pituitary gland.

APKD, abbreviation for *adult polycystic kidney disease.*

aplasia /əplā′zhə/ [Gk *a, plassein* not to form] **1.** a developmental failure resulting in the absence of an organ or tissue. **2.** in hematology, a failure of the normal process of cell generation and development.

aplasia cutis congenita [Gk *a, plassein;* L *cutis* skin; *congenitus* born with], the congenital absence of a localized area of skin. The defect is usually covered by a thin, translucent membrane or scar tissue, or it may be raw and ulcerated.

aplastic [Gk *a, plassein* not to form], **1.** pertaining to the absence or defective development of a tissue or organ. **2.** failure of a tissue to produce normal daughter cells by mitosis.

aplastic anemia, a deficiency of all of the formed elements of the blood, representing a failure of the cell-generating capacity of the bone marrow. It may be caused by neoplastic disease of the bone marrow or by destruction of the bone marrow by exposure to toxic chemicals, ionizing radiation, or medications.

APMA, abbreviation for *American Podiatric Medical Society.*

apnea /apnē′ə, ap′nē-ə/ [Gk *a, pnein* not to breath], an absence of spontaneous respiration. Kinds of apnea include **cardiac apnea, deglutition apnea, periodic apnea of the newborn, primary apnea, reflex apnea, secondary apnea,** and **sleep apnea.** –**apneic,** *adj.*

apnea alarm mattress, a mattress for infants, designed to sound an alarm if the child stops breathing for a given period of time.

apnea monitoring, the act of closely observing the respiratory activity of individuals, particularly infants. The procedure may involve the use of electronic devices that detect changes in thoracic or abdominal movements and heart rate. Apneic detection devices may include an alarm that sounds if breathing stops.

apneic oxygenation [Gk *a, pnein* + *oxys* sharp + *genein* to produce], the maintenance of oxygen flow to the upper airway of patients with breathing difficulty.

apneustic breathing /apnōō′stik/,[Gk *a, pneusis* not breathing], a pattern of respirations characterized by a prolonged inspiratory phase followed by expiration apnea.

apneustic center, an area of nerve tissue in the lower portion of the pons that controls the inspiratory phase of respiration.

apocrine /ap′əkrin/ [Gk *apo* from + *krinein* to separate], **1.** pertaining to a gland that loses part of its substance while secreting. **2.** pertaining to sweat glands, which are generally located in areas covered with hair.

apocrine secretion [Gk *apo* + *krinein; L secernere* to separate], a mammary gland type of secretion in which the end of the secreting cell is broken off and its contents expelled. The secretion thus contains cellular granules in addition to fluid.

apocrine sweat gland [Gk *apo* from, *krinein* to separate], one of the large, deep exocrine glands located in the axillary, anal, genital, and mammary areas of the body. The apocrine glands become functional after puberty, and they secrete sweat.

apodial symmelia. See **sirenomelia.**

apoenzyme [Gk *apo* + *en* into, *zyme* ferment], an enzyme without any associated cofactors or with less than the entire amount of cofactors or prosthetic groups.

apogee /ap′əjē/ [Gk *apo* + *ge* earth], the climax of a disease or the period of greatest severity of signs and symptoms, usually followed by a crisis.

apolipoprotein [Gk *apo* + *lipos* fat, *pro-* tos first], the protein component of lipoprotein complexes.

aponeurosis /ap′ōnŏŏrō′sis/, *pl.* **aponeuroses** [Gk *apo* + *neuron* nerve, sinew], a strong sheet of fibrous connective tissue that serves as a tendon to attach muscles to bone or as fascia to bind muscles together.

aponeurosis of the obliquus externus abdominis, the strong membrane that covers the entire ventral surface of the abdomen and lies superficial to the rectus abdominis. Fibers from both sides of the aponeurosis interlace in the midline to form the linea alba.

aponeurotic fascia [Gk *apo* from + *neuron* tendon], a thickened layer of connective tissue that provides attachment to a muscle.

apophyseal fracture, a fracture that separates an apophysis of a bone from the main osseous tissue at a point of strong tendinous attachment.

apophysis /əpof′isis/ [Gk, a growing away], any small projection, process, or outgrowth, usually on a bone. –**apophyseal,** *adj.*

apophysitis /əpof′əsī′tis/, a condition characterized by the inflammation of an outgrowth or swelling, especially a bony outgrowth that is not separated from the bone.

apoprotein, a polypeptide chain not yet complexed to its specific prosthetic group.

apothecaries′ measure /əpoth′əker′ēz/ [Gk *apotheke* a store], a system of graduated liquid volumes originally based on the minim, formerly equal to one drop of water but now standardized to 0.06 ml; 60 minims equals 1 fluid dram, 8 fluid drams equals 1 fluid ounce, 16 fluid ounces equals 1 pint, 2 pints equals 1 quart, 4 quarts equals 1 gallon.

apothecaries′ weight, a system of graduated amounts arranged in order of heaviness and based on the grain, formerly equal to the weight of a plump grain of wheat but now standardized to 65 mg; 20 grains equals one scruple, 3 scruples equals 1 dram, 8 drams equals 1 ounce, 12 ounces equals 1 pound.

apothecary [Gk *apotheke* store], a pharmacist.

apparatus [L *ad* toward, *parare* to make ready], a device or a system composed of different parts that act together to perform some special function, as the attachment apparatus or tissues that support the teeth.

apparent death. See **death.**

appendage [L *appendere* to add something], an accessory structure attached to another part or organ.

appendectomy /ap'əndek'təmē/ [L *appendere* + Gk *ektome* excision], the surgical removal of the vermiform appendix through an incision in the right lower quadrant of the abdomen. The operation is performed in acute appendicitis to remove an inflamed appendix before it ruptures and prophylactically at the time of other abdominal surgery.

appendiceal /ap'endish'əl/, of or pertaining to the vermiform appendix. Also **appendicial, appendical** /əpen'dikəl/.

appendiceal abscess, [L *appendere* to hang upon, *abscedere* to go away], an abscess of the vermiform appendix.

appendicitis /əpen'disī'tis/ [L *appendere* + Gk *itis*], inflammation of the vermiform appendix, usually acute, which if undiagnosed leads rapidly to perforation and peritonitis. The most common symptom is constant pain in the right lower quadrant of the abdomen around McBurney's point, which the patient describes as having begun as intermittent pain in midabdomen. To decrease the pain, the patient keeps his knees bent to avoid tension of abdominal muscles. Appendicitis is characterized by vomiting, a low-grade fever of 99° F to 102° F, an elevated white blood count, rebound tenderness, a rigid abdomen, and decreased or absent bowel sounds. Appendicitis is most apt to occur in teenagers and young adults and is more frequent in males. A kind of appendicitis is **chronic appendicitis.**

appendicitis pain, severe general abdominal pain that develops rapidly and usually becomes localized in the lower right quadrant. It is accompanied by extreme tenderness over the right rectus muscle with rebound pain at McBurney's point. Occasionally, the pain is on the left side.

appendicular /ap'əndik'yələr/, 1. pertaining to the vermiform appendix. 2. pertaining to the limbs of the skeleton.

appendicular abscess, 1. an abscess on a limb. 2. an abscess of the vermiform appendix.

appendicular skeleton, the bones of the limbs and their girdles, attached to the axial skeleton.

appendix, pl. **appendixes, appendices,** 1. an accessory part of a main structure. 2. See **vermiform appendix.**

appendix dyspepsia [L *appendere* + Gk *dys* difficult, *peptein* to digest], an abnormal condition characterized by the impairment of the digestive function associated with chronic appendicitis.

appendix epididymidis /ep'ididim'idis/, a cystic structure sometimes found on the head of the epididymis. It represents a remnant of the mesonephros.

appendix epiploica, pl. **appendices epiploicae** [L *appendere* + Gk *epiploon* caul], one of the fat pads scattered through the peritoneum along the colon and the upper part of the rectum, especially along the transverse and the sigmoid parts of the colon.

appendix vermiformis. See **vermiform appendix.**

apperception [L *ad* toward, *percipere* to perceive] 1. mental perception or recognition. 2. (in psychology) a conscious process of understanding or perceiving in terms of a person's previous knowledge, experiences, emotions, and memories. –**apperceptive,** *adj.*

appetite [L *appetere* to long for], a natural or instinctive desire, such as for food.

appliance [L *applicare* to apply], a device or instrument designed for a specific purpose, such as a dental orthodontic device.

application, a computer procedure or problem to be processed, such as payroll, inventory, data about patients, scheduling of procedures and activities, pharmacy requisition and control, recording of nursing notes, or care planning.

applied anatomy, the study of the structure and morphology of the organs of the body as it relates to the diagnosis and treatment of disease. Kinds of applied anatomy are **pathologic anatomy, radiologic anatomy,** and **surgical anatomy.**

applied chemistry, the application of the study of chemical elements and compounds to industry and the arts.

applied psychology, 1. the interpretation of historical, literary, medical, or other data according to psychologic principles. 2. any branch of psychology that emphasizes practical rather than theoretic approaches and objectives, such as clinical psychology, child psychology, industrial psychology, and educational psychology.

applied science. See **science.**

AP portable chest radiograph, a radiographic examination of the chest performed in the room of an immobilized patient with a portable x-ray machine. The film holder is placed behind the patient with the x-ray tube in front.

apposition /ap'əsish'ən/ [L *apponere* to put to], the placing of objects in close proximity, as in the layering of tissue cells or juxtapositioning facing surfaces side-byside.

appositional growth, an increase in size by the addition of new tissue or similar material at the periphery of a particular part or structure, as in the addition of new layers in bone and tooth formation.

approach-approach conflict [L *ad, propiare* to draw near], a conflict resulting from the simultaneous presence of two or more incompatible impulses, desires, or goals, each of which is desirable.

approach-avoidance conflict, a conflict resulting from the presence of a single goal or desire that is both desirable and undesirable.

appropriate for gestational age (AGA) infant [L *ad* toward, *proprius* ownership], a newborn infant whose size, growth, and maturation are normal for gestational age, whether delivered prematurely, at term, or later than term.

approximate [L *ad, proximare* to come near], to bring two tissue surfaces close together, as in the repair of a wound or to bring the bones of a joint together, as in physical therapy.

approximator, a medical instrument used to draw together the edges of divided tissues, as in closing a wound or in repairing a fractured rib.

apraxia /əprak′sē·ə/ [Gk *a, pressein* not to act], an impairment in the ability to perform purposeful acts or to manipulate objects. The condition is primarily neurologic but occurs in several forms. **Ideational apraxia** is characterized by impairment caused by a loss of the perception of the use of an object. **Motor apraxia** is characterized by an inability to use an object or perform a task without any loss of perception of the use of the object or the goal of the task. **Amnestic apraxia** is characterized by an inability to perform the function because of an inability to remember the command to perform it. **Apraxia of speech** is an articulatory disorder caused by brain damage and resulting in an inability to program the position of speech muscles and the sequence of muscle movements necessary to produce understandable speech. –**apraxic,** *adj.*

aprobarbital /ap′rōbär′bital/, an intermediate-acting barbiturate prescribed as a sedative-hypnotic for sedation and induction of sleep on a short-term basis.

aprosody /āprəs′odē/ [Gk *a, prosodia* not modulated voice], a speech defect characterized by the absence of the normal variations in pitch, intonation, and rhythm of word formation.

aprosopia /ā′prəsō′pē·ə/ [Gk *aprosopos* faceless], a congenital anomaly characterized by the absence of part or all of the facial structures. The condition is usually associated with other malformations.

APTA, abbreviation for *American Physical Therapy Association.*

aptitude [L *aptitudo* ability], a natural ability, tendency, talent, or capability to learn, understand, or acquire a particular skill; mental alertness.

aptitude test, any of a variety of standardized tests for measuring an individual's ability to learn certain skills.

apyrexia [Gk *a* without, *pyrexis* fever], an absence or remission of fever. –**apyretic,** *adj.*

AQ, abbreviation for **achievement quotient.**

aqua (aq), the Latin word for water.

aqua amnii. See **amniotic fluid.**

aquaphobia [L *aqua* + Gk *phobos* fear], fear of water.

aquapuncture [L *aqua* + *punctura* puncture], the injection of water under the skin or spraying of a fine jet of water on the surface of the skin to relieve a mild irritation.

aquathermia pad /-thur′mē·ə/, a waterproof plastic or rubber pad that can be applied to areas of muscle sprain, edema, or mild inflammation. The pad contains channels through which heated or cooled water flows. It is connected by hoses to a bedside control unit that contains a temperature regulator, a motor for circulating the water, and a reservoir of distilled water.

aqueduct [L *aqua* water, *ductus* act of leading], any canal, channel, or passage through or between body parts, as the aqueduct of Sylvius in the brain.

aqueduct of Sylvius. See **cerebral aqueduct.**

aqueductus /ak′wəduk′təs/, the Latin word for canal.

aqueous /ā′kwē·əs, ak′wē·əs/ [L *aqua*], **1.** watery or waterlike. **2.** a medication prepared with water.

aqueous chambers [L *aqua* + Gk *kamara* something with an arched cover], the anterior and posterior chambers of the eye, containing the aqueous humor.

aqueous humor, the clear, watery fluid circulating in the anterior and posterior chambers of the eye.

aqueous solution [L *aqua* + *solutus* dissolved], a homogenous liquid preparation of any substance dissolved in water.

Ar, symbol for the element **argon.**

AR, abbreviation for *assisted respiration.*

arabinosylcytosine. See **cytarabine.**

arachidonic acid /ar′əkidon′ik/ [L *arachos* a legume], an essential fatty acid that is a component of lecithin and a basic material for the biosynthesis of some prostaglandins.

arachnid [Gk *arachne* spider], pertaining to the animal class of Arachnida, which includes spiders, scorpions, mites, and ticks.

arachnodactyly /ərak′nōdak′tilē/ [Gk *arachne* spider, *dactylos* finger], a congenital condition of having long, thin, spiderlike fingers and toes, which is seen in Marfan's syndrome.

arachnoid /ərak′noid/ [Gk *arachne* + *eidos* form], a delicate, fibrous structure resembling a cobweb or spiderweb, such as the arachnoid membrane. **–arachnoidal,** *adj.*

arachnoidea encephali /ar′aknoi′dē·ə ensef′əlē/ [Gk, spiderweb; *enkephalos* brain], the arachnoid membrane surrounding the brain.

arachnoidea spinalis [Gk, spiderweb; L *spina* spine], a continuation of the arachnoid membrane of the brain, extending along the spinal cord as far as the cauda equina with sheaths that cover the various spinal nerves as they pass outward to the intervertebral foramina.

arachnoidism /ərak′noidiz′əm/ [Gk *arachne* + *eidos* form], the condition produced by the bite of a venomous spider.

arachnoid membrane, a thin, delicate membrane enclosing the brain and the spinal cord, interposed between the pia mater and the dura mater.

arachnoid of the brain. See **arachnoidea encephali.**

arachnoid of the spinal cord. See **arachnoidea spinalis.**

arachnoid sheath [Gk *arachne* + *eidos* AS *scaeth*], pertaining to the arachnoid membrane that lies under the dura mater and over the pia mater, enveloping the brain and spinal cord.

arachnoid villi [Gk *arachne* + *villus* shaggy hair], projections of fibrous tissue from the arachnoid membrane.

Aran-Duchenne muscular atrophy /aran′dŌŌshen′/ [Francois A. Aran, French physician, b. 1817; Guillaume B. A. Duchenne, French neurologist, b. 1806], a form of amyotrophic lateral sclerosis affecting the hands, arms, shoulders, and legs at the onset before becoming more generalized.

arbitrary inference, a form of cognitive distortion in which a judgment based on insufficient evidence leads to an erroneous conclusion.

arbitrator [L *arbiter* umpire], an impartial person appointed to resolve a dispute between parties. **–arbitration,** *n.*

arborization test. See **ferning test.**

arbovirus /är′bōvī′rəs/, any one of more than 300 arthropod-borne viruses that cause infections characterized by a combination of two or more of the following: fever, rash, encephalitis, and bleeding into the viscera or skin. Dengue, yellow fever,

and equine encephalitis are arboviral infections.

ARC. See **AIDS-wasting syndrome.**

arch, any anatomic structure that is curved or has a bowlike appearance.

arch bar, any one of various types of wires, bars, or splints that conform to the arch of the teeth, used in the treatment of fractures of the jaws and in the stabilization of injured teeth.

archenteric canal. See **neurenteric canal.**

archenteron /ärken′təron/, *pl.* **archentera** [Gk *arche* beginning, *enteron* intestine], the primitive digestive cavity formed by the invagination into the gastrula in the embryonic development of many animals. **–archenteric,** *adj.*

arches of the foot [L *arcus* bow + AS *fot*], the bony arches of the instep, including the longitudinal, or anteroposterior, and the transverse arches.

archetype /är′kətīp′/ [Gk *arche* + *typos* type], **1.** an original model or pattern from which a thing or group of things is made or evolves. **2.** (in analytic psychology) an inherited primordial idea or mode of thought derived from the experiences of the human race and present in the unconscious of the individual in the form of drives, moods, and concepts. **–archetypal, archetypic, archetypical,** *adj.*

archiblastoma /är′kiblastō′mə/, *pl.* **archiblastomas, archiblastomata** [Gk *arche* + *blastos* germ, *oma*], a tumor composed of cells derived from the layer of tissue surrounding the germinal vesicle.

archigaster. See **archenteron.**

archinephric canal, archinephric duct. See **pronephric duct.**

archinephron. See **pronephros.**

archistome. See **blastopore.**

architectural barriers, architectural features of homes and public buildings that limit access and mobility of disabled persons.

architis [Gk *archos* anus, *itis* inflammation], an inflammation of the anus.

arch length, the length of a dental arch, usually measured through the points of contact between adjoining teeth.

arch length deficiency, the difference in any dental arch between the required length to accommodate all the natural teeth and the actual space available.

arch of the aorta, one of the four portions of the aorta, giving rise to three arterial branches called the innominate (brachiocephalic), left common carotid, and left subclavian arteries.

arch width, the width of a dental arch, which varies in all diameters between the left and right opposite teeth and is deter-

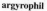

mined by direct measurement between the canines, the first molars, and the second premolars.

arch wire, an orthodontic wire fastened to two or more teeth through fixed attachments used to cause or guide tooth movement.

arcing spring contraceptive diaphragm /är′king/, a kind of contraceptive diaphragm in which the flexible metal spring that forms the rim is a combination of a flexible coil spring and a flat band spring made of stainless steel.

arcuate [L *arcuare* to bow], an arch or bow-shape.

arcuate scotoma /är′ky o͞o·at/ [L *arcuatus* bowed; Gk *skotoma* darkness], an arc-shaped blind area that may develop in the field of vision of a person with glaucoma. It is caused by damage to nerve fibers in the retina.

arcus. See **arch.**

arcus senilis [L, bow, aged], an opaque ring, gray to white in color, that surrounds the periphery of the cornea. The condition is caused by deposits of fat granules in the cornea or hyaline degeneration and occurs primarily in older persons.

ARDS, abbreviation for **acute respiratory distress syndrome.**

area [L, space], (in anatomy) a limited anatomic space that contains a specific structure of the body or within which certain physiologic functions predominate, such as the aortic area and the association areas of the cerebral cortex.

area under the concentration curve (AUC), a method of measurement of the bioavailability of a drug based on a plot of blood concentrations sampled at frequent intervals. It is directly proportional to the total amount of unaltered drug in the patient's blood.

areflexia /ā′rēflek′sē·ə/, the absence of the reflexes.

Arenavirus /er′inəvī′rəs/, a genus of viruses usually transmitted to humans by oral or cutaneous contact with the excreta of wild rodents. Individual arenaviruses are identified with specific geographic areas, such as **Bolivian hemorrhagic fever** and **Argentine hemorrhagic fever.**

areola /erē′ōlə/, *pl.* **areolae, 1.** a small space or a cavity within a tissue. **2.** a circular area of a different color surrounding a central feature, such as the discoloration about a pustule or vesicle. **3.** the part of the iris around the pupil. **–areolar,** *adj.*

areola mammae /mam′ē/, the pigmented, circular area surrounding the nipple of each breast.

areolar gland /erē′ələr/, one of the large sebaceous glands in the areolae encircling the nipples on the breasts of women. The areolar glands secrete a lipoid fluid that lubricates and protects the nipple.

areolar tissue, a kind of connective tissue having little tensile strength and consisting of loosely woven fibers and areolae.

ARF, abbreviation for **acute respiratory failure.**

Arg, abbreviation for **arginine.**

argentaffin cell /är′jentaf′in/ [L *argentum* silver, *affinitas* affinity], a cell containing serotonin-secreting granules that stain readily with silver and chromium parts. Such cells occur in most regions of the GI tract and are especially abundant in the crypts of Lieberkühn.

argentaffinoma /är′jentaf′inō′mə/, *pl.* **argentaffinomas, argentaffinomata,** a carcinoid tumor arising most often from argentaffin cells in epithelium of the crypts of Lieberkühn in the GI tract.

argentaffinoma syndrome. See **carcinoid syndrome.**

Argentine hemorrhagic fever, an infectious disease caused by an arenavirus transmitted to humans by the ingestion of food contaminated by the excreta of infected rodents and by personal contact.

arginase /är′ginās/, an enzyme that catalyzes the hydrolysis of arginine during the urea cycle, producing urea and ornithine.

arginine (Arg) /är′ginin/, an amino acid produced by the digestion or hydrolysis of proteins formed during the urea cycle by the transfer of a nitrogen atom from aspartate to citrulline.

argininemia /är′jininē′mē·ə/, an autosomal recessive disorder characterized by an increased amount of arginine in the blood caused by a deficiency of arginase. Without arginase, ammonia cannot be metabolized into urea.

argininosuccinic acidemia, an inherited amino acid metabolism disorder in which the lack of an enzyme, argininosuccinase, results in an excess of argininosuccinic acid in the blood. The condition is characterized by seizures and mental retardation.

argon (Ar) /är′gon/ [Gk *argos* inactive], a colorless, odorless, chemically inactive gas and one of the six rare gases in the atmosphere. Its atomic weight is 39.95; its atomic number is 18. It forms no compounds.

Argyll Robertson pupil [Douglas M. C. L. Argyll Robertson, Scottish physician, b. 1837], a pupil that constricts on accommodation but not in response to light. It is most often seen with miosis and in advanced neurosyphilis.

argyrophil /ärji′rəfil/ [Gk *argyros* silver, *philein* to love], a cell or other object that is easily stained or impregnated with silver.

arhythmia. See **arrhythmia.**

ariboflavinosis /ārī′bōflā′vinō′sis/ [Gk *a* not, ribose; L *flavus* yellow; Gk *osis*], a condition caused by deficiency of vitamin B₂ in the diet and characterized by lesions at the corners of the mouth, on the lips, and around the nose and eyes by seborrheic dermatitis and by various visual disorders.

Arica therapy, a mental health treatment that focuses on altered states of consciousness with a goal of increasing the powers of the mind.

arithmetic mean. See **mean.**

Arkansas stone, a fine-grained stone of novaculite used for making hones with which surgical instruments may be sharpened.

arm [L *armus*], **1.** a portion of the upper limb of the body between the shoulder and the elbow. **2.** *nontechnical.* the arm and the forearm.

armamentarium [L *armamentum* implement], the total therapeutic assets of a physician or medical facility, including medicines and equipment.

arm board, 1. a board used to position the affected arm of a hemiplegic. It fastens to the arm rest of a wheelchair, supporting the arm in correct position for subluxation of the shoulder and flaccid arm, and to prevent edema. **2.** a board used to keep the arm still to permit the drawing of blood or for starting an intravenous needle.

arm bone. See **humerus.**

arm cylinder cast Arica, an orthopedic device of plaster of paris or fiberglass, used for immobilizing the upper limb from the wrist to the upper arm. It is most often applied to immobilize or position the elbow.

armpit. See **axilla.**

Army Nurse Corps (ANC), a branch of the U.S. Army, founded Feb. 2, 1901, with headquarters in Falls Church, Virginia.

Arnold-Chiari malformation /är′nəld-kē·är′ē/ [Julius Arnold, German pathologist, b. 1835; Hans Chiari, French pathologist, b. 1851], a congenital herniation of the brain stem and lower cerebellum through the foramen magnum into the cervical vertebral canal.

AROM, abbreviation for **active range of motion.**

aroma [Gk, spice], any agreeable odor or pleasing fragrance, especially of food, drink, spices, or medication.

aromatic [Gk *aroma* spice], **1.** pertaining to a strong but agreeable odor such as a

spicy odor. **2.** a stimulant or spicy medicine.

aromatic alcohol, a fatty alcohol in which part of the hydrogen of the alcohol radical is replaced by a phenyl hydrocarbon.

aromatic ammonia spirit [Gk *aroma* + *Ammon* temple ancient source of ammonium chloride salt, *spiritus* breath], a strongly fragrant solution of ammonium carbonate in dilute liquid ammonia, oils, alcohol, and water. It is used as a reflex stimulant, antacid, and carminitive.

aromatic bath, a medicated bath in which aromatic substances or essential oils are added to the water.

aromatic compounds, organic compounds that contain a benzene, naphthalene, or analogous ring. Many of these compounds have agreeable odors, which accounts for the origin of this term for such compounds.

aromatic hydrocarbon [Gk *aroma* + *hydor* water; L *carbo* coal], an organic compound that has a benzene or quinoid ring, as distinguished from open-chain aliphatic compounds.

arousal [OE, to rise], to awaken from sleep, or to excite, or evoke action or response to sensory stimuli.

arrest [L *ad, resistare* to withstand], to inhibit, restrain, or stop, as to arrest the course of a disease.

arrested dental caries, dental caries in which the area of decay has stopped progressing and infection is not present but in which the demineralized area in the tooth remains as a cavity.

arrested development, the cessation of one or more phases of the developmental process in utero before normal completion, resulting in congenital anomalies.

arrested labor [L *ad, restare* to withstand + *labor* work], an interruption in the labor process that may be caused by an obstruction in the pelvis or lack of uterine contractions.

arrhenoblastoma /erē′nōblastō′mə/ [Gk *arrhen* male, *blastos* germ, *oma* tumor], an ovarian neoplasm whose cells mimic those in testicular tubules and secrete male sex hormone, causing virilization in females.

arrhenogenic /erē′nōjen′ik/, producing only male offspring.

arrhenokaryon /erē′nōker′ē·on/ [Gk *arrhen* male, *karyon* nucleus], an organism that is produced from an egg that has only paternal chromosomes.

arrhenoma. See **arrhenoblastoma.**

arrhythmia /ərith′mē·ə, ərith′mē·ə/ [Gk *a, rhythmos* not rhythm], any deviation from the normal pattern of the heartbeat.

Kinds of arrhythmias include **atrial fibrillation, atrial flutter, heart block, premature atrial contraction,** and **sinus arrhythmia.** Also spelled **arhythmia.** **–arrhythmic, arrhythmical,** *adj.*

ARRT, abbreviation for **American Registry of Radiologic Technologists.**

arsenic (As) /är'sənik/ [Gk *arsen* strong], an element that occurs throughout the earth's crust in metal arsenides, arsenious sulfides, and arsenious oxides. Its atomic number is 33; its atomic weight is 74.91. This element has been used for centuries as a therapeutic agent and as a poison and continues to have limited use in some trypanocidal drugs. The environmental distribution of arsenic ensures its concentration in the food chain. **–arsenic** /ärsen'ik/, *adj.*

arsenic poisoning, poisoning caused by the ingestion or inhalation of arsenic or a substance containing arsenic, an ingredient in some pesticides, herbicides, dyes, and medicinal solutions. Small amounts absorbed over a period of time may result in chronic poisoning, producing nausea, headache, coloration and scaling of the skin, hyperkeratoses, anorexia, and white lines across the fingernails. Ingestion of large amounts of arsenic results in severe GI pain, diarrhea, vomiting, and swelling of the extremities.

arsenic stomatitis [Gk *arsen* strong; *stoma* mouth, *itis* inflammation], an abnormal oral condition associated with arsenic poisoning, characterized by dry, red, and painful oral mucosa, ulceration, purpura, and mobility of teeth.

ART, abbreviation for **active resistance training.**

artefact, See **artifact.**

arteria alveolaris inferior. See **inferior alveolar artery.**

arterial [Gk *arteria* airpipe], of or pertaining to an artery.

arterial bleeding [Gk *arteria;* ME *blod*], pertaining to loss of blood from an artery, an event usually characterized by blood that is bright red and spurting.

arterial blood gas (ABG), the oxygen and carbon dioxide in arterial blood, measured by various methods to assess the adequacy of ventilation and oxygenation, and the acid base status.

arterial blood pressure (ABP), the pressure of the blood in the arterial system, which depends on the pumping pressure of the heart, the resistance of the arterial walls, the amount of blood, and its viscosity.

arterial capillaries, microscopic blood vessels (capillaries) extending beyond the terminal ends of arterioles.

arterial catheter [Gk *arteria* + *katheter* a thing lowered into], a catheter that can be inserted into an artery either to draw blood or to measure blood pressure directly.

arterial circle of Willis. See **circle of Willis.**

arterial circulation [Gk *arteria* + L *circulare* to go around], the movement of blood through the arteries directed away from the heart, as opposed to venous circulation.

arterial insufficiency, inadequate blood flow in arteries caused by occlusive atherosclerotic plaques or emboli, by damaged, diseased, or intrinsically weak vessels, by arteriovenous fistulas, by aneurysms, by hypercoagulability states, or by heavy use of tobacco. Signs of arterial inadequacy include pale, cyanotic, or mottled skin over the affected area, absent or decreased sensations, tingling, diminished sense of temperature, muscle pains, reduced or absent peripheral pulses, and, in advanced disease, atrophy of muscles of the involved extremity.

arterial insufficiency of lower extremities, a condition characterized by hardening, thickening, and loss of elasticity of the walls of peripheral arteries causing decreased circulation, sensation, and function. Symptoms include sharp, cramping pain during exercise or rest at night, numbness, skin changes ranging from pallor to ulceration, and loss of hair on the legs. Pedal and popliteal pulses may be diminished or absent.

arterial line, an arterial blood monitoring system consisting of a catheter inserted into an artery and connected to pressure tubing and a transducer. The device permits continuous direct blood pressure readings as well as access to the blood supply when samples are needed for analysis.

arterial nephrosclerosis [Gk *arteria* + *nephros* kidney, *sklera* hard, *osis* condition], arteriosclerosis of the kidney arteries, leading to deprivation of oxygenated blood to the kidney tissues and their destruction.

arterial palpitation [Gk *arteria* + L *palpitare* to flutter], a palpitation felt in an artery.

arterial pH, the hydrogen ion concentration of arterial blood. Normal range is 7.35 to 7.45. The figure represents a ratio of 20:1 between bicarbonate ions and carbon dioxide dissolved in the blood.

arterial pressure, the stress exerted by the circulating blood on the walls of the arteries. It is the product of the cardiac output and the systemic vascular resistance.

arterial rete [Gk *arteria* + L *rete*, net], a network of arteries and arterioles.

arterial sclerosis [Gk *arteria* + *sklerosis* hardening], a thickening of the arteries.

arterial tension, the pressure on artery walls caused by the force of blood being squeezed into the systemic circulation by contraction of the heart's left ventricle.

arterial wall, the fibrous muscular enclosure of the many vessels that carry oxygenated blood from the heart to structures throughout the body, and of the pulmonary arteries that carry venous blood from the heart to the lungs. The arteries, like the veins, are cylindric tubes enclosed by layers of different kinds of tissue. The inner layer is composed of a membrane of endothelium, a subendothelial layer of delicate connective tissue, and an internal elastic membrane. The endothelium of the inner layer is composed of a single layer of simple squamous cells and is continuous with the endothelium of the capillaries and the endocardium of the heart. The middle layer of tissue around each artery comprises most of the arterial wall and is composed of circular sheets of smooth muscle cells and elastic tissue. The outer layer consists of areolar connective tissue with a fine network of collagenous and elastic fibers.

arteriectomy /ärtir′ē·ek′təmē/ [Gk *arteria* + *ektome* cutting out], the surgical removal of a portion of an artery.

arteriogram /ärtir′ē·əgram′/, an x-ray film of an artery injected with a radiopaque medium.

arteriography /ärtir′ē·og′rəfē/ [Gk *arteria* airpipe, *graphein* to record], a method of radiologic visualization of arteries performed after a radiopaque contrast medium is introduced into the bloodstream or into a specific vessel by injection or through a catheter. –**arteriographic,** *adj.*

arteriole /ärtir′ē·ōl/ [L *arteriola* little artery], the smallest vascular branch of the arterial circulation. Blood flowing from the heart is pumped through the arteries to the arterioles to the capillaries into the veins and returned to the heart. The muscular wall of the arterioles constricts and dilates in response to neurochemical stimuli; thus, arterioles play a significant role in peripheral vascular resistance and in regulation of blood pressure.

arteriopathy /ärtir′ē·op′əthē/, [Gk *arteria* + *pathos* suffering], a disease of an artery.

arterioplasty [Gk *arteria* + *plassein* to mold], plastic surgery of an artery. The procedure is often performed to correct an aneurysm.

arteriosclerosis [Gk *arteria* + *sklerosis* hardening], a common arterial disorder characterized by thickening, loss of elasticity, and calcification of arterial walls, resulting in a decreased blood supply, especially to the cerebrum and lower extremities. The condition often develops with aging and in hypertension, nephrosclerosis, scleroderma, diabetes, and hyperlipidemia. Kinds of arteriosclerosis are **atherosclerosis** and **Mönckeberg's arteriosclerosis.** –**arteriosclerotic,** *adj.*

arteriosclerosis obliterans [Gk *arteria, skleros* + L *obliterare* efface], a gradual narrowing of the arteries with degeneration of the intima and thrombosis. The condition may lead to complete occlusion of the artery and subsequent gangrene.

arteriosclerotic heart disease (ASHD), a thickening and hardening of the walls of the coronary arteries.

arteriosclerotic retinopathy [Gk *arteria* + *sklerosis* hardening; L *rete* net; Gk *pathos* disease], a disorder of the retina associated with hardening and thickening of the arteries supplying that part of the eye. The condition often accompanies hypertension.

arteriospasm [Gk *arteria* + *spasmos* spasm], a spasm of an artery.

arteriovenous /ärtir′ē·ōvē′nəs/ [Gk *arteria* + L *vena* vein], of or pertaining to arteries and veins.

arteriovenous anastomosis [Gk *arteria* + L *vena;* Gk *anastomoein* to form a mouth], a communication between an artery and a vein, either as a congenital anomaly or a surgically produced link between vessels.

arteriovenous aneurysm, an aneurysm affecting both an artery and a vein, often as an abnormal linkage between a vein and artery.

arteriovenous angioma of the brain, a congenital tumor consisting of a tangle of coiled, usually dilated arteries and veins, islets of sclerosed brain tissue, and, occasionally, cartilaginous cells.

arteriovenous fistula, an abnormal communication between an artery and vein occurring congenitally or resulting from trauma, infection, arterial aneurysm, or a malignancy.

arteriovenous oxygen (a-vo$_2$) difference, the arterial oxygen content minus the central venous oxygen content.

arteriovenous shunt, a passageway, artificial or natural, that allows blood to flow from an artery to a vein without going through a capillary network.

arteritis /är′tərī′tis/ [Gk *arteria* + *itis*], an inflammatory condition of the inner layers or the outer coat of one or more arteries, occurring as a clinical entity or accompanying another disorder, such as rheumatoid arthritis, rheumatic fever, polymyositis, or systemic lupus erythematosus. Kinds of arteritis include **infantile arteritis, rheumatic arteritis, Takayasu's arteritis,** and **temporal arteritis.**

arteritis obliterans. See **Friedländer's disease.**

arteritis umbilicalis, a septic inflammation of the umbilical artery in newborn infants, usually by the bacteria of the species *Clostridium tetani.*

artery [Gk *arteria* airpipe], one of the large blood vessels carrying blood in a direction away from the heart. The wall of an artery has three layers: the **tunica adventitia,** the outer coat; the **tunica media,** the middle coat; and the **tunica intima,** the inner coat.

artery forceps, any forceps used for grasping, compressing, and holding the end of an artery during ligation. Generally self-locking, its handles are scissorlike.

arthralgia /ärthral'jə/ [Gk *arthron* joint, *algos* pain], joint pain. **–arthralgic,** *adj.*

arthritis /ärthrī'tis/ [Gk *arthron* joint, *itis*], any inflammatory condition of the joints characterized by pain and swelling.

arthritis deformans. See **rheumatoid arthritis.**

arthrocentesis /är'thrōsintē'sis/ [Gk *arthron* + *kentesis* pricking], the puncture of a joint with a needle and the withdrawal of fluid performed to obtain samples of synovial fluid for diagnostic purposes.

arthrodesis. See **ankylosis.**

arthrodia. See **gliding joint.**

arthrogram /är'thrəgram/, a radiogram of a joint after injection of a contrast medium.

arthrography [Gk *arthron* + *graphein* to record], a method of radiographically visualizing the inside of a joint by injecting air or a contrast medium.

arthrogryposis multiplex congenita [Gk *arthron, gryposis* joint curve; L *multus* many, *plica* fold; *congenitus* born with], fibrous stiffness of one or more joints, present at birth, often associated with incomplete development of the muscles that move the involved joints and degenerative changes of the motor neurons that innervate those muscles.

arthrokinematic /är'thrəkin'əmat'ik/, pertaining to the movement of joint surfaces.

arthron /är'thron/ [Gk, a joint, including its various components of bones, cartilaginous inserts, all soft tissue structures intervening between the rigid skeletal parts, and the adjacent muscular elements.

arthropathy /ärthrop'əthē/ [Gk *arthron* + *pathos* suffering], any disease or abnormal condition affecting a joint. **–arthropathic,** *adj.*

arthroplasty /är'thrəplast'ē/ [Gk *arthron* + *plassein* to shape], the surgical reconstruction or replacement of a painful, degenerated joint to restore mobility to a joint in osteoarthritis or rheumatoid arthritis or to correct a congenital deformity. Either the bones of the joint are reshaped and soft tissue or a metal disk is placed between the reshaped ends, or all or part of the joint is replaced with a metal or plastic prosthesis.

arthropod /är'thrəpod'/ [Gk *arthron* + *pous* foot], a member of the Arthropoda, a large phylum of animal life that includes crabs and lobsters as well as mites, ticks, spiders, and insects. They bite, sting, cause allergic reactions, and carry viruses and other disease agents.

arthroscope /-skōp'/, [Gk *arthron* + *skopein* to watch], a type of endoscope used to examine joints.

arthroscopy /ärthros'kəpē/ [Gk *arthron* + *skopein* to watch], the examination of the interior of a joint, performed by inserting a specially designed endoscope through a small incision. The procedure, used chiefly in knee problems, permits biopsy of cartilage or synovium, the diagnosis of a torn meniscus, and, in some instances, the removal of loose bodies in the joint space. **–arthroscopic,** *adj.*

arthrous /är'thrəs/ [Gk *arthron*], **1.** pertaining to joints or articulation of bones. **2.** pertaining to a disease of a joint.

Arthus reaction /ärtoos'/ [Nicholas M. Arthus, French physiologist, b. 1862], a rare, severe, immediate hypersensitivity reaction to injection of a foreign substance, which is usually not irritating but in certain individuals is antigenic.

articular /ärtik'yələr/ [L *articulare* to divide into joints], relating to a joint or the involvement of joints.

articular capsule [L *articulare*], an envelope of tissue that surrounds a freely moving joint composed of an external layer of white fibrous tissue and an internal synovial membrane.

articular cartilage [L *articulare* + *cartilago*], a type of hyaline connective tissue that covers the articulating surfaces of bases within synovial joints.

articular disk, the platelike end of certain bones in movable joints developed from unabsorbed mesoderm and sometimes closely associated with surrounding muscles or with cartilage.

articular fracture, a fracture involving the articular surfaces of a joint.

articulatio cubiti. See **elbow joint.**

articulatio ellipsoidea. See **condyloid joint.**

articulatio genus. See **knee joint.**

articulation. See **joint.**

articulation of the pelvis, any one of the connections between the bones of the pelvis, involving four groups of ligaments. The first group connects the sacrum and the ilium; the second, the sacrum and the ischium; the third, the sacrum and the coccyx; and the fourth, the two pubic bones.

articulatio plana. See **gliding joint.**

articulatio sellaris. See **saddle joint.**

articulator [L *articulare* to divide into joints], (in dentistry) a mechanical device used in the fabrication and testing of dentures. It represents the temporomandibular joints and jaw members to which maxillary and mandibular casts may be attached.

artifact [L *ars* skill, *facere* to make], anything extraneous, irrelevant, or unwanted, such as a substance, structure, or piece of data or information. In radiologic imaging, an artifact may confuse the radiologist and the results of any examination.

artifactual modification, a change in protein structure caused by in vitro manipulation.

artificial airway [L *artificiosum* skillfully made], a plastic or rubber device that can be inserted into the upper or lower respiratory tract to facilitate ventilation or the removal of secretions.

artificial alimentation, See **parenteral nutrition.**

artificial assists, any prosthetic device or contrivance that may enable a physically challenged person to function. Examples include heart pacemakers, crutches, and artificial limbs.

artificial blood. See **perfluorocarbons.**

artificial classification of cavities, any cavity that may be classified in one of six groups, the first five of which are those proposed by G.V. Black, Class 1: cavities associated with structural tooth defects in the occlusal surfaces of posterior teeth, such as pits and fissures; Class 2: cavities in the proximal surfaces of premolars and molars; Class 3: cavities in the proximal surfaces of the canines and incisors that do not involve removal and restoration of the incisal angle; Class 4: cavities in the proximal surfaces of premolars and molars that require the removal and restoration of the incisal angle; Class 5: cavities, except pit cavities, in the gingival third of the labial, buccal, or lingual surfaces of the teeth; Class 6: cavities on the incisal edges and cusp tips of the teeth.

artificial crown, a dental prosthesis that restores part or all of the coronal portion of a natural tooth.

artificial fever, an elevated body temperature produced by artificial means, such as the injection of malarial parasites or of a vaccine known to produce fever symptoms, or by applying heat to the body. An artificial fever may be prescribed for a patient to arrest a disease that is sensitive to elevated body temperatures.

artificial heart, a mechanical device of molded polyurethane, consisting of two ventricles implanted in the body and powered by an air compressor located outside the body. The first artificial heart for humans was implanted in December 1982.

artificial insemination, the introduction of semen into the vagina or uterus by mechanical or instrumental means rather than by sexual intercourse. The procedure is planned to coincide with the expected time of ovulation so that fertilization can occur. Kinds of artificial insemination are **artificial insemination-donor** and **artificial insemination-husband.**

artificial insemination-donor (AID), artificial insemination in which the semen specimen is provided by an anonymous donor. The procedure is used primarily in cases where the husband is sterile.

artificial insemination-husband (AIH), artificial insemination in which the semen specimen is provided by the husband. The procedure is used primarily in cases of impotency, low sperm count, a vaginal disorder, or when the husband is incapable of sexual intercourse because of some physical disability.

artificial intelligence (AI), a system that makes it possible for a machine to perform functions similiar to human intelligence, such as learning, reasoning, self-correcting, and adapting. Computer technology produces many instruments and systems that mimic and surpass some human capabilities, as speed of counting, correlating, sensing, and deducing.

artificial kidney, a device used to rid blood, circulated outside of the body, of substances commonly excreted in urine. It usually consists of a set of tubes or catheters that pass the blood through a dialysate solution where wastes are removed by osmosis and diffusion.

artificial labor [L *artificiosus* + *labor* work], induced labor, such as started with drugs or mechanical devices.

artificial limb. See **prosthesis.**

artificial lung. See **Drinker respirator.**

artificially acquired immunity. See **acquired immunity.**

artificial menopause [L *artificiosus* + *mensis* month; Gk *pauein* to cease], the termination of menstrual periods by surgery, radiation, or other methods.

artificial pacemaker. See **pacemaker.**

artificial respiration. See **artificial ventilation.**

artificial saliva, a mixture of carboxymethylcellulose, sorbitol, sodium and potassium chloride in an aqueous solution. It is available in a spray container for the treatment of xerostomia, or dry mouth.

artificial selection, the process by which the genotypes of successive plant and animal generations are determined through controlled breeding.

artificial stone, a calcined gypsum derivative similar to but stronger than plaster of paris, used for making dental casts and dies.

artificial ventilation, the process of supporting respiration by manual or mechanical means when normal breathing is inefficient or has stopped. Effective ventilation of the lungs may fail because of bronchial obstruction by swelling, a foreign body, increased secretions, neuromuscular weakness, status asthmaticus, exhaustion, pharmacologic depression, or trauma to the chest wall. Before an attempt to administer artificial ventilation, the airway is tested and any obstruction removed.

art therapy, a type of mental health treatment in which the patient is encouraged to express his or her feelings through various forms of artwork.

aryepiglottic folds /er´ē·ep·iglot´ik/, folds of mucous membrane that extend around the margins of the larynx from a junction with the epiglottis. They function as a sphincter during swallowing.

aryl hydrocarbon hydroxylase (AHH), an enzyme that converts carcinogenic chemicals in tobacco smoke and in polluted air into active carcinogens within the lungs.

As, symbol for the element **arsenic.**

AS, 1. abbreviation for **auris sinistra** (left ear). 2. abbreviation for **aortic stenosis.**

ASA, 1. abbreviation for *American Society of Anesthesiologists.* 2. abbreviation for **aspirin** (acetylsalicylic acid).

ASAHP, abbreviation for *American Society of Allied Health Professionals.*

ASAP, abbreviation for *as soon as possible.*

asbestos [Gk *asbestos* unquenchable], a group of fibrous impure magnesium silicate minerals. Inhalation of the fibers can lead to pulmonary fibrosis if the fibers accumulate in terminal bronchioles. Continued exposure to asbestos fibers can result in lung cancer.

asbestosis [Gk *asbestos* inextinguishable, *osis* condition], a chronic lung disease caused by the inhalation of asbestos fibers that results in the development of alveolar, interstitial, and pleural fibrosis. Asbestos miners and workers are most frequently affected, but the disease sometimes occurs in other people who have been exposed to asbestos building materials.

ASC, abbreviation for **altered state of consciousness.**

ascariasis /as´kərī´əsis/ [Gk *askaris* intestinal worm, *osis* condition], an infection caused by a parasitic worm, *Ascaris lumbricoides,* that migrates through the lungs in its larval stage. The eggs are passed in human feces, contaminating the soil and allowing transmission to the mouths of others through hands, water, or food. After hatching in the small intestine, the larvae travel through the wall of the intestine, whence they are carried by the lymphatics and blood to the lungs.

Ascaris /as´kəris/, a genus of large parasitic intestinal roundworms, such as *Ascaris lumbricoides,* a cause of ascariasis, found throughout temperate and tropic regions.

ascending aorta [L *ascendere* to climb], one of the four main sections of the aorta, branching into the right and left coronary arteries, rising from the semilunar valve of the heart, curving to the right near the cranial border of the second right costal cartilage, and lying about 6 cm deep to the dorsal surface of the sternum.

ascending colon, the segment of the colon that extends from the cecum in the lower right side of the abdomen to the transverse colon at the hepatic flexure on the right side, usually at the level of the umbilicus.

ascending current. See **centripetal current.**

ascending neuritis [L *ascendere;* Gk *neuron* nerve, *itis* inflammation], a nerve inflammation that begins on the periphery and moves upward along a nerve trunk.

ascending neuropathy, a disease of the nervous system that begins at a lower place in the body and spreads upward.

ascending oblique muscle. See **obliquus internus abdominis.**

ascending paralysis, a condition in which there is successive flaccid paralysis of the legs, then the trunk and arms, and finally the muscles of respiration. Causes may include poliomyelitis, infectious polyneuritis, or exposure to toxic chemicals.

ascending pharyngeal artery, one of the smallest arteries that branch from the external carotid artery, deep in the neck, supplying various organs and muscles of the head, such as the tympanic cavity, the longus capitis, and the longus colli.

ascending poliomyelitis [L *ascendere;* Gk *polios* gray, *myelos* marrow, *itis* inflammation], poliomyelitis that begins in the legs and spreads upward to involve the trunk and respiratory muscles.

ascending tract [L, *tractus*], a nervous system pathway found in the spinal cord that carries impulses toward the brain.

ascending urography. See **urography.**

asceticism /aset'isiz'əm/ [Gk *askein* to exercise], (in psychiatry) a defense mechanism that involves repudiation of all instinctual impulses.

Ascheim-Zondek (AZ) test /ash'hīmt-son'dek/, an obsolete biologic test for pregnancy.

Aschoff bodies [Karl Albert Ludwig Aschoff, German pathologist, b. 1866; AS, *bodig*], tiny rounded or spindle-shaped nodules containing multinucleated giant cells, fibroblasts, and basophilic cells found in joints, tendons, the pleura, and the cardiovascular system of rheumatic fever patients.

ascites /əsī'tēz/ [Gk *askos* bag], an abnormal intraperitoneal accumulation of a fluid containing large amounts of protein and electrolytes. The condition may be accompanied by general abdominal swelling, hemodilution, edema, or a decrease in urinary output. Ascites is a complication of cirrhosis, congestive heart failure, nephrosis, malignant neoplastic disease, peritonitis, or various fungal and parasitic diseases. –**ascitic,** *adj.*

ascites adiposus. See **chylous ascites.**

ascites praecox [Gk *askos* + L, premature], an abnormal accumulation of fluid within the peritoneal cavity preceding the development of generalized edema associated with pericarditis.

ascitic fluid [Gk *askos*], a watery fluid containing albumin, glucose, and electrolytes that accumulates in the peritoneal cavity in association with certain disease conditions, such as liver disease or congestive heart failure. The fluid occurs as leakage from the veins and lymphatics into extravascular spaces.

ascorbemia /as'kôrbē'mē·ə/ [Gk *a* not; AS *scurf* scurvy; Gk *haima* blood], the presence of ascorbic acid in the blood in amounts greater than normal, usually reflecting only an excess of ascorbic acid in the diet.

ascorbic acid /əskôr'bik/ [Gk *a* not; AS *scurf* scurvy], a water-soluble, white crystalline vitamin present in citrus fruits, tomatoes, berries, potatoes, and fresh, green, leafy vegetables. It is essential for the formation of collagen and fibrous tissue for normal intercellular matrices in teeth, bone, cartilage, connective tissue, and skin, and for the structural integrity of capillary walls. Severe deficiency results in scurvy.

ascorburia /as'kôrby ŏŏr'ē·ə/ [Gk *a* not; AS *scurf* scurvy; Gk *ouron* urine], the presence of ascorbic acid in the urine in amounts greater than normal, usually reflecting only an excess of ascorbic acid in the diet.

ascribed role, an assigned role in society based on age, sex, or other factors about which the individual has no choice.

ASD, abbreviation for **atrial septal defect.**

asepsis /āsep'sis/ [Gk *a, sepsis* not decay] **1.** the absence of germs. **2. medical asepsis,** the removal or destruction of disease organisms or infected material. **3. surgical asepsis,** protection against infection before, during, or after surgery by the use of sterile technique. –**aseptic,** *adj.*

aseptic body image, an awareness by operating room personnel of body, hair, makeup, clothing, jewelry, and placement with regard for maintenance of a sterile environment and changing proximities between sterile and contaminated areas as a field becomes progressively contaminated.

aseptic bone necrosis, a type of bone and joint damage that may occur in workers exposed to repeated compressed-air environments, as in diving or tunneling occupations. It may be asymptomatic or, if joint surfaces are involved, marked by severe pain and joint collapse.

aseptic fever, a fever not associated with infection. Mechanical trauma, as in a crushing injury, can cause fever even when no pathogenic microorganism is present.

aseptic gauze, 1. sterile gauze prepared and packed for surgical use. **2.** any gauze that is free of microorganisms.

aseptic meningitis, an inflammation of the meninges that is caused by one of a number of viruses, including coxsackieviruses, nonparalytic polio viruses, echoviruses, and mumps.

aseptic necrosis [Gk *a, sepsis* + *nekros* dead, *osis* condition], cystic and sclerotic degenerative changes in tissues, as may follow an injury in the absence of infection.

aseptic peritonitis [Gk *a, sepsis* + *peri* near, *teinein* to stretch, *itis* inflammation], peritonitis in which inflammation of the peritoneum is caused by chemicals, radiation, or injury, rather than by an infectious agent.

aseptic surgery [Gk *a, sepsis* + *cheirourgos* surgeon], the avoidance of contamination during surgical procedures.

aseptic technique, any health care procedure in which added precautions are used to prevent contamination of a person, object, or area by microorganisms.

asexual /āsek'shōō·əl/ [Gk *a* not; L *sexus* male or female], **1.** not sexual. **2.** of or pertaining to an organism that has no sexual organs. **3.** of or pertaining to a process that is not sexual. **–asexuality,** *n.*

asexual dwarf, an adult dwarf whose genital organs are underdeveloped.

asexual generation, any type of reproduction that occurs without the union of male and female gametes, such as fission, budding, sporulation, or parthenogenesis.

asexualization /āsek'shōō·əlīzā'shən/, the process of making one incapable of reproduction; sterilization of an individual or animal by castration, vasectomy, removal of the ovaries, or other means.

asexual reproduction, a type of reproduction found in plants and lower animals in which new organisms are formed without the union of gametes, as occurs in budding, fission, and spore formation.

ASHA, abbreviation for **American Speech, Language, and Hearing Association.**

ASHD, abbreviation for **arteriosclerotic heart disease.**

Asherman syndrome, secondary amenorrhea in a hormonally normal woman, caused by obliteration of the endometrial cavity by adhesions that form as a result of curettage or infection.

asialorrhea. See **hyposalivation.**

Asian flu. See **influenza.**

asiderosis /ā'sidərō'sis/, an iron deficiency and a cause of anemia.

ASLT, abbreviation for **antistreptolysin-O test.**

ASMT, abbreviation for *American Society for Medical Technology.*

Asn, abbreviation for **asparagine.**

asocial [Gk *a;* L *socius* companion], withdrawn or disengaged from normal contacts with other individuals.

ASOT, abbreviation for **antistreptolysin-O test.**

asparaginase /aspar'əjinās/ [Gk *asparagos* asparagus], an enzyme that catalyzes the hydrolysis of asparagine to asparaginic acid and ammonia.

asparagine (Asn) /aspar'əjin/, a nonessential amino acid found in many proteins in the body.

aspartame, a white, almost odorless crystalline powder with an intensely sweet taste that is used as an artificial sweetener. Excessive use of aspartame should be avoided by patients with phenylketonuria (PKU) because the substance hydrolyzes to form aspartylphenylalanine.

aspartate aminotransferase (AST) /aspär'tāt/, an enzyme normally present in body serum and in certain body tissues that affects the intermolecular transfer of an amino group from aspartic acid to alpha-ketoglutaric acid, forming glutamic acid and oxaloacetic acid.

aspartate kinase, an enzyme that catalyzes the transfer of a phosphate group from adenosine triphosphate to aspartate to produce phosphoaspartate.

aspartate transaminase. See **aspartate aminotransferase.**

aspartic acid (Asp) /aspär'tik/, a nonessential amino acid present in sugar cane, beet molasses, and the breakdown products of many proteins.

ASPEN, abbreviation for **American Society of Parenteral and Enteral Nutrition.**

aspergillic acid /as'pərjil'ik/, an antibiotic substance derived from *Aspergillus flavus,* an aflatoxin-producing mold found on corn, grain, and peanuts.

aspergillosis /as'pərjilō'sis/ [L *aspergere* to sprinkle; Gk *osis* condition], an infection caused by a fungus of the genus *Aspergillus,* most commonly affecting the ear but capable of causing inflammatory, granulomatous lesions on or in any organ.

Aspergillus /as'pərjil'əs/ [L *aspereger* to sprinkle], a genus of fungi that is a common contaminant in the laboratory and a cause of nosocomial infection.

aspermia /āspur'mē·ə/ [Gk *a, sperma* not seed], lack of formation or ejaculation of semen.

asphyxia /asfik'sē·ə/ [Gk *a, sphyxis* not pulse], severe hypoxia leading to hypoxemia and hypercapnia, loss of consciousness, and, if not corrected, death. Some of the more common causes of asphyxia are drowning, electric shock, aspiration of vomitus, lodging of a foreign body in the respiratory tract, inhalation of toxic gas or smoke, and poisoning. **–asphyxiate,** *v.,* **asphyxiated,** *adj.*

asphyxia livida /liv'ədə/, an abnormal condition in which a newborn infant's skin is cyanotic, the pulse is weak and slow, and the reflexes are slow or absent.

asphyxia neonatorum, a condition in which a newborn does not breath spontaneously. The asphyxia may develop before or during labor or occur immediately after delivery.

asphyxia pallida /pal'ədə/, an abnormal condition in which a newborn infant appears pale and limp, shows signs of apnea, and suffers from bradycardia as marked by a heartbeat of 80 beats per minute or less.

asphyxiate /asfik'sē·āt/ [Gk *a* + *sphyxis* pulse], to induce an inability to breathe.

Causes may include circulatory congestion, chemical poisoning, electrical shock, or physical suffocation.

asphyxiation, a state of asphyxia or inability to breathe.

aspirant /as'pirənt/, the fluid, gas, or solid particles that are withdrawn from the body by aspiration methods.

aspirant maneuver, a procedure used in making x-ray films of the laryngopharyngeal area. The patient exhales completely, then slowly inhales while making a harsh, high-pitched sound.

aspirate [L *aspirare* to breathe upon], to withdraw fluid or air from a cavity. The process is usually aided by the use of a syringe or a suction device.

aspirating needle, a long hollow needle used to remove fluid from a cavity, vessel, or structure of the body.

aspirating syringe, (in dentistry) a hypodermic syringe used in the injection of local anesthetics. It can be checked by aspirating to ensure that the anesthetic solution is not being deposited in a blood vessel.

aspiration, **1.** the act of taking a breath, inhaling. **2.** the act of withdrawing a fluid, such as mucus or serum, from the body by a suction device. **–aspirate,** *n.*

aspiration biopsy, the removal of living tissue for microscopic examination by suction through a fine needle attached to a syringe. The procedure is used primarily to obtain cells from a lesion containing fluid or when fluid is formed in a serous cavity.

aspiration biopsy cytology (ABC), a microscopic examination of cells obtained directly from living body tissue by aspiration through a fine needle.

aspiration drug abuse, the inhalation of a liquid, solid, or gaseous chemical into the respiratory system for nontherapeutic purposes.

aspiration of vomitus, the inhalation of regurgitated gastric contents into the pulmonary system.

aspiration pneumonia, an inflammatory condition of the lungs and bronchi caused by the inhalation of foreign material or vomitus containing acid gastric contents.

aspiration, high risk for, a NANDA-accepted nursing diagnosis of the risk for entry of gastric secretions, oropharyngeal secretions, or exogenous food or fluids into tracheobronchial passages caused by dysfunction or absence of normal protective mechanisms. Risk factors include reduced level of consciousness, depressed cough and gag reflexes, the presence of a tracheostomy or endotracheal tube, an overinflated tracheostomy or endotracheal tube cuff, inadequate inflation of a trache-

ostomy or endotracheal tube cuff, GI tubes, and bolus tube feedings or medication administration.

aspirator [L *aspirare* to breathe upon], any instrument that removes a substance from body cavities by suction, such as a bulb syringe, piston pump, or hypodermic syringe.

aspirin, an analgesic, antipyretic, and antirheumatic. It is prescribed to reduce fever and for the relief of pain and inflammation.

aspirin poisoning. See **salicylate poisoning.**

asplenia [Gk *a* without, *spleen*], absence of a spleen. The condition may be congenital or the result of surgical removal.

ASRT, abbreviation for *American Society of Radiologic Technologists.*

Assam fever. See **kala-azar.**

assault [L *assilirere* to leap upon], **1.** an unlawful act that places another person, without that person's consent, in fear of immediate bodily harm or battery. The act must be apparently possible, thus causing well-founded apprehension in the victim of the assault. **2.** the act of committing an assault. **3.** to threaten a person with bodily harm or injury.

assay /asā'/ [Fr *essayer* to try], the analysis of the purity or effectiveness of drugs and other biologic substances, including laboratory and clinical observations.

assertiveness, a form of behavior that is directed toward claiming one's rights without denying the rights of others.

assertive training [L *asserere* to join to oneself], a technique used in behavior therapy to help individuals become more self-assertive and self-confident in interpersonal relationships.

assessing [L *assidere* to sit beside], (in five-step nursing process) a category of nursing behavior that includes the gathering, verifying, and communicating of information relative to the client. The nurse collects information from verbal interactions with the patient, the patient's family and significant others; examines standard data sources for information; systematically checks for symptoms and signs; determines the patient's ability to perform self-care activities; assesses the patient's environment; and identifies reactions of the staff (including the nurse who is performing the assessment) to the patient and to the patient's family and significant others.

assessment [L *assidere* to sit beside], (in medicine and nursing) **1.** an evaluation or appraisal of a condition. **2.** the process of making such an evaluation. **3.** (in a problem-oriented medical record) an examiner's evaluation of the disease or condition based on the patient's subjective report of the symptoms and course of the illness or condition and the examiner's objective findings, including data obtained through laboratory tests, physical examination, and medical history. **–assess,** *v.*

assessment of the aging patient, an evaluation of the changes characteristic of advancing years exhibited by an elderly person.

assimilate [L *assimilare* to make alike], a phase of anabolism in which nutritive substances are absorbed from the digestive tract to the circulatory system and consequently converted into living tissues.

assimilation, 1. the process of incorporating nutritive material into living tissue; the end stage of the nutrition process, after digestion and absorption or occurring simultaneously with absorption. 2. (in psychology) the incorporation of new experiences into a person's pattern of consciousness. 3. (in sociology) the process in which a person or a group of people of a different ethnic background become absorbed into a new culture. **–assimilate,** *v.*

assist-control mode, a system of mechanical ventilation in which the patient is allowed to establish an acceptable rate of breathing, but the ventilator delivers a set volume with each breath.

assisted breech [L *assistere* to stand by], an obstetric operation in which a baby being born feet or buttocks first is permitted to deliver spontaneously as far as its umbilicus and is then extracted.

assisted circulation [L *assistere* to stand, *circulare* to go around], a method of treating patients with severe circulatory deficiencies by introducing a mechanical pumping system to aid the blood flow.

assisted death, a form of euthanasia in which an individual expressing a wish to die prematurely is helped to accomplish that goal by another person, either by counseling and/or providing a poison or other lethal instrument. The assisted death may be regarded as a homicide or suicide by local authorities and the person giving assistance may be held responsible for the death. In most cases, the deceased was a terminally ill patient.

assisted suicide, a form of euthanasia in which a person wishes to commit suicide but feels unable to perform the act alone because of a physical disability or lack of knowledge about the most effective means. An individual who assists a suicide victim in accomplishing that goal may or may not be held responsible for the death, depending on local laws.

assisted ventilation, the use of mechanical or other devices to help maintain respiration, usually by delivering air or oxygen under positive pressure.

Associate Degree in Nursing (ADN) [L *associare* to unite], an academic degree awarded on satisfactory completion of a 2-year course of study, usually at a community or junior college. The recipient is eligible to take the national licensing examination to become a registered nurse.

associate nurse, *U.S.* 1. (in primary nursing) a nurse who is responsible for implementing a primary nurse's care plans. 2. in some states, a registered nurse who holds a diploma from a hospital school of nursing or an associate degree.

associated antagonist, one of a pair of muscles or group of muscles that pull in opposite directions but whose combined action results in moving a part in one direction.

association [L *associare* to unite], 1. a connection, union, joining, or combination of things. 2. (in psychology) the connection of remembered feelings, emotions, sensations, thoughts, or perceptions with particular persons, things, or ideas. Kinds of association are **association of ideas, clang association, controlled association, dream association,** and **free association.**

association area, any part of the cerebral cortex involved in the integration of sensory information.

Association for Practitioners of Infection Control (APIC), a national professional organization of nurses who work in the field of infection control.

Association for the Advancement of Medical Instrumentation (AAMI), a nonprofit organization involved in education and standards relating to biomedical engineering.

Association for the Care of Children's Health (ACCH), an international, interdisciplinary organization concerned with the psychosocial needs of children and their families in health care settings.

Association of Canadian Medical Colleges (ACMC), a Canadian organization of the deans and faculty members of the nation's 16 medical schools.

association of ideas, a mental connection established between similar or simultaneously occurring ideas, feelings, or perceptions.

Association of Operating Room Nurses (AORN), a national organization of operating room nurses.

association test, a technique used in psychiatric diagnosis and in educational and psychologic evaluation in which a person is asked to respond to a stimulus word with the first word that comes to mind.

associationist model of learning, a theory that defines learning as behavioral change that is a result of reinforced practice.

association paralysis, a motor neuron disease in which wasting, weakness, and fasciculation of the tongue, facial muscles, pharynx, and larynx occur.

associative looseness, a form of thought disorder in which relationships among ideas are determined in an autistic manner.

associative play, a form of play in which a group of children participate in similar or identical activities without formal organization, group direction, group interaction, or a definite goal.

assortive mating, the matching of males and females for reproduction in a manner that avoids random selection.

assumed role, a role in life that an individual usually selects or achieves by choice, such as one's role in marriage or employment.

AST, 1. abbreviation for **angiotensin sensitivity test.** 2. abbreviation for **aspartate aminotransferase.**

astasia /astā′zhə/, a motor nerve disorder marked by an inability to stand without assistance.

astasia-abasia [Gk *a, stasis* not stand + *a, basis* not step], a form of ataxia in which the patient is unable to stand or walk due to lack of motor coordination although able to carry out natural leg movements when sitting or lying down.

astatine (At) [Gk *astasis* unsteady], a very unstable, radioactive element that occurs naturally in tiny amounts. Its atomic number is 85; its atomic weight is 210.

asteatosis /as′tē·ətō′sis/ [Gk *a, stear* not tallow, *osis* condition], a dry skin condition caused by a deficiency of sebaceous gland secretions. There may be scales and fissures as a result of the dryness.

astereognosis /əstir′ē·og·nō′sis/ [Gk *a, stereos* not solid, *gnosis* knowledge], a neurologic disorder characterized by an inability to identify objects by touch.

asterixis /as′tərik′sis/ [Gk *a, sterixis* not fixed position], a hand-flapping tremor, often accompanying metabolic disorders.

asteroid body [Gk *aster* star, *eidos* form], an irregular star-shaped structure that develops in the giant cells in certain diseases, including sarcoidosis, actinomycosis, and nocardiosis.

asthenia /asthē′nē·ə/ [Gk *a, sthenos* not strength], 1. the lack or loss of strength or energy; weakness; debility. 2. (in psychiatry) lack of dynamic force in the personality. Kinds of asthenia include **myal-**gic asthenia and **neurocirculatory asthenia.** –**asthenic,** *adj.*

asthenic habitus [Gk *a, sthenos* not strength; L *habere* to have], a body structure characterized by a slender build with long limbs, an angular profile, and prominent muscles or bones.

asthenic personality, a personality characterized by low energy, lack of enthusiasm, and oversensitivity to physical and emotional strain.

asthenopia /as′thənō′pē·ə/ [Gk *a, sthenos* + *ops* eye], a condition in which the eyes tire easily because of weakness of the ocular or ciliary muscles. Symptoms include pain in or around the eyes, headache, dimness of vision, dizziness, and slight nausea.

asthma /az′mə/ [Gk, panting], a respiratory disorder characterized by recurring episodes of paroxysmal dyspnea, wheezing on expiration due to constriction of the bronchi, coughing, and viscous mucoid bronchial secretions. The episodes may be precipitated by inhalation of allergens or pollutants, infection, cold air, vigorous exercise, or emotional stress.

asthma crystal. See **Charcot-Leyden crystal.**

asthma in children, an obstructive respiratory condition characterized by recurring attacks of paroxysmal dyspnea, wheezing, prolonged expiration, and an irritative cough that is a common, chronic illness in childhood. Onset usually occurs between 3 and 8 years of age. Asthmatic attacks are caused by constriction of the large and small airways, resulting from bronchial smooth muscle spasm, edema or inflammation of the bronchial wall or excessive production of mucus. It is a complex disorder involving biochemical, immunologic, infectious, endocrinologic, and psychologic factors. Asthma in children is usually extrinsic; that is, most attacks are associated with an allergenic hypersensitivity to a foreign substance, such as airborne pollen, mold, house dust, certain foods, animal hair and skin, feathers, insects, smoke, and various chemicals or drugs. In infants, especially those born into a family with a history of allergic reactions, food allergy is a common precipitating factor. There is a strong hereditary factor associated with the disease and the child usually has other allergic manifestations, such as hay fever, eczema, or urticaria. The disease occurs twice as often in boys as in girls before puberty, but both boys and girls are affected equally during adolescence.

asthmatic breathing [Gk *asthma* panting; AS *braeth*], breathing marked by prolonged wheezing upon exhalation due to spasmodic contractions of the bronchi.

asthmatic cough [Gk *asthma;* AS *cohhetan*], a wheezing cough accompanied by signs of breathing difficulty.

asthmatic eosinophilia, a form of eosinophilic pneumonia, characterized by allergic bronchospasm, by expectoration of bronchial casts containing eosinophils and mycelium, and by cough and fever. The condition usually occurs in the fourth or fifth decade of life, and is twice as common in women as in men. It is a result of hypersensitivity to *Aspergillus fumigatus* or *Candida albicans.*

astigmatism /əstig′mətiz′əm/ [Gk *a, stigma* not point], an abnormal condition of the eye in which the light rays cannot be focused clearly in a point on the retina because the spheric curve of the cornea is not equal in all meridians. Vision is blurred, and use of the eyes causes discomfort. The person cannot accommodate to correct the problem. The condition usually may be corrected with contact lenses or with eye glasses ground to neutralize the defect. **–astigmatic,** *adj.*

astragalus. See talus.

astringent /əstrin′jənt/ [Gk *astringere* to tighten] **1.** a substance that causes contraction of tissues upon application, usually used locally. **2.** having the quality of an astringent. **–astringency,** *n.*

astringent bath, a bath in which alum, tannic acid, or another astringent is added to the water.

astroblastoma /as′trōblastō′mə/, *pl.* **astroblastomas, astroblastomata** [Gk *aster* star, *blastos* germ, *oma* tumor], a malignant neoplasm of the brain and spinal cord. Cells of an astroblastoma lie around blood vessels or, in some cases, around connective tissue septa.

astrocyte /as′trōsīt′/ [Gk *aster* + *kytos* cell], a large, star-shaped cell found in certain tissues of the nervous system.

astrocytoma /as′trōsītō′mə/, *pl.* **astrocytomas, astrocytomata** [Gk *aster, kytos* + *oma*], a primary tumor of the brain composed of astrocytes and characterized by slow growth, cyst formation, invasion of surrounding structures, and, often, the development of a highly malignant glioblastoma within the tumor mass.

astrocytosis /as′trōsītō′sis/ [Gk *aster, kytos* + *osis* condition], an increase in the number of neuroglial cells with fibrous or protoplasmic processes frequently observed in an irregular area adjacent to degenerative lesions, such as abscesses, certain brain neoplasms, and encephalomalacia.

asymmetric, asymmetrical /ā′simet′rik,

as′imet′rik/ [Gk *a, symmetria* not proportion], (of the body or parts of the body) unequal in size or shape; different in placement or arrangement about an axis. **–asymmetry** /āsim′itrē, asim′-/, *n.*

asymmetric tonic neck reflex. See tonic neck reflex.

asymptomatic [Gk *a* without, *symptom*], absence of symptoms.

asymptomatic neurosyphilis [Gk, *a,* without, *symptoma* + *neuron* nerve; Fr *syphilide*], a form of neurosyphilis that shows pathologic changes in the cerebrospinal fluid although there are no symptoms of nervous system damage. Asymptomatic neurosyphilis may occur many years before actual nervous system damage is noticeable.

asynchronous /āsing′krənəs/ [Gk *a, synchronos,* not simultaneous], (of an event or device) not synchronized with the timing circuit of the cental processing unit of a computer.

asynclitism /āsing′klitiz′əm/ [Gk *a, syn* not together, *kleisis* to lean], presentation of a parietal aspect of the fetal head to the maternal pelvic inlet in labor, the sagittal suture being parallel to the transverse diameter of the pelvis but anterior or posterior to it. **Anterior asynclitism,** in which the anterior parietes present, is called Nägele's obliquity. **Posterior asynclitism** is called Litzmann's obliquity.

asyndesis /əsin′dəsis/, a mental disorder marked by an inability to assemble related ideas or thoughts into one coherent concept.

asynergy /āsin′ərjē/ [Gk *a, syn* + *ergein* to work] **1.** a condition characterized by faulty coordination among groups of organs or muscles that normally function harmoniously. **2.** the state of muscle antagonism found in cerebellar disease.

asyntaxia /ā′sintak′sē-ə/ [Gk *a, syn* + *taxis* arrangement], any interference with the orderly sequence of growth and differentiation of the fetus during embryonic development, resulting in one or more congenital anomalies. A kind of asyntaxia is **asyntaxia dorsalis.**

asyntaxia dorsalis, failure of the neural tube to close during embryonic development.

asystole /āsis′təlē/ [Gk *a, systole* not contraction], the absence of a heartbeat, as distinguished from fibrillation, in which electric activity persists but contraction ceases. Cardiotoxic asystole is characterized by a brief period of cardiac arrest caused by an acceleration in the heart rate. **–asystolic** /ā′sistol′ik/, *adj.*

At, symbol for the element **astatine.**

Atabrine stomatitis, an abnormal oral

condition that may be associated with the use of Atabrine, (quinacrine hydrochloride), characterized by oral changes simulating lichen planus.

ataractic /at'ərak'tik/ [Gk *ataraktos* quiet], pertaining to a drug or other agent that has a tranquilizing or sedating effect.

atavism /at'əviz'əm/ [L *atavus* ancestor], the appearance in an individual of traits or characteristics more like those of a grandparent or earlier ancestor than of the parents. Atavistic data may offer clues to an examining physician of genetic or familial health factors. **–atavistic,** *adj.*

ataxia /ətak'sē·ə/ [Gk, disorder], an abnormal condition characterized by impaired ability to coordinate movement. A staggering gait and postural imbalance are caused by a lesion in the spinal cord or cerebellum. **–ataxial, ataxic,** *adj.*

ataxia-telangiectasia [Gk *ataxia* + *telos* end, *aggeion* vessel, *ektasis* expansion], a rare genetic disease involving immunoglobulin metabolism that is transmitted as an autosomal recessive trait. The onset usually occurs in infancy and progresses slowly with increasing cerebellar degeneration and recurrent sinopulmonary infections. Telangiectasias are most prominent on the skin and conjunctiva.

ataxic aphasia. See **motor aphasia.**

ataxic breathing, a type of breathing associated with a lesion in the medullary respiratory centers and characterized by a series of inspirations and expirations.

ataxic speech, abnormal speech characterized by faulty formation of the sounds because of neuromuscular dysfunction.

ATCC, abbreviation for **American Type Culture Collection.**

atelectasis /at'ilek'təsis/ [Gk *ateles* incomplete, *ektasis* expansion], an abnormal condition characterized by the collapse of lung tissue, preventing the respiratory exchange of carbon dioxide and oxygen.

atelectatic rale /at'iləktat'ik/ [Gk *ateles, ektasis* + Fr *rale* rattle], an abnormal intermittent crackling sound heard during auscultation of the chest. It usually disappears after the individual being examined coughs or breathes deeply several times.

ateliotic dwarf /at'əlē·ot'ik/, a dwarf whose skeleton is incompletely formed, resulting from the nonunion of the epiphyses and diaphyses during bone development.

atelorachidia /at'əlôr'əkidid'ē·ə/ [Gk *ateles* incomplete, *rhachis* spine], a defective, incomplete formation of the spinal column.

atenolol /aten'əlôl/, a beta-blocker prescribed for the treatment of hypertension.

ATG, abbreviation for **antithymocyte globulin.**

atherectomy catheter /ath'ərek'təmē/, a specially designed catheter for cutting away atheromatous plaque from the lining of an artery. The catheter is positioned and monitored by fluoroscopy.

atheroembolic renal disease /ath'ərō·embol'ik/, a condition of gradual or rapid kidney failure resulting from obstruction of the renal arteries by atheromas and emboli.

atherogenesis [Gk *athere* porridge, *oma* tumor, *genein* to produce], the formation of subintimal plaques in the lining of arteries.

atheroma /ath'ərō'mə/, *pl.* **atheromas, atheromata** [Gk *athere* meal, *oma* tumor], an abnormal mass of fat or lipids, as in a sebaceous cyst or in deposits in an arterial wall. **–atheromatous,** *adj.*

atheromatosis /ath'ərōmətō'sis/, the development of many atheromas.

atheromatous plaque, a yellowish raised area on the lining of an artery formed by fatty deposits.

atherosclerosis /ath'ərōsklərō'sis/ [Gk *athere* meal, *sklerosis* hardening], a common arterial disorder characterized by yellowish plaques of cholesterol, lipids, and cellular debris in the inner layers of the walls of large and medium-sized arteries. With the formation of the plaques, the vessel walls become thick, fibrotic, and calcified, and the lumen narrows, resulting in reduced circulation in organs and areas normally supplied by the artery. Atheromatous lesions are major causes of coronary heart disease, angina pectoris, myocardial infarction, and other cardiac disorders. Atherosclerosis usually occurs with aging and is often associated with obesity, hypertension, and diabetes.

atherosclerotic aneurysm [Gk *athere, skleros* hard, *aneurysma* a widening], an aneurysm that develops as a result of atherosclerotic weakening of an arterial wall.

athetoid /ath'ətoid/, pertaining to athetosis.

athetosis /ath'ətō'sis/ [Gk *athetos* not fixed], a neuromuscular condition characterized by slow, writhing, continuous, and involuntary movement of the extremities, as seen in some forms of cerebral palsy and in motor disorders resulting from lesions in the basal ganglia.

athiaminosis /əthī'əminō'sis/, a condition resulting from lack of thiamine in the diet.

athlete's foot. See **tinea pedis.**

athlete's heart, the typical, normal but enlarged heart of an athlete trained for endurance, characterized by a slow rate of contractions, an increased pumping capacity, and greater than average ability to deliver oxygen to skeletal muscles.

athletic habitus, a physique characterized by a well-proportioned, muscular body with broad shoulders, thick neck, deep chest, and flat abdomen.

athletic heart syndrome. See **athlete's heart.**

athletic trainer, an allied health professional career who, with the consultation and supervision of attending physicians, is an integral part of the health care system associated with sports. Through preparation in both academic and practical experience, the athletic trainer provides a variety of services including injury prevention, recognition, immediate care, treatment, and rehabilitation of athletic trauma. Standards for recognition of athletic training as an allied health occupation were approved by the American Medical Association in 1990.

atlantal /ətlan'təl/, pertaining to the atlas, the first cervical vertebra.

atlantoaxial /ətlan'tō·ak'sē·əl/ [Gk *atlas* bear + *axis pivot*], pertaining to the first two cervical vertebrae.

atlantooccipital joint /-oksip'itəl/ [Gk *Atlas, theni* to bear; L *ob* against, *caput* head], one of a pair of condyloid joints formed by the articulation of the atlas of the vertebral column with the occipital bone of the skull. It permits nodding and lateral movements of the head.

atlas [Gk *Atlas* a mythical king-giant], the first cervical vertebra, articulating with the occipital bone and the axis.

atm, 1. abbreviation for **atmosphere.** 2. abbreviation for **atmospheric.**

atman /ät'män/, (in psychiatry) a concept derived from Eastern Indian philosophy that the highest value is to know one's true self.

atmosphere (atm) [Gk *atmos* vapor, *sphaira* sphere] 1. the natural body of air, composed of approximately 20% oxygen, 78% nitrogen, and 2% carbon dioxide and other gases, that covers the surface of the earth. 2. an envelope of gas, which may or may not duplicate the natural atmosphere in chemical components. 3. a unit of gas pressure that is usually defined as being equivalent to the average pressure of the earth's atmosphere at sea level, or about 14.7 pounds per square inch. **–atmospheric,** *adj.*

atmospheric pressure, the pressure exerted by the weight of the atmosphere. The atmospheric pressure at sea level is approximately 15 pounds per square inch. With increasing altitude the pressure decreases.

ATN, abbreviation for **acute tubular necrosis.**

atom [Gk *atmos* indivisible], 1. (in physics) the smallest division of an element that exhibits all the properties and characteristics of the element. It comprises neutrons, electrons, and protons. 2. *nontechnical.* the mass of any substance that is so small further division is not possible. 3. *informal.* a minute amount of any substance. **–atomic,** *adj.*

atomic mass unit (amu), the mass of a neutral atom of an element, expressed as 1/12 of the mass of carbon, which has an arbitrarily assigned value of 12. The energy equivalent of 1 amu is 931. 2 MeV. The mass equivalent of 1 amu is $1.66(10^{-24}$ g).

atomic number, the number of protons, or positive charges, in the nucleus of an atom of a particular element. The atomic number equals the number of electrons, and their number and arrangement determine the chemical characteristics of the atom, with the exception of its atomic weight and radioactivity.

atomic theory [Gk *atmos* indivisible, *theoria* speculation], a concept that all matter is composed of submicroscopic atoms, which are in turn composed of protons, electrons, and neutrons. A chemical element is identified by the number of protons in its atoms.

atomic weight (A, at. wt.), the relative average mass of an atom based on the mass of carbon 12 isotope.

atomize. See **nebulize.**

atomizer, a device for reducing a liquid and ejecting it as a fine spray or vapor.

atonia /ātō'nē·ə/ [Gk *a, tonos* not tone], an abnormal lack of muscle tone.

atonia constipation, constipation caused by the failure of the colon to respond to the normal stimuli for evacuation. It may occur in elderly or bedridden patients or after prolonged dependence on laxatives.

atonic /əton'ik/, 1. weak. 2. lacking normal tone, as in the case of a muscle that is flaccid. 3. lacking vigor, such as an atonic ulcer, which heals slowly. **–atony** /at'onē/, *n.*

atonic bladder. See **flaccid bladder.**

atonic impotence. See **impotence.**

atonicity [Gk *a* without, *tonos* tone], a condition of atony, or lack of muscle tone or tension.

atony. See **atonic.**

atopic /ātop'ik/ [Gk *a, topos* not place], of or pertaining to a hereditary tendency to develop immediate allergic reactions, such as asthma, atopic dermatitis, or vasomotor rhinitis, because of the presence of an antibody (atopic reagin) in the skin and sometimes the bloodstream. **–atopy** /at′ope̅/, *n.*

atopic asthma. See **allergic asthma.**

atopic dermatitis, an intensely pruritic, often excoriated, maculopapular inflammation commonly found on the face and antecubital and popliteal areas of allergy-prone individuals.

atopic reagin. See **reagin.**

atopognosia /ătop′əgnō′zhə/ [Gk *a, topos* not place, *gnosis* knowledge], a form of corporeal agnosia in which a person is unable to locate a sensation properly.

atopy. See **atopic.**

atoxic. See **nontoxic.**

ATP, abbreviation for **adenosine triphosphate.**

ATPase, abbreviation for **adenosine triphosphatase.**

ATPD, abbreviation for *ambient temperature, ambient pressure, dry.*

ATPS, abbreviation for *ambient temperature, ambient pressure, saturated* (with water vapor).

atransferrinemic anemia /ā′transfer′ine̅′ mik/, an iron-transport deficiency disease characterized by a failure of iron to move from the liver or other storage sites to tissues in which erthyrocytes develop.

atraumatic [Gk *a* without + *trauma*], pertaining to therapies or therapeutic instruments and devices that are unlikely to cause tissue damage.

atresia /ətre̅′zhə/ [Gk *a, tresis* not perforation], the absence of a normal body opening, duct, or canal, such as the anus, vagina, or external ear canal. **–atresic, atretic,** *adj.*

atresic teratism /ətre̅′sik/ [Gk *a, tresis + tera* monster], a congenital anomaly in which any of the normal openings of the body, such as the mouth, nares, anus, or vagina, fail to form.

atrial appendix. See **auricle.**

atrial fibrillation, a condition characterized by rapid, random contractions of the atria, causing irregular ventricular beats at the rate of 130 to 150 a minute. The atria may discharge more than 350 impulses a minute, but some do not pass the atrioventricular junction. The ventricles cannot contract in response to all the stimuli that are received, and ventricular contractions become disordered.

atrial flutter, a condition characterized by rapid, regular contractions of the atria, approximately 300 beats per minute. The ventricles cannot respond to the stimuli and contract at a submultiple of the atrial rate, usually about 150 beats per minute.

atrial gallop, an abnormal cardiac rhythm in which a low-pitched, extra sound is heard late in diastole on auscultation of the heart.

atrial myxoma, a benign, pedunculated gelatinous tumor that originates in the interatrial septum of the heart. It may cause palpitations, disseminated neuritis, nausea, weight loss, fatigue, dyspnea, fever, and, occasionally, sudden loss of consciousness because of obstruction of the flow of blood through the heart.

atrial septal defect (ASD), a congenital cardiac anomaly characterized by an abnormal opening between the two atria. The severity of the condition depends on the size and location of the defect, which depend on the stage at which embryonic development of the septum structures was arrested. The defects are classified as ostium secundum defect, in which the aperture in the septum secundum, or second septum, of the fetal heart fails to close; ostium primum defect, in which there is inadequate development of the endocardial cushions of the first septum of the heart; and sinus venosus defect, in which the superior portion of the atrium fails to develop.

atrial septum [L *atrium* hall + *saeptum* fence], a partition between the left and right atria of the heart.

atrial standstill, a condition of complete failure of the atria to contract. Generally, a junctional pacemaker maintains continuation of ventricular activity during atrial standstill. P waves are absent in all ECG surface leads and A waves are absent in the jugular venous pulse and right atrial pressure tracings.

atrial systole, the contraction of the atria of the heart, which precedes ventricular contraction by a fraction of a second.

atrial tachycardia [L *atrium* hall; Gk *tachys* quick + *kardia* heart], rapid contraction of the atria due to an ectopic focus that may increase the beat to more than 200 per minute. The ventricles usually respond to each atrial contraction. When an attack begins or ends suddenly it is referred to as **paroxysmal atrial tachycardia (PAT)** and may be influenced by impulses from the vagus nerve. Attacks are often terminated by stimulation of the vagus nerve.

atrichosis [Gk *a, trichia* without hair + *osis* condition], a congenital absence of hair.

atrioventricular (AV) [L *atrium* hall, *ventriculum*], pertaining to an atrium and a ventricle.

atrioventricular (AV) block /ā′tre̅-ōven-trik′yələr/ [L *atrium + ventriculus* little belly], the slowed conduction or stoppage of the cardiac excitatory impulse, occurring at the atrioventricular node, bundle of His, or its branches. Kinds of AV block include first-degree block, with prolonged AV conduction, second-degree block, with partial AV block, and third-degree block, with complete atrioventricular block.

atrioventricular bundle. See **bundle of His.**

atrioventricular (AV) node, an area of specialized cardiac muscle that receives the cardiac impulse from the sinoatrial (SA) node and conducts it to the atrioventricular bundle of His and thence to the walls of the ventricles. The AV node is located in the septal wall of the right atrium.

atrioventricular rhythm, an obsolete term for a heart beat in control of the atrioventricular node.

atrioventricular septum, a small portion of membrane that separates the atria from the ventricles of the heart.

atrioventricular valve, a valve in the heart through which blood flows from the atria to the ventricles. The valve between the left atrium and left ventricle is the mitral valve; the right atrioventricular valve is the tricuspid valve.

at risk, the state of an individual or population being vulnerable to a particular disease or injury. The factors determining risk may be environmental or physiologic.

atrium /ā'trē-əm/, *pl.* **atria** [L, hall], a chamber or cavity, such as the right and left atria of the heart or the nasal cavity.

atrium of the heart, one of the two upper chambers of the heart. The right atrium receives deoxygenated blood from the superior vena cava, the inferior vena cava, and the coronary sinus. The left atrium receives oxygenated blood from the pulmonary veins.

atrophic arthritis. See **rheumatoid arthritis.**

atrophic catarrh [Gk *a, trophe* not nourishment; *kata* down, *rhoia* flow], an abnormal condition characterized by inflammation and discharge from the mucous membranes of the nose, accompanied by the loss of mucosal and submucosal tissue.

atrophic cirrhosis [Gk *a, trophe* atrophy, *kirrhos* yellowish coloration], a form of advanced portal cirrhosis with massive shrinkage of the liver.

atrophic fracture, a spontaneous fracture caused by atrophy, as in the bones of an elderly person.

atrophic gastritis, a chronic inflammation of the stomach, associated with degeneration of the gastric mucosa.

atrophic glossitis, a pathologic condition in which the various papillae are lost from the dorsum of the tongue resulting in a very sore and highly sensitive surface that makes eating difficult.

atrophic rhinitis [Gk *a, trophe* + *rhis* nose + *itis,* inflammation], a nasal condition in which there is atrophy of the mucous membrane of the nose, resulting in failure of the ciliary function and drying and crusting of the lining of the nasal passages. This may alter olfactory sensation.

atrophic vaginitis [Gk *a, trophe;* L *vagina* sheath; Gk *itis* inflammation], a condition of degeneration of the vaginal mucous membrane following menopause.

atrophied, decreased size of an organ, tissue, or body part due to disuse or disease.

atrophoderma [Gk *a, trophe* + *derma* skin], the wasting away or decrease in size of the skin. The atrophy may affect the entire body surface or only localized areas.

atrophy /at'rəfē/ [Gk *a, trophe* not nourishment], a wasting or diminution of size or physiologic activity of a part of the body because of disease or other influences. A skeletal muscle may undergo atrophy because of lack of physical exercise or as a result of neurologic or musculoskeletal disease. Cells of the brain and central nervous system may atrophy in old age because of restricted blood flow to those areas. **–atrophic,** *adj.,* **atrophy,** *v.*

atrophy of disuse [Gk *a, trophe;* L *dis* opposite of, *usus*], a shrinkage of tissues resulting from immobility or lack of exercise.

atropine /at'rōpēn/ [Gk *Atropos* one of the three Fates], an alkaloid from *Atropa belladonna* and *Datura stramonium* plants.

atropine sulfate, an antispasmodic and anticholinergic prescribed in the treatment of GI hypermotility, inflammation of the iris or the uvea, cardiac dysrhythmias, parkinsonism, and certain kinds of poisoning and as an adjunct to anesthesia.

atropine sulfate poisoning [Gk *Atropos;* L *sulphur, potio* drink], toxic effects of an overdose of a drug sometimes used as an adjunct to general anesthesia. Symptoms include tachycardia, hot and dry flushed skin, dry mouth with thirst, restlessness and excitement, urinary retention, constipation, and a burning pain in the throat. Treatment includes gastric lavage and administration of barbiturates, and pilocarpine if the eyes are involved.

attachment [Fr *attachement*], **1.** the state or quality of being affixed or attached. **2.** (in psychiatry) a mode of behavior in which one individual relates in an affiliative or dependent manner to another; a feeling of affection or loyalty that binds one person to another. **3.** See **bonding. 4.** (in dentistry) any device, such as a retainer or artificial crown, used to secure a partial denture to a natural tooth in the mouth.

attachment apparatus, the combination of tissues that invest and support the teeth, such as the cementum, the periodontal ligament, and the alveolar bone.

attending physician [L *attendere* to stretch], the physician who is responsible for a particular, usually private, patient. In a university setting, an attending physician often also has teaching responsibilities and holds a faculty appointment.

attention [L *attendere* to stretch], the element of cognitive functioning in which the mental focus is maintained on a specific issue, object, or activity.

attention deficit disorder, a syndrome affecting children, adolescents, and, rarely, adults characterized by learning and behavior disabilities. Symptoms include impairment in perception, conceptualization, language, memory, and motor skills, decreased attention span, increased impulsivity and emotional lability, and usually, but not always, hyperactivity.

attenuated /əten'yōō·ā'tid/ [L *attenure* to make thin], pertaining to the dilution of a solution or the reduction in virulence or toxicity of a microorganism or a drug by weakening it.

attenuated virus [L *attenuare* + *virus* poison], a strain of virus whose virulence has been lowered by physical or chemical processes or by repeated passage through the cells of another species. Vaccines made by attenuated strains are used to prevent tuberculosis, small pox, measles, mumps, rubella, polio, and yellow fever.

attenuation [L *attenuare* to make thin], the process of reduction, such as the attenuation of an x-ray beam by reducing its intensity or the weakening of the degree of virulence of a disease organism.

attenuation coefficient, (in positron emission tomography) a number that represents the difference between the number of photons that enter a body part being studied and the number that are not detected.

attic. See **epitympanic recess.**

attitude, 1. a body position or posture, particularly the fetal position in the uterus as determined by the degree of flexion of the head and extremities. 2. (in psychiatry) any of the major integrative forces in the development of personality that gives consistency to an individual's behavior.

attitudinal isolation [L *attitudo* posture], a type of social isolation that results from a person's own cultural or personal values.

attitudinal reflex, any reflex initiated by a change in position of the head or by a change in position of the head with respect to the position of the body. Kinds of attitudinal reflexes include **tonic neck reflex** and **tonic labyrinthine reflex.**

attraction [L *attrahere* to draw to], a tendency of the teeth or other maxillary or mandibular structures to elevate above their normal position.

attrition [L *atterere* to wear away], the process of wearing away or wearing down by friction.

at. wt, abbreviation for **atomic weight.**

atypia [Gk *a, typos* not type], a condition of being irregular or not standard.

atypical [Gk *a* not, *typos* type], a condition or object that is not of a usual or standard type.

atypical measles syndrome (AMS), a form of measles (rubeola) that tends to infect persons previously immunized by either killed measles vaccine or live, attenuated measles vaccine that may have been stored improperly. Symptoms vary somewhat from typical measles.

atypical *Mycobacterium* [Gk *a, typos* + *mykes* fungus, *bakterion* small staff], a group of mycobacteria, including both pathogenic and nonpathogenic forms, that are classified according to their ability to produce pigments, growth characteristics, and reactions to chemical tests.

atypical pneumonia [Gk *a, typos* + *peumon* lung, *ia* condition], a group of relatively mild symptoms of chills, headache, muscular pains, moderate fever, and coughing, but without evidence of a bacterial infection. Chest x-rays may show mottling at the bases. Eaton's agent, or *Mycoplasma pneumoniae,* may be the cause of the symptoms.

atypical somatoform disorder, an abnormal condition marked by physical symptoms and complaints that appear related to a preoccupation with an imagined defect in one's personal appearance or ability.

Au, symbol for the element **gold.**

audible [L *audire* to hear], capable of being heard. Some animals are able to hear sounds of higher or lower frequencies and different intensities than those audible to most humans.

audioanalgesia [L *audire* to hear; Gk *a, algos* not pain], the use of music to enhance relaxation and to distract a patient's mind from pain, as during dentistry.

audiogram /ô′dē·əgram′/ [Gk *audire* + Gk *gramma* record], a chart showing the acuteness of hearing of an individual as indicated by the ability to hear sounds and to distinguish different speech sounds.

audiologist [L *audire* + Gk *logos* science], a health professional with at least a masters degree who studies the sense of hearing, detects and diagnoses hearing loss,

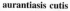

and works to provide rehabilitation of individuals with hearing loss.

audiology [L *audire* + Gk *logos* science], a field of research devoted to the study of hearing, especially impaired hearing that cannot be corrected by medical means. –**audiologic,** *adj.*

audiometer /ô′dē·om′ətər/ [L *audire* + Gk *metron* measure], an electric device for testing hearing.

audiometry /ô′dē·om′ətrē/, the testing of the sense of hearing. Various audiometric tests determine the lowest intensity of sound at which an individual can perceive an auditory stimulus (hearing threshold), hear different frequencies, and distinguish different speech sounds. –**audiometric,** *adj.*

audit, a review and evaluation of health care procedures.

auditory [L *auditorius* hearing], pertaining to the sense of hearing and the hearing organs involved.

auditory amnesia, [L *auditorius;* Gk *amnesia* forgetfulness], a loss of memory for the meaning of sounds.

auditory canal, one of two passageways for sound impulses passing through the ear. One leads from the outer ear to the tympanic membranes. The other, located in the temporal bone, contains the auditory nerve, which transmits impulses from the inner ear to the brain.

auditory hair [L *audire;* AS *haer*], one of the cells with hairlike processes in the spiral organ of Corti. The hairs, or cilia, function as sensory receptors.

auditory hallucination [L, *audire* + *alucinari* a wandering mind], a subjective experience of hearing voices or other sounds despite the absence of a real world stimulus to account for the phenomenon.

auditory meatus [L *audire* + *meatus* passage], **1.** external auditory meatus, a tubelike channel of the external ear extending from the auricle to the tympanum of the middle ear. **2.** internal auditory meatus, a short channel extending from the petrous part of the temporal bone to the fundus near the vestibule. It contains the eighth cranial nerve.

auditory ossicles [L *audire* + *ossiculum* little bone], the incus, the malleus, and the stapes, small bones in the middle ear that articulate with each other and the tympanic membrane. Sound waves are transmitted through them as the tympanic membrane vibrates.

auditory system assessment, an evaluation of the patient's ears and hearing and an investigation of present and past diseases or conditions that may be responsible for an auditory impairment.

auditory threshold [L *audire;* AS *therscold*], the lowest intensity at which a sound may be heard.

auditory tube. See **eustachian tube.**

auditory vertigo [L *audire* + *vertigo* dizziness], a form of vertigo that is associated with ear disease, with sensations of gyration, and when severe, prostration and vomiting.

Auerbach's plexus [Leopold Auerbach, Polish anatomist, b. 1828; L, *plexus,* plaited], the myenteric plexus, a group of autonomic nerve fibers and ganglia located in the muscle tissue of the intestinal tract.

Auer rod /ou′ər/ [John Auer, American physiologist, b. 1875], an abnormal, needle-shaped or round, pink-staining inclusion in the cytoplasm of myeloblasts and promyelocytes in acute myelogenous or myelomonocytic leukemia. These inclusions contain enzymes such as acid phosphatase, peroxidase, and esterase and may represent abnormal derivatives of cytoplasmic granules.

augmentation /ôg′məntā′shən/ [L *augmentare* to increase], a process in which a substance or mechanism can stimulate an increased rate of biologic activity, such as faster cell division or heart beat.

aura /ôr′ə/ [L, breath], **1.** *pl.* **aurae** /ôr′ē/, a sensation, as of light or warmth, that may precede an attack of migraine or an epileptic seizure. **2.** *pl.* **auras,** an emanation of light or color surrounding a person as seen in Kirlian photography and studied in healing techniques.

aural[1] /ôr′əl/, of or pertaining to the ear or hearing. –**aurally,** *adv.*

aural[2], of or pertaining to an aura.

aural forceps, a dressing forceps with fine, bent tips, used in aural surgery.

aural rehabilitation, a form of therapy in which hearing-impaired individuals are taught to improve their ability to communicate. Methods taught include, but are not limited to, speech-reading, auditory training, use of hearing aids, and use of assistive listening devices such as telephone amplifiers.

auramine /ôr′əmēn/, a yellow aniline dye used in the manufacture of paints, textiles, and rubber products. The experimental carcinogen in animals has been identified as a cause of bladder cancer in humans.

auranofin /ôr′ənof′in/, an oral antiarthritic drug prescribed for the treatment of rheumatoid arthritis.

aurantiasis cutis /ôr′əntī′əsis/ [L *aurantium* orange; Gk *osis* condition; L *cutis* skin], a yellowish skin pigmentation that results from eating excessive amounts of foods containing carotene, such as carrots.

auricle /ôr'ikəl/ [L *auricula* little ear], **1.** also called **pinna**. the external ear. **2.** the left or right cardiac atrium, so named because of its earlike shape.

auricular, 1. of or pertaining to the auricle of the ear. **2.** otic.

auricularis anterior, one of three extrinsic muscles of the ear. Arising from the anterior portion of the fascia in the temporal area and inserting into a projection in front of the helix, it functions to move the auricula forward and upward.

auricularis posterior, one of three extrinsic muscles of the ear. Arising from the mastoid area of the temporal bone by short aponeurotic fibers and inserting into the lower part of the cranial surface of the concha, it serves to draw the auricula backward.

auricularis superior, a thin, fan-shaped muscle that is one of three extrinsic muscles of the ear. It arises in the fascia of the temporal area and converges to insert with a thin, flattened tendon into the cranial surface of the auricula. It acts to draw the auricula upward.

auricular line, a hypothetical line passing through the external auditory meatuses and perpendicular to the Frankfort horizontal plane.

auricular point, the center of the external auditory meatus.

auriculin, a hormonelike substance with diuretic activity produced in the atria of the heart.

auriculoventriculostomy /ôrik'yŏōlōventrik'yŏōlos'təmē/ [L *auricula* + *ventriculus* little belly; Gk *stoma* opening], a surgical procedure that directs cerebrospinal fluid into the general circulation in the treatment of hydrocephalus. A polyethylene tube is passed from the lateral ventricle through a burr hole in the parietal skull area under the scalp and into the jugular vein for the discharge of cerebrospinal fluid into the superior vena cava or the right atrium.

auriosis. See chrysiasis.

auris dextra (a.d.), the Latin term for right ear.

auris sinistra (a.s.), the Latin term for left ear.

aurothioglucose /ôr'ōthī'ōglŏō'kōs/, an organic gold antiarthritic used in chrysotherapy for adjunctive treatment of adult and juvenile rheumatoid arthritis.

auscultation /ôs'kəltā'shən/ [L *auscultare* to listen], the act of listening for sounds within the body to evaluate the condition of the heart, lungs, pleura, intestines, or other organs or to detect the fetal heart sound. Auscultation may be performed directly, but most commonly a stethoscope is used to determine the frequency, intensity, duration, and quality of the sounds. **–auscultate,** *v.*

auscultatory percussion. See auscultation, percussion.

Austin Flint murmur, a presystolic murmur, similar to a mitral stenosis murmur, which may be detected at the apex of the heart.

Australia antigen, hepatitis B surface antigen (HBsAG), found in the serum of a person who has acute or chronic serum hepatitis or who is a carrier for that virus. Extremely dilute concentrations of the antigen can cause the disease.

Australian lift, a type of shoulder lift used to move a patient who is unable to assume a sitting position on a bed or other surface.

Australian Q fever. See Q fever.

autacoid /ô'təkoid/, any of a group of substances, as hormones, that are produced in one organ and are transported via blood or lymph as a means to control a physiologic process in another part of the body.

authenticity, (in psychiatry) emotional and behavioral openess; a quality of being genuine and trustworthy.

authoritarian personality, a group of behavioral traits characteristic of one who advocates obedience and strict adherence to the rules.

authority, a relationship between two or more persons or groups characterized by the influence one may exercise over the other through ideas, commands, suggestions, or instructions.

authority figure, a person who by virtue of status, strength, knowledge, or other recognized superiority exerts influence over others.

autism [Gk *autos* self], a mental disorder characterized by extreme withdrawal and an abnormal absorption in fantasy, accompanied by delusion, hallucination, and an inability to communicate verbally or to otherwise relate to people. **–autistic,** *adj.*

autistic disorder [Gk *autos* self], a severe pervasive developmental disorder with onset in infancy or childhood, characterized by impaired social interaction, impaired communication, and a remarkably restricted repertoire of activities and interests.

autistic phase, a period of preoedipal development, according to Mahler's system of personality stages. It lasts from birth to around 1 month and is considered normal.

autistic thought, a form of thinking in which the ideas have a private meaning to the individual. Fantasy life may be interpreted as reality.

autoactivation [Gk *autos* + *activus* active], a process of self-activation, as when a gland is stimulated by its own secretions.

autoagglutination [Gk *autos* + L *agglutinare* to glue], **1.** the agglutination or clumping of red blood cells by the serum of the same individual. **2.** the agglutination or clumping together of certain antigens such as bacteria.

autoamputation, the spontaneous detachment of a body part, usually the fourth or fifth toe, as occurs among the males of some African peoples. The condition is usually painless and has no other symptoms.

autoantibody /ô′tō·an′tibod′ē/ [Gk *autos* + *anti* against; AS *bodig* body], an immunoglobulin that reacts against a normal constituent in a person's body, such as nuclear material in the patient with systemic lupus erythematosus. Autoantibodies are found against gastric parietal cells in pernicious anemia, against platelets in autoimmune thrombocytopenia, and against antigens on the surface of erythrocytes in autoimmune hemolytic anemia.

autoantigen /ô′tō·an′tijin/ [Gk *autos* + *anti* against, *genein* to produce], an endogenous body constituent that stimulates the production of autoantibody and a resulting autoimmune reaction against one or more tissues of the person in whom the abnormal reaction occurs.

autochthonous idea /ôtok′thənəs/ [Gk *autos* + *chthon* earth], an idea that originates in the unconscious and arises spontaneously in the mind, independent of the conscious train of thought.

autoclave /ô′təklāv/, an appliance used to sterilize medical instruments or other objects with steam under pressure.

autodiploid /ô′tōdip′loid/ [Gk *autos* + *diploos* double, *eidos* form], **1.** also **autodiploidic.** of or pertaining to an individual, organism, strain, or cell containing two genetically identical or nearly identical chromosome sets that are derived from the same ancestral species and result from the duplication of the haploid set. **2.** such an individual, organism, strain, or cell.

autodiploidy /ô′tōdip′loidē/, the state or condition of having two genetically identical or nearly identical chromosome sets from the same ancestral species. Such a state enables cell division to occur in a normal manner.

autoeroticism [Gk *autos* + *eros* love], **1.** sensual, usually sexual, gratification of the self, usually obtained through the stimulus of one's own body without the participation of another person. **2.** sexual feeling or desire occurring without any external stimulus. **3.** (in Freudian psychoanalytic theory) an early phase of psychosexual development, occurring in the oral and the anal stages. **–autoerotic,** *adj.*

autoerythrocyte sensitization /ô′tō·ərith′rəsīt/ [Gk *autos* + *erythros* red, *kytos* cell], an unusual disorder characterized by the spontaneous appearance of painful, hemorrhagic spots on the anterior aspects of the arms and legs, resulting from hypersensitivity to the patient's own red blood cells. Psychoneurotic disorders may be associated with the disorder.

autoerythrocyte sensitization syndrome. See **Gardner-Diamond syndrome.**

autogenesis /ô′tōjen′əsis/ [Gk *autos* + *genein* to produce], **1.** abiogenesis. **2.** self-produced condition; a condition originating from within the organism. **–autogenetic, autogenic,** *adj.*

autogenic therapy, a mental health therapy based on the concept that natural forces in the brain are able to remove disturbing influences so that functional harmony can be restored in the mind and body.

autogenous /ôtoj′ənəs/, **1.** self-generating. **2.** originating from within the organism, as a toxin or vaccine.

autogenous graft [Gk *autos* + *genein* to produce, *graphion* stylus], a self-produced skin graft transplanted from one site to another in the same individual.

autogenous vaccine [Gk *autos* + *genein* to produce; L *vaccinus* cow], a vaccine prepared from cultures of the microorganism taken from a lesion of the patient to be treated.

autogeny. See **autogenesis.**

autograft [Gk *autos* + *graphion* stylus], surgical transplantation of any tissue from one part of the body to another location in the same individual. Autografts are commonly used to replace skin lost in severe burns.

autographism. See **dermatographia.**

autohemolysis /-hēmol′isis/ [Gk *autos* + *haima* blood, *lysein* to loosen], the destruction of erythrocytes by hemolytic agents found in the blood serum of the individual.

autohexaploid, autohexaploidic. See **autopolyploid.**

autohypnosis [Gk *autos* + *hypnos* sleep], the self-induction of hypnosis by an individual who concentrates on one subject to attain an altered state of consciousness. It may also occur in a person who has become sensitized to the process by undergoing hypnosis a number of times.

autoimmune [Gk *autos* + L *immunus* exempt], pertaining to the development of an immune response (autoantibodies or cellular immune response) to one's own tissues.

autoimmune disease, one of a large group of diseases characterized by the subversion or alteration of the function of the immune system of the body. Antigens normally present in the internal cells stimulate the development of antibodies, and the antibodies, unable to distinguish antigens of the internal cells from external antigens, act against the internal cell to cause localized and systemic reactions. These reactions affect the epithelial and the connective tissues of the body, causing a variety of diseases that can be divided into two general categories: the collagen diseases (including systemic lupus erythematosus, dermatomyositis, periarteritis nodosa, scleroderma, and rheumatoid arthritis) and the autoimmune hemolytic disorders (including idiopathic thrombocytopenic purpura, acquired hemolytic anemia, and autoimmune leukopenia).

autoimmunity, an abnormal characteristic or condition in which the body reacts against constituents of its own tissues. Autoimmunity may result in hypersensitivity and autoimmune disease.

autoimmunization, the process whereby an individual's immune system develops antibodies against one or more of the person's own tissues.

autoinoculation [Gk *autos* + L *inoculare* to graft], the inoculation of a microorganism obtained by contact with a lesion on one's own body, producing a secondary infection.

autointoxication [Gk *autos* + L *in*; Gk *toxikon* poison], a condition of poisoning by substances generated by one's own body, such as toxins resulting from a metabolic disorder.

autolet /ô′tōlet/, a small, sharp instrument, as a lancet, that is used to obtain a capillary blood specimen.

autologous [Gk *autos* + *logos* ratio], pertaining to a tissue or structure occurring naturally and derived from the same individual.

autologous graft [Gk *autos, logos, graphion* stylus], the transfer of tissue from one site to another on the same body.

autologous transfusion /ôtol′əgəs/, a procedure in which blood is removed from a donor and stored for a variable period before it is returned to the donor's own circulation.

automatic behavior. See **automatism.**

automatic bladder. See **spastic bladder.**

automatic infiltration detector [Gk *automatismos* self-action], a temperature-sensitive device that activates an alarm and automatically stops an intravenous infusion when infiltration of the intravenous fluid occurs. The device detects any cooling of the skin at the intravenous site, a common sign of infiltration.

automaticity /ô′tōmatis′itē/, a property of specialized excitable tissue that allows self-activation through spontaneous development of an action potential, as in the pacemaker cells of the heart.

automatic mallet condenser. See **mechanical condenser.**

automatic speech, speech composed of or containing words or phrases spoken without voluntary control, often consisting of expletives, profanities, and greetings.

automation, use of a machine designed to follow repeatedly and automatically a predetermined sequence of individual operations.

automatism /ôtom′ətiz′əm/ [Gk *automatismos* self-action], **1.** (in physiology) involuntary function of an organ system independent of apparent external stimuli, such as the beating of the heart, or dependent on external stimuli but not consciously controlled, such as the dilatation of the pupil of the eye. **2.** (in philosophy) the theory that the body acts as a machine and that the mind, whose processes depend solely on brain activity, is a noncontrolling adjunct of the body. **3.** (in psychology) mechanical, repetitive, and undirected behavior that is not consciously controlled, as seen in psychomotor epilepsy, hysteric states, and such acts as sleepwalking. Kinds of automatism include **ambulatory, command,** and **immediate posttraumatic automatism.**

autonomic /ô′tənom′ik/ [Gk *autos* + *nomos* law] **1.** having the ability to function independently without outside influence. **2.** of or pertaining to the autonomic nervous system.

autonomic-active bronchodilators, a category of drugs with actions that dilate bronchiolar smooth muscle tissue by acting on the autonomic nervous system. Examples include adrenergic drugs, such as epinephrine, and anticholinergic products, such as atropine sulfate.

autonomic drug, any of a large group of drugs that mimic or modify the function of the autonomic nervous system.

autonomic dysreflexia, a dysreflexia that is the result of impaired function of the autonomic nervous system caused by simultaneous sympathetic and parasympathetic activity.

autonomic ganglion [Gk *autos* + *nomos* law; *gagglion* knot], a group of autonomic neuron cell bodies with a common function.

autonomic hyperreflexia, a neurologic

disorder characterized by a discharge of sympathetic nervous system impulses as a result of stimulation of the bladder, large intestine, or other visceral organs.

autonomic imbalance [Gk *autos* + *nomos;* L *in* not, *bilanx* having two scales], a disruption of a segment of the autonomic nervous system, as in autonomic ataxia.

autonomic nerve [Gk *autos* + *nomos* + *neuron* nerve], a nerve of the autonomic nervous system, which includes both the sympathetic and parasympathetic nervous systems, with the ability to function independently and spontaneously as needed to maintain optimum status of bodily activities.

autonomic nervous system, the part of the nervous system that regulates involuntary vital function, including the activity of the cardiac muscle, the smooth muscle, and the glands. It has two divisions: The **sympathetic nervous system** accelerates heart rate, constricts blood vessels, and raises blood pressure; the **parasympathetic nervous system** slows heart rate, increases intestinal peristalsis and gland activity, and relaxes sphincters.

autonomic neuropathy, self-controlling, functionally independent disturbances in the peripheral nervous system.

autonomic reflex, any of a large number of normal reflexes governing and regulating the functions of the viscera. Autonomic reflexes control such activities of the body as blood pressure, heart rate, peristalsis, sweating, and urination.

autonomous bladder /ôton'məs/. See flaccid bladder.

autonomy /ôton'əmē/ [Gk *autos* + *nomos* law], the quality of having the ability or tendency to function independently. –**autonomous,** *adj.*

autonomy drive, a behavioral trait characterized by the attempt of an individual to master the environment and to impose the person's purposes on it.

autopentaploid, autopentaploidic. See autopolyploid.

autoplastic maneuver, (in psychology) a process that is part of adaptation, involving an adjustment within the self.

autoplasty /ô'təplas'tē/ [Gk *autos* + *plassein* to shape], a plastic surgery procedure in which autografts, or parts of the patient's own tissues, are used to replace or repair body areas damaged by disease or injury.

autopolyploid /ô'tōpol'iploid/ [Gk *autos* + *polyploos* many times, *eidos* form], **1.** also **autopolyploidic.** of or pertaining to an individual, organism, strain, or cell that has more than two genetically identical or nearly identical sets of chromosomes that

are derived from the same ancestral species. **2.** such an individual, organism, strain, or cell.

autopolyploidy /ô'tōpol'iploi'dē/, the state or condition of having more than two identical or nearly identical sets of chromosomes.

autopsy /ô'topsē/ [Gk *autos* + *opsis* view], a postmortem examination performed to confirm or determine the cause of death. –**autopsic, autopsical,** *adj.,* **autopsist,** *n.*

autopsy pathology, the study of disease by the examination of the body after death by a pathologist.

autoregulation [Gk *autos* + L *regula* rule], an intrinsic capacity of tissues to regulate their own blood flow due to the self-excitable contractile process of smooth muscle that acts to constrict and dilate vessels. It allows organ systems to maintain constant blood flow despite variations in systemic arterial pressure and is an essential mechanism to meet the metabolic needs of an organ.

autosensitization [Gk *autos* + L *sentire* to feel], the sensitization of an individual by humoral antibodies or a delayed cellular reaction to substances in his or her own body tissues.

autoserous treatment /ô'təsir'əs/ [Gk *autos* + L *serum* whey], therapy of an infectious disease by inoculating the patient with the patient's own serum.

autosite /ô'təsīt/ [Gk *autos* + *sitos* food], the larger, more normally formed member of unequal or asymmetric, conjoined twins on whom the other smaller fetus depends for various physiologic functions and for nutrition and growth. –**autositic.** *adj.*

autosomal /ô'təsō'məl/ [Gk *autos* + *soma* body], **1.** pertaining to or characteristic of an autosome. **2.** pertaining to any condition transmitted by an autosome.

autosomal dominant inheritance, a pattern of inheritance in which the transmission of a dominant gene on an autosome causes a characteristic to be expressed. Affected individuals have an affected parent unless the condition is the result of a fresh mutation. Half of the children of a heterozygous affected parent are affected. All of the children of a homozygous affected parent are affected.

autosomal inheritance, a pattern of inheritance in which the transmission of traits depends on the presence or absence of certain genes on the autosomes. The pattern may be dominant or recessive. Kinds of autosomal inheritance are **autosomal dominant inheritance** and **autosomal recessive inheritance.**

autosomal recessive inheritance, a pattern of inheritance in which the transmission of a recessive gene on an autosome results in a carrier state if the person is heterozygous for the trait and in the affected state if the person is homozygous for the trait. One fourth of the children of two unaffected heterozygous parents are affected. All of the children of two homozygous affected parents are affected.

autosome /ô'təsōm/, any chromosome that is not a sex chromosome and that appears as a homologous pair in the somatic cell. Humans have 22 pairs of autosomes, which are involved in transmitting all genetic traits and conditions other than those that are sex-linked.

autosplenectomy /ô'tōsplinek'təmē/ [Gk *autos* + *splen* spleen, *ektome* excision], a progressive shrinking of the spleen that may occur in sickle cell anemia. The spleen is replaced by fibrous tissue and becomes nonfunctional.

autosuggestion [Gk *autos* + L *suggerere* to suggest], an idea, thought, attitude, or belief suggested to oneself, often as a formula or incantation, as a means of controlling one's behavior.

autotetraploid,   autotetraploidic. See **autopolyploid.**

autotopagnosia /ô'tōtop'əg·nō'zhə/ [Gk *autos* + *topos* place, *a, gnosis* not knowledge], the inability to recognize or localize the various parts of the body because of organic brain damage.

autotransfusion, the collection, anticoagulation, filtration, and reinfusion of blood from an active bleeding site. It may be used in cases of major trauma or in major surgery when blood can be collected from a sterile site.

autotriploid,   autotriploidic. See **autopolyploid.**

autumn fever. See **leptospirosis.**

auxanology /ôks'ənol'əjē/ [Gk *auxein* to grow, *logos* science], the scientific study of growth and development. –**auxanologic,** *adj.*

auxesis /ôksē'sis/, *pl.* **auxeses** [Gk *auxein* + *osis* condition], an increase in size or volume because of cell expansion rather than of an increase in the number of cells or tissue elements; hypertrophy. –**auxetic,** *adj., n.*

auxiliary [L *auxilium* aid], an individual or group serving in helpful, supporting, or complementary tasks in a clinical setting.

auxilliary enzyme, in a coupled assay system, an enzyme that links the enzyme being measured with an indicator enzyme.

auxiliary storage, a storage device for adding to the main storage of the computer, employing such media as floppy disks, hard disks, cassette tapes, magnetic tapes, or cartridge tapes.

AV, abbreviation for **arteriovenous, atrioventricular,** *auriculoventricular.*

available arch length [ME *availen* to be of use], the length or space in a dental arch that is available for all the natural teeth of an individual.

avalvular / āvalv'yələr/ [Gk *a* without + L *valva* valve], an absence of one or more valves.

avantin. See **isopropyl alcohol.**

avascular /āvas'kyŏōlər/ [Gk *a* not; L *vasculum* vessel], **1.** (of a tissue area) not receiving a sufficient supply of blood. **2.** (of a kind of tissue) not having blood vessels.

avascular graft [Gk *a* without + L *vasculum* vessel; Gk *graphion* stylus], a tissue graft in which there is no infiltration of blood vessels.

avascularization [Gk *a* without + L *vasculum* vessel], pertaining to a diversion of blood flow away from tissues.

AVB, abbreviation for **atrioventricular block.**

aversion therapy [L *aversus* a turning away], a form of behavior therapy in which punishment or unpleasant or painful stimuli, such as electric shock or drugs that induce nausea, are used in the suppression of undesirable behavior.

aversive stimulus, a stimulus, as electric shock, that causes psychic or physical pain.

aviation medicine, a branch of medicine that is concerned with the health effects of travel by aircraft, including such aspects as jetlag, restricted body movement for long periods, and reaction to violent aircraft movement in turbulent weather.

aviation physiology, a branch of physiology that is concerned with the effects on humans and animals exposed for long periods in pressurized cabins, radiation hazards at high altitudes, weightlessness, disturbances of biological rhythms, acceleration, and mental functions under stressful flying conditions.

avidin, a glycoprotein in raw egg white with strong affinity for biotin.

avidity /avid'itē/ [L *avidus* eager], a measure of the binding strength of antibodies to multiple antigenic determinants on natural antigens.

A-V interval [L *intervallum* space between ramparts], the time or space that separates an atrial systole and a ventricular systole in producing an electrocardiogram.

avirulent [Gk *a* not + L *virus* poison], not virulent; not pathogenic.

avitaminosis /āvī'təminō'sis/ [Gk *a* not; L *vita* life, amine, *osis* condition], a condition resulting from a deficiency of or the lack of absorption or use of one or more essential vitamins in the diet.

AV nicking, a vascular abnormality on the retina of the eye, visible on ophthalmologic examination, in which a vein is compressed by an arteriovenous crossing. The vein appears "nicked" because of constriction or spasm.

Avogadro's law /av'ōgad'rōz/ [Count Amedeo Avogadro, Italian physicist, b. 1776], a law in physics stating that equal volumes of all gases at a given temperature and pressure contain the identical number of molecules.

Avogadro's number, the number of atoms in exactly 12 grams of the isotope of carbon C_{12}, or 6.02×10^{23}. One mole of any monoatomic element contains this number of atoms and one mole of any polyatomic element or molecule contains this number of molecules. The mass of a mole of any element or compound is a mass in grams numerically equal to the relative atomic mass of the atoms or molecules.

avoidance [ME *avoiden* to empty], (in psychiatry) a conscious or unconscious defense mechanism, physical or psychologic, by which an individual tries to avoid or escape from unpleasant stimuli, conflicts, or feelings, such as anxiety, fear, pain, or danger.

avoidance-avoidance conflict, a conflict resulting from the confrontation of two or more alternative goals or desires that are equally aversive and undesirable.

avoidance conditioning, the establishment of certain patterns of behavior to avoid unpleasant or painful stimuli.

avoidant personality, a personality disorder characterized by hypersensitivity to rejection and a reluctance to start a relationship because of a fear of not being accepted uncritically.

avoirdupois weight /av'ərdəpoiz'/ [OF *avoir de pois* property of weight], the English system of weights in which there are 7,000 grains, 256 drams, or 16 ounces to 1 pound. One ounce in this system equals 28.35 g, and 1 pound equals 453.59 g.

avulsed teeth /əvulst/ [L *avulsio* a pulling away], teeth that have been forcibly displaced from their normal position. Also spelled **evulsed teeth.**

avulsion [L *avulsio* a pulling away], the separation, by tearing, of any part of the body from the whole, such as an umbilical cord torn in the process of delivering the placenta. **–avulse,** *v.*

avulsion fracture, a fracture caused by the tearing away of a fragment of bone where a strong ligamentous or tendinous attachment forcibly pulls the fragment away from osseous tissue.

awake anesthesia [ME *awakenen*], an anesthetic procedure in which analgesia and anesthesia are accomplished without loss of consciousness and the concomitant need for life support equipment, personnel, and expertise. Dental procedures and certain kinds of surgery are performed using awake anesthesia.

AWOL /ā'wôl/, abbreviation for **absent without leave.**

axial (A) [Gk *axon* axle], **1.** pertaining to or situated on the axis of a structure or part of the body. **2.** (in dentistry) relating to the long axis of a tooth.

axial current, the central part of the blood current.

axial gradient, 1. the variation in metabolic rate in different parts of the body. **2.** the development toward the body axis or its parts in relation to the metabolic rate in the various parts.

axial illumination. See **illumination.**

axial neuritis. See **parenchymatous neuritis.**

axial skeleton [L *axis* axle; Gk *skeletos* dried up], the bones forming the axis of the skeleton, including the skull, vertebrae, ribs, and sternum.

axial spillway, a groove that crosses a cusp ridge or a marginal ridge and extends onto an axial surface of a tooth.

axilla /aksil'ə/, *pl.* **axillae** [L, wing], a pyramid-shaped space forming the underside of the shoulder between the upper part of the arm and the side of the chest. **–axillary,** *adj.*

axillary abscess [L *axilla* + *abscedere* to go away], an abscess in the armpit.

axillary anesthesia. See **brachial plexus anesthesia.**

axillary artery /ak'sələr'ē/ [L *axilla* wing], one of a pair of continuations of the subclavian arteries that starts at the outer border of the first rib and ends at the distal border of the teres major, where it becomes the brachial artery.

axillary nerve, one of the last two branches of the posterior cord of the brachial plexus before the posterior cord becomes the radial nerve.

axillary node, one of the lymph glands of the axilla that help fight infections in the chest, armpit, neck, and arm and drain lymph from those areas. The 20 to 30 axillary nodes are divided into the lateral group, the anterior group, the posterior group, the central group, and the medial group.

axillary temperature [L *axilla* wing + *temperatura*], the body temperature as recorded by a thermometer placed in the armpit. The reading is generally 0.5 to 1.0 degree less than the oral temperature.

axillary vein, one of a pair of veins of the upper limb that begins at the junction of the basilic and the brachial veins near the distal border of the teres major and becomes the subclavian vein at the outer border of the first rib.

axis, *pl.* **axes** /ak'sēz/ [Gk *axon* axle] **1.** (in anatomy) a line that passes through the center of the body, or a part of the body, such as the frontal axis, binauricular axis, and basifacial axis. **2.** the second cervical vertebra about which the atlas rotates, allowing the head to be turned, extended, and flexed.

axis artery, one of a pair of extensions of the subclavian arteries, running into and supplying the upper limb, continuing into the forearm as the palmar interosseous artery.

axis cylinder. See **axon.**

axis traction, 1. the process of pulling a baby's head with obstetric forceps in a direction in line with the path of least resistance, following the curve of Carus through the mother's birth canal. **2.** *informal.* any mechanical device attached to obstetric forceps to facilitate pulling in the proper direction.

axoaxonic synapse /ak'sō·akson'ik/ [Gk *axon* axle (to) *axon* axle], a type of synapse in which the axon of one neuron comes in contact with the axon of another neuron.

axodendritic synapse /ak'sōdendrit'ik/ [Gk *axon* + *dendron* tree], a type of synapse in which the axon of one neuron comes in contact with the dendrites of another neuron.

axodendrite [Gk *axon* axle, *dendron* tree], a nonmedullated fibril appendage of the main axon of a nerve cell.

axodendrosomatic synapse /ak'sōden'drō-sōmat'ik/, a type of synapse in which the axon of one neuron comes in contact with both the dendrites and the cell body of another neuron.

axon /ak'son/ [Gk, axle], the cylindric extension of a nerve cell that conducts impulses away from the neuron cell body. Axons may be bare or sheathed in myelin.

axon flare, vasodilatation, reddening, and increased sensitivity of skin surrounding an injured area, caused by an axon reflex.

axonotmesis /ak'sənotmē'sis/ [Gk *axon* + *temnein* to cut], an interruption of the axon with subsequent wallerian degeneration of the distal nerve segment.

axon reflex, a neuron reflex in which an afferent impulse travels along a nerve fiber away from the cell body until it reaches a branching, where it is diverted to an end organ without entering the cell body. It does not involve a complete reflex arc, and therefore it is not a true reflex (vasodilation that occurs when the skin is stimulated).

axon sheath [Gk *axle;* AS *scaeth*], a laminated myelin sheath that is interrupted at intervals by nodes of Ranvier.

axoplasmic flow /ak'sōplaz'mik/ [Gk *axon* + *plassein* to shape], the continuous pulsing, undulating movement of the cytoplasm between the cell body of a neuron, where protein synthesis occurs, and the axon fiber to supply it with the substances vital for the maintenance of activity and for repair.

axosomatic synapse /ak'sōsōmat'ik/ [Gk *axon* + *soma* body], a type of synapse in which the axon of one neuron comes in contact with the cell body of another neuron.

azatadine maleate /azat'ədēn/, an antihistamine with antiserotonin, anticholinergic, and sedative effects used in the treatment of allergic rhinitis and chronic urticaria.

azathioprine /az'əthī'ōprēn/, an immunosuppressive prescribed to prevent organ rejection after transplantation and in the treatment of lupus erythematosus and other systemic inflammatory diseases.

azidothymidine /az'ədōthī'midēn/. See **zidovudine.**

azlocillin /az'lōsil'in/ **sodium,** a semisynthetic penicillin antibiotic prescribed for lower respiratory tract, urinary tract, skin, and bone and joint infections and bacterial septicemia caused by susceptible strains of microorganisms, mainly *Pseudomonas aeruginosa.*

azo compounds [Fr *azote* nitrogen], one of many organic aromatic compounds containing the divalent chromophore, -N=N-. They are produced by the alkaline reduction of nitro compounds.

azo dye /ā'zō/, a type of nitrogen-containing compound used in commercial coloring materials. Some forms of the chemical are potential carcinogens.

azoospermia /āzō'əspur'mē·ə/ [Gk *a, zoon* not animal, *sperma* seed], lack of spermatozoa in the semen. It may be caused by testicular dysfunction or by blockage of the tubules of the epididymis, or it may be induced by vasectomy.

azotemia /az'ōtē'mē·ə/ [Fr *azote* nitrogen; Gk *haima* blood], the retention in the blood of excessive amounts of nitrogenous compounds. The condition is caused by failure of the kidneys to remove urea from the blood. **–azotemic,** *adj.*

azoturia /az'ōtŏŏr'ē·ə/ [Fr *azote* nitrogen + Gk *ouron* urine], an excess of nitrogenous compounds including urea in the urine.

AZT, a trademark for an HIV virus inhibitor (zidovudine).

AZ test. See **Ascheim-Zondek test.**

azul, azula. See **pinta.**

azygos. See **azygous.**

azygospore /az′igəspôr′/ [Gk *a, zygon* not yoke, *sporos* seed], a spore that is produced directly from a gamete that does not undergo conjugation, as in certain algae and fungi.

azygous /az′əgəs/ [Gk *a, zygon* not yoke], occurring as a single entity or part, such as any unpaired anatomic structure; not part of a pair. Also **azygos.** **–azygous** /az′əgos′/, *n.*

azygous lobe, a congenital anomaly of the lung caused by a fold of pleural tissue carried by the azygous vein during descent into the thorax during embryonic development. This produces an extra lobe in the right upper lung.

azygous vein, one of the seven veins of the thorax. Beginning opposite the first or second lumbar vertebra, it ends in the superior vena cava.

B, symbol for the element **boron.**

Ba, symbol for the element **barium.**

BA, abbreviation for *Bachelor of Arts.*

babbling, a stage in speech development characterized by the production of strings of speech sounds in vocal play.

Babcock's operation [William W. Babcock, American surgeon, b. 1872], the extirpation of a varicosed saphenous vein by inserting an acorn-tipped sound, tying the vein to the sound, and drawing it out.

babesiosis /bəbē′sē·ō′sis/[Victor Babès, Rumanian bacteriologist, b. 1854], an infection caused by protozoa of the genus *Babesia.* The infective organism is introduced into the host through the bite of ticks of the species *Ixodes dammini.*

Babinski's reflex /babin′skēz/ [Josef F.F. Babinski, French neurologist, b. 1857], dorsiflexion of the big toe with extension and fanning of the other toes elicited by firmly stroking the lateral aspect of the sole of the foot. The reflex is normal in newborn infants and abnormal in children and adults.

babymain [ME *babe*], **1.** an infant or young child, especially one who is not yet able to walk or talk. **2.** to treat gently or with special care.

Baby bottle tooth decay, a dental condition that occurs in children between 12 months and 3 years of age as a result of being given a bottle at bedtime, resulting in prolonged exposure of the teeth to milk or juice. Caries are formed because pools of milk or juice in the mouth break down to lactic acid and other decay-causing substances. Preventive measures include elimination of the bedtime feeding or substitution of water for milk or juice in the nighttime bottle.

Baby Jane Doe regulations, rules established in 1984 by the U.S. Health and Human Services Department requiring state governments to investigate complaints about parental decisions involving the treatment of handicapped infants. The controversial regulations have been held illegal by a federal court. The popular name for the federal rules was taken from the name "Jane Doe" given to an infant born in New York and who became the object of a campaign to force life-saving surgery for the child over the objections of the parents.

baby talk, 1. the speech patterns and sounds of young children learning to talk, characterized by mispronunciation, imperfect syntax, repetition, and phonetic modifications, such as lisping or stuttering. **2.** the intentionally oversimplified manner of speech, imitative of young children learning to talk, used by adults in addressing children or pets. **3.** the speech patterns characteristic of regressive stages of various mental disorders, especially schizophrenia.

bacampicillin hydrochloride, a semisynthetic penicillin prescribed in the treatment of respiratory tract, urinary tract, skin, and gonococcal infections.

Bachelor of Science in Nursing (BSN), an academic degree awarded on satisfactory completion of a 4-year course of study in an institution of higher learning. The recipient is eligible to take the national certifying examination to become a registered nurse.

Bacillaceae /bas′əlā′si·ē/ [L *bacillum* small rod], a family of *Schizomycetes* of the order *Eubacteriales,* consisting of gram-positive, rod-shaped cells that can produce cylindric, ellipsoid, or spheric endospores. Some are parasitic on insects and animals and are pathogenic.

bacillary dysentery. See **shigellosis.**

bacille Calmette-Guérin (BCG) /kalmet′-gäraN′/ [Léon C.A. Calmette, French bacteriologist, b. 1863; Camille Guérin, French bacteriologist, b. 1872], an attenuated strain of tubercle bacilli, used in many countries as a vaccine against tuberculosis, most often administered intradermally, with a multiple-puncture disk. It appears to prevent the more serious forms of tuberculosis and to give some protection to persons living in areas where tuberculosis is prevalent.

bacilli /basil′ī/ *sing.* **bacillum** [L *bacillum* small rod], any rod-shaped bacteria.

bacilliform /bəsil′ifôrm/, rod-shaped, like a bacillus.

bacilluria /bas′əlŏŏr′ē·ə/ [L *bacillum* + Gk *ouron* urine], the presence of bacilli in the urine.

Bacillus /basil′as/ [L *bacillum* small rod],

a genus of aerobic, gram-positive spore-producing bacteria in the family Bacillaceae, order Eubacteriales, including 33 species, three of which are pathogenic.

Bacillus anthracis, a species of gram-positive, facultative anaerobe that causes anthrax.

bacillus Calmette-Guérin vaccine. See **BCG vaccine.**

bacitracin /bas'itrā'sin/ [L *bacillum* + *Tracy* surname of patient in whom toxin-producing bacillus species was isolated], an antibacterial prescribed for skin infections sensitive to bacitracin.

back [AS *baec*], the posterior portion of the trunk of the body between the neck and the pelvis. The back is divided by a middle furrow that lies over the tips of the spinous processes of the vertebrae. The upper cervical vertebrae cannot be felt in this furrow, but the seventh cervical vertebra is easily distinguished just above the more prominent first thoracic vertebra. The skeletal portion of the back includes the thoracic and the lumbar vertebrae and both scapulas. The root of the spine of the scapula is on a level in the back with the spine of the third thoracic vertebra, and the inferior angle of the scapula is on a level with the spine of the seventh thoracic vertebra.

backache [AS *baec* + ME *aken*], pain in the lumbar, lumbosacral, or cervical regions of the back, varying in sharpness and intensity. Causes may include muscle strain or other muscular disorders or pressure on the root of a nerve, such as the sciatic nerve, caused in turn by a variety of factors, including a ruptured vertebral disk. Treatment may include heat, ultrasound, devices to provide support for the affected area, bed rest, surgical intervention, and medications to relieve pain and relax spasm of the muscle of the affected area.

back-action condenser, (in dentistry) an instrument for compacting amalgams that has a U-shaped shank to develop the condensing force from a pulling motion rather than the more common pushing motions.

backcross [AS *baec* + *cruc* cross], **1.** (in genetics) the cross of a first filial generation hybrid with one of the parents or with a genotype that is identical to the parental strain. **2.** the organism or strain produced by such a cross.

background radiation [AS *baec* + OE *grund* ground], naturally occurring radiation emitted by materials in the soil, ground waters, and building material, radioactive substances in the body, especially potassium 40 (^{40}K), and cosmic rays from outer space. Each year the average

person is exposed to 44 millirads (mrad) of cosmic radiation, 44 mrads from external terrestrial radiation, and 18 mrads from naturally occurring internal radioactive sources.

back pressure [AS *baec*; L *premere* to press], pressure that builds in a vessel or a cavity as fluid is accumulated.

backscatter radiation. See **scattered radiation.**

baclofen, an antispastic agent prescribed for the alleviation of spasticity.

bacteremia /bak'tirē'mē·ə/ [Gk *bakterion* small staff, *haima* blood], the presence of bacteria in the blood. **–bacteremic,** *adj.*

bacteremic shock. See **septic shock.**

bacteria /baktir'ē·ə/, *sing.* **bacterium** [Gk *bakterion* small staff], any of the small unicellular microorganisms of the class Schizomycetes. The genera vary morphologically, being spheric (cocci), rod-shaped (bacilli), spiral (spirochetes), or comma-shaped (vibrios).

bacterial aneurysm, a localized dilatation in the wall of a blood vessel caused by the growth of bacteria, often following septicemia or bacteremia and usually occurring in peripheral vessels.

bacterial endocarditis, an acute or subacute bacterial infection of the endocardium or the heart valves or both. The condition is characterized by heart murmur, prolonged fever, bacteremia, splenomegaly, and embolism.

bacterial food poisoning, a toxic condition resulting from the ingestion of food contaminated by certain bacteria. Acute infectious gastroenteritis caused by various species of *Salmonella* is characterized by fever, chills, nausea, vomiting, diarrhea, and general discomfort beginning 8 to 48 hours after ingestion and continuing for several days. Food poisoning caused by the neurotoxin of *Clostridium botulinum* is characterized by GI symptoms, disturbances of vision, weakness or paralysis of muscles, and, in severe cases, respiratory failure.

bacterial inflammation [L *bacterium* + *inflammare* to set afire], any inflammation that is part of a body's response to a bacterial infection.

bacterial kinase, **1.** a kinase of bacterial origin. **2.** a bacterial enzyme that activates plasminogen, the precursor of plasmin.

bacterial meningitis. See **meningitis.**

bacterial plaque, a film comprised of microorganisms that attaches to the teeth and often causes caries and infections of the gums. Mucin secreted by the salivary glands is also a component of plaque.

bacterial protein, a protein produced by a bacterium.

bacterial resistance, the ability of certain strains of bacteria to develop a tolerance toward specific antibiotics.

bacterial toxin, any poisonous substance produced by a bacterium. Kinds of bacterial toxins include **endotoxins** and **exotoxins.**

bacterial vaginosis, a chronic inflammation of the vagina caused by a bacterium, *Gardnerella vaginalis.*

bactericidal /baktir′isĭ′dəl/, destructive to bacteria.

bactericidal antibiotic [L *bacterium* + *caedere* to kill, Gk, *anti,* against, *bios,* life], an antibiotic drug that kills bacteria.

bactericide /baktir′əsīd/, any drug or other agent that kills bacteria.

bactericidin [Gk *bakterion* + L *caedere* to kill], an antibody that kills bacteria in the presence of complement.

bacteriologic sputum examination, a laboratory procedure to determine the presence or absence of bacteria in a specimen of a patient's sputum. Part of the specimen is examined microscopically and part is mixed with culture media and allowed to incubate for more specific examination later.

bacteriologist, a specialist in bacteriology.

bacteriology [Gk *bakterion* + *logos* science], the scientific study of bacteria. **–bacteriologic, bacteriological,** *adj.*

bacteriolysin /baktir′ē·ŏlĭ′sin/ [Gk *bakterion* + *lyein* to loosen], an antibody that causes the breakdown of a particular species of bacterial cell.

bacteriolysis /baktir′ē·ŏl′əsis/, the breakdown of bacteria intracellularly or extracellularly. **–bacteriolytic,** *adj.*

bacteriophage /baktir′ē·əfāj′/ [Gk *bakterion* + *phagein* to eat], any virus that causes lysis of host bacteria, including the blue-green "algae." Bacteriophages resemble other viruses in that each is composed of either ribonucleic acid or deoxyribonucleic acid. **–bacteriophagic,** *adj.,* **bacteriophagy** /-of′əjē/, *n.*

bacteriophage typing, the process of identifying a species of bacteria according to the type of virus that attacks it.

bacteriostasis /baktir′ē·ŏs′təsis/ [L *bacterium;* Gk *stasis* standing still], a state of suspended growth and/or reproduction of bacteria.

bacteriostatic /baktir′ē·əstat′ik/ [Gk *bakterion* + *statikos* standing], tending to restrain the development or the reproduction of bacteria.

bacteriuria /baktir′ēyŏŏr′ē·ə/, the presence of bacteria in the urine.

bacteroid /bak′təroid/, **1.** of, pertaining to, or resembling bacteria. **2.** a structure that resembles a bacterium. Also **bacterioid** /baktir′ē·oid/. **–bacteroidal, bacterioidal,** *adj.*

Bacteroides /bak′təroi′dēz/ [Gk *bakterion* small staff, *eidos* form], a genus of obligate anaerobic bacilli normally found in the colon, mouth, genital tract, and upper respiratory system. Severe infection may result from the invasion of the bacillus through a break in the mucous membrane.

BAEP, abbreviation for **brainstem auditory-evoked potential.**

baffling, the process of removing large water particles from suspension in a jet nebulizer so that the particles entering the patient's airways are of a uniform therapeutic size.

bag [AS *baelg*], a flexible or dilatable sac or pouch to contain gas, fluid, or semisolid material such as crushed ice. Several types of bags are used in medical or surgical procedures to dilate the anus, vagina, or other body openings.

bagasse /bəgas′/ [Fr, cane trash], the crushed fibers or the residue of sugar cane.

bagassosis /bag′əsō′sis/, a self-limited lung disease caused by an allergic response to bagasse, the fungi-laden, dusty debris left after the syrup has been extracted from sugar cane.

bagging, *informal.* the artificial respiration performed with a ventilator or respirator bag, such as an Ambu bag or Hope resuscitator. The bag is squeezed to deliver air to the patient's lungs as the mask is held over the mouth.

bag of waters. the membranous sac of amniotic fluid surrounding the fetus in the uterus of a pregnant woman.

bag-valve-mask resuscitator, a device consisting of a manually compressible container with a plastic bag of oxygen at one end and at the other a one-way valve and mask that fit over the mouth and nose of a person to be resuscitated.

Bain Breathing Circuit, a continuous-flow anesthetic system that does not require a soda-lime absorber.

Bainbridge reflex [Francis A. Bainbridge, English physiologist, b. 1874], a cardiac reflex consisting of an increased pulse rate, resulting from stimulation of stretch receptors in the wall of the left atrium.

Baker's cyst, a cyst that forms at the back of the knee. It is often associated with rheumatoid arthritis and may appear only when the leg is straightened.

baker's itch [OE *becan* to bake; AS *giccan*], a rash that may develop on the hands and forearms of bakery workers, probably as an allergic reaction to flours or other ingredients in bakery products.

BAL, abbreviation for **British antilewisite.**

balance [L *bilanx* having two scales], **1.** an instrument for weighing. **2.** a normal state of physiologic equilibrium. **3.** a state of mental or emotional equilibrium. **4.** to bring into equilibrium.

balanced articulation, the simultaneous contacting of the upper and lower teeth as they glide over each other when the mandible is moved from centric relation to various eccentric relations.

balanced diet, a diet containing all of the essential nutrients that cannot be synthesized in adequate quantities by the body, in amounts adequate for growth, energy needs, nitrogen equilibrium, repair of wear, and maintenance of normal health.

balanced occlusion, 1. an occlusion of the teeth that presents a harmonious relation of the occluding surfaces in centric and eccentric positions within the functional range of mandibular positions and tooth size. **2.** the simultaneous contacting of the upper and lower teeth on both sides and in the anterior and posterior occlusal areas of the jaws.

balanced polymorphism, in a population, the recurrence of an equalized mixture of homozygotes and heterozygotes for specific genetic traits, which are maintained from generation to generation by the forces of natural selection.

balanced suspension, a system of splints, ropes, slings, pulleys, and weights for suspending the lower extremities of the body, used as an aid to healing and recuperation from fractures or from surgical operations.

balanced traction, a system of balanced suspension that supplements traction in the treatment of fractures of the lower extremities or after various operations affecting the lower parts of the body.

balanced translocation, the transfer of segments between nonhomologous chromosomes in such a way that there are changes in the configuration and total number of chromosomes, but each cell or gamete contains no more or no less than the normal amount of diploid or haploid genetic material.

balancing side, (in dentistry) the side of the mouth opposite the working side of a dentition or denture.

balanic /bəlan'ik/ [Gk *balanos* acorn], of or pertaining to the glans penis or the glans clitoridis.

balanitis /bal'ənī'tis/ [Gk *balanos + itis*], inflammation of the glans penis.

balanitis xerotica obliterans /zirot'ikə oblit'ərans/ [Gk *balanos, itis; xeros* dry, *tokos* labor; L *obliterare* to efface], a chronic skin disease of the penis, characterized by a white indurated area surrounding the meatus.

balanoplasty /bal'ənōplas'tē/ [Gk *balanos + plassein* to shape], an operation involving plastic surgery of the glans penis.

balanoposthitis /bal'ənōposthī'tis/ [Gk *balanos + posthe* foreskin, *itis*], a generalized inflammation of the glans penis and prepuce, characterized by soreness, irritation, and discharge, occurring as a complication of bacterial or fungal infection.

balanopreputial /bal'ənōpripyoo'shəl/ [Gk *balanos + L praeputium* foreskin], of or pertaining to the glans penis and the prepuce.

balanorrhagia /bal'ənōrā'jē·ə/ [Gk *balanos + thegnynai* to gush], balanitis in which pus is discharged copiously from the penis.

balantidiasis /bal'əntidī'əsis/, an infection caused by ingestion of cysts of the protozoan *Balantidium coli*. In some cases the organism is a harmless inhabitant of the large intestine, but infection with *B. coli* usually causes diarrhea.

Balantidium coli /bal'əntid'ē·əm/ [Gk *balantidion* little bag; *kolon* colon], the largest and the only ciliated protozoan species that is pathogenic to humans, causing balantidiasis.

baldness [ME *balled*], absence of hair, especially from the scalp.

Balkan frame, an overhead rectangular frame, attached to the bed of an orthopedic patient for use in attaching splints, suspending or changing the position of immobilized limbs, and for continuous traction involving weights and pulleys.

Balkan tubulointerstitial nephritis /tōō'byələ·in·tərstish'əl/, a chronic kidney disorder marked by renal insufficiency, proteinuria, tubulointerstitial nephritis, and anemia. The disease is endemic in the Balkans but is not hereditary.

ball [ME *bal*], a relatively spheric mass, such as one of the chondrin balls imbedded in hyaline cartilage.

ball-and-socket joint, a synovial joint in which the globular head of an articulating bone is received into a cuplike cavity, such as in hip and shoulder joints.

ball-catcher position, a position of the hands for the purpose of making a radiograph to diagnose rheumatoid arthritis. The hands are held with the palms upward and the fingers cupped, as if to catch a ball.

ballism /bôl'izəm/ [Gk *ballismo* dancing],

an abnormal neuromuscular condition characterized by uncoordinated swinging of the limbs and jerky movements.

ballistic movement, a high-velocity musculoskeletal movement, such as a tennis serve, requiring reciprocal organization of agonistic and antagonistic synergies.

ballistics [Gk, *ballein*, to throw], the study of the motion, trajectory, and impact of projectiles, including bullets and rockets.

ballistocardiogram /bəlis′tōkär′′de-əgram′/ [Gk *ballein* to throw, *kardia* heart, *graphein* to record], a record of the motion of the body caused by the thrust of the heart during systolic ejection of the blood into the aorta and the pulmonary arteries. The ballistocardiogram is a sensitive tool that is useful in measuring cardiac output and the force of contraction of the heart.

ball of the foot, the part of the foot composed of the heads of the metatarsals and their surrounding fatty fibrous tissue pad.

balloon angioplasty, a method of dilating or reopening an obstructed blood vessel by threading a small catheter, followed by a balloon, into the vessel. The balloon is then inflated to widen the blood vessel.

balloon bezoar [Fr *ballon* ball; Ar *bazahr* counter-poison], a balloon that is inserted into the stomach and inflated to create a sensation of fullness, used as a therapy for obesity.

balloon septostomy. See **Rashkind procedure.**

balloon-tip catheter, a catheter bearing a nonporous inflatable sac around its distal end. After insertion of the catheter the sac can be inflated with air or sterile water, introduced via injection into a special port at the proximal end of the catheter. Kinds of balloon-tip catheters include **Foley catheter, Swan-Ganz catheter.**

ballottable /bəlot′əbəl/ [Fr *ballotage* a shaking about], pertaining to a use of palpation to detect the movement of objects suspended in fluid, such as the body of a fetus in its amniotic fluid.

ballottable head, a fetal head that has not descended and has become fixed in the maternal bony pelvis.

ballottement /bä′lôtmäN′, bəlot′ment/ [Fr, tossing], a technique of palpating an organ or floating structure by bouncing it gently and feeling it rebound.

ball thrombus, a relatively round, coagulated mass of blood containing platelets, fibrin, and cellular fragments that may obstruct a blood vessel or an orifice, usually the mitral valve of the heart.

ball-valve action, the intermittent opening and closing of an orifice by a buoy-ant, ball-shaped mass, which acts as a valve. Some kinds of objects that may act in this manner are kidney stones, gallstones, and blood clots.

balm /bäm/ [Gk *balsamon* balsam], **1.** a healing or a soothing substance, such as any of various medicinal ointments. **2.** an aromatic plant of the genus *Melissa* that relieves pain.

balneology /bal′nē·ol′əjē/ [L *balneum* bath; Gk *logos* science], a field of medicine that deals with the chemical compositions of various mineral waters and their healing characteristics, especially in baths. **–balneologic,** *adj.*

balneotherapy /bal′nē·other′əpē/ [L *balneum* + Gk *therapeia* treatment], a use of baths in the treatment of many diseases and conditions.

balsam [Gk *balsamon*], any of a variety of resinous saps, generally from evergreens, usually containing benzoic or cinnamic acid.

Baltimore Longitudinal Study of Aging, a long-range examination of the interrelations between cerebral physiologic changes of advancing age and psychologic capacities and psychiatric symptoms of men over the age of 65. Men selected for the original study in 1955 were of varied backgrounds in categories of religion, country of birth, education, occupation, retired and working, and householder status ranging from independent to nursing home to explore uncontrolled factors that might lead to new areas of geriatric knowledge.

bamboo spine [Malay *bambu*], the characteristically rigid spine of advanced ankylosing spondylitis.

band [ME *bande* strip], **1.** (in anatomy) a bundle of fibers, as seen in striated muscle, that encircles a structure or binds one part of the body to another. **2.** (in dentistry) a strip of metal that fits around a tooth and serves as an attachment for orthodontic components. **3.** *informal;* the immature form of a segmented granulocyte characterized by a sausage-shaped nucleus.

band adapter, an instrument for aiding in the fitting of an orthodontic band to a tooth.

bandage [ME *bande* strip], **1.** a strip or roll of cloth or other material that may be wound around a part of the body in a variety of ways to secure a dressing, maintain pressure over a compress, or immobilize a limb or other part of the body. **2.** to apply a bandage.

bandage shears, a sturdy pair of scissors used to cut through bandages. The blades of most bandage shears are angled to the shaft of the instrument, and the lower blade has a rounded blunt protuberance to facilitate insertion under the bandage without harming the patient's skin.

band cell, any one of the developing granular leukocytes in circulating blood, characterized by a curved or indented nucleus.

banding [ME *bande* strip], (in genetics) any of several techniques of staining chromosomes with fluorescent stains or chemical dyes that produce a series of lateral light and dark areas whose intensity and position are characteristic for each chromosome.

Bandl's ring. See **pathologic retraction ring.**

bandpass, (in radiology) a measure of the number of times per second an electron beam can be modulated. It is a factor that influences horizontal resolution on a cathode-ray tube.

band pusher, an instrument used for adapting metal orthodontic bands to the teeth.

band remover, an instrument used for removing orthodontic bands from the teeth.

Bangkok hemorrhagic fever. See **dengue fever.**

bank blood [It *banca* bench; AS *blod*], anticoagulated, preserved blood collected from donors in units of 500 ml and stored under refrigeration for future use.

Banti's syndrome /ban'tēz/ [Guido Banti, Italian pathologist, b. 1852], a serious, progressive disorder involving several organ systems, characterized by portal hypertension, splenomegaly, anemia, leukopenia, GI tract bleeding, and cirrhosis of the liver.

BAO, abbreviation for **basal acid output.**

bar, a measure of air pressure. It is equal to 1,000 millibars, or 10^6 dynes/cm², or approximately 1 standard atmosphere (1 atm).

baralyme (BL) /ber'əlīm/ [Gk *barys* heavy; AS *lim* lime], a mixture of calcium and barium compounds used to absorb exhaled carbon dioxide in an anesthesia rebreathing system.

Bárány's test. See **caloric test.**

barber's itch. See **sycosis barbae.**

barbiturate /bärbich'əōōrāt, -ərit/ [Saint Barbara, drug discovered on day of the saint, 1864], a derivative of barbituric acid that acts as a sedative or hypnotic. These derivatives act by depressing the respiratory rate, blood pressure, temperature, and central nervous system.

barbiturate coma [Ger, Saint Barbara's Day; Gk *koma* deep sleep], an effect of barbituric acid or its derivatives, which may be rapid-acting sedatives, hypnotics, and respiratory depressants. Death may re-

sult from intentional or accidental overdosage.

barbiturism /bärbich'əriz'əm/, 1. acute or chronic poisoning by any of the derivatives of barbituric acid. 2. addiction to a barbiturate.

Bard-Pic syndrome /bärd'pik'/ [Louis Bard, French anatomist, b. 1857; Adrian Pic, French physician, b. 1863], a condition characterized by progressive jaundice, enlarged gallbladder, and cachexia, associated with advanced pancreatic cancer.

Bard's sign [Louis Bard], the increased oscillations of the eyeball in organic nystagmus when the patient tries to visually follow a target moved from side to side across the line of sight.

bar graph [OF *barre*], a graph in which frequencies are represented by bars extending from the ordinate or the abscissa, allowing the distribution of the entire sample to be seen at once.

bariatrics /ber'ē·at'riks/ [Gk *baros* weight, *iatros* physician], the field of medicine that focuses on the treatment and the control of obesity and diseases associated with obesity.

baritosis /ber'ətō'sis/, a benign form of pneumoconiosis caused by an accumulation of barium dust in the lungs. The condition is most likely to affect persons involved in the mining and processing of barite, a barium product used in the manufacture of paints.

barium (Ba) /ber'ē·əm/ [Gk *barys* heavy], a pale yellow, metallic element classified with the alkaline earths. Its atomic number is 56; its atomic weight is 137.36. Fine, milky barium sulfate is used as a contrast medium in roentgenography of the digestive tract.

barium enema, a rectal infusion of barium sulfate, a radiopaque contrast medium, which is retained in the lower intestinal tract during roentgenographic studies for diagnosing obstruction, tumors, or other abnormalities.

barium meal, the ingestion of barium sulfate, a radiopaque contrast medium, for the radiographic examination of the esophagus, stomach, and intestinal tract in the diagnosis of such conditions as dysphagia, peptic ulcer, and fistulas.

barium sulfate, a radiopaque medium used as a diagnostic aid in roentgenology. It is prescribed for x-ray examination of the GI tract.

barium swallow [Gk *barys* heavy; AS *swelgan* to swallow], the oral administration of a radiopaque barium sulfate solution in order to radiographically demonstrate possible defects in the esophagus and abnormal borders of the posterior aspects of the heart. See also **barium meal.**

barium test [Gk *barys* heavy; L *testum* crucible], the administration of barium sulfate, which is opaque to x-rays, as a meal or enema for radiographic studies of the digestive tract.

Barlow's disease. See **infantile scurvy.**

Barlow's syndrome, an abnormal cardiac condition characterized by an apical systolic murmur, a systolic click, and an electrocardiogram indicating inferior ischemia.

barognosis /ber'əgnō'sis/, *pl.* **barognoses** [Gk *baros* weight, *gnosis* knowledge], the ability to perceive and evaluate weight, especially that held in the hand.

barograph /ber'əgraf'/ [Gk *baros* + *graphein* to record], an instrument that continuously monitors barometric pressure and provides a record on paper of pressure changes.

barometer /bərom'ətər/ [Gk *baros* + *metron* measure, an instrument for measuring atmospheric pressure, commonly consisting of a slender tube filled with mercury, sealed at one end, and inverted into a reservoir of mercury. At sea level the normal height of mercury in the tube is 760 mm. **–barometric,** *adj.*

barometric pressure. See **atmospheric pressure.**

baroreceptor /ber'ōrisep'tər/ [Gk *baros* + L *recipere* to receive], one of the pressure-sensitive nerve endings in the walls of the atria of the heart, the vena cava, the aortic arch, and the carotid sinus. Baroreceptors stimulate central reflex mechanisms that allow physiologic adjustment and adaptation to changes in blood pressure via vasodilatation or vasoconstriction.

barosinusitis. See **aerosinusitis.**

barotitis. See **aerotitis.**

barotitis media. See **aerotitis media.**

barotrauma /ber'ōtrô'mə, -trou'mə/ [Gk *baros* + *trauma* wound], physical injury sustained as a result of exposure to increased environmental pressure, such as may occur among deep-sea divers or caisson workers.

Barr body. See **sex chromatin.**

barrel chest, a large, rounded thorax, considered normal in some stocky individuals and certain others who live in high-altitude areas and consequently develop increased vital capacities. Barrel chest may also be a sign of pulmonary emphysema.

Barr-Epstein virus. See **Epstein-Barr virus.**

Barré's pyramidal sign /bäräz'/ [Jean A. Barré, French neurologist, b. 1880], a diagnostic sign of a prefrontal brain lesion observed as a phenomenon in which the lateral or vertical movement of one leg of a recumbent patient is followed by a similar movement of the other leg.

Barrett's syndrome [Norman R. Barrett, English surgeon, b. 1903], a disorder of the lower esophagus marked by a benign ulcerlike lesion in columnar epithelium, resulting most often from chronic irritation of the esophagus by gastric reflux of acidic digestive juices.

barrier [ME *barrere*], **1.** a wall or other obstacle that can restrain or block the passage of substances. **2.** something nonphysical that obstructs or separates, as barriers to communication or compliance. **3.** (in radiography) any device that intercepts beams of x-rays.

barrier creams, ointments, lotions, and similar preparations applied to exposed areas of the skin to protect skin cells from exposure to various allergens, irritants, and carcinogens, including sunlight.

barrier-free design [ME *barrere;* AS *freo,* barreres; L *designare* to mark out], the design of homes, workplaces, and public buildings so that physically challenged individuals can make normal use of such structures.

Barsony-Koppenstein method, a procedure for making x-ray images of the cervical intervertebral foramina.

Barthel Index (BI), a disability profile scale developed by D.W. Barthel in 1965 to evaluate a patient's self-care abilities in 10 areas including bowel and bladder control. The patient is scored from 0 to 15 points in various self-care categories, depending on his or her need for help.

bartholinitis /bär'təlinī'tis/ [Caspar T. Bartholin, Danish anatomist, b. 1655; Gk *itis*], an inflammatory condition of one or both Bartholin's glands, caused by bacterial infection. The condition is characterized by swelling of one or both glands, pain, and the development of an abscess in the infected gland.

Bartholin's abscess [Caspar T. Bartholin; L *abscedere* to go away], an abscess of the greater vestibular gland of the vagina.

Bartholin's cyst /bär'təlinz/ [Caspar T. Bartholin], a cyst that arises from one of the vestibular glands or from its ducts, filling with clear fluid that replaces the suppurative exudate characteristic of chronic inflammation.

Bartholin's duct, the major duct of the sublingual gland.

Bartholin's gland, one of two small, mucus-secreting glands located on the posterior and lateral aspect of the vestibule of the vagina.

Barton, Clara (1821–1912), an American humanitarian and founder of the American National Red Cross. During the Civil War, she was a volunteer nurse and at its end she organized a bureau of records to help in the search for missing men. When the Franco-Prussian War erupted, she assisted in the organization of military hospitals in Europe in association with the International Red Cross. This led to her advocacy of an American Red Cross organization, of which she became the first president.

Bartonella /bär′tənel′ə/ [Alberto Barton, Peruvian bacteriologist, b. 1871], a genus of small, gram-negative flagellated pleomorphic coccobacilli. Members of the genus are intracellular parasites that infect red blood cells and the epithelial cells of the lymph nodes, liver, and spleen. They are transmitted at night by the bite of a sandfly of the genus *Phlebotomus.*

bartonellosis /bär′tənəlō′sis/, an acute infection caused by *Bartonella bacilliformis,* transmitted by the bite of a sandfly. It is characterized by fever, severe anemia, bone pain, and skin lesions. Untreated, the infection is often fatal.

Barton forceps. See **obstetric forceps.**

Barton's fracture [John R. Barton, American surgeon, b. 1794], a fracture of the distal articular surface of the radius, which may be accompanied by the dorsal dislocation of the carpus on the radius.

Bartter's syndrome /bär′tərz/ [Frederick C. Bartter, American physiologist, b. 1914], a rare hereditary disorder, characterized by hyperplasia of the juxtaglomerular apparatus and secondary hyperaldosteronism.

barye /ber′ē/, a measure of atmospheric pressure equal to 1 dyne/cm², or 1/1,000 of a millibar.

basal /bā′səl/ [Gk *basis* foundation], of or pertaining to the fundamental or the basic, as basal anesthesia, which produces the first stage of unconsciousness, and the basal metabolic rate, which indicates the lowest metabolic rate.

basal acid output (BAO), the minimum volume of gastric fluid produced by an individual in a given period of time, used in the diagnosis of various diseases of the stomach and intestines.

basal anesthesia [Gk *basis* foundation; *anaisthesia* absence of feeling], **1.** a state of unconsciousness just short of complete surgical anesthesia in depth, in which the patient does not respond to words but still reacts to pinprick or other noxious stimuli. **2.** narcosis produced by injection or infusion of potent sedatives alone, without added narcotics or anesthetic agents.

3. any form of anesthesia in which the patient is completely unconscious, in contrast to awake anesthesia.

basal body temperature, the temperature of the body taken in the morning, orally or rectally, after at least 8 hours of sleep and before doing anything else, including getting out of bed, smoking a cigarette, moving around, talking, eating, or drinking.

basal-body-temperature method of family planning, a natural method of family planning that relies on the identification of the fertile period of the menstrual cycle by noting the progesterone-mediated rise in basal body temperature of 0.5° F to 1° F that occurs with ovulation. The fertile period is considered to continue until the temperature is above the baseline for 5 days; the rise occurs slowly during all 5 days or increases rapidly, reaching a plateau at which it remains for 3 or 4 days. The days after that period are considered "safe" unfertile days.

basal bone, 1. (in prosthodontics) the osseous tissue of the mandible and the maxillae, except for the rami and the processes, which provides support for artificial dentures. **2.** (in orthodontics) the fixed osseous structure that limits the movement of teeth in the creation of a stable occlusion.

basal cell, any one of the cells in the base layer of stratified epithelium.

basal cell acanthoma. See **basal cell papilloma.**

basal cell carcinoma [Gk *basis* + L *cella* storeroom; Gk *karkinos* crab, *oma* tumor], a malignant, epithelial cell tumor that begins as a papule and enlarges peripherally, developing a central crater that erodes, crusts, and bleeds. The primary cause of the cancer is excessive exposure to the sun or to x-rays.

basal cell papilloma [Gk *basis* + L *cella* storeroom, *papilla* nipple; Gk *oma* tumor], a benign, epidermal neoplasm characterized by multiple yellow or brown raised oval lesions that usually develop in middle age.

basal ganglia [Gk *basis* + *ganglion* knot], the islands of gray matter within each cerebral hemisphere, the most important being the caudate nucleus, the putamen, and the pallidium.

basal lamina [Gk *basis* + L, thin plate], a thin, noncellular layer of ground substance lying just under epithelial surfaces.

basal layer. See **stratum basale.**

basal membrane, a sheet of tissue that forms the outer layer of the choroid and lies just under the pigmented layer of the retina.

basal metabolic rate (BMR), the amount of energy used in a unit of time by a fasting, resting subject to maintain vital functions. The rate, determined by the amount of oxygen used, is expressed in calories consumed per hour per square meter of body surface area or per kilogram of body weight.

basal metabolism [Gk *basis* + *metabole* change], the amount of energy needed to maintain essential basic body functions, such as respiration, circulation, temperature, peristalsis, and muscle tone, measured when the subject is awake and at complete rest, has not eaten for 14 to 18 hours, and is in a comfortable, warm environment.

basal narcosis [Gk *basis* + *narkosis* a benumbing], a complete unconsciousness that is induced in a surgical patient before general anesthetic is administered. The state of induced unsconsciousness is less profound than that of general anesthesia. The patient is unresponsive to verbal stimuli but may respond to noxious stimuli.

basaloid carcinoma [Gk *basis* + *eidos* form; *karkinos* crab, *oma* tumor], a rare, malignant neoplasm of the anal canal containing areas that resemble basal cell carcinoma of the skin.

basaloma. See **basal cell carcinoma.**

basal seat, (in dentistry) the oral tissues and structures that support a denture.

basal seat area, the portion of the oral structures that is available to support a denture.

basal seat outline, (in dentistry) a profile on the mucous membrane or on a cast of the entire oral area to be covered by a denture.

basal temperature. See **basal body temperature.**

basal temperature chart [Gk *basis;* L *temperatura* + *charta* paper], a daily temperature chart, usually including the temperature on awakening. A basal temperature chart is sometimes used by women to establish a date of ovulation, when the temperature may show a sudden increase.

base [Gk *basis* foundation], **1.** a chemical compound that combines with an acid to form a salt. **2.** a molecule or radical that takes up or accepts protons. **3.** the major ingredient of a compounded material, particularly one that is used as a medication. **4.** (in radiology) the rigid but flexible foundation of a sheet of x-ray film.

base analog [Gk *basis* + *analogos* proportionate], an analog of one of the purine or the pyrimidine bases normally found in ribonucleic acid or deoxyribonucleic acid.

Basedow's goiter /bä′sədōz/ [Karl A. von Basedow, German physician, b. 1799], an enlargement of the thyroid gland, characterized by the hypersecretion of thyroid hormone after iodine therapy.

base excess, a measure of metabolic alkalosis or metabolic acidosis.

base-forming food, a food that increases the pH of the urine. Base-forming foods include mainly fruits, vegetables, and dairy products, which are sources of sodium and potassium.

baseline [Gk *basis* + L *linea*], **1.** a known value or quantity with which an unknown is compared when measured or assessed. **2.** (in radiology) any of several basic anatomic planes or locations used for positioning purposes.

baseline behavior, a specified frequency and form of a particular behavior during preexperimental or pretherapeutic conditions.

baseline condition, an environmental condition during which a particular behavior reflects a stable rate of response before the introduction of experimental or therapeutic conditions.

baseline fetal heart rate, the fetal heart rate pattern between uterine contractions.

basement lamina. See **basal lamina.**

basement membrane [Fr *soubassement* under base], the fragile, noncellular layer of tissue that secures the overlying layers of stratified epithelium.

base of the heart, the portion of the heart opposite the apex, directed to the right side of the body. It forms the upper border of the heart, lies just below the second rib, and involves primarily the left atrium, part of the right atrium, and portions of the great vessels.

base of the skull, the floor of the skull, containing the anterior, middle, and posterior cranial fossae and numerous foramina, such as the optic foramen, foramen ovale, foramen lacerum, and foramen magnum.

base pair, a pair of nucleotides in a nucleic acid. One of the pair must be a purine, the other a pyrimidine.

base pairing, (in molecular genetics) the association in nucleic acids of the purine bases adenine and guanine with the pyrimidine bases cytosine, thymine, and uracil.

baseplate [Gk *basis* + ME *plate*], a temporary form that represents the base of a denture, used for making records of maxillomandibular relationships, arranging artificial teeth, or for trial placement in the mouth to ensure a precise fit of a denture.

base ratio, the ratio of molar quantities of

the bases in ribonucleic and deoxyribonucleic acids.

bas-fond /bäfôN'/ [Fr, bottom], the bottom or fundus of any structure, especially the fundus of the urinary bladder.

basic amino acid, an amino acid that has a positive electric charge in solution. The basic amino acids are arginine, histidine, and lysine.

basic group identity, (in psychiatry) the shared social characteristics, such as world view, language, and value and ideologic system, that evolve from membership in an ethnic group.

basic health services, the minimum degree of health care considered to be necessary to maintain adequate health and protection from disease.

basic human needs, the things required for survival and normal mental and physical health, such as food, water, shelter, and love.

basic life support (BLS) [Gk *basis;* AS *lif;* L *supportare* to bring up to], the role of cardiopulmonary resuscitation (CPR) and emergency cardiac care (ECC) in reinstituting either circulatory or respiratory function, or both, in the emergency treatment of a victim of cardiac or respiratory arrest.

basic salt, a salt that contains an unreplaced hydroxide ion from the base generating it, such as Ca(OH)Cl.

basifacial /bā'sifā'shəl/ [Gk *basis* + L *facies* face], pertaining to the lower portion of the face.

basilar /bas'ilər/ [Gk *basis* foundation], of or pertaining to a base or a basal area.

basilar artery, the single arterial trunk formed by the junction of the two vertebral arteries at the base of the skull, extending from the inferior to the superior border of the pons, dividing into the left and right cerebral arteries.

basilar artery insufficiency syndrome, the composite of clinical indicators associated with insufficient blood flow through the basilar artery, a condition that may be caused by arterial occlusion.

basilar artery occlusion, an obstruction of the basilar artery, resulting in dysfunction involving cranial nerves III through XII, cerebellar dysfunction, hemiplegia or quadriplegia, and loss of proprioception.

basilar membrane, the cellular structure that forms the floor of the cochlear duct and is supported by bony and fibrous projections from the cochlear wall.

basilar plexus [Gk *basis* + L, braided, the venous network interlaced between the layers of the dura mater over the basilar portion of the occipital bone.

basilar sulcus [Gk *basis* + L, furrow], the sulcus that cradles the basilar artery, in the midline of the pons.

basilic vein /bəsil'ik/, one of the four superficial veins of the arm, beginning in the ulnar part of the dorsal venous network and running proximally on the posterior surface of the ulnar side of the forearm. It is joined by the median cubital vein, then ascends to join the brachial vein to form the axillary vein.

basiloma. See **basal cell carcinoma.**

basiloma terebrans /ter'əbranz/ [Gk *basis, oma* + L *terebare* to bore], an invasive basal cell epithelioma.

basioccipital [Gk *basis* + L *occiput* back of the head], of or pertaining to the basilar process of the occipital bone.

basion /bā'sē·on/ /ā'sē·on/ [Gk *basis* foundation], the midpoint on the anterior margin of the foramen magnum of the occipital bone, opposite the opisthion in the middle of the posterior margin.

basis pedunculi cerebri. See **crus cerebri.**

basket cell [L *bascauda*], a cerebral cotex cell with a horizontal axon that sends out branches. Each branch breaks up into a basketlike mesh that surrounds a Purkinje cell.

Basle Nomina Anatomica (BNA), an international system of anatomic terminology adopted at Basel, Switzerland.

basophil /bā'səfil/ [Gk *basis* + *philein* to love], a granulocytic white blood cell characterized by a segmented nucleus that contains granules that stain blue when exposed to a basic dye. Basophils represent 1% or less of the total white blood cell count.

basophilic adenoma [Gk *basis* + *philein, aden* gland, *oma*], a tumor of the pituitary gland composed of cells that can be stained with basic dyes.

basophilic erythrocyte [Gk *basis* + *philein, erythros* red, *kytos* cell], a red blood cell that contains basophilic material. resulting in the appearance of blue stippling in the erythrocyte. The effect can be a sign of lead poisoning.

basophilic leukemia [Gk *basis* + *philein, leukos* white, *haima* blood], an acute or chronic malignant neoplasm of blood-forming tissues, characterized by large numbers of immature basophilic granulocytes in peripheral circulation and in tissues.

basophilic stippling [Gk *basis* + *philein;* D *stippen* to prick], the abnormal presence of punctate, basophilic granules in the red blood cells, observed under the microscope on a gram-stained smear of the blood. Stippling is characteristic of lead poisoning.

basosquamous cell carcinoma /bā′sō-skwä′məs/ [Gk *basis* + L *squamosus* scaly], a malignant epidermal tumor composed of basal and squamous cells.

Bassen-Kornzweig syndrome. See **abetalipoproteinemia.**

bath [AS *baeth*], (in the hospital) a cleansing procedure performed daily by or for almost all patients to help prevent infection, preserve the unbroken condition of the skin, stimulate circulation, promote oxygen intake, maintain muscle tone and joint mobility, and provide comfort.

bath blanket, a thin, lightweight blanket used to cover a patient during a bath.

bathesthesia /bath′əsthē′zhə/ [Gk *bathys* deep, *anaisthesia* loss of feeling], a loss of deep feeling, such as that associated with organs or structures beneath the surface of the body, such as muscles and joints.

bathmic evolution. See **orthogenic evolution.**

Batten's disease [Frederick E. Batten, English neurologist, b. 1865], a progressive childhood encephalopathy with disturbed metabolism of polyunsaturated fatty acids.

battered baby. See **child abuse.**

battered woman syndrome (BWS), repeated episodes of physical assault on a woman by the man with whom she lives, often resulting in serious physical and psychologic damage to the woman.

battery [Fr *batterie*], **1.** a complex of two or more electrolytic cells connected together to form a single source providing direct current or voltage. **2.** a series or a combination of tests to determine the cause of a particular illness or the degree of proficiency in a particular skill or discipline. **3.** the unlawful use of force on a person.

Battey bacillus /bat′ē/ [Battey Hospital, in Rome, Georgia, where bacteria strain first isolated], any of a group of atypical mycobacteria, including *Mycobacteria avium* and *M. intracellulare,* that cause a chronic pulmonary disease resembling tuberculosis.

battledore placenta /bat′əldôr′/ [ME *batyldoure* a beating instrument; L, flat cake], a placenta to which the umbilical cord is attached at the periphery.

Battle's sign [William H. Battle, English surgeon, b. 1855], a small hemorrhagic spot behind the ear that appears in cases may indicate a fracture of a bone of the lower skull.

batyl alcohol, an alcohol found in fish liver oil that is used to treat bracken poisoning in cattle.

Baudelocque's diameter. See **external conjugate.**

Baudelocque's method /bô′dəlok′s/ [Jean L. Baudelocque, French obstetrician, b. 1746], (in obstetrics) a maneuver used to convert a face presentation to a vertex presentation. The operator flexes the fetal head vaginally and applies counterpressure to the back of the head abdominally while an assistant rotates the fetus in the direction of flexion until the vertex is fixed in the pelvis.

Bayley Scales of Infant Development, a three-part scale for assessing the development of children between the ages of two months and two and a half years. Using boards, blocks, and utensils, the infants are tested for perception, memory, and vocalization on the mental scale; sitting, stair-climbing, and manual manipulation on the motor scale, and attention span, social behavior, and persistence on the behavioral scale.

Baynton's bandage /bān′tənz/ [Thomas Baynton, English surgeon, b. 1761], a spiral adhesive wrap applied to the leg over a dressing used in the treatment of indolent ulcers of the leg.

bayonet angle former [Fr *baionette* a steel blade], a hoe-shaped paired cutting instrument for accenting angles in a Class 3 tooth cavity.

bayonet condenser [Fr *baionette*], (in dentistry) an instrument for compacting restorative material. It has an offset nib device and a shank with right angle bends for varying the line of force.

BBB, abbreviation for **blood-brain barrier.**

B cell, a type of lymphocyte that originates in the bone marrow. A precursor of the plasma cell on suitable antigenic stimulation, it is one of the two lymphocytes that play a major role in the body's immunologic response.

BCG, abbreviation for **bacille Calmette-Guérin.**

BCG vaccine, an active immunizing agent prepared from bacille Calmette-Guérin. It is prescribed most commonly for immunization against tuberculosis.

BCNU. See **carmustine.**

B complex vitamins, a large group of water-soluble substances that includes **vitamin B$_1$** (thiamine), **vitamin B$_{12}$** (cyanocobalamin), biotin, folic acid, **vitamin B$_3$** (niacin), **B$_6$** (pyridoxal, pyridoxine, pyridoxamine, riboflavin, and pantothenic acid.) The B complex vitamins are essential in converting carbohydrates into glucose to provide energy for metabolism of fats and proteins, for normal functioning of the nervous system, for maintenance of muscle tone in the GI tract, and for the health of skin, hair, eyes, mouth, and liver. They are found in brewer's yeast, liver, whole grain cereals, nuts, eggs, meats, fish, and vegetables and are produced by the intestinal bacteria. Maintaining milk-free diets or taking antibiotics may destroy these bacteria. Symptoms of vitamin B deficiency include nervousness, depression, insomnia, neuritis, anemia, alopecia, acne or other skin disorders, and hypercholesterolemia.

b.d. See **b.i.d.**

Be, symbol for the element **beryllium.**

beaded [ME *bede*], **1.** of or having a resemblance to a row of beads. **2.** of or pertaining to bacterial colonies that develop along the inoculation line in various stab cultures. **3.** of or pertaining to stained bacteria that develop more deeply stained beadlike granules.

beaker cell. See **goblet cell.**

beam [ME *beem* tree], a bedframe fitting for pulleys and weights, used in the treatment of patients requiring weight traction. See **Balkan frame.**

beam [ME *beem* tree], **1.** a bedframe fitting for pulleys and weights, used in the treatment of patients requiring weight traction. **2.** (in radiology), the primary beam of radiation emitted from the x-ray tube.

BEAM /bēm, bē′ē′ā′em′/, abbreviation for **brain electric activity map.**

beam alignment, the process of locating the radiographic tube head so it is focused properly on the x-ray film.

beam collimation, the restriction of x-radiation to only the area being examined or treated by confining the beam with collimators or metal diaphragms or shutters with high radiation absorption power.

beam hardening, the process of increasing the energy level of the x-ray beam spectrum by filtering out the low-energy photons.

BE amputation, an amputation of the arm below the elbow.

beam quality, (in radiology) the energy of the x-ray beam.

beam restrictors, devices that reduce scatter radiation from x-ray equipment.

beam-splitting mirror, a device that allows a radiologist to view a fluoroscopic examination of a patient while the same view is being recorded on film.

bean [ME *bene*], the pod-enclosed flattened seed of numerous leguminous plants. Beans used in pharmacologic preparations are alphabetized by specific name.

bearing down [OE *beran* to bear, *adune*

down], a voluntary effort by a woman in in the second stage of labor to aid in the expulsion of a fetus. By applying the Valsalva maneuver, the mother increases intraabdominal pressure.

bearing down pains [OE *beran* + *adune;* L *poena* penalty], the pains experienced by a woman during the second stage of labor while performing the Valsava maneuver to help expel the fetus.

beat, the force of contraction of the heart muscle, which may be detected and recorded as the pulse.

Becker's muscular dystrophy, a chronic degenerative disease of the muscles, characterized by progressive weakness. It occurs in childhood between 8 and 20 years of age. It is transmitted genetically as an autosomal recessive trait.

Beck's Diagnostic Inventory (BDI), a system of classifying a total of 18 criteria of depressive illness. It was developed by A.T. Beck in the 1970s as a diagnostic and therapeutic tool for the treatment of childhood affective disorders.

Beck's triad [Claude S. Beck, American surgeon, b. 1894], a combination of three symptoms that characterize cardiac compression: high venous pressure, low arterial pressure, and a small, quiet heart.

Beckwith's syndrome [John B. Beckwith, American pathologist, b. 1933], an hereditary disorder of unknown cause associated with neonatal hypoglycemia and hyperinsulinism. Clinical manifestations include gigantism, macroglossia, omphalocele or umbilical hernia, visceromegaly, and other abnormalities.

Beckwith-Wiedemann syndrome. See **EMG syndrome.**

beclomethasone dipropionate, a glucocorticoid prescribed in an inhaler in the treatment of bronchial asthma.

becquerel (Bq) /bekrel′, bek′ərel′/ [Antoine H. Becquerel, French physicist, b. 1852], the SI unit of radioactivity, equal to one radioactive decay per second.

bed [AS *bedd*], (in anatomy) a supporting matrix of tissue, as the nail beds of modified epidermis over which the fingernails and the toenails move as they grow.

bedbug [AS *bedd* + ME *bugge* hobgoblin], a blood-sucking arthropod of either the species *Cimex lectularius* or the species *C. hemipterus* that feeds on humans and other animals. The bite causes itching, pain, and redness.

Bedford finger stall, a removable finger splint that holds the injured finger in a brace or cast, along with the adjacent finger.

Bednar's aphthae /bed′närz/ [Alois Bednar, Austrian pediatrician, b. 1816], the small, yellowish, slightly elevated ulcerated patches that occur on the posterior portion of the hard palate of infants who place infected objects in their mouths.

bed pan, a vessel, usually made of metal, used to collect feces and urine of bedridden patients.

bed rest, the restriction of a patient to bed for therapeutic reasons for a prescribed period.

bedside manner, the behavior of a nurse or doctor as perceived by a patient.

bedsore. See decubitus ulcer.

bedwetting. See enuresis.

Bee cell pessary. See pessary.

beef tapeworm. See *Taenia saginata.*

beef tapeworm infection [OF *buef* cow; AS *taeppe, wyrm*], an infection caused by the tapeworm *Taenia saginata,* transmitted to humans when they eat contaminated beef. The infection is rarely found in North America and Western Europe, where beef is carefully inspected and is thoroughly cooked before eating.

bee sting [AS *beo, stingan*], an injury caused by the venom of bees, usually accompanied by pain and swelling. The stinger of the honeybee usually remains implanted and should be removed. Pain may be alleviated by application of an ice pack or a paste of sodium bicarbonate and water. Hypersensitive individuals are encouraged to carry emergency treatment supplies with them when the possibility of bee sting exists.

behavior [ME *behaven*], **1.** the manner in which a person acts or performs. **2.** any or all of the activities of a person, including physical actions, which are observed directly, and mental activity, which is inferred and interpreted. Kinds of behavior include **abnormal, automatic, invariable,** and **variable behavior.**

behavioral isolation, social isolation that occurs because of a person's socially unacceptable behavior.

behavioral objective, a goal in therapy or research that concerns an act or a specific behavior or pattern of behaviors.

behavioral science, any of the various interrelated disciplines, such as psychiatry, psychology, sociology, and anthropology, that observes and studies human activity, including psychologic and emotional development, interpersonal relationships, values, and mores.

behavior disorder, any of a group of antisocial behavior patterns occurring primarily in children and adolescents, such as overaggressiveness, overactivity, destructiveness, cruelty, truancy, lying, disobedience, perverse sexual activity, criminality, alcoholism, and drug addiction.

behaviorism, a school of psychology founded by John B. Watson that studies and interprets behavior by observing measurable responses to stimuli without reference to consciousness, mental states, or subjective phenomena, such as ideas and emotions.

behaviorist, a disciple of the school of behaviorism.

behavioristic psychology. See behaviorism.

behavior modification. See behavior therapy.

behavior systems model, a conceptual framework describing factors that may affect the stability of a person's behavior. The model examines systems of behavior, not the behavior of an individual at any particular time.

behavior therapy, a kind of psychotherapy that attempts to modify observable, maladjusted patterns of behavior by the substitution of a new response or set of responses to a given stimulus.

Behçet's disease /bā'sets/ [Hulusi Behçet, Turkish dermatologist, b. 1889] a rare and severe illness of unknown cause, mostly affecting young males and characterized by severe uveitis and retinal vasculitis.

Behla's bodies. See Plimmer's bodies.

BEI, abbreviation for butanol extractable iodine.

BEIR-III Report, a report, *"The Biological Effects of Low Doses of Ionizing Radiation,"* by the National Academy of Sciences; it estimates the risk of cancer deaths from exposure to radiation at various dose levels.

bejel /bej'əl/ [Ar *bajal*], a nonvenereal form of syphilis prevalent among children in the Middle East and North Africa, caused by the spirochete *Treponema pallidum II.* The primary lesion is usually on or near the mouth, appearing as a mucus patch, followed by the development of pimplelike sores on the trunk, arms, and legs.

Békésy audiometry /bek'əsē/ [George von Békésy, Hungarian-American physicist, b. 1899], a type of hearing test in which the subject controls the intensity of the stimulus by pressing a button while listening to a pure tone whose freqency slowly moves through the entire audible range.

bel [Alexander G. Bell, Canadian inventor, b. 1847], a unit that expresses intensity of sound. It is the logarithm (to the base 10) of the ratio of the power of any specific sound to the power of a reference sound. The most common reference sound has a power of 10^{-16} watts per cm^2, or the approximate minimum intensity of

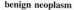

sound at 1,000 cycles per second, that is perceptible to the human ear.

belching. See **eructation.**

belladonna [It, fair lady], the dried leaves, roots, and flowering or fruiting tops of *Atropa belladonna,* a common perennial called deadly nightshade, containing the alkaloids hyoscine and hyoscyamine. Hyoscyamine is a source of atropine.

belladonna and atropine poisons [It *belladonna;* Gk *Atropos,* fate; L *potio* drink], two powerful poisons obtained from solanaceous plants. Atropine, derived from *Atropa belladonna,* blocks the effects of acetylcholine in effector organs supplied by post-ganglionic cholinergic nerves. Belladonna is obtained from the dried leaves of *Atropa belladonna,* also known as deadly nightshade, or of *Atropa acuminata,* a source of alkaloids that are converted to atropine. Atropine is commonly used in ophthalmology and as an antispasmodic.

bellows murmur[AS *belg* bag; L, humming], a blowing sound, such as air moving in and out of a bellows.

bellows ventilator, a respiratory care device in which oxygen and other gases are mixed in a bellows that contracts and expands as system pressure is increased or decreased in the chamber surrounding the bellows.

Bell's law [Charles Bell, Scottish surgeon, b. 1774], an axiom stating that the ventral spinal roots are motor and the dorsal spinal roots are sensory.

Bell's palsy [Charles Bell, Scottish surgeon, b. 1774], a paralysis of the facial nerve, resulting from trauma to the nerve, compression of the nerve by a tumor, or, possibly, an unknown infection. The person may not be able to open an eye or close the mouth. Plastic surgery may reduce the deformity.

Bell's phenomenon, a sign of peripheral facial paralysis, manifested by the upward and outward rolling of the eyeball when the affected individual tries to close the eyelid.

belly. See **abdomen.**

belly button. See **umbilicus.**

belonephobia /bel'ənəfō'bē·ə/[Gk *belone* needle, *phobos* fear], a morbid fear of sharp-pointed objects, especially needles and pins.

belt restraint, a device used to secure a patient on a stretcher or in a chair.

Benassi method /bänas'ē/, a positioning procedure for producing x-ray images of the liver.

Bence Jones protein /bens/ [Henry Bence Jones, English physician, b. 1813], a protein found almost exclusively in the urine of patients with multiple myeloma.

bench research, *informal.* (in medicine) any research done in a controlled laboratory setting using other than human subjects.

Bender's Visual Motor Gestalt test [Lauretta Bender, American psychiatrist, b. 1897], a standard psychologic test in which the subject copies a series of patterns.

bending fracture, a fracture indirectly caused by the bending of an extremity, such as of the foot or the big toe.

bendrofluazide. See **bendroflumethiazide.**

bendroflumethiazide /ben'drōflōō'məthī'-əzīd/, a diuretic and antihypertensive prescribed in the treatment of hypertension and edema.

bends. See **decompression sickness.**

Benedict's qualitative test [Stanley R. Benedict, American biochemist, b. 1884], a test for sugar in the urine based on the reduction by glucose of cupric ions. Formation of an orange or red precipitate indicates more than 2% sugar (called 4+), yellow indicates 1% to 2% sugar (called 3+), olive green indicates 0.5% to 1% sugar (called 2+), and green indicates less than 0.5% sugar (called 1+).

benign [L *benignare* to bless], (of a tumor) noncancerous and therefore not an immediate threat, even though treatment eventually may be required for health or cosmetic reasons.

benign familial chronic pemphigus [L *benignare* to bless, *familia* household; Gk *pemphix* bubble], a hereditary condition of the skin characterized in the early stages by blisters which break, leaving red, eroded areas followed by crusts.

benign hypertension, a misnomer implying an innocent elevation of blood pressure.

benign intracranial hypertension. See **pseudotumor cerebri.**

benign juvenile melanoma, a benign, pink or fuchsia raised papule with a scaly surface, usually on a cheek and occurring most commonly in children between 9 and 13 years of age.

benign mesenchymoma [L *benignare* + Gk *meso* middle, *egchyma* infusion, *oma* tumor], a benign neoplasm that has two or more definitely recognizable mesenchymal elements in addition to fibrous tissue.

benign neoplasm [L *benignare* + Gk *neos* new, *plasma* formation], a localized tumor that has a fibrous capsule, limited potential for growth, a regular shape, and cells that are well differentiated. A benign neoplasm does not invade surrounding tissue or metastasize to distant sites. Some kinds of benign neoplasms are **adenoma, fibroma, hemangioma,** and **lipoma.**

benign nephrosclerosis, a renal disorder marked by arteriolosclerotic lesions in the kidney. It is associated with hypertension.

benign prostatic hypertrophy, enlargement of the prostate gland, common among men after the age of 50. The condition is not malignant or inflammatory but is usually progressive and may lead to obstruction of the urethra and to interference with the flow of urine, possibly causing frequency of urination, the need to urinate during the night, pain, and urinary tract infections.

benign pseudohypertrophic muscular dystrophy. See **Becker's muscular dystrophy.**

benign stupor, a state of apathy or lethargy, such as occurs in severe depression.

benign thrombocytosis. See **thrombocytosis.**

benign tumor [L *benignare* to bless; L, swelling], a neoplasm that does not invade other tissues or metastasize in other sites. A benign tumor is usually well encapsulated, and its cells exhibit less anaplase than those of a malignant growth.

Bennet's small corpuscle. See **Drysdale's corpuscle.**

Bennett angle [Norman G. Bennett, English dentist, b. 1870], (in dentistry) the angle formed by the sagittal plane and the path of the advancing condyle during lateral mandibular movement.

Bennett hand tool test, a test used in occupational therapy and prevocational testing to measure hand function and coordination and speed in performance.

Bennett's fracture [Edward H. Bennett, Irish surgeon, b. 1837], a fracture that runs obliquely through the base of the first metacarpal bone and into the carpometacarpal joint, detaching the greater part of the articular facet.

bent fracture [ME *benden*], an incomplete greenstick fracture.

bentonite [Fort Benton, Montana], colloidal, hydrated aluminum silicate used as a bulk laxative and as a base for skin care preparations.

bentonite test, a flocculation test for the presence of rheumatoid factor in patient blood samples. After sensitized bentonite particles are added to the serum, the test is considered positive for rheumatoid arthritis if adsorption has occurred with 50% of the particles.

benz, abbreviation for a *benzoate carboxylate anion.*

benzalkonium chloride, a disinfectant

and fungicide prepared in an aqueous solution in various strengths.

benzathine penicillin G. See **penicillin G benzathine.**

benzene poisoning, a toxic condition caused by ingestion of benzene, the inhalation of benzene fumes, or exposure to benzene-related products such as toluene or xylene, characterized by nausea, headache, dizziness, and incoordination. In acute cases respiratory failure or ventricular fibrillation may cause death.

benzethonium chloride /ben′zəthō′nē·əm/, a topical antiinfective used for disinfecting the skin and for treating some infections of the eye, nose, and throat. It is also used as a preservative in some pharmaceutic preparations.

benzhexol hydrochloride. See **trihexyphenidyl hydrochloride.**

benzo(a)pyrene dihydrodiol epoxide (BPDE-I), a carcinogenic derivative of benzo(a)pyrene associated with tobacco smoke.

benzocaine /ben′zəkān/, a local anesthetic agent derived from aminobenzoic acid, used in many over-the-counter compounds for pruritus and pain.

benzodiazepine derivative /ben′zōdī·a-z′əpin/, one of a group of psychotropic agents, including the tranquilizers chlordiazepoxide, diazepam, oxazepam, and chlorazepate, prescribed to alleviate anxiety, and the hypnotics flurazepam and nitrazepam, prescribed in the treatment of insomnia. Diazepam is also prescribed to relieve spasm of the muscles and to increase the seizure threshold.

benzoic acid /benzō′ik/, a keratolytic agent, usually used with salicylic acid as an ointment in the treatment of athlete's foot and ringworm of the scalp.

benzonatate /benzō′nənāt/, a nonopiate antitussive prescribed to suppress the cough reflex.

benzoyl peroxide /benzō′il/, an antibacterial, keratolytic, drying agent prescribed in the treatment of acne.

benzphetamine hydrochloride /benzfet′əmēn/, a sympathomimetic used as an anorexic agent prescribed to decrease the appetite in the treatment of obesity.

benzquinamide /benzkwin′əmīd/, an antiemetic prescribed in the treatment of postoperative nausea and vomiting.

benzthiazide /benzthī′əzīd/, a diuretic and antihypertensive prescribed in the treatment of hypertension and edema.

benztropine mesylate /benztrō′pēn/, an anticholinergic and antihistaminic agent prescribed as adjunctive therapy in the treatment of all forms of parkinsonism.

benzyl alcohol /ben′zil/, a clear, colorless, oily liquid, derived from certain balsams, used as a topical anesthetic and as a bacteriostatic agent in solutions for injection.

benzyl benzoate /benzō′āt/, a clear, oily liquid with a pleasant, aromatic odor. It is used as an agent to destroy lice and scabies, as a solvent, and as a flavor for gum.

benzyl carbonol. See **phenylethyl alcohol.**

benzylpenicillin. See **penicillin G.**

bereavement [ME *bereven* to rob], a form of depression with anxiety symptoms that is a common reaction to the loss of a loved one. It may be accompanied by insomnia, hyperactivity, and other effects.

Berger's disease, a kidney disorder characterized by recurrent episodes of macroscopic hematuria, proteinuria, and a granular deposition of IgA from the glomerular mesangium. The onset of disease is usually in childhood or early adulthood, and males are affected twice as often as females.

Berger's paresthesia [Oskar Berger, German neurologist, b. 1844; Gk *para* near, *aisthesia* sensation], a condition of tingling, prickliness, or weakness and a loss of feeling in the legs without evidence of organic disease. The condition affects young people.

Bergonié-Tribondeau law /ber′gônē′trā′-bônō′/ [Jean A. Bergonié, French radiologist, b. 1857; Louis Frédéric A. Tribondeau, French physician, b. 1872], (in radiotherapy) a rule stating that the radiosensitivity of tissue depends on the number of undifferentiated cells, their mitotic activity, and the length of time they are actively proliferating.

beriberi /ber′ēber′ē/ [Singhalese *beri* weakness], a disease of the peripheral nerves caused by a deficiency of or an inability to assimilate thiamine. It is frequently the result of a diet limited to polished white rice. Symptoms are fatigue, diarrhea, appetite and weight loss, disturbed nerve function causing paralysis and wasting of limbs, edema, and heart failure. Kinds of beriberi include alcoholic beriberi, atrophic beriberi, cardiac beriberi, and cerebral beriberi.

berkelium (Bk) /burk′lē·əm/ [Berkeley, California], an artificial radioactive transuranic element. Its atomic number is 97; its atomic weight is 247.

berlock dermatitis [Fr *breloque* bracelet charm], an abnormal skin condition, characterized by hyperpigmentation and skin lesions, caused by a unique reaction to psoralen-type photosynthesizers, commonly used in perfumes, colognes, and pomades, such as oil of bergamot. This condition affects mostly women and children and may result from the use of products containing psoralens and from exposure to ultraviolet light.

Bernard-Soulier syndrome /bernär′sŏŏl-yā′/, a coagulation disorder characterized by an absence of or a deficiency in the ability of the platelets to aggregate because of the relative lack of an essential glycoprotein in the membranes of the platelets. The use of aspirin may provoke hemorrhage in people who have this condition.

Bernoulli's principle /bərnoo′lēz/ [Daniel Bernoulli, Swiss scientist, b. 1700], (in physics) a principle stating that the sum of the velocity, and the kinetic energy of a fluid flowing through a tube is constant. The greater the velocity, the less the lateral pressure on the wall of the tube. Thus, if an artery is narrowed by an atherosclerotic plaque, the flow of blood through the constriction increases in velocity and decreases in lateral pressure.

Bernstein test. See **acid-perfusion test.**

berry aneurysm [ME *berye*; Gk *aneurysma* widening], a small, saccular dilatation of the wall of a cerebral artery, occurring most frequently at the junctures of vessels in the circle of Willis.

Bertel method /bur′təl/, a positioning procedure for producing x-ray images of the inferior orbital fissures.

berylliosis /bəril′ē·ō′sis/, poisoning that results from the inhalation of dusts or vapors containing beryllium or beryllium compounds. It is characterized by granulomas, pulmonary fibrosis, dry cough, shortness of breath, and chest pain.

beryllium (Be), a steel-gray, lightweight metallic element. Its atomic number is 4; its atomic weight is 9.012. Beryllium occurs naturally as beryl and is used in metallic alloys and in fluorescent powders.

bestiality [L *bestia* beast], **1.** a brutal or animal-like character or nature. **2.** conduct or behavior characterized by beastlike appetites or instincts. **3.** sexual relations between a human being and an animal. **4.** sodomy.

besylate, a contraction for benzenesulfonate.

beta, β, the second letter of the Greek alphabet, employed as a combining form with chemical names to distinguish one of two or more isomers or to indicate the position of substituted atoms in certain compounds.

beta-adrenergic blocking agent. See **antiadrenergic.**

beta-adrenergic receptor. See **beta receptor.**

beta-adrenergic stimulating agent. See **adrenergic.**

beta-alaninemia /-al'əninē'mē-ə/, an inherited metabolic disorder marked by a deficiency of an enzyme, beta-alanine-alpha-ketoglutarate amino transferase. The clinical signs include seizures, somnolence, and, if uncorrected, death.

beta-carotene [Gk, beta; L *carota* carrot], an ultraviolet screening agent prescribed to ameliorate photosensitivity in patients with erythropoetic protoporphyria.

beta cells, 1. insulin-producing cells situated in the islets of Langerhans. The insulin-producing function of the beta cells tends to accelerate the movement of glucose, amino acids, and fatty acids out of the blood and into the cellular cytoplasm, countering glucagon function of alpha cells. **2.** the basophilic cells of the anterior lobe of the pituitary gland.

beta decay, a type of radioactivity that results in the emission of beta particles, such as electrons or positrons.

beta fetoprotein, a protein found in fetal liver and in some adults with liver disease. It is identical with normal liver ferritin.

beta-galactosidase. See **lactase.**

beta hemolysis, the development of a clear zone around a bacterial colony growing on blood agar medium, characteristic of certain pathogenic bacteria.

beta-hemolytic streptococci, the pyogenic streptococci of groups A, B, C, E, F, G, H, K, L, M, and O that cause hemolysis of red blood cells in blood agar in the laboratory. These organisms cause most of the acute streptococcal infections seen in humans.

beta-hydroxyisovaleric aciduria, an inherited metabolic disease caused by a deficiency of an enzyme needed to metabolize the amino acid leucine.

beta-ketobutyric acid. See **acetoacetic acid.**

beta-lactamase /-lak'təmāz\ [*lactam*, a cyclic amide + *ase* enzyme], an enzyme that catalyzes the hydrolysis of the beta-lactam ring of some penicillins and cephalosporins, producing penicilloic acid and rendering the antibiotic ineffective.

beta-lactamase resistance, See **beta-lactamase-resistant antibiotics.**

beta-lactamase-resistant antibiotics, antibiotcs that are resistant to the enzymatic effects of **beta-lactamase.**

beta-lactamase-resistant penicillin, See **beta-lactamase-resistant antibiotics.**

beta-naphthylamine /-nafthil'əmēn/, an aromatic amine used in aniline dyes and a cause of bladder cancer in humans.

beta-oxidation, a catabolic process in which fatty acids are used by the body as a source of energy.

beta particle, an electron or positron emitted from the nucleus of an atom during radioactive decay of the atom. Beta particles have a range of 10 meters in air and 1 mm in soft tissue.

beta phase, the period immediately following the alpha, or redistribution, phase of drug administration. During the beta phase the blood level of the drug falls more slowly as it is metabolized and excreted from the body.

beta rays [Gk *beta;* L *ray* radius], a stream of beta particles, as emitted from atoms of disintegrating radioactive elements. Normally, when the element is a nuclide with a high ratio of neutrons to protons, the beta particle is an electron; when the nuclide has a higher proportion of protons to neutrons, the beta particle is a positron.

beta receptor, any one of the adrenergic components of receptor tissues that responds to epinephrine. Activation of beta receptors causes various physiologic reactions, as relaxation of the bronchial muscles and an increase in the rate and force of cardiac contraction.

beta rhythm. See **beta wave.**

beta wave, one of the four types of brain waves, characterized by relatively low voltage and a frequency of more than 13 Hz. Beta waves are the "busy waves" of the brain, recorded by electroencephalograph from the frontal and the central areas of the cerebrum when the patient is awake and alert with eyes open.

betatron /bā'tətron/, a cyclic accelerator that produces high-energy electrons for radiotherapy treatment.

betaxolol hydrochloride /betak'səlol/, a topical drug prescibed for the relief of ocular hypertension and chronic open-angle glaucoma.

bethanechol chloride /bethan'əkol/, a cholinergic prescribed in the treatment of fecal and urinary retention and neurogenic atony of the bladder.

Betz cells [Vladimir Aleksandrovich Betz, Russian anatomist, b. 1834; L *cella* storeroom], large pyramidal neurons of the motor cortex with axons that form part of the pyramidal tract associated with voluntary movements.

bevel /bev'əl/ [OFr *baif* open mouth angle], **1.** any angle, other than a right angle, between two planes or surfaces. **2.** (in dentistry) any angle other than 90 degrees between a tooth cut and a cavity wall in the preparation of a tooth cavity.

bezoar /bē'zôr/ [Ar *bazahr* protection against poison], a hard ball of hair and vegetable fiber that may develop within the intestines of humans but more often is found in the stomachs of ruminants.

B/F, a symbol for *black female,* often used in the initial identifying statement in a patient record.

B-galactosidase. See **lactase.**

bhang /bang/ [Hindi *bag*], an Asian Indian hallucinogenic, composed of dried leaves and the young stems of uncultivated *Cannabis sativa.* It produces euphoria.

Bi, symbol for the element **bismuth.**

BIA, abbreviation for **bioelectrical impedance analysis.**

bias [MFr *biais*], **1.** an oblique or a diagonal line. **2.** a prejudiced or subjective attitude. **3.** (in statistics) the systematic distortion of a statistic caused by a particular sampling process. **4.** (in electronics) a voltage applied to an electronic device, such as a vacuum tube or a transistor, to control operating limits.

biased sample [OFr *biais* slant; L *exemplum* sample], (in research), a sample of a group in which all factors or participants were not equally balanced or objectively represented.

biasing, a method of treating neuromuscular dysfunction by contracting a muscle against resistance, causing the muscle spindles to readjust to the shorter length.

bibliotherapy, a type of group therapy in which books, poems, and newspaper articles are read in the group to help stimulate thinking about events in the real world and to foster relations between group members.

bicarbonate [L *bis* two, *carbo* coal], any salt of carbonic acid in which only one of the hydrogen atoms has been replaced by a metal or radical, as sodium bicarbonate ($NaHCO_3$).

bicarbonate of soda. See **sodium bicarbonate.**

bicarbonate precursor, an injection of sodium lactate used in the treatment of metabolic acidosis. It is metabolized in the body to sodium bicarbonate.

bicarbonate therapy, a procedure to increase a patient's stores of bicarbonate when there are signs of severe acidosis.

bicarbonate transport, the route by which most of the carbon dioxide is carried in the bloodstream. Once dissolved in the blood plasma, the carbon dioxide combines with water to form carbonic acid, which immediately ionizes into hydrogen and bicarbonate ions.

biceps brachii /bī′seps brā′kē-ī/ [L *bis* twice, *caput* head; *bracchii* arm], the long fusiform muscle of the upper arm on the anterior surface of the humerus arising in two heads from the scapula. The short head arises in a tendon from the corocoid process, the long head arises in the glenoid cavity. Both parts of the muscle converge in a flattened tendon that inserts into the radius of the forearm. It flexes the arm and the forearm and supinates the hand. The long head draws the humerus toward the glenoid fossa, strengthening the shoulder joint.

biceps femoris [L *bis* twice, *caput* head; thigh], one of the posterior femoral muscles. It has two heads at its origin. The long head arises from the tuberosity of the ischium and from the inferior part of the sacrotuberous ligament; the short head arises from the linea aspera and from the lateral intermuscular septum. The fibers passing from both heads join in a tendon that inserts into the lateral side of the fibula, and by a few fibers, into the lateral condyle of the tibia. The tendon of insertion forms the lateral hamstring. The biceps femoris flexes the leg and rotates it laterally and extends the thigh and tends to rotate it laterally.

biceps flexor cubiti. See **biceps brachii.**

biceps reflex, a contraction of a biceps muscle produced when the tendon is tapped with a percussor in testing deep tendon reflexes.

bicipital groove [L *bis* + *caput* heads; D *groove*], a groove between the greater and lesser tubercles of the humerus for passage of the tendon of the long head of the biceps muscle.

Bickerdyke /bik′ərdīk/, **Mary Ann** (1817–1901), an American nurse who, after taking a short course in homeopathy, cared for the sick and wounded on the battlefields during the Civil War. She insisted on cleanliness, good food, and the best of medical care for her patients.

biclor /bī′klôr/, abbreviation for a *bichloride noncarboxylate anion.*

biconcave [L *bis* twice, *concavare* to make hollow], concave on both sides, especially as applied to a lens. **−biconcavity,** *n.*

biconvex [L *bis* + *convexus* vaulted], convex on both sides, especially as applied to a lens. **−biconvexity,** *n.*

bicornate /bīkôr′nāt/ [L *bis* + *cornu* horn], having two horns or processes.

bicornate uterus, an abnormal uterus that may be either a single or a double organ with two horns or branches.

bicuspid /bīkus′pid/ [L *bis* + *cuspis* point] **1.** having two cusps or points. **2.** one of the two teeth between the molars and canines of the upper and lower jaw.

bicuspid valve. See **mitral valve.**

bicycle ergometer [L *bis;* Gk *kyklos* circle, *ergon* work, *metron* measure], a stationary bicycle dynamometer that measures the power of the contraction of the muscles of an individual.

b.i.d., (in prescriptions) abbreviation for *bis in die* /bĭ′dē′ā/, a Latin phrase meaning "twice a day." The times of administration are commonly 9 AM and 7 PM.

bidactyly /bīdak′tilē/ [L *bis* + Gk *daktylos* finger], an abnormal condition in which the second, third, and fourth digits on the same hand are missing and only the first and fifth are represented. **–bidactylous,** *adj.*

bidermoma /bī′dərō′mə/, *pl.* **bidermomas, bidermomata** [L *bis* + Gk *derma* skin, *oma* tumor], a teratoid neoplasm composed of cells and tissues originating in two germ layers.

bidet /bidā′/[Fr, pony], a fixture resembling a toilet bowl, with a rim to sit on and usually equipped with plumbing implements, for cleaning the genital and rectal areas of the body.

biduotertian fever [L *bis* + *dies*, day, *tertius* three], a form of malaria characterized by overlapping paroxysms of chills, fever, and other symptoms caused by infection with two strains of *Plasmodium*, each having its own cycle of symptoms, such as in quartan and tertian malaria.

bifid [L *bis* + *findere* to cleave], split into two parts.

bifid tongue [L *bis* + *findere*; AS *tunge*], a tongue divided by a longitudinal furrow. Also called **cleft tongue.**

bifocal [L *bis* + *focus* hearth], **1.** of or pertaining to the characteristic of having two foci. **2.** (of a lens) having two areas of different focal lengths.

bifocal glasses [L *bis* + *focus*; AS *glaes*], eyeglasses in which each lens has two foci to permit both near and far vision.

bifrontal suture [L *bis* + *frons* front + *sutura*], the interlocking lines of fusion between the frontal and parietal bones of the skull.

bifurcate /bifur′kāt/ [L *bis* + *furca* fork], the division or branching of an object into two forks, as the branching of blood vessels or bronchi.

bifurcation [L *bis* + *furca*], a splitting into two branches, such as the trachea, which branches into the two bronchi at about the level of the fifth thoracic vertebra.

Bigelow's lithotrite /big′əlōz/ [Henry J. Bigelow, American surgeon, b. 1818; Gk *lithos* stone; L *terere* to rub], a long-jawed lithotrite, passed through the urethra, for crushing a calculus in the bladder.

bigeminal pulse /bījem′inəl/, an abnormal pulse in which two beats in close succession are followed by a pause during which no pulse is felt.

bigeminal rhythm [L *bis* + *geminus* twin; Gk *rhythmos*], a coupled heart beat with ventricular or atrial ectopic beats alternating with sinus beats or ventricular ectopics occurring in pairs, such as ventricular tachycardia with 3:2 exit block.

bigeminy /bījem′inē/ [L *bis* + *geminus*] **1.** an association in pairs. **2.** a cardiac arrhythmia characterized by two beats in rapid succession followed by a longer interval. **–bigeminal,** *adj.*

bilabe /bī′lāb/ [L *bis* + *labium* lip], a narrow forceps used to remove small calculi from the bladder.

bilaminar /bīlam′ənər/ [L *bis* + *lamina* thin plate], pertaining to or having two layers.

bilaminar blastoderm, the stage of embryonic development before mesoderm formation in which only the ectoderm and entoderm primary germ layers have formed.

bilateral [L *bis* + *lateralis* side], **1.** having two sides. **2.** occurring or appearing on two sides. A patient with bilateral hearing loss may have partial or total deafness in both ears. **3.** having two layers.

bilateral carotid [L *bis* + *latus* side; Gk *karos* heavy sleep], a main artery to the head and neck that divides into left and right branches and again into external and internal branches.

bilateral lithotomy [L *bis* + *latus;* Gk *lithos* stone, *temnein* to cut], a surgical procedure for removing urinary tract stones from the bladder by making transverse perineal incisions through the lateral lobes of the prostate.

bilateral long-leg spica cast, an orthopedic device of plaster of paris, fiberglass, or other casting material that encases and immobilizes the trunk cranially as far as the nipple line and both legs caudally as far as the toes. A horizontal crossbar to improve immobilization connects the parts of the cast encasing both legs at ankle level.

bilateral strabismus [L *bis* + *latus;* Gk *strabismos*], an eye disorder characterized by bilateral squint in which the condition is due to a failure of ocular accommodation.

bilateral symmetry [L *bis* + *latus;* Gk *syn* together + *metron* measure], the symmetry of two halves of an organism.

Bilbao tube /bilbō′ə/, a long, thin, flexible tube that is used to inject barium into the small intestine. The tube is guided with a stiff wire to the end of the duodenum under fluoroscopic control.

bile [L *bilis*], a bitter, yellow-green secretion of the liver. Stored in the gallbladder, bile receives its color from the presence of bile pigments, such as bilirubin. Bile passes from the gallbladder through the common bile duct in response to the presence of a fatty meal in the duodenum. Bile emulsifies these fats, preparing them for further digestion and absorption in the small intestine. **–biliary,** *adj.*

bile acid, a steroid acid of the bile produced during the metabolism of cholesterol. On hydrolysis bile acid yields glycine and cholic acid.

bile duct. See **biliary duct.**

bile pigments, a group of substances that contribute to the colors of bile, which may range from a yellowish green to brown. A common bile pigment is bilirubin.

bile salts [L *bilis* bile; AS *sealt*], a mixture of sodium salts of the bile acids and cholic and chendoxychoic acids synthesized in the liver as a derivative of cholesterol. Their low surface tension contributes to the emulsification of fats in the intestine.

bile solubility test, a bacteriologic test used in the differential diagnosis of pneumococcal and streptococcal infection.

Bilharzia. See *Schistosoma.*

bilharziasis. See **schistosomiasis.**

biliary /bil′ē·er′ē/, of or pertaining to bile or to the gallbladder and its ducts, which transport bile. These are often called the **biliary tract** or the **biliary system.**

biliary atresia, congenital absence or underdevelopment of one or more of the biliary structures, causing jaundice and early liver damage.

biliary calculus [L *bilis* bile, *calculus* pebble], a stone formed in the biliary tract consisting of bile pigments and calcium salts. Biliary calculi may cause jaundice, right upper quadrant pain, obstruction, and inflammation of the gallbladder.

biliary cirrhosis [L *bilis* + *kirrhos* yellow, *osis* condition], an inflammatory condition in which the flow of bile through the ductules of the liver is obstructed.

biliary colic [L *bilis* + *kolikos* colon pain], a type of smooth muscle or visceral pain specifically associated with the passing of stones through the bile ducts.

biliary duct, a muscular duct through which bile passes from the liver to the duodenum.

biliary fistula, an abnormal passage from the gallbladder, a bile duct, or the liver to an internal organ or the surface of the body.

biliary obstruction, blockage of the common or cystic bile duct, usually caused by one or more gallstones. It impedes bile drainage and produces an inflammatory reaction.

biliary tract [L *bilis* + *tractus*], the pathway for bile flow from the canaliculi in the liver to the opening of the bile duct into the duodenum.

biliary tract cancer, a rare adenocarcinoma in an extrahepatic bile duct, occurring more often in men than in women, characterized by progressive jaundice, pruritus, weight loss, and severe pain. The lesion may be papillary or flat and ulcerated. Transhepatic cholangiography and x-ray examination are used to identify and determine the site of the lesion.

bilingulate /bīling′gyəlit/ [L *bis* twice, *lingula* little tongue], having two tongues or two tonguelike structures.

bilious /bil′yəs/ [L *bilis* bile], **1.** of or pertaining to bile. **2.** characterized by an excessive secretion of bile. **3.** characterized by a disorder affecting the bile.

bilirubin /bil′ir̄oo′bin/ [L *bilis* + *ruber* red], the orange-yellow pigment of bile, formed principally by the breakdown of hemoglobin in red blood cells after termination of their normal lifespan. In a healthy person about 250 mg of bilirubin are produced daily, and the majority of that is eventually excreted from the body in the stool. The characteristic yellow pallor of jaundice is caused by the accumulation of bilirubin in the blood and in the tissues of the skin.

bilirubinemia [L *bilis* + *ruber*; Gk, *haima*, blood], the presence of biirubin in the blood.

bilirubinuria, the presence of bilirubin in urine.

biliuria /bil′iy ŏŏr′ē·ə/ [L *bilis* + Gk *ouron* urine], the presence of bile in the urine.

biliverdin /bil′ivur′din/ [L *bilis* + *virdis* green], a greenish bile pigment formed in the breakdown of hemoglobin and converted to bilirubin.

Billings method, a way of estimating ovulation time by changes in the cervical mucus that occur during the menstrual cycle.

Billroth's operation I [Christian A. Billroth, Austrian surgeon, b. 1829], the surgical removal of the pylorus in the treatment of gastric cancer. The proximal end of the duodenum is anastomosed to the stomach.

Billroth's operation II, the surgical removal of the pylorus and duodenum. The cut end of the stomach is anastomosed to the jejunum through the transverse mesocolon.

bilobate /bīlō′bāt/ [L *bis* twice, *lobus* lobe], having two lobes.

bilobate placenta [L *bis* + *lobus* lobe, *placenta* a flat cake], a placenta with two connected lobes.

bilobulate /bīlob′yəlāt/, having two lobules. Also **bilobular.**

bilocular [L *bis* + *loculus* compartment], **1.** divided into two cells. **2.** containing two cells. Also **biloculate.**

bimanual [L *bis* + *manus* hand], of or pertaining to the functioning of both hands.

bimanual palpation, the examination of a woman's pelvic organs conducted by the examiner placing one hand on the abdomen and one or two fingers of the other hand in the vagina.

bimanual percussion [L *bis* + *manus* hand, *percutere* to strike through], a diagnostic technique of producing sound vibrations in body cavities by the use of two hands, one serving as the plexor and the other as the pleximeter.

bimaxillary [L *bis* + *maxilla* jawbone], of or pertaining to the right and left maxilla.

bimodal distribution [L *bis* + *modus* measure], the distribution of quantitative data around two separate modes. It is suggestive of two separate normally distributed populations from which the data are drawn.

bimolecular reaction (E²), an elimination reaction in which more than one kind of molecule is involved. It may follow first-order, second-order, or more complicated chemical kinetics.

binangle /bin'ang·gəl/ [L *bini* twofold, *angulus* angle], a surgical instrument that has a shank with two offsetting angles to keep the cutting edge of the instrument within 3 mm of the shaft axis.

binary fission /bī'nərē/ [L *bini* twofold; *fissionis* splitting], direct division of a cell or nucleus into two equal parts. It is the common form of asexual reproduction of bacteria, protozoa, and other lower forms of life.

binaural stethoscope /bīnôr'əl/ [L *bini* + *auris* ear], a stethoscope having two earpieces.

bind [AS *binden*], **1.** to bandage or wrap in a band. **2.** to join together with a band or with a ligature. **3.** (in chemistry) to combine or unite molecules by employing reactive groups within the molecules or by using a binding chemical.

binder, a bandage made of a large piece of material to fit and support a specific body part.

binding energy, the amount of energy required to remove a particle from the orbit or nucleus of an atom.

binding site [ME *binden;* L *situs*], the location on the surface of a cell or a molecule where other cell fragments or molecules attach to initiate a chemical or physiologic action.

Binet age /binā'/ [Alfred Binet, French psychologist, b. 1857], the mental age of an individual, especially a child, as determined by the Binet-Simon tests, which are evaluated on the basis of tested intelligence of the "normal" individual at any given age. The Binet age corresponding to "profoundly retarded" is 1 to 2 years; to "severely retarded," 3 to 7 years; and to "mildly retarded," 8 to 12 years.

binocular /bīnok'yələr/ [L *bini* + *oculus* eye], **1.** pertaining to both eyes, especially regarding vision. **2.** a microscope, telescope, or field glass that can accommodate viewing by both eyes.

binocular fixation, the process of having both eyes directed at the same object at the same time.

binocular ophthalmoscope, an ophthalmoscope having two eyepieces through which stereoscopic examination of the eye may be made.

binocular parallax /par'əlaks/ [L *bini, oculus;* Gk *parallax* in turn], the difference in the angles formed by the sight lines to two objects situated at different distances from the eyes. Binocular parallax is a major factor in depth perception.

binocular perception, the visual ability to judge depth or distance by virtue of having two eyes.

binocular vision, the use of both eyes simultaneously so that the images perceived by each eye are combined to appear as a single image.

binomial /bīnō'mē·əl/, containing two names or terms.

binomial nomenclature [L *bis;* Gk *nomos* law; L *nomenclatio* calling by name], a system of classification of animals and plants by assigning Latinized genus and species names to each, as *Homo sapiens* for humans.

binovular /bīnov'yələr/ [L *bini* + *ovum* egg], developing from two distinct ova, as in dizygotic twins. Also **diovular.**

binovular twins. See dizygotic twins.

binuclear [L *bis* + *nucleus* nut], having two nuclei, as in the example of a heteroakryon or binucleate hybrid cell.

bioactive [Gk *bios* life; L *activus* with energy], of or pertaining to a substance that has an effect on or causes a reaction in living tissue.

bioactivity, any response from or reaction in living tissue.

bioassay /bī'ō·as'ā, -əsā'/[Gk *bios* + Fr *assayer* to try], the laboratory determination of the concentration of a drug or other substance in a specimen by comparing its effect on an organism, an animal, or an isolated tissue with that of a standard preparation.

bioavailability [Gk *bios* + ME *availen* to

serve], the degree of activity or amount of an administered drug or other substance that becomes available for activity in the target tissue.

biochemical genetics. See *molecular genetics.*

biochemical marker [Gk *bios* + *chemeia* alchemy], any hormone, enzyme, antibody, or other substance that is detected in the urine or other body fluids or tissues that may serve as a sign of a disease or other abnormality.

biochemistry, the chemistry of living organisms and life processes.

biochromatic analysis /-krōmat′ik/ [Gk *bios* + *chroma* color], the spectrophotometric monitoring of a reaction at two wavelengths. It is used to correct for background color.

biodegradable [Gk *bios;* L *de* away, *gradus* step], the natural ability of a chemical substance to be broken down into less complex compounds, or compounds having fewer carbon atoms by bacteria or other microorganisms.

bioelectric impedance analysis (BIA), a method of measuring the fat composition of the body, compared to other tissues, by its resistance to electricity.

bioelectricity [Gk *bios* + *elektron* amber], electric current that is generated by living tissues, such as nerves and muscles.

bioenergetics [Gk *bios* + *energein* to be active], a system of exercises based on the concept that natural healing will be enhanced by bringing into harmony the patient's body rhythms and the natural environment.

bioequivalent /bī′ō·ikwiv′ələnt/ [Gk *bios* + L *aequus* equal, *valere* to be strong], **1.** (in pharmacology) of or pertaining to a drug that has the same effect on the body as another drug, usually one nearly identical in its chemical formulation. **2.** a bioequivalent drug. **–bioequivalence,** *n.*

biofeedback [Gk *bios* + AS *faedan* food, *baec* back], a process providing a person with visual or auditory information about the autonomic physiologic functions of his or her body, such as blood pressure, muscle tension, and brain wave activity, usually through use of instrumentation.

bioflavonoid /bī′ōflā′vənoid/ [Gk *bios* + L *flavus* yellow; Gk *eidos* form, a generic term for any of a group of colored flavones found in many fruits and essential for the absorption and metabolism of ascorbic acid.

biogenesis /bī′ōjen′əsis/ [Gk *bios* + *genein* to produce], **1.** the doctrine that living material can originate only from preexisting life and not from inanimate matter. **2.** the origin of life and living organisms;

ontogeny and phylogeny. **–biogenetic,** *adj.*

biogenetic law. See **recapitulation theory.**

biogenic /bī′ōjen′ik/, **1.** produced by the action of a living organism, such as fermentation. **2.** essential to life and the maintenance of health, such as food, water, and proper rest.

biogenic amine, one of a large group of naturally occurring biologically active compounds most of which act as neurotransmitters. The most dominant, norepinephrine, is involved in such physiologic functions as emotional reactions, memory, sleep, and arousal from sleep.

biogenous /bī·oj′ənəs/ **1.** biogenetic. **2.** biogenic.

biogeny. See **biogenesis.**

biohazard [Gk *bios;* OFr *hasard*], anything that is a risk to living organisms, as exposure to ionizing radiation.

biokinetics /-kinet′iks/ [Gk *bios* + *kinetikos* moving], a branch of science that deals with movements within developing organisms.

biologic [Gk *bios* + *logos* science], **1.** pertaining to living organisms and their products. **2.** any preparation made from living organisms or the products of living organisms and used as diagnostic, preventive, or therapeutic agents. Kinds of biologics are **antigens, antitoxins, serums,** and **vaccines.**

biologic activity, the inherent capacity of a substance, such as a drug or toxin, to alter one or more of the chemical or physiologic functions of a cell. The capacity has relationships not only to the physical and chemical nature of the substance but also to its concentration and the duration of cellular exposure to the substance.

biologic armature, the connective-tissue-rich aggregate of larger ducts, vessels, and autonomic nerves that in many mammalian exocrine glands serve as an internal framework whose function of support, and often of anchorage, resembles that of the armature within a clay sculpture.

biologic assay. See **bioassay.**

biologic half-life, the time required for the body to eliminate one half of an administered dose of any substance by regular physiologic processes.

biologic monitoring, 1. a process of measuring the levels of various physiologic substances, drugs, or metabolites within a patient during diagnosis or therapy. **2.** the measurement of toxic substances in the environment and the identification of health risks to the population.

biologic plausibility, a method of reasoning used to establish a cause and effect relationship between a biologic factor and a particular disease.

biologic psychiatry, a school of psychiatric thought that stresses the physical, chemical, and neurologic causes of and treatments for mental and emotional disorders.

biologic rhythm [Gk *bios* + *logos* science + *rhythmos*], the periodic recurrence of certain biologic phenomena, such as circadian rhythms.

biologic vector. See **vector.**

biologist [Gk *bios* + *logos*], a person who studies the science of life.

biology, the scientific study of plants and animals. Some branches of biology are **biometry, ecology, molecular biology,** and **paleontology.**

biome /bī′ōm/ [Gk *bios* + *oma* tumor, mass, the total group of biologic communities existing in and characteristic of a given geographic region, such as a desert, woodland, or marsh.

biomechanical adaptation, a process in the use of orthotic treatment to enable a disabled person to resume normal function of a body part with the aid of a device, such as an ankle-foot brace. The process of adaptation includes the central nervous system input received during therapeutic exercises with the orthotic appliance.

biomechanics [Gk *bios* + *mechane* machine], the study of mechanical laws and their application to living organisms, especially the human body and its locomotor system. **–biomechanic, biomechanical,** *adj.*

biomedical engineering [Gk *bios* + L *medicare* to heal], a system of techniques in which knowledge of biologic processes is applied to solve practical medical problems and to answer questions in biomedical research.

bionics /bī·on′iks/, the science of applying electronic principles and devices, such as computers and solid state miniaturized circuitry, to medical problems, such as artificial pacemakers used to correct abnormal heart rhythms. **–bionic,** *adj.*

biophore /bī′əfôr′/ [Gk *bios* + *phora* bearer], a theoretical basic hereditary unit contained in the germ plasm from which all living cells develop and all inherited characteristics are transmitted.

biopotentials, electric charges produced by various tissues of the body, particularly muscle tissue during contractions.

biopsy /bī′opsē/ [Gk *bios* + *opsis* view], **1.** the removal of a small piece of living tissue from an organ or other part of the body for microscopic examination to confirm or establish a diagnosis, estimate prognosis, or follow the course of a disease. **2.** the tissue excised for examination. **3.** *informal.* to excise tissue for examination. Kinds of biopsy include **aspiration, needle, punch,** and **surface biopsy.** **–bioptic,** *adj.*

biopsychic [Gk *bios* + *psyche* mind], of or pertaining to psychic factors as they relate to living organisms.

biopsychology. See **psychobiology.**

biopsychosocial [Gk *bios* + *psyche* mind; L *socius* companion], of or pertaining to the complex of biologic, psychologic, and social aspects of life.

bioptome tip catheter /bī·op′tōm/, a catheter with a special tip designed for obtaining endomyocardial biopsy samples. The bioptome tip device is used to monitor heart transplant patients for early signs of tissue rejection.

biorhythm /bī′ōrithm/ [Gk *bios* + *rhythmos* rhythm], any cyclic, biologic event or phenomenon, such as the sleep cycle, the menstrual cycle, or the respiratory cycle. **–biorhythmic,** *adj.*

biostatistics, numeric data on births, deaths, diseases, injuries, and other factors affecting the general health and condition of human populations.

biosynthesis [Gk *bios* + *synthesis* putting together], any one of thousands of chemical reactions continually occurring throughout the body in which molecules form more complex biomolecules. **–biosynthetic,** *adj.*

biotaxis /bī′ōtak′sis/ [Gk *bios* + *taxis* arrangement], the ability of living cells to develop into certain forms and arrangements. **–biotactic,** *adj.*

biotaxy /bī′ōtak′sē/, **1.** biotaxis. **2.** the systematic classification of living organisms according to their anatomic characteristics; taxonomy.

biotechnology [Gk *bios* + *techne* art, *logos* science] **1.** the study of the relationships between humans or other living organisms and machinery, such as the ability of airplane pilots to perform tasks when traveling at supersonic speeds. **2.** the industrial application of the results of biologic research, particularly in fields such as recombinant DNA or gene splicing.

biotelemetry /bī′ōtələm′ətrē/, the transmission of physiologic data, such as ECG and EEG recordings, heart rate, and body temperature by radio or telephone systems.

biotic potential /bī·ot′ik/, the possible growth rate of a population of organisms under ideal conditions, including absence of predators and maximum nutrients and space for expansion.

biotin /bī′ətin/ [Gk *bios* life], a colorless, crystalline, water-soluble B complex vitamin that acts as a coenzyme in fatty acid production and in the oxidation of fatty acids and carbohydrates.

biotin deficiency syndrome, an abnormal condition caused by a deficiency of biotin, characterized by dermatitis, hyperesthesia, muscle pain, anorexia, slight anemia, and changes in electrocardiographic activity of the heart.

biotope /bī′ətōp/ [Gk *bios* + *topos* place], a specific biologic habitat or site.

biotransformation [Gk *bios* + L *trans* across, *formare* to form], the chemical changes a substance undergoes in the body, such as by the action of enzymes.

Biot's respiration /bē-ōz′/ [Camille Biot, French physician, b. 1878], an abnormal respiratory pattern, characterized by irregular breathing with periods of apnea.

biovular twins. See **dizygotic twins.**

bipara /bip′ərə/, a woman who has given birth twice in separate pregnancies.

biparental inheritance. See **amphigenous inheritance.**

biparietal /bīpərī′ətəl/ [L *bis* twice, *paries* wall], of or pertaining to the two parietal bones of the head, such as the biparietal diameter.

biparietal diameter, the distance between the protuberances of the two parietal bones of the skull.

biparietal suture [L *bis* + *paries* wall + *sutura*], the interlocking lines of fusion between two parietal bones of the skull.

biparous [L *bis* twice, *parere* to produce], pertaining to the birth of two infants in a single pregnancy.

bipartite /bīpär′tīt/, having two parts.

biped /bī′ped/, **1.** having two feet. **2.** any animal with only two feet.

bipedal [L *bis* twice, *pes* foot], capable of locomotion on two feet.

bipenniform /bīpen′ifôrm′/ [L *bis* + *penna* feather, *forma* form], (of bodily structure) having the bilateral symmetry of a feather, such as the pattern formed by the fasciculi that converge on both sides of a muscle tendon in the rectus femoris.

biperiden /bīper′iden/, a synthetic anticholinergic agent prescribed in the treatment of Parkinson's disease and drug-induced extrapyramidal disorders. Biperiden hydrochloride is administered orally, and biperiden lactate is administered intramuscularly or intravenously.

biphasic /bīfā′zik/ [L *bis* + Gk *phasis* appearance], having two phases, parts, aspects, or stages.

bipolar /bīpo′lər/ [L *bis* + *polus* pole], **1.** having two poles, such as in certain electrotherapeutic treatments using two poles or in certain bacterial staining that affects only the two poles of the microor-

ganism under study. **2.** (of a nerve cell) having an afferent and an efferent process.

bipolar disorder, a major psychologic disorder characterized by episodes of mania, depression, or mixed mood. One or the other phase may be predominant at any given time, one phase may appear alternately with the other, or elements of both phases may be present simultaneously. Characteristics of the manic phase are excessive emotional displays, excitement, euphoria, hyperactivity accompanied by elation, boisterousness, impaired ability to concentrate, decreased need for sleep, and seemingly unbounded energy, often accompanied by delusions of grandeur. In the depressive phase, marked apathy and underactivity are accompanied by feelings of profound sadness, loneliness, guilt, and lowered self-esteem.

bipolar lead /lēd/, **1.** an electrocardiographic conductor having two electrodes placed on different body regions, with each electrode contributing significantly to the record. **2.** *informal.* a tracing produced by such a lead on an electrocardiograph.

bipotentiality [L *bis* + *potentia* power], the characteristic of acting or reacting according to either of two potentials.

bird breeder's lung. See **pigeon breeder's lung.**

bird face retrognathism, an abnormal facial profile with an undeveloped mandible, which may be caused by interference of condylar growth associated with trauma or condylar infection.

bird headed dwarf, a person affected with Seckel's syndrome, a congenital disorder characterized by a proportionate shortness of stature; a proportionately small head with hypoplasia of the jaws, large eyes, and a beaklike protrusion of the nose; mental retardation; and various other defects.

birth [ME *burth*], **1.** the event of being born, the coming of a new person out of its mother into the world. Kinds of birth are **breech birth, live birth,** and **stillbirth. 2.** the child-bearing event, the bringing forth by a mother of a baby. **3.** a medical event, the delivery of a fetus by an obstetric attendant.

birth canal, *informal.* the passage that extends from the inlet of the true pelvis to the vaginal orifice through which an infant passes during vaginal birth.

birth control. See **contraception.**

birth defect. See **congenital anomaly.**

birth injury, trauma suffered by a baby while being born. Some kinds of birth injury are **Bell's palsy, cerebral palsy,** and **Erb's palsy.**

birth mother, the biological mother or

woman who bears a child. The child may have been conceived in a surrogate mother with sperm of the biological father.

birth palsy [ME *burth;* Gk *paralyein* to be palsied], a loss of motor or sensory nerve function in some part of the body because of a nerve injury during the birth process.

birth paralysis, paralysis, usually of an arm, due to a brachial plexus injury during the birth process.

birth parents, the biological parents, or the combined source of the entire genetic information of a child.

birth rate, the proportion of the number of births in a specific area during a given period to the total population of that area, usually expressed as the number of births per 1,000 of population.

birth trauma, 1. any physical injury suffered by an infant during the process of delivery. **2.** the supposed psychic shock, according to some psychiatric theories, that an infant suffers during delivery.

birth weight, the measured heaviness of a baby when born, usually about 3,500 g (7.5 pounds). In the United States, 97% of newborns weigh between 2,500 g (5.5 pounds) and 4,500 g (10 pounds).

birthmark. See nevus.

birthing chair, a chair used in labor and delivery to promote the comfort of the mother and the efficiency of parturition. The birthing chair allows the woman to sit straight up or to recline. The upright position appears to shorten the time in labor, particularly the second or expulsive stage of labor, probably because of gravity and increased participation of the mother.

bisacodyl /bisak′ōdil/, a cathartic prescribed in the treatment of acute or chronic constipation, to empty the bowel preoperatively or postoperatively or before diagnostic radiographic procedures.

bisect /bīsekt′/ [L *bis* + *secare* to cut], to divide into two equal lengths or parts.

bisexual /bīsek′shōo·əl/ [L *bis* + *sexus* male or female], **1.** hermaphroditic; having gonads of both sexes. **2.** possessing physical or psychologic characteristics of both sexes. **3.** engaging in both heterosexual and homosexual activity. **4.** desiring sexual contact with persons of both sexes.

bisexual libido, (in psychoanalysis) the tendency in a person to seek sexual gratification with people of either sex.

bisferial pulse /bisfer′ē·əs/ [L *bis* + *ferire* to beat], an arterial pulse that has two palpable peaks, the second of which is slightly weaker than the first. It may be detected in cases of aortic regurgitation and obstructive cardiomyopathy.

bishydroxycoumarin. See dicumarol.

bis in die (b.d., b.i.d.) /dē′ā/, a Latin phrase, used in prescriptions, meaning "twice a day." It is more commonly used in its abbreviated form.

bismuth (Bi) [Ger *wismut* white mass], a reddish, crystalline, trivalent metallic element. Its atomic number is 83; its atomic weight is 209. It is combined with various other elements, such as oxygen, to produce numerous salts used in the manufacture of many pharmaceutical substances.

bismuth gingivitis, a symptom of metallic poisoning caused by bismuth administered in the treatment of systemic disease. It is characterized by a dark bluish line along the gingival margin.

bismuth stomatitis, an abnormal oral condition caused by systemic use of bismuth compounds over prolonged periods, characterized by a blue-black line on the inner aspect of the gingival sulcus or pigmentation of the buccal mucosa, a sore tongue, metallic taste, and a burning sensation in the mouth.

bitart, abbreviation for a *bitartrate carboxylate anion.*

bite [AS *bitan*], **1.** the act of cutting, tearing, holding, or gripping with the teeth. **2.** the lingual portion of an artificial tooth between its shoulder and incisal edge. **3.** an occlusal record or relationship.

bite block. See occlusion rim.

bitegage /bīt′gāj′/ [AS *bitan* + OFr *gauge* measure], a prosthetic dental device that helps attain proper occlusion of the teeth rooted in the maxilla and the mandible.

biteguard [AS *bitan* + OFr *garder* to defend], a resin appliance that covers the occlusal and incisal surfaces of the teeth. It is designed to stabilize the teeth and provide a platform for the excursive glides of the mandible.

biteguard splint, a device for covering the occlusal and incisal surfaces of the teeth and for protecting them from traumatic occlusal forces during immobilization and stabilization processes.

bitelock /bīt′lok′/, a dental device for retaining the occlusion rims in the same relation outside the mouth as inside the mouth.

bitemporal /bītem′pərəl/ [L *bis* twice, *tempora* temples], of or pertaining to both temples or both temporal bones.

bitemporal hemianopia [L *bis* + *tempora;* Gk *hemi* half, *opsis* vision], a loss of the temporal half of the vision in each eye, usually due to a lesion in the chiasmal area, such as pituitary tumors.

biteplane /bīt′plān/, **1.** a plane formed by the biting surfaces of the teeth. **2.** a metal sheet laid across the biting surfaces of either mandibular or maxillary teeth to determine the relationship of the teeth to this predetermined plane. **3.** an orthodontic appliance worn over the maxillary occlusal surfaces and used to treat pain of the temporomandibular joint and adjacent muscles.

biteplate, a device used in dentistry as a diagnostic or a therapeutic aid for prosthodontics or for orthodontics.

bite reflex, a swift, involuntary biting action that may be triggered by stimulation of the oral cavity.

bite wing film [AS *bitan* + ME *winge*], a type of dental x-ray film that has a central tab or wing on which the teeth close to maintain film position during radiographic examination.

bite wing radiograph, a kind of dental radiograph that reveals approximately the coronal portions of maxillary and mandibular teeth and portions of the interdental septa on the same film.

bithionol (TBP) /bithī′ənôl/, a pale gray powder, soluble in acetone, alcohol, or ether, used as a local antiseptic and administered orally in the treatment of infestations of the giant liver fluke and of the lung fluke.

Bithynia /bəthin′ē·ə/, a genus of snails, species of which act as intermediate hosts to *Opisthorchis.*

biting in childhood, a natural behavior trait and reflex action in infants, acquired at about 5 to 6 months of age in response to the introduction of solid foods in the diet and the beginning of the teething process. The activity represents a significant modality in the psychosocial development of the child, because it is the first aggressive action the infant learns, and through it the infant learns to control the environment.

bitolterol mesylate /bitol′tərol mes′ilāt/, an orally inhaled bronchodilator used in the treatment of bronchial asthma and reversible bronchospasm.

Bitot's spots /bitōz′/ [Pierre Bitot, French surgeon, b. 1822], white or gray triangular deposits on the bulbar conjunctiva adjacent to the lateral margin of the cornea, a clinical sign of vitamin A deficiency.

bitrochanteric lipodystrophy /bī′trōkənter′ik/ [L *bis* + Gk *trochanter* runner; *lipos* fat, *dys* bad, *trophe* nourishment], an abnormal and excessive deposition of fat on the buttocks and the outer aspect of the upper thighs, occurring most commonly in women.

biuret test /bī′yŏŏret/ [L *bis* + Gk *ouron* urine], a method for detecting urea and other soluble proteins in serum.

bivalent /bīvā′lənt/ [L *bis* + *valere* to be powerful], **1.** (in genetics) a pair of synapsed homologous chromosomes that are attached to each other by chiasmata during the early first meiotic prophase of gametogenesis. **–bivalence,** *n.*

bivalent chromosome, a pair of synapsed homologous chromosomes during the early stages of gametogenesis.

bivalve cast [L *bis* + *valva* valve], an orthopedic cast used for immobilizing a section of the body for the healing of one or more broken bones or for correction or the maintenance of correction of an orthopedic deformity. The cast is cut in half to monitor and detect pressure under the cast.

bizarre leiomyoma. See **epithelioid leiomyoma.**

BK, abbreviation for *below the knee,* a term referring to amputations, amputees, prostheses, and orthoses.

Bk, symbol for the element **berkelium.**

BL, abbreviation for **baralyme.**

black damp. See **damp.**

black death. See **bubonic plague.**

Blackett-Healy method, a procedure for positioning a patient for making radiographs of the subscapularis area. The affected shoulder joint is centered to the midline of the film, the arm abducted, and the elbow flexed.

black eye, an eyelid contusion. It is usually treated for the first 24 hours with ice packs to reduce swelling, then treated with hot compresses to aid in resorption of blood from the hematoma.

black fever. See **kala-azar.**

black hairy tongue [AS *blac* + *haer* + *tunge*], a black or brown patch on the back of the tongue accompanied by filiform papillae. The condition is associated with heavy smoking or the use of broad spectrum antibiotics.

blackhead. See **comedo.**

black light. See **Wood's light.**

black lung disease. See **anthracosis, pneumoconiosis.**

black measles [AS *blac;* OHG *masala*], hemorrhagic measles characterized by a darkened rash due to bleeding into the skin and mucous membranes.

blackout, *informal.* a temporary loss of vision or consciousness resulting from cerebral ischemia.

black plague. See **bubonic plague.**

black spots film fault, a defect in a radiograph, seen as dark spots throughout the image area.

black tongue. See **parasitic glossitis.**

blackwater fever, a serious complication of chronic falciparum malaria, characterized by jaundice, hemoglobinuria, acute renal failure, and the passage of bloody dark red or black urine because of massive intravascular hemolysis.

Blackwell, Elizabeth (1821–1910), a British-born American physician, the first woman to receive a medical degree. She established the New York Infirmary, a 40-bed hospital staffed entirely by women. Her influence helped establish nursing schools to improve patient care.

black widow spider [AS blac, widewe], a poisonous arachnid found in many parts of the world. The venom injected with its bite causes perspiration, abdominal cramps, nausea, headaches, and dizziness of various levels of intensity.

black widow spider bite [AS *blac* + *widewe*; ME *spithre*; AS *bitan*], the bite of the spider species *Lactrodectus mactans*, causing generalized spastic contractions and localized tissue necrosis. Black widow venom contains some enzymatic proteins, including a peptide that affects neuromuscular transmission. The bite is perceived as a sharp pinprick pain, followed by a dull pain in the area of the bite, muscular rigidity in the shoulders, back, and abdomen, restlessness, anxiety, sweating, weakness, and drooping eyelids.

black widow spider antivenin, a passive immunizing agent prescribed in the treatment of black widow spider bite.

bladder [AS *blaedre*], **1.** a membranous sac serving as a receptacle for secretions. **2.** the urinary bladder.

bladder cancer, the most common malignancy of the urinary tract, characterized by multiple growths that tend to recur in a more aggressive form. Bladder cancer occurs 2.3 times more often in men than in women and is more prevalent in urban than in rural areas. The risk of bladder cancer is increased with cigarette smoking and exposure to aniline dyes, beta-naphthylamine, mixtures of aromatic hydrocarbons, or benzidine and its salts, used in chemical, paint, plastics, rubber, textile, petroleum, wood industries, and in medical laboratories. Other predisposing factors are chronic urinary tract infections, calculous disease, and schistosomiasis. Early symptoms of bladder cancer include hematuria, frequent urination, dysuria, and cystitis. Urinalysis, excretory urography, cystoscopy, or transurethral biopsy are performed for diagnosis. The majority of bladder malignancies are transitional cell carcinomas; a small percentage are squamous cell carcinomas or adenocarcinomas.

bladder flap, *informal.* the vesicouterine fold of peritoneum that is incised during low cervical cesarean section so that the bladder can be separated from the uterus to expose the lower uterine segment for incision. The flap is reapproximated with sutures during closure.

bladder irrigation [AS *blaedre;* L *irrigare* to conduct water], the washing out of the bladder by a continuous or intermittent flow of water or a medicated solution. The bladder also may be irrigated by an oral intake of fluid.

bladder retraining [AS *blaedre;* L *trahere* to draw], a system of therapy for incontinence in which a patient in a hospital setting practices withholding urine for intervals that begin with one hour and increase over a period of 10 days while maintaining a normal intake of fluid. The patient also learns to recognize and react to the urge to void.

bladder sphincter [AS *blaedre;* Gk *sphigkter* one that binds], a circular muscle surrounding the opening of the urinary bladder into the urethra.

bladder stone. See vesicle calculus.

Blakemore-Sengstaken tube. See Sengstaken-Blakemore tube.

Blalock-Taussig procedure /blä'loktô'sig/ [Alfred Blalock, American surgeon, b. 1899; Helen B. Taussig, American physician, b. 1898], surgical construction of a shunt as a temporary measure to overcome congenital pulmonary stenosis and atrial septal defect, such as in an infant born with tetralogy of Fallot. The subclavian artery is joined end to end with the pulmonary artery, directing blood from the systemic circulation to the lungs. Thrombosis of the shunt is the major postoperative complication.

blame placing, the process of placing responsibility for one's behavior on others.

blanch [Fr *blanchir* to become white], **1.** to cause to become pale, as a spider angiomata may be blanched using digital pressure. **2.** to whiten or bleach a surface or substance. **3.** to become white or pale, as from vasoconstriction accompanying fear or anger.

blanch test [Fr *blanchir;* L *testum* crucible], a test of blood circulation in the fingers or toes. Pressure is applied to the nail over a finger or toe until normal color is lost. The pressure is then removed and, if the circulation is normal, color will return within about five seconds.

bland [L *blandus*], mild or having a soothing effect.

bland aerosols, aerosols that consist of water, saline solutions, or similar substances that lack important pharmacologic action. They are primarily used for humidification and liquefaction of secretions.

bland diet, a diet that is mechanically, chemically, physiologically, and, sometimes, thermally nonirritating. It is often prescribed in the treatment of peptic ulcer, ulcerative colitis, gallbladder disease, diverticulosis and diverticulitis, gastritis, idiopathic spastic constipation, and mucous colitis and after abdominal surgery. The diet may include eggs, meat, poultry, fish, and enriched fine cereals; milk is usually an important ingredient. Highly seasoned foods, carbonated beverages, raw fruits and vegetables, and rich desserts are avoided.

blanket bath [OFr *blanchet* a white garment], the procedure of wrapping the patient in a wet pack and then in blankets.

blast cell [Gk *blastos* germ], any immature cell, such as an erythroblast, a lymphoblast, or a neuroblast.

blastema /blastē′mə/, *pl.* **blastemas, blastemata** [Gk, bud], **1.** any mass of living protoplasm capable of growth and differentiation, specifically the primordial undifferentiated cellular material from which a particular organ or tissue develops. **2.** in certain animals, a group of cells capable of regenerating a lost or damaged part or of giving rise to a complete organism in asexual reproduction. **3.** the budding or sprouting area of a plant. –**blastemal, blastematic, blastemic,** *adj.*

blastic transformation, a late stage in the progress of chronic granulocytic leukemia. There are signs of anemia and blood platelet deficiency. Blastic transformation indicates that the patient has developed resistance to therapy and has entered a terminal stage of leukemia.

blastid /blas′tid/ [Gk *blastos* germ], the site in the fertilized ovum where the pronuclei fuse and the nucleus forms.

blastin /blas′tin/ [Gk *blastanein* to grow], any substance that provides nourishment for or stimulates the growth or proliferation of cells, such as allantoin.

blastocoele /blas′təsēl′/ [Gk *blastos* germ, *koilos* hollow], the fluid-filled cavity of the blastocyst in mammals and the blastula or discoblastula of lower animals. The cavity increases the surface area of the developing embryo for better absorption of nutrients and oxygen.

blastocyst /blas′təsist/ [Gk *blastos* + *kystis* bag], the embryonic form that follows the morula in human development. It is a spheric mass of cells having a central, fluid-filled cavity (blastocele) surrounded by two layers of cells. The outer layer (trophoblast) later forms the placenta; the inner layer (embryoblast) later forms the embryo. Implantation in the wall of the uterus usually occurs at this stage on approximately the eighth day after fertilization.

blastocyte /blas′təsīt/ [Gk *blastos* + *kytos* cell], an undifferentiated embryonic cell before germ layer formation. –**blastocytic,** *adj.*

blastocytoma. See **blastoma.**

blastoderm /blas′tədurm′/ [Gk *blastos* + *derma* skin], the layer of cells forming the wall of the blastocyst in mammals and the blastula in lower animals during early embryonic development. It is produced by the cleavage of the fertilized ovum and gives rise to the primary germ layers, the ectoderm, mesoderm, and endoderm. Kinds of blastoderm are **bilaminar, embryonic, extraembryonic,** and **trilaminar blastoderm.** –**blastodermal, blastodermic,** *adj.*

blastodisk, the disklike nonyolk area of the protoplasm surrounding the animal pole where cleavage occurs in a fertilized ovum containing a large amount of yolk, such as in birds and reptiles.

blastogenesis /blas′tōjen′əsis/ [Gk *blastos* + *genein* to produce], **1.** asexual reproduction by budding. **2.** the theory of the transmission of hereditary characteristics by the germ plasm, as opposed to the theory of pangenesis. **3.** the early development of the embryo during cleavage and formation of the germ layers. **4.** the process of transforming small lymphocytes in tissue culture into large blastlike cells by exposure to phytohemagglutin or other substances, often for the purpose of inducing mitosis. –**blastogenetic,** *adj.*

blastogenic, 1. originating in the germ plasm. **2.** initiating tissue proliferation. **3.** relating to or characterized by blastogenesis.

blastogeny /blastoj′ənē/, the early stages in ontogeny; the germ plasm history of an organism or species, which traces the history of the inherited characteristics.

blastokinin /blas′təki′nin/ [Gk *blastos* + *kinein* to move], a globulin, secreted by the uterus in many mammals, that may stimulate and regulate the implantation process of the blastocyst in the uterine wall.

blastolysis /blastol′isis/ [Gk *blastos* + *lysis* loosening], destruction of a germ cell or blastoderm. –**blastolytic,** *adj.*

blastoma /blastō′mə/, *pl.* **blastomas, blastomata** [Gk *blastos* + *oma* tumor], a neoplasm of embryonic tissue developing from the blastema of an organ or tissue. **blastomatous,** *adj.*

blastomatosis /blast′tōmətō′sis/ [Gk *blastos* + *oma* tumor, *osis* condition], the development of many tumors derived from embryonic tissue.

blastomere /blas′təmēr/ [Gk *blastos* + *meros* part], one of a pair of cells that develops in the first mitotic division of the segmentation nucleus of a fertilized ovum. The two blastomeres divide and subdivide to form the morula in the first several days of pregnancy. **–blastomeric,** *adj.*

blastomerotomy [Gk *blastos* + *meros* part, *tome* cut], the destruction or the separation of blastomeres, either caused naturally or induced artificially. **–blastomerotomic,** *adj.*

Blastomyces /blas′tōmī′sēz/ [Gk *blastos* + *mykes* fungus], a genus of yeastlike fungus, usually including the species *Blastomyces dermatitidis,* which causes North American blastomycosis, and *Paracoccidioides brasiliensis,* which causes South American blastomycosis.

blastomycosis /blas′tōmīkō′sis/ [Gk *blastos* + *mykes* fungus, *osis* condition], an infectious disease caused by a yeastlike fungus, *Blastomyces dermatitidis,* which usually affects only the skin but may invade the lungs, kidneys, central nervous system, and bones. Skin infections often begin as small papules on the hand, face, neck, or other exposed areas where there has been a cut, bruise, or other injury and spread into surrounding areas. When the lungs are involved, x-ray films of the chest show tumors resembling cancer.

blastopore /blas′təpôr/ [Gk *blastos* + *poros* opening], (in embryology) the invagination into a blastula that occurs in the process of the blastula becoming a gastrula.

blastoporic canal. See **neurenteric canal.**

blastosphere. See **blastula.**

blastotomy. See **blastomerotomy.**

blastula /blas′tyələ/ [Gk *blastos* germ], an early stage of the process through which a zygote develops into an embryo, characterized by a fluid-filled sphere formed by a single layer of cells called a blastoderm. The blastula develops from the morula stage.

blastulation, the transformation of the morula into a blastocyst or blastula by the development of a central cavity, the blastocoele.

BLB mask, abbreviation for **Boothby-Lovelace-Bulbulian mask.**

bleb /bleb/ [ME, blob], an accumulation of fluid under the skin.

bleed [AS *blod* blood], **1.** to lose blood from the blood vessels of the body. **2.** to cause blood to flow from a vein or an artery.

bleeder, *informal.* **1.** a person who has hemophilia or any other vascular or hematologic condition associated with a tendency to hemorrhage. **2.** blood vessel that

bleeds, especially one cut during a surgical procedure.

bleeding, the release of blood from the vascular system as a result of damage to or inadequacy of one or more blood vessels.

bleeding diasthesis, a predisposition to abnormal blood clotting.

bleeding time, the time required for blood to stop flowing from a tiny wound.

blended family [ME *blenden* to mix], a family formed when parents bring together children from previous marriages.

blending inheritance, the apparent fusion in the offspring of distinct, dissimilar characteristics of the parents, usually of a quantitative nature, such as height, with segregation of the specific traits failing to appear in successive generations.

blennorrhea /blen′ərē′ə/ [Gk *blennos* mucus, *rhoia* flow], excessive discharge of mucus.

bleomycin sulfate /blē′əmī′sin/, an antineoplastic antibiotic prescribed in the treatment of a variety of neoplasms.

blepharal /blef′ərəl/ [Gk *blepharon* eyelid], of or pertaining to the eyelids.

blepharitis /blef′ərī′tis/ [Gk *blepharon* + *itis*], an inflammatory condition of the lash follicles and meibomian glands of the eyelids characterized by swelling, redness, and crusts of dried mucus on the lids. **Ulcerative blepharitis** is caused by bacterial infection. **Nonulcerative blepharitis** may be caused by psoriasis, seborrhea, or an allergic response.

blepharoadenoma /blef′ərō·ad′inō′mə/, *pl.* **blepharoadenomas, blepharoadenomata,** a glandular epithelial tumor of the eyelid.

blepharoatheroma /blef′ərō·ath′ərō′mə/, *pl.* **blepharoatheromas, blepharoatheromata,** a tumor of the eyelid.

blepharoncus /blef′əron′kəs/ [Gk *blepharon* + *onkos* swelling], a tumor of the eyelid.

blepharoplasty /blef′əroplas′tē/ [Gk, *blepharon,* eyelid, *plassein,* to mold], the use of plastic surgery to restore or repair the eyelid and eyebrow.

blepharoplegia /blef′əröplē′jē·ə/ [Gk *blepharon* + *plege* stroke], paralysis of the eyelid.

blepharospasm /blef′ərōspaz′əm/, the involuntary contraction of eyelid muscles.

blight, any disease of plants caused by fungus.

blighted ovum, a fertilized ovum that fails to develop.

blind [AS *blind*], the absence of sight. The term may indicate a total loss of vision or may be applied in a modified manner to describe certain visual limitation, as in yellow color blindness (tritanopia) or word blindness (dyslexia).

blind fistula [AS *blind*; L, pipe], an abnormal passage with only one open end; the opening may be on the body surface or on or within an internal organ or structure.

blindgut. See **cecum.**

blind intubation. See **intubation.**

blind loop [AS *blind*; ME *loupe*], a redundant segment of intestine. Blind loops may be created inadvertently by surgical procedures, such as side to side ileotransverse colostomy.

blindness. See **blind.**

blind spot, 1. a normal gap in the visual field occurring when an image is focused on the space in the retina occupied by the optic disc. **2.** an abnormal gap in the visual field because of a lesion on the retina or in the optic pathways or because of hemorrhage or choroiditis, often perceived as light spots or flashes.

blink reflex, [ME *blenken*; L *reflectere* to bend back], the automatic closure of the eyelid when an object is perceived to be approaching the eye rapidly.

blister, a vesicle or bulla.

bloat [ME *blout*], a swelling or filling with gas, as the distention of the abdomen from swallowing air or from intestinal gas.

blockade, an agent that interferes with or prevents a specific action in an organ or tissue, such as a cholinergic blockade that inhibits transmission of acetylcholine-stimulated nerve impulses along fibers of the autonomic nervous system.

block anesthesia. See **conduction anesthesia.**

blocked communication, a situation in which communication with a patient is difficult because of incongruent verbal and nonverbal messages, and messages that contain discrepancies and inconsistencies.

blocking [ME *blok*], **1.** preventing the transmission of an impulse, such as by an antiadrenergic agent or by the injection of an anesthetic. **2.** interrupting an intracellular biosynthetic process. **3.** being unable to remember or involuntarily interrupting a train of thought or speech, usually because of emotional or mental conflict. **4.** repressing an idea or emotion to keep it from obtruding into the consciousness.

blocking antibody, an antibody that fails to cross-link and cause agglutination.

blood [AS *blod*], the liquid pumped by the heart through all the arteries, veins, and capillaries. It consists of a clear yellow fluid called plasma and the formed elements, a series of different cell types, all with varying functions. The major function of the blood is to transport oxygen and nutrients to the cells and to remove from the cells carbon dioxide and other waste products for detoxification and elimination.

blood agar, a culture medium consisting of blood and nutrient agar, used in bacteriology to cultivate certain microorganisms, including *Staphylococcus epidermidis, Diplococcus pneumoniae,* and *Clostridium perfringens.*

blood albumin [AS *blod*; L *albus*], the albumin circulating in blood serum.

blood bank, an organizational unit responsible for collecting, processing, and storing blood to be used for transfusion and other purposes. It is usually a subdivision of a laboratory in a hospital.

blood bank technology specialist, an allied health professional who performs both routine and specialized tests in blood bank immunohematology in technical areas of the modern blood bank and perform transfusion services using methodology that conforms to the *Standards for Blood Banks and Transfusion Services* of the American Association of Blood Banks.

blood-borne pathogens, pathogenic microorganisms that are present in human blood and cause disease in humans.

blood-brain barrier (BBB) [AS *blod; bragen;* ME *barrere*], an anatomic-physiologic feature of the brain thought to consist of walls of capillaries in the central nervous system and surrounding glial membranes. The blood-brain barrier functions in preventing or slowing the passage of various chemical compounds, radioactive ions, and disease-causing organisms from the blood into the central nervous system.

blood buffers [AS *blod*; ME *buffe* to cushion], a system of buffers, composed primarily of dissolved carbon dioxide and bicarbonate ions that functions in maintaining the proper pH of the blood.

blood capillaries [AS *blod*; L *capillaris* hairlike], the hairlike vessels that convey blood between the arterioles and the venules. The capillary wall generally has a thickness of one cell, and occasional tiny openings permit the distribution of oxygen and nutrients to the tissues supplied by the capillary network and the collection of waste products released by the cells.

blood cell, any one of the formed elements of the blood, including red cells (erythrocytes), white cells (leukocytes), and platelets (thrombocytes). Together they normally constitute about 50% of the total volume of the blood.

blood cell casts [AS *blod*; L *cella* storeroom; ONorse *kasta*], a mass of blood debris released from a diseased body surface or excreted in the urine.

blood circulation [AS *blod;* L *circulare* to go around], the circuit of blood through the body, from the heart through the arteries, arterioles, capillaries, venules, veins, and back to the heart.

blood clot [AS *blod; clott* lump], a semisolid, gelatinous mass, the end result of the clotting process in blood. It ordinarily consists of red cells, white cells, and platelets enmeshed in an insoluble fibrin network.

blood clotting, the conversion of blood from a free-flowing liquid to a semisolid gel. The process usually starts with tissue damage and exposure of the blood to air. Within seconds of injury to the vessel wall, platelets clump at the site. If normal amounts of calcium, platelets, and tissue factors are present, prothrombin will be converted to thrombin. Thrombin then acts as a catalyst for the conversion of fibrinogen to a mesh of insoluble fibrin, in which all the formed elements are immobilized.

blood corpuscle [AS *blod;* L *corpusculum* little body], a blood cell, either an erythrocyte or leukocyte.

blood count, See **complete blood count.**

blood culture medium, a liquid enrichment medium for the growth of bacteria in the diagnosis of blood infections.

blood donor, anyone who donates his or her blood to a blood bank or directly to another person.

blood dyscrasia [AS *blod;* Gk *dys* bad, *krasis* mingling], a pathologic condition in which any of the constituents of the blood are abnormal or are present in abnormal quantity, such as in leukemia or hemophilia.

blood fluke, a parasitic flatworm of the class Trematoda, genus *Schistosoma,* including the species *S. haematobium, S. japonicum,* and *S. mansoni.*

blood gas, gas dissolved in the liquid part of the blood. Blood gases include oxygen, carbon dioxide, and nitrogen.

blood gas determination, an analysis of the pH of the blood and the concentration and pressure of oxygen, carbon dioxide, and hydrogen ion in the blood.

blood gas tension, the partial pressure of a gas in the blood.

blood glucose. See **blood sugar.**

blood group, the classification of blood based on the presence or absence of genetically determined antigens on the surface of the red cell. Several different grouping systems have been described. These include ABO, Duffy, highfrequency antigens, I, Kell, Kidd, Lewis, low-frequency antigens, Lutheran, MNS, P, Rh, and Xg.

blood island, one of the clusters of mesodermal cells that proliferate on the outer surface of the embryonic yolk sac and give it a lumpy appearance.

blood lactate, lactic acid that appears in the blood as a result of anaerobic metabolism when oxygen delivery to the tissues is insufficient to support normal metabolic demands.

blood lavage [AS *blod;* L *lavere* to wash], the removal of toxic elements from the blood by the injection of serum into the veins.

bloodless phlebotomy [AS *blod;* ME *les;* Gk *phleps* vein, *tomos* cutting], a technique of trapping blood in a body region by the application of tourniquet pressure that is less than needed to interrupt arterial blood flow.

blood level, the concentration of a drug or other substance in a measured amount of plasma, serum, or whole blood.

blood level of glucose [AS *blod;* OFr *livel;* Gk *glykys* sweet], the amount of glucose found in the bloodstream, normally about 80 to 120 mg/dl. Concentrations higher or lower than normal can be a sign of a variety of diseases, such as diabetes mellitus or pancreatic cancer.

blood osmolality [AS *blod;* Gk *osmos* impulsion], the osmotic pressure of blood. The normal values in serum are 280 to 295 mOsm/L.

blood patch. See **epidural blood patch.**

blood pH, the hydrogen ion concentration of the blood, or a measure of its acidity or alkalinity. The normal pH values for arterial whole blood are 7.38 to 7.44; for venous whole blood, 7.36 to 7.41; for venous serum or plasma, 7.35 to 7.45.

blood plasma [AS *blod;* Gk *plassein* to mold], the liquid portion of the blood, free of its formed elements and particles. Plasma represents approximately 50% of the total volume of the blood and contains glucose, proteins, amino acids and other nutritive materials, urea and other excretory products, as well as hormones, enzymes, vitamins, and minerals.

blood platelet. See **platelet.**

blood poisoning. See **septicemia.**

blood pressure (BP) [AS *blod;* L *premere* to press], the pressure exerted by the circulating volume of blood on the walls of the arteries, the veins, and the chambers of the heart. Overall blood pressure is maintained by the complex interaction of the homeostatic mechanisms of the body, moderated by the volume of the blood, the lumen of the arteries and arterioles, and the force of the cardiac contraction. The pressure in the aorta and the large arteries of a healthy young adult is approximately 120 mm Hg during systole and 70 mm Hg in diastole. The pulse pressure is approximately 50 mm Hg.

blood pressure monitor [AS *blod;* L *premere* to press *monere* to warn], a device that automatically measures blood pressure and records the information continuously. Automatic monitorng of blood pressure may be required in surgery or in an intensive care unit.

blood proteins [AS *blod;* Gk *proteios* of first rank], the proteins normally in the blood, such as albumin, globulin, hemoglobin, proteins bound to hormones or other compounds.

blood pump, 1. a pump for regulating the flow of blood into a blood vessel during transfusion. **2.** a component of a heart-lung machine that pumps the blood through the machine for oxygenation and then through the peripheral circulatory system of the body.

blood serum. See **serum.**

bloodshot, a reddening of the conjunctiva or sclera of the eye caused by dilation of blood vessels in the tissues.

blood smear, a small specimen of blood that is smeared or spread onto a glass microscope slide for examination.

blood substitute, a substance used as a replacement for circulating blood or for extending its volume. Plasma, human serum albumin, packed red cells, platelets, leukocytes, and concentrates of clotting factors are often administered in place of whole blood transfusions in the treatment of various disorders. Substances that are sometimes used in solution to expand blood volume include dextran, hetastarch, albumin solutions, or plasma protein fraction.

blood sugar, 1. one of a group of closely related substances, as glucose, fructose, and galactose, which are normal constituents of the blood and are essential for cellular metabolism. **2.** *nontechnical.* the concentration of glucose in the blood, represented in milligrams of glucose per deciliter of blood.

blood test, any test that determines something about the characteristics or properties of the blood.

blood transfusion [AS *blod;* L *transfundere* to pour through], the administration of whole blood or a component, such as packed red cells, to replace blood lost through trauma, surgery, or disease. Blood for transfusion is obtained from a healthy donor or donors whose ABO blood group and antigenic subgroups match those of the recipient and who have an adequate hemoglobin level (above 13.5 g/100 ml for men and above 12.5 g/100 ml for women). Each 500 ml of blood collected from a donor is stored in a plastic bag containing citrate-dextrose or citrate-phosphate. A unit can be stored under refrigeration for only 3 weeks; at that time the leukocytes, platelets, and 20% to 30% of the red cells are nonviable, and the levels of clotting factors V and VIII are low.

blood typing, identification of genetically determined antigens on the surface of the red blood cell used to determine a person's blood group. Usually, a blood bank procedure, it is the first step in testing donor's and recipient's blood to be used in transfusion and is followed by crossmatching.

blood urea nitrogen (BUN) [AS *blod;* Gk *ouron* urine; *nitron* soda, *genein* to produce], nitrogen in the blood in the form of urea. The urea is formed in the liver as the end product of protein metabolism and is deposited in the blood to be excreted through the kidney. The BUN, determined by a blood test, is directly related to the metabolic function of the liver and the excretory function of the kidney.

blood vessel, any one of the network of tubes that carries blood. Kinds of blood vessels are **arteries, arterioles, capillaries, veins,** and **venules.**

blood warming coil, a device constructed of coiled plastic tubing, used for the warming of reserve blood before massive transfusions, such as those often required for patients who develop extensive GI bleeding.

bloody show. See **vaginal bleeding.**

bloody sputum [AS *blod;* L *sputum* spittle], blood-tinged material expelled from the respiratory passages. The amount and color of blood in sputum expelled by coughing or clearing the throat may indicate the cause and location of the bleeding.

Bloom's syndrome [David Bloom, American physician, b. 1892], a rare genetic disease occuring mainly in Ashkenazi Jews. It is transmitted as an autosomal recessive trait and is characterized by growth retardation, telangiectatic erythema of the face and arms, sensitivity to sunlight, and an increased risk of leukemia.

blow bottles, a device used in respiratory care to provide resistance to expiration. The bottles are partially filled with water, and the patient is encouraged to blow the water from one bottle to another.

blow-out fracture, a fracture of the floor of the orbit caused by a blow that suddenly increases the intraocular pressure.

BLS, abbreviation of **basic life support.**

blue asphyxia. See **asphyxia livida.**

blue baby [OFr *blou;* ME *babe*], an infant born with cyanosis caused by a congenital heart lesion, such as transposition of the great vessels, by tetralogy of Fallot, or by incomplete expansion of the lungs (congenital atelectasis).

blue fever, *informal.* Rocky Mountain spotted fever, so named for the dark cyanotic discoloration of the skin after the initial rickettsial infection.

blue nevus [OFr *blou;* L *naevus* mole], a sharply circumscribed, usually benign, steel blue skin nodule. It is found on the face or upper extremities, grows very slowly, and persists throughout life. Any sudden change in the size of such a lesion demands surgical attention and biopsy. The dark color is caused by large, densely packed melanocytes deep in the dermis of the nevus.

blue phlebitis. See **phlegmasia cerulea dolens.**

blue spot, 1. one of a number of small grayish blue spots that may appear near the armpits or around the groins of individuals infested with lice, such as in pediculosis corporis and pediculosis pubis. **2.** one of a number of dark blue or mulberry hued round or oval spots that may appear as a congenital condition in the sacral regions of certain children and usually disappear spontaneously as the affected individual matures.

blunt dissection [ME *blunt;* L *dissecare* to cut apart], a dissection performed by separating tissues along natural lines of cleavage, without cutting.

blunthook [ME *blunt* + AS *hoc*], **1.** a sturdy hook-shaped bar used in obstetrics for traction between the abdomen and the thigh in cases of difficult breech deliveries. **2.** a hook-shaped device with a blunt end used in embryotomy.

blunting, a decrease in the intensity of emotional expression from the level one would normally expect as a reaction to a specific situation.

blurred film fault, a defect in a photograph or radiograph that appears as an indistinct or blurred image.

blush [ME *blusshen* to redden], a brief, diffuse erythema of the face and neck, commonly the result of dilation of superficial small blood vessels in response to heat or sudden emotion.

B lymphocyte. See **B cell.**

B/M, symbol for black male, often used in the initial identifying statement in a patient record.

BMA, abbreviation for **British Medical Association.**

BMD, abbreviation for **Bureau of Medical Devices.**

B-mode, brightness modulation, an imaging technique used in ultrasound scanning in which bright dots on an oscilloscope screen represent echoes and the intensity of the brightness indicates the strength of the echo.

BMR, abbreviation for *basal metabolic rate.*

BNA, abbreviation for *Basle Nomina Anatomica.*

BOA, abbreviation for **born out of asepsis.**

board certification, a process in which an individual is certified in a medical specialty or subspecialty. Certification is provided by the member boards of the American Board of Medical Specialties and is given following completion of accredited training and examination, as well as fulfilling individual requirements of the individual board.

board certified, denoting a physician who has completed the certification requirements established by a medical specialty board and has been certified as a specialist in a particular field of medicine.

board eligible, pertaining to a physician who has completed all of the requirements for admission to a medical specialty board.

boarder baby, an infant abandoned to a hospital because the mother is unable to care for him or her.

board of health, an administrative body acting on a municipal, county, state, provincial, or national level. Among the tasks of most boards of health are prevention of disease, health education, and implementation of laws pertaining to health.

Boas' test /bō′az/ [Ismar I. Boas, German physician, b. 1858], **1.** a test for hydrochloric acid in the contents of the stomach. **2.** a test for free hydrochloric acid in the contents of the stomach in which filtered stomach fluid is boiled with a special reagent. **3.** a test for lactic acid in a sample of gastric juice that depends on the oxidation of the lactic acid to aldehyde and formic acid by sulfuric acid and manganese. **4.** a test for gastric motility in which a fasting patient drinks 400 ml of water that has been tinted green by the addition of 20 drops of chlorophyll solution.

Bodansky unit [Aaron Bodansky, American biochemist, b. 1887], the quantity of phosphatase in 100 ml of serum needed to liberate 1 mg of phosphorous as phosphate ion from sodium betaglycerophosphate in 1 hour at 37° C. It is used to express the measure of certain enzymes, such as acid phosphatase in the body.

body [AS *bodig*], **1.** the whole structure of an individual with all the organs. **2.** a cadaver or a corpse. **3.** the largest or the main part of any organ, such as the body of the tibia or the body of the vastus lateralis.

body cast [AS *bodig* body; ONorse *kasta*], a molded cast that may extend from the chest to the groin to immobilize the spine.

body cavity, any of the spaces in the chest and abdomen that contain body organs.

body fluid [AS *bodig*; L *fluere* to flow], a fluid contained in the three fluid compartments of the body: the blood plasma of the circulating blood, the interstitial fluid between the cells, and the cell fluid within the cells. Blood plasma and interstitial fluid make up the extracellular fluid; the cell fluid is the intracellular fluid. The chemical constituents of the fluids vary greatly; for example, sodium is present in large amounts in both compartments of the extracellular fluid but is nearly absent in the intracellular fluid; protein is present in the blood plasma and cell fluid but not in the interstitial fluid.

body image [AS *bodig*; L *imago* likeness], a person's subjective concept of his or her physical appearance. The mental representation, which may be realistic or unrealistic, is constructed from self-observation, the reactions of others, and a complex interaction of attitudes, emotions, memories, fantasies, and experiences, both conscious and unconscious.

body image agnosia. See **autotopagnosia.**

body image disturbance, a NANDA-accepted nursing diagnosis of a disruption in the way one perceives one's body image. Defining characteristics include verbal or nonverbal responses to a real or perceived change in structure or function, a missing body part, personalization of the missing part by giving it a name, refusal by the client to look at a part of the body, negative feelings about the body, trauma to a nonfunctioning part, a change in general social involvement or life-style, and a fear of rejection by others.

body jacket, an orthopedic cast that encases the trunk of the body but does not extend over the cervical area. It is used to help immobilize the trunk for the healing of spinal injuries and scoliosis and for postoperative positioning and immobilization after spinal surgery.

body language [AS *bodig*; L *lingua* tongue], a set of nonverbal signals, including body movements, postures, gestures, spatial positions, facial expressions, and bodily adornment, that give expression to various physical, mental, and emotional states.

body mechanics, the field of physiology that studies muscular actions and the func-

tion of muscles in maintaining the posture of the body.

body movement, motion of all or part of the body, especially at a joint or joints. Some kinds of body movements are **abduction, adduction, extension, flexion,** and **rotation.**

body odor, a fetid smell associated with stale perspiration. Freshly secreted perspiration is odorless, but after exposure to the atmosphere and bacterial activity at the surface of the skin, chemical changes occur to produce the odor.

body of Retzius /ret′sē·əs/ [Magnus G. Retzius, Swedish anatomist, b. 1842], any one of the masses of protoplasm containing pigment granules at the lower end of a hair cell of the organ of Corti in the internal ear.

body plethysmograph [AS *bodig*; Gk *plethynein* to increase, *graphein* to record], a device for studying alveolar pressures, lung volumes, and airway resistance. The patient sits or reclines in an airtight compartment and breathes normally. The pressure changes in the alveoli are reciprocated in the compartment and are recorded automatically.

body position, attitude or posture of the body. Some kinds of body position are **anatomic position, decubitus, Fowler's position, prone, supine,** and **Trendelenburg position.**

body righting reflex [AS *bodig*; L *rectus* straight; *reflectere* to bend back], any one of the neuromuscular responses to restore the body to its normal upright position when it has been displaced.

body scheme, a Piagetian term for a cognitive structure that develops in infants in the sensorimotor period during the first 2 years of life as they learn to differentiate between themselves and the world around them.

body-scheme disorder. See **autotopagnosia.**

body-section radiography, a radiographic technique used to produce a more distinct image of a selected body plane by moving the film and x-ray tube in opposite directions.

body stalk, the elongated part of the embryo that is connected to the chorion.

body surface area. See **surface area.**

body systems model, (in nursing education) a conceptual framework in which illness is studied in relation to the functional systems of the body. In this model, nursing care is directed toward manipulating the patient's environment in such a way that the signs and symptoms of the health problem are alleviated.

body temperature, the level of heat produced and sustained by the body processes. Variations and changes in body temperature are major indicators of disease and other abnormalities. Heat is generated within the body through metabolism of food and lost from the body surface through radiation, convection, and evaporation of perspiration. Heat production and loss are regulated and controlled in the hypothalamus and brainstem. Diseases of the hypothalamus or interference with the other regulatory centers may produce abnormally low body temperatures. Normal adult body temperature, as measured orally, is 98.6° F. Oral temperatures ranging from 96.5° F to 99° F are consistent with good health, depending on the physical activity of the person, the ambient temperature, and the particular normal body temperature for that person. Axillary temperature is usually 1° F lower than the oral temperature. Rectal temperatures may be 0.5° F to 1° F higher than oral readings. Body temperature appears to vary 1° F to 2° F throughout the day, with lows recorded early in the morning and peaks between 6 PM and 10 PM.

body temperature, altered, high risk for, a NANDA-accepted nursing diagnosis of an individual's risk for failure to maintain body temperature within normal range. Risk factors include extremes of age or weight; exposure to cool-to-cold or warm-to-hot environments; dehydration; inactivity or vigorous activity; medications causing vasoconstriction or vasodilation; altered metabolic rate; sedation; inappropriate clothing for environmental temperature; and illness or trauma affecting temperature regulations.

body type, the general physical appearance of an individual human body.

Boeck's sarcoid. See **sarcoidosis.**

Boerhaave's syndrome [Hermann Boerhaave, Dutch physician, b. 1668], a condition marked by spontaneous rupture of the esophagus, leading to mediastinitis and pleural effusion. Emergency care is needed, with surgery and drainage, to save the life of the patient.

Bohr effect [Christian Bohr, Danish physiologist, b. 1855], the effect of CO_2 and H^+ on the affinity of hemoglobin for molecular O_2. Increasing P_{CO_2} and H^+ decrease oxyhemoglobin saturation, whereas decreasing concentrations have the opposite effect.

boil [AS *byle* sore], a skin abscess.

boiling point [ME *boilen* to make bubbles; L *pungere* to prick], the temperature at which a substance passes from the liquid to the gaseous state at a particular atmospheric pressure.

bole /bōl/, any of a variety of soft, friable clays of various colors, although usually red from iron oxide.

Bolivian hemorrhagic fever, an infectious disease caused by an arenavirus, generally transmitted from infected rodents to humans through contamination of food by rodent urine, though direct transmission between people has also been observed. The patient experiences chills, fever, headache, muscle ache, anorexia, nausea, and vomiting.

bolus /bō′ləs/ [Gk *bolos* lump], **1.** a round mass, specifically a masticated lump of food ready to be swallowed. **2.** a large round preparation of medicinal material for oral ingestion, usually soft and not prepackaged. **3.** a dose of a medication or a contrast material, radioactive isotope, or other pharmaceutic preparation injected all at once intravenously. **4.** in radiotherapy, material used to fill in irregular body surfaces to get a better dose distribution for hyperthermia or to increase the dose to the skin when high-energy photon beams are used.

Bombay phenotype, a rare genetic trait involving the phenotypic expression of the ABO blood groups. Cells of such individuals are phenotypically of blood type O, even though they are genotype AB, and the serum contains anti-A, anti-B, and anti-H antigens. The trait is named for the city in which it was first reported.

bonding[1] [ME *band* to bind], **1.** the attachment process that occurs between an infant and the parents, especially the mother, and is significant in the formation of affectionate ties that later influence both the physical and psychologic development of the child. Especially important in initiating bonding is eye to eye contact, fondling of the infant, soothing talk, and other affectionate behavior that begins to create positive emotional ties. Mothers are more concerned with physically touching and holding the infant, whereas fathers are more intent on forming a sense of absorption, preoccupation, and visual interest in the child--what has been called paternal engrossment. Although bonding is considered primarily an emotional response, it is theorized that there may be some biochemical and hormonal interaction in the mother that may stimulate the response, but studies are still inconclusive.

bonding[2], (in dentistry) a technique of joining orthodontic brackets or other attachments directly to the enamel surface of a tooth, using orthodontic adhesives.

bond specificity, the nature of enzyme action that causes the disruption of only certain bonds between atoms.

bone [AS *ban*],   **1.** the dense, hard, and slightly elastic connective tissue, comprising the 206 bones of the human skeleton. It is composed of compact osseous tissue surrounding spongy cancelous tissue permeated by many blood vessels and nerves and enclosed in membranous periosteum. Long bones contain yellow marrow in longitudinal cavities and red marrow in their articular ends. Red marrow also fills the cavities of the flat and the short bones, the bodies of the vertebrae, the cranial diploe, the sternum, and the ribs. Blood cells are produced in active red marrow. Osteocytes form bone tissue in concentric rings around an intricate haversian system of interconnecting canals that accommodates blood vessels, lymphatic vessels, and nerve fibers. **2.** any single element of the skeleton, such as a rib, the sternum, or the femur.

bone age [AS *ban*; L *aetas*],   the stage of development or decline of the skeleton or its segments, as seen in radiographic examination, when compared with x-ray views of the bone structures of other individuals of the same chronologic age.

bone cancer [AS *ban*; Gk *karkinos* crab],   a skeletal malignancy occurring primarily as a sarcoma in an area of rapid growth or, secondarily, as a metastasis from cancer elsewhere in the body. Primary bone tumors are rare; the incidence peaks during adolescence, decreases, and then rises slowly after the age of 35. In adults, bone cancer is linked to exposure to ionizing radiation. Paget's disease, hyperparathyroidism, chronic osteomyelitis, old bone infarcts, and fracture callosities increase the risk of many bone tumors. Most osseous malignancies are metastatic lesions found most often in the spine or pelvis and less often in sites away from the trunk. Bone cancers progress rapidly but are often difficult to detect; pain that increases at night may be the only symptom. The most common osseous malignancies are osteosarcomas, followed by chrondrosarcomas, fibrosarcomas, and Ewing's sarcoma.

bone cell [AS *ban*; L *cella* storeroom],   an osteocyte, a cell resembling a melon seed, but with myriad spidery processes.

bone cutting forceps,   a kind of forceps that has long handles, single or double joints, and heavy blades.

bone cyst [AS *ban*; Gk *kytis* cyst],   **1.** an aneurysmal vascular bone cyst, usually eccentrically placed. **2.** osteitis fibrosa cystica, a parathyroid disorder characterized by cyst formation and replacement of bone by fibrous tissue.

bone graft,   the transplantation of a piece of bone from one part of the body to another to repair a skeletal defect.

bone lamella [AS *ban* + *lamella* small plate],   a thin plate of bone matrix, a basic structural unit of mature bone.

bone marrow [AS *ban*; ME *marowe*],   specialized, soft tissue filling the spaces in cancelous bone of the epiphyses. Fatty, **yellow marrow** is found in the compact bone of most adult epiphyses. **Red marrow** is found in many bones of infants and children and in the spongy bone of the proximal epiphyses of the humerus and femur and in the sternum, ribs, and vertebral bodies of adults. It is composed of myeloid tissue and is essential in the manufacture and maturation of red blood cells.

bone marrow transplant,   the transplantation of bone marrow from healthy donors to stimulate the production of formed blood cells. The bone marrow is removed from the donor by aspiration and infused intravenously into the recipient.

bone plate [AS *ban*; OFr *plate*],   a metal plate used to reconstruct a bone that has been fractured. The plate is designed to hold fragments in apposition.

bone recession [AS *ban*; L *recedere* to recede],   apical progression of the level of the alveolar crest, associated with inflammatory or dystrophic periodontal disease and resulting in decreased bone support for the teeth.

bone tissue [AS *ban*; OFr *tissu*],   a hard form of connective tissue composed of osteocytes and a calcified collagenous intercellular substance arranged in thin plates.

Bonnevie-Ullrich syndrome. See **Turner's syndrome.**

Bonwill's triangle [William G. A. Bonwill, American dentist, b. 1833],   an equilateral triangle with 4 inch (10 cm) sides formed by lines from the contact points of the lower central incisors (or the median line of the residual ridge of the mandible) to the condyle on either side and from one condyle to the other.

bony landmark [AS *ban*; AS *land, meark*],   a groove or prominence on a bone that serves as a guide to the location of other body structures.

bony palate. See **hard palate.**

bony thorax [AS *ban*; Gk, *thorax* chest],   the skeletal part of the chest, including the thoracic vertebrae, ribs, and sternum.

booster injection,   the administration of an antigen, such as a vaccine or toxoid, usually in a smaller amount than the original immunization, given to maintain the immune response at an appropriate level.

Boothby-Lovelace-Bulbulian   **(BLB) mask,**   an apparatus for the administration of oxygen, consisting of a mask fitted with an inspiratory-expiratory valve and a rebreathing bag.

boracic acid. See **boric acid.**

borate /bôr´āt/, any salt of boric acid. Borate salts and boric acid, although formerly used as mild antiseptic irrigant solutions, especially for ophthalmic conditions, are highly poisonous when taken internally or absorbed through a cut, abrasion, or other wound in the skin.

borax bath [Ar *bauraq*; AS *baeth*], a medicated bath in which borax and glycerin are added to the water.

borborygmus /bôr´bərig´məs/, pl. **borborygmi** [Gk *borborygmos* bowel rumbling], an audible abdominal sound produced by hyperactive intestinal peristalsis. Borborygmi are rumbling, gurgling, and tinkling noises heard in auscultation.

borderline [OFr *bordure*; L *linea*], pertaining to a state of health in which the patient has some of the signs and symptoms of a disease, but not enough to justify a definite diagnosis.

borderline personality [OFr *bordure*; L *linea, personalis*], a personality that is difficult to classify because it shows characteristics of both a normal and abnormal personality. The borderline personality, for example, may display a consistent stable mood but it also may be replaced suddenly by an irritable, impulsive, antisocial persona.

Bordetella /bôr´ditel´ə/ [Jules J.B.V. Bordet, Belgian bacteriologist, b. 1870], a genus of gram-negative coccobacilli, some species of which are pathogens of the respiratory tract of humans, including *Bordetella bronchiseptica, B. parapertussis,* and *B. pertussis.*

boric acid /bôr´ik/, a white, odorless powder or crystalline substance used as a buffer and formerly used as a topical antiseptic and eye wash.

Bornholm disease. See **epidemic pleurodynia.**

born out of asepsis (BOA), (in a hospital) denoting a newborn infant who was not delivered in the usual place in an obstetric unit. Depending on the policy of the institution, a BOA-designated infant may have been born on the way to the hospital or in the hospital, on the way to the delivery suite or in a labor room.

boron (B) /bôr´on/, a nonmetallic element, similar to aluminum. Its atomic number is 5; its atomic weight is 10.8. Elemental boron occurs in the form of dark crystals and as a greenish yellow amorphous mass. Certain concentrations of this element are toxic to plant and animal life, but plants need traces of boron for normal growth. It is the characteristic element of

boric acid, used chiefly as a dusting powder and ointment for minor skin disorders.

Borrelia /bərel´ē·ə/ [Amédée Borrel, French bacteriologist, b. 1867], a genus of coarse, unevenly coiled, helical spirochetes, several species of which cause tickborne and louseborne infections. Many animals serve as reservoirs and hosts for *Borrelia.*

Borrelia burgdorferi /burg´dərfer´ī/, the etiologic agent in Lyme disease. The organism is transmitted to humans by tick vectors, particularly *Ixodes dammini.*

boss [ME *boce*], a swelling, eminence, or protuberance on an organ, such as a tumor or overgrowth on a bone surface.

Boston exanthem [Boston; Gk *ex* out, *anthema* blossoming], an epidemic disease characterized by scattered, pale red maculopapules on the face, chest, and back, occasionally accompanied by small ulcerations on the tonsils and soft palate. It is caused by echovirus 16 and requires no treatment.

bottle feeding [OFr *bouteille*; AS *faeden*], feeding an infant or young child from a bottle with a rubber nipple on the end as a substitute for or supplement to breastfeeding.

botulinus toxin /boch´əlī´nəs/ [L *botulus* sausage; Gk *toxikon* poison], any of a group of potent bacterial toxins produced by different strains of *Clostridium botulinum.* The strains are sometimes identified by letters of the alphabet, as A, B, C, and so on.

botulism /boch´əliz´əm/ [L *botulus* sausage], an often fatal form of food poisoning caused by an endotoxin produced by the bacillus *Clostridium botulinum.* The toxin is ingested in food contaminated by *C. botulinum,* although it is not necessary for the live bacillus to be present if the toxin has been produced. In rare instances, the toxin may be introduced into the human body through a wound contaminated by the organism. Botulism develops without gastric distress and may not occur for up to 1 week after the contaminated food has been ingested. Botulism is characterized by a period of lassitude and fatigue followed by visual disturbances. Muscles may become weak, and the victim often develops dysphagia.

bouba. See **yaws.**

Bouchard's node /booshärz´/ [Charles J. Bouchard, French physician, b. 1837], an abnormal cartilaginous or bony enlargement of a proximal interphalangeal joint of a finger, usually occurring in degenerative diseases of the joints.

bougie /boo´zhē, boozhē´/ [Fr, candle], a thin, cylindric instrument made of rubber, waxed silk, or other flexible material for insertion into canals of the body in order to dilate, examine, or measure them.

boulimia. See **bulimia.**

boundary, (in psychology) an aspect of family health in which the generations are clearly defined and issues dealt with by the appropriate generation.

boundary lubrication, a coating of a thin layer of molecules on each weight-bearing surface of a joint to facilitate a sliding action by the opposing bone surfaces.

boundary maintenance mechanisms, (in psychology) behavior and practices that exclude members of some groups from the customs and values of another group.

bound carbon dioxide, carbon dioxide that is transported in the bloodstream as part of a sodium bicarbonate molecule, as distinguished from dissolved carbon dioxide, or bicarbonate ion.

bounding pulse [OFr *bondir* to leap; L *pulsare* to beat], a pulse that, on palpation, feels full and springlike because of an increased thrust of cardiac contraction or an increased volume of circulating blood within the elastic structures of the vascular system.

bouquet fever. See **dengue fever.**

Bourdon regulator, a commonly used adjustable regulator with an attached pressure gauge for cylinders of oxygen or other medical gases.

Bourneville's disease. See **tuberous sclerosis.**

boutonneuse fever /bōō'tanōōz'/ [Fr *bouton* pustule; L *febris*], an infectious disease caused by *Rickettsia conorii,* transmitted to humans through the bite of a tick. The onset of the disease is characterized by a lesion called a *tache noire* /tāshnô·är'/, or black spot, at the site of the infection, fever lasting from a few days to 2 weeks, and a papular erythematous rash that spreads over the body to include the skin of the palms and soles.

boutonnière deformity /bōō'tônyer'/ [Fr, buttonhole], an abnormality of a finger marked by the fixed flexion of the proximal interphalangeal joint and the hyperextension of the distal interphalangeal joint.

bovine tuberculosis /bō'vin/ [L *bos* ox + *tuber* swelling; Gk *osis* condition], a form of tuberculosis caused by Mycobacterium tuberculosis that primarily affects cattle. Mastitis and pulmonary symptoms can occur.

Bowditch's law. See **all-or-none law.**

bowel. See **intestine.**

bowel training [OFr *boel*], a method of establishing regular evacuation by reflex conditioning, used in the treatment of fe-

cal incontinence, impaction, chronic diarrhea, and autonomic hyperreflexia. In patients with autonomic hyperreflexia, distention of the rectum and bladder causes paroxysmal hypertension, restlessness, chills, diaphoresis, headache, elevated temperature, and bradycardia.

Bowen's disease, Bowen's precancerous dermatosis. See **intraepidermal carcinoma.**

bowleg. See **genu varum.**

Bowman's capsule /bō'manz/ [Sir William Bowman, English surgeon, b. 1816], the cup-shaped end of a renal tubule containing a glomerulus.

Bowman's glands [Sir William Bowman; L *glans* acorn], glands in the mucous membrane of the mouth.

Bowman's lamina [Sir William Bowman; L *lamina* thin plate], a tough membrane beneath the corneal epithelium.

bowtie filter, (in radiology) a special bowtie-shaped filter that may be used in computed tomography procedures to compensate for the shape of the patient's head or body.

box bath. See **cabinet bath.**

boxer's fracture [Dan *bask* a blow; L *fractura* break], a fracture of one or more metacarpal bones, usually the fourth or fifth, caused by punching a hard object. Such a fracture is often distal, angulated, and impacted.

boxing, (in dentistry) the forming of vertical walls, most commonly made of wax, to produce the desired shape and size of the base of a cast.

Boyle's law [Robert Boyle, English scientist, b. 1627], (in physics) a law stating that the product of the volume and pressure of a gas compressed at a constant temperature remains constant.

BP, abbreviation for **blood pressure.**

BPDE-I, abbreviation for **benzo-(a)pyrene dihydrodiol epoxide.**

Br, symbol for the element **bromine.**

brace [OFr *bracier* to embrace], an orthotic device, sometimes jointed, to support and hold any part of the body in the correct position to allow function, such as a leg brace that permits walking and standing.

brachial /brā'kē·əl/ [Gk *brachion* arm], of or pertaining to the arm.

brachial artery, the principal artery of the upper arm that is the continuation of the axillary artery. It has three branches and terminates at the radial and the ulnar arteries.

brachialgia [Gk *brachion* + *algos* pain], a severe pain in the arm, often related to a disorder involving the brachial plexus.

brachialis /brā'kē·al'is/ [Gk *brachion* arm],

a muscle of the upper arm, covering the anterior part of the elbow joint and the distal half of the humerus. It functions to flex the forearm.

brachial paralysis, paralysis of an arm or hand.

brachial plexus [Gk *brachion;* L, braided], a network of nerves in the neck, passing under the clavicle and into the axilla, originating in the fifth, sixth, seventh, and eighth cervical and first two thoracic spinal nerves and innervating the muscles and skin of the chest, shoulders, and arms.

brachial plexus anesthesia, an anesthetic block of the region innervated by the anterior divisions of the last four cervical and first two thoracic nerves. The plexus extends from the transverse processes to the apex of the axilla, where the terminal nerves are formed.

brachial plexus paralysis. See **Erb's palsy.**

brachial pulse [Gk *brachion;* L *pulsare* to beat], the pulse of the brachial artery, palpated in the antecubital space.

brachiocephalic, of or relating to the arm and head.

brachiocephalic arteritis. See *Takayasu's arteritis.*

brachiocephalic artery, brachiocephalic trunk. See **innominate artery.**

brachiocephalic vein. See **innominate vein.**

brachiocubital [Gk *brachion;* L *cubitus* elbow], pertaining to the arm and forearm.

brachioradialis /brā′kē-ôrā′dē-al′is/, the most superficial muscle on the radial side of the forearm. It functions to flex the forearm.

brachioradialis reflex [Gk *brachion;* L, radial; *reflectare* to bend backward], a deep tendon reflex, elicited by striking the lateral surface of the forearm proximal to the distal head of the radius, characterized by normal slight elbow flexion and forearm supination.

brachycardia [Gk *brachys* short, *kardia* heart], slowness of the heart.

brachycephaly /brak′isef′əlē/ [Gk *brachys* short, *kephale* head], a congenital malformation of the skull in which premature closure of the coronal suture results in excessive lateral growth of the head, giving it a short, broad appearance with a cephalic index of between 81 and 85. –**brachycephalic, brachycephalous,** *adj.*

brachydactyly /brak′idak′təlē/, a condition of abnormally short fingers or toes.

brachytherapy [Gk *brachys* + *therapeia* treatment], the use of radioactive materials in the treatment of malignant neoplasms by placing the radioactive sources in contact with or implanted into the tissues to be treated.

Bradford frame [Edward H. Bradford, American surgeon, b. 1848], a rectangular orthopedic frame made of pipes to which heavy movable straps of canvas are attached, running from side to side to support a patient in a prone or supine position. The straps can be removed to permit the patient to urinate or defecate while remaining immobile.

Bradford solid frame, a rectangular orthopedic device of metal covered with canvas to aid in immobilization, especially of children in traction. The main purpose of the device is to assist in maintaining proper immobilization, positioning, and alignment by controlling movement.

Bradford split frame, a rectangular orthopedic device of metal covered with two separate pieces of canvas fastened at both ends of the frame. Used especially in pediatrics to aid in the immobilization of children in traction, it is divided in the middle by a large opening designed to accommodate the excretory functions of an incontinent patient in a hip spica cast. The division also allows for the upper and lower extremities of the patient to be elevated separately and for the maintenance of a clean and dry cast. For an incontinent child, a plastic funnel leading into the bedpan is positioned below the opening in the frame.

Bradley method, a method of psychophysical preparation for childbirth developed by Robert Bradley, MD, comprising education about the physiology of childbirth, exercise and nutrition during pregnancy, and techniques of breathing and relaxation for control and comfort during labor and delivery. The father is extensively involved in the classes and acts as the mother's "coach" during labor. Among the advantages of the method are its simplicity, the involvement of the father, and the realistic approach to the efforts and discomfort of labor.

bradyarrhythmia, an abnormally slow heart rhythm.

bradycardia /brad′ikär′dē-ə/ [Gk *bradys* slow, *kardia* heart], a circulatory condition in which the myocardium contracts steadily but at a rate of less than 60 contractions a minute. The heart normally slows during sleep, and in some physically fit people the pulse may be quite slow. Cardiac output is decreased, causing faintness, dizziness, chest pain, and eventually syncope and circulatory collapse.

bradycardia-tachycardia syndrome [Gk *bradys, kardia* + *tachys* fast, *kardia; syn* together, *dromos* course], a heart disorder characterized by a heart rate that alternates between abnormally slow and abnormally rapid rhythms.

bradydiastole [Gk *bradys* + *dia* through, *stellein* to set], a diastolic phase that is abnormally long. It is associated with myocardial infarction.

bradyesthesia /-esthē′zhə/ [Gk *bradys* + *aisthesis* feeling], a slowness in perception.

bradykinesia /brad′ikinē′zhə, -kīnē′zhə/ [Gk *bradys* + *kinesis* motion], an abnormal condition characterized by slowness of all voluntary movement and speech, such as caused by parkinsonism, and extrapyramidal disorders, and certain tranquilizers.

bradykinin /-kī′nin/ [Gk *bradys* + *kinein* to move], a peptide of nonprotein origin containing nine amino acid residues. It is produced from $α_2$-globulin by kallikrein, and it is a potent vasodilator.

bradypnea /brad′ipnē′ə/ [Gk *bradys* + *pnein* to breath], an abnormally slow rate of breathing.

bradytachycardia [Gk *bradys* + *tachy* fast, *kardia*, heart], a heart rate that alternates between abnormally slow and abnormally fast, as in *sick sinus syndrome.*

Bragg curve [Sir William H. Bragg, English physicist, b. 1862], in radiation therapy, the path followed by ionizing particles used in a treatment. Because certain particles reach a peak of potential near the end of their path, the Bragg curve can be used to direct the radiation so that it reaches deep-seated tumors while significantly sparing the normal overlying tissues.

Braille /brāl, brä′yə/ [Louis Braille, French teacher of blind, b. 1809], a system of printing for the blind consisting of raised dots or points that can be read by touch.

brain [AS *bragen*], the portion of the central nervous system contained within the cranium. It consists of the cerebrum, cerebellum, pons, medulla, and midbrain.

brain abscess [AS *bragen*; L *abscedere* to go away], a pocket of infection in a part of the brain, usually as a result of the spread of an infection from another source, such as the skull, sinuses, or other structures in the head. The infection also may be secondary to a disease in the bones, the nervous system outside the brain, or the heart.

brain concussion [AS *bragen*; L *concussus* a shaking], a violent jarring or shaking, or other blunt, nonpenetrating injury to the brain caused by a sudden change in momentum of the head. After a mild concus-

sion there may be a transient loss of consciousness followed, on awakening, by a headache. Severe concussion may cause prolonged unconsciousness and disruption of certain vital functions of the brainstem, such as respiration and vasomotor stability.

brain death [AS *bragen, daeth*], an irreversible form of unconsciousness characterized by a complete loss of brain function while the heart continues to beat. The legal definition of this condition varies from state to state. The usual clinical criteria for brain death include the absence of reflex activity, movements, and respiration. The pupils are dilated and fixed. A diagnosis of brain death requires that the electric activity of the brain be evaluated and shown to be absent on two electroencephalograms performed 12 to 24 hours apart.

brain edema. See **cerebral edema.**

brain electric activity map (BEAM), a topographic map of the brain areas that show electric potentials evoked by a flash of light. Potentials recorded at 4-millisecond intervals are converted into a many-colored map of the brain, showing them to be positive or negative.

brain fever, *informal.* any inflammation of the brain or meninges.

brain scan [AS *bragen*; L *scandere* to climb], a diagnostic procedure using radioisotope imaging techniques to localize and identify intracranial masses, lesions, tumors, or infarcts. Radioisotopes are injected intravenously to circulate to the brain, where they accumulate in abnormal tissue. The radioisotopes are traced and photographed by a scintillator, or scanner, and the size and location of the abnormality are determined.

Brain's reflex [Walter Russell Brain, English physician, b. 1895; L, *reflectere,* to bend back], the reflexive extension of the flexed paralyzed arm of a hemiplegia patient upon assuming a quadripedal posture.

brainstem [AS *bragen, stemm*], the portion of the brain comprising the medulla oblongata, the pons, and the mesencephalon. It performs motor, sensory, and reflex functions and contains the corticospinal and the reticulospinal tracts. The 12 pairs of cranial nerves from the brain arise mostly from the brainstem.

brainstem auditory evoked potential (BAEP), the electric activity that may be recorded from the brainstem in the first 10 msec following presentation of an auditory stimulus. A delayed, normally shaped waveform may indicate a hearing loss caused by middle or inner ear pathology, while one or more missing peaks may indicate neural pathology.

brain swelling, See **cerebral edema.**

brain syndrome, a group of symptoms resulting from impaired function of the brain. It may be acute and reversible or chronic and irreversible.

brain tumor, an invasive neoplasm of the intracranial portion of the central nervous system. Brain tumors cause significant morbidity and mortality, but are treated successfully. Intracranial tumors in children are usually the result of a developmental defect. In adults 20% to 40% of malignancies in the brain are metastatic lesions from cancers in the breast, lung, GI tract, kidney, or any site of a malignant melanoma. The origin of primary brain tumors is not known. Symptoms of a brain tumor are often those of increased intracranial pressure, such as headache, nausea, vomiting, papilledema, lethargy, and disorientation. Localizing signs, such as loss of vision on the side of an occipital neoplasm may occur. Gliomas, chiefly astrocytomas, are the most common malignancies. Surgery is the initial treatment for most primary tumors of the brain.

brain wave [AS *bragen* + *wafian*], any of a number of patterns of rhythmic electric impulses produced in different parts of the brain. Most patterns, identified by the Greek letters alpha, beta, delta, gamma, kappa, and theta, are similar for all normal persons and are relatively stable for each individual. Alpha waves are produced when the person is awake but resting while beta waves signal an active phase of cerebral function and delta waves are emitted during deep sleep. Brain waves also help in the diagnosis of certain neurologic disorders, such as epilepsy or brain tumors.

bran bath [OFr *bren;* AS *baeth*], a bath in which bran has been boiled in the water; used for the relief of skin irritation.

branched chain ketoaciduria. See **maple syrup urine disease.**

branched tubular gland [OFr *branche*], one of the many multicellular glands with one excretory duct from two or more tube-shaped secretory branches, such as some of the gastric glands.

branchial /brang′kē-əl/ [Gk *branchia* gills], pertaining to body structures of the neck and throat area, particularly the muscles.

branchial arches, arched structures in the embryonic pharynx. In aquatic vertebrates, the arches develop into gills.

branchial cleft [Gk *brachial* gills; ME *clift*], a linear depression in the pharynx of the early embryo opposite a branchial, or pharyngeal, pouch.

branchial cyst, a cyst derived from a branchial remnant in the neck.

branchial fistula, a congenital, abnormal passage from the pharynx to the external surface of the neck, resulting from the failure of a branchial cleft to close during fetal development.

branching canal. See **collateral pulp canal.**

branchiogenic /brang′kē-ōjen′ik/ [Gk *bragchia* gills, *genein* to produce], pertaining to any tissues originating in the branchial cleft or arch.

Brandt-Andrews maneuver [M.L. Brandt, American obstetrician, b. 1894; C.J. Andrews, American surgeon], a method of expressing the placenta from the uterus in the third stage of labor.

brassfounder's ague. See **metal fume fever.**

brassy cough [AS *brase* brassy, *cohhetan* to cough], a high-pitched cough caused by irritation of the recurrent pharyngeal nerve or by pressure on the trachea.

brassy eye. See **chalkitis.**

Braun's canal. See **neurenteric canal.**

Braxton Hicks contraction /brak′stən-hiks′/ [John Braxton Hicks, English physician, b. 1823], irregular tightening of the pregnant uterus that begins in the first trimester and increases in frequency, duration, and intensity as pregnancy progresses. Near term, strong Braxton Hicks contractions are often difficult to distinguish from the contractions of true labor.

Braxton Hicks version, one of several types of maneuvers sometimes used to turn the fetus from an undesirable position to one that is more likely to facilitate delivery.

Brazelton assessment, a system for assessing the interactional behavior of newborns with a series of 27 reaction tests, including response to inanimate objects, to a pinprick, to light, and to the sound of a rattle or bell.

Brazilian trypanosomiasis. See **Chagas' disease.**

breach of contract, the failure to perform as promised or agreed in a contract.

breach of duty, 1. the failure to perform an act required by law. **2.** the performance of an act in an unlawful way.

breakbone fever. See **dengue fever.**

break test, a test of muscle strength of a patient by applying resistance after the patient has reached the end of a range of motion. Resistance is applied gradually in a direction opposite to the line of pull of the muscle or muscle group being tested.

breakthrough bleeding [AS *brecan;* ME *thurh* across], the escape of uterine blood between menstrual periods, a side effect experienced by some women using oral contraceptives.

breast [AS *braest*], **1.** the anterior aspect of the surface of the chest. **2.** a mammary gland.

breast cancer, a malignant neoplastic disease of breast tissue, the most common malignancy in women in the United States. The incidence increases exponentially with age from the third to the fifth decade and reaches a second peak at age 65, suggesting that breast cancer in premenopausal women may be related to ovarian hormonal function and in postmenopausal patients to adrenal function. Based on the great prevalence of breast cancer in affluent countries, especially in high socioeconomic groups, it is thought that a high-fat diet may be a causative factor. Risk factors include a family history of breast cancer, nulliparity, exposure to ionizing radiation, early menarche, late menopause, obesity, diabetes, hypertension, chronic cystic disease of the breast, and, possibly, postmenopausal estrogen therapy. Initial symptoms, detected in most cases by self-examination, include a small painless lump, thick or dimpled skin, or nipple retraction. As the lesion progresses, there may be nipple discharge, pain, ulceration, and enlarged axillary glands. Metastasis through the lymphatic system to axillary lymph nodes and to bone, lung, brain, and liver is common. Surgical treatment, depending on the assessment of the tumor, may be a radical, modified radical, or simple mastectomy, with dissection of axillary nodes, or a lumpectomy. Postoperative radiotherapy, chemotherapy, or both are usually prescribed.

breast examination, a process in which the breasts and their accessory structures are observed and palpated in assessing the presence of changes or abnormalities that could indicate malignant disease.

breastfeeding [AS *braest*; ME *feden*], **1.** suckling or nursing, such as giving a baby milk from the breast. Breastfeeding encourages postpartum uterine involution and slows the natural return of the menses, providing a measure of contraception. **2.** taking milk from the breast.

breastfeeding, effective, a NANDA-accepted nursing diagnosis of a state in which a mother-infant dyad/family exhibits adequate proficiency and satisfaction with the breastfeeding process. The defining characteristics include the mother's ability to position the infant at the breast to promote a successful latch-on response, regular and sustained suckling/swallowing at the breast, and infant content after feeding.

breastfeeding, ineffective, a NANDA-accepted nursing diagnosis of dissatisfaction or difficulty with the breastfeeding process that a mother, infant, and/or family experiences. The major defining characteristic is the unsatisfactory breastfeeding process. Other characteristics include an actual or perceived inadequate milk supply, no observable signs of oxytocin release, persistence of sore nipples beyond the infant's first week of life, and maternal reluctance to put the infant to breast as necessary.

breastfeeding, interrupted, a NANDA-accepted nursing diagnosis of a break in the continuity of the breastfeeding process as a result of inability or inadvisability to put the baby to breast for feeding. The defining characteristics include the infant not receiving nourishment at the breast for some or all feedings, separation of mother and infant, and lack of knowledge about expression and storage of breast milk.

breast milk [AS *braest; meoluc*], human milk. The nurse should counsel mothers that it is easily digested, clean, and warm and that it confers some immunities (bronchiolitis and gastroenteritis are rare in breastfed babies). Infants fed breast milk are less likely to become obese or to develop dental malocclusions.

breast milk jaundice, jaundice and hyperbilirubinemia in breastfed infants that occur in the first weeks of life as a result of a metabolite in the mother's milk that inhibits the infant's ability to conjugate bilirubin to protein for excretion.

breast pump, a device for withdrawing milk from the breast.

breast self-examination. See **self-breast examination.**

breast shadows, artifacts on chest radiographs of women caused by breast tissue. The shadows accentuate the underlying tissue and may cause the appearance of an interstitial disease process.

breast transillumination [AS *braest*; L *trans* through, *illuminare* to light up], a method of examining the inner structures of the breast by directing light through the outer wall.

Breathalyzer /breth′əlī′zər/, trademark for a device that analyzes exhaled air. It is commonly used to test for blood alcohol levels, based on a relationship between alcohol in the breath and alcohol in the blood circulating through the lungs.

breath-holding [AS *braeth*; ME *holden*], a form of voluntary apnea that is usually performed with a closed glottis. Although breath-holding may be prolonged for several minutes, it is invariably terminated by an involuntary breaking point.

breathing. See **respiration.**

breathing cycle, a ventilatory cycle consisting of an inspiration followed by the expiration of a volume of gas called the tidal volume. The duration of a breathing cycle is the breathing or ventilatory period.

breathing frequency (f), the number of breathing cycles per a given unit of time.

breathing nomogram [AS *braeth;* Gk *nomos* law, *gramma* a record], a chart that presents scales of data for body weight, breathing frequency, and predicted basal tidal volume arranged in a pattern. It allows calculation of an unknown value on one scale by drawing a line that connects known values on two other scales.

breathing pattern, ineffective, a NANDA-accepted nursing diagnosis of an inhalation and/or exhalation pattern that does not enable adequate pulmonary inflation or emptying. Defining characteristics include dyspnea, shortness of breath, tachypnea, fremitus, abnormal concentrations of arterial blood gases, cyanosis, cough, nasal flaring, change in depth of respiration, pursed lip breathing or prolonged expiratory phase, increased anteroposterior diameter of the chest, use of accessory muscles of breathing, and altered excursion of the chest wall with respiration.

breathing tube, a device inserted into the trachea through the mouth or nose to ensure a patent airway for adequate respiration during artificial or assisted ventilation.

breathing work, the energy required for breathing movements. It is the cumulative product of instantaneous pressure developed by the respiratory muscles and the volume of air moved during a breathing cycle.

breathlessness. See **dyspnea.**

breath odor, an odor usually produced by substances or diseases in the lungs or mouth. Certain specific odors are associated with some diseases, such as diabetes, liver failure, uremia, or a lung abscess.

breath sound [AS *braeth;* L *sonus*], the sound of air and carbon dioxide passing in and out of the respiratory system as heard with a stethoscope.

Breckinridge, Mary (1881–1965), an American nurse who founded the Frontier Nursing Service in Kentucky. The Service was designed to improve the obstetric care of women living in the remote mountainous area. The nurses in the Service had training in midwifery. The Service began training midwives and stimulated the increase of other midwifery schools.

breech birth [ME *brech, burth*], parturition in which the baby emerges feet, knees, or buttocks first. Breech birth is often hazardous: The body may deliver easily, but the aftercoming head may become trapped by an incompletely dilated cervix because babies' heads are usually larger than their bodies.

breech extraction [ME *brech;* L *ex* out, *trahere* to pull], an obstetric operation in which a baby being born feet or buttocks first is grasped before any part of the trunk is born and delivered by traction.

breech presentation [ME *brech;* L *praesentare* to show], intrauterine position of the fetus in which the buttocks or feet present, occurring in approximately 3% of labors. Kinds of breech presentation are **complete breech, footling breech,** and **frank breech.**

bregma /breg′mə/ [Gk, the front of the head], the junction of the coronal and sagittal sutures on the top of the skull. **–bregmatic,** *adj.*

bremsstrahlung radiation /brems′shträ-′lŏŏng/, [Ger, braking radiation], a type of x-ray in which there is a loss of kinetic energy from interaction with the nucleus of a target atom, resulting in an x-ray photon.

Brenner tumor [Fritz Brenner, German pathologist, b. 1877], an uncommon, benign ovarian neoplasm consisting of nests or cords of epithelial cells containing glycogen that are enclosed in fibrous connective tissue. The tumor may be solid or cystic.

bretylium tosylate /britil′ē-əm/, an antiarrhythmic agent prescribed in the treatment of life-threatening ventricular arrhythmias when other measures have not been effective.

brewer's yeast [ME *brewen* to boil, *yest* foam], a preparation containing the dried pulverized cells of a yeast, such as *Saccharomyces cerevisiae,* that is used as a leavening agent and as a dietary supplement. It is a source of the B complex vitamins, many minerals, and a high grade of protein.

brick dust urine, a sign of precipitated urates in acidic urine in a urinalysis sample.

bridge of Varolius. See **pons.**

bridgework, a fixed prosthetic appliance that is cemented permanently to abutment teeth.

bridging [AS *brycg*], **1.** a nursing technique of positioning a patient so that bony prominences are free of pressure on the mattress by using pads, bolsters of foam rubber, or pillows to distribute body weight over a larger surface. **2.** a nursing technique for supporting a part of the body, such as the testicles in treating orchitis using a Bellevue bridge made of a towel or other material.

brief psychotherapy, (in psychiatry) treatment directed toward the active resolution of personality or behavioral problems rather than toward the speculative analysis of the unconscious.

brief reactive psychosis, a short episode, usually less than 2 weeks, of psychotic behavior that occurs in response to a significant psychosocial stressor.

brightness gain, (in radiology) the ability of an image intensifier to increase the illumination level of an image.

Brill-Symmers disease. See **giant follicular lymphoma.**

Brill-Zinsser disease /bril′zin′sər/ [Nathan E. Brill, American physician, b. 1860; Hans Zinsser, American bacteriologist, b. 1878], a mild form of typhus that recurs in a person who appears to have completely recovered from a severe case of the disease. Some rickettsiae remain in the body after the symptoms of the disease abate, causing the recurrence of symptoms.

brim, the edge of the upper border of the true pelvis, or the pelvic inlet.

Brinnell hardness test, a means of determining the surface hardness of a material by measuring the amount of resistance to the impact of a steel ball. The test result is recorded as the Brinnell hardness number (BHN). It is commonly used to measure this quality in various materials used in dental restorations, such as amalgams, cements, and porcelains.

Briquet's syndrome. See **somatization disorder.**

Brissaud's dwarf /brisōz′/ [Edouard Brissaud, French physician, b. 1852], a person affected with infantile myxedema in which short stature is associated with hypothyroidism.

British antilewisite. See **dimercaprol.**

British Medical Association (BMA), a national professional organization of physicians in the United Kingdom.

British Pharmacopoeia (BP), the official British reference work setting forth standards of strength and purity of medications and containing directions for their preparation to ensure that the same prescription written by different doctors and filled by different pharmacists will contain exactly the same ingredients in the same proportions.

British thermal unit (BTU), a unit of heat energy. The amount of thermal energy that must by absorbed by one pound of water to raise its temperature by one degree Fahrenheit at 39.2° F. It is also equivalent to 1,055 joules or 252 calories.

brittle bones. See **osteogenesis imperfecta.**

brittle diabetes. See **insulin-dependent diabetes mellitus.**

broach, an elongated, tapering dental instrument used for shaping and enlarging holes, particularly in removing pulp or cleansing of a root canal.

broad beta disease, a familial type of hyperlipoproteinemia in which a lipoprotein, high in cholesterol and triglycerides, accumulates in the blood. The condition is characterized by yellowish nodules (xanthomas) on the elbows and knees, peripheral vascular disease, and elevated serum cholesterol levels.

broad ligament [ME *brood;* L *ligare* to tie], a folded sheet of peritoneum draped over the uterine tubes, the uterus, and the ovaries.

broad ligament of the liver [ME *brod;* L *ligare* to bind; AS *lifer*], a crescent-shaped fold of peritoneum attached to the lower surface of the diaphragm, connecting with the liver and the anterior abdominal wall.

broad-spectrum antibiotic, an antibiotic that is effective against a wide range of infectious microorganisms.

Broca's area /brō′kəz/ [Pierre P. Broca, French surgeon, b. 1824], an area involved in speech production situated on the inferior frontal gyrus of the brain.

Broca's plane [Pierre P. Broca], a plane that extends from the tip of the interalveolar septum between the upper central incisors to the lowest point of the occipital condyle.

Brodie's abscess [Sir Benjamin Brodie, English surgeon, b. 1783], a form of osteomyelitis consisting of an indolent staphylococcal infection of bone, usually in the metaphysis of a long bone of a child, characterized by a necrotic cavity surrounded by dense granulation tissue.

Brodmann's areas /brod′manz, brōt′mons/ [Korbinian Brodmann, German anatomist, b. 1868], the 47 different areas of the cerebral cortex that are associated with specific neurologic functions and distinguished by different cellular components.

brom, abbreviation for a *bromide noncarboxylate anion.*

bromhidrosis /brō′midrō′sis/ [Gk *bromos* stench, *hidros* sweat], an abnormal condition in which the apocrine sweat has an unpleasant odor.

bromide /brō′mīd/ [Gk *bromos* stench], a compound in which the negative element is bromine, especially a salt of hydrobromic acid. Bromides, once widely prescribed as sedatives, are now seldom used for that purpose.

bromine (Br) /brō'mēn/, a toxic, red-brown, liquid element of the halogen group. Its atomic number is 35; its atomic weight is 79.909. Bromides are binary compounds of bromine; they have been used as sedatives, hypnotics, and analgesics.

bromocriptine mesylate /brō'mōkrip'tēn/, a dopamine receptor agonist prescribed for the treatment of amenorrhea and galactorrhea associated with hyperprolactinemia, female infertility, and Parkinson's disease.

bromoderma /brō'mōdur'mə/[Gk *bromos* stench, *derma* skin], an acneiform, bullous, or nodular skin rash, occurring as a hypersensitivity reaction to ingested bromides.

brompheniramine maleate /brom'fənir'-əmin/, an antihistamine prescribed in the treatment of a variety of hypersensitivity reactions, including rhinitis, skin reactions, and itching.

Brompton's cocktail, an analgesic solution containing alcohol, morphine or heroin, and, in some cases, a phenothiazine. The cocktail is administered in the control of pain in the terminally ill patient.

bronchial [Gk, *brogchos*, windpipe], pertaining to the bronchi or bronchioles.

bronchial asthma. See **asthma.**

bronchial breath sound [Gk *bronchos* windpipe], an abnormal sound heard with a stethoscope over the lungs, indicating consolidation because of pneumonia or compression. Expiration and inspiration produce loud, high-pitched sounds of equal duration.

bronchial drainage. See **postural drainage.**

bronchial fremitus, a vibration that can be palpated or auscultated on the chest wall over a bronchus congested by secretions that rattle as the air passes during respiration.

bronchial hyperreactivity [Gk *bronchos; hyper* excess; L *re* again, *agere* to act], an abnormal respiratory condition characterized by reflex bronchospasm in response to histamine or a cholinergic drug. It is a universal feature of asthma and is used in the differential diagnosis of asthma and heart disease.

bronchial pneumonia. See **bronchopneumonia.**

bronchial secretion, a substance produced in the bronchial tree that consists of mucus, protein salts, plasma fluid, and proteins, including fibrinogen.

bronchial spasm, an excessive and prolonged contraction of the involuntary muscle fibers in the walls of the bronchi and bronchioles. The contractions may be localized or general.

bronchial toilet, special care that is given patients with tracheostomies and respiratory disorders, including stimulation of coughing, deep breathing, and the suctioning of the respiratory tract.

bronchial tree, an anatomic complex of the bronchi and the bronchial tubes. The bronchi branch from the trachea, and the bronchial tubes branch from the bronchi.

bronchial washing [Gk *bronchos* windpipe; ME *wasshen* to wash], the irrigation of the bronchi and bronchioles to cleanse them and to collect specimens for laboratory examination.

bronchiectasis /brong'kē·ek'təsis/ [Gk *bronchos* + *ektasis* stretching], an abnormal condition of the bronchial tree, characterized by irreversible dilatation and destruction of the bronchial walls. The condition is sometimes congenital but is more often a result of bronchial infection or of obstruction by a tumor or an aspirated foreign body. Symptoms include a constant cough productive of copious purulent sputum, hemoptysis, chronic sinusitis, clubbing of fingers, and persistent moist, coarse rales.

bronchiolar. See **bronchiole.**

bronchiolar carcinoma. See **alveolar cell carcinoma.**

bronchiolar collapse [L *bronchiolus* little windpipe; *colabor* to fall], a condition in which bronchioles become compressed by the pressure of surrounding structures and the lack of inflowing air needed to keep them inflated. The condition occurs in such disorders as emphysema, cystic disease, and bronchiectasis.

bronchiole /brong'kē·ōl/ [L *bronchiolus* little windpipe], a small airway of the respiratory system extending from the bronchi into the lobes of the lung. There are two divisions of bronchioles: terminal bronchioles and respiratory bronchioles. –**bronchiolar** /brongkē'ələr/, *adj.*

bronchiolitis /brong'kē·ōli'tis/ [L *bronchiolus* little windpipe + Gk *itis* inflammation], an acute viral infection of the lower respiratory tract that occurs primarily in infants under 18 months of age, characterized by expiratory wheezing, respiratory distress, inflammation, and obstruction at the level of the bronchioles. The most common causative agents are the respiratory syncytial viruses (RSV) and the parainfluenza viruses. *Mycoplasma pneumoniae*, the rhinoviruses, enteroviruses, and measles virus are less common causative agents. Transmission occurs by infection with airborne particles or by contact with infected secretions.

bronchiospasm. See *bronchial spasm.*

bronchitis /brongkī'tis/ [Gk *bronchos* windpipe + *itis* inflammation], an acute or chronic inflammation of the mucous membranes of the tracheobronchial tree. **Acute bronchitis** is characterized by a productive cough, fever, hypertrophy of mucus-secreting structures, and back pain. Caused by the spread of upper respiratory viral infections to the bronchi, it is often observed with or after childhood infections like measles, whooping cough, diphtheria, and typhoid fever. **Chronic bronchitis** is distinguished by an excessive secretion of mucus in the bronchi with a productive cough for at least 3 consecutive months in at least 2 successive years. Predisposing factors for chronic bronchitis include cigarette smoking, air pollution, chronic infections, and abnormal physical development of the bronchi that interferes with bronchial drainage. Most common in adults, it is often a complication of cystic fibrosis in children.

bronchoalveolar [Gk *bronchos*; L *alveolus* little hollow], pertaining to the terminal air sacs at the ends of the bronchioles.

bronchoconstriction [Gk *bronchos*; L *constringere* to draw tight], a constriction of the bronchi, resulting in a narrowing of the airway lumen.

bronchodilatation [Gk *bronchos*; L *dilatare* to widen], an increase in the diameter or lumen of the bronchi, allowing increased airflow to and from the lungs.

bronchodilator, a substance, especially a drug, that relaxes contractions of the smooth muscle of the bronchioles to improve ventilation to the lungs. Pharmacologic bronchodilators are prescribed to improve aeration in asthma, bronchiectasis, bronchitis, and emphysema.

bronchofibroscopy. See **fiberoptic bronchoscopy.**

bronchogenic [Gk *bronchos* + *genein* to produce], originating in the bronchi.

bronchogenic carcinoma, one of the malignant lung tumors that originate in bronchi. Lesions, usually associated with cigarette smoking, may cause coughing and wheezing, fatigue, chest tightness, aching joints, and, in the late stages, bloody sputum, clubbing of the fingers, weight loss, and pleural effusion.

bronchography /brongkog'rəfē/, an x-ray examination of the bronchi after they have been coated with a radiopaque substance.

bronchomotor tone, the state of contraction or relaxation of smooth muscle in the bronchial walls that regulates the caliber of the airways.

bronchophony /brongkof'ənē/ [Gk *bronchos* + *phone* voice], an increase in intensity and clarity of vocal resonance that may result from an increase in lung tissue density, such as in the consolidation of pneumonia.

bronchopneumonia [Gk *bronchos* + *pneumon* lung], an acute inflammation of the lungs and bronchioles, characterized by chills, fever, high pulse and respiratory rates, bronchial breathing, cough with purulent bloody sputum, severe chest pain, and abdominal distension. The disease is usually a result of the spread of bacterial infection from the upper respiratory tract to the lower respiratory tract. The condition results in pleural effusion, empyema, lung abscess, peripheral thrombophlebitis, respiratory failure, congestive heart failure, and jaundice.

bronchopulmnary [Gk *bronchos* + L *pulmonis* lung], of or pertaining to the bronchi and the lungs of the respiratory system.

bronchopulmonary hygiene, the care and cleanliness of the respiratory tract, including ventilatory equipment and natural air passages. Hygienic care also allows for complete assessment of the patient's respiratory condition and of any equipment or devices used to support his or her breathing.

bronchopulmonary lavage [Gk *bronchos*; L *pulmonis* lung; Fr, *lavage* washing out], the irrigation or washing out of the bronchi and bronchioles to remove pulmonary secretions.

bronchoscope /brong'kəskōp'/, a curved, flexible tube for visual examination of the bronchi. It contains fibers that carry light down the tube and project an enlarged image up the tube to the viewer. **–bronchoscopic,** *adj.*

bronchoscopy /brongkos'kəpē/, the visual examination of the tracheobronchial tree, using a bronchoscope. The patient is in a fasting state and is usually sedated before the examination, which is routinely performed under topical anesthesia. In addition to visualization, the procedure can be used for suctioning, for obtaining a biopsy and fluid or sputum for examination, and for removal of foreign bodies.

bronchospasm, an abnormal contraction of the smooth muscle of the bronchi, resulting in an acute narrowing and obstruction of the respiratory airway. A cough with generalized wheezing usually indicates this condition.

bronchospirometry /brong'kōspīrom'ətrē/, a technique for the study of the ventilation and gas exchange of each lung separately by the introduction of a catheter into either the left or the right mainstem bronchus.

bronchotomogram /-tom′əgram/, an image of the upper respiratory system, from the trachea to the lower bronchi, produced by tomography.

bronchovesicular, pertaining to the bronchial tubes and the alveoli.

bronchovesicular sound [Gk *bronchos;* L *vesicula* small bladder + *sonus* sound], normal breath sounds that are between sounds of the bronchial tubes and those of the alveoli, or a combination of the two sounds.

bronchus /brong′kəs/, *pl.* **bronchi** [L; Gk *bronchos* windpipe], any one of several large air passages in the lungs through which pass inhaled air and exhaled waste gases. Each bronchus has a wall consisting of three layers. The outermost is made of dense fibrous tissue, reinforced with cartilage. The middle layer is a network of smooth muscle. The innermost layer consists of ciliated mucous membrane. Kinds of bronchi are **lobar, primary, secondary,** and **segmental bronchus.** –**bronchial,** *adj.*

Bronsted-Lowry base, any chemical compound that accepts a proton.

broth, **1.** a fluid culture medium used to support the growth of bacteria for laboratory analysis. **2.** a beverage or other fluid made with meat extract and water.

brow, the forehead, particularly the eyebrow or ridge above the eye.

brown fat [ME *broun;* AS *faett* filled], a type of fat present in newborn infants and rarely found in adults. Brown fat is a unique source of heat energy for the infant because it has greater thermogenic activity than ordinary fat.

brownian movement /brou′nyən/ [Robert Brown, Scottish botanist, b. 1773], a random movement of microscopic particles suspended in a liquid or gas. The movement is produced by the natural kinetic activity of molecules of the fluid striking the foreign particles.

brown recluse spider bite [OE *brun;* L *recludere* to shut off; ME *spithre;* AS *bitan*], the bite of the brown or violin spider, *Loxosceles reclusa,* producing a characteristic necrotic lesion. There is little or no initial pain but localized pain develops about an hour later. A bleb forms, sometimes in a target or bull's eye pattern. The blood-filled bleb increases in size and eventually ruptures, leaving a black scar. The patient may also experience systemic symptoms.

Brown-Séquard's treatment. See **organotherapy.**

Brown-Séquard syndrome /broun′sākär′/

[Charles E. Brown-Séquard, French physiologist, b. 1817], a traumatic neurologic disorder resulting from compression of one side of the spinal cord, above the tenth thoracic vertebrae, characterized by spastic paralysis on the injured side of the body, loss of postural sense, and loss of the senses of pain and heat on the other side of the body.

brown spider, a poisonous insect, also known as the brown recluse or violin spider, found in both North and South America. The venom from its bite usually creates a blister surrounded by concentric white and red circles. Pain, nausea, fever, and chills are common, but the reaction is usually self-limited.

brow presentation, an obstetric situation in which the brow, or forehead, of the fetus is the first part of the body to enter the birth canal. Because the diameter of the fetal head at this angle may be greater than the mother's pelvic outlet, a cesarean section may be recommended.

Brucella abortus. See **abortus fever.**

brucellosis /broo͞′səlo͞′sis/ [Sir David Bruce, English pathologist, b. 1855], a disease caused by any of several species of the gram-negative coccobacillus *Brucella.* Brucellosis is primarily a disease of animals (including cattle, pigs, and goats), and humans usually acquire it by ingesting contaminated milk or milk products or through a break in the skin. It is characterized by fever, chills, sweating, malaise, and weakness. Although brucellosis itself is rarely fatal, treatment is important because serious complications such as pneumonia, meningitis, and encephalitis can develop.

Bruch's disease. See **Marseilles fever.**

Brudzinski's sign /broodzin′skēz/ [Josef Brudzinski, Polish physician, b. 1874], an involuntary flexion of the arm, hip, and knee when the neck is passively flexed, seen in patients with meningitis.

bruise. See **contusion, ecchymosis.**

bruit /broo͞′ē/ [Fr, noise], an abnormal sound or murmur heard while auscultating an organ or gland, such as the liver or thyroid. The specific character of the bruit, its location, and the time of its occurrence in a cycle of other sounds are all of diagnostic importance.

Brunnstrom hemiplegia classification, an evaluation procedure that assesses muscle tone and voluntary control of movement patterns in a stroke patient. Results indicate the patient's progress through stages of recovery.

brush border, microvilli on the free surfaces of certain epithelial cells, particularly the absorptive surfaces of the intestine and the proximal convoluted tubules of the kidney. The tiny cylindric processes increase the surface area of the tissues.

Brushfield's spots [Thomas Brushfield, English physician, b. 1858; ME *spotte* stain], pinpoint, white or light yellow spots on the iris of a child with Down syndrome.

Bruton's agammaglobulinemia [Ogden C. Bruton, American physician, b. 1908], a sex-linked, inherited condition characterized by the absence of gamma globulin in the blood. Patients with this syndrome are deficient in antibodies and susceptible to repeated infections.

bruxism /bruk'sizəm/ [Gk *brychein* to gnash the teeth], the compulsive, unconscious grinding of the teeth, especially during sleep or as a mechanism for the release of tension during periods of extreme stress in the waking hours.

Bryant's traction [Sir Thomas Bryant, English physician, b. 1828; L *trahere* to pull], an orthopedic mechanism used only with infants to immobilize both lower extremities in the treatment of a fractured femur or in the correction of the congenital dislocation of the hip. This mechanism consists of a traction frame supporting weights, connected by ropes that run through pulleys to traction foot plates worn by the infant.

BSA, 1. abbreviation for **body surface area. 2.** abbreviation for *bovine serum albumin.*

BSE, abbreviation for **breast self-examination.**

BSN, abbreviation for **Bachelor of Science in Nursing.**

BSP, abbreviation for *Bromsulphalein.*

BT, abbreviation for **bleeding time.**

BTPD, abbreviation for *body temperature, ambient pressure, dry.*

BTPS, abbreviation for *body temperature, ambient pressure, saturated* (with water vapor).

BTU, abbreviation for **British thermal unit.**

bubbling rale [ME *bubblen* to make bubbles; Fr *ralement* a rattling], an abnormal chest sound characteristic of moisture moving in the lungs.

bubble-diffusion humidifier, a device that provides humidified oxygen or other therapeutic gases by allowing the gas to bubble through a reservoir of water.

bubble oxygenator, a heart-lung device that oxygenates the blood while it is diverted outside the patient's body.

bubo /byoo'bō/, *pl.* buboes [Gk *boubon* groin], a greatly enlarged, inflamed lymph node usually in the axilla or groin,

associated with such diseases as chancroid, lymphogranuloma venereum, bubonic plague, and syphilis.

bubonic plague /byoobon'ik/ [Gk *boubon* groin; L *plaga* stroke], the most common form of plague, characterized by painful buboes in the axilla, groin, or neck, fever often rising to 106° F (41.11° C), prostration with a rapid, thready pulse, hypotension, delirium, and bleeding into the skin from the superficial blood vessels. The symptoms are caused by an endotoxin released by a bacillus, *Yersinia pestis,* usually introduced into the body by the bite of a rat flea that has bitten an infected rat. Inoculation with plague vaccine confers partial immunity; infection provides lifetime immunity. Conditions favor a plague epidemic when a large infected rodent population lives with a large nonimmune human population in a damp, warm climate.

buccal /buk'əl/ [L *bucca* cheek], of or pertaining to the inside of the cheek, the surface of a tooth, or the gum next to the cheek.

buccal administration of medication, oral administration of a drug, usually in the form of a tablet, by placing it between the cheek and the teeth or gum until it dissolves.

buccal bar, an orthodontic appliance auxillary that consists of a rigid metal wire extending anteriorly from the buccal side of a molar band anteriorly.

buccal contour [L *bucca; cum* together with, *tornare* to turn], the shape of the buccal side of a posterior tooth, usually characterized by a slight occlusocervical convexity with its largest prominence at the gingival third of the clinical buccal surface.

buccal fat pad, a fat pad in the cheek under the subcutaneous layer of the skin, over the buccinator. It is particularly prominent in infants and is often called a sucking pad.

buccal flange [L *bucca;* OFr *flanche* flank], the portion of a denture flange that occupies the buccal vestibule of the mouth and extends distally from the buccal notch.

buccal glands [L *bucca, glans* acorn], small salivary glands located between the buccinator muscle and the mucous membrane in the vestibule of the mouth.

buccal notch, a depression in a denture flange that accommodates the buccal frenum.

buccal smear, a sample of cells removed from the buccal mucosa for purposes of obtaining a karyotype to determine the genetic sex of an individual.

buccal splint, any material, usually plaster, placed on the buccal surfaces of fixed partial denture units to hold the units in position for assembly.

buccinator /buk´sinā´tər/ [L *buccina* trumpet], the main muscle of the cheek, one of the 12 muscles of the mouth. It arises from the maxilla above and the mandible below, inserting in the lips; its superficial surface is covered by the buccopharyngeal fascia and the buccal fat pad. The buccinator compresses the cheek, acting as an important accessory muscle of mastication by holding food under the teeth.

buccogingival /buk´ōjinjī´vəl/, pertaining to the internal mouth structures, particularly the cheeks and gums.

buccolinguomasticatory triad /buk´ōling´wōmas´təkatôr´e/ [L *bucca* cheek, *lingua* tongue, *masticare* to gnash the teeth], a complex of involuntary lip, tongue, jaw, and head movements seen in tardive dyskinesia.

buccopharyngeal /buk´ōfərin´jē·əl/, of or pertaining to the cheek and the pharynx or to the mouth and the pharynx.

bucket. See **socket.**

bucket handle fracture [OFr *buket* tub; ME *handel* part grasped; L *fractura* break], a fracture that produces a tear in a semilunar cartilage along the medial side of the knee joint.

bucking, *informal.* **1.** gagging on an endotracheal tube. **2.** involuntarily resisting insufflation by a positive pressure respirator.

buck knife, a periodontal surgical knife with a spear-shaped cutting point, used for interdental incision associated with a gingivectomy.

Buck's skin traction, an orthopedic procedure that applies traction to the lower extremity with the hips and the knees extended. It is used in the treatment of hip and knee contractures, in postoperative positioning and immobilization, and in disease processes of the hip and the knee.

Buck's traction [Gurdon Buck, American surgeon, b. 1807; L *trahere* to pull], one of the most common orthopedic mechanisms by which pull is exerted on the lower extremity with a system of ropes, weights, and pulleys. Buck's traction is used to immobilize, position, and align the lower extremity in the treatment of contractures and diseases of the hip and knee.

Bucky diaphragm [Gustav P. Bucky, American radiologist, b. 1880; Gk *diaphragma* partition], (in radiology) a device consisting of a moving grid that limits the amount of scattered radiation and thus obtains finer x-ray film contrast and detail.

buclizine hydrochloride /bōō´kləzēn/,

an antiemetic drug derived from piperazine but with antihistamine properties. It is also used to treat allergies and vertigo.

Budd-Chiari syndrome /bud´kē·är´ē/ [George Budd, English physician, b. 1880; Hans Chiari, Czech-French pathologist, b. 1851], a disorder of hepatic circulation, marked by venous obstruction, that leads to liver enlargement, ascites, extensive development of collateral vessels, and severe portal hypertension.

budding [ME *budde*], a type of asexual reproduction in which the cell produces a budlike projection containing chromatin that eventually separates from the parent and develops into an independent organism. It is a common form of reproduction in the lower animals and plants, such as sponges, yeasts, and molds.

buddy splint, a splinting technique commonly used after a finger injury requiring immobilization. The injured finger and the adjacent finger are typically taped together to limit the range of motion of the affected finger.

Buerger's disease. See **thromboangiitis obliterans.**

Buerger's postural exercises [Leo Buerger, American physician, b. 1879; L *ponere* to place, *exercere* to continue working], a set of special exercises designed to maintain circulation in a limb.

buffalo hump, an accumulation of fat on the back of the neck associated with the prolonged use of large doses of glucocorticoids or the hypersecretion of cortisol caused by Cushing's syndrome.

buffer [ME *buffe* to cushion], a substance or group of substances that tends to control the hydrogen ion concentration in a solution by absorbing hydrogen ions when an acid is added to the system and releasing hydrogen ions upon the addition of a base. Buffers minimize significant changes of pH in a chemical system.

buffer anions, the negatively charged bicarbonate, protein, and phosphate ions that comprise the buffer systems of the body.

buffer cations, the positively charged ions of the body's electrolytes, including sodium, calcium, potassium, and magnesium.

buffer solution [ME *buffet*; L *solutus* dissolved], a solution that will maintain or will maintain a given pH value despite dilution or the addition of a small amount of base or acid.

buffy coat [ME *buffet*; Fr *cote*], a grayish white layer of white blood cells and platelets, mixed with some red blood cells, that accumulates on the surface of sedimented erythrocytes when blood plasma is allowed to stand.

buffy coat transfusion. See **granulocyte transfusion.**

bulb [L *bulbus* swollen root], any rounded structure, such as the eyeball, hair roots, and certain sensory nerve endings.

bulbar [L *bulbus*], **1.** pertaining to a bulb. **2.** pertaining to the medulla oblongata of the brain and the cranial nerves.

bulbar ataxia, a loss of motor coordination because of a lesion in the medulla oblongata or pons.

bulbar myelitis, an inflammation of the central nervous system involving the medulla oblongata.

bulbar palsy, a form of paralysis resulting from a defect in the motor centers of medulla oblongata.

bulbar paralysis, a degenerative neurologic condition characterized by progressive paralysis of the lips, tongue, mouth, pharynx, and larynx.

bulbar poliomyelitis, a form of poliomyelitis that involves the medulla oblongata and gradually progresses to bulbar paralysis, with respiratory and circulatory failure.

bulbocavernosus, a muscle that covers the bulb of the penis in the male and the bulbus vestibuli in the female.

bulbourethral gland, one of two small glands located on each side of the prostate, draining to the urethra. Bulbourethral glands secrete a fluid component of the seminal fluid.

bulbous, pertaining to a structure that resembles a bulb or that originates in a bulb.

bulb syringe, a blunt-tipped, flexible syringe usually made of rubber or plastic. Bulb syringes are used primarily for irrigating external orifices, such as the auditory canal.

bulbus oculi. See **eye.**

bulimia /byo͞olim′ē·ə/ [Gk *bous* ox, *limos* hunger], an insatiable craving for food, often resulting in episodes of continuous eating followed by periods of depression and self-deprivation. –**bulemic,** *n., adj.*

bulk. See **dietary fiber.**

bulk cathartic [ME *bulke* heap; Gk *kathartikos* evacuation of bowels], a cathartic that acts by softening and increasing the mass of fecal material in the bowel.

bulla /bo͞ol′ə, bul′ə/, *pl.* **bullae** [L, bubble], a thin-walled blister of the skin or mucous membranes greater than 1 centimeter in diameter containing clear, serous fluid.

bulldog forceps, short, spring forceps for clamping an artery or vein for hemostasis. The jaws may be padded to avoid injury to vascular tissue.

bullet forceps, a kind of forceps that has thin, curved, serrated blades designed for extracting a foreign object, such as a bullet, from the base of a puncture wound.

bullous disease /bo͞ol′əs/, any disease marked by eruptions of blisters filled with fluid, or bullae, on the skin or mucous membranes. An example is pemphigus.

bullous myringitis [L *bulla; myringa* eardrum], an inflammatory condition of the ear, characterized by fluid-filled vesicles on the tympanic membrane and the sudden onset of severe pain in the ear.

bullous pemphigoid [L *bulla;* Gk *pemphix* bubble, *eidos* form], a condition characterized by chronic eruptions of skin blisters over multiple body areas.

bumetanide, a diuretic prescribed in the treatment of edema caused by cardiac, hepatic, or renal disease.

BUN, abbreviation for **blood urea nitrogen.**

bundle branch [Dan *bondel;* Fr *branche*], a segment of a network of specialized muscle fibers that conduct electrical impulses within the heart. It is a continuation of the bundle of His, extending from the upper part of the intraventricular septum of the heart.

bundle branch block (BBB), an abnormal conduction of the cardiac impulse within the ventricles, resulting in an abnormally shaped QRS complex. Bundle branch block is commonly caused by ischemia or necrosis of the bundle branches, trauma (as in surgical manipulation), or mechanical compression of the branches by a tumor. Pacemaker insertion may be performed if further deterioration in conduction is anticipated.

bundle of His /his/ [Dan *bondel;* Wilhelm His, German physician, b. 1863], a band of atypical cardiac muscle fibers with few contractile units. It arises from the distal portion of the AV node and extends across the AV groove to the top of the intraventricular septum where it divides into the bundle branches.

bunion /bun′yən/ [Gk *bounion* turnip], an abnormal enlargement of the joint at the base of the great toe. It is caused by inflammation of the bursa and characterized by soreness, swelling, thickening of the skin, and lateral displacement of the great toe.

bunionectomy /bun′yənek′təmē/, excision of a bunion.

bunionette /bun′yənet′/, an abnormal enlargement and inflammation of the joint at the base of the small toe.

Bunnell block, a small wooden block used in exercise of the fingers after surgery. The exercises with the block allow each joint to be exercised individually with full tendon excursion while the other joints are held extended.

Bunyamwera arbovirus /bun'yəmwir'ə/, one of a group of arthropod-borne viruses that infect humans, carried by mosquitoes from rodent hosts causing California encephalitis, Rift Valley fever, and other diseases characterized by headache, weakness, low-grade fever, myalgia, and a rash.

buphthalmos. See congenital glaucoma.

bupivacaine hydrochloride /byōōpiv'ə-kān/, a local anesthetic prescribed for caudal, epidural, peripheral, or sympathetic anesthetic block.

buprenorphine hydrochloride /bōō'prən-ôr'fēn/, a parenteral analgesic prescribed for the relief of moderate to severe pain.

Bureau of Medical Devices (BMD), an agency of the Food and Drug Administration organized in 1976 with the responsibility of providing standards for and regulation of the manufacture and uses of medical devices.

buret /byōōret'/ [Fr, small jug], a laboratory utensil used to deliver a wide range of volumes accurately.

buried suture [OE byrgan protect; L sutura], a suture that is inserted to bring together soft tissues between the viscus and the skin.

Burkitt's lymphoma /bur'kits/ [Denis P. Burkitt, English physician, b. 1911], a malignant neoplasm composed of undifferentiated lymphoreticular cells that form a large osteolytic lesion in the jaw or, in children, an abdominal mass. The tumor, which is seen chiefly in Central Africa, is characteristically a gray-white mass with a branlike consistency, sometimes containing areas of hemorrhage and necrosis.

burn [AS baernan], any injury to tissues of the body caused by heat, electricity, chemicals, radiation, or gases in which the extent of the injury is determined by the amount of exposure of the cell to the agent and to the nature of the agent. The treatment of burns includes pain relief, careful asepsis, prevention of infection, maintenance of the balance in the body of fluids and electrolytes, and good nutrition.

burn center, a health care facility that is designed to care for patients who have been severely burned. A network of burn centers established throughout the United States and Canada provide sophisticated advanced techniques of care for burn victims.

burning feet syndrome, a neurologic disorder characterized by symptoms of a burning sensation in the sole of the foot. The burning tends to be more intense at night and may also involve the hands.

burning pain [AS baernan; L poena penalty], the pain experienced as a result of a thermal burn.

burnisher [ME burnischen to make brown], a dental instrument with a blade or beveled nib used to smooth out rough edges of restorations.

burnout, a popular term for the condition of having mental or physical energy depletion after a period of chronic, unrelieved job-related stress characterized sometimes by physical illness.

burn therapy, the management of a patient burned by flames, a hot liquid, or explosive, chemical, or electric current. Partial thickness burns may be first degree, involving only the epidermis, or second degree, involving the epidermis and corium, whereas full-thickness or third-degree burns involve all skin layers. Second-degree burns covering more than 30% of the body and third-degree burns on the face and extremities, or more than 10% of the body surface, are critical. In the first 48 hours of a severe burn, vascular fluid, sodium chloride, and protein rapidly pass into the affected area causing local edema, blister formation, hypovolemia, hypoproteinemia, hyponatremia, hyperkalemia, hypotension, and oliguria. The initial hypovolemic stage is followed by a shift of fluid in the opposite direction resulting in diuresis, increased blood volume, and decreased serum electrolytes. Potential complications in serious burns include circulatory collapse, renal damage, gastric atony, paralytic ileus, infections, septic shock, pneumonia, and stress ulcer (Curling's ulcer), characterized by hematemesis and peritonitis.

Burow's solution /byōōr'ōz/ [Karl A. von Burow, German physician, b. 1809], a liquid preparation containing aluminum sulfate, acetic acid, precipitated calcium carbonate, and water, used as a topical astringent, antiseptic, and antipyretic for a wide variety of skin disorders.

burp, informal. **1.** to belch, or eructate. **2.** a belch, or eructation.

burr cell [ME burre; L cella storeroom], a form of mature erythrocyte in which the cells or cell fragments have spicules, or tiny projections, on the surface.

burrowing flea. See chigoe.

bursa /bur'sə/, pl. **bursae** [Gk byrsa wineskin] **1.** a fibrous sac between certain tendons and the bones beneath them. Lined with a synovial membrane that secretes synovial fluid, the bursa acts as a small cushion that allows the tendon as it contracts and relaxes to move over the bone. **2.** a sac or closed cavity.

bursa of Achilles, bursa separating the tendon of Achilles and the calcaneus.

bursectomy [Gk *byrsa* + *ektome* cutting out], the excision of a bursa.

bursitis /bursī'tis/, an inflammation of the bursa, the connective tissue structure surrounding a joint. Bursitis may be precipitated by arthritis, infection, injury, or excessive or traumatic exercise or effort. The chief symptom is severe pain of the affected joint, particularly on movement. The goals of treatment for bursitis include the control of pain and the maintenance of joint motion. Some kinds of bursitis are **housemaid's knee, miner's elbow,** and **weaver's bottom.**

bursting fracture [ME *bersten;* L *fractura* break], any fracture that disperses multiple bone fragments, usually at or near the end of a bone.

Buschke's disease. See **cryptococcosis.**

buspirone hydrochloride, an oral antianxiety drug prescribed for anxiety disorders and the short-term relief of anxiety symptoms.

busulfan, an alkylating agent prescribed in the treatment of chronic myelocytic leukemia.

butabarbital sodium /by oo'təbär'bitôl/, a sedative prescribed for the relief of anxiety, nervous tension, and insomnia.

butaconazole nitrate /by oo'təkō'nəzōl/, an intravaginal antifungal cream prescribed for the treatment of vulvovaginal fungal infections caused by *Candida* species.

butamben picrate /by ootam'bən pik'rāt/, a local anesthetic for the temporary relief of pain from minor burns.

butanoic acid. See **butyric acid.**

butanol. See **butyl alcohol.**

butanol-extractable iodine (BEI) /by oo'-tənôl/, iodine that can be separated from plasma proteins by a solvent, as butanol, and measured for analyzing thyroid function.

butaperazine maleate /by oo'təper'əzēn ma'ē-āt/, an antipsychotic prescribed in the treatment of schizophrenia and chronic brain syndrome.

butorphanol tartrate /by ootôr'fənôl/, a parenteral agonist/antagonist narcotic of the phenanthrene family, given for surgical premedication and as an analgesic component of balanced anesthesia. It provides almost immediate relief from pain when given intravenously and begins to take effect within 10 minutes when given intramuscularly.

butterfly bandage [AS *buttorfleoge*], a narrow adhesive strip with broader wing-like ends used to approximate the edges of a superficial wound and to hold the sides together as they heal. It is used in place of a suture in certain cases.

butterfly fracture, a bone break in which the center fragment contained by two cracks forms a triangle.

butterfly rash, an erythematous, scaling eruption of both cheeks joined by a narrow band of rash across the nose. It is seen in lupus erythematosus, rosacea, and seborrheic dermatitis.

buttermilk [Gk *boutyron* butter; AS *meoluc*], **1.** the slightly sour-tasting liquid residue remaining after the solids in cream have been churned into butter. **2.** cultured milk made by the addition of certain organisms to fat-free milk.

buttock. See **nates.**

buttonhole [OFr *boton;* AS *hol*], a small slitlike hole in the wall of a structure or a cavity of the body.

buttonhole fracture, any fracture caused by the perforation of a bone by a bullet.

buttonhook, any of a variety of devices designed to help patients with limited finger range of motion or amputations to fasten clothing.

button suture, a technique in suturing in which the ends of the suture material are passed through buttons on the surface of the skin and tied. It is used to prevent the suture from cutting through the skin.

butyl /by oo'til/ [Gk *boutyron* butter, *hyle* matter], a hydrocarbon radical (C_4H_9), the compounds of which are obtained from petroleum. Butyl compounds, some of which are toxic and irritating, are used in a variety of industrial and medical applications, including anesthesia.

butyl alcohol, a clear, toxic liquid used as an organic solvent. It is one of four isomers, the others being isobutyl, secondary butyl, and tertiary butyl alcohol.

butyric acid /by ootir'ik/, a fatty acid occurring in rancid butter, feces, urine, perspiration, and, in trace amounts, in the spleen and blood. Butyric acid is used in the preparation of flavorings, emulsifying agents, and pharmaceutics.

butyric fermentation, the conversion of carbohydrate to butyric acid.

butyrophenone /by oo'tərōfē'nōn/, one of a small group of major tranquilizers used in treating psychosis to decrease the choreic symptoms of Huntington's chorea and the tics and coprolalia of Gilles de la Tourette's syndrome.

BWS, abbreviation for **battered woman syndrome.**

bypass [AS *bi* alongside; Fr *passer*], **1.** any one of various surgical procedures to divert the flow of blood or other natural fluids from normal anatomic courses. A bypass may be either temporary or permanent. Bypass surgery is commonly performed in the treatment of cardiac and GI disorders. **2.** a term used by some hospitals to signal that its emergency department lacks the personnel and equipment to handle additional cases, thereby advising that ambulances transporting new cases be diverted to other hospitals.

byssinosis /bis′inō′sis/ [Gk *byssos* flax, *osis* condition], an occupational respiratory disease characterized by shortness of breath, cough, and wheezing. The condition is an allergic reaction to dust or fungi in cotton, flax, and hemp fibers.

c, 1. symbol for *capillary blood.* **2.** abbreviation for **curie.**

C, 1. symbol for **compliance** in respiratory physiology. **2.** symbol for concentration of gas in the blood.

Ca, symbol for the element **calcium.**

CABG, abbreviation for *coronary artery bypass graft.*

cabinet bath [ME *cabane* cabin], a bath in which the patient is enclosed in a cabinet, except for the head, heated by hot air or radiant heat.

Cabot rings /kab′ot/ [Richard C. Cabot, American physician, b. 1868], threadlike figures, often appearing as loops or rings, observed in red blood cells of patients with severe anemia.

Cabot's splint [Arthur T. Cabot, American surgeon, b. 1852], a metal splint worn behind the thigh and leg for support.

cacao [Mex *caca*], **1.** cocoa. **2.** the substance *Theobroma cacao.* **3.** the seeds of *Theobroma cacao.*

cacesthesia /kak′əsthē′zhə/ [Gk *kakos* bad, *aisthesis* feeling], any morbid feeling or disordered sensibility. **–cacesthetic,** *adj.*

cachet /käshā′/ [Fr, tablet], any lenticular edible capsule that encloses a dose of medicine.

cachexia /kəkek′sē·ə/ [Gk *kakos + hexis* state], general ill health and malnutrition marked by weakness and emaciation, usually associated with serious disease, as tuberculosis or cancer. **–cachectic,** *adj.*

cachinnation /kak′ənā′shən/ [L *cachinnare* to laugh aloud], an excessive laughter for no apparent reason, often part of the behavioral pattern in schizophrenia. **–cachinnate,** *v.*

cacodemonomania /kak′ōdē′mənōmā′nē·ə/ [Gk *kakos + daimon* spirit, *mania* madness], an abnormal mental condition in which the patient claims to be possessed by an evil spirit.

cacophony /kəkof′ənē/, *pl.* **cacophonies** [Gk *kakos + phone* voice], a harsh or discordant sound or a mixture of confused, different sounds. **–cacophonic, cacophonous,** *adj.*

cacosmia [Gk *kakos + osme* odor], the perception of foul odors or stench when none exists. In most instances the condition results from psychologic factors, as in olfactory hallucinations.

CAD, abbreviation for **coronary artery disease.**

cadaver [L, dead body], a dead body used for dissection and study. **–cadaveric,** *adj.*

cadaver graft, the transfer of tissue from the body of a dead individual to repair a defect in a living body.

cadence, [L, *cadere,* to fall], a rhythm as in voice, music, or movement.

cadmium /kad′mē·əm/ **(Cd)** [Gk *kadmeia* zinc ore], a metallic, bluish white element that resembles tin. Its atomic number is 48; its atomic weight is 112.40. Cadmium was formerly used in medications. Such medications have been replaced by less toxic drugs.

cadmium poisoning, poisoning resulting from the inhalation of cadmium in fumes created by welding, smelting, or other industrial processes involving solder. The effects may include vomiting, dyspnea, headache, prostration, pulmonary edema, and possibly, years later, cancer.

caduceus /kədoo′sē·əs/ [L; Gk *karykeion* herald], the wand of the god Hermes or Mercury, used as the symbol for the U.S. Army Medical Corps. It is represented as a staff with two serpents coiled around it and is often confused with the staff of Æsculapius, a rod with one snake entwined about it.

caenogenesis. See **cenogenesis.**

Caesarean hysterectomy. See **cesarean hysterectomy.**

Caesarean section. See **cesarean section.**

café-au-lait spot /kaf′ä·ōlā′/ [Fr, coffee with milk], a pale tan macule the color of coffee with milk. Several café-au-lait spots developing simultaneously are associated with neurofibromatosis, but occasional café-au-lait spots occur normally.

caffeine /kafēn′, kaf′ē·in/ [Ar *gahwah* coffee], a central nervous system stimulant. It is prescribed to counteract migraine, drowsiness, and mental fatigue.

caffeine poisoning [Ar, *qahwah,* coffee, L, *potio,* drink], a state of toxic poisoning characterized by palpitations, nervousness, anxiety, and insomnia. It results from ingestion of an excessive amount of caffeine found in coffee, tea, cola beverages, or certain stimulant drugs.

caffeinism, See **caffeine poisoning.**

Caffey's disease. See **infantile cortical hyperostosis.**

Caffey's syndrome, the battered baby syndrome, first described by American pediatrician John Caffey in 1946.

CAH, **1.** abbreviation for **chronic active hepatitis. 2.** abbreviation for **congenital adrenal hyperplasia.**

CAHEA, abbreviation for *Committee on Allied Health Education and Accreditation.*

caisson disease. See **decompression sickness.**

cajeputol. See **eucalyptol.**

caked [ONorse *kaka*], formed into a compact mass or crust, as the scab of coagulated blood on a healing wound.

caked breast, an accumulation of milk in the secreting ducts of the breast after child delivery, causing all or a part of the breast to become hardened and the tissues to become engorged.

cal, **1.** abbreviation for **small calorie. 2.** abbreviation for a *calcium cation.*

Cal, abbreviation for **large calorie.**

calabar swelling /kal'əbär/ [Calabar, a Nigerian seaport], an abnormal condition characterized by fugitive, swollen lumps of subcutaneous tissue caused by a parasitic, filarial worm endemic to Africa. The swollen areas migrate with the worm through the body. At times the worm may move under the conjunctiva of the eye and may live in the anterior chamber of the eye.

calamine /kal'əmīn/ [Gk *kadmeia* zinc ore], a pink, odorless, powdered concoction used as a protectant or as an astringent and sometimes prepared as a lotion. It is composed of zinc oxide with 0.5% ferric oxide.

calcaneal /kalkā'nē·əl/ [L *calcaneum* heel], of or pertaining to the calcaneus at the back of the tarsus.

calcaneal epiphysitis, a painful disorder involving the calcaneus at its epiphysis. The condition tends to affect mainly children who are physically active and whose heel bones are still divided by a layer of cartilage.

calcaneal spurs, abnormal often painful bony outgrowths on the lower surface of the calcaneus, resulting from chronic traumatic pressure on the heel.

calcaneal tendon. See **Achilles tendon.**

calcaneal tuberosity, a transverse elevation on the plantar surface of the calcaneus to which are attached the abductor digiti

minimi, the long plantar ligament, and various other muscles.

calcaneodynia /kalkā'nē·ōdin'ē·ə/ [L *calcaneum;* Gk *odyne* pain], a painful condition of the heel.

calcaneus /kalkā'nē·əs/ [L *calcaneum* heel], the heel bone. The largest of the tarsal bones, it articulates proximally with the talus and distally with the cuboid. **–calcaneal, calcanean,** *adj.*

calcar /kal'kär/, *pl.* **calcaria,** a spur or a structure that resembles a spur.

calcar avis [L *calcar* spur; *avis* bird], a projection on the medial wall of the posterior horn of the lateral ventricle of the brain. It is associated with the lateral extension of the calcarine fissure.

calcareous /kalker'ē·əs/ [L *calcar* spur], of or pertaining to calcium or lime.

calcarine /kal'kərīn/, **1.** having the shape of a spur. **2.** of or pertaining to the calcar.

calcarine fissure, a fissure between the cuneus and the lingual gyrus on the medial surface of the occipital lobe of the brain.

calcemia. See **hypercalcemia, hypocalcemia.**

calcifediol /kal'sife'dē·ol/, a physiologic form of vitamin D prescribed in the treatment of metabolic bone disease associated with chronic renal failure.

calciferol /kalsif'ərôl/ [L *calx* lime, *ferre* to bear], a type of fat-soluble, crystalline, unsaturated alcohol produced by ultraviolet irradiation of ergosterol and used as a dietary supplement in the prophylaxis and treatment of rickets, osteomalacia, and other hypocalcemic disorders. It occurs naturally in milk and fish-liver oils.

calcific [L, *calx,* lime, *facere,* to make], pertaining to the formation of chalk, lime, or calcium.

calcific aortic disease [L *calx* lime], an abnormal condition characterized by small deposits of calcium in the aorta.

calcification [L *calx* + *facere* to make], the accumulation of calcium salts in tissues. Normally, about 99% of all the calcium entering the human body is deposited in the bones and teeth; the remaining 1% is dissolved in body fluids such as the blood.

calcific tendinitis [L, *calx,* lime, *facere,* to make, *tendo,* tendon; Gk, *itis,* inflammation], a chronic inflammation of a tendon as a result of an accumulation of calcium depositsin the tissue.

calcified fetus. See **lithopedion.**

calcination /kal'sinā'shən/ [L *calcinare* to burn lime], (in dentistry) a process of removing water by heat, used in the manufacture of plaster and stone from gypsum.

calcinosis /kal'sənō'sis/, a condition characterized by abnormal deposits of calcium salts in various tissues of the body.

calcitonin /kal'sitō'nin/ [L *calx* + Gk *tonos* tone], a hormone produced in parafollicular cells of the thyroid that participates in regulating the blood level of calcium and also stimulates bone mineralization. A synthetic preparation of the hormone is used in the treatment of certain bone disorders.

calcitriol /kalsit'rē·ôl/, a regulator of calcium metabolism. It is prescribed in the management of hypocalcemia occurring in patients undergoing chronic renal dialysis.

calcium (Ca) [L *calx* lime], an alkaline earth metal element. Its atomic number is 20; its atomic weight is 40. Its metallic form is a white, flammable solid, somewhat harder than lead. Calcium is the fifth most abundant element in the human body and occurs mainly in the bone. The body requires calcium ions for the transmission of nerve impulses, muscle contraction, blood coagulation, cardiac functions, and other processes. It is a component of extracellular fluid and of soft tissue cells. Abnormally high levels of ionized calcium in the extracellular fluid can produce muscle weakness, lethargy, and coma. A relatively small decrease from the normal level of this element can produce tetanic seizures.

calcium channel blocker, a drug that inhibits the flow of calcium ions across the membranes of smooth muscle cells. By reducing the calcium flow, smooth muscle tone is relaxed and the risk of muscle spasms is diminished. Calcium channel blockers are used primarily in the treatment of coronary artery spasms.

calcium chloride, a concentrated solution of the chloride salt of calcium used to replenish calcium in the blood. It is prescribed for hypocalcemic tetany and as an antidote for magnesium poisoning or an overdose of magnesium sulfate.

calcium gluconate ($C_{12}H_{22}CaO_{14}$), a white, odorless, tasteless powder or granules administered orally or intravenously to replenish the body's calcium stores, as after a transfusion.

calcium phosphate [$Ca_3(PO_4)_2$], an odorless, tasteless white powder used as a calcium supplement, laxative, and antacid.

calcium pump, a theoretical, energy-requiring mechanism for transmitting calcium ions across a cell membrane from a region of low calcium ion concentration to one of higher concentration.

calciuria /kal'si ŏŏr'ē·ə/ [L, *calx,* lime; Gk, *ouron,* urine], the presence of calcium in the urine.

calculation for children dosage, See **Clark's rule, Cowling's rule, pediatric dosage, Young's rule.**

calculus /kal'kyələs/, *pl.* **calculi** /kal'kyəlī/ [L, little stone], an abnormal stone formed in body tissues by an accumulation of mineral salts. Kinds of calculi include **biliary calculus** and **urinary calculus.**

calculus anuria, the cessation of urine production caused by renal calculi.

Caldwell-Moloy pelvic classification /kôl'dwelmələoi'/ [William E. Caldwell, American obstetrician, b. 1880; Howard C. Moloy, American gynecologist, b. 1903], a system for classifying the structure of the bony pelvis of the female. The types in this system are android, anthropoid, gynecoid, and platypelloid. The sacrum, sidewalls, sacrosciatic notch, ischial spines, pubic arch, and ischial tuberosities are the anatomic points of reference used to determine pelvic type.

calefacient /kal'əfā'shənt/ [L *calare* to be warm, *facere* to make], **1.** making or tending to make anything warm or hot. **2.** an agent that imparts a sense of warmth when applied, such as a hot-water bottle or a hot compress.

calendar method of family planning. See **rhythm method.**

calf, *pl.* **calves** [ONorse *kalfi*], the fleshy mass at the back of the leg below the knee, composed chiefly of the gastrocnemius muscle.

calf bone. See **fibula.**

caliber [Fr *calibre* bore of a gun], the diameter of a tube or a canal, as any of the blood vessels.

calibration [Fr, *calibre,* the bore of a gun], the process of measuring or calibrating against a standardized known, such as a deciliter or kilogram.

California encephalitis, a common, acute viral infection that affects the central nervous system. The mild form is characterized by headache, malaise, GI symptoms, and a fever that may reach 104° F. The more severe form may be marked by a sudden onset of fever, vomiting, headaches, lethargy, and signs of neurologic involvement such as loss of reflexes, disorientation, seizure, loss of consciousness, and flaccid paralysis.

californium (Cf) [State of California], an artificial element in the actinide group. Its atomic number is 98; its atomic weight is 251. Californium 252 isotope is a potent source of neutrons.

calipers [Fr *calibre* bore of a gun], an instrument with two hinged, adjustable, curved legs, used to measure the thickness or the diameter of a convex body or solid.

caliper splint, a splint for the leg consisting of two metal rods running from the back of a band around the thigh or from a cushioned ring around the lower portion of the pelvis. The rods are attached to a metal plate under the shoe below the arch of the foot.

calix /kā′liks/. See **calyx.**

Calliphoridae /kal′əfôr′ədē/ [Gk *kallos* beauty, *pherein* to bear], a family of medium-sized to large flies that belong to the order Diptera, serve as pathogenic vectors, and may cause intestinal or nasopharyngeal myiasis in humans.

callomania [Gk *kallos* beauty, *mania* madness], an abnormal psychologic condition characterized by delusions of personal beauty.

callosal fissure [L *callosus* hard; *fissura* cleft], a groove following the convex aspect of the corpus callosum.

callosity. See **callus.**

callosomarginal fissure /kəlō′sō/, a long, irregular groove on the medial surface of a cerebral hemisphere. It divides the cingulate gyrus from the medial frontal gyrus and from the paracentral lobule.

callosum [L, *callosus*, hard], pertaining to the **corpus callosum.**

callous ulcer [L, *callosus*, hard + *ulcus*, ulcer], an ulcer with a hard, indurated base and thick inelastic margins. It lacks a blood supply and is frequently associated with edema of the legs.

callus [L, hard skin], **1.** a common, usually painless thickening of the epidermis at locations of external pressure or friction. **2.** bony deposit formed between and around the broken ends of a fractured bone during healing. **–callous,** *adj.*

calmodulin, a calcium-binding protein that mediates a variety of biochemical and physiologic processes, including the contraction of muscles and the release of norepinephrine.

calor /kal′ôr/ [L, warmth], heat, as that generated by inflammation of tissues or that from the normal metabolic processes of the body.

caloric, of or pertaining to heat or calories.

caloric test, a procedure in which the ears are alternately irrigated with warm water or air and cold water or air. If the ear is normal, warm irrigation produces a rotatory nystagmus toward the irrigated side. Cold irrigation produces a rotatory nystagmus away from the irrigated side. If the ear is normal, all irrigations will produce nystagmus of approximately equal intensity. If the ear is diseased, irrigation may produce less nystagmus than the normal ear.

calorie [L *calor* warmth], **1. gram calorie, small calorie,** the amount of heat required to raise 1 g of water 1° C at atmospheric pressure. **2. large calorie,** a quantity of heat equal to 1,000 small calories. **3.** a unit, equal to the large calorie, used to denote the heat expenditure of an organism and the fuel or energy value of food. –**caloric,** *adj.*

calorific /kal′ərif′ik/, pertaining to the production of heat.

calorigenic /kəlôr′ijen′ik/ [L *calor* warmth; Gk *genein* to produce], of or pertaining to a substance or process that produces heat or energy or that increases the consumption of oxygen.

calorimeter /kal′ərim′ətər/, a device used for measuring quantities of heat generated by friction, by chemical reaction, or by the human body. –**calorimetric,** *adj.*

calorimetry /kal′ərim′ətrē/ [L *calor* warmth; Gk *metron* measure], the measurement of the amounts of heat radiated and the amounts of heat absorbed. –**calorimetric,** *adj.*

calvaria /kalver′ē·ə/, the skull cap or superior portion of the skull, which varies greatly in shape among individuals. In some persons the calvaria is relatively oval; in others it is more circular.

Calve-Perthes disease, See **Perthes' disease.**

calvities /kalvish′ī·ēz/ [L *calvus* without hair], the condition of baldness. –**calvous,** *adj.*

calyx /kā′liks/, *pl.* **calyces** /kal′isēz/, **calyxes** [Gk *kalyx* shell], **1.** a cup-shaped organ. **2.** a renal calyx. **3.** the wall of an ovarian follicle after expulsion of the ovum at ovulation. Also spelled **calix.**

cambium layer [L *cambire* to exchange], **1.** the loose, inner cellular layer of the periosteum that develops during ossification. **2.** a cellular layer of formative tissue that lies between the wood and the bark in plants.

camera [L, vaulted chamber], (in anatomy) any cavity or chamber, as those of the eye or the heart.

camisole restraint. See **straitjacket.**

cAMP, abbreviation for **cyclic adenosine monophosphate.**

camphor /kam′fər/ [L *camphora*], a colorless or white crystalline substance with a penetrating odor and pungent taste, occuring naturally in certain plants, especially *Cinnamomum camphora.*

camphorated oil [Malay, *kapur,* chalk; L, *oleum,* oil], a colorless to yellowish liquid with the penetrating, pungent odor of camphor. It is derived from a combination of a dozen organic chemicals, including terpenes, safrole, and acetaldhehyde obtained from the camphor laurel plant. It is used mainly as a liniment, counter-irritant, and rubefacient.

camphor bath, an air bath in which the air is filled with camphor vapor.

camphor poisoning, a severe toxic condition resulting from the accidental ingestion of camphorated oils. Symptoms may include headache, hallucinations, nausea, vomiting, diarrhea, convulsions, and kidney failure.

camphor salicylate, a crystalline substance formed by the fusion of 84 parts of camphor and 65 parts of salicylic acid, previously used in skin ointments and administered internally for diarrhea.

camptodactyly /kamp'tədak'təlē/ [Gk kamptos bent, daktylos finger], the permanent flexion of one or more fingers. **–campodactylic,** adj.

camptomelia /kamp'təmē'lyə/ [Gk kamptos bent, melos arm], a congenital anomaly characterized by bending of one or more limbs, causing permanent bowing or curving of the affected area. **–camptomelic,** adj.

Campylobacter [Gk campylos curved, bacterion rod], a genus of bacteria found in the family Spirillaceae. The type species is *C. fetus,* which consists of several subspecies that cause human infections, as well as abortion and infertility in cattle.

camsylate, a contraction for camphorsulfonate.

Camurati-Engelmann disease, an inherited disorder of bone development marked by an onset of symptoms of muscular pain, weakness, and wasting, mainly in the legs, during childhood. The symptoms vary individually from mild to disabling. In some cases there may be compression of nerve tissue. The symptoms usually subside during early adulthood.

Canadian Association of University Schools of Nursing (CAUSN), a national Canadian organization of nursing schools affiliated with institutions of higher learning.

Canadian Association of University Teachers (CAUT), a national Canadian organization representing the interests of all who teach in the universities of the provinces and territories of Canada.

Canadian crutch, a wooden or a metal device that helps a disabled patient stand or walk. It consists of two uprights with a crosspiece to accommodate the hand and a concave crosspiece that fits the armpit for support.

Canadian Journal of Public Health (CJPH), the official publication of the Canadian Public Health Association.

Canadian Medical Association Journal (CMAJ), the official publication of the Canadian Medical Association.

Canadian Nurses' Association (CNA), the official national organization for the professional registered nurses of Canada who are members of the 10 provincial nurses' associations and the Northwest Territory's association.

Canadian Nurses' Association Testing Service (CNATS), the organizational affiliate of the Canadian Nurses' Association that is concerned with testing the graduates of approved schools of nursing to qualify them as registered nurses.

Canadian Nurses' Foundation (CNF), a national Canadian foundation organized to support scholarship in nursing.

Canadian Nurses' Respiratory Society (CNRS), an organization of nurses working with or interested in alleviating the problems of respiratory disease.

Canadian Orthopedic Nurses' Association (CONA), a national Canadian organization concerned with the nursing care of orthopedic patients and the continuing education of nurses working in orthopedics.

Canadian Public Health Association (CPHA), a national Canadian organization concerned with issues in public health and epidemiology.

canal [L canalis channel], **1.** (in anatomy) a narrow tube or channel. Some kinds of canals are **adductor canal, Alcock's canal,** and **alveolar canal. 2.** (in dentistry) one of the accessory root canals and collateral pulp canals in the teeth.

canaliculus /kan'əlik'yələs/, *pl.* **canaliculi** [L, little channel], a very small tube or channel, like the tiny haversian canaliculi throughout bone tissue.

canalization /kan'əlīzā'shən/, the formation of canals or of passages through any tissue.

canal of Schlemm /shlem/ [Friedrich Schlemm, German anatomist, b. 1795], a tiny vein at the angle of the anterior chamber of the eye that connects with the pectinate villi, draining the aqueous humor and funneling it into the bloodstream.

canavanine /kan'əvan'in/, an amino acid antagonist present in alfalfa sprouts in concentrations of about 15,000 ppm, or 1.5% by weight. Canavanine can displace arginine in cellular proteins.

cancellous /kan'siləs/ [L cancellus lattice], (of tissue) latticelike, porous, spongy. Cancellous tissue is normally present in the interior of many bones, where the spaces are usually filled with marrow.

cancer [L, crab], **1.** a neoplasm characterized by the uncontrolled growth of anaplastic cells that tend to invade surrounding tissue and to metastasize to distant body sites. **2.** any of a large group of malignant neoplastic diseases characterized by the presence of malignant cells. Each cancer is distinguished by the nature, site, or clinical course of the lesion. The basic origin of cancer is undetermined, but many potential causes are recognized. More than 80% of cases of cancer are attributed to cigarette smoking, exposure to carcinogenic chemicals, ionizing radiation, and ultraviolet rays. Many viruses induce malignant tumors in animals, and viral particles are detected in some human tumors. The high incidence of various kinds of cancer in certain families suggests that genetic susceptibility is an important factor. An excess rate of malignant tumors in organ transplant recipients after immunosuppressive therapy indicates that the immune system plays a major role in controlling the proliferation of anaplastic cells. The age-adjusted death rate for oral cancer is almost 10 times higher in Hong Kong than in Denmark, and that for prostate cancer is more than 10 times greater in Sweden than in Japan, but leukemia mortality is similar throughout the world. In the United States, cancer is second only to heart disease as a cause of mortality. Surgery remains the major form of treatment, but irradiation is widely used as preoperative, postoperative, or primary therapy; chemotherapy, with single or multiple antineoplastic agents, is often highly effective.

cancer bodies. See **Russell's bodies.**

cancericidal /kan'sərisī'dəl/ [L, crab, *caedere* to kill], of or pertaining to a substance or procedure capable of destroying cancer cells.

cancer in situ. See **carcinoma in situ.**

cancer of the small intestine, a neoplastic disease of the duodenum, jejunum, or ileum. Its characteristics vary, depending on the kind of tumor and the site, but may include abdominal pain, vomiting, weight loss, diarrhea, intermittent bowel obstruction, GI bleeding, or a mass deep in the right abdomen. Adenocarcinomas, the most common tumors, occur more frequently in the duodenum or upper jejunum and form polypoid or constricting napkin-ring growths. Lymphomas, found most often in the lower small intestine, are associated with a malabsorption syndrome. Surgery, including a wide resection of mesenteric lymph nodes, is indicated for adenocarcinomas. Irradiation is not effective in ablation of these tumors but is recommended postoperatively for lymphomas to treat metastatic lesions.

cancerous [Gk, *karkinos,* crab, *oma,* tu-

mor], pertaining to or resembling a cancer.

cancer staging, a system for describing the size and extent of spread of a malignant tumor used to plan treatment and predict prognosis. Staging may involve a physical examination, diagnostic procedures, surgical exploration, and histologic examination. The system developed by the American Joint Committee for Cancer Staging and End Results Reporting uses the letter T to represent the tumor, N for the regional lymph node involvement, M for distant metastases, and numeric subscripts in each category to indicate the degree of dissemination. According to this system $T_1N_0M_0$ designates a small, localized tumor; $T_2N_1M_0$ is a larger primary tumor that has extended to regional nodes; and $T_4N_3M_3$ is a very large lesion involving regional nodes and distant sites. Other systems may be used for staging breast carcinoma, colorectal cancer, and cutaneous melanoma.

cancriform /kang'krifôrm'/ [L, crab, *forma* form], of or pertaining to a lesion resembling a cancer.

cancroid [L, crab; Gk *eidos* form], **1.** of or pertaining to a lesion resembling a cancer. **2.** a moderately malignant skin cancer.

candela. See **candle.**

Candida /kan'didə/ [L *candidus* white], a genus of yeastlike fungi including the common pathogen, *Candida albicans.*

Candida albicans /al'bəkanz/, a common, budding, yeastlike, microscopic fungal organism normally present in the mucous membranes of the mouth, intestinal tract, and vagina and on the skin of healthy people. Under certain circumstances, it may cause superficial infections of the mouth or vagina and, less commonly, serious invasive systemic infection and toxic reaction.

Candida vaginitis. See **candidiasis.**

candidiasis /kan'didī'əsis/ [L *candidus* + Gk *osis* condition], any infection caused by a species of *Candida,* usually *Candida albicans,* characterized by pruritus, a white exudate, peeling, and easy bleeding. Diaper rash, intertrigo, vaginitis, and thrush are common topical manifestations of candidiasis.

Candiru fever /kan'dirōō'/, an arbovirus infection transmitted to humans by the bite of a sandfly, characterized by an acute fever, headache, and muscle aches.

candle [L *candela* light], (in optics) the basic unit of measurement for luminous intensity, equal to ⅟₆₀ of the luminous intensity of a square centimeter of a black body heated to 1773.5° C or the solidification temperature of platinum, adopted in 1948 as the international standard of luminous intensity.

candy-striper, *informal;* a hospital volunteer, named for the striped pink and white uniforms traditionally worn by the young people who perform this service.

cane [Ar *qanah* reed], a sturdy wooden or metal shaft, or walking stick, used to give support and mobility to an ambulatory but partially disabled person.

cane-cutter's cramp. See **heat cramp.**

canefield fever. See **field fever.**

canine fossa /kā′nīn/ [L *canis* dog; L, ditch], (in dentistry) either of the wide depressions on the external surface of each maxilla, superolateral to the canine tooth socket.

canine tooth, any one of the four teeth, two in each jaw, situated immediately lateral to the incisor teeth in the human dental arches. The canine teeth are larger and stronger than the incisors, and they project beyond the level of the other teeth in both arches. Their roots sink deeply into the bones, causing marked prominences on the alveolar arch. The canines erupt as deciduous teeth about 16 to 20 months after birth. The eruption of the permanent canines occurs during the eleventh or the twelfth year of life.

canker /kang′kər/ [L *cancer* crab], an ulcer or sore, especially in the mouth.

canker sore, an ulcerous lesion of the mouth, characteristic of aphthous stomatitis.

cannabis /kan′əbis/ [Gk *kannabis* hemp], a psychoactive drug derived from the flowering tops of hemp plants. It has no currently acceptable clinical use in the United States but has been used in the treatment of glaucoma and as an antiemetic in some cancer patients to counter the nausea and vomiting associated with chemotherapy. Cannabis is controlled under Schedule I of the Comprehensive Drug Abuse Prevention and Control Act of 1970. The common hemp from which cannabis is obtained is an herbaceous annual of which *Cannabis sativa* is the sole species. All parts of the plant contain psychoactive substances or cannabinoids, the highest concentrations of which are in the resin of the flowering tops of the plant.

cannabism /kan′əbiz′əm/, a condition associated with excessive or extended use of cannabis drugs. It is characterized by anxiety, disorientation, hallucinations, memory defects, and paranoia.

cannon wave [L *cane* tube; AS *wafian*], a powerful "a" wave in the jugular pulse, characteristic of a complete heart block and of premature ventricular beats of the heart. Cannon waves are caused by the contraction of the right atrium of the heart immediately after contraction of the right ventricle has closed the tricuspid valve.

cannula /kan′yələ/, *pl.* **cannulas, cannulae** [L, small tube], a flexible tube containing a stiff, pointed trocar that may be inserted into the body, guided by the trocar. As the trocar is removed, a body fluid may be passed through the cannula to the outside. **–cannular, cannulate,** *adj.*

cannulation /kan′yəlā′shən/, the insertion of a cannula into a body duct or cavity, as into the trachea, bladder, or a blood vessel. **–cannulate, cannulize,** *v.*

cantering rhythm [*Canterbury gallop;* Gk, *rhythmos,* beat], a pattern of three heart sounds in each cardiac cycle, resembling the canter of a horse.

cantharis /kan′thäris/, *pl.* **cantharides** /kanther′idēz/ [Gk *kantharis* beetle], the dried insects *Cantharis vesicatoria* containing cantharidin, formerly used as a topical vesicant.

canthus /kan′thəs/, *pl.* **canthi** [Gk *kanthus* corner of the eye], the angle at the medial and the lateral margins of the eyelids. **–canthic,** *adj.*

CAOT, abbreviation for *Canadian Association of Occupational Therapists.*

cap, abbreviation for Latin *capiat,* "let him or her take," used in prescriptions.

CAP, 1. abbreviation for **College of American Pathologists. 2.** (in molecular genetics) abbreviation for **catabolic activator protein.** CAP participates in initiating the transcription of RNA in organisms without a true nucleus, as bacteria.

capacitance vessels /kəpas′ətəns/ [L *capacitas* capacity], **1.** the blood vessels that hold the major portion of the intravascular blood volume. **2.** the veins that are downstream from the arterioles, capillaries, and venules.

capacitation /kəpas′itā′shən/, the process in which the spermatozoon, after it reaches the ampulla of the fallopian tube, undergoes a series of changes that lead to its ability to fertilize an ovum.

capacity factor [L *capacitas; factum* to make], the ratio of the elution volume of a substance to the void volume in the column.

CAPD, abbreviation for **continuous ambulatory peritoneal dialysis.**

capeline bandage /kap′əlin/ [Fr, hooded cape], a caplike covering used for protecting the head, shoulder, or a stump.

capillaritis /kap′ilərī′tis/ [L *capillaris* hairlike; Gk *itis* inflammation], an abnormal condition characterized by a progressive pigmentary disorder of the skin without inflammation but with dilatation.

capillarity. See **capillary action.**

capillary /kap'iler'ē/ [L *capillaris* hairlike], one of the tiny blood vessels (about 0.008 mm in diameter) joining arterioles and venules. Through their walls, which consist of a single layer of endothelial cells, blood and tissue cells exchange various substances.

capillary action, the action involving molecular adhesion by which the surface of a liquid in a tube is either elevated or depressed, depending on the cohesiveness of the liquid molecules.

capillary angioma. See **cherry angioma.**

capillary attraction, See **capillary action.**

capillary bed, a capillary network.

capillary flames. See **telangiectatic nevus.**

capillary fracture, any thin hairlike fracture.

capillary hemangioma, a blood-filled birthmark or a benign tumor consisting of closely packed, small blood vessels. Commonly found in infants, it first grows, then spontaneously disappears in early childhood without treatment.

capillary permeability [L, *capillaris,* hairlike, *permeare,* to pass through], a condition of the capillary wall structure that allows blood elements and waste products to pass through them.

capillary pressure [L, *capillaris,* hairlike, *premere,* to press], the blood pressure within a capillary.

capillary pulse. See **Quincke's pulse.**

capillary refilling, the process of blood returning to a portion of the capillary system after being interrupted briefly. A capillary refill of more than 3 seconds is considered a sign of sluggish digital circulation, and a time of 5 seconds is regarded as abnormal.

capillary tufting, an abnormal condition in which pulmonary capillaries project as tufts, or small masses, into the alveoli.

capillus /kəpil'əs/, *pl.* **capilli** [L, filament], one of the hairs of the body, especially one of the hairs of the scalp.

capitate, having the shape of a head.

capitate bone [L *caput* head; AS *ban*], one of the largest carpal bones, located at the center of the wrist and having a rounded head that fits the concavity of the scaphoid and the lunate bones.

capitation fee [L, *caput,* head; ME, *fief,* payment], a method of paying a physician for annual services based on a fee per patient.

capitulum /kəpich'ələm/, *pl.* **capitula** [L, small head], a small, rounded prominence on a bone where it articulates with another bone.

capitulum humeri /hy oo'mərī, h oo'-mərē/[L, small head; *humerus* shoulder], a rounded eminence at the distal end of the humerus. It articulates with the radius.

capnograph /kap'nəgraf'/ [Gk *kapnos* smoke, *graphein* to record], an instrument used in anesthesia, respiratory physiology, and respiratory therapy to produce a tracing, or capnogram, which shows the proportion of carbon dioxide in expired air.

capnometry /kapnom'ətrē/, the measurement of carbon dioxide in a volume of gas, usually by methods of infrared absorption or mass spectrometry.

capotement /käpōtmäN'/, a splashing sound made by fluid movements in a dilated stomach.

capreomycin /kap'rē·ōmī'sin/, an antibiotic prescribed in the treatment of pulmonary infections caused by capreomycin-susceptible strains of *Mycobacterium tuberculosis* when the primary agents are ineffective or cannot be used.

capric acid /kap'rik/[L *caper* goatlike], a white, crystalline substance with a rancid odor, occurring as a glyceride in natural oils.

caproic acid /kaprō'ik/, a fatty acid that occurs in milk fat and some plant oils. It is used in the production of artificial flavors.

capsid /kap'sid/ [L *capsa* box], the layer of protein enveloping a virion.

capsomere /kap'səmir/, one of the building blocks of a viral capsid. It consists of groups of identical protein molecules and is visible in an electron microscope.

capsula. See **capsule.**

capsular /kap'sələr/ [L, *capsula,* little box], pertaining to or resembling a small container.

capsular cataract [L *capsula;* Gk *katarrhaktes* waterfall], a visual opacity caused by a thickening of the epithelial cells lining the capsule. The condition is frequently the result of the aging process or a disease involving surrounding eye tissues.

capsular pattern, a series of limitations of joint movement when the joint capsule is a limiting structure. It occurs only in synovial joints that are controlled by muscles.

capsular swelling test. See **quellung reaction.**

capsule [L *capsula* little box], **1.** a small, soluble container, usually made of gelatin, used for enclosing a dose of medication for swallowing. **2.** a membranous shell surrounding certain microorganisms, such as the pneumococcus bacterium. **3.** a well-defined anatomic structure that encloses an organ or part, such as the capsule of the adrenal gland.

capsulectomy /kap'səlek'təmē/, the surgical excision of a capsule, usually the capsule of a joint or the capsule of the lens of the eye.

capsule of Tenon. See **fascia bulbi.**

capsule of the kidney, the fatty enclosure of the kidney, consisting of adipose tissue continuous at the hilus with the fat of the renal sinus.

capsule of the lens. See **lens capsule.**

capsulitis [L *capsula* + Gk *itis* inflamation], an inflammation involving any anatomic capsule.

capsuloma /kap'səlō'mə/, *pl.* **capsulomas, capsulomata** [L *capsula* + Gk *oma* tumor], a neoplasm of the renal capsule or the subcapsular area.

capsulotomy /kap'səlot'əmē/ [L *capsula* + Gk *temnein* to cut], an incision into the capsule of the eye, such as in an operation to remove a cataract.

captain-of-the-ship doctrine, the medicolegal principle that the physician is ultimately responsible for all patient-care activities and thus may be held accountable and may be sued for negligence or malpractice when the act at issue is performed by an employee or other person under the physician's control, even if not ordered by the physician.

captopril /kap'tōpril/, an angiotensin-converting enzyme inhibitor prescribed for the treatment of severe hypertension.

caput /kā'pət, kap'ət/, *pl.* **capita** /cap'itə/ [L, head], **1.** the head. **2.** the enlarged or prominent extremity of an organ or part.

caput costae [L, head; *costa* rib], the head of a rib; it articulates with a vertebral body.

caput epididymidis, the head of the epididymus.

caput femoris, the head of the femur; it fits into the acetabulum.

caput fibulae, the head of the fibula; it articulates with the lateral condyle of the tibia.

caput humeri, the head of the humerus; it fits into the glenoid cavity of the scapula.

caput mallei, the head of the malleus.

caput mandibulae, the articular process of the ramus of the mandible.

caput ossis metacarpalis, the metacarpal head; it articulates with the proximal phalanx of the same digit.

caput phalangis, the articular head at the distal end of the proximal and middle phalanges.

caput radii, the head of the radius; it articulates with the capitulum of the humerus.

caput stapedis, the head of the stapes.

caput succedaneum [L, head; *succeder* to replace], a localized pitting edema in the scalp of a fetus that may overlie sutures of the skull. It is usually formed during labor as a result of the circular pressure of the cervix on the fetal occiput.

caramiphen edisylate /kəram'ifen' ēdis'i-lāt/, an antitussive prescribed in the treatment of coughs.

carapace /kar'əpās/ [Sp *carapacho* hard shell], a horny shield or shell covering the dorsal surface of an animal, such as a turtle.

carate. See **pinta.**

carb, abbreviation for a carbonate noncarboxylate anion.

carbam, abbreviation for a carbamate carboxylate anion.

carbamate /kär'bəmāt/, any of a group of anticholinesterase enzymes that cause reversible inhibition of cholinesterase. They are used in certain medications and insecticides. Some carbamates are toxic and may cause convulsions and death through ingestion or skin contact.

carbamate kinase, a liver enzyme that catalyzes the transfer of a phosphate group from adenosine triphosphate, associated with ammonia and carbon dioxide, to form adenosine diphosphate and carbamoylphosphate.

carbamazepine /kär'bəmaz'əpin/, an analgesic and anticonvulsant prescribed in the treatment of trigeminal neuralgia and certain seizure disorders.

carbamide peroxide /kärbam'īd/, a topical antiinfective and ceruminolytic prescribed in the treatment of canker sores and other minor inflammatory conditions of the gums and mouth and to soften impacted earwax.

carbamino compound, a chemical complex formed by the binding of carbon dioxide molecules to plasma proteins.

carbamino-hemoglobin, a chemical complex formed by carbon dioxide and hemoglobin after the release of oxygen by the hemoglobin to a tissue cell. The action is similar to that of the formation of a carbamino compound. It accounts for nearly 25% of the carbon dioxide released in the lung.

carbenicillin disodium /kär'bənəsil'in/, a semisynthetic penicillin antibiotic prescribed in the treatment of certain infections.

carbidopa /kär'bidō'pə/, a decarboxylase inhibitor prescribed in combination with levodopa in the treatment of idiopathic Parkinson's disease.

carbinoxamine maleate /kär'bənok'sə-mēn/, an antihistamine prescribed in the treatment of a variety of hypersensitivity reactions, including rhinitis, skin reactions, and itching.

carbocyclic. See **closed-chain.**

carbohydrate [L *carbo* coal; Gk *hydor* water], any of a group of organic compounds, the most important being sugar, starch, cellulose, and gum. They are classified according to molecular structure as mono-, di-, tri-, poly-, and heterosaccharides. Carbohydrates constitute the main source of energy for all body functions and are necessary for the metabolism of other nutrients. They are synthesized by all green plants and in the body are either absorbed immediately or stored in the form of glycogen. They can also be manufactured in the body from some amino acids and the glycerol component of fats.

carbohydrate loading, a dietary practice of some endurance athletes, such as marathon runners, intended to increase glycogen stores in the muscle tissue. A period of carbohydrate abstinence designed to deplete stored glycogen is followed by a diet high in complex carbohydrates. The practice is controversial and not universally practiced.

carbohydrate metabolism, the sum of the anabolic and catabolic processes of the body involved in the synthesis and breakdown of carbohydrates, principally galactose, fructose, and glucose. Energy-rich phosphate bonds are produced in many metabolic reactions requiring carbohydrates.

carbolated camphor [L *carbo* coal; *camphora*], a mixture of 1.5 parts camphor with 1 part each of alcohol and phenol, used as an antiseptic dressing for wounds.

carbol-fuchsin solution /kär′bolfŏŏk′sin/ [L *carbo* coal; Leonard Fuchs, German botanist, b. 1501], a preparation used in the treatment of superficial fungal infections. It contains boric acid, phenol, resorcinol, fuchsin, acetone, and alcohol in water.

carbol-fuchsin stain, a solution of dilute phenol and basic fuchsin used on microorganisms and cell nuclei for microscopic examination.

carbolic acid /kärbol′ik/ [L *carbo* coal; *acidus* sour], a poisonous, colorless to pale pink crystalline compound obtained from coal tar distillation and converted to a clear liquid with a strong odor and burning taste by the addition of water.

carbolic acid poisoning. See **phenol poisoning.**

carbon (C) /kär′bən/ [L *carbo* coal], a nonmetallic, chiefly tetravalent element. Its atomic number is 6; its atomic weight is 12.011. Carbon occurs in pure form in diamond and graphite and is a component of all living tissue. Most of the study of organic chemistry focuses on the vast number of carbon compounds. Carbon is essential to the chemistry of the body, participating in many metabolic processes and acting as a component of carbohydrates, amino acids, triglycerides, deoxyribonucleic and ribonucleic acids, and many other compounds. Carbon dioxide produced in glycolysis is important in the acid-base balance of the body and in controlling respiration.

carbon 11, a radioisotope of carbon with a half-life of 20 minutes. It is produced by a cyclotron and emits positrons.

carbon 14, a beta-emitter with a half-life of 5,760 years. It occurs naturally, arising from cosmic rays, and is used as a tracer in studying various aspects of metabolism and in dating relics that contain natural carbonaceous materials.

carbon arc lamp, an electric lamp producing a strong white light of adjustable intensity from an arc of current between carbon electrodes.

carbonate /kär′bənāt/, a CO_3^{2-} anion. Carbonates are in equilibrium with bicarbonates in water and frequently occur in compounds as insoluble salts, such as calcium carbonate.

carbon cycle, the steps by which carbon in the form of carbon dioxide is extracted from and returned to the atmosphere by living organisms. The process starts with the photosynthetic production of carbohydrates by plants, progresses through the consumption of carbohydrates by animals and human beings, and ends with the exhalation of carbon dioxide and also with the release of carbon dioxide during the decomposition of plants and animals.

carbon damp. See **damp.**

carbon dioxide (CO_2) [L *carbo*; Gk *dis* twice, *oxys* sharp], a colorless, odorless gas produced by the oxidation of carbon. Carbon dioxide, as a product of cell respiration, is carried by the blood to the lungs and is exhaled. The acid-base balance of body fluids and tissues is affected by the level of carbon dioxide and its carbonate compounds. Solid carbon dioxide (dry ice) is used in the treatment of some skin conditions.

carbon dioxide acidosis, a condition in which carbon dioxide retained in the lungs increases the acidity of body fluids.

carbon dioxide bath, a bath taken in water that is saturated with carbon dioxide.

carbon dioxide narcosis, a condition of severe hypercapnia, with symptoms of confusion, tremors, convulsions, and coma, which may occur if blood levels of carbon dioxide are increased to 70 mg Hg or higher.

carbon dioxide poisoning, toxic effects of inhaling excessive amounts of carbon dioxide. Carbon dioxide is a respiratory stimulant, but it is also an asphyxiant. Concentrations of 10% or greater can cause unconsciousness and death from ventilatory failure. Particularly vulnerable are persons who work in confined spaces with poor air circulation, such as mine shafts, silos, or holds of ships.

carbon dioxide pressure. See **carbon dioxide tension.**

carbon dioxide retention, any increased partial pressure and body stores of carbon dioxide resulting from impaired carbon dioxide elimination. Respiratory acidosis may result from carbon dioxide retention.

carbon dioxide response, the ventilatory reaction to increased concentrations of carbon dioxide gas. Responses normally increase in a linear curve up to a concentration of 8% to 10%. It flattens slightly near the peak and falls off at concentrations of about 20%. At concentrations around 25%, the person is conscious but is unable to perform simple tasks.

carbon dioxide stores, the volume of carbon dioxide contained in the body as a gas and also in the form of carbonic acid, carbonate, bicarbonate, and carbaminohemoglobin. During a steady state of respiration and circulation, the quantity of carbon dioxide stores remains constant.

carbon dioxide tension, the partial pressure of carbon dioxide gas, expressed as P_{CO_2}, which is proportional to its percentage in the blood or lungs. A high rate of ventilation causes a lower alveolar P_{CO_2}; a lower rate of breathing leads to higher amounts of alveolar and blood carbon dioxide.

carbon dioxide therapy, the therapeutic inhalation of a low concentration of carbon dioxide gas. Such therapy may be used to dilate the blood vessels, stimulate the cardiovascular brain centers, and overcome hyperventilation.

carbon dioxide titration curve, a line plotted on a graph showing the blood pH and total carbon dioxide concentration changes that result from the addition or removal of carbon dioxide.

carbon fiber, a material consisting of graphite fibers in a plastic matrix used in radiologic devices to reduce patient exposure to x-rays.

carbonic acid (H_2CO_3) [L, *carbo,* coal, *acidus,* acid], an unstable acid formed by dissolving carbon dioxide in water. It is the basis of carbonated beverages and is related to the carbonate group of compounds.

carbonic anhydrase, an enzyme that assists in the hydration of carbon dioxide to carbonic acid in the red blood cell so that it can be transported from the tissue cell to the lungs.

carbonic anhydrase inhibitor, a substance that decreases the rate of carbonic acid and H^+ production in the kidney, thereby increasing the excretion of solutes and the rate of urinary output.

carbon monoxide [L *carbo;* Gk *monos* single, *oxys* sharp], a colorless, odorless, poisonous gas produced by the combustion of carbon or organic fuels in a limited oxygen supply. Carbon monoxide combines irreversibly with hemoglobin, preventing the formation of oxyhemoglobin and reducing the oxygen supply to the tissues.

carbon monoxide poisoning, a toxic condition in which carbon monoxide gas has been inhaled and absorbed by erythrocytes in the circulation, displacing oxygen from the red blood cells and decreasing the capacity of the blood to carry oxygen to the cells of the body. Headache, dyspnea, drowsiness, confusion, cherry-pink skin, unconsciousness, and apnea occur in sequence as the level of carbon monoxide in the blood increases. Treatment includes removal of the victim from the toxic environment, resuscitation, and administration of oxygen.

carbon tetrachloride [L *carbo;* Gk *tetra* four, *chloros* greenish], a colorless, volatile, toxic liquid used as a solvent and in fire extinguishers. Ingestion of the liquid or inhalation of the fumes usually results in headaches, nausea, depression, abdominal pain, and convulsions. In poisoning by inhalation, ventilatory assistance and oxygen may be necessary.

carbon tetrachloride poisoning [L *carbo;* Gk *tetra* + *chloros;* L *potio* drink], toxic effects of exposure to carbon tetrachloride, a colorless commercial dry cleaning fluid also used in fire extinguishers and industrial solvents. It may attack both liver and kidneys. Symptoms include persistent headache, nausea, vomiting, diarrhea, uremia, lethargy, confusion from CNS depression, and degeneration of the liver and kidneys.

carboxyfluoroquinolone /kärbok′sē-floo′ōrōkwī′nəlōn/, any of a group of oral quinolone antibiotics that is generally effective against Enterobacteriaceae and shows varying activity against *Pseudomonas* and other species. The drugs differ in their oral absorption.

carboxyhemoglobin /kärbok′sēhē′məglo'bin, -hem'-/[L *carbo* + Gk *oxys* sharp, *haima* blood; L *globus* ball], a compound produced by the exposure of hemoglobin to carbon monoxide.

carboxyl /kärbok'sil/, a monovalent radical COOH characteristic of organic acids. The hydrogen of the radical can be replaced by metals to form salts.

carboxylation, a chemical process in which a carboxyl group (-COOH) replaces a hydrogen atom.

carbuncle /kär'bungkəl/ [L *carbunculus* little coal], a large staphylococcal infection containing purulent matter in deep, interconnecting, subcutaneous pockets. Eventually pus discharges to the skin surface through openings. Common sites for carbuncles are the back of the neck and the buttocks.

carbunculosis /kärbung'kyəlō'sis/, an abnormal condition characterized by a cluster of deep painful abscesses that drain through multiple openings onto the skin surface, usually around hair follicles. Carbunculosis is a form of folliculitis, most commonly caused by the coagulase-positive *Staphylococcus aureus*. The lesions caused by this condition may result in fever and malaise.

carcinoembryonic antigen (CEA) /kär'sənō-em'brē-on'ik/ [Gk *karkinos* crab, *en* into, *bryein* to grow; *anti* against, *genein* to produce], an antigen present in very small quantities in adult tissue. A greater than normal amount is suggestive of cancer.

carcinogen /kärsin'əjin/ [Gk *karkinos* + *genein* to produce], a substance or agent that causes the development or increases the incidence of cancer.

carcinogenesis /kär'sinəjen'əsis/, the process of initiating and promoting cancer.

carcinogenic /kär'sinəjen'ik/, of or pertaining to the ability to cause the development of a cancer.

carcinoid /kär'sinoid/ [Gk *karkinos* + *eidos* form], a small yellow tumor derived from argentaffin cells in the GI mucosa that secrete serotonin, other catecholamines, and similar compounds.

carcinoid syndrome, the systemic effects of serotonin-secreting carcinoid tumors manifested by flushing, diarrhea, cramps, skin lesions resembling pellagra, labored breathing, palpitations, and valvular heart disease, especially of the pulmonary valve. Treatment includes surgical excision of the tumor.

carcinolysis /kär'sinol'isis/ [Gk *karkinos* + *lysis* loosening], the destruction of cancer cells, as by the action of an antineoplastic drug. **–carcinolytic,** *adj.*

carcinoma /kär'sinō'mə/, *pl.* **carcinomas,**

carcinomata [Gk *karkinos* + *oma* tumor], a malignant epithelial neoplasm that tends to invade surrounding tissue and to metastasize to distant regions of the body. It develops most frequently in the skin, large intestine, lungs, stomach, prostate gland, cervix, or breast. The tumor is characteristically firm, irregular, and nodular, with a well-defined border in some places. It usually cannot be clearly dissected and excised without removing normal surrounding tissue. Macroscopically, it is whitish with diffuse, dark hemorrhagic patches, and it has yellow areas of necrosis in the center. **–carcinomatous,** *adj.*

carcinoma basocellulare. See **basal cell carcinoma.**

carcinoma cutaneum. See **basal cell carcinoma, squamous carcinoma.**

carcinoma en cuirasse /äN'kēräs'/ [Gk *karkinos, oma;* Fr, breastplate], a rare neoplasm accompanying advanced breast cancer and characterized by progressive extensive fibrosis and rigidity of the skin of the chest, neck, back, and, occasionally, abdomen.

carcinoma fibrosum. See **scirrhous carcinoma.**

carcinoma gigantocellulare. See **giant cell carcinoma.**

carcinoma in situ [Gk *karkinos, oma;* L, in position], a premalignant neoplasm that has not invaded the basement membrane but shows cytologic characteristics of invasive cancer. Such neoplastic changes in stratified squamous or glandular epithelium are frequently seen on the uterine cervix and also occur in the anus, bronchi, buccal mucosa, esophagus, eye, lip, penis, uterine endometrium, vagina, and lesions of senile keratosis.

carcinoma lenticulare /len'tic oōlär'ə/ [Gk karkinos, oma; L, lens], a form of carcinoma tuberosum or scirrhous skin cancer characterized by the development of many small, relatively flat nodules that often coalesce to form larger areas resembling a fungus infection.

carcinoma medullare, carcinoma molle. See **medullary carcinoma.**

carcinoma mucocellulare. See **Krukenberg's tumor.**

carcinoma scroti /skrō'tī/, an epithelial cell carcinoma of the scrotum.

carcinoma spongiosum /spon'jē-ō'səm/, a carcinoma that is soft and spongy with small and large cavities in it.

carcinoma telangiectaticum /telan'jē--ektat'ikəm/ [Gk *karkinos, oma; telos* end, *aggeion* vessel, *ektasis* dilatation], a neoplasm of the capillaries of the skin causing dilatation of the vessels and red spots on the skin that blanch with pressure.

carcinomatoid /kär′sinō′mətoid/, resembling a carcinoma.

carcinomatosis, an abnormal condition characterized by the extensive spread of carcinoma throughout the body.

carcinomatous, pertaining to carcinoma.

carcinoma tuberosum. See **tuberous carcinoma.**

carcinoma villosum. See **villous carcinoma.**

carcinophilia /kär′sinōfil′yə/ [Gk *karkinos* + *philein* to love], the property in which there is an affinity for carcinomatous tissue. **–carcinophilic,** *adj.*

carcinosarcoma /kär′sinōsärkō′mə/, *pl.* **carcinosarcomas, carsinosarcomata** [Gk *karkinos* + *sarx* flesh, *oma* tumor], a malignant neoplasm composed of carcinomatous and sarcomatous cells. Tumors of this type may occur in the esophagus, thyroid gland, and uterus.

carcinosis /kär′sinō′sis/, *pl.* **carcinoses,** a condition characterized by the development of many carcinomas throughout the body. Kinds of carcinoses are **carcinosis pleurae, miliary carcinosis, pulmonary carcinosis.**

carcinosis pleurae /plo͞o′rē/, a secondary malignancy of the pleura in which nodules develop throughout the membranes.

carcinostatic /kär′sinōstat′ik/ [Gk *karkinos* + *statikos* causing to stand], of or pertaining to the tendency to slow or halt the growth of a carcinoma.

carcinous /kär′sinəs/, carcinomatous.

cardia /kär′dē·ə/ [Gk *kardia* heart], **1.** the opening between the esophagus and the cardiac portion of the stomach. **2.** the portion of the stomach surrounding the esophagogastric connection, characterized by the absence of acid cells. **3.** an obsolete term formerly and vaguely used to describe the heart and the region around the heart. **–cardiac,** *adj.*

cardiac [Gk *kardia* heart], **1.** of or pertaining to the heart. **2.** pertaining to a person with heart disease. **3.** of or pertaining to the proximal part of the stomach.

cardiac aneurysm. See **ventricular aneurysm.**

cardiac angiography [Gk *kardia, aggeion* vessel, *graphein* to record], the radiographic study of the heart and coronary vessels after being injected with medium.

cardiac apnea [Gk *kardia* + *a, pnein* not to breathe], abnormal, temporary absence of respiration, as in Cheyne-Stokes respiration.

cardiac arrest [Gk *kardia* + L *ad, restare* to withstand], a sudden cessation of cardiac output and effective circulation, usually precipitated by ventricular fibrillation and, in some instances, by ventricular

asystole. When cardiac arrest occurs, delivery of oxygen and removal of carbon dioxide stop, tissue cell metabolism becomes anaerobic, and metabolic and repiratory acidosis ensue.

cardiac arrhythmia [Gk *kardia* + *a, rhythmos* not rhythm], an abnormal rate or rhythm of atrial or ventricular myocardial contraction. The condition may be caused by a defect in the ability of the sinoatrial node to maintain its pacemaker function, or by a failure of the bundle of His, the bundle branches, or the Purkinje network to conduct the contractile impulse. Kinds of arrhythmia include **bradycardia, extrasystole, heart block, premature atrial contraction, premature ventricular contraction, tachycardia.**

cardiac asthma, an attack of asthma associated with heart disease, such as ventricular failure, and characterized by predominant pulmonary congestion with some bronchoconstriction.

cardiac catheter, a long, fine catheter designed to be passed into the heart through a blood vessel.

cardiac catheterization, a diagnostic procedure in which a catheter is introduced into a large vein or artery, usually of an arm or a leg, and threaded through the circulatory system to the heart.

cardiac cirrhosis [Gk, *kardia,* heart, *kirrhos,* yellowish orange, *osis,* condition], an increase of fibrous tissue in the liver resulting from congestive heart failure, chronic myocarditis, or cardiac fibrosis.

cardiac compression. See **cardiac tamponade.**

cardiac conduction defect, any impairment of the electrical pathways and the specialized muscular fibers that conduct action impulses to contract the atria and the ventricles.

cardiac cycle [Gk *kardia* + *kyklos* circle], the cycle of events during which an electrical impulse is conducted through special fibers over the muscle of the myocardium, from the sinoatrial (SA) node to the atrioventricular (AV) node, to the bundle of His and the bundle branches, and to the Purkinje fibers, causing contraction of the atria followed by contraction of the ventricles. Contraction occurs with depolarization of the muscle fibers. Deoxygenated blood enters the right atrium of the heart from the inferior and superior venae cava and is pumped through the tricuspid valve into the right ventricle. From the right ventricle, blood is pumped through the pulmonary valve into the pulmonary artery and the lungs for oxygenation. Oxygen-rich blood is returned to the heart through the branches of the pulmonary veins to the left rium and pumped through the mitral valve into the left ventricle. The blood is pumped through the aortic valve into the aorta for peripheral circulation. The contractions of the left and the right atria are nearly simultaneous; they precede the nearly simultaneous contractions of the ventricles. Structural, chemical, or electric abnormalities may cause a large variety of anomalies in electric conduction, muscular contraction, and blood flow in the heart.

cardiac decompensation, a condition of heart failure in which the heart is unable to fulfill its normal function of ensuring adequate cellular perfusion to all parts of the body without assistance. Causes may include myocardial infarction, increased work load, infection, toxins, or defective heart valves.

cardiac depressant [L, *deprimere,* to press down], an agent that decreases the heart rate and contractility.

cardiac dyspnea [Gk, *dys,* difficult, *pnoia,* breath], breathing distress that is caused by heart disease, most commonly the result of pulmonary venous congestion.

cardiac edema [Gk, *oidema,* swelling], an accumulation of serum fluid from blood plasma in the interstitial tissues as a result of congestive heart failure. In severe cases, the fluid may also accumulate in serous cavities.

cardiac electrical axis, the angle the mean cardiac vector in the frontal plane makes with a horizontal plane drawn through the center of Einthoven's triangle and left hip.

cardiac failure. See **heart failure.**

cardiac hypertrophy, an abnormal enlargement of the heart muscle.

cardiac impulse [Gk *kardia* + L *impellere* to set in motion], the movement of the thorax, caused by the beating of the heart. It is readily palpable and easily recorded.

cardiac index, a measure of the cardiac output of a patient per square meter of body surface area. It is obtained by dividing the cardiac output in liters per minute by the body surface area.

cardiac insufficiency, the inability of the heart to perform its normal functions properly.

cardiac massage, repeated, rhythmic compression of the heart applied directly, during surgery, or through the intact chest wall in an effort to maintain circulation after cardiac arrest or ventricular fibrillation.

cardiac monitor, a device for the continuous observation of cardiac function.

cardiac monitoring, a continuous check on the functioning of the heart with an electronic instrument that provides an electrocardiographic reading on an oscilloscope.

cardiac murmur, an abnormal sound heard during auscultatory examination of the heart, caused by the flow of blood into a chamber or through a valve or by a valve opening or closing. A murmur is classified by the time of its occurrence during the cardiac cycle, the duration, and the intensity of the sound on a scale of I to V.

cardiac muscle, a special striated muscle of the myocardium, containing dark intercalated disks at the junctions of abutting fibers. Cardiac muscle is an exception among involuntary muscles, which are characteristically smooth. Its contractile fibrillae resemble those of skeletal muscle but are only one third as large in diameter, are richer in sarcoplasm, and contain centrally located instead of peripheral nuclei.

cardiac output, the volume of blood expelled by the ventricles of the heart, equal to the amount of blood ejected at each beat (the stroke output), multiplied by the number of beats in the period of time used in the computation. A normal heart in a resting adult ejects from 4 to 8 L of blood per minute. A decreased output at rest is usually indicative of a late stage in abnormal cardiac performance; its failure to increase during exercise occurs much earlier in a malfunctioning heart.

cardiac output, decreased, a NANDA-accepted nursing diagnosis of a state in which the amount of blood pumped by an individual's heart is sufficiently reduced that it is inadequate to meet the needs of the body's tissues. Defining characteristics include variations in blood pressure, arrhythmias, fatigue, jugular vein distention, color changes of the skin and mucous membranes, oliguria, decreased peripheral pulses, cold and clammy skin, rales, dyspnea, orthopnea, and restlessness.

cardiac pacemaker. See **pacemaker.**

cardiac pain, See **angina pectoris.**

cardiac plexus [Gk *kardia* + L, pleated], one of several nerve complexes situated close to the arch of the aorta. The cardiac plexuses contain sympathetic and parasympathetic nerve fibers that leave the plexuses, accompany the right and the left coronary arteries, and enter the heart to terminate in the sinoatrial and atrioventricular nodes and in the atrial myocardium.

cardiac radionuclide imaging [Gk *kardia* + L *radiare* to shine, *nucleus* kernel; *imago* image], the noninvasive examination of the heart, using a radiopharmaceutical, such as thallium 201, and a detection device, such as a gamma camera, positron camera, or rectilinear scanner.

cardiac reflex [L, *reflectere,* to bend back],

a pair of stimuli that automatically increase or reduce the heart rate. Stimulation of vagus fibers in the right side of the heart by increased venous return accelerate increase the heart rate while increased arterial blood pressure stimulates nerve endings in the carotid sinus to slow the heart rate.

cardiac regurgitation [Gk *kardia* + L *re, gurgitare* to flow], a backward flow of blood through one or more defective heart valves.

cardiac rehabilitation [Gk *kardia;* L *re, habilitas* ability], a supervised program of progressive exercise, psychologic support, and education or training to enable a myocardial infarction patient to resume the activities of daily living on an independent basis. Special training may be needed to adapt the patient to a new occupation and life-style.

cardiac reserve, the potential capacity of the heart to function well beyond its basal level, responding to the demands of various physiologic and psychologic changes.

cardiac rhythm [Gk *kardia* + *rhythmos*], the recurring beat of the heart.

cardiac souffle [Gk *kardia;* Fr, puff], a heart murmur.

cardiac sphincter [Gk *kardia* + *sphigkter* binder], a ring of muscle fibers at the juncture of the esophagus and stomach.

cardiac standstill, the complete cessation of ventricular contractions and ejection of blood by the heart.

cardiac stenosis [Gk *kardia;* Gk *stenos* narrow + *osis* condition], an obstruction of blood flow through any of the chambers of the heart that is not valvular in origin. The cause may be a thrombosis or tumor.

cardiac stimulant, a pharmacologic agent that increases the action of the heart. Cardiac glycosides, such as digitalis, digitoxin, digoxin, deslanoside, lanatoside, acetyldigitoxin, and ouabain, increase the force of myocardial contractions and decrease the heart rate and conduction velocity, allowing more time for the ventricles to relax and become filled with blood. They are used in the treatment of congestive heart failure, atrial flutter and fibrillation, paroxysmal atrial tachycardia, and cardiogenic shock. Epinephrine, a potent vasopressor and cardiac stimulant, is sometimes used to restore heart rhythm in cardiac arrest. Isoproterenol hydrochloride may be used in treating heart block. Dobutamine hydrochloride and dopamine are used in the short-term treatment of cardiac decompensation resulting from depressed contractility.

cardiac syncope [Gk *kardia* + *syncope* fainting], a temporary loss of consciousness caused by inadequate cerebral blood flow due, in turn, to a sudden failure in cardiac output for any reason.

cardiac tamponade, compression of the heart produced by the accumulation in the pericardial sac of fluid or of blood resulting from the rupture of a blood vessel of the myocardium, as by a penetrating wound.

cardiac thrombosis [Gk *kardia* + *thrombos* lump + *osis* condition], a blood clot located at a heart valve or in one of the heart chambers. A left ventricular thrombosis may follow a large infarct.

cardiasthenia [Gk *kardia* + *a, sthenos* strength], a form of neurasthenia in which cardiovascular symptoms are prominent.

cardinal [L *cardo* hinge], pertaining to something so fundamental that other things hinge on it, such as a cardinal trait that influences one's total behavior.

cardinal frontal plane [L *cardo; frons* forehead; *planum* level ground], the plane that divides the body into front and back portions.

cardinal horizontal plane. See **transverse plane.**

cardinal ligament [L *cardo; ligare* to bind], a sheet of subserous fascia extending across the female pelvic floor as a continuation of the broad ligament. It is embedded in the adipose tissue on each side of the vagina and is formed by the fasciae of the vagina and the cervix converging at the lateral borders of these organs.

cardinal movements of labor, the typical sequence of positions assumed by the fetus as it descends through the pelvis during labor and delivery, usually designated as engagement, flexion, descent, internal rotation, extension, and external rotation or restitution.

cardinal position of gaze, (in ophthalmology) one of six positions to which the normal eye may be turned. Each position requires the function of a specific ocular muscle and a cranial nerve.

cardinal sagittal plane. See **median plane.**

cardinal symptom. See **symptom.**

cardioangiography, See **cardiac angiography.**

cardiocatheterization /kär'dē·ōkath'ər-īzā'shən/ [Gk *kardia* heart + *katheter* a thing lowered into], the introduction of a flexible radiopaque catheter through a saphenous or median basilic vein and the superior vena cava to the heart chambers. It may be used to collect samples of blood in the heart and to measure blood pressure in various heart chambers as well as illuminate the coronary arteries.

cardiocirculatory /kär′dē·ōsur′kyōōlə-tôr′ē/ [Gk *kardia*; L *circulare* to go around], of or pertaining to the heart and the circulation.

cardioesophageal reflux [Gk *kardia* + *oisophagos* gullet; L *refluere* to flow back], a backward flow or regurgitation of stomach contents into the esophagus. Repeated episodes of reflux can lead to esophagitis. Among factors contributing to the condition are stomach pressure greater than pressure in the esophagus, hiatus hernia, and incompetence of the lower esophageal sphincter.

cardiogenic shock /kär′dē·ōjen′ik/ [Gk *kardia* + *genein* to produce; Fr *choc*], an abnormal condition often characterized by low cardiac output in association with acute myocardial infarction and congestive heart failure. Cardiogenic shock is fatal in about 80% of cases, and immediate therapy is necessary to save affected individuals. Depending on the signs, therapy may include the administration of fluids, diuretics, or vasoactive drugs and the application of various devices.

cardiogram, an electronically recorded tracing of cardiac activity.

cardiograph, See **electrocardiogram, electrocardiograph.**

cardiography /kär′dē·og′rəfē/, the technique of graphically recording the movements of the heart by means of a cardiograph.

cardiologist, a physician specializing in the diagnosis and treatment of disorders of the heart.

cardiology [Gk *kardia* + *logos* science], the study of the anatomy, normal functions, and disorders of the heart.

cardiolysis /kär′dē·ol′isis/ [Gk *kardia* + *lysein* to loosen], an operation that separates the heart and the pericardium from the sternal periosteum in a procedure to correct adhesive mediastinopericarditis.

cardiomegaly /kär′dē·ōmeg′əlē/ [Gk *kardia* + *megas* large], enlargement of the heart caused hypertrophy (thickening) of the walls of the heart. In athletes an enlarged, well-functioning heart is a normal finding.

cardiomyopathy /kär′dē·ōmī·op′əthē/ [Gk *kardia* + *mys* muscle, *pathos* disease], any disease that affects the myocardium, as alcoholic cardiomyopathy.

cardiomyopexy /kär′dē·ōmī′əpeksē/ [Gk *kardia* + *mys* muscle, *pexis* fixation], a surgical procedure in which the blood supply from the nearby pectoral muscles of the chest is diverted directly to the coronary arteries of the heart.

cardiopathy /kär′dē·op′əthē/ [Gk *kar-dia* + *pathos* disease], a disease of the heart.

cardioplasty /kär′dē·ōplas′tē/, a surgical procedure to correct a defect in the cardiac sphincter of the esophagus that frequently leads to cardiospasm.

cardioplegia /kär′dē·ōplē′jə/ [Gk *kardia* + *plege* stroke], 1. paralysis of the heart. 2. the arrest of myocardial contractions by injection of chemicals, hypothermia, or electrical stimuli for the purpose of performing surgery on the heart.

cardiopulmonary [Gk *kardia* + L *pulmoneus* lungs], of or pertaining to the heart and the lungs.

cardiopulmonary arrest. See **cardiac arrest.**

cardiopulmonary bypass, a procedure used in heart surgery in which the blood is diverted from the heart and lungs by means of a pump oxygenator and returned directly to the aorta.

cardiopulmonary murmur [Gk *kardia;* L *pulmo* lung, *murmur* humming], a sound heard over the heart during breathing and during the heart beat. It is caused by vibrations resulting from the heart striking the lung tissue with every beat.

cardiopulmonary resuscitation (CPR), a basic emergency procedure for life support, consisting of artificial respiration and manual external cardiac massage. It is used in cases of cardiac arrest to establish effective circulation and ventilation to prevent irreversible cerebral damage resulting from anoxia. External cardiac massage compresses the heart between the lower sternum and the thoracic vertebral column. During compressions, blood is forced into systemic and pulmonary circulation, and venous blood refills the heart when the compression is released. Mouth-to-mouth breathing or a mechanical form of ventilation is used concomitantly with CPR to oxygenate the blood being pumped through the circulatory system.

cardiorrhaphy /kär′dē·ôr′əfē/ [Gk *kardia* + *rhaphe* suture], an operation in which the heart muscle is sutured.

cardioscope, an obsolete device for inspecting and manipulating the internal structures of the heart.

cardiospasm /kär′dē·ōspaz′əm/ [Gk *kar-dia* + *spasmos* pull], a form of achalasia characterized by a failure of the cardia at the distal end of the esophagus to relax, causing dysphagia and regurgitation, and sometimes requiring surgical division of the muscle.

cardiotachometer /kär′dē·ōtəkom′ətər/ [Gk *kardia* + *tachos* speed, *metron* measure], an instrument that continuously monitors and records the heartbeat.

cardiotomy /kär′dē-ot′əmē/ [Gk *kardia* + *temnein* to cut], **1.** an operation in which the heart is incised. **2.** an operation in which the cardiac end of the stomach or cardiac orifice is incised.

cardiotonic /kär′dē-ōton′ik/ [Gk *kardia* + *tonos* tone], **1.** of or pertaining to a substance that tends to increase the efficiency of contractions of the heart muscle. **2.** a pharmacologic agent that increases the force of heart contractions.

cardiotoxic [Gk *kardia* + *toxikon* poison], having a toxic or injurious effect on the heart.

cardiovascular /kär′dē-ōvas′kyələr/ [Gk *kardia* + L *vasculum* small vessel], of or pertaining to the heart and blood vessels.

cardiovascular assessment, an evaluation of the condition, function, and abnormalities of the heart and circulatory system.

cardiovascular disease, any abnormal condition characterized by dysfunction of the heart and blood vessels. Some common kinds of cardiovascular disease are **atherosclerosis, cor pulmonale, rheumatic heart disease, syphilitic heart disease,** and **systemic hypertension.**

cardiovascular shunt [Gk *kardia*; L, *vasculum* little vessel; ME *shunten*], any abnormal passage between chambers of the heart or between systemic and pulmonary circulatory systems.

cardiovascular system, the network of structures, including the heart and the blood vessels, that pump and convey the blood throughout the body. The system includes thousands of miles of vessels, capillaries, and venules and is vital to maintaining homeostasis. Numerous control mechanisms of the system assure that the blood is delivered to the structures where it is most needed and at the proper rate. The system delivers nutrients and other essential materials to the fluids surrounding the cells and removes waste products, which are conveyed to excretory organs, such as the kidneys and the intestine. The cardiovascular system functions in close association with the respiratory system, transporting oxygen inhaled into the lungs and conveying carbon dioxide to the lungs for expiration.

cardiovascular technologist, an allied health professional who performs diagnostic examinations at the request or direction of a physician in one or more of the following three areas: (1) invasive cardiology, (2) noninvasive cardiology, and (3) massive peripheral vascular study. Through subjective sampling and/or recording, the technologist creates an easily definable foundation of data from which a correct anatomic and physiologic diagnosis may be established for each patient.

cardioversion [Gk *kardia* + L *vertere* to turn], the restoration of the heart's normal sinus rhythm by delivery of a synchronized electric shock through two metal paddles placed on the patient's chest. Cardioversion is used in the treatment of atrial fibrillation and in ventricular, nodal, and atrial arrhythmias.

carditis /kärdī′tis/, an inflammatory condition of the muscles of the heart, usually resulting from infection. In most cases more than one layer of muscles is involved. Chest pain, cardiac arrhythmia, circulatory failure, and damage to the structures of the heart may occur. Kinds of carditis are **endocarditis, myocarditis,** and **pericarditis.**

career ladder, (in nursing education) a pathway for upward mobility that begins with a course of study in practical nursing or a program that grants an associate degree in nursing. On completion of this basic level, the candidate may continue up the ladder, taking a baccalaureate program in nursing and continue on to a masters and a doctoral program.

caregiver, one who contributes the benefits of medical, economic, or environmental resources to a dependent or partially dependent individual, such as a critically ill person.

caregiver role strain, a NANDA-accepted nursing diagnosis of a state in which a caregiver perceives difficulty in performing the family caregiver role. Defining characteristics include the caregiver's report of difficulty in providing specific caregiving activities, inadequate resources to provide required care, worry about the care receiver, the feeling that caregiving interferes with important roles in the caregiver's life, feeling of loss, family conflict, stress, and depression.

caregiver role strain, high risk for, a NANDA-accepted nursing diagnosis of a state of vulnerability for feeling difficulty in performing the family caregiver role. Risk factors may be physiologic, such as severity of the care receiver's illness or caregiver health impairment; developmental, such as a developmental inability to fulfill the caregiver role; psychosocial, such as psychologic or cognitive problems in the care receiver; and situational, such as the presence of abuse or violence.

care of the chronically ill, a pattern of medical and nursing care that focuses on long-term care of people with chronic diseases or conditions, either at home or in a medical facility. It includes care specific to the problem, as well as other measures to encourage self-care, to promote health, and to prevent loss of function.

care of the sick, (in public health nursing) the care of sick patients in their homes, as distinguished from health supervision. Public health nursing agencies are reimbursed for the nursing services rendered by the nurses according to the kind of service rendered, such as a sick visit or a health supervision visit.

care plan. See **nursing care plan.**

CARF, abbreviation for *Commission on Accreditation of Rehabilitation Facilities.*

caries /ker′ēz/ [L, decay], an abnormal condition of a tooth or a bone characterized by decay, disintegration, and destruction of the structure. Kinds of caries include **dental caries, radiation caries,** and **spinal caries.**

carina /kərē′nə/, *pl.* **carinae** [L, keel], any structure shaped like a ridge or keel, such as the carina of the trachea, that projects from the lowest tracheal cartilage.

caring behaviors, behaviors associated with concern for the well-being of the patient, such as sensitivity, comforting, attentive listening, and honesty.

cariocas /kär′ē·ō′kəs/, a form of lateral movement in a gait cycle in which the side-stepping leg is brought successively behind and then in front of the stance leg.

cariogenic /ker′ē·ōjen′ik/, tending to produce caries.

carisoprodol /kər′isōprō′dol/, a skeletal muscle relaxant prescribed for the relief of muscle spasm.

carmalum. See **carmine dye.**

carminative /kärmin′ətiv/ [L *carminare* to cleanse] **1.** of or pertaining to a substance that relieves flatulence and abdominal distention. **2.** a carminative agent that relieves gaseous distention and painful spasms, especially after meals.

carmine dye /kär′min/ [AR *qirmize*; AS *deag*], a red coloring substance, produced by the addition of alum to an extract of cochineal, used for staining specimens in histology.

carmustine /kärmus′tin/, a lipid-soluble nitrosourea, 1,3-bis(2-chloroethyl)-1-nitrosourea, used as a single antineoplastic agent or with other approved chemotherapeutic agents in the treatment of brain tumors, multiple myeloma, Hodgkin's disease, and non-Hodgkin's lymphomas.

carnal /kär′nəl/ [L, *caro,* flesh], pertaining to the flesh or body, or worldly things, as distinguished from the spiritual.

carneous /kär′nē·əs/, having the quality of flesh.

carnitine /kär′nitin/, a substance found in skeletal and cardiac muscle and certain other tissues that functions as a carrier of fatty acids across the membranes of the mitochondria. It is used therapeutically in treating heart diseases.

carnivore /L *caro* flesh, *vorare* to devour], an animal belonging to the order *Carnivora,* classified as a flesheater, with appropriate teeth and a characteristically simple stomach and a short intestine for such a diet. **–carnivorous,** *adj.*

carotene /kar′ətin/ [L *carota* carrot], a red or orange hydrocarbon found in carrots, sweet potatoes, milk fat, egg yolk, and leafy vegetables, as beet greens, spinach, and broccoli. Carotene is a provitamin and in the body is converted into vitamin A.

carotenemia /kar′ətinē′mē·ə/, the presence of high levels of carotene in the blood resulting in an abnormal yellow appearance of the plasma and skin.

carotenoid /kərot′ənoid/, any of a group of red, yellow, or orange highly unsaturated pigments that are found in some animal tissue and in foods, such as carrots, sweet potatoes, and leafy green vegetables. Many of these substances are necessary for the formation of vitamin A in the body.

carotenosis. See **carotenemia.**

carotid /kərot′id/ [Gk *karos* heavy sleep], of or pertaining to the carotid artery.

carotid arch [Gk *karos;* L, *arcus,* bow], the third arch of the aorta, the source of the common carotid arteries.

carotid body [Gk *karos;* AS *bodig*], a small structure containing neural tissue at the bifurcation of the carotid arteries. It monitors the oxygen content of the blood and assists in regulating respiration.

carotid-body reflex [Gk *karos* + AS *bodig;* L *reflecere* to bend backward], a normal chemical reflex initiated by a decrease in oxygen concentration in the blood and, to a lesser degree, by increased carbon dioxide and hydrogen ion concentrations that act on chemoreceptors at the bifurcation of the common carotid arteries and result in nerve impulses that cause the respiratory center in the medulla to increase respiratory activity.

carotid-body tumor, a benign, round, firm growth that develops at the bifurcation of the common carotid artery. The tumor sometimes may cause dizziness, nausea, and vomiting, especially if it impedes the flow of blood because pressure is increased in the vascular system.

carotid plexus [Gk *karos* + L, pleated], any one of three nerve plexuses associated with the carotid arteries.

carotid pulse, the pulse of the carotid artery, palpated by gently pressing a finger in the groove between the larynx and the sternocleidomastoid muscle in the neck.

carotid sinus [Gk *karos* + L, curve], a dilatation of the arterial wall at the bifurcation of the common carotid artery. It contains sensory nerve endings from the vagus nerve that respond to changes in blood pressure.

carotid sinus reflex, the decrease in the heart rate as a reflex reaction from pressure on or within the carotid artery at the level of its bifurcation.

carotid sinus syndrome, a temporary loss of consciousness that sometimes accompanies convulsive seizures because of the intensity of the carotid sinus reflex when pressure builds in one or both carotid sinuses.

carotodynia /kərot'ōdin'ē·ə/ [Gk *karos* + *odyne* pain], a pain along the length of the common carotid artery, caused by pressure.

carpal /kär'pəl/ [Gk *karpos* wrist], of or pertaining to the carpus, or wrist.

carpal tunnel [Gk *karpos* + Fr *tonnel*], a conduit for the median nerve and the flexor tendons, formed by the carpal bones and the flexor retinaculum.

carpal tunnel syndrome, a common painful disorder of the wrist and hand, induced by compression on the median nerve between the inelastic carpal ligament and other structures within the carpal tunnel. The median nerve innervates the palm and the radial side of the hand; compression of the nerve causes weakness, pain with opposition of the thumb, and burning, tingling, or aching, sometimes radiating to the forearm and to the shoulder joint.

carpometacarpal (CMC) joint /kär'pōmet'əkär'pəl/ [Gk *karpos* wrist, *meta* next, *karpos*], any of the joints formed by the distal row of carpal bones and the bases of the metacarpals. The joints are essential for prehensile patterns.

carpopedal spasm [Gk *karpos* + L *pes* foot], a spasm of the hand, or thumbs, or foot, or toes that sometimes accompanies tetany.

carpus /kär'pəs/ [L; Gk *karpos*], the wrist, made up of eight bones arranged in two rows. The proximal row consists of the scaphoid, lunate, triangular, and pisiform. The distal row consists of the trapezium, trapezoid, capitate, and hamate.

Carrel-Lindbergh pump. See **Lindbergh pump.**

carrier [OFr *carier*], **1.** a person or animal who harbors and spreads an organism causing disease in others but who does not become ill. **2.** one whose chromosomes carry a recessive gene.

Carrión's disease. See **bartonellosis.**

Carroll Quantitative Test of Upper Extremity Function, a six-part test of the ability of the patient to grasp and lift objects of different shapes and sizes.

carrying angle, the angle at which the humerus and radius articulate.

carry-over [L *carrus* wagon; AS *ofer*], contamination of a specimen by the previous one.

car sickness [L *carrum* chariot; AS *seoc*], nausea and vomiting due to the motion of the vehicle.

cartilage /kär'tilij/ [L *cartilago*], a nonvascular supporting connective tissue composed of various cells and fibers, found chiefly in the joints, the thorax, and various rigid tubes, such as the larynx, trachea, nose, and ear. Temporary cartilage, such as that comprising most of the fetal skeleton at an early stage, is later replaced by bone. Permanent cartilage remains unossified, except in certain diseases and, sometimes, in advanced age. Kinds of permanent cartilage are **hyaline cartilage, white fibrocartilage,** and **yellow cartilage. –cartilaginous,** *adj.*

cartilage graft, the transplantation of cartilage. It is used to correct congenital ear and nose defects in children and to treat severe injuries in adults.

cartilage-hair hypoplasia [L *cartilago* + AS *haer*; Gk *hypo* under, *plasis* forming], a genetic disorder, inherited as an autosomal recessive trait, characterized by dwarfism caused by hypoplasia of the cartilage, multiple skeletal abnormalities, and excessively sparse, short, fine, brittle hair that is usually light colored.

cartilaginous [L, *cartilago*, cartilage], pertaining to cartilage.

cartilaginous joint [L *cartilago* + *junger* to join], a slightly movable joint in which cartilage unites bony surfaces. Two types of articulation involving cartilaginous joints are synchondrosis and symphysis.

cartilaginous skeleton [L, *cartilago*; Gk, *skeletos*, dried up], the parts of the skeleton that are formed by cartilage.

caruncle /kär'ungkəl/ [L *caruncula* small piece of flesh], a small, fleshy projection, as one of the lacrimal caruncles at the inner canthus of the eye or the hymenal caruncles that are the hymenal remnants.

carunculae hymenales [L *caruncula* + Gk *hymen* membrane], remnants of a ruptured hymen that appear as irregular projections of normal skin around the introitus to the vagina.

cascade [L *cadere* to fall], any process that develops in stages, with each stage dependent on the preceding one, often producing a cumulative effect.

cascade humidifier, a bubbling respiratory care device in which gases travel down a tower and pass through a grid into a chamber of heated water.

cascara sagrada /kasker'ə səgrä'də/ [Sp, sacred bark], a stimulant cathartic prepared from the bark of the *Rhamnus purshianus* tree prescribed for constipation.

case [L *casus* a happening], **1.** an episode of illness or injury. **2.** a container.

caseation /kā'sē-ā'shən/ [L *caseus* cheese], a form of tissue necrosis in which there is loss of cellular outline and the appearance is that of crumbly cheese. It is typical of tuberculosis. —**caseate,** *v.*

caseation necrosis [L *caseus* cheese; Gk *nekros* dead, *osis* condition], necrosis that transforms tissue into a dry cheeselike mass.

case-control study, a retrospective type of scientific investigation in which a group of patients with a particular disease or disorder, such as myocardial infarction, is compared with a control group of persons who have not developed that medical problem.

case fatality rate [L *casus, fatum* fate, *(pro) rata*], the number of registered deaths caused by any specific disease, expressed as a percentage of the total number of reported cases of a specific disease.

casefinding, the act of locating individuals with a disease.

case history [L *casus, historia*], a complete medical record of a patient before a current illness or injury. The history includes any infectious diseases experienced by the person; all immunizations, hospitalizations or therapies; information relating to deaths or illnesses of parents and other close family members; allergies; and congenital or acquired physical defects.

case management, the assignment of a health care provider to assist a patient in assessing health and social service systems and to assure that all required services are obtained.

case nursing [L *casus, nutrix* nourish], a health care system in which one nurse is assigned to a single patient for delivery of total nursing care.

caseous /kā'sē-əs/, cheeselike; describing the mixture of fat and protein that appears in some body tissues undergoing necrosis.

caseous fermentation [L *caseus* cheese; *fermentum* yeast], the coagulation of soluble casein through the action of rennin.

cassette [Fr, little box], a device used in radiography for holding a sheet of x-ray film and a set of screens. A cassette also may have a grid to absorb scattered radiation.

cast [ONorse *kasta*], **1.** a stiff, solid dressing formed with plaster of paris or other material around a limb or other body part to immobilize it during healing. **2.** a mold of a part or all of a patient's teeth and internal jaw area for fitting prostheses or dentures. **3.** a tiny structure formed by deposits of mineral or other substances on the walls of renal tubules, bronchioles, or other organs. Casts often appear in samples of urine or blood collected for laboratory examination. **4.** the deviation of an eye from the normal parallel lines of vision, such as in strabismus.

cast brace, a combination of a brace within a cast at a joint.

cast core [ONorse *kasta;* L *cor* heart], a metal casting that uses a post in the root canal for retaining an artificial tooth crown.

Castellani's paint. See **carbol-fuchsin solution.**

casting, 1. the act of encasing a body part in a cast. **2.** (in dentistry) the process by which crowns, inlays, and other metallic restorations are produced.

casting tape, an adhesive or resin-impregnated tape used for shaping lightweight casts.

castor oil [L, beaver, *oleum* olive oil], an oil derived from *Ricinus communis,* used as a stimulant cathartic. It is prescribed for constipation and for a cleansing preparation of the bowel or colon before examination.

castration /kastrā'shən/ [L *castrare* to castrate], the surgical excision of one or both testicles or ovaries, performed most frequently to reduce the production and secretion of certain hormones that may stimulate the proliferation of malignant cells in women with breast cancer or in men with cancer of the prostate.

castration anxiety, 1. the fantasized fear of injury or loss of the genital organs, often as the reaction to a repressed feeling of punishment for forbidden sexual desires. **2.** a general threat to the masculinity or femininity of a person or an unrealistic fear of bodily injury or loss of power.

castration complex. See **castration anxiety.**

cast saw, a saw used to cut through a plaster cast.

cast shoe, a shoe worn over a foot that is encased in a plaster cast.

cast stabilization, the use of rods, pins, broom handles, or other devices to lend stability to a cast.

casuistics /kazh'əwis'tiks/ [L *casus* a happening], the recording and the study of the cases of any disease.

CAT /kat/, abbreviation for *computerized*

axial tomography. See **computed tomography.**

catabasis /kətab′əsis/, *pl.* **catabases** [Gk *kata* down, *bainein* to go], the phase in which a disease declines. −**catabatic**, *adj.*

catabiosis /kat′əbī·ō′sis/, the normal aging of cells. −**catabiotic**, *adj.*

catabolic activator protein. See **CAP.**

catabolism /kətab′əliz′əm/ [Gk *kata + ballein* to throw], a complex, metabolic process in which energy is liberated for use in work, energy storage, or heat production by the destruction of complex substances by living cells to form simple compounds. −**catabolic**, *adj.*

catacrotism /kətak′rətiz′əm/ [Gk *kata + krotein* to strike], an anomaly of the pulse, characterized by one or more small additional waves in the descending limb of the pulse tracing. −**catacrotic**, *adj.*

catagen. See **hair.**

catagenesis /kat′əjen′əsis/ [Gk, *kata,* down, *genein,* to produce], a form of evolution that is retrogressive.

catalase [Gk *katalein* to dissolve], a heme enzyme, found in almost all biologic cells, that catalyzes the decomposition of hydrogen peroxide to water and oxygen.

catalepsy /kat′əlep′sē/ [Gk *kata + lambanein* to seize], an abnormal state characterized by a trancelike level of consciousness and postural rigidity. It occurs in hypnosis and in certain organic and psychologic disorders, such as schizophrenia, epilepsy, and hysteria.

catalysis /kətal′əsis/ [Gk *katalein* to dissolve], an increase in the rate of any chemical reaction caused by a chemical material that is neither part of the process itself nor consumed or affected by the reaction. −**catalytic**, *adj.*

catalyst /kat′əlist/ [Gk *katalein* to dissolve], a substance that influences the rate of a chemical reaction without being permanently altered by the process. Most catalysts, including enzymes in living organisms, accelerate chemical reactions; negative catalysts retard such reactions.

catamenia. See **menses.**

catamnesis /kat′amnē′sis/ [Gk *kata + men* month], the medical history of a patient from the onset of an illness.

cataphylaxis /kat′əfəlak′sis/ [Gk /kata + *phylax* guard], **1.** the migration of leukocytes and antibodies to the site of an infection. **2.** the deterioration of the natural defense system of the body. −**cataphylactic**, *adj.*

cataplexy /kat′əplek′sē/ [Gk *kata + plexis* stroke], a condition characterized by sudden muscular weakness and hypotonia, caused by emotions, as anger, fear or sur-

prise, often associated with narcolepsy. −**cataplectic**, *adj.*

cataract /kat′ərakt/ [Gk *katarrhakies* waterfall], an abnormal progressive condition of the lens of the eye, characterized by loss of transparency. A gray-white opacity can be seen within the lens, behind the pupil. Most cataracts are caused by degenerative changes, occurring most often after 50 years of age. The tendency to develop cataracts is inherited. **Congenital cataracts** are usually hereditary but may be caused by viral infection during the first trimester of gestation. If cataracts are untreated, sight is eventually lost. At first vision is blurred; then, bright lights glare diffusely, and distortion and double vision may develop. Uncomplicated cataracts of old age (**senile cataracts**) are usually treated with excision of the lens and prescription of special contact lenses or glasses.

catarrh /katär′/ [Gk *kata + rhoia* flow], *obsolete.* inflammation of the mucous membranes with discharge, especially inflammation of the air passages of the nose and the trachea. −**catarrhal**, **catarrhous**, *adj.*

catarrhal conjunctivitis [Gk *kata + rhoia;* L *conjunctivus* connecting; Gk *itis* inflammation], a simple form of inflammation of the conjunctiva, usually associated with an infection, allergy, exposure to pollution, or physical irritation as by an eyelash in the eye and accompanied by a discharge.

catarrhal croup, a severe laryngitis acompanied by a croupy cough.

catarrhal dysentery. See **sprue.**

catarrhal ophthalmia [Gk *kata + rhoia, ophthalmos* eye], a catarrhal inflammation of the conjunctiva with a discharge.

catarrhal pneumonia, See **bronchial pneumonia.**

catastrophic care [Gk *katastrophe* sudden downturn; L *garrire* to babble], a pattern of medical and nursing care that involves intensive, highly technical life-support care of an acutely ill or severely traumatized patient.

catastrophic health insurance, health insurance that awards benefits to pay for the cost of severe or lengthy disability or illness. Most policies have a limit in total benefits paid, and payment for certain kinds of services may either be precluded or limited to a maximum indemnity.

catastrophic illness, any illness that requires lengthy hospitalization, extremely expensive therapies, or other care that would deplete a family's financial resources, unless covered by special medical insurance policies.

catastrophic reaction [Gk *katastrophe*

sudden downturn; L *re* again, *agere* to act], the uncoordinated response to a drastic shock or a sudden threatening condition, such as often occurs in the victims of car crashes and disasters.

catatonia /kat'ətō'nē·ə/ [Gk *kata* + *tonos* tension], a state or condition characterized by conspicuous motor disturbance, manifested usually as immobility with extreme muscular rigidity or, less commonly, as excessive, impulsive activity. **–catatonic,** *adj.*

catatonic excitement, a state of extreme agitation that may occur when a patient is unable to maintain catatonic immobility.

catatonic schizophrenia [Gk *kata, tonos* + *schizein* to split, *phren* mind], a form of schizophrenia characterized by alternating periods of extreme withdrawal and extreme excitement. During the withdrawal stage stupor, muscular rigidity, mutism, blocking, negativism, and catalepsy (cerea flexibilitas) may be seen; during the period of excitement, purposeless and impulsive activity may range from mild agitation to violence.

catatonic stupor, a form of catatonia marked by a lack of response; it may be related to a patient's fear of losing the ability to control his or her impulses.

cat-bite fever. See **cat-scratch fever.**

CAT-CAM, abbreviation for **contoured adducted trochanteric controlled alignment method.**

catchment area [L *capere* to take; *area* space], the specific geographic area for which a particular institution, especially a mental health center, is responsible.

catch-up growth [L *capere* + As *uf, gruowan*], an acceleration of the growth rate following a period of growth retardation caused by a secondary deficiency, such as acute malnutrition or severe illness. The phenomenon, which is routinely seen in premature infants, involves rapid increase in weight, length, and head circumference and continues until the normal individual growth pattern is resumed.

cat-cry syndrome [L *catta* cat, *quiritare* to cry out; Gk *syndromos* course], a rare, congenital disorder recognized at birth by a kittenlike cry caused by a laryngeal anomaly. The condition is associated with a defect in chromosome 5. Other characteristics include low birth weight, microcephaly, "moon face," wide-set eyes, strabismus, and low-set misshaped ears. Infants are hypotonic; heart defects and mental and physical retardation are common.

catecholamine /kat'əkəlam'in/, any one of a group of sympathomimetic compounds composed of a catechol molecule and the aliphatic portion of an amine. Some catecholamines are produced naturally by the body and function as key neurologic chemicals. Catecholamines are also synthesized as drugs used in the treatment of various disorders, such as anaphylaxis, asthma, cardiac failure, and hypertension. Some important endogenous catecholamines are dopamine, epinephrine, and norepinephrine.

catechol-o-methyl transferase (COMT) /kat'əkol'ōmeth'il/, an enzyme that deactivates the catecholamines epinephrine and norepinephrine.

cat-eye syndrome [L *catta* + AS *eage*; Gk *syndromos* course], a rare, congenital autosomal anomaly, marked by the presence of an extra, small chromosome 22 and pupils that resemble the vertical pupils of a cat.

categoric data [Gk *kategorikos* affirmation; L *datus* giving], (in research) any data that are classified by name rather than by number, such as race, religion, ethnicity, or marital status.

catgut [L *catta* + AS *guttas*], a nonabsorbable suture material, prepared from the intestines of sheep, used to close surgical wounds.

catharsis /kəthär'sis/, 1. a cleansing or purging. **–cathartic,** *n.* 2. the therapeutic release of pent-up feelings and emotions by open discussion of ideas and thoughts. 3. the process of bringing repressed ideas and feelings into the consciousness by the technique of free association, often in conjunction with hypnosis and the use of hypnotic drugs.

cathartic /kəthär'tik/ [Gk *katharsis* cleansing] 1. of or pertaining to a substance that causes evacuation of the bowel. 2. a cathartic agent that promotes bowel evacuation by stimulating peristalsis, increasing the fluidity or bulk of intestinal contents, softening the feces, or lubricating the intestinal wall. **–catharsis,** *n.*

catheter /kath'ətər/ [Gk *katheter* something lowered], a hollow, flexible tube that can be inserted into a vessel or cavity of the body to withdraw or to instill fluids. Kinds of catheters include **acorn-tipped catheter, Foley catheter,** and **intrauterine catheter.**

catheter hub, a threaded plastic connection at the end of an intravenous catheter.

catheterization /kath'ətərizā'shən/, the introduction of a catheter into a body cavity or organ to inject or remove a fluid. The most common procedure is the insertion of a catheter into the bladder through the urethra for the relief of urinary retention and for emptying the bladder completely before surgery. Sterile, aseptic techniques are necessary to prevent infection. For indwelling catheters, attention is given to maintaining continuous free drainage and to the increased possibility of infection. Kinds of catheterization are **cardiac catheterization, hepatic vein catheterization,** and **laryngeal catheterization.** —**catheterize,** v.

cathexis /kəthek′sis/ [Gk *kathexis* retention], the conscious or unconscious attachment of emotional feeling and importance to a specific idea, person, or object. —**cathectic,** adj.

cathode /kath′ōd/ [Gk *kata* down, *hodos* way], the electrode at which reduction occurs.

cathode ray, a stream of electrons emitted by the negative electrode of a gaseous discharge device when the cathode is bombarded by positive ions, such as in a cathode ray tube or an oscilloscope. The ray is usually focused by electromagnets that control its direction and position on a screen coated with a phosphor to create a visible pattern.

cathode ray oscilloscope [Gk *kata, hodos*; L *radius*; *ocillare* to swing; Gk *skopein* to view], an instrument that produces a visual representation of electric variations by means of the fluorescent screen of a cathode ray tube. Oscilloscopes are used to display patients' brain waves and heart beats for monitoring and diagnostic purposes.

cathode ray tube (CRT), a vacuum tube that focuses a beam of electrons onto a spot on a screen coated with a phosphor, creating a visible image of information on the face of the tube.

cation /kat′ī·on/ [Gk *kata* down, *ion* going], a positively charged ion that in solution is attracted to the negative electrode.

cation-exchange resin, any one of various insoluble organic polymers with high molecular weights that exchange their cations for other ions in solution.

catling, a long, sharp, double-edged knife used in amputation.

catoptric /kətop′trik/ [Gk *katoptron* mirror], of or pertaining to a reflected image or reflected light, such as from a mirror.

CAT scan. See **computed tomography.**

cat-scratch disease, See **cat-scratch fever.**

cat-scratch fever, a disease that results from the scratch or bite of a healthy cat. Inflammation and pustules are found on the scratched skin, and lymph nodes in the neck, head, groin, or axilla swell 2 weeks later.

cat's eye amaurosis [L *catta*; AS *aege*; Gk *amauroin* to darken], a monocular blindness, with a bright reflection from the pupil caused by a white mass in the vitreous humor resulting from inflammation or a malignant lesion.

Caucasian, pertaining to a person whose ancestors were believed to have in ancient times inhabited the geographic region of the Caucasus, in Southeastern Europe, or whose ancestors were members of the hypothetical Indo-European cultures identified with the Caucuses.

caudad /kô′dad/ [L *cauda* tail], toward the tail or end of the body, away from the head.

cauda equina [L *cauda* + *equinus* horse], the lower end of the spinal cord at the first lumbar vertebra and the bundle of lumbar, sacral, and coccygeal nerve roots that descend through the spinal canal of the sacrum and coccyx.

caudal /kô′dəl/, signifying a position toward the distal end of the spine.

caudal anesthesia, the injection of a local anesthetic agent into the caudal portion of the spinal canal through the sacrum. It is performed in labor and in such procedures as culdoscopy and anorectal and genitourinary surgery.

caudate /kô′dāt/, having a tail.

caudate lobe of the liver [L *cauda*; Gk, *lobos,* lobe; AS, *lifer*], a part of the right lobe of the liver that lies near the vena cava.

caudate nucleus [L *cauda* + *nucleus* nut], a crescent-shaped mass of gray matter lateral to the thalamus in the floor of the anterior horn and body of the lateral ventricle.

caudate process [L *cauda* + *processus* projection], a small elevation of tissue that extends obliquely from the lower extremity of the caudate lobe of the liver to the visceral surface of the right lobe.

caudocephalad /kô′dōsef′əlad/ [L, *cauda;* Gk, *kephale* head; L *ad* toward], movement from the tail toward the head.

caul [ME *cawel* basket], the intact amniotic sac surrounding the fetus at birth. The sac usually ruptures or is ruptured during the course of labor or delivery; when it remains intact, it must be torn or cut to allow the baby to breathe.

cauliflower ear [L *caulis* cabbage, *fiore* flower; AS *eare*], a thickened, deformed ear caused by repeated trauma, such as that suffered by boxers.

caumesthesia /kô′məsthē′zhə/ [Gk *kauma* heat, *aisthesis* feeling], an abnormal condition in which a patient has a low temperature but experiences a sense of intense heat. —**caumesthetic,** adj.

causalgia /kôzal′jə/ [Gk *kausis* burning, *algos* pain], a severe sensation of burning pain, often in an extremity, sometimes with local erythema of the skin. It is the result of injury to a peripheral sensory nerve.

causal hypothesis [L *causa* cause; Gk *hypotithenia* foundation], (in research) a hypothesis that predicts a cause-and-effect relationship among the variables to be studied.

causal hypothesis testing study, (in nursing research) an experimental design used in testing a hypothesis that predicts a cause-and-effect relationship within the data to be studied.

causality /kôsal′itē/, (in research) a relationship between one phenomenon or event (A) and another (B) in which A precedes and causes B and the direction of influence and the nature of the effect are predictable and reproducible and may be empirically observed.

causal treatment. See **treatment.**

causation /kôsā′shən/ [L *causa*], (in law) the existence of a reasonable connection between the misfeasance, malfeasance, or nonfeasance of the defendant and the injury or damage suffered by the plaintiff.

cause [L *causa*], any process, substance, or organism that produces an effect or condition.

CAUSN, abbreviation for **Canadian Association of University Schools of Nursing.**

caustic /kôs′tik/ [Gk *kaustikos* burning], **1.** any substance that is destructive to living tissue, such as silver nitrate, nitric acid, or sulfuric acid. **2.** exerting a burning or corrosive effect.

caustic poisoning, the accidental ingestion of strong acids or alkalis, resulting in burns and tissue damage to the mouth, esophagus, and stomach. The victim experiences immediate pain, swelling, and edema. The pulse may be weak and rapid. Respirations become shallow, and edema may close the airway. Administration of "neutralizing" substances is not recommended because of the risk of a heat-producing chemical reaction.

CAUT, abbreviation for **Canadian Association of University Teachers.**

cauterization /kô′tərīzā′shən/ [Gk, *kauterion,* branding iron], the process of burning a part of the body by cautery.

cauterize /kô′tərīz/ [Gk, *kauterion,* branding iron], to burn tissues by thermal heat, including steam, hot metal, solar radiation, electricity, or other agent, including dry ice, usually with the objective of destroying damaged or diseased tissues.

cautery /kô′tərē/ [Gk *kauterion* branding iron] **1.** a device or agent that scars and burns the skin, such as in the coagulation

of tissue by heat or caustic substances. **2.** a destructive effect produced by a cauterizing agent.

cautery knife, a surgical knife that cuts tissue and cauterizes it to prevent bleeding. The knife is connected to an electric source that generates the heat necessary for cauterization.

cavalry bone. See **rider's bone.**

Cavell, Edith, (1865-1915), an English nurse who trained at London Hospital. In 1907 she became the head of a nurses' training school in Brussels, with the task of raising nursing standards to match those of Britain. After the Germans occupied Belgium in World War I, she nursed or sheltered more than 200 fleeing soldiers and helped them reach Holland. She was arrested by the Germans, tried, and shot on October 12, 1915. Her execution brought her widespread fame.

cavernoma See **cavernous hemangioma.**

cavernous /kav′ərnəs/. [L *caverna* hollow place], containing cavities or hollow spaces.

cavernous angioma. See **cavernous hemangioma.**

cavernous body of the clitoris, cavernous body of the penis. See **corpus cavernosum.**

cavernous hemangioma [L *caverna* hollow place; Gk *haima* blood, *oma* tumor], a benign, congenital tumor consisting of large, blood-filled, cystic spaces. The scalp, face, and neck are the most common sites.

cavernous lymphangioma. See **lymphangioma cavernosum.**

cavernous rale [L *caverna* + Fr, rattle], an abnormal hollow, metallic sound heard during auscultation of the thorax. It is caused by contraction and expansion of a pulmonary cavity during respiration and indicates a pathologic condition.

cavernous sinus [L *caverna* + *sinus* curve], one of a pair of irregularly shaped, bilateral venous channels between the sphenoid bone of the skull and the dura mater. It is one of the five anterior inferior venous sinuses that drain the blood from the dura mater into the internal jugular vein.

cavernous sinus syndrome, an abnormal condition characterized by edema of the conjunctiva, the upper eyelid, and the root of the nose and by paralysis of the third, the fourth, and the sixth nerves. It is caused by a thrombosis of the cavernous sinus.

cavernous sinus thrombosis, a syndrome, usually secondary to infections near the eye or nose, characterized by orbital edema, venous congestion of the eye, and palsy of the nerves supplying the extraocular muscles.

cavitary [L *cavus* hollow], **1.** denoting the presence of one or more cavities. **2.** any entozoon having a body cavity or an alimentary canal.

cavitate /kav'itāt/ [L *cavus* hollow], the act of rapidly forming and collapsing vapor pockets or bubbles in a flowing fluid with low pressure areas, often causing damage to surrounding structures.

cavitation, 1. the formation of cavities within the body, such as those formed in the lung by tuberculosis. **2.** any cavity within the body, such as the pleural cavities.

cavity [L *cavus*], **1.** a hollow space within a larger structure, such as the peritoneal cavity or the oral cavity. **2.** *nontechnical.* a space in a tooth formed by dental caries.

cavity classification, the taxonomy of carious lesions according to the tooth surfaces on which they occur, such as labial, buccal, or occlusal; and type of surface, such as pitted or smooth.

cavogram /kav'əgram'/ [L *cavus* + Gk *gramma* record], an angiogram of the inferior or superior vena cava.

cavosurface angle, (in dentistry) the angle formed by the junction of the wall of a prepared cavity with the external surface of the tooth.

cavosurface bevel [L cavus + *superficies* surface; OFr *baif* open mouth], the incline of the cavosurface angle of a prepared tooth cavity wall relative to the enamel wall.

cavum /kā'vəm/, *pl. cava,* **1.** any hollow or cavity. **2.** the inferior or superior vena cava.

cavus [L, *cavum,* cavity], an abnormally high arch of the foot.

Cb, symbol for the chemical element **columbium.**

CBC, abbreviation for **complete blood count.**

CBF, abbreviation for *cerebral blood flow.*

CC, 1. abbreviation for **chief complaint. 2.** abbreviation for *Commission Certified.*

CCK, abbreviation for **cholecystokinin.**

CCPD, abbreviation for **continuous cycling peritoneal dialysis.**

CCRN, 1. abbreviation for *Certified Critical Care Registered Nurse;* **2.** trademark of **American Association of Critical-Care Nurses Certified Corporation.**

CCU, abbreviation for **coronary care unit.**

Cd, symbol for the chemical element **cadmium.**

CDCP, abbreviation for **Centers for Disease Control and Prevention.**

CDE, the major symbols used in one system for the nomenclature of the Rh system, in which D is the same as Rh_0, the major determining factor of Rh positivity.

CD8, symbol for peripheral lymphocyte T cells that secrete large amounts of gamma-interferon, a lymphokine involved in the body's defense against viruses. Whereas, CD4 T cells produce mainly lymphokine interleukin 2 (IL2), an autocrine and paracrine T-cell growth factor, preactivated or memory CD4 T cells secrete a much larger array of lymphokines upon restimulation. CD4 and CD8 lymphocytes carry out different functions during immune reactions partly because of distinct patterns of lymphokines secreted upon stimulation.

CD4, symbol for a glycoprotein expressed on the surface of most thymocytes and some lymphocytes, including helper T cells. Human CD4 is the receptor that serves as a docking site for HIV viruses on certain lymphocyte cells. Binding of the viral glycoprotein gp120 to CD4 is the first step in viral entry, leading to the fusion of viral and cell membranes.

CD4 cell count, a method of analyzing the prognosis of HIV-infected patients. As the virus binds to CD4 and kills T cells bearing this antigen, the level of CD4 helper T cells in the blood is an indicator of the progress of the infection. The CD4 cell count also helps measure the effectiveness of clinical trials of HIV antiviral drugs and the CD4 count in a patient can be reinforced by administering doses of the antigen.

Ce, symbol for the chemical element **cerium.**

CEA, abbreviation for **carcinoembryonic antigen.**

ceasmic /sē·az'mik/ [Gk *keazein* to split], pertaining to or characterized by a persistent embryonic fissure or abnormal cleavage of parts.

ceasmic teratism [Gk *keazein* + *teras* monster], a congenital anomaly, caused by developmental arrest, in which parts of the body that should be fused remain in their fissured embryonic state, such as in cleft palate.

cecal /sē'kəl/ [L *caecus* blind (gut)], **1.** of or pertaining to the cecum. **2.** of or pertaining to the optic disc or the blind spot in the retina.

cecal appendix. See **vermiform appendix.**

cecocolostomy /sē'kōkəlos'təmē/ [L *caecus* blind (gut); Gk *kolon* colon, *stoma* mouth], **1.** a surgical operation that creates an anastomosis between the cecum and the colon. 2. the anastomosis produced by this operation.

cecofixation. See **cecopexy.**

cecoileostomy /sē′kō·il′ē·os′təmē/ [L *caecus* + *ilia* intestine, *stoma* mouth], a surgical operation that connects the ileum with the cecum.

cecopexy /sē′kōpek′sē/ [L caecus/ + Gk *pexis* fix], a surgical operation that fixes or suspends the cecum to correct its excessive mobility.

cecostomy /sēkos′təmē/ [L *caecus* + Gk *stoma* mouth], the surgical construction of an opening into the cecum, performed as a temporary measure to relieve intestinal obstruction in a patient who cannot tolerate major surgery.

cecum /sē′kəm/ [L *caecus* blind (gut)], a cul-de-sac constituting the first part of the large intestine.

CED, abbreviation for *Certified Diabetes Educator.*

cefaclor /sē′fəklôr/, a cephalosporin antibiotic prescribed in the treatment of certain infections.

cefadroxil monohydrate /sē′fədrok′sil/, a cephalosporin antibiotic prescribed in the treatment of certain bacterial infections.

cefamandole nafate /sē′fəman′dōlnaf′ā/, a cephalosporin antibiotic prescribed in the treatment of certain bacterial infections.

cefazolin sodium /sēfaz′ōlin/, a cephalosporin antibacterial prescribed in the treatment of a variety of infections.

cefonicid sodium /sēfon′isid/, a parenteral cephalosporin-type antibiotic prescribed for infections of the lower respiratory or urinary tract, skin, bones and joints, septicemia, and surgical prophylaxis.

cefoperazone sodium /sē′fōper′əzōn/, a cephalosporin antibiotic prescribed in the treatment of respiratory tract, intraabdominal, skin, and female genital tract infections and bacterial septicemia.

cefmandole /sēfôr′ənīd/, a parenteral cephalosporin-type antibiotic prescribed for infections of the lower respiratory or urinary tract, skin, or bones and joints, septicemia, endocarditis, and surgical prophylaxis.

cefotaxime sodium /sē′fōtak′zēm/, a cephalosporin antibiotic prescribed for lower respiratory tract, genitourinary, gynecologic, intraabdominal, skin, bone and joint, and central nervous system infections and bacterial septicemia caused by susceptible strains of microorganisms.

cefotetan disodium /sē′fōtet′ən/, a cephalosporin antibiotic prescribed for parenteral administration of infections of the lower respiratory tract, urinary tract, skin,

abdomen, bones or joints, reproductive organs, or surgical prophylaxis.

cefoxitin sodium /sēfok′sitin/, a cephalosporin antibiotic prescribed in the treatment of certain bacterial infections.

ceftazidime /seftaz′idēm/, a cephalosporin-type parenteral antibiotic prescribed for treatment of infections of the lower respiratory tract, urinary tract, skin, abdomen, blood, bones and joints, and central nervous system.

ceftizoxime sodium /sef′tizok′zēm/, a cephalosporin antibiotic prescribed in the treatment of several bacterial infections.

ceftriaxone sodium /sef′trī·ak′sōn/, a cephalosporin-type parenteral antibiotic prescribed for infections of the lower respiratory tract, urinary tract, skin, abdomen, bones, and joints. It is also used to treat gonorrhea, septicemia, and meningitis, and for surgical prophylaxis, particularly in coronary bypass operations.

cefuroxime sodium, a cephalosporin antibiotic prescribed in the treatment of lower respiratory tract, urinary tract, skin, and gonococcal infections, bacterial septicemia, meningitis, and for the prevention of postoperative infections.

celiac /sē′lē·ak/ [Gk, *koilia,* belly], pertaining to the abdominal cavity.

celiac artery [Gk *koilia* belly; *arteria* air pipe], a thick visceral branch of the abdominal aorta, arising caudal to the diaphragm, usually dividing into the left gastric, the common hepatic, and the splenic arteries.

celiac disease [Gk *koilia* + L *dis* opposite of; Fr *aise* ease], an inborn error of metabolism characterized by the inability to hydrolyze peptides contained in gluten. The disease affects adults and young children, who suffer from abdominal distention, vomiting, diarrhea, muscle wasting, and extreme lethargy. Most patients respond well to a high-protein, high-calorie, gluten-free diet.

celiac plexus. See **solar plexus.**

celiac rickets [Gk *koilia* + *rhachis* spine, *itis* inflammation], arrested growth and osseous deformities resulting from malabsorption of fat and calcium.

celiocolpotomy /sē′lē·ōkəlpot′əmē/ [Gk *koilia* + *kolpos* vagina, *temnein* to cut], an incision into the abdomen through the vagina.

celioma /sēlē·ō′mə/, *pl.* **celiomas, celiomata** [Gk *koilia* + *oma* tumor], an abdominal neoplasm, especially a mesothelial tumor of the peritoneum.

celioscope. See **laparoscope.**

celiothelioma /sē′lē·ōthē′lē·ō′mə/, *pl.* **celiotheliomas, celiotheliomata,** a mesothelioma of the abdomen.

cell [L *cella* storeroom], the fundamental unit of all living tissue. Eukaryotic cells consist of a nucleus, cytoplasm, and organelles surrounded by a cytoplasmic membrane. Within the nucleus are the nucleolus and chromatin granules that develop into chromosomes. Organelles within the cytoplasm include the endoplasmic reticulum, ribosomes, the Golgi complex, mitochondria, lysosomes, and the centrosome. Prokaryotic cells are similar but lack a nucleus. The specialized nature of body tissue reflects the specialized structure and function of its constituent cells.

cella /sel'ə/, *pl.* **cellae** [L, storeroom, an enclosed space.

cell biology, the science that deals with the structures, living processes, and functions of cells, especially human cells.

cell body [L *cella* + AS *bodig*], the part of a cell that contains the nucleus and surrounding cytoplasm exclusive of any projections or processes, such as the axon and dendrites of a neuron or the tail of a spermatozoon. It is concerned more with the metabolism of the cell than with a specific function.

cell culture [L, *cella,* storeroom, *colere,* to cultivate], living cells that are maintained *in vitro* in an artificial media of serum and nutrients for the study and growth of certain strains or for experiments in controlling diseases, such as cancer.

cell cycle, the sequence of events that occurs during the growth and division of tissue cells.

cell death, **1.** terminal failure of a cell to maintain the essential life functions. **2.** the point in the process of dying at which vital functions have ceased at the cellular level.

cell division, the continuous process by which a cell divides in four stages: prophase, metaphase, anaphase, and telophase. Preliminary to prophase, the centrosome of the cell divides into two parts, which become oriented at opposite poles of the nucleus. During the prophase, previously dispersed chromatin condenses into chromomeres strung along a threadlike chromonema composed of deoxyribonucleic acid. During metaphase, the chromosomes become oriented in the equatorial plane with a clear area directed toward the two centrosomes. Each centromere divides during late metaphase and early anaphase. In telophase, the chromosomes form a compact mass, lose their individuality, and disperse into the chromatin of the intermitotic nucleus.

Cellector, trademark for a device that modifies human blood cells by circulating them through a box containing a number of polystyrene plates. Genetically engineered monclonal antibodies are permanently attached to the polystyrene plates which capture specifically targeted cells while the rest of the cells are transfused back into the patient's body. The device is used in bone marrow transplant cases.

cell inclusion [L, *cella,* storeroom + *in, claudere,* to shut], pertaining to any foreign matter that is enclosed within a cell.

cell line [L *cella* + *linea*], a colony of animal cells developed as a subculture from a primary culture.

cell mass [L, *cella,* storeroom, *massa*], the embryonic cluster of cells that develops into an individual or a part of an organism.

cell-mediated immune response, a delayed type IV hypersensitivity reaction, mediated primarily by sensitized T cell lymphocytes as opposed to antibodies.

cell-mediated immunity. See **cellular immunity.**

cell membrane, the outer covering of a cell, often having projecting microvilli and containing the cellular cytoplasm. The cell membrane controls the exchange of materials between the cell and its environment.

cell organelle [L, *cella,* storeroom; Gk, *organon,* instrument], any of a number of membrane-bound structures within a cell that have specific functions, such as reproduction or metabolism. Examples include mitochondria and Golgi bodies.

cells of Paneth [Josef Paneth, Austrian physiologist, b. 1857], large granular epithelial cells found in intestinal glands. They secrete digestive enzymes.

cell theory, the proposition that cells are the basic units of all living substance and that cellular function is the essential process of life.

cellular [L, *cella,* storeroom], pertaining to or consisting of cells.

cellular hypersensitivity reaction. See **cell-mediated immune response.**

cellular immunity [L *cellula* little cell; *immunis* exempt], the mechanism of acquired immunity characterized by the dominant role of small T-cell lymphocytes, such as in resistance to infectious diseases, in delayed hypersensitivity reactions, resistance to cancer, autoimmune diseases, graft rejection, and certain allergies.

cellular infiltration, the migration and grouping of cells within tissues throughout the body.

cellulitis /sel'yəlī'tis/ [L *cellula* little cell; Gk *itis* inflammation], an infection of the skin characterized most commonly by local heat, redness, pain, and swelling, and occasionally by fever, malaise, chills, and headache. Abscess and tissue destruction usually follow if antibiotics are not taken.

cellulose /sel'yŏolōs/ [L *cellula* little cell], a colorless, insoluble, nondigestible, transparent solid carbohydrate that is the primary constituent of the skeletal substances of the cell walls of plants.

cell wall, the structure that covers and protects the cell membrane in some kinds of cells, such as certain bacteria and all plant cells.

celom. See **coelom.**

celosomia /sē'ləsō'mē·ə/ [Gk *kele* hernia, *soma* body], a congenital malformation characterized by a fissure or absence of the sternum and ribs and protrusion of the viscera.

celosomus /sē'ləsō'məs/, a fetus with celosomia.

celothelioma. See **mesothelioma.**

Celsius (C) /sel'sē·əs/ [Anders Celsius, Swedish scientist, b. 1701], denoting a temperature scale in which 0° C is the freezing point of water and 100° C is the boiling point of water at sea level.

Celsius thermometer. See **Celsius.**

cement [L *caementum* rough stone], **1.** a sticky or mucilaginous substance that helps neighboring tissue cells stick together. **2.** any of a variety of dental materials used to fill cavities or to hold bridgework or other dental prostheses in place. **3.** a material used in the fixation of a prosthetic joint in adjacent bone, such as methyl methacrylate.

cemental fiber [L *caementum* rough stone; *fibra*], any one of the many fibers of the periodontal membrane that extend from the cementum to the intermediate plexus.

cement base, (in dentistry) a layer of insulated dental cement, sometimes medicated, pressed into the bottom of a prepared cavity to protect the pulp, to reduce the bulk of metallic restoration, or eliminate undercuts in a tapered preparation.

cementifying fibroma [L *caementum* + *facere* to make; *fibra* fiber; Gk *oma* tumor], **1.** an intrabony lesion that is not associated with the teeth, composed of fibrous connective tissue enclosing foci of calcified material resembling cementum. **2.** a rare odontogenic tumor composed of varying amounts of fibrous connective tissue resembling cementum. **3.** a central lesion of the jaws.

cementoblast, (in dentistry), a large squamous or cuboidal cell that is responsible for the formation of cementum on the root dentin of a developing tooth.

cementoblastoma /simen'tōblastō'mə/, *pl.* **cementoblastomas, cementoblastomata** [L *caementum* + Gk *blastos* germ, *oma* tumor], an odontogenic fibrous tumor consisting of cells developing into cementoblasts but containing only a small amount of calcified tissue.

cementoma /sē'mentō'mə/, *pl.* **cementomas, cementomata** [L *caementum* + Gk *oma* tumor], an accumulation of cementum existing free at the apex of a tooth, probably caused by trauma rather than neoplastic growth.

cementopathia [L *caementum* + Gk *pathos* disease], an abnormal condition of the teeth caused by necrotic cementum and insufficient cementogenesis.

cementum /simen'təm/, the bonelike connective tissue that covers the roots of the teeth and helps to support them.

cen, abbreviation for **centromere.**

CEN, abbreviation for *Certified Emergency Nurse.*

cenesthesia /sē'nesthē'zhə/ [Gk *kenos* empty, *aisthesis* feeling], the general sense of existing, derived as the aggregate of all the various stimuli and reactions throughout the body at any specific moment to produce a feeling of health or of illness.

cenogenesis /sē'nōjen'əsis/ [Gk *kenos* empty, *genein* to produce], the development of physical characteristics that are absent in earlier forms of a species, as an adaptive response to environmental conditions.

cenophobia. See **kenophobia.**

censor [L *censere* to assess], **1.** a person who monitors or evaluates books, newspapers, plays, works of art, speech, or other means of expression in order to suppress certain kinds of information. **2.** (in psychoanalysis) a psychic suppression that allows unconscious thoughts to rise to consciousness only if they are heavily disguised.

center [Gk *kentron*], **1.** the middle point of the body or geometric entity, equidistant from points on the periphery. **2.** a group of neurons with a common function, such as the accelerating center in the brain that controls the heartbeat.

center of gravity, the midpoint or center of the weight of a body or object. In the standing adult human the center of gravity is in the midpelvic cavity, between the symphysis pubis and the umbilicus.

Centers for Disease Control and Prevention (CDCP), a federal agency of the U.S. government that provides facilities and services for the investigation, identification, prevention, and control of disease. It is concerned with all aspects of the epidemiology and the laboratory diagnosis of disease. Immunization programs, quarantine regulations and programs, laboratory standards, and community surveillance for disease are among the activities of the CDC, located in Atlanta. Formerly, the Communicable Disease Center.

centesis /sentē′sis/ [Gk *kentesis* pricking], a perforation or a puncture, such as a paracentesis, abdominocentesis, or thoracocentesis.

centigrade. See **Celsius.**

centimeter (cm) /sen′timē′tər/ [L *centum* hundred; Gk *metron* measure], the metric unit of measurement equal to one hundredth of a meter, or 0.3937 inches.

centimeter-gram-second system (cgs, CGS), the internationally accepted scientific system of expressing length, mass, and time in basic units of centimeters, grams, and seconds. The CGS system is gradually being replaced by the Système International d'Unités (SI) or the International System of Units, based on the meter, kilogram, and second.

centipede bite [L *centum* hundred, *pes* foot], a wound produced by the poison claws and the first body segment of a centipede, an elongate arthropod with many pairs of legs. The bite of a few species may cause painful local inflammation, fever, headache, vomiting, and dizziness.

centipoise /sen′təpois/ [Jean L. M. Poiseuille, French physiologist, b. 1799], a measure of the viscosity of a liquid, equal to one hundredth of a poise.

central [Gk *kentron* center], pertaining to or situated at a center.

central amaurosis [Gk *kentron; amauroein* to darken], blindness caused by a disease of the central nervous system.

central auditory processing disorder (CAPD), difficulty in processing and interpreting auditory stimuli in the absence of a peripheral hearing loss, usually resulting from a problem in the brainstem or cerebral cortex. Children with CAPD often have difficulty reading and may exhibit other learning disabilities as well.

central canal of spinal cord [Gk *kentron;* L *canalis* channel], the conduit that runs the entire length of the spinal cord and contains most of the 140 ml of cerebrospinal fluid in the body of the average individual. The central canal of the spinal cord lies in the center of the cord between the ventral and the dorsal gray commissures and extends cranialward into the medulla oblongata, where it opens into the fourth ventricle of the brain.

central catheter [Gk, *kentron,* central, *katheter,* a thing lowered into], a catheter inserted into either a central artery or a central vein for diagnostic or therapeutic procedures.

central chemoreceptor, any of the sensory nerve cells or chemical receptors that are located in the medulla of the brain.

central chondrosarcoma [Gk *kentron; chondros* cartilage, *sarx* flesh, *oma* tumor], a malignant cartilaginous tumor that forms inside a bone.

central deafness. See **central auditory processing disorder (CAPD).**

central electrode, a key part of a radiation detection instrument. It consists of a positively charged rigid wire in the center of a gas-filled cylinder.

central fissure. See **central sulcus.**

central implantation. See **superficial implantation.**

central line, an intravenous line inserted for continuous access to a central vein for administering fluids and medicines and for obtaining diagnostic information. Keeping the central line in place ensures accessibility to the venous system in case the veins collapse.

central lobe, one of the lobes constituting each of the cerebral hemispheres, lying hidden in the depths of the lateral sulcus. The central lobe can be seen only if the lips of the sulcus are parted or cut away.

central necrosis [Gk, *kentron,* central, *nekros,* dead, *osis,* condition], death of the central part of a tissue or organ.

central nervous system (CNS) [Gk *kentron;* L *nervus* nerve; Gk *systema*], one of the two main divisions of the nervous system of the body, consisting of the brain and the spinal cord. The central nervous system processes information to and from the peripheral nervous system and is the main network of coordination and control for the entire body. The spinal cord extends various types of nerve fibers from the brain and acts as a switching and relay terminal for the peripheral nervous system. The 12 pairs of cranial nerves emerge directly from the brain. Sensory nerves and motor nerves of the peripheral system leave the spinal cord separately between the vertebrae but unite to form 31 pairs of spinal nerves containing sensory fibers and motor fibers. More than 10 billion neurons constitute but one tenth of the brain cells, the other cells consisting of neuroglia. Flowing through various cavities of the central nervous system, such as the ventricles of the brain, the subarachnoid spaces of the brain and spinal cord, and the central canal of the spinal cord is the cerebrospinal fluid. The brain and the spinal cord are composed of gray matter and white matter. The gray matter contains primarily nerve cells and associated processes; the white matter consists of bundles of predominantly myelinated nerve fibers.

central nervous system depressant, any drug that decreases the function of the central nervous system, such as alcohol, barbiturates, and hypnotics. Such drugs can depress excitable tissue throughout the central nervous system by stabilizing neural membranes, decreasing the amount of transmitter released by the nerve impulse, and generally depressing postsynaptic responsiveness and ion movement. Central nervous system depressants elevate the seizure threshold and can produce physical dependence in a relatively short period of time. Sudden withdrawal of general central nervous system depressants that have been used in high doses for prolonged periods can be fatal to some individuals.

central nervous system stimulant, a substance that quickens the activity of the central nervous system by increasing the rate of neuronal discharge or by blocking an inhibitory neurotransmitter. Many natural and synthetic compounds stimulate the central nervous system, but only a few are used therapeutically.

central nervous system syndrome (CNS syndrome), a constellation of neurologic and emotional signs and symptoms that results from a massive whole-body dosage of radiation.

central nervous system tumor, a neoplasm of the brain or spinal cord that characteristically does not spread beyond the cerebrospinal axis, although it may be highly invasive locally and have widespread effects on body functions. Many brain tumors are metastatic lesions from primary cancer in the breast, lung, GI tract, kidney, or a site of melanoma.

central neurogenic hyperventilation (CNHV) [Gk *kentron; neuron* nerve, *genein* to produce], a pattern of breathing marked by rapid and regular respirations at a rate of about 25 per minute. Increasing regularity, rather than rate, is an important diagnostic sign because it indicates an increasing depth of coma.

central pain [Gk, *kentron;* L, *poena,* penalty], pain caused by a lesion in centrally located nerve tissue.

central paralysis [Gk, *kentron, paralyein,* to be palsied], paralysis caused by a lesion in the central nervous system.

central placenta previa [Gk *kentron;* L, flat cake; *praevius* preceding], placenta previa in which the placenta is implanted in the lower segment of the uterus and completely covers the internal os of the uterine cervix. In labor, as the cervix dilates, the placenta is gradually separated from the underlying blood vessels in the uterine lining, resulting in bleeding.

central ray (CR), the portion of the x-ray beam that is directed toward the center of the film or of the object being radiographed.

central scotoma Gk *kentron; skotos* darkness, *oma* tumor, an area of blindness or site of depressed vision involving the macula of the retina.

central sleep apnea, a form of sleep apnea resulting from a decreased respiratory center output. It may involve primary brainstem medullary depression.

central stimulant. See **central nervous system stimulant.**

central sulcus [Gk *kentron;* L, furrow], a cleft separating the frontal from the parietal lobes of brain.

central tendon, a broad connective tissue sheet that forms the diaphragm. It is composed of interlacing fibers that arise from the lumbar vertebrae, the costal margin, and the xiphoid process of the sternum.

central venous catheter, a catheter that is threaded through the internal jugular, antecubital, or subclavian vein, usually with the tip resting in the superior vena cava or the right atrium.

central venous oxygen saturation (CVSo$_2$), the oxygen saturation in the vena cava. The CVSo$_2$ is measured through a central venous catheter and is useful in measuring cardiac output.

central venous pressure (CVP), the blood pressure in the large veins of the body, as distinguished from peripheral venous pressure in an extremity. It is measured with a water manometer that may be attached to the head of a patient's bed and to a central venous catheter inserted into the vena cava.

central venous pressure (CVP) monitor, a device for measuring and recording the venous blood pressure by means of an indwelling catheter and a pressure manometer.

central venous return, the blood from the venous system that flows into the right atrium through the vena cava.

central vertigo [Gk *kentron;* L *vertigo* dizziness], vertigo that is caused by a central nervous system disorder.

central vision, vision that results from images falling on the macula of the retina.

centrencephalic /sen'trensif'ik/ [Gk *kentron + enkephalos* brain], of, pertaining to, or involving the center of the encephalon.

centrifugal /sentrif'ŏŏgəl/ [Gk *kentron +* L *fugere* to flee], **1.** denoting a force that is directed outward, away from a central point or axis, such as the force that keeps

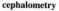

the moon in its orbit around the earth. **2.** a direction away from the head.

centrifugal analyzer, equipment that uses centrifugal force to mix the sample aliquot with reagent and a spinning rotor to pass the reaction mixture through a detector.

centrifugal current, an electric current in the body with the positive pole near the nerve center and the negative pole at the periphery.

centrifugal force [Gk, *kentron,* L, *fugere,* to flee, *fortis,* strong], a natural force that affects objects undergoing circular motion. The force is the product of the mass and its radial acceleration. In centrifugation, heavier components of a mixture are separated from other components by being thrown to the periphery of the orbit.

centrifuge /sen′trifyo̅o̅j′/ [Gk *kentron* + L *fugere* to flee], a device for separating components of different densities contained in liquid by spinning them at high speeds. Centrifugal force causes the heavier components to move to one part of the container, leaving the lighter substances in another. **–centrifugal,** *adj.,* **centrifuge,** *v.*

centrilobular /sen′trəlob′yələr/ [Gk *kentron* + L *lobulus* small lobe], pertaining to, or situated at the center of a lobule.

centriole /sen′trē-ōl′/ [Gk *kentron*], an intracellular organelle, usually as a component of the centrosome. Often occurring in pairs, centrioles are associated with cell division. They appear to aid in the formation of the spindle that develops during mitosis.

centripetal /sentrip′ətəl/ [Gk *kentron* + L *petere* to seek], **1.** denoting an afferent direction, such as that of a sensory nerve impulse traveling toward the brain. **2.** denoting the direction of a force pulling an object toward an axis of rotation or constraining an object to a specific curved path.

centripetal current, an electric current passing through the body from a peripheral positive electrode to a negative pole near the nerve center.

centripetal force, (in radiology) a "center-seeking" electrical force that holds electrons in their orbits about the nucleus of an atom.

centromere /sen′trəmir/ [Gk *kentron* + *meros* part], the specialized, constricted region of the chromosome that joins the two chromatids to each other and attaches to the spindle fiber in mitosis and meiosis. During cell division the centromeres split longitudinally, half going to each of the new daughter chromosomes.

centrosome [Gk *kentron* + *soma* body], a

self-propagating cytoplasmic organelle, which consists of the centrosphere and the centrioles. It is located near the nucleus and functions as the dynamic center of the cell, especially during mitosis.

centrosphere [Gk *kentron* + *sphaira* ball], the differentiated, condensed area of cytoplasm surrounding the centrioles in the centrosome of the cell.

centrum, *pl.* **centra** [L; Gk *kentron*], any kind of center, especially one related to a structure of the body, as the centrum semiovale of a cerebral hemisphere.

CEO, abbreviation for **Chief Executive Officer.**

cephalad /sef′əlad/ [Gk *kephale* head], toward the head, away from the end, or tail.

cephalalgia /sef′əlal′jə/ [Gk *kephale* head, *algos* pain], headache, often combined with another word to indicate a specific type of headache, such as histamine cephalalgia.

cephalexin /sef′əlek′sin/, a cephalosporin antibacterial prescribed orally in the treatment of certain infections.

cephalgia. See **cephalalgia, headache.**

cephalhematoma /sef′əlhē′mətō′mə, -hem′ətō′mə/, swelling caused by subcutaneous bleeding and accumulation of blood.

cephalic /sifal′ik/, of or pertaining to the head.

cephalic index [Gk *kephale, index* pointer], a ratio between the breadth and length of the head. It is calculated as 100 times the maximum breadth of the head measured at the greatest diameter of the cranial vault above the supramastoid crest divided by the maximum length measured from the most prominent point on the glabella to the opisthocranion.

cephalic presentation, a classification of fetal position in which the head of the fetus is at the uterine cervix. Cephalic presentation is usually further qualified by an indication of the part of the head presenting, such as the occiput, bregma, or mentum.

cephalic vein, one of the four superficial veins of the upper limb. It receives deoxygenated blood from the dorsal and the palmar surfaces of the forearm.

cephalocaudal [Gk *kephale* + L *cauda* tail], pertaining to the long axis of the body, or the relationship between the head and the base of the spine.

cephalomelus /sef′əlom′ələs/ [Gk *kephale* + *melos* limb], a deformed individual with a structure resembling an arm or a leg protruding from the head.

cephalometry /sef′əlom′ətrē/, scientific measurement of the head, such as that performed in dentistry to determine appropriate orthodontic procedures for correcting malocclusions and other abnormal conditions. **–cephalometric,** *adj.*

cephalopagus. See **craniopagus.**

cephalopelvic, pertaining to a relationship between the fetal head and the maternal pelvis.

cephalopelvic disproportion (CPD) [Gk *kephale* + L *pelvis* basin; *dis* opposite of, *proportio* similarity], an obstetric condition in which a baby's head is too large or a mother's birth canal too small to permit normal labor or birth. In **relative CPD,** the size of the baby's head is within normal limits but larger than average or the size of the mother's birth canal is within normal limits but smaller than average, or both. In **absolute CPD,** the baby's head is markedly or abnormally enlarged or the mother's birth canal is markedly or abnormally contracted, making vaginal delivery impossible.

cephaloridine /sef′əlôr′idēn/, a cephalosporin antibiotic prescribed in the treatment of a variety of infections.

cephalosporin /sef′əlōspôr′in/ [Gk *kephale* + *sporos* seed], a semisynthetic derivative of an antibiotic originally derived from the microorganism *Cephalosporium acremonium.* Cephalosporins are similar in structure to penicillins except for a beta-lactam-dihydrothiazine ring in place of beta-lactam-thiazolidin in penicillin.

cephalothin sodium /sef′əlōthin/, a cephalosporin antibacterial prescribed in the treatment of a variety of infections.

cephalothoracoiliopagus. See **synadelphus.**

cephalothoracopagus /sef′əlōthôr′əkop′ə-gəs/ [Gk *kephale* + *thorax* chest, *pagos* joined], a conjoined twin fetal monster united at the head, neck, and thorax.

cephapirin /sef′əprin/, an antibiotic prescribed in the treatment of infections caused by cephapirin-susceptible strains of a wide variety of microorganisms causing septicemia, endocarditis, osteomyelitis, and infections of the respiratory tract, urinary tract, and skin.

cephradine /sef′rədēn/, a cephalosporin antibacterial prescribed in the treatment of certain bacterial infections.

ceramics, (in dentistry) the technology of making dental restorations from fused porcelain and other glasses.

cercaria /sərker′ē·ə/, *pl.* **cercariae** [Gk *kerkos* tail], a wormlike form of trematode. It develops in a freshwater snail and is released into the water. Cercariae enter the body of the next host by ingestion, by direct invasion through the skin, or through a cut or other break in the skin. They en-

cyst and complete their development in various organs of the body. Each species tends to migrate to one organ, such as *Fasciola hepatica,* which becomes a liver fluke.

cerclage /serkläzh′/ [Fr, cask hooping], **1.** an orthopedic procedure in which the ends of an oblique bone fracture or the chips of a broken patella are bound together with a wire loop or a metal band to hold the bone fragments in position until healed. **2.** a procedure in which a taut silicone band is applied around the sclera to restore contact between the retina and the choroid when the retina is detached. **3.** an obstetric procedure in which a nonabsorbable suture is used for holding the cervix closed to prevent spontaneous abortion in a woman who has an incompetent cervix.

cerea flexibilitas /sirē′ə flek′sibil′itas/ [L, waxlike flexibility], a cataleptic state, frequently observed in catatonic schizophrenia, in which the limbs retain for an indefinite period of time the positions in which they are placed.

cerebellar /ser′əbel′ər/ [L *cerebellum* small brain], of or pertaining to the cerebellum.

cerebellar angioblastoma [L *cerebellum;* Gk *aggeion* vessel, *blastos* germ, *oma*], a tumor in the cerebellum composed of a mass of blood vessels. It may be cystic and is frequently associated with von Hippel-Lindau disease.

cerebellar artery occlusion, an obstruction of one of the arteries supplying the cerebellum.

cerebellar ataxia [L, *cerebellum,* small brain, Gk, *ataxia,* lack of order], a loss of muscle coordination caused by a lesion in the cerebellum.

cerebellar atrophy [L *cerebellum;* Gk *a, trophe* not nourishment], any of several diseases characterized by deterioration and wasting of tissues of the cerebellum.

cerebellar cortex, the superficial gray matter of the cerebellum covering the white substance in the medullary core and consisting of two layers, an external molecular layer and an internal granule cell layer. The layers are separated by an incomplete stratum of Purkinje cells.

cerebellar gait [L, *cerebellum,* small brain, ONorse, *geta,* a way], a staggering gait in which the person walks with a wide base and has difficulty turning. The feet are thrown outward and the person comes down first on the heel and then on the toes. The condition is caused by a lesion in the cerebellum or cerebellar pathways.

cerebellar inferior peduncle [L, *cerebellum,* small brain, *inferior,* lower, *pes,* foot], a band of nerve fibers that forms the lateral boundary of the bottom part of the fourth ventricle and carries afferent fibers into the cerebellum.

cerebellar middle peduncle [L, *cerebellum,* small brain, *medius, pes,* foot], a lateral extension of the transverse nerve fibers of the pons. It consists mainly of fibers from the pontine nuclei to the neocerebellum.

cerebellar speech [L *cerebellum;* AS *spaec*], abnormal speech seen in diseases of the cerebellum. It is characterized by slow, jerky, and slurred articulation that may be intermittent and explosive or monotonous and unvaried in pitch.

cerebellar superior peduncle [L, *cerebellum,* small brain, *superior, pes,* foot], a band of nerve fibers that pass from the cerebellum on either side of the superior medullary velum. It includes nerve tracts linking the dentate nucleus to the red nucleus of the midbrain and to the thalamus.

cerebellar tremor [L, *cerebellum,* small brain + *tremor,* shaking], an intention tremor or trembling during voluntary movements due to lesions in the cerebellum.

cerebellopontine /ser′əbel′ōpon′tīn/ [L *cerebellum* + *pons* bridge], leading from the cerebellum to the pons varolii.

cerebellospinal /ser′əbel′ōspī′nəl/ [L *cerebellum* + *spina* backbone], leading from the cerebellum to the spinal cord.

cerebellum /ser′əbel′əm/, *pl.* **cerebellums, cerebella** [L, small brain], the part of the brain located in the posterior cranial fossa behind the brainstem. It consists of two lateral cerebellar hemispheres, or lobes, and a middle section called the vermis. Three pairs of peduncles link it with the brainstem. Its functions are concerned with coordinating voluntary muscular activity.

cerebral, of or pertaining to the cerebrum.

cerebral aneurysm [L *cerebrum* brain; Gk *aneurysma* widening], an abnormal localized dilatation of a cerebral artery, most commonly the result of congenital weakness of the media or muscle layer of the vessel wall. Cerebral aneurysms may also be caused by infection, such as subacute bacterial endocarditis or syphilis, and by neoplasms, arteriosclerosis, and trauma. Cerebral aneurysms may occur in infancy or old age and may be fusiform dilatations of the entire circumference of an artery or saccular outcroppings of the side of a vessel, which may be as small as a pinhead or as large as an orange but are usually the size of a pea.

cerebral angiography L *cerebrum;* Gk *aggeion* vessel, *graphein* to record, an

x-ray procedure for visualizing the vascular system of the brain by injecting a radiopaque contrast material into a carotid, subclavian, brachial, or femoral artery and taking x-ray films at specific intervals in a series.

cerebral aqueduct [L *cerebrum; aqueductus* water canal], the narrow conduit between the third and fourth ventricles in the midbrain that conveys the cerebrospinal fluid.

cerebral compression [L, *cerebrum,* brain, *comprimere,* to press together], any abnormal condition, such as hemorrhage, abscess, or tumor, that increases intracranial pressure. If untreated, the compression destroys the brain tissues and causes herniation of the brain.

cerebral cortex [L *cerebrum; cortex* bark], a thin layer of gray matter on the surface of the cerebral hemisphere, folded into gyri with about two thirds of its area buried in fissures. It integrates higher mental functions, general movement, visceral functions, perception, and behavioral reactions. It has been classified many different ways, with reference according to supposed phylogenetic and ontogenetic differences, structure, cell, and fiber layers, and function areas. Research has described more than 200 areas on the basis of differences in myelinated fiber patterns and has defined 47 separate function areas with different cell designs.

cerebral deafness. See **central auditory processing disorder.**

cerebral depressant [L *cerebrum, deprimere* to press down], a drug or other agent that has a sedating effect on the brain, reducing activity and alertness, and, in some instances, causing a loss of consciousness.

cerebral dominance, the specialization of each of the two cerebral hemispheres in the integration and control of different functions. In 90% of the population, the left cerebral hemisphere specializes in or dominates the ability to speak and write and the ability to understand spoken and written words. In the other 10% of the population, either the right hemisphere or both hemispheres dominate the speech and writing abilities. The right cerebral hemisphere perceives tactual stimuli and visual spatial relationships better than the left cerebral hemisphere.

cerebral edema [L *cerebrum;* Gk *oidema* swelling], an accumulation of fluid in the brain tissues. Causes can include an infection, tumor, and trauma. Brain tissues are compressed. Early symptoms are involuntary muscle contractions, dilated pupils, and a gradual loss of consciousness. Cerebral edema can be fatal.

cerebral embolism [L *cerebrum; embolos* plug], an embolus that blocks the flow of blood through the vessels of the cerebrum, resulting in tissue ischemia distal to the occlusion.

cerebral gigantism [L *cerebrum;* Gk *gigas* giant], an abnormal condition characterized by excessive weight and size at birth, accelerated growth during the first 4 or 5 years after birth without any increase in the level of growth hormone, and then reversion to normal growth.

cerebral hemiplegia [L *cerebrum;* Gk *hemi* half, *plege* stroke], paralysis of one side of the body caused by a lesion in the brain.

cerebral hemisphere [L *cerebrum;* Gk *hemi* half, *sphaira* ball], one of the halves of the cerebrum. The two cerebral hemispheres are divided by a deep longitudinal fissure and are connected medially at the bottom of the fissure by the corpus callosum. Prominent grooves subdivide each hemisphere into four major lobes. The hemispheres consist of external gray substance, internal white substance, and internal gray substance and are covered by cerebral cortexes at the surface.

cerebral hemorrhage [L *cerebrum;* Gk *haima* blood, *rhegnynei* to gush], a hemorrhage from a blood vessel in the brain. Three criteria used to classify cerebral hemorrhages are location (subarachnoid, extradural, subdural), the kind of vessel involved (arterial, venous, capillary), and origin (traumatic, degenerative). Each kind of cerebral hemorrhage has its own clinical characteristics. Most cerebral hemorrhages occur in the region of the basal ganglia and are caused by the rupture of a sclerotic artery as a result of hypertension. Other causes of rupture include congenital aneurysm, cerebrovascular infarction, and head trauma.

cerebral infarction [L *cerebrum, infarcire* to stuff], an area of brain tissue that undergoes necrosis secondary to an interruption of the blood supply, with or without hemorrhage. An infarct may be the result of thrombosis, an embolism, or vasospasm.

cerebral localization, 1. the determination of various areas in the cerebral cortex associated with specific functions, such as the 47 areas of Brodmann. 2. the diagnosis of a cerebral condition, such as a brain lesion, by determining the area of the brain affected, a determination made by analysis of the signs manifested by the patient and of electroencephalograms.

cerebral nerve. See **cranial nerves.**

cerebral palsy [L *cerebrum;* Gk *para* beyond, *lysis* loosening], a motor function disorder caused by a permanent, nonpro-gressive brain defect or lesion present at birth or shortly thereafter. The neurologic deficit may result in spastic hemiplegia, monoplegia, diplegia, or quadriplegia, athetosis or ataxia, seizures, paresthesia, varying degrees of mental retardation, and impaired speech, vision, and hearing. The disorder is usually associated with premature or abnormal birth and intrapartum asphyxia, causing damage to the nervous system. Walking is usually delayed, and, when attempted, the child manifests a typical scissors gait. The arms may be affected only slightly, but the fingers are often spastic. Deep-tendon reflexes are exaggerated, and there may be slurred speech, delay in acquiring sphincter control, and athetotic movements of the face and hands. Treatment is individualized and may include the use of braces, surgical correction of deformities, speech therapy, and various muscle relaxants and anticonvulsants.

cerebral peduncle [L, *cerebrum,* brain, *pes,* foot], a pair of cylindrical masses of nerve fibers at the upper border of the pons that disappears into the left and right hemispheres. It includes corticopontine and pyramidal-tract fibers.

cerebral perfusion pressure (CPP), a measure of the amount of blood flow to the brain. It is calculated by subtracting the intracranial pressure from the mean systemic arterial blood pressure.

cerebral thrombosis [L *cerebrum;* Gk *thrombos* lump, *osis* condition], a clotting of blood in any cerebral vessel, such as the middle cerebral artery or the ascending parietal artery.

cerebral vertigo [L *cerebrum + vertigo* dizziness], vertigo that is caused by organic brain disease.

cerebriform carcinoma. See **medullary carcinoma.**

cerebrocerebellar atrophy [L *cerebrum* brain, *cerebellum* small brain; Gk *a, trophe* without nourishment], a deterioration of the cerebellum caused by certain abiotrophic diseases.

cerebroid /ser'əbroid/ [L *cerebrum +* Gk *eidos* form], resembling the substance of the brain.

cerebroma /ser'əbrō'mə/, pl. **cerebromas, cerebromata,** any unusual mass of brain tissue.

cerebromedullary tube. See **neural tube.**

cerebropathia psychia toxemia. See **Korsakoff's psychosis.**

cerebroretinal angiomatosis /ser'əbrō-ret'ənəl, sərē'brō-/ [L *cerebrum + rete* net; Gk *aggeion* vessel, *oma* tumor, *osis* condition], a hereditary disease characterized by congenital, tumorlike vascular nodules in the retina and cerebellum.

cerebroside /ser'əbrōsīd'/, any of a group of glycolipids found in the brain and other tissue of the nervous system, especially the myelin sheath.

cerebroside sulfatase [L, *cerebrum,* brain, *sulfur,* brimstone, *ase,* enzyme], an enzyme of the hydrolase class that catalyzes the reaction of cerebroside 3-sulfate + H_2O. A deficiency of the enzyme, which is transmitted as an autosomal recessive gene, is a cause of metachromatic leukodystrophy.

cerebrospinal /ser'əbrōspī'nəl, sərē'brō-/, pertaining to or involving the brain and the spinal cord.

cerebrospinal axis [L *cerebrum, spina* spine, *axle*], a line formed by the brain and spinal cord about which the body turns.

cerebrospinal fluid (CSF), the fluid that flows through and protects the four ventricles of the brain, the subarachnoid space, and the spinal canal. It is composed mainly of secretions of the choroid plexi in the lateral ventricles and in the third and the fourth ventricles of the brain. Openings in the roof of the fourth ventricle allow the fluid to flow into the subarachnoid spaces around the brain and the spinal cord. Samples of the fluid may be removed by lumbar puncture between the third and fourth lumbar vertebrae.

cerebrospinal nerves, the 12 pairs of cranial nerves and 31 pairs of spinal nerves that originate in the brain and spinal cord.

cerebrospinal pressure [L *cerebrum, spina, premere,* to press], the pressure of cerebrospinal fluid in the central nervous system. It usually measures between 100 and 150 mm of water and is measured by a manometer attached to the end of a needle after it has been inserted into the subarachnoid space.

cerebrospinal rhinorrhea [L *cerebrum, spina;* Gk *rhis* nose + *rhoia* flow], a discharge of cerebrospinal fluid from the nose.

cerebrotendinous xanthomatosis. See **van Bogaert's disease.**

cerebrovascular /ser'əbrōvas'kyələr, sərē'brō-/ [L *cerebrum* + *vasculum* little vessel], of or pertaining to the vascular system and blood supply of the brain.

cerebrovascular accident (CVA), an abnormal condition of the blood vessels of the brain characterized by occlusion by an embolus or cerebrovascular hemorrhage, resulting in ischemia of the brain tissues normally perfused by the damaged vessels.

cerebrum /ser'əbrəm, sərē'brəm/, *pl.* **cerebrums, cerebra** [L, brain], the largest and uppermost section of the brain, divided by a central sulcus into the left and the right cerebral hemispheres, and connected by the corpus callosum. The internal structures of the hemispheres merge with those of the diencephalon and further communicate with the brain stem through the cerebral peduncles. The cerebrum performs sensory functions, motor functions, and less easily defined integration functions associated with various mental activities. Some of the processes that are controlled or affected by the cerebrum are memory, speech, writing, and emotional response. **–cerebral,** *adj.*

cerium (Ce) [L *Ceres* Roman goddess of agriculture], a ductile, gray rare-earth element. Its atomic number is 58; its atomic weight is 140.13. A compound of cerium, cerium oxalate, is used as a sedative, an antiemetic, and an antitussive.

cerium nitrate, a topical antiseptic used to control bacterial and fungal infections in the treatment of burns.

ceroid /sir'oid/ [L *cera* wax; Gk *eidos* form], a golden, waxy pigment appearing in the cirrhotic livers of some individuals, in the GI tract, in the nervous system, and in the muscles.

ceroma /sirō'mə/, *pl.* **ceromas, ceromata** [L *cera* wax; Gk *oma* tumor], a neoplasm that has undergone waxy degeneration.

certifiable [L, *certus,* certain, *facere,* to make], **1.** a legal term pertaining to a patient with a mental illness who has been found incompetent and requires care by a guardian or in a hospital. **2.** pertaining to infectious diseases or dangerous conditions that must be reported to local health authorities.

certificate-of-need or -necessity, a statement or certificate issued by a governmental agency to the effect that a proposed construction or modification of a health facility will be needed at the time of its completion.

certification [L *certus* certain, *facere* to make], **1.** a process in which an individual, an institution, or an educational program is evaluated and recognized as meeting certain predetermined standards. Certification is usually made by a nongovernmental agency. **2.** (in nursing) a process in which the professional organization or association verifies the fact that a person who is licensed to practice has met the standards for specialty practice specified by the profession.

certification for excellence, (in nursing) certification that recognizes professional achievement, advanced training, and superior performance in a special or subspecial field of practice.

certification in nursing, one of two processes in which a professional organization formally recognizes the right of a nurse to practice a subspecialty of nursing. One process, certification for excellence, bases recognition on professional achievement, advanced training, and superior performance. The second process, entry level certification, bases recognition on advanced training in a program approved by the certifying organization.

certified dental assistant, a person who has successfully completed the education, training, and testing of the Certification Board of the American Dental Assistant Association.

certified medical transcriptionist. See **medical transcriptionist.**

certified milk, raw milk that is obtained, handled, and marketed in compliance with state health laws. The milk must be produced by disease-free cows, which are regularly inspected by a veterinarian and are milked by sterilized equipment in hygienic surroundings, contain less than a specified low bacterial count, and be less than 36 hours old when delivered.

Certified Nurse-Midwife (CNM), (according to the American College of Nurse-Midwives) "an individual educated in the two disciplines of nursing and midwifery, who possesses evidence of certification according to the requirements of the American College of Nurse-Midwives."

Certified Occupational Therapy Assistant (COTA), an allied health professional who, under the direction of an occupational therapist, directs an individual's participation in selected tasks to restore, reinforce, and enhance performance; facilitates learning of skills and functions essential for adaptation and productivity; diminishes or corrects pathology; and promotes and maintains health.

certified registered nurse anesthetist. See **nurse anesthetist.**

certified respiratory therapy technician (CRTT), a health care professional who performs routine care, management, and treatment of patients with respiratory disorders under the supervision of a respiratory therapist. Certification requires completion of an approved 1-year training course and examination by the National Board for Respiratory Care.

certify, **1.** to guarantee formally that certain requirements have been met based on expert knowledge of significant, pertinent facts. **2.** to attest, by a legal process, that someone is insane. **3.** to attest to the fact of someone's death in writing, usually on a form as required by local authority. **4.** to declare that a person has satisified certain requirements for membership or acceptance into a professional or other group. –**certification,** *n.,* **certifiable,** *adj.*

cerulean /sirōō'lē-ən/ [L *caelum* sky], sky-blue.

ceruloplasmin /sirōō'lōplaz'min/ [L *caelum* sky; Gk *plassein* to shape], a glycoprotein in plasma that transports 96% of the plasma copper.

cerumen /sirōō'mən/ [L *cera* wax], a yellowish or brownish waxy secretion produced by vestigial apocrine sweat glands in the external ear canal.

ceruminolytic /sirōō'mənōlit'ik/, pertaining to a drug or other agent that dissolves cerumen.

ceruminolytic agent [L *cera;* Gk *lysis* a loosening; L *agere* to do], a medication that dissolves or loosens cerumen (earwax) to allow for removal.

ceruminosis /sirōō'minō'sis/, excessive buildup of cerumen or earwax in the external auditory canal. It can cause discomfort, symptoms of hearing loss, and irritation leading to the development of infection.

ceruminous gland /sirōō'minəs/, one of a number of tiny structures in the external ear canal, believed to be modified sweat glands. They secrete a waxy cerumen instead of watery sweat.

cervical /sur'vikəl/ [L *cervix* neck], **1.** of or pertaining to the neck or the region of the neck. **2.** of or pertaining to the constricted area of a necklike structure, such as the neck of a tooth or the cervix of the uterus.

cervical abortion [L *cervix; ab* away from, *oriri* to be born], spontaneous expulsion of a cervical pregnancy.

cervical adenitis [L *cervix;* Gk *aden* gland, *itis* inflammation], an abnormal condition characterized by enlarged, tender lymph nodes of the neck.

cervical amputation, the removal of the neck of the uterus.

cervical canal, the canal within the uterine cervix, which protrudes into the vagina. The uterine end of the canal is closed at the internal os and, in the nullipara, at the distal end by the external os. The canal is a passageway through which the menstrual flow escapes and, vastly dilated and effaced by labor, through which the infant must come to be delivered vaginally. Sperm must travel upward through the canal to reach the uterus and fallopian tubes.

cervical cancer, a neoplasm of the uterine cervix that can be detected in the early, curable stage by the Papanicolaou (Pap) test. Factors associated with the development of cervical cancer are coitus at an early age, many sexual partners, genital herpesvirus infections, multiparity, and poor obstetric and gynecologic care. Early cervical neoplasia is usually asymptomatic, but there may be a watery vaginal discharge or occasional spotting of blood; advanced lesions may cause a dark, foul-smelling vaginal discharge, leakage from bladder or rectal fistulas, anorexia, weight loss, and back and leg pains. About 90% of cervical tumors are squamous cell carcinomas, fewer than 10% are adenocarcinomas, and others are mixtures of these kinds, or, in rare cases, sarcomas. Tumors on the surface of the cervix may be huge, polypoid masses whereas endophytic lesions tend to be small and hard; ulcerative lesions may cause extensive erosion. Cervical cancer invades the tissues of adjacent organs and may metastasize through lymphatic channels to distant sites, including the lungs, bone, liver, brain, and paraaortic nodes.

cervical cap, a contraceptive device consisting of a small rubber cup fitted over the uterine cervix to prevent spermatozoa from entering the cervical canal. In some studies, its contraceptive effectiveness equals or exceeds that of the diaphragm. It may be more comfortable than the diaphragm and may be left safely on the cervix for days or weeks and remain effective.

cervical cauterization, the destruction, usually by heat or electric current, of the superficial tissues of the cervix.

cervical conization, the excision of a cone-shaped section of tissue from the endocervix.

cervical cyst [L, *cervix,* neck; Gk, *kystis,* bag], a mucus cyst of the uterine cervix.

cervical dilatation, [L *dilatare,* to widen], the diameter of the opening of the cervix in labor as measured on vaginal examination, expressed in centimeters. At full dilatation the diamter of the cervical opening is 10 cm.

cervical disk syndrome, an abnormal condition characterized by compression or irritation of the cervical nerve roots in or near the intervertebral foramina before the roots divide into the anterior and the posterior rami. Cervical disk syndrome may be caused by ruptured intervertebral disks, degenerative cervical disk disease, or cervical injuries. The form caused by ruptured cervical intervertebral disks or by degenerative disease may produce varying degrees of malalignment, causing nerve root compression. Most cervical disk syndromes are caused by injuries that involve

hyperextension, which results in compression of the anatomic structures. Flexion injuries in the cervical area do not result in nerve compression. Pain, the most common symptom, usually emanates from the cervical area but may radiate down the arm to the fingers and increase with cervical motion. Other signs and symptoms associated with cervical disk syndrome may be paresthesia, headache, blurred vision, decreased skeletal function, and weakened hand grip. Examination may reveal varying degrees of muscular atrophy, sensory abnormalities, muscular weakness, and decreased reflexes.

cervical endometritis, an inflammation of the inner lining of the cervix uteri.

cervical erosion [L *cervix; erodere* to consume], a condition in which the squamous epithelium of the cervix is abraded as a result of irritation caused by infection or trauma, such as childbirth, and is replaced by columnar epithelium.

cervical fistula, an abnormal passage from the cervix to the vagina or bladder that may be caused by a malignant lesion, radiotherapy, surgical trauma, or injury during childbirth. A cervical fistula communicating with the bladder permits leakage of urine, causing irritation, odor, and embarrassment. When surgical repair is not possible, the patient is advised to take sitz baths, use a deodorizing douche or powder, such as sodium borate, and wear plastic pants or a protective apron.

cervical mucus, a secretion of the columnar epithelium lining the upper portion of the cervical canal of the uterus.

cervical mucus method of family planning. See **ovulation method of family planning.**

cervical nerves [L, *cervix,* neck, *nervus,* nerve], the eight pairs of spinal nerves that arise from the neck area of the spinal cord, from above the atlas to below the seventh vertebra. The first four supply the head and neck and the other four mainly innervate the upper limbs, scalp, and back.

cervical os. See **external cervical os, internal cervical os.**

cervical plexus, the network of nerves formed by the ventral primary divisions of the first four cervical nerves. The plexus is located opposite the cranial aspect of the first four cervical vertebrae. It communicates with certain cranial nerves and numerous muscular and cutaneous branches.

cervical plexus anesthesia, nerve block at any point below the mastoid process from C_2 to the second cervical vertebra transverse process of the sixth cervical vertebra. This method is used for operations on the area between the jaw and clavicle.

cervical polyp [L *cervix;* Gk *polys* mean, *pous* foot], an outgrowth of columnar epithelial tissue of the endocervical canal, usually attached to the wall of the canal by a slender pedicle. Often there are no symptoms, but multiple or abraded polyps may cause bleeding, especially with contact during coitus. Polyps are most common in women over 40 years of age. The cause is not known.

cervical smear [L *cervix;* AS *smero* grease], a small amount of the secretions and superficial cells of the cervix, secured with a sterile applicator or special small wooden or plastic spatula from the external os of the uterine cervix. For a Pap smear, it is obtained from the squamocolumnar junction of the uterine cervix and from the vaginal vault and endocervical canal. The specimen is spread on a specially labeled glass slide and sent for cytologic examination by a special laboratory.

cervical spondylosis [L *cervix;* Gk *spondylos* vertebra, *osis* condition], a form of degenerative joint and disk disease affecting the cervical vertebrae and resulting in compression of the associated nerve roots. Symptoms include pain or loss of feeling in the affected arm and shoulder, and stiffness of the cervical spine.

cervical stenosis [L *cervix;* Gk *stenos* narrow, *osis* condition], a narrowing of the canal between the body of the uterus and the cervical os.

cervical tenaculum. See **tenaculum.**

cervical triangle, one of two triangular areas formed in the neck by the oblique course of the sternocleidomastoideus. The anterior triangle is bounded by the midline of the throat anteriorly, the sternocleidomastoideus laterally, and the body of the mandible superiorly. The posterior triangle is bounded by the clavicle inferiorly and by the borders of the sternocleidomastoideus and the trapezius superiorly.

cervical vertebra, one of the first seven segments of the vertebral column. They differ from the thoracic and the lumbar vertebrae by the presence of a foramen in each transverse process. The first cervical vertebra has no body, supports the head, and contains a smooth, oval facet for articulation with the dens of the second cervical vertebra. The seventh cervical vertebra has a very long, prominent spinous process that is nearly horizontal in direction and is often used as a palpable reference for locating the other cervical spines.

cervicitis /sur′visi′tis/, acute or chronic inflammation of the uterine cervix. **Acute**

cervicitis is infection of the cervix marked by redness, edema, and bleeding on contact. Symptoms do not always occur but may include any or all of the following: copious, foul-smelling discharge from the vagina, pelvic pressure or pain, scant bleeding with intercourse, and itching or burning of the external genitalia. **Chronic cervicitis** is a persistent inflammation of the cervix usually occurring among women in their reproductive years. Symptoms include a thick, irritating, malodorous discharge that may in severe cases be accompanied by significant pelvic pain. The cervix looks congested and enlarged, nabothian cysts are often present, and there are signs of eversion of the cervix and often old lacerations from childbirth. The most effective treatments are hot or cold cautery.

cervicodynia /sur′vikōdin′ē·ə/, pain in the neck.

cervicofacial actinomycosis. See **actinomycosis.**

cervicolabial /sur′vikōlā′bē·əl/ [L *cervix* + *labium* lip], pertaining to or situated in the labial area of the neck of an incisor or a canine tooth.

cervicouterine /sur′vikōyōō′tərin/, pertaining to or situated at the cervix of the uterus.

cervicovaginitis, an inflammation of the cervix and vagina.

cervicovesical /sur′vikōves′ikəl/ [L *cervix* + *vesica* bladder], of or pertaining to the cervix of the uterus and the bladder.

cervix /sur′viks/ [L, neck], the part of the uterus that protrudes into the cavity of the vagina. The cervix is divided into the supravaginal portion and the vaginal portion. The supravaginal portion is separated ventrally from the bladder by the parametrium. The vaginal portion of the cervix projects into the cavity of the vagina and contains the cervical canal.

ceryl alcohol /sē′ril/ [L *cera* wax; Ar *alkohl* essence], a fatty alcohol present in many waxes.

cesarean hysterectomy [L *Caesar lex* Roman law; Gk *hystera* womb, *ektome* excision], a surgical operation in which the uterus is removed at the time of cesarean section. It is performed most often for complications of cesarean section, usually intractable hemorrhage.

cesarean postmortem section [Caesar's law; L, *post,* after + *mors,* death + *sectio*], the surgical removal of the fetus immediately after the death of the mother.

cesarean section [L *Caesar lex* Roman law, *sectio*], a surgical procedure in which the abdomen and uterus are incised and a baby is delivered transabdominally. It is performed when abnormal maternal or fetal conditions exist that are judged likely to make vaginal delivery hazardous. Maternal indications for the operation include hemorrhage from placenta previa or abruptio placenta, severe preeclampsia, and dysfunctional labor. Delivery by cesarean section at a prior parturition is no longer considered an absolute indication for repeating it in future deliveries. The incision in the skin of the abdomen may be horizontal or vertical, regardless of the kind of internal incision into the uterus.

cesium (Cs) /sē′zē·əm/ [L *caesius* sky blue], an alkali metal element. Its atomic number is 55; its atomic weight is 132.9.

cesium 137, a radioactive material with a half-life of 30.2 years that is used in radiotherapy as a sealed source of gamma rays intended for application to various malignancies that are treated by brachytherapy.

cesspool fever, *informal.* typhoid fever.

cestode. See tapeworm.

cestode infection, cestodiasis. See tapeworm infection.

cestoid /ses′toid/ [Gk *kestos* girdle, *eidos* form] **1.** resembling a tapeworm. **2.** a tapeworm of the Cestoda subclass.

CET, abbreviation for *Certified Enterostomal Therapist.*

cetyl alcohol /sē′til/ [L *cetus* whale; Ar *alkohl* essence], a fatty alcohol, derived from spermaceti, used as an emulsifier and stiffening agent in creams and ointments.

cetylpyridinium chloride /sē′təlpī′ridin′ē·əm/, an antiinfective used as a preservative in pharmaceutical preparations and as a topical cleanser.

CEU, abbreviation for **continuing education unit.**

cevitamic acid. See ascorbic acid.

Cf, symbol for the chemical element **californium.**

CF test, abbreviation for **complement-fixation test.**

CGC, abbreviation for *Certified Gastrointestinal Clinician.*

cGMP, abbreviation for **cyclic guanosine monophosphate.**

cgs, CGS, abbreviation for **centimeter-gram-second system.**

Ch¹, symbol for **Christchurch chromosome.**

Chaddock reflex [Charles G. Chaddock, American neurologist, b. 1861], an abnormal reflex, induced by firmly stroking the ulnar surface of the forearm, characterized by flexion of the wrist and extension of the fingers in fanlike position.

Chaddock's sign [Charles G. Chaddock], a variation of Babinski's reflex, elicited by firmly stroking the side of the foot just dis-

tal to the lateral malleolus, characterized by extension of the great toe and fanning of the other toes.

Chadwick's sign /chad′wiks/ [James R. Chadwick, American gynecologist, b. 1844], the bluish coloration of the vulva and vagina that develops after the sixth week of pregnancy as a normal result of local venous congestion. It is an early sign of pregnancy.

chafe [L *calefacere* to make warm], an irritation of the skin by friction, such as when rough material rubs against an unprotected area of the body.

chafing, superficial irritation of the skin by friction.

Chagas-Cruz disease. See Chagas' disease.

Chagas' disease /chag′əs/ [Carlos Chagas, Brazilian physician, b. 1879], a parasitic disease transmitted to humans by the bite of bloodsucking insects. The acute form is marked by a lesion at the site of the bite, fever, weakness, enlarged spleen and lymph nodes, edema of the face and legs, and tachycardia. The chronic form may be manifested by cardiomyopathy or by dilation of the esophagus or colon.

Chagres fever /chag′ris/ [Chagres River, Panama; L *febris*], a phlebotomus arbovirus infection transmitted to humans through the bite of a sandfly. The disease is rarely fatal and is characterized by fever, headache, and muscle pains of the chest or abdomen.

chain [L *catena*], **1.** a length of several units linked together in a linear pattern, such as a polypeptide chain of amino acids or a chain of atoms forming a chemical molecule. **2.** a group of individual bacteria linked together, such as streptococci formed by a chain of cocci. **3.** the serial relationship of certain structures essential to function, such as the chain of ossicles in the middle ear.

chain ligature [L *catena; ligare* to bind], an interlocking ligature that ties off a pedicle at several places by passing a long thread through the pedicle at different points.

chain reaction, **1.** (in chemistry) a reaction that produces a compound needed for the reaction to continue. **2.** (in physics) a reaction that perpetuates itself by the proliferating fission of nuclei and the release of atomic particles that cause more nuclear fissions.

chain reflex, a series of reflexes, each stimulated by the preceding one.

chain-stitch suture, a continuous surgical stitch in which each loop of the suture is secured by the next loop.

chalasia /kəlā′zhə/ [Gk *chalasis* relaxation], abnormal relaxation or incompetence of the cardiac sphincter of the stomach, resulting in reflux of the gastric contents into the esophagus with subsequent regurgitation.

chalazion /kəlā′zion/ [Gk, hailstone], a small, localized swelling of the eyelid resulting from obstruction and retained secretions of the meibomian glands.

chalice cell. See **goblet cell.**

chalicosis /kal′ikō′sis/, a type of fibrosis that results from the inhalation of calcium dusts. Respiratory impairment is generally caused by the presence of free silica in the calcium dust.

chalkitis /kalkī′tis/ [Gk *chalkos* brass, *itis* inflammation], an abnormal condition characterized by inflammation of the eyes, caused by rubbing the eyes with the hands after touching or handling brass.

challenge, a method of testing the sensitivity of an individual to a hormone, allergen, or other substance by administering a sample. To challenge the person's sensitivity to a particular antigen, a small amount may be injected to determine whether the immune system will react by producing appropriate antibodies.

chalone /kā′lōn/ [Gk *chalan* to relax], any one of numerous polypeptide inhibitors that is elaborated by a tissue and functions like a hormone on specific target organs.

chamaeprosopy /kam′əpros′əpē/ [Gk *chamai* low, *prosopon* face], a facial appearance characterized by a low brow and a broad face with a facial index of 90 or less. **–chamaeprosopic,** *adj.*

chamber [Gk *kamara* vaulted enclosure], **1.** a hollow but not necessarily empty space or cavity in an organ, as in the anterior and posterior chambers of the eye or the atrial and ventricular chambers of the heart. **2.** a room or closed space used for research or therapeutic purposes, such as a decompression chamber or hyperbaric oxygen chamber.

Chamberlain's line [W.E. Chamberlain, American radiologist, b. 1891], a line that extends from the posterior of the hard palate to the dorsum of the foramen magnum.

Chamberlen forceps [Peter Chamberlen, English obstetrician, b. 1560], one of the earliest kinds of obstetric forceps, introduced in the seventeenth century.

CHAMPUS, abbreviation for **Civilian Health and Medical Programs for Uniformed Services.**

chancre /shang′kər/ [Fr, canker], **1.** a skin lesion, usually of primary syphilis, that begins at the site of infection as a papule and develops into a red, bloodless, painless ulcer with a scooped-out appear-

ance. The chancre teems with *Treponema pallidum* spirochetes and is highly contagious. **2.** a papular lesion or ulcerated area of the skin that marks the point of infection of a nonsyphilitic disease, such as tuberculosis.

chancroid /shang′kroid/ [Fr *chancre* canker; Gk *eidos* form], a highly contagious, sexually transmitted disease caused by infection with a bacillus, *Haemophilus ducreyi.* It characteristically begins as a papule, usually on the skin of the external genitalia; it then grows and ulcerates, other papules form, and, if untreated, the bacillus spreads, causing buboes in the groin.

change agent, a role in which communication skills, education, and other resources are applied to help a client adjust to changes caused by illness or disability.

change of life, *informal;* the female climacteric; menopause.

channel [L *canalis* pipe], a passageway or groove that conveys fluid, such as the central channels that connect the arterioles with the venules.

channel ulcer [L *canalis* pipe, *ulcus* sore], a rare type of peptic ulcer found in the pyloric canal between the stomach and the duodenum.

chaotic atrial tachycardia, an atrial rhythm of more than 100 beats per minute due to multifocal atrial activity with at least three different shapes of P waves on the electrocardiogram. The condition is often associated with chronic obstructive lung disease.

chapped [ME *chappen* cracked], pertaining to skin that is roughened, cracked, or reddened by exposure to cold or excessive surface evaporation. Stinging or burning sensations often accompany the disorder. Prevention is by protection against exposure to cold and wind.

character [Gk *charassein* to engrave], **1.** the integrated composite of traits and behavioral tendencies that enable a person to react in a relatively consistent way to the customs and mores of society. **2.** any letter, number, symbol, or punctuation mark, usually composed of eight bits or one byte, that can be transmitted as output by a computer.

character analysis, a systematic investigation of the personality of an individual with special attention to psychologic defenses and motivations, usually undertaken to improve behavior.

character disorder, a chronic, habitual, maladaptive, and socially unacceptable pattern of behavior and emotional response.

characteristic curve, (in radiology) the pattern of a plot on a graph representing the relationship between the density, or degree of blackness of an x-ray film, and the exposure.

characteristic radiation, radiation produced when a projectile electron interacts with an inner-shell electron of a target atom, causing total removal of the electron. It is one of the principles of x-ray production.

character neurosis. See **character disorder.**

charcoal. See **activated charcoal.**

Charcot-Bouchard aneurysm /shärkō'booshär'/ [Jean M. Charcot, French neurologist, b. 1825; Charles J. Bouchard, French physician, b. 1837], a small, round aneurysm of a small artery of the cerebral cortex or basal ganglia, which some authorities believe is the cause of massive cerebral hemorrhage.

Charcot-Leyden crystal /shärkō'lī'dən/ [Jean M. Charcot; Ernst V. von Leyden, German physician, b. 1832], any one of the crystalline structures shaped like narrow, double pyramids found in the sputum of individuals suffering from bronchial asthma. They are also found in the feces of dysentery patients.

Charcot-Marie-Tooth atrophy /shärkō'-mərē'tooth'/ [Jean M. Charcot; Pierre Marie, French neurologist, b. 1853; Howard H. Tooth, English neurologist, b. 1856], a progressive hereditary disorder characterized by degeneration of the peroneal muscles of the fibula, resulting in clubfoot, foot drop, and ataxia.

Charcot's fever /shärköz'/ [Jean M. Charcot], a syndrome characterized by a recurrent fever, jaundice, and abdominal pain in the right upper quadrant occurring with inflammation of the bile ducts.

Charcot's joint, See **neuropathic joint disease.**

Charcot's triad [Jean M. Charcot; Gk *trias* three], a set of three signs of brainstem involvement in multiple sclerosis. They are intention tremor, nystagmus, and scanning speech.

charlatan [Fr, imposter], a totally unqualified individual posing as an expert, especially an individual pretending to be a physician. **–charlatanical,** *adj.*

Charles' law. See **Gay-Lussac's law.**

charley horse [Fr, *Charley* slang for an old, lame horse; ME *hors*], a painful condition of the quadriceps or hamstring muscles characterized by soreness and stiffness. It is the result of a strain, tear, or bruise of the muscle.

chart [L *charta* paper], **1.** *informal.* a patient record. **2.** to note data in a patient record, usually at prescribed intervals.

charta /kär'tə/, *pl.* **chartae** [L, paper], a

piece of paper, especially one treated with medicine, as for external application, or with a chemical for a special purpose, such as litmus paper.

chauffeur's fracture [Fr, stoker; L *fractura* break], any fracture of the radial styloid, produced by a twisting or a snapping type injury.

Chaussier's areola /shôsyāz'/ [Francois Chaussier, French anatomist, b. 1746; L, little space], an areola of indurated tissue surrounding a malignant pustule.

CHB, abbreviation for **complete heart block.**

CHC, abbreviation for *community health center.*

CHD, abbreviation for *coronary heart disease.*

check ligament. See **alar ligament.**

check-up [Fr *eschec* acquire; AS *uf*], a thorough study or examination of the health of an individual.

Chediak-Higashi syndrome /ched'ē·ak·-higä'shē/ [Moises Chediak, twentieth century French physician; Ototaka Higashi, twentieth century Japanese physician], a congenital, autosomal disorder, characterized by partial albinism, photophobia, massive leukocytic inclusions, psychomotor abnormalities, recurrent infections, and early death.

cheek [AS *ceace*], a fleshy prominence, especially the fleshy protuberances on both sides of the face between the eye and the jaw and the ear and the nose and mouth.

cheekbone. See **zygomatic bone.**

cheesy abscess [AS *cese*; L *abscedere* to go away], an abscess that contains a yellowish semisolid, cheeselike, material. It is found in tuberculous abscesses.

cheilitis /kīlī'tis/ [Gk *cheilos* lip, *itis* inflammation], an abnormal condition of the lips characterized by inflammation and cracking of the skin.

cheilocarcinoma /kī'lōkär'sinō'mə/, *pl.* **cheilocarcinomas, cheilocarcinomata,** a malignant epithelial tumor of the lip.

cheiloplasty /kī'ləplas'tē/ [Gk *cheilos* lip, *plassein* to mold], surgical correction of a defect of the lip.

cheilorraphy /kīlôr'əfē/ [Gk *cheilos* lip, *raphe* suture], a surgical procedure that sutures the lip, such as in the repair of a congenitally cleft lip or a lacerated lip.

cheilosis /kīlō'sis/, a disorder of the lips and mouth characterized by scales and fissures, resulting from a deficiency of riboflavin in the diet.

cheiralgia /kəral'jə/ [Gk *cheir* + *algos* pain], a pain in the hand, especially the pain associated with arthritis. **–cheiralgic,** *adj.*

cheiromegaly /kī'rōmeg'əlē/ [Gk *cheir* + *megas* large], an abnormal condition characterized by excessively large hands. **–cheiromegalic,** *adj.*

cheiroplasty /kī'rōplas'tē/, an operation involving plastic surgery of the hand. **–cheiroplastic,** *adj.*

chelate /kē'lāt/ [Gk *chele* claw], **1.** (of a metal ion and two or more polar groups of a single molecule) to form a bond, thus creating a ringlike complex. **2.** (in medicine) a compound composed of a central metal ion and an organic molecule with multiple bonds, arranged in ring formations, used especially in chemotherapeutic treatments for metal poisoning. **3.** of or pertaining to chelation.

chelating agent /kē'lāting/, a substance that promotes chelation. Chelating agents are used in the treatment of metal poisoning.

chelation /kēlā'shən/, a chemical reaction in which there is a combination with a metal to form a ring-shaped molecular complex in which the metal is firmly bound and sequestered.

cheloid. See **keloid.**

cheloidosis. See **keloidosis.**

chemabrasion /kem'əbrā'zhən/ [Gk *chemeia* alchemy; L *ab, radere* to scrape off], a method of treating scars, chromatosis, or other skin disorders by applying chemicals that remove the surface layers of skin cells.

chemical [Gk *chemeia* alchemy], **1.** a substance composed of chemical elements or a substance produced by or used in chemical processes. **2.** pertaining to chemistry.

chemical action, any process in which natural elements and compounds react with each other to produce a chemical change or a different compound; for example, hydrogen and oxygen combine to produce water.

chemical affinity [Gk, *chemeia,* alchemy; L, *affinis,* related], an attraction that results in the formation of molecules from atoms.

chemical agent, any chemical power, active principle, or substance that can produce an effect in the body by interacting with various body substances, such as aspirin, which produces an analgesic effect.

chemical antidote [Gk *chemeia; anti* against, *dotos* that which is given], any substance that reacts chemically with a poison to form a compound that is harmless.

chemical burn, tissue damage caused by exposure to a strong acid or alkali, such as phenol, creosol, mustard gas, or phosphorus. Emergency treatment includes washing the surface with copious amounts of water to remove the chemical and, if the damage is more than slight and superficial, immediate transport to a medical facility.

chemical carcinogen [Gk, *chemeia,* alchemy, *karkinos,* crab, *oma,* tumor, *genein,* to produce], any chemical agent that can induce the development of cancer in living tissue.

chemical cauterization [Gk *chemeia; kauterion* branding iron], the corroding or burning of living tissue by a caustic chemical substance, such as potassium hydroxide.

chemical diabetes. See **impaired glucose tolerance.**

chemical energy. See **energy.**

chemical equivalent, a drug or chemical containing similar amounts of the same ingredients as another drug or chemical.

chemical fog, a dull gray discoloration on x-ray film, usually caused by chemical contamination of the developer used.

chemical gastritis, inflammation of the stomach caused by the ingestion of a chemical compound.

chemical indicator, a commercially prepared device that monitors all or part of the physical conditions of the sterilization cycle. It usually consists of a sensitive ink dye that changes colors under certain conditions.

chemical mediator, a neurotransmitter chemical, such as acetylcholine.

chemical name, the exact designation of the chemical structure of a drug as determined by the rules of accepted systems of chemical nomenclature. For example, N,N-bis-(2-chloroethyl)-N'-(3-hydroxypropyl) phosphordiamidic acid cyclic acid monohydrate is the chemical name of cyclophosphamide, a drug used in cancer chemotherapy.

chemical peritonitis [Gk, *chemeia,* alchemy, *peri,* near, *teinein,* to stretch, *itis,* inflammation], an inflammation of the peritoneum resulting from chemicals, including digestive substances, in the peritoneum.

chemical shift, the slight departure in the nuclear magnetic resonance spectrum of an element, such as hydrogen, when it is a constituent in a complex biomolecule, from the spectrum for a sample containing that element in pure form.

chemical warfare, the waging of war with poisonous chemicals and gases.

cheminosis /kem'ənō'sis/ [Gk *chemeia* + *osis* condition], any disease caused by a chemical substance.

chemistry [Gk *chemeia* alchemy], the science dealing with the elements, their compounds, and the chemical structure

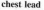

and interactions of matter. Kinds of chemistry include **inorganic chemistry** and **organic chemistry**.

chemistry, normal values, the amounts of various substances in the normal human body, determined by testing a large sample of people presumed to be healthy. Normal values are expressed in ranges of numbers and can vary from laboratory to laboratory.

chemocautery. See **chemical cauterization.**

chemodifferentiation /kē′mō-, kem′ō-/, a stage in embryonic development that precedes and controls specialization and differentiation of the cells into rudimentary organs.

chemonucleolysis /kē′mōn̄oo′klē·ol′isis, kem′-/ [Gk *chemeia* + L *nucleus* kernel; Gk *lysein* to loosen], a method of dissolving the nucleus pulposus of an intervertebral disk by the injection of a chemolytic agent, such as the enzyme chymopapain.

chemoprophylaxis [Gk *chemeia* + *prophylax* advance guard], the use of antimicrobial drugs to prevent the acquisition of pathogens in an endemic area or to prevent their spread from one body area to another.

chemoreceptor [Gk *chemeia* + L *recipere* to receive], a sensory nerve cell activated by chemical stimuli, such as a chemoreceptor in the carotid that is sensitive to the Pco_2 in the blood, signaling the respiratory center in the brain to increase or decrease respiration.

chemoreflex, any reflex initiated by the stimulation of chemical receptors, such as the carotid and aortic bodies, which respond to changes in carbon dioxide, hydrogen ion, and oxygen concentrations in the blood.

chemosis /kimō′sis/ [Gk *cheme* cockle, *osis* condition], an abnormal edematous swelling of the mucous membrane covering the eyeball and lining the eyelids that is usually the result of local trauma or infection.

chemostat /kē′məstat′/, a device that assures a steady rate of cell division in bacterial populations by maintaining a constant environment.

chemosurgery [Gk *chemeia* + *cheirourgos* surgeon], the destruction of malignant, infected, or gangrenous tissue by the application of chemicals. The technique is used successfully to remove skin cancers.

chemotaxis /kē′mətak′sis/ [Gk *chemeia* + *taxis* arrangement], a response involving movement that is positive (toward) or negative (away from) to a chemical stimulus. —**chemotactic** *adj.*

chemotherapeutic agent, a chemical

agent used to treat diseases. The term usually refers to a medication used to treat cancer because it can alter the growth of cancer cells.

chemotherapy, the treatment of infections and other diseases with chemical agents. In modern usage, chemotherapy usually refers to the use of chemicals to destroy cancer cells on a selective basis. The cytotoxic agents used in cancer treatments generally function in the same manner as ionizing radiation; they do not kill the cancer cells directly but instead impair their ability to replicate. Chemotherapeutic agents are often used in combination with radiation treatments for their synergistic effect.

chemotherapy (unsealed radioactive), the oral or parenteral administration of a radioisotope, such as iodine 131 (^{131}I) for the treatment of hyperthyroidism or thyroid cancer, phosphorus 32 (^{32}P) for leukemia or polycythemia vera, or gold 198 (^{198}Au) for lung cancer or peritoneal ascites resulting from widely disseminated carcinoma.

chenodeoxycholic acid /ken′ōdē·ok′si-kō′lik/, a secondary bile acid. It is used in vivo to dissolve cholesterol gallstones, particularly in the elderly and poor-risk patients.

cherry angioma [L *cerasus; aggeion* vessel, *oma* tumor], a small, bright red, clearly circumscribed vascular tumor on the skin. It occurs most often on the trunk but may be found anywhere on the body. The lesion is very common.

cherry red spot, an abnormal red circular area of the choroid, seen through the fovea centralis of the eye and surrounded by a contrasting white edema. It is associated with cases of infantile cerebral sphingolipidosis and sometimes appears in the late infantile form of amaurotic familial idiocy.

cherubism /cher′əbiz′əm/ [Heb *kerubh*], an abnormal hereditary condition characterized by progressive bilateral swelling at the angle of the mandible, especially in children.

chest. See **thorax.**

chest cavity. See **body cavity.**

chest lead 1. an electrocardiographic conductor in which the exploring electrode is placed on the chest or precordium. The indifferent electrode is placed on the patient's back for a CB (chest back) lead, on the front of the chest for a CF (chest front) lead, on the left arm for a CL (chest left) lead, and on the right arm for a CR (chest right) lead. **2.** *informal;* the tracing produced by such a lead on an electrocardiograph.

chest pain [AS *cest* box; L *poena* punishment], a physical complaint that requires immediate diagnosis and evaluation. Chest pain may be symptomatic of cardiac disease, such as angina pectoris, myocardial infarction, or pericarditis, or of disease of the lungs, such as pleurisy, pneumonia, or pulmonary embolism or infarction. The source of chest pain may also be musculoskeletal, GI, or psychogenic. Over 90% of severe chest pain is caused by coronary disease, spinal root compression, or psychologic disturbance. Specific cardiovascular conditions associated with chest pain are myocardial infarction, angina pectoris, pericarditis, and a dissecting aneurysm of the thoracic aorta. Musculoskeletal conditions include rib fractures, swelling of the rib cartilage, and muscle strain. GI conditions associated with chest pain include esophagitis, peptic ulcers, hiatus hernia, and pancreatitis.

chest physiotherapy. See **cupping and vibrating, percussion.**

chest thump [AS, *cest,* box; thump = echoic], a sharp blow to the chest in the precordial area to restore a normal heart beat after cardiac arrest.

chest tube, 1. a catheter inserted through the thorax into the chest cavity for removing air or fluid. **2.** radiographic artifacts caused by the presence of oral or tracheal tubes, or a pulmonary artery catheter, in the body of a patient.

chest wall percussion. See **percussion.**

chewing gum diarrhea. See **osmotic diarrhea.**

chewing reflex, a pathologic sign in brain-damaged adults, characterized by repetitive chewing motions when the mouth is stimulated.

Cheyne-Stokes respiration (CSR) /chān-′stōks′/ [John Cheyne, Scottish physician, b. 1777; William Stokes, Irish physician, b. 1804; L *respirare* to breathe], an abnormal pattern of respiration, characterized by alternating periods of apnea and deep, rapid breathing. The respiratory cycle begins with slow, shallow breaths that gradually increase to abnormal depth and rapidity. Respiration gradually subsides as breathing slows and becomes shallower, climaxing in a 10- to 20-second period without respiration before the cycle is repeated.

CHF, abbreviation for **congestive heart failure.**

ch'i, a Chinese concept of a fundamental life energy that flows in orderly ways along meridians, or channels, in the body.

Chiari-Frommel syndrome /kē·är′ē-from′əl/ [Johann B. Chiari, German physician, b. 1817; Richard Frommel, German gynecologist, b. 1854], a hormonal disorder that occurs after a pregnancy in which weaning does not spontaneously end lactation.

Chiari's syndrome. See **Budd-Chiari syndrome.**

chiasm /kī′azəm/ [Gk *chiasma* lines that cross] **1.** the crossing of two lines or tracts, as the crossing of the optic nerves at the optic chiasm. **2.** (in genetics) the crossing of two chromatids in the prophase of meiosis. **–chiasmal, chiasmic,** *adj.*

chiasma /kī·az′mə/, *pl.* **chiasmata** [Gk, lines that cross], (in genetics), the visible point of connection between homologous chromosomes during the first meiotic division in gametogenesis. The X-shaped configurations form during the late prophase stage and provide the means by which exchange of genetic material occurs. **–chiasmatic, chiasmic.** *adj.*

chiasmatypy. See **crossing over.**

chiasmic. See **chiasm, chiasma.**

chickenpox [AS *cicen;* ME *pokke*], an acute, highly contagious viral disease caused by a herpesvirus, varicella zoster virus (VZV). It occurs primarily in young children and is characterized by crops of pruritic vesicular eruptions on the skin. The disease is transmitted by direct contact with skin lesions or, more commonly, by droplets spread from the respiratory tract of infected persons, usually in the prodromal period or the early stages of the rash. The vesicular fluid and the scabs are infectious until entirely dry. Indirect transmission through uninfected persons or objects is rare. The diagnosis is usually made by physical examination and by the characteristic appearance of the disease. The virus may be identified by culture of the vesicle fluid.

chiclero's ulcer /chikler′ōz/ [Mex *tzictli* chicle; L *ulcus*], a kind of leishmaniasis endemic among the workers in the Yucatan and Central America who harvest chicle from the forest. The disease is characterized by cutaneous ulcers on the head that usually heal spontaneously by 6 months, except for those on the pinna of the ear, which may last for years and cause scarring and deformities.

chief cell [Fr *chef*; L *cella* storeroom], **1.** any one of the columnar epithelial cells or the cuboidal epithelial cells that line the gastric glands and secrete pepsinogen and intrinsic factor, which is needed for the absorption of vitamin B_{12} and the normal development of red blood cells. Anemia is caused by the absence of intrinsic factor. **2.** any one of the epithelioid cells with pale-staining cytoplasm and a large nucleus containing a prominent nucleolus.

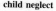

3. any one of the polyhedral epithelial cells, within the parathyroid glands.

chief complaint (CC), a subjective statement made by a patient describing the patient's most significant or serious symptoms or signs of illness or dysfunction.

Chief Executive Officer (CEO), the most senior official of an organization or institution.

chief resident, a senior resident physician who acts temporarily as the clinical and administrative director of the house staff in a department of the hospital.

chief surgeon, a surgeon appointed or elected head of the surgeons on the staff of a health care facility.

chigger /chig´ər/ [Fr *chique*], the larva of *Trombicula* mites found in tall grass and weeds. It sticks to the skin and causes irritation and severe itching.

chigoe /chig´ō/, a flea found in tropical and subtropical America and Africa. The pregnant female flea burrows into the skin of the feet, causing an inflammatory condition that may lead to spontaneous amputation of a toe.

chikungunya encephalitis /chik´ən-gun´yə/ [Bantu, to bend upward; Gk *enkephalos* brain, *itis* inflammation], an arbovirus infection characterized by a high fever that begins abruptly, muscle aches, a rash, and pain in the joints. It is transmitted by the bite of a mosquito and occurs mainly in Africa, Asia, and on some Pacific islands.

chilblain /chil´blān/ [AS *cele* cold, *bleyn* blister], redness and swelling of the skin because of excessive exposure to cold. Burning, itching, blistering, and ulceration, similar to a thermal burn, may occur. Treatment includes protection against cold and injury, gentle warming, and avoidance of tobacco.

child [AS *cild*], **1.** a person of either sex between the time of birth and adolescence. **2.** an unborn or recently born human being; fetus, neonate, infant. **3.** an offspring or descendant; a son or daughter or a member of a particular tribe or clan. **4.** one who is like a child or immature.

child abuse, the physical, sexual, or emotional maltreatment of a child. It may be overt or covert and often results in permanent physical or psychiatric injury, mental impairment, or sometimes death. Child abuse is the result of multiple and complex factors involving both the parents and the child, compounded by various stressful environmental circumstances, such as poor socioeconomic conditions, inadequate physical and emotional support within the family, and any major life change or crisis, especially those crises arising from marital strife. Parents at high risk for abuse are characterized as having unsatisfied needs, difficulty in forming adequate interpersonal relationships, unrealistic expectations of the child, and a lack of nurturing experience, often involving neglect or abuse in their own childhoods. Obvious physical marks on a child's body, as burns, welts, or bruises, and signs of emotional distress, including symptoms of failure to thrive, are common indications of some degree of neglect or abuse. Often, x-ray film to detect healed or new fractures of the extremities or diagnostic tests to identify sexual molestation are necessary.

childbearing period [AS *cild* + *beran* to bear; Gk *peri* around, *hodos* way], the reproductive period in a woman's life, from puberty to menopause. It is the time during which she is physiologically able to conceive children.

childbed fever. See **puerperal fever.**

childbirth. See **birth.**

childbirth center, a health facility where prenatal care and delivery services are made available to low-risk pregnant women by a team of nurse-midwives, obstetricians, pediatricians, and ancillary health professionals.

child development, the various stages of physical, social, and psychologic growth that occur from birth through adulthood.

childhood, 1. the period in human development that extends from birth until the onset of puberty. **2.** the state or quality of being a child.

childhood aphasia, an inability to process language because of a brain dysfunction in childhood.

childhood myxedema [AS *cildhad;* Gk *myxa* mucus, *oidema* swelling], a juvenile form of hypothyroidism characterized by atrophy of the thyroid gland following a severe infection of the gland.

childhood-onset pervasive developmental disorders, disturbances in thought, affect, social relatedness, and behavior that emerge between the ages of 30 months and 12 years.

childhood polycystic disease. See **polycystic kidney disease.**

childhood triad, three types of behavior—fire setting, bedwetting, and cruelty to animals—that may predict emerging sociopathy when they occur consistently and in combination.

child neglect, the failure by parents or guardians to provide for the basic needs of a child by physical or emotional deprivation that interferes with normal growth and development or that places the child in jeopardy.

child psychology, the study of the mental, emotional, and behavioral development of infants and children.

child welfare, any service sponsored by the community or special organizations that provide for the physical, social, or psychologic care of children in need of it.

chill [AS *cele*], **1.** the sensation of cold caused by exposure to a cold environment. **2.** an attack of shivering with pallor and a feeling of coldness, often occurring at the beginning of an infection and accompanied by a rapid rise in temperature.

Chilomastix /kī'lōmas'tiks/, a genus of flagellate protozoa, as *Chilomastix mesnili,* a nonpathogenic intestinal parasite of humans.

chimera /kimir'ə, kīmir'ə/ [Gk *khimaros* fire-breathing monster], an organism carrying cell populations derived from two or more different zygotes of the same or of different species. It may be a natural phenomenon, such as in a bone marrow graft.

chimerism /kimir'izəm/, a state in bone marrow transplantation in which bone marrow and host cells exist compatibly without signs of graft-versus-host rejection disease.

chimney-sweeps' cancer. See **scrotal cancer.**

chin, the raised triangular portion of the mandible below the lip. It is formed by the mental protuberance.

Chinese restaurant syndrome, a syndrome consisting of tingling and burning sensations of the skin, facial pressure, headache, and chest pain that occurs immediately after eating food containing monosodium glutamate, frequently used in Chinese cooking.

chip [AS *kippen* to slice], **1.** a relatively small piece of a bone or tooth. **2.** to break off or cut away a small piece.

chip fracture, any small fragmental fracture, usually one involving a bony process near a joint.

chiralgia /kəral'jə/, a pain in the hand, particularly one that does not result from a nerve injury or disease.

chirality. See **handedness.**

chiroplasty /kir'əplas'tē/ a surgical procedure to restore an injured or congenitally deformed hand to normal use.

chiropodist /kirop'ədist, shir-/, a health professional trained to diagnose and treat diseases and other disorders of the feet. A chiropodist may be awarded a degree of DSC (Doctor of Surgical Chiropody) or PodD (Doctor of Podiatry) after completing 4 years of study in an accredited college of podiatry. After a refresher course, a DSC or a PodD may be granted the postgraduate degree DPM (Doctor of Podiatric Medicine).

chiropody /kirop'ədē, shir-/ [Gk *cheir* hand, *pous* foot], the study of minor disorders of the feet and the practice of treating these disorders. Practitioners trained in chiropody are licensed to practice by the various states.

chiropractic /kī'rōprak'tik/ [Gk *cheir* hand, *practikos* efficient], a system of therapy based on the theory that the state of a person's health is determined in general by the condition of his nervous system. In most cases treatment provided by chiropractors involves the mechanical manipulation of the spinal column. Some practitioners use radiology for diagnosis and use physiotherapy and diet in addition to spinal manipulation. Chiropractic does not use drugs or surgery, the primary basis of treatment used by medical physicians. A chiropractor is awarded the degree of Doctor of Chiropractic, or DC, after completing 4 years of training in an approved chiropractic school.

chiropractor /-prak'tər/, a practitioner of **chiropractic.**

chirospasm. See **writer's cramp.**

chisel fracture, any fracture in which there is an oblique detachment of a bone fragment from the head of the radius.

chi square (χ_2) /kī/, (in statistics) a statistical test for an association between observed data and expected data represented by frequencies. The test yields a statement of the probability of the obtained distribution having occurred by chance alone.

Chlamydia /kləmid'ē·ə/ [Gk *chlamys* cloak] **1.** a microorganism of the genus *Chlamydia.* **2.** a genus of microorganisms that live as intracellular parasites, have a number of properties in common with gramnegative bacteria, and are currently classified as specialized bacteria. *Chlamydia trachomatis,* an organism that lives in the conjunctiva of the eye and the epithelium of the urethra and cervix, is responsible for inclusion conjunctivitis, lymphogranuloma venereum, and trachoma. *Chlamydia psittaci* is an organism that infects birds and causes a type of pneumonia in humans.

chloasma /klō·az'mə/ [Gk *chloazein* to be green], tan or brown pigmentation, particularly of the forehead, cheeks, and nose, commonly associated with pregnancy or the use of oral contraceptives.

chloracne /klôrak'nē/ [Gk *chloros* green, *akme* point], a skin condition characterized by small, black follicular plugs and papules on exposed surfaces, especially on the arms, face, and neck of workers in contact with chlorinated compounds, such as cutting oils, paints, varnishes, and lacquers.

chloral camphor /klôr′əl/, a mixture of equal parts of camphor and chloral hydrate, used externally as a sedative.

chloral hydrate, a sedative and hypnotic prescribed for the relief of insomnia, anxiety, or tension.

chlorambucil /klôr′ambōo′sil/, an alkylating agent prescribed in the treatment of a variety of malignant neoplastic diseases, including chronic lymphocytic leukemia and Hodgkin's disease.

chloramphenicol /-amfē′nikol/, an antibacterial and antirickettsial prescribed in the treatment of a wide variety of serious infections.

chlorcyclizine hydrochloride /klôrsī′klizin/, an antihistamine that has been used for rhinitis, sinusitis, and hayfever. As a cream, it is also used for skin conditions.

chlordane poisoning. See **chlorinated organic insecticide poisoning.**

chlordiazepoxide /klôr′dī·az′əpok′sīd/, a minor tranquilizer prescribed in the treatment of anxiety and nervous tension and alcohol withdrawal symptoms.

chlorhexidine /-hek′sidēn/ an antimicrobial agent used as a surgical scrub, hand rinse, and topical antiseptic.

chlorhydria /-hī′drē·ə/, an excessive level of hydrochloric acid in the stomach.

chloride /klôr′īd/ [Gk *chloros* green], a compound in which the negative element is chlorine. Chlorides are salts of hydrochloric acid, the most common being sodium chloride (table salt).

chloride shift, an exchange of chloride ions in red blood cells in peripheral tissues in response to Pco_2 of blood. The shift reverses in the lungs.

chloriduria, an excessive level of chlorides in the urine.

chlorinated [Gk, *chloros,* greenish], pertaining to material that contains or has been treated with chlorine.

chlorinated organic insecticide poisoning, poisoning resulting from the inhalation, ingestion, or absorption of DDT and other insecticides containing chlorophenothane, as heptachlor, dieldrin, and chlordane. It is characterized by vomiting, weakness, malaise, convulsions, tremors, ventricular fibrillation, respiratory failure, and pulmonary edema.

chlorination [Gk, *chloros,* greenish], the disinfection or treatment of water or other substances with free chlorine.

chlorine (**Cl**) /klôr′ēn/, a yellowish green, gaseous element of the halogen group. Its atomic number is 17; its atomic weight is 35.453. It has a strong, distinctive odor, is irritating to the respiratory tract, and is poisonous if ingested or inhaled. It occurs in nature chiefly as a component of sodium chloride in sea water and in salt deposits. It is used as a bleach and as a disinfectant to purify water for drinking or for use in swimming pools.

chlormezanone /-mez′ənōn/, an antianxiety agent prescribed for mild anxiety and for nervous tension.

chloroform /klôr′əfôrm′/ [Gk *chloros* + L *formica* ant], a nonflammable, volatile liquid that was the first inhalation anesthetic to be discovered. Chloroform is a dangerous anesthetic drug: A difference of only 10% in drug-plasma levels can result in hypotension, myocardial and respiratory depression, cardiogenic shock, ventricular fibrillation, coma, and death.

chloroformism, 1. the habit of inhaling chloroform for its narcotic effect. **2.** the anesthetic effect of chloroform.

chloroleukemia /klôr′ōlōokē′mē·ə/ [Gk *chloros* green, *leukos* white, *haima* blood], a kind of myelogenous leukemia in which specific tumor masses are not seen at autopsy but body fluids and organs are green.

chlorolymphosarcoma /klôr′ōlim′fōsärkō′mə/, *pl.* **chlorolymphosarcomas, chlorolymphosarcomata** [Gk *chloros* + L *lympha* water; Gk *sarx* flesh, *oma* tumor], a greenish neoplasm of myeloid tissue occurring in patients with myelogenous leukemia. The mononuclear cells in the peripheral blood are believed to be lymphocytes rather than myeloblasts, such as found with chloroma.

chloroma /klôrō′mə/, *pl.* **chloromas, chloromata,** a malignant, greenish neoplasm of myeloid tissue occurring anywhere in the body in patients with myelogenous leukemia.

chloromyeloma. See **chloroma.**

chlorophyll /klôr′əfil/ [Gk *chloros* + *phyllon* leaf], a plant pigment capable of absorbing light and converting it to energy for the oxidation and reduction involved in the photosynthesis of carbohydrates.

chlorophyll test. See **Boas′ test.**

chloroprocaine /klôr′ōprō′kān/, a local anesthetic with a chemical structure similar to procaine.

chloroquine /klôr′əkwin′/, an antimalarial prescribed in the treatment of malaria, extraintestinal amebiasis, rheumatoid arthritis, some forms of lupus erythematosus, and photoallergic reactions.

chlorosis /klôrō′sis/, *archaic.* an iron deficiency anemia of young women characterized by hypochromic, microcytic erythrocytes and a small reduction in the total number of erythrocytes.

chlorothiazide /-thī′əzīd/, a diuretic and antihypertensive prescribed in the treatment of hypertension and edema.

chlortrianisene /-trī·an′isēn/, an estrogen prescribed in the treatment of postpartum breast engorgement, menopausal symptoms, and prostatic cancer.

chlorpheniramine maleate /-fenir′əmēn/, an antihistamine prescribed in the treatment of a variety of hypersensitivity reactions, including rhinitis, skin rash, and pruritus.

chlorpromazine /klôrprō′məzēn/, a phenothiazine tranquilizer and antiemetic prescribed in the treatment of psychotic disorders, severe nausea and vomiting, and intractable hiccups.

chlorpropamide /-prō′pəmīd/, an oral antidiabetic prescribed in the treatment of mild, stable non-insulin-dependent diabetes mellitus.

chlorprothixene /klôr′prōthik′sēn/, a thioxanthine antipsychotic agent prescribed in the treatment of psychotic disorders.

chlortetracycline hydrochloride, /-tet′rəsī′klēn/ an antibiotic prescribed in the treatment of a variety of infections.

chlorthalidone /-thal′idōn/, a diuretic and antihypertensive prescribed in the treatment of high blood pressure and edema.

chlorzoxazone /klôrzok′səzōn/, a skeletal muscle relaxant prescribed for the relief of muscle spasm.

CHN, abbreviation for *Certified Hemodialysis Nurse.*

choana /kō′ənə/, *pl.* **choanae, 1.** a funnel-shaped channel. **2.** See **posterior nares.**

choanal atresia /kō′ənəl/ [Gk *choane* funnel, *a, tresis* not hole], a congenital anomaly in which a bony or membranous occlusion blocks the passageway between the nose and pharynx.

chocolate cyst [Mex, *chocolatl,* Gk, *kystis,* bag], a darkly pigmented cyst sometimes found in the endometrium.

choke [ME *choken*], to interrupt respiration by compression or obstruction of larynx or trachea.

choke damp. See **damp.**

choked disc. *informal.* papilledema.

chokes, a respiratory condition, occurring in decompression sickness, characterized by shortness of breath, substernal pain, and a nonproductive cough caused by bubbles of gas in the blood vessels of the lungs.

choking, the condition in which a respiratory passage is blocked by constriction of the neck, an obstruction in the trachea, or swelling of the larynx. It is characterized by sudden coughing and a red face that rapidly becomes cyanotic. The person cannot breathe and clutches his throat.

cholangeostomy /kōlan′jē·os′təmē/ [Gk *chloe* bile, *aggeion* small vessel, *stoma* mouth], a surgical operation to form an opening in a bile duct.

cholangiocarcinoma /kōlan′jē·okär′sinō′mə/, a cancer of the biliary epithelium in the liver. It tends to occur mainly in patients who have had ulcerative colitis or an infestation of liver flukes.

cholangiogram /kōlan′jē·əgram′/, an x-ray film of the bile ducts produced after injection of a radiopaque contrast medium.

cholangiography /kōlan′jē·og′rəfē/, a special roentgenographic test procedure for outlining the major bile ducts by the intravenous injection or the direct instillation of a radiopaque contrast material.

cholangiohepatoma /kōlan′jē·ōhep′ətō′mə/, *pl.* **cholangiohepatomas, cholangiohepatomata,** a neoplasm in which there is an abnormal mixture of liver cord cells and bile ducts.

cholangiolitis /kōlan′jē·əlī′tis/, an abnormal condition characterized by inflammation of the fine tubules of the bile duct system, which may cause cholangiolitic cirrhosis. **–cholangiolitic,** *adj.*

cholangioma /kōlan′jē·ō′mə/, *pl.* **cholangiomas, cholangiomata,** a neoplasm of the bile ducts.

cholangitis /kō′lanjī′tis/, inflammation of the bile ducts, caused either by bacterial invasion or by obstruction of the ducts by calculi or a tumor. The condition is characterized by severe right upper quadrant pain, jaundice (if an obstruction is present), and intermittent fever.

cholecalciferol. See **vitamin D₃.**

cholecystectomy /kō′lisistek′təmē/ [Gk *chole* + *kystis* bag, *ektome* excision], the surgical removal of the gallbladder, performed to treat cholelithiasis and cholecystitis. The gallbladder is excised and the cystic duct ligated; the common duct is searched, and any stones found are removed. A T tube is left in place to ensure adequate bile drainage; a Penrose drain may be left in a separate stab wound to prevent the formation of an abscess.

cholecystitis /kō′lisistī′tis/ [Gk *chole* + *kystis* bag, *itis* inflammation], acute or chronic inflammation of the gallbladder. **Acute cholecystitis** is usually caused by a gallstone that cannot pass through the cystic duct. Pain is felt in the right upper quadrant of the abdomen, accompanied by nausea, vomiting, eructation, and flatulence. **Chronic cholecystitis,** the more common type, has an insidious onset. Pain, often felt at night, may follow a fatty meal.

cholecystogram

213

Complications include biliary calculi, pancreatitis, and carcinoma of the gallbladder.

cholecystogram /kō'lisis'təgram'/, an x-ray film of the gallbladder, made after the ingestion or injection of a radiopaque substance, usually a contrast material containing iodine.

cholecystography /kō'lisistog'rəfē/, an x-ray examination of the gallbladder. At least 12 hours before the study the patient has a fat-free meal and ingests a contrast material containing iodine. The iodine, which is opaque to x-rays, is excreted by the liver into the bile in the gallbladder. After the procedure, the patient consumes a fatty meal or cholecystokinin, which stimulates the gallbladder to contract, expelling bile and contrast material into the bile duct.

cholecystoileostomy /kō'lisis'tō·il'ē·os'təmē/ [Gk *chole, kystis* + *eilein* to twist, *stoma* mouth], a surgical procedure performed to connect the gallbladder to the ileum.

cholecystokinin /kol'isis'təkī'nin/ [Gk *chole* + *kystis* bag, *kinein* to move], a hormone, produced by the mucosa of the upper intestine, that stimulates contraction of the gallbladder and the secretion of pancreatic enzymes.

choledochal /-dok'əl/ [Gk *chole, dochus* containing], pertaining to the common bile duct.

choledochojejunostomy /-dok'ōjē·jōōno·s'təmē/ [Gk *chole, dochus;* L *jejunus* empty; Gk *stoma* mouth], a surgical procedure in which the bile duct is connected to the jejunum.

choledocholithiasis. See **biliary calculus.**

choledocholithotomy /kōled'ōkō'lithot'əmē/ [Gk *chole* + *dochus* + *lithos* stone, *temnein* to cut], a surgical operation to make an incision in the common bile duct to remove a stone.

cholelithiasis /kō'lilithī'əsis/ [Gk *chole* + *lithos* stone, *osis* condition], the presence of gallstones in the gallbladder. The condition affects about 20% of the population over 40 years of age and is more prevalent in women and in persons with cirrhosis of the liver. Patients complain of abdominal discomfort, eructation, and intolerance to certain foods.

cholelithic dyspepsia /kō'lilith'ik/ [Gk *chole* + *lithos* stone; *dys* bad, *peptein* to digest], an abnormal condition characterized by sudden attacks of indigestion associated with the dysfunction of the gallbladder.

cholelithotomy /kō'lilithot'əmē/, a surgical operation to remove gallstones through an incision in the gallbladder.

cholera /kol'ərə/ [Gk *chole* + *rhein* to flow], an acute bacterial infection of the small intestine, characterized by severe diarrhea and vomiting, muscular cramps, dehydration, and depletion of electrolytes. The symptoms are caused by toxic substances produced by the infecting organism, *Vibrio cholerae.* The profuse, watery diarrhea, as much as a liter an hour, depletes the body of fluids and minerals.

choleragen /kol'ərəjin/, an exotoxin, produced by the cholera vibrio, that stimulates the secretion of electrolyte and water into the small intestine in Asiatic cholera.

cholera vaccine, an active immunizing agent prescribed as an immunization against cholera.

choleretic /kō'ləret'ik/ [Gk *chole* + *eresis* removal] **1.** stimulating the production of bile either by cholepoiesis or by hydrocholeresis. **2.** a choleretic agent.

choleric /kol'ərik, kəler'ik/, having a hot temper or an irascible nature.

cholestasis /kō'ləstā'sis/ [Gk *chole* + *stasis* standing still], interruption in the flow of bile through any part of the biliary system, from liver to duodenum. It is essential to discover whether the cause is within the liver (intrahepatic) or outside it (extrahepatic). Symptoms of both types include jaundice, pale and fatty stools, dark urine, and intense itching over the skin. –**cholestatic,** *adj.*

cholestatic hepatitis /kō'listat'ik/, inflammation of the liver caused by hepatitis infection that produces interruption of the flow of bile in the intrahepatic ducts.

cholesteatoma /kōles'tē·ətō'mə/ [Gk *chole* + *stear* fat, *oma* tumor], a cystic mass composed of epithelial cells and cholesterol that is found in the middle ear and occurs as a congenital defect or as a serious complication of chronic otitis media.

cholesterase /kəles'tərās'/ [Gk *chole* + *aither* air; Ger *Saure* acid; *ase* enzyme suffix], an enzyme in the blood and other tissues that forms cholesterol and fatty acids by hydrolyzing cholesterol esters.

cholesteremia. See **cholesterolemia.**

cholesterol /kəles'tərôl/ [Gk *chole* + *steros* solid], a fat-soluble crystalline steroid alcohol found in animal fats and oils, and egg yolk, and widely distributed in the body, especially in the bile, blood, brain tissue, liver, kidneys, adrenal glands, and myelin sheaths of nerve fibers. It facilitates the absorption and transport of fatty acids and acts as the precursor for the synthesis of vitamin D at the surface of the skin, as well as for the synthesis of the various steroid hormones. Increased levels of serum cholesterol may be associated with the pathogenesis of atherosclerosis.

cholesterolemia /-ē′mē-ə/, **1.** the presence of excessive amounts of cholesterol in the blood. **2.** the abnormal condition of having excessive amounts of cholesterol in the blood.

cholesteroleresis /kəles′tərōler′isis/ [Gk *chole, steros* + *eresis* removal], the increased elimination of cholesterol in the bile.

cholesterol metabolism, the anabolic and catabolic processes in the synthesis and degradation of cholesterol in the body. Ingested cholesterol is quickly absorbed. It is also synthesized in the liver and by most other tissues of the body.

cholesterolopoiesis /kəles′tərōlōpō·ē′sis/ [Gk *chole, steros* + *poiesis* producing], the elaboration of cholesterol by the liver.

cholesterolosis /kəles′tərəlō′sis/, an abnormal condition in which there are deposits of cholesterol within large macrophages in the submucosa of the gallbladder.

cholesteryl ester storage disease /kōles′təril/, an inherited disorder in which there is an accumulation of neutral lipids, such as cholesterol esters and glycerides, in body tissues. A form of the disorder affecting infants, with symptoms in the first weeks after birth, is Wolman's disease.

cholestyramine /-tir′əmēn/, a substance that acts on the liver's bile acids, interrupting the bile-acid cycle and increasing the function of LDL receptors, thereby increasing cellular cholesterol uptake and lowering blood cholesterol levels.

cholestyramine resin, an ion-exchange resin and antihyperlipoproteinemic agent prescribed for hyperlipoproteinemia and for pruritus resulting from partial biliary obstruction.

choline /kō′lēn/ [Gk *chole* bile], a lipotropic substance sometimes included in the B complex vitamins as essential for the metabolism of fats in the body. It is a primary component of acetylcholine, the neurotransmitter, and functions with inositol as a basic constituent of lecithin. The richest sources of choline are liver, kidneys, brains, wheat germ, brewer's yeast, and egg yolk.

choline esters, a group of cholinergic drugs that act in body sites where acetylcholine is the neurotransmitter. Examples include bethanechol, carbachol, and methacholine.

cholinergic [Gk *chole* + *ergon* to work], **1.** of or pertaining to nerve fibers that elaborate acetylcholine at the myoneural junctions. **2.** the tendency to transmit or to be stimulated by or to stimulate the elaboration of acetylcholine.

cholinergic blocking agent, any agent that blocks the action of acetylcholine and substances similar to acetylcholine. Such agents, in effect, block the action of cholinergic nerves that transmit impulses by the release of acetylcholine at their synapses.

cholinergic crisis, a pronounced muscular weakness and respiratory paralysis caused by excessive acetylcholine, often apparent in patients suffering from myasthenia gravis as a result of overmedication with anticholinesterase drugs.

cholinergic fibers [Gk *chole, ergon,* work; L *fibra*], nerve fibers of the autonomic nervous system that release the neurotransmitter acetylcholine. They include all preganglionic fibers, all postganglionic sympathetic fibers to sweat glands, and efferent fibers innervating skeletal muscle.

cholinergic nerve, a nerve that releases the neurotransmitter acetylcholine at its synapse. The cholinergic nerves include all the preganglionic sympathetic and the preganglionic parasympathetic nerves, the postganglionic parasympathetic nerves, the somatic motor nerves to skeletal muscles, and some nerves to sweat glands and to certain blood vessels.

cholinergic receptor [Gk *chole* + *ergon;* L *recipere* to receive], a specialized sensory nerve ending that responds to the stimulation of acetylcholine.

cholinergic stimulant. See **cholinergic.**

cholinergic urticaria [Gk *chole* + *ergon;* L *urtica* nettle], an abnormal and usually transient vascular reaction of the skin, often associated with sweating in susceptible individuals subjected to stress, strong exertion, or hot weather.

cholinesterase /kō′lines′tərās/, an enzyme that acts as a catalyst in the hydrolysis of acetylcholine to choline and acetate.

choliopancreatography /kōlē·ōpan′krē·ətog′rəfē/ [Gk *chole* + *pan* all, *kreas* flesh, *graphein* to record], the x-ray visualization of the bile and pancreatic ducts.

chondral /kon′drəl/, of or pertaining to cartilage.

chondrectomy /kondrek′təmē/, the surgical excision of a cartilage.

chondrial bone [Gk *chondros* cartilage; AS *ban* bone], pertaining to bone that forms under the periostial membrane.

chondriocont /kon′drē·ōkont′/, a threadlike or rod-shaped mitochondrion.

chondriome /kon′drē·ōm/ [Gk *chondros* cartilage], the total mitochondria content of a cell, taken as a unit.

chondriomite /kon′drē·ōmīt′/ [Gk *chondros* + *mitos* thread], a single granular mitochondrion or a group of such organelles appearing in a chain formation.

chondriosome. See **mitochondrion.**

chondritis /kondrī'tis/, any inflammatory condition affecting the joints.

chondroadenoma. See **adenochondroma.**

chondroangioma /kon'drō·an'jē·ō'mə/, pl. **chondroangiomas, chondroangiomata** [Gk *chondros* + *aggeion* little vessel, *oma* tumor], a benign, mesenchymal tumor containing vascular and cartilaginous elements.

chondroblast /kon'drōblast/ [Gk *chondros* + *blastos* germ], any one of the cells that develops from the mesenchyma and forms cartilage.

chondroblastoma /kon'drōblastō'mə/, pl. **chondroblastomas, chondroblastomata,** a benign tumor, derived from precursors of cartilage cells, that develops most frequently in epiphyses of the femur and humerus.

chondrocalcinosis /kon'drōkal'sinō'sis/ [Gk *chondros* + L *calyx* lime; Gk *osis* condition], an arthritic disease in which calcium deposits are found in the peripheral joints. It resembles gout and is often found in patients over 50 years of age who have osteoarthritis or diabetes mellitus.

chondrocarcinoma /kon'drōkär'sinō'mə/, pl. **chondrocarcinoma, chondrocarcinomata** [Gk *chondros* + *karkinos* crab, *oma* tumor], a malignant epithelial tumor in which there is cartilaginous metaplasia.

chondroclast /kon'drōklast/ [Gk *chondros* + *klasis* breaking], a giant multinucleated cell associated with the resorption of cartilage. **–chondroclastic,** adj.

chondrocostal /kon'drōkos'təl/ [Gk *chondros* + L *costa* rib], of or pertaining to the ribs and the costal cartilages.

chondrocyte /kon'drəsīt/ [Gk *chondros* + *kytos* cell], any one of the polymorphic cells that form the cartilage of the body. **–chondrocytic,** adj.

chondrodysplasia /kon'drōdisplā'zhə/ [Gk *chondros* + *dys* bad, *plassein* to form], an inherited disease characterized by abnormal growth at the ends of bones, particularly the long bones of the arms and legs.

chondrodysplasia punctata, an inherited form of dwarfism characterized by ichthyotic skin lesions, radiographic epiphyseal stippling, and a pug nose. There are two types of the anomaly, a benign Conradi-Hunermann form and a lethal rhizomelic form.

chondrodystrophia calcificans congenita [Gk *chondros* + *dys* bad, *trophe* nourishment; L *calyx* lime; *congenitus* born with], an inherited defect characterized by many small opacities in the epiphyses of the long bones. Dwarfism, contractures, cataracts,

mental retardation, and short stubby fingers develop as the infant grows into childhood.

chondrodystrophy /kon'drōdis'trəfe/ [Gk *chondros* + *dys* bad, *trophe* nourishment], a group of disorders in which there is abnormal conversion of cartilage to bone, particularly in the epiphyses of the long bones.

chondroectodermal dysplasia /kon'drō·ek'tədur'məl/, an inherited form of dwarfism marked by distal limb shortening, postaxial polydactyly, and cardiovascular abnormalities.

chondroendothelioma /kon'drō·en'dōthē'lē·ō'mə/, pl. **chondroendotheliomas, chondroendotheliomata** [Gk *chondros* + *endon* within, *thele* nipple, *oma* tumor], a benign mesenchymal tumor containing cartilaginous and endothelial components.

chondrofibroma /kon'drōfibrō'mə/, pl. **chondrofibromas, chondrofibromata,** a fibrous tumor containing cartilaginous components.

chondrogenesis /kon'drōjen'əsis/, the development of cartilage. **–chondrogenetic,** adj.

chondroid /kon'droid/, resembling cartilage.

chondrolipoma /kon'drōlipō'mə/, pl. **chondrolipomas, chondrolipomata,** a benign mesenchymal tumor containing fatty and cartilaginous components.

chondroma /kondrō'mə/, pl. **chondromas, chondromata,** a benign, fairly common tumor of cartilage cells that grows slowly within cartilage (enchondroma) or on the surface (ecchondroma). Kinds of chondromas are **joint chondroma** and **synovial chondroma. –chondromatous,** adj.

chondromalacia /kon'drōmälä'shə/ [Gk *chondros* + *malakia* softness], a softening of cartilage. **Chondromalacia fetalis** is a lethal congenital form of the condition in which the stillborn infant is born with soft and pliable limbs. **Chondromalacia patellae** occurs in young adults after knee injury and is characterized by swelling and pain and by degenerative changes, which are revealed on examination by x-ray.

chondroma sarcomatosum. See **chondrosarcoma.**

chondromatosis /kon'drōmatō'sis/, a condition characterized by the presence of many cartilaginous tumors. A kind of chondromatosis is **synovial chondromatosis.**

chondromere /kon'drōmir/ [Gk *chondros* + *meros* part], a cartilaginous, embryonic vertebra and its costal component.

chondromyoma /kon'drōmī·ō'mə/, pl. **chondromyomas, chondromyomata** [Gk chondros + mys muscle, oma tumor], a benign mesenchymal tumor containing myomatous and cartilaginous tissue.

chondromyxofibroma /kon'drōmik'sōfī-brō'mə/ [Gk chondros + myxa mucus; L fibra fiber; oma tumor], a benign tumor that develops from cartilage-forming connective tissue. The lesion, typically a firm, grayish white, somewhat rubbery mass, tends to occur in the knee and small bones of the foot.

chondromyxoid /kon'drōmik'soid/ [Gk chondros + myxa mucus, eidos form], composed of cartilaginous and myxoid elements.

chondromyxoid fibroma. See chondromyxofibroma.

chondrophyte /kon'drōfīt'/ [Gk chondros + phyton growth], an abnormal mass of cartilage. —chondrophytic, adj.

chondroplasia /-plā'zhə/ [Gk, chondros, cartilage, plassein, to form], the formation of cartilage.

chondroplast. See chondroblast.

chondroplasty /kon'drōplas'tē/ [Gk chondros + plassein to form], the surgical repair of cartilage.

chondrosarcoma /kon'drōsärkō'mə/, pl. **chondrosarcomas, chondrosarcomata** [Gk chondros + sarx flesh, oma tumor], a malignant neoplasm of cartilaginous cells or their precursors that occurs most frequently on long bones, the pelvic girdle, and the scapula. Kinds of chondrosarcomas are **central chondrosarcoma** and **mesenchymal chondrosarcoma.** —chondrosarcomatous, adj.

chondrosarcomatosis /kon'drōsär'kōmə-tō'sis/, a condition characterized by multiple, malignant cartilaginous tumors.

chondrosis /kondrō'sis/, 1. the development of the cartilage of the body. 2. a cartilaginous tumor.

chondrotomy /kondrot'əmē/, a surgical procedure for dividing a cartilage.

CHOP, an anticancer drug combination of cyclophosphamide, doxorubicin, vincristine, and prednisone.

chopping, a therapeutic exercise to improve the strength and coordination of upper trunk nerves and muscles by lifting the arms overhead and bringing them down in a chopping or slashing movement.

chordae tendineae /kô'dētendin'i-ē/, sing. **chorda tendinea,** the strands of tendon that anchor the cusps of the mitral and the tricuspid valves to the papillary muscles of the ventricles of the heart, preventing prolaspe of the valves into the atria during ventricular contraction.

chordal canal. See notochordal canal.

chorda spinalis. See spinal cord.

chorda umbilicalis. See umbilical cord.

chordee /kôr'dē, kôr'dā/ [Gk chorde cord], a congenital defect of the genitourinary tract resulting in a ventral curvature of the penis, caused by a fibrous band of tissue instead of normal skin along the corpus spongiosum.

chordencephalon /kôrd'ensef'əlon/ [Gk chorde + enkephalos brain], the portion of the central nervous system that develops in the early weeks of pregnancy from the neural tube and includes the mesencephalon, the rhombencephalon, and the spinal cord. —chordencephalic, adj.

chorditis /kôrdī'tis/, 1. inflammation of a spermatic cord. 2. inflammation of the vocal cords or of the vocal folds.

chordoid /kôr'doid/ [Gk chorde + eidos form], resembling the notocord or notochordal tissue.

chordoma /kôrdō'mə/, pl. **chordomas, chordomata,** a rare, congenital tumor of the brain developing from the fetal notochord.

chordotomy /kôrdot'əmē/ [Gk chorde + temnein to cut], an operation in which the anterolateral tracts of the spinal cord are surgically divided to relieve pain.

chorea /kôrē'ə/ [Gk choreia dance], a condition characterized by involuntary, purposeless, rapid motions, as flexing and extending the fingers, raising and lowering the shoulders, or grimacing.

chorea gravidarum /kôr'ē-əgrav'idär'əm/, a form of chorea occurring during a first pregnancy subsequent to an episode of Sydenham's chorea in childhood.

chorea minor. See Sydenham's chorea.

choreic ataxia [Gk, choreia, dance, ataxia, lack of order], a form of ataxia in which patients lack muscular coordination and movements are marked by involuntary twitchng and abrupt jerking.

choreiform /kərē'əfôrm'/, resembling the rapid jerky movements associated with chorea.

choreiform spasm [Gk choreia; L forma; Gk spasmos], a condition of involuntary muscle contractions that result in dancing motions. One type of dancing spasm involves powerful contractions of the leg muscles, resulting in a leaping, jumping action. It can also involve arm, shoulder, and neck muscles.

choreoathetoid cerebral palsy /kôr'ē-ō-ath'ətoid/, a form of cerebral palsy characterized by both choreiform (jerky, ticlike twitching) and athetoid (slow, writhing) movements.

chorioadenoma /kərē'ō-ad'inō'mə/, pl. **chorioadenomas, chorioadenomata** [Gk chorion skin, aden gland, oma tumor], an epithelial cell tumor of the outermost fetal membrane that is intermediate in the malignant development of a hydatid mole to invasive choriocarcinoma.

chorioadenoma destruens /-ad′ənō′mə-des′troo·ons/ [Gk *chorion, aden, oma* + L *destruere* to pull down], an invasive hydatidiform mole in which the chorionic villi of the mole penetrate into the myometrium and parametrium of the uterus and metastasize to distant parts of the body.

chorioallantoic graft [Gk *chorion* + *allas* sausage, *eidos* form; *graphion* stylus], the grafting of tissue onto the chorioallantoic membrane of the egg of a hen to improve the environment for embryonic growth.

chorioamnionic /kôr′ē·ō·am′nē·ot′ik/, of or pertaining to the chorion and the amnion.

chorioamnionitis /-am′nē·ōnī′tis/ [Gk *chorion* + *amnion* fetal membrane, *itis* inflammation], an inflammatory reaction in the amniotic membranes caused by organisms in the amniotic fluid.

choriocarcinoma /kôr′ē·ōkär′sinō′mə/, pl. **choriocarcinomas, choriocarcinomata**, an epithelial malignancy of fetal origin that develops from the chorionic portion of the products of conception, usually from a hydatidiform mole. The primary tumor usually appears in the uterus as a soft, dark red, crumbling mass.

choriocele /kôr′ē·əsēl′/ [Gk *chorion* + *kele* hernia], a hernia or protrusion of the tissue of the choroid layer of the eye.

chorioepithelioma. See **choriocarcinoma.**

choriogenesis /kôr′ē·ōjen′əsis/, the development of the chorion after the trophoblast anchors to the uterine tissue and extends primary villi into the intervillous space. —**choriogenetic,** *adj.*

choriomeningitis. See **lymphocytic choriomeningitis.**

chorion /kôr′ē·on/ [Gk, a skin], (in biology) the outermost extraembryonic membrane composed of trophoblast lined with mesoderm. It develops villi about 2 weeks after fertilization and is vascularized by allantoic vessels 1 week later. It gives rise to the placenta and persists until birth as the outer of the two layers of membrane containing the amniotic fluid and the fetus.

chorionic carcinoma, chorionic epithelioma. See **choriocarcinoma.**

chorionic gonadotropin (CG) /kôr′ē·on′ik gon′ədōtrōp′in/ [Gk *chorion; gone* seed, *trophe* nutrition], a chemical component of the urine of pregnant women and pregnant mares. This glycoprotein hormone is secreted by the placental trophoblastic cells. It is composed of two subunits, alpha and beta human cho-

rionic gonadotropin. The alpha subunit is nearly identical to similar subunits of the follicle-stimulating, luteinizing, and thyroid-stimulating hormones. The specific hormonal effects of chorionic gonadotropin are activated by the beta portion. They include stimulation of the corpus luteum to secrete estrogen and progesterone and to decrease lymphocyte activation.

chorionic plate [Gk *chorion; platys* flat], the part of the fetal placenta that gives rise to chorionic villi, which attach to the uterus during the early stage of formation of the placenta.

chorionic sac [Gk *chorion* + *sakkos* sack], the saclike membrane that develops from the blastocyst wall to envelop the embryo.

chorionic villi [Gk *chorion;* L *villus* shaggy hair], tiny vascular fibrils on the surface of the chorion that infiltrate the maternal blood sinuses of the endometrium and help form the placenta.

chorionic villi sampling [Gk *chorion;* L *villus* shaggy hair, *exemplum* sample], a procedure for obtaining prenatal evaluation data early in a pregnancy by withdrawing a chorionic villi sample from the fetal membranes. The sample is obtained through a catheter inserted into the uterus.

chorioretinitis /kôr′ē·ōret′inī′tis/, an inflammatory condition of the choroid and retina of the eye, usually as a result of parasitic or bacterial infection. It is characterized by blurred vision, photophobia, and distorted images.

chorioretinopathy /kôr′ē·ōret′ənop′əthē/ [Gk *chorion* + L *rete* net; Gk *pathos* disease], a noninflammatory process caused by disease that involves the choroid and the retina.

choroid /kôr′oid/ [Gk *chorion* + *eidos* form], a thin, highly vascular membrane covering the posterior five sixths of the eye between the retina and sclera.

choroidal malignant melanoma [Gk *chorion, eidos* + L *malignus* ill-disposed; Gk *melas* black, *oma* tumor], a tumor of the choroid coat that grows into the vitreous humor, causing detachment and degeneration of the overlying retina.

choroiditis /kôr′oidī′tis/, an inflammatory condition of the choroid membrane of the eye.

choroidocyclitis /kôroi′dōsikli′tis/ [Gk *chorion, eidos* + *kyklos* circle, *itis* inflammation], an abnormal condition characterized by inflammation of the choroid and the ciliary processes.

choroidoretinitis. See **chorioretinopathy.**

choroid plexectomy /pleksek′təmē/ [Gk *chorion, eidos;* L *plexus* pleated; Gk *ek-*

tome excision], a surgical procedure for the reduction of cerebrospinal fluid production in the ventricles of the brain in hydrocephalus, usually in the newborn.

choroid plexus [Gk *chorion, eidos*; L, pleated], any one of the tangled masses of tiny blood vessels contained within the ventricles of the brain.

Christchurch chromosome (Ch¹), [Christchurch, city on South Island of New Zealand], an abnormally small acrocentric chromosome of the G group, involving any members of chromosome pairs 21 or 22, in which the short arms are missing or partially deleted.

Christian-Weber disease [Henry Asbury Christian, American physician, b. 1876; Frederick Parkes Weber, English physician, b. 1863], a rare form of panniculitis characterized by nodular formations in the subcutaneous tissues and prolonged intermittent relapsing fever.

Christmas disease. See **hemophilia B.**

Christmas factor. See **factor IX.**

chromaffin /krō'məfin/ [Gk *chroma* color; L *affin* affinity], having an affinity for strong staining with chromium salts, especially strong staining of the cells of the adrenal, the coccygeal, and the carotid glands, certain cells of the adrenal medulla, and the cells of the paraganglions. Also **chromaphil** /krō'məfil/.

chromaffin body. See **paraganglion.**

chromaffin cell, any one of the special cells comprising the paraganglia and connected to the ganglia of the celiac, the renal, the suprarenal, the aortic, and the hypogastric plexuses. The chromaffin cells of the adrenal medulla secrete two catecholamines, epinephrine and norepinephrine, which affect smooth muscle, cardiac muscle, and glands in the same way as sympathetic stimulation, increasing and prolonging sympathetic effects.

chromaffinoma. See **pheochromocytoma.**

chromaphil. See **chromaffin.**

chromatic /krōmat'ik/ [Gk *chroma* color], 1. of or pertaining to color. 2. stainable by a dye. 3. of or pertaining to chromatin. Also **chromatinic.**

chromatic asymmetry of iris [Gk, *chroma,* color, *a, symmetria,* commensurability, *iris,* rainbow], a difference in color of the two irides.

chromatic dispersion [Gk *chroma* + L *dis* apart, *spargere* to scatter], the splitting of light into its various component wavelengths or frequencies, such as with a prism.

chromatid /krō'mətid/ [Gk *chroma* color], one of the two identical threadlike filaments of a chromosome.

chromatid deletion, the breakage of a chromatid. The breakage may be caused by a single-hit effect produced by radiation. The fragments are isochromatids.

chromatin /krō'mətin/ [Gk *chroma* color], the material within the cell nucleus from which the chromosomes are formed. It consists of fine, threadlike strands of deoxyribonucleic acid attached to a protein base, usually histone. During cell division, portions of the chromatin condense and coil to form the chromosomes. A kind of chromatin is **sex chromatin, –chromatinic,** *adj.*

chromatin-negative, pertaining to or descriptive of the nuclei of cells that lack sex chromatin, specifically characteristic of the normal male, but also occurring in certain chromosomal abnormalities.

chromatin nucleolus. See **karyosome.**

chromatin-positive, pertaining to or descriptive of the nuclei of cells that contain sex chromatin, specifically characteristic of the normal female, but occurring also in certain chromosomal abnormalities.

chromatism /krō'mətiz'əm/, 1. an abnormal condition characterized by hallucinations in which the affected individual sees colored lights. 2. abnormal pigmentation.

chromatogram /krōmat'əgram'/, 1. the record produced by the separation of gaseous substances or dissolved chemical substances moving through a column of absorbent material that filters out the various absorbates in different layers. 2. any graphic record produced by any chromatographic method.

chromatography /krō'mətog'rəfē/, any one of several processes for separating and analyzing various gaseous or dissolved chemical materials according to differences in their absorbency with respect to a specific substance and according to their different pigments. Some kinds of chromatography are **column, displacement, gas, ion-exchange,** and **paper chromatography. –chromatographic,** *adj.*

chromatopsia /krō'mətop'sē·ə/ [Gk *chroma* + *opsis* vision], 1. an abnormal condition characterized by a visual defect that makes colorless objects appear tinged with color. 2. a form of color blindness characterized by the imperfect perception of various colors. It may be caused by a deficiency in one or more of the retinal cones or from defective nerve circuits that convey color-associated impulses to the cerebral cortex. The most common defect in color sense is the inability to distinguish red from green.

chromatosis, a condition of abnormal skin pigmentation in any part of the body.

chromaturia [Gk, *chroma,* color, *ouron,* urine], urine that has an abnormal color.

chromesthesia /krō′misthē′zhə/ [Gk *chroma* + *aisthesis* feeling], **1.** the color sense that depends on the mixture of wavelengths in the light that enters the eye and the response of the different types of retinal cones associated with color vision. **2.** an abnormal condition characterized by the confusion of other senses, such as taste and smell, with imagined sensations of color.

chromhidrosis /krō′midrō′sis/ [Gk *chroma* + *hidros* sweat], a rare, functional disorder in which apocrine sweat glands secrete colored sweat.

chromic catgut /krō′mik/ [Gk, *chroma,* color; L, *catta;* AS, *guttas*], surgical catgut that has been treated with chromium trioxide to strengthen it.

chromic myopia, a kind of color blindness characterized by the ability to distinguish colors only of those objects that are close to the eye.

chromium (Cr) /krō′mē·əm/ [Gk *chroma* color], a hard, brittle, metallic element. Its atomic number is 24; its atomic weight is 51.9. Traces of chromium occur in plants and animals, and there is evidence this element may be important in human nutrition, especially in carbohydrate metabolism. Chromium 51 isotope is used in blood studies.

chromium alum, a chemical commonly used to fix, or harden, the emulsion of an x-ray film during manual processing.

chromobacteriosis /krō′məbaktir′ē·ō′sis/, an extremely rare, usually fatal systemic infection caused by a bacillus *Chromobacterium violaceum,* found in fresh water in tropic and subtropic regions, which enters the body through a break in the skin.

chromoblastomycosis /krō′mōblas′tōmī-kō′sis/ [Gk *chroma* + *blastos* germ, *mykes* fungus, *osis* condition], an infectious skin disease caused by any of a variety of fungi and characterized by the appearance of pruritic, warty nodules that develop in a cut or other break in the skin.

chromocenter. See **karyosome.**

chromogen /krō′mōjən/, a substance that absorbs light, producing color.

chromolipid, chromolipoid. See **lipochrome.**

chromomere /krō′əmir/ [Gk *chroma* + *meros* part], any of the series of beadlike structures that lie along the chromonema of a chromosome during the early stages of cell division.

chromomycosis. See **chromoblastomycosis.**

chromonema /krō′mənē′mə/, *pl.* **chromonemata** [Gk *chroma* + *nema* thread], the coiled filament along which the chromomeres lie that forms the central part of the chromatid of the chromosome during cell division.

chromophilic /krō′məfil′ik/ [Gk *chroma* + *philein* to love], denoting a cell, tissue, or microorganism that is easily stained, particularly certain leukocytes.

chromophobe adenoma. See **chromophobic adenoma.**

chromophobia /krō′mə-/ [Gk *chroma* + *phobos* fear] **1.** the resistance of certain cells and tissues to stains. **2.** a morbid aversion to colors. **–chromophobe,** *n.*

chromophobic /krō′məfō′bik/, denoting a cell, tissue, or microorganism that is not easily stained, particularly certain cells of the anterior lobe of the pituitary gland.

chromophobic adenoma, a tumor of the pituitary gland composed of cells that do not stain with acid or basic dyes.

chromoplasm. See **chromatin.**

chromosomal aberration [Gk *chroma* + *soma* body; L *aberrare* to wander], any change in the structure or number of any of the chromosomes for a given species, which can result in anomalies of varying severity. In humans, a number of disorders are directly associated with chromosomal defects, including Down syndrome, Turner's syndrome, and Kleinfelter's syndrome.

chromosomal nomenclature, a standard nomenclature that serves to identify the complement of chromosomes in an individual according to the number of chromosomes, sex, and the deletion or addition of a specific chromosome or part of a chromosome. Complement in a normal female is recorded as 46,XX, and for a normal male, 46,XY. Chromosomal aberrations are designated by indicating the total chromosomal number, sex complement, and the group or specific chromosome in which the addition or deletion occurs. The short arm of a chromosome is designated "p," the long arm is "q," and a translocation is "t".

chromosomal sex [Gk, *chroma,* color + *soma,* body; L, *sexus,* male or female], in mammals, the sex of an individual as determined by the presence or absence of the Y chromosome.

chromosome /krō′məsōm/ [Gk *chroma* + *soma* body, any one of the threadlike structures in the nucleus of a cell that function in the transmission of genetic information. Each consists of a double strand of the nucleoprotein deoxyribonucleic acid (DNA), which is coiled in a helix formation and attached to a protein base, usually a histone. The genes, which contain the genetic material that controls the inheritance of traits, are arranged in a linear pattern along the entire length of each DNA strand. Each species has a characteristic number of chromosomes in the somatic cell, which in humans is 46 and includes 22 homologous pairs of autosomes and one pair of sex chromosomes, with one member of each pair being derived from each parent. Kinds of chromosomes include **accessory, Christchurch, daughter, gametic, giant, homologous, Philadelphia, sex, somatic, W,** and **Z chromosome.** –**chromosomal,** *adj.*

chromosome banding. See **banding.**

chromosome coil, the spiral formed by the coiling of two or more chromonemata of the chromatid within the chromosome.

chromosome complement, the normal number of chromosomes found in the somatic cell of any given species. In humans it is 46, consisting of 22 pairs of homologous autosomes and one pair of sex chromosomes.

chromosome 5p–syndrome. See **cat-cry syndrome.**

chromosome mapping. See **mapping.**

chromosome puff, a band of accumulated chromatic material located at a specific site on a giant chromosome. It is indicative of gene activity, specifically DNA and RNA synthesis, for the particular locus.

chromosome walking, the process by which overlapping molecular clones that span large chromosomal intervals are isolated.

chromotrope /krō′mətrōp/ [Gk *chroma* + *trepein* to turn], **1.** a component of tissue that stains metachromatically with metachromatic dyes. **2.** any one of several dyes differentiated by numeric suffixes. –**chromotropic,** *adj.*

chronaxie /krō′naksē/ [Gk *chronos* time, *axia* value], (in electroneuromyography) a measure of the shortest duration of an electric stimulus needed to excite nerve or muscle tissue.

chronic /kron′ik/ [Gk *chronos* time], (of a disease or disorder) developing slowly and persisting for a long period of time, often for the remainder of the lifetime of the individual.

chronic abscess [Gk, *chronos,* time; L, *abscedere,* to go away], a slowly developing abscess that produces pus but shows little or no inflammation, redness, or pain. It is usually a tuberculous abscess.

chronic airway obstruction, a type of respiratory disorder in which the patient, when at rest, appears to breathe at a normal rate and does not show signs of respiratory distress. However, there may be prolongation of the expiratory phase with pursed-lip breathing.

chronic alcoholic delirium. See **Korsakoff's psychosis.**

chronic alcoholism, a pathologic condition resulting from the habitual use of alcohol in excessive amounts. Symptoms include anorexia, diarrhea, weight loss, neurologic and psychiatric disturbances (most notably depression), and fatty deterioration of the liver, sometimes leading to cirrhosis.

chronic appendicitis, a type of appendicitis characterized by thickening or scarring of the vermiform appendix, caused by previous inflammation.

chronic bronchitis, a very common debilitating respiratory disease, characterized by greatly increased production of mucus by the glands of the trachea and bronchi and resulting in a cough with expectoration for at least 3 months of the year for more than 2 consecutive years.

chronic care, a pattern of medical and nursing care that focuses on long-term care of people with chronic diseases or conditions, either at home or in a medical facility.

chronic carrier, an individual who acts as host to pathogenic organisms for an extended period of time without displaying any signs of disease.

chronic cervicitis. See **cervicitis.**

chronic cholecystitis. See **cholecystitis.**

chronic chorea. See **Huntington's chorea.**

chronic cystic mastitis. See **fibrocystic disease.**

chronic delirium [Gk, *chronos,* time; L, *delirare,* to rave], a form of delirium in which the patient shows signs of psychosis but is afebrile. The condition is sometimes associated with exhaustion, malnutrition, and wasting.

chronic disease, a disease that persists over a long period of time as compared with the course of an acute disease. The symptoms of chronic disease are usually less severe than those of the acute phase of the same disease.

chronic endoarteritis [Gk *chronos, endon* within, *arteria* windpipe, *itis,* inflammation], an inflammatory condition of the tunica intima lining of an artery wall. It may be accompanied by fatty degeneration of arterial tissue and calcium deposits.

chronic endocarditis [Gk *chronos, endon* + *kardia* heart, *itis* inflammation], an inflammatory condition of the endocardium lining the heart, usually following an attack of acute endocarditis, syphilis, or an atheroma. It frequently involves the cardiac valves, making them incompetent.

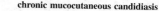

chronic fatigue syndrome (CFS), a condition characterized by the onset of disabling fatigue after an initial viral-like illness. The fatigue is accompanied by a constellation of symptoms including myalgias, arthralgias without frank arthritis, low-grade fevers, painful cervical adenopathy, sore throat, headache, memory deficits, and sleep disturbances. The diagnosis is one of exclusion; the cause remaining obscure. Therapy is directed toward the relief of symptoms. Psychiatric intervention is frequently helpful in support of depression which frequently accompanies the condition. The disorder usually resolves spontaneously.

chronic gastritis. See **gastritis.**

chronic glaucoma. See **glaucoma.**

chronic glomerulonephritis, a noninfectious disease of the glomerulus of the kidney characterized by proteinuria, hematuria, edema, and decreased production of urine.

chronic gout [Gk *chronos;* L *gutta* drop], a persistent condition of purine metabolism, characterized by abnormally high levels of serum uric acid and attacks of arthritis, with deposits of urates in the joints. The disorder may be familial and if untreated can lead to renal failure.

chronic hepatitis [Gk *chronos, hepar* liver *itis*], a state in which the symptoms continue for several months and may increase in severity. In some cases of hepatitis B, the patient may become a lifelong carrier of the antigen and may show prolonged evidence of the infection.

chronic hyperplastic rhinitis [Gk *chronos* + *hyper* excess + *plassein* to form + *rhis* nose + *itis*], chronic inflammation of the mucous membranes of the nose, with polyp formation.

chronic hyperplastic sinusitis [Gk *chronos* + *hyper* + *plassein;* L *sinus* hollow; Gk *itis* inflammation], chronic sinus inflammation, with polyp formation in the nose and sinuses.

chronic hypertrophic rhinitis [Gk *chronos* + *hyper* + *trophe* nourishment + *rhis,* nose + *itis*], a condition of chronic inflammation of the nasal mucosa associated with enlargement of the mucous membrane.

chronic hypoxia, a usually slow, insidious reduction in oxygen flow to the tissue cells resulting from gradually destructive or fibrotic lung diseases, congenital or acquired heart disorders, or chronic blood loss. There is usually an absence of acute symptoms; but the person develops persistent mental and physical fatigue, shows sluggish mental responses, and complains

of a loss of ability to perform physical tasks.

chronic idiopathic thrombocytopenic purpura. See **idiopathic thrombocytopenic purpura.**

chronic illness, any illness that persists over a long period of time and affects physical, emotional, intellectual, social, or spiritual functioning.

chronic intestinal ischemia. See **intestinal angina.**

chronic interstitial nephritis. See **interstitial nephritis.**

chronic intractable pain [Gk, *chronos,* time; L, *intractabilis* + *poena,* penalty], persistent pain that fails to respond to nonnarcotic analgesics and other treatment measures.

chronicity /krōnis′itē/, pertaining to a state of being chronic.

chronic leg ulcer [Gk *chronos;* ONorse *leggr;* L *ulcus* ulcer], a slow-healing ulcer of the leg, usually associated with varicose veins or a similar circulatory obstacle.

chronic lingual papillitis [Gk *chronos* + L *lingua* tongue; *papilla* nipple; Gk *itis*], an inflammatory disorder of the tongue, sometimes extending to the buccal mucosa and palate, characterized by irregularly scattered red patches, thinning of the lingual papillae, severe burning pain, and shedding of epidermal tissue.

chronic lymphocytic leukemia (CLL) [Gk *chronos* + L *lympha* water; Gk *kytos* cell; *leukos* white, *haima* blood], a neoplasm of blood-forming tissues, characterized by a proliferation of small, long-lived lymphocytes, chiefly B cells, in bone marrow, blood liver, and lymphoid organs. No treatment is curative, but remissions may be induced by chemotherapy with chlorambucil and glucocorticoids or by thymic, splenic, or total body irradiation.

chronic mastitis. See **mastitis.**

chronic mountain sickness [Gk *chronos;* L *montana;* AS *soec*], a form of altitude sickness in which the increased production of red cells results in polycythemia. Some symptoms of mountain sickness such as headache, weakness, and limb aches occasionally develop in indigenous mountain dwellers as well as persons who had become acclimatized to the higher altitudes.

chronic mucocutaneous candidiasis, an abnormal condition and rare form of candidiasis, characterized by lesions of the skin, viral infections, and recurrent respiratory tract infections. This disease usually occurs during the first year of life but can develop as late as the 20s. It affects both men and women and is associated with an inherited defect of the cell-mediated immune system and apparently allows autoantibodies to develop against target organs. The humoral immune system functions normally in this disease. The onset of infections associated with the disease may precede endocrinopathy.

chronic myelocytic leukemia (CML), a malignant neoplasm of blood-forming tissues, characterized by a proliferation of granular leukocytes and, often, of megakaryocytes. The disease is marked by malaise, fatigue, heat intolerance, bleeding gums, purpura, skin lesions, weight loss, hyperuricemia, abdominal discomfort, and massive splenomegaly.

chronic myocarditis [Gk *chronos, mys* muscle, *kardia* heart, *itis* inflammation], an inflammatory condition of the myocardium that persists after an acute bacterial attack. Chronic myocarditis is characterized by degeneration of muscle tissue and fibrosis or infiltration of interstitial tissues.

chronic nephritis [Gk *chronos, nephros* kidney, *itis*], a form of kidney inflammation usually secondary to another disease, such as chronic pyelonephritis. In chronic interstitial nephritis, the kidney becomes small and granular with thickening of arteries and arterioles and proliferation of interstitial tissue. There may be functional abnormalities, such as urea retention, hematuria, and casts.

chronic nephropathy, a kidney disorder characterized by generalized or local damage to the tubulointerstitial areas of the kidney. The condition frequently results from more than a single cause, such as diabetes and a bacterial infection. Symptoms include polyuria, renal acidosis, edema, proteinuria, and blood in the urine.

chronic obstructive pulmonary disease (COPD), a progressive and irreversible condition characterized by diminished inspiratory and expiratory capacity of the lungs. The person complains of dyspnea with physical exertion, of difficulty in inhaling or exhaling deeply, and sometimes of a chronic cough.

chronic (open-angle) glaucoma. See **glaucoma.**

chronic pain, pain that continues or recurs over a prolonged period, caused by various diseases or abnormal conditions, as rheumatoid arthritis. Chronic pain is often less intense than the acute pain. The person with chronic pain does not display increased pulse and rapid respiration because these autonomic reactions to pain cannot be sustained for long periods.

chronic pancreatitis [Gk *chronos + pan* all + *kreas* flesh + *itis*], chronic inflammation of the pancreas with fibrosis and calcification of the gland. It may follow repeated acute attacks and can lead to diabetes.

chronic peritonitis [Gk *chronos, peri* near, *tenein* to stretch, *itis*], a form of peritonitis in which the peritoneum thickens and ascites develop. The condition is usually associated with another disorder, such as pericarditis or polyserositis.

chronic pharyngitis [Gk *chronos, pharynx* throat, *itis*], a form of throat inflammation that may be associated with the lymphoid granules in the pharyngeal mucosa.

chronic prostatitis [Gk *chronos, prostates* one standing before, *itis*], a persistent inflammatory condition of the prostate gland characterized by a dull, aching pain in the lower back or perineal area, dysuria, fever, and discharge from the penis.

chronic pyelonephritis. See **pyelonephritis.**

chronic rheumatism [Gk *chronos + rheumatismos* that which flows], a chronic nonspecific painful condition of the musculoskeletal tissues, including nonarticular forms of arthritis.

chronic synovitis [Gk *chronos + syn* together; L *ovum* egg; Gk *itis* inflammation], chronic inflammation of the synovial membrane of a joint. Kinds of chronic synovitis include **chronic purulent synovitis, chronic serous synovitis.**

chronic tetanus [Gk *chronos + tetanos* convulsive tension], **1.** a form of tetanus with a delayed onset, slow progress of the disease, and milder than usual symptoms. **2.** a reactivated tetanus infection in a healed wound.

chronic tuberculous mastitis, a rare infection of the breast resulting from extension of tuberculosis of underlying ribs.

chronic undifferentiated schizophrenia, a condition marked by the symptoms of more than one of the classic types of schizophrenia--simple, paranoid, catatonic, or hebephrenic.

chronograph /kron'əgraf/ [Gk *chronos + graphein* to record], a device that records small intervals of time, such as a stopwatch. **–chronographic,** *adj.*

chronologic, chronological [Gk *chronos + logos* reason] **1.** arranged in time sequence. **2.** of or pertaining to chronology.

chronologic age, the age of an individual expressed as a period of time that has elapsed since birth, as the age of an infant, which is expressed in hours, days, or months, and the age of children and adults, expressed in years.

chronopsychophysiology /kron'ō'sīkofis'-ē·ol'əjē/, the science of physiologic cyclic processes in the body.

chronotropism /krənot'rəpiz'əm/ [Gk *chronos + trepein* to turn], the act or process of affecting the regularity of a periodic function, especially interference with the rate of heartbeat. **–chronotropic,** *adj.*

chrysarobin /kris′ərō′bin/, a substance obtained from the wood of araboa trees and used as an irritant in the treatment of parasitic skin diseases and psoriasis.

chrysiasis /krəsī′əsis/ [Gk *chrysos* gold, *osis* condition], an abnormal condition characterized by the deposition of gold in the tissues of the body.

chrysotherapy /kris′ōther′əpē/ [Gk *chrysos* + *therapeia* treatment], the treatment of any disease with gold salts. **–chrysotherapeutic,** *adj.*

Chua K'a, a holistic counseling system of muscle tension release that emphasizes clarification and cleansing of the mind and emotions.

Churg-Strauss syndrome /churg′strous′/, an allergic disorder marked by granulomatosis, usually of the lungs, and often involving the circulatory system.

Chvostek's sign /khvôsh′teks/ [Franz Chvostek, Austrian surgeon, b. 1835], an abnormal spasm of the facial muscles elicited by light taps on the facial nerve in patients who are hypocalcemic. It is a sign of tetany.

Chvostek-Weiss sign. See **Chvostek's sign.**

chyle /kīl/ [Gk *chylos* juice], the cloudy liquid products of digestion taken up by the small intestine. Consisting mainly of emulsified fats, chyle passes through fingerlike projections in the small intestine. **–chylous,** *adj.*

chyliform ascites. See **chylous ascites.**

chyloid /kī′loid/, resembling the chyle that fills the lacteals of the small intestine during the digestion of fatty foods.

chylomediastinum /kī′lōmēdē·astī′nəm/ [Gk, *chylos*, juice; L, *mediastinus*, midway], the presence of chyle in the mediastinum.

chylomicron /kī′lōmī′kron/ [Gk *chylos* + *mikros* small], minute droplets of the lipoproteins measuring less than 0.5 μm in diameter. Chylomicrons consist of about 90% triglycerides with small amounts of cholesterol, phospholipids, and protein. They are synthesized in the GI tract and carry dietary glycerides from the intestinal mucosa into the plasma.

chylosus ascites. See **chylous ascites.**

chylothorax /kī′lōthôr′aks/ [Gk *chylos* + *thorax* chest], a condition marked by the effusion of chyle from the thoracic duct into the pleural space.

chylous ascites, an abnormal condition characterized by an accumulation of chyle in the peritoneal cavity.

chyluria /kīlŏŏr′ē·ə/ [Gk *chylos* + *ouron* urine], a condition characterized by the milky appearance of the urine because of the presence of chyle.

chylus. See **chyle.**

chyme /kīm/ [Gk *chymos* juice], the viscous, semifluid contents of the stomach present during digestion of a meal.

chymopapain /kīmōpəpā′ēn/ [Gk *chymos* + Sp *papaya*], a proteolytic enzyme isolated from the fruit of *Carica papaya* and related to papain.

chymosin. See **rennin.**

chymotrypsin /kī′mōtrip′sin/ [Gk *chymos* + *tryein* to rub, *pepsin* digestion], **1.** a proteolytic enzyme, produced by the pancreas, that catalyzes the hydrolysis of casein and gelatin. **2.** a yellow crystalline powder prepared from an extract of ox pancreas, used in treating digestive disorders.

chymotrypsinogen /kī′mōtripsin′əjən/, a substance, produced in the pancreas, that is the zymogen precursor to the enzyme chymotrypsin. It is converted to chymotrypsin by trypsin.

Ci, abbreviation for **curie.**

CI, abbreviation for **color index.**

CI, abbreviation for *Colour Index.*

cibophobia /sē′bə-/ [L *cibus* food; Gk *phobos* fear], an abnormal or morbid aversion to food or to eating.

CIC, abbreviation for *Certified Infection Control.*

cicatricial entropion. See **cicatrix, entropion.**

cicatrical scar /sik′ətrish′əl/ [L *cicatrix* scar; Gk *eschara* scab], a fibrous scar that remains after a wound has healed.

cicatricial stenosis [L *cicatrix*; Gk *stenos* narrow, *osis* condition], the narrowing of a duct or tube because of the formation of scar tissue.

cicatrix /sik′ətriks, sikā′triks/, *pl.* **cicatrices** /sik′ətrī′sēz/ [L, scar], scar tissue that is avascular, pale, contracted, and firm after the earlier phase of skin healing characterized by redness and softness. **–cicatricial** /sik′ətrish′əl/, *adj.* **cicatrize,** *v.*

cicatrize [L *cicatrix* scar], to heal so as to form a scar.

ciclopirox /sī′kləpī′roks/, an antifungal agent prescribed in the treatment of tinea and candidiasis.

ciclosporin. See **cyclosporine.**

cicutism /sik′yōōtiz′əm/ [L *Cicuta* hemlock; Gk *ismos* process], poisoning caused by water hemlock, resulting in cyanosis, dilated pupils, convulsions, and coma.

CID, abbreviation for **cytomegalic inclusion disease.**

cigarette drain [Sp *cigarro;* AS *dranen*], a

surgical drain fashioned from a section of gauze or surgical sponge drawn into a tube of gutta-percha.

cigarette smoking, the inhalation of the gases and hydrocarbon vapors generated by slowly burning tobacco in cigarettes. The practice is partly due to the effect on the nervous system of the nicotine contained in the smoke. In addition to nicotine, nearly 1,000 other chemicals have been identified in cigarette smoke.

ciguatera poisoning /sē′gwɔter′ə/ [Sp *cigua* sea snail; L *potio* drink], a nonbacterial food poisoning that results from eating fish contaminated with the ciguatera toxin. Characteristics of ciguatera poisoning are vomiting, diarrhea, tingling or numbness of extremities and the skin around the mouth, itching, muscle weakness, and pain.

cilia /sil′ē·ə/, *sing.* **cilium** [L, eyelids] **1.** the eyelids or eyelashes. **2.** small, hairlike processes on the outer surfaces of some cells, aiding metabolism by producing motion, eddies, or current in a fluid. **–ciliary,** *adj.*

ciliary /sil′ē·er′ē/ [L, *cilium,* eyelash], pertaining to the eyelashes or eyelids.

ciliary body [L *cilium* eyelid], the thickened part of the vascular tunic of the eye that joins the iris with the anterior portion of the choroid.

ciliary canal, the spaces of the iridocorneal angle.

ciliary gland, one of the numerous tiny, modified sweat glands arranged in several rows near the free margins of the eyelids.

ciliary margin, the peripheral border of the iris, continuous with the ciliary body.

ciliary movement, the waving motion of the hairlike processes projecting from the epithelium of the respiratory tract and from certain microorganisms.

ciliary mucus transport, the movement of particles from the upper respiratory tract by means other than exhalation, particularly through the wave motion of cilia lining the tract and the mucus layer.

ciliary muscle, a semitransparent, circular band of smooth muscle fibers attached to the choroid of the eye, the chief agent in adjusting the eye to view near objects.

ciliary process, any one of about 80 tiny fleshy projections on the posterior surface of the iris, forming a frill around the margin of the crystalline lens of the eye.

ciliary reflex. See **accommodation reflex.**

ciliary ring, a small grooved band of tissue, about 4 mm wide, that forms the posterior part of the ciliary body of the eye.

ciliary zone, an outer circular area on the anterior surface of the iris, separated from the inner circular area by the angular line. The ciliary zone contains the stroma of the iris.

Ciliata /sil′ē·ā′tə/, a class of protozoa of the subphylum Ciliophora, characterized by cilia throughout the life cycle.

ciliate /sil′ē·it/, of or having cilia, as certain epithelial cells of the body or protozoa of the class Ciliata.

ciliated epithelium [L *cilium* eyelid; Gk *epi* upon, *thele* nipple], any epithelial tissue that projects cilia from its surface, such as portions of the epithelium in the respiratory tract.

ciliospinal reflex /sil′ē·ōspī′nəl/ [L *cilium* + *spina* backbone, *reflectere* to bend backward], a normal brainstem reflex initiated by scratching or pinching the skin of the back of the neck, resulting in dilatation of the pupil.

cimetidine /simet′idēn/, a histamine H$_2$-receptor antagonist prescribed to inhibit the production and secretion of acid in the stomach in the treatment of duodenal ulcer, pancreatitis, and hypersecretory conditions.

Cimex lectularius. See **bedbug.**

cinchona /singkō′nə, sinchō′nə/ [Countess of Chinchon, Peru], the dried bark of the stem or root of species of *Cinchona,* containing the alkaloids quinine and quinidine.

cinchonism /sin′kōniz′əm/, a condition resulting from excessive ingestion of cinchona bark or its alkaloid derivatives. Cinchonism is characterized by deafness, headache, ringing in the ears, and signs of cerebral congestion.

cineangiocardiogram /sin′ē·an′jē·ōkär′-dē·əgram′/, a radiograph of the cardiovascular system obtained by special instruments that use a combination of x-ray, fluoroscopic, and motion-picture techniques.

cineangiocardiography /sin′ē·an′jē·ōkär′-dē·og′rəfē/ [Gk *kinesis* movement, *aggeion* vessel, *kardia* heart, *graphein* to record], the filming of fluorescent images of the cardiovascular system combining use of fluoroscopic, x-ray, and motion-picture techniques.

cineangiogram /sin′ē·an′jē·əgram′/, a movie film record of a blood vessel or of a portion of the cardiovascular system, obtained by injecting a patient with a nontoxic radiopaque medium and filming the action of the vessels through which it courses.

cineangiograph /sin′ē·an′jē·əgraf′/, a special movie camera for recording fluorescent images of the cardiovascular system.

cine film /sin′ē/, a special type of motion

picture film used in cineradiography, usually in cardiac catheterization or GI studies.

cinefluorography. See **cineradiography.**

cinematics. See **kinematics.**

cineradiography /sin′irā′dē·og′rəfē/ [Gk *kinesis* movement; L *radiere* to shine; Gk *graphein* to record], the filming with a movie camera of the images that appear on a fluorescent screen.

cingulate /sing′gyəlit/ [L *cingulum* girdle] **1.** having a zone or a girdle, usually with transverse markings. **2.** of or pertaining to a cingulum.

cingulate sulcus. See **callosomarginal fissure.**

cingulectomy /sing′gyo͞olek′təmē/ [L *cingulum* + Gk *ektome* excision], the surgical excision of a portion of the cingulate gyrus in the frontal lobe of the brain and the immediately surrounding tissue.

cingulotomy /sing′gyo͞olot′əmē/ [L *cingulum* + temnein to cut], a procedure in brain surgery to alleviate intractable pain by producing lesions in the tissue of the cingulate gyrus of the frontal lobe.

cinnamon [Gk *kinnamomon*], the aromatic inner bark of several species of *Cinnamomum*, a tree native to the East Indies and China. Saigon cinnamon is commonly used as a carminative, an aromatic stimulant, or a spice. **–cinnamic,** *adj.*

CIPM, abbreviation for **Comité International des Poids et Mesures.**

circadian dysrhythmia [L *circa* about, *dies* day; Gk *dys* bad, *rhythmos*], the biologic and psychologic stress effects of jet lag, or rapid travel through several time zones. In addition to a shift in normal eating and sleeping patterns, medication schedules and other therapies may be disrupted.

circadian rhythm /sərkā′dē·ən, sur′kədē′ən/ [L *circa* about, *dies* day; Gk *rhythmos*], a pattern based on a 24-hour cycle, especially the repetition of certain physiologic phenomena, as sleeping and eating.

circinate /sur′sināt/ [L *circinare* to make round], having a ring-shaped outline or formation; annular.

circle [L *circulus*], (in anatomy) a circular or nearly circular structure of the body, as the circle of Willis and circle of Zinn.

circle of Carus. See **curve of Carus.**

circle of Willis [Thomas Willis, English physician, b. 1621], a vascular network at the base of the brain, formed by the interconnection of the internal carotid, anterior cerebral, posterior cerebral, anterior communicating, and posterior communicating arteries.

Circolectric (COL) bed, a trademark for an electronically controlled bed that can be vertically rotated 210 degrees and permits vertical alteration of the position of the bed patient from prone to supine. This type of bed is used especially in orthopedics and in the treatment of patients with severe burns. The patient is "sandwiched" and secured between the two straight frames during rotation.

circuit [L *circuitus* going around], a course or pathway, particularly one through which an electric current passes. Current passes through a closed or continuous circuit and stops if the circuit is open, interrupted, or broken.

circuit training, a method of physcial exercise in which activities are arranged in sets so that the participant moves quickly from one activity to another with a minimum of rest between sets.

circular bandage [L *circularis* round], a bandage wrapped around an injured part, usually a limb.

circular fiber, any one of the many fibers in the free gingiva that encircle the teeth.

circular fold, one of the numerous annular projections in the small intestine. They vary in size and frequency and are formed by mucous and submucous tissue.

circulation [L *circulatio* to follow a circuit], movement of an object or substance through a circular course so that it returns to its starting point, such as the circulation of blood through the circuitous network of arteries and veins.

circulation rate, the velocity of blood flow, usually measured in the amount of blood pumped through the heart per minute. The rate varies with such factors as blood volume and cardiac contractility.

circulation time, normal, the time required for blood to flow from one part of the body to another. It involves injecting a traceable dye or radioisotope into a vein and timing its reappearance in an artery at the point of injection [L *circulatio* + *fallere* to deceive], failure of the cardiovascular

circulatory failure [L *circulatio* + *fallere* to deceive], failure of the cardiovascular system to supply the cells of the body with a volume of blood adequate to meet the metabolic demands of the cells.

circulatory fluid. See **blood, lymph.**

circulatory overload [L *circulatio;* AS *ofer;* ME *lod*], an effect of increased blood volume, as by transfusion, that raises the blood pressure. The condition can lead to heart failure or pulmonary edema.

circulatory system, the network of channels through which the nutrient fluids of the body circulate.

circulus arteriosus minor [L, circle; Gk *arteria* air pipe; L, less], the small artery encircling the outer circumference of the iris.

circumanal /sur′kəmā′nəl/ [L *circum* around, *anus*], of or pertaining to the area surrounding the anus.

circumcision [L *circum* around, *cadere* to cut], a surgical procedure in which the prepuce of the penis or, rarely, the prepuce of the clitoris is excised. Ritual circumcision is required by the religions of approximately one sixth of the population of the world.

circumcorneal, pertaining to the area of the eye surrounding the cornea.

circumduction /sur′kəmduk′shən/ [L *circum* + *ducere* to lead], **1.** the circular movement of a limb or of the eye. **2.** the motion of the head of a bone within an articulating cavity, as the hip joint. Circumduction is a combination of abduction, adduction, extension, and flexion.

circumferential fibrocartilage [L *circum* + *ferre* to bring; *fibra* fiber, *cartilago*], a structure made of fibrocartilage, in which fibrocartilaginous rims surround the margins of various articular cavities, as the glenoid labra of the hip and the shoulder.

circumferential implantation. See **superficial implantation.**

circumflex /sur′kəmfleks/ [L, *circum,* around, *flextere,* to bend], pertaining to blood vessels or nerve that wind around other body structures.

circumlocution, the use of pantomime or nonverbal communication or word substitution by a patient to avoid revealing that a word has been forgotten.

circumoral /sur′kəmôr′əl/ [L *circum* + *os* mouth], of or pertaining to the area of the face around the mouth.

circumoral pallor [L *circum* + *os, pallor,* paleness], a pale skin area around the mouth, a possible sign of scarlet fever.

circumscribed [L *circum, scribere* to draw], pertaining to a well defined area, or one with definite boundaries or limits.

circumscribed abscess [L *circum, scribere* + *abscedere* to go away], an abscess separated from surrounding tissues by a wall of fibroblasts.

circumscribed scleroderma. See **morphea.**

circum-speech [L *circum* + AS *spaec*], (in psychiatry) behavioral characteristics associated with conversation. They include body language, maintenance of personal space between individuals, handsweeps, head nods, and task-oriented activities such as walking or knitting while carrying on a conversation.

circumstantiality [L *circum* + *stare* to stand], (in psychiatry) a speech pattern in which a patient has difficulty in separating relevant from irrelevant information while describing an event. Circumstantiality may be a sign of chronic brain dysfunction.

circumvallate papilla. See **papilla.**

circus movement, 1. an unusual and involuntary rolling or somersaulting because of injured neurologic mechanisms that control body posture, such as the cerebral pedicles or the vestibular apparatus. **2.** an unusual circular gait caused by injury to the brain or to basal nerve centers. **3.** a mechanism associated with the excitatory wave of the atrium of the heart that travels a circular path characterized by a gap between the refractory and the excitatory tissue.

cirrhosis /sirō′sis/ [Gk *kirrhos* yellowish-orange, *osis* condition], a chronic degenerative disease of the liver in which the lobes are covered with fibrous tissue, the parenchyma degenerates, and the lobules are infiltrated with fat. Gluconeogenesis, detoxification of drugs and alcohol, bilirubin metabolism, vitamin absorption, GI function, hormonal metabolism, and other functions of the liver deteriorate. Cirrhosis is most commonly the result of chronic alcohol abuse but can be the result of nutritional deprivation or hepatitis or other infection. The symptoms of cirrhosis are the same regardless of the cause: nausea, flatulence, anorexia, weight loss, ascites, light-colored stools, weakness, abdominal pain, varicosities, and spider angiomas. Kinds of cirrhosis are **biliary, fatty,** and **posthepatic cirrhosis.**

cirsoid aneurysm. See **racemose aneurysm.**

cis configuration /sis/, **1.** the presence of the dominant alleles of two or more pairs of genes on one chromosome and the recessive alleles on the homologous chromosome. **2.** the presence of the mutant genes of a pair of pseudoalleles on one chromosome and the wild-type genes on the homologous chromosome. **3.** (in chemistry) a form of isomerism in which two substituent groups are on the same side of a double bond.

cisplatin /sisplat′in/, an antineoplastic prescribed in the treatment of a wide variety of neoplasms, as metastatic testicular, prostatic, and ovarian tumors.

cistern /sistərn/ [L, *cisterna,* a vessel], a storage reservoir for fluids.

cisterna /sistur′nə/, *pl.* **cisternae** [L, a vessel], a cavity that serves as a reservoir for lymph or other body fluids. Kinds of cisternae include **cisterna chyli** and **cisterna subarachnoidea.**

cisterna chyli [L, vessel; *chylos* juice], a dilatation at the beginning of the thoracic duct. It receives the two lumbar lymphatic trunks and the intestinal lymphatic trunk.

cisternal puncture [L, vessel; *punctura* a piercing], the insertion of a needle into the cerebellomedullary cistern to withdraw cerebrospinal fluid for examination. The puncture is made between the atlas and the occipital bone.

cisterna subarachnoidea [L, vessel; *sub* under; Gk *arachne* spider, *eidos* form], any one of many small subarachnoid spaces that serve as reservoirs for cerebrospinal fluid.

cistron /sis′tron/ [L *cis* this side, *trans* across], a fragment or portion of DNA that codes for a specific polypeptide. It is the smallest unit functioning as a transmitter of genetic information. **–cistronic,** *adj.*

cisvestitism /sisves′titiz′əm/ [L *cis* this side, *vestis* garment], the practice of wearing attire appropriate to the sex of the individual involved but not suitable to the age, occupation, or status of the wearer.

cit, abbreviation for a *citrate carboxylate anion.*

citrate /sit′rāt, sī′trāt/ [L *kitron* citron] **1.** any salt or ester of citric acid. **2.** the act of treating with a citrate or citric acid. **–citration,** *n.*

citric acid /sit′rik/ [Gk *kitron* citron; L *acidus* sour], a white, crystalline, organic acid soluble in water and alcohol. It is extracted from citrus fruits or obtained by fermentation of sugars and is used as a flavoring agent in foods, carbonated beverages, and certain pharmaceutical products.

citrin /sit′rin/ [Gk *kitron* citron], a crystalline flavonoid concentrate that is used as a source of bioflavonoid.

citrovorum factor. See **folinic acid.**

citrulline /sitrul′ēn/ [*Citrullus* watermelon], an amino acid that is produced from ornithine during the urea cycle and is subsequently transformed to arginine by the transfer of a nitrogen atom from aspartate.

citrullinemia, a disorder of amino acid metabolism caused by a deficiency of an enzyme, argininosuccinic acid synthetase. The clinical features include vomiting, convulsions, and coma.

Civilian Health and Medical Programs for Uniformed Services (CHAMPUS), a health care insurance system for military dependents and members of the military services when certain kinds of care are not available through the usual military medical service.

CJPH, abbreviation for *Canadian Journal of Public Health.*

C/kg, a unit of radiation exposure in the SI system. It represents coulombs per kilogram of air, as in the relationship, 1 roentgen (R) = 2.58×10^{-4} C/kg of air.

Cl, symbol for the chemical element chlorine.

claims-made policy [L *clamere* to cry out; ME *maken;* L *politicus* the state], a professional liability-insurance policy that covers the holder for the period in which a claim of malpractice is made.

clairvoyance /klervoi′əns/, the alleged power or ability to perceive or to be aware of objects or events without the use of the physical senses.

clam poisoning. See **shellfish poisoning.**

clamp [AS *clam* to hold together], an instrument with serrated tips and locking handles, used for gripping, holding, joining, supporting, or compressing an organ or vessel.

clamp forceps. See **pedicle clamp.**

clang association [L *clangere* to resound; *associare* to unite], the mental connection between dissociated ideas made because of similarity in the sounds of the words used to describe the ideas.

clapping [AS *cloeppan* to beat], (in massage) the procedure of making percussive movements on the body of a patient by lowering the cupped palms alternately in a series of rapid, stimulating blows.

clarification [L *clarus* clear, *facere* to make], (in psychology) an intervention technique designed to guide the patient in focusing on and recognizing gaps and inconsistencies in his or her statements.

clarify, (in chemistry) to clear a turbid liquid by allowing any suspended matter to settle, by adding a substance that precipitates any suspended matter, or by heating. **–clarification,** *n.*

Clark's rule [Cecil Clark, twentieth-century English chemist; L *regula* model], a method of calculating the approximate pediatric dosage of a drug for a child using this formula: weight in pounds/150 ′ adult dose.

clasp [ME *clippen* to embrace], **1.** (in dentistry) a sleevelike fitting that is fastened over a tooth to hold a partial denture in place. **2.** (in surgery) any device for holding tissues together, especially bones.

clasp-knife reflex, an abnormal sign in which a spastic limb resists passive motion and then suddenly gives way, similar to the blade of a jackknife.

clasp torsion, the twisting of a dental retentive clasp arm on its long axis.

Class II biological safety cabinet, a vertical or other container that recirculates air through a high-efficiency filter. It is used to prepare chemotherapeutic agents in an environment that protects personnel from exposure to potentially hazardous materials.

classic cesarean section [L *classicus* the highest class, *Caesar lex* Roman law; *sectio* a cutting], a method for surgically delivering a baby through a vertical midline incision of the upper segment of the uterus.

classic conditioning, a form of learning in which a previously neutral stimulus comes to elicit a given response through associative training.

classic tomography [L *classicus* + Gk *tome* section, *greaphein* to record], a method that moves the x-ray source and the x-ray plate during an exposure to produce an image in which all but a particular plane is blurred out.

classic typhus. See **epidemic typhus.**

classification [L *classis* collection, *facere* to make], (in research) a process in data collection and analysis in which data are grouped according to previously determined characteristics. **–classify,** v.

classification of caries [L *classis, facere* to make, *caries* decay], a system of defining dental caries according to the part of the tooth. The system, devised by G.V. Black, defines Class I caries as pits and fissures in the occlusal surfaces of molars and premolars (bicuspids), in facial and lingual surfaces of molars and in the lingual surfaces of maxillary incisors; Class II, proximal surfaces of premolars and molars, not broken through from proximal to occlusal; Class III, proximal surfaces of incisors and canines not including the incisal angles; Class IV, proximal surfaces of incisors and canines which include the incisal angles; and Class V, cervical one third of facial or lingual surfaces, not pits and fissures.

classification of malocclusion [L *classis, mallus* bad, *occludere* to close up], a system developed by E.H. Angle for defining malposition and contact of the maxillary and mandibular teeth. The system: Class I (neutroclusion), a normal anteroposterior relationship of the jaws, but with crowding of maxillary or mandibular teeth; protruded or retruded maxillary incisors; anterior and/or posterior crossbite, and mesial drift of molars in cases of premature loss of teeth. Class II (distoclusion), the buccal groove of the first mandibular molar is distal to the mesiobuccal cusp of the maxillary first permanent molar by at least the width of a premolar. Class III (mesiocclusion), the lower arch is anterior to the upper in one or both lateral segments, and the lower first molar is mesial to the upper first molar, and Class IV, the occlusal relations of the dental arches present the peculiar condition of being in distal occlusion upon one lateral half and in mesial occlusion upon the other half of the mouth.

classification schemes, systems of organizing data or information, usually involving categories of items with similar characteristics. Examples include the *International Classification of Diseases (ICD)* compiled by the World Health Organization (WHO), the North American Nursing Diagnoses Association (NANDA) and the *Diagnostic and Statistical Manual of Mental Disorders (DSM)*, prepared by the American Psychiatric Association.

claudication /klô′dikā′shən/ [L *claudicatio* a limping], cramplike pains in the calves caused by poor circulation of the blood to the leg muscles.

claustrophobia /klôs′trə-/ [L *claustrum* a closing; Gk *phobos* fear], a morbid fear of being in or becoming trapped in enclosed or narrow places.

claustrum /klôs′trəm/, *pl.* **claustra** [L, a closing] **1.** a barrier, as a membrane that partially closes an aperture. **2.** a thin sheet of gray matter, composed chiefly of spindle cells, situated lateral to the external capsule of the brain and separating the internal capsule from white matter of the insula.

clavicle /klav′ikəl/ [L *clavicula* little key], a long, curved, horizontal bone just above the first rib, forming the ventral portion of the shoulder girdle. It articulates medially with the sternum and laterally with the acromion of the scapula and accommodates the attachment of numerous muscles.

clavicular notch /kləvik′yələr/ [L *clavicula* + OFr *enochier*], one of a pair of oval depressions at the superior end of the sternum.

clavus. See **corn.**

clawfoot. See **pes cavus.**

clawhand [AS *clawu,* hand], an abnormal condition of the hand characterized by extreme flexion of the middle and distal phalanges and hyperextension of the metacarpophalangeal joints.

claw-type traction frame, an orthopedic apparatus that holds various pieces of traction equipment, such as the pulleys, the ropes, and the weights by which traction is applied to various parts of the body or by which various parts of the body are suspended.

clean-catch specimen, a urine specimen that is as free from bacterial contamination as possible without the use of a catheter.

cleansing enema, an enema, usually composed of soapsuds, administered to remove all formed fecal material from the colon.

clearance [L *clarus* clear], the removal of a substance from the blood via the kidneys. Kidney function can be tested by measuring the amount of a specific substance excreted in the urine in a given length of time.

clear cell [L *clarus* + *cella* storeroom], **1.** a type of cell found in the parathyroid gland that does not take on a color with the ordinary tissue stains used for microscopic examination. **2.** the principal cell of most renal cell carcinomas and, occasionally, of ovarian and parathyroid tumors. **3.** a specific type of epidermal cell, probably of neural origin, that has a dark-staining nucleus but clear cytoplasm with hematoxylin and eosin stain.

clear cell carcinoma, 1. a malignant tumor of the tubular epithelium of the kidney that contain abundant clear cytoplasm. **2.** an uncommon ovarian neoplasm characterized by cells with clear cytoplasm.

clear cell carcinoma of the kidney. See **renal cell carcinoma.**

clearing agent, a chemical, such as ammonium thiosulfate, used in the processing of exposed x-ray film to remove unexposed and undeveloped silver halide from the emulsion.

clearing test, a range of motion test that moves the joint to its limits, stretching the capsule and other soft tissues in an attempt to reproduce symptoms. If no symptoms are produced, the joint is cleared as a cause of a musculoskeletal disorder.

clear-liquid diet [L *clarus* + *liquere* to flow], a diet that supplies fluids and provides minimal residue. The diet is nutritionally inadequate and is usually prescribed for a limited amount of time, as 1 day, postoperatively.

cleavage [AS *cleofan* to split], **1.** the series of repeated mitotic cell divisions occurring in the ovum immediately after fertilization to form a mass of cells that transforms the single-celled zygote into a multicellular embryo capable of growth and differentiation. At this initial stage, as the zygote remains uniform in size, the cleavage cells, or blastomeres, become smaller with each division. **2.** the act or process of cleaving or splitting, primarily the splitting of a complex molecule into two or more simpler molecules. Kinds of cleavage include **determinate, equal, indeterminate, partial, total,** and **unequal cleavage.**

cleavage cavity. See **blastocoele.**

cleavage cell. See **blastomere.**

cleavage fracture, any fracture that splits cartilage with the avulsion of a small piece of bone from the distal portion of the lateral condyle of the humerus.

cleavage line, any one of a number of linear striations in the skin that delineate the general structural pattern and tension of the subcutaneous fibrous tissue. They correspond closely to the crease lines on the surface of the skin and are present in all areas of the body but are visible only in certain sites, such as the palms of the hands and soles of the feet.

cleavage nucleus. See **segmentation nucleus.**

cleavage plane, 1. the area in a fertilized ovum where cleavage takes place; the axis along which any cell division occurs. **2.** any plane within the body where organs or structures can be separated with minimal damage to surrounding tissue.

cleave [AS, *cleofan*], segmentation or division, as in cell division or the splitting of a complex molecule into simpler molecules.

cleft [ME *clift*], **1.** divided. **2.** a fissure, especially one that originates in the embryo, as the branchial cleft or the facial cleft.

cleft foot, an abnormal condition in which the division between third and fourth toes extends into the metatarsum of the foot.

cleft lip, a congenital anomaly consisting of one or more clefts in the upper lip resulting from the failure in the embryo of the maxillary and median nasal processes to close.

cleft-lip repair, the surgical correction of a unilateral or bilateral congenital interruption of the upper lip, usually resulting from the embryologic failure of the median nasal and maxillary processes to unite.

cleft palate, a congenital defect characterized by a fissure in the midline of the palate, resulting from the failure of the two sides to fuse during embryonic development. The fissure may be complete, extending through both the hard and soft palates into the nasal cavities, or it may show any degree of incomplete or partial cleft.

cleft-palate repair, the surgical correction of a congenital fissure in the midline of the partition separating the oral and nasal cavities. Palatine clefts range from a simple separation in the uvula to an extensive fissure involving the soft and hard palate and extending forward unilaterally or bilaterally through the alveolar ridge. A cleft lip often accompanies a cleft palate. Repair of a cleft palate is usually undertaken in the child's second year.

cleft tongue [ME *clift;* AS *tunge*], a tongue divided by a longitudinal fissure.

cleft uvula, an abnormal congenital condition in which the uvula is split into halves because of the failure of the posterior palatine folds to unite.

cleidocranial dysostosis /klē′dōkrā′nē-əl/ [Gk *kleis* key, *kranion* skull; *dys* bad, *osteon* bone], a rare, abnormal hereditary condition characterized by defective ossification of the cranial bones and by the complete or partial absence of the clavicles. The defective ossification of the cranial bones delays the closing of the cranial sutures and results in large fontanelles.

cleidocranial dystrophia. See **cleidocranial dysostosis.**

clemastine /klemas′tēn/, an antihistaminic agent prescribed in the treatment of symptoms of allergic rhinitis, as sneezing, rhinorrhea, pruritus, or lacrimation.

cleptomania. See **kleptomania.**

click [Fr *cliquer* to clash], (in cardiology) an extra heart sound that occurs during systole.

client [L *clinare* to lean], **1.** a person who is recipient of a professional service. **2.** a recipient of health care regardless of the state of health. **3.** a recipient of health care who is not ill or hospitalized. **4.** a patient.

client-centered therapy, a nondirective method of group or individual psychotherapy in which the role of the therapist is to listen to and then reflect or restate without judgment or interpretation the words of the client.

client interview. See **patient interview.**

climacteric. See **menopause.**

climacteric melancholia. See **involutional melancholia.**

climate [Gk *klima* inclination], a composite of the prevailing weather conditions that characterizes any particular geographic region. **–climatic,** *adj.*

climax [Gk *klimax* ladder], a peak of intensity, such as a sexual orgasm or the high point of a fever.

climbing fiber [ME *climben*; L *fibra*], a type of nerve fiber that carries impulses to the Purkinje cells of the cerebellar cortex.

clindamycin hydrochloride, an antibacterial prescribed in the treatment of certain serious infections.

clinic [Gk *kline* bed], **1.** a department in a hospital where persons not requiring hospitalization may receive medical care. Formerly it was called a dispensary. **2.** a group practice of doctors. **3.** a meeting place for doctors and medical students where instruction can be given at the bedside of a patient or in a similar setting. **4.** a seminar or other scientific medical meeting. **5.** a detailed published report of the diagnosis and treatment of a health care problem.

clinical [Gk *kline* bed], **1.** of or pertaining to a clinic. **2.** of or pertaining to di-

rect, bedside medical care. **3.** of or pertaining to materials or equipment used in the care of a sick person.

clinical crown, 1. the portion of a tooth that is covered by enamel and visible in the mouth. **2.** the portion of a tooth that is occlusal to the deepest part of the gingival crevice.

clinical-crown/clinical-root ratio, the proportion between the length of the portion of the teeth lying coronal to the epithelial attachment and the length of the portion of the root lying apical to the epithelial attachment. The ratio is useful in the diagnosis and prognosis of periodontal disease.

clinical cytogenetics, the branch of genetics that studies the relationship between chromosomal abnormalities and pathologic conditions.

clinical diagnosis, a diagnosis made on the basis of knowledge obtained by medical history and physical examination alone, without benefit of laboratory tests or x-rays films.

clinical disease, a stage in the history of a pathologic condition that begins with anatomic or physiologic changes that are sufficient to produce recognizable signs and symptoms of a disease.

clinical genetics, a branch of genetics that studies inherited disorders and investigates the possible genetic factors that may influence the occurrence of any pathologic condition.

clinical horizon, the imaginary line above which detectable signs and symptoms of a disease first begin to appear.

clinical humidity therapy, respiratory therapy in which water is added to the therapeutic gases to make them more comfortable to breathe.

clinical laboratory, a laboratory in which tests directly related to the care of patients are performed.

clinical nurse specialist (CNS), a registered nurse who holds a master-of-science degree in nursing (MSN) and who has acquired advanced knowledge and clinical skills in a specific area of nursing and health care.

clinical-pathologic conference, a teaching conference in which a case is presented to a clinician who then demonstrates the process of reasoning that leads to his or her diagnosis. A pathologist then presents an anatomic diagnosis, based on the study of tissue removed at surgery or obtained in autopsy.

clinical pathology, the laboratory study of disease by a pathologist using techniques appropriate to the specimen being studied.

clinical pelvimetry, a process used to assess the size of the birth canal by means of the systematic vaginal palpation of specific bony landmarks in the pelvis and an estimation of the distances between them. Findings are commonly recorded in terms such as "adequate,""borderline," or "inadequate," rather than in centimeters or inches.

clinical psychology, the branch of psychology concerned with the diagnosis, treatment, and prevention of personality and behavioral disorders.

clinical research center, an organization, often associated with a medical school or a teaching hospital, that studies, analyzes, correlates, and describes medical cases. Such centers usually have extensive laboratory facilities and specialized staffs of physicians and medical technicians.

clinical specialist, a physician or nurse having advanced training in a particular field of practice, as a nurse-midwife, pediatrician, or radiologist.

clinical thermometer, [Gk, *kline,* bedside + *therme,* heat + *metron,* measure], a thermometer designed for measuring the body temperature of patients.

clinical thermometry, a method for determining temperature in heated tissue.

clinical trials, organized studies to provide large bodies of clinical data for statistically valid evaluation of treatment.

Clinitron bed, a special bed containing an air-fluidization mattress that conforms to the body shape of the patient.

clinocephaly /klī′nōsef′əlē/ [Gk *klinein* to bend, *kephale* head], a congenital anomaly of the head in which the upper surface of the skull is saddle-shaped or concave. –**clinocephalic, clinocephalous,** *adj.*

clinodactyly /klī′nōdak′təlē/ [Gk *klinein* + *daktylos* finger], a congenital anomaly characterized by abnormal lateral or medial bending of one or more fingers or toes. –**clinodactylic, clinodactylous,** *adj.*

clinoid processes /klī′noid/ [Gk *kline, eidos* form; L *processus*], the anterior, middle, and posterior processes of the sphenoid bone at the base of the skull.

clinometer /klīnom′ətər/, an instrument used to measure angular convergence of the eyes or the degree of paralysis of extraocular muscles.

clioquinol. See **iodochlorhydroxyquin.**

clip [AS *clyppan* to embrace], a surgical device used for grasping the skin to align the edges of a wound and to stop bleeding, especially of the smaller blood vessels.

clipped speech. See **scamping speech.**

clitoris /klit′əris/ [Gk *kleitoris*], the vaginal erectile structure homologous to the corpora cavernosa of the penis. It consists of two corpora cavernosa within a dense layer of fibrous membrane, joined along their inner surfaces by an incomplete fibrous septum.

CLL, abbreviation for **chronic lymphocytic leukemia.**

cloaca /klō·ā′kə/, *pl.* **cloacae** [L, sewer] **1.** (in embryology) the end of the hindgut before the developmental division into the rectum, the bladder, and the primitive genital structures. **2.** (in pathology) an opening into the sheath of tissue around a necrotic bone.

cloacal membrane, a thin sheath that separates the internal and external portions of the cloaca in the developing embryo.

cloacal septum. See **urorectal septum.**

clobetasol propionate /klōbet′əsol prō′pyōnāt/, a topical corticosteroid prescribed for the short-term treatment of inflammation and pruritis associated with certain moderate to severe types of dermatitis.

clocortolone pivalate /klōkôr′təlōn piv′əlāt/, a topical corticosteroid used topically as an antiinflammatory agent.

clofibrate /klō′fəbrāt/, an antihyperlipoproteinemic prescribed in the treatment of high blood levels of cholesterol, triglycerides, or both.

clomiphene citrate /klō′məfēn/, a nonsteroidal antiestrogen that acts to stimulate ovulation. It is prescribed principally in the treatment of anovulation and oligoovulation in women.

clomiphene stimulation test, a test used to evaluate gonadal function in males who show signs of abnormal pubertal development. Clomiphene, a nonsteroidal analog of estrogen, stimulates the hypothalamic-pituitary system to raise FSH and LH levels of the blood.

clonal selection theory. See **antibody specific theory.**

clonazepam /klōnaz′əpam/, an anticonvulsant prescribed in the prevention of seizures in petit mal epilepsy and other convulsive disorders.

clone [Gk *klon* a plant cutting], a group of genetically identical cells or organisms derived from a single common cell or organism through mitosis.

clonic /klon′ik/ [Gk *klonos* tumult], pertaining to increased reflex activity, as in upper motor neuron lesions when repetitive muscular contractions and relaxations in rapid succession are induced by stretching.

clonic convulsion [Gk *klonos*; L *convulsio* cramp], a form of convulsion characterized by rhythmic alternate involuntary contraction and relaxation of muscle groups.

clonic spasm [Gk *klonos* + *spasmos*], involuntary alternate contractions and relaxations of muscles.

clonidine hydrochloride /klō′nədēn/, an antihypertensive prescribed for the reduction of high blood pressure.

clonorchiasis /klō′nôrkī′əsis/, an infestation of liver flukes.

Clonorchis sinensis /klōnôr′kis sinen′sis/, the Chinese or Oriental liver fluke, a form of tapeworm that is acquired by humans who eat raw or imperfectly cooked fish that is the intermediate host of the parasite.

clonus /klō′nəs/ [Gk *klonos* tumult], an abnormal pattern of neuromuscular activity, characterized by rapidly alternating involuntary contraction and relaxation of skeletal muscle.

C-loop, a surgically formed loop of bowel with a C-shape.

clor, abbreviation for a chloride noncarboxylate anion.

clorazepate dipotassium /klôraz′əpāt/, a minor tranquilizer prescribed in the treatment of anxiety, nervous tension, and alcohol withdrawal.

closed amputation [L *claudere* to shut; *amputare* to cut away], a kind of amputation in which one or two broad flaps of muscular and cutaneous tissue are retained to form a cover over the end of the bone. It is performed only when no infection is present.

closed-angle glaucoma. See **glaucoma.**

closed bite [L *claudere* + AS *bitan*], **1.** an abnormal overbite. **2.** a decrease in the occlusal vertical dimension produced by various factors, such as tooth abrasion and insufficient eruption of supportive posterior teeth.

closed-chain, (in organic chemistry) of or pertaining to a compound in which the carbon atoms are bonded together to form a closed ring.

closed-circuit breathing, any breathing system in which a contained gas mixture is rebreathed, either directly or after recirculation through a water or carbon dioxide absorbing unit. An example is a spirometer.

closed-circuit helium dilution, a technique for measuring residual lung volume and functional residual capacity by having a patient breathe through a spirometer containing a known concentration of helium.

closed dislocation [L *claudere* + *dis* apart, *locare* to place], a dislocation that is not accompanied by a skin break at the joint.

closed drainage. See **drainage.**

closed fracture [L *claudere* + *fractura*], a bone fracture that is not accompanied by a break in the skin.

closed group, a group in which all members are admitted at the same time and vacancies that occur in the membership are unfilled.

closed reduction of fractures [L *claudere* + *reducere* to lead back + *fractura*], the manual reduction of a fracture without incision.

closed system, a system that does not interact with its environment.

closed-system helium dilution method, a technique for measuring functional residual capacity and residual volume.

closed-wound suction, any one of several techniques for draining potentially harmful fluids, such as blood, pus, serosanguineous fluid, and tissue secretions from surgical wounds. The technique is used as an aid to many operations, such as mastectomies, augmentations, plastic and reconstructive procedures, and urologic and urogenital procedures. Closed-wound suction devices usually consist of disposable transparent containers attached to suction tubes and portable suction pumps. Closed-wound suction also allows irrigation of the wound with special flow controls to permit a periodic change in the flow direction of solutions.

closing capacity (CC), (in respiratory therapy) the sum of the closing volume and the residual volume of gas in the lungs.

closing volume (CV), the volume of gas remaining in the lungs when the small airways begin to close during a controlled maximum exhalation.

clostridial /klostrid′ē·əl/ [Gk *kloster* spindle], of or pertaining to anaerobic spore-forming bacteria of the genus *Clostridium.*

clostridial myonecrosis. See **myonecrosis.**

Clostridium [Gk *kloster* spindle], a genus of spore-forming, anaerobic bacteria of the Bacillaceae family involved in gas gangrene, botulism, food poisoning, cellulitis, wound infections, and tetanus.

Clostridium botulinum [Gk *kloster*], a species of anaerobic bacteria that cause botulism in humans and botulism-like diseases in other animals. Botulinus food poisoning results from ingesting food containing preformed toxins produced by the species. It is a proteolytic pathogen commonly present in soil, where its endospores can survive for years. Their resistance to heat makes the spores an important cause of poisoning in improperly cooked or canned foods.

Clostridium perfringens [Gk, *kloster*, spindle], a species of anaerobic gram-positive bacteria capable of causing gas gangrene in humans and various digestive and urinary tract disease in livestock. The oval spores of the bacteria are found in the soil and in the intestinal tracts of humans and animals.

closure /klō′zhər/ [L *claudere* to shut] **1.** the surgical closing of a wound by suture. **2.** a visual phenomenon in which the mind "sees" an entire figure when only a portion is actually visible.

closylate /klos′ilāt/, a contraction for *p*-chlorobenzenesulfonate.

clot. See **blood clot.**

clotrimazole /klōtrim′əzōl/, a broad-spectrum antifungal agent of the imidazole group used in topical applications to treat fungal and yeast infections.

clotting. See **blood clotting.**

clotting time [AS *clott*], the time required for blood to form a clot, tested by collecting 4 ml of blood in a glass tube and examining it for clot formation.

cloud baby [AS *clud; babe*], a newborn who appears well and healthy but is a carrier of infectious bacterial or viral organisms. The infant may contaminate the surrounding environment with airborne droplets from the respiratory tract forming clouds of the organisms.

clouding of consciousness, a mental state in which a patient is confused about or is not fully aware of the immediate surroundings.

clove [L *clavus* nail], the dried flower bud of *Eugenia caryophyllata.* It contains the lactone caryophyllin and a volatile oil used as a dental analgesic, a germicide, and a salve.

cloverleaf nail [AS *clafre, leaf; nagel*], a surgical nail shaped in cross-section like a cloverleaf, used especially in the repair of fractures of the femur.

cloverleaf skull deformity, a congenital defect characterized by a trilobed skull resulting from the premature closure of multiple cranial sutures during embryonic development.

cloxacillin sodium /klok′səsil′in/, an antibacterial prescribed in the treatment of certain serious infections, primarily those caused by penicillin-resistant strains of staphylococci.

clubbed penis, [ME *clubbe;* L *penis*], a penis that is curved or twisted, or both. The abnormality may be accompanied by epispadias or hypospadias.

clubbing [ME *clubbe*], an abnormal enlargement of the distal phalanges, usually associated with cyanotic heart disease or advanced chronic pulmonary disease but sometimes occurring with biliary cirrhosis, colitis, chronic dysentery, and thyrotoxicosis. Clubbing occurs in all the digits but is most easily seen in the fingers.

clubfoot [ME *clubbe;* AS *fot*], a congenital deformity of the foot, sometimes resulting from intrauterine constriction and characterized by unilateral or bilateral deviation of the metatarsal bones of the forefoot. Ninety-five percent of clubfoot deformities are **equinovarus,** characterized by medial deviation and plantar flexion of the forefoot, but a few are **calcaneovalgus,** or **calcaneovarus,** characterized by lateral deviation and dorsiflexion either outward from or inward toward the midline of the body.

club hair, a hair in the resting, or final, stage of the growth cycle.

clubhand, a congenital disorder in which the hand develops abnormally as a widened stump at the end of the wrist with stunted fingers.

cluster analysis [AS *clyster* growing together; Gk *analyein* to loosen], (in statistics) a complex technique of data analysis of numeric scale scores that produces clusters of variables related to one another. The technique is performed with a computer.

cluster breathing, a breathing pattern in which a closely grouped series of respirations is followed by apnea. The activity is associated with a lesion in the lower pontine region of the brainstem.

cluster headache. See **histamine headache.**

cluttering [ME *clotter*], a speech defect characterized by a rapid, confused, nervous delivery with uneven rhythmic patterns and the omission or transposition of various letters or syllables.

clysis /klī′sis/ [Gk *klyster* washout], the administration of an enema.

cm, symbol for **centimeter.**

cm², symbol for **square centimeter.**

cm³, symbol for **cubic centimeter.**

Cm, symbol for the chemical element **curium.**

CMA, abbreviation for *Canadian Medical Association.*

CMAJ, abbreviation for *Canadian Medical Association Journal.*

CMC, abbreviation for **carpometacarpal.**

CMF, an anticancer drug combination of cyclophosphamide, methotrexate, and fluorouracil.

CMHC, abbreviation for **community mental health center.**

CML, abbreviation for **chronic myelocytic leukemia.**

CMRNG, abbreviation for *chromosom-*

ally mediated resistant Neisseria gonorrhea.

CMT, abbreviation for *Certified Medical Transcriptionist.*

CMV, abbreviation for **cytomegalovirus.**

CNA, abbreviation for **Canadian Nurses' Association.**

CNATS, abbreviation for **Canadian Nurses' Association Testing Service.**

CNF, abbreviation for **Canadian Nurses' Foundation.**

CNM, abbreviation for **Certified Nurse-Midwife.**

CNOR, abbreviation for *Certified Nursing, Operating Room.*

CNP, abbreviation for **community nurse practitioner.**

CNRN, abbreviation for *Certified Neuroscience Registered Nurse.*

CNRS, abbreviation for **Canadian Nurses' Respiratory Society.**

CNS, 1. abbreviation for **central nervous system. 2.** abbreviation for **clinical nurse specialist.**

CNSN, abbreviation for *Certified Nutrition Support Nurse.*

CNS sympathomimetic, a drug, such as cocaine or amphetamine, whose effects mimic those of sympathetic nervous system stimulation.

CNS syndrome. See **central nervous system syndrome.**

Co, symbol for the chemical element **cobalt.**

CO, 1. symbol for **carbon monoxide. 2.** abbreviation for **cardiac output.**

CO₂, symbol for **carbon dioxide.**

CoA, abbreviation for **coenzyme A.**

coagglutination [L *cum, agglutinare* to glue], a clumping of red blood cells by mixtures of protein antigens and their antisera.

coaguability [L *coagulare* to curdle], the state of being able to coagulate or form blood clots.

coagulant /kō·ag′yələnt/ [L *coagulare*], an agent that causes a coagulum, or blood clot, to form.

coagulase /kō·ag′yəlās/ [L *coagulare*], an enzyme produced by bacteria, particularly the *Staphylococcus aureus*, that promotes the formation of thrombi.

coagulation /kō·ag′yəlā′shən/ [L *coagulare*] **1.** the process of transforming a liquid into a solid, especially of the blood. **2.** (in colloid chemistry) the transforming of the liquid dispersion medium into a gelatinous mass. **3.** the hardening of tissue by some physical means, as by electrocoagulation or photocoagulation.

coagulation current, an electric current delivered by a needle ball or other variously shaped points that coagulates tissue.

coagulation factor, one of 13 factors in the blood, the interactions of which are responsible for the process of blood clotting. The factors, using standardized numeric nomenclature, are factor I, fibrinogen; factor II, prothrombin; factor III, tissue thromboplastin; factor IV, calcium ions; factors V and VI, proaccelerin or labile factors; factor VII, proconvertin or stable factor; factor VIII, antihemophilic globulin; factor IX, plasma thromboplastin component (PTC); factor X, Stuart factor; factor XI, plasma thromboplastin antecedent (PTA); factor XII, Hageman factor or glass factor; factor XIII, fibrin stabilizing factor or Laki-Lorand factor.

coagulation necrosis. See **necrosis.**

coagulation time. See **clotting time.**

coagulopathy /kō·ag′yəlop′əthē/, a pathologic condition affecting the ability of the blood to coagulate.

coalesce /kō′əles′/ [L, *coalescere,* to grow together], to grow together.

coal tar, a topical antieczematic prescribed in the treatment of chronic skin diseases, as eczema and psoriasis.

coal worker's pneumoconiosis. See **anthracosis.**

Coanda effect, a phenomenon of fluid movement similar to the Bernoulli effect in which passage of a stream of gas next to a wall results in a pocket of turbulence that makes the gas stream adhere to the wall. The principle is used in fluidic ventilators.

coaptation splint /kō′aptā′shən/ [L *coaptare* to fit together; ME *splinte*], a small splint fitted to a fractured limb to prevent overriding of the fragments of bone.

coarct /kō·ärkt′/ [L *coarctare* to press together], the act of narrowing or constricting, especially the lumen of a blood vessel.

coarctate retina /kō·ärk′tāt/ [L, *coartare,* to press together + *rete,* net], a funnel-shaped retina caused by a leakage of fluid between the retina and the choroid.

coarctation /kō′ärktā′shən/, a stricture or contraction of the walls of a vessel as the aorta.

coarctation of the aorta, a congenital cardiac anomaly characterized by a localized narrowing of the aorta, which results in increased pressure proximal to the defect and decreased pressure distal to it. Symptoms of the condition are directly related to the pressure changes created by the constriction. Clinical manifestations include dizziness, headaches, fainting, epistaxis, reduced or absent femoral pulses, and muscle cramps in the legs from tissue anoxia during increased exercise.

coarse [ME *cors* common], (in physiol-

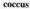

ogy) involving a wide range of movements, such as those associated with tremors and other involuntary movements of the skeletal muscle.

coarse fremitus, a rough, loud, tremulous vibration of the chest wall noted on palpation of the chest during a physical examination as the person inhales and exhales.

coarse rale, an abnormal breathing sound caused by air moving through an excessive amount of fluid present in an airway, as in pulmonary edema.

coarse tremor, a tremor in which the movements are relatively slow and may involve larger muscle groups.

coat [ME *cote*], **1.** a membrane that covers the outside of an organ or part. **2** .one of the layers of a wall of an organ or part, especially a canal or a vessel.

coated tablet [OFr *cote;* Fr *tablette*], a solid disc of one or more pharmaceutical agents coated with sugar or a flavoring to mask the taste or by a substance that resists dissolution in the stomach but allows release of the medication in the intestine.

coated tongue [OFr *cote;* AS *tunge*], a tongue with a white, yellow, or brown furred surface, representing a possible accumulation of mycelia, bacteria, food debris, or desquamated epithelial cells. There are many possible causes, ranging from a fungal infection to sleeping with the mouth open.

cobalamin /kōbôl′əmin/ [Ger *kobold* mine goblin], a generic term for a chemical portion of the vitamin B_{12} group.

cobalt (Co) /kō′bôlt/ [Ger *kobold* mine goblin], a metallic element that occurs in the minerals cobaltite, smaltite, and linnaeite. Its atomic number is 27; its atomic weight is 58.9. Cobalt is a component of vitamin B_{12}, is found in most common foods, and is readily absorbed by the GI tract. Certain amounts of cobalt stimulate the production of erythropoietin.

cobalt 60 (^{60}Co), (in radiotherapy) a radioactive isotope of the silver-white metallic element cobalt with a mass number of 60 and a half-life of 5.2 years. ^{60}Co emits high-energy gamma rays and is frequently used in radiotherapy.

cobra venom solution [L *colubra* snake, *venenum* venom, *solutus* dissolved], a sterile physiologic salt solution containing minute amounts of cobralysin, the hemolytic substance in cobra venom.

coca, a species of South American shrubs, native to Bolivia and Peru and cultivated in Indonesia. It is a natural source of cocaine.

cocaine babies /kōkān′/, infants with birth defects caused by exposure to cocaine in utero.

cocaine hydrochloride, a white crystalline powder used as a local anesthetic. It was originally derived from coca leaves but can also be prepared synthetically. In solution the drug is an effective topical anesthetic commonly used in the examination and treatment of the eye, ear, nose, and throat. The vasoconstrictive action of the drug slows bleeding and limits absorption. Prolonged or frequent use may damage the mucous membranes. Cocaine is a Schedule II drug under the Controlled Substances Act.

cocaine hydrochloride poisoning, toxic effects of exposure to the colorless crystalline alkaloid derived from coca leaves. Although used as a local analgesic for a century, cocaine is highly toxic with moderate vasoconstrictor activity and serious psychotropic effects. Symptoms include nervous excitement, restlessness, incoherent speech, fever, hypertension, cardiac arrhythmias, leading to convulsions, collapse, respiratory arrested, and death. The euphoric effect of cocaine lasts about 30 minutes.

cocarcinogen /kōkär′sənəjən/ [L *cum* together with; Gk *karkinos* crab, *genein* to produce], an agent that, by itself, does not transform a normal cell into a cancerous state but in concert with another can effect the transformation.

coccidioidomycosis /kôksid′ē·oi′dōmīkō′sis/ [Gk *kokkos* berry, *eidos* form, *mykes* fungus, *osis* condition], an infectious fungal disease caused by the inhalation of spores of the bacterium *Coccidioides immitis,* which is carried on windborne dust particles. The disease is endemic in hot, dry regions of North and South America. Primary infection is characterized by symptoms resembling those of the common cold or influenza. Secondary infection, occurring after a period of remission, is marked by low-grade fever, anorexia and weight loss, cyanosis, dyspnea, hemoptysis, focal skin lesions resembling erythema nodosum, and arthritic pain in the bones and joints.

coccidiosis /kok′sidē·ō′sis/ [Gk *kokkos* + *osis* condition], a parasitic disease of tropical and subtropical regions caused by the ingestion of oocysts of the protozoa *Isospora belli* or *I. hominis.* Symptoms include fever, malaise, abdominal discomfort, and watery diarrhea.

coccus /kok′əs/, *pl.* **cocci** [Gk *kokkos* berry], a bacterium that is round, spheric, or oval, as gonococcus, pneumococcus, staphylococcus, streptococcus. **–coccal,** *adj.*

coccygeal body [Gk *kokkyx* cuckoo's beak; AS *bodig*], the coccyx.

coccygeal vertebra, one of the four segments of the vertebral column that fuse to form the adult coccyx. They are considered rudimentary vertebrae and have no pedicles, laminae, or spinous processes.

coccygeus /koksij′ē·əs/ [Gk *kokkyx*], one of two muscles in the pelvic diaphragm. Stretching across the pelvic cavity like a hammock, it is a triangular sheet of muscle and tendinous fibers, dorsal to the levator ani, arising from the spine of the ischium and from the sacrospinous ligament. It acts to draw the coccyx ventrally, helping to support the pelvic floor.

coccygodynia /kok′sigōdin′ē·ə/, a pain in the coccygeal area of the body.

coccyx /kok′siks/, *pl.* **coccyges** /koksī′jēz, kok′sijēz/ [Gk *kokkyx*], the beaklike bone joined to the sacrum by a disk of fibrocartilage at the base of the vertebral column. It is formed by the union of three to five rudimentary vertebrae. **–coccygeal** /koksij′ē·əl/, *adj.*

cochineal /koch′inēl′/ [L *coccineus* bright red], a red dye prepared from the dried female insects of the species *Coccus cacti* containing young larvae.

cochlea /kok′lē·ə/ [L, snail shell], a conic bony structure of the inner ear, perforated by apertures for passage of fibers of the acoustic nerve. Part of the osseous labyrinth, it is a spiral tunnel about 30 mm long with two full and three quarter-turns, resembling a tiny snail shell. **–cochlear,** *adj.*

cochlear canal [L *cochlea* + *canalis* channel], a bony spiral tunnel within the cochlea of the internal ear. It contains one opening that communicates with the tympanic cavity, a second that connects with the vestibule, and a third that leads to a tiny canal opening on the inferior surface of the temporal bone.

cochlear duct. See **cochlear canal.**

cochlear implant, an electronic device that is surgically implanted into the cochlea of a deaf individual. It allows the individual to be aware of sounds that would not otherwise be heard.

cochlear nerve [L, *cochlea*, snail shell, *nervus*, nerve], one of the main divisions of the eighth cranial nerve, with fibers that arise in spiral ganglion cells and terminate in the dorsal and ventral cochlear nuclei of the brainstem.

cochlear toxicity, toxic effects of drugs that may result in hearing disorders, such as tinnitus.

cochlear window. See **round window.**

cockroach, the common name of members of the Blattidae family of insects that infest homes, workplaces, and other areas inhabited by humans. Cockroaches transmit a number of disease agents, including bacteria, protozoa, and eggs of parasitic worms.

cockscomb papilloma [AS *cocc, camb;* L *papilla* nipple; Gk *oma* tumor], a benign, small red lesion that may project from the uterine cervix during pregnancy; it regresses after delivery.

cocktail [AS *cocc, toegel*], *informal.* an unofficial mixture of drugs, usually in solution, combined to achieve a specific purpose.

cockup splint, a splint used to immobilize the wrist and leave the fingers free.

cocontraction, the simultaneous contraction of agonist and antagonist muscles around a joint to hold a position.

code [L *caudex* book], **1.** (in law) a published body of statutes, as a civil code. **2.** a collection of standards and rules of behavior, as a dress code. **3.** a symbolic means of representing information for communication or transfer, as a genetic code. **4.** a system of notation that allows information to be transmitted rapidly, such as Morse code, or in secrecy, such as a cryptographic code. **5.** *informal.* a discreet signal used to summon a special team to resuscitate a patient without alarming patients or visitors. **6.** to enter data by use of a given programing language into a computer.

codeine /kō′dēn/ [Gk *kodeia* poppyhead], a narcotic analgesic used to treat mild to moderate pain, to treat diarrhea, and as an antitussive.

codeine phosphate, a narcotic analgesic and antitussive prescribed to suppress cough and to relieve pain.

code of ethics, a statement encompassing the set of rules by which practitioners of a profession are expected to conform.

code team, a specially trained and equipped team of physicians, nurses, and technicians that is available to provide cardiopulmonary resuscitation when summoned by a code set by the institution.

coding [L *caudex* book], the process of organizing information into categories, which are assigned codes for the purposes of sorting, storing, and retrieving the data.

cod-liver oil, a pale yellow, fatty oil extracted from the fresh livers of the codfish and other related species. It is a rich source of vitamins A and D.

Codman's exercise [Ernest Amory Codman, American surgeon, b. 1869; L *exercere* to keep at work], mild exercises for restoring range of motion and function in the arms after immobilization of the limbs. The patient flexes the trunk over a surface to create a pendulum. The arm then hangs free and can be moved through the motions of the trunk without active contraction of the shoulder muscle.

Codman's tumor. See *chondroblastoma*.

codominant /kōdom'ənənt/ [L *cum* together with, *dominari* to rule], of or pertaining to the alleles or to the trait resulting from the full expression of both alleles of a pair in a heterozygote, as the AB or MNS blood group antigens. **–codominance,** *n.*

codominant inheritance, the transmission of a trait or condition in which both alleles of a pair are given full expression in a heterozygote, such as in the AB blood group antigens.

codon /kō'don/, a unit of three adjacent nucleotides in a DNA or messenger RNA molecule that designates a specific amino acid in the polypeptide chain during protein synthesis.

coefficient [L *cum* together with, *efficere* to effect], a mathematic relationship between factors that can be used to measure or evaluate a characteristic under specified conditions.

Coelenterates /sēlen'tərā'tēz/, a phylum of marine animals that includes jellyfish, sea anemones, hydroids, and corals.

coelenteron, /sēlen'təron/ *pl.* coelentera [Gk *koilos* hollow, *enteron* intestine], the digestive cavity of those animals having only two germ layers, such as the hydra and jellyfish.

coelom /sē'ləm/ [Gk *koilos* hollow], the body cavity of the developing embryo. A kind of coelom is **extraembryonic coelom. –coelomic, celomic,** *adj.*

coelosomy /sē'ləsomē/ [Gk *koilos* + *soma* body], a congenital anomaly characterized by the protrusion of the viscera from the body cavity.

coenesthesia, coenesthesis, coenogenesis. See *cenesthesia*.

coenzyme /kō·en'zīm/ [L *cum* together with, *en* in, *zyme* ferment], a nonprotein substance that combines with an apoenzyme to form a complete enzyme or holoenzyme. Coenzymes include some of the vitamins.

coenzyme A (CoA) [L *cum, en,, zyme* ferment], an important metabolite in the citric acid cycle. Although not a true enzyme, it plays a significant role in the transfer of acetyl groups and the metabolism of acids and amino acids.

coffee [Ar *qahwah*], the dried and roasted ripe seeds of *Coffea arabica, C. liberica,* and *C. robusta* trees that grow in tropical areas. Coffee contains the alkaloid caffeine.

coffee-ground vomitus, dark brown vomitus the color and consistency of coffee grounds, composed of gastric juices and old blood and indicative of slow upper GI bleeding.

cognition /kognish'ən/ [L *cognoscere* to know], the mental process characterized by knowing, thinking, learning, and judging. **–cognitive,** *adj.*

cognitive /kog'nitiv/, pertaining to the mental processes of comprehension, judgment, memory, and reasoning, as contrasted with emotional and volitional processes.

cognitive development, the developmental process by which an infant becomes an intelligent person, acquiring, with growth, knowledge and the ability to think, learn, reason, and abstract.

cognitive dissonance [L *cognoscere* to know, *dis* opposite of, *sonare* to sound], a state of tension resulting from a discrepancy in a person's emotional and intellectual frame of reference for interpreting and coping with his or her environment.

cognitive function, an intellectual process by which one becomes aware of, perceives, or comprehends ideas.

cognitive learning, 1. learning that is concerned with acquisition of problem-solving abilities and with intelligence and conscious thought. 2. a theory that defines learning as behavioral change based on the acquisition of information about the environment.

cognitive psychology, the study of the development of thought, language, and intelligence in infants and children.

cognitive restoration, an intervention technique designed to restore cognitive functioning.

cognitive restructuring, a change in attitudes, values, or beliefs that limit a person's self-expression; it occurs as a result of insight or behavioral achievement.

cognitive structuring, the process of reviewing with a patient the changes that have occurred in the patient's thinking to show a sense of change and a sense of playing an active role in bringing about that change.

cognitive therapy, any of the various methods of treating mental and emotional disorders that help a person change attitudes, perceptions, and patterns of thinking.

cogwheel rigidity [ME *cugge* tooth on a gear; AS *hweol*; L *rigiditas* unbending], an abnormal rigor in muscle tissue, characterized by jerky movements when the muscle is passively stretched.

cohabitate /kōhab'itāt/, to live together in a sexual relationship when not married.

cohere /kōhir'/ [L *cohaerere* to cling together], to stick together, as similar molecules of a common substance.

coherence, 1. the property of sticking together, as the molecules within a common substance. 2. (in psychology) the logical pattern of expression and thought evident in the speech of a normal, stable individual. **–coherent,** *adj.*

cohesiveness [L *cohaerere* to cling together], 1. (in psychiatry) a force that attracts members to a group and causes them to remain in the group. 2. (in dentistry) a property of annealed pure gold that allows it to be used as a filling material.

cohesive termini, (in molecular genetics) the complementary single-stranded ends projecting from a double-stranded DNA segment that can be joined to introduced fragments.

COHN, abbreviation for *Certified Occupational Health Nurse.*

cohort /kō′hôrt/ [L *cohortem* large group], (in statistics) a collection or sampling of individuals who share a common characteristic, such as members of the same age or the same sex.

cohort study, (in research) a study concerning a specific subpopulation, such as the children born between May and December in 1975 and the children born in the same months in 1955.

coil. See **intrauterine device.**

coiled tubular gland [L *colligere* to gather together; *tubulus* small tube; *glans* acorn], one of the many multicellular glands that contain a coiled, tube-shaped secretory portion, such as the sweat glands.

coil-spring contraceptive diaphragm, a kind of contraceptive diaphragm in which the flexible metal spring that forms the rim is a coiled, circular spring.

coincidence counting [L *coincidere* to occur together], (in radiotherapy) the detection of two photons that arrive at separate counters simultaneously as the result of annihilation of a positron (created during a radioactive decay) and an electron. As an imaging technique, the coincidence counting of two photons greatly reduces the significance of any background radiation.

coinnervation. See **cocontraction.**

coitus /kō′itəs/ [L *coire* to come together], the sexual union of two people of opposite sex in which the penis is introduced into the vagina, typically resulting in mutual excitation and usually orgasm. **–coital,** *adj.*

coitus interruptus. See **withdrawal method.**

colation /kōlā′shən/ [L *colare* to strain], the act of filtering or straining, as urine is often strained for medical examination.

COL bed. See **Circolectric (COL) bed.**

colchicine /kol′chəsēn/ [Gk *kolchikon*], a gout suppressant prescribed in the treatment of acute gout and prophylaxis of recurrent gouty arthritis.

cold [AS *kald*], 1. the absence of heat. 2. also called **common cold,** a contagious viral infection of the upper respiratory tract, usually caused by a strain of rhinovirus. It is characterized by rhinitis, tearing, low-grade fever, and malaise and is treated symptomatically with rest, mild analgesia, decongestants, and an increased intake of fluids.

cold abscess, a site of infection that does not show common signs of heat, redness, and swelling.

cold agglutinin, a nonspecific antibody, found on the surface of red blood cells in certain diseases, that may cause clumping of the cells at temperatures below 4° C and may cause hemolysis.

cold agglutinin disease [AS, *kald;* L, *agglutinare,* to glue, *dis,* without; Fr, *aise,* ease], a disorder characterized by circulating antibodies that can agglutinate red cells at less than normal body temperatures. They occur in the sera of patients with atypical pneumonia and blood diseases, particularly hemolytic anemia. The disease also tends to affect elderly patients.

cold bath, a bath in which the water temperature is approximately 50° F (10° C) to 65° F (18° C), used primarily to reduce body temperature.

cold-blooded, unable to regulate body heat, as fishes, reptiles, and amphibians that have internal temperatures that are close to the temperatures of the environments in which they live.

cold cautery. See **cryocautery.**

cold caloric irrigation, a procedure for testing the integrity of brain stem function by irrigating the external auditory canal of the patient with a cold saline solution while the head is flexed at approximately 30 degrees. The stimulus results in jerky but regular eye movements in a normal patient.

cold compress [AS *kald;* L *comprimere* to press together], a pad of damp, thickly folded, soft absorbent cloth, dipped in cold water, wrung out, and applied to a body part for the relief of pain or reduction of inflammation.

cold environment, a human environment arbitrarily designated as one in which the temperature is below 10° C (50° F). The human body generally begins to experience some functional impairment when unprotected in temperatures below 15° C (59° F). The body's hemostatic mechanism reacts with vasoconstriction, reducing heat loss to the environment. When vasoconstriction no longer eases the thermal strain between the skin and the environment, muscular hypertonus and shivering become mechanisms for maintaining body temperature.

cold hemoglobinuria. See **hemoglobinuria.**

cold injury, any of several abnormal and often serious physical conditions caused by exposure to cold temperatures.

cold pack [AS, *kald;* ME, *pakke*], a method, now generally obsolete, of lowering body temperature by wrapping the patient in a blanket or sheet that has been dipped in cold water and wrung out.

cold-pressor test, a test for the tendency to develop essential hypertension. One hand of the individual is immersed in ice water for about 60 seconds. An excessive rise in the blood pressure or an unusual delay in the return of normal blood pressure when the hand is removed from the water is believed to indicate that the individual is at risk for hypertension.

cold-sensitive mutation, a genetic alteration resulting in a gene that functions at a high temperature and not at a low temperature.

cold sore. See **herpes simplex (HSV-I).**

cold urticaria [AS, *kald;* L, *urtica*, nettle], wheals caused by exposure to cold temperatures.

cold-wet-sheet pack, a form of somatic therapy for agitated patients. The patient is swathed in cold, wet sheets, which are then warmed by body heat.

colectomy /kəlek′təmē/ [Gk *kolon* colon, *ektome* excision], surgical excision of part or all of the colon, performed to treat cancer of the colon or severe chronic ulcerative colitis.

colestipol hydrochloride /kōles′tipol/, an antihyperlipoproteinemic that acts by sequestering bile acids in the intestine, thus reducing plasma levels of cholesterol. It is prescribed in the treatment of hypercholesterolemia and xanthoma.

colic /kol′ik/ [Gk *kolikos* colon pain], **1.** sharp visceral pain resulting from torsion, obstruction, or smooth muscle spasm of a hollow or tubular organ, such as a ureter or the intestines. Kinds of colic include **biliary, infantile,** and **renal colic. 2.** of or pertaining to the colon. **–colicky,** *adj.*

colicinogen /kol′isin′əjən/ [(E.) *coli* + L *caedere* to kill; Gk *genein* to produce], an episome in some strains of *Escherichia coli* that induces secretion of a colicin, a

protein lethal to other strains of the bacterium.

coliform /kol′ifôrm/ [(E.) *coli* + L *forma* form] **1.** of or pertaining to the colon-aerogenes group, or the *Escherichia coli* species of microorganisms, constituting most of the intestinal flora in humans and other animals. **2.** having the characteristic of a sieve or cribriform structure, such as some of the porous bones of the skull.

colistimethate sodium /kō′listim′əthāt/, an antibacterial prescribed in the treatment of GI infections caused by certain gram-negative microorganisms and as a topical medication.

colistin sulfate, an antibacterial prescribed topically in the treatment of infections of the outer ear and systemically for serious gram-negative infections and for the treatment of gastroenteritis caused by *Escherichia coli* infections.

colitis, an inflammatory condition of the large intestine, either one of the episodic, functional, irritable bowel syndromes or one of the more serious chronic, progressive, inflammatory bowel diseases. Irritable bowel syndrome is characterized by bouts of colicky pain and diarrhea or constipation, often resulting from emotional stress. **–colitic,** *adj.*

collaborative power structure, an arrangement whereby adult family members of a functional family make major decisions and are in agreement about power distribution.

collagen /kol′əjən/ [Gk *kolla* glue, *genein* to produce], a protein consisting of bundles of tiny reticular fibrils, which combine to form the white glistening inelastic fibers of the tendons, the ligaments, and the fascia. **–collagenous** /kəlaj′ənəs/, *adj.*

collagenase ointment /kəlaj′ənās/, a medication used in the treatment of decubitus ulcers, burns, and other epidermal lesions. It is an enzyme preparation derived from the fermentation of *Clostridium histolyticum.*

collagen disease, any of the various abnormal conditions characterized by extensive disruption of the connective tissue, as inflammation and fibrinoid degeneration. Some collagen diseases are polyarteritis nodosa, rheumatoid coronary arteritis, and ankylosing spondylitis.

collagenoblast /kəlaj′ənōblast′/ [Gk *kolla, genein* + *blastos* germ], a cell that differentiates from a fibroblast and functions in the formation of collagen. It can also transform into cartilage and bone tissue by metaplasia.

collagenous fiber, any one of the tough, white fibers that constitute much of the intercellular substance and the connective tissue of the body.

collagen vascular disease, any of a group of acquired disorders that have in common diffuse immunologic and inflammatory changes in small blood vessels and connective tissue. Common features of most of these entities include arthritis, skin lesions, iritis and episcleritis, pericarditis, pleuritis, subcutaneous nodules, myocarditis, vasculitis, and nephritis.

collapse [L *collabi* to fall], **1.** *nontechnical.* a state of extreme depression or a condition of complete exhaustion because of physical or psychosomatic problems. **2.** an abnormal condition characterized by shock. **3.** the abnormal sagging of an organ or the obliteration of its cavity.

collapse of the lung [L, *collabi,* to fall together; AS, *lungen*], a reduction in the volume of the lung and the amount of air in it as a result of increased intrapleural pressure from accumulating air or fluid in the pleural cavity or because of a loss of internal pressure and elastic recoil of the lung.

collar [L *collum* neck], any structure that encircles another, usually around its neck, such as the periosteal bone collars that form around the diaphyses of young bones.

collarbone. See **clavicle.**

collateral /kōlat′ərəl/ [L *cum* together with, *lateralis* side] **1.** secondary or accessory. **2.** (in anatomy) a small branch, such as any one of the arterioles or venules in the body.

collateral circulation [L *cum, latus + circulare* to go around], a redundant blood pathway developed through enlargement of secondary vessels following obstruction of a main channel.

collateral fissure, a fissure separating the subcalcarine and the subcollateral gyri of the cerebral hemisphere.

collateral pulp canal, (in dentistry) a branch of the pulp canal that emerges from the root at a place other than the apex.

collateral ventilation, the ventilation of pulmonary air spaces through indirect pathways, such as pores in alveolar septa.

collateral vessel [L cum, latus + *vascellum* small vase], a branch of an artery or vein used as an accessory to the blood vessel from which it arose.

collecting tubule [L *colligere* to gather; *tubulus* small tube], any one of the many relatively large straight tubules of the kidney that funnel urine into the renal pelvis. The collecting tubules play an important role in maintaining the fluid balance of the body by allowing water to osmose through

their membranes into the interstitial fluid in the renal medulla.

collective bargaining, the use of collective action by employees in negotiating working conditions and economic issues with their employer.

collective unconscious [L *colligere* to gather; AS *un* not; L *conscious* aware], (in analytic psychology) that portion of the unconscious common to all mankind.

collector, (in medicine) a device with various modifications, used for collecting secretions from the bronchi and esophagus for bacteriologic and cytologic examination.

college [L *collegium* society], **1.** an organization of individuals with common professional training and interests, as the American College of Nurse-Midwives, the American College of Cardiology, or the American College of Surgeons. **2.** an institution of higher learning.

College of American Pathologists (CAP), a national professional organization of physicians who specialize in pathology.

Colles' fascia /kol′ēz/ [Abraham Colles, Irish surgeon, b. 1773; L, *band*], the deep layer of the subcutaneous fascia of the perineum, constituting a distinctive structure in the urogenital region of the body. It is a strong, smooth sheet of tissue containing elastic fibers.

Colles' fracture [Abraham Colles], a fracture of the radius at the epiphysis within 1 inch of the joint of the wrist, easily recognized by the dorsal and lateral position of the hand that it causes.

colligative /kol′igā′tiv/ [L *colligere* to gather], (in physical chemistry) of or pertaining to those properties of matter that depend on the concentration of particles, such as molecules and ions, rather than the chemical properties of any substance.

collimator /kol′imā′tər/ [L *collinare* to bring into alignment], a device for limiting particles of radiation to parallel paths, used to restrict the beam of a radiotherapy machine to a specified area.

colliquation /kol′ikwā′shən/ [L *cum* together with, *liquifacere* to make liquid], the degeneration of a tissue of the body to a liquid state, usually associated with necrotic tissue.

colliquative /kol′ikwā′tiv/, characterized by the profuse discharge of fluid, as in suppurating wounds and structures of the body that are infected.

collision tumor [L *cum* together with, *laedere* to strike], a tumor formed as two separate growths, developing close to each other, join.

collodion /kəlō′dē·ən/ [Gk *kolla* glue, *eidos*

form], a clear or a slightly opaque, highly inflammable liquid composed of pyroxylin, ether, and alcohol. It dries to a strong, transparent film.

collodion baby, an infant whose skin at birth is covered with a scaly, parchment-like membrane.

colloid /kol′oid/ [Gk *kolla* glue, *eidos* form], a state or division of matter in which large molecules or aggregates of molecules that do not precipitate, and that measure between 1 and 100 nm, are dispersed in another medium.

colloidal solution /koloi′dəl/ [Gk *kolla* + *eidos*; L, *solutus,* dissolved], a solution in which small particles, such as large polymeric molecules, are homogenously dispersed through a liquid medium. See also **colloid.**

colloidal sulfur, a form of very finely divided sulfur that is used in the treatment of acne and other skin disorders.

colloid bath, a bath taken in water that contains such substances as bran, gelatin, and starch, used to relieve irritation and inflammation.

colloid carcinoma, a former term for mucinous carcinoma.

colloid chemistry, the science dealing with the composition and nature of chemical colloids.

colloid cyst [Gk *kolla, eidos* + *kystis* bag], **1.** a thyroid gland follicle distended with thyroid secretion. **2.** a cyst in the third ventricle, leading to hydrocephalus.

colloid goiter, a greatly enlarged, soft thyroid gland in which the follicles are distended with colloid.

colloid suspension [Gk *kolla, eidos*; L *suspendere* to hang], a system of solids dispersed in a liquid medium, with particles generally smaller than 100 nm.

collyrium /kolir′ē·əm/, an ophthalmic liquid containing medications to be instilled into the eye.

coloboma /kol′əbō′mə/, *pl.* **colobomas, colobomata** [Gk *koloboma* defect], a congenital or pathologic defect in the ocular tissue of the body, usually affecting the iris, ciliary body, or choroid by forming a cleft that extends inferiorly. —**colobomatous,** *adj.*

coloenteritis. See **enterocolitis.**

colon /kō′lən/ [Gk *kolon*], the portion of the large intestine extending from the cecum to the rectum. It has four segments: ascending colon, transverse colon, descending colon, and sigmoid colon. —**colonic** /kəlon′ik/, *adj.*

colonic /kəlon′ik/. See **colon.**

colonic fistula [Gk *kolon;* L, pipe], an abnormal passage from the colon to the surface of the body or an internal organ or structure.

colonic irrigation, a procedure for washing the inner wall of the colon by filling it with water, then draining it. It is not considered an enema, but rather a technique for removing any material that may be present high in the colon.

colonization, the presence and multiplication of microorganisms without tissue invasion or damage.

colonoscope /kō′lənōskōp′/ [Gk *kolon, skopein* to watch], a long instrument with a light and lens that permits examination of the interior of the colon.

colonoscopy /kō′lənos′kəpē/, the examination of the mucosal lining of the colon using a colonoscope, an elongated endoscope.

colon stasis. See **atonia constipation.**

colony [L *colonia*], **1.** (in bacteriology) a mass of microorganisms in a culture that originates from a single cell. Some kinds of colonies, according to different configurations, are smooth colonies, rough colonies, and dwarf colonies. **2.** (in cell biology) a mass of cells in a culture or in certain experimental tissues, such as a spleen colony.

colony counter, a device used for counting colonies of bacteria growing in a culture and usually consisting of an illuminated, transparent plate that is divided into sections of known area.

coloproctitis /kōləpraktī′tis/, an inflammation of both the colon and rectum.

coloptosis /kō′loptō′sis/ [Gk *kolon* + *ptosis* fall], the prolapse or downward displacement of the colon.

Colorado tick fever, a relatively mild, self-limited arbovirus infection transmitted to humans by the bite of a tick. Symptoms, occurring in two phases separated by a period of remission, include chills, fever, headache, pain in the eyes, legs, and back, and sensitivity to light.

color blindness [L, color; AS *blint*], an abnormal condition characterized by an inability to clearly distinguish colors of the spectrum. In most cases it is not a blindness but a weakness in perceiving them distinctly. There are two forms of color blindness. **Daltonism** is the most common form and is characterized by an inability to distinguish reds from greens. It is an inherited, sex-linked disorder. **Total color blindness,** or **achromatic vision,** is characterized by an inability to perceive any color at all. Only white, gray, and black are seen. It may be the result of a defect in or the absence of the cones in the retina.

color dysnomia /disnō′mē·ə/ [L, color; Gk *dys* difficult, *onoma* name], an inability to name colors despite an ability to match and distinguish them. It may be caused by expressive dysphasis.

colorectal cancer /kō′lərek′təl/ [Gk kolon colon; L rectus straight], a malignant neoplastic disease of the large intestine, characterized by melena, a change in bowel habits, and the passing of blood. The high incidence of colorectal cancer in the Western world, as contrasted with the low incidence in Japan and rural Africa, suggests that a diet high in refined carbohydrates and beef and low in roughage may be a causative factor. Most lesions of the large bowel are adenocarcinomas; one half arise in the rectum, one fifth in the sigmoid colon, approximately one sixth in the cecum and ascending colon, and the rest in other sites.

colorimetry /kol′ərim′ətrē/ 1. measurement of the intensity of color in a fluid or substance. 2. measurement of color in the blood by use of a colorimeter to determine hemoglobin concentration. –**colorimetric,** adj.

color index (CI), the ratio between the concentration of hemoglobin and the number of red blood cells in any given sample of blood. The color index is computed by dividing the concentration of hemoglobin by the approximate number of red blood cells.

color vision, a recognition of color as the result of changes in the pigments of the cones in the retina that react to varying intensities of red, green, and blue light.

colosigmoidoscopy /kō′ləsig′moidos′kəpē/ [Gk kolon + sigma, S-shaped, eidos form, skopein to look], the direct examination of the sigmoid portion of the colon with a sigmoidoscope.

colostomate /kəlos′təmāt/ [Gk kolon + stoma mouth; L atum one acted upon], a person who has undergone a colostomy.

colostomy /kəlos′təmē/ [Gk kolon + stoma mouth], surgical creation of an artificial anus on the abdominal wall by incising the colon and bringing it out to the surface, performed for cancer of the colon and benign obstructive tumors, and severe abdominal wounds. A colostomy may be single-barreled, with one opening, or double-barreled, with distal and proximal loops open onto the abdomen. A type of colostomy is **loop colostomy.**

colostomy irrigation, a procedure used by colostomates to clear the bowel of fecal matter and to help establish an evacuation schedule.

colostrum /kəlos′trəm/ [L, first milk after calving], the fluid secreted by the breast during pregnancy and the first days postpartum before lactation begins, consisting of immunologically active substances and white blood cells, water, protein, fat, and carbohydrate in a thin, yellow, serous fluid.

colotomy /kōlot′əmē/, a surgical incision into the colon, usually performed through the abdominal wall.

Colour Index (CI), a publication of dyers, colorists, and textile chemists that specifies all the standard industrial pigments and stains according to five-digit numbers. For example, methylene blue is assigned number 52015.

colovaginal /kō′lōvaj′inəl/ [Gk, kolon, colon; L, vagina, sheath], pertaining to the colon and vagina, or to a communication between the two structures.

colpalgia /kolpal′jə/, a pain in the vagina.

colpectomy /kolpek′təmē/, the surgical excision of the vagina.

colpitis /kolpī′tis/, a vaginal inflammation.

colpocystitis /kol′pōsistī′tis/, an inflammation of the vagina and urinary bladder.

colpocystocele /kol′pəsis′təsēl/ the prolapse of the urinary bladder into the vagina, usually through the anterior vaginal wall.

colphysterectomy [Gk kolpos vagina, hystera womb, ektome excision], vaginal hysterectomy.

colporrhaphy /kolpôr′əfē/ [Gk kolpos + raphe suture], a surgical procedure in which the vagina is sutured, as for the purpose of narrowing the vagina.

colposcope /kol′pəskōp/, a lighted instrument with lenses for direct examination of the surfaces of the vagina and cervix.

colposcopy /kolpos′kəpē/ [Gk kolpos + skopein to watch], an examination of the vagina and cervix with a colposcope.

colpotomy /kolpot′əmē/ [Gk kolpos + temnein to cut], any surgical incision into the wall of the vagina.

columbium, former name for **niobium.**

columnar cell [L, columna, column, cella, storeroom], an epithelial cell that appears long and narrow when sectioned along its long axis.

columnar epithelium [L, columna, column; Gk, epi, upon, thele, nipple], a type of epithelial cell that resembles a hexagonal prism and approximately rectangular when sectioned along its long axis.

columnar layer [L, columna, column; AS, lecgan], the layer of rods and cones in the retina.

column chromatography [L columna; Gk chroma color, graphein to record], the process of separating and analyzing a group of substances according to the differences in their absorption affinities for a given absorbent as evidenced by pigments

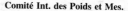

deposited during filtration through the same absorbent contained in a glass cylinder or tube. The substances are dissolved in a liquid that is passed through the absorbent. The absorbates move down the column at different rates and leave behind a band of pigments that is subsequently washed with a pure solvent to "develop" discrete pigmented bands that constitute a chromatograph.

coma [Gk *koma* deep sleep], a state of profound unconsciousness, characterized by the absence of spontaneous eye movements, response to painful stimuli, and vocalization. The person cannot be aroused. Coma may be the result of trauma, brain tumor, hematoma, toxic condition, acute infectious disease with encephalitis, vascular disease, poisoning, diabetic acidosis, or intoxication.

comatose, pertaining to a state of coma, or abnormally deep sleep, caused by illness or injury.

combat fatigue [L *com* together, *battuere* to beat; *fatigare* to tire], any of a variety of psychoneurotic disorders resulting from exhaustion, the stress of combat, or the cumulative emotions and psychologic strain of warfare or similar situations. It is characterized by anxiety, depression, memory and sleep disorders, and various related symptoms.

combination chemotherapy, the use of two or more anticancer drugs at the same time.

combined anesthesia. See **balanced anesthesia.**

combined carbon dioxide [L *com* together, *bini* twofold], the portion of the total carbon dioxide that is contained in blood carbonate and can be calculated as the difference between the total and dissolved carbon dioxide.

combined cycling ventilator, a mechanical ventilator that has more than one cycling mechanism, such as equipment that may have time cycling or pressure cycling as a backup to a volume cycling control device.

combined modality treatment, the use of chemotherapy in combination with surgery or radiation or both in the treatment of cancer.

combined oxygen, the oxygen that is physically bound to hemoglobin as oxyhemoglobin (HbO_2) One gram-molecular weight of oxygen can combine with 16,700 g of hemoglobin, and each gram of hemoglobin can take up and carry 1.34 ml of oxygen.

combined patterns, pertaining to a method of evaluating the neuromuscular functions of a patient through tests that re-

veal the degree of coordination between movement patterns of the trunk and the extremities.

combined system disease, a disorder of the nervous system caused by a deficiency of vitamin B_{12} that results in pernicious anemia and degeneration of the spinal cord and peripheral nerves, marked by increased difficulty in walking, a feeling of vibration in the legs, and a loss of sense of position.

combining sites, **1.** concave features on antibody molecules that serve as locations for binding antigens. Because of possible variations, each kind of antibody can provide combining sites for a specific antigen. **2.** locations on protein molecules where drugs or other substances may become bound by electrochemical attraction.

combustion, the process of burning or oxidation, which may be accompanied by light and heat. Oxygen itself does not burn, but oxygen supports combustion. The rate of combustion is influenced by both oxygen concentration and its partial pressure.

comedo /kom′idō/, *pl.* **comedones** /komidō′nēz/ [L *comedere* to consume], blackhead, the basic lesion of acne vulgaris, caused by an accumulation of keratin and sebum within the opening of a hair follicle. It is dark because of the effect of oxygen on sebum, not because of the presence of dirt.

comedocarcinoma /kom′idōkär′sinō′mə/, *pl.* **comedocarcinomas, comedocarcinomata** [L *comedere* to consume; Gk *karkinos* crab, *oma* tumor], a malignant intraductal neoplasm of the breast, in which the central cells degenerate and may be easily expressed from the cut surface of the tumor.

comedogenicity /kom′idōjənis′itē/, the ability of certain drugs or agents, such as anabolic steroids, to produce acne comedones.

COMDU, abbreviation for *cardiac monitor and diagnostic unit.*

comfort measure [L *com* together, *fortis* strong], any action taken to promote comfort of the patient, as a back rub, a change in position, or the prewarming of a stethoscope or a bedpan.

comfort zone [ME *comforten;* Gk *zone* belt], the boundaries of temperature, humidity, wind velocity, and solar radiation within which a person dressed in a specified manner can perform certain tasks without discomfort.

Comité International des Poids et Mesures (CIPM) /kômitā′ aNternäsyōnäl′ dā pô·ä′ ā mesYr′/, a group of scientists that meets periodically to define the international (SI) units of physical quantities, as the volume of a liter, the length of a meter, or the precise amount of time in a minute.

command automatism, a condition characterized by an abnormal mechanical responsiveness to commands, usually followed without critical judgment, such as may be seen in hypnosis and certain psychotic states.

command hallucination, a psychotic condition in which the patient hears and obeys voices that command him or her to perform certain acts.

commensal /kəmen'səl/ [L *com* together, *imensa* table], (of two different organisms) living together in an arrangement that is not harmful to either and may be beneficial to both.

comminuted /kom'inyo͞o'tid/ [L *comminuire* to break into pieces], crushed or broken into a number of pieces.

comminuted fracture, a fracture in which there are several breaks in the bone, creating numerous fragments.

commissure /kom'iso͞or, -syo͞or/ **1.** a band of nerve fiber or other tissue that crosses from one side of the body to the other, usually connecting two structures or masses of tissue. **2.** a site of union of two anatomic parts, as the corner of the eye, lips, or labia.

commissurotomy /kom'isho͞orot'əmē/ [L *commissura* a joining together; Gk *temnein* to cut], the surgical division of a fibrous band or ring connecting corresponding parts of a body structure.

commitment [L *committere* to put in charge], **1.** the placement or confinement of an individual in a specialized hospital or other institutional facility. **2.** the legal procedure of admitting a mentally ill person to an institution for psychiatric treatment. **3.** a pledge or contract to fulfill some obligation or agreement, used especially in some forms of psychotherapy or marriage counseling.

common bile duct [L *communis* community, *bilis* bile, *ducere* to lead], the duct formed by the juncture of the cystic duct and hepatic duct.

common carotid artery [L *communis* + Gk *karos* heavy sleep, *arteria* air pipe], one of the major arteries supplying blood to the head and neck. Each divides into an external common carotid and an internal common carotid. Branches supply the face, scalp, neck, throat, brain, and other tissues.

common carotid plexus, a network of nerves on the common carotid artery, supplying sympathetic fibers to the head and the neck, with branches that accompany the cranial blood vessels.

common cold. See **cold.**

common hepatic artery, the visceral branch of the celiac trunk of the abdominal aorta, passing to the pylorus and dividing into five branches.

common iliac artery, a division of the abdominal aorta, starting to the left of the fourth lumbar vertebra and dividing into external and internal iliac arteries.

common iliac node, a node in one of the seven groups of parietal lymph nodes serving the abdomen and the pelvis.

common iliac vein, one of the two veins that are the sources of the inferior vena cava, formed by the union of the internal and the external iliac veins.

communicability period, the usual time span during which contact with an infected person is most likely to result in spread of the infection.

communicable /kəmyo͞o'nəkəbəl/ [L *communis* common], contagious; transmissible by direct or indirect means, as a communicable disease.

communicable disease, any disease transmitted from one person or animal to another directly, by contact with excreta or other discharges from the body; or indirectly, via substances or inanimate objects, such as contaminated drinking glasses, toys, or water; or via vectors, as flies, mosquitoes, ticks, or other insects. Many communicable diseases, by law, must be reported to the local health department.

Communicable Disease Center, former name of the **Centers for Disease Control and Prevention.**

communicating hydrocephalus [L *communicans*; Gk *hydor* water, *kephale* head], a form of hydrocephalus in which there is an increase in cerebrospinal fluid that involves the entire ventricle system and the subarachnoid space because of an abnormality in the ability to absorb fluid in the subarachnoid space.

communication [L *communis* common], any process in which a message containing information is transferred, especially from one person to another, via any of a number of media.

communication channels, (in communication theory) any gesture, action, sound, written word, or visual image used in transmitting messages.

communication, impaired verbal, a NANDA-accepted nursing diagnosis of a state in which an individual experiences a decreased or absent ability to use of understand language in human interaction. Defining characteristics include an inability to speak the dominant language of the culture, slurring, stuttering, difficulty in forming words or sentences, difficulty in expressing thoughts verbally, inappropriate verbalization, dyspnea, disorientation, and the absence of speech.

communication theme, (in psychiatry) a recurrent concept or idea that ties together components of communication. Kinds of communication themes include **content theme,** in which a single concept links varied topics of discussion; **mood theme,** in which the underlying idea is the emotion communicated by the individual; and **interaction theme,** in which a particular idea best describes the dynamics between communicating participants.

communication theory, a theory that describes a model of a system of communication consisting of a source of information (the sender), a transmitter, a communication channel, a source of noise (interference), a receiver, and a purpose for the message.

community [L *communis* common], a group of people who reside in a designated geographic area and who share common interests or bonds.

community-acquired infection, an infection acquired from the environment, including infections acquired indirectly from the use of medications. Community-acquired infections are distinguished from nosocomial, or hospital-acquired, diseases by the types of organisms that affect patients who are recovering from a disease or injury.

community health nursing, a field of nursing that is a blend of primary health care and nursing practice with public health nursing. The community health nurse conducts comprehensive health programs that pay special attention to social and ecologic influences and specific populations at risk.

community medicine, a branch of medicine that is concerned with the health of the members of a community, municipality, or region.

community mental health, a treatment philosophy based on the social model of psychiatric care that advocates a comprehensive range of mental health services to be made readily available to all members of the community.

community mental health center (CMHC), a community-based center that provides comprehensive mental health services, including ambulatory and inpatient care. The specific services to be provided are defined in an act of Congress, the Community Mental Health Centers Act.

community nurse practitioner (CNP), a nurse who has completed a postbaccalaureate program in community nursing.

community psychiatry, the branch of psychiatry concerned with the development of an adequate and coordinated program of mental health care for residents of specified catchment areas.

community reintegration, the return and acceptance of a disabled person as a participating member of the community.

compact bone [L *compingere* to put together], hard, dense bone that is usually found at the surface of skeletal structures, as distinguished from spongy cancellous bone.

companionship [L *com* together, *panis* food], (in psychiatric nursing) the assignment of a staff member or of another patient to stay with a disturbed patient to provide support and to protect the patient from self-harm or the harming of others.

comparative anatomy [L *com* + *par* equal], the study of the morphology and function of all living animals from the simplest to the most highly specialized animals.

comparative embryology, the study of the similarities and differences among various organisms during the embryologic period of development.

comparative method, the analytic method to which the test method is compared in the comparison-of-methods experiment.

comparative physiology, the study of the similarities and differences of the vital processes found in various species of living organisms to determine fundamental physiologic relationships.

comparative psychology, 1. the study of human behavior as it relates to or differs from animal behavior. 2. the study of the psychologic and behavioral differences among various peoples.

compartment model, a mathematical representation of the body or an area of the body created to study physiologic or pharmacologic kinetics. A compartment model can simulate all of the biologic processes involved in the kinetic behavior of a drug after it has been introduced into the body, leading to a better understanding of the drug's pharmacodynamic effects.

compartment syndrome [L *com* + *partiri* to share], a pathologic condition caused by the progressive development of arterial compression and reduced blood supply.

compatibility /kompat'əbil'itē/ [L *compatibilis* agreeable], 1. the quality or state of existing together in harmony; congruity. 2. the orderly, efficient integration of the elements of one system with those of another. 3. the formation of a stable chemical or biochemical system, specifically in medication, so that two or more drugs can be administered at the same time without producing undesired side effects or without canceling or changing the therapeutic effects of the others. **4.** (in immunology) the degree to which the body's defense system will tolerate the presence of foreign material, such as transfused blood, grafted tissue, or transplanted organs, without an immune reaction. Usually, complete compatibility exists between identical twins. **5.** (in blood grouping or crossmatching) the lack of reaction between blood groups so that there is no agglutination when the red blood cells of one sample are mixed with the serum of another sample; no reaction from transfused blood. **–compatible,** *adj.*

compendium /kəmpen'dē·əm/, *pl.* **compendia** [L *compendere* to weigh together], a collected body of information on the standards of strength, purity, and quality of drugs. The official compendia in the United States are the *United States Pharmacopoeia,* the *Homeopathic Pharmacopoeia of the United States,* the *National Formulary,* and their supplements.

compensated acidosis [L *compensare* to weigh together, *acidus* sour; Gk *osis* condition], a condition in which the pH of the blood is maintained within normal limits, although the blood bicarbonate level is below normal.

compensated alkalosis, a condition in which the blood bicarbonate is increased but buffering keeps the blood pH within the normal range.

compensated flow meter [L *compensare* to balance], a gas therapy device with a scale that is calibrated against a constant pressure of 50 psi instead of the atmosphere.

compensated gluteal gait, one of the more common abnormal gaits associated with a weakness of the gluteus medius. It is a variation of the Trendelenburg gait and involves the dropping of the pelvis on the unaffected side of the body during the walking cycle between the moment of heelstrike on the affected side and the moment of heelstrike on the unaffected side.

compensated heart failure, an abnormal cardiac condition in which heart failure is compensated for by such mechanisms as increased sympathetic adrenergic stimulation of the heart, fluid retention with increased venous return, increased end-diastolic ventricular volume and fiber length, and hypertrophy.

compensating current, an electric current that neutralizes the intensity of a muscle current.

compensating curve, the curvature of alignment of the occlusal surfaces of the teeth, developed to compensate for the paths of the condyles as the mandible moves from centric to eccentric positions.

compensating filter, (in radiology) a device, such as a wedge fashioned from aluminum or plastic, that is positioned over a body area to compensate for differences in radiopacity.

compensation /kom'pənsā'shən/ [L *compensare* to balance], **1.** the process of counterbalancing any defect in bodily structure or function. **2.** (in cardiology) the process of maintaining an adequate blood flow through such normal cardiac and circulatory mechanisms as tachycardia, fluid retention with increased venous return, and hypertrophy. Failure of the heart to compensate and to provide the required cardiac output indicates a diseased heart muscle. **3.** (in psychiatry) a complex defense mechanism that allows one to avoid the unpleasant or painful emotional stimuli that result from a feeling of inferiority or inadequacy. A kind of compensation is **dosage compensation.**

compensation neurosis, an unconscious process by which one prolongs the symptoms resulting from an injury or disease to receive secondary gains, especially money.

compensator /kom'pənsā'tər/, a device used in radiotherapy to correct for irregularities in body surfaces by providing a differential attenuation of the beam before it reaches the patient.

compensatory hypertrophy [L *compensare* to balance], an increase in the size or the function of an organ or part to counterbalance a structural or functional defect.

compensatory pause, a longer than normal period between heartbeats. This increased refractory period may be associated with premature ventricular contractions. Because the stimulus is out of phase, it interferes with the usual sequence of excitability and refractoriness, resulting in a lag before the next contraction.

competence [L *competentia* capable], **1.** (in embryology) the total capacity of an embryonic cell to react to determinative stimuli in various ways of differentiation. **2.** the ability of bacteria to take up donor DNA molecules.

competent community, a population that is aware of resources, that can make decisions about issues facing the group, and that can cope adaptively with problems. It parallels the concept of positive mental health.

competitive antagonist. See **antimetabolite.**

competitive-binding assay [L *competere* to come together], an analytic procedure based on the reversible binding of a ligand to a binding protein.

competitive displacement, the tendency of one drug to displace another at a protein-binding site when both drugs are taken at the same time. The bound drug becomes less pharmacologically active than the free drug.

competitive identification, the unconscious modeling of one's personality on that of another as a means of outdoing or bettering the other person.

competitive inhibitor, an inhibitor of an enzyme reaction that competes with the substrate by binding at the active site.

complaint [L *complangere* to beat the breast], **1.** (in law) a pleading by a plaintiff made under oath to initiate a suit. It is a statement of the formal charge and the cause for action against the defendant. **2.** *informal.* any ailment, problem, or symptom identified by the client, patient, member of the person's family, or other knowledgeable person.

complement [L *complementum* that which completes], one of 11 complex, enzymatic serum proteins. In an antigen-antibody reaction, complement causes lysis.

complement abnormality, an unusual condition characterized by deficiencies or by dysfunctions of any of the nine functional components of the enzymatic proteins of blood serum. The components are labeled C1 through C9. Theoretically, any of the nine complement components may be lacking. The most common abnormalities are C2 and C3 deficiencies and C5 familial dysfunction. Patients with complement deficiencies or with complement dysfunctions may be more susceptible to infections and to collagen vascular diseases. Some patients with lupus erythematosus or dermatomyositis have displayed complement abnormalities. Studies indicate that primary complement deficiencies may be inherited. Secondary complementary deficiencies may stem from immunologic reactions, such as drug-induced serum disease, which depletes complement.

complemental inheritance, the acquisition or expression of a trait or condition from the presence of two independent pairs of nonallelic genes. Both of the genes must be present for the characteristic to appear in the phenotype.

complementarity, pertaining to a relationship in which differences are maximal.

complementary feeding [L *complementum* that which completes], a supplemental feeding given an infant that is still hungry after breast feeding.

complementary gene, either member of two or more nonallelic gene pairs that interact to produce an effect not expressed in the absence of any of the pairs.

complement cascade, a biochemical process involving the C1 to C9 complement components in which one complement interacts with another in a specific sequence called a complement pathway. The reaction sequence is C1, 4, 2, 3, 5, 6, 7, 8, 9 (the first complements being out of numerical sequence for historical reasons). The cascade effect leads to an accumulation of fluid in a cell and finally lysis of the membrane, causing the cell to rupture.

complement fixation, an immunologic reaction in which an antigen combines with an antibody and its complement, causing the complement factor to become inactive or "fixed."

complement-fixation test (C-F test), any serologic test in which complement fixation is detected, indicating the presence of a particular antigen. Specific C-F tests are used to aid in the diagnosis of amebiasis, Rocky Mountain spotted fever, trypanosomiasis, and typhus.

complement protein molecule [L *complementum, proteios* first rank], any of the proteins molecules that are chief humoral mediators of antigen-antibody reactions in the immune system. Nine are involved in the "classical pathway" cascade resulting in the lysis of antibody-coated bacteria. They are designated C1 to C9.

complete abortion [L *complere* to fill up], termination of pregnancy in which the conceptus is expelled or removed in its entirety.

complete bed bath, a bath in which the entire body of a patient is washed while the person is in bed.

complete blood count (CBC), a determination of the number of red and white blood cells per cubic millimeter of blood. Many electronic blood counters automatically determine hemoglobin or hematocrit and include this value in the complete blood count.

complete breech, a fetal presentation in which the nates present with the legs folded on the thighs and the thighs on the abdomen.

complete dislocation [L *complere,* to fill up, *dis* apart, *locare* to place], a dislocation in which the articular surfaces of the joint are completely separated.

complete fistula, an abnormal passage from an internal organ or structure to the surface of the body or to another internal organ or structure.

complete fracture, a bone break that completely disrupts the continuity of osseous tissue across the entire width of the bone involved.

complete health history, a health history that includes a history of the present illness, a health history, social history, occupational history, sexual history, and a family health history.

complete heart block (CHB) [L *complere;* Gk *kardia* heart; OFr *bloc*], a condition of complete failure of the conduction of all impulses from the atria to the ventricles so that they beat independently.

complete hernia [L *complere, hernia* rupture], a hernia characterized by protrusion of the hernial sac and abdominal contents through the abdominal wall.

complete paralysis [L *complere;* Gk *paralyein* to be palsied], paralysis characterized by a complete loss of motor function.

complete rachischisis, a rare congenital fissure of the entire vertebral column and spinal cord, resulting from the failure of the embryonic neural tube to close.

complete response (CR), the total disappearance of a tumor.

complex [L *complexus* an embrace], **1.** a group of items, as chemical molecules, that are related in structure or function as are the iron and protein portions of hemoglobin or the cobalt and protein portions of vitamin B$_{12}$. **2.** a combination of signs and symptoms of disease that forms a syndrome. **3.** (in psychology) a group of associated ideas with strong emotional overtones affecting a person's attitudes.

complex carbohydrate, a polysaccharide, such as a carbohydrate that is composed of a large number of glucose molecules, so called to distinguish it from simple sugars.

complex cavity, a cavity that involves more than one surface of a tooth.

complex ectopic beat [L *complexus* an embrace; Gk *ektos* outside, *topos* place], a heart contraction impulse that originates from some point other than the sinoatrial node.

complex fracture, a closed fracture in which the soft tissue surrounding the bone is severely damaged.

complex odontoma. See **composite odontoma.**

complex protein, a protein that contains a simple protein and at least one molecule of another substance, as a glycoprotein, nucleoprotein, or hemoglobin.

complex spatial relations, the perceptual relationship of one figure or part of a figure to another.

complex sugars, sugar molecules that can be hydrolyzed or digested to yield two molecules of the same or different simple sugars, as sucrose, lactose, and maltose.

compliance [L *complere* to complete], **1.** fulfillment by the patient of the caregiver's prescribed course of treatment. **2.** (in respiratory physiology) a measure of distensibility of the lung volume produced by a unit pressure change.

compliance factor, a measure of the amount of trapped tidal volume in a mechanical ventilating system associated with expansion of the flexible tubing when pressure is applied.

complicated dislocation [L *complicare* to fold together, *dis* apart, *locare* place], a dislocation complicated by damage to other tissues.

complicated labor [L *complicare* + *labor* work], any labor that is complicated by a deviation from the normal procedure.

complication [L *com* + *plicare* to fold], a disease or injury that develops during the treatment of an earlier disorder. The complication frequently alters the prognosis.

component [L *componere* to assemble], a significant part of a larger unit.

component drip set, a device used for delivering intravenous fluids, especially whole blood. It includes plastic tubing and a combination drip-chamber and filter.

component syringe set, a device used for delivering intravenous fluids. It includes plastic tubing, two slide clamps, a Y-connector, and a syringe.

component therapy, a kind of transfusion in which specific blood components are administered instead of whole blood. Packed red cells or platelet-rich plasma suspensions may be transfused in larger quantities than would be possible if whole blood were used.

composite core [L *componere* to assemble], a buildup of composite resin, designed and installed to retain an artificial tooth crown.

composite odontoma, an odontogenic tumor composed of abnormally arranged calcified enamel and dentin.

compos mentis, the quality of having a sound mind.

compound [L *componere* to assemble], **1.** (in chemistry) a substance composed of two or more different elements, chemically combined in definite proportions, that cannot be separated by physical means. **2.** any substance composed of two or more different ingredients. **3.** to make a substance by combining ingredients, such as a pharmaceutical. **4.** denoting an injury characterized by multiple factors, such as a compound fracture.

compound aneurysm, a localized dilatation of an arterial wall in which some of the layers are distended and others are ruptured or dissected.

compound dislocation [L *componere, dis* apart, *locare* place], a dislocation in which there is a break in the skin associated with the affected joint.

compound fracture, a fracture in which the broken end or ends of the bone have torn through the skin.

compound joint [L, *componere,* to put together, *jungere,* to join], any joint that involves more than two bones.

compound melanocytoma. See **benign juvenile melanoma.**

compound microscope [L *componere;* Gk *mikros* small, *skopein* to view], a microscope with two or more simple or complex lens systems.

compound monster, a fetus in which some of the parts or organs are duplicated but not fully developed.

compound tubuloalveolar gland, one of the many multicellular glands with more than one secretory duct that contains both tube-shaped and sac-shaped portions, as the salivary glands.

comprehensive care. See **holistic health care.**

Comprehensive Health Manpower Act of 1971, legislation passed by the U.S. Congress providing educational funding for nurse-practitioner (NP) and physician-assistant (PA) programs.

Comprehensive Health Planning (CHP) and Public Health Services Amendments, legislation passed by the U.S. Congress in 1966 that emphasized regional planning and established for the first time the concept that each person has a "right to health care."

compress [L *comprimere* to press together], a soft pad, usually made of cloth, used to apply heat, cold, or medications to the surface of a body area. A compress also may be applied over a wound to help control bleeding.

compressed air hazards. See **decompression sickness.**

compressibility factor, a measure of the amount of tidal volume that may be trapped in a mechanical ventilator system in relation to the water pressure applied. It is expressed in milliliters of gas per centimeter of water pressure.

compressible volume, a part of the tidal volume of gas produced by a mechanical ventilator that does not reach the patient because of compression of the gas and expansion of the flexible tubing in the equipment.

compression [L *comprimere* to press together], the act of pressing, squeezing, or otherwise applying pressure to an organ, tissue, or body area. Kinds of pathologic compression include **compression fracture,** in which bone surfaces are forced against each other, causing a break, and **compression paralysis,** marked by paralysis of a body area caused by pressure on a nerve.

compression fracture, a bone break, especially in a short bone, that disrupts osseous tissue and collapses the affected bone.

compression neuropathy, any of several disorders involving damage to sensory nerve roots or peripheral nerves, caused by mechanical pressure or localized trauma and characterized by paresthesia, weakness, or paralysis.

compression paralysis [L *comprimere;* Gk *paralyein* to be palsied], a paralysis that is caused by sustained pressure on a peripheral nerve. The condition can be temporary or permanent, depending on the duration and intensity of the pressure.

compressive atelectasis, a loss of the ability of the lung to move air in and out of the atelectatic region because of intrathoracic pressures that compress the alveoli. The condition may result from a pulmonary embolism.

compressor naris /kompres′ ôrnär′is/, the transverse part of the nasalis muscle that depresses the cartilage of the nose and draws the ala toward the septum.

compromise [L *com* together, *promittere* to promise], an action that may involve a change in a person's behavior, as in substituting goals or delaying satisfaction of needs in one area to reduce stress in another.

compromise body image, a new body image acquired by a patient as part of his or her adjustment to a physical dysfunction. A compromise body image incorporates and modifies unacceptable features of the condition through psychologic defense mechanisms.

compromised host, a person who is less-than-normally able to resist infection, because of immunosuppressive therapy, immunologic defect, severe anemia, or concurrent disease or condition, including AIDS, metastatic malignancy, cachexia, or severe malnutrition.

Compton scatter [Arthur H. Compton, American physicist, b. 1892], the principal interaction process of photons with tissue in the diagnostic and therapeutic radiology energy range.

compulsion [L *compellere* to urge], an irresistible, repetitive, irrational impulse to perform an act that is usually contrary to one's ordinary judgments or standards yet results in overt anxiety if it is not completed. A kind of compulsion is **repetition compulsion.**

compulsion need [L *compellere;* Gk *neuron* nerve, *osis* condition], a need characterized by a compulsion to perform certain acts repeatedly in spite of conscious recognition that it is abnormal behavior. The compulsive act may have symbolic significance to the patient.

compulsive [L *compellere*], pertaining to an act repeatedly performed under the stress of compulsion.

compulsive idea [L *compellere*], a recurring, irrational idea that persists in the mind, usually resulting in an irresistible urge to perform some inappropriate act.

compulsive personality, a type of character structure in which there is a pattern of chronic and obsessive adherence to rigid standards of conduct. The compulsive person is likely to follow repetitive patterns of behavior, such as snapping the fingers, crossing the legs, or refusing to walk on cracks in the sidewalk.

compulsive personality disorder, a condition in which an irrational preoccupation with order, rules, ritual, and detail interferes with everyday functioning and normal behavior.

compulsive polydipsia, a neurotic, compelling urge to drink excessive amounts of liquid. Extreme cases can result in death from water intoxication and electrolyte imbalance.

compulsive ritual, a series of acts a person feels must be carried out even though he recognizes the behavior to be useless and inappropriate.

computed tomography (CT), an x-ray technique that produces a film representing a detailed cross section of tissue structure. The procedure uses a narrowly collimated beam of x-rays that rotates in a continuous 360-degree motion around the patient to image the body in cross-sectional slices. An array of detectors, positioned at several angles, records those x-rays that pass through the body. The image is created by computer.

CONA, abbreviation for **Canadian Orthopedic Nurses' Association.**

conation [L *conari* to attempt], the mental process characterized by desire, impulse, volition, and striving.

concanavalin A, a hemagglutinin, isolated from the meal of the jack bean, that reacts with polyglucosans in the blood of mammals causing agglutination.

concatenates /kənkat'ənāts/, long molecules formed by continuous repeating of the same molecular subunit.

concave-convex joint relationship, the relative shape of each component of a

joint's articulating surfaces. One surface is usually concave and the other convex.

concave spherical lens [L *concavare* to make hollow; Gk *sphaira* ball; L *lentil*], a lens that has curved, depressed surfaces to diverge the rays of light. It is used for the management of myopia.

concavity /kənkav'itē/, a deep depression or inward curving surface of an organ or body structure.

concealed accessory pathway [L *con* together, *celare* to hide], (in cardiology) an extramuscular tract between the atria and ventricles that conducts only in a retrograde direction.

concealed junctional extrasystole, a junctional impulse that arises in and discharges the atrioventricular junction but fails to reach either atria or ventricles.

conceive [L *concipere* to take together], to become pregnant.

concentrate [L *con* + *centrum* center], **1.** to decrease the bulk of a liquid and increase its strength per unit of volume by the removal of inactive ingredients through evaporation or other means. **2.** a substance, particularly a liquid, that has been strengthened and reduced in volume through such means.

concentration gradient, a gradient that exists across a membrane separating a high concentration of a particular ion from a low concentration of the same ion.

concentric /kənsen'trik/ [L *con* + *centrum* center], describing two or more circles that have a common center.

concentric contraction, a common form of muscle contraction that occurs in rhythmic activities when the muscle fibers shorten as tension develops.

concentric fibroma, a fibrous tumor surrounding the uterine cavity.

concentric hypertrophy, a type of tissue overgrowth in which the walls of an organ continue to increase in size but the exterior size remains the same while the internal size is diminished.

concept [L *concipere* to take together], a construct or abstract idea or thought that originates and is held within the mind. **–conceptual,** *adj.*

conception [L *concipere* to take together], **1.** the beginning of pregnancy, usually taken to be the instant that a spermatozoon enters an ovum and forms a viable zygote. **2.** the act or process of fertilization. **3.** the act or process of creating an idea or notion. **4.** the idea or notion created; a general impression resulting from the interpretation of a symbol or set of symbols.

conceptional age, in fetal development, the number of weeks since conception.

conception control. See **contraception.**

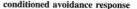

conceptive [L *concipere*], 1. able to become pregnant. 2. pertaining to or characteristic of the mental process of forming ideas or impressions.

conceptual disorder [L *concipere*], a disturbance in thought processes, in cognitive activities, or in the ability to formulate concepts.

conceptual framework, a group of concepts that are broadly defined and systematically organized to provide a focus, a rationale, and a tool for the integration and interpretation of information.

conceptus /kənsep′təs/ [L *concipere* to take together], the product of conception; the fertilized ovum and its enclosing membranes at all stages of intrauterine development, from the time of implantation to birth.

concha /kong′kə/, a body structure that is shell-shaped, as the cavity in the external ear that surrounds the external auditory canal meatus.

concoction [L *con* + *coquere* to cook], a remedy prepared from a mixture of two or more drugs or substances that have been heated.

concomitant /konkom′itənt/ [L *con* + *comitari* to accompany], designating one or more of two or more things, occurring simultaneously, that may or may not be interrelated or produced as a result of the others; accompanying.

concomitant symptom, any symptom that accompanies a primary symptom.

concordance [L *concordare* to agree], (in genetics) the expression of one or more specific traits in both members of a pair of twins. —**concordant,** *adj.*

concreteness [L *concrescere* to be formed], pertaining to the content of a communication that is not vague, but which includes specific feelings, behaviors, and experiences or situations.

concrete operation, a thought process based on concrete rather than abstract points of reference.

concrete thinking, a stage in the development of the cognitive thought processes in the child. During this phase, thought becomes increasingly logical and coherent so that the child is able to classify, sort, order, and organize facts while still being incapable of generalizing or dealing in abstractions.

concretion. See **calculus.**

concurrent disinfection [L *concurrere* to meet at one place; *dis* opposite of, *inficere* to taint], the daily handling and disposal of contaminated material or equipment.

concurrent infection [L *concurrere* + *inficere* to stain], a condition during which a person has two or more infections at the same time.

concurrent nursing audit. See **nursing audit.**

concurrent sterilization, a method of preparing an infant-feeding formula in which all ingredients and equipment are sterilized before mixing the formula.

concurrent validity, validity of a test or a measurement tool that is established by concurrently applying a previously validated tool or test to the same phenomena, or data base, and comparing the results.

concussion /konkush′ən/ [L *concutere* to shake violently], 1. a violent jarring or shaking, as caused by a blow or an explosion. 2. *informal;* brain concussion.

condensation [L *condensare* to make denser], 1. a reduction to a denser form, such as from water vapor to a liquid. 2. (in psychology) a process often present in dreams in which two or more concepts are fused so that a single symbol represents the multiple components.

condensation nuclei, neutral particles, such as dust, in the atmosphere that are able to absorb or adsorb water and grow in size. At relatively high humidities, they form fogs or hazes. Condensation nuclei consisting of sulfuric or nitric acid vapors or nitrogen oxides may be a source of respiratory irritants.

condensed milk, a thick liquid prepared by the evaporation of half of the water content of cow's milk and the addition of sugar.

condenser, (in dentistry) an instrument for compacting restorative material into a prepared tooth cavity. It has a working end, or nib, with a flat or serrated face.

condition [L *condicere* to make arrangements], 1. a state of being, specifically in reference to physical and mental health or well-being. 2. anything that is essential for or that restricts or modifies the appearance or occurrence of something else. 3. to train the body or mind, usually through specific exercises and repeated exposure to a particular state or thing. 4. (in psychology) to subject a person or animal to conditioning or associative learning so that a specific stimulus will always elicit a particular response.

conditional discharge, a specified leave of absence or liberty from a psychiatric hospital in which certain behaviors are expected from the patient and the original commitment order remains in effect.

conditioned avoidance response, a learned reaction that is performed either consciously or unconsciously to avoid an unpleasant or painful stimulus or to prevent such stimuli from occurring.

conditioned escape response, a learned reaction that is performed either consciously or unconsciously to stop or to escape from an aversive stimulus.

conditioned orientation response (COR), the desired response in an audiometry technique used in hearing tests for children under the age of 2 years. A toy mounted on a loudspeaker moves or lights up after presentation of a test tone. If later test sounds are audible to the child, he or she will look toward the toy after hearing a tone.

conditioned reflex, a reflex developed gradually by training in association with a specific, repeated external stimulus.

conditioned response, an automatic reaction to a stimulus that does not normally elicit such response but which has been learned through training. Such responses are produced by repeated association of some physiologic function or behavioral pattern with an unrelated stimulus or event.

conditioned stimulus [L, *conditio* + *stimulus,* goad], any stimulus to which a reflex response has become conditioned by previous training or experience.

conditioning [L *condicere* to make arrangements], a form of learning based on the development of a response or set of responses to a stimulus or series of stimuli. Kinds of conditioning are **classical, instrumental,** and **operant conditioning.**

condom /kon'dəm/ [Doctor Condon, eighteenth-century English physician], a soft, flexible sheath that covers the penis and prevents semen from entering the vagina in sexual intercourse, used to avoid the transmittal of an infection and to prevent conception.

conduct disorder, (in psychiatry) behavior in an adolescent that is unacceptable in the social environment and could be considered criminal in an adult.

conduction [L *conducere* to lead], 1. (in physics) a process in which heat is transferred from one substance to another because of a difference in temperature; a process in which energy is transmitted through a conductor. 2. (in physiology) the process by which a nerve impulse is transmitted.

conduction anesthesia, a loss of sensation, especially pain, in a region of the body, produced by injecting a local anesthetic along the course of a nerve or nerves to inhibit the conduction of impulses to and from the area supplied by that nerve or nerves.

conduction aphasia, a dissociative speech phenomenon in which there is no difficulty in comprehending words seen or heard and in which there is no dysarthria, yet the patient has problems in self-expression. The patient may substitute words similar in sound or meaning for the correct ones but is unable to repeat from dictation, to spell, and to read aloud.

conduction deafness. See **conductive hearing loss.**

conduction system, specialized tissue that carries electrical impulses, such as bundle branches and Purkinje fibers.

conduction system of the heart, the network of nervous tissue that transmits the electrical impulses needed for a heart beat. It includes the sinoatrial and atrioventricular nodes, the bundle of His, the Purkinje fibers, and the left and right bundle branches.

conduction velocity, the speed with which an electrical impulse can be transmitted through excitable tissue, as in the movement of a contraction impulse through His-Purkinje fibers of the heart.

conductive hearing loss [L *conducere* to lead], a form of hearing loss in which sound is inadequately conducted through the external or middle ear to the sensorineural apparatus of the inner ear. Sensitivity to sound is diminished, but clarity is not changed.

conductor, 1. any substance through which electrons flow easily. 2. (in psychiatry) a family therapist who uses his or her own personality to give direction to a family in therapy.

conduit /kon'do͞o·it/, 1. an artificial channel or passage that connects two organs or different parts of the same organ. 2. a tube or other device for conveying water or other fluids from one region to another.

condylar fracture /kon'dilər/ [Gk *kondylos* knuckle], any fracture of the round end of a hinge joint, usually occurring at the distal end of the humerus or at the distal end of the femur, frequently detaching a small bone fragment that includes the condyle.

condylar guide, a mechanical device on a dental articulator designed to guide articular movement similar to that produced by the paths of the condyles in the temporomandibular joints.

condyle /kon'dīl/ [Gk *kondylos* knuckle], a rounded projection at the end of a bone that anchors muscle ligaments and articulates with adjacent bones.

condyloid /kon'diloid/ [Gk, *kondylos,* knuckle], resembling a knuckle.

condyloid joint [L *kondylos* + *eidos* form], a synovial joint in which a condyle is received into an elliptic cavity, as the wrist joint. A condyloid joint permits no axial rotation but allows flexion, extension, adduction, abduction, and circumduction.

condyloma /kon´dilō´mə/, pl. **condylomata** [Gk kondyloma a knob], a wartlike growth on the anus, vulva, or glans penis.

condyloma acuminatum, pl. **condylomata acuminata,** a soft, wartlike or papillomatous growth common on warm and moist skin and the mucous membrane of the genitalia.

condyloma latum, pl. **condylomata lata,** a flat, moist, papular growth that appears in secondary syphilis in the coronal sulcus of the perineum or on the glans penis.

cone /kōn/ [Gk konos cone], **1.** a photoreceptor cell in the retina of the eye that enables a person to visualize colors. There are three kinds of retinal cones, one for each of the colors, blue, green, and red; other colors are seen by stimulation of more than one type of cone. **2.** a cone-shaped device attached to radiologic equipment to focus x-rays on a small target of tissue. **–conic, conical,** adj.

cone biopsy, surgical removal of a cone-shaped segment of the cervix, including both epithelial and endocervical tissue.

cone cutting, the interference by a radiographic cone with an x-ray beam caused by misalignment of the tube, cone, and film.

cone of light, 1. a triangular reflection observed during an ear examination when the light of an otoscope is focused on the image of the malleus. **2.** the group of light rays entering the pupil of the eye and forming an image on the retina.

confabulation /kənfab´yəlā´shən/ [L con + fabulari to speak], the fabrication of experiences or situations, often recounted in a detailed and plausible way to fill in and cover up gaps in the memory.

confession, an act of seeking expiation through another from guilt for a real or imagined transgression.

confidentiality, the nondisclosure of certain information except to another authorized person.

configuration [L configuare to form from], the hardware, software, and peripherals assembled to work as a computer unit in a specific situation.

configurationism. See **Gestalt psychology.**

confinement [L confinis common boundary], **1.** a state of being held or restrained within a specific place in order to hinder or minimize activity. **2.** the final phase of pregnancy during which labor and childbirth occur; parturition.

confinement deprivation, an emotional disorder that may result when an individual is separated from familiar surroundings or denied contact with familiar persons or objects.

conflict [L conflictere to strike together], **1.** a mental struggle, either conscious or unconscious, resulting from the simultaneous presence of opposing or incompatible thoughts, ideas, goals, or emotional forces, such as impulses, desires, or drives. **2.** a painful state of consciousness caused by the arousal of such opposing forces and the inability to resolve them. **3.** (in psychoanalysis) the unconscious emotional struggle between the demands of the id and those of the ego and superego or between the demands of the ego and the restrictions imposed by society. Kinds of conflict include **approach-approach, approach-avoidance, avoidance-avoidance, extrapsychic,** and **intrapsychic conflict.**

confluence of the sinuses [L confluere to flow together], the wide junction of the superior sagittal, the straight, and the occipital sinuses with the two large transverse sinuses of the dura mater.

confluent /kon´flōō-ənt/ [L, confluere, to flow together], running together, such as the sinuses of the dura mater, or skin eruptions that are confluent.

confrontation test [L con + frons forehead], a method of assessing the visual field of a patient by moving an object into the periphery of each of the visual quadrants. The test is conducted while one eye is covered and the vision of the other is fixed on a point straight ahead. The patient reports when the moving object is first detected.

confusion [L confundere to mingle], a mental state characterized by disorientation regarding time, place, or person, causing bewilderment, perplexity, lack of orderly thought, and inability to choose or act decisively. **–confusional,** adj.

confusional insanity. See **amentia.**

confusional state, a mild form of delirium that may be experienced by an elderly person or a patient with preexisting brain disease. The confusional state may be triggered by a sudden or unexpected change in the person's environment.

congener /kon´jənər/ [L con + genus origin], one of two or more things that are similar or closely related in structure, function, or origin. Examples of congeners are muscles that function identically and chemical compounds similar in composition and effect. **–congenerous** /kənjen´ərəs/, adj.

congenital /kənjen´itəl/ [L congenitus born with], present at birth, as a congenital anomaly or defect.

congenital absence of sacrum and lumbar vertebrae, an abnormal condition present at birth and characterized by varying degrees of deformity, ranging from the absence of the lower segment of the coccyx to the absence of the entire sacrum and all lumbar vertebrae.

congenital adrenal hyperplasia, a group of disorders that have in common an enzyme defect resulting in low levels of cortisol and increased secretion of ACTH. The disorder leads to pseudohermaphroditism in female infants and macrogenitosomia in male infants.

congenital amputation, the absence of a fetal limb or part at birth, previously attributed to amputation by constricting bands in utero but now regarded as a developmental defect.

congenital anomaly, any abnormality present at birth, particularly a structural one, which may be inherited genetically, acquired during gestation, or inflicted during parturition.

congenital aspiration pneumonia [L congenitus born with, aspirare to breathe upon; Gk pneumon lung], a neonatal lung inflammation caused by the aspiration of fluid or meconium during labor.

congenital cardiac anomaly, any structural or functional abnormality or defect of the heart or great vessels existing from birth. Congenital heart disease is a major cause of neonatal distress and is the most common cause of death in the newborn other than problems related to prematurity. Kinds of congenital cardiac anomalies include **atrial septal defect, coarctation of the aorta, tetralogy of Fallot, transposition of the great vessels, tricuspid atresia,** and **ventricular septal defect.**

congenital cloaca. See **persistent cloaca.**

congenital cyanosis [L congenitus; Gk kyanos blue, osis condition], cyanosis present at birth because of a congenital heart disease or atelectasis of the lungs.

congenital cyst [L congenitus; Gk kystis bag], a cyst present at birth, as a dermoid cyst resulting from an embryonic defect in the skin or midline structures.

congenital cytomegalovirus (CMV) disease. See **cytomegalic inclusion disease.**

congenital dermal sinus, a channel present at birth, extending from the surface of the body and passing between the bodies of two adjacent lumbar vertebrae to the spinal canal.

congenital dislocation of the hip, a congenital orthopedic defect in which the head of the femur does not articulate with the acetabulum because of an abnormal shallowness of the acetabulum.

congenital erythropoietic porphyria [L congenitus; Gk erythros red, poein to make, porphyros purple], a rare autosomal recessive trait caused by a defect in hemoglobin synthesis in erythrocytes and release of porphyrin from normoblasts in the bone marrow. The porphyrin is excreted in the urine. Symptoms may include dermatitis, enlarged spleen, and hemolytic anemia.

congenital facial diplegia. See **Möbius' syndrome.**

congenital glaucoma, a rare form of glaucoma affecting infants and young children, resulting from a congenital closure of the iridocorneal angle by a membrane that obstructs the flow of aqueous humor and increases the intraorbital pressure. The condition is progressive, usually bilateral, and may damage the optic nerve.

congenital goiter, an enlargement of the thyroid gland at birth. It may be caused by a deficiency of enzymes required for the production of thyroxine.

congenital heart disease. See **congenital cardiac anomaly.**

congenital hernia [L congenitus + hernia, rupture], a hernia caused by a defect present at birth, as with an umbilical hernia.

congenital hypogammaglobulinemia [L congenitus; Gk hypo deficiency, gamma; L globus small globe, haima blood], a genetic disease characterized by a deficiency of gamma globulin and antibody in the serum. The cause may be a genetic defect leading to a failure to develop a normal beta-lymphocyte system and immune responses.

congenital hypoplastic anemia. See **Diamond-Blackfan syndrome.**

congenital immunity [L congenitus, immunis free from], the immunity one has at birth that is acquired from the mother's antibodies as they pass through the placenta.

congenital jaundice [L congenitus; Fr jaune yellow], jaundice found at birth or during the first 24 hours of life. It is usually caused by poorly developed bile ducts.

congenital laryngeal stridor [L congenitus; Gk larynx; L stridens a grating noise], a harsh respiratory sound that some infants make the first weeks after birth.

congenital megacolon. See **Hirschsprung's disease.**

congenital nonspherocytic hemolytic anemia, a large group of blood disorders made up of a number of similar inherited diseases, each with a deficiency of one of the enzymes of red-cell glycolysis. Most are associated with varying degrees of hemolysis.

congenital oculofacial paralysis. See Möbius' syndrome.

congenital polycystic disease. See polycystic kidney disease.

congenital pulmonary arteriovenous fistula, a direct connection between the arterial and venous systems of the lung present at birth that results in a right-to-left shunt and permits unoxygenated blood to enter systemic circulation. The fistula may be single or multiple and may occur in any part of the lung.

congenital scoliosis, an abnormal condition present at birth, characterized by a lateral curvature of the spine, resulting from specific congenital rib and vertebral anomalies. The etiologic and the pathologic characteristics of congenital scoliosis are divided into six categories. Category I is associated with partial unilateral failure of the formation of a vertebra. Category II is associated with complete unilateral failure of the formation of a vertebra. Category III is associated with bilateral failure of segmentation with the absence of disk space. Category IV is associated with the unilateral failure of segmentation with the unsegmented bar. Category V is associated with the fusion of ribs. Category VI is associated with any condition not covered in the other categories. Category IV scoliosis seems to progress more rapidly and cause the greatest degree of deformity.

congenital short neck syndrome, a rare congenital malformation of the cervical spine in which the cervical vertebrae are fused, usually in pairs, into one mass of bone, resulting in decreased neck motion and decreased cervical length, sometimes with neurologic involvement. When the deformity involves nerve-root compression, symptoms of peripheral nerve involvement, as pain or a burning sensation, may be evident, accompanied by paralysis, hyperesthesia, or paresthesia.

congenital subluxation of the hip. See congenital dislocation of the hip.

congenital syphilis [L congenitus; Gk syn together + philein to love], a form of syphilis acquired in utero and generally characterized by osteitis, rashes, coryza, and wasting in the first months of life. Later childhood signs of the infection include interstitial keratitis, deafness, and notches in the incisor teeth. Some infected infants may appear disease-free at birth but develop typical signs of the disease in adolescence. Infants are treated with penicillin; all infected infants require an ophthalmic examination. If left untreated, the infection may result in deafness, blindness, crippling or death.

congestion [L congerere to accumulate], abnormal accumulation of fluid in an organ or body area. The fluid is often blood, but it may be bile or mucus.

congestive atelectasis [L congerere + Gk ateles incomplete, ektasis stretching], severe pulmonary congestion characterized by diffuse injury to alveolar-capillary membranes, resulting in hemorrhagic edema, stiffness of the lungs, difficult ventilation, and respiratory failure.

congestive cardiomyopathy [L congerere to heap together; Gk kardia heart, mys muscle, pathos disease], a heart muscle disease characterized by heart failure and enlargement.

congestive dysmenorrhea [L congerere; Gk dys difficult, mens month, rhein to flow], a form of secondary dysmenorrhea caused by pelvic congestion, arising in turn from an increased blood supply in the area due to a pelvic disease.

congestive heart failure (CHF), an abnormal condition that reflects impaired cardiac pumping, caused by myocardial infarction, ischemic heart disease, or cardiomyopathy. Failure of the ventricle to eject blood efficiently results in volume overload, chamber dilatation, and elevated intracardiac pressure. Retrograde transmission of increased hydrostatic pressure from the left heart causes pulmonary congestion; elevated right heart pressure causes systemic venous congestion and peripheral edema.

congestive splenomegalia [L congerere; Gk splen + megas large], an enlarged spleen associated with gastric hemorrhages, anemia, portal hypertension, and cirrhosis of the liver.

conglomerate silicosis [L con + glomerare to wind into a ball], a severe form of silicosis marked by conglomerate masses of mineral dust in the lungs, causing acute shortness of breath, coughing, and production of sputum. The patient usually develops cor pulmonale.

Congolese red fever. See murine typhus.

Congress for Nursing Practice, a unit of the American Nurses' Association whose activities concern the scope of nursing practice, legal aspects of nursing practice, public recognition of the significance of nursing practice in health care, and implications of health care trends for nursing practice.

congruent communication, a communication pattern in which the person sends the same message on both verbal and nonverbal levels.

conic papilla.   See **papilla.**

conization,   the removal of a cone-shaped sample of tissue, as in a cone biopsy.

conjoined manipulation /kənjoind'/ [L con + jungere to join],   the use of both hands in obstetric and gynecologic procedures, with one positioned in the vagina and the other on the abdomen.

conjoined tendon.   See **inguinal falx.**

conjoined twins,   two fetuses developed from the same ovum who are physically united at birth. Conjoined twins result when separation of the blastomeres in early embryonic development does not occur until a late cleavage phase and is incomplete, causing the fused condition.

conjoint family therapy,   a form of psychotherapy in which a single nuclear family is seen, and the issues and problems raised by family members are addressed by the therapist.

conjugate /kon'jəgit/ [L con + jungere to join],   (in pelvimetry) the measurement of the female pelvis to determine whether the presenting part of a fetus can enter the birth canal.

conjugated estrogen,   a mixture of sodium salts of estrogen sulfates, chiefly those of estrone, equilin, and 17-alpha-dihydroequilin, blended to approximate the average composition of estrogenic substances in the urine of pregnant mares. Conjugated estrogens may be prescribed to relieve postmenopausal vasomotor symptoms such as hot flushes, for the treatment of atrophic vaginitis, female hypogonadism, primary ovarian failure, and palliation in advanced prostatic carcinoma and metastatic breast cancer.

conjugate deviation [L conjugare to yoke together, deviare to turn aside],   pertaining to movements of the two eyes in which their visual axes function in parallel. The cause is a dysfunction of the ocular muscles, allowing the eyes to diverge to the same side when at rest.

conjugated protein,   a compound that contains a protein molecule united to a nonprotein substance.

conjugate paralysis [L conjugere; Gk paralyein to be palsied],   a condition of paralysis of the conjugate movements of the two eyes, up or down, or to the right or left. There is no diplopia. The cause is a cranial nerve lesion.

conjugation /kon'jəgā'shən/,   (in genetics) a form of sexual reproduction in unicellular organisms in which the gametes temporarily fuse so that genetic material can transfer from the donor male to the recipient female, where it is incorporated, recombined, and then passed on to the progeny through replication.

conjugon /kon'jōōgon/,   an episome that induces bacterial conjugation.

conjunctiva /kon'jungktī'və/[L conjunctivus connecting],   the mucous membrane lining the inner surfaces of the eyelids and anterior part of the sclera. The **palpebral conjunctiva** lines the inner surface of the eyelids and is thick, opaque, and highly vascular. The **bulbar conjunctiva** is loosely connected, thin, and transparent, covering the sclera of the anterior third of the eye.

conjunctival burns,   chemical burns of the conjunctiva. Emergency treatment involves bathing the eye with copious amounts of water until the chemical has been neutralized. The injured eye should be examined and treated by an ophthalmologist to prevent complications.

conjunctival edema.   See **chemosis.**

conjunctival fornix.   See **inferior conjunctival fornix, superior conjunctival fornix.**

conjunctival reflex,   a protective mechanism for the eye in which the eyelids close whenever the conjunctiva is touched.

conjunctival sac [L conjunctivus connecting; Gk sakkos],   the space enclosed by the conjunctiva and the eyelids.

conjunctival test,   a procedure used to identify offending allergens by instilling the eye with a dilute solution of the allergenic extract.

conjunctivitis /kənjungk'tivī'tis/,   inflammation of the conjunctiva caused by bacterial or viral infection, allergy, or environmental factors. Red eyes, a thick discharge, sticky eyelids in the morning, and inflammation without pain are characteristic.

conjunctivitis of newborn [L conjunctivus, itis, inflammation; ME newe, borne],   a condition characterized by a purulent discharge from the eyes of an infant during the first three weeks of life. A frequent cause is a gonococcal infection, which may lead to blindness if untreated.

connecting fibrocartilage [L con + nectere to bind],   a disk of fibrocartilage found between many joints, especially those with limited mobility, such as the spinal vertebrae. Each disk is composed of concentric rings of fibrous tissue separated by cartilaginous laminae.

connective,   pertaining to a binding or connection.

connective tissue,   tissue that supports and binds other body tissue and parts. It derives from the mesoderm of the embryo and is dense, containing large numbers of cells and large amounts of intercellular material. The intercellular material is composed of fibers in a matrix or ground substance that may be liquid, gelatinous, or solid, such as in bone and cartilage. Kinds of connective tissue are **bone, cartilage,** and **fibrous connective tissue.**

connective tissue disease. See **collagen vascular disease.**

Conn's syndrome [Jerome W. Conn, American physician, b. 1907, Gk *syn* together, *dromos* course], primary hyperaldosteronism, characterized by excessive secretion of aldosterone with symptoms of headache, fatigue, nocturia, and polyuria. The patient may also experience hypertension, hypokalemic alkalosis potassium depletion, and hypervolemia.

Conor's disease. See **Marseilles fever.**

Conradi's disease. See **chondrodystrophia calcificans congenita.**

consanguinity /kon′sang·gwin′itē/ [L *con* + *sanguis* blood], a hereditary or "blood" relationship between persons, by having a common parent or ancestor.

conscience [L *conscientia* to be privy to information] **1.** the moral, self-critical sense of what is right and wrong. **2.** (in psychoanalysis) the part of the superego system that monitors thoughts, feelings, and actions and measures them against internalized values and standards.

conscious [L *conscire* to be aware], **1.** (in neurology) capable of responding to sensory stimuli; awake, alert; aware of one's external environment. **2.** (in psychiatry) that part of the psyche or mental functioning in which thoughts, ideas, emotions, and other mental content are in complete awareness.

consciousness, a clear state of awareness of self and the environment in which attention is focused on immediate matters.

conscious proprioception, the conscious awareness of body position and movement of bodily segments. It is regulated by the lemniscal system through pathways that begin in joint receptors and end in the parietal lobe of the cerebral cortex; it enables the cortex to refine voluntary movements.

conscious sedation. See **awake anesthesia.**

consensual [L *con* + *sentire* to feel], pertaining to a reflex action in which stimulation of one part of the body results in a response into another part.

consensual light reflex, a normally present crossed reflex in which light directed at one eye causes the opposite pupil to contract. In monocular blindness the pupil of the blind eye reacts consensually with stimulation of the seeing eye but does not cause constriction of the pupil of either eye.

consensually validated symbols, symbols that are accepted by enough people that they have an agreed-upon meaning.

consensual reaction to light. See **consensual light reflex.**

consensual validation, a mutual agreement by two or more persons about a particular meaning that is to be attributed to verbal or nonverbal behavior.

consensus sequence, (in molecular genetics) a sequence in a strand of RNA nucleotides that is used as a site for the insertion of a splice of an RNA sequence from another source into the segment.

consent [L *consentire* to agree], to give approval, assent, or permission.

consenting adult, an adult who willingly agrees to participate in an activity with one or more other adults. The term is usually applied to sexual activity.

consequences, stimulus events following a behavior that strengthen or weaken the behavior. They may be either reinforcers or punishers.

conservation of energy [L *conservare* to preserve], (in physics) a law stating that in any closed system the total amount of energy is constant.

conservation of matter, (in physics) a law stating that matter can neither be created nor destroyed and that the amount of matter in the universe is finite.

conservation principles of nursing, a conceptual framework for nursing that is directed toward maintaining the wholeness or integrity of the patient when the normal ability to cope is disturbed or exceeded by stress. Nursing intervention is determined by the patient's need to conserve energy and to maintain structural, personal, and social integrity. The nurse acts as a "conservationist."

conservative treatment. See **treatment.**

consolidation [L *consolidare* to make solid], **1.** the combining of separate parts into a single whole. **2.** a state of solidification. **3.** (in medicine) the process of becoming solid, as when the lungs become firm and inelastic in pneumonia.

consolidation of individuality and emotional constancy, (in psychiatry) the fourth and final subphase in Mahler's system of the separation-individuation phase of preoedipal development. It begins toward the end of the second year.

constancy, an absence of variation in quality of distinctive features despite location, rotation, size, or color of an object.

constant positive airway pressure. See **continuous positive airway pressure (CPAP).**

constant positive pressure ventilation. See **continuous positive pressure ventilation (CPPV).**

constant pressure generator, a generator that provides or generates a constant gas pressure throughout the inspiratory cycle of breathing. The pressure may range from a low value, such as 12 cm H_2O, to a high value of as much as 3,500 cm H_2O, as required.

constant region, an area of an immunoglobulin molecule in which the amino acid sequence is relatively constant.

constant touch, a technique to diagnose of the sensibility of an injured body part by pressing the eraser end of a pencil or another object in various areas to determine the ability of the person to detect the pressure.

constipation [L *constipare* to crowd together] **1.** difficulty in passing stools or an incomplete or infrequent passage of hard stools. Among the organic causes are intestinal obstruction, diverticulitis, and tumors. Functional impairment of the colon may occur in elderly or bedridden patients who fail to respond to the urge to defecate. **2.** a NANDA-accepted nursing diagnosis. The defining characteristics include decreased frequency of elimination; a hard, formed stool; a palpable rectal mass; straining at stool; decreased bowel sounds; reported feeling of abdominal or rectal fullness or pressure; less than useful amount of stool; and nausea. Abdominal pain, appetite impairment, back pain, headache, and interference with daily living may also be present. **–constipated,** *adj.*

constipation, colonic, a NANDA-accepted nursing diagnosis of a pattern of elimination that is characterized by hard, dry stool that results from a delay in passage of food residue. Defining characteristics include decreased frequency, hard dry stool, straining at stool, painful defecation, abdominal distention, a palpable mass, rectal pressure, headache, appetite impairment, and abdominal pain.

constipation, perceived, a NANDA-accepted nursing diagnosis of a state in which an individual makes a self-diagnosis of constipation and ensures a daily bowel movement through use of laxatives, enemas, and suppositories. The defining characteristic is an expectation of a daily bowel movment, which may be expected at the same time every day, with the resulting overuse of laxatives, enemas, and suppositories.

constipation, rectal, a NANDA-accepted nursing diagnosis of a pattern of elimination that is characterized by stool retention, normal stool consistency, and delayed elimination, which results from biopsychosocial disruptions. There is also abdominal discomfort, rectal fullness, and a change in flatus.

constitutional delay [L *constituere* to establish], a period in the development of a child during which growth may be interrupted. In some cases constitutional delay may be associated with an illness or stressful event.

constitutional disease [L *constituere;* Gk *dis* without; Fr *aise* ease], any disease associated with the inborn physical condition of the client, such as a hereditary susceptibility.

constitutional psychology, the study of the relationship of individual psychologic makeup to body morphology and organic functioning.

constitutional symptom. See **symptom.**

constitutive resistance, the bacterial resistance to antibiotics that is contained in the DNA molecules of the organism. The trait can be passed on to daughter cells through cell division.

constriction [L *constringere* to draw tight], an abnormal closing or reduction in the size of an opening or passage of the body, as in vasoconstriction of a blood vessel.

constriction ring, a band of contracted uterine muscle that forms a stricture around part of the fetus during labor, usually after premature rupture of the membranes and sometimes impeding labor.

constrictive cardiomyopathy [L *constringere;* Gk *kardia* heart, *mys* muscle, *pathos* disease], a heart disorder in which there is decreased diastolic compliance of the ventricles, imitating constrictive pericarditis.

constrictive pericarditis, a fibrous thickening of the pericardium caused by gradual scarring or fibrosis of the membrane that resists the normal dilation of the heart chambers during the blood-filling phases of the cardiac cycle.

constrictor, a muscle that causes a narrowing of an opening, as the ciliary body fibers that control the size of the pupil.

constructional apraxia [L *construere* to build], a form of apraxia characterized by the inability to copy drawings or to manipulate objects to form patterns or designs. It is caused by a right hemisphere lesion.

constructive aggression, an act of self-assertiveness in response to a threatening action for purposes of self-protection and preservation.

constructive interference, (in ultrasonography) an increase in amplitude of sound waves that results when multiple waves of equal frequency are transmitted precisely in phase.

construct validity, validity of a test or a

measurement tool that is established by demonstrating its ability to identify the variables that it proposes to identify.

consultant [L, *consultare,* to deliberate], a person who by training and experience has acquired a special knowledge in a subject area which has been recognized by a peer group.

consultation [L *consultare* to deliberate], a process in which the help of a specialist is sought to identify ways to handle problems in patient management or in the planning and implementation of health care programs.

consultee-centered communication, expert guidance that is given a consultee (health care worker) to improve the consultee's capacity to function more effectively in working with patients.

consumption, an obsolete term for tuberculosis.

consumption coagulopathy. See **disseminated intravascular coagulation (DIC).**

contact [L *contingere* to touch], **1.** the touching or bringing together of two surfaces, as those of upper and lower teeth. **2.** the bringing together either directly or indirectly, as through the handling of food or clothing, of two individuals so as to allow the transmission of an infectious organism from one to the other. **3.** a person who has been exposed to an infectious disease.

contact dermatitis, skin rash resulting from exposure to a primary irritant or to a sensitizing antigen. In the nonallergic type, a primary irritant, such as an alkaline detergent or an acid, causes a lesion similar to a thermal burn. In the allergic type, sensitizing antigens, on first exposure, result in an immunologic change in certain lymphocytes. Poison ivy and nickel dermatitis are common examples of delayed hypersensitivity reaction.

contact factor. See **factor XII.**

contact lens, a small, curved, glass or plastic lens shaped to fit the person's eye and to correct refraction. Contact lenses float on the precorneal tear film.

contactor, a switching device that is part of the timer for the control of voltage across an x-ray tube.

contact shield, a protective device constructed of metal or other material that is positioned directly over the eyes or gonads of a patient to be exposed to an x-ray beam.

contagion /kəntā′jən/ [L *contingere* to touch], the transmission of a disease by direct contact with a person who has the disease or by indirect contact through handling of clothing, bedding, dishes, or other objects the person has used.

contagious [L *contingere* to touch], communicable, such as a disease that may be transmitted by direct or indirect contact. **–contagion,** *n.*

contagious disease. See **communicable disease.**

contagious pustular dermatitis [L *contingere* to touch, *pustula* pustules; Gk *derma* skin, *itis* inflammation], a skin disease normally affecting sheep but transmitted to humans who handle infected animals. It is caused by a pox virus and results in lesions on the hands, and occasionally on the face. The lesions resolve spontaneously, but slowly.

contaminant [L *contaminare* to pollute], to bring in contact, an agent that causes contamination, pollution, or spoilage, such as a mold spore that makes food unsafe to eat.

contamination [L *contaminare*], a condition of being soiled, stained, touched, or otherwise exposed to harmful agents, making an object potentially unsafe for use as intended or without barrier techniques.

content validity, validity of a test or a measurement as a result of the use of previously tested items or concepts within the tool.

context [L *contexere* to weave together], (in communications theory) the setting, meaning, and language of a message.

continence [L *continere* to contain], **1.** the ability to control bladder or bowel function. **2.** the use of self-restraint, particularly in regard to sexual intercourse.

continent ileostomy, an ileostomy that drains into a surgically created pouch or reservoir in the abdomen. Involuntary discharge of intestinal contents is prevented by a nipple valve created from the ileum.

contingency contracting [L *contingere* to touch], a formal agreement between a psychotherapist and a patient undergoing behavior therapy regarding the consequences of certain actions by both parties.

contingency management, any of a group of techniques used in behavior therapy that attempts to modify a behavioral response by controlling the consequences of that response. Kinds of contingency management include **contingency contracting, shaping,** and **token economy.**

continuing care nurse [L *continuare* to unite], a nurse specializing in coordination of the overall needs of the patient with the potential health care resources of the community. Continuing care nursing responsibilities ideally begin at the time a patient is admitted to a hospital.

continuing education, (in nursing) formal, organized, educational programs designed to promote the knowledge, skills, and professional attitudes of nurses. Continuing education is required for relicensure in many states. It is not to be confused with academic, degree-granting programs, such as advanced education or postgraduate education.

continuing education unit (CEU), a point awarded to a professional person by a professional organization for having attended an educational program relevant to the goals of the organization.

continuity theory, a concept that an individual's personality does not change as the person ages, with the result that his or her behavior becomes more predictable.

continuous ambulatory peritoneal dialysis (CAPD) [L *continuare* + *ambulare* to walk about; Gk *peri* near, *tenein* to stretch, *dia* through, *lysis* loosening], a maintenance system of peritoneal dialysis in which an indwelling catheter permits fluid to drain into and out of the peritoneal cavity by gravity.

continuous anesthesia [L *continuare* to unite], a method for maintaining regional nerve block in anesthesia for surgical operations or labor in which an anesthetic solution drips either at intervals or at a low rate of flow. The procedure is named according to the area infiltrated: continuous spinal, caudal, epidural, peridural, or lumbar.

continuous bath. See **continuous tub bath.**

continuous cycling peritoneal dialysis (CCPD), a type of dialysis in which the patient is attached to an automatic cycler for short exchanges while sleeping at night.

continuous fever, a fever that persists steadily for a prolonged period of time.

continuous murmur, a heart or venous murmur that characteristically begins in systole and spills into diastole. The cause may be a patent ductus arteriosus.

continuous negative chest wall pressure, a negative pressure (below ambient pressure) that is applied to the chest wall during the entire respiratory cycle, thus providing increased transpulmonary pressure.

continuous passive motion (CPM), a technique for maintaining or increasing the amount of movement in a joint with the use of a mechanical device that applies force to bring about motion in a joint without normal muscle function.

continuous phase [L *continuare;* Gk *phasis* appearance], the phase of a colloidal solution corresponding to that of the solvent of a true solution.

continuous positive airway pressure (CPAP), (in respiratory therapy) ventilation assisted by a flow of air delivered at a constant pressure throughout the respiratory cycle. It is performed for patients who can initiate their own respirations but who are not able to maintain adequate arterial oxygen levels without assistance. CPAP may be given through a ventilator and endotracheal tube, through a nasal cannula, or into a hood over the patient's head.

continuous positive pressure ventilation (CPPV), a positive pressure above ambient pressure maintained at the upper airway throughout the breathing cycle. The term is usually applied to positive end-expiratory pressure (PEEP) and mechanical ventilation.

continuous reinforcement, a schedule of reinforcement in which omission of a response is followed by the reinforcer.

continuous tremor, fine, rhythmic, purposeless movements that persist during rest but sometimes disappear briefly during voluntary movements.

continuous tub bath, a therapeutic bath, usually prescribed in the treatment of some dermatologic conditions, in which the patient lies supported in a medicated solution of tepid water.

continuum /kəntin'yo͞o·əm/, *pl.* **continua** **1.** a continuous series or whole. **2.** (in mathematics) a system of real numbers.

contoured adducted trochanteric controlled alignment method (CAT-CAM), a design for an artificial lower limb for persons who have undergone above the knee (AK) amputations.

contra bevel [L *contra* against; OFr *baif* open mouth] **1.** (in dentistry) the angle between a cutting blade and the base of the periodontal pocket when the blade is held so that it separates the sulcular epithelium from the external epithelium of the gingiva. **2.** (in dentistry) an external bevel of a tooth preparation extending onto a buccal or lingual cusp from an intracoronal restoration.

contraception [L *contra* + *concipere* to take in], a process or technique for the prevention of pregnancy by means of a medication, device, or method that blocks or alters one or more of the processes of reproduction in such a way that sexual union can occur without impregnation. Kinds of contraception include **cervical cap, condom, contraceptive diaphragm, intrauterine device, natural family-planning method, oral contraceptive, spermatocide,** and **sterilization.**

contraceptive [L *contra* + *concipere* to take in], any device or technique that prevents conception.

contraceptive diaphragm, a contraceptive device consisting of a hemisphere of thin rubber bonded to a flexible ring, inserted in the vagina together with spermaticidal jelly or cream so that spermatozoa cannot enter the uterus, thus preventing conception. Kinds of diaphragms are **arcing spring, coil spring,** and **flat spring.**

contraceptive diaphragm fitting, a procedure, performed in an office or clinic, in which a contraceptive diaphragm is selected according to the clinical assessment of certain anatomic factors specific to the woman being fitted.

contraceptive effectiveness, the effectiveness of a method of contraception in preventing pregnancy. It is sometimes represented as a percentage but more accurately as the number of pregnancies per 100 woman-years. A contraceptive method that results in a pregnancy rate of less than 10 pregnancies per 100 woman-years is considered highly effective.

contraceptive jelly [L *contra* opposed, *concipere* to take in, *gelare* to congeal], a gelatinous preparation containing a spermicide for introduction into the vagina to prevent conception.

contraceptive method, any act, device, or medication for avoiding conception or a viable pregnancy.

contract [L *con* + *trahere* to draw], **1.** an agreement or a promise that meets certain legal requirements, including competence of both or all parties to the contract, proper lawful subject matter, mutuality of agreement, mutuality of obligation, and consideration (the giving of something of value in payment for the obligation undertaken). **2.** to make such an agreement or promise. –**contractual,** *adj.*

contractile [L, *cum,* with, *trahere,* to draw], capable of becoming reduced in size or length or of being drawn together in response to some stimulus.

contractile ring dysphagia [L *con* + *trahere* to draw; AS *hring*], an abnormal condition characterized by difficulty in swallowing because of an overreactive interior esophageal sphincteric mechanism that induces painful sticking sensations under the lower sternum.

contractility, (in cardiology) the force of a heart contraction when preload and afterload are constant.

contraction [L *con* + *trahere* to draw], **1.** a reduction in size, especially of muscle fibers. **2.** an abnormal shrinkage. **3.** (in labor) a rhythmic tightening of the musculature of the upper uterine segment that begins mildly and becomes very strong late in labor, occurring as frequently as every 2 minutes, and lasting over 1 minute.

4. abnormal smallness of the birth canal or part of it, a cause of dystocia. **Inlet contraction** exists if the anteroposterior diameter is 10 cm or less or if the transverse diameter is 11.5 cm or less. **Midpelvic contraction** exists if the sum of the measurements in centimeters of the interspinous diameter (normally 10.5 cm) and the posterior sagittal diameter (normally 5 cm) is 13.5 cm or less. **Outlet contraction** exists if the intertuberous diameter is 8 cm or less.

contracture /kontrak′chər/ [L *contractura* a pulling together], an abnormal, usually permanent condition of a joint, characterized by flexion and fixation and caused by atrophy and shortening of muscle fibers or by loss of the normal elasticity of the skin, such as from the formation of extensive scar tissue over a joint.

contraindicate /kon′trə·in′dicāt/ [L *contra* + *indicare* to make known], to report the presence of a disease or physical condition that makes it impossible or undesirable to treat a particular patient in the usual manner or to prescribe medicines that might otherwise be suitable.

contraindication /kon′trə·in′dikā′shən/ [L *contra* against, *indicare* to make known], a factor that prohibits the administration of a drug or the performance of a procedure in the care of a specific patient.

contralateral [L *contra* + *lateralis* side], affecting or originating in the opposite side of a point or reference, such as a point on a body.

contralateral reflexes [L *contra* + *latus* side, *reflectere* to bend back], an overflow phenomenon of the nervous system in which a reflex is elicited on one side of the body by a stimulus to the opposite side.

contrast [L *contra* + *stare* to stand], a measure of the differences between two adjacent areas in an image. Contrast may be based on differences in optic density or differences in radiation transmission, or other parameters.

contrast bath, a bath in which the patient alternately immerses a part of the body, usually the hands or feet, in hot and cold water for a specified period of time.

contrast enema. See **barium enema.**

contrast examination, the use of radiopaque materials, such as iodine and barium, to make internal organs visible on x-ray film.

contrast medium, a radiopaque substance injected into the body to facilitate roentgen imaging of internal structures that otherwise are difficult to visualize on x-ray films.

contrecoup injury /kôNtrek oo′/ [L *contra;* Fr *coup* blow; L *injuria*], an injury, usually involving the brain, in which the tissue damage is on the side opposite the site of the trauma, as when a blow to the left side of the head results in brain damage on the right side.

control [Fr *controler* to register], to exercise restraint or maintain influence over a situation, as in self-control, the conscious limitation or suppression of impulses.

control cable, a stainless steel wire, usually contained in a flexible stainless steel housing, used to move a prosthesis, such as an artificial arm.

control gene, (in molecular genetics) a gene, such as the operator gene or regulator gene, that controls the transcription of the amino-acid sequence in the structural gene by either inducing or repressing protein synthesis.

control group. See **group.**

controlled area, a part of a hospital or other health facility that is occupied primarily by personnel who work with radioactive materials. It is designed with barrier shielding to confine the radiation exposure rate.

controlled association, 1. a direct connection of relevant ideas as the result of a specific stimulus. 2. a process of bringing repressed ideas into the consciousness in response to words spoken by a psychoanalyst.

controlled hypotension. See **deliberate hypotension.**

controlled oxygen therapy, the administration of oxygen to a patient on a dose-response basis in which oxygen is regarded as a drug and only the smallest amount of gas is used to obtain a desired therapeutic effect.

controlled substance [Fr, *contrôle,* check; L, *substantia,* essence], any drug as defined in the five categories of the federal **Controlled Substances Act of 1970.** The categories, or schedules, cover opium and its derivatives, hallucinogens, depressants, and stimulants.

Controlled Substances Act, a United States law enacted in 1970 that regulates the prescribing and dispensing of psychoactive drugs, including stimulants, depressants, and hallucinogens. The Act lists five categories of restricted drugs, depending on their medical acceptance, abuse potential, and ability to produce dependence.

controlled ventilation, the use of an intermittent positive pressure breathing unit or other respirator that has an automatic cycling device that replaces spontaneous respiration.

control of hemorrhage, the limitation of the flow of blood from a break in the wall of a blood vessel, as by direct pressure, use of a tourniquet, or application of pressure on pressure points proximal to the wound. Direct pressure with a thick compress is applied in such a way that the edges of the wound are brought together. A tourniquet is applied proximal to the site of bleeding only in the most drastic emergency, for the limb may then have to be sacrificed because of tissue anoxia stemming from the use of the tourniquet. Pressure is applied to a pressure point by using firm manual pressure over the main artery supplying the wound. Points used to obtain the pulse may be used as pressure points to stop hemorrhage.

control process, a system of establishing standards, objectives, and methods, and measuring actual performance, comparing results, reinforcing strengths, and taking necessary corrective action.

contusion [L *contundere* to bruise], an injury that does not break the skin, caused by a blow to the body and characterized by swelling, discoloration, and pain. The immediate application of cold may limit the development of a contusion.

convalescence [L *convalescere* to grow strong], the period of recovery after an illness, injury, or surgery.

convalescent home. See **extended care facility.**

convection [L *convehere* to bring together], (in physics) the transfer of heat through a gas or liquid by the circulation of heated particles.

convergence [L *convegere* to bend together], the movement of two objects toward a common point, such as the turning of the eyes inward to see an object close to the face.

convergent evolution, the development of similar structures or functions within widely differing phylogenetic species in response to similar environmental conditions.

convergent squint [L *convergere;* ME *squint*], a visual disorder in which a deviating eye looks inward toward the nose.

convergent strabismus. See **esotropia.**

conversion [L *convertere* to turn around], 1. changing from one form to another, transmutation. 2. (in obstetrics) the correction of a fetal position during labor. 3. (in psychiatry) an unconscious defense mechanism by which emotional conflicts ordinarily resulting in anxiety are repressed and transformed into symbolic physical symptoms having no organic basis.

conversion disorder, a kind of hysteric neurosis in which emotional conflicts are repressed and converted into sensory, motor, or visceral symptoms having no underlying organic cause, such as blindness, anesthesia, hypesthesia, hyperesthesia, paresthesia, involuntary muscular movements, paralysis, aphonia, mutism, hallucinations, catalepsy, choking sensations, and respiratory difficulties.

conversion reaction, an ego defense mechanism whereby intrapsychic conflict is expressed symbolically through physical symptoms.

convoluted kidney tubules [L *convolvere* to roll together; ME *kidenei*; L *tubulus*], pertaining to the convoluted portion of the nephron that leads from the glomerulus to the connecting ducts. The proximal and distal sections are convoluted while the ascending and descending limbs of the loop of Henle are relatively straight.

convoluted seminiferous tubules, the long, threadlike tubes in the aerolar tissue of the testes. The testes also contain straight segments of seminiferous tubules.

convulsive seizure [L, *convulsio,* cramp; OFr, *seisir*], a sudden onset of a disease characterized by convulsions, palpitations, and other symptoms. The term is sometimes applied to an attack of an epileptic disorder.

convulsive tic, a disorder of the facial nerve, causing involuntary spasmodic contractions of the facial muscles supplied by that nerve.

Cooley's anemia. See **thalassemia.**

Coolidge tube, a basic type of hot-cathode x-ray tube that, with modern refinements, has been used by radiologists since it was invented in 1913.

cooling [AS *colian* cool], reducing body temperature by the application of a hypothermia blanket, cold moist dressings, ice packs, or an alcohol bath.

cooling rate, the rate at which temperature decreases with time (°C/minute) immediately after the completion of hyperthermia treatment.

Coombs' positive hemolytic anemia /kōomz/ [Robin R. A. Coombs, British immunologist, b. 1921], a form of anemia resulting from premature destruction of circulating red blood cells.

Coombs' test. See **antiglobulin test.**

cooperative play, any organized play among a group of children in which activities are planned for the purpose of achieving some goal.

coordinated reflex [L *coordinare* to arrange], a sequence of muscular actions occurring in a purposeful, orderly progression, such as the act of swallowing.

COPD, abbreviation for **chronic obstructive pulmonary disease.**

coping [Gk *kolaphos* buffet], a process by which a person deals with stress, solves problems, and makes decisions. The process has two components, cognitive and noncognitive. The cognitive component includes the thought and learning necessary to identify the source of the stress. The noncognitive components are automatic and focus on relieving the discomfort.

coping, defensive, a NANDA-accepted nursing diagnosis of a falsely positive self-evaluation based on a self-protective pattern that defends against undelying perceived threats to positive self-regard. Defining characteristics include denial of obvious problems, projection of blame, rationalization of failures, hypersensitivity to criticism, a superior attitude toward others, difficulty in relationships, ridicule of others, difficulty in reality testing perceptions, and lack of follow through or participation in treatment or therapy.

coping, family: potential for growth, a NANDA-accepted diagnosis of the need for self-actualization that occurs when a person's basic needs have been satisfied and the adaptive tasks required by the client's health problem have been mastered. Defining characteristics include the family's expressed wish to discuss the impact of the situation on the client's own life and values, interest in meeting with others in similar situations, and choice of healthful options available to the client.

coping, ineffective family: compromised, a NANDA-accepted nursing diagnosis of a lack or absence of emotional and psychologic support for the client that is usually available from a family member or other supportive person, a deficiency that causes further difficulty for the client in coping with the current health problem. Defining characteristics include expression by the client that support is lacking or expression by the supportive person that fear, anticipatory grief, anxiety, or other reaction is interfering with the ability to give support to the client.

coping, ineffective family: disabling, a NANDA-accepted nursing diagnosis of the detrimental attitudes and behavior of a family, a family member, or other person who is important to the client. Defining characteristics include neglect in the care of the client, intolerance, rejection or abandonment, adoption of the symptoms of the client, disregard of the client's needs, and marked distortion of reality in regard to the client's health problem.

coping, ineffective individual, a NANDA-accepted nursing diagnosis of an individual's problem with situational crises, maturational crises, or personal vulnerability. Defining characteristics include an inability to ask for help, an inability to solve problems, verbalization of the inability to cope, an inability to meet the expectations of a role, an inability to meet one's basic needs, or an alteration in ability to participate in society.

coping mechanism, any effort directed toward stress management, including task-oriented and ego-defense mechanisms; the factors that enable an individual to regain emotional equilibrium after a stressful experience.

coping resources, the characteristics of a person, group, or environment that are helpful in assisting individuals in adapting to stress.

coping style, the cognitive, affective, or behavioral responses of a person to problematic or traumatic life events.

COPP, an anticancer drug combination of cyclophosphamide, procarbazine, and prednisone.

copper (Cu) [L *cuprum*], a malleable, reddish brown, metallic element. Its atomic number is 29; its atomic weight is 63.54. Copper is a component of several important enzymes in the body and is essential to good health. Copper deficiency in the body is rare because only 2 to 5 mg daily, easily obtained from a variety of foods, is sufficient for a proper balance. Copper accumulates in individuals with Wilson's disease, primary biliary cirrhosis, and, occasionally, chronic extrahepatic biliary tract obstruction.

copperhead [L *cuprum* + ME *hed*], a poisonous pit viper found mainly in the southeastern United States. The reddish-brown, darkly banded snake is responsible for nearly 40% of the snake bites in the United States; few bites are fatal. Pain, swelling, fang marks, and a bruise are usually present.

Copper Kettle, a trademark for a kind of vaporizer used in the circuits of an anesthesia machine to mix the carrier gas and the volatile anesthetic liquid to form an anesthetizing vapor.

copper T, a trademark for an intrauterine device (IUD). It is recommended only for women over 25 who have been pregnant, have a monogamous relationship, and have not had pelvic inflammatory disease.

coprogogue. See **cathartic.**

coprolalia /kop′rōlā′lyə/ [Gk *kopros* dung, *lalein* to babble], the excessive use of obscene language.

coproporphyria /kop′rōpôrfir′ē·ə/ [Gk *kopros* + *porphyros* purple], a rare, hereditary, metabolic disorder in which large quantities of nitrogenous substances, called porphyrins, are excreted in the urine. Attacks, with varying GI and neu-

rologic symptoms, may be precipitated by certain drugs.

coproporphyrin /kop′rōpôr′firin/ [Gk *kopros* + *porphyros* purple], any of the nitrogenous organic substances normally excreted in the feces that are products of the breakdown of bilirubin from hemoglobin decomposition.

copulation. See **coitus.**

cor, 1. the heart. 2. relating to the heart.

coracobrachialis /kôr′əkōbrā′kē·al′is/, a muscle with its origin on the scapula and its insertion on the inner side of the humerus. It functions by adducting the shoulder.

coracoid process [Gk *korax* crow, *eidos* form; L *processus*], the thick, curved extension of the superior border of the scapula, to which the pectoralis minor is attached.

coral snake, a poisonous snake with transverse red, black, and yellow bands that is native to the southern United States. Bites are rare; pain is not always present, but neuromuscular and respiratory effects may be severe.

cord [Gk *chorde* string], any long, rounded, flexible structure. The body contains many different cords, such as the spermatic, vocal, spinal, nerve, umbilical, and hepatic cords. –**cordal,** *adj.*

corditis /kôrdī′tis/ [Gk *chorde* + *itis* inflammation], an abnormal inflammation of the spermatic cord, accompanied by pain in the testis, often caused by an infection originating in the urethra or by tumor, hydrocele, or varicocele.

core [L *cor* heart], (in dentistry) a section of a mold, usually of plaster, made over assembled parts of a dental restoration to record and maintain their relationships so that the parts can be reassembled in their original position.

core gender identity. See **gender identity.**

core temperature [L *cor* + *temperatura*], the temperature of deep structures of the body, such as the liver, as compared to temperatures of peripheral tissues.

Cori's disease /kôr′ēz/ [Carl F. Cori, b. 1896; Gerty T. Cori, b. 1896; American biochemists], a rare type of glycogen storage disease, in which a missing enzyme results in abnormally large deposits of glycogen in the liver, skeletal muscles, and heart. Signs are an enlarged liver, hypoglycemia, acidosis, and, occasionally, stunted growth.

corium See **dermis.**

corkscrew esophagus [ME *cork* bark; L *scrofa* sow]; Gk *oisophagos* gullet, a neurogenic disorder in which normal peristaltic contractions of the esophagus are replaced by spastic movements occurring spontaneously or with swallowing or gastric acid reflux.

corn [L *cornu* horn], a horny mass of condensed epithelial cells overlying a bony prominence. Corns result from chronic friction and pressure.

cornea /kôr′nē·ə/ [L *corneus* horny], the convex, transparent, anterior part of the eye, comprising one sixth of the outermost tunic of the eye bulb. It is a fibrous structure with five layers: the anterior corneal epithelium, continuous with that of the conjunctiva; the anterior limiting layer (Bowman's membrane); the substantia propria; the posterior limiting layer (Descemet's membrane); and the endothelium of the anterior chamber (keratoderma). It is dense, uniform in thickness, and nonvascular.

corneal abrasion /kôr′nē·əl/ [L *corneus* horny; *abrasio* scraping], the rubbing off of the outer layers of the cornea.

corneal grafting, transplantation of corneal tissue from one human eye to another, performed to improve vision in corneal scarring or distortion or to remove a perforating ulcer. Under local anesthesia the affected area is excised; an identical section of clear cornea is cut from the donor eye and sutured in place, using an operating microscope. Postoperatively, the eye is covered with a protective metal shield, and the patient is cautioned to avoid coughing, sneezing, sudden movement, or lifting.

corneal loupe, (in ophthalmology) a loupe designed especially for examining the cornea.

corneal reflex, a protective mechanism for the eye in which the eyelids close when the cornea is touched.

cornification /kôr′nifikā′shən/, thickening of the skin by a buildup of dead, keratinized epithelial cells.

corn pad, a device that helps relieve the pressure and the pain of a corn by transferring the pressure to surrounding, unaffected areas.

cornual pregnancy /kôr′nyoo·əl/ [L *cornu* horn; *praegnans* child bearing], an ectopic pregnancy in one of the straight or curved extensions of the body of the uterus. The cornu of the uterus usually ruptures between 12 and 16 weeks of the pregnancy unless the condition is treated surgically to remove the products of conception.

corona /kərō′nə/ [L, crown], **1.** a crown. **2.** a crownlike projection or encircling structure, such as a process extending from a bone. **–coronal, coronoid,** *adj.*

coronal plane. See **frontal plane.**

coronal section [L *corona* + *sectio*], a section of the body cut in the plane of the coronal suture, or parallel to it.

coronal suture, the serrated transverse suture between the frontal bone and the parietal bone on each side of the skull.

corona radiata, *pl.* **coronae radiatae** [L, crown; *radiare* to emit rays], **1.** a network of fibers that weaves through the internal capsule of the cerebral cortex and intermingles with the fibers of the corpus callosum. **2.** an aggregate of cells that surrounds the zona pellucida of the ovum.

coronary /kôr′əner′ē/ [L *corona*], **1.** (in anatomy) of or pertaining to encircling structures, such as the coronary arteries; of or pertaining to the heart. **2.** *nontechnical.* myocardial infarction or occlusion.

coronary arteriovenous fistula, an unusual congenital abnormality characterized by a direct communication between a coronary artery, usually the right, and the right atrium or ventricle, the coronary sinus, or the vena cava. A large shunt may result in growth failure, limited exercise tolerance, dyspnea, and anginal pain.

coronary artery, one of a pair of arteries that branch from the aorta, including the left and the right coronary arteries. Since these vessels and their branches supply the heart, any dysfunction or disease that affects them can cause serious, sometimes fatal complications. The branches of the coronary arteries are affected by many different disorders, such as embolic, neoplastic, inflammatory, and noninflammatory diseases.

coronary artery disease, any one of the abnormal conditions that may affect the arteries of the heart and produce various pathologic effects, especially the reduced flow of oxygen and nutrients to the myocardium. Any of the coronary artery diseases, such as coronary atherosclerosis, coronary arteritis, or fibromuscular hyperplasia of the coronary arteries, may produce the common characteristic symptom of angina pectoris, which, however, may also be associated with cardiomyopathy, in which the coronary arteries are normal. The most common kind of coronary artery disease is coronary atherosclerosis, now the leading cause of death in the Western world. Coronary atherosclerosis occurs most frequently in populations with regular diets high in calories, total fat, saturated fat, cholesterol, and refined carbohydrates. The risk is also greater among cigarette smokers than nonsmokers and appears to be proportional to the number of cigarettes smoked per day. Atherosclerosis develops with the formation of fatty fibrous plaques that narrow the lumen of the coronary arteries and may lead to thrombosis and myocardial infarction. Treatment of the patient with coronary artery disease concentrates on reducing myocardial oxygen demand or on increasing oxygen supply. Therapy commonly includes the administration of nitrates, such as nitroglycerin, isosorbide dinitrate, or propranolol, a beta-adrenergic blocker.

coronary artery fistula, a congenital anomaly characterized by an abnormal communication between a coronary artery and the right side of the heart or the pulmonary artery.

coronary bypass, open-heart surgery in which a prosthesis or a section of a blood vessel is grafted onto one of the coronary arteries and connected to the ascending aorta, bypassing a narrowing or blockage in a coronary artery. The operation is performed in coronary artery disease to improve the blood supply to the heart muscle, to reduce the workload of the heart, and to relieve anginal pain.

coronary care nursing, the nursing care provided in a hospital in a coronary care unit.

coronary care unit (CCU), a specially equipped hospital area designed for the treatment of patients with sudden, life-threatening cardiac conditions, as acute coronary thrombosis. Such units contain resuscitation and monitoring equipment and are staffed by personnel especially trained and skilled in recognizing and immediately responding to cardiac emergencies with cardiopulmonary resuscitation techniques, the administration of antiarrhythmic drugs, and other appropriate therapeutic measures.

coronary collateralization, the spontaneous development of new blood vessels in or around areas of restricted blood flow to the heart.

coronary occlusion, an obstruction of any one of the coronary arteries, usually caused by progressive atherosclerosis and sometimes complicated by thrombosis. Coronary occlusions are usually caused by an obstruction of a coronary artery that develops gradually from the accumulation of fatty, fibrous plaques that narrow the arterial lumen, reduce the blood flow, and lead to myocardial infarction. In certain heart diseases arterial spasms may narrow the lumen of a coronary artery, blocking blood flow. Occlusion of the circumflex branch of the left coronary artery causes a lateral wall infarction. Occlusion of the anterior descending branch of the left coronary artery causes an infarction of the anterior heart wall. Occlusion of the right coronary artery or one of its branches causes a posterior wall infarction. Many patients who

suffer coronary occlusions recover because of fast treatment and collateral circulation provided by extensive arterial anastomoses of the heart.

coronary plexus [L *corona* crown, *plexus* plaited], a network of autonomic nerve fibers located near the base of the heart.

coronary sinus, the wide venous channel, about 2.25 cm long, situated in the coronary sulcus and covered by muscular fibers from the left atrium. It drains five coronary veins through a single semilunar valve.

coronary thrombosis, a development of a thrombus that blocks a coronary artery, often causing myocardial infarction and death. Coronary thromboses commonly develop in segments of arteries with atherosclerotic lesions.

coronary valve [L *corona* + *valva* leaf of a door], the valve of the coronary sinus, a semicircular fold of endocardium, leading into the right atrium.

coronary vein, one of the veins of the heart that drains blood from the capillary beds of the myocardium through the coronary sinus into the right atrium.

coronavirus /kôr′ənəvī′rəs/ [L *corona* + *virus* poison], a member of a family of viruses that includes several types capable of causing acute respiratory illnesses.

coroner /kôr′ənər/ [L *corona* crown], a public official who investigates the causes and circumstances of a death occurring within a specific legal jurisdiction or territory, especially a death that may have resulted from unnatural causes.

coronoid fossa /kô′rənoid/ [L *corona* + Gk *eidos* form; L *fossa* ditch], a small depression in the distal, dorsal surface of the humerus that receives the coronoid process of the ulna when the forearm is flexed.

coronoid process of mandible, a prominence on the anterior surface of the ramus of the mandible to which each temporal muscle attaches.

coronoid process of ulna, a wide, flaring projection of the proximal end of the ulna. The proximal surface of the process forms the lower part of the trochlear notch.

corpse /kôrps/ [L *corpus* body], the body of a dead human.

cor pulmonale /kôr po͞ol′mənal′ē/ [L, heart; *pulmoneus* pertaining to the lungs], an abnormal cardiac condition characterized by hypertrophy of the right ventricle of the heart as a result of hypertension of the pulmonary circulation. Pulmonary hypertension associated with this condition is caused by some disorder of the pulmonary parenchyma or of the pulmonary vascular system between the origin of the left pulmonary artery and the entry of the pulmonary veins into the left atrium. Approximately 85% of patients with cor pulmonale have chronic obstructive pulmonary disease; 25% of patients with emphysema eventually develop cor pulmonale. Pulmonary capillary destruction and pulmonary vasoconstriction decrease the cross-sectional area of the pulmonary vascular bed, increasing pulmonary vascular resistance and causing pulmonary hypertension. The right ventricle dilates and hypertrophies to compensate for the extra work required in forcing blood through the lungs. Some of the early signs of cor pulmonale include chronic cough, exertional dyspnea, fatigue, wheezing, and weakness.

corpus. See **body.**

corpus cavernosum /kôr′pəs/ [L, body; *caverna* hollow place], a type of spongy erectile tissue within the penis or clitoris. The tissue becomes engorged with blood during sexual excitement.

corpuscle /kôr′pəsəl/ [L *corpusculum* little body] 1. any cell of the body. 2. a red or white blood cell. **–corpuscular,** *adj.*

corpuscular radiation /kôrpus′kyələr/ [L *corpusculum; radiare* to emit rays], the radiation associated with subatomic particles, such as electrons, protons, neutrons, or alpha particles, that travel in streams at various velocities.

corpus luteum, /kôr′pəs lōō′tē·əm/ *pl.* **corpora lutea** [L, body; *luteus* yellow], an anatomic structure on the surface of the ovary, consisting of a spheroid of yellowish tissue 1 to 2 cm in diameter that grows within the ruptured ovarian follicle after ovulation. It acts as a short-lived endocrine organ that secretes progesterone, which maintains the decidual layer of the endometrium in the richly vascular state necessary for implantation and pregnancy. If conception occurs, the corpus luteum grows and secretes increasing amounts of progesterone.

corpus spongiosum /kôr′pəs spon′jē·ō′səm/, one of the cylinders of spongy tissue that, with the corpora cavernosa, form the penis.

corpus vitreum. See **vitreous humor.**

corrected pressure [L *corrigere* to make straight], a method of applying Boyle's law of gas pressures to adjust simultaneously for changes in both pressure and humidity.

corrective emotional experience, a process by which a patient gives up old patterns of behavior and learns or relearns new patterns by reexperiencing early unresolved feelings and needs.

corrective exercise. See **therapeutic exercise.**

correlation [L *com* + *relatio* a carrying back], (in statistics) a relationship between variables that may be negative (inverse), positive, or curvilinear.

correlative differentiation, (in embryology) specialization or diversification of cells or tissues caused by an inductor or other external factor.

Corrigan's pulse [Dominic J. Corrigan, Irish physician, b. 1802], a bounding pulse in which a great surge is felt followed by a sudden and complete absence of force or fullness in the artery. It occurs in excited emotional states, in various abnormal cardiac conditions and as a result of systemic arteriosclerosis.

corrosion of surgical instruments [L *corrodere* to gnaw away], the rusting of surgical instruments or the gradual wearing away of their polished surfaces because of oxidation and the action of contaminants. It usually occurs because of inadequate cleaning and drying of surgical instruments after use, the use of sterilizing solutions that eat into the surface, overexposure to such solutions, or a faulty autoclave.

corrosive [L *corrodere* to gnaw away], 1. eating away a substance or tissue, especially by chemical action. 2. an agent or substance that eats away a substance or tissue. **–corrode,** *v.,* **corrosion,** *n.*

corrosive gastritis, an acute inflammatory condition of the stomach caused by the ingestion of an acid, alkali, or other corrosive chemical in which the lining of the stomach is eaten away by the corrosive substance.

corrugator supercilii /kôr′əgā′tər sōō′pərsil′ē·ī/ [L *corrugare* to wrinkle; *super* above, *cilium* eyelash], one of the three muscles of the eyelid. It functions to draw the eyebrow downward and inward, as if to frown.

cortex, *pl.* **cortices** /kôr′tisēz/ [L, bark], the outer layer of a body organ or other structure, as distinguished from the internal substance.

cortical audiometry. See **audiometry.**

cortical blindness [L *cortex* + AS *blind*], blindness that results from a lesion in the visual center of the cerebral cortex of the brain.

cortical bone, bone that is 70% to 90% mineralized.

cortical fracture [L *cortex* + *fractura* break], any fracture that involves the cortex of the bone.

cortical substance of cerebellum. See **cerebellar cortex.**

corticosteroid /kôr′tikōstir′oid/ [L *cortex* + *steros* solid], any one of the natural or the synthetic hormones associated with the adrenal cortex, which influences or controls key processes of the body, such as carbohydrate and protein metabolism, electrolyte and water balance, and the functions of the cardiovascular system, the skeletal muscle, the kidneys, and other organs. The corticosteroids synthesized by the adrenal glands include the glucocorticoids and the mineralocorticoids. The principal glucocorticoids are cortisol and corticosterone. The only physiologically important mineralocorticoid in humans is aldosterone.

corticotropin. See **adrenocorticotropic hormone.**

corticotropin-releasing factor (CRF) /kôr'tikōtrop'in/, a polypeptide secreted by the hypothalamus into the bloodstream. It triggers the release of ACTH from the pituitary gland.

cortisol /kôr'təsôl/, a steroid hormone occurring naturally in the body and produced synthetically for pharmacologic use. It is prescribed as an antiinflammatory agent.

cortisone /kôr'təsōn/, a glucocorticoid produced in the liver and also made synthetically. It is prescribed as an antiinflammatory agent.

Corti's organ. See **organ of Corti.**

Corynebacterium /kôr'inēbaktir'ē-əm/ [Gk *koryne* club, *bakterion* small staff], a common genus of rod-shaped, curved bacilli having many species. The most common pathogenic species are *Corynebacterium acnes,* commonly found in acne lesions, and *C. diphtheriae,* the cause of diphtheria.

coryza. See **rhinitis.**

coryza spasmodica. See **hay fever.**

cosmetic surgery [Gk *kosmesis* adornment], reconstruction of cutaneous or underlying tissues performed to correct a structural defect or to remove a scar, birthmark, or some normal evidence of aging. Kinds of cosmetic surgery include **rhinoplasty, rhytidoplasty.**

cosmic radiation, high-energy particles with great penetrating power originating in outer space and reaching the earth as normal background radiation. The rays consist partly of high-energy atomic nuclei.

costal /kos'təl/ [L *costa* rib], **1.** of or pertaining to a rib. **2.** situated near a rib or on a side close to a rib.

costal arch [L *costa* + *arcus,* bow], an arch formed by the shafts of the ribs.

costal cartilage, the cartilage at the anterior end of each rib.

costalgia /kostal'jē-ə/ [L *costa* rib; Gk *algos* pain], a pain in the ribs.

cost analysis [L *costare* to stand firm; Gk *ana* again, *lyein* to loosen], an analysis of the disbursements of a given activity, agency, department, or program.

cost-benefit ratio, a ratio that represents the relationship of the cost of an activity to the benefit of its outcome or product.

cost cap, *informal;* a limit on the amount of money that an agency, department, or institution may spend.

cost center, a department, division, or other subunit of an institution established within its accounting system so that the income and expenses of the subunit can be separated from the income or expenses of other centers and monitored for cost and benefit.

cost control, the process of monitoring and regulating of the expenditure of funds by an agency or institution.

cost effectiveness, the extent to which an activity is thought to be as valuable as it is expensive, such as a public-assistance program that gives vouchers for nutritious foods in pregnancy being cost-effective if it were to prevent the costly incidence of perinatal morbidity.

Costen's syndrome. See **temporomandibular joint pain-dysfunction syndrome.**

costocervical /kos'tōsur'vikəl/ [L *costa* rib, *cervix* neck], pertaining to or involving the ribs and the neck.

costochondral /kos'təkon'drəl/ [L *costa* + Gk *chondros* cartilage], of or pertaining to a rib and its cartilage.

costoclavicular /kos'tōklavik'yələr/ [L *costa* + *clavicula,* little key], pertaining to or involving the ribs and the clavicle.

costophrenic (CP) angle /kos'tōfren'ik/ [L *costa* + *phrenicus* diaphragm], the angle at the bottom of the lung where the diaphragm and chest wall meet.

costosternal /kos'tostur'nəl/, pertaining to or involving the ribs and the sternum.

costotransverse articulation [L *costa* + *transversus* a cross direction], any one of 20 gliding joints between the ribs and associated vertebrae, except for the eleventh and twelfth ribs.

costovertebral, of or relating to a rib and the vertebral column.

costovertebral angle (CVA), one of two angles that outline a space over the kidneys. The angle is formed by the lateral and downward curve of the lowest rib and the vertical column of the spine itself.

cosyntropin /kō'sintrop'in/, a synthetic form of ACTH that is used in the diagnosis and treatment of adrenal hypofunction disorders, such as Addison's disease.

COTA, abbreviation for **Certified Occupational Therapy Assistant.**

cot death. See **sudden infant death syndrome.**

cotton-mill fever. See byssinosis.

cottonmouth, a poisonous pit viper commonly found near water and swamps of the southeastern part of the United States. The symptoms of the bite of a cottonmouth are rapid swelling, severe pain, skin discoloration at bite marks, and weakness.

Cotton's fracture, a trimalleolar fracture involving medial, lateral, and posterior malleoli.

cotton-wool exudate [Ar, *qutun,* AS, *wull,* ME, *spot*], a soft-white exudate seen on the retina of patients with certain systemic conditions, such as AIDS, hypertension, and lupus erythematosus. It can also be observed in retinal infections.

cotyledon /kat′ilē′don/ [Gk *kotyledon* cup-shaped], one of the visible segments on the maternal surface of the placenta. A typical placenta may have 15 to 28 cotyledons, each consisting of fetal vessels, chorionic villi, and intervillous space.

cotyloid cavity. See acetabulum.

cough [AS *cohhetan*], a sudden, audible expulsion of air from the lungs. Coughing is preceded by inspiration, the glottis is partially closed, and the accessory muscles of expiration contract to expel the air forcibly from the respiratory passages. Coughing is an essential protective response that serves to clear the lungs, bronchi, or trachea of irritants and secretions or to prevent aspiration of foreign material into the lungs. It is a common symptom of diseases of the chest and larynx. Antitussive medications are sometimes prescribed in the treatment of a cough in the absence of mucus or congestion.

cough fracture, any fracture of a rib, usually the fifth or the seventh rib, caused by violent coughing.

cough syncope [As, *cohhetan;* Gk, *syncope,* fainting], a temporary loss of consciousness due to an interruption in cerebral blood flow during coughing.

coulomb /kōō′lōm/ [Charles A. de Coulomb, French physicist, b. 1736], the SI unit of electricity equal to the quantity of charge transferred in 1 second across a conductor in which there is a constant current of 1 ampere, or 1 ampere-second.

Coulomb's law, (in physics) a law stating that the force of attraction or repulsion between two electrically charged bodies is directly proportional to the strength of the electric charges and inversely proportional to the square of the distance between them.

coulometry /kōōlom′ətrē/, a type of electroanalytic chemistry in which a reagent generated at the surface of an electrode reacts with a substance to be measured. The substance, usually a metal ion, is measured in terms of the coulombs required for the reaction.

Coulter counter /kōl′tər/ [W. H. Coulter, twentieth-century American engineer], a trademark for an electric device that rapidly identifies, sorts, and counts the various kinds of cells present in a small specimen of blood.

coumarin /kōō′mərin/, an anticoagulant prescribed for prophylaxis and treatment of thrombosis and embolism.

counseling [L *consulere* to consult], the act of providing advice and guidance to a patient or the patient's family. It helps the patient recognize and manage stress and facilitates interpersonal relationships.

count [L *computere* to calculate], a computation of the number of objects or elements present per unit of measurement. Kinds of counts include **Addis count, bacteria count, blood count,** and **platelet count.**

counterclaim [L *contra* + *clamere* to cry out], (in law) a claim made by a defendant establishing a cause for action in his favor against the plaintiff.

counterconditioning, a process used in behavioral therapy in which a learned response is replaced by an alternative response that is less disruptive.

countercurrent, a change in the direction of the flow of a fluid, such as occurs in the ascending branch of a kidney tubule where osmolality undergoes a reversal after a gradual change in sodium chloride concentrations.

counterinjunction, (in transactional analysis) an overt message from the parent ego state of the mother or father that may be difficult to follow if the message conflicts with earlier parental instructions.

counterphobic behavior, an expression of reaction to a phobia by a patient who actively seeks exposure to the type of situation that precipitates phobic symptoms.

counterpulsation [L *contra* + *pulsare* to beat], **1.** the action of a circulatory-assist pumping device synchronized counter to the normal action of the heart. **2.** the process of increasing the intraaortic pressure in diastole by inflation of an intraaortic balloon and deflation of the balloon immediately preceding the next systole.

countershock [L *contra* + Fr *choc*], (in cardiology) a high-intensity, short-duration electric shock applied to the area of the heart, resulting in total cardiac depolarization.

countertraction [L *contra* + *trahere* to pull], a force that counteracts the pull of traction, especially in orthopedics, such as the force of body weight resulting from the pull of gravity.

countertransference, the conscious or unconscious emotional response of a psychotherapist or psychoanalyst to a patient.

countertransport [L *contra* + *trans* across, *portare* carry], the simultaneous transport of two different substances across the same membrane, each in the opposite direction.

counting cell hemocytometer [OFr *conter;* L *cella* storeroom; Gk *haima* blood, *metron* measure], a device for counting the number of cells in a volume of blood or other fluid. It consists of a microscope slide with a counting chamber. The chamber has a known volume and the slide has a ruled area to help count the cells.

coup /kōō/ [Fr, blow], any blow or stroke or the effects of such a blow to the body, usually used with a French word identifying a type of stroke: **1. coup de sabre** /kōōdəsäb'r(ə)/, a wound resembling a sword cut. **2. coup de soleil.** See **sunstroke. 3. coup sur coup** /kōōsYrkōō'/, administration of a drug in small amounts over a short period of time rather than in a single larger dose. **4. contre coup** /kôNtrəkōō'/, an injury most often associated with a blow to the skull in which the force of the impact is transmitted through the skull bones to the opposite side of the head where the bruise, fracture, or other sign of injury appears.

couples therapy, psychotherapy in which couples, who may be married or unmarried but living together, undergo therapy together.

coupling [L *copula* bonding], **1.** the act of coming together, joining, or pairing. **2.** (in genetics) the situation in linked inheritance in which the nonalleles of two or more mutant genes are located on the same chromosome and are close enough so that they are likely to be inherited together. **3.** (in radiation therapy) the efficiency of transfer of power from an applicator to the treatment site.

coupling interval, the interval between the dominant heartbeat and a coupled extrasystole.

Courvoisier's law /kōōrvô·äze̅·äz'/ [Ludwig Courvoisier, Swiss surgeon, b. 1843], a statement that the gallbladder is smaller than usual if a gallstone blocks the common bile duct but is dilated if the common bile duct is blocked as a result of a cause other than a gallstone, such as pancreatic cancer.

couvade /kōōväd'/, a custom in some non-Western cultures whereby the husband goes through mock labor while his wife is giving birth.

Couvelaire uterus /kōōver'/ [Alexandre Couvelaire, French obstetrician, b. 1873], a hemorrhagic process in uterine musculature that may accompany severe abruptio placenta. Extravasated blood effuses between the muscle fibrils and under the uterine peritoneum and the uterus does not contract well.

Cowling's rule /kou'lings/, a method of calculating the approximate pediatric dosage of a drug for a child using this formula: (age at next birthday/24) $\times$ adult dose.

Cowper's gland /kou'pərz/ [William Cowper, English surgeon, b. 1666], either of two round, pea-sized glands embedded in the urethral sphincter of the male.

cowpox [AS *cu;* ME *pokkes*], a mild infectious disease characterized by a pustular rash, caused by the vaccinia virus transmitted to humans from infected cattle. Cowpox infection usually confers immunity to smallpox because of the similarity of the variola and vaccinia viruses.

coxa /kok'sə/, *pl.* **coxae** [L, hip], the hip joint; the head of the femur and the acetabulum of the innominate bone.

coxa adducta, coxa flexa. See **coxa vara.**

coxal articulation [L *coxa* + *articularis* relating to the joints], the ball-and-socket joint of the hip, formed by the articulation of the head of the femur into the cupshaped cavity of the acetabulum.

coxa magna, an abnormal widening of the head and neck of the femur.

coxa plana. See **Perthes' disease.**

coxa valga, a hip deformity in which the angle formed by the axis of the head and neck of the femur and the axis of its shaft is significantly increased.

coxa vara, a hip deformity in which the angle formed by the axis of the head and neck of the femur and the axis of its shaft is decreased.

coxa vara luxans, a fissure or crack in the neck of the femur with dislocation of the head, caused by coxa vara.

coxsackievirus /koksak'ē-/ [Coxsackie, New York; L *virus* poison], any of 30 serologically different enteroviruses associated with a variety of symptoms and primarily affecting children during warm weather. Among the diseases associated with coxsackievirus infections are herpangina, hand, foot, and mouth disease, epidemic pleurodynia, myocarditis, pericarditis, aseptic meningitis, and several exanthems.

CP, 1. abbreviation for **candle power. 2.** abbreviation for **cerebral palsy. 3.** abbreviation for **chemically pure.**

CPAN, abbreviation for **Certified Post-Anesthesia Nurse.**

CPAP, abbreviation for **continuous positive airway pressure.**

CPD, **1.** abbreviation for **cephalopelvic disproportion. 2.** abbreviation for **childhood polycystic disease. 3.** abbreviation for **congenital polycystic disease.**

C-peptide, a biologically inactive residue of insulin formation in the beta cells of the pancreas.

CPHA, abbreviation for the **Canadian Public Health Association.**

CPK, abbreviation for *creatine phosphokinase.* See **creatine kinase.**

CPK isoenzyme fraction, one of several blood-borne enzymes that are released after myocardial necrosis. The isoenzyme of CPK (creatine phosphokinase) is a diagnostic clue to heart damage.

CPNP/A, abbreviation for *Certified Pediatric Nurse Practitioner/Associate.*

CPPB, abbreviation for *continuous positive pressure breathing.*

CPPD, abbreviation for *calcium pyrophosphate dihydrate.*

CPPV, abbreviation for **continuous positive pressure ventilation.**

CPR, abbreviation for **cardiopulmonary resuscitation.**

CPRAM, abbreviation for *controlled partial rebreathing anesthesia method.*

CPT, abbreviation for **Current Procedural Terminology.**

Cr, symbol for the chemical element **chromium.**

CR, abbreviation for *controlled respiration.*

crab louse [AS *crabba, lus*], a species of body louse, *Phthirus pubis,* that infests the hairs of the genital area and is often transmitted between persons by venereal contact.

crack [ME, *craken*], a street drug made by chemically converting cocaine hydrochloride to a form that can be smoked. Smoking crack is a faster, more direct way of getting cocaine molecules into the brain. Because larger amounts of the drug reach the brain more quickly, the effects are more intense than when cocaine, in the white-powder form, is injected, ingested, or inhaled.

crack baby, an infant who was exposed to effects of cocaine in utero by a mother who used the "crack" form of the drug while pregnant.

cracked-pot sound [ME *craken, pott*; L *sonus* sound], a sound sometimes heard on percussion over a cavity with an opening to a bronchus.

crackle, a fine, bubbling sound heard on auscultation of the lung. It is produced by air entering distal airways and alveoli that contain serous secretions.

crackling rale [AS, *cracian;* Fr, rattle], an abnormal breathing sound produced by fluid in the bronchioles during inspiration.

cradle cap [AS *cradel, caeppe*], a common seborrheic dermatitis of infants consisting of thick, yellow, greasy scales on the scalp. Treatment includes oil or ointment to soften the scales, and frequent shampoos.

cramp [AS *crammian* to fill], **1.** a spasmodic and often painful contraction of one or more muscles. **2.** a pain resembling a muscular cramp. Kinds of cramps include **cane-cutter's cramp, fireman's cramp, miner's cramp, stoker's cramp,** and **writer's cramp.**

cranial arachnoid. See **arachnoidea encephali.**

cranial arteritis. See **temporal arteritis.**

cranial bones /krā′nē·əl/ [Gk, *kranion,* cranium, AS, *ban*], the bones of the skull, particularly the part of the cranium that encloses the brain.

cranial nerves [Gk *kranion* skull; L *nervus*], the 12 pairs of nerves emerging from the cranial cavity through various openings in the skull. Beginning with the most anterior, they are designated by Roman numerals and named (I) olfactory, (II) optic, (III) oculomotor, (IV) trochlear, (V) trigeminal, (VI) abducens, (VII) facial, (VIII) acoustic, (IX) glossopharyngeal, (X) vagal, (XI) accessory, (XII) hypoglossal. The cranial nerves are attached to the base of the brain and carry impulses for such functions as smell, vision, ocular movement, pupil contraction, muscular sensibility, general sensibility, mastication, facial expression, glandular secretion, taste, cutaneous sensibility, hearing, equilibrium, swallowing, phonation, tongue movement, head movement, and shoulder movement.

craniectomy [Gk *kranion, ektome* cutting out], the surgical removal of a portion of the cranium.

craniocele. See **encephalocele.**

craniocervical [Gk *kranion* + L *cervix* neck], pertaining to the junction of the skull and neck, particularly the area of the foramen magnum.

craniodidymus /krā′nē·ōdid′iməs/ [Gk *kranion* + *didymos* twin], a two-headed fetal monster in which the bodies are fused.

craniofacial [Gk *kranion;* L *facies* face], pertaining to the cranium and the face.

craniofacial dysostosis [Gk *kranion* + L *facies* face; Gk *dys* bad, *osteon* bone], an abnormal hereditary condition characterized by acrocephaly, exophthalmos, hypertelorism, strabismus, parrot-beaked nose, and hypoplastic maxilla with relative mandibular prognathism.

craniohypophyseal xanthoma /krā′nē·ō-hī′pōfiz′ē·əl/ [Gk *kranion* + *hypo* deficient, *phyein* to grow; *xanthos* yellow, *oma* tumor], a condition in which cholesterol deposits are formed around the hypophyses of the bones, as in Hand-Schüller-Christian disease.

craniometaphyseal dysplasia /kran′ē·ō-met′əfiz′ē·əl/, an inherited bone disorder characterized by paranasal overgrowth, thickening of the skull and jaw, and entrapment of cranial nerves. The patient may experience nasorespiratory infections, associated with bone overgrowth at the sinuses, and malocclusion of the jaws.

craniopagus /krā′nē·op′əgəs/ [Gk *kranion* + *pagos* fixed], conjoined twins that are united at the heads. Fusion can occur at the frontal, occipital, or parietal regions.

craniopharyngeal /krā′nē·ōfərin′jē·əl/ [Gk *kranion* + *phyarynx* throat], of or pertaining to the cranium and the pharynx.

craniopharyngioma /krā′nē·ōfərin′jē·ō′mə/, pl. **craniopharyngiomas, craniopharyngiomata**, a congenital pituitary tumor, appearing most often in children and adolescents, that arises in cells derived from Rathke's pouch or the hypophyseal stalk. The tumor may interfere with pituitary function, damage the optic chiasm, disrupt hypothalamic control of the autonomic nervous system, and result in hydrocephalus.

craniostenosis /krā′nē·ōstənō′sis/ [Gk *kranion* + *stenos* narrow, *osis* condition], a congenital deformity of the skull resulting from premature closure of the sutures between the cranial bones.

craniostosis /krā′nē·ostō′sis/ [Gk *kranion* + *osteon* bone, *osis* condition], premature ossification of the sutures of the skull, often associated with other skeletal defects. The sutures close before or soon after birth. If no surgical correction is made, the growth of the skull is inhibited, the head is deformed, and the eyes and brain are often damaged.

craniotabes /krā′nē·ōtā′bēz/ [Gk *kranion* + L *tabes* wasting], benign, congenital thinness of the top and back of the skull of a newborn, common because the rate of brain growth exceeds the rate of calcification of the skull during the last month of gestation.

craniotomy /kran′ē·ot′əmē/ [Gk *kranion* skull, *temnein* to cut], any surgical opening into the skull, performed to relieve intracranial pressure, to control bleeding, or to remove a tumor.

craniotubular /kran′ē·ōtōō͞b′yələr/, pertaining to a bossing, or overgrowth, of bone that results in an abnormal contour and increased bone density.

cranium /krā′nē·əm/ [Gk *kranion* skull], the bony skull that holds the brain. It is composed of eight bones: frontal, occipital, sphenoid, and ethmoid bones, and paired temporal and parietal bones. – **cranial,** *adj.*

crankcase-spool catheter, a special, elastic catheter stored within a plastic spool to facilitate its insertion, especially for hyperalimentation. The crankcase-spool catheter is usually lodged in the subclavian vein. It is highly flexible, and each revolution of the crankcase spool feeds about 5 inches of the catheter into the vein involved.

crash cart, a cart carrying emergency equipment, such as analgesics, antiseptics, suction devices, sutures, scalpels, surgical needles, sponges, swabs, retractors, hemostats, forceps, trachea tubes, and often a defibrillator. Hospital emergency rooms and intensive care units usually have several crash carts equipped according to prescribed specifications.

cravat bandage /krəvat′/ [Fr *cravate* scarf; *bande* strip], a triangular bandage, folded lengthwise. It may be used as a circular, figure-of-eight, or spiral bandage to control bleeding or to tie splints in place.

crawling reflex. See **symmetric tonic neck reflex.**

C-reactive protein (CRP), a protein not normally detected in the serum but present in many acute inflammatory conditions and with necrosis. CRP appears in the serum within 24 to 48 hours of the onset of inflammation. After a myocardial infarction, it is present in 24 hours. CRP disappears when an inflammatory process is suppressed by salicylates and steroids, or both.

cream [Gk *chrima* oil], **1.** the portion of milk rich in butterfat. **2.** any fluid mixture of thick consistency, such as used to apply medication to the surface of the body.

crease [ME *creste* crest], an indentation or margin formed by a doubling back of tissue, such as the folds or creases on the palm of the hand and sole of the foot.

creatine /krē′ətēn, -tin/ [Gk *kreas* flesh], an important nitrogenous compound produced by metabolic processes in the body. Combined with phosphorus, it forms high-energy phosphate.

creatine kinase, an enzyme in muscle, brain, and other tissues that catalyzes the transfer of a phosphate group from adenosine triphosphate to creatine, producing adenosine diphosphate and phosphocreatine.

creatine phosphate [Gk *kreas;* Du *potass-*

chen], an enzyme that increases in blood levels when there has been muscle damage, as in pseudohypertrophic muscular dystrophy.

creatinine /krē·at′inēn, -nin/, a substance formed from the metabolism of creatine, commonly found in blood, urine, and muscle tissue.

creatinine clearance test, a diagnostic test for kidney function, as a measure of the filtration rate of creatinine, the end product of muscle metabolism. It is calculated on the basis of a urine volume in milliliters per minute times the amount of milligrams per liter of urinary creatinine excreted in 24 hours. The resulting figure is divided by the amount of serum creatinine in milligrams per deciliter.

creatinine height index (CHI), a measurement of a 24-hour urinary excretion of creatinine, which is generally related to the patient's muscle mass and an indicator of malnutrition, particularly in young males.

credentials, a predetermined set of standards, such as certification, establishing that a person or institution has achieved professional recognition in a specific field of health care.

Credé's method /kredāz′/ [Karl S. Credé, German physician, b. 1819], a technique for promoting the expulsion of urine by manual compression of the bladder through pressure on the lower abdominal wall.

Credé's prophylaxis [Karl S. Credé], the instillation of a 1% silver-nitrate solution into the conjunctiva of newborn infants to prevent ophthalmia neonatorum.

creep, a rheologic effect of metals and other solid materials that may become elongated or deformed as a result of a load being applied for a long period of time.

creeping eruption [AS *creopan* bent; L *erumpere* to burst forth], a skin lesion characterized by irregular, wandering red lines made by the burrowing larvae of hookworms and certain roundworms.

cremaster /krimas′tər/ [Gk *kremastos* hanging], a thin, muscular layer spreading out over the spermatic cord in a series of loops. It is a continuation of the obliquus internus. It functions to draw the testis up toward the superficial inguinal ring in response to cold or to stimulation of the nerve.

cremasteric reflex /krē′məster′ik/, a superficial neural reflex elicited by stroking the skin of the upper inner aspect of the thigh in a male. This normally results in a brisk retraction of the testis on the side of the stimulus.

crenation /krinā′shən/ [L *crena* notch], the formation of notches or leaflike, scalloped edges on an object. Red blood cells exposed to a hypertonic saline solution acquire a notched, shriveled surface because of the osmotic effect of the solution. They are then called crenated red blood cells. **–crenate, crenated,** *adj.*

creosol /krē′əsol/, an oily liquid that is one of the active constituents (phenol) of creosote. It should not be confused with cresol.

creosote /krē′əsōt/, a flammable, oily liquid with a smoky odor that is used primarily as a wood preservative. It can be a cause of a wide variety of health problems, ranging from cancer and corneal damage to convulsions.

crepitant /krep′itənt/ [L *crepitans* crackling], pertaining to a sound of crackling or rattling, or of rough surfaces being rubbed together.

crepitant rale [L *crepitans;* Fr, rattle], an abnormal breathing sound produced at the end of inspiration and caused by air entering collapsed alveoli that contain fibrous exudate. It is heard in cases of pneumonia, tuberculosis, and pulmonary edema.

crepitus /krep′itəs/ [L, crackling], **1.** flatulence or the noisy discharge of fetid gas from the intestine through the anus. **2.** a sound like a crackling noise associated with gas gangrene, the rubbing of bone fragments, or the rales of a consolidated area of the lung in pneumonia.

crescendo angina [L *crescere* to increase], a form of anginal discomfort associated with ischemic electrocardiographic changes, marked by increased frequency, provocation, intensity, or character.

crescendo murmur [L *crescere* + *murmur* humming], a murmur of steadily increasing intensity to a sudden termination.

cresol /krē′sol/, a mixture of three isomers in a liquid with a phenolic odor. It is derived from coal tar and used in synthetic resins and disinfectants. Symptoms of chronic poisoning include skin eruptions, digestive disorders, uremia, jaundice, nervous disorders, vertigo, and mental changes.

CREST syndrome /krest/, abbreviation for **calcinosis, Raynaud's phenomenon, esophageal dysfunction, sclerodactyly,** and **telangiectasis,** which may occur for varying periods of time in patients with scleroderma.

cretin dwarf /krē′tən/, a person in whom short stature is caused by infantile hypothyroidism and severe deficiency of thyroid hormone.

cretinism /krē′təniz′əm/ [Fr *cretin* idiot], a condition characterized by severe congenital hypothyroidism and often associated with other endocrine abnormalities.

ical signs of cretinism include dwarfism, mental deficiency, puffy facial features, dry skin, a large tongue, umbilical hernia, and muscular incoordination. The disorder occurs usually in areas where the diet is deficient in iodine and where goiter is endemic. **–cretinoid, cretinous,** *adj.,* **cretin,** *n.*

Creutzfeldt-Jakob disease /kroits'feltyä-'kôp/ [Hans G. Creutzfeldt, German neurologist, b. 1885; Alfons M. Jakob, German neurologist, b. 1884], a rare, fatal encephalopathy caused by a slow virus. The disease occurs in middle age, and symptoms are progressive dementia, dysarthria, muscle wasting, and various involuntary movements, such as myoclonus and athetosis. Deterioration is obvious week to week. Death ensues, usually within a year.

CRF, abbreviation for **corticotropin-releasing factor.**

crib death. See **sudden infant death syndrome.**

cribriform carcinoma. See **adenocystic carcinoma.**

cricoid /krī'koid/ [Gk *krikos* ring, *eidos* form] **1.** having a ring shape. **2.** a ring-shaped cartilage connected to the thyroid cartilage by the cricothyroid ligament at the level of the sixth cervical vertebra.

cricoid cartilage, a ring-shaped cartilage of the larynx, consisting of a narrow anterior arch and a wide quadrilateral lamina posteriorly.

cricoidectomy /krī'koidek'təmē/ [Gk *krikos* + *eidos* + *ektome* cutting out], a surgical procedure for removing the cricoid cartilage.

cricoid pressure, a technique to reduce the risk of the aspiration of stomach contents during induction of general anesthesia. The cricoid cartilage is pushed against the esophagus to prevent passive regurgitation.

cricopharyngeal /krī'kōfərin'jē·əl/ [Gk *krikos* + *pharynx* throat], of or pertaining to the cricoid cartilage and the pharynx.

cricopharyngeal incoordination, a defect in the normal swallowing reflex. The cricopharyngeus muscle ordinarily serves as a sphincter to keep the top of the esophagus closed except when the person is swallowing, vomiting, or belching. The trachea remains open for breathing, but air normally does not enter the esophagus during respiration. When the series of neuromuscular actions is not properly coordinated, the patient may choke, swallow air, regurgitate fluid into the nose, or experience discomfort in swallowing food.

cricothyroid membrane, a fibroelastic membrane including the cricothyroid ligament that connects the cricoid and thyroid cartilages.

cricothyrotomy /krī'kōthīrot'əmē/ [Gk *krikos* + *thyreos* shield, *eidos* form, *temnein* to cut], an emergency incision into the larynx, performed to open the airway in a person who is choking. A small vertical midline cut is made just below the Adam's apple and above the cricoid cartilage. The incision is opened further with a transverse cut through the cricothyroid membrane, and the wound is held open with a tube that is open at both ends to allow air to move in and out.

cri-du-chat syndrome. See **cat-cry syndrome.**

Crigler-Najjar syndrome /krig'lərnaj'är/ [John F. Crigler, Jr., American pediatrician, b. 1919; Victor A. Najjar, American pediatrician, b. 1914], a congenital, familial, autosomal anomaly, in which glucuronyl transferase, an enzyme, is deficient or absent. The condition is characterized by nonhemolytic jaundice, an accumulation of unconjugated bilirubin in the blood, and severe disorders of the central nervous system.

crime [L *crimen*], any act that violates a law and may include criminal intent.

Crimean-Congo hemorrhagic fever /krīmē'ən/, an arbovirus infection transmitted to humans through the bite of a tick, characterized by fever, dizziness, muscle ache, vomiting, headache, and other neurologic symptoms.

criminal abortion, the intentional termination of pregnancy under any condition prohibited by law.

criminal psychology, the study of the mental processes, motivational patterns, and behavior of criminals.

crisis [Gk *krisis* turning point], **1.** a turning point for better or worse in the course of a disease, usually indicated by a marked change in the intensity of signs and symptoms. **2.** a turning point in events affecting the emotional state of a person, such as death or divorce.

crisis intervention, (in psychiatry) therapeutic intervention to help resolve a particular and immediate problem. The goal is to restore in the person the level of functioning that existed before the current crisis.

crisis-intervention unit, a group trained in emergency medical treatment and in various methods for rendering psychiatric therapeutic assistance to a person or group of persons during a period of crisis, especially instances involving suicide attempts or drug abuse.

crisis resolution, (in psychiatry) the development of effective adaptive and coping devices to resolve a crisis.

crisis theory, a conceptual framework for defining and explaining the phenomena that occur when a person faces a problem that appears to be insoluble.

crisscross inheritance [*Christcross* mark of a cross; L *in, hereditas* in heredity], the acquisition of genetic characteristics or conditions from the parent of the opposite sex.

crista supraventricularis /kris′tə s o͞o′prə-ven′trik′yələr′is/ [L *crista* ridge; *supra* above, *ventriculum* belly], the muscular ridge on the interior dorsal wall of the right ventricle of the heart.

criterion /krītir′ē-ən/, *pl.* **criteria** [Gk *kriterion* a means for judging], a standard or rule by which something may be judged, such as a health condition, or a diagnosis established. Usually plural, criteria refers to a set of rules or principles against which something may be measured, such as health care practices.

critical care. See **intensive care.**

critical organs [Gk *krisis* turning point; *organon* instrument], tissues that are the most sensitive to irradiation, such as the gonads, lymphoid organs, and intestine. The skin, cornea, oral cavity, esophagus, vagina, cervix, and optic lens are the next most sensitive organs to irradiation.

critical pathway, a schedule of critical care medical and nursing procedures, including diagnostic tests, medications, and consultations designed to effect an efficient, coordinated program of treatment.

critical period [Gk *kritikos* + *peri* near, *hodos* way], a period of time during a developmental or rehabilitation crisis. Examples are the brief period in which a zygote may be formed, a patient may survive a myocardial infarction, or when an embryo is most vulnerable to effects of medications used by the mother.

critical period of development, a specific time during which the environment has its greatest impact on an individual's development.

critical point, the temperature and pressure at which, in a sealed system, the densities of the liquid and gas forms of a substance will be equal and the two are not visibly separated.

critical pressure, the pressure exerted by a vapor in a closed system at the critical temperature.

critical temperature, the highest temperature at which a substance can exist as a liquid outside a sealed system.

CRNA, abbreviation for **Certified Registered Nurse Anesthetist.**

CRNI, abbreviation for *Certified Registered Nurse, Intravenous.*

Crohn's disease /krōnz\ [Burrill B. Crohn, American physician, b. 1884], a chronic inflammatory bowel disease of unknown origin, usually affecting the ileum, the colon, or both structures. Diseased segments may be separated by normal bowel segments. Crohn's disease is characterized by frequent attacks of diarrhea, severe abdominal pain, nausea, fever, chills, weakness, anorexia, and weight loss.

cromoglicic acid. See **cromolyn sodium.**

cromolyn sodium /krom′olin/, an antiasthmatic that acts by decreasing allergic bronchospasm resulting from an inhaled allergen. It is prophylactically prescribed in the treatment of bronchial asthma. The drug has no effect after an attack has begun.

Cronkhite-Canada syndrome [Leonard W. Cronkhite, American physician, b. 1919; Wilma J. Canada, American radiologist], an abnormal familial condition characterized by GI polyposis accompanied by ectodermal defects, such as nail atrophy, alopecia, and excessive skin pigmentation. In some individuals it is also accompanied by protein-losing enteropathy, malabsorption, and deficiency of blood calcium, potassium, and magnesium.

cross [L *crux*], (in genetics) any method of crossbreeding or any individual, organism, or strain produced from crossbreeding. Kinds of crosses include **dihybrid cross, monohybrid cross, polyhybrid cross,** and **trihybrid cross.**

cross-bite tooth [L *crux* + AS *bitan, toth*], any of the posterior teeth that allow the modified buccal cusps of the upper teeth to be positioned in the central fossae of the lower teeth.

crossbreeding [L *crux* + *bredan*], the production of offspring by the mating of plants and animals from different varieties, strains, or species; hybridization.

crossed amblyopia [L *crux;* Gk *amblys* dull, *ops* eyes], a visual disorder in which the patient is unable to see on one side of the visual field, associated with hemianesthesia of the opposite side of the body.

crossed extension reflex, one of the spinal-mediated reflexes normally present in the first 2 months of life. It is demonstrated by the flexion, adduction, and extension of one leg when the foot of the other leg is stimulated.

crossed grid, (in radiography) an assembly of two parallel x-ray grids that may be rotated at right angles to each other.

...ed reflex, any neural reflex in which ...mulation of one side of the body results in a response on the other side, such as the consensual light reflex.

cross-eye. See esophoria.

cross fertilization, 1. (in zoology), the union of gametes from different species or varieties to form hybrids. **2.** (in botany) the fertilization of the flower of one plant by the pollen from a different plant, as opposed to self-fertilization.

cross infection [L crux; L, inficere to stain], the transmittal of an infection from one patient in a hospital or health care setting to another patient in the same environment.

crossing over, the exchange of sections of chromatids between homologous pairs of chromosomes during the prophase stage of the first meiotic division.

crossmatching of blood [L crux + AS gemaecca matching], a procedure used to determine compatibility of a donor's blood with that of a recipient after the specimens have been matched for major blood type. Serum from the donor's blood is mixed with red cells from the recipient's blood, and cells from the donor are mixed with serum from the recipient. If agglutination occurs, an antigenic substance is present and the bloods are not compatible.

crossover [L crux + AS ofer], the result of the recombination of genes on homologous pairs of chromosomes during meiosis.

cross-reacting antibody [L crux, re, agere; Gk anti; AS bodig body], an antibody that reacts with antigens that are similar but different than the specific antigens with which it originally reacted.

cross resistance, the resistance to a particular antibiotic that also results in resistance against a different antibiotic to which the bacteria may not have been exposed.

cross-sectional [L crux + secare to cut], (in statistics) pertaining to the comparative data of two groups of persons at one point in time.

cross-sectional anatomy, the study of the relationship of the structures of the body by the examination of cross sections of the tissue or organ.

cross sensitivity, a sensitivity to one substance that predisposes an individual to sensitivity to other substances that are related in chemical structure.

cross-sequential [L crux + sequi to follow], (in statistics) pertaining to data that compare several cohorts at different points in time.

cross tolerance, a tolerance to other drugs that develops after exposure to only one agent. An example is the cross tolerance that develops between alcohol and barbiturates.

crotamiton /krōtam'iton/, a scabicide prescribed in treating scabies and other pruritic skin diseases.

croup /kroop/ [Scot, to croak], an acute viral infection of the upper and lower respiratory tract that occurs primarily in infants and young children 3 months to 3 years of age after an upper respiratory tract infection. It is characterized by hoarseness, fever, a distinctive harsh, brassy cough, persistent stridor during inspiration, and varying degrees of respiratory distress resulting from obstruction of the larynx. The most common causative agents are the parainfluenza viruses, especially type 1, followed by the respiratory syncytial viruses (RSV) and influenza A and B viruses. **–croupous, croupy,** adj.

Croupette /kroopet'/, a trademark for a device that provides cool humidification with the administration of oxygen or of compressed air, used especially in the treatment of pediatric patients. It consists of a nebulizer with attached tubing that connects with a canopy to enclose the patient and contain the humidifying mist.

Crouzon's disease /kroozonz'/ [Octave Crouzon, French neurologist, b. 1874; L dis; Fr aise ease], a familial disease characterized by a malformed skull and various ocular disorders, including exophthalmos, divergent squint, and optic atrophy.

crowing inspiration [ME crouen; L inspirare to breathe in], a harsh noise heard on inhalation caused by an acute obstruction in the larynx.

crown [L corona], **1.** the upper part of an organ or structure, such as the top of the head. **2.** the portion of a human tooth that is covered by enamel.

crown-heel length [L corona; AS hela, lengthu], the length of an embryo, fetus, or newborn as measured from the crown of the head to the heel. It is compared to the standing height of an older individual.

crowning [L corona], (in obstetrics) the phase at the end of labor in which the fetal head is seen at the introitus of the vagina. The labia are stretched in a crown around the head.

crown/root ratio, the relation of the clinical crown to the clinical root of a tooth.

crown-rump length, the length of an embryo, fetus, or newborn as measured from the crown of the head to the prominence of the buttocks.

crown static, an x-ray film artifact caused by a buildup of electrons in the film emul-

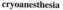

sion. It is most likely to occur during periods of low environmental humidity.

CRP, abbreviation for **C-reactive protein.**

CRRN, abbreviation for *Certified Rehabilitation Registered Nurse.*

CRT, abbreviation for **cathode-ray tube.**

CRTT, abbreviation for **Certified Respiratory Therapy Technician.**

crucial anastomosis [L *crux* cross; Gk *anastomoein* to provide a mouth], an anastomosis in the upper part of the thigh, formed between the first perforating branch of the profunda femoris artery, the inferior gluteal artery, and the lateral and medial circumflex arteries.

crucial bandage. See **T bandage.**

cruciate ligament of the atlas [L *crux* cross; *ligare* to bind], a crosslike ligament attaching the atlas to the base of the occipital bone above and the posterior surface of the body of the axis below.

crude birth rate [L *crudus* raw; ME *burth;* L *reri* to reckon], the number of births per 1,000 people in a population during 1 year.

crura anthelicis /krŏŏr'ə anthel'isis/ [L *crus* leg; Gk *anti* against, *helix* coil], the two ridges on the external ear marking the superior termination of the anthelix and bounding the triangular fossa.

crural /krŏŏrəl/, pertaining to the leg, particularly the upper leg or thigh.

crural hernia [L *crus* + *hernia* rupture], a hernia that protrudes behind the posterior layer of the femoral sheath.

crureus. See **vastus intermedius.**

crus /krus/, *pl.* **crura** /krŏŏr'ə/ [L, leg] **1.** the leg, from knee to foot. **2.** a structure resembling a leg, such as crura anthelicis.

crus cerebri /ser'əbrī, -brē/ [L *crus* + *cerebrum* brain], the ventral part of the cerebral peduncle, composed of the descending fiber tracts passing from the cerebral cortex to form the longitudinal fascicles of the pons.

crushing wound [ME *crushen;* AS *wund*], a break in the external surface of the body due to a severe force applied against the tissues. The body structures may be crushed without signs of external bleeding.

crush syndrome [OFr *cruisir* to crush], **1.** a severe, life-threatening condition caused by extensive crushing trauma, characterized by destruction of muscle and bone tissue, hemorrhage, and fluid loss resulting in hypovolemic shock, hematuria, renal failure, and coma. **2.** a severe complication of heroin-induced coma characterized by edema, vascular occlusion, and lymphatic obstruction.

crust [L *crusta* shell], a solidified, hard outer layer formed by the drying of a bodily exudate, common in such dermatologic conditions as eczema, impetigo, seborrhea, and favus, and during the healing of burns and lesions; a scab.

crutch [AS *cryce*], a wooden or metal staff, the most common kind of which reaches from the ground almost to the axilla, to aid a person in walking. A padded, curved surface at the top fits under the arm; a grip in the form of a crossbar is held in the hand at the level of the palms to support the body. Kinds of crutches include **axillary crutches, forearm crutches.**

Crutchfield tongs [W. Gayle Crutchfield, American surgeon, b. 1900; ME *tonges*], an instrument inserted into the skull to hyperextend the head and neck of patients with fractured cervical vertebrae. The tongs are inserted into small bur holes drilled in each parietal region of the skull; the surrounding skin is sutured and covered with a collodion dressing. A weight is suspended from a rope extending from the center of the tongs, over a pulley attached to head of the bed.

crutch gait, a gait achieved by a person on crutches by alternately bearing weight on one or both legs and on the crutches. In a three-point gait, weight is borne on the noninvolved leg, then on both crutches, then on the noninvolved leg. Four-point gait gives stability but requires bearing weight on both legs. Each leg is used alternately with each crutch. Two-point gait characteristically uses each crutch with the opposing leg. The swing-to and swing-through gaits are often used by paraplegic patients with weight-supporting braces on the legs. Weight is borne on the supported legs; the crutches are placed one stride in front of the person who then swings to that point or through the crutches to a spot in front of them.

crutch palsy, the temporary or permanent loss of sensation or muscle control resulting from pressure on the radial nerve by a crutch.

Cruz trypanosomiasis. See **Chagas' disease.**

cry [OFr *crier*], **1.** a sudden, loud, voluntary, or automatic vocalization in response to pain, fear, or a startle reflex. **2.** weeping because of pain or as an emotional response to depression or grief.

crying vital capacity (CVC), a measurement of the tidal volume while an infant is crying. The CVC may be valuable in monitoring infants with lung diseases that cause changes in functional residual capacity.

cryoanesthesia /krī'ō·an'isthē'zhə/ [Gk *kryos* cold, *aisthesis* feeling], the freezing of a part to achieve adequate deadening of neural sensitivity to pain during brief minor surgical procedures.

cryocautery /krī'ōkô'tərē/ [Gk *kryos* + *kauterion* branding iron], the application of any substance, such as solid carbon dioxide, that destroys tissue by freezing.

cryogen /krī'əjən/ [Gk *kryos* + *genein* to produce], a chemical that induces freezing, used to destroy diseased tissue without injury to adjacent structures. Cell death is caused by dehydration. Kinds of cryogens include **carbon dioxide, freon, liquid nitrogen,** and **nitrous oxide.** –**cryogenic,** *adj.*

cryoglobulin /krī'ōglob'yŏolin/ [Gk *kryos* + L *globulus* small sphere], an abnormal plasma protein that precipitates and coalesces at low temperatures and dissolves and disperses at body temperature.

cryoglobulinemia /krī'ōglob'yŏolin-ē'mē-ə/ [Gk *kryos* + L *globulus* small sphere; Gk *haima* blood], an abnormal condition in which cryoglobulins are present in the blood.

cryonics /krī-on'iks/ [Gk *kryos* cold], the techniques in which cold is applied for a variety of therapeutic goals, including brief local anesthesia, destruction of superficial skin lesions, and preservation of cells, tissue, organs, or the entire body. –**cryonic,** *adj.*

cryoprecipitate /krī'ō·prisip'itāt/. **1.** any precipitate formed upon cooling a solution. **2.** a preparation rich in factor VIII collected from fresh human plasma that has been frozen and thawed.

cryostat [Gk *kryos* + *statos* standing], a device used in surgical pathology that consists of a special microtome used for freezing and slicing sections of tissue for study by a surgical pathologist.

cryosurgery [Gk *kryos* + *cheirourgos*], use of subfreezing temperature to destroy tissue, such as in the destruction of the ganglion of nerve cells in the thalamus in the treatment of Parkinson's disease. The coolant is circulated through a metal probe, chilling it to as low as −160° C, depending on the chemical used. The moist tissues adhere to the cold metal of the probe and freeze.

cryotherapy /krī-ōther'əpē/ [Gk *kryos* + *therapeia*], a treatment using cold as a destructive medium for some common skin disorders. Solid carbon dioxide or liquid nitrogen is applied briefly with a sterile cotton-tipped applicator.

crypt /kript/ [Gk *kryptos* hidden], a blind pit or tube on a free surface. Some kinds of crypts are **anal crypt, dental crypt,** and **synovial crypt.**

cryptic [Gk *kryptos*], pertaining to something concealed.

cryptocephalus /krip'tōsef'ələs/ [Gk *kryptos* + *kephale* head], a malformed fetus that has a small, underdeveloped head. –**cryptocephalic, cryptocephalous,** *adj.* **cryptocephaly,** *n.*

cryptococcosis /krip'tōkokō'sis/, an infectious disease caused by a fungus, *Cryptococcus neoformans,* which spreads through the lungs to the brain and central nervous system, skin, skeletal system, and urinary tract. Initial symptoms may include coughing or other respiratory effects because the lungs are a primary site of infection. After the fungus spreads to the meninges, neurologic symptoms may develop, including headache, blurred vision, and difficulty in speaking.

Cryptococcus /krip'tōkok'əs/, a genus of yeastlike fungi that reproduces by budding rather than by producing spores. Certain pathogenic species exist; *C. neoformans* is the most important.

Cryptococcus neoformans, a species of yeastlike fungus that causes cryptococcosis, a potentially fatal infection that can affect the lungs, skin, and brain.

cryptodidymus /krip'tōdid'əməs/ [Gk *kryptos* + *didymos* twin], conjoined twins in which one fetus is small, underdeveloped, and concealed within the body of the other, more fully formed autosite.

crypt of iris, any one of the small pits in the iris along its free margin encircled by the circulus arteriosus minor.

cryptogenic /krip'tōjen'ik/ [Gk *kryptos* + *genein* to produce], **1.** pertaining to a disease of unknown etiology. **2.** a parasitic organism living within another organism.

cryptomenorrhea /krip'tōmenôrē'ə/ [Gk *kryptos* + L *mensis* month; Gk *rhoia* flow], an abnormal condition in which the products of menstruation are retained within the vagina because of an imperforate hymen, or, less often, within the uterus because of an occlusion of the cervical canal. –**cryptomenorrheal,** *adj.*

cryptophthalmos /krip'təfthal'məs/ [Gk *kryptos* + *ophthalmos* eye], a developmental anomaly characterized by complete fusion of the eyelids, usually with defective formation or lack of the eyes.

cryptorchid [Gk *kryptos* + *orchis* testis], a developmental defect characterized by failure of the testicles to descend into the scrotum. They are retained in the abdomen or inguinal canal.

cryptorchidism /kriptôr'kidiz'əm/ [Gk *kryptos* + *orchis* testis], failure of one or both of the testicles to descend into the scrotum.

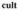

cryptorchis. See **cryptorchid, cryptorchidism.**

cry reflex, a normal infantile reaction to pain, hunger, or need for attention. The reflex may be absent in an infant born prematurely or one in poor health.

crystal /kris'təl/ [Gk *krystallos*], a solid inorganic substance, the atoms or molecules of which are arranged in a regular, repeating three-dimensional pattern, which determines the shape of a crystal. **—crystalline,** *adj.*

crystalline lens /kris'təlin, -līn/ [Gk *krystallos;* L, lentil], a transparent structure of the eye, enclosed in a capsule, situated between the iris and the vitreous humor, and slightly overlapped at its margin by the ciliary processes. The capsule of the lens is a transparent, elastic membrane that touches the free border of the iris anteriorly and is secured by the suspensory ligament of the lens. The posterior surface is more convex than the anterior. It is composed of a soft, cortical material, a firm nucleus, and concentric laminae.

crystallization /kris'təlīzā'shən/ [Gk *krystallos* rock crystal], the production of crystals, either by cooling a liquid or gas to a solid state or by cooling a solution until the solute precipitates as a crystalline deposit.

crystalloid /kris'təloid/ [Gk *krystallos* + *eidos* form], a substance in a solution that can be diffused through a semipermeable membrane.

crystalluria /kris'təloor'ē·ə/, the presence of crystals in the urine. The condition may be a source of urinary tract irritation.

Cs, symbol for the element **cesium.**

CS, abbreviation for **cesarean section.**

c-section, see **cesarean section.**

CSF, abbreviation for **cerebrospinal fluid.**

CSN, abbreviation for *Certified School Nurse.*

CSR, abbreviation for **Cheyne-Stokes respiration.**

CT, abbreviation for **computed tomography.**

C3 nephritic factor, a C3 complement protein molecule that may be deposited in glomerular capillary walls and mesangial tissues, precipitating or contributing to local immune inflammatory injury and kidney damage.

Cu, symbol for the element **copper.**

Cuban itch. See **alastrim.**

cubic centimeter (cm³) [Gk *kybos;* L *centum* hundred; Gk *metron* measure], a theoretical cube or its equivalent, each edge of which is 1 cm long. One cubic centimeter is equivalent to 1 milliliter (ml).

cubital /kyoo'bitəl/, pertaining to the elbow or the forearm.

cuboidal epithelium [Gk *kybos* + *eidos* form, *epi* above, *thele* nipple], simple epithelial cells that are generally cube-shaped and one layer in thickness.

cuboid bone [Gk *kybos* + *eidos* form], the cuboidal tarsal bone on the lateral side of the foot. It articulates with the calcaneus, lateral cuneiform, and fourth and fifth metatarsal bones.

cucm, abbreviation for **cubic centimeter.**

cue, a stimulus that determines or may prompt the nature of a person's response.

cuff, an inflatable elastic tube that is placed about the upper arm and expanded with air to restrict arterial circulation during blood pressure examination.

cuffed endotracheal tube, an endotracheal tube with a balloon at one end that may be inflated to tighten the fit of the tube in the lumen of the airway. The balloon forms a cuff that prevents gastric contents from passing into the lungs and gas from leaking back from the lungs.

cuirass /kwitas'/ [Fr *cuirasse* breastplate], **1.** a negative-pressure full-body respirator. An electric-driven pump is adjusted to match the timing of the patient's spontaneous breathing. **2.** a tightly fitted chest bandage.

cul-de-sac /kul'dəsak, kYdesok'/, *pl.* **culs-de-sac, cul-de-sacs** [F, bottom of the bag], a blind pouch or cecum, such as the conjunctival cul-de-sac and the dural cul-de-sac.

cul-de-sac of Douglas, a pouch formed by the caudal portion of the parietal peritoneum.

culdocentesis /kul'dōsentē'sis/, the use of needle puncture or incision through the vagina to remove intraperitoneal fluid, including purulent material.

culdotomy /kuldot'əmē/, incision or needle puncture of the cul-de-sac of Douglas by way of the vagina.

Culex /koo'leks/, a genus of humpbacked mosquitoes. It includes species that transmit viral encephalitis and filariasis.

Cullen's sign [Thomas S. Cullen, American gynecologist, b. 1868], the appearance of faint, irregularly formed hemorrhagic patches on the skin around the umbilicus. It may appear 1 to 2 days after the onset of anorexia and the severe, poorly localized abdominal pains that are characteristic of acute pancreatitis.

cult, a specific complex of beliefs, rites, and ceremonies maintained by a group in association with some particular person or object.

cultural assimilation, a process by which members of an ethnic minority group lose cultural characteristics that distinguish them from the dominant cultural group.

cultural event, a communication of meaning that takes place each time one member of a society interacts with another member.

cultural healer, a member of an ethnic or cultural group who uses traditional methods of healing rather than modern scientific methods to provide health care for other members of the group.

cultural relativism, a concept that health and normality emerge within a social context, and that the content and form of mental health will vary greatly from one culture to another.

culturally relativistic perspective, an ability to understand the behavior of transcultural patients (those who move from one culture to another) within the context of their own culture.

culture [L *colere* to cultivate], **1.** (in microbiology) a laboratory test involving the cultivation of microorganisms or cells in a special growth medium. **2.** (in psychology) a set of learned values, beliefs, customs, and behavior that is shared by a group of interacting individuals.

culture-bound, pertaining to a health condition that is specific to a particular culture, such as a belief in the effects of certain kinds prayer or the "evil eye."

culture medium. See **medium.**

culture procedure, (in bacteriology) any of several techniques for growing colonies of microorganisms to identify a pathogen and to determine which antibiotics are effective in combating the infection caused by the organism.

culture shock, the psychologic effect of a drastic change in the cultural environment of an individual. The person may exhibit feelings of helplessness, discomfort, and disorientation in attempting to adapt to a different cultural group with dissimilar practices, values, and beliefs.

cumm, abbreviation for **cubic millimeter.**

cumulative /kyōō′myəlā′tiv/ [L *cumulare* to pile on], increasing by incremental steps with an eventual total that may exceed the expected result.

cumulative action, 1. the increased activity of a therapeutic measure or agent when administered repeatedly. **2.** increased activity demonstrated by a drug when repeated doses accumulate in the body and exert a greater biologic effect than the initial dose.

cumulative dose, the total dose that accumulates from repeated exposure to radiation or a radiopharmaceutic product.

cumulative gene. See **polygene.**

cuneate /kyōō′nē·āt/ [L *cuneus* wedge], (of tissue) wedge-shaped, used especially in describing cells of the nervous system.

cuneiform /kyōōnē′əfôrm′/ [L *cuneus* wedge, *forma*], (of bone and cartilage) wedge-shaped.

cuneiform bone. See **triangular bone.**

cuneiform cartilage [L, *cuneus,* wedge-shaped, *forma, cartilago*], an elongated elastic laryngeal cartilage at the edge of the aryepiglottic fold, above and anterior to the corniculate cartilage.

cunnilingus /kun′əling′gəs/, the oral stimulation of the female genitalia.

cup arthroplasty of the hip joint [L *cupa* cask; Gk *arthron* joint, *plassein* to form], the surgical replacement of the head of the femur by a metal or plastic mold to relieve pain and increase motion in arthritis or to correct a deformity. The damaged or diseased bone is removed under general anesthesia, and the acetabulum and the head of the femur are reshaped. A metal Vitallium cup is inserted between the two and becomes the articulating surface of the femur. Postoperatively, the patient's leg is suspended in traction to hold it in a position of abduction and internal rotation to keep the disk in place in the acetabulum. Continued abduction is necessary for 6 weeks. Possible complications include infection, thrombophlebitis, pulmonary embolism, and fat embolism. The patient receives extensive physical therapy; crutches are necessary to avoid bearing of full weight for 6 months, and an exercise program must be followed for several years.

cupping, a counterirritant technique of applying a suction device to the skin to draw blood to the surface of the body.

cupping and vibrating, the procedures to help remove mucus and fluid from the lungs by the use of the clinical nursing techniques of manual percussion and vibration to dislodge and mobilize the secretions. Cupping is performed by the rhythmic percussion of the affected segments of the lungs or bronchi by the cupped hands of the nurse. Vibration is done by placing the nurse's hands over the affected area and tensing and contracting the muscles of the hand, arm, and, mainly, shoulder, as if having a shaking chill. The movements are transmitted to the patient's chest, which increases the turbulence and velocity of exhaled air in the small bronchi.

cupric /kyōō′prik/ [L *cuprum* copper], of or pertaining to copper in its divalent form, such as cupric sulfate.

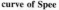

cupulolithiasis /kyo͞o′pyo͞olōlithī′əsis/ [L *cupula* little cup; Gk *lithos* stone], a severe, long-lasting vertigo brought on by movement of the head to certain positions. There are many possible causes, among them otitis media, ear surgery, or injury to the inner ear. In addition to extreme dizziness, signs are nausea, vomiting, and ataxia.

curare /kyo͞orä′rē/ [S.Am. Indian *ourari*], a substance derived from tropic plants of the genus *Stryknos*. It is a potent muscle relaxant that acts by preventing transmission of neural impulses across the myoneural junctions. Large dosage can cause complete paralysis, but action is usually reversible with anticholinergics.

curariform /kyo͞orä′rifôrm/ [*curare* + L *forma*] 1. chemically similar to curare. 2. having the effect of curare.

curative treatment. See **treatment.**

cure [L *cura*], 1. restoration to health of a person afflicted with a disease or other disorder. 2. the favorable outcome of the treatment of a disease or other disorder. 3. a course of therapy, a medication, a therapeutic measure, or another remedy used in treatment of a medical problem, as faith healing, fasting, rest cure, or work cure.

curet /kyo͞oret′/ [Fr *curette* scoop], 1. a surgical instrument shaped like a spoon or scoop for scraping and removing material or tissue from an organ, cavity, or surface. 2. to remove tissue or debris with such a device. Kinds of curets include **Hartmann's curet.**

curettage /kyo͞or′ətäzh′/ [Fr *curette* scoop], scraping of material from the wall of a cavity or other surface, performed to remove tumors or other abnormal tissue or to obtain tissue for microscopic examination. Curettage also refers to clearing unwanted material from fistulas and areas of chronic infection.

curie (c, Ci) /kyo͞or′ē/ [Marie S. Curie, Polish-born chemist, b. 1867; Pierre Curie, French scientist, b. 1859], a unit of radioactivity used before adoption of the becquerel (Bq) as the SI unit. It is equal to 3.70×10^{10} Bq.

curium (Cm) [Marie S. Curie; Pierre Curie], a radioactive metallic element. Its atomic number is 96; its atomic weight is 247.

Curling's ulcer [Thomas B. Curling, English surgeon, b. 1811], a duodenal ulcer that develops in people who have severe burns on the surface of the body.

CURN, abbreviation for *Certified Urological Registered Nurse.*

currant jelly clot [ME *corauns*; L *gelare* to congeal; AS *clott*], a red, jellylike blood clot that is rich in hemoglobin from erythrocytes in the clot.

current [L *currere* to run], 1. a flowing or streaming movement. 2. a flow of electrons along a conductor in a closed circuit; an electric current. 3. certain physiologic electric activity and characteristics of blood circulation. Physiologic currents include abnerval current, action current, axial current, centrifugal current, centripetal current, compensating current, demarcation current, and electrotonic current.

current of injury. an abnormal current flow to and from injured myocardium resulting from reduced membrane potential in the injured area conpared to that of the normal fibers.

Current Procedural Terminology (CPT), a system developed by the American Medical Association for standardizing the terminology and coding used to describe medical services and procedures.

curriculum vitae (CV) /kərik′ələm wē′tī, vē′tē/, *pl.* **curricula vitae** [L *curriculum* course; *vita* life], a summary of educational and professional experiences, including activities and honors, to be used in seeking employment, for biographic citations on professional meeting programs, or for related purposes.

Curschmann spiral /ko͞orsh′mon/ [Heinrich Curschmann, German physician, b. 1846; Gk *speira* coil], one of the coiled fibrils of mucus occasionally found in the sputum of persons with bronchial asthma.

curtain effect, (in radiology) an x-ray film artifact caused by chemical processing stains that were not properly squeezed from the film during development.

curvature myopia, a type of nearsightedness caused by refractive errors associated with an excessive curvature of the cornea.

curve [L *curvare* to bend], (in statistics) a straight or curved line used as a graphic method of demonstrating the distribution of data collected in a study or survey.

curve of Carus [Karl G. Carus, German physician, b. 1789], the normal axis of the pelvic outlet.

curve of occlusion, 1. a curved occlusal surface that simultaneously contacts the major portion of the incisal and occlusal prominances of the existing teeth. 2. the curve of dentition on which lie the occlusal surfaces of the teeth.

curve of Spee [Ferdinand Graf von Spee, German embryologist, b. 1855], 1. the anatomic curvature of the occlusal alignment of the teeth, beginning at the tip of the lower canine, following the buccal cusps of the natural premolars and molars, and continuing to the anterior border of the ramus. 2. the curve of the occlusal surfaces of the arches in vertical dimension, produced by a downward dipping of the mandibular premolars, with a corresponding adjustment of the upper premolars.

curvilinear [L *curvus* bent, *linea* line], pertaining to a curved line.

curvilinear trend [L *curvus* + *linea*; AS *trendan* to turn], (in statistics) a trend in which a graphic representation of the data yields a curved line.

cushingoid /kŏŏsh′ingoid/ [Harvey W. Cushing, American surgeon, b. 1869; Gk *eidos* form], having the habitus and facies characteristic of Cushing's disease: fat pads on the upper back and face, striae on the limbs and trunk, and excess hair on the face.

Cushing's disease /kŏŏsh′ingz/ [Harvey W. Cushing], a metabolic disorder characterized by the abnormally increased secretion of adrenocortical steroids caused by increased amounts of adrenocorticotropic hormone (ACTH) secreted by the pituitary, such as by a pituitary adenoma. Excess adrenocortical hormones result in accumulations of fat on the chest, upper back, and face and in edema, hyperglycemia, increased gluconeogenesis, muscle weakness, purplish striae on the skin, decreased immunity to infection, osteoporosis with susceptibility to fracture of bones, acne, and facial hirsutism.

Cushing's syndrome [Harvey W. Cushing], a metabolic disorder resulting from the chronic and excessive production of cortisol by the adrenal cortex or by the administration of glucocorticoids in large doses for several weeks or longer. When occurring spontaneously, the syndrome represents a failure in the body's ability to regulate the secretion of cortisol or adrenocorticotropic hormone (ACTH). (Normally cortisol is produced only in response to ACTH, and ACTH is not secreted in the presence of high levels of cortisol.) The most common cause of the syndrome is a pituitary tumor that causes an increased secretion of ACTH. The patient with Cushing's syndrome has a decreased glucose tolerance, central obesity, round "moon" face, supraclavicular fat pads, a pendulous, striae-covered pad of fat on the chest and abdomen, oligomenorrhea or decreased testosterone levels, muscular atrophy, edema, hypokalemia, and some degree of emotional change. The skin may be abnormally pigmented and fragile; minor infections may become systemic and long-lasting.

cusp [L *cuspis* point], **1.** a sharp projection or a rounded eminence that rises from the chewing surface of a tooth, such as the two pyramidal cusps that arise from the

premolars. **2.** any one of the small flaps on the valves of the heart, as the ventral, dorsal, and medial cusps attached to the right atrioventricular valve.

cuspid [L *cuspis* point], **1.** having but one cusp, or point. **2.** canine tooth.

cuspid valve. See **atrioventricular valve.**

cuspless tooth, a tooth without cuspal prominences on its masticatory surface.

custodial care [L *custodia* guarding; *garrire* to chatter], services and care of a nonmedical nature provided on a long-term basis, usually for convalescent and chronically ill individuals. Kinds of custodial care include **board, room,** and **personal assistance.**

cut, (in molecular genetics) a fissure or split in a double strand of DNA in contrast to a nick in a single strand.

cutaneous /kyŏŏtā′nē·əs/ [L *cutis* skin], of or pertaining to the skin.

cutaneous absorption, the taking up of substances through the skin.

cutaneous anaphylaxis, a localized, exaggerated reaction of hypersensitivity in the form of a wheal and flare caused by an antigen injected into the skin of a sensitized individual, generally used as a test of sensitivity to various allergens.

cutaneous horn, a hard, skin-colored projection of the epidermis, usually on the head or face.

cutaneous larva migrans, a skin condition caused by a hookworm, *Ancylostoma braziliense,* a parasite of cats and dogs. Its ova are deposited in the ground with the feces of infected animals, develop into larvae, and invade the skin of people, particularly bare feet, but any skin may be involved. Secondary infections often occur if the skin has been broken by scratching.

cutaneous leishmaniasis. See **oriental sore.**

cutaneous lupus erythematosus. See **discoid lupus erythematosus.**

cutaneous membrane. See **skin.**

cutaneous nerve, a nerve that enters the skin.

cutaneous nevus [L *cutis* skin, *naevus* a mole on the body], a congenital discoloration of a skin area, such as a strawberry birthmark.

cutaneous papilloma, a small brown or flesh-colored outgrowth of skin, occurring most frequently on the neck of an older person.

cutaneous sensation [L *cutis* + *sentire* to feel], a sensation experienced in or arising from receptors of the skin.

cutdown [ME *cutten, doun*], an incision into a vein with insertion of a catheter for intravenous infusion. It is performed when an infusion cannot be started by venipuncture and in hyperalimentation therapy, when highly concentrated solutions are given via catheter into the superior vena cava.

cuticle /kyōō′təkəl/ [L *cuticula* little skin] **1.** epidermis. **2.** the sheath of a hair follicle. **3.** the thin edge of cornified epithelium at the base of a nail.

cutis. See **skin.**

cutis laxa /kyōō′təs/ [L, skin; *laxus* loose], abnormally loose, relaxed skin resulting from an absence of elastic fibers in the body, usually a hereditary condition.

cutis marmorata. skin that has a "marbled" appearance due to conspicuous veining and dilatation of small vessels.

cutting oil dermatitis, a skin disorder that affects people who use cutting oils as coolants and lubricants. Exposure to the oil obstructs hair follicles, sweat ducts, and sebaceous glands, leading to development of comedones and folliculitis.

cuvette /kyōōvet′/ [Fr *cuva* tub], a small transparent tube or container with specific optical properties that is used in laboratory research and analyses, such as photometric evaluations, colorimetric determinations, and turbidity studies.

CVA, 1. abbreviation for **cerebrovascular accident. 2.** abbreviation for **costovertebral angle.**

CVP, 1. abbreviation for **central venous pressure. 2.** an anticancer drug combination of cyclophosphamide, vincristine, and prednisone.

CVP monitor. See **central venous pressure monitor.**

cyanide poisoning /sī′ənīd/ [Gk *kyanos* blue], poisoning resulting from the ingestion or inhalation of cyanide from such substances as bitter almond oil, wild cherry syrup, prussic acid, hydrocyanic acid, or potassium or sodium cyanide. Characterized by tachycardia, drowsiness, convulsion, and headache, cyanide poisoning may result in death within 1 to 15 minutes.

cyanocobalamin /sī′ənōkōbal′əmin/ [Gk *kyanos* + Ger *kobald* mine goblin], a red, crystalline, water-soluble substance with activity similar to that of vitamin B₁₂. It is involved in the metabolism of protein, fats, and carbohydrates, normal blood formation, and neural function. Deficiency is usually caused by the absence of intrinsic factor, which is necessary for the absorption of cyanocobalamin from the GI tract and which results in pernicious anemia and brain damage. Symptoms of deficiency include nervousness, neuritis, numbness and tingling in the hands and feet, poor muscular coordination, unpleasant body odor, and menstrual disturbances.

cyanogenetic glycosides /sī′ənōjənet′ik/, chemical compounds contained in foods that release hydrogen cyanide when chewed or digested. This disrupts the structure of the substances, causing cyanide to be released. Although human poisoning from cyanogenetic glycosides is rare, cases have been reported of cyanide poisoning from certain varieties of lima beans, cassava, and bitter almonds.

cyanomethemoglobin /sī′ənōmethē′məglō′bin/ [Gk *kyanos* + *meta* together with, *haima* blood; L *globus* ball], a hemoglobin derivative formed during nitrite therapy for cyanide poisoning.

cyanosis /sī′ənō′sis/ [Gk *kyanos* blue, *osis* condition], bluish discoloration of the skin and mucous membranes caused by an excess of deoxygenated hemoglobin in the blood or a structural defect in the hemoglobin molecule, such as in methemoglobin. **–cyanotic,** *adj.*

cyanotic congenital defect, a congenital heart defect that allows the mixing of unsaturated (venous) blood with saturated (arterial) blood to produce cyanosis.

cyclacillin /sī′kləsī′lin/, a penicillin antibiotic prescribed in the treatment of certain bacterial infections.

cyclamate /sī′kləmāt/, an artificial, nonnutritive sweetener formerly used in the form of calcium or sodium salt.

cyclandelate /sīklan′dəlāt/, a vasodilator prescribed in the treatment of muscular ischemia and peripheral vascular obstruction or spasm.

cyclencephaly /sīk′lənsef′əlē/ [Gk *kyklos* circle, *enkephalos* brain], a developmental anomaly characterized by the fusion of the two cerebral hemispheres. **–cyclencephalic, cyclencephalous,** *adj.,* **cyclencephalus,** *n.*

cyclic adenosine monophosphate (cAMP) /sik′lik, sī′klik/, a cyclic nucleotide formed from adenosine triphosphate by the action of adenyl cyclase. This cyclic compound, known as the "second messenger," participates in the action of catecholamines, vasopressin, adrenocorticotropic hormone, and many other hormones.

cyclic guanosine monophosphate (cGMP), a substance that mediates the action of certain hormones in a manner similar to that of cyclic adenosine monophosphate (cAMP).

cyclitis /siklī′tis/ [Gk *kyklos* + *itis*], inflammation of the ciliary body causing redness of the sclera adjacent to the cornea of the eye.

cyclizine hydrochloride /sī′klizēn/, an

antihistamine prescribed in the treatment or prevention of motion sickness.

cyclobenzaprine hydrochloride /sī'klə-ben'zəprēn/, a muscle relaxant prescribed in the short-term treatment of muscle spasm.

cyclocephalic, cyclocephalous, cyclocephaly. See cyclopia.

cyclomethycaine sulfate /si'klōmeth'ikān/, a local anesthetic agent for use on nontraumatized mucous membranes before clinical examination or instrumentation.

cyclophosphamide /si'klōfos'fəmīd/, an alkylating agent prescribed in the treatment of a variety of neoplasms and as an immunosuppressant in organ transplants.

cyclopia /sīklō'pē·ə/ [Gk *Cyclops* mythic one-eyed giant], a developmental anomaly characterized by fusion of the orbits into a single cavity containing one eye.

cycloplegia /sī'kləplē'jə/ [Gk *kyklos* + *plege* stroke], paralysis of the ciliary muscles, as induced by certain ophthalmic drugs to allow examination of the eye.

cycloplegic /sī'kləplē'jik/, **1.** of or pertaining to a drug or treatment that causes paralysis of the ciliary muscles of the eye. **2.** one of a group of anticholinergic drugs used to paralyze the ciliary muscles of the eye for ophthalmologic examination or surgery. Any of the cycloplegics may cause adverse effects in persons sensitive to anticholinergics.

cyclopropane /sī'klōprō'pān/, a highly flammable and explosive potent anesthetic gas that gives good analgesia and skeletal muscle relaxation, with low toxicity, minimal adverse effects, and rapid induction and emergence. It has been replaced by the nonflammable halogenated hydrocarbons and is no longer used because of its high flammability and explosion potential.

cycloserine /sī'klōser'ēn/, an antibiotic prescribed in the treatment of active pulmonary and extrapulmonary tuberculosis.

cyclosporin /si'klō·spôr'in/, any of a group of biologically active metabolites of *Tolypocladium inflatum Gams* and certain other fungi. The major forms are cyclosporin A and C, which are cyclic oligopeptides with immunosuppressive, antifungal, and antipyretic effects. As immunosuppressants, cyclosporins affect primarily the T cell lymphocytes.

cyclosporine /si'klō·spôr'ēn/, an alternative term for cyclosporin A.

cyclothymic disorder /si'klō·thim'ik/ [Gk *kyklos* + *thymos* mind], a disorder of mood, whereby the essential feature is a chronic mood disturbance of at least 2 years' duration, involving numerous periods of depression and hypomania, but not of sufficient severity and duration to meet the criteria for a major depressive or manic episode.

cyclothymic personality, a personality characterized by extreme swings in mood from elation to depression.

cyclotomy /sīklot'əmē/, a surgical procedure for the correction of a defect in the ciliary muscle of the eye.

cyclotron /sī'klətron/ [Gk *kyklos* + *electron* amber], a device used to accelerate charged particles or ions. The particles bombard special targets where they create radioactive species to be used as radiopharmaceutical or to make neutrons that can be used for radiotherapy.

cyesis [Gk *kyesis* pregnancy], pregnancy.

cylindrical grasp, the normal position of the hand and fingers when holding cylindrical objects, such as a glass tumbler. The fingers close around the object, which is stabilized against the palm of the hand. It occurs as a reflex action in infants and later is developed into a voluntary gross grasp.

cylindroma /sil'indrō'mə/, *pl.* **cylindromas, cylindromata** [Gk *kylindros* cylinder], a benign neoplasm of the skin, usually of the scalp or face, developing from a hair follicle or sweat gland.

cylindromatous carcinoma. See adenocystic carcinoma.

cylindromatous spiradenoma. See cylindroma.

cyma line /sī'mə/, an S-shaped line seen on radiographs at the articulation of the talonavicular and calcaneocuboid bones of the foot.

cyproheptadine hydrochloride /sī'prōhep'tədēn/, an antihistamine prescribed in the treatment of a variety of hypersensitivity reactions, including rhinitis, skin rash, and pruritus.

cypionate /sī'pyōnāt/, a contraction for cyclopentanepropionate.

Cyprus fever. See brucellosis.

Cys, abbreviation for cysteine.

cyst /sist/ [Gk *kystis* bag], a closed sac in or under the skin lined with epithelium and containing fluid or semisolid material, such as a **sebaceous cyst.**

cystadenocarcinoma /sis'tədē'nəkär'-sinō'mə/, a pancreatic tumor that evolves from a mucus cystadenoma. Clinical features include epigastric pain and a palpable abdominal mass.

cystadenoma /sis'tədinō'mə/, *pl.* **cystadenomas, cystadenomata** [Gk *kystis* + *aden* gland, *oma* tumor], **1.** an adenoma associated with a cystoma. **2.** an adenoma containing multiple cystic structures.

cystathioninemia /sis'təthīəninē'mē·ə/, an inherited metabolic disorder caused by a deficiency of the enzyme cystathionase.

It results in an excess of the amino acid methionine. Some patients may be asymptomatic, whereas others show signs of mental retardation.

cystectomy /sistek′təmē/ [Gk kystis + ektome excision], a surgical procedure in which all or a part of the bladder is removed, as may be required in treating cancer of the bladder.

cysteine (Cys) /sis′tēn/, a nonessential amino acid found in many proteins in the body, including keratin. It is a metabolic precursor of cystine and an important source of sulfur for various body functions.

cystic /sis′tik/ [Gk kystis bag], **1.** pertaining to a cyst. **2.** pertaining to a fluid-filled sac, such as the gallbladder or urinary bladder.

cystic acne. See acne conglobata.

cystic carcinoma, a malignant neoplasm containing cysts or cystlike spaces. Tumors of this kind occur in the breast and ovary.

cystic duct, the duct through which bile from the gallbladder passes into the common bile duct.

cysticercosis /sis′tisərkō′sis/ [Gk kystis + kerkos tail, osis condition], an infection and infestation by the larval stage of the pork tapeworm Taenia solium or the beef tapeworm T. saginata. The eggs are ingested and hatch in the intestine; the larvae invade the subcutaneous tissue, brain, eye, muscle, heart, liver, lung, and peritoneum. The invasive, early phase of the infection is characterized by fever, malaise, muscle pain, and eosinophilia. Epilepsy and personality change may appear if the brain is affected.

cysticercus /sis′tiser′kəs/, a larval form of tapeworm. It consists of a single scolex enclosed in a bladderlike cyst.

cystic fibroma, a fibrous tumor in which cystic degeneration has occurred.

cystic fibrosis, an inherited disorder of the exocrine glands, causing those glands to produce abnormally thick secretions of mucus, elevation of sweat electrolytes, increased organic and enzymatic constituents of saliva, and overactivity of the autonomic nervous system. The glands most affected are those in the pancreas, the respiratory system, and the sweat glands. Cystic fibrosis is usually recognized in infancy or early childhood. When present in infancy, the earliest manifestation is meconium ileus, an obstruction of the small bowel by viscid stool. Other early signs are a chronic cough, frequent, foul-smelling stools, and persistent upper respiratory infections. The most reliable diagnostic tool is the sweat test, which shows elevations of both sodium and chloride.

cystic goiter, an enlargement of the thyroid gland containing cysts resulting from mucoid or colloid degeneration.

cystic kidney [Gk kystis; ME kidenei], pertaining to any of several cystic disorders of the kidney, including congenital polycystic disease, solitary renal cysts, or cortical cysts associated with nephroslcerosis.

cystic lymphangioma, a cystic growth formed by lymph vessels; usually congenital, it most frequently occurs in the neck, axilla, or groin of children.

cystic mastitis, a form of mammary dysplasia with inflammation and the formation of nodular cysts in the breast tissue. The cysts contain a turbid fluid. Symptoms may vary with individual breast changes that occur during the menstrual cycle.

cystic mole. See hydatid mole.

cystic myxoma, a tumor of the connective tissue that has undergone cystic degeneration.

cystic neuroma, a neoplasm of nerve tissue that has degenerated and become cystic.

cystic tumor, a tumor with cavities or sacs containing a semisolid or a liquid material.

cystine /sis′tin/, a nonessential amino acid found in many proteins in the body, including keratin and insulin. Cystine is a product of the oxidation of two cysteine molecules.

cystinosis /sis′tinō′sis/ [cystine + Gk osis condition], a congenital disease characterized by glucosuria, proteinuria, cystine deposits in the liver, spleen, bone marrow, and cornea, rickets, excessive amounts of phosphates in the urine, and retardation of growth.

cystinuria /sis′tinŏŏr′ē·ə/ [cystine + Gk ouron urine], **1.** abnormal presence in the urine of the amino acid cystine. **2.** an inherited defect of the renal tubules, characterized by excessive urinary excretion of cystine and several other amino acids. In high concentration, cystine tends to precipitate in the urinary tract and form kidney or bladder stones.

cystitis /sistī′tis/ [Gk kystis + itis inflammation], an inflammatory condition of the urinary bladder and ureters, characterized by pain, by urgency and frequency of urination, and by hematuria. It may be caused by a bacterial infection, calculus, or tumor.

cystocele /sis′təsēl′/ [Gk kystis + kele hernia], a herniation or protrusion of the urinary bladder through the wall of the vagina.

cystogram /sis′təgram′/ [Gk kystis + gramma record], a graphic record, usually a series of x-ray films, obtained as a part of any excretory urographic procedure, such as in retrograde pyelography or retrograde cystoscopy.

cystoid /sis′toid/ [Gk *kystis* + *eidos* form], pertaining to or resembling a cyst or bladder.

cystolith. See **vesicle calculus.**

cystoma /sistō′mə/, pl. **cystomas, cystomata** [Gk *kystis* + *oma* tumor], any tumor or growth containing cysts, especially one in or near the ovary.

cystometry /sistom′ətrē/ [Gk *kystis* + *metron* measure], the study of bladder function by use of a **cystometer** /sistom′ətər/, an instrument that measures capacity in relation to changing pressure. The urologic procedure, **cystometography** /sis′tōmətog′rəfē/,/ measures the amount of pressure exerted on the bladder at varying degrees of capacity. The results of the measurements are traced graphically on a **cystometogram** /sis′tōmet′əgram′/.

cystosarcoma phyllodes /sis′tōsärkō′ma filō′dēs/, a benign breast tumor that grows rapidly and tends to recur if not adequately excised.

cystoscope /sis′təskōp′/ [Gk *kystis* + *skopein* to look], an instrument for examining and treating lesions of the urinary bladder, ureter, and kidney. It consists of an outer sheath with a lighting system, a viewing obturator, and a passage for catheters and operative devices.

cystoscopic urography. See **retrograde cystoscopy.**

cystoscopy /sistos′kəpē/, the direct visualization of the urinary tract by means of a cystoscope inserted in the urethra. The procedure is usually performed under sedation or anesthesia with the patient in the lithotomy position. The bladder is distended with air or water and the patient is in a fasting state. **—cystoscopic,** *adj.*

cystourethrogram /sis′tə·y o͞ore′thrəgram′/, a radiograph of the urinary bladder and urethra usually performed with use of an iodinated contrast medium to make the structures visible.

cysts of liver, small, single, simple watery cysts, usually secondary to another disorder, such as cystic kidney disease.

cytarabine /siter′əbēn/, an antineoplastic agent prescribed in the treatment of acute and chronic myelocytic leukemia, acute lymphocytic leukemia, and erythroleukemia.

cytoarchitectonic /sī′tō·är′är′kitekton′ik/ [Gk *kytos* cell; L *architectura* architecture], pertaining to the cellular arrangement within a tissue or structure.

cytoarchitecture, the typical pattern of cellular arrangement within a particular tissue or organ, as in the cerebral cortex. **—cytoarchitectural,** *adj.*

cytobiotaxis. See **cytoclesis.**

cytocentrum. See **centrosome.**

cytocerastic. See **cytokerastic.**

cytochemism /sī′tōkem′izəm/ [Gk *kytos* + *chemeia* alchemy], the chemical activity within the living cell, specifically the various reactions to and affinity for chemical substances.

cytochemistry, the study of the various chemicals within a living cell and their actions and functions.

cytochrome [Gk *kytos* + *chroma* color], **1.** a class of hemoproteins whose function is electron transport. These proteins have the ability to reverse the valence of hemeiron compounds, alternating between ferrous and ferric states. **2.** proteins involved in mitochondrial exudative electron transport systems associated with ATP production.

cytochrome P-450, a cytochrome protein involved with extramitochondrial electron transport in the liver and in drug detoxification.

cytocide /sī′tosīd/ [Gk *kytos* + L *caedere* to kill], any substance that is destructive to cells. **—cytocidal,** *adj.*

cytoclesis /sī′tōklē′sis/ [Gk *kytos* + *klesis* calling for], the influence exerted by one cell on the action of other cells; the vital principle of all living tissue.

cytoctony /sītok′tənē/ [Gk *kytos* + *ktonos* killing], the destruction of cells, specifically the killing of cells in culture by viruses.

cytode /sī′tōd/[Gk *kytos* + *eidos* form], the simplest type of cell, consisting of a protoplasmic mass without a nucleus, such as a bacterium.

cytodieresis /sī′tōdī·er′isis/, pl. **cytodiereses** [Gk *kytos* + *diairesis* separation], cell division, especially the phenomena involving the division of the cytoplasm. **—cytodieretic,** *adj.*

cytodifferentiation [Gk *kytos* + L *differentia* difference] **1.** a process by which embryonic cells acquire biochemical and morphologic properties essential for specialization and diversification. **2.** the total and gradual transformation from an undifferentiated to a fully differentiated state.

cytofluorograph /sī′toflôr′əgraf′/, a diagnostic instrument used to measure the level of CD4 T lymphocytes in HIV-positive patients. The lymphocytes are stained with specific monoclonal antibodies. The normal value of the CD4 count is 800 per mm^3. Antiretroviral therapy may begin when the CD4 level drops below 500 per mm^3.

cytogene /sī′təjēn/ [Gk *kytos* + *genein* to

produce], a particle within the cytoplasm of a cell that is self-replicating, derived from the genes in the nucleus, and capable of transmitting hereditary information.

cytogenesis /sī'tōjen'əsis/ [Gk *kytos* + *genein* to produce], the origin, development, and differentiation of cells. **–cytogenetic, cytogenic,** *adj.*

cytogeneticist /sī'tōjənet'isist/, one who specializes in cytogenetics.

cytogenetics /sī'tōjənet'iks/, the branch of genetics that studies the cellular constituents concerned with heredity, primarily the structure, function, and origin of the chromosomes. One kind of cytogenetics is **clinical cytogenetics. –cytogenetic,** *adj.*

cytogenic gland, a glandular organ that secretes living cells, specifically the testes and ovary.

cytogenic reproduction, the formation of a new organism from a unicellular germ cell, either sexually through the fusion of gametes to form a zygote or asexually by means of spores.

cytogenics. See **cytogenetics.**

cytogeny /sītoj'ənē/, **1.** cytogenetics. **2.** the origin and development of the cell. **–cytogenous, cytogenic,** *adj.*

cytogony /sītog'ənē/, cytogenic reproduction.

cytohistogenesis /sī'tōhis'tōjen'əsis/ [Gk *kytos* + *histos* tissue, *genein* to produce], the structural development and formation of cells. **–cytohistogenetic,** *adj.*

cytohyaloplasm. See **hyaloplasm.**

cytoid /sī'toid/ [Gk *kytos* + *eidos* form], like or resembling a cell.

cytoid body, a small white spot on the retina of each eye that is seen by using an ophthalmoscope in examining the eyes of a patient affected with systemic lupus erythematosus.

cytokerastic /sī'tōkəras'tik/ [Gk *kytos* + *kerastos* mixed], pertaining to or characteristic of cellular development from a lower to a higher form or from a simple to more complex arrangement. Also **cytocerastic** /-səras'tik/.

cytokinesis /sī'tōkinē'sis, -kīnē'sis/ [Gk *kytos* + *kinesis* movement], the division of the cytoplasm, exclusive of nuclear division, that occurs during the final stages of mitosis and meiosis to form daughter cells; the total of all the changes that occur in the cytoplasm during mitosis, meiosis, and fertilization. **–cytokinetic,** *adj.*

cytologic map /sī'tōloj'ik/ [Gk *kytos* + *logos* science; L *mappa* table napkin], the graphic representation of the location of genes on a chromosome, based on correlating genetic recombination test-crossing results with the structural analysis of chromosomes that have undergone such changes as deletions or translocations as detected by banding techniques.

cytologic sputum examination, a microscopic examination of a specimen of bronchial secretions, including a search for cells that may be cancerous or otherwise abnormal.

cytologist /sītol'əjist/, one who specializes in the study of cells, specifically one who uses cytologic techniques in the differential diagnosis of neoplasms.

cytology /sītol'əjē/ [Gk *kytos* + *logos* science], the study of cells, including their formation, origin, structure, function, biochemical activities, and pathology. Kinds of cytology are **aspiration biopsy cytology** and **exfoliative cytology. –cytologic, cytological,** *adj.*

cytolymph. See **hyaloplasm.**

cytolysin /sītol'isin/ [Gk *kytos* + *lyein* to loosen], an antibody that dissolves antigenic cells. Kinds of cytolysin are **bacteriolysin** and **hemolysin.**

cytolysis /sītol'isis/, *pl.* **cytolyses** [Gk *kytos* + *lyein* to loosen], the destruction or breakdown of the living cell, primarily by the disintegration of the outer membrane. A kind of cytolysis is **immune cytolysis. –cytolytic,** *adj.*

cytomegalic inclusion disease (CID) /sī'tōmegal'ik/ [Gk *kytos* + *megas* large; L *in, claudere* in enclosure], a viral infection caused by the cytomegalovirus (CMV), a virus related to the herpesviruses, characterized by malaise, fever, lymphadenopathy, pneumonia, hepatosplenomegaly, and superinfection with various bacteria and fungi as a result of the depression of immune response characteristic of herpesviruses. It is primarily a congenitally acquired disease of newborn infants, transmitted in utero from the mother to the fetus. Results may range from spontaneous abortion or fatal neonatal illness to birth of a normal infant.

cytomegalovirus (CMV) /sī'tōmeg'əlōvī'rəs/ [Gk *kytos* + *megas* large; L *virus* poison], a member of a group of large species-specific herpes-type viruses with a wide variety of disease effects.

cytomegalovirus (CMV) disease. See **cytomegalic inclusion disease.**

cytometer /sītom'ətər/ [Gk *kytos* + *metron* measure], a device for counting and measuring the number of cells within a given amount of fluid, as blood, urine, or cerebrospinal fluid.

cytometry /sītom'ətrē/, the counting and measuring of cells, specifically blood cells. **–cytometric,** *adj.*

cytomitome /sī'təmī'tōm/ [Gk *kytos* + *mitos* thread], the fibrillary network within the cytoplasm of a cell, as contrasted with that in the nucleoplasm.

cytomorphology /sī′tōmôrfol′əjē/ [Gk *kytos* + *morphe* shape, *logos* science], the study of the various forms of cells and the structures contained within them. **–cytomorphologic, cytomorphological,** *adj.,* **cytomorphologist,** *n.*

cytomorphosis /sī′tōmôr′fəsis/, *pl.* **cytomorphoses** [Gk *kytos* + *morphosis* shaping], the various changes that occur within a cell during the course of its life cycle.

cyton /sī′ton/ [Gk *kytos* cell], the cell body of a neuron or that portion containing the nucleus and its surrounding cytoplasm from which the axon and dendrites are formed.

cytopenia /sī′tōpē′nē·ə/, [Gk *kytos* + *penes* poor], a deficiency of cells in the blood.

cytopheresis /sī′tōfôr′əsis/ [Gk *kytos* + *pherein* to bear], **1.** a therapeutic technique to remove red or white blood cells or platelets from patients with certain blood disorders. **2.** a laboratory procedure for separating specific components, such as white blood cells or platelets, from donor blood by centrifugation.

cytophotometer /sī′tōfətom′ətər/ [Gk *kytos* + *phos* light, *metron* measure], an instrument for measuring light density through stained portions of cytoplasm, used for locating and identifying chemical substances within cells.

cytophotometry /sī′tōfətom′ətrē/, the identification of chemical substances within cells, using a cytophotometer.

cytophysiology /sī′tōfis′ē·ol′əjē/ [Gk *kytos* + *physis* nature, *logos* science], the study of the biochemical processes involved in the functioning of an individual cell, as contrasted with the functioning of organs or tissues. **—cytophysiologic, cytophysiological,** *adj.,* **cytophysiologist,** *n.*

cytoplasm /sī′təplaz′əm/ [Gk *kytos* + *plassein* to mold], all of the substance of a cell other than the nucleus.

cytoplasmic bridge. See **intercellular bridge.**

cytoplasmic inheritance /sī′tōplaz′mik/, the acquisition of traits or conditions controlled by self-replicating substances within the cytoplasm, such as mitochondria or chloroplasts, rather than by the genes. The phenomenon occurs in plants and lower animals but has not yet been demonstrated in humans.

cytoscopy /sītos′kapē/ [Gk, *kytos* + *skopein* to watch], the diagnostic study of cells obtained from patient specimens with the aid of microscopes and other laboratory equipment.

cytosine /sī′təsin/, a major pyrimidine base found in nucleotides and a fundamental constituent of DNA and RNA. In free or uncombined form it occurs in trace amounts in most cells.

cytosine arabinoside. See **cytarabine.**

cytoskeleton [Gk *kytos* + *skeletos* dried body], the cytoplasmic elements, including the tonofibrils, keratin, and other microfibrils, that function as a supportive system within a cell, especially an epithelial cell.

cytosome /sī′təsōm/, a multilayered membrane-bound lamellar body found in type II pneumocytes. It is a precursor of pulmonary surfactant.

cytotechnologist, an allied health professional who specializes in the study of the structure and function of cells. Cytotechnologists prepare cellular samples for study under the microscope and assist in the diagnosis of disease by the examination of the samples. Using the findings of the cytotechnologist, the physician is able to detect cancer and other diseases at a very early stage.

cytotoxic /sī′tōtok′sik/ [Gk *kytos* + *toxikon* poison], pertaining to a pharmacologic compound or other agent that destroys or damages tissue cells.

cytotoxic anaphylaxis, an exaggerated reaction of hypersensitivity to an injection of antibodies specific for antigenic substances that occur normally on surfaces of body cells.

cytotoxic drug, any pharmacologic compound that inhibits the proliferation of cells within the body. Such compounds as the alkylating agents and the antimetabolites are designed to destroy abnormal cells selectively; they are commonly used in chemotherapy.

cytotoxic hypersensitivity [Gk *kytos* + *toxikon* poison; *hyper* above; L *sentire* to feel], an IgG or an IgM complement-dependent, immediate-acting hypersensitive humoral response to foreign cells or to alterations of surface antigens on the cells.

cytotoxic T cells. See **CD8.**

cytotoxin /sī′tōtok′sin/ [Gk *kytos* + *toxikon* poison], a substance that has a toxic effect on certain cells. An antibody may act as a cytotoxin. **–cytotoxic,** *adj.*

cytotrophoblast /sī′tōtrof′əblast′/ [Gk *kytos* + *trophe* nutrition, *blastos* germ], the inner layer of cells of the trophoblast of the early mammalian embryo that gives rise to the outer surface and villi of the chorion. **—cytotrophoblastic,** *adj.*

Cytovene, trademark for a brand of ganciclovir, an antiviral drug active against the retinitis of cytomegalovirus.

CY-VA-DIC, an anticancer drug combination of cyclophosphamide, vincristine, doxorubicin, and dacarbazine.

D

d, symbol for one tenth.

D, 1. symbol for *dead space gas.* **2.** symbol for **diffusing capacity. 3.** abbreviation for *diopter.* **4.** abbreviation for *dexter,* meaning "right."

da, symbol for the multiple 10.

DA, abbreviation for **developmental age.**

dacarbazine /dekär′bəzēn/, an alkylating agent used as an antineoplastic prescribed primarily in the treatment of malignant melanoma, sarcoma, and Hodgkin's disease.

Dacron cuff, a sheath of Dacron surrounding an atrial or venous catheter to prevent ascending infections and accidental displacement of the catheter.

dacryoadenitis /dak′rē·ō·ad′ənī′tis/, an inflammation of the lacrimal gland.

dacryocyst /dak′rē·ōsist′/ [Gk *dakryon* tear, *kytis* bag], a lacrimal sac at the medial angle of the eye, a normal anatomic feature.

dacryocystectomy /dak′rē·ōsistek′təmē/ [Gk *dakryon* + *kytis* bag, *ektome* excision], partial or total excision of the lacrimal sac.

dacryocystitis /dak′rē·ōsistī′tis/, an infection of the lacrimal sac caused by obstruction of the nasolacrimal duct, characterized by tearing and discharge from the eye.

dacryocystorhinostomy /dak′rē·ōsis′-tôrīnos′təmē/ [Gk *dakryon* + *kytis, rhis* nose, *stoma* nouth], a surgical procedure for restoring drainage into the nose from the lacrimal sac when the nasolacrimal duct is obstructed.

dacryostenosis /dak′rē·ōstinō′sis/ [Gk *dakryon* + *stenos* narrow, *osis* condition], an abnormal stricture of the nasolacrimal duct, occurring either as a congenital condition or as a result of infection or trauma. Dacryocystorhinostomy may be required to correct this condition.

dactinomycin /dak′tinōmī′sin/, an antibiotic used as an antineoplastic agent prescribed in the treatment of a variety of malignant neoplastic diseases, including Wilms' tumor and rhabdomyosarcoma in children.

dactyl /dak′til/ [Gk *dactylos* finger], a digit (finger or toe). **–dactylic,** *adj.*

dactylitis /dak′tilī′tis/, a painful inflammation of the fingers or toes, usually associated with sickle cell anemia or certain infectious diseases, particularly syphilis or tuberculosis.

daily adjusted progressive resistance exercise (DAPRE), a program of isotonic exercises that allows for individual differences in the rate at which a patient regains strength in an injured or diseased body part.

Dakin's solution [Henry D. Dakin, American biochemist, b. 1880; L *solutus* dissolved], an antiseptic solution containing boric acid and 0.4% to 0.5% of sodium hypochlorite.

daltonism /dôl′təniz′əm/ [John Dalton, English chemist, b. 1766], *informal;* a form of red-green color blindness. It is genetically transmitted as a sex-linked autosomal recessive trait.

Dalton's law of partial pressures /dôl′tənz/ [John Dalton], (in physics) a law stating that the total pressure exerted by a mixture of gases is equal to the sum of the pressures that could be exerted by the gases if they were present alone in the container.

damages [L *damnum* loss], (in law) a sum of money awarded to a plaintiff by a court as compensation for any loss, detriment, or injury to the plaintiff's person, property, or rights caused by the malfeasance or negligence of the defendant. **Actual damages** are awarded to reimburse the plaintiff for the loss or injury sustained. **Nominal damages** are awarded to show that a legal wrong has been committed, although no recoverable loss can be determined. **Punitive damages** exceed the actual cost of injury or damage and are awarded when the defendant has acted maliciously or in reckless disregard of the plaintiff's rights.

damp [AS, vapor], a potentially lethal atmosphere in caves and mines. **Black damp** or **choke damp** is caused by absorption of the available oxygen by coal seams. **Fire damp** is composed of methane and other explosive hydrocarbon gases. **White damp** is another name for carbon monoxide.

damping [AS, vapor], (in cardiology) pertaining to a diminishing of the amplitude of a series of waves or oscillations, as in damping of the arterial pressure wave form.

danazol /dan'əzol/, a synthetic androgen that acts to suppress the output of gonadotropins from the pituitary prescribed in the treatment of endometriosis.

dance reflex [ME *dauncen;* L *reflectere* to look backward], a normal response in the neonate to simulate walking by a reciprocal flexion and extension of the legs when held in an erect position with the soles touching a hard surface.

dance therapy, (in psychology) the use of rhythmic body movements or dance to release expression of feelings.

dander, dry scales shed from the scalp.

dandruff /dan'druf/, an excessive amount of scaly material composed of dead, keratinized epithelium shed from the scalp that may be a mild form of seborrheic dermatitis. Treatment with a keratolytic shampoo is usually recommended.

dandy fever. See **dengue fever.**

Dandy-Walker cyst [Walter E. Dandy, American neurosurgeon, b. 1886; Arthur E. Walker, American surgeon, b. 1907], a cystic malformation of the fourth ventricle of the brain, resulting from hydrocephalus.

danthron /dan'thron/, a stimulant laxative prescribed in the treatment of constipation or for bowel evacuation before radiologic or surgical procedures.

dantrolene sodium /dan'trəlēn/, a skeletal muscle relaxant prescribed in the treatment of muscle spasticity resulting from injury to the spinal cord or cerebrum. It is not indicated in treatment of spasm from rheumatic disorders.

DAP, abbreviation for **Draw-A-Person Test.**

DAPRE, abbreviation for **daily adjusted progressive resistance exercise.**

dapsone (DADPS) /dap'sōn/, a bacteriostatic sulfone derivative prescribed in the treatment of lepromatous leprosy and dermatitis herpetiformis.

Darier's disease. See **keratosis follicularis.**

dark adaptation, a normal increase in sensitivity of the retinal rod cells of the eye to detect any light that may be available for vision in a dimly lighted environment. The process is accompanied by an adjustment of the pupils to allow more light to enter the eyes.

darkfield microscopy [AS *deorc* hidden, *feld* field; Gk *mikros* small, *skopein* to look], examination with a darkfield microscope, in which the specimen is illuminated by a peripheral light source. Organisms in specimens that have been prepared for use with a darkfield microscope appear to glow against a dark background.

dark-film fault [AS *deorc* hidden, *filmen* skin; L *fallere* to disappoint], a defect in a photograph or radiograph, which appears as an excessively darkened image and image area.

darkroom, a room in a hospital or similar facility for the storage and processing of light-sensitive materials, such as x-ray film.

darwinian reflex. See **grasp reflex.**

darwinian theory /därwin'ē-ən/ [Charles R. Darwin, English naturalist, b. 1809], the theory postulated by Charles Darwin that organic evolution results from the process of natural selection of those variants of plants and animals best suited to survive in their environmental surroundings. **–darwinian,** *adj., n.*

DASE, abbreviation for **Denver Articulation Screening Examination.**

data /d,ā'tə, dat'ə, dä'tə/ *sing.* **datum** [L *datum* giving], **1.** pieces of information, especially those that are part of a collection of information to be used in an analysis of a problem, such as the diagnosis of a health problem. **2.** information stored and processed by a computer.

data acquisition system (DAS), a radiation detection system that measures the amount of radiation passing through a patient.

data analysis, (in research) the phase of a study that includes classifying, coding, and tabulating information needed to perform statistic or qualitative analyses according to the research design and appropriate to the data.

data clustering, the grouping of related information from the patient's health history, physical examination, and laboratory results as part of the process of making a diagnosis.

data collection, (in research) the phase of a study that includes the gathering of information and identification of sampling units as directed by the research design.

data source, the origin of information relevant to a patient's level of wellness and health patterns.

data validation, the process of determining if information gathered during a patient health evaluation is complete and accurate.

date/acquaintance rape, a sexual assault or rape by a person known to the victim, such as a date, employer, friend, or casual acquaintance.

datum. See **data.**

daughter cell [ME *doughter;* L *cella* storeroom], one of the cells produced by the division of a parent cell.

daughter chromosome [AS *tohter* female child; Gk *chroma* color, *soma* body], either of the paired chromatids that during the anaphase stage of mitosis separate and migrate to opposite ends of the cell before division. Each contains the complete genetic information of the original chromosome.

daughter element, an element that results from the radioactive decay of a parent element. An example is technetium 99, which is the daughter element created by the decay of an atom of molybdenum 99.

daughter product. See **decay product.**

daunorubicin hydrochloride /dô′nōrōo̅′-bisin/, an anthracycline antibiotic antineoplastic agent prescribed in the treatment of cancer, particularly the leukemias and neuroblastoma.

Davidson regimen [Edward C. Davidson, American physician, b. 1894; L, direction], a method of treating chronic constipation in children, of developing regular bowel habits, and of identifying those with functional bowel disease or obstructive disorders. The child is then given mineral oil in increasing doses, until four or five loose bowel movements occur daily. Some children, especially those under 2 years of age, require supplemental, fatsoluble vitamins to maintain proper nutrition. The child is placed on a potty-chair at a specific time each day for 5 to 15 minutes, and, as regular habits develop, the mineral oil is gradually withdrawn over a period of several weeks.

dawn phenomenon [ME *daunen;* Gk *phainomenon* anything seen], a tendency for patients with insulin-dependent diabetes mellitus to require an increased insulin dose in the early morning hours because of an increase in plasma glucose concentration.

day blindness. See **hemeralopia.**

day care [OE *doeg;* L *garrire* to chatter], a specialized program or facility that provides care for preschool children, usually within a group framework, either as a substitute for or extension of home care, particularly for single parents or for parents who are both employed outside the home.

daydream, a usually nonpathologic reverie that occurs while a person is awake. The content is usually the fulfillment of wishes that are not disguised, and fulfillment is imagined as direct.

day health care services, the provision of hospitals, nursing homes, or other facilities for health-related services to adult patients who are ambulatory or can be transported and who regularly use such services for a certain number of daytime hours but do not require continuous inpatient care.

day hospital [OE *doeg;* L *hospes* guest], a psychiatric facility that offers a therapeutic program during daytime hours for formerly institutionalized patients.

day patient. See **inpatient.**

day sight. See **nyctalopia.**

dB, abbreviation for **decibel.**

DC, abbreviation for **direct current.**

d/c, abbreviation for *discontinue.*

D & C, abbreviation for **dilatation and curettage.**

DD, abbreviation for **developmental disability.**

ddC, symbol for 2′3-dideoxycytidine, an antiretroviral drug used in the treatment of AIDS. It is related chemically to DDI.

DDI, abbreviation for 2′,3′-dideoxyinosine, an antiretroviral medication.

DDS, abbreviation for *Doctor of Dental Surgery.*

DDST, abbreviation for **Denver Developmental Screening Test.**

DDT (dichlorodiphenyltrichloroethane), a nondegradable water-insoluble chlorinated hydrocarbon once used worldwide as a major insecticide, especially in agriculture. In recent years, knowledge of its adverse impact on the environment has led to restrictions in its use.

DDT poisoning. See **chlorinated organic insecticide poisoning.**

DEA, abbreviation for **dose equivalent.**

DEA, **1.** abbreviation for *Drug Enforcement Administration.* **2.** abbreviation for **Drug Enforcement Agency.**

deactivation [L *de* from, *activus* active], the process of becoming or making something inactive or inoperable.

dead-end host [AS *dead, ende;* L *hospes* guest], any animal from which a parasite cannot escape to continue its life cycle. Humans are dead-end hosts for trichinosis because the larvae encyst in muscle and human flesh is unlikely to be a source of food for other animals susceptible to this parasite.

dead fetus syndrome, a condition in which the fetus has died but has remained in the uterus for more than 6 weeks. The condition leads to a blood coagulation disorder, and eventual delivery is usually accompanied by massive bleeding.

dead pulp. See **nonvital pulp.**

dead space [AS; L *spatium*], **1.** a cavity that remains after the incomplete closure of a surgical or traumatic wound, leaving an area in which blood can collect and delay healing. **2.** the amount of lung in contact with ventilating gases but not in contact with pulmonary blood flow. **Alveolar dead space** refers to alveoli that are ventilated by the pulmonary circulation but are not perfused. The condition may exist when pulmonary circulation is obstructed, as by a thromboembolus. **Anatomic dead space** is an area in the trachea, bronchi, and air passages containing air that does not reach the alveoli during respiration. As a general rule, the volume of air in the anatomic dead space in milliliters is approximately equal to the weight in pounds of the involved individual. Certain lung disorders, as emphysema, increase the amount of anatomic dead space. **Physiologic dead space** is an area in the respiratory system that includes the anatomic dead space together with the space in the alveoli occupied by air that does not contribute to the oxygen-carbon dioxide exchange.

dead space effect, any of several potential adverse effects of dead space resulting from mechanical ventilation, particularly when there is alveolar dead space. In hospitalized patients it can be responsible for producing hypoxemia and hypercarbia. A pulmonary embolism can also produce a dead space effect; blood flow in the pulmonary arteries is reduced without impeding ventilation.

deaf [AS], **1.** unable to hear; hard of hearing. **2.** people who are unable to hear or who suffer hearing impairment. **–deafness,** *n.*

deafferentation /dē·af′ərəntā′shən/ [L *de* from, *ad, ferre* to bear], an interruption in an afferent nerve system.

deafness, a condition characterized by a partial or complete loss of hearing. In assessing deafness, the patient's ears are examined for drainage, crusts, accumulation of cerumen, or structural abnormality. It is determined if the deafness is conductive or sensory, temporary or permanent, and congenital or acquired in childhood, adolescence, or adulthood. The effect of aging, when applicable, is evaluated, and a psychosocial assessment is conducted to ascertain if the individual is well adjusted to deafness or reacts to the handicap with fear, anxiety, frustration, depression, anger, or hostility. In all cases the degree of loss and the kind of impairment causing the loss are determined.

deaminase /dē·am′ināts/ [L *de* away, *amine* ammonia; Fr *diastase* enzyme], an enzyme that catalyses the hydrolysis of the NH_2 bond in amino compounds. The enzymes are usually named according to the substrate, such as **adenosine deaminase,** or **guanosine deaminase.**

deamination /dē′amǐnā′shən/, the removal, usually by hydrolysis, of the NH_2 radical from an amino compound.

dean [L *decanus* chief of ten], the chief executive and educational officer of a unit of a university, school, or college.

deanol /dē′ənol/, a psychostimulant prescribed in the treatment of learning problems and hyperkinetic-behavior problems.

death [AS], **1. apparent death,** the cessation of life as indicated by the absence of heartbeat or respiration. **2. legal death,** the total absence of activity in the brain and central nervous system, the cardiovascular system, and the respiratory system as observed and declared by a physician.

death instinct, instinctive behavior that tends to be self-destructive.

death mask [AS *déath;* Fr *masque*], a mask made from a plaster of paris cast of the face of a dead person.

death rate, the number of deaths occurring within a specified population during a particular time period, usually expressed in terms of deaths per 1,000 persons per year.

death rattle, a sound produced by air moving through mucus that has accumulated in the throat of a dying person after loss of the cough reflex.

death trance, a state in which a person appears to be dead.

"death with dignity" [AS *déath;* L *dignus* worthy], a philosophical concept that a terminally ill patient should be allowed to die naturally, rather than experience a comatose, vegetative life prolonged needlessly by mechanical support systems.

debilitating /dibi′itā′ting/, pertaining to a disease or injury that enfeebles, weakens, or otherwise disables a person.

debility /dibil′itē/, feebleness, weakness, or loss of strength.

debride /dibrēd′/ [Fr *debridle* remove], to remove dirt, foreign objects, damaged tissue, and cellular debris from a wound or a burn to prevent infection and to promote healing. In treating a wound, debridement is the first step in cleansing it. **–debridement** /debrēdmäN′/, *n.*

debris /dəbrē′/, the dead, diseased, or damaged tissue and any foreign material that is to be removed from a wound or other area being treated.

decalcification /dēkal′sifikā′shən/ [L *de* + *calyx* lime, *facere* to make], loss of calcium salts from the teeth and bones caused by malnutrition, malabsorption, or other dietary or physiologic factors. It may result from a diet that lacks adequate calcium. Malabsorption may be caused by a lack of vitamin D necessary for the absorption of calcium from the intestine, by an excess of dietary fats that can combine with calcium, by the presence of oxalic acid that can combine with calcium, or by a relative lack of acid in the digestive tract.

Other factors include the parathyroid hormone control of the calcium level in the bloodstream, the ratio of calcium to phosphorus in the blood, and the relative activity of osteoblast cells that form calcium deposits in the bones and teeth and osteoclast cells that absorb calcium from bones and teeth.

decannulation /dēkan'yəlā'shən/ [L *de* from, *cannula* small reed], the removal of a cannula or tube that may have been inserted during a surgical procedure.

decanoic acid. See **capric acid.**

decay product /dika'/[L *de* + *cadere* to fall; *producere* to produce], (in radiology) a stable or radioactive nuclide formed directly from the radioactive disintegration of a radionuclide or as a result of successive transformation in a radioactive series.

deceleration /dēsel'ərā'shən/ [L *de* + *accelerare* to hasten], a decrease in the speed or velocity of an object or reaction.

deceleration phase, (in obstetrics) the latter part of active labor characterized by a decreased rate of dilatation of the cervical os on a Friedman curve.

decerebrate posture /dēser'əbrāt/ [L *de* + *cerebrum* brain; *ponere* to place], the position of a patient, who is usually comatose, in which the arms are extended and internally rotated and the legs are extended with the feet in forced plantar flexion. The posture is usually observed in patients afflicted by compression of the brainstem at a low level.

decerebration /dēser'abrā'shən/ [L *de* + *cerebrum,*], the process of removing the brain or of cutting the brainstem above the level of the red nucleus, thus eliminating cerebral function.

decibel (dB) /des'əbəl/ [L *decimus* one tenth, *bel* Alexander G. Bell], a unit of measure of the intensity of sound. A decibel is 0.1 of 1 bel; an increase of 1 bel is perceived as an approximate doubling of loudness, based on a sound-pressure reference level of 0.0002 dyn/cc.

decidua /disij'oo-ə/ [L *decidere* to fall off], the epithelial tissue of the endometrium lining the uterus. It envelops the conceptus during gestation and is shed in the puerperium. It is also shed periodically during menstruation.

decidua basalis, the decidua of the endometrium in the uterus that lies beneath the implanted ovum.

decidua capsularis, the decidua of the endometrium of the uterus covering the implanted ovum.

decidual endometritis /disij'oo-əl/, an inflammation or infection of any portion of the decidua during pregnancy.

decidua menstrualis, the endometrium shed during menstruation.

decidua parietalis. See **decidua vera.**

decidua reflexa. See **decidua capsularis.**

decidua serotina. See **decidua basalis.**

decidua vera, the decidua of the endometrium lining the uterus except for those areas beneath and above the implanted and developing ovum called, respectively, the decidua basalis and the decidua capsularis.

deciduoma /disij'oo-ō'mə/, a tumor of the endometrial tissue of the uterus. A deciduoma tends to develop after a pregnancy, regardless of the outcome of the pregnancy. It may be benign or malignant.

deciduous dentition. See **deciduous tooth.**

deciduous tooth /disij'oo-əs/ [L *decidere* to fall off; AS *toth*], any one of the set of 20 teeth that appear normally during infancy, consisting of four incisors, two canines, and four molars in each jaw. Deciduous teeth start developing at about the sixth week of fetal life. In most individuals the first deciduous tooth erupts through the gum about 6 months after birth. Thereafter, one or more deciduous teeth erupt about every month until all 20 have appeared. The deciduous teeth are usually shed between the ages of 6 and 13.

decisional conflict, a NANDA-accepted nursing diagnosis of uncertainty about the course of action to be taken when choice among competing actions involves risk, loss, or challenge to personal life values. The focus of conflict is to be specified, such as choices regarding health, family relationships, career, or finances. Defining characteristics include verbalized feelings of distress related to uncertainty about choices or undesired consequences of alternative actions being considered, vacillation between alternative choices, delayed decision making, and physical signs of distress, such as increased heart rate, increased muscle tension, and restlessness.

decoction /dikok'shən/ [L *de* + *coquere* to cook], a liquid medicine made from an extract of water-soluble substances, usually with the aid of boiling water. Herbal remedies are usually decoctions.

decode, to interpret coded information into a form usable by people.

decoded message, (in communication theory) a message as translated by a receiver.

decoic acid. See **capric acid.**

decompensation /dē'kəmpənsā'shən/ [L *de* + *compensare* to weigh together], the failure of a system, as cardiac decompensation in heart failure.

decomposition /dē'kəmpəsish'ən/ [L *de* + *componere* to put together], the dissolution of a substance into simpler chemical forms.

decompression /dē'kəmpresh'ən/ [L *de* + *comprimere* to press together], **1.** a technique used to readapt an individual to normal atmospheric pressure after exposure to higher pressures, as in diving. **2.** the removal of pressure caused by gas or fluid in a body cavity, as the stomach or intestinal tract.

decompression sickness, a painful, sometimes fatal syndrome caused by the formation of nitrogen bubbles in the tissues of divers, caisson workers, and aviators who move too rapidly from environments of higher to those of lower atmospheric pressures. Gaseous nitrogen then accumulates in the joint spaces and peripheral circulation, impairing tissue oxygenation. Disorientation, severe pain, and syncope follow. Treatment is by rapid return of the patient to an environment of higher pressure followed by gradual decompression.

decongestant /dē-konjes'tənt/ [L *de* + *congerere* to pile up], **1.** of or pertaining to a substance or procedure that eliminates or reduces congestion or swelling. **2.** a decongestant drug. Antihistaminic agents and adrenergic drugs that cause bronchodilatation or vasoconstriction of nasal mucosa are used as decongestants.

decontamination /dē'kəmtam'inā'shən/, the process of making a person, object, or environment free of microorganisms, radioactivity, or other contaminants.

decorticate posture /dēkôr'tikāt/ [L *de* + *cortex* bark; *ponere* to place], the position of a comatose patient in which the upper extremities are rigidly flexed at the elbows and at the wrists. The decorticate posture indicates a lesion in a mesencephalic region of the brain.

decortication /dēkôr'tikā'shən/ [L *de* + *cortex* bark], (in medicine) the removal of the cortical tissue of an organ or structure, such as the kidney, the brain, and the lung. **–decorticate,** *v., adj.*

decrement /dek'rəmənt/ [L *de* + *crescere* to grow], a decrease or stage of decline, as of a uterine contraction.

decremental conduction /dek'rəmen'təl/, (in cardiology) conduction that slows progressively as the effectiveness of the propagating impulse gradually decreases.

decrudescence /dē'krŏŏdes'əns/ [L *de* + *crudescere* to become bad], a decrease in the severity of symptoms.

decubital /dikyŏŏ'bitəl/ [L *decumbere* to lie down], pertaining to bedsores.

decubitus /dikyŏŏ'bitəs/ [L *decumbere*], a recumbent or horizontal position, as lateral decubitus, which is lying on one side.

decubitus care, the management and prevention of decubitus ulcers that occur most frequently on the sacrum, elbows, heels, outer ankles, inner knees, hips, shoulder blades, and ear rims of immobilized patients, especially those who are obese, elderly, or suffering from infections, injuries, or a poor nutritional state. Decubiti may be prevented by repositioning the immobile patient every 2 hours, keeping the skin dry, and inspecting pressure areas every 4 to 6 hours for signs of redness.

decubitus posture, the position acquired by a bedridden patient to rest on his or her side to relieve the pressure of body weight on the sacrum, heels, or other body areas vulnerable to decubitus ulcers.

decubitus projection, (in radiology) a position for producing a radiograph of the chest or abdomen of a patient who is lying down, with the central ray parallel to the horizon. Variations of the position include left and right AP oblique, dorsal decubitus, ventral decubitus, and left and right lateral decubitus.

decubitus ulcer, an inflammation, sore, or ulcer in the skin over a bony prominence. It results from ischemic hypoxia of the tissues because of prolonged pressure on the part. The sores are graded by stages of severity. Stage I: The skin is red; with massage and relief of pressure, the color of the skin does not return to normal. Stage II: The skin is blistered, peeling, or cracked, although damage is still superficial. Stage III: The skin is broken; a full thickness of skin is lost, subcutaneous tissue may also be damaged, and a serous or bloody drainage may be seen. Stage IV: A deep, craterlike ulcer has formed. The full thickness of skin and the subcutaneous tissues are destroyed. Fascia, connective tissue, bone, or muscle underlying the ulcer are exposed and may be damaged.

decussate /dəcus'āt/ [L *decussis* intersection], to cross in the form of an "X," as certain nerve fibers from the retina cross at the optic chiasm. **–decussation,** *n.*

decussation /di'kusā'shən/ [L *decussare* to make a cross], a crossing of central nervous system fibers in the brain, with some fibers on the left side crossing to the right side and vice versa.

decussation of pyramids, the crossing of nerve fibers of the corticospinal motor tract at the ventral side on the lower portion of the medulla oblongata.

deduction [L *deducere* to lead], a system of reasoning that leads from a known principle to an unknown, or from the general to the specific. Deductive reasoning is used to test diagnostic hypotheses.

deemed status [AS *deman* to judge; L, a

standing], a status conferred on a hospital by a professional standards review organization (PSRO) in formal recognition that the hospital's review, continued-stay review, and medical care evaluation programs meet certain effectiveness criteria.

deep brachial artery [As *dyppan* to dip; Gk *brachion* arm; *arteria* air pipe], a branch of each of the brachial arteries arising at the distal border of the teres major and supplying the humerus and the muscles of the upper arm.

deep breathing and coughing exercises, the exercises taught to a person to improve aeration or to maintain respiratory function, especially after prolonged inactivity or after general anesthesia. Incisional pain after surgery in the chest or abdomen often inhibits normal respiratory excursion.

deep fascia, the most extensive of three kinds of fascia comprising an intricate series of connective sheets and bands that hold the muscles and other structures in place throughout the body, wrapping the muscles in gray, feltlike membranes.

deep heat, the application of heat in the treatment of deep body tissues, particularly muscles and tendons. The thermal effects may be produced with shortwave therapy, phonophoresis, or ultrasound.

deep palmar arch, the termination of the radial artery, joining the deep palmar branch of the ulnar artery in the palm of the hand.

deep reflexes [ME *dep* hollow; L *reflectere* to bend back], any reflex caused by stimulation of a deep body structure, such as a tendon reflex.

deep sensation, the awareness or perception of pain, pressure, or tension in the deep layers of the skin, the muscles, tendons, or joints.

deep structure, (in neurolinguistics) the deeper experience and meaning to which surface structures in a communication may refer.

deep temporal artery, one of the branches of the maxillary artery on each side of the head. It branches into the anterior portion and the posterior portion to supply the temporalis.

deep tendon reflex (DTR), a brisk contraction of a muscle in response to a sudden stretch induced by a sharp tap on the tendon of insertion of the muscle. Absence of the reflex may have been caused by damage to the muscle, the peripheral nerve, nerve roots, or the spinal cord at that level. Kinds of deep tendon reflexes include **Achilles tendon, biceps, brachioradialis, patellar,** and **triceps reflex.**

deep vein, one of the many systemic veins that accompany the arteries, usually enclosed in a sheath that wraps both the vein and the associated artery. The larger arteries are usually accompanied by only one deep vein. The deep veins accompanying the smaller arteries occur usually in pairs, one vein on each side of the artery.

deep vein thrombosis, a disorder involving a thrombus in one of the deep veins of the body. Symptoms include tenderness, pain, swelling, warmth, and discoloration of the skin. A deep vein thrombus is potentially life threatening, and treatment is directed toward prevention of movement of the thrombus toward the lungs.

deep x-ray therapy, the treatment of internal neoplasms, such as Wilms' tumor of the kidney, Hodgkin's disease, and other cancers, with ionizing radiation from an external source. Deep x-ray therapy is beamed directly to the site, reducing side scatter.

deerfly fever. See **tularemia.**

defamation [L *diffamare* to discredit], any communication, written or spoken, that is untrue and that injures the good name or reputation of another or that in any way brings that person into disrepute.

default judgment [L *defallere* to lack; *judicare* to decide], (in law) a judgment rendered against a defendant because of the defendant's failure to appear in court or to answer the plaintiff's claim within the proper time.

defecation /def′ikā′shən/ [L *defaecare* to clean], the elimination of feces from the digestive tract through the rectum.

defecation reflex. See **rectal reflex.**

defecography /def′əkog′rəfē/, a radiographic procedure for evaluating the rectum and anal canal of children with fecal incontinence. The child is examined while sitting on a radiolucent toilet seat or potty.

defective [L *defectus* a failing], pertaining to something that is imperfect, or, as in an outdated term, to an individual who may be suffering from a any disorder.

defendant, (in law) the party that is named in a plaintiff's complaint and against whom the plaintiff's allegations are made. The defendant must respond to the allegations.

defense mechanism [L *defendere* to repulse; *mechanicus* machine], an unconscious, intrapsychic reaction that offers protection to the self from a stressful situation. Kinds of defense mechanisms include **compensation, conversion, dissociation, displacement,** and **sublimation.**

defensin /difen′sin/, a peptide with natural antibiotic activity found within human neutrophils. Three types of defensins have been identified, each consisting of a chain of about 30 amino acids.

defensive radical therapy, (in psychology) a therapeutic technique intended as a survival tactic. The therapist begins at the patient's present state and uses encouragement to help the patient avoid self-defeating behavior.

deferent duct. See **vas deferens.**

deferoxamine mesylate /dē'fərok'səmēn/, a chelating agent prescribed in the treatment of acute iron intoxication and chronic iron overload.

defervescence /di'fərves'əns/ [L *defervescere* to reduce heat], the diminishing or disappearance of a fever. **–defervescent,** *adj.*

defibrillate /difi'brilāt, difib'-/ [L *de* + *fibrilla* little thread], to stop fibrillation of the ventricles by delivering an electric shock through the chest wall.

defibrillation /difi'brilā'shən/, the termination of ventricular fibrillation by delivering an electric shock to the patient's precordium.

defibrillator /difi'brilā'tər, difib'-/, a device that delivers an electric shock at a preset voltage to the myocardium through the chest wall. It is used for restoring the normal cardiac rhythm and rate when the heart has stopped beating or is fibrillating.

deficiency disease [L *de* + *facere* to make; *dis* opposite of; Fr *aise* ease], a condition resulting from the lack of one or more essential nutrients in the diet, from metabolic dysfunction, or from impaired digestion or absorption, excessive excretion, or increased biological requirements.

deficiency of sweating [AS *swaetan*], a failure of the sweat glands to secrete perspiration in normal amounts. The condition may be the result of a congenital defect, a blockage of the sweat ducts as a sequel to prickly heat, excessive heat, or conditions such as hemorrhage or diarrhea that cause a loss of body fluid.

deficit, any deficiency or difference from what is normal, such as an oxygen deficit, a cause of hypoxia.

definitive /difin'ətiv/ [L *definitivus* a limiting], **1.** final; clearly established without doubt or question. **2.** (in embryology) fully formed in the final differentiation of a tissue, structure, or organ. **3.** (in parasitology) of or pertaining to the host in which the parasite undergoes the sexual phase of its reproductive cycle.

definitive host, any animal in which the reproductive stages of a parasite develop. The female *Anopheles* mosquito is the definitive host for malaria. Humans are definitive hosts for pinworms, schistosomes, and tapeworms.

definitive prosthesis, a permanent prosthetic device that replaces an immediate-fit appliance, such as a pylon.

definitive treatment, any therapy generally accepted as a specific cure of a disease.

defloration /def'lôrā'shən/ [L *de* + *flos* flower, *atio* process], the rupture of the vaginal hymen. Defloration may occur during sexual intercourse, during a gynecologic examination, or by surgery if necessary to remove an obstruction to menstrual flow.

deformity [L *deformis* misshapen], a condition of being distorted, disfigured, flawed, malformed, or misshapen that may affect the body in general or any part of it and may be the result of disease, injury, or birth defect.

degeneration [L *degenerare* to become unlike others], the gradual deterioration of normal cells and body functions.

degenerative [L *degenerare*], pertaining to or involving degeneration or changing to a lower form or dysfunctional form.

degenerative chorea. See **Huntington's chorea.**

degenerative disease /dijen'ərətiv/, any disease in which there is deterioration of structure or function of tissue. Some kinds of degenerative disease are **arteriosclerosis, cancer,** and **osteoarthritis.**

degenerative joint disease. See **osteoarthritis.**

degenerative lesion [L *degenerare* + *laesio* hurting], an injury or disease state that results in loss of function.

degenerative neuralgia [L *degenerare*; Gk *neuron* nerve, *algos* pain], a form of neuralgia caused by degenerative changes in nervous tissue, usually affecting older individuals.

degenerative neuritis [L *degenerare*; Gk *neuron* nerve, *itis* inflammation], an inflammation caused by degenerative changes in nervous tissue.

degloving [L *de* + AS *glof*], **1.** an injury to a finger in which the soft tissue down to the bone, including neurovascular bundles and sometimes tendons, is peeled off the finger. **2.** (in dentistry) the exposure of the bony mandibular anterior or posterior regions by oral surgery.

deglutition /di'glōōtish'ən/ [L *deglutire* to swallow], swallowing.

deglutition apnea, the normal absence of respiration during swallowing.

degradation [L *de* + *gradus* step], the reduction of a chemical compound to a compound less complex, usually by splitting off one or more groups or subgroups of atoms, such as deamination.

dehiscence /dihis'əns/ [L *dehiscere* to

gape], the separation of a surgical incision or rupture of a wound closure.

dehumanization [L *de* + *humanitas* human nature], the process of losing altruistic qualities, as may occur in some psychotic states.

dehydrate /dihī′drāt/ [L *de* + Gk *hydor* water], **1.** to remove or lose water from a substance. **2.** to lose excessive water from the body. **–dehydration** *n.*

dehydrated alcohol, a clear, colorless, highly hygroscopic liquid with a burning taste, containing at least 99.5% ethyl alcohol by volume.

dehydration, 1. excessive loss of water from the body tissues. Dehydration is accompanied by a disturbance in the balance of essential electrolytes, particularly sodium, potassium, and chloride. Signs of dehydration include poor skin turgor, flushed dry skin, coated tongue, oliguria, irritability, and confusion. **2.** rendering a substance free from water.

dehydration fever, a fever that frequently occurs in newborns, thought to be caused by dehydration.

dehydration of gingivae, the drying of gingival tissue, often the result of mouth breathing, which lowers the resistance of the gingival tissue to infection.

deinstitutionalization [L *de* + *instituere* to put in place], the transfer to a community setting of a patient who has been hospitalized for an extended period, generally many years.

Deiters' nucleus /dī′tərz, dē′[tərz/ [Otto F. C. Deiters, German anatomist, b. 1834], one of the vestibular nuclei located in the brainstem.

déjà vu /dāzhävY′, -vē′, -vōō′/ [Fr, previously seen], the sensation or illusion that one is encountering a set of circumstances or a place that was previously experienced. The phenomenon results from some unconscious emotional connection with the present experience.

Déjérine-Sottas disease /dezh′ərinsot′əz/ [Joseph J. Déjérine, French neurologist, b. 1849; Jules Sottas, French neurologist, b. 1866], a rare, congenital spinocerebellar disorder characterized by the development of palpable thickenings along peripheral nerves, degeneration of the peripheral nervous system, pain, paresthesia, ataxia, diminished sensation, and deep tendon reflexes.

del, (in cytogenetics) abbreviation for **deletion.**

Delano, Jane A. (1862–1919), an American nurse who organized the American Red Cross Nursing Service, an organization formed to supply nurses to the military forces.

delayed echolalia [Fr *delai* time extension; Gk *echo* sound, *lalein* to babble], a phenomenon, commonly seen in schizophrenia, involving the meaningless, automatic repetition of overheard words and phrases. It occurs hours, days, or even weeks after the original stimulus.

delayed graft, a type of skin graft that is partially elevated and replaced for use in a later transfer.

delayed hypersensitivity reaction. See **cell-mediated immune response.**

delayed postpartum hemorrhage, hemorrhage occurring later than 24 hours after delivery. It is most often caused by retained fragments of the placenta, a laceration of the cervix or vagina that was not discovered or that was not completely sutured, or by subinvolution of the placental site within the uterus.

delayed sensation, a feeling or impression that is not experienced immediately after a stimulus.

delayed symptom [Fr *délai;* Gk *symptoma* that which happens], a symptom, such as shock, that may not appear until after the precipitating cause.

delayed treatment seeker, (in psychology) a person who delays seeking treatment for a problematic life event until months or years after the event, usually following a precipitating event such as an anniversary reaction.

Delecato-Doman theory, a therapeutic concept that full neurologic organization of a disabled or mentally retarded child requires that the child pass through developmental patterns covering progressively higher anatomic levels of the nervous system.

deleterious /del′itir′ē-əs/ [Gk *deleterios* destroyer], pertaining to something that is harmful or dangerous.

deletion (del) [L *deletionum* destruction], (in cytogenetics) the loss of a piece of a chromosome because it has broken away from the genetic material.

deletion syndrome, any of a group of congenital autosomal anomalies that result from the loss of chromosomal genetic material because of breakage of a chromatid during cell division, as the cat-cry syndrome, which results from the absence of the short arm of chromosome 5.

Delhi boil. See **oriental sore.**

deliberate biologic programing [L *deliberare* to weigh carefully], the Hayflick theory of aging based on studies showing that human cells contain biologic clocks that predetermine death after undergoing mitosis a finite number of times.

deliberate hypotension, an anesthetic process in which a short-acting hypotensive agent such as sodium nitroprusside or trimethaphan camsylate is given to reduce blood pressure and thus bleeding during surgery.

delinquency [L *delinquere* to fail], **1.** negligence or failure to fulfill a duty or obligation. **2.** an offense, fault, misdemeanor, or misdeed; a tendency to commit such acts.

delinquent, 1. characterized by neglect of duty or violation of law. **2.** one whose behavior is characterized by persistent antisocial, illegal, violent, or criminal acts; a juvenile delinquent.

délire de toucher /dālir'dət ōōshā'/ [Fr], an abnormal desire or irresistable urge to touch or handle objects.

delirious mania, an extreme form of the manic state in which activity is so frenzied, confused, and incoherent that it is difficult to discern any link between affect and behavior.

delirium /dilir'ē·əm/ [L *delirare* to rave], **1.** a state of frenzied excitement or wild enthusiasm. **2.** an acute organic mental disorder characterized by confusion, disorientation, restlessness, clouding of the consciousness, incoherence, fear, anxiety, excitement, and often illusions, hallucinations, usually of visual origin, and at times delusions. The condition is caused by disturbances in cerebral functions that may result from a wide range of metabolic disorders, including nutritional deficiencies and endocrine imbalances; postpartum or postoperative stress; the ingestion of toxic substances, as various gases, metals, or drugs, including alcohol; and other causes of physical and mental shock or exhaustion. Kinds of delirium include **acute delirium, delirium tremens, exhaustion delirium, senile delirium,** and **traumatic delirium. –delirious,** *adj.*

delirium of persecution [L *delirare + persecutor* to pursue], a state of clouded consciousness in which the patient believes others are threatening or conspiring against the person.

delirium tremens (DTs), an acute and sometimes fatal psychotic reaction caused by excessive intake of alcoholic beverages over a long time. The reaction may follow a prolonged alcoholic binge without an adequate intake of food, occur during a period of abstinence, be precipitated by a head injury or infection, or result from the partial or total withdrawal of alcohol after prolonged drinking. Initial symptoms include loss of appetite, insomnia, and general restlessness, followed by agitation, excitement, disorientation, mental confusion, vivid and often frightening hallucinations, acute fear and anxiety, illusions and delusions, coarse tremors of the hands, feet, legs, and tongue, fever, increased heart rate, extreme perspiration, GI distress, and precordial pain.

delivery [L *de + liberare* to free], (in obstetrics) the birth of a child; parturition.

delivery room, a unit of a hospital utilized for obstetric delivery and infant resuscitation.

DeLorme technique, a method of physical exercise with weights in which sets of repetitions are repeated with rests between sessions. The technique involves the use of heavier weights and fewer repetitions in successive sets.

delousing /dēlous'sing/ [L *de;* AS *lus*], to rid a person or object of an infestation of lice.

delta /del'ta/, Δ, δ, fourth letter of the Greek alphabet.

delta agent hepatitis [Gk *delta;* L *agere* to do; Gk *hepar* liver, *itis* inflammation], an infection caused by an RNA virus (δ Ag) associated with the hepatitis B surface antigen (HBsAg) in cases of chronic hepatitis and progressive liver damage. The delta agent apparently is able to induce the infection when it is present along with the B surface antigen.

delta-1-testolactone. See **testolactone.**

delta-9-tetrahydrocannabinol (THC), a pharmacologically active ingredient of cannabis that has been used in treating some cases of nausea and vomiting associated with cancer chemotherapy.

delta optical density analysis [Gk *delta; optikos* of sight; L *densus* thick; Gk, a loosening], a technique used to diagnose anemia in a fetus by measuring the proportion of bilirubin decomposition products in the amniotic fluid. The method involves spectrographic examination of a fluid sample. The data are sometimes expressed in terms of δOD_{450}, representing the wavelength in nm at which maximum absorption of light by bilirubin occurs.

delta wave, 1. the slowest of the four types of brain waves, characterized by a frequency of 4 Hz and a relatively high voltage. Delta waves are "deep-sleep waves" associated with a dreamless state. **2.** (in cardiology) a slurring of the QRS portion of an ECG tracing caused by preexcitation.

deltoid /del'toid/ [Gk *delta* (triangular), *eidos* form], **1.** triangular. **2.** of or pertaining to the deltoid muscle that covers the shoulder.

deltoid ligament [Gk *delta + eidos;* L *ligamentum*], the medial ligament of the ankle joint.

deltoid muscle, a large, thick triangular muscle that covers the shoulder joint and abducts, flexes, extends, and rotates the arm.

delusion /dilo͞o′zhən/ [L *deludere* to deceive], a persistent, aberrant belief or perception held inviolable by a person even though it is illogical, unique, and probably wrong.

delusion of being controlled, the false belief that one's feelings, beliefs, thoughts, and acts are governed by some external force, as seen in various forms of schizophrenia.

delusion of grandeur, the gross exaggeration of one's importance, wealth, power, or talents, as seen in such disorders as megalomania, general paresis, and paranoid schizophrenia.

delusion of persecution, a morbid belief that one is being mistreated and harassed by unidentified enemies, as seen in paranoia and paranoid schizophrenia.

delusion of poverty, (in psychology) a false belief by a person that he or she is impoverished.

delusion of reference. See **idea of reference.**

delusion stupor, the state of lethargy and unresponsiveness observed in catatonic schizophrenia.

demand pacemaker [L *demandere* to give in charge, *passus* step; ME *maken*], a device used to stimulate the heart electrically when the heart's own impulses are not sufficient. Pacemakers can be set to produce a heart beat when the heart's own impulses are not fast enough.

demarcation /dē′märkā′shən/ [L *de* + *marcare* to mark], the process of setting limits or boundaries.

demarcation current, an electric current that flows from an uninjured to an injured end of a muscle.

deme /dēm/ [Gk *demos* common population], a small, closely related, interbreeding population of organisms or individuals, usually occupying a circumscribed area.

demecarium bromide /dē′maker′ē·əm/, an ophthalmic anticholinesterase agent prescribed in the treatment of open-angle glaucoma.

demeclocycline hydrochloride /dēmek′lōsī′klēn/, a tetracycline antibiotic prescribed in the treatment of a variety of infections, including infections in which use of penicillin is contraindicated.

dementia /dimen′shə/ [L *de* + *mens* mind], a progressive, organic mental disorder characterized by chronic personality disintegration, confusion, disorientation, stupor, deterioration of intellectual capacity and function, and impairment of control of memory, judgment, and impulses. Demen-

tia may be caused by drug intoxication, hyperthyroidism, pernicious anemia, paresis, subdural hematoma, benign brain tumor, hydrocephalus, insulin shock, and tumor of islet cells of the pancreas. Kinds of dementia include **Alzheimer's disease, dementia paralytica, Pick's disease, secondary dementia, senile dementia,** and **toxic dementia.**

dementia paralytica. See **general paresis.**

demigauntlet bandage /dem′igônt′lit/ [L *demidus* half; Fr *gant* glove], a glovelike bandage covering only the hand and leaving the fingers free.

demineralization /dēmin′əral′īzā′shən/ [L *de* + *minera* mine], a decrease in the amount of minerals or inorganic salts in tissues, as occurs in certain diseases.

demise [OFr *démettre* to put away], death, destruction, or ceasing to exist.

democratic style, a people-centered leadership style in which the group participates openly in decision making for group goals.

demography /dəmog′rəfē/ [Gk *demos* people, *graphein* to record], the study of human populations, particularly the size, distribution, and characteristics of members of population groups. Demography is applied in studies of health problems involving ethnic groups, populations of a specific geographic region, or religious groups with special dietary restrictions.

demonstrative, an action, such as indicating the size of an object with the hands, that accompanies and illustrates speech.

De Morgan's spots. See **cherry angioma.**

demulcent /dimul′sənt/ [L *demulcere* to stroke down] **1.** any of several oily substances used for soothing and reducing irritation of surfaces that have been abraded or irritated. **2.** soothing, as a counterirritant or balm.

demyelination /dimī′əlinā′shən/ [L *de* + Gk *myelos* marrow], the process of destruction or removal of the myelin sheath from a nerve or nerve fiber.

denaturation /dēnach′ərā′shən/ [L *de* + *natura* natural], **1.** the alteration of the basic nature or structure of a substance. **2.** the process of making a potential food or beverage substance unfit for human consumption, although it may still be used for other purposes, such as a solvent.

denatured alcohol /dēnach′ərātid/, ethyl alcohol made unfit for ingestion by the addition of acetone or methanol, used as a solvent and in chemical processes.

denatured protein [L *de* + *natura* + *proteios* first rank], a protein that has undergone change so that its original properties are lost. A protein can be denatured by radiation, heat, strong acids, or alcohol.

dendrite /den'drīt/ [Gk *dendron* tree], a branching process that extends from the cell body of a neuron. Each neuron usually possesses several dendrites.

dendritic /dendrit'ik/, **1.** treelike, with branches that spread toward or into neighboring tissues, as dendritic keratitis. **2.** of or pertaining to a dendrite.

dendritic calculus [Gk *dendron* tree, *calculus* pebble], a large calculus lodged in the pelvis of the kidney and shaped to fit the branches of the calyx.

dendritic keratitis, a serious herpes virus infection of the eye, characterized by an ulceration of the surface of the cornea resembling a tree with knobs at the ends of the branches. Untreated dendritic keratitis may result in permanent scarring of the cornea with impaired vision or blindness.

dendrodendritic /den'drōdendrit'ik **synapse** [Gk *dendron, dendron* + *synaptein* to join], a type of synapse in which a dendrite of one neuron comes in contact with a dendrite of another neuron.

denervated /dēnur'vātid/ [L *de* + *nervus* nerve], a condition of having a nerve impulse route interrupted, as by excision or administration of a drug that blocks the pathway. This results in decreased or no transmission of impulses through this pathway.

dengue fever /deng'gē, den'gā/ [Sp, influenza; L *febris* fever], an acute arbovirus infection transmitted to humans by the *Aedes* mosquito and occurring in tropic and subtropic regions. The disease usually produces a triad of symptoms: fever, rash, and severe head, back, and muscle pain. Dengue is a self-limited illness, though it may take patients several weeks to recover.

dengue hemorrhagic fever shock syndrome (DHFS), a grave form of dengue fever characterized by shock with collapse or prostration; cold, clammy extremities; a weak, thready pulse; respiratory distress; and all of the symptoms of dengue fever. Hemorrhage, bruises, small reddish spots indicating bleeding from skin capillaries, and bloody vomit, urine, and feces may occur and precede circulatory collapse.

denial /dinī'əl/ [L *denegare* to negate], **1.** refusal or restriction of something requested, claimed, or needed, often resulting in physical or emotional deficiency. **2.** an unconscious defense mechanism in which emotional conflict and anxiety are avoided by refusing to acknowledge those thoughts, feelings, desires, impulses, or external facts that are consciously intolerable.

denial, ineffective, a NANDA-accepted nursing diagnosis of a conscious or unconscious attempt to disavow the knowledge or meaning of an event to reduce anxiety or fear to the detriment of health. The individual delays or refuses medical attention and does not perceive personal relevance of symptoms or danger. Defining characteristics include self-treatment to relieve symptoms, minimizing of symptoms, displacement of the source of symptoms to other organs, and displacement of fear of impact of the condition.

Denis Browne splint [Sir Denis J. W. Browne, English surgeon, b. 1892], a splint for the correction of talipes equinovarus (clubfoot), composed of a curved bar attached to the soles of a pair of high-top shoes.

denitrogenation /dēnī'trōjənā'shən/, the elimination of nitrogen from the lungs and body tissues during a period of breathing pure oxygen.

Denman's spontaneous evolution [Thomas Denman, English physician, b. 1733; L *sponte* voluntarily; *evolvere* to roll forth], a natural, unassisted turning of the fetus from the transverse presentation. The head rotates back and, as the breech descends, the shoulder ascends in the pelvis.

dens, *pl.* **dentes** /den'tēz/ [L, tooth], **1.** a tooth or toothlike structure or process. The term is sometimes modified to identify a particular tooth, such as dens caninus. **2.** the cone-shaped odontoid process of the axis, or second cervical vertebra.

dens deciduus. See **deciduous tooth.**

dense fibrous tissue [L *densus* thick], a fibrous connective tissue consisting of compact, strong, inelastic bundles of parallel collagenous fibers that have a glistening white color.

dens in dente /den'tə/, an anomaly of the teeth, found chiefly in the maxillary lateral incisors and characterized by invagination of the enamel.

densitometer /den'sitom'ətər/ [L *densus* + Gk *metron* measure], a device that uses a photoelectric cell to detect differences in the density of light transmitted through a liquid.

density [L *densus* thick], **1.** the amount of mass of a substance in a given volume. The greater the mass in a given volume, the greater the density. **2.** (in radiology) the degree of x-ray film blackening.

density gradient, the variation of the concentration of a solute in a confined solution.

dens serotinus. See **wisdom tooth.**

dental [L *dens* tooth], of or pertaining to a tooth or teeth.

dental abscess, an abscess that forms in bone or soft tissues of the jaw as a result of an infection that may follow dental caries or injury to a tooth. Symptoms include pain that may be continuous and exacerbated by hot or cold foods or the pressure of closing the jaws firmly.

dental alveolus /alvē´ələs/, a tooth socket in the mandible or maxilla.

dental amalgam, an alloy of silver, tin, and mercury with small amounts of copper and sometimes zinc, used for filling tooth cavities.

dental anesthesia, any of several anesthetic procedures used in dental surgery.

dental anomaly, an aberration in which one or more teeth deviate from the normal in form, function, or position.

dental appliance, any device used by a dentist for a specific purpose, such as an orthodontic appliance used to correct malocclusion.

dental arch, the curving shape formed by the arrangement of a normal set of teeth.

dental assistant, a person who assists a dentist in the performance of generalized tasks, including chairside assistance, clerical work, reception, and some radiography and dental laboratory work.

dental biomechanics, the field of biomechanics that deals with the biologic effects of dental restoration on oral structures.

dental calculus, a salivary deposit of calcium phosphate and calcium carbonate with organic matter on the teeth or a dental prosthesis.

dental caries, a plaque disease caused by the complex interaction of food, especially starches and sugars, with bacteria that form dental plaque. This material adheres to the surfaces of the teeth and provides the medium for the growth of bacteria and the production of organic acids that cause breaks in the enamel sheath of the tooth. Enzymes produced by the bacteria then attack the protein component of the tooth. This process, if untreated, ultimately leads to the formation of deep cavities and bacterial infection of the pulp chamber and nerves. The term is also applied to any lesion caused by demineralization of a tooth. Kinds of dental caries include **active caries, arrested caries, primary caries,** and **secondary caries.**

dental crypt, the space occupied by a developing tooth.

dental engine, an apparatus consisting of a hand instrument to which various rotating tools or drills can be fitted. It is driven by an electric motor.

dental erosion, the chemical or mechanicochemical destruction of a tooth substance that causes variously shaped con-cavities at the cementoenamel junctions of teeth. The surfaces of these depressions, unlike those of carious cavities, are hard and smooth.

dental ethics, a sense of moral obligation and a system of moral principles governing the professional conduct of dental and dental hygiene practices.

dental extracting forceps, a type of forceps used for grasping teeth in extractions.

dental film, a type of x-ray film made for either intraoral or extraoral exposure. Intraoral films are small, double-emulsion films without screens but with a lead foil backing to reduce patient dose. Extraoral films are large single-emulsion screen films.

dental fistula, an abnormal passage from the apical periodontal area of a tooth to the surface of oral mucous membrane.

dental floss, a waxed or unwaxed thread used to clean tooth surfaces and spaces between the teeth.

dentalgia /dental´jē·ə/ [L *dens* tooth; Gk *algos* pain], toothache.

dental granuloma, a pathologic condition characterized by a mass of granulation tissue which is surrounded by a fibrous capsule attached to the apex of a pulp-involved tooth.

dental hygienist, a person with special training to provide dental services under the supervision of a dentist. Services supplied by a dental hygienist include dental prophylaxis, radiography, application of medications, and provision of dental education at chairside and in the community.

dental identification, the process of establishing the unique characteristics of the teeth and dental work of an individual, thereby leading to the identification of an individual by comparison with the person's dental charts and records.

dental implant, a plastic or metal device that is implanted in the jaw bones to provide permanent support for fixed bridges or dentures when there is insufficient bony ridge to support a denture.

dental jurisprudence [L *dens* + *juris prudentia,* knowledge of the law], the application of the principles of law as they relate to the practice of dentistry, and the relations of dentists to patients, to society, and to each other.

dental laboratory technician, a person who makes dental prostheses and orthodontic appliances as prescribed by a dentist. The dental laboratory technician may have a private laboratory or work in the premises of a dentist.

dental operculum [L *dens* + *operculum* a covering structure], a hood or flap of gingival tissue overlying the crown of an erupting tooth. This tissue disappears as the tooth erupts by being chewed away.

dental papilla [L *dens* + *papilla* a nipple-shaped projection], a small mass of mesenchymal tissue in the enamel organ, which differentiates into dentin and dental pulp. The innermost layer consists of a cell-free zone of reticular fibers that form the basement membrane.

dental pathology. See **oral pathology, pathodontia.**

dental plaque. See **bacterial plaque.**

dental plate, a dental prosthesis made to the shape of the maxillary or mandibular jaw to support artificial teeth.

dental probe. See **periodontal probe.**

dental prosthesis [L *dens;* Gk *prosthesis* an addition], a fixed or removable appliance to replace one or more lost natural teeth.

dental pulp, a small mass of connective tissue, blood vessels, and nerves located in a chamber within the dentin and enamel layers of a tooth.

dental radiograph [L *dens, radire* to shine; Gk, *graphein,* to record], an intraoral and extraoral x-ray of teeth and the bone surrounding them.

dental restoration. See **restoration.**

dental root cyst. See **periodontal cyst.**

dental sealants, plastic film coatings that are applied and adhere to the chewing surfaces of teeth to seal pits and grooves where food and bacteria usually become trapped.

dental stone. See **artificial stone.**

dental surgeon [L *dens;* Gk, *cheirourgos,* surgeon], a dentist who specializes in the teeth and surrounding oral tissues. An **operative dental surgeon** is concerned with the restoration of teeth that have been damaged. An **oral and maxillofacial surgeon** specializes in surgically reconstructing facial malformations due to diseases of the head and neck or traumatic accidents. An **oral surgeon** specializes in the surgical removal of the teeth and surrounding oral tissues.

dental technician. See **dental laboratory technician.**

dentate fracture /den′tāt/ [L *dens*], any fracture that causes serrated bone ends that fit together like the teeth of gears.

dentate nucleus, a deep cerebellar nucleus that receives fibers from the lateral zone of the cerebellar cortex and appears to act as a trigger for the motor cortex, governing intentional movements as well as properties of ongoing movements.

denticle /den′tikəl/, a calcified body in the pulp chamber of a tooth.

dentifrice /den′tifris/ [L *dens* + *fricare* to rub], a pharmaceutic compound used with a toothbrush for cleaning and polishing the teeth. It typically contains a mild abrasive, a detergent, flavoring agent, and a binder.

dentigerous cyst /dentij′ərəs/ [L *dens* + *gerere* to bear], one of three kinds of follicular cyst, consisting of an epithelium-lined sac, filled with fluid or viscous material that surrounds the crown of an unerupted tooth or odontoma.

dentin /den′tin/ [L *dens*], the chief material of teeth, surrounding the pulp and situated inside of the enamel and cementum. Harder and denser than bone, it consists of solid organic substratum infiltrated with lime salts.

dentin eburnation /ē′burnā′shən/, a change in carious teeth in which softened and decalcified dentin develops a hard, brown, polished appearance.

dentin globule, a small spheric body in peripheral dentin, created by early calcification.

dentinoenamel /den′tinō·inam′əl/ [L *dens* + OFr *enesmail* enamel], pertaining to both the dentin and the enamel of the teeth.

dentinoenamel junction, the interface of enamel and dentin of a tooth crown, generally conforming to the shape of the crown.

dentinogenesis /den′tinōjen′əsis/ [L *dens* + Gk *genein* to produce], the formation of the dentin of the teeth. **–dentinogenic,** *adj.*

dentinogenesis imperfecta, hereditary dysplasia of dentin of deciduous and permanent teeth in which brown, opalescent dentin overgrows and obliterates the pulp cavity. The teeth have short roots and wear rapidly.

dentist [L *dens*], a person who is qualified by training and licensed by the state to practice dentistry. Training requires a minimum of 2 years, preferably 4, in an undergraduate college and a satisfactory score on a Dental Aptitude Test (DAT), followed by 4 years at an ADA-accredited dental college. After completing dental college, a dentist is awarded a degree of either Doctor of Dental Surgery (DDS) or Doctor of Dental Medicine (DMD), which are equivalent degrees.

dentistry [L *dens*], the art and science of practicing the prevention and treatment of diseases and disorders of the teeth and surrounding structures of the oral cavity. Responsibilities include the repair and restoration of teeth and replacement of missing teeth, as well as the detection of signs of diseases, such as tumors, that would require treatment by a physician. There are eight recognized specialties, each requiring additional training after graduation from a dental college: **endodontics, oral pathology, maxofacial surgery, orthodontics, pediatric dentistry, periodontics, prosthodontics,** and **public health dentistry.**

dentition /dentish′ən/ [L *dentire* to cut teeth], **1.** the development and eruption of the teeth. **2.** the arrangement, number, and kind of teeth as they appear in the dental arch of the mouth. **3.** the teeth of an individual or species as determined by their form and arrangement. Kinds of dentition include **artificial, deciduous, mixed, natural, permanent, precocious, predeciduous,** and **retarded dentition.**

dentoalveolar abscess /den′tō·alvē′ələr/ [L *dens* + *alveolus* little hollow; *abscedere* to go away], the formation and accumulation of pus in a tooth socket or the jawbone around the base of a tooth.

dentoalveolar cyst. See **periodontal cyst.**

dentoenamel junction. See **dentinoenamel junction.**

dentofacial, of or pertaining to an oral or gnathic structure.

dentofacial anomaly, an abnormality in which an oral or gnathic structure deviates from the normal in form, function, or position.

dentogenesis imperfecta /den′tōjen′əsis/, **1.** a genetic disturbance of the dentin, characterized by early calcification of the pulp chambers, marked attrition, and an opalescent hue to the teeth. **2.** a localized form of mesodermal dysplasia affecting the dentin of the teeth. It may be hereditary and associated with osteogenesis imperfecta. **3.** a genetic condition that produces defective dentin but normal tooth enamel.

dentogingival fiber /den′tōjinjī′vəl/ [L *dens* + *gingiva* gum], any one of the many fibers that spread like a fan, emerge from the supraalveolar portion of the cementum, and terminate in the free gingiva.

dentogingival junction, the junction between the gingival attachment, a nonkeratinized epithelium, and the surface of the teeth.

dentoperiosteal fiber /den′tōper′ē·os′tē·əl/ [L *dens* + Gk *peri* around, *osteon* bone], any one of the many fibers that emerge from the supraalveolar part of the cementum of a tooth and extend into the mucoperiosteum of the attached gingiva.

dentulous /den′tyələs/ [L *dens* + *-ulosus* characterized by], possessing one or more natural teeth.

dentulous dental arch, a dental arch that contains natural teeth.

denture /den′chər/ [L *dens*], an artificial tooth or a set of artificial teeth not permanently fixed or implanted.

denture base, 1. the portion of a denture that fits the oral mucosa of the basal seat and supports artificial teeth. **2.** the part of a denture that covers the soft tissue of the mouth, commonly made of resin or a combination of resins and metal.

denture flask, a sectional metal case in which plaster of paris or artificial stone is molded to process dentures or other resin restorations.

denture packing, the laboratory procedure of filling and compressing a denturebase material into a mold in a flask.

denturist /den′chərist/, a person who performs the same type of work as a dental technician but without a dentist's prescription, providing dental prostheses directly to clients.

denucleated /dēnyo͞o′klē·ā′tid/ [L *de* + *nucleus* nut], a condition in which the nucleus has been removed.

Denver Articulation Screening Examination (DASE), a test for evaluating the clarity of pronunciation in children between 2 ½ and 6 years of age. Each child's performance may be compared with a standardized norm for the age.

Denver classification, the system of identifying and classifying human chromosomes according to the criteria established at the Denver (1960), London (1963), and Chicago (1966) conferences of cytogeneticists. It is based on chromosome size and position of the centromere as determined during mitotic metaphase and is divided into seven major groups, designated A through G, which are arranged according to decreasing length.

Denver Developmental Screening Test (DDST), a test for evaluating development in children from 1 month to 6 years of age. The developmental level of motor, social, and language skills is expressed as a ratio in which the child's age is the denominator and the age at which the norm possesses skills equal to those of the child being tested is the numerator.

deodorant [L *de* + *odor* smell], **1.** destroying or masking odors. **2.** a substance that destroys or masks odors. Underarm deodorants contain an antiperspirant, as aluminum chloride, aluminum hydroxyl, aluminum sulfate, or aluminum zirconyl hydroxychloride. These aluminum salts form an obstructive hydroxide gel in sweat ducts. Some underarm deodorants contain antibacterial agents or fragrances. Vaginal deodorant sprays contain a fatty ester emollient, a masking fragrance, and an antimicrobial agent, such as benzethonium chloride, chlorhexidine hydrochloride, or triacetin.

deodorized alcohol, a liquid, free of organic impurities, containing 92.5% absolute alcohol.

deontologism /dē'ontol'əgiz'əm/ [Gk *deon* obligation, *logos* science], a doctrine of ethics that states that moral duty or obligation is binding.

deossification /dē·os'ifikā'shən/, the loss of mineral matter from bones.

deoxygenation /dē·ok'sijənā'shən/ [L *de;* Gk *oxys* sharp, *genein* to produce], the removal of oxygen from a chemical compound.

deoxyribonucleic acid (DNA) /dē·ok'sirī'-bōn ōōklē'ik/, a large nucleic acid molecule, found principally in the chromosomes of the nucleus of a cell, that is the carrier of genetic information. The genetic information is coded in the sequence of the nitrogenous, molecular subunits of the molecule.

Department of Health and Human Services (HHS), a cabinet-level department of the U.S. government with the responsibility for functions of various federal social welfare and health delivery agencies, such as the Food and Drug Administration (FDA). It also directs the U.S. Office of Consumer Affairs, Office of Civil Rights, Administration on Aging, Public Health Service, Indian Health Service, Social Security Administration, and National Institutes of Health.

Department of Transportation (DOT), a cabinet-level department of the U.S. government responsible for national transportation policies, including maritime, aviation, railroad, and highway safety and regulation of the transport of hazardous materials, such as medical gases.

dependence [L *de* + *pendere* to hang upon], **1.** the state of being dependent. **2.** the total psychophysical state of one addicted to drugs or alcohol who must receive an increasing amount of the substance to prevent the onset of abstinence symptoms.

dependency needs, the sum of the physical and emotional requirements of an infant for survival, including parenting, love, affection, shelter, protection, food, and warmth. Reliance on others to satisfy these needs normally decreases with age and maturity.

dependent, of or pertaining to a condition of being reliant on someone or something else for help, support, favor, and other need, as a child is dependent on a parent, a narcotics addict is dependent on a drug, or one variable is dependent on another variable. **–depend,** *v.*

dependent differentiation. See correlative differentiation.

dependent edema [L *de* + *pendere;* Gk *oidema* swelling], a fluid accumulation in the tissues influenced by gravity. It is usually greater in the lower part of the body than in tissues above the level of the heart.

dependent intervention, a therapeutic action based on the written or verbal orders of another health professional.

dependent personality, behavior characterized by excessive or compulsive needs for attention, acceptance, and approval from other people to maintain security and self-esteem.

dependent personality disorder, a mental state characterized by a lack of self-confidence and an inability to function independently.

dependent variable, (in research) a factor that is measured to learn the effect of one or more independent variables.

depersonalization [L *de* + *persona* mask], a feeling of strangeness or unreality concerning oneself or the environment, often resulting from anxiety.

depersonalization disorder, an emotional disturbance characterized by depersonalization feelings in which a dreamlike atmosphere pervades the consciousness. The body may not feel like one's own, and important events may be watched with equanimity.

depilation /dep'ilā'shən/ [L *de* + *pilum* hair], the removal or extraction of hair from the body, either temporarily by mechanical or chemical means or permanently, by electrolysis, which destroys the hair follicle. **–depilate,** *v.*

depilatory /dipil'ətôrē/, **1.** of or pertaining to a substance or procedure that removes hair. **2.** a depilatory agent.

depilatory techniques [L *depilare* to deprive of hair; Gk *technikos* skillful], methods of removing unwanted body hair, such as by plucking, external application of chemicals, electrolysis, or the application of melted wax.

depolarization /dēpō'lərizā'shən/ [L *de* + Gk *polos* pilot], the reduction of a membrane potential to a less negative value.

deposition [L *deponere* to lay down], (in law) a sworn pretrial testimony given by a witness in response to oral or written questions and cross-examination.

depot /dē'pō, dep'ō/ [Fr, depository], **1.** any area of the body in which drugs or other substances, as fat, are stored and from which they can be distributed. **2.** (of a drug) injected or implanted to be slowly absorbed into the circulation.

depot injection, an intramuscular injec-

depressant /dipres′ənt/ [L *deprimere* to press down], **1.** (of a drug) tending to decrease the function or activity of a system of the body. **2.** such a drug; for example, a cardiac depressant or a respiratory depressant.

depressed [L *deprimere*], **1.** pertaining to a body structure that has been forced below the surface of surrounding parts, as in a fracture. **2.** pertaining to a condition in which general bodily activity is diminished, often accompanied by emotional dejection, loss of initiative, listlessness, loss of appetite, and concentration difficulty.

depressed fracture, any fracture of the skull in which fragments are depressed below the normal surface of the skull.

depression /dipresh′ən/ [L *deprimere* to press down], **1.** a depressed area, hollow, or fossa; downward or inward displacement. **2.** a decrease of vital functional activity. **3.** a mood disturbance characterized by feelings of sadness, despair, and discouragement resulting from and normally proportionate to some personal loss or tragedy. **4.** an abnormal emotional state characterized by exaggerated feelings of sadness, melancholy, dejection, worthlessness, emptiness, and hopelessness that are inappropriate and out of proportion to reality. Kinds of depression include **agitated, anaclitic, endogenous, involutional melancholia, reactive,** and **retarded depression,** and **involutional melancholia. –depressive,** *adj.*

depression with psychotic features [L *deprimere;* Gk *psyche* mind, *osis* condition], a psychosis in which a major diagnostic sign is depression.

depressor /dipres′ər/ [L *deprimere*], any agent that reduces activity when applied to nerves and muscles.

depressor reflex [L *deprimere + reflectere* to bend back], a reflexive vasodilatation, or fall in arterial blood pressure, as may result from stimulation of the carotid sinus.

depressor septi /sep′tī/, one of the three muscles of the nose. It lies between the mucous membrane and the muscular structure of the lip and draws the ala down, constricting the nostril.

deprivation /dep′rivā′shən/ [L *deprivare* to deprive], the loss of something considered valuable or necessary by taking it away or denying access to it. In experimental psychology, animal or human subjects may be deprived of something desired or expected for study of their reactions.

deprivation of sleep effects [L *de + privare* to deprive; ME *slep;* L *efficere* to accomplish], the deliberate prevention of sleep resulting in progressive mental aberrations after 30 to 60 continuous hours. After this point, boring tasks become intolerable, speech begins to become slurred, and performance becomes increasingly poor. After a week of sleep deprivation, symptoms of psychosis may begin to appear.

depth dose [AS *diop;* Gk *dosis* giving], (in radiotherapy) the relationship between dose at any depth from a beam of radiation compared with the dose at the entrance from that beam.

depth   electroencephalography. See **electroencephalography.**

depth perception, the ability to judge depth or the relative distance of objects in space and to orient one's position in relation to them. Binocular vision is essential to this ability.

depth psychology, any approach to psychology that emphasizes the study of personality and behavior in relation to unconscious motivation.

de Quervain's fracture /də kərvānz′/ [Fritz de Quervain, Swiss surgeon, b. 1868], fracture of the navicular bone of the hand, with dislocation of the lunate bone.

de Quervain's thyroiditis [Fritz de Quervain; Gk *thyreos* shield, *itis* inflammation], an inflammatory condition of the thyroid, characterized by swelling and tenderness of the gland, fever, dysphagia, fatigue, and severe pain in the neck, ears, and jaw. The disorder often occurs after a viral infection of the upper respiratory tract and tends to remit spontaneously and to recur several times.

der, (in cytogenetics) abbreviation for **derivative chromosome.**

derailment /dirāl′mənt/, a pattern of speech in which incomprehensible, disconnected, and unrelated ideas replace logical and orderly thought.

derby hat fracture. See **dishpan fracture.**

dereflection /dē′rəflek′shən/ [L *de + reflectere* to bend backward], a technique of logotherapeutic psychology that is directed toward taking a person's mind off a certain goal through a positive redirection to another goal, with emphasis on assets and abilities rather than the problems at hand.

dereistic thought /dē′rē·is′tik/ [L *de + res* thing], a type of mental activity in which fantasy is not modified by logic, experience, or reality.

derivative /dəriv′ativ/ [L *derivare* to turn

away], anything that is derived or obtained from another substance or object; for example, organs and tissues are derivatives of the primordial germ cells.

derived protein /dirīvd′/, a metabolic product of protein hydrolysis, as proteose, peptone, or peptide.

derived quantity, any secondary quantity derived from a combination of base quantities, such as mass, length, and time.

dermabrasion /dur′məbrā′zhən/ [Gk *derma* skin; L *abradere* to scrape], a treatment for the removal of scars on the skin by the use of revolving wire brushes or sandpaper. An aerosol spray is used to freeze the skin for this procedure.

Dermacentor /dur′məsen′tər/, a genus of ticks. It includes species that transmit Rocky Mountain spotted fever, tularemia, brucellosis, and other infectious diseases.

dermal /dur′məl/ [Gk *derma* skin], pertaining to the skin.

dermal graft [Gk *derma, graphion* stylus], the transplantation of any living skin tissue that contains dermis and thus is capable of regenerating and secreting sweat and sebum and generating new hair growth.

dermal papilla [Gk *derma;* L *papilla* nipple], any small elevation in the skin, as the elongated alpine papilla seen in psoriasis.

dermatitis /dur′mətī′tis/ [Gk *derma* + *itis* inflammation], an inflammatory condition of the skin, characterized by erythema and pain or pruritus. Various cutaneous eruptions occur and may be unique to a particular allergen, disease, or infection. Some kinds of dermatitis are **actinic, contact, rhus,** and **seborrheic dermatitis.**

dermatitis exfoliativa neonatorum. See Ritter's disease.

dermatitis herpetiformis, a chronic, severely pruritic skin disease with symmetrically located groups of red, papulovesicular, vesicular, bullous, or urticarial lesions that leave hyperpigmented spots.

dermatitis medicamentosa. See **drug rash.**

dermatitis venenata. See **contact dermatitis.**

dermatocele /dur′mətōsēl′/ [Gk *derma* + *kele* hernia], an overgrowth of skin and subcutaneous tissue that hangs in pendulous folds.

dermatocyst /dur′mətōsist′/, a cystic tumor of cutaneous tissues.

dermatofibroma /dur′mətōfĭbrō′mə/, *pl.* **dermatofibromas, dermatofibromata** [Gk *derma* + L *fibra* fiber, *oma* tumor], a cutaneous nodule that is painless, round, firm, gray or red, and elevated. It is most commonly found on the extremities.

dermatofibrosarcoma /dur′mətōfī′brō-särkō′mə/ [Gk *derma* + L *sarx* flesh, *oma* tumor], a fibrosarcoma or fibrous tumor of the skin.

dermatoglyphics /dur′mətōglif′iks/ [Gk *derma* + *glyphe* a carving], the study of the skin ridge patterns on fingers, toes, palms of hands, and soles of feet. The patterns are used as a basis of identification and also have diagnostic value because of associations between certain patterns and chromosomal anomalies.

dermatographia /dur′mətōgraf′ē·ə/ [Gk *derma* + *graphein* to record], an abnormal skin condition characterized by wheals that develop from tracing on the skin with the fingernail or a blunted instrument.

dermatologist, a physician specializing in disorders of the skin.

dermatology [Gk *derma* + *logos* science], the study of the skin, including the anatomy, physiology, and pathology of the skin and the diagnosis and treatment of skin disorders.

dermatome /dur′mətōm/ [Gk *derma* + *temnein* to cut] **1.** (in embryology) the mesodermal layer in the early developing embryo that gives rise to the dermal layers of the skin. **2.** (in surgery) an instrument used to cut thin slices of skin for grafting. **3.** an area on the surface of a body innervated by afferent fibers from one spinal root.

dermatomycosis /dur′mətōmīkō′sis/ [Gk *derma* + *mykes* fungus, *osis* condition], a superficial, fungal infection of the skin, characteristically found on parts that are moist and protected by clothing, as the groin or feet. It is caused by a dermatophyte. —**dermatomycotic,** *adj.*

dermatomyositis /dur′mətōmī·ōsī′tis/ [Gk *derma* + *mys* muscle, *itis* inflammation], a disease of the connective tissues, characterized by pruritic or eczematous inflammation of the skin and tenderness and weakness of the muscles. Muscle tissue is destroyed, and loss is often so severe that the person may become unable to walk or to perform simple tasks.

Dermatophagoides farinae /dur′mətō-fagoi′dēz/ [Gk *derma* + *phagein* to eat, *eidos* form], a ubiquitous species of household dust mite responsible for allergic reactions in sensitive individuals.

dermatophyte /dur′mətōfīt′, dərmat′əfīt/, any of several fungi that cause parasitic skin disease in humans.

dermatophytid /dur′mətof′itid, dur′mət-ōfī′-tid/ [Gk *derma* + *phyton* plant], an allergic skin reaction characterized by small vesicles and associated with dermatomycosis.

dermatophytosis /dur′mətō′fītō′sis/ [Gk *derma* + *phyton* plant, *osis* condition], a superficial fungus infection of the skin, caused by *Microsporum, Epidermophyton,* or *Trichophyton* species of dermatophyte. On the trunk and upper extremities it is commonly called "ringworm" infection and is characterized by round or oval, scaly patches with slightly raised borders and clearing centers. On the feet small vesicles, cracking, itching, scaling, and often secondary bacterial infections occur and are commonly called "athlete's foot."

dermatoplasty /dur′mətōplas′tē/, a surgical procedure in which skin tissue is transplanted to a body surface damaged by disease or injury.

dermatosclerosis /dur′mətōskların′sis/ [Gk *derma* + *sklerosis* hardening], a skin disease characterized by fibrous infiltration of the fatty subcutaneous tissue, leading to patches of thick, leatherlike skin.

dermatosis /dur′mətō′sis/ [Gk *derma* + *osis* condition], any disorder of the skin, especially those not associated with inflammation.

dermatosis papulosa nigra, a common abnormal skin condition in blacks consisting of multiple, tiny, benign, skin-colored or hyperpigmented papules on the cheeks.

dermis, the layer of skin, just below the epidermis, consisting of papillary and reticular layers and containing blood and lymphatic vessels, nerves and nerve endings, glands, and hair follicles.

dermographism. See **dermatographia.**

dermoid /dur′moid/ [Gk *derma* + *eidos* form], **1.** of or pertaining to the skin. **2.** *informal.* a dermoid cyst.

dermoid cyst, a tumor, derived from embryonal tissues. It consists of a fibrous wall lined with epithelium and a cavity containing fatty material, and frequently hair, teeth, bits of bone, and cartilage. Kinds of dermoid cysts are **implantation dermoid cyst, inclusion dermoid cyst, thyroid dermoid cyst,** and **tubal dermoid cyst.**

derotation brace /dē′rōtā′shən/, a customized orthosis that provides stability at the knee joint. It consists of a single-joint hinged bar on one side and a rotating dial pad on the opposite side.

DES, abbreviation for *diethylstilbestrol.*

desalination /dēsal′inā′shən/ [L *de* + *sal* salt], the process of removing salt from water or other substances.

desaturation /dēsat′yərā′shən/ [L *de* + *saturare* to fill], the formation of an unsaturated chemical compound from a saturated one.

descending aorta /disen′ding/ [L *descendere* to descend; Gk *aerein* to raise], the main portion of the aorta, consisting of the thoracic aorta and the abdominal aorta, that continues from the aortic arch into the trunk of the body and supplies many parts, such as the esophagus, lymph glands, ribs, and stomach.

descending colon, the segment of the colon that extends from the end of the transverse colon at the splenic flexure on the left side of the abdomen down to the beginning of the sigmoid colon in the pelvis.

descending current. See **centrifugal current.**

descending myelitis [L *descendere;* Gk *myelos* marrow, *itis* inflammation], a form of myelitis in which the pathologic changes spread downward along the spinal cord.

descending neuritis [L *descendere;* Gk *neuron* nerve, *itis* inflammation], a form of neuritis that spreads downward from the upper part of the nervous system.

descending neuropathy [L *descendere;* Gk *neuron* nerve, *pathos* disease], a disease of the peripheral nervous system that spreads downward from the upper part of the body.

descending oblique muscle. See **obliquus externus abdominis.**

descending tract [L *descendere* + *tractus*], a nerve tract found in the spinal cord that carries impulses away from the brain axis of the body or body part.

descending urography. See **intravenous pyelography.**

descensus /disen′səs/, the process of falling or descending; prolapse.

descent of testis [L *descendere* + *testis* testicle], the normal prenatal movement of the testis from the abdomen to the adult position in the scrotum. Incomplete descent is typically due to hormonal or mechanical defects that may be surgically corrected in early childhood.

descriptive anatomy [L *describere* to write], the study of the morphology and structure of the body by systems, such as the vascular system and the nervous system.

descriptive embryology, the study of the changes that occur in cells, tissues, and organs during the progressive stages of prenatal development.

descriptive epidemiology, the first stage of epidemiologic investigation. It focuses on describing disease distribution by characteristics relating to time, place, and person.

descriptive psychiatry, the study of external, readily observable behavior.

DES daughters, a group of women with increased susceptibility to cancer of the vagina and other reproductive organs because their mothers were given an estrogen medication, diethylstilbestrol (DES), from the 1940s through the 1960s to prevent miscarriage. Sons of women who took DES have an increased risk of undescended testes or other genital disorders.

desensitization. See **systemic desensitization.**

desensitize /dēsen'sitīz/ [L *de* + *sentire* to feel], **1.** (in immunology) to render an individual insensitive to any of the various antigens. **2.** (in psychiatry) to relieve an emotionally disturbed person of the stress of phobias and neuroses by encouraging discussion of the anxieties and the stressful experiences that cause the emotional problems involved. **3.** (in dentistry) to remove or reduce the painful response of vital, exposed dentin to irritating substances and temperature changes.

deserpidine /disur'pədēn/, a rauwolfia alkaloid prescribed for mild hypertension and for mild anxiety.

desert fever. See **coccidioidomycosis.**

desert rheumatism. See **coccidioidomycosis.**

desiccant /des'ikənt/ [L *desiccare* to dry thoroughly], any agent or procedure that promotes drying or causes a substance to dry up.

desiccate /des'ikāt/, **1.** to dry thoroughly. **2.** to preserve by drying, especially food.

designer drugs [L *de* + *signare* to mark], synthetic organic compounds that are designed as analogs of illicit drugs, with the same narcotic or other dangerous effects. Because designer drugs are generally not listed as controlled substances by the United States Drug Enforcement Agency, prosecution of manufacturers, distributors, or users is frequently difficult.

desipramine hydrochloride /desip'rəmēn/, a tricyclic antidepressant prescribed in the treatment of mental depression.

deslanoside /dislan'əsīd/, a cardiotonic prescribed for congestive heart failure and certain arrhythmias.

desmocyte. See **fibroblast.**

desmoid tumor /dez'moid/ [Gk *desmos* band, *eidos* form], a neoplasm in skeletal muscle and fascia. The tumor is usually a firm, circumscribed, rubbery mass, which is often regarded as overproliferation of scar tissue.

desmopressin acetate /dez'mōpres'in/, an antidiuretic analog of vasopressin prescribed in the treatment of diabetes insipidus.

desmosis /dezmō'sis/, any disease of the connective tissue.

desmosome /dez'məsōm/ [Gk *desmos* band, *soma* body], a small, circular, dense area within the intercellular bridge that forms the site of adhesion between certain epithelial cells, especially the stratified epithelium of the epidermis.

desonide /des'ənīd/, a topical corticosteroid prescribed as an antiinflammatory agent.

desoximetasone /desok'simet'əsōn/, a topical corticosteroid prescribed as an antiinflammatory agent.

desoxycorticosterone acetate /desok'-sikôr'təkōstē'rōn/, a mineralocorticoid hormone prescribed in replacement therapy, in congenital adrenal hyperplasia, and in chronic primary adrenocortical insufficiency to prevent the excess loss of salt from the body.

desoxyribonucleic acid. See **deoxyribonucleic acid.**

desquamation /des'kwəmā'shən/ [L *desquamare* to take off scales], a normal process in which the cornified layer of the epidermis is sloughed in fine scales. –**desquamate,** *v.,* **desquamative** /deskwam'ətiv/, *adj.*

desquamative gingivitis, a gingival inflammation, characterized by peeling of the surface epithelium. It is frequently associated with menopause and may also be associated with biologic stress.

desquamative interstitial pneumonia, a respiratory disease characterized by an accumulation of cellular matter in the alveoli and bronchial tubes. It leads to a fibrotic condition with symptoms of coughing, chest pain, weight loss, and dyspnea.

destructive aggression [L *destruere* to destroy; *aggresio* an attack], an act of hostility unnecessary for self-protection or preservation that is directed toward an external object or person.

destructive interference, (in ultrasonography) a phenomenon that results when propagated waves are out of phase so that maximum molecular compression for one wave occurs at the same point as the maximum rarefaction for the second wave.

destructive lesion [L *destruere* + *laesio* a hurting], a disorder that leads to the damage or necrosis of an organ or tissue.

detached retina. See **retinal detachment.**

detection bias, a potential artifact in epidemiologic data resulting from the use of a particular diagnostic technique or equipment.

detergent [L *detergere* to cleanse], **1.** a cleansing agent. **2.** cleansing. **3.** (in respiratory therapy) a wetting agent that is administered to mediate the removal of respiratory tract secretions from airway walls.

deterioration [L *deterior* worse], pertaining to a condition that is gradually worsening.

determinant evolution [L *determinare* to limit], the theory that evolution progresses according to a predetermined course.

determinants of occlusion, (in dentistry) the classifiable factors that influence proper closure of the teeth. The common fixed factors are the intercondylar distance, anatomy, mandibular centricity, and relationship of the jaws. The common changeable factors are tooth shapes, tooth positions, and vertical dimensions of occlusion, cusp height, and fossa depth.

determinate cleavage, mitotic division of the fertilized ovum into blastomeres that are each destined to form a specific part of the embryo. Damage to or destruction of any of these cells results in a malformed organism.

detoxification /dētok'sifikā'shən/ [L *de* + Gk *toxikon* poison; L *facere* to make], the removal of a poison or its effects from a patient.

detoxification service, a hospital service providing treatment to diminish or remove from a patient's body the toxic effects of chemical substances, such as alcohol, drugs, or poisonous substances to which a person may have been exposed.

detoxify /dētok'sifī/ [L *de* + Gk *toxikon* poison], to make a poisonous substance harmless or to overcome the effects of a poison.

detrusor urinae muscle /ditr oo'zər/ [L *detruder* to thrust; Gk *ouron* urine; L *musculus*], a complex of longitudinal fibers that form the external layer of the muscular coat of the bladder.

deuterium (^{2}H) /dy oootir'ē·əm/ [Gk *deuteros* second], a radioactive isotope of the hydrogen atom, used as a tracer.

deuteroplasm. See **deutoplasm.**

deutoplasm /doo'təplaz'əm/ [Gk *deuteros* + *plasma* something formed], the inactive elements of the protoplasm, primarily the stored nutritive material contained in the yolk.

DEV, abbreviation for **duck embryo vaccine.**

devascularization /dēvas'kyəler'īzō'shən/ [L *de* + *vasculum* small vessel], the drawing away of blood from a body part or stopping the flow of blood to the part.

development [Fr *developper* to unfold], **1.** the gradual process of change and differentiation from a simple to a more advanced level of complexity. Kinds of development include **arrested, mosaic, psychomotor, psychosexual, psychosocial,** and **regulative development. 2.** (in biol-

ogy) the series of events that occur within an organism from the time of fertilization of the ovum to the adult stage. **–developmental,** *adj.*

developmental age (DA), an expression of a child's developmental progress stated in age and determined by standardized measurements, as of body size and dimensions, by social and psychologic functioning, by observations of motor skills, and by the giving of mental and aptitude tests.

developmental agraphia, a deficiency in a child's ability to learn to form letters and to write.

developmental anatomy, the study of the differentiation and the growth of an organism from one cell to birth.

developmental anomaly, any congenital defect that results from the interference with the normal growth and differentiation of the fetus. Such defects can arise at any stage of embryonic development, vary greatly in type and severity, and are caused by a wide variety of determining factors, including genetic mutations, chromosomal aberrations, teratogenic agents, and environmental factors.

developmental apraxia [L *développer* development; Gk *a* not, *prassein* to do], a condition of ineffective motor planning and execution in children because of immaturity of the child's central nervous system.

developmental arrest. See **arrested development.**

developmental crisis, severe, usually transient, stress that occurs when a person is unable to complete the tasks of a psychosocial stage of development and is therefore unable to move on to the next stage.

developmental disability (DD), a pathologic condition that starts developing before 18 years of age.

developmental disorder, a form of mental retardation that develops in some children after they have progressed normally for the first 3 or 4 years of life.

developmental dyspraxia, a disorder of sensory integration characterized by an impaired ability to plan skilled nonhabitual movements.

developmental fog, (in radiology) an x-ray film that is dull, washed out, and lacking in contrast. Causes include temperature, timing, and developer concentration.

developmental groove, a fine recessed line in the enamel of a tooth that marks the union of the lobes of the crown in its development.

developmental guidance, (in dentistry) the comprehensive dentofacial orthopedic control over the growth of the jaws and the eruption of the teeth. The control may be needed throughout the entire growth and maturation of the face, beginning at the earliest detection of a developing malformation.

developmental horizon, any one of 25 stages in the development of the human embryo from the one-cell stage at conception to the morphologically and physiologically complex organism at the end of the seventh week of gestation.

developmental model, 1. a conceptual framework devised to be used as a guide in making a diagnosis, in understanding a developmental process, and in forming a prognosis for continued development. **2.** (in nursing) a conceptual framework describing four stages, or processes, of patient therapy. In the first stage, called orientation, the patient begins a relationship with the nurse or other therapist and begins to clarify the problem with the help of the therapist. In the second stage, called identification, the patient develops a sense of closeness and attachment to the therapist. In the third stage, called exploitation, the patient makes full use of the nursing services offered, begins to assume some control of interactions, and becomes more independent. During the last stage, called resolution, the therapeutic relationship is terminated; the patient is independent and no longer needs the nurse or therapist.

developmental physiology, the study of the physiologic processes as they relate to embryonic development.

developmental quotient (DQ), the numeric expression of a child's developmental level as measured by dividing the developmental age by the chronologic age and multiplying by 100.

developmental sequence [Fr *développer;* L *sequi* to follow], the order in which structure and function change during the process of growth and development of an organism.

developmental task, a physical or cognitive skill that a person must accomplish during a particular age period to continue developing, such as walking, which precedes the development of a sense of autonomy in the toddler period.

developmental theory of aging, a concept based on the premise that traits and characteristics developed early in life tend to continue into the later years.

deviance /dē'vē·əns/ [L *deviare* to turn aside], behavior that is contrary to the accepted standards of a community or culture.

deviant [L *deviare*], pertaining to a person or object that departs from what is considered normal or standard.

deviant behavior, actions that exceed the usual limits of accepted behavior and involve failure to comply with the social norm of the group.

deviate /dē'vē·it/ [L *deviare* to turn aside,] **1.** a person or an act that varies from that which is considered standard, such as a social or sexual deviate, or that which is within a statistic norm. **2.** to vary from that which is considered standard or within a statistic norm. **–deviant,** *adj.,* **deviation,** *n.*

deviated septum, a shifted medial partition of the nasal cavity, a condition affecting many adults. The nasal septum more commonly shifts to the left during normal growth, but severe deflection of the septum may significantly obstruct the nasal passages and result in infection, sinusitis, shortness of breath, headache, or recurring nosebleeds.

deviation, axis, in electrocardiography, deviation of the mean electrical axis of the heart.

deviation from normal, a quality, characteristic, symptom, or clinical finding that is different from what is commonly regarded as normal, such as an elevated temperature, multiple gestation, or an extra digit.

deviation of tongue [L *deviare;* AS *tunge*], a tendency of the tongue to turn away from the midline when extended or protruded. The condition is associated with a hypoglossal nerve defect.

device [OFr *deviser* to divide], an item other than a drug that has application in the healing arts. The term is sometimes restricted to items used directly by, on, or in the patient and not surgical instruments or other equipment used for diagnosis and treatment. Devices include orthopedic appliances, crutches, artificial heart valves, pacemakers, and prostheses.

devil's grip. See **epidemic pleurodynia.**

devitalized /dēvī'təlīzd/, pertaining to tissues with a reduced oxygen supply and blood flow.

devital tooth. See **pulpless tooth.**

dewar /dyoo'ər/, (in nuclear magnetic resonance imaging) a double chamber used to maintain the temperature of superconducting magnet coils at near absolute zero.

dew point, the temperature at which air becomes saturated with water vapor and the water vapor condenses to liquid. In aerosol therapy, water may condense on containers, tubing, and other surfaces when the dew point is reached.

dexamethasone /dek'səmeth'əsōn/, a glucocorticoid prescribed in the treatment of a variety of inflammatory conditions.

dexchlorpheniramine maleate /deks'-klôrfənir'əmēn mal'ē·it/, an antihistamine prescribed in the treatment of a variety of hypersensitivity reactions, including rhinitis, skin rash, and pruritus.

dexter /deks'tər/, pertaining to the right side.

dexterity [L dexteritas], skillfulness in the use of one's hands or body.

dextrad writing /deks'trad/ [L dexter right; ME writen], writing that moves from left to right.

dextrality. See **right-handedness.**

dextran fermentation /dek'stran/ [L dexter right side; fermentare to cause to rise], the conversion of dextrose to dextran by the action of Leuconostoc mesenteroides dextran (LMD) bacteria.

dextran preparation, any of a group of solutions containing polysaccharides, water, and, in some preparations, electrolytes. These solutions are used as plasma volume extenders in cases of hypovolemia from hemorrhage, dehydration, or another cause.

dextroamphetamine sulfate /deks'trō·amfet'əmēn/, a central nervous system stimulant prescribed in the treatment of narcolepsy and in the treatment of hyperkinetic disorders in children. It has also been prescribed as an anorexiant in treating exogenous obesity.

dextrocardia /deks'trōkär'dē·ə/, pertaining to the location of the heart in the right hemithorax, either as a result of displacement by disease or as a congenital defect.

dextrocardiogram [L dexter; Gk kardia heart, gramma record], an electrocardiogram made from a unipolar electrode facing the right ventricle, producing a complex of a small R wave and a large S wave.

dextromethorphan hydrobromide /deks'-trōmethôr'fən/, an antitussive derived from morphine, but lacking narcotic effects. It is prescribed for the suppression of nonproductive cough.

dextrose /dek'strōs/ [L dexter right side], a glucose available in various solutions for intravenous administration. It is prescribed to provide calories and fluid and to correct hypoglycemia.

dextrose and sodium chloride injection, a fluid, nutrient, and electrolyte replenisher. It is available for parenteral use in a variety of concentrations.

dextrothyroxine sodium, an antihyperlipidemic prescribed in the treatment of hyperlipidemia.

DHFS, abbreviation for **dengue hemorrhagic fever shock syndrome.**

dhobie itch /dō'bē/ [Hindi dhobie laundryman; AS giccan], a form of contact dermatitis associated with the use of laundry marking fluids.

diabetes /dī'əbē'tēz/ [Gk diabainein to pass through], a clinical condition characterized by the excessive excretion of urine. The excess may be caused by a deficiency of antidiuretic hormone (ADH), as in diabetes insipidus, or it may be the polyuria resulting from the hyperglycemia occurring in diabetes mellitus.

diabetes insipidus /insip'idəs/, a metabolic disorder, characterized by extreme polyuria and polydipsia, caused by deficient production or secretion of the antidiuretic hormone (ADH) or an inability of the kidney tubules to respond to ADH. Rarely, the symptoms are self-induced by an excessive water intake. The condition may be acquired, familial, idiopathic, or nephrogenic. The patient is usually well and comfortable except for the annoyance of frequent urination and a constant need to drink.

diabetes mellitus (DM) /məli'təs/, a complex disorder of carbohydrate, fat, and protein metabolism that is primarily a result of a relative or complete lack of insulin secretion by the beta cells of the pancreas or of defects of the insulin receptors. The disease is often familial but may be acquired, such as in Cushing's syndrome, as a result of the administration of excessive glucocorticoid. The various forms of diabetes have been organized into a series of categories developed by the National Diabetes Data Group of the National Institutes of Health. Type I diabetes in this classification scheme includes patients dependent on insulin to prevent ketosis. The category is also known as the insulin-dependent diabetes mellitus (IDDM) subclass. This group was previously called juvenile-onset diabetes, brittle diabetes, or ketosis-prone diabetes. Patients with Type II, or non-insulin-dependent diabetes mellitus (NIDDM), are those previously designated as having maturity-onset diabetes, adult-onset diabetes, ketosis-resistant diabetes, or stable diabetes. Type II patients are further subdivided into obese NIDDM and nonobese NIDDM groups. Those with gestational diabetes (GDM), usually identified as Type III, are in a separate subclass composed of women who developed glucose intolerance in association with pregnancy. Type IV, also identified as Other Types of Diabetes, includes patients whose diabetes is associated with a pancreatic disease, hormonal changes, adverse effects of drugs, or genetic or other anomalies. A fifth subclass, the impaired glucose tolerance (IGT) group, includes persons whose plasma glucose levels are abnormal, although not sufficiently beyond the normal range to be diagnosed as diabetic. The onset of diabetes mellitus is sudden in children and usually insidious in non-insulin-dependent diabetes mellitus (Type II). Characteristically, the course is progressive and includes polyuria, polydipsia, weight loss, polyphagia, hyperglycemia, and glycosuria. The eyes, kidneys, nervous system, skin, and circulatory system may be affected, infections are common, and atherosclerosis often develops. Kinds of diabetes mellitus are **gestational diabetes, insulin-dependent diabetes,** and **non-insulin-dependent diabetes.**

diabetic /dī′əbet′ik/, **1.** of or pertaining to diabetes. **2.** affected with diabetes. **3.** a person who has diabetes mellitus.

diabetic acidosis [Gk *diabainein* to pass through; L *acidus* acid; Gk *osis* condition], a type of acidosis that may occur in diabetes mellitus as a result of excessive production of ketone bodies during oxidation of fatty acids.

diabetic amaurosis [Gk *diabainein* to pass through; *amauroein* to darken], blindness associated with diabetes, caused by a proliferative, hemorrhagic form of retinopathy that is characterized by capillary microaneurysms and hard or waxy exudates. Cataracts are also common.

diabetic coma, a life-threatening condition occurring in diabetic patients, caused by inadequate treatment, by failure to take prescribed insulin, excessive food intakes, or, most frequently, by infection, surgery, trauma, or other stressors that increase the body's need for insulin. Without insulin to metabolize glucose, fats are burned for energy, resulting in ketone waste accumulation and acidosis. Warning signs of diabetic coma include a dull headache, fatigue, inordinate thirst, epigastric pain, nausea, vomiting, parched lips, a flushed face, and sunken eyes. The temperature usually rises and then falls; the systolic blood pressure drops, and circulatory collapse may occur.

diabetic diet, a diet prescribed in the treatment of diabetes mellitus, usually containing limited amounts of sugar or readily available carbohydrates and increased amounts of proteins, complex carbohydrates, and unsaturated fats. Dietary regulation depends on the severity of the disease and on the type and extent of insulin therapy.

diabetic foot and leg care, the special attention given to prevent the circulatory disorders and infections that frequently occur in the lower extremities of diabetic patients. The patient's legs and feet are examined daily for signs of dry, scaly, red, itching, or cracked skin, blisters, corns, calluses, abrasions, infection, blueness and swelling around varicosities, and thickened, discolored nails. The feet are bathed daily in tepid water with mild or superfatted soap and are dried gently but thoroughly with a soft towel. A lanolin-based lotion is then applied.

diabetic gangrene [Gk *diabainein, gaggraina*], gangrene, usually involving the lower extremities, that develops secondary to peripheral vascular disease complications related to the diabetic disease process.

diabetic glycosuria [Gk *diabainein* + *glykys* sweet, *ouron* urine], excessive excretion of sugar into the urine as an effect of diabetes mellitus.

diabetic ketoacidosis (DKA), an acute, life-threatening complication of uncontrolled diabetes mellitus in which urinary loss of water, potassium, ammonium, and sodium results in hypovolemia, electrolyte imbalance, extremely high blood-glucose levels, and the breakdown of free fatty acids causing acidosis, often with coma. The person appears flushed; has hot, dry skin; is restless, uncomfortable, agitated, and diaphoretic; and has a fruity odor to the breath. Coma, confusion, and nausea are often noted. Untreated, the condition invariably proceeds to coma and death.

diabetic retinopathy, a disorder of retinal blood vessels characterized by capillary microaneurysms, hemorrhage, exudates, and the formation of new vessels and connective tissue. The disorder occurs most frequently in patients with long-standing, poorly controlled diabetes. Repeated hemorrhage may result in permanent opacity of the vitreous humor, and blindness may eventually set in.

diabetic treatment, therapy of diabetes mellitus by means of a low carbohydrate diet, insulin injections, or oral hypoglycemic agents, such as chlorpropamide, acetohexamide, tolbutamide, and tolazamide.

diabetic vulvovaginitis [Gk *diabainein;* L *vulva* wrapper + *vagina* sheath; Gk *itis* inflammation], a form of mycotic inflammation of the vulva and vagina that is associated with diabetes.

diabetic xanthoma, an eruption of yellow papules or plaques on the skin in uncontrolled diabetes mellitus. The lesion disappears as the metabolic functions are stabilized and the disease is brought under control.

diabetogenic state /dī′əbet′ōjen′ik/, a health condition manifested by signs and symptoms of diabetes.

diacet, abbreviation for a *carboxylate diacetate anion.*

diacetic acid. See **acetoacetic acid.**

diacondylar fracture /dī′əkon′dīlər/ [Gk *dia* through, *kondylos* knuckle; L *fractura* break], any fracture that runs across the line of a condyle.

diadochokinesia /dī·ad′əkōkīnē′zhə/ [Gk *diadochos* successor, *kinesis* motion], the normal ability of the muscles to move a limb alternately in opposite directions by flexion and extension.

diagnose, to determine the type and cause of a health condition based on the signs and symptoms of the patient, data obtained from laboratory analysis of fluid, tissue specimens, and other tests, and family and occupational background information.

diagnosis, *pl.* **diagnoses** [Gk *dia* + *gnosis* knowledge] **1.** identification of a disease or condition by a scientific evaluation of physical signs, symptoms, history, laboratory tests, and procedures. Kinds of diagnoses are **clinical, differential, laboratory, nursing,** and **physical diagnosis. 2.** the art of naming a disease or condition. –**diagnostic,** *adj.,* **diagnose,** *v.*

diagnosis by exclusion [Gk *dia* + *gnosis;* L *excludere* to shut out], making a diagnosis by eliminating other possible causes of disease symptoms.

diagnosis-related group (DRG), groups of patients classified for measuring a medical facility's delivery of care. The classifications, used to determine Medicare payments for inpatient care, are based on primary and secondary diagnosis, primary and secondary procedures, age, and length of hospitalization.

diagnostic, pertaining to a diagnosis.

Diagnostic and Statistical Manual of Mental Disorders (DSM), a manual, published by the American Psychiatric Association, listing the official diagnostic classifications of mental disorders. The *DSM* recommends the use of a multiaxial evaluation system as a holistic diagnostic approach. It consists of five axes, each of which refers to a different class of information, including both mental and physical data. Axes I and II include all of the mental disorders, classified broadly as clinical syndromes and personality disorders; axis III contains physical disorders and conditions; and axes IV and V provide a coded outline of supplemental information which may be useful for planning individual treatment and predicting its outcome. Each of the classifications of the mental disorders contains a code that pro-

vides a reference to the WHO *International Classification of Diseases (ICD).*

diagnostic anesthesia, a procedure in which analgesia is induced to a depth adequate to comfortably permit performance of moderately painful diagnostic procedures of short duration. Awake anesthesia is often used for this purpose.

diagnostician, a person skilled and trained in making diagnoses.

Diagnostic Medical Sonographer, an allied health professional who provides patient services, using diagnostic ultrasound under the supervision of a doctor of medicine or osteopathy responsible for the use and interpretation of ultrasound procedures. The sonographer assists the physician in gathering sonographic data necessary to reach diagnostic decisions.

diagnostic position of gaze. See **cardinal position of gaze.**

diagnostic process, the act of determining a patient's health status and evaluating the factors influencing that status.

diagnostic radiology, medical imaging using external sources of radiation.

diagnostic radiopharmaceutical, a radioactive drug administered to a patient as a diagnostic tracer to differentiate normal from abnormal anatomic structures or biochemical or physiologic functions. Most diagnostic radioactive tracers indicate their position within the body by emitting gamma rays. Tracers prepared with tritium, carbon 14, or phosphorus 32, which do not emit gamma rays, are used diagnostically by analyzing the concentration of the isotope in a metabolic end product in the patient's blood, urine, breath, or biopsy samples.

diagnostic services, services related to the diagnosis made by a physician but which may be performed also by nurses or other health professionals.

diagonal conjugate, a radiographic measurement of the distance from the inferior border of the symphysis pubis to the sacral promontory. The measurement averages around 12.5 to 13.0 cm.

diakinesis /dī′əkinē′sis, dī′əkī-/ [Gk *dia* + *kinesis* motion], the final stage in the first meiotic prophase in gametogenesis in which the chromosomes achieve maximum contraction and are ready to separate.

dialect, a variation of a language different from other forms of the same language in pronunciation, syntax, and word meanings.

dialysate /dī·al′isāt/, a solution used in dialysis.

dialysis /dī·al′isis/ [Gk *dia* + *lysis* a loosening] **1.** the process of separating colloids and crystalline substances in solution by the difference in their rate of diffusion through a semipermeable membrane. **2.** a medical procedure for the removal of certain elements from the blood or lymph by virtue of the difference in their rates of diffusion through an external semipermeable membrane or, in the case of peritoneal dialysis, through the peritoneum.

dialysis dementia, a neurologic disorder that occurs in some patients undergoing dialysis. The precise cause is unknown, but the effect is believed to be related to chemicals in the dialyzing fluid, drugs administered to the dialysis patient, or both.

dialysis disequilibrium syndrome, a disorder caused by a rapid change in extracellular fluid composition during dialysis. The syndrome may be marked by cerebral or neurologic disturbances, cardiac arrhythmias, and pulmonary edema.

dialysis fluid, the solution that flows on the opposite side of a semipermeable membrane to blood.

dialysis shunt [Gk *dia* + *lysis* loosening; ME *shunten*], an external artificial link between a peripheral artery and vein, either in an arm or leg, for use in hemodialysis.

dialysis technician [Gk *dia* + *lysis* + *technikos* skilful], an allied health professional who operates and maintains dialysis equipment for patients with kidney diseases.

dialyzer /dī′əlī′zər/ [Gk *dia* + *lysis* a loosening], **1.** a machine used in dialysis. **2.** a semipermeable membrane or porous diaphragm in a dialysis machine.

diameter of fetal skull [Gk *diametros;* L *fetus;* AS *skulle* bowl], the average distances between certain landmarks of the fetal skull as measured at term, such as biparietal, the fetal head between the two parietal eminences, 9.25 cm; occipitofrontal, from the external occipital protuberance to the most prominent point of the frontal midline, 11 cm; occipitomental, from the external occipital protuberance to the midpoint of the chin, 13 cm; and suboccipitobregmatic, from the lowest posterior point of the occipital bone to the center of the anterior fontanel, 9.5 cm.

Diameter-Index Safety System (DISS), a system of standardized connections between cylinders of medical gases and flow meters or pressure regulators. Each type of gas and connector is assigned a DISS number, such as 1040 for nitrous oxide.

Diamond-Blackfan syndrome, a rare congenital disorder evident in the first 3 months of life, characterized by severe anemia, very low reticulocyte count, but normal numbers of platelets and white cells.

diamond stone, (in dentistry) any of the rotary devices that contain diamond chips as an abrasive.

diapedesis /dī′əpidē′sis/ [Gk *dia* + *pedesis* an oozing], the passage of red or white blood corpuscles through the walls of the vessels that contain them without damage to the vessels.

diaper rash [ME *diapre* patterned fabric], a maculopapular and occasionally excoriated eruption in the diaper area of infants caused by irritation from feces, moisture, heat, or ammonia produced by the bacterial decomposition of urine. Secondary infection by *Candida albicans* is common.

diaper restraint, a therapeutic device used especially in orthopedics for countertraction with lower extremity traction when other methods of countertraction are not effective. Diaper restraints are commonly used in treating children with orthopedic diseases and abnormalities and are designed to fit over the pelvic area like a diaper, with rings incorporated at each of four corners. A webbing strap is threaded through the rings and attached to the top side of the bedspring frame.

diaphanography /dī′af′ənog′rəfē/ [Gk *diaphanes* shining through, *graphein* to record], a type of transillumination used to examine the breast, using selected wavelengths of light and special imaging equipment.

diaphanoscopy /dī′af′ənos′kəpē/, examination of an internal structure with a **diaphanoscope,** an instrument that transilluminates body tissues. It is sometimes used in the diagnosis of breast tumors.

diaphoresis /dī′əfərē′sis/ [Gk *dia* + *pherein* to carry], the secretion of sweat, especially the profuse secretion associated with an elevated body temperature, physical exertion, exposure to heat, and mental or emotional stress.

diaphoretic. See sudorific.

diaphragm /dī′əfram/ [Gk *diaphragma* a partion] **1.** (in anatomy) a dome-shaped musculofibrous partition that separates the thoracic and the abdominal cavities. The convex cranial surface of the diaphragm forms the floor of the thoracic cavity, and the concave surface forms the roof of the abdominal cavity. This partition is pierced by various openings through which pass the aorta, esophagus, and vena cava. **2.** *informal.* a contraceptive diaphragm. **3.** (in optics) an opening that controls the amount of light passing through an optical network. **4.** a thin, membranous partition, as that used in dialysis. **5.** (in radiography) a metal plate with a small opening that limits the diameter of the radiographic beam. **–diaphragmatic,** *adj.*

diaphragmatic breathing [Gk *diaphragma* partition], deliberate use of the diaphragm to control breathing. The technique is taught to patients with COPD to facilitate respiration.

diaphragmatic hernia [Gk *diaphragma* partition; L, rupture], the protrusion of part of the stomach through an opening in the diaphragm, most commonly an abnormally enlarged esophageal hiatus. In some cases the intestines may also herniate into the chest. The enlargement of the normal opening for the esophagus may be caused by trauma, congenital weakness, increased abdominal pressure, or relaxation of ligaments of skeletal muscles, and permits part of the stomach to slide into the thorax. A sliding hiatus hernia, one of the most common pathologic conditions of the upper GI tract, may occur at any age but is most frequent in elderly and middle-aged people. A kind of diaphragmatic hernia is **hiatus hernia.**

diaphragmatic node, a node in one of three groups of thoracic parietal lymph nodes, situated on the thoracic side of the diaphragm and consisting of the anterior set, the middle set, and the posterior set.

diaphragm pessary. See **pessary.**

diaphragm stethoscope, an instrument for auscultation of bodily sounds. Originally designed by René Laënnec, it consists of a vibrating disk, or diaphragm, which transmits sound waves through tubing to two earpieces.

diaphyseal aclasis /dī′əfiz′ē·əl ak′ləsis/ [Gk *dia* + *phyein* to grow; *a, klasis* not breaking], a relatively rare abnormal condition that affects the skeletal system. Characterized by multiple exostoses or bony protrusions, it is hereditary. The characteristic exostoses are radiographically and microscopically similar to osteochondromas.

diaphyseal dysplasia. See **Camurati-Engelmann disease.**

diaphysis /dī·af′isis/ [Gk *dia* + *phein* to grow], the shaft of a long bone, consisting of a tube of compact bone enclosing the medullary cavity.

diapositive. See **reversal film.**

diarrhea /dī′ərē′ə/ [Gk *dia* + *rhein* to flow], **1.** the frequent passage of loose, watery stools, generally the result of increased motility in the colon. The stool may also contain mucus, pus, blood, or excessive amounts of fat. Conditions in which diarrhea is an important symptom are dysenteric diseases, malabsorption syndrome, lactose intolerance, irritable bowel syndrome, GI tumors, and inflammatory bowel disease. Untreated, diarrhea may lead to rapid dehydration and electrolyte imbalance. and should be treated symptomatically until proper diagnosis can be made. **2.** a NANDA-accepted nursing diagnosis. The defining characteristics include abdominal pain, cramping, increased frequency of elimination, increased frequency of bowel sounds, loose or liquid stools, urgency of defecation, and a change in the color of the feces. **–diarrheal, diarrheic,** *adj.*

diarthrosis. See **synovial joint.**

diarticular /dī′ärtik′yələr/ [Gk *di* twice; L *articulare* to divide into joints], biarticular, or having two joints.

diastasis /dī·as′təsis/ [Gk, separation], the forcible separation of two parts that normally are joined together, such as the separation of parts of a bone at an epiphysis or the separation of two bones that lack a synovial joint.

diastasis recti abdominis, the separation of the two rectus muscles along the median line of the abdominal wall. In an adult woman, the abnormality is often caused by repeated pregnancies.

diastatic fermentation /dī′əstat′ik/ [Gk *diastasis* separation; L *fermentare* to cause to rise], the conversion of starch to glucose by the enzyme ptyalin.

diastole /dī·as′təlē/ [Gk *dia* + *stellein* to set], the period of time between contractions of the atria or the ventricles during which blood enters the relaxed chambers from the systemic circulation and the lungs. Ventricular diastole begins with the onset of the second heart sound and ends with the first heart sound. **–diastolic** /dī′əstol′ik/, *adj.*

diastolic /dī′əstol′ik/, pertaining to diastole, or the blood pressure at the instant of maximum cardiac relaxation.

diastolic augmentation, an increase in arterial diastolic pressure caused by the counterpulsation of a circulatory assist device, such as an intraaortic balloon pump.

diastolic blood pressure, the minimum level of blood pressure measured between contractions of the heart. Diastolic pressures for an individual may vary with age, sex, body weight, emotional state, and other factors.

diastolic filling pressure, the blood pressure in the ventricle during diastole.

diastolic murmur [Gk *dia* + *stellein* to set, L *murmur* humming], a murmur heard during ventricular diastole. It may indicate aortic or pulmonary valve incompetence, tricuspid or mitral valve stenosis.

diastrophic /dī′əstrof′ik/ [Gk *diastrephein* to distort], pertaining to a bent or curved condition of bones or distortion of other structures.

diastrophic dwarf, a person in whom short stature is caused by osteochondrodysplasia and is associated with various deformities of the bones and joints, including scoliosis, clubfoot, micromelia, hand defects, multiple joint contractures and subluxations, ear deformities, and cleft palate.

diathermy /dī′əthur′mē/ [Gk dia + therme heat], the production of heat in body tissues for therapeutic purposes by high-frequency currents that are insufficiently intense to destroy tissues or to impair their vitality. Diathermy is used in treating chronic arthritis, bursitis, fractures, gynecologic diseases, sinusitis, and other conditions.

diathesis /dī·ath̄ē′sis/, pl. **diatheses** [Gk, arrangement], an inherited physical constitution predisposing to certain diseases or conditions, many of which are believed associated with the Y chromosome, because males appear to be more susceptible than females.

diazepam /dī·az′əpam/, a sedative and tranquilizer prescribed in the treatment of anxiety, nervous tension, and muscle spasm, and as an anticonvulsant.

diazoxide /dī′əzok′sīd/, a vasodilator used as an antihypertensive. It is prescribed for the emergency reduction of blood pressure in malignant hypertension when drastic reduction of the diastolic blood pressure is required and in some cases of hypoglycemia.

dibromodulcitol. See **mitolactol.**

dibucaine /dī′bəkān/, a topical anesthetic ointment.

dic, (in cytogenetics) abbreviation for dicentric.

DIC, abbreviation for **disseminated intravascular coagulation.**

dicalcium phosphate and calcium gluconate with vitamin D /dikal′sē·əm/, a source of calcium and phosphorus. It is prescribed for hypocalcemia, especially in pregnancy and lactation.

dicephaly /dīsef′əlē/ [Gk di twice, kephale head], a developmental anomaly in which the fetus has two heads. **–dicephalous, dicephalic,** adj., **dicephalus,** n.

dichlorodiphenyltrichloroethane. See **DDT.**

dichlorphenamide /dī′klôrfen′əmīd/, a carbonic anhydrase inhibitor prescribed in the treatment of chronic glaucoma.

dichorial twins, dichorionic twins. See **dizygotic twins.**

dichroic stain /dīkrō′ik/, a radiographic film artifact caused by a colored chemical stain. The color may range from yellow to purple and is usually the result of improper processing.

dichromatic vision /dī′krōmat′ik/ [Gk di + chroma color; L visio], a form of color vision in which only two of the three primary colors are perceived.

dichotomy /dīkot′əmē/ [Gk dicha in two, temnein to cut], a division or separation into two equal parts.

Dick-Read method. See **Read method.**

Dick test [George F. Dick, b. 1881; Gladys R. H. Dick, b. 1881; American physicians], a skin test for determining sensitivity to an erythrotoxin produced by the group A streptococci that cause scarlet fever.

dicloxacillin sodium /dī′kloksəsil′in/, an antibacterial prescribed in the treatment of staphylococcal infections, especially those caused by penicillinase-producing strains of staphylococci.

dicrotic notch /dīkrot′ik/, a phenomenon observed on the downstroke of the arterial pressure waveform. It represents closure of the aortic valve at the onset of ventricular diastole. Also observed on the pulmonary artery pressure waveform, the interval represents closure of the pulmonic valve.

dicrotic pulse, a pulse with two separate peaks, the second usually weaker than the first.

dicumarol /dīkyoo′mərol/, a synthetic anticoagulant prescribed for the prophylaxis and treatment of thrombosis and embolism.

dicyclomine hydrochloride /dīsī′kləmīn/, an anticholinergic prescribed as an adjunct to ulcer therapy.

didactic /dīdak′tik/ [Gr didaskein to teach], pertaining to materials to be used for teaching or instruction.

didanosine. See **dideoxyinosine (DDI).**

dideoxycytidine (ddC) /dī′dē·ok′sēsī′-tidēn/, an antiretroviral drug that prevents the HIV virus from multiplying. It is chemically related to **dideoxyinosine (DDI).**

dideoxyinosine (DDI) /dī′dē·oksē·in′ōsēn/, an antiretroviral drug, also called didanosine, used in the treatment of HIV infections. DDI inhibits the enzyme reverse transcriptase, thereby restricting viral replication activity. Inside the body, DDI is converted to dideoxyadenosine, which becomes incorporated into the DNA chain, interrupting its normal sequence and making viral replication impossible.

didymitis /did′əmī′tis/, an inflammation in a testicle.

didymus /did′iməs/, a testis.

diecious /dī·ē′shəs/ [Gk di + oikos house],

an animal or plant that is sexually distinct, having either male or female reproductive organs.

dieldrin /dī·el'drin/, a highly toxic pesticide that is also poisonous to humans and animals if ingested, inhaled, or absorbed through the skin. It causes dysfunction of the central nervous system and is a possible carcinogen.

diencephalon /dī'ənsef'əlon/ [Gk di + enkephalon brain], the division of the brain between the cerebrum and the mesencephalon. It consists of the hypothalamus, thalamus, metathalamus, and the epithalamus and includes most of the third ventricle.

diener /dē'nər/ [Ger, man-servant], an individual who maintains the hospital laboratory or equipment and facilities.

dienestrol /dī'ines'trōl/, an estrogen prescribed in the treatment of atrophic vaginitis and kraurosis vulvae.

diet [Gk diaita a way of living], **1.** food and drink considered with regard to their nutritional qualities, composition, and effects on health. **2.** nutrients prescribed, regulated, or restricted as to kind and amount for therapeutic or other purposes. **3.** the customary allowance of food and drink regularly provided or consumed. –**dietetic,** adj.

dietary allowances, the recommended allowances of essential nutrients formulated by the Food and Nutrition Board of the National Research Council to serve as a guide for planning the diet to maintain good nutrition in healthy individuals. In general the recommended allowances exceed average nutritional requirements and are lower than the amounts needed in disease or deficiency states.

dietary amenorrhea [Gk diaita way of living, a absence, men month, rhoia to flow], an interruption of menstruation because of malnutrition, starvation, or excessive voluntary dieting.

dietary fiber, a generic term for nondigestible chemical substances found in plant cell walls and surrounding cellular material, each with a different effect on the various GI functions, such as colon transit time, water absorption, and lipid metabolism. The main dietary fiber components are cellulose, lignin, hemicellulose, pectin, and gums.

dietetic assistant, a person who assists in providing food-service supervision and nutritional-care services under the guidance of a registered or consultant dietitian or administrator. A dietetic assistant is usually required to complete a training pro-

gram approved by the American Dietetic Association.

dietetic food, 1. a specially prepared low-calorie food, often containing artificial sweeteners. **2.** a food prepared for any specific dietary need or restriction, such as salt-free or vegetarian foods.

dietetic food diarrhea. See osmotic diarrhea.

dietetics /dī'itet'iks/, the science of applying nutritional principles to the planning and preparation of foods and regulation of the diet in relation to both health and disease.

dietetic technician, a person qualified by an associate degree program approved by the American Dietetic Association who may assist in providing food service management or nutritional-care services under the supervision of a dietitian or administrator.

diethylcarbamazine citrate /dī·eth'-əlkärbam'əzēn/, an anthelmintic prescribed in the treatment of ascariasis, filariasis, onchocerciasis, loiasis, and tropic eosinophilia.

diethyl ether. See ether.

diethylpropion hydrochloride /dī·eth'-ilprō'pē·on/, an appetite depressant prescribed in the treatment of exogenous obesity.

diethylstilbestrol (DES) /dī·eth'ilstilbes'trol/, a synthetic hormone with estrogenic properties.

diethylstilbestrol diphosphate, an antineoplastic agent prescribed for inoperable, progressing prostatic cancer.

dietitian, a person who meets all the requirements for active membership in the American Dietetic Association after completing special educational training in the nutritional care of groups and individuals. A registered dietitian is one who has successfully completed an examination and maintains continuing education requirements of the Commission on Dietetic Registration.

Dietl's crisis /dē'təlz/ [Joseph Dietl, Polish physician, b. 1804; Gk krisis turning point], a sudden, excruciating pain in the kidney, caused by distention of the renal pelvis, by the rapid ingestion of very large amounts of liquid, or by a kinking of a ureter that produces temporary occlusion of the flow of urine from the kidney.

differential absorption [L differentia difference], (in radiology), the difference between those x-rays absorbed photoelectrically and those not absorbed at all, resulting in the x-ray image.

differential diagnosis, the distinguishing between two or more diseases with similar symptoms by systematically comparing their signs and symptoms.

differential growth, a comparison of the various increases in size or the different rates of growth of dissimilar organisms, tissues, or structures.

differential white blood cell count, an examination and enumeration of the distribution of leukocytes in a stained blood smear. The different kinds of white cells are counted and reported as percentages of the total examined.

differentiation [L *differentia* difference], **1.** (in embryology) a process in development in which unspecialized cells or tissues are systemically modified and altered to achieve specific and characteristic physical forms, physiologic functions, and chemical properties. Kinds of differentiation are **correlative, functional, invisible,** and **self-differentiation. 2.** progressive diversification leading to complexity. **3.** the acquisition of functions and forms different from those of the original. **4.** the distinguishing of one thing or disease from another, as in differential diagnosis. **5.** (in psychology) a mental autonomy or separation of intellect and emotions so that one is not dominated by reactive anxiety of a family or group emotional system. **6.** the first subphase of the separation-individuation phase in Mahler's system of preoedipal development. **–differentiate,** *v.*

diffraction [L *dis* opposite of, *frangere* to break], the bending and scattering of wavelengths of light or other radiation, such as the radiation that passes around obstacles in its path. X-ray diffraction is used in the study of the internal structure of cells. The x-rays are diffracted by cell parts into patterns that are indicative of chemical and physical structure.

diffuse [L *diffundere* to spread out], becoming widely spread, such as through a membrane or fluid.

diffuse fibrosing alveolitis. See **interstitial pneumonia.**

diffuse goiter, an enlargement of all parts of the thyroid gland.

diffuse hypersensitivity pneumonia, an immunologically mediated inflammatory reaction in the lungs induced by exposure to an allergen or by an adverse reaction to a drug. The disorder is characterized by cough, fever, dyspnea, malaise, pulmonary edema, and infiltration of the alveoli with eosinophils and large mononuclear cells.

diffuse idiopathic skeletal hyperostosis, a form of degenerative joint disease in which the ligaments along the spinal column become calcified and lose their flexibility.

diffuse lipoma, diffuse lipomatosis. See **multiple lipomatosis.**

diffuse myocardial fibrosis, a type of heart disease characterized by a generalized distribution of fibrous tissue that replaces normal heart muscle cells.

diffuse peritonitis [L *diffundere*; Gk *peri* near, *teinein* to stretch, *itis* inflammation], widespread peritonitis, affecting most of the peritoneum, usually caused by a ruptured stomach or appendix.

diffuse sclerosis [L *diffundere*; Gk *sklerosis* hardening], a form of sclerosis that extends through much of the central nervous system.

diffusing capacity, the rate of gas transfer through a unit area of a permeable membrane per unit of gas pressure difference across it. It is affected by specific chemical reactions that may occur in the blood.

diffusing capacity of lungs (D_L), the number of milliliters of a gas that diffuse from the lung across the alveolar-capillary (A-C) membrane into the bloodstream each minute, for each 1 mm Hg difference in the pressure gradient across the membrane.

diffusion [L *diffundere* to spread out], the process in which solid, particulate matter in a fluid moves from an area of higher concentration to an area of lower concentration, resulting in an even distribution of the particles in the fluid.

diffusion constant, a mathematical constant relating to the ability of a substance to spread widely.

diffusion defect, any impairment of alveolar-capillary diffusion caused by pathologic changes in any of the structures of the alveolar-capillary membrane and resulting in fewer molecules of oxygen crossing the membrane.

diffusion deposition, the impaction of an aerosol particle on the surface of an alveolar membrane or other airway structure, causing it to settle out of a vapor or gas.

diffusion of gases, a natural process, essential in respiration, in which molecules of a gas pass from an area of high concentration to one of lower concentration.

diflorasone diacetate /dīflôr′əsōn dī·as-′ətāt/, a topical corticosteroid prescribed as an antiinflammatory agent.

diflunisal /dīflōo′nisal/, a nonsteroidal antiinflammatory agent prescribed for mild to moderate pain and inflammation in osteoarthritis and other musculoskeletal disorders.

digastricus /dīgas′trikəs/ [Gk *di* twice, *gaster* stomach], one of four suprahyoid muscles having two parts, an anterior belly and a posterior belly. The anterior belly acts to open the jaw and to draw the hyoid bone forward. The posterior belly draws back and raises the hyoid bone.

DiGeorge's syndrome /dijôrj'əz/ [Angelo M. DiGeorge, American physician, b. 1821], a congenital disorder characterized by severe immunodeficiency and structural abnormalities, including hypertelorism, notched, low-set ears, small mouth, downward slanting eyes, cardiovascular defects, and the absence of the thymus and parathyroid glands.

digest [L *digere* to digest], **1.** /dijest'/ to soften by heat and moisture. **2.** /dijest'/ to break into smaller parts and simpler compounds by mastication, hydrolysis, and the action of intestinal secretions and enzymes. **3.** /dī'jəst/ any material that results from digestion or hydrolysis.

digestant /dijes'tant/, a substance, such as pepsin, that is added to the diet as an aid to the digestion of food.

digestion [L *digere* to digest], the conversion of food into absorbable substances in the GI tract. Digestion is accomplished through the mechanical and chemical breakdown of food into smaller and smaller molecules, with the help of glands located both inside and outside the gut. –**digestive,** *adj.*

digestive enzyme [L, *digere,* to separate; Gk, *en, zyme,* ferment], any digestive system enzyme that hydrolyzes fats, proteins, and carbohydrates for absorption.

digestive fever, a slight rise in body temperature that normally accompanies the digestive process.

digestive gland, any one of the many structures that secretes reactive agents involved in the breaking down of food into the constituent absorbable substances needed for metabolism. Some kinds of digestive glands are the salivary glands, gastric glands, intestinal glands, liver, and pancreas.

digestive system, the organs, structures, and accessory glands of the digestive tube of the body through which food passes from the mouth to the esophagus, stomach, and intestines. The accessory glands secrete the digestive enzymes, used by the digestive system to break down food substances in preparation for absorption into the bloodstream before carrying the waste to the intestines for excretion.

digestive tract, a musculomembranous tube, about 9 m long, extending from the mouth to the anus and lined with mucous membrane. Its various portions are the mouth, pharynx, esophagus, stomach, small intestine, and large intestine. The tube, which is part of the digestive system

of the body, includes numerous accessory organs.

digital /dij'itəl/ [L *digitus* finger], **1.** of or pertaining to a digit, that is, a finger or toe. **2.** resembling a finger or toe. **3.** the characterization or measurement of a signal in terms of a series of numbers rather than in terms of some continuously varying value.

digital angiography, a technique of producing enhanced x-ray images of the heart with computerized fluoroscopy equipment.

digital compression [L *digitus* + *comprimere* to press together], the act of pressing with the fingers, as when arresting the blood flow from a wound.

digital fluoroscopy, a method of conducting fluoroscopic examinations with an image intensifier–television system combined with a high-speed digital video image processor.

digitalis /dij'ital'is/ [L *digitus* finger], a cardiotonic prescribed in the treatment of congestive heart failure and certain cardiac arrhythmias.

digitalis glycoside. See **glycoside.**

digitalis poisoning [L *digitus* + *potio* drink], the toxic effects of digitalis medications prescribed for heart disorders such as heart failure and atrial fibrillation. Toxicity may develop as a result of a cumulative effect of the drug. Symptoms include vomiting, headache, heart beat abnormalities, and visual color distortions.

digitalis therapy, the administration of a digitalis preparation to a person with a heart disorder to increase the force of myocardial contractions, produce a slower, more regular apical rate, and slow the transmission of impulses through the conduction system. Digitalis may be used in treating many cardiac disorders, including atrial fibrillation, atrial septal defect, coarctation of the aorta, congenital heart block, congestive heart failure, endocardial fibroelastosis, great vessel transposition, malformation of the tricuspid valve, myocarditis, paroxysmal atrial tachycardia, and patent ductus arteriosus.

digitalization, the administration of digitalis in doses sufficient to achieve maximum pharmacologic effects without also producing toxic symptoms.

digitalized, the state of having a therapeutic total body level of a cardiac glycoside.

digitalizing dose, the amount of a cardiac glycoside needed to digitalize a patient.

digital radiography (DR), any method of x-ray image formation that uses a computer to store and manipulate data.

digital subtraction angiography (DSA), a method by which x-ray images of blood vessels filled with contrast material are digitized and then subtracted from images stored before the administration of contrast. Thus the background is eliminated and only the vessels appear.

digital tomosynthesis, a system of tomography using a computer and digital fluoroscopy unit, making it possible to synthesize any tomographic plane from a single tomographic pass.

digitate /dij′itāt/ [L *digitatus* having fingers], having fingers or fingerlike projections.

digitate wart, a fingerlike, horny projection that arises from a pea-shaped base and occurs on the scalp or near the hairline. Like other warts, it is a benign viral infection of the skin and the adjacent mucous membrane.

digitoxin /dij′itok′sin/, a cardiac glycoside obtained from leaves of *Digitalis purpurea.* It is prescribed in the treatment of congestive heart failure and certain cardiac arrhythmias.

diglyceride /dīglis′ərīd/, a chemical compound, an ester of glycerol in which the hydrogen in two of the hydroxyl groups is replaced by an acyl radical.

digoxin /dijok′sin/, a cardiac glycoside obtained from leaves of *Digitalis lanata.* It is prescribed in the treatment of congestive heart failure and certain cardiac arrhythmias.

digoxin immune Fab, ovine, a parenteral antidote prescribed for life-threatening digoxin or digitoxin toxicity.

diGuglielmo's disease, diGuglielmo's syndrome. See **erythroleukemia.**

dihybrid /dī′hī′brid/ [Gk *di* twice; L *hybrida* mongrel offspring], (in genetics) pertaining to or describing a person, organism, or strain that is heterozygous for two specific traits.

dihybrid cross, (in genetics) the mating of two individuals, organisms, or strains that have different gene pairs that determine two specific traits or in which two particular characteristics or gene loci are being followed.

dihydric alcohol /dīhī′drik/, an alcohol containing two hydroxyl groups.

dihydroergotamine mesylate /dīhī′drō··urgot′əmēn me′silat/, an alpha-adrenergic blocking agent prescribed for migraine and for vascular headache.

dihydrotachysterol /dīhī′drōtəkis′tərol/, a rapid-acting form of vitamin D. It is prescribed in the treatment of hypocalcemia resulting from hypoparathyroidism and pseudohypoparathyroidism.

diiodohydroxyquin. See **iodoguinol.**

dilatation /dil′ətā′shən/ [L *dilatare* to widen], an artificial increase in the diameter of an opening either by medication, as in the use of cycloplegic eyedrops to open the pupil wide for examination of the retina, or by instrumentation as in the use of a dilator to open the uterine cervix to facilitate curettage. –**dilatate,** /dī′lāt/, *v.,* **dilatator, dilator,** *n.*

dilatation and curettage (D & C), dilatation of the uterine cervix and scraping of the endometrium of the uterus, performed to diagnose disease of the uterus, to correct heavy or prolonged vaginal bleeding, or to empty uterine contents of the products of conception. It is also done to remove tumors, to rule out carcinoma of the uterus, to remove retained placental fragments postpartum or after an incomplete abortion, and to find the cause of infertility.

dilatation of the heart [L *dilatare;* AS *heorte*], an enlargement of the heart caused by stretching the muscle tissue in the walls, due to a weakening of the myocardium. The condition is associated with acute pulmonary embolism and heart failure.

dilatator naris, the alar portion of the nasalis muscle that dilates the nostril.

dilatator pupillae, a muscle that contracts the iris of the eye and dilates the pupil.

dilate, to make wider.

dilation. a natural physiologic increase in the diameter of a body opening, blood vessel, or tube, such as the widening of the pupil of the eye in response to decreased light.

dilation and evacuation (D & E) [L, *dilatare* + *evacuare* to empty], the removal of the products of conception, using suction curretage and forceps, during the second trimester of pregnancy.

dilator [L *dilatare* to widen], a device for expanding a body opening or cavity.

diltiazem /diltī′azəm/, a slow channel blocker or calcium antagonist. It is prescribed for the treatment of vasospastic and effort-associated angina.

diluent /dil′ōō·ənt, dil′yōō·ənt/ [L *diluere* to wash], a substance, generally a fluid, that makes a solution or mixture thinner, less viscous, or more liquid.

dilute /dilōōt′, dī′loot/ [L *diluere* to wash], pertaining to a solution in which there is a relatively small amount of solute in proportion to solvent.

diluting agent, (in respiratory therapy) a substance that can modify the viscosity of secretions so that they can be removed easily. Examples include water and hypotonic saline, which can be aerosolized or nebulized.

dimenhydrinate /dim'ənhī'drināt/, an antihistamine prescribed in the treatment of nausea and motion sickness.

dimensional stability, (in radiology) the rigidity of the polyester base used for radiographic film and its resistance to image distortion from warping or changing size or shape during processing.

dimer /dī'mər/ [Gk *di* twice, *meros* parts], a compound formed by the union of two radicals or two molecules of a simpler compound, as a polymer formed from two or more molecules of a monomer.

dimercaprol /dī'mərkap'rol/, a heavy-metal antagonist. It is prescribed in the treatment of Wilson's disease and in the treatment of acute arsenic, mercury, or gold poisoning, as from an overdosage with mercurial diuretics, arsenics, or gold salts or from an accidental ingestion of mercury, gold, or arsenic.

dimethindene maleate /dīmeth'indēn/, an antihistamine prescribed in the treatment of a variety of hypersensitivity reactions, including rhinitis, skin reactions, and itching.

dimethoxymethylamphetamine (DOM) /dī'məthok'sēmeth'iləmfet'əmēn/, a psychoactive or hallucinogenic agent.

dimethyl carbinol. See **isopropyl alcohol.**

dimethyl sulfoxide (DMSO) /dīmeth'il/, an antiinflammatory agent prescribed in the treatment of interstitial cystitis and is being investigated as a topical antiinflammatory agent in orthopedic sports injuries.

dimethyl tubocurarine iodide. See **metocurine iodide.**

Dimitri's disease. See **Sturge-Weber syndrome.**

dimorphous /dīmôr'fəs/ [Gk *di* + *morphe* form], in biology, chemistry, and genetics, an organism or substance that exists in two distinct forms.

dimpling [ME, *dympull*], small, abnormal indentations or depressions on the surface of a body or organ.

dinitrochlorobenzene (DNCB) /dīnī'trōklôr'ōben'zēn/, a substance applied topically as a test for delayed hypersensitivity reactions.

diode /dī'od/, (in radiology) an x-ray tube with two electrodes.

diolamine /dī·ol'əmēn/, a contraction for *diethanolamine.*

Dionysian /dē·onis'ē·ən/ [Gk *Dionysos* Greek god of wine], the personal attitude of one who is uninhibited, mystic, sensual, emotional, and irrational and who may seek to escape from the boundaries imposed by the limits of one's senses.

diopter /dī·op'tər/ [Gk *dioptra* optical measuring instrument], a metric measure of the refractive power of a lens. It is equal to the reciprocal of the focal length of the lens in meters. For example, a lens with a focal length of 0.5 m has a diopter measure of 2.0 (1/2.0) and when prescribed as a corrective lens for the eye should make printed matter most clearly focused when held 0.5 m from the eyes.

dioptric power /dī·op'trik/, the refractive power of an optic lens as measured in diopters.

diovular. See **binovular.**

diovulatory /dī·ov'yələtôr'ē/ [Gk *di* twice; L *ovum* egg], routinely releasing two ova during each ovarian cycle.

dioxide /dī·ok'sīd/ [Gk *di* + *oxys* sharp, *genein* to produce], an oxide that contains two oxygen atoms.

dioxin /dī·ok'sin/, a contaminant of the herbicide 2,4,5-trichlorophenoxyacetic acid (2,4,5-T), widely used throughout the world for weed control. Exposure to dioxin is associated with chloracne and porphyria cutanea tarda (PCT). Dioxin was a contaminant of the jungle defoliant Agent Orange.

dioxyline phosphate/ dī·ok'silēn/, a synthetic antispasmodic and vasodilator. It is prescribed for the relief of angina pectoris and for spasm of blood vessels in arms, legs, or lungs.

DIP, abbreviation for **desquamative interstitial pneumonia.**

diphasic /dīfā'zik/ [Gk *di* + *phasis* appearance], pertaining to or involving something that occurs in two stages or phases.

diphemanil methylsulfate /dīfē'mənil/, an anticholinergic prescribed as an adjunct to ulcer therapy.

diphenadione /dī'fənad'ē·ōn/, an anticoagulant prescribed in the treatment of thrombosis and embolism.

diphenhydramine hydrochloride /dī'fənhī'drəmēn/, an antihistamine prescribed in the treatment of a variety of hypersensitivity reactions, including rhinitis, skin rash, and pruritus, and in the treatment of motion sickness.

diphenidol /dīfē'nidol/, an antiemetic, antivertigo agent prescribed in the treatment of vertigo and to control nausea and vomiting.

diphenoxylate hydrochloride /dīfənok'silāt/, an antidiarrheal prescribed in the treatment of diarrhea and intestinal cramping.

diphenylhydantoin. See **phenytoin.**

diphenylpyraline hydrochloride /dī'fenəlpī'rəlēn/, an antihistamine prescribed in the treatment of a variety of hypersensitivity reactions, including rhinitis, skin rash, and pruritus.

2,3-diphosphoglyceric acid (DPG) /dīfos'fōgliser'ik/, a substance in the erythrocyte that affects the affinity of hemoglobin for oxygen. It is a chief end product of glucose metabolism.

diphtheria /difthir'ē·ə, dipthir'ē·ə/ [Gk *diphthera* leather membrane], an acute, contagious disease caused by the bacterium *Corynebacterium diphtheriae,* characterized by the production of a systemic toxin and a false membrane lining of the mucous membrane of the throat. The toxin is particularly damaging to the tissues of the heart and central nervous system, and the dense pseudomembrane in the throat may interfere with eating, drinking, and breathing. Untreated, the disease is often fatal, causing heart and kidney failure.

diphtheria and tetanus toxoids (DT), an active immunizing agent prescribed for immunization against diphtheria and tetanus.

diphtheria and tetanus toxoids and pertussis vaccine (DTP), an active immunizing agent prescribed for the routine immunization of children under 6 years of age against diphtheria, tetanus, and pertussis.

diphtheria antitoxin [Gk *diphthera* + *anti, toxikon* poison], an antitoxin prepared by immunizing horses with diphtheria toxoid and extracting. The serum is standardized for strength and quality.

diphtheria toxin [Gk, *diphthera* + *toxikon* poison], a filtrate of a broth culture used to prepare an intradermal injectable form of toxin for Schick tests.

diphtheritic croup /dif'thirit'ik/ [Gk *diphthera;* Scot *croak* to speak hoarsely], a diphtheritic inflammation of the larynx.

diphtheritic laryngitis [Gk *diphthera, larynx, itis*], an inflammation of the larynx caused by the Klebs-Loeffler bacillus *(Corynebacterium diphtheriae).* A serious complication is formation of a false membrane.

diphtheritic pharyngitis [Gk *diphthera, pharynx, itis*], an inflammation of the pharynx caused by an infection of the Klebs-Loeffler bacillus *(Corynebacterium diphtheriae)* and associated with the formation of a false membrane.

diphtheroid /dif'thəroid'/ [Gk *diphthera* leather membrane, *eidos* form], **1.** of or pertaining to diphtheria. **2.** resembling the bacillus *Corynebacterium diphtheriae.*

diphyllobothriasis. See *fish tapeworm infection.*

Diphyllobothrium /dəfil'ōboth'rē·əm/ [Gk *di* twice, *phyllon* leaf, *bothrion* pit], a genus of large, parasitic, intestinal flatworms having a scolex with two slitlike grooves.

dipivefrin /dī'pivef'rin/, an ophthalmic adrenergic prescribed in the treatment of open-angle glaucoma.

diplegia /dīplē'jē·ə/ [Gk *di* twice, *plege* stroke], bilateral paralysis of both sides of any part of the body or of like parts on the opposite sides of the body. A kind of diplegia is **facial diplegia. –diplegic,** *adj.*

diplococcus /dip'lōkok'əs/, *pl.* **diplococci** /-kok'sī/ [Gk *diploos* double, *kokkos* berry], a coccus that occurs in pairs.

diploë /dip'lō·ē/, the loose tissue filled with red bone marrow between the two tables of the cranial bones.

diploid /dip'loid/ [Gk *diploos* + *eidos* form], of or pertaining to an individual, organism, strain, or cell that has two complete sets of homologous chromosomes. In humans the normal diploid number is 46. **–diploidic,** *adj.*

diploidy /dip'loidē/, the state or condition of having two complete sets of homologous chromosomes.

diplokaryon /dip'lōker'ē·on/ [Gk *diploos* + *karyon* nut], a nucleus that contains twice the diploid number of chromosomes.

diploma program in nursing, an educational program that trains nurses in a hospital setting, usually in 2 or 3 years. The recipient of a diploma is eligible to take the national certifying examination to become a registered nurse.

diplomate /dip'ləmāt/, an individual who has earned a diploma or certificate, especially a physician who has been certified by a specialty board.

diplonema /dip'lənē'mə/ [Gk *diploos* + *nema* thread], the looplike formation of the chromosomes in the diplotene stage of the first meiotic prophase of gametogenesis.

diplopagus /diplop'əgəs/ [Gk *diploos* + *pagos* something fixed], conjoined twins that are more or less equally developed, although one or several internal organs may be shared.

diplopia /diplō'pē·ə/ [Gk *diploos* + *opsis* vision], double vision caused by defective function of the extraocular muscles or a disorder of the nerves that innervate the muscles.

diplornavirus /dī'plôrnəvī'rəs/, a double-stranded RNA virus that is the cause of Colorado tick fever. It is related to the reoviruses that are associated with various respiratory infections.

diplosomatia /dip'lōsōmā'shə/ [Gk *diploos* + *soma* body], a congenital anomaly in which fully formed twins are joined at one or more areas of their bodies.

diplotene /dip'lətēn/ [Gk *diploos* + *tainia* ribbon], the fourth stage in the first meiotic prophase in gametogenesis in which the tetrads exhibit chiasmata between the chromatids of the paired homologous chromosomes and genetic crossing-over occurs.

dipodia /dīpō'dē·ə/ [Gk *di* twice, *pous* foot], a developmental anomaly characterized by the duplication of one or both feet.

dipolar ion. See **zwitterion.**

dipole /dī'pol/, a molecule with areas of opposing electric charges, as hydrogen chloride with a predominance of electrons about the chloride portion and a positive charge on the hydrogen side.

diprop, abbreviation for a *carboxylate dipropionate anion.*

diprosopus /dīpros'əpəs, dī'prəsō'pəs/ [Gk *di* twice, *prosopon* face], a malformed fetus that has a double face showing varying degrees of development.

dipsomania /dip'sōmā'nē·ə/ [Gk *dipsa* thirst, *mania* madness], an uncontrollable, often periodic craving for and indulgence in alcoholic beverages; alcoholism.

dipstick, a chemically treated strip of paper used in the analysis of urine or other fluids.

dipus /dī'pəs/, conjoined twins that have only two feet.

dipygus /dīpī'gəs, dip'əgəs/ [Gk *di* twice, *pyge* rump], a malformed fetus that has a double pelvis, one of which is usually not fully developed.

dipyridamole /dī'pirid'əmōl/, a coronary vasodilator prescribed for the long-term treatment of angina.

direct antagonist [L *diregere* to direct; Gk *antagonisma* struggle], one of a pair or a group of muscles that pull in opposite directions and whose combined action keeps the part from moving.

direct calorimetry, the measurement of the amount of heat directly generated by any oxidation reaction, especially one involving a living organism.

direct causal association, a cause-and-effect relationship between a causative factor and a disease with no other factors intervening in the process.

direct contact, mutual touching of two individuals or organisms. Many communicable diseases may be spread by the direct contact between an infected and a healthy person.

direct current (DC), an electric current that flows in one direction only and is substantially constant in value.

direct endometriosis [L *diregire* to direct; Gk *endon* within, *metra* womb, *osis* condition], an invasion of the myometrium of the uterus by the mucous membrane lining.

direct-exposure film, a type of x-ray film sometimes used to produce images of thin body parts, such as the hands and feet, that have a high subject contrast.

direct fracture, any fracture occurring at a specific point of injury that is a direct result of that injury.

direct generation. See **asexual generation.**

direct gold, any form of pure gold that may be compacted directly into a prepared tooth cavity to form a restoration.

direct illumination. See **illumination.**

directive therapy [L *diregere; therapeia* treatment], a psychotherapeutic approach in which the psychotherapist directs the course of therapy by intervening to ask questions and offer interpretations.

direct laryngoscopy [L *diregire;* Gk *larynx, skopein* to watch], an examination of the larynx by means of a lighted tube inserted through the mouth.

direct lead, 1. an electrocardiographic conductor in which the exploring electrode is placed directly on the surface of the exposed heart. **2.** *informal.* a tracing produced by such a lead on an electrocardiograph.

direct light reflex, the constriction of a pupil receiving increased illumination, as by a flashlight during an ophthalmologic examination.

direct measurement of blood pressure [L *diregire, mensura* to measure; ME *blod;* L *premere* to press], measurement of blood pressure in an artery by inserting a catheter into the blood vessel and recording the pressure directly, as opposed to the indirect method of using a pressure cuff, stethoscope, and sphygmomanometer.

direct nursing care functions, liaison nursing activities that are focused on a particular patient, patient's family, or a group for whom the nurse is directly responsible and accountable.

direct patient care, (in nursing) care of a patient provided in person by a member of the staff.

direct percussion. See **percussion.**

direct provider reimbursement, a method of direct payment for health care services, as fee-for-service.

direct-question interview, an inquiry that usually requires simple one- or two-word responses.

direct relationship. See **positive relationship.**

direct retainer, a clasp, attachment, or assembly fastened to an abutment tooth for the purpose of maintaining a removable restoration in its planned position in relation to oral structures.

direct self-destructive behavior (DSDB), any form of suicidal activity, such as suicide threats, attempts, or gestures and the act of suicide itself. The intent of the behavior is death, and the person is aware of this as the desired outcome.

direct transfusion [L *dirigere, transfundere* to pour through], the transfer of whole blood directly from a vein of the donor to a vein of the recipient.

dirofilariasis /dī'rōfil'ərī'əsis/, a rare human infestation of the dog heartworm, *Dirofilaria immitis,* which may be transmitted through the bite of any of several species of mosquitoes.

disability [L *dis* opposite of, *habilis* fit], the loss, absence, or impairment of physical or mental fitness that is observable and measurable.

disaccharidase deficiency. See **lactase deficiency.**

disaccharide /dīsak'ərīd/ [Gk *di* two, *sakcharon* sugar], a general term for simple carbohydrates formed by the union of two monosaccharide molecules.

disadvantaged [L *dis* + *abante* superior position] **1.** any group of people who lack money, education, literacy, or another status advantage. **2.** a euphemism for "poor."

disarticulation /dis'ärtik'yəlā'shən/ [L *dis* + *articulare* to divide into joints], the separation of a joint without cutting through a bone.

disaster-preparedness plan [L *dis* + *astrum* favorable stars; *praeparare* to prepare], a formal plan of action, usually prepared in written form, for coordinating the response of a hospital staff in the event of a disaster within the hospital or the surrounding community.

disc. See **disk.**

discharge [OFr *deschargier* to expel], **1.** to release a substance or object. **2.** to release a patient from a hospital. 3. to release an electric charge, which may be manifested by a spark or surge of electricity, from a storage battery, condenser, or other source. **4.** to release a burst of energy from or through a neuron. **5.** a release of emotions, often accompanied by a wide range of voluntary and involuntary reflexes, weeping, rage, or other emotional displays, called **affective discharge** in psychology. **6.** a substance or object discharged.

discharge abstract, items of information compiled from medical records of patients discharged from a hospital, organized and recorded in a uniform format to provide data for statistic studies, reports, or research.

discharge coordinator, an individual who arranges with community agencies and institutions for the continuing care of patients after their discharge from a hospital.

discharge planning, the activities that facilitate a client's movement from one health care setting to another. It is a multidisciplinary process involving physicians, nurses, social workers, and possibly other health professionals and its goal is to enhance continuity of care.

discharge summary, a clinical report prepared by a physician or other health professional at the conclusion of treatment, outlining the patient's chief complaint, the diagnostic findings, the therapy administered, and the patient's response to it.

discharging lesion [OFr *deschargier;* L *laesio* hurting], an injury or infection of the central nervous system that causes sudden abnormal episodes of discharging nerve impulses.

disciform keratitis /dis'ifôrm/ [Gk *diskos* flat plate; L *forma* form; Gk *keras* horn, *itis* inflammation], an inflammatory condition of the eye that often follows an attack of dendritic keratitis and is believed to be an immunologic response to an ocular herpes simplex infection. The condition is characterized by disclike opacities in the cornea, usually with inflammation of the iris.

disclosing solution [L *dis* + *claudere* to close; *solutus* dissolved], a topically applied dye, used in aqueous solution to stain and reveal plaque and other deposits on teeth.

discoblastula /dis'kōblas'tyələ/ [Gk *diskos* flat plate, *blastos* germ], a blastula formed from the partial cleavage that occurs in a fertilized ovum containing a large amount of yolk.

discocyte /dis'kəsīt/ [Gk *diskos* + *kytos* cell], a mature, normal, erythrocyte, exhibiting one of its many steady-state configurations. It is a biconcave disk without a nucleus.

discoid lupus erythematosus (DLE) /dis'koid/ [Gk *diskos* + *eidos* form; L *lupus* wolf; Gk *erythema* redness, *osis* condition], a chronic, recurrent disease, primarily of the skin, characterized by red macules that are covered with scales and extend into follicles. The lesions are typically distributed in a butterfly pattern covering the cheeks and bridge of the nose but may also occur on other parts of the body. The cause of the disease is not established, but there is evidence that it may be an autoimmune disorder, and some cases seem to be induced by certain drugs.

discoid meniscus, an abnormal condition characterized by a discoid rather than semilunar shape of the cartilaginous meniscus of the knee. Common complaints are that a "clicking" occurs in the knee joint or that the knee joint gives way. These characteristics are often associated with an injury to the knee but occur also without any history of trauma.

discoid placenta [Gk *diskos* quoit, *eidos* form; L *placenta* flat cake], a round placenta.

disconfirmation, a dysfunctional communication that negates, discounts, or ignores information received from another person.

discordance /diskôr′dəns/ [L *discordare* to disagree], (in genetics) the expression of one or more specific traits in only one member of a pair of twins. –**discordant,** *adj.*

discordant twins, twins showing a marked difference in size (greater than 10% in weight) at birth.

discovery [L *dis* + *coopiere* to cover], (in law) a pretrial procedure allowing one party to examine vital witnesses and documents held exclusively by the adverse party.

discrete x-rays. See **x-ray.**

discrimination [L *discrimen* division], the act of distinguishing or differentiating. The ability to distinguish between touch or pressure at two nearby points on the body is known as two-point discrimination.

discriminator, (in nuclear medicine) an electronic device capable of accepting or rejecting a pulse of energy according to the pulse height of voltage. It is used to separate low-energy from high-energy radionuclides.

discus. See **disk.**

discus articularis /dis′kəs/, a small oval plate between the condyle of the mandible and the mandibular fossa.

discus interpubicus. See **interpubic disk.**

discus nervi optici. See **optic disc.**

disdiadochokinesia /dis′dī·ad′əkōkīnē′-zhə/ [L *dis* apart, *diadochos* successor, *kinesis* movement], an inability to quickly make fine coordinated motor movements.

disease [L *dis* + Fr *aise* ease], 1. a condition of abnormal vital function involving any structure, part, or system of an organism. 2. a specific illness or disorder characterized by a recognizable set of signs and symptoms, attributable to heredity, infection, diet, or environment.

disease prevention, activities designed to protect patients or other members of the public from actual or potential health threats and their harmful consequences.

disengagement [Fr *disengager* to release from engagement], 1. an obstetrical manipulation in which the presenting part of

the baby is dislodged from the maternal pelvis as part of an operative delivery. 2. the release or detachment of oneself from other persons or responsibilities. 3. (in transactional family therapy) a role assumed by a therapist in observing and restructuring intervention without becoming actively and directly involved in the problem.

disengagement theory, the psychosocial concept that aging individuals and society normally withdraw from active engagement with each other.

disequilibrium /disē′kwilib′rē·əm/ [L *dis* + *aequilibrium*], the loss of balance or adjustment, particularly mental or psychologic balance.

dishpan fracture [AS *disc* plate; L *patina* dish; *fractura* break], a fracture that depresses the skull.

disinfect [L *dis* + *inficere* to stain], to remove pathogens.

disinfectant [L *dis* + *inficere* to corrupt], a chemical that can be applied to objects to destroy microorganisms.

disinfection, the process of killing pathogenic organisms or of rendering them inert.

disinfection of thermometer [L *dis* + *inficere;* Gk *therme* heat, *metron* measure], the destruction of infectious organisms that may be present on a clinical glass thermometer. The process usually involves the use of chemical germicides after thorough washing, following the Centers for Disease Guidelines for cleaning, disinfection, and sterilization of hospital equipment.

disinfestation [L *dis* + *infestare* to attack], eliminating a threat of infestation by vermin, rodents, lice, or other noxious organisms.

disinhibition [L *dis* + *inhibere* to restrain], the removal of inhibition.

disintegrative psychosis, a mental disorder of childhood that usually has an onset after the age of 3 years and following normal development of speech, social behavior, and other traits. After a vague illness, the child undergoes mental deterioration, eventually reaching a stage of severe mental retardation.

disjunction [L *disjungere* to disjoint], (in genetics) the separation of the paired homologous chromosomes during the anaphase stage of the first meiotic division or of the chromatids during anaphase of mitosis and the second meiotic division.

disk [Gk *diskos* flat plate], 1. also spelled (chiefly in ophthalmology) **disc.** a flat, circular platelike structure, as an articular disk or an optic disc. 2. *informal.* an intervertebral disk.

diskography, the radiologic examination

of individual intervertebral disks. It involves the injection of a small amount of water-soluble iodinated media into the center of the disk by a double-needle entry.

dislocation [L *dis* + *locare* to place], the displacement of any part of the body from its normal position, particularly a bone from its normal articulation with a joint. **–dislocate,** *v.*

dislocation of clavicle [L *dis* + *locare, clavicula little key*], displacement of the collarbone. It may occur at the sternal end or the acromial or scapular extremity.

dislocation of finger [L *dis* + *locare; AS finger*], displacement of a finger at a joint, as a result of trauma. In the absence of an accompanying fracture, the dislocated finger can usually be reduced by steadying the hand at the femur and maneuvering the dislocated bone into place. After the dislocation has been reduced, a splint should be applied from the fingertip to the palm of the hand and a post-reduction x-ray obtained.

dislocation of hip [L *dis* + *locare; AS hype*], a displacement of the femoral head out of the hip joint, usually accompanied by pain, rigidity, shortening of the leg, and loss of function. The dislocation can occur as an **obturator dislocation,** in which the head of the femur lies in the obturator foramen; a **perineal dislocation,** in which the head of the femur is displaced into the perineum; a **sciatic dislocation,** in which the head of the femur is lying in the sciatic notch; or a **subpubic dislocation,** in which there is anterior displacement of the femoral head.

dislocation of jaw [L *dis* + *locare; ME jowel*], a displacement of the jaw, which may be unilateral or bilateral, as a result of a blow, a fall, or yawning. The mandible will appear fixed in an open position with only the back teeth in contact. If the mandible appears deviated to one side, the dislocation involves only one side. The dislocation is reduced manually, with or without injection of a local anesthetic.

dislocation of knee [L *dis* + *locare; AS cneow*], a displacement of one of the bones of the knee joint. First aid treatment for the dislocation is the same as for a fracture: the joint is immobilized with splints and the patient is moved quickly to a medical facility.

dislocation of shoulder [L *dis* + *locare; AS sculder*], any of several kinds of displacement of the shoulder joint, including acromial joint disruption and separation and dislocation of the glenohumeral joint with the humeral head displaced anteriorly and inferiorly.

dismiss [L *dis* + *mittere* to send], (in law) to discharge or dispose of an action, suit, or motion trial. **–dismissal,** *n.*

disodium edetate. See **edetate disodium.**

disopyramide phosphate /dī'sōpir'əmīd/, a cardiac depressant prescribed in the treatment of premature ventricular contractions and ventricular tachycardia.

disorder [L *dis* apart, *ordo* rank], a disruption or interference with normal functions or established systems, as a mental disorder or nutritional disorder.

disorders of movement [L *dis* + *ordo* rank, *movere* to move], any perverse or abnormal functions of muscular action that may result from infection, injury, or congenital disability, such as ataxia, involuntary grimacing, or chorea.

disorders of sleep [L *dis* + *ordo; AS slaep*], any condition that interferes with normal sleep patterns, such as sleep apnea, phase shift, use of alcohol and certain drugs, excessive sleepiness, sleep walking, nightmares, Ekbom's syndrome, sleep paralysis, and narcolepsy. Treatment may include medications and therapy offered at sleep disorder clinics.

disorganized schizophrenia [L *dis* + Gk *organon* organ], a form of schizophrenia characterized by an earlier age of onset, usually at puberty, and a more severe disintegration of the personality than occurs in other forms of the disease. Symptoms include inappropriate laughter and silliness; peculiar mannerisms, such as grimaces; talking and gesturing to oneself; regressive, bizarre, and often obscene behavior.

disorient, to cause to lose awareness or perception of space, time, or personal identity and relationships.

disorientation [L *dis* + *orienter* to proceed from], a state of mental confusion characterized by inadequate or incorrect perceptions of place, time, or identity.

disparate twins /dis'pərāt, disper'it/, twins who are distinctly different from each other in weight and other features.

dispense [L *dis* + *pensare* to weigh], to prepare and issue drugs or drug mixtures from a pharmaceutical outlet or department.

dispersing agent [L *dis* + *spargere* to scatter; *agere* to do], a chemical additive used in pharmaceuticals to cause the even distribution of the ingredients throughout the product, such as in dermatologic emulsions containing both oil and water.

dispersion, the scattering or dissipation of finely divided material, as when particles of a substance are scattered throughout the volume of a fluid.

dispersion medium. See **continuous phase, medium.**

displaced fracture [Fr *deplacement* to remove], a traumatic bone break in which two ends of a fractured bone are separated from each other. The ends of broken bones in displaced fractures often pierce surrounding skin, as in an open fracture, or may be contained within the skin, as in a closed fracture.

displaced testis [Fr *deplacement; L testis* testicle], a testis that is located in the pelvis, inguinal canal, or elsewhere after it normally would have descended into the scrotum.

displacement [Fr *deplacement* to remove], **1.** the state of being displaced or the act of displacing. **2.** (in chemistry) a reaction in which an atom, molecule, or radical is removed from combination and replaced by another. **3.** (in physics) the displacing in space of one mass by another, such as the weight or volume of a fluid being displaced by a floating or submerged body. **4.** (in psychiatry) an unconscious defense mechanism for avoiding emotional conflict and anxiety by transferring emotions, ideas, or wishes from one object to a substitute that is less anxiety-producing.

DISS, abbreviation for **Diameter-Index Safety System.**

dissect [L *dissecare* to cut apart], to cut apart tissues for visual or microscopic study using a scalpel, a probe, or scissors. **–dissection,** *n.*

dissecting aneurysm [L *dissecare* to cut apart; Gk *aneurysma* a widening], a localized dilatation of an artery, most commonly the aorta, characterized by a longitudinal dissection between the outer and middle layers of the vascular wall. Blood entering a tear in the intimal lining of the vessel causes a separation of weakened elastic and fibromuscular elements in the medial layer and leads to the formation of cystic spaces filled with ground substance. Rupture of a dissecting aneurysm may be fatal in less than 1 hour.

disseminated intravascular coagulation (DIC) [L *dis + seminare* to sow; *intra* within, *vasculum* little vessel; *coagulare* to curdle], a grave coagulopathy resulting from the overstimulation of the body's clotting and anticlotting processes in response to disease or injury, such as septicemia, poisonous snake bites, severe trauma, or hemorrhage. The primary disorder initiates generalized intravascular clotting, which in turn overstimulates fibrinolytic mechanisms; as a result the initial hypercoagulability is succeeded by a deficiency in clotting factors with hypocoagulability and hemorrhaging.

disseminated lupus erythematosus. See **systemic lupus erythematosus.**

disseminated multiple sclerosis. See **multiple sclerosis.**

dissent [L *dis + sentire* to feel], (in law) a statement written by a judge who disagrees with the decision of the majority of the court. The dissent explicitly states the reasons for the dissenting judge's contrary opinion. **–dissenting,** *adj.*

dissimilar twins. See **dizygotic twins.**

dissociation [L *dis + sociare* to unite], **1.** the act of separating into parts or sections. **2.** an unconscious defense mechanism by which an idea, thought, emotion, or other mental process is separated from the consciousness and thereby loses emotional significance. **–dissociative** /disō´shē·ōtiv/, *adj.*

dissociative anesthesia, an anesthetic procedure characterized by analgesia and amnesia without loss of respiratory function or pharyngeal and laryngeal reflexes. This form of anesthesia may be used to provide analgesia during brief, superficial operative procedures or diagnostic processes.

dissociative disorder, a condition in which emotional conflicts are so repressed that a separation or split in the personality occurs, resulting in an altered state of consciousness or a confusion in identity. Symptoms include amnesia, somnambulism, fugue, dream state, or multiple personality.

dissolution [L *dissolvere* to loose], **1.** the separation of a complex chemical compound into simpler molecules. **2.** the liquifaction of organic substances. **3.** the loss of mental powers.

dissolved gas [L *dis + solvere* to loosen], gas in a simple physical solution, as distinguished from gas that has reacted chemically with a solvent or other solutes and is chemically combined.

distal /dis´təl/ [L *distare* to be distant] **1.** away from or being the farthest from a point of origin. **2.** away from or being the farthest from the midline or a central point, as a distal phalanx.

distal latency, (in electroneuromyography) the time interval between the stimulation of a compound muscle and the observed response.

distal muscular dystrophy, a rare form of muscular dystrophy, usually affecting adults, characterized by moderate weakness and by wasting that begins in the arms and legs and then extends gradually to the proximal and facial muscles.

distal phalanx, any one of the small distal bones in the third row of phalanges of the hand or the foot. Each distal phalanx of the toes is smaller and more flattened than that of a finger.

distal radioulnar articulation, the pivot-like articulation of the head of the ulna and the ulnar notch on the lower end of the radius, involving two ligaments.

distal renal tubular acidosis (distal RTA), an abnormal condition characterized by excessive acid accumulation and bicarbonate excretion. It is caused by the inability of the distal tubules of the kidney to secrete hydrogen ions, thus decreasing the excretion of titratable acids and ammonium and increasing the urinary loss of potassium and bicarbonate. **Primary distal RTA** occurs mostly in females, adolescents, older children, and young adults. It may occur sporadically or as the result of hereditary defects. **Secondary distal RTA** is associated with numerous disorders, such as cirrhosis of the liver, malnutrition, starvation, and various genetic problems.

distal sparing, a condition in which the spinal cord remains intact below a lesion. The reflex arc remains but is not modified by supraspinal influences. As a result there may be spastic movements distal to the level of the lesion.

distance regulation [L *distantia; regula* rule], behavior that is related to the control of personal space. Most humans establish a quantum of space between themselves and others that offers security from either psychologic or physical threat while not creating a feeling of isolation.

distance vision, the ability to see objects clearly, usually from more than 20 feet or 6 m away.

distemper [L *dis* + *temperare* to regulate], **1.** any disorder or indisposition, mentally or physically. **2.** a potentially fatal viral disease of animals, characterized by rhinitis, fever, and a loss of appetite.

distend [L *distendere* to stretch], to make something enlarged or dilated.

distensibility [L *distendere* to stretch], pertaining to the ability of something to become stretched, dilated, or enlarged.

distension, the state of being distended or swollen.

distillate /distil'it/ [L *distillare* to drop down], the product of distillation.

distillation, the process of vaporization followed by condensation in another part of the system.

distilled water [L *distillare*; AS *waeter*], water that has been purified by being heated to a vapor form and then condensed into another container as liquid water free of nonvolatile solutes.

distortion [L *dis* + *torquere* to twist], **1.** (in psychology) the process of shifting experience in one's perceptions. The distortions of patients tend to influence their views of the world and themselves. **2.** (in radiology) x-ray image artifacts that may be caused by variations in the size and shape or the position of the object.

distractibility [L *dis* + *trahere* to draw apart], a mental state in which attention does not remain fixed on any one subject but wavers or wanders.

distraction [L *distrahere* to pull apart], **1.** procedures that prevent or lessen the perception of pain by focusing attention on sensations unrelated to pain. **2.** a method of straightening a spinal column by the forces of axial tension pulling on the joint surfaces, such as applied by a Milwaukee brace.

distraught [OFr *destrait* inattentive], a mental state of confusion, distraction, or absent-mindedness.

distress [ME *distressen* to cause sorrow], an emotional or physical state of pain, sorrow, misery, suffering, or discomfort.

distress of the human spirit. See **spiritual distress.**

distributive analysis and synthesis, the system of psychotherapy used by the psychobiologic school of psychiatry.

distributive care, a pattern of health care that is concerned with environment, heredity, living conditions, life-style, and early detection of pathologic effects.

district [L *distringere* to draw apart], **1.** (in hospital nursing) a group of patients in an area of the unit for whom a head nurse or primary nurse is responsible, usually a subdivision of a ward unit. **2.** the area of a city or town assigned to a public health nurse.

district nurse. See **public health nursing.**

disulfiram /dīsul'firam/, an alcohol-use deterrent prescribed in the treatment of chronic alcoholism. It causes severe intestinal cramping, diaphoresis, and nausea if alcohol is ingested.

disuse phenomena [L *dis* + *usus* to make use of; Gk *phainein* to show], the physical and the psychologic changes, usually degenerative, that result from the lack of use of a part of the body or a body system. Disuse phenomena are associated with confinement and immobility, especially in orthopedics. The physical changes often induced by continued bed rest constitute problems affecting many key areas and systems of the body, such as the skin, the musculoskeletal system, the GI tract, the cardiovascular system, and the respiratory system. Unused muscles lose size and strength, often wasting away until they are unable to perform their vital functions of support and contraction. Another disuse phenomenon is contracture, which may result from constant flexion or extension of a body part by the patient on prolonged bed rest. The immobilized patient may experience bone demineralization because of a restricted diet and decreased motility.

disuse syndrome, high risk for, a NANDA-accepted nursing diagnosis of a state in which an individual is at risk for deterioration of body systems as the result of prescribed or unavoidable inactivity. Risk factors include paralysis, mechanical immobilization, prescribed immobilization, severe pain, and altered level of consciousness.

diuresis /dī´yo͝ore͞´sis/ [Gk *dia* through, *ouron* urine], increased formation and secretion of urine. Diuresis occurs in conditions such as diabetes mellitus and diabetes insipidus.

diuretic /dī´yo͝oret´ik/, **1.** (of a drug or other substance) tending to promote the formation and excretion of urine. **2.** a drug that promotes the formation and excretion of urine. The more than 50 diuretic drugs available in the United States and Canada are classified by chemical structure and pharmacologic activity into these groups: aldosterone antagonists, carbonic anhydrase inhibitors, loop diuretics, mercurials, osmotics, potassium-sparing diuretics, and thiazides. A diuretic medication may contain drugs from one or more of these groups.

diurnal /dīyo͝or´nəl/ [L *diurnalis* of a day], happening daily, as sleeping and eating.

diurnal enuresis [L *diurnalis* daily; Gk *enourein* to urinate], an involuntary voiding of urine during the daylight hours.

diurnal mood variation, a change in mood that is related to the time of day. Examples are commonly found in differences between "night people" and "morning people."

diurnal rhythm [L *diurnalis;* Gk *rhythmos*], patterns of activity or behavior that follow day-night cycles, such as breakfast-lunch-dinner schedules.

diurnal variation, the range of the output or excretion rate of a substance in a specimen being collected for laboratory analysis over a 24-hour period.

divalent. See **bivalent.**

divergence [L *dis + vergere* to incline], a separation or movement of objects away from each other, as in the simultaneous turning of the eyes outward due to an extraocular muscle defect.

divergent squint [L *di + vergere;* ME *squint*], a visual disorder in which a de-

viating eye looks outward. The outward looking eye often is blind or has defective vision.

diversional activity deficit, a NANDA-accepted nursing diagnosis of a lack of diversion in the environment, long-term hospitalization, or frequent or prolonged treatments. Defining characteristics include statements from the client that there is nothing to do or that everything is boring, but the usual diversions or hobbies pursued at home are not undertaken.

diverticular disease. See **diverticulitis, diverticulosis.**

diverticulitis /dī´vurtik´yo͝olī´tis/ [L *diverticulare* to turn aside; Gk *itis* inflammation], inflammation of one or more diverticula. The penetration of fecal matter through the thin-walled diverticula causes inflammation and abcess formation in the tissues surrounding the colon. With repeated inflammation, the lumen of the colon narrows and may become obstructed. During periods of inflammation, the patient will experience crampy pain, particularly over the sigmoid colon, fever, and leukocytosis. Barium enemas and proctoscopy are performed to rule out carcinoma of the colon, which exhibits some of the same symptoms. Conservative treatment includes bed rest, intravenous fluids, antibiotics, and nothing taken by mouth. In acute cases, bowel resection of the affected part greatly reduces mortality and morbidity.

diverticulosis /dī´vurtik´yo͝olō´sis/ [L *diverticulare* to turn aside; Gk *osis* condition], the presence of pouchlike herniations through the muscular layer of the colon, particularly the sigmoid colon.

diverticulum /dī´vurtik´yo͝oləm/, *pl.* **diverticula** [L *diverticulare* to turn aside], a pouchlike herniation through the muscular wall of a tubular organ. A diverticulum may be present in the stomach, in the small intestine, or, most commonly, the colon. **–diverticular,** *adj.*

diving, the act of work or recreation in an underwater environment. The main health effects are related to the increased pressure to which the person is subjected as the ambient pressure generally increases by 1 atm (14.7 pounds per square inch) for each 33 feet of descent below the water surface.

diving goiter [AS *dyypan* to dip; L *guttur* throat], a large movable thyroid gland located at times above the sternal notch and at other times below the notch.

diving reflex, an automatic change in the cardiovascular system that occurs when the face and nose are immersed in water. The heart rate decreases and the blood pressure remains stable or increases slightly, while blood flow to all parts of the body except the brain is reduced.

division [L *dividere* to divide], **1.** an administrative subunit in a hospital, such as a division of medical nursing or a division of surgical nursing. **2.** (in public health nursing) an area that encompasses several geographic districts. **3.** the separation of something into two or more parts or sections, such as **cell division.**

divorce therapy, a type of counseling that attempts to help couples disengage from their former relationship and malicious behavior toward each other or their children.

Dix, Dorothea Lynde (1802–87), an American humanitarian who achieved fame as a social reformer, primarily for her work in improving prison conditions and care of the mentally ill. During her lifetime, she helped to establish mental institutions in 30 states and in Canada. During the Civil War, she was appointed superintendent of army nurses for government hospitals.

dizygotic /dī'zīgot'ik/ [Gk *di* twice, *zygotos* yolked together], of or pertaining to twins from two fertilized ova.

dizygotic twins, two offspring born of the same pregnancy and developed from two ova that were released from the ovary simultaneously and fertilized at the same time. They may be of the same or opposite sex, differ both physically and in genetic constitution, and have two separate and distinct placentas and membranes, both amnion and chorion.

dizziness [AS *dysig* stupid], a sensation of faintness or an inability to maintain normal balance in a standing or seated position, sometimes associated with giddiness, mental confusion, nausea, and weakness. A patient who experiences dizziness should be carefully lowered to a safe position because of the danger of injury from falling.

DKA, abbreviation for **diabetic ketoacidosis.**

DLE, abbreviation for **discoid lupus erythematosus.**

DM, abbreviation for **diabetes mellitus.**

DMD, abbreviation for *Doctor of Dental Medicine.* It is equivalent to a **DDS** degree.

DMSO, abbreviation for **dimethyl sulfoxide.**

DNA, abbreviation for **deoxyribonucleic acid.**

DNA chimera /kīmē'rə/, (in molecular genetics) a recombinant molecule of DNA composed of segments from more than one source.

DNA ligase, an enzyme that can repair

breaks in a strand of DNA by synthesizing a bond between adjoining nucleotides. Under some circumstances the enzyme can join together loose ends of DNA strands, and in some cases it can repair breaks in RNA.

DNA polymerase /pol'imərās/, (in molecular genetics) an enzyme that catalyzes the assembly of deoxyribonucleoside triphosphates into DNA, with single-stranded DNA serving as the template.

DNCB, abbreviation for **dinitrochlorobenzene.**

DNR, abbreviation for *do not resuscitate.*

DO, abbreviation for *Doctor of Osteopathy.*

DOA, abbreviation for *dead on arrival.*

Dobie's globule /dō'bēz/ [William M. Dobie, English physician, b. 1828], a very small stainable body in the transparent disk of a striated muscle fiber.

dobutamine hydrochloride /dōbyoo'təmēn/, a beta-adrenergic stimulating agent prescribed to increase cardiac output in severe chronic congestive heart failure and as an adjunct in cardiac surgery.

Dock, Lavinia Lloyd (1858–1956), an American public health nurse. She advocated an international public health movement and the improvement of education for nurses. With M. Adelaide Nutting, she wrote *History of Nursing,* a classic in nursing literature.

doctoral program in nursing, an educational program of study that offers preparation for a doctoral degree in the field of nursing designed to prepare nurses for advanced practice and research. Upon successful completion of the course of study, the degree PhD or EdD in nursing or DSN (Doctor of Science in Nursing) is awarded.

Doctor of Medicine, Doctor of Osteopathy. See **physician.**

docusate /dok'yoosāt/, a stool softener prescribed in the treatment of constipation.

δOD, abbreviation for **delta optic density.**

Doederlein's bacillus /dā'dərlinz, dōdərlēnz/ [Albert S. Doederlein, German physician, b. 1860], a gram-positive bacterium present in normal vaginal secretions.

Doehle bodies /dā'lə, dōll/ [Karl G. P. Doehle, German pathologist, b. 1855], blue inclusions in the cytoplasm of some leukocytes in May-Hegglin anomaly and in blood smears from patients with acute infections.

Döhle-Heller disease. See **syphilitic aortitis.**

dolichocephaly. See **scaphocephaly.**

doll's-eye reflex, a normal response in newborns to keep the eyes stationary as the head is moved to the right or left. The reflex disappears as ocular fixation develops.

dolor /dō'lôr/ [L, pain], any condition of physical pain, mental anguish, or suffering from heat. It is one of the four signs of inflammation. The others are calor (heat), rubor (redness), and tumor (swelling).

DOM, abbreviation for **dimethoxymethylamphetamine.**

dome fracture [L *domus* house; *fractura* break], any fracture of the acetabulum, specifically involving a weight-bearing surface.

dominance [L *dominari* to rule], (in genetics) a basic principle stating that not all genes determining a given trait operate with equal vigor. If two genes at a given locus produce a different effect, the gene that is manifest is dominant. **–dominant,** *adj.*

dominant gene [L *dominari* to rule; Gk *genein* to produce], one that produces a phenotypic effect regardless of whether its allele is the same or different.

dominant group, a social group that controls the value system and rewards in a particular society.

dominant trait, an inherited characteristic, such as eye color, that is likely to appear in an offspring although it may occur in only one parent.

Donath-Landsteiner syndrome /dō'notland'stīnər/ [Julius Donath, Austrian physician, b. 1870; Karl Landsteiner, Austrian-American pathologist, b. 1868], a rare blood disorder, marked by hemolysis minutes or hours after exposure to cold. Systemic symptoms include the passage of dark urine, severe pain in the back and legs, headache, vomiting, diarrhea, and moderate reticulocytosis.

Don Juan, a seductive and sexually promiscuous man.

donor [L *donare* to give], **1.** a human or other organism that gives living tissue to be used in another body, for example, blood for transfusion or a kidney for transplantation. **2.** a substance or compound that gives part of itself to another substance.

donor card [L *donare, charta*], a document in which a person offers to make an anatomic gift of body parts, at the time of death, for transplantation to recipients needing replacement of vital organs or tissues. The card is often incorporated into a state driver's license so the authorization will be immediately available if the donor dies in a traffic accident.

do not attempt resuscitation (DNAR), an advisory instruction that resuscitation of a patient should not be attempted. The order is more strictly defined than the **DNR** (do not re-

suscitate), which may be interpreted as authorizing an attempt at resuscitation.

Donovan bodies [Charles Donovan, Irish physician, b. 1863], encapsulated gram-negative rods of the species *Calymmatobacterium granulomatis,* present in the cytoplasm of mononuclear phagocytes obtained from the lesions of granuloma inguinale.

donut pad, a pad designed to protect an injured joint. It is cut to fit over the site of the injury and cause force on the body part to be transferred to surrounding areas.

dopa /dō'pə/, an amino acid derived from tyrosine that occurs naturally in plants and animals. It is a precursor of dopamine, epinephrine, and norepinephrine.

dopamine hydrochloride /dō'pəmin/, a sympathomimetic catecholamine prescribed in the treatment of shock, hypotension, and low cardiac output.

dopaminergic /dō'pəminur'jik/, having the effect of dopamine.

dope [AS *dyppan* to dip], *slang.* morphine, heroin, or another narcotic, or marijuana or another substance illicitly bought, or sold, and often self-administered for sedative, hypnotic, euphoric, or other mood-altering purpose.

Doppler effect /dop'lər/ [Christian J. Doppler, Austrian scientist, b. 1803; L *effectus*], the apparent change in frequency of sound, light, or radio waves emitted by a source as it moves away from or toward an observer. The frequency increases as the source moves toward the observer and decreases as it moves away.

Doppler scanning [Christian J. Doppler; L *scandere* to climb], a technique used in ultrasound imaging to monitor the behavior of a moving structure, such as flowing blood or a beating heart.

dornase /dôr'nās/, a natural proteolytic substance that depolymerizes DNA molecules. Because as much as 70% of the solid matter of purulent material consists of DNA, dornase is used in respiratory therapy to help break off sputum accumulation in the airways.

dorsal /dôr'səl/ [L *dorsum* the back], pertaining to the back or posterior. **–dorsum,** *n.*

dorsal carpal ligament. See **retinaculum extensorum manus.**

dorsal cutaneous nerve, a nerve that is close to the surface of the foot and ankle, where it may be both visible and palpable.

dorsal decubitus position. See **supine.**

dorsal digital vein, one of the communicating veins along the sides of the fingers.

dorsal flexure [L *dorsalis* back, *flectere* to

bend], the dorsal convexity of the thoracic region of the spine.

dorsal horn [L *dorsalis;* AS, horn], a crescent-shaped projection of gray matter within the spinal cord, appearing as a horn in transverse sections.

dorsal inertia posture, a tendency of a debilitated or weak person to slip downward in bed when the head of the bed is raised.

dorsal interventricular artery, the arterial branch of the right coronary artery, branching to supply both ventricles.

dorsalis pedis artery, the continuation of the anterior tibial artery, starting at the ankle joint, dividing into five branches, and supplying various muscles of the foot and toes.

dorsalis pedis pulse, the pulse of the dorsalis pedis artery, palpable between the first and second metatarsal bones on the top of the foot.

dorsal lip, the marginal fold of the blastopore during gastrulation in the early stages of embryonic development of many animals.

dorsal recumbent [L *dorsalis, recumbere* to lie down], lying on the back, as in a supine position.

dorsal recumbent position [L *dorsalis, positio*], the supine position with the person lying on the back, head, and shoulders.

dorsal rigid posture, a position in which a patient lying in bed holds one or both legs drawn up to the chest. It often involves only the right leg and is intended to relieve abdominal pain.

dorsal root [L *dorsalis;* AS *rot*], the sensory component or root of a spinal nerve.

dorsal root ganglion [L *dorsalis;* AS *rot;* Gk *gagglion* knot], a swelling consisting of sensory neuron cell bodies located on the dorsal root of a spinal nerve.

dorsal scapular nerve, one of a pair of supraclavicular branches from the roots of the brachial plexus. It supplies the rhomboideus major and the rhomboideus minor and sends a branch to the levator.

dorsiflect /dôr′siflekt/ [L *dorsum* + *flectere* to bend], to bend or flex backward as in the upward bending of the fingers, wrist, foot, or toes.

dorsiflexion /dôr′siflek′shən/, flexion toward the back, as accomplished by a muscle.

dorsiflexor /dôr′siflek′sər/, a muscle causing backward flexion of a part of the body, as the hand or foot.

dorsiflexor gait, an abnormal gait caused by the weakness of the dorsiflexors of the ankle. It is characterized by footdrop during the entire gait cycle and excessive

knee and hip flexion to allow clearance of the involved extremity during the swing phase.

dorsodynia /dôr′sōdin′ē·ə/, a pain in the back, particularly in the muscles of the upper back area.

dorsosacral position. See **lithotomy position.**

dorsum /dôr′səm/ [L *dorsalis* back], the back of the body, the posterior or upper surface of a body part.

dorsum sellae /dôr′səm sel′ē/, the posterior boundary of the sella turcica of the sphenoid bone. It bears the posterior clinoid process and is an anatomic marker for the location of the pituitary gland at the base of the skull.

dosage [L *dosis* a giving], the regimen governing the size, frequency, and number of doses of a therapeutic agent to be administered to a patient.

dosage compensation, (in genetics) the mechanism that counterbalances the number of X-linked gene doses in the sex chromosomes so that they are equal in both the male, which has one X chromosome, and the female, which has two. In mammals this is accomplished by genetic activation of only one of the X chromosomes in the somatic cells of females.

dose [L *dosis* a giving], the amount of a drug or other substance to be administered at one time.

dose equivalent (DE), a quantity used in radiation-safety work that equates on a unified scale the amount of radiation dose and the physical damages that it might produce. The unit of dose equivalent is the sievert (Sv) or the rem.

dose fractionation. See **fractionation.**

dose-limiting recommendations, maximum permissible dose (MPD) of radiation exposure, which may vary for different body or organ exposures. For example, the MPD for the skin or forearms of a radiation worker is much higher than the whole-body exposure MPD.

dose rate, (in radiotherapy) the amount of delivered radiation absorbed per unit of time.

dose ratemeter, (in radiotherapy) an instrument for measuring the dose rate of radiation.

dose response, a range of drug effects between the minimum dose needed to reach the threshold level, at which an effect is first observed, and a toxic dose level, where adverse effects result.

dose-response relationship, (in radiology) a mathematical relationship between the dose of radiation and the body's reaction to it. In a linear dose-response relationship, the response is proportional to the dose.

dose threshold, (in radiotherapy) the minimum amount of absorbed radiation that produces a detectable degree of a given effect.

dose to skin, (in radiotherapy) the amount of absorbed radiation at the center of the irradiation field on the skin. It is the sum of the dose in the air and the scatter from body parts.

dosimeter /dōsim′ətər/ [L *dosis* + Gk *metron* measure], an instrument to detect and measure accumulated radiation exposure.

dosimetry /dōsim′ətrē/, **1.** the determination of the amount, rate, and distribution of radiation or radioactivity from a source of ionizing radiation. **2.** the accurate determination of medicinal doses, based on body size, sex, age, and other factors.

double-approach   conflict. See **approach-approach conflict.**

double-avoidant   conflict. See **avoidance-avoidance conflict.**

double bind [L *duplus* double; AS *bindan* to bind], a "no win" situation resulting from two conflicting messages from a person who is crucial to one's survival, as a verbal message that differs from a nonverbal message.

double-blind study, an experiment designed to test the effect of a treatment or substance using groups of experimental and control subjects in which neither the subjects nor the investigators know which treatment or substance is being administered to which group. In a test of a new drug, the substance may be identified to the investigators by only a code. A double-blind study may be augmented by a **crossover experiment,** in which experimental subjects unknowingly become control subjects, and vice versa, at some point in the study.

double-blind test [L *duplus* double; AS *blind; testum* crucible], an experimental design for drug testing in which neither the clients receiving the drugs nor the persons conducting the test know which subjects are receiving a new drug and which are getting a placebo, or sugar pill.

double-channel catheter [L *duplus; ME chanel; Gk katheter* a thing lowered into], a double-lumen catheter used to irrigate an internal cavity, with fluid entering one lumen and draining through the other.

double-contrast arthography, a method of making an x-ray image of a joint by injecting two contrast agents into the capsular space. The technique is most commonly used in radiography of the knee joint.

double-contrast barium enema [L *duplus* + *contra* against; Gk *barys* heavy, *enienai* to send in], an enema of radiopaque barium followed by evacuation and injection of air. The purpose is to radiographically detail the mucosal lining of the large intestine.

double-emulsion film, x-ray film that is coated with gelatin emulsion on both sides.

double-flap amputation [L *duplus;* ME *flappe* flap; L *amputare*], an amputation in which two flaps are made from the soft tissues to cover an area that has lost its integument in surgery or accident.

double fracture, a fracture consisting of breaks or cracks in two places in a bone, resulting in more than two bone segments.

double gel diffusion. See **immunodiffusion.**

double innervation, innervation of effector organs by fibers of the sympathetic and parasympathetic divisions of the autonomic nervous system. The pelvic viscera, bronchioles, heart, eyes, and digestive system are all doubly innervated.

double monster, a fetus that has developed from a single ovum but has two heads, trunks, and multiple limbs.

double-needle entry, a technique for injecting a contrast medium or other agent with two needles, one with a larger bore. In diskography, a 20-gauge needle is used to perform a spinal puncture, after which a longer, 26-gauge needle is passed through the guide needle to the injection target area.

double personality [L *duplus, personalis* of a person], a state of dissociation in which the individual presents personas to associates at different times as two different persons, each with different names and personality traits. The two personalities are generally independent, contrasting, and unaware of the existence of the other.

double quartan fever, a form of malaria in which paroxysms of fever occur in a repeating pattern of 2 consecutive days followed by 1 day of remission. The pattern is usually the result of concurrent infections by two species of the genus *Plasmodium,* one causing paroxysms every 72 hours and the other every 48 hours.

double setup, a nursing procedure in which an obstetric operating room is prepared for both vaginal delivery and cesarean section. The circulating and scrub nurses lay out the equipment required for both procedures.

double vision. See **diplopia.**

double-void, a urinalysis procedure in which the first specimen is discarded and a second, obtained 30 to 45 minutes later, is tested. This method gives a more accurate measure of the amount of glucose in the urine at that particular time.

douche /dŏŏsh/ [Fr, shower-bath], **1.** a procedure in which 1 liter or more of a solution of a medication or cleansing agent in warm water is introduced into the vagina under low pressure. The woman often performs the procedure herself, sitting on a toilet seat or semisitting in a bathtub. **2.** to perform a douche.

doughnut pessary. See **pessary.**

Douglas' cul-de-sac [James Douglas, Scottish anatomist, b. 1675; Fr, bottom of the bag], a rectouterine pouch or recess formed by a fold of peritoneum that extends between the rectum and the uterus.

Downey cells [Hal Downey, American physician, b. 1877], lymphocytes identified in one system of classification of the blood cells of patients with infectious mononucleosis. The cells are designated as Downey I, II, or III lymphocytes.

Down syndrome [John L. Down, English physician, b. 1828], a congenital condition characterized by varying degrees of mental retardation and multiple defects. It is the most common chromosomal abnormality of a generalized syndrome and is caused by the presence of an extra chromosome 21 in the G group or, in a small percentage of cases, by the translocation of chromosomes 14 or 15 in the D group and chromosomes 21 or 22. Infants with the syndrome are small and hypotonic, with characteristic microcephaly, brachycephaly, a flattened occiput, and typical facies with a mongoloid slant to the eyes, depressed nasal bridge, low-set ears, and a large, protruding tongue that is furrowed and lacks the central fissure. The hands are short and broad with a transverse palmar or simian crease; the fingers are stubby and show clinodactyly, primarily of the fifth finger. The feet are broad and stubby with a wide space between the first and second toes and a prominent plantar crease. The most significant feature of the syndrome is mental retardation, which varies considerably, although the average IQ is in the range of 50 to 60, so that the child is generally trainable and in most instances can be reared at home. The mortality rate is high within the first few years, especially in children with cardiac anomalies.

doxapram hydrochloride /dok′səpram/, a respiratory stimulant prescribed to improve respiratory function after anesthesia, in drug-induced central nervous system depression, and for chronic pulmonary disease associated with acute hypercapnia.

doxepin hydrochloride /dok′səpin/, a tricyclic antidepressant prescribed in the treatment of depression.

doxorubicin hydrochloride /dok′sərŏŏ′-bisin/, an anthracycline antibiotic prescribed in the treatment of a variety of malignant neoplastic diseases.

doxycycline /dok′sisī′klēn/, a tetracycline antibacterial prescribed in the treatment of a variety of infections.

doxylamine succinate /dok′silam′ēn/, an antihistamine prescribed for the treatment of acute allergic symptoms produced by the release of histamine.

dp/dt, (in cardiology) the rate of pressure change per unit of time.

DPG, abbreviation for **2,3-diphosphoglyceric acid.**

DPH, abbreviation for *Diploma in Public Health.*

DPT vaccine, abbreviation for **diphtheria, tetanus toxoids, and pertussis vaccine.**

DQ, abbreviation for **developmental quotient.**

dr., 1. abbreviation for **drachm. 2.** abbreviation for **dram.**

drachm (dr.) [Gk *drachme* a weight of equal value]. See **dram.**

dracunculiasis /drakun′kyŏŏlī′əsis/ [Gk *drakontion* little dragon, *osis* condition], a parasitic infection caused by infestation by the nematode *Dracunculus medinensis.* It is characterized by ulcerative skin lesions on the legs and feet that are produced by gravid female worms. People are infected by drinking contaminated water or eating contaminated shellfish.

Dracunculus medinensis /drakun′kyŏŏləs/, a parasitic nematode of the Mediterranean area that causes dracunculiasis. An American species is *Dracunculus insignis.*

drag-to gait [ME *dragen* + *gate* path], a method of walking with crutches in which the feet are dragged rather than lifted with each step.

drain, a tube or other opening used to remove air or a fluid from a body cavity or wound. The drain may be a closed system, designed to provide complete protection against contamination, or an open system.

drainage [AS *drachen* teardrop], the removal of fluids from a body cavity, wound, or other source of discharge by one or more methods. **Closed drainage** is a system of tubing and other apparatus attached to the body to remove fluid in an airtight circuit that prevents environmental contaminants from entering the wound or cavity. **Open drainage** is drainage in which discharge passes through an open-ended tube into a receptacle. **Suction**

drainage utilizes a pump or other mechanic device to assist in extracting a fluid. **Tidal drainage** is drainage in which a body area is washed out by alternately flooding and then emptying it with the aid of gravity, a technique that may be used in treating a urinary bladder disorder.

drainage tube, a heavy-gauge catheter used for the evacuation of air or a fluid from a cavity or wound in the body.

draining sinus [AS *drachen* teardrop; L *sinus* hollow], an abnormal channel or fistula permitting the escape of exudate to the outside of the body.

Draize test /drāz/, a controversial method of testing the toxicity of pharmaceutical and other products to be used by humans by placing a small amount of the substance in the eyes of rabbits. The eye-irritancy potential of a substance is considered a measure of the possible effect the product could have on similar human tissues.

dram (dr.) [Gk *drachme* weight of the same value], a unit of mass equivalent to an apothecaries' measure of 60 grains or ⅛ ounce and to 1⁄16 ounce or 27.34 grains avoirdupois.

dramatic play [Gk *drama* deed; AS *plegan* game], an imitative activity in which a child fantasizes and acts out various domestic and social roles and situations, as rocking a doll, pretending to be a doctor or nurse, or teaching school.

drape [ME *drap* cloth], a sheet of fabric or paper, usually the size of a small bed sheet, for covering all or a part of a person's body during a physical examination or treatment. **–drape,** *v.*

Draw-a-Person Test (DAP) [AS *dragan;* L *personalis* + *testum* crucible], a test developed by Karen Machover [American psychologist, b. 1902] based on the interpretation of drawings of human figures of both sexes. Interpretation depends on the subject's verbalizations, self-image, anxiety, sexual conflicts, and other factors.

drawer sign [AS *dragan* to drag], a diagnostic sign of a ruptured or torn knee ligament. It is tested by having the patient flex the knee at a right angle while the examiner grasps the lower leg just below the knee and moves the leg first toward, then away from himself. The test is positive for the knee injury if the head of the tibia can be moved more than a half inch from the joint.

drawing, *informal;* a vague sensation of muscle tension.

drawsheet, a sheet that is smaller than a bottom or top sheet of a bed and is usually placed to keep the mattress and bottom linens dry or used to turn or move a patient in bed.

dream [ME *dreem* joyful noise], **1.** a sequence of ideas, thoughts, emotions, or images that pass through the mind during the rapid-eye-movement stage of sleep. **2.** the sleeping state in which this process occurs. **3.** a visionary creation of the imagination experienced during wakefulness. **4.** (in psychoanalysis) the expression of thoughts, emotions, memories, or impulses repressed from the consciousness. **5.** (in analytic psychology) the wishes, emotions, and impulses that reflect the personal unconscious and the archetypes that originate in the collective unconscious.

dream analysis, a process of gaining access to the unconscious mind by means of examining the content of dreams, usually through the method of free association.

dream association, a relationship of thoughts or emotions discovered or experienced when a dream is remembered or analyzed.

dream state, a condition of altered consciousness in which a person does not recognize the environment and reacts in a manner opposed to his or her usual behavior, as by flight or an act of violence.

drepanocytic anemia /drep′ənōsit′ik/ [Gk *drepane* sickle, *kytos* cell], sickle cell anemia.

dress code [OFr *dresser* to arrange; L *codex* book], the standards set by an institution for the dress of the members of the institution.

dressing [OFr *dresser* to arrange], a clean or sterile covering applied directly to wounded or diseased tissue for absorption of secretions, for protection from trauma, for administration of medications, to keep the wound clean, or to stop bleeding. Kinds of dressings include **absorbent, antiseptic, occlusive, pressure,** and **wet dressing.**

dressing forceps, a kind of forceps that has narrow blades and blunt or notched teeth, designed for dressing wounds, removing drainage tubes, or extracting fragments of necrotic tissue.

Dressler's syndrome /dres′lərz/, an autoimmune disorder that may occur several days after acute coronary infarction, characterized by fever, pericarditis, pleurisy, pleural effusions, and joint pain. It results from the body's immunologic response to a damaged myocardium and pericardium.

DRG, abbreviation for **diagnostis related groups.**

drift [AS *drifan* to move forward], **1. antigenic drift,** a change that occurs in a strain of virus so that variations appear periodically with alterations in antigenic qualities. **2. genetic drift,** random variations in gene frequency of a population from one generation to the next.

drifting tooth, any one of the teeth that migrate from normal position in the associated dental arch.

Drinker respirator [Philip Drinker, American engineer, b. 1893], an airtight respirator consisting of a metal tank that encloses the entire body, except for the head. Used for long-term therapy, it alternates positive and negative air pressure within the tank, providing artificial respiration.

drip [AS *dryppan* to fall in drops], **1.** the process of a liquid or moisture forming and falling in drops. Kinds of drip are **nasal drip** and **postnasal drip. 2.** the slow but continuous infusion of a liquid into the body, as into the stomach or a vein. **3.** to infuse a liquid continuously into the body.

drip gavage, a method of feeding a liquid formula diet through a tube inserted through the nostrils to the stomach.

drip system, (in intravenous therapy) an apparatus for delivering specific volumes of intravenous solutions within predetermined periods of time and at a specific flow rate.

drive [AS *drifan* to move forward], a basic, compelling urge. **Primary drive** refers to one that is innate and in close contact with physiologic processes. A **secondary drive** is one that evolves during the process of growth and that incites and directs behavior.

dromostanolone propionate /drō′mostan′əlōn/, a synthetic androgen prescribed for female breast cancer.

dronabinal /drōnab′inol/, an oral antiemetic prescribed for refractory nausea and vomiting caused by cancer chemotherapy.

drop [AS *dropa*], a small spherical mass of liquid. A drop may vary in size with differences in temperature, viscosity, and other factors. For therapeutic purposes, a drop is regarded as having a volume of 0.06 to 0.1 ml, or 1 to 1.5 minims.

drop arm test, a diagnostic test for a tear in the supraspinatus tendon. It is positive if the patient is unable to slowly and smoothly lower the affected arm from a position of 90 degrees of abduction.

drop attack, a form of transient ischemic attack (TIA) in which a brief interruption of cerebral blood flow results in a person falling to the floor without losing consciousness. The episode may affect the person's sense of balance or leg muscle tone.

droperidol /drəper′ədol/, an antipsychotic, sedative drug of the butyrophenone group, used most commonly with a narcotic analgesic (fentanyl) in neuroleptanesthesia.

drop foot. See footdrop.

droplet infection [AS *dropa;* L *inficere* to taint], an infection acquired by the inhalation of pathogenic microorganisms suspended in particles of liquid exhaled, sneezed, or coughed by another infected person or animal.

dropper, a glass or plastic tube narrowed at one end so it will dispense a liquid medication one drop at a time.

dropsy. See hydrops.

Drosophila /drōsof′ilə/ [Gk *drosos* dew, *philein* to love], a genus of fly, including *Drosophila melanogaster,* the Mediterranean fruit fly, useful in genetic experiments because of the large chromosomes found in its salivary glands and its sensitivity to environmental effects, such as exposure to radiation.

drowning [ME *drounen*], asphyxiation because of submersion in a liquid.

drox, abbreviation for a *noncarboxylate hydroxide anion.*

drug [Fr *drogue*], **1.** any substance taken by mouth, injected into a muscle, the skin, a blood vessel, or a cavity of the body, or applied topically to treat or prevent a disease or condition. **2.** *informal;* a narcotic substance.

drug absorption, the process whereby a drug moves from the muscle, digestive tract, or other site of entry into the body toward the circulatory system and the target organ or tissue.

drug abuse, the use of a drug for a nontherapeutic effect, especially one for which it was not prescribed or intended. Some of the most commonly abused drugs are alcohol, amphetamines, barbiturates, cocaine, methaqualone, and opium alkaloids.

drug action, the means by which a drug exerts a desired effect.

drug addiction, a condition characterized by an overwhelming desire to continue taking a drug to which one has become habituated through repeated consumption because it produces a particular effect, usually an alteration of mental activity, attitude, or outlook. Addiction is usually accompanied by a compulsion to obtain the drug, a tendency to increase the dose, a psychologic or physical dependence, and detrimental consequences for the individual and society.

drug administration, the giving by a nurse or other authorized person of a single dose of a drug to a patient.

drug agonist, one of two similar drugs that may affect the same target organ or tissue, producing the same or a similar effect.

drug allergy, hypersensitivity to a pharmacologic agent, manifested by reactions ranging from a mild rash to anaphylactic shock, depending on the individual, the allergen, and the dose.

drug clearance, the elimination of a drug from the body. The rate of clearance helps determine the size and frequency of a dosage of a particular medication.

drug compliance, the reliability of the patient to use a prescribed medication exactly as ordered by the physician. Noncompliance occurs when a patient neglects to take the prescribed dosages at the recommended times or discontinues the drug without consulting the physician.

drug dependence, a psychologic craving for or a physiologic reliance on a chemical agent, resulting from habituation, abuse, or addiction.

drug dispensing, the preparation, packaging, labeling, record keeping, and transfer of a prescription drug to a patient or an intermediary, such as a nurse, who is responsible for administration of the drug.

drug distribution, the pattern of absorption of drug molecules by various tissues after the chemical enters the circulatory system. Because of differences in pH, cell membrane functions, and other individual tissue factors, most drugs are not distributed equally in all parts of the body.

drug-drug interaction, a modification of the effect of a drug when administered with another drug. The effect may be an increase or a decrease in the action of either substance, or it may be an adverse effect that is not normally associated with either drug.

Drug Enforcement Agency (DEA), an agency of the Drug Enforcement Administration of the federal government, empowered to enforce regulations regarding the import or export of narcotic drugs and certain other substances or the traffic of these substances across state lines.

drug eruption. See **drug rash.**

drug fever, a fever caused by the pharmacologic action of a medication, its thermoregulatory action, a local complication of parenteral administration, or, most commonly, an immunologic reaction mediated by drug-induced antibodies. The onset of fever occurs usually between 7 and 10 days after the medication is begun; a return to normal is seen within 2 days of the discontinuance of the drug.

drug-food interaction, the effect produced when some drugs and certain foods or beverages are taken at the same time, as in the example of monoamine oxidase inhibitors that can react dangerously with foods containing the amino acid tyramine.

drug-induced parkinsonism, a reversible syndrome with the clinical features of Parkinson's disease, but caused by the dopamine-blocking actions of antipsychotic drugs.

drug metabolism, the transformation of a drug by the body tissues into a metabolite. Examples include aspirin, which is metabolized to salicylic acid, an analgesic, and codeine, which is converted to morphine.

drug monograph, a statement that specifies the kinds and amounts of ingredients a drug or class of drugs may contain, the directions for the drug's use, the conditions in which it may be used, and contraindications for its use.

drug overdose (OD) [Fr *drogue;* AS *ofer;* Gk *dosis* giving], an accidental or purposeful dose of a drug large enough to cause severe adverse reactions.

drug potency, a measure of the effect of one drug as compared to a similar medication of the same dosage. The drug that produces the maximum effect with the smallest dose has the greater potency.

drug psychosis [Fr *drogue;* Gk *psyche* mind, *osis* condition], a psychotic state induced by excessive dosage of certain therapeutic drugs as well as drugs of abuse. Therapeutic drugs often associated with drug-induced psychosis include belladonna, chloral hydrate, paraldehyde, steroids, and isoniazid.

drug rash, a skin eruption, usually an allergic reaction, that is caused by a particular drug. When a drug rash occurs as a sensitivity reaction, the skin rash does not occur the first time the drug is taken, but the effect is observed with subsequent uses of the same drug.

drug reaction [Fr *drogue;* L *re* + *agere* to act], any adverse effect of the body to therapeutic drugs, drugs of abuse, or by the interaction of two or more pharmacologically active agents within a short time span. Drugs most likely to cause adverse reactions include hypnotics, central nervous system stimulants, antidepressants, tranquilizers, and muscle relaxants.

drug receptor, any part of a cell, usually an enzyme or large protein molecule, with which a drug molecule interacts to trigger its desired response or effect.

drug rehabilitation center, an agency that provides long-term care for a gradual return to the community of a person with a chemical or drug dependency.

drug-seeking behavior (DSB), a pattern of seeking narcotic pain medication or tranquilizers with forged prescriptions, false identification, repeatedly asking for replacement of "lost" drugs or prescriptions, complaining of severe pain without an organic basis, and being abusive or threatening when denied drugs.

drug sequestration, the process by which certain drugs are stored in the body tissues. Examples include tetracycline, which may be stored in bone tissue, and chloroquine, which is stored in the liver.

drug tolerance, a condition of cellular adaptation to a pharmacologically active substance so that increasingly larger doses are required to produce the same physiologic or psychologic effect as obtained earlier with smaller doses.

drug trial, the process of determining an adequate and effective therapeutic dose of a specific drug for a particular patient. The trial culminates with (1) an acceptable clinical result, (2) intolerable adverse effects, (3) a poor response after an appropriate blood level is reached, or (4) the drug is administered for a specific time.

drusen /droo′zən, drē′zən/ [Ger *Druse* stony granule], small, white hyaline deposits that develop beneath the retinal pigment epithelium, sometimes appearing as nodules within the optic nerve head. They tend to occur most frequently in persons over the age of 60.

dry catarrh [AS *dryge;* Gk *kata* down, *rhoia* flow], a dry cough, accompanied by almost no expectoration that occurs in severe coughing spells. It is associated with asthma and emphysema in older people.

dry dressing, a plain dressing containing no medication, applied directly to an incision or a wound to prevent contamination or trauma or to absorb secretions.

dry eye syndrome, a dryness of the cornea and conjunctiva caused by a deficiency in tear production. The condition results in a sensation of a foreign body in the eye, burning eyes, keratitis, and erosion of the epithelial layers of the cornea and conjunctiva.

dry gangrene. See **gangrene.**

dry gas (D), (in respiratory therapy) a gas that contains no water vapor.

dry heat sterilization [AS *dryge* + *haetu;* L *sterilis*], a method of sterilization utilizing heated dry air at a temperature of 160° C-180° C for 90 minutes to 3 hours.

dry ice, solid carbon dioxide, with a temperature of about −140° F. It is used in cryotherapy of various skin disorders.

dry labor, *informal;* labor in which the amniotic fluid has already escaped.

dry pleurisy [AS *dryge* dry; Gk *pleuritis*], an inflammation of the pleura without sig-nificant effusion. The cause may be a localized injury or an early sign of tuberculosis.

Drysdale's corpuscle /drīz′dālz/ [Thomas M. Drysdale, American gynecologist, b. 1831], one of a number of transparent cells in the fluid of some ovarian cysts.

dry skin, epidermis lacking moisture or sebum, often characterized by a pattern of fine lines, scaling, and itching. Causes include too frequent bathing, low humidity, decreased production of sebum in aging skin, and ichthyosis.

dry tooth socket, an inflamed condition of a tooth socket (alveolus) after extraction. Normally, a blood clot forms over the alveolar bone at the base of the tooth socket after an extraction. If the clot fails to form properly or becomes dislodged, the bone tissue is exposed to the environment and can become infected.

dry vomiting [AS *dryge;* L *vomere* to vomit], nausea with retching that does not result in vomitus.

DSB, abbreviation for **drug-seeking behavior.**

DSDB, abbreviation for **direct self-destructive behavior.**

DSM, abbreviation for *Diagnostic and Statistical Manual of Mental Disorders. DSM-III-R* identifies the revised version of the third edition of the manual.

DSN, abbreviation for *Doctor of Science in Nursing.*

DSR, abbreviation for **dynamic spatial reconstructor.**

DT, abbreviation for **diphtheria and tetanus toxoids.**

dTc, abbreviation for *d-tubocurarine.*

DTP vaccine, a combination of diphtheria and tetanus toxoids and killed pertussis vaccine that is administered intramuscularly for active immunization against those diseases.

DTR, abbreviation for **deep tendon reflex.**

DTs, abbreviation for **delirium tremens.**

dual-energy imaging, an x-ray imaging technique in which two radiographs are taken of the same target area using two different kilovoltages. One image isolates bone contrast and the other isolates soft tissue contrast. The combined x-ray films can help to make a more precise identification of an abnormality.

dual-focus tube, an x-ray tube used for diagnostic imaging. A large focal spot is used when techniques that produce high heat are required, and a small focal spot is used to produce fine, detailed images.

duality of central nervous system control, a theory that the normal central nervous system is regulated by a check-and-balance feedback program. The theory is based on studies of posture-movement, mobility-stability, flexion-extension synergies, and similar action-reaction examples.

dual personality. See **double personality.**

DUB, 1. abbreviation for **dysfunctional uterine bleeding.** 2. a genetically determined human blood factor that is associated with immunity to certain diseases.

Dubin-Johnson syndrome /dōo'bin-jon'sən/ [Isadore N. Dubin, American pathologist, b. 1913; Frank B. Johnson, American pathologist, b. 1919], a rare, chronic, hereditary hyperbilirubinemia, characterized by nonhemolytic jaundice, abnormal liver pigmentation, and abnormal function of the gallbladder.

DuBois formula /dōoboiz'/, a logarithmic method of calculating the number of square meters of body surface area (BSA) of an individual from the height in centimeters, the weight in kilograms, and a constant, 0.007184.

Dubowitz assessment, a system of estimating the gestational age of a newborn child according to such factors as posture, ankle dorsiflexion, and arm and leg recoil.

Duchenne-Erb paralysis. See **Erb's palsy.**

Duchenne's disease /dōoshenz'/ [Guillame B. A. Duchenne, French neurologist, b. 1806], a series of three different neurologic conditions: **spinal muscular atrophy, bulbar paralysis,** and **tabes dorsalis.**

Duchenne-Aran disease /dōoshen'äräN/, muscular atrophy caused by degeneration of the anterior horn cells of the spinal cord and affecting primarily the upper extremities. There is chronic muscle wasting and weakness that first appears in the hands and advances progressively to the arms and shoulders, eventually affecting the legs and other body areas.

Duchenne's muscular dystrophy [Guillame B. A. Duchenne], an abnormal congenital condition characterized by progressive symmetric wasting of the leg and pelvic muscles. It is an X-linked recessive disease that appears insidiously between 3 and 5 years of age and spreads from the leg and pelvic muscles to the involuntary muscles. Associated muscle weakness produces a waddling gait and pronounced lordosis. Muscles rapidly deteriorate, and calf muscles become firm and enlarged from fatty deposits. Affected children develop contractures, have difficulty climbing stairs, often stumble and fall, and display wing scapulae when they raise their arms.

Duchenne's paralysis [Guillame B. A. Du-

chenne; Gk *paralyein* to be palsied], a form of motor neuron disease characterized by wasting and weakness in the laryngeal, pharyngeal, tongue, and facial muscles, leading to dysarthria and dysphagia. There may also be pyramidal tract involvement.

duck embryo vaccine. See **rabies vaccine.**

duck walk. See **metatarsus valgus.**

duct [L *ducere* to lead], a narrow tubular structure, especially one through which material is secreted or excreted.

duct carcinoma, a neoplasm developed from the epithelium of ducts, especially in the breast or pancreas.

duct ectasia, an abnormal dilation of a duct by lipids and cellular debris.

ductility /duktil'itē/, the property of a material that has a large elastic range and tends to deform before failing from stress.

duction /duk'shən/, the movement of an individual eyeball from the primary to secondary or tertiary positions of gaze.

ductless gland, a gland lacking an excretory duct, such as an endocrine gland, which secretes hormones into blood or lymph.

duct of Rivinus /rivē'nəs/ [L *ducere* to lead; Augustus Q. Rivinus. German anatomist, b. 1652], one of the minor sublingual ducts.

duct of Wirsung. See **pancreatic duct.**

ductus /duk'təs/, *pl.* **ductus** /duk'tōos/, a duct.

ductus arteriosus, a vascular channel in the fetus that joins the pulmonary artery directly to the descending aorta.

ductus deferens. See **vas deferens.**

ductus epididymidis, a tube into which the efferent ductules of the testes empty.

ductus venosus, the vascular channel in the fetus passing through the liver and joining the umbilical vein with the inferior vena cava.

Duke diet. See **rice diet.**

Duke longitudinal study, a long-range, in-depth research into the normal aging process of middle-aged and older men and women conducted at Duke University Medical Center. The Duke studies led to development of the "longevity quotient" (LQ) used to evaluate an individual's rate of aging. It is calculated by the number of years a person survives beyond a given point in time divided by the expected number of years derived from actuarial tables.

Dukes' classification, a system of identifying stages of colorectal tumors, from A to D, according to the degree of tissue invasion and metastasis. A Dukes' A tumor is one that is confined to the mucosa and submucosa. A B tumor is one that has invaded the musculature but has not involved the lymphatic system. C tumors have invaded the musculature with metastatic involvement of the regional lymph nodes. D tumors are those that have metastasized to distant organ tissues.

dull pain [ME *dul* not sharp; L *poena* penalty], a mildly throbbing acute or chronic pain.

dumdum fever. See **kala-azar.**

dumping syndrome [ME *dumpen* to throw down], the combination of profuse sweating, nausea, dizziness, and weakness experienced by patients who have had a subtotal gastrectomy. Symptoms are felt soon after eating, when the contents of the stomach empty too rapidly into the duodenum.

Duncan's mechanism [James M. Duncan, English obstetrician, b. 1826; Gk *mechane* machine], a technique for delivery of the placenta with the maternal rather than the fetal surface presenting.

Dunlop skeletal traction, an orthopedic mechanism that helps immobilize the upper limb in the treatment of the contracture or the supracondylar fracture of the elbow. The mechanism uses a system of traction weights, pulleys, and ropes. The system is attached to the bone involved with a pin or wire.

Dunlop skin traction, an orthopedic mechanism that helps immobilize the upper limb in the treatment of contracture and supracondylar fracture of the elbow. The mechanism uses a system of traction weights, pulleys, and ropes and may be applied as adhesive skin traction or nonadhesive skin traction.

duodenal /dōō'ədē'nəl/ [L *duodeni* twelve each], of or pertaining to the duodenum.

duodenal bulb, the first part of the superior portion of the duodenum, which has a bulblike appearance on x-ray views of the small intestine.

duodenal digestion [L *duodeni* 12 fingers long, *digere* to separate], digestion that occurs in the first intestinal segment beyond the pylorus, where secretions of the liver and pancreas are received and mixed with the partially digested food from the stomach. Chyle is formed, fats are emulsified, starch is hydrolyzed, and proteolytic enzymes begin to break down proteins.

duodenal ulcer, an ulcer in the duodenum, the most common type of peptic ulcer.

duodenectomy [L *duodeni;* Gk *ektome* cutting out], the total or partial excision of the duodenum.

duodenitis [L *duodeni;* Gk *itis* inflammation], a condition of inflammation of the duodenum.

duodenography /dōō'ədənog'rəfē/ [L *duodeni;* Gk *graphein* to record],/ the process of making an x-ray image of the duodenum and pancreas.

duodenojejunal flexure. See **angle of Treitz.**

duodenoscope /dōō'ədē'nəskōp'/, an endoscopic instrument, usually fiberoptic, for the visual examination of the duodenum.

duodenoscopy /dōō'ədənos'kəpē/, the visual examination of the duodenum by means of an endoscope.

duodenostomy [L *duodeni;* Gk *stoma* mouth], the surgical creation of a direct opening to the duodenum through the abdominal wall.

duodenum /dōō'ədē'nəm, dōō·od'inəm/, *pl.* **duodena, duodenums** [L *duodeni* twelve each], the shortest, widest, and most fixed portion of the small intestine, taking an almost circular course from the pyloric valve of the stomach so that its termination is close to its starting point. It is about 25 cm long and is divided into superior, descending, horizontal, and ascending portions.

dup, (in cytogenetics) abbreviation for *duplication.*

duplex inheritance. See **amphigenous inheritance.**

duplex transmission [L *duoplex* twofold], the passage of a neural impulse in both directions along a nerve fiber.

duplicating film, a single-emulsion film used to copy an existing x-ray image by exposing it through ultraviolet light.

Dupuytren's contracture /dYpȲ·itraNs', dēpē·itranz'/ [Baron Guillame Dupuytren, French surgeon, b. 1777; L *contractura* drawing together], a progressive, painless thickening and tightening of subcutaneous tissue of the palm, causing the fourth and fifth fingers to bend into the palm and resist extension. Tendons and nerves are not involved. An incision is made into the palm, and the thickened tissue is excised carefully to avoid injury to adjacent ligaments.

Dupuytren's fracture. See **Galeazzi's fracture.**

dura /dōō'rə, dyōō'rə/ [L *durare* to make hard], a thick, tough membrane that surrounds the brain and spinal cord.

durable power of attorney for health, a document that designates an agent or proxy to make health-care decisions.

dural sac, the blind pouch formed by the lower end of the dura mater, at the level of the second sacral segment.

dura mater /dōō'rə mā'tər, dyōō'rə/ [L

dura hard; *mater* mother], the outermost and most fibrous of the three membranes surrounding the brain and spinal cord. The **dura mater encephali** covers the brain, and the **dura mater spinalis** covers the cord.

duress [L *durus* hardness], (in law) an action compelling another person to do what otherwise would not be done voluntarily. A consent form signed under duress is not valid.

Duroziez's murmur /dy′rōzyās′, dir′-, dōō′r-/, [Paul Louis Duroziez, French physician, b. 1826; L *murmur* humming], a systolic murmur heard over the femoral or another large artery when the artery is compressed. The phenomenon is associated with high arterial pulse pressure and aortic insufficiency. A diastolic murmur may also be heard by increasing pressure on the artery distal to the stethoscope.

dust [AS], any fine, particulate, dry matter. Kinds of dust are **inorganic dust** and **organic dust.**

dust fever. See brucellosis.

Dutton's relapsing fever [Joseph E. Dutton, English pathologist, b. 1877], an infection caused by a spirochete, *Borrelia duttonii,* which is transmitted by a soft tick, *Ornithodoros moubata,* found in human dwellings in tropical Africa. The spirochete enters the lesion through a tick bite, producing a high fever, chills, rapid heartbeat, headache, joint and muscle pain, vomiting, and neurologic disorders.

duty [ME *duete* conduct], (in law) an obligation owed by one party to another. Duty may be established by statute or other legal process or it may be voluntarily undertaken.

Duverney's fracture /dōō′vərnāz′/ [Joseph G. Duverney, French anatomist, b. 1648], fracture of the ilium just below the anterior superior spine.

dv/dt, (in cardiology) the rate of change of voltage with respect to time.

DVM, abbreviation for *Doctor of Veterinary Medicine.*

dwarf [AS *dweorge*], **1.** an abnormally short, undersized person, especially one whose bodily parts are not proportional. Kinds of dwarfs include **achondroplastic, Amsterdam, asexual, ateliotic, birdheaded, Brissaud's, cretin, diastrophic, phocomelic, pituitary, primordial, rachitic, renal, Russell, sexual, Silver,** and **thanatophoric dwarf. 2.** to prevent or retard normal growth.

dwarfism, the abnormal underdevelopment of the body, characterized predominantly by extreme shortness of stature. Dwarfism has multiple causes, including genetic defects, endocrine dysfunction in-

volving either the pituitary or thyroid glands, chronic diseases, such as rickets, renal failure, and intestinal malabsorption defects, and psychosocial stress.

dwarf tapeworm infection, a type of intestinal parasitic disease caused by an infestation of *Hymenolepia nana.* It occurs mainly in the southern United States and usually affects children who ingest eggs by placing contaminated materials in the mouth.

Dwayne-Hunt law /dwān′hunt′/, (in radiology) a principle that x-ray energy is inversely proportional to the photon wavelength. As the photon wavelength increases, photon energy decreases, and vice versa. The minimum x-ray wavelength is associated with the maximum x-ray energy.

dwindles, *informal.* a condition of physical deterioration involving several systems of the body, usually in an elderly person.

Dwyer instrumentation /dwī′ər/, one of the two most common surgical methods for correcting the spinal curvature associated with scoliosis. The Dwyer cable method uses a mechanical device that is inserted to assist in maintaining the corrected curvature while the fusion heals.

Dy, symbol for the element **dysprosium.**

dyad /dī′ad/ [Gk *dyas* two], (in genetics) one of the paired homologous chromosomes, consisting of two chromatids, which result from the division of a tetrad in the first meiotic division of gametogenesis. **–dyadic,** *adj.*

dyadic interpersonal communication /dī·ad′ik/, a process in which two people interact face to face as senders and receivers, as in a conversation.

dyclonine hydrochloride /dī′klōnīn/, a local anesthetic, with bactericidal and fungicidal properties, for oral pain, pruritis, insect bites, and minor skin burns and injuries.

dydrogesterone /dī′drəjes′tərōn/, a synthetic oral progestin prescribed in the treatment of abnormal uterine bleeding, menopausal vasomotor symptoms, pickwickian syndrome, and endometrial cancer, and for contraception.

dye /dī/ [AS *deag*], **1.** to apply coloring matter to a substance. **2.** a chemical compound capable of imparting color to a substance to which it is applied as stains for tissues, as test reagents, as therapeutic agents, and to color pharmaceutic preparations.

dynamic [Gk *dynamis* force], **1.** tending to change or to encourage change, such as a dynamic nurse-patient relationship.

2. (in respiratory therapy) a condition of changing volume.

dynamic cardiac work, the energy transfer that occurs during the process of ventricular ejection of blood.

dynamic compliance, the distensibility of the lung, as measured by plethysmography during the breathing cycle.

dynamic equilibrium, the ability of a patient to adjust to displacements of the body's center of gravity by changing the body's base of support.

dynamic ileus, an intestinal obstruction with associated recurrent and continuous muscle spasma.

dynamic imaging, (in ultrasonography) the imaging of an object in motion at a frame rate that does not cause significant blurring of any one image and at a repetition rate sufficient to adequately represent the movement pattern.

dynamic nurse-patient relationship, a conceptual framework in which the interpersonal aspects of the nurse-patient relationship are analyzed. The relationship is affected by the behavior of the patient, the reaction of the nurse, and the actions of the nurse that are intended to aid the patient.

dynamic psychiatry, the study of motivational, emotional, and biologic factors as determinants of human behavior.

dynamic range, 1. (in radiology) the range of voltage or input signals that result in a digital output. **2.** (in audiology) the range of decibels from the faintest sound a person can hear to the level of sound that causes pain.

dynamic response, the accuracy with which a physiologic monitoring system, such as an electrocardiograph, will simulate the actual event being recorded.

dynamic spatial reconstructor (DSR), a kind of roentgenographic machine used in research permitting moving three-dimensional images of human organs to be examined visually and from any direction.

dynamic splint [Gk *dynamis* force; D, *splinte*], any splint that incorporates springs, elastic bands, or other materials that produce a constant active force to counteract deforming forces of a splint.

dynamometer /dī'nəmom'ətər/ [Gk *dynamis* force, *metron* measure], a device for measuring the degree of force expended in the contraction of a group of muscles, such as a squeeze dynamometer, which measures the gross grip strength of the hand muscles.

dyne /dīn/, a unit of force, specifically the force required to accelerate a free mass of 1 g at 1 cm per second. One dyne equals 10^{-5} newton.

dynode /dī'nōd/, one of a series of plate-like elements that amplify electron pulses in a photomultiplier tube. For each electron that strikes each dynode, several secondary electrons are emitted. The dynode gain is the ratio of secondary electrons to incident electrons.

dyphylline /dīfil'in/, a bronchodilator prescribed in the treatment of bronchospasm in acute bronchial asthma, bronchitis, and emphysema.

dysacusis /dis'əkōō'sis/ [Gk *dys* difficult, *akouein* to hear], a condition in which loud sounds or noises can cause pain or discomfort; usually caused by damage to the cochlea.

dysadrenia /dis'adrē'nē·ə/ [Gk *dys* bad; L *ad* to, *ren* kidney], abnormal adrenal function characterized by decreased production of hormones, as in hypoadrenalism or hypoadrenocorticism, or by increased secretion of the products of the gland, as in hyperadrenalism or hyperadrenocorticism.

dysarthria /disär'thrē·ə/ [Gk *dys* + *arthroun* to articulate], difficult, poorly articulated speech, resulting from interference in the control over the muscles of speech, usually because of damage to a central or peripheral motor nerve.

dysarthrosis /dis'ärthrō'sis/ [Gk *dys* + *arthron* joint], any disorder of a joint, including disease, dislocation, or deformity, that makes movement of the joint difficult.

dysautonomia /disô'tənō'mē·ə/ [Gk *dys* + *autonomia* self-government], a dysfunction of the autonomic nervous system that can be a clinical feature of diabetes, parkinsonism, Adie's syndrome, Shy-Drager syndrome, or Riley-Day syndrome. A fairly common effect is orthostatic hypotension with syncope and drop attacks.

dysbarism /dis'bäriz'əm/, a reaction to a sudden change in ambient pressure, such as rapid exposure to the lower atmospheric pressures of high altitudes. It is marked by symptoms similar to those of decompression sickness.

dysbetalipoproteinemia /disbet'əlip'əprō'tinē'mē·ə/, an accumulation of abnormal beta-lipoprotein in the blood.

dyscholia /diskō'lē·ə/ [Gk *dys* + *chole* bile], any abnormal condition of the bile, either regarding the quantity secreted or the condition of the constituents.

dyschondroplasia. See **enchondromatosis.**

dyschroic film fault /diskrō'ik/, a defect in a radiograph that appears as a pinkish coloration when the film is viewed by transmitted light and as a green coloration when the film is viewed by reflected light.

dyscrasia /diskrā'zhə/ [Gk *dys* + *krasis* mingling], an abnormal blood or bone marrow condition, such as leukemia, aplastic anemia, or prenatal Rh incompatibility.

dyscrasic fracture /diskraz′ik/, any fracture caused by the weakening of a specific bone as a result of a debilitating disease.

dysdiadochokinesia /dis′dī·ədō′kōkinē′-zhə/ [Gk *dys* + *diadochos* working in turn, *kinesis* movement], an inability to perform rapidly alternating movements, such as rhythmically tapping the fingers on the knee. The cause is a cerebellar lesion and is related to dysmetria.

dysentery /dis′inter′ē/ [Gk *dys* + *entron* intestine], an inflammation of the intestine, especially of the colon, that may be caused by chemical irritants, bacteria, protozoa, or parasites. It is characterized by frequent and bloody stools, abdominal pain, and tenesmus. **–dysenteric,** *adj.*

dysergia /disur′jē·ə/ [Gk *dys* + *ergon* work], a condition in which the muscles, because of an efferent nerve irregularity, fail to function normally in certain voluntary movements.

dysesthesia /dis′esthē′zhə/, a common effect of spinal cord injury characterized by sensations of numbness, tingling, burning, or pain felt below the level of the lesion.

dysfunctional [Gk *dys* + L *functio* performance], (of a body organ or system) unable to function normally. **-dysfunction,** *n.*

dysfunctional communication, a communication that results from inaccurate perceptions, faulty internal filters (personal interpretations of information), and social isolation.

dysfunctional stereotype, a stereotype in which the dysfunctional aspects of a culture are emphasized.

dysfunctional uterine bleeding (DUB), abnormal uterine bleeding that is not caused by a tumor, inflammation, or pregnancy. It may be characterized by painless, irregular, heavy bleeding or intermenstrual spotting or periods of amenorrhea. The condition is associated with anovulation and unopposed estrogen stimulation.

dysgammaglobulinemia /disgam′əglob′y-linē′mē·ə/, an inherited immune deficiency disease characterized by blood disorders and a tendency to experience repeated infections. The cause is a deficiency of immunoglobulins needed to produce antibodies.

dysgenesis /disjen′əsis/ [Gk *dys* + *genein* to produce], **1.** defective or abnormal formation of an organ or part, primarily during embryonic development. **2.** impairment or loss of the ability to procreate. A kind of dysgenesis is **gonadal dysgenesis. –dysgenic,** *adj.*

dysgenics /disjen′iks/, the study of those factors or situations that are genetically detrimental to the future of a race or species.

dysgenitalism /disjen′itəliz′əm/ [Gk *dys* + L *genitalis* belonging to birth], any condition involving the abnormal development of the genital organs.

dysgerminoma /dis′jərminō′mə/, *pl.* **dysgerminomas, dysgerminomata** [Gk *dys* + L *germen* germ; Gk *oma* tumor], a rare malignant tumor of the ovary, believed to arise from the undifferentiated germ cells of the embryonic gonad.

dysgeusia /disgoō′zhə/ [Gk *dys* + *geusis* taste], an abnormal or impaired sense of taste.

dysgnathic anomaly /disnath′ik/ [Gk *dys* + *gnathos* jaw], (in dentistry) an abnormality that extends beyond the teeth, affecting the maxilla, the mandible, or both.

dysgraphia /disgraf′ē·ə/ [Gk *dys* + *graphein* to write], an impairment of the ability to write, caused by a pathologic disorder. **–dysgraphic,** *adj.*

dyshidrosis /dis′hidrō′sis, dis′hī-/ [Gk *dys* + *hidrosis* sweating], a condition in which abnormal sweating occurs. Kinds of dyshidrosis are **hyperhidrosis** and **miliaria.**

dyskeratosis /dis′kerətō′sis/ [Gk *dys* + *keras* horn, *osis* condition], an abnormal or premature keratinization of epithelial cells.

dyskinesia /dis′kinē′zhə/ [Gk *dys* + *kinesis* movement], an impairment of the ability to execute voluntary movements. Dyskinesia can be an adverse effect of prolonged use of phenothiazine medications in elderly patients or those with brain injuries. **–dyskinetic,** /-et′ik/, *adj.*

dyskinetic syndrome /dis′kinet′ik/, a form of cerebral palsy involving a basal ganglia disorder. Clinical features include athetoid movements of the extremities and sometimes the trunk. The movements tend to increase with emotional tension and diminish during sleep.

dyslexia /dislek′sē·ə/ [Gk *dys* + *lexis* word], an impairment of the ability to read, as a result of a variety of pathologic conditions, some of which are associated with the central nervous system. Dyslexic persons often reverse letters and words, cannot adequately distinguish the letter sequences in written words, and have difficulty determining left from right. **–dyslexic,** *adj.*

dysmaturity /dis′machoōr′itē/ [Gk *dys* + L *maturare* to make ripe] **1.** the failure of an organism to develop, ripen, or otherwise achieve maturity in structure or function. **2.** the condition of a fetus or newborn being abnormally small or large for its age of gestation. Kinds of dysmaturity are **small for gestational age** and **large for gestational age.** **–dysmature,** *adj.*

dysmegalopsia /dis′megəlop′sē·ə/ [Gk *dys* + *megas* large, *opsis* appearance], an inability to judge accurately the size or measure of an object.

dysmelia /disme′lyə/ [Gk *dys* + *melos* limb], an abnormal congenital condition characterized by missing or shortened extremities of the body and associated with abnormalities of the spine in some individuals. It is caused by abnormal metabolism during the development of the embryonic limbs.

dysmenorrhea /dis′menərē′ə/ [Gk *dys* + *men* month, *rhein* to flow], pain associated with menstruation. Primary dysmenorrhea is menstrual pain that results from factors intrinsic to the uterus and the process of menstruation. It is extremely common, occurring at least occasionally in almost all women. If the painful episode is mild and brief, it is considered functional and normal and requires no treatment. In approximately 10% of women, dysmenorrhea is sufficiently severe to cause episodes of partial or total disability. Pain occurs typically in the lower abdomen or back and is crampy, coming in successive waves—apparently in conjunction with intense uterine contractions and slight cervical dilatation. Pain usually begins just before, or at the onset of, menstrual flow and lasts from a few hours to 1 day or more. Pain is frequently associated with nausea, vomiting, and frequent bowel movements with intestinal cramping. Dizziness, fainting, pallor, and obvious distress may also be observed. Secondary dysmenorrhea is menstrual pain that occurs secondary to specific pelvic abnormalities, such as endometriosis, adenomyosis, chronic pelvic infection, chronic pelvic congestion, or degenerating fibroid tumors.

dysmetria /disme′trē·ə/ [Gk *dys* + *metron* measure], an abnormal condition that prevents the affected individual from properly measuring distances associated with muscular acts and from controlling muscular action. It is associated with cerebellar lesions and typically characterized by overestimating or underestimating the range of motion needed to place the limbs correctly during voluntary movement.

dysmnesic syndrome /disne′sik/, a memory disorder characterized by an inability to learn simple new skills, although the person can still perform highly complex skills learned before the onset of the condition. The cause is a disease or injury that affects only certain brain tissues associated with memory.

dysmorphogenesis /dis′môrfōjen′əsis/, the development of ill-shaped or otherwise malformed body structures.

dysmorphophobia /dis′môrfō′bē·ə/ [Gk *dys* + *morphe* form, *phobos* fear], **1.** a fundamental delusion of body image. **2.** the morbid fear of deformity.

dysostosis /dis′ostō′sis/ [Gk *dys* + *osteon* bone, *osis*], an abnormal condition characterized by defective ossification, especially by defects in the normal ossification of fetal cartilages. Kinds of dysostoses include **cleidocranial, craniofacial, mandibulofacial, metaphyseal,** and **Nager's acrofacial dysostosis.**

dyspareunia /dis′pəroo͞o′nē·ə/ [Gk *dys* + *pareunos* mating], an abnormal condition of pain during sexual intercourse. The pain may result from abnormal conditions of the genitalia, dysfunctional psychophysiologic reaction to sexual union, forcible coition, or incomplete sexual arousal.

dyspepsia /dispep′sē·ə/ [Gk *dys* + *peptein* to digest], a vague feeling of epigastric discomfort, felt after eating. There is an uncomfortable feeling of fullness, heartburn, bloating, and nausea. **–dyspeptic,** *adj.*

dysphagia /disfā′jē·ə/ [Gk *dys* + *phagein* to swallow], difficulty in swallowing, commonly associated with obstructive or motor disorders of the esophagus. Patients with obstructive disorders such as esophageal tumor or lower esophageal ring are unable to swallow solids but can tolerate liquids. Persons with motor disorders are unable to swallow solids or liquids.

dysphagia lusoria, an abnormal condition, characterized by difficulty in swallowing, caused by the compression of the esophagus from an anomalous right subclavian artery that arises from the descending aorta and courses behind or in front of the esophagus.

dysphasia /disfā′zhə/ [Gk *dys* + *phasis* speaking], an impairment of speech, not as severe as aphasia, usually the result of an injury to the speech area in the cerebral cortex of the brain.

dysphonia /disfō′nē·ə/ [Gk *dys* + *phone* voice], any abnormality in the speaking voice, such as hoarseness. Dysphonia puberum identifies the voice changes that occur in adolescent boys.

dysphoria /disfôr′ē·ə/, a disorder of affect characterized by depression and anguish.

dysplasia /displā′zhə/ [Gk *dys* + *plassein* to form], any abnormal development of tissues or organs.

dyspnea /dispnē′ə/ [Gk *dys* + *pnoia* breathing], a shortness of breath or a difficulty in breathing that may be caused by certain heart conditions, strenuous exercise, or anxiety. **–dyspneal, dyspneic,** *adj.*

dyspraxia /disprak′sē·ə/ [Gk *dys* + *prassein* to do], a partial loss of the ability to perform skilled, coordinated movements in the absence of any associated defect in motor or sensory functions.

dysprosium (Dy) /disprō′sē·əm/ [Gk *dys* + *prositos* to approach], a rare-earth metallic element. Its atomic number is 66; its atomic weight is 162.50. Radioactive isotopes of dysprosium are used in radioisotope scanning.

dysproteinemia /disprō′tēnē′mē·ə/[Gk *dys* + *protos* first, *haima* blood], an abnormality of the protein content of the blood, usually involving the immunoglobulins.

dysraphia /disrā′fē·ə/ [Gk *dys* + *raphe* seam], failure of a raphe to fuse completely, as in incomplete closure of the neural tube.

dysraphic syndrome /disrat′ik/, a developmental disorder, usually involving the spinal cord, such as encephalocele or myelomenigocele.

dysreflexia /dis′riflek′sē·ə/ [Gk *dys* + L *reflectere* to bend backward], a NANDA-accepted nursing diagnosis of a condition in which an individual with a spinal cord injury at T7 or above experiences or is at risk to experience a life-threatening uninhibited sympathetic response of the nervous system to a noxious stimulus. Defining characteristics include paroxysmal hypertension, bradycardia or tachycardia, diaphoresis above the injury, red splotches on the skin above the injury, pallor below the injury, a headache that is a diffuse pain, chilling, conjunctival congestion, blurred vision, chest pain, a metallic taste in the mouth, nasal congestion, and pilomotor reflex. **–dysreflexic,** *adj.*

dysrhythmia /disrith′mē·ə/, any disturbance or abnormality in a normal rhythmic pattern, specifically, irregularity in the brain waves or cadence of speech.

dyssebacea /disibā′shē·ə/ [Gk *dys* + L *sevum* suet], a skin condition characterized by red, scaly, greasy patches on the nose, eyelids, scrotum, and labia.

dyssynergia /dis′inur′jē·ə/ [Gk *dys* + *syn* together, *ergein* work], any disturbance in muscular coordination, such as in cases of ataxia.

dystaxia /distak′sē·ə/ [Gk *dys* + *taxis* order], partial ataxia, such as dystaxia agitans in which there is a tremor caused by a spinal cord irritation but there is no paralysis.

dysthymia /disthim′ē·ə/ [Gk *dys* + *thymos* mind], a form of chronic unipolar depression that tends to occur in elderly persons with debilitating physical disorders, multiple interpersonal losses, and chronic marital difficulties. Several depressive episodes may merge into a low-grade chronic depressive state.

dysthymic disorder [Gk *dys* + *thymos* mind], a disorder of mood whereby the essential feature is a chronic disturbance of mood of at least two years duration, involving either depressed mood or loss of interest or pleasure in all or almost all usual activities and pastimes, and associated symptoms, but not of sufficient severity and duration to meet the criteria for a major depressive episode.

dystocia /distō′shə/ [Gk *dys* + *tokos* birth], pathologic or difficult labor, which may be caused by an obstruction or constriction of the birth passage or an abnormal size, shape, position, or condition of the fetus.

dystonia /distō′nē·ə/ [Gk *dys* + *tonos* tone], any impairment of muscle tone. The condition commonly involves the head, neck, and tongue and often occurs as an adverse effect of a medication.

dystonia musculorum deformans /distō′nē·ə/, a rare abnormal condition characterized by intense, irregular torsion muscle spasms that contort the body. The muscles of the trunk, shoulder, and pelvis are commonly involved. Muscle power and tone appear normal, but convulsive spasms make the involved muscles relatively useless.

dystonic /diston′ik/, referring to an excessive increase in muscle tone, often resulting in postural abnormalities.

dystrophic calcification /distrof′ik/ [Gk *dys* + *trophe* nourishment; L *calx* lime, *facere* to make], the pathologic accumulation of calcium salts in necrotic or degenerated tissues.

dystrophy /dis′trəfē/ [Gk *dys* + *trophe* nourishment], any abnormal condition caused by defective nutrition, often applied to a developmental change in muscles that does not involve the nervous system, such as fatty degeneration associated with increased size but decreased strength. **–dystrophic** /distrof′ik/, *adj.*

dysuria /disyōōr′ē·ə/ [Gk *dys* + *ouron* urine], painful urination, usually the result of a bacterial infection or obstructive condition in the urinary tract. The patient complains of a burning sensation when passing urine, and laboratory examination may reveal the presence of blood, bacteria, or white blood cells.

E, symbol for **expired gas.**

E¹, symbol for **monomolecular elimination reaction.**

E², symbol for **bimolecular elimination reaction.**

E and GW, abbreviation for **Economic and General Welfare.**

ear [AS *eare*], the organ of hearing, consisting of the internal, middle, and external ear. The external ear includes the skin-covered cartilaginous auricle visible on either side of the head and the portion of the external auditory canal that is outside the skull. The middle ear contains three very small bones, the malleus, incus, and stapes, which transmit vibrations caused by sound waves reaching the tympanic membrane to the oval window of the inner ear. The inner ear contains two separate organs: the vestibular apparatus, which provides the sense of balance, and the organ of Corti, which receives vibrations from the middle ear and translates them into nerve impulses, which are again interpreted by brain cells as specific sounds.

earache [AS *eare* + *acan* to hurt], a pain in the ear, sensed as sharp, dull, burning, intermittent, or constant. The cause is not necessarily a disease of the ear, because infections and other disorders of the nose, oral cavity, larynx, and temporomandibular joint can produce referred pain in the ear.

eardrop instillation, the instillation of a medicated solution into the external auditory canal of the ear. The patient is asked to turn the head to the side so that the ear being treated faces upward. The drops of medicine are directed toward the internal wall of the canal.

eardrops [AS *eare* + *dropa*], a topical, liquid form of medication for the local treatment of various conditions of the ear, such as inflammation or infection of the lining of the external auditory canal or impacted cerumen.

eardrum. See **tympanic membrane.**

Early and Periodic Screening Diagnosis and Treatment (EPSDT), a section of the Medicaid program that requires all states to maintain a program to determine the physical and mental defects of persons under age 21 who are covered by the program and to provide short- and long-range treatment.

ear oximeter /oksim'ətrē/, a device placed over the ear lobe that transmits a beam of light through the ear tissue to a receiver. It is a noninvasive method of measuring the level of saturated hemoglobin in the blood. The amount of saturated hemoglobin in the blood alters the wavelengths of light transmitted.

ear speculum [AS *eare*; L *speculum* mirror], a short, funnel-shaped tube attached to an otoscope for examining the ear canal.

earth bath, the covering of a part of the body with warm sand or earth.

ear thermometry, the measurement of the temperature of the tympanic membrane by detection of infrared radiation from the eardrum.

earwax. See **cerumen.**

East African Sleeping Sickness. See **Rhodesian trypanosomiasis.**

eastern equine encephalitis. See **equine encephalitis.**

eating disorders, any of a group of dysfunctional behaviors of nutrition, including anorexia, bulimia, or cravings for such nonfood items as ice, clay, or starch.

Eaton agent, an alternative name for *Mycoplasma pneumoniae*, a common cause of atypical pneumonia in humans.

Eaton agent pneumonia. See **mycoplasma pneumonia.**

Eaton-Lambert syndrome, a form of myasthenia that tends to be associated with lung cancer.

Ebbecke's reaction. See **dermatographia.**

EBP, abbreviation for **epidural blood patch.**

Ebstein's anomaly [Wilhelm Ebstein, German physician, b. 1836; Gk, *anomalia*, irregularity], a congenital heart defect in which the tricuspid valve is displaced downward into the right ventricle. The abnormality is often associated with right-to-left atrial shunting and Wolff-Parkinson-White syndrome.

EBV, abbreviation for **Epstein-Barr virus.**

ECC, 1. abbreviation for **emergency car-**

diac care. 2. abbreviation for *external cardiac compression.*

eccentric [Gk *ek* out, *centre* center], **1.** pertaining to an object or activity that departs from the usual course or practice. **2.** behavior that may appear to be odd or unconventional but is not necessarily a disorder.

eccentric contraction, a type of muscle contraction that involves lengthening of the muscle fibers, such as when a weight is lowered through a range of motion. The muscle yields to the resistance, allowing itself to be stretched.

eccentric implantation [Gk *ek* out, *centre* center], (in embryology) the embedding of the blastocyst within a fold or recess of the uterine wall, which then closes off from the main cavity.

eccentricity, behavior that is regarded as odd or peculiar for a particular culture or community, although not unusual enough to be considered pathologic.

eccentric jaw relation, (in dentistry) any jaw relation other than centric relation.

eccentric occlusion [Gk *ek* + *centre*; L *occludere* to close up], an occlusion of the teeth in which the habitual voluntary closure pattern of the mandible does not coincide with centric relation, resulting in premature tooth contacts.

ecchondroma /ek'əndrō'mə/ [Gk *ek* + *chondros* cartilage, *oma* tumor], a benign cartilaginous tumor that develops on the surface of a cartilage or under the periosteum of bone.

ecchondrosis. See **ecchondroma.**

ecchymosis /ek'imō'sis/, *pl.* **ecchymoses** [Gk *ek* + *chymos* juice], discoloration of an area of the skin or mucous membrane caused by the extravasation of blood into the subcutaneous tissues as a result of trauma to the underlying blood vessels or by fragility of the vessel walls. —**ecchymotic,** *adj.*

ecchymotic mask /ek'imot'ik/ [Gk *ek* + *chymous*; Fr *masque*], a cyanotic or bluish discoloration of the face of a victim of traumatic asphyxia, as in strangulation or choking. The color is the result of petechial hemorrhages.

ecchymotic rash [Gk *ek* + *chymos* juice; OFr *rasche* scurf], a skin eruption characterized by black-blue spots caused by extravasation of blood into the tissues, usually the result of a contusion.

eccrine /ek'rin/ [Gk *ekkrinein* to secrete, of or pertaining to a sweat gland that secretes outwardly through a duct to the surface of the skin.

eccrine gland, one of two kinds of sweat glands in the corium of the skin. Such glands promote cooling by evaporation of their secretion.

eccyesis. See **ectopic pregnancy.**

ECF, 1. abbreviation for **extended care facility. 2.** abbreviation for **extracellular fluid.**

ECG, 1. abbreviation for **electrocardiogram. 2.** abbreviation for **electrocardiograph.**

ecgonine /ek'gōnēn/ the principal part of the cocaine molecule.

echinococcosis /ekī'nōkokō'sis/ [Gk *echinos* prickly husk, *kokkos* berry, *osis* condition], an infestation, usually of the liver, caused by the larval stage of a tapeworm of the genus *Echinococcus*. Humans, especially children, can become infested with larvae by ingesting eggs shed in the stool of infected dogs. Clinical manifestations and prognosis vary, depending on the tissue invaded and the extent of infestation.

Echinococcus /ekī'nōkok'əs/ [Gk *echinos* prickly husk, *kokkos* berry], a genus of small tapeworms that infects primarily canines.

echinocyte. See **burr cell.**

echo, *informal.* echoradiography.

echo beat [Gk; sound; AS *beatan* to throb], a reciprocal heart beat, or one that results from the return of an impulse to an atrium or ventricle to reactivate a contraction.

echocardiogram /ek'ōkärdē·əgram'/ [Gk *echo* sound, *kardia* heart, *gramma* record], a graphic outline of movements of the heart structures compiled from ultrasound vibrations echoed from the heart structures.

echocardiography /ek'ōkär'dē·og'rəfē/ [Gk *echo* + *kardia* heart, *graphein* to record], a diagnostic procedure for studying the structure and motion of the heart. Ultrasonic waves directed through the heart are reflected backward, or echoed, when they pass from one type of tissue to another.

echoencephalogram /ek'ō·ensef'ələgram'/ [Gk *echo* + *enkephalos* brain, *gramma* record], a recording produced by an echo-encephalograph.

echoencephalography /ek'ō·ensef'ələg'rəfē/, the use of ultrasound to study the intracranial structures of the brain. —**echoencephalographic,** *adj.*

echogram /ek'ōgram/ [Gk *echo* + *gramma* record], a recording of ultrasound echo patterns of body structures, such as a gravid uterus.

echography. See **ultrasonography.**

echolalia /ek'ōlā'lyə/ [Gk *echo* + *lalein* to babble], **1.** (in psychiatry) the automatic and meaningless repetition of another's words or phrases, especially as seen in schizophrenia. A kind of echolalia is **delayed echolalia**. 2. (in pediatrics) a baby's imitation or repetition of sounds or words produced by others. It occurs normally in early childhood development. –**echolalic**, *adj.*

echopraxia /ek′ōprak′sē·ə/ [Gk *echo* + *prassein* to practice], imitation or repetition of the body movements of another person, a behavior exhibited by some schizophrenic patients.

echoradiography /ek′ōrā′dē·og′rəfē/ [Gk *echo* + L *radius* ray; Gk *graphein* to record], a diagnostic procedure using ultrasonography and various devices for the visualization of internal structures of the body.

echo speech. See **echolalia**.

echothiophate iodide, /ek′ōthī′ōfāt/ an anticholinesterase used for ophthalmic purposes. It is prescribed for chronic open-angle glaucoma and accommodative esotropia.

ECHO virus /ek′ōvī′rəs/ [enteric *cyto-pathic human orphan* + L *virus* poison], a picornavirus associated with many clinical syndromes but not identified as the causative organism of any specific disease. There are many echoviruses; most are harmless.

eclampsia /iklamp′sē·ə/ [Gk *ek* out, *lampein* to flash], the gravest form of toxemia of pregnancy, characterized by grand mal convulsion, coma, hypertension, proteinuria, and edema. The symptoms of impending convulsion often include anxiety, epigastric pain, headache, and blurred vision. Convulsions may be prevented by bed rest in a quiet, dimly lit room and parenteral administration of magnesium sulfate.

eclamptogenic toxemia /iklamp′tōjen′ik/ [Gk *ek* + *lampein* to flash, *genein* to produce, *toxikon* poison, *haima* blood], a form of blood poisoning accompanied by convulsions that may occur during pregnancy.

eclectic /iklek′tik/ [Gk *eklektikos* selecting], pertaining to a therapy that selects, combines, and incorporates diverse techniques from several systems or theories into an integrated approach.

eclipse scotoma [Gk *ekleipsis* abandoning, *skotos* darkness, *oma* tumor], a small central area of depressed or lost vision due to looking directly at the sun without adequate protection.

ECM, abbreviation for **erythema chromicum migrans**.

ECMO, abbreviation for **extracorporeal membrane oxygenator**.

E. coli, an abbreviation for *Escherichia coli*.

ecologic chemistry, the study of chemical compounds synthesized by plants that influence ecology because of their toxic effects.

ecologic fallacy, a false assumption that the presence of a pathogenic factor and a disease in a population can be accepted as proof that the agent is the cause of the disease in a particular individual.

ecology [Gk *oekos* house, *logos* science], the study of the interaction between living organisms and the various influences of their environment.

econazole, /ikon′əzōl/ an antifungal agent prescribed in the treatment of tinea and candidiasis.

Economic and General Welfare (E and GW), a unit of the American Nurses' Association that works to upgrade the salaries, benefits, and working conditions of nurses.

ecosystem, the sum total of all living and nonliving things that support a chain of life events within a particular area.

ecstasy [Gk *ekstasis* derangement], an emotional state characterized by exultation, rapturous delight, or frenzy. –**ecstatic**, *adj.*

ECT, abbreviation for **electroconvulsive therapy**.

ecthyma /ek′thimə/ [Gk *ek* out, *thyein* to rush], a deep, burrowing form of impetigo characterized by large pustules, crusts, and ulcerations surrounded by erythema. Staphylococci and streptococci are the offending bacteria.

ectoderm /ek′tədurm/ [Gk *ektos* outside, *derma* skin], the outermost of the three primary cell layers of an embryo. The ectoderm gives rise to the nervous system; the organs of special sense, such as the eyes and ears; the epidermis and epidermal tissue, such as fingernails, hair, and skin glands; and the mucous membranes of the mouth and anus. –**ectodermal, ectodermic**, *adj.*

ectodermal cloaca, a part of the cloaca in the developing embryo that lies external to the cloacal membrane and eventually gives rise to the anus and anal canal.

ectomorph /ek′təmôrf′/ [Gk *ektos* + *morphe* form], a person whose physique is characterized by slenderness, fragility, and a predominance of structures derived from the ectoderm.

ectoparasite /ek′tōper′əsīt/ [Gk *ektos* + *parasitos* guest], (in medical parasitology) an organism that lives on the outside of the body of the host, as a louse.

ectopic /ektop′ik/ [Gk *ektos* + *topos* place], 1. (of an object or organ) situated in an unusual place, away from its normal location; for example, an ectopic pregnancy is a pregnancy that occurs outside the uterus. **2.** (of an event) occurring at the wrong time, as a premature heart beat or premature ventricular contraction.

ectopic beat, [Gk *ek* + *topos*; AS *beatan*], a heart beat that had its origin at some place other than the sinoatrial node.

ectopic focus, an abnormal cardiac impulse that produces abnormal, or ectopic, beats. Ectopic foci may occur in both healthy and diseased hearts and are usually associated with irritation of a small area of myocardial tissue.

ectopic myelopoiesis. See **extramedullary myelopoiesis.**

ectopic pacemaker, [Gk *ek* + *topos*; L *passus* step; ME *maken*], an abnormally located group of cardiac nerve cells that initiate a heart impulse and override the sinoatrial node. The ectopic sites may be in an atrium, ventricle, or atrioventricular node.

ectopic pregnancy, an abnormal pregnancy in which the conceptus implants outside the uterine cavity. Kinds of ectopic pregnancy are **abdominal pregnancy, ovarian pregnancy,** and **tubal pregnancy.**

ectopic rhythm [Gk *ek* + *topos*, *rhythmos* beat], an abnormal heart rhythm caused by formation of the impulse in a focus outside the usual pacemaker. An ectopic focus usually develops when the natural sinus node pacemaker is depressed or an ectopic focus develops.

ectopic tachycardia [Gk *ek* + *topos*, *tachys* swift + *kardia* heart], an abnormally rapid heart beat due to a stimulus from an ectopic focus, or one outside the sinoatrial node.

ectopic teratism, a congenital anomaly in which one or more parts are misplaced, as dextrocardia, palatine teeth, and transposition of the great vessels.

ectopy /ek'təpē/ [Gk *ek* + *topos* place], a condition in which an organ or substance is not in its natural or proper place, as an ectopic pregnancy that develops outside the uterus or ectopic heart beats.

ectotoxin. See **exotoxin.**

ectrodactyly /ek'trōdak'təlē/ [Gk *ektrosis* miscarriage, *daktylos* finger], a congenital anomaly characterized by the absence of part or all of one or more of the fingers or toes.

ectrogenic teratism /ek'trōjen'ik/ [Gk *ektrosis* + *genein* to produce; *teras* monster], a congenital anomaly caused by developmental failure in which one or more parts or organs are missing.

ectrogeny /ektroj'ənē/ [Gk *ektrosis* + *genein* to produce], the congenital absence or

defect of any organ or part of the body. — **ectrogenic,** *adj.* ectromelia /ek'trōmē'lyə/ [Gk *ektrosis* + *melos* limb], the congenital absence or incomplete development of the long bones of one or more of the limbs. Kinds of ectromelia are **amelia, hemimelia,** and **phocomelia.** –**ectromelic,** *adj.,* **ectromelus,** *n.*

ectropion /ektrō'pē·on/ [Gk *ek* + *trepein* to turn], eversion, most commonly of the eyelid, exposing the conjunctival membrane lining the eyelid and part of the eyeball. The condition may involve only the lower eyelid or both eyelids.

ectrosyndactyly /ek'trōsindak't əlē/ [Gk *ektrosis* + *syn* together, *daktylos* finger], a congenital anomaly characterized by the absence of some but not all of the digits, with those that are formed being webbed so as to appear fused.

ECU, abbreviation for *extended care unit.*

eczema /ek'simə/ [Gk *ekzein* to boil over], superficial dermatitis of unknown cause. In the early stage it may be pruritic, erythematous, papulovesicular, edematous, and weeping. –**eczematous,** *adj.*

eczema herpeticum, a generalized vesiculopustular skin disease caused by herpes simplex virus or vaccinia virus infection of a preexisting rash such as atopic dermatitis.

eczema marginatum. See **tinea cruris.**

eczematous conjunctivitis, /eksem'ətəs/ conjunctival and corneal inflammation associated with multiple, tiny, ulcerated vesicles.

ED, abbreviation for **effective dose.**

ED, abbreviation for **emergency department.**

ED50, symbol for **median effective dose.**

edaphon /ed'əfon/, the composite of organisms that live in the soil. –**edaphic,** *adj.*

EDB, abbreviation for **ethylene dibromide.**

EDC, abbreviation for *expected date of confinement.*

edema /idē'mə/ [Gk *oidema* swelling], the abnormal accumulation of fluid in interstitial spaces of tissues, such as in the pericardial sac, intrapleural space, peritoneal cavity, or joint capsules. –**edematous, edematose,** *adj.*

edema of glottis [Gk *oidema* swelling, *glossa* tongue], a swelling due to fluid accumulation in the soft tissues of the larynx. The condition, usually inflammatory, may be due to an infection, injury, or inhalation of toxic gases.

edematous /ēdem'ətəs/ [Gk, *oidema,* swelling], pertaining to or resembling edema, or excessive fluid accumulation in the tissues, causing swelling.

edentulous /ēden′chələs/, toothless.

edetate (EDTA) /ed′ətāt/, one of several salts of edetic acid, including calcium disodium edetate and edetate disodium, used as a chelating agent in treating poisoning with heavy metals.

edetate disodium, a parenteral chelating agent. It is prescribed for hypercalcemic crisis, for ventricular arrhythmia and heart block resulting from digitalis toxicity, and for lead poisoning.

edetic acid (EDTA) /idet′ik/, a chelating agent.

EDG, abbreviation for **electrodynograph.**

edge response function (ERF), the ability of a computed tomography system to reproduce accurately a high-contrast edge, as in the scanning of a structure such as the heart.

edgewise fixed orthodontic appliance, an orthodontic appliance characterized by tooth attachment brackets with a rectangular slot that engages a round or rectangular arch wire. It is used to correct or improve malocclusion.

edrophonium chloride, /ed′rōfō′nē·əm/ a cholinesterase inhibitor that acts as an antidote to curare and is an aid in the diagnosis of myasthenia gravis. It is also used to terminate paroxysmal supraventricular tachycardia.

edrophonium test, a test for myasthenia gravis by the injection of an IV solution of edrophonium chloride into a patient.

Edsall's disease [David L. Edsall, American physician, b. 1869], a cramping condition that is the result of excessive exposure to heat.

EDTA, 1. abbreviation for **edetate.** 2. abbreviation for **edetic acid.**

educational psychology [L *educatus* to rear; Gk *psyche* mind, *logos* science], the application of psychologic principles, techniques, and tests to educational problems.

Edwards' syndrome. See trisomy 18.

EEE, abbreviation for **eastern equine encephalitis.** See **equine encephalitis.**

EEG, 1. abbreviation for **electroencephalogram.** 2. abbreviation for **electroencephalography.**

EENT, abbreviation for *eyes, ears, nose, and throat.*

EEOC, abbreviation for **Equal Employment Opportunity Commission.**

EFA, abbreviation for **essential fatty acid.**

effacement /ifās′mənt/ [Fr *effacer* to erase], the shortening of the vaginal portion of the cervix and thinning of its walls as it is stretched and dilated by the fetus during labor.

effective compliance [L *effectus* performance], the ratio of tidal volume to peak airway pressure.

effective dose (ED), the dosage of a drug that may be expected to cause a specific intensity of effect in the people to whom it is given.

effective half-life (ehl), (in radiotherapy) the time required for a radioactive element in an animal body to be diminished 50% as a result of the combined action of radioactive decay and biological elimination.

effective refractory period, the period after the firing of an impulse during which a fiber may respond at the cellular level to a stimulus but the response will not be propagated.

effector /ifek′tər/ [L *efficere* to accomplish], 1. an organ that produces an effect, such as glandular secretion, as a result of nerve stimulation. 2. a molecule, such as an enzyme, that can start or stop a chemical reaction.

effects of sleep deprivation [L *effectus*; AS *slaep*; L *deprivare* to deprive], interference with a basic physiologic urge to sleep, which appears to be governed by sleep centers in the hypothalamus and reticular activating system. The loss of sleep for 24 hours usually has no significant effect on physical or mental functioning. Subjects kept awake for 30 or more hours, however, have difficulty handling boring tasks and performance on tests becomes increasingly poor. After several continuous sleepless days, subjects begin to show symptoms of psychoses, such as paranoid reactions and detachment from reality.

effeminate [L *effeminare* to make womanish], the state of being womanly or female in physical and mental characteristics, regardless of the biological sex of the person.

efferent /ef′ərənt/ [L *effere* to carry out], directed away from a center, as certain arteries, veins, nerves, and lymphatics.

efferent duct, any duct through which a gland releases its secretions.

efferent nerve, a nerve that transmits impulses away or outward from a nerve center, such as the brain or spine, usually resulting in a muscle contraction, release of a glandular secretion, or other activity.

efferent pathway [L *effere* to bear out; ME *paeth weg*], 1. the route of nerve fibers carrying impulses away from a nerve center. 2. the system of blood vessels that conveys blood away from a body part.

effervescence [L *effervescere* to foam up], the production of small bubbles or foam associated with the escape of gas from a fluid.

effervescent, producing and releasing gas bubbles.

efficacy /ef'əkəsē/ [L *effectus* performance], (of a drug or treatment) the maximum ability of a drug or treatment to produce a result, regardless of dosage.

effleurage /ef'ləräzh'/ [Fr, skimming the surface], a technique in massage in which long, light, or firm strokes are used, usually over the spine and back.

effluent /ef'lōō·ənt/, a liquid, solid, or gaseous emission, as the discharge or outflow from a machine or industrial process.

effluvium /iflōō'vē·əm/ [L *effluvium* a flowing out], an outflow of gas or vapor, usually malodorous or toxic.

effort syndrome [Fr, exertion; Gk *syn* together, *dromos* course], an abnormal condition characterized by chest pain, dizziness, fatigue, and palpitations. This condition is often associated with soldiers in combat but occurs also in other individuals. The symptoms of effort syndrome often mimic angina pectoris but are more closely connected to anxiety states.

effraction /ifrak'shən/, a breaking open or weakening.

effusion /ify oo'zhən/ [L *effundere* to pour out], **1.** the escape of fluid from blood vessels because of rupture or seepage, usually into a body cavity. The condition is usually associated with a circulatory or renal disorder and is often an early sign of congestive heart disease. **2.** the outward spread of a bacterial growth.

eflornithine hydrochloride /eflôr'nithēn/, a drug used to treat *Pneumocystis carinii* pneumonia (PCP). It blocks the activity of ornithine decarboxylase, an enzyme required for polyamine synthesis in normal cell division and differentiation.

EFM, abbreviation for **electronic fetal monitor.**

egest /ijest'/ [L *egerere* to expel], to discharge or evacuate a substance from the body, especially to evacuate unabsorbed residue of foods from the intestines. −**egesta,** *n. pl.,* **egestive,** *adj.*

ego /ē'gō, eg'ō/ [Gk, I or self], **1.** the conscious sense of the self; those elements of a person, such as thinking, feeling, willing, and emotions, that distinguish the person as an individual. **2.** (in psychoanalysis) the part of the psyche that experiences and maintains conscious contact with reality and which tempers the primitive drives of the id and the demands of the superego with the social and physical needs of society.

ego-alien. See **ego-dystonic.**

ego analysis, (in psychoanalysis) the intensive study of the ego, especially the defense mechanisms.

ego boundary, (in psychiatry) a sense or awareness that there is a distinction between the self and others.

egocentric [Gk *ego* + *kentron* center], **1.** regarding the self as the center, object, and norm of all experience and having little regard for the needs, interests, ideas, and attitudes of others. **2.** a person possessing these characteristics.

ego-defense mechanism. See **defense mechanism.**

ego-dystonic /ē'gōdiston'ik/, describing the elements of a person's behavior, thoughts, impulses, drives, and attitudes that are at variance with the standards of the ego and inconsistent with the total personality.

ego-dystonic homosexuality, a psychosexual disorder in which there is a persistent desire to change sexual orientation from homosexuality to heterosexuality.

ego ideal, the image of the self to which a person aspires both consciously and unconsciously and against which he measures himself and his performance.

egoism /ē'gō·iz'əm, eg'-/, **1.** an overvaluation of the importance of the self, expressed as a willingness to gain an advantage at the expense of others. **2.** the belief that individual self-interest is, or ought to be, the basic motive for all conscious behavior.

egoist /ē'gō·ist, eg'-/, **1.** a person who seeks to satisfy his own interests at the expense of others. **2.** a person who believes in or follows the concept that all conscious action is justifiably motivated by self-interest. −**egoistic, egoistical,** *adj.*

ego libido, (in psychoanalysis) concentration of the libido on the self; self-love, narcissism.

egomania [Gk *ego* I, madness], a pathologic preoccupation with the self and an exaggerated sense of one's own importance.

egophony, /ēgof'ənē/ (in respiratory therapy) a change in the voice sound as heard on auscultation of a patient with pleural effusion.

ego strength, (in psychotherapy) the ability to maintain the ego by a cluster of traits that together contribute to good mental health.

ego-syntonic /ē'gōsinton'ik/, those elements of a person's behavior, thoughts, impulses, drives, and attitudes that agree with the standards of the ego and are consistent with the total personality.

egotism /ē'gətiz'əm, eg'-/, the overvaluation of the importance of the self and undervaluation or contempt of others. **–egotistic, egotistical,** *adj.*

egotist /ē′gətist, eg′-/, one who places too much importance on the self and is boastful, egocentric, and arrogant.

egress /ē′gres/, the act of emerging or moving forward.

Egyptian ophthalmia. See **trachoma.**

EHD, abbreviation for **electrohemodynamics.**

ehl, abbreviation for **effective half-life.**

Ehlers-Danlos syndrome /ā′lərzdan′ləs/ [Edward Ehlers, Danish physician, b. 1863; Henri A. Danlos, French physician, b. 1844], a hereditary disorder of connective tissue, marked by hyperplasticity of skin, tissue fragility, and hypermotility of joints.

eicosanoic acid /ī′kōsənō′ik/ [Gk *eikosa* twenty], a fatty acid containing 20 carbon atoms in a straight chain, such as arachidic acid found in peanut oil, butter, and other fats.

eidetic /īdet′ik/ [Gk *eidos* a form of shape seen] **1.** pertaining to or characterized by the ability to visualize and reproduce accurately the image of objects or events previously seen or imagined. **2.** a person possessing such ability.

eidetic image, an unusually vivid, elaborate, and apparently exact mental image resulting from a visual experience and occurring as a fantasy, dream, or memory.

eighth cranial nerve. See **auditory nerve.**

einsteinium (Es) /īnstī′nē·əm/ [Albert Einstein, German-born scientist, b. 1879], a synthetic transuranic metallic element. Its atomic number is 99; its atomic weight is 254.

Einthoven's formula /int′hōvənz/ [Willem Einthoven, Dutch physician, b. 1860; L *forma* pattern], a theory that the heart lies in the center of an equilateral triangle (Einthoven's triangle) in the frontal plane of the body, defined by the right shoulder, left shoulder, and symphysis pubis (left leg). The potential difference in bipolar electrocardiograph lead II (right arm-left leg) is subtracted from the sum of the potential differences of the other bipolar leads.

Eisenmenger's complex /ī′sənmeng′ərz/ [Victor Eisenmenger, German physician, b. 1864; L *complexus* encirclement], a congenital heart disease in which there is a defect of the ventricular septum, a malpositioned aortic root that overrides the interventricular septum, and a dilated pulmonary artery.

ejaculate /ijak′yəlit/, the semen discharged in a single emission. **–ejaculate** /ijak′yəlāt/, *v.*

ejaculation [L *ejaculari* to hurl out], the sudden emission of semen from the male urethra, usually occurring during copulation, masturbation, and nocturnal emission. It is a reflex action. The sensation of ejaculation is commonly also called orgasm. **–ejaculatory** /ijak′yələtôr′ē/, *adj.*

ejaculatory duct, the passage through which semen enters the urethra.

ejection [L *ejicere* to cast out], the forceful expulsion of something, such as blood from a ventricle of the heart.

ejection clicks, sharp clicking sounds from the heart, which may be caused by the sudden swelling of a pulmonary artery, the abrupt dilatation of the aorta, or the forceful opening of the aortic cusps.

ejection fraction (EF), the proportion of blood that is ejected during each ventricular contraction compared with the total ventricular volume.

ejection murmur. See **systolic murmur.**

ejection sounds, sharp clicking sounds heard early in systole, coinciding with the onset of either right or left ventricular systolic ejection and reflecting either dilatation of the pulmonary artery or aorta or the presence of valvular abnormalities.

Ekbom syndrome. See **restless legs syndrome.**

EKC, abbreviation for **epidemic keratoconjunctivitis.**

EKG, abbreviation for **electrocardiogram.**

elaborate [L *elaborare* to work out], (in endocrinology) a process by which a gland synthesizes a complex substance from simpler substances and secretes it, usually under the stimulation of a tropic hormone from the pituitary gland. **–elaboration,** *n.*

elastance /ilas′təns/ [Gk *elaunein* to drive], **1.** the quality of recoiling or returning to an original form after the removal of pressure. **2.** the degree to which an air-filled or fluid-filled organ, such as a lung, bladder, or blood vessel, can return to its original dimensions when a distending or compressing force is removed. **3.** the measurement of the unit volume of change in such an organ per unit of decreased pressure change. **4.** the reciprocal of compliance.

elastic bandage [Gk *elaunein* to drive; Fr *bande* strip], a bandage of elasticized fabric that provides support and allows movement.

elastic-band fixation, a method of treatment of fractures of the jaw using rubber bands to connect metal splints or wires that are attached to the maxilla and mandible.

elastic bougie, a flexible bougie that can

be passed through angular or winding channels.

elastic cartilage. See **yellow cartilage.**

elasticity, the ability of tissue to regain its original shape and size after being stretched, squeezed, or otherwise deformed.

elastic recoil, the difference between intrapleural pressure and alveolar pressure at a given lung volume under static conditions.

elastic tissue [Gk *elaulnein* to drive; OFr *tissu*], a type of connective tissue containing elastic fibers. It is found in ligaments of the spinal column and in the walls of some large blood vessels.

elastic traction [Gk *elaunein*; L *trahere* to draw], any therapeutic apparatus that uses an elastic device to pull on a limb.

elastin /ilas'tin/ [Gk *elaunein* to drive], a protein that forms the principal substance of yellow elastic tissue fibers.

elation [L *elatus* a lifting up], an emotional reaction characterized by euphoria, excitement, extreme joyfulness, optimism, and self-satisfaction.

elbow [AS *elboga*], the bend of the arm at the joint that connects the arm and forearm.

elbow bone. See **ulna.**

elbow jerk [AS *elboga* elbow], a triceps reflex induced by tapping the triceps tendon near the insertion into the olecranon when the elbow is semiflexed. The reflex results in extension at the elbow joint.

elbow joint, the hinged articulation of the humerus, the ulna, and the radius. The elbow joint allows flexion and extension of the forearm.

elbow reflex. See **triceps reflex.**

elderly primagravida, a woman who beomces pregnant for the first time after the age of 34.

elective [L *eligere* to choose], of or pertaining to a procedure that is performed by choice but which is not essential, such as elective surgery.

elective abortion, induced termination of a pregnancy, usually before the fetus has developed enough to live if born. Commonly called **therapeutic abortion.**

elective induction of labor. See **induction of labor.**

Electra complex /ilek'trə/, (in psychiatry) the libidinous desire of a daughter for her father.

electrically stimulated osteogenesis [Gk *elktron* amber; L *stimulare* to incite; Gk *osteon* bone, *genein* to produce], a bone regeneration process induced by surgically implanted electrodes conveying electric current, especially at nonunion fracture sites. The process is effective because of

the different electrical potentials within bone tissue.

electric blood warmer, a device for heating blood before infusions, especially massive transfusions in which cold blood might put the patient into shock.

electric burns, the tissue damage resulting from heat of up to 5,000° C generated by an electric current. The point of contact on the skin is burned, and the muscle and subcutaneous tissues may be damaged.

electric cautery. See **electrocautery.**

electricity [Gk *elektron* amber], a form of energy expressed by the activity of electrons and other subatomic particles in motion, as in dynamic electricity, or at rest, as in static electricity. Electricity can be produced by heat, generated by a voltaic cell, produced by induction, by rubbing nonconductors with dry materials, or by chemical activity. Electricity may be negative, when there is a surplus of electrons, or positive, when there is a surplus of protons or a deficiency of electrons.

electric potential gradient, the net difference in electric charge across the membrane of a cell.

electric shock, a traumatic physical state caused by the passage of electric current through the body. It usually involves accidental contact with exposed parts of electric circuits in home appliances and domestic power supplies but may also result from lightning or contact with high-voltage wires. The damage electricity does in passing through the body depends on the intensity of the electric current, the type of current, and the duration and the frequency of current flow. Severe electric shock commonly causes unconsciousness, respiratory paralysis, muscle contractions, bone fractures, and cardiac disorders.

electric shock therapy. See **electroconvulsive therapy.**

electric spinal orthosis, an electric device that helps control curvature of the spine by stimulating back muscles.

electroanalgesia /ilek'trō·an'əljē'sē·ə/, the use of an electric current, applied to the spinal cord or a peripheral nerve to relieve pain.

electroanalytic chemistry [Gk *elektron* + *analysis* a loosening; *chemeia* alchemy], the branch of chemistry concerned with the analysis of compounds using electric current to produce characteristic, observable change in the substance being studied.

electroanesthesia /ilek'trō·an'esthē'zhə/, the use of an electric current to produce local or general anesthesia.

electrocardiogram (ECG, EKG) /ilek'-

trōkär′dē·əgram′/ [Gk *elektron* + *kardia* heart, *gramma* record], a graphic record produced by an electrocardiograph.

electrocardiograph /ilek′trōkär′dē·əgraf′/, a device used for recording the electric activity of the myocardium to detect transmission of the cardiac impulse through the conductive tissues of the muscle. Electrocardiography allows diagnosis of specific cardiac abnormalities. –**electrocardiographic,** *adj.*

electrocardiographic-auscultatory syndrome. See **Barlow's syndrome.**

electrocardiographic technician, an allied health professional with special training and experience in operating and maintaining electrocardiographic equipment and providing recorded data for diagnostic review by a physician.

electrocardiograph lead /lēd/, **1.** an electrode placed on part of the body and connected to an electrocardiograph. **2.** a record, made by the electrocardiograph, that varies depending on the site of the electrode. Electrocardiography is generally performed with the use of three peripheral leads and six leads placed on the precordium. The peripheral or extremity leads are designated I, II, and III, and the chest leads are designated V_1, V_2, V_3, V_4, V_5, and V_6 to indicate the points on the precordium on which the electrodes are placed.

electrocardiography /ilek′trōkär′dē·og′rəfē/ [Gk *elektron* + *kardia* heart, *graphein* to record], a method of recording electrical activity generated by the heart muscle.

electrocautery /ilek′trōkô′tərē/ [Gk *elektron* + *kauterion* branding iron], the application of a needle or snare heated by electric current for the destruction of tissue, such as for the removal of warts or polyps.

electrocoagulation /ilek′trōko·ag′yŏōlā′-shən/ [Gk *elektron* + L *coagulare* to curdle], a therapeutic, destructive form of electrosurgery in which tissue is hardened by the passage of high-frequency current from an electric cautery device.

electroconvulsive therapy (ECT), /ilek′-trōkənvul′siv/ the induction of a brief convulsion by passing an electric current through the brain for the treatment of affective disorders. The patient loses consciousness and undergoes tonic contractions for approximately 10 seconds, followed by a somewhat longer period of clonic convulsions accompanied by apnea; on awakening the individual has no memory of the shock.

electrocution, death caused by the passage of electric current through the body.

electrode /ilek′trōd/ [Gk *elektron* + *hodos* way], **1.** a contact for the induction or detection of electric activity. **2.** a medium for conducting an electric current from the body to physiologic monitoring equipment.

electrodermal audiometry /ilek′trō-dur′məl/ [Gk *elektron* + *derma* skin; L *audire* to hear; Gk *metron* measure], a method of testing hearing in which a harmless electric shock is used to condition the subject to a pure tone; thereafter the tone, coupled with the anticipation of a shock, elicits a brief electrodermal response, which is recorded, and the lowest intensity of the sound producing the skin response is considered the subject's hearing threshold.

electrodesiccation /ilek′trōdes′ikā′shən/ [Gk *elektron* + *desiccare* to dry up], a technique in electrosurgery in which tissue is destroyed by burning with an electric spark. It is used primarily for eliminating small superficial growths.

electrodiagnosis [Gk *elektron* + *dia* twice, *gnosis* knowledge], the diagnosis of disease or injury by applying electrical stimulation to various nerves and muscles.

electrodynamics, the study of electrostatic charges in motion, as in the flow of electrons in an electric current.

electrodynograph (EDG) /ilek′trōdin′əgraf′/ [Gk *elektron* + *dynamis* force, *graphein* to record], an electronic device used to measure pressures exerted in biologic activity, such as the pressures exerted by the human foot in walking, running, jogging, or climbing stairs.

electroencephalogram (EEG) /ilek′trō·en-sef′ələgram′/ [Gk *elektron* + *enkephalos* brain, *gramma* record], a graphic chart on which is traced the electric potential produced by the brain cells, as detected by electrodes placed on the scalp. The resulting brain waves are called alpha, beta, delta, and theta rhythms, according to the frequencies they produce.

electroencephalograph /ilek′trō·ensef′ələgraf′/, an instrument for receiving and recording the electric potential produced by the brain cells.

electroencephalographic technologist, a person trained in the management of an electroencephalographic laboratory.

electroencephalography (EEG) /ilek′trō·ensef′əlog′rəfē/, the process of recording brain-wave activity. –**electroencephalographic,** *adj.*

electrogram /ilek′trōgram′/ [Gk *elektron* + *gramma* record], a unipolar or bipolar record of electric activity of the heart as recorded from electrodes within the cardiac chambers or on the epicardium. Examples are atrial electrogram (AEG), ventricular electrogram (VEG), and His bundle electrogram (HBE).

electrohemodynamics (EHD) /ilek'trōhē-'mōdīnam'iks/ [Gk *elektron* + *haima* blood, *dynamis* force], a technique for noninvasively measuring the mechanical properties and hemodynamic characteristics of the vascular system, including arterial blood pressure, electric impedance, blood flow, and resistance to blood flow.

electroimmunodiffusion. See **immunodiffusion.**

electrolysis /il'ektrol'isis/ [Gk *elektron* + *lysis* loosening], a process in which electric energy causes a chemical change in a conducting medium, usually a solution or a molten substance. Electrodes, usually pieces of metal, induce the flow of electric energy through the medium. Electrons enter the solution through the cathode and leave the solution through the anode. Negatively charged ions, or anions, are attracted to the anode; positively charged ions, or cations, are attracted to the cathode. **–electrolytic,** *adj.*

electrolyte /ilek'trōlīt/ [Gk *elektron* + *lytos* soluble], an element or compound that, when melted or dissolved in water or other solvent, dissociates into ions and is able to conduct an electric current. Electrolytes differ in their concentrations in blood plasma, interstitial fluid, and cell fluid and affect the movement of substances between those compartments. Proper quantities of principal electrolytes and balance among them are critical to normal metabolism and function. **–electrolytic,** *adj.*

electrolyte balance, the equilibrium between electrolytes in the body.

electrolyte solution, any solution containing electrolytes prepared for oral, parenteral, or rectal administration for the replacement or supplementation of ions necessary for homeostasis. Electrolyte solutions containing combinations of calcium, sodium, phosphate, chloride, or magnesium may be given to treat acid-base disturbance, as seen in chronic renal dysfunction or diabetic ketoacidosis.

electromagnetic [Gk *elektron* + *Magnesia* ancient source of lodestone], pertaining to magnetism that is induced by an electric current.

electromagnetic induction [Gk *elektron* + *magnes* lodestone; L *inducere* to bring in], the production in tissue of electric fields and associated eddy currents by magnetic fields generated by coils carrying an electric current.

electromagnetic radiation, every kind of electric and magnetic radiation, regarded as a continuous spectrum of energy that includes energy with the shortest wavelength (gamma rays, with a wavelength of 0.0011) to that with the longest wavelength (long radio waves, with a wavelength of more than 1 million kilometers).

electromallet condenser /ilek'trōmal'ət/ [Gk *elektron* + Ofr *mail* maul; L *condensare* to make dense], an electromechanic device for compacting direct-filling gold in prepared tooth cavities.

electromotive force (EMF), the electric potential, or ability of electric energy to perform work. EMF is usually measured in joules per coulomb, or volts (V). The higher the voltage, the greater the potential of electric energy.

electromyogram (EMG) /ilek'trōmī'ə-gram'/, a record of the intrinsic electric activity in a skeletal muscle. Such data help in diagnosing neuromuscular problems and are obtained by applying surface electrodes or by inserting a needle electrode into the muscle.

electron /ilek'tron/ [Gk *elektron* amber], **1.** a negatively charged elementary particle that has a specific charge, mass, and spin. The number of electrons circling the nucleus of an atom is equal to the atomic number of the substance. Electrons may be shared or exchanged by two atoms; after the exchange the atom becomes an ion. **2.** a negative beta particle emitted from a radioactive substance.

electronarcosis /ilek'trōnärkō'sis/ [Gk *elektron* + *narkosis* numbness], general anesthesia without the use of anesthetic gases or drugs. Narcosis is produced by passing an electric current through the brain.

electron capture, a radioactive decay process in which a nucleus with an excess of electrons brings one of them into the nucleus, creating a neutron out of a proton, thus decreasing the atomic number of the atom by 1.

Electroneurodiagnostic Technologist, an allied health professional who specializes in recording and studying the electrical activity of the brain. Working in collaboration with an electroencephalographer, the electroneurodiagnostic technologist takes and abstracts medical histories, applies adequate recording electrodes using EEG and EP techniques, and understands the interface between EEG and EP equipment and other electrophysiologic devices. The responsibilities may also include laboratory management and supervision of EEG technicians.

electroneuromyography /ilek'trōn ōōr'ō-mī·og'rəfē/ [Gk *elektron* + *neuron* nerve, *mys* muscle, *graphein* to record], a procedure for testing and recording neuro-muscular activity by the electric stimulation of nerves.

electronic fetal monitor (EFM) [Gk *elektron* + L *fetus; monere* to warn], a device that allows observation of the fetal heart rate and the maternal uterine contractions. It may be applied externally, in which case the fetal heart is detected by an ultrasound transducer on the abdomen. Internal monitoring of the fetal heart rate is accomplished via an electrode clipped to the fetal scalp.

electronic thermometer, a thermometer that registers temperature rapidly by electronic means.

electron microscope, an instrument, similar to an optic microscope, that scans cell surfaces with a beam of electrons, instead of visible light.

electron microscopy, a technique, using an electron microscope, in which a beam of electrons is focused by an electromagnetic lens and directed onto an extremely thin specimen.

electron scanning microscope. See **scanning electron microscope.**

electron volt (eV), a unit of energy equal to the energy acquired by an electron in falling through a potential difference of one volt. One eV equals 1.6×10^{-12} erg or 1.6×10^{-19} J.

electronystagmography /ilek′trōnis′tag-mog′rəfē/ [Gk *elektron* + *nystagmos* nodding, *graphein* to record], a method of assessing and recording eye movements by measuring the electric activity of the extraocular muscles.

electrophoresis /ilek′trōfərē′sis/ [Gk *elektron* + *pherein* to bear], the movement of charged suspended particles through a liquid medium in response to changes in an electric field. The pattern of migration can be recorded in bands on an **electrophoretogram** /ilek′trōfəret′ōgram/. The technique is widely used to separate and identify serum proteins and other substances. **–electrophoretic,** *adj.*

electrophysiology /ilek′trōfis′ē·ol′əjē/ [Gk *elektron* + *physis* nature, *logos* science], a branch of medical science concerned with the relationship between electrical phenomena and human health.

electroporation /ilek′trōpōrā′shən/, a type of osmotic transfection in which an electric current is used to produce holes in cell membranes so the alien DNA molecules can enter the cells.

electroresection [Gk *elektron* + L *re* again, *secare* to cut], a technique for the removal of bladder tumors by the insertion of an electric wire through the urethra.

electroshock [Gk *elektron*; Fr *choc*], a condition of shock caused by accidental contact with an electric current. The symptoms are similar to those of shock by thermal burns, trauma, or coronary thrombosis.

electroshock therapy. See **electroconvulsive therapy (ECT).**

electrosleep therapy [Gk *elektron* + AS *slaep;* Gk *therapeia* treatment], a technique designed to induce sleep, especially in psychiatric patients, by administering a low-amplitude pulsating current to the brain. The cathode is placed supraorbitally, and the anode is placed over the mastoid process. The current, which is discharged for 15 to 20 minutes, produces a tingling sensation, but does not always induce sleep.

electrostatic imaging [Gk *elektron* + *stasis* standing still; L *imago* image], techniques for producing radiographic images in which the ionic charge liberated during the irradiation process is converted to a visible image.

electrosurgery [Gk *elektron* + *cheiourgos* surgeon], surgery performed with various electric instruments that operate on high-frequency electric current. Kinds of electrosurgery include **electrocoagulation, electrodesiccation.**

electrotherapy. See **electroconvulsive therapy (ECT).**

electrotonic current [Gk, *electron* + *tonos,* tension], a current induced in a nerve sheath by an action potential within the nerve or an adjacent nerve.

eleidin /əlē′ədin/ [Gk *elaia* olive tree], a transparent protein substance, resembling keratin, found in the stratum lucidum of the epidermis.

element [L *elementum* first principle], one of more than 100 primary, simple substances that cannot be broken down by chemical means into any other substance. Each atom of any element contains a specific number of electrons orbiting the nucleus. The nucleus contains a variable number of neutrons. A **stable element** contains an equal number of neutrons and electrons and does not easily give up neutrons. A **radioactive element** does not contain a balanced number of electrons and neutrons and gives off neutrons readily.

element 104, a synthetic, radioactive element, the twelfth transuranic element, and the first transactinide element. It is called **rutherfordium** (Rf) and **kurchatovium** (Ku).

element 105, a synthetic element, and the thirteenth transuranic element. It is called **hahnium** (Ha).

element 106, a synthetic element, with a half-life of 0.9 seconds. It was first synthesized in 1974 by scientists working independently in the United States and the former USSR.

element 107, an element reportedly synthesized in 1976 by Soviet scientists who bombarded isotopes of bismuth with heavy nuclei of chromium 54. The finding was not confirmed by scientists of other nations.

elephantiasis /el'əfəntī'əsis/ [Gk *elephas* elephant, *osis* condition], the end-stage lesion of filariasis, characterized by tremendous swelling, usually of the external genitalia and the legs. Elephantiasis results from filariasis that has lasted for many years.

elephantoid fever. See **elephantiasis, filariasis.**

eleventh nerve. See **accessory nerve.**

elimination diet [L *eliminare* to expel; Gk *diata* way of living], a procedure for identifying a food or foods to which a person is allergic by successively omitting from the diet certain foods in order to detect those responsible for the symptoms.

ELISA /əī'zə/, abbreviation for **enzyme-linked immunosorbent assay.**

elixir /ilik'sər/ [Ar *el-iksir* philosopher's stone], a clear liquid containing water, alcohol, sweeteners, or flavors, used primarily as a vehicle for the oral administration of a drug.

Elliot forceps. See **obstetric forceps.**

Elliot's position [John W. Elliott, American surgeon, b. 1852], a supine posture assumed by the patient on the operating table, with a support placed under the lower costal margin to elevate the chest. The position is used in gallbladder surgery.

elliptocyte /ilip'təsīt/ [Gk *elleipsis* ellipse, *kytos* cell], an oval red blood cell.

elliptocytosis /ilip'tōsītō'sis/ [Gk *elleipsis, kytos* + *osis* condition], a mild abnormal condition of the blood that is characterized by increased numbers of elliptocytes or oval erythrocytes.

Ellis-van Creveld syndrome. See **chondroectodermal dysplasia.**

elongation /i'longā'shən/ [L *elongatio* a prolonging], a state of being lengthened or extended.

elope [ME *gantlopp* to run away], *informal.* to leave a locked psychiatric institution without notice or permission.

eluate /el'yoō·āt/ [L *eluere* to wash out], a solution or substance that results from an elution process.

eluent /el'yoō·ənt/, a solvent or solution used in the elution process, as in column chromatography.

elution /eloō'shən/, the removal of an ab-

sorbed substance from a porous bed or chromatographic column by means of a stream of liquid or gas or by the application of heat. The term is also applied to the removal of antibodies or radioactive tracers from erythrocytes.

emaciation /imā'shi·ā'shən/ [L *emaciare* to make lean], excessive leanness caused by disease or lack of nutrition.

emancipated minor [L *mancipare* to set free], a person who is not legally an adult but because of marriage, being in the military, or otherwise no longer dependent on the parents, may not require parental permission for medical or surgical care. State and national laws vary in specific interpretations of the rule.

emasculation, a loss of the testes or penis or both.

embalming, the practice of applying antiseptics and preservatives to a corpse to retard the natural decomposition of tissues.

Embden-Meyerhof defects /emb'den-mī'ərhof/ [Gustav G. Embden, German biochemist, b. 1874; Otto F. Meyerhof, German biochemist, b. 1884], a group of hereditary hemolytic anemias caused by enzyme deficiencies. The most common form of the disorder is a pyruvate kinase deficiency.

Embden-Meyerhof pathway, a sequence of enzymatic reactions in the anaerobic conversion of glucose to lactic acid, producing energy in the form of adenosine triphosphate.

embedded tooth, an unerupted tooth, usually completely covered with bone.

embolectomy /em'bəlek'təmē/ [Gk *embolos* plug, *ektome* excision], a surgical incision into an artery for the removal of an embolus or clot, performed as emergency treatment for arterial embolism.

embolic gangrene /embol'ik/ [Gk *embolos, gaggraina*], the death and putrifaction of body tissues caused by an embolus blocking the blood supply to that part.

embolic thrombosis [Gk *embolos, thrombos* lump + *osis* condition], a thrombosis that develops at the site of an impacted embolus in a blood vessel.

embolism /em'bəliz'əm/, an abnormal circulatory condition in which an embolus travels through the bloodstream and becomes lodged in a blood vessel. Kinds of embolism include **air embolism** and **fat embolism.** –**embolic,** *adj.*

embolization agent, a substance used to occlude or drastically reduce blood flow within a vessel. Examples include vasoconstrictors and silicone beads.

embolized atheroma, an embolized fat particle lodged in a blood vessel.

embolotherapy /em'bōlōther'əpē/, a

technique of blocking a blood vessel with a balloon catheter. It is used for treating bleeding ulcers and blood vessel defects and, during surgery, to stop blood flow to a tumor.

embolus /em'bələs/, *pl.* **emboli** [Gk *embolos* plug], a foreign object, a quantity of air or gas, a bit of tissue or tumor, or a piece of a thrombus that circulates in the bloodstream until it becomes lodged in a vessel. Kinds of emboli include **air embolus** and **fat embolus.** **–embolic, emboloid,** *adj.*

embrasure /embrā'zhər/, a normally occurring space formed between adjacent teeth because of variations in positions and contours.

embryatrics. See **fetology.**

embryectomy /em'brē·ek'təmē/ [Gk *en, bryein* to grow, *ektome* excision], the surgical removal of an embryo, most commonly in an ectopic pregnancy.

embryo /em'brē·ō/ [Gk *en, bryein* to grow], **1.** any organism in the earliest stages of development. **2.** in humans, the stage of prenatal development between the time of implantation of the fertilized ovum about 2 weeks after conception until the end of the seventh or eighth week. **–embryonal, embryonoid, embryonic,** *adj.*

embryoctony /em'brē·ok'tənē/ [Gk *en, bryein* + *kteinein* to kill], the intentional destruction of the living embryo or fetus in utero.

embryogenesis /em'brē·ōjen'əsis/ [Gk *en, bryein* + *genein* to produce], the process in sexual reproduction in which an embryo forms from the fertilization of an ovum.

embryologic development, the various intrauterine stages and processes involved in the growth and differentiation of the conceptus from the time of fertilization of the ovum until the eighth week of gestation. The stages are related to the biological status of the unborn child and are divided into two distinct periods. The first is embryogenesis, or the formation of the embryo, which occurs during the 10 days to 2 weeks after fertilization until implantation. The second period, organogenesis, involves the differentiation of the various cells, tissues, and organ systems and the development of the main external features of the embryo; it occurs from approximately the end of the second week to the eighth week of intrauterine life. The fetal stage follows these stages, beginning at about the ninth week of gestation.

embryologist /em'brē·ol'əjist/, one who specializes in the study of embryology.

embryology /em'brē·ol'əjē/[Gk *en, bryein* + *logos* science], the study of the origin, growth, development, and function of an organism from fertilization to birth. Kinds of embryology include **comparative, descriptive,** and **experimental embryology.** **–embryologic, embryological,** *adj.*

embryoma /em'brē·ō'mə/, *pl.* **embryomas, embryomata** [Gk *en, bryein* + *oma* tumor], a tumor arising from embryonic cells or tissues.

embryoma of the ovary. See **dysgerminoma**

embryomorph /embrē'əmôrf'/ [Gk *en, bryein* + *morphe* form], any structure that resembles an embryo, especially a mass of tissue that may represent an aborted conceptus. **–embryomorphous,** *adj.*

embryonal adenomyosarcoma, embryonal adenosarcoma. See **Wilms' tumor.**

embryonal carcinoma /em'brē·ənəl/, an extremely malignant neoplasm derived from germinal cells, which usually develops in gonads, especially the testes.

embryonal leukemia. See **stem cell leukemia.**

embryonate /em'brē·ənāt'/ [Gk *en, bryein* + L *atus* shaped like], **1.** impregnated; containing an embryo. **2.** of, pertaining to, or resembling an embryo.

embryonic abortion, /em'brē·on'ik/ **1.** termination of pregnancy before the twentieth week of gestation. **2.** expelled products of conception before the twentieth week.

embryonic anideus [Gk *en, bryein* + *an* not, *eidos* form], a blastoderm in which the axial elongation of the primitive streak and primitive groove fail to develop.

embryonic blastoderm, the area of the blastoderm that gives rise to the primitive streak from which the embryonic body develops.

embryonic competence, the ability of an embryonic cell to react normally to the stimulation of an inductor, allowing continued, normal growth or differentiation of the embryo.

embryonic disk, the thickened plate from which the embryo develops in the second week of pregnancy.

embryonic layer, one of the three layers of cells in the embryo, the endoderm, the mesoderm, and the ectoderm. From these layers of cells arise all of the structures and organs and parts of the body.

embryonic rest, a portion of embryonic tissue that remains in the adult organism. Such tissue may act as organ-specific indicators in certain types of cancer.

embryonic stage, (in embryology) the interval of time from the end of the germinal stage, at 10 days of gestation, to the eighth week.

embryonic tissue [Gk *en* + *bryein* to grow;

OFr *tissu*], a loose, gelatinous mass of connective tissue cells. The gelatinous matrix is due to the presence of mucopolysaccharides.

embryoniform /em'brē·on'ifôrm'/ [Gk *en, bryein* + L *forma* form], resembling an embryo.

embryopathy /em'brē·op'əthē/ [Gk *en, bryein* + *pathos* disease], any anomaly occurring in the embryo or fetus as a result of interference with normal intrauterine development. A kind of embryopathy is **rubella embryopathy.**

embryoplastic /em'brē-ōplas'tik/ [Gk *en, bryein* + *plassein* to mold], of or pertaining to the formation of an embryo, usually with reference to cells.

embryoscopy /em'brē·os'kəpē/, the examination of an embryo directly by insertion of a lighted instrument through the mother's abdominal wall and uterus.

embryotome /em'brē·ətōm'/ [Gk *en, bryein* + *temnein* to cut], an instrument used in embryotomy.

embryotomy /em'brē·ot'əmē/ [Gk *en, bryein* + *temnein* to cut], **1.** the dismemberment or mutilation of a fetus for removal from the uterus when normal delivery is not possible. **2.** the dissection of an embryo for examination and analysis.

embryotoxon. See **arcus juvenilis.**

embryotroph /em'brē·ətrof'/ [Gk *en, bryein* + *trophe* nourishment], the liquefied uterine nutritive material, composed of glandular secretions and degenerative tissue, that nourishes the mammalian embryo until placental circulation is established.

embryotrophy /em'brē·ot'trəfē/, the nourishment of the embryo. **–embryotrophic,** *adj.*

embryulcia /em'brē·ul'sē·ə/ [Gk *en, bryein* + *elkein* to draw], the surgical extraction of the embryo or fetus from the uterus.

emergence /imur'jəns/ [L *emergere* to come forth], a stage in the process of recovery from general anesthesia that includes spontaneous respiration, voluntary swallowing, and consciousness.

emergency [L *emergere* to come forth], a serious situation that arises suddenly and threatens the life or welfare of a person or a group of people, as a natural disaster or a medical crisis.

emergency cardiac care (ECC), the concentration of personnel and facilities organized to sustain the cardiovascular and pulmonary systems when a heart attack occurs. The interventions assure prompt availability of basic life support (BLS), monitoring and treatment facilities, prevention of complications, and psychologic reassurance. If a heart attack occurs out-

side a hospital, efforts are devoted to stabilizing the client's cardiovascular and pulmonary systems before removing the individual to a hospital.

emergency childbirth, a birth that occurs accidentally or precipitously in or out of the hospital, without standard obstetric preparations and procedures. Signs and symptoms of impending delivery include increased bloody show, frequent strong contractions, a desire on the part of the mother to bear down forcibly or her report that she feels as though she is going to defecate, visible bulging of the bag of waters, or crowning of the baby's head at the vaginal introitus.

emergency department (ED), (in a health care facility) a section of an institution that is staffed and equipped to provide rapid and varied emergency care, especially for those stricken with sudden and acute illness or those who are the victims of severe trauma.

emergency doctrine, (in law) a doctrine that assumes a person's consent to medical treatment when the person is in imminent danger and unable to give informed consent to treatment. Emergency doctrine assumes that the person would consent if able to do so.

emergency handling of radiation accidents, first aid treatment of a person who has received external body radiation through exposure to radioactive material or internal radiation contamination by inhaling or ingesting radioactive material. External radiation exposure is treated initially by cleansing and surgical isolation to protect others. One who has inhaled or ingested radioactive material should be given emergency treatment similiar to a person who has been exposed to chemical poisons. But body wastes should be collected and checked for radiation levels. If the victim has also suffered a wound, care must be taken to avoid cross-contamination of exposed surfaces. In general, except for taking special precautions to control the spread of radiation effects, the patient should be given any lifesaving emergency treatment needed and personnel handling the patient should wear surgical gowns, caps, and gloves.

Emergency Medical Service (EMS), a national network of services coordinated to provide aid and medical assistance from primary response to definitive care, involving personnel trained in the rescue, stabilization, transportation, and advanced treatment of traumatic or medical emergencies.

Emergency Medical Technician (EMT), a person trained in and responsible for the administration of specialized emergency care and the transportation to a medical facility of victims of acute illness or injury.

Emergency Medical Technician-Advanced Life Support (EMT-ALS), a third-level EMT. The EMT-ALS is locally certified in all the skills of the basic-level EMT and EMT-IV. Additionally, the EMT-ALS may administer certain medications following the orders of the hospital physician, with whom radio contact is maintained. An EMT-ALS is also trained in the use of advanced life-support systems, including electric defibrillation equipment.

Emergency Medical Technician-Intermediate (EMT-I), a second-level emergency medical technician nationally certified as both an EMT-ALS and an EMT-IV.

Emergency Medical Technician-Intravenous (EMT-IV), a second-level emergency medical technician. The EMT-IV is trained and locally certified in intravenous therapy, endotracheal intubation, and the use of other antishock techniques.

Emergency Medical Technician-Paramedic (EMT-P), an advanced-level emergency medical technician. The EMT-P is nationally certified in all the skills of EMTs of other levels, and has additional training in pharmacology and the administration of emergency drugs.

emergency medicine, a branch of medicine concerned with the diagnosis and treatment of conditions resulting from trauma or sudden illness.

Emergency Nurses' Association, a national professional organization of emergency department nurses that defines and promotes emergency nursing practice.

emergency nursing, nursing care provided to prevent imminent severe damage or death or to avert serious injury. Activities that exemplify emergency nursing are basic life support, cardiopulmonary resuscitation, and control of hemorrhage.

emergency preparation of safe drinking water, methods of purifying unclean water for drinking purposes. The three basic techniques include boiling the water and straining it through a cloth, adding three drops of tincture (alcoholic solution) of iodine per each quart of the water, or adding 10 drops of 1% chlorine bleach per each quart of water. When purifying chemicals are added, they should be thoroughly mixed with the water and the mixture allowed to stand for 30 minutes.

emergency room (ER), a hospital area specially designed to receive and initially treat patients suffering from sudden trauma or medical problems, as accidental hemorrhage, poisoning, fracture, heart attack, and respiratory failure.

emergent /imur'jənt/ [L *emergens* emerging], something that arises unexpectedly or that improves or modifies an existing thing.

emergent evolution, the theory that evolution occurs in a series of major changes at certain critical stages and results from the total rearrangement of existing elements so that completely new and unpredictable characteristics appear within the species.

Emery-Dreifuss syndrome /em'ərē-drī'fəs/, an X-linked recessive form of scapuloperoneal dystrophy that begins in early childhood and is characterized by joint contractures and cardiac conduction disorders.

emesis. See vomit.

emesis basin /em'əsis, əmē'sis/ [Gk *emesis* vomiting; Fr *bassin* hollow vessel], a kidney-shaped bowl or pan that fits against the neck to collect vomitus.

emetic /imet'ik/, **1.** of or pertaining to a substance that causes vomiting. **2.** an emetic agent, such as apomorphine hydrochloride and syrup of ipecac.

EMG, 1. abbreviation for **electromyogram. 2.** abbreviation for *exophthalmos, macroglossia, and gigantism.*

EMG syndrome, a hereditary disorder transmitted as an autosomal recessive trait. Clinical manifestations include exophthalmos, macroglossia, and gigantism, often accompanied by visceromegaly, dysplasia of the renal medulla, and enlargement of the cells of the adrenal cortex.

emissary veins /em'əser'ē/ [L *emittere* to send forth], the small vessels in the skull that connect the sinuses of the dura with the veins on the exterior of the skull through a series of anastomoses.

emission [L *emittere* to send out], a discharge or release of something, as a fluid from the body, electronic signals from a radio transmitter, or an alpha or beta particle from an atomic nucleus during radioactive decay.

emission computed tomography (ECT) [L *emittere* to send forth; *computare* to count; Gk *tome* section, *graphein* to record], a form of tomography in which the emitted decay products, as positrons or gamma rays, of an ingested radioactive pharmaceutic are recorded in detectors outside the body.

emmetropia /em'ətrō'pē·ə/ [Gk *emmetros* proportioned, *opsis* vision], a state of normal vision characterized by the proper relationship between the refractive system of the eyeball and its axial length. This correlation ensures that light rays entering the eye parallel to the optic axis are focused exactly on the retina. **—emmetropic,** *adj.*

Emmet's operation, a surgical procedure for repair of a lacerated perineum or ruptured uterine cervix.

emollient /imol'yənt/ [L *emolliere* to soften], a substance that softens tissue, particularly the skin and mucous membranes.

emollient bath, a bath taken in water containing an emollient, such as bran, to relieve irritation and inflammation.

emotion [L *emovere* to disturb], the affective aspect of consciousness as compared with volition and cognition.

emotional abuse, the debasement of a person's feelings so that he perceives himself as inept, uncared for, and worthless.

emotional age [L *emovere*; L *aetas* age], the age of an individual as determined by the stage of emotional development reached.

emotional amalgam, an unconscious effort to deny or counteract anxiety.

emotional care of the dying patient, the compassionate, consistent support offered to help the terminally ill patient and the family cope with impending death.

emotional deprivation [L *emovere, deprivare* to deprive], a lack of adequate warmth, affection, and interest, especially on the part of a parent or significant other. It is a relatively common problem among institutionalized persons or children from broken homes.

emotional illness. See **mental disorder.**

emotional need, a psychologic or mental requirement of intrapsychic origin, usually centering on such basic feelings as love, fear, anger, sorrow, anxiety, frustration, and depression and involving the understanding, empathy, and support of one person for another. Such needs normally occur in everyone but usually are increased during periods of excessive stress or physical and mental illness and during various stages of life, as infancy, early childhood, and old age. If these needs are not routinely met by appropriate, socially accepted means, they can precipitate psychopathologic conditions.

emotional response, a reaction to a particular intrapsychic feeling or feelings, accompanied by physiologic changes that may or may not be outwardly manifest but that motivate or precipitate some action or behavioral response.

emotional support, the sensitive, understanding approach that helps patients accept and deal with their illnesses, communicate their anxieties and fears, derive comfort from a gentle, sympathetic, caring

person, and increase their ability to care for themselves.

empathic /empath'ik/ [Gk, *en*, into, *pathos*, feeling], pertaining to or involving the entering of one person into the emotional state of another while remaining objective and distinctly separate.

empathy /em'pəthē/ [Gk *en* in, *pathos* feeling], the ability to recognize and to some extent share the emotions and states of mind of another and to understand the meaning and significance of that person's behavior. It is an essential quality for effective psychotherapy. **—empathic,** *adj.,* **empathize,** *v.*

emphysema /em'fəsē'mə/ [Gk *en* + *physema* a blowing], an abnormal condition of the pulmonary system, characterized by overinflation and destructive changes of alveolar walls, resulting in a loss of lung elasticity and decreased gases. When emphysema occurs early in life, it is usually related to a rare genetic deficiency of serum alpha-1-antitrypsin, which inactivates the enzymes leukocyte collagenase and elastase. Acute emphysema may be caused by the rupture of alveoli by severe respiratory efforts, as in acute bronchopneumonia, suffocation, and whooping cough, and occasionally during labor. Chronic emphysema usually accompanies chronic bronchitis, a major cause of which is cigarette smoking. Emphysema is also seen after asthma or tuberculosis, conditions in which the lungs are overstretched until the elastic fibers of the alveolar walls are destroyed. In old age, the alveolar membranes atrophy and may collapse, resulting in large air-filled spaces with decreased total surface area of the pulmonary membranes. **—emphysematous,** *adj.*

emphysematous chest /em'fisem'ətəs/ [Gk *en* + *physema*; AS *cest* box], an atrophic type of emphysema accompanied by breathlessness but without a change in chest contour.

empiric /empir'ik/ [Gk *empeirikos* experimental], of or pertaining to a method of treating disease based on observations and experience without an understanding of the cause or mechanism of the disorder or the way the employed therapeutic agent or procedure effects improvement or cure. The empiric treatment of a new disease may be based on observations and experience gained in the management of analogous disorders. **—empirical,** *adj.*

empiricism /empir'isiz'əm/, a form of therapy based on personal experience and the experience of other practitioners. **—empiricist,** *n.*

empiric treatment. See **treatment.**

emprosthotonos /em'prosthot'ənəs/ [Gk

emprosthen forward, *tenein* to cut], a position of the body characterized by a forward, rigid flexure of the body at the waist. The position is the result of a prolonged, involuntary, muscle spasm that is most commonly associated with tetanus infection or strychnine poisoning.

empty sella syndrome [AS *oemettig* unoccupied; L *sella* saddle], an abnormal enlargement of the sella turcica in which no pituitary tumor is present; the gland may be smaller than normal, or it may be absent. Signs and symptoms of hormonal imbalance may be present, but some patients show no evidence of hypopituitarism or of any other endocrine abnormality. The condition is especially frequent in overweight, middle-aged, multiparous women.

empyema /em′pī·ē′mə, em′pē·ē′mə/ [Gk *en* + *ipyon* pus], an accumulation of pus in a body cavity, especially the pleural space, as a result of bacterial infection, as pleurisy or tuberculosis.

EMS, 1. abbreviation for **Emergency Medical Service.** 2. abbreviation for **eosinophilia-myalgia syndrome.**

EMT, abbreviation for **Emergency Medical Technician.**

EMT-A, abbreviation for *emergency medical technician-ambulance,* a basic member of an emergency medical services crew.

EMT-ALS, abbreviation for **Emergency Medical Technician-Advanced Life Support.**

EMT-D, abbreviation for *emergency medical technician-defibrillator,* a member of an emergency medical services crew with special training in the use of cardiac defibrillating equipment.

EMT-I, abbreviation for **Emergency Medical Technician-Intermediate.**

EMT-IV, abbreviation for **Emergency Medical Technician-Intravenous.**

EMT-P, abbreviation for **Emergency Medical Technician-Paramedic.**

emulsifier /imul′sifi′ər/ [L *emulgere* to milk out, *facere* to make], a substance such as egg yolk or gum arabic that can cause oil to be suspended in water.

emulsify [L *emulgere* to drain, *facere* to make], to disperse a liquid into another liquid, making a colloidal suspension. Soaps and detergents emulsify by surrounding small globules of fat, preventing them from settling out. Bile acts as an emulsifying agent in the digestive tract by dispersing ingested fats into small globules. **–emulsification,** n.

emulsion /imul′shən/ [L *emulgere* to drain], 1. a system consisting of two immiscible liquids, one of which is dispersed in the

other in the form of small droplets. 2. (in photography) a composition sensitive to actinic rays of light, consisting of one or more silver halides suspended in gelatin applied in a thin layer to film.

ENA, abbreviation for **Emergency Nurses' Association.**

enabler, a significant other of a substance abuser who provides covert support of substance-abusing behavior.

enalapril maleate, /enal′əpril/ an angiotensin-converting enzyme (ACE) inhibitor used as an oral antihypertensive drug.

enamel [OFr, *esmail*], a hard white substance that covers the dentin of the crown of a tooth.

enamel hypocalcification, a hereditary dental defect in which the enamel of the teeth is soft and undercalcified in context yet normal in quantity, caused by defective maturation of the ameloblasts.

enamel hypoplasia, a developmental dental defect in which the enamel of the teeth is hard in context but thin and deficient in amount, caused by defective enamel matrix formation with a deficiency in the cementing substance.

enanthema /en′anthē′mə/ [Gk *en* + *anthema* blossoming], an eruptive lesion from the surface of a mucous membrane.

enarthrosis. See **ball-and-socket joint.**

en bloc /enblok′, äNblôk′/ [Fr, in a block], all together, or as a whole.

encainide /en′kānīd/, a sodium channel antagonist used as an antiarrhythmic agent. It is prescribed in the treatment of life-threatening ventricular arrhythmias and other symptomatic ventricular arrhythmias.

encapsulated [Gk *en* + L *capsula* little box], (of arteries, muscles, nerves, and other body parts) enclosed in fibrous or membranous sheaths.

encephalitis /ensef′əlī′tis/, *pl.* **encephalitides** /-tidēz/ [Gk *enkephalos* brain, *itis* inflammation], an inflammatory condition of the brain. The cause is usually an arbovirus infection transmitted by the bite of an infected mosquito, but it may be the result of lead or other poisoning or of hemorrhage. **Postinfectious encephalitis** occurs as a complication of another infection, such as chickenpox, influenza, or measles, or after smallpox vaccination. The condition is characterized by headache, neck pain, fever, nausea, and vomiting. Severe inflammation with destruction of nerve tissue ay result in a seizure disorder, loss of a special sense or other permanent neurologic problem, or death. Usually, the inflammation involves the spinal cord and brain; hence, in most

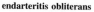

cases, a more accurate term is *encephalomyelitis.*

encephalitis lethargica. See **epidemic encephalitis.**

encephalitis periaxialis diffusa. See **Schilder's disease.**

encephalocele /ensef'ələsēl'/ [Gk *enkephalos* + *koilia* cavity], protrusion of the brain through a congenital defect in the skull; hernia of the brain.

encephalodysplasia, any congenital anomaly of the brain.

encephalogram /ensef'ələgram'/ [Gk *enkephalos* + *gramma* record], a radiograph of the brain made during encephalography.

encephalography /ensef'əlog'rəfē/, radiographic delineation of the structures of the brain containing fluid after the cerebrospinal fluid is withdrawn and replaced by a gas, as air, helium, or oxygen. Kinds of encephalography are **pneumoencephalography** and **ventriculography.** **–encephalographic,** *adj.*

encephaloid carcinoma. See **medullary carcinoma.**

encephalomeningitis /ensef'əlōmen'inji'tis/ [Gk *enkephalos* brain, *menigx* membrane, *itis,* inflammation], an inflammation of the brain and meninges.

encephalomeningocele. See **meningoencephalocele.**

encephalomyelitis /ensef'əlōmī'əlī'tis/ [Gk *enkephalos* + *myelos* marrow, *itis*], an inflammatory condition of the brain and spinal cord characterized by fever, headache, stiff neck, back pain, and vomiting. Depending on the cause, the age and condition of the person, and the extent of the inflammation and irritation to the central nervous system, seizures, paralysis, personality changes, a decreased level of consciousness, coma, or death may occur.

encephalomyocarditis /ensef'əlōmī'ōkärdī'tis/ [Gk *enkephalos* + *mys* muscle, *kardia* heart, *itis* inflammation], an infectious disease of the central nervous system and heart tissue caused by a group of small RNA picornaviruses. Symptoms are generally similar to those of poliomyelitis. Most victims recover promptly without sequelae.

encephalon /ensef'əlon/ [Gk *enkephalos* brain], 1. the cerebrum and its related structures of cerebellum, pons, medulla oblongata. 2. the contents of the cranium.

encephalopathy /ensef'əlop'əthē/ [Gk *enkephalos* + *pathos* disease], any abnormal condition of the structure or function of tissues of the brain, especially chronic, destructive, or degenerative conditions, as Wernicke's encephalopathy or Schilder's disease.

encephalotrigeminal angiomatosis. See **Sturge-Weber syndrome.**

enchondroma /en'kəndrō'mə/, pl. **enchondromas, enchondromata** [Gk *en* + *chondros* cartilage, *oma* tumor], a benign, slowly growing tumor of cartilage cells that arises in the extremity of the shaft of tubular bones in the hands or feet.

enchondromatosis /en'kəndrō'mətō'sis/ [Gk *en, chondros* + *oma* tumor, *osis* condition], a congenital disorder characterized by the proliferation of cartilage within the extremity of the shafts of bones, causing thinning of the cortex and distortion in length.

enchondromatous myxoma /en'kondrō'mətəs/, a tumor of the connective tissue, characterized by the presence of cartilage between the cells of connective tissue.

enchondrosarcoma. See **central chondrosarcoma.**

enchondrosis. See **enchondroma.**

enchylema. See **hyaloplasm.**

encoded message, (in communication theory) a message as transmitted by a sender to a receiver.

encopresis /en'kōprē'sis/, fecal incontinence. **–encopretic,** *adj.*

encounter [Gk *en* + L *contra* against], (in psychotherapy) the interaction between a patient and a psychotherapist, such as occurs in existential therapy, or among several members of a small group, such as encounter or sensitivity training groups, in which emotional change and personal growth are brought about by the expression of strong feelings by the participants.

encounter group, (in psychology) a small group of people who meet to increase self-awareness, promote personal growth, and improve interpersonal communication.

enculturation /enkul'chərā'shən/ [Gk *en* + L *cultura* cultivation], the process of learning the concepts, values, and behavioral standards of a particular culture.

encyst /ensist'/, to form a cyst or capsule. **–encysted,** *adj.*

endarterectomy /en'därtərek'təmē/ [Gk *endon* within, *arteria* air pipe, *ektome* excision], the surgical removal of the intimal lining of an artery. The procedure is performed to clear a major artery that may be blocked by an accumulation of plaque.

endarteritis /en'därtərī'tis/ [Gk *endon, arteria* + *itis* inflammation], an inflammatory disorder of the inner layer of one or more arteries, which may become partially or completely occluded.

endarteritis obliterans, an inflammatory condition of the lining of the arterial walls in which the intima proliferates, narrowing the lumen of the vessels and occluding the smaller vessels.

end bud [AS *ende;* Gk *bolbos* onion], a mass of undifferentiated cells produced from the remnants of the primitive node and the primitive streak at the caudal end of the developing embryo after the formation of the somites is completed.

end bulbs of Krause. See **Krause's corpuscles.**

end-diastolic pressure /end'dī'əstol'ik/ [AS *ende;* Gk *dia* + *stellein* to set; L, *premere,* to press], the pressure of the blood in the ventricles at the end of diastole and just before the next ventricular systole.

endemic /endem'ik/ [Gk *endemos* native], (of a disease or microorganism) indigenous to a geographic area or population.

endemic goiter, an enlargement of the thyroid gland caused by the intake of inadequate amounts of dietary iodine. Iodine deprivation leads to diminished production and secretion of thyroid hormone by the gland. Initially, the goiter is diffuse; later, it becomes multinodular. Endemic goiter occurs occasionally in adolescents at puberty and widely in population groups in geographic areas in which limited amounts of iodine are present in the soil, water, and food. A large goiter may cause dysphagia, dyspnea, tracheal deviation, and cosmetic problems.

endemic typhus. See **murine typhus.**

end-feel, the sensation imparted to the examiner's hands at the end point of the available range of motion. Types of end-feel include capsular, bone-on-bone, spasm, and springy block.

endobronchial anesthesia /en'dobrong'kē·əl/ [Gk *endon* + *bronchos* windpipe], a procedure, rarely performed, in which anesthetic gas is administered into the bronchi.

endocardial cushion defect /en'dōkär'dē·əl/, any cardiac defect resulting from the failure of the endocardial cushions in the embryonic heart to fuse and form the atrial septum.

endocardial cushions, a pair of thickened tissue sections in the embryonic atrial canal.

endocardial fibroelastosis /fī'brō·ē'lastō'sis/ [Gk *endon* + *kardia* heart; L *fibra* fiber; Gk *elaunein* to drive, *osis* condition], an abnormal condition characterized by the development of a thick, fibroelastic endocardium that can result in pump failure.

endocarditis /en'dōkärdī'tis/ [Gk *endon kardia* heart, *itis* inflammation], an abnormal condition that affects the endocardium and the heart valves and is characterized by lesions caused by a variety of diseases. The kinds of endocarditis are

bacterial endocarditis, nonbacterial thrombotic endocarditis, and Libman-Sacks endocarditis. Untreated, all types of endocarditis are rapidly lethal.

endocardium /en'dōkär'dē·əm/, pl. **endocardia,** the lining of the heart chambers, containing small blood vessels and a few bundles of smooth muscle. It is continuous with the endothelium of the great blood vessels.

endocervical /en'dōsur'vikal/ [Gk *endon* + L *cervix* neck], pertaining to the interior of the cervix and uterus.

endocervicitis /en'dōsur'visī'tis/, an abnormal condition characterized by inflammation of the epithelium and glands of the canal of the uterine cervix.

endocervix /en'dōsur'viks/, **1.** the membrane lining the canal of the uterine cervix. **2.** the opening of the cervix into the uterine cavity.

endochondral /en'dōkon'drəl/ [Gk *endon* within, *chondros* cartilage], pertaining to something within the cartilage.

endocrine /en'dəkrēn, en'dəkrīn/ [Gk *endon* + *krinein* to secrete], pertaining to a process in which a group of cells secrete into the blood or lymph circulation a substance that has a specific effect on tissues in another part of the body.

endocrine diabetes mellitus [Gk *endon* + *krinein, diabainein* to pass through, *mellitus* honeyed], a form of diabetes associated with diseases of other glands, such as the adrenals, pituitary, or thyroid.

endocrine fracture /en'dōkrīn, -krēn/, any fracture that results from weakness of a specific bone because of an endocrine disorder, such as hyperparathyroidism.

endocrine system [Gk *endon* + *krinein* to secrete; *systema*], the network of ductless glands and other structures that elaborate and secrete hormones directly into the bloodstream, affecting the function of specific target organs. Glands of the endocrine system include the thyroid and the parathyroid, the anterior pituitary, the posterior pituitary, the pancreas, the suprarenal glands, and the gonads. The pineal gland is also considered an endocrine gland because it is ductless.

endocrine therapy. See **hormone therapy.**

endocrinologist /en'dōkrinol'əjist/, a physician who specializes in endocrinology.

endocrinology /en'dōkrinol'əjē/ [Gk *endon* + *krinein* to secrete, *logos* science], the study of the anatomy, physiology, and pathology of the endocrine system and of the treatment of endocrine problems.

endocrinopathy /en'dōkrinop'əthē/ [Gk *endon* + *krinein, pathos* disease], a disease involving an endocrine gland or the quality or quantity of its secretion.

endoderm /en′dədurm/ [Gk *endon* + *derma* skin], (in embryology) the innermost of the cell layers that develop from the embryonic disk of the inner cell mass of the blastocyst. The endoderm comprises the lining of the cavities and passages of the body and the covering for most of the internal organs.

endodermal /en′dōdur′məl/ [Gk *endon* + *derma* skin], pertaining to the inner of the three layers of the embryo, the epithelial lining of the respiratory system, the digestive tract, and other tissues.

endodermal cloaca, a part of the cloaca in the developing embryo that lies internal to the cloacal membrane and gives rise to the bladder and urogenital ducts.

endodontia /en′dōdon′tē·ə/ [Gk *endon* + *odous* tooth], the diagnosis, treatment, and prevention of disorders of dental pulp, tooth root, periapical tissues, and the associated practice of root canal therapy.

endodontics, a branch of dentistry that specializes in the diagnosis and treatment of diseases in the dental pulp and its surrounding tissues, including root canal therapy.

endodontist, a dentist who specializes in the etiology, diagnosis, and treatment of diseases of the dental pulp, tooth root, and periapical tissues and performs root canal therapy.

endogenous /endoj′ənəs/ [Gk *endon* + *genein* to produce], **1.** growing within the body. **2.** originating from within the body or produced from internal causes, such as a disease caused by the structural or functional failure of an organ or system. **–endogenic,** *adj.*

endogenous carbon dioxide, carbon dioxide produced within the body by metabolic processes.

endogenous depression, a major disorder of mood characterized by a persistent dysphoric mood, anxiety, irritability, fear, brooding, appetite and sleep disturbances, weight loss, psychomotor agitation or retardation, decreased energy, feelings of worthlessness or guilt, difficulty in concentrating or thinking, occasional delusions and hallucinations, and thoughts of death or suicide.

endogenous infection, an infection caused by the reactivation of previously dormant organisms, as in coccidioidomycosis, histoplasmosis, and tuberculosis.

endogenous obesity, obesity resulting from dysfunction of the endocrine or metabolic systems.

endogenous uric acid [Gk *endon* + *genein* to produce, *ouron* urine; L *acidus*], uric acid produced by the metabolism of purines in the body's own nucleoproteins, as distinguished from metabolism of purine products in foods.

endolith. See **denticle.**

endolymph /en′dəlimf/ [Gk *endon* + *lympha* water], the fluid in the membranous labyrinth (cochlear duct) of the internal ear.

endolymphatic duct /en′dəlimfat′ik/, a labyrinthine passage joining an endolymphatic sac with a utricle and saccule.

endometrial /en′dōmē′trē·əl/ [Gk *endon* + *metra* womb], **1.** of or pertaining to endometrium. **2.** of or pertaining to the uterine cavity.

endometrial cancer, a malignant neoplastic disease of the endometrium of the uterus most often occurring in the fifth or sixth decade of life. Some of the factors associated with an increased incidence of the disease are a medical history of infertility, anovulation, administration of exogenous estrogen, uterine polyps, and a combination of diabetes, hypertension, and obesity. Abnormal vaginal bleeding, especially in a postmenopausal woman, is the cardinal symptom. There also may be lower abdominal and low back pain; a large, boggy uterus is often a sign of advanced disease.

endometrial cyst [Gk *endon* + *metra* womb, *kystis* bag], **1.** an endometrial tumor. **2.** an ovarian cyst that develops as a distention of an endometrial gland.

endometrial hyperplasia, an abnormal condition characterized by overgrowth of the endometrium resulting from sustained stimulation by estrogen (of endogenous or exogenous origin) that is not opposed by progesterone. Endometrial hyperplasia often results in abnormal uterine bleeding; such bleeding, particularly in older women, constitutes an indication for biopsy or curettage of the endometrium to establish histopathologic diagnosis and to rule out malignancy.

endometrial polyp, a pedunculated overgrowth of endometrium, usually benign. Polyps are a common cause of vaginal bleeding in perimenopausal women and are often associated with other uterine abnormalities, such as endometrial hyperplasia or fibroids.

endometrioma /en′dōmē′trē·ō′mə/ [Gk *endon* + *metra* + *oma* tumor], a tumor or mass of ectopic endometrial tissue that has no function in the uterus.

endometriosis /en′dōmē′trē·ō′sis/ [Gk *endon* + *metra* womb, *osis* condition], an abnormal gynecologic condition characterized by ectopic growth and function of endometrial tissue. Precise incidence of the disease is unknown, but evidence of it is found in approximately 15% of women who undergo pelvic laparotomy for other indications. Women of higher socioeconomic status and women who defer pregnancy are more likely to contract the disease. The average age of women found to have endometriosis is 37 years. The disease is uncommon among black women. Pregnancy has a definite but inconsistent influence in preventing or ameliorating the disease. The causes of endometriosis are unknown.

endometritis /en'dōmitrī'tis/ [Gk *endon* + *metra* womb, *itis* inflammation], an inflammatory condition of the endometrium, usually caused by bacterial infection, commonly gonococci or hemolytic streptococci. It is characterized by fever, abdominal pain, malodorous discharge, and enlargement of the uterus. It occurs most frequently after childbirth or abortion and in women fitted with an intrauterine contraceptive device. A kind of endometritis is **decidua endometritis.**

endometritis dessicans, *obsolete.* endometritis characterized by ulceration and shedding of the endometrium of the uterus.

endometrium /en'dōmē'trē·əm/ [Gk *endon* + *metra* womb], the mucous membrane lining of the uterus, consisting of the stratum compactum, the stratum spongiosum, and the stratum basale. The endometrium changes in thickness and structure with the menstrual cycle.

endomorph /en'dəmôrf'/ [Gk *endon* + *morphe* form], a person whose body build is characterized by a soft, round physique with a large trunk and thighs, tapering extremities, an accumulation of fat throughout the body, and a predominance of structures derived from the endoderm.

endomyocarditis /en'dōmī'ōkärdī'tis/ [Gk *endon* + *mys* muscle, *kardia* heart, *itis*, inflammation], an inflammation of the lining of the heart.

endoparasite /en'dōper'əsīt/ [Gk *endon* + *parasitos* guest], (in medical parasitology) an organism that lives within the body of the host, such as a tapeworm.

endophthalmitis /endof'thalmī'tis/ [Gk *endon* + *ophthalmos* eye, *itis*], an inflammatory condition of the internal eye in which the eye becomes red, swollen, painful, and, sometimes, filled with pus. This condition may blur the vision and cause vomiting, fever, and headache.

endophthalmitis phacoanaphylactica /fak'ō·an'əfilak'təkə/, an abnormal condition characterized by an acute autoimmune reaction of the eye. It is caused by hypersensitivity of the eye to the protein of the crystalline lens and commonly oc-

curs after trauma to the crystalline lens or after a cataract operation. Associated symptoms include swelling and inflammation of the eye, severe pain, and blurred vision.

endophytic /en'dōfit'ik/ [Gk *endon* + *phyton* plant], of or pertaining to the tendency to grow inward, such as an endophytic tumor that grows on the inside of an organ or structure.

endoplasm /en'dəplaz'əm/ [Gk *endon* + *plasma* plasm], the inner portion of cytoplasm.

endoplasmic reticulum [Gk *endon* + *plassein* to mold], an extensive network of membrane-enclosed tubules in the cytoplasm of cells. The structure functions in the synthesis of proteins and lipids and in the transport of these metabolites within the cell.

endoprosthesis /en'dōprosthē'sis, en'dōpros'thəsis/ [Gk *endon* + *prosthesis* addition], a prosthetic device installed within the body, such as dentures or an internal cardiac pacemaker.

end-organ [AS *ende*; Gk *organon* instrument], a nerve ending in which the terminal nerve filaments are encapsulated.

endorphin /endôr'fin/ [Gk *endon* + L *Morpheus* god of dreams], any one of the neuropeptides composed of many amino acids, elaborated by the pituitary gland and acting on the central and the peripheral nervous systems to reduce pain. Endorphins isolated by researchers are alpha-endorphin, beta-endorphin, and gamma-endorphin, all chemicals producing pharmacologic effects similar to morphine.

endorsement [Gk *en* + L *dorsum* the back], a statement of recognition of the license of a health practitioner in one state by another state.

endoscope /en'dōskōp'/ [Gk *endon* + *skopein* to look], an illuminated optic instrument for the visualization of the interior of a body cavity or organ. Although the endoscope is generally introduced through a natural opening in the body, it may also be inserted through an incision. **–endoscopic,** *adj.*

endoscopic retrograde cholangiography, (in radiology) a diagnostic procedure for outlining the common bile duct. A flexible fiberoptic duodenoscope is placed in the common bile duct.

endoscopy /endos'kəpē/, the visualization of the interior of organs and cavities of the body with an endoscope.

endoskeletal prosthesis [Gk *endon* + *skeletos* dried up; *prosthesis* addition], a prosthetic device in which an internal pylon provides the actual support of the body.

endoskeleton, the internal network of bones to which muscles are attached. Compare **exoskeleton.**

endosteal hyperostosis /endos'tē·əl/, an inherited bone disorder characterized by an overgrowth of the mandible and brow areas. The excessive bone growth can lead to entrapment of cranial nerves.

endostomy therapist. See **enterostomal therapist.**

endothelial /en'dōthē'lē·əl/ [Gk, *endon*, within, *thele*, nipple], pertaining to or resembling endothelium.

endothelial cell [Gk *endon* + *thele* nipple; L *cella* storeroom], a lining cell of a body cavity or of the cardiovascular system. It is usually seen as a flat nucleated cell.

endothelial myeloma /en'dōthē'lē·əl/ [Gk *endon* + *thele* nipple; *myelos* marrow, *oma* tumor], a malignant myeloma that develops in the bone marrow, occurring most frequently in the long bones.

endothelin (ET), /en'dōthē'lin/ any of a group of vasoconstrictive peptides produced by endothelial cells from pre-pro-endothelin by a cleavage performed by an **endothelin converting enzyme (ACE).** Three known endothelins designated as **ET-1, ET-2,** and **ET-3** are chemically related to asp venom. ET-1 is the most potent vasopressor compound yet discovered, being 10 times greater than **angiotensin-II,** previously believed to be the most powerful vasopressor.

endothelium /en'dōthē'lē·əm/ [Gk *endon* + *thele* nipple], the layer of simple squamous epithelial cells that lines the heart, the blood and the lymph vessels, and the serous cavities of the body. **–endothelial** *adj.*

endotoxin /en'dōtok'sin/ [Gk *endon* + *toxikon* poison], a toxin contained in the cell walls of some microorganisms, especially gram-negative bacteria, that is released when the bacterium dies and is broken down in the body.

endotoxin shock [Gk *endon* + *toxikon* poison; Fr *choc*], a septic shock in response to the release of endotoxins produced by gram-negative bacteria. The toxin is released upon the death of the bacterial cell.

endotracheal /en'dōtrā'kē·əl/ [Gk *endon* + *tracheia, arteria* rough air pipe], within or through the trachea.

endotracheal anesthesia, inhalation anesthesia that is achieved by the passage of an anesthetic gas or mixture of gases through an endotracheal tube into the respiratory tract.

endotracheal intubation, the management of the patient with an airway catheter inserted through the mouth or nose into the trachea. An endotracheal tube may be used to maintain a patent airway, to prevent aspiration of material from the digestive tract in the unconscious or paralyzed patient, to permit suctioning of tracheobronchial secretions, or to administer positive-pressure ventilation that cannot be given effectively by a mask.

endotracheal tube, a large-bore catheter inserted through the mouth or nose and into the trachea to a point above the bifurcation of the trachea proximal to the bronchi. It is used for delivering oxygen under pressure when ventilation must be totally controlled and in general anesthetic procedures. Endotracheal tubes may be made of rubber or plastic and usually have an inflatable cuff to maintain a closed system with the ventilator.

endoxin /endok'sin/, an endogenous analog of digoxin, occurring naturally in humans. It is a hormone that may regulate the excretion of salt.

end plate [AS *ende*; ME *plat*], in the nervous system, the motor end plate, located at the terminal membrane of an axon and the postjunctional membrane of the adjoining muscle tissue.

end-stage disease [AS *ende*; OFr *estage*; L *dis*; Fr *aise* ease], a disease condition that is essentially terminal because of irreversible damage to vital tissues or organs. Kidney or renal end-stage disease is defined as a point at which the kidney is so badly damaged or scarred that hemodialysis or transplantation is required for patient survival.

end-tidal capnography, /end'tīdəl/ (in respiratory therapy) the process of continuously recording the concentration or percentage of carbon dioxide in expired air. It is used in continuous monitoring of critically ill patients and also in pulmonary function testing.

end-tidal CO_2 determination, the concentration of carbon dioxide in a patient's end-tidal breath.

endurance, the ability to continue an activity despite increasing physical or psychologic stress. Although endurance and strength are different qualities, weaker muscles tend to have less endurance than strong muscles.

enema /en'əmə/ [Gk *enienai* injection], a procedure in which a solution is introduced into the rectum for cleansing or therapeutic purposes. Enemas may be commercially packed disposable units or reusable equipment prepared just before use.

energy [Gk *energia*], the capacity to do work or to perform vigorous activity. Energy may occur in the form of heat, light, movement, sound, or radiation. Human energy is usually expressed as muscle contractions and heat production. Chemical energy refers to the energy released as a result of a chemical reaction. **–energetic,** *adj.*

energy conservation, a principle that energy cannot be created or destroyed, although it can be changed from one form into another, as when heat energy is converted to light energy.

energy cost of activities, the metabolic cost in calories or kilojoules of various forms of physical activity. For example, the average metabolic equivalent of walking at a rate of 3 km/hr is 2 METS per minute while the energy cost of walking at a speed of 6 km/hr is 5 METs per minute.

energy-protein malnutrition, a wasting condition resulting from a diet deficient in both calories and proteins.

energy subtraction, (in digital x-ray imaging) a technique in which two different x-ray beams are used alternately to provide a subtraction image resulting from differences in photoelectric interaction.

enervation /en'ərvā'sh[ə]n/ [L *enervare* to weaken], **1.** the reduction or lack of nervous energy; weakness; lassitude; languor. **2.** removal of a complete nerve or of a section of nerve.

en face /äNfäs', enfäs'/, "face-to-face"; a position in which the mother's face and the infant's face are approximately 8 inches apart and on the same plane, as when the mother holds the infant up in front of her face or when she nurses the child.

enflurane /en'floŏrān/, a nonflammable anesthetic gas belonging to the ether family, used for induction and maintenance of general anesthesia in cases in which ethers are the drugs of choice.

engagement [Fr, a bonding], **1.** fixation of the presenting part of the fetus in the maternal true pelvis. The largest diameter of the presenting part is at or below the level of the ischial spines. **2.** fixation of the fetal head in the maternal midpelvis with the biparietal diameter of the head level with the ischial spines.

English position. See **lateral recumbent position.**

engorgement [Fr *engorger* to fill up], distention or vascular congestion of body tissues, such as the swelling of breast tissue caused by an increased flow of blood and lymph preceding true lactation.

engram /en'gram/, **1.** a hypothetical neurophysiologic storage unit in the cerebrum that is the source of a particular memory. **2.** an interneuronal circuit involving specific neurons and muscle fibers that can be

coordinated to perform specific motor activity patterns.

engrossment. See **bonding.**

enhancement [ME *enhauncen* to raise], to improve, heighten, or augment.

enkephalin /enkef'əlin/ [Gk *enkepalos* brain, *in* within], one of two pain-relieving pentapeptides produced in the body. Researchers have isolated enkephalins in the pituitary gland, brain, and GI tract. The enkephalins are methionine-enkephalin and isoleucine-enkephalin, each composed of five amino acids, four of which are identical in both compounds. It is believed that these two neuropeptides can depress neurons throughout the central nervous system.

enol /ē'nol/, an organic compound with an alcohol or hydroxyl group adjacent to a double bond.

enophthalmos /en'əfthal'məs/ [Gk *en* in, *ophthalmos* eye], backward displacement of the eye in the bony socket, caused by traumatic injury or developmental defect. **–enophthalmic,** *adj.*

ensiform process. See **xiphoid process.**

ENT, abbreviation for *ear, nose, and throat.*

Entameba. See *Entamoeba.*

entamebiasis. See **amebiasis.**

Entamoeba /en'təmē'bə/ [Gk *entos* within, *amoibe* change], a genus of intestinal amebic parasites of which several species are pathogenic to humans. Also spelled *Entameba.*

Entamoeba histolytica /his'təlit'ikə/, a pathogenic species of ameba that causes amebic dysentery and hepatic amebiasis in humans.

entamoebiasis. See **amebiasis.**

enteral /enter'əl/ [Gk *enteron* bowel], within the small intestine, or via the small intestinal.

enteral nutrition, the provision of nutrients through the GI tract when the client cannot inject, chew, or swallow food, but can digest and absorb nutrients.

enteral tube feeding [Gk *enteron* bowel; L *tubus*; AS *faedan*], the introduction of food or nutritive material directly into the digestive tract by nasogastric or gastric tube.

enterectomy /en'tərek'təmē/ [Gk *enteron* intestine, *ektome* excision], the surgical removal of a portion of intestine.

enteric /enter'ik/ [Gk *enteron* bowel], pertaining to the intestine.

enteric coating, a coating added to oral medications that are designed to be absorbed from the intestinal tract. The coating resists the effects of stomach juices.

enteric cytopathogenic human orphan virus. See **ECHO virus.**

enteric fever. See **typhoid fever.**

enteric infection, a disease of the intestine caused by any infection. Symptoms similar to those caused by pathogens may be produced by chemical toxins in ingested foods and by allergic reactions to certain food substances. Among bacteria commonly involved in enteric infections are *Escherichia coli, Vibrio cholerae,* and several species of *Salmonella, Shigella,* and anaerobic streptococci. Enteric infections are characterized by diarrhea, abdominal discomfort, nausea and vomiting, and anorexia.

entericoid fever /enter'ikoid/ [Gk *enteron* + *eidos* form], a typhoidlike febrile disease characterized by intestinal inflammation and dysfunction.

enteric orphan virus [Gk *enteron* + *orphanos* bereft; L *virus* poison], a GI disease virus that has been identified and isolated but was not originally associated with the disease.

enteritis /en'tərī'tis/, inflammation of the mucosal lining of the small intestine, resulting from a variety of causes—bacterial, viral, functional, and inflammatory. Involvement of small and large intestine is called **enterocolitis.**

Enterobacter cloacae /en'tirōbak'tər klō·ā' kē, klō·ā'sē/ [Gk *enteron* + *bakterion* small staff; L *cloaca* sewer], a common species of bacteria found in human and animal feces, dairy products, sewage, soil, and water.

Enterobacteriaceae /en'tirōbaktir'ē·ā'si·ē/ [Gk *enteron* + *bakterion* small staff], a family of aerobic and anaerobic bacteria that includes both normal and pathogenic enteric microorganisms. Among the significant genera of the family are *Escherichia, Klebsiella, Proteus,* and *Salmonella.*

enterobacterial /en'tirōbaktir'ē·əl/ [Gk *enteron* + *bakterion* small staff], of or pertaining to a species of bacteria found in the digestive tract.

enterobiasis /en'tirōbī'əsis/ [Gk *enteron* + *bios* life, *osis* condition], a parasitic infestation with *Enterobius vermicularis,* the common pinworm. The worms infect the large intestine, and the females deposit eggs in the perianal area, causing pruritus and insomnia.

Enterobius vermicularis /en'tərō'bē·əs/ [Gk *enteron* + *bios* life; L *vermiculus* small worm], a common parasitic nematode that resembles a white thread between 0.5 and 1 cm long.

enterochromaffin cell. See **argentaffin cell.**

enteroclysis /en'tərok'lisis/, a radiographic procedure in which a contrast medium is injected into the duodenum to examine the small intestine.

enterococcus /en'tərōkok'əs/, *pl. enterococci* /en'tərōkok'sī, en'tərōkôk'ē/ [Gk *enteron* + *kokkos* berry], any *Streptococcus* that inhabits the intestinal tract.

enterocolitis /en'tərōkōlī'tis/ [Gk *enteron* + *kolon* bowel, *itis*], an inflammation involving both the large and small intestines.

enteroenterostomy /en'tərō·en'təros' təmē/, the surgical creation of an artificial connection between two segments of the intestine.

enterohepatic circulation /en'tərōhə pat'ik/, a route by which part of the bile produced by the liver enters the intestine to be reabsorbed by the liver and recycled back into the intestine. The remainder of the bile is excreted in feces.

enterokinase /en'tirōkī'nās/ [Gk *enteron* + *kinesis* movement, *ase* enzyme], an intestinal juice enzyme that activates the proteolytic enzyme in pancreatic juice as the enzymes enter the duodenum.

enterolith /en'tərōlith'/ [Gk *enteron* + *lithos* stone], a stone consisting of ingested material found in the intestine.

enterolithiasis /en'tərōlithī'əsis/, the presence of enteroliths in the intestine.

enteropathy /en'tərop'əthē/, a disease or other disorder of the intestines.

enterostomal therapist /en'tərōstō'məl/, a registered nurse who is qualified by education in an accredited program in enterostomal therapy to provide care for patients.

enterostomy /en'təros'təmē/ [Gk *enteron* + *stoma* mouth], a surgical procedure that produces an artificial anus or fistula in the intestine by incision through the abdominal wall.

enterotoxigenic /en'tirōtok'sijen'ik/, pertaining to an organism or other agent that produces a toxin causing an adverse reaction by cells of the intestinal mucosa. Examples include bacteria that produce enterotoxins, resulting in intestinal reactions such as vomiting, diarrhea, and other symptoms of food poisoning.

enterotoxin, /en'tirōtok'sin/ a toxic substance specific for the cells of the intestinal mucosa, produced usually by certain species of bacteria, such as *Staphylococcus.*

enterovirus /en'tirōvī'rəs/ [Gk *enteron* + L *virus* poison], a virus that multiplies primarily in the intestinal tract. Kinds of enteroviruses are **coxsackievirus, echovirus,** and **poliovirus.** –**enteroviral,** *adj.*

enthesitis /en'thəsī'tis/, an inflammation of the insertion of a muscle with a strong tendency toward fibrosis and calcification.

It is usually only painful when the involved muscle is activated.

entoderm. See **endoderm.**

entrainment /entrān′mənt/ [Fr *entrainer* to drag along], a phenomenon observed in the microanalysis of sound films in which the speaker moves several parts of the body and the listener responds to the sounds by moving in ways that are coordinated with the rhythm of the sounds. Entrainment is thought to be an essential factor in the process of maternal-infant bonding.

entrance block [Fr *entrer* to enter; AS *blok*], (in cardiology) a theoretic zone surrounding the heart's natural pacemaker focus, protecting it from discharge by an extraneous impulse that might trigger ectopic ventricular contractions.

entrance exposure, (in radiology) the skin dose of radiation. It may be expressed in milliroentgens.

entrapment neuropathy [OFr *entraper* to catch in a trap; Gk *neuron* nerve, *pathos* disease], injury or inflammation of single nerves due to pressure from surrounding tissues, such as ligaments and fascia.

entropion /entrō′pē·on/ [Gk *en* + *tropos* a turning], turning inward or turning toward, usually a condition in which the eyelid turns inward toward the eye. **Cicatricial entropion** can occur in either the upper or lower eyelid as a result of scar tissue formation. **Spastic entropion** results from an inflammation or other factor that affects tissue tone. An inflammation of the eyelid may be the result of an infectious disease or irritation from an inverted eyelash.

entropy /en′trəpē/ [Gk *en* + *tropos* a turning], the tendency of a system to go from a state of order to a state of disorder, expressed in physics as a measure of the part of the heat or energy in a thermodynamic system that is not available to perform work.

ENT specialist, a physician who specializes in the treatment of the eye, nose, and throat.

enucleation /inoo̅ ̅′klē·ā′shən/ [L *e* out of, *nucleus* nut] **1.** removal of an organ or tumor in one piece. **2.** removal of the eyeball, performed for malignancy, severe infection, or extensive trauma or to control pain in glaucoma.

enucleator /inoo̅ ̅′klē·ā′tər/ [L *e* + *nucleus* nut], a procedure or device for removing a nucleus from a cell.

enuresis /en′yŏŏrē′sis/ [Gk *enourein* to urinate], incontinence of urine, especially in bed at night.

environment [Gk *en* in; L *viron* circle], all of the many factors, as physical and psychologic, that influence or affect the life and survival of a person. **–environmental,** *adj.*

environmental carcinogen, any of many natural or synthetic substances that can cause cancer. Such agents, or oncogens, may be divided into chemical agents, physical agents, and certain hormones and viruses.

environmental control units, control units that regulate various devices for handicapped persons from remote positions such as a bed or wheelchair. Examples include units (often with switches that can be manipulated by the lips, chin, or other functional body parts) that control lamps, television, radio, telephone, and alarm systems.

environmental health, the total of various aspects of substances, forces, and conditions in and about a community that affect the health and well-being of the population.

environmental services, a housekeeping function of a hospital or other health care facility.

enzygotic twins. See **monozygotic twins.**

enzymatic detergent asthma, a type of allergic reaction experienced by persons who have become sensitized to alcalase, an enzyme contained in some laundry detergents.

enzyme /en′zīm/ [Gk *en* in, *zyme* ferment], a protein produced by living cells that catalyzes chemical reactions in organic matter. Most enzymes are produced in minute quantities and catalyze reactions that take place within the cells.

enzyme induction [Gk *en* + *zyme* ferment; L *inducere* to lead in], the increase in the rate of a specific enzyme synthesis from basal to maximum level due to the presence of a substrate or substrate analog that acts as an inducer. The inducer may be a substance that inactivates a repressor chemical in the cell.

enzyme-linked immunosorbent assay (ELISA), a laboratory technique for detecting specific antigens or antibodies, using enzyme-labeled immunoreactants and a solid-phase binding support, such as a test tube. ELISA is nearly as sensitive as radioimmunoassay and more sensitive than complement-fixation, agglutination, and other techniques. It is commonly used in the diagnosis of AIDS infections.

eosin /ē′əsin/, a group of red, acidic xanthine dyes often used in combination with a blue-purple, basic dye, such as hematoxylin, to stain tissue slides in the laboratory.

eosinophil /ē′əsin′əfil/ [Gk *eos* dawn, *philein* to love], a granulocytic, bilobed leukocyte somewhat larger than a neutrophil characterized by the large number of coarse, refractile, cytoplasmic granules that stain intensely with the acid dye, eosin. **–eosinophilic,** *adj.*

eosinophilia /ē′əsin′ōfil′ē·ə/, an increase in the number of eosinophils in the blood, accompanying many inflammatory conditions. Substantial increases are considered a reflection of an allergic response.

eosinophilia-myalgia syndrome, tryptophan-induced, a potentially fatal disorder characterized by a symptom complex of severe muscle pain, tenosynovitis, muscle edema, and skin rash lasting several weeks. The cause has been associated with a contaminant in L-tryptophan taken for sedation or psychotropic support.

eosinophilic /ē′əsin′əfil′ik/ **1.** the tendency of a cell, tissue, or organism to be readily stained by the dye eosin. **2.** of or pertaining to an eosinophilic leukocyte.

eosinophilic adenoma. See **acidophilic adenoma.**

eosinophilic enteropathy, a rare form of food allergy that is characterized by nausea, crampy abdominal pain, diarrhea, urticaria, an elevated eosinophil count in the blood, and eosinophilic infiltrates in the intestine.

eosinophilic granuloma, a growth characterized by numerous eosinophils and histiocytes, usually occurring as a single or multiple lesion in bone.

eosinophilic leukemia, a malignant neoplasm of leukocytes in which eosinophils are the predominant cells.

eosinophilic pneumonia, inflammation of the lungs, characterized by infiltration of the alveoli with eosinophils and large mononuclear cells, pulmonary edema, fever, night sweats, cough, dyspnea, and weight loss.

EP, abbreviation for **evoked potential.**

ependyma /ipen′dimə/ [Gk, an upper garment], a layer of ciliated epithelium that lines the central canal of the spinal cord and the ventricles of the brain. **–ependymal,** *adj.*

ependymal glioma, a large, vascular, fairly solid glioma in the fourth ventricle.

ependymoblastoma /ipen′dimōblastō′mə/, a malignant neoplasm composed of primitive cells of the ependyma.

ependymoma /ipen′dimō′mə/ [Gk *ependyma* an upper garment, *oma* tumor], a neoplasm composed of differentiated cells of the ependyma.

ephapse /ef′aps/ [Gk *ephasis* a touching], a point of lateral contact between nerve fibers across which impulses may be transmitted directly through the membranes of the cells rather than across a synapse. **–ephaptic,** *adj.*

ephaptic transmission /ifap′tik/, the passage of a neural impulse from one nerve fiber, axon, or dendrite to another through the membranes.

ephebiatrics /ēfeb′ē·at′riks/ [Gk *ephebos* puberty, *iatros* physician], a branch of medicine that specializes in the health of adolescents.

ephedrine /ef′ədrēn/, an adrenergic bronchodilator prescribed in the treatment of asthma and bronchitis and is used topically as a nasal decongestant.

ephemeral /ifem′ərəl/ [Gk *epi* above, *hemera* day], pertaining to a short-lived condition, such as a fever.

ephemeral fever, any febrile condition lasting only 24 to 48 hours that is uncomplicated and of unknown origin.

epiblast /ep′iblast′/ [Gk *epi* upon, *blastos* germ], the primordial outer layer of the blastocyst or blastula, before differentiation of the germ layers, that gives rise to the ectoderm and contains cells capable of forming the endoderm and mesoderm. **–epiblastic,** *adj.*

epicanthus /ep′ikan′thəs/ [Gk *epi* + *kanthos* lip of a vessel], a vertical fold of skin over the angle of the inner canthus of the eye. It is normal in Asian people and is of no clinical significance. **–epicanthal, epicanthic,** *adj.*

epicardia /ep′ikär′dē·ə/ [Gk *epi* + *kardia* heart], the part of the esophagus that lies between the cardiac orifice of the stomach and the esophageal opening of the diaphragm.

epicardium /ep′ikär′dē·əm/ [Gk *epi* + *kardia* heart], one of the three layers of tissue that form the wall of the heart. It is the visceral portion of the serous pericardium and folds back on itself to form the parietal portion of the serous pericardium. **–epicardial,** *adj.*

epicondylar fracture /ep′ikon′dilər/, any fracture that involves the medial or the lateral epicondyle of a specific bone, such as the humerus.

epicondyle /ep′ikon′dəl/ [Gk *epi* + *kondylos* knuckle], a projection on the surface of a bone above its condyle. **–epicondylar,** *adj.*

epicondylitis /ep′ikon′dilī′tis/, a painful and sometimes disabling inflammation of the muscle and surrounding tissues of the elbow, caused by repeated strain on the forearm near the lateral epicondyle of the humerus, such as from violent extension or supination of the wrist against a resisting force.

epicranial aponeurosis /ep′ikrā′nē·əl/ [Gk

epi + kranion skull; apo away, neuron tendon], a fibrous membrane that covers the cranium between the occipital and frontal muscles of the scalp.

epicranium /ep′ikrā′nē·əm/ [Gk epi + kranion skull], the complete scalp, including the integument, the muscular sheets, and the aponeuroses. –**epicranial,** adj.

epicranius [Gk epi + kranion skull], the broad, muscular, and tendinous layer of tissue covering the top and the sides of the skull from the occipital bone to the eyebrows.

epicritic /ep′ikrit′ik/, pertaining to the somatic sensations of fine discriminative touch, vibration, two-point discrimination, stereognosis, and conscious and unconscious proprioception.

epidemic [Gk epi + demos people] **1.** affecting a significantly large number of people at the same time. **2.** a disease that spreads rapidly through a demographic segment of the human population, such as everyone in a given geographic area. **3.** a widespread disease that tends to occur periodically.

epidemic diarrhea in newborn [Gk epi + demos the people, dia through, rhein flow; ME newe, beren], any severe gastroenteritis epidemic among a community of newborns, as may occur in a hospial nursery.

epidemic encephalitis, any diffuse inflammation of the brain occurring in epidemic form. Two kinds of epidemic encephalitis are **Japanese encephalitis** and **St. Louis encephalitis.**

epidemic hemoglobinuria. See **hemoglobinuria.**

epidemic hemorrhagic conjunctivitis [Gk epi + demos, haima blood, rhegnynei, to gush; L conjunctivus connecting; Gk itis inflammation], a highly contagious infection, commonly involving an enterovirus, that begins with eye pain, accompanied by swollen eyelids, hyperemia of the conjunctiva. It is a self-limiting disorder and there is no specific remedy.

epidemic hemorrhagic fever, a severe viral infection marked by fever and bleeding. The disorder develops rapidly, characterized initially by fever and muscle ache, possibly followed by hemorrhage, peripheral vascular collapse, hypovolemic shock, and acute kidney failure. The arbovirus or other pathogen is believed transmitted by mosquitoes, ticks, or mites. Among the various forms of epidemic hemorrhagic fevers are **Argentine hemorrhagic, Bolivian hemorrhagic, dengue hemorrhagic, Lassa,** and **yellow fever.**

epidemic keratoconjunctivitis (EKC) [Gk

epi + demos, keras horn; L conjunctivus; Gk itis inflammation], an acute complex of keratitis and conjunctivitis transmitted by an adenovirus. A highly contagious form of keratoconjunctivitis, it is often with lymph node involvement. It is commonly spread by handling contaminated materials in eye clinics, particularly offices that handle emergency care of eye injuries.

epidemic myalgia, a disease caused by coxsackie B virus, characterized by sudden, acute chest or epigastric pain and fever lasting a few days, followed by complete, spontaneous recovery.

epidemic myositis. See **epidemic myalgia, epidemic pleurodynia.**

epidemic parotitis. See **mumps.**

epidemic pleurodynia, an infection caused by a coxsackievirus, affecting mainly children. It is characterized by severe intermittent pain in the abdomen or lower chest, fever, headache, sore throat, malaise, and extreme myalgia.

epidemic typhus, an acute, severe rickettsial infection characterized by prolonged high fever, headache, and a dark maculopapular rash that covers most of the body. The causative organism, Rickettsia prowazekii, is transmitted indirectly as a result of the bite of the human body louse. The pathogen is contained in feces of the louse and enters the body tissues as the bite is scratched. An intense headache and a fever reaching 40° C (104° F) begin after an incubation period of 10 days to 2 weeks. The rash follows.

epidemiologist /ep′idē′mē·ol′əjist/, a physician or medical scientist who studies the incidence, prevalence, spread, prevention, and control of disease in a community or a specific group of individuals.

epidemiology /ep′idē′mē·ol′əjē/ [Gk epi + demos people, logos science], the study of the occurrence, distribution, and causes of disease in humankind. –**epidemiologic,** adj., **epidemiologist,** n.

epidermal nevus [Gk epi + derma the skin; L naevus birthmark], a discrete, discolored lesion caused by an overgrowth of epidermis. It may be seen in newborns.

epidermis /ep′idur′mis/ [Gk epi + derma skin], the superficial, avascular layers of the skin, made up of an outer, dead, cornified portion and a deeper, living, cellular portion. –**epidermal, epidermoid,** adj.

epidermoid carcinoma [Gk epi, derma + eidos form], a malignant neoplasm in which the tumor cells tend to differentiate in the manner of epidermal cells, then form horny cells called prickle cells.

epidermoid cyst, a common, benign,

variable, subcutaneous swelling lined by keratinizing epithelium and filled with a cheesy material composed of sebum and epithelial debris.

epidermolysis bullosa /ep'idərmol'isis/ [Gk *epi, derma* + *lysis* loosening], a group of rare, hereditary or acquired skin diseases in which vesicles and bullae develop, usually at sites of trauma.

epidermophytosis, a superficial fungus infection of the skin.

epididymis /ep'idid'imis/, *pl.* **epididymides** [Gk *epi* + *didymos* pair], one of a pair of long, tightly coiled ducts that carry sperm from the seminiferous tubules of the testes to the vas deferens.

epididymitis /ep'idid'imī'tis/ [Gk *epi, didymos* + *itis* inflammation], acute or chronic inflammation of the epididymis. Symptoms include fever and chills, pain in the groin, and tender, swollen epididymis.

epididymoorchitis /ep'idid'imō-ôrki'tis/ [Gk *epi, didymos* + *orchis* testis, *itis*], inflammation of the epididymis and of the testis.

epididymovesiculography /ep'idid'imōves'ikyəlog'rəfē/, a radiologic examination of the seminal ducts usually performed in cases of sterility, cysts, tumors, abscesses, and inflammation.

epidural /ep'idŏŏr'əl/ [Gk *epi* + *dura* hard], outside the dura mater.

epidural anesthesia, the process of achieving regional anesthesia of the pelvic, abdominal, genital, or other area by the injection of a local anesthetic into the epidural space of the spinal column.

epidural blood patch, a patch repairing a tear or a hole in the dura mater around the spinal cord. The tear is usually the result of needle puncture during spinal anesthesia or lumbar puncture.

epidural hemorrhage, a hemorrhage that results in a collection of blood outside the dura mater of the brain or spinal cord.

epidural space, the space immediately surrounding the dura mater of the brain or spinal cord, beneath the periosteum of the cranium and the spinal column.

epigastric [Gk *epi* + *gaster* stomach], pertaining to the epigastrium.

epigastric node [Gk *epi* + *gaster* stomach; L *nodus* knot], a node in one of the seven groups of parietal lymph nodes serving the abdomen and the pelvis, comprising about four nodes along the caudal portion of the inferior epigastric vessels.

epigastric pain [Gk *epi* + *gaster* stomach; L *poena* penalty], pain in the epigastric region of the abdomen.

epigastric reflex [Gk *epi* + *gaster*; L *reflectere* to bend back], a contraction of the rectus abdominis muscle that occurs when the skin surface in the upper and middle abdominal region is stimulated. The reflex also may be induced when the axillary region of the fifth and sixth dorsal nerves is stimulated.

epigastric region, the part of the abdomen in the upper zone between the right and left hypochondriac regions.

epigastric sensation, a weak, sinking feeling of undefined nature that is usually localized in the pit of the stomach but may occur throughout the abdominal region.

epigastrium. See epigastric region.

epigenesis /ep'ijen'əsis/ [Gk *epi* + *genein* to produce], (in embryology) a theory of development in which the organism grows from a simple to more complex form through the progressive differentiation of an undifferentiated cellular unit. **–epigenesist,** *n.* **epigenetic,** *adj.*

epiglottiditis. See epiglottitis.

epiglottis /ep'iglot'is/ [Gk *epi* + *glossa* tongue], the cartilaginous structure that overhangs the larynx like a lid and prevents food from entering the larynx and the trachea while swallowing.

epiglottitis /ep'iglotī'tis/ [Gk *epi* + *glossa* tongue, *itis* inflammation], an inflammation of the epiglottis. It is characterized by fever, sore throat, stridor, croupy cough, and an erythematous, swollen epiglottis. The child may become cyanotic and require an emergency tracheostomy to maintain respiration.

epilating forceps /ep'ilā'ting/ [L *e, pilus* without hair], a kind of small spring forceps used for removing unwanted hair.

epilation. See depilation.

epilepsy /ep'ilep'sē/ [Gk *epilepsia* seizure], a group of neurologic disorders characterized by recurrent episodes of convulsive seizures, sensory disturbances, abnormal behavior, loss of consciousness, or all of these. Common to all types of epilepsy is an uncontrolled electric discharge from the nerve cells of the cerebral cortex. Although most epilepsy is of unknown cause, it may sometimes be associated with cerebral trauma, intracranial infection, brain tumor, vascular disturbances, intoxication, or chemical imbalance. **–epileptic,** *adj., n.*

epileptic dementia [Gk *epilepsia* seizure; L *de* + *mens* mind], a loss of cognitive and intellectual functions that develops in some cases of incompletely controlled epilepsy. Symptoms include slowness and circumstantiality of speech and narrowed attention span.

epileptic stupor, the state of unawareness and unresponsiveness after an epileptic seizure.

epileptic vertigo [Gk *epilepsia*; L *vertigo*

dizziness], an aura of dizziness that may precede, accompany, or follow an epileptic seizure.

epiloia. See **tuberous sclerosis.**

epimysium /ep'imiz'ē·əm/ [Gk *epi* + *mys* muscle], a fibrous sheath that enfolds a muscle and extends between the bundles of muscle fibers, such as the perimysium.

epinephrine /ep'ənef'rin/ [Gk *epi* + *nephros* kidney], an adrenal hormone and synthetic adrenergic vasoconstrictor. It is prescribed in the treatment of anaphylaxis, acute bronchial spasm, and nasal congestion and to increase the effectiveness of a local anesthetic.

epinephryl borate /ep'inef'ril/, an adrenergic prescribed in the treatment of primary open-angle glaucoma.

epiphora. See **tearing.**

epiphyseal fracture /ep'ifiz'ē·əl/ [Gk *epi* + *phyein* to grow; *fractura* break], a fracture involving the epiphyseal growth plate of a long bone, resulting in separation or in fragmentation of the plate.

epiphyseal plate [Gk *epi* + *phyein* to grow, *platys* flat], a thin layer of cartilage between the epiphysis, a secondary bone-forming center, and the bone shaft. The new bone forms along the plate.

epiphysis /ipif'isis/, *pl.* **epiphyses** [Gk *epi* + *phyein* to grow], the head of a long bone that is separated from the shaft of the bone by the epiphyseal plate until the bone stops growing, the plate is obliterated, and the shaft and the head become united. —**epiphyseal** /ipif'əsē'əl/, *adj.*

epiphysis cerebri. See **pineal body.**

epiphysitis /ipif'isī'tis/, an inflammation of the epiphysis, usually of a long bone, such as the femur or humerus.

epiploic foramen /ep'iplō'ik/ [Gk *epiploon* caul; L *foramen* a hole], a passage between the peritoneal cavity and the omental bursa. It is lined with peritoneum and is approximately 3 cm in diameter.

epipygus. See **pygomelus.**

episcleritis /ep'isklərī'tis/, inflammation of the outermost layers of the sclera and of the tissues overlying the posterior portions of this tough, white outer coat of the eyeball.

episiotomy /epē'zē·ot'əmē/ [Gk *episeion* pubic region, *temnein* to cut], a surgical procedure, usually required for forceps delivery, in which an incision is made in a woman's perineum to enlarge her vaginal opening for delivery, performed most often electively to prevent tearing of the perineum, to hasten or facilitate delivery of the baby.

episode [Gk *episodion* coming in besides], an incident or event that stands out from the continuity of everyday life, such as an episode of illness or a traumatic episode in the course of a child's development. —**episodic,** *adj.*

episode of hospital care, the services provided by a hospital in the continuous course of care for a patient with a medical problem or other health condition.

episodic care, a pattern of medical and nursing care in which care is given to a person for a particular problem, without an ongoing relationship being established between the person and health care professionals. Emergency rooms provide episodic care.

episome /ep'isōm/ [Gk *epi* + *soma* body], (in bacterial genetics) an extrachromosomal replicating unit that exists autonomously or functions with a chromosome.

epispadias /ep'ispā'dē·əs/ [Gk *epi* + *spadon* a rent], a congenital defect in which the urethra opens on the dorsum of the penis at some point proximal to the glans. The corresponding defect in women, fissure of the upper wall of the urethra, is quite rare.

epistasis /epis'təsis/ [Gk, a standing], (in genetics) a type of interaction between genes at different loci on a chromosome in which one is able to mask or suppress the expression of the other. —**epistatic,** *adj.*

epistaxis /ep'istak'sis/ [Gk, a dropping], bleeding from the nose caused by local irritation of mucous membranes, violent sneezing, fragility of the mucous membrane or of the arterial walls, chronic infection, trauma, hypertension, leukemia, vitamin K deficiency, or, most often, picking of the nose.

epistropheus. See **axis.**

epithalamus /ep'ithal'əməs/ [Gk *epi* + *thalamos* chamber], one of the portions of the diencephalon. It includes the trigonum habenulae, the pineal body, and the posterior commissure. —**epithalamic,** *adj.*

epithelial /ep'ithē'lē·əl/ [Gk *epi* + *thele* nipple], pertaining to or involving the outer layer of the skin.

epithelial cancer [Gk *epi* + *thele*; L *cancer* crab], a carcinoma that develops from squamous or transitional epithelium, or related tissues in the skin, esophagus, and other organs.

epithelial debridement [Gk *epi* + *thele*; Fr *débridement* an incision], the removal of the entire inner lining and the attachment from the gingival or periodontal pocket in gingival curettage.

epithelialization /ep'ithē'lē·al·īzā'shən/ [Gk *epi* + *thele*; L *ization* process], the regrowth of skin over a wound.

epithelial peg [Gk *epi* + *thele* nipple], any of the papillary projections of the epithelius that penetrate the underlying stroma of connecting tissue and normally develop in mucous membranes and dermal tissues.

epithelial rest. See **embryonic rest.**

epithelial tissue [Gk *epi* + *thele*; OFr *tissu*], a closely packed single or stratified layer of cells covering the body and lining its cavities, with the exception of the blood and lymph vessels.

epitheliofibril. See **tonofibril.**

epithelioid leiomyoma /ep′ithē′lē·oid/ [Gk *epi*, *thele* + *eidos* form], an uncommon neoplasm of smooth muscle in which the cells are polygonal in shape. It usually develops in the stomach.

epithelioma /ep′ithē′lē·ō′mə/ [Gk *epi*, *thele* + *oma* tumor], a neoplasm derived from the epithelium.

epithelioma adamantinum. See **ameloblastoma.**

epithelioma adenoides cysticum. See **trichoepithelioma.**

epithelium /ep′ithē′lē·əm/ [Gk *epi* + *thele* nipple], the covering of the internal and the external organs of the body, including the lining of vessels. It consists of cells bound together by connective material and varies in the number of layers and the kinds of cells. Epithelium in different parts of the body is made of simple squamous cells, simple cuboidal cells, and stratified columnar cells. **–epithelial,** *adj.*

epitope /ep′itōp/ [Gk *epi* + *topos* place], an antigenic determinant that causes a specific reaction by an immunoglobulin. It consists of a group of amino acids on the surface of the antigen.

epitympanic recess /ep′itimpan′ik/ [Gk *epi* + *tympanon* drum], a recess cranial to the tympanic membrane. It contains the upper half of the malleus and greater part of the incus.

epizootic /ep′izō·ot′ik/, a disease or condition that occurs at about the same time in many of the animals of a species in a geographic area.

EPO, abbreviation for **erythropoietin.**

eponychium. See **cuticle.**

eponym /ep′ənim/ [Gk *epi* above, *onyma* name], a name for a disease, organ, procedure, or body function that is derived from the name of a person, usually a physician or scientist who first identified the condition or devised the object bearing the name. Examples include fallopian tube, Parkinson's disease, and Billing's method.

epoophorectomy /ep′ō·of′ərek′təmē/ [Gk *epi* + *oophoron* ovary, *temnein* to cut], surgical removal of the epoophoron.

epoophoron /ep′ō·of′əron/ [Gk *epi* + *oophoron* ovary], a structure that is situated in the mesosalpinx between the ovary and the uterine tube.

epoxy, 1. a prefix for terms relating to epoxide group chemicals. 2. an organic chemical formula formed by the union of an oxygen atom and two other atoms, usually carbon. Epoxy resins are used as bonding agents.

EPSDT, abbreviation for **Early and Periodic Screening Diagnosis and Treatment.**

epsilon /ep′silon/, E, ϵ, the fifth letter of the Greek alphabet.

Epsom salt. See **magnesium sulfate.**

EPSP, abbreviation for *excitatory postsynaptic potential.*

Epstein-Barr virus (EBV) /ep′stīnbär′/ [Michael A. Epstein, English pathologist, b. 1921; Yvonne M. Barr, twentieth-century English virologist; L *virus* poison], the herpesvirus that causes infectious mononucleosis.

Epstein's pearls [Alois Epstein, Czechoslovakian physician, b. 1849; L *perla* a mussel], small, white, pearl-like epithelial cysts that occur on both sides of the midline of the hard palate of the newborn baby.

e.p.t., a trademark for a human pregnancy test kit using monoclonal antibody technology to detect the presence of human chorionic gonadotropin (HCG) in urine.

epulis /epyōō′lis/, *pl.* **epulides** [Gk *epi* + *oulon* gum], any tumor or growth on the gingiva.

equal cleavage [L *aequare* to make alike; AS *cleofan*], mitotic division of the fertilized ovum into blastomeres of identical size, such as occurs in humans and most mammals.

Equal Employment Opportunity Commission (EEOC), a commission appointed by the President of the United States to administer the Civil Rights Act of 1964, particularly to investigate complaints of discrimination in employment in businesses engaged in interstate commerce. Discrimination based on race, color, creed, or national origin is forbidden; but certain kinds of employers and certain conditions of employment allow exceptions to the act.

equatorial plate [L *aequare* to make alike; Fr *flat vessel*], the platelike configuration formed by the chromosomes at the center of the spindle during the metaphase stage of mitosis and meiosis.

equianalgesic dose, a dose of one analgesic that is equivalent in pain-relieving effects to another analgesic, permitting the substitution of medications in order to avoid possible adverse effects of one of the drugs. The term is also applied to equivalent alternative dose sizes and routes of administration.

equilibration /ē'kwilibrā'shən/ [L *aequus* equal, *libra* balance], the balancing and integrating of new experiences with those of the past in the psychologic development of an individual.

equilibrium /ā'kwilib'rē·əm/ [L *aequilibrium*], **1.** a state of balance or rest resulting from the equal action of opposing forces, such as calcium and phosphorus in the body. **2.** (in psychiatry) a state of mental or emotional balance. **3.** (in radiotherapy) a point at which the rate of production of a daughter element is equal to the rate of decay of the parent element and the activities of parent and daughter are identical.

equilibrium reaction, any of several reflexes that enable the body to recover balance.

equine encephalitis /ē'kwīn, ek'wīn/ [L *equinus* horse; Gk *enkephalon* brain, *itis* inflammation], an arbovirus infection, characterized by inflammation of the nerve tissues of the brain and spinal cord, with high fever, headache, nausea, vomiting, myalgia, and neurologic symptoms, such as visual disturbances, tremor, lethargy, and disorientation. The virus is transmitted by the bite of an infected mosquito. Horses are the primary host of the viruses. **Eastern equine encephalitis (EEE)** is a severe form of the infection. It occurs along the eastern seaboard of the United States and lasts longer and causes more deaths and residual morbidity than **western equine encephalitis (WEE),** which occurs throughout the United States and results in a mild, brief illness, as does **Venezuelan equine encephalitis (VEE),** which is common in Central and South America, Florida, and Texas.

equine gait [L *equus* horse; ONorse *gata* a way], a manner of walking characterized by drop foot. The condition is the result of damage to the peroneal nerve, causing the foot to hang in a toes-downward position.

equinus /ēkwī'nəs/ [L, horse], a condition characterized by tiptoe walking on one or both feet. It is usually associated with clubfoot.

equivalent weight [L *aequus* equal, *valere* value; AS *gewiht*], **1.** the weight of an element in any given unit (such as grams) that will displace a unit weight of hydrogen from a compound or combine with or replace a unit weight of hydrogen. **2.** the weight of an acid or base that will produce or react with 1.008 grams of hydrogen ion. **3.** the weight of an oxidizing or reducing agent that will produce or accept one electron in a chemical reaction.

equivocal symptom [L *aequus* + *vocare* to

call; Gk *symptoma* that which happens], a symptom that may be attributed to more than one cause or that may occur in several diseases.

Er, symbol for the chemical element **erbium.**

ER, abbreviation for **emergency room.**

Erb-Duchenne paralysis. See **Erb's palsy.**

erbium (Er) /ur'bē·əm/ [Ytterby, Sweden], a rare-earth, metallic element. Its atomic number is 68; its atomic weight is 167.26.

Erb's muscular dystrophy [Wilhelm H. Erb, German neurologist, b. 1840], a form of muscular dystrophy that first affects the shoulder girdle and later often involves the pelvic girdle. It is a progressively crippling disease.

Erb's palsy [Wilhelm H. Erb], a kind of paralysis caused by traumatic injury to the upper brachial plexus. It occurs most commonly in childbirth from forcible traction during delivery, with injury to one or more cervical nerve roots.

Erb's point, a landmark of the brachial plexus on the upper trunk, located about 1 inch (2.5 cm) above the clavicle at about the level of the sixth cervical vertebra.

erectile /irek'til, -tīl/ [L *erigere* to erect], capable of being erected or raised to an erect position. The term is usually applied in the description of spongy tissue of the penis or clitoris that becomes turgid and erectile when filled with blood.

erectile myxoma, an angioma that contains areas of myxomatous tissue.

erection /irek'shən/ [L *erigere* to erect], the condition of hardness, swelling, and elevation observed in the penis and to a lesser degree in the clitoris, usually caused by sexual arousal but also occurring during sleep or as a result of physical stimulation. It is needed to enable the penis to enter the vagina and to emit semen.

erector spinae. See **sacrospinalis.**

erector spinae reflex [L *erigere* to erect, *spina* spine, *reflectere* to bend back], a reflex characterized by contraction of the sacrospinalis and other back muscles when the overlying skin is stimulated.

erg /urg, erg/, a unit of energy in the CGS (centimeter-gram-second) system equal to the work done by a force of 1 dyne through a distance of 1 cm.

ergastoplasm [Gk *ergaster* worker, *plassein* to mold], a network of cytoplasmic structures that show basophilic staining properties; granular endoplasmic reticulum.

ergocalciferol. See **calciferol.**

ergoloid mesylates /ur'gōloid/, an adrenergic with psychotropic actions. It is prescribed in the treatment of symptomatic decline in mental capacity for an unknown cause, as in senile dementia.

ergometry /ergom'ətrē/, the study of physical work activity, including work performed by specific muscles or muscle groups. The studies may involve testing with equipment such as stationary bicycles, treadmills, or rowing machines.

ergonomics /ur'gōnom'iks/ [Gk *ergon* work, *nomos* law], a scientific discipline devoted to the study and analysis of human work, especially as it is affected by individual anatomy, psychology, and other human factors. −**ergonomic,** *adj.*

ergonovine maleate /ur'gōnō'vēn/, an oxytocic ergot alkaloid prescribed to contract the uterus in the treatment or prevention of postpartum or postabortion hemorrhage.

ergosome. See **polysome.**

ergosterol /ərgos'tərôl/, an unsaturated hydrocarbon of the vitamin D group isolated from yeast, mushrooms, ergot, and other fungi. When treated with ultraviolet irradiation it is converted into vitamin D_2.

ergot /ur'gət/ [L *ergota* a plant disease], (in pharmacology) the food storage body of a fungus, *Claviceps purpurea,* which commonly infects rye and other cereal grasses. It contains ergot alkaloids.

ergot alkaloid, one of a large group of alkaloids derived from a common fungus, *Claviceps purpurea,* that grows on rye and other grains throughout the temperate areas of the world. The alkaloids are divided into three groups: the amino acid alkaloids, typified by ergotamine; the dihydrogenated amino acid alkaloids, such as dihydroergotamine; and the amine alkaloids, such as ergonovine.

ergotamine tartrate /ərgot'əmēn/, a vasoconstrictor and oxytocic prescribed in the treatment of migraine and postpartum uterine atony.

ergotherapy /ur'gōther'[ə]pē/ [Gk *ergon* work, *therapeia* treatment], the use of physical activity and exercise in the treatment of disease. By extension, the therapy includes any procedure that increases the blood supply to a diseased or injured part, such as massage or various types of hot baths. −**ergotherapeutic,** *adj.*

ergotism /ur'gətiz'əm/ [Fr *argot* a grain fungus], **1.** an acute or chronic disease caused by excessive dosages of medications containing ergot. Symptoms may include cerebrospinal symptoms such as spasms, cramps, and dry gangrene. **2.** a chronic disease caused by eating cereal products made with rye flour contaminated by ergot fungus.

ergot poisoning, the toxic effects of in-

gesting food or medications containing ergot alkaloids, particularly ergotamine.

ergotropic, /ur'gōtrop'ik/ **1.** pertaining to an activity or work state involving somatic muscle, sympathetic nervous system, and cortical alpha rhythm activity. **2.** pertaining to the administration of medications or other therapies to energize the power of the body's blood and other tissues to resist infections.

erogenous /iroj'ənəs/ [Gk *eros* love, *genein* to produce], pertaining to the production of erotic sensations or sexual excitement.

erogenous zones, areas of the body in which sexual tension tends to become concentrated and can be relieved by manipulation of the region. The areas include the mouth, anus, and genitals.

Eros /ir'os, er'os/ [Gk, mythic love-inciting son of Aphrodite], a Freudian term for the drive or instinct for survival, including self-preservation and survival of the species through reproduction.

erosion [L *erodere* to consume], the wearing away or gradual destruction of a surface, such as a mucosal or epidermal surface as a result of inflammation, injury, or other effects.

erosive gastritis, an inflammatory condition characterized by multiple erosions of the mucous membrane lining the stomach.

erosive osteoarthritis. See **Kellgren's syndrome.**

eroticism /irot'isiz'əm/ [Gk *erotikos* sexual love], 1. sexual impulse or desire. **2.** the arousal or attempt to arouse the sexual instinct through suggestive or symbolic means. **3.** the expression of sexual instinct or desire. **4.** an abnormally persistent sexual drive.

erratic [L *erraticus* wandering], deviating from the normal but with no apparent fixed course or purpose.

error [L *errare* to wander], (in research) a defect in the design of a study, in the development of measurements or instruments, or in the interpretation of the findings.

ERT, abbreviation for **external radiation therapy.**

erucic acid /erōō'sik/, a fatty acid that has been associated with heart disease. It is present in rapeseed oil and is used in some countries as a vegetable oil for salad dressings, margarines, and mayonnaise.

eructation /ē'ruktā'ən/ [L *eructare* to belch], the act of bringing up air from the stomach with a characteristic sound.

eruption [L *eruptio* bursting forth], the rapid development of a skin lesion, especially of a viral exanthem or of the rash commonly accompanying a drug reaction.

eruptive fever [L *eruptio* bursting forth;

febris], any disease characterized by fever and a rash.

eruptive gingivitis, a gingival inflammation that may occur concurrently with the eruption of the permanent teeth.

eruptive xanthoma, a skin disorder associated with elevated triglyceride levels in the blood. Erythematous or pale raised papules suddenly appear in large numbers.

ERV, abbreviation for **expiratory reserve volume.**

erysipelas /er′isip′ələs/ [Gk *erythros* red, *pella* skin], an infectious skin disease characterized by redness, swelling, vesicles, bullae, fever, pain, and lymphadenopathy.

erysipeloid /er′isip′əloid/ [Gk *erhthros, pella + eidos* form], an infection of the hands characterized by blue-red nodules or patches and, occasionally, by erythema. It is acquired by handling meat or fish infected with *Erysipelothrix rhusiopathiae.*

erythema /er′ithē′mə/ [Gk *erythros* red], redness or inflammation of the skin or mucous membranes that is the result of dilatation and congestion of superficial capillaries. Examples of erythema are nervous blushes and mild sunburn. **–erythematous,** *adj.*

erythema chronicum migrans (ECM), a skin lesion that begins as a small papule and spreads peripherally, extending by a raised, red margin and clearing in the center. It marks the site of a deer tick bite, and is a diagnostic sign of **Lyme disease.**

erythema infectiosum, an acute, benign infectious disease, mainly of children, characterized by fever and an erythematous rash beginning on the cheeks and appearing later on the arms, thighs, buttocks, and trunk.

erythema marginatum, a variant of **erythema multiforme** seen in acute rheumatic fever, characterized by transient, disk-shaped, nonpruritic, reddened macules that fade in the center, leaving raised margins.

erythema multiforme /mul′tifôr′mē, mōōl′-tēfôr′mä/, a hypersensitivity syndrome characterized by polymorphous eruption of skin and mucous membranes. Macules, papules, nodules, vesicles or bullae, and target, or bull's-eye-shaped, lesions are seen. A severe form of this condition is known as **Stevens-Johnson syndrome.**

erythema neonatorum, a common skin condition of neonates characterized by a pink papular rash frequently superimposed with vesicles or pustules. The rash appears within 48 hours after birth, covers the thorax, abdomen, back, and diaper area, and disappears after several days.

erythema nodosum, a hypersensitivity vasculitis characterized by bilateral, reddened, tender, subcutaneous nodules on the shins and, occasionally, on other parts of the body. The nodules may be seen with streptococcal infections, tuberculosis, sarcoidosis, drug sensitivity, ulcerative colitis, and pregnancy.

erythema perstans, a persistent local redness of the skin, often caused by a fixed-combination drug eruption.

erythematous eczema /er′ithem′ətəs/ [Gk *erythema* redness, *ekzein* to boil over], a scaly red skin eruption frequently accompanied by edema.

erythematous pemphigus [Gk *erythema, pemphix* bubble], a type of skin eruption characterized by bullous eruptions on the trunk and a facial eruption that resembles lupus erythematosus. The condition may be accompanied by sebhorrheic dermatitis.

erythralgia /er′ithral′jə/ [Gk *erythema + algos* pain], a skin disorder characterized by a painful burning sensation, raised skin temperature, and redness, generally of the lower limbs.

erythrasma /er′ithraz′mə/ [Gk *erythros* red], a bacterial skin infection of the axillary or inguinal regions, characterized by irregular, reddish brown, raised patches.

erythremia /er′ithrē′mē·ə/ [Gk *erythros + haima* blood], an abnormal increase in the number of red blood cells.

erythrityl tetranitrate, /erith′rĭtil/ a coronary vasodilator prescribed in the treatment of angina pectoris.

erythroblast /erith′rəblast′/, an immature form of a red blood cell. It is normally found only in bone marrow.

erythroblastoma /erith′rōblastō′mə [Gk *erythros + blastos* germ, *oma* tumor], a myeloma tumor (osteolytic neoplasm) in which the cells resemble erythroblasts.

erythroblastosis fetalis /erith′rōblastō′sis/ [Gk *erythros + blastos* germ, *osis* condition; L *fetus* bringing forth], a type of hemolytic anemia that occurs in newborns as a result of maternal-fetal blood group incompatibility, specifically involving the Rh factor and the ABO blood groups. The condition is caused by an antigen-antibody reaction in the bloodstream of the infant resulting from the placental transmission of maternally formed antibodies against the incompatible antigens of the fetal blood. In Rh factor incompatibility, the hemolytic reaction occurs only when the mother is Rh negative and the infant is Rh positive. The isoimmunization process rarely occurs with the first pregnancy, but there is increased risk with each succeeding pregnancy.

erythrocyte /erith´rəsīt´/ [Gk *erythros* + *kytos* cell], the major cellular element of the circulating blood; a reddish biconcave disk about 7 μm in diameter that contains hemoglobin confined within a lipoid membrane. Its principal function is to transport oxygen. Erythrocytes originate in the marrow of the long bones. Maturation proceeds from a stem cell (promegaloblast) through the pronormoblast stage to the normoblast, the last stage before the mature adult cell develops. Kinds of erythrocytes include **burr cell, discocyte, macrocyte, meniscocyte,** and **spherocyte.**

erythrocyte sedimentation rate (ESR), the rate at which red blood cells settle out in a tube of unclotted blood, expressed in millimeters per hour. Blood is collected in an anticoagulant and allowed to form a sediment in a calibrated glass column.

erythrocythemia /erith´rōsīthē´mē-ə/ [Gk *erythros, kytos* + *haima* blood], an increase in the number of erythrocytes circulating in the blood.

erythrocytopenia /erith´rōsī´təpē´nē-ə/ [Gk *erythros* + *kytos* + *penes* poor], a condition characterized by a deficiency of erythrocytes.

erythrocytosis /erith´rōsītō´sis/ [Gk *erythros, kytos* + *osis* condition], an abnormal increase in the number of circulating red cells.

erythroderma /erith´rōdur´mə/ [Gk *erythros* + *derma* skin], any dermatosis associated with abnormal redness of the skin.

erythroleukemia /erith´rōl ook´mē-ə/ [Gk *erythros* + *leukos* white, *haima* blood], a malignant blood disorder characterized by a proliferation of erythropoietic elements in bone marrow, erythroblasts with bizarre lobulated nuclei, and abnormal myeloblasts in peripheral blood. The disease may have an acute or chronic course.

erythromelalgia /erith´rōmilal´jə/ [Gk *erythros* + *melos* limb, *algos* pain], a rare disorder characterized by a paroxysmal dilatation of the peripheral blood vessels. **–erythromelalgic,** *adj.*

erythromycin /erith´rōmī´sin/, an antibacterial antibiotic prescribed in the treatment of many bacterial and mycoplasmic infections, particularly infections that cannot be treated with penicillins.

erythromyeloblastic leukemia. See **erythroleukemia.**

erythrophobia /erith´rōfō´bē-ə/ [Gk *erythros* + *phobos* fear], **1.** an anxiety disorder characterized by an irrational fear of blushing or of displaying embarrassment. **2.** a neurotic symptom manifested by blushing at the slightest provocation. **3.** a morbid fear of or aversion to the color red. **–erythrophobic,** *adj.*

erythroplasia of Queyrat /erith´rōplā´zhə/ [Gk *erythros* + *plasis* forming; Auguste Queyrat, French dermatologist, b. 1872], a premalignant lesion on the glans or corona of the penis. It is a well-circumscribed reddish patch.

erythropoiesis /erith´rōpō-ē´sis/ [Gk *erythros* + *poiein* to make], the process of erythrocyte production involving the maturation of a nucleated precursor into a hemoglobin-filled, nucleus-free erythrocyte that is regulated by erythropoietin, a hormone produced by the kidney. **–erythropoietic,** *adj.*

erythropoietic porphyria. See **porphyria.**

erythropoietin (EPO) /erith´rōpō-ē´tin/ [Gk *erythros* + *poiein* to make], a glycoprotein hormone synthesized mainly in the kidneys and released into the bloodstream in response to anoxia.

Es, symbol for the chemical element **einsteinium.**

escape beat [ME *escapen* to flee; *beten* to beat], an automatic beat of the heart that occurs after an interval longer than the duration of the dominant heart beat cycle. Escape beats function as safety mechanisms, and anything that produces a pause in the prevailing heart cycle may allow an escape to occur. Some kinds of pauses in which escape beats occur are caused by sinoatrial (SA) block, atrioventricular (AV) block, extrasystole, and the completion of a paroxysm of tachycardia.

escape phenomenon. See **Marcus Gunn pupil sign.**

escape rhythm [OFr *escaper*; Gk *rhythmos* beat], a heart rhythm that occurs when the atrioventricular junction or any ventricular muscle fiber assumes control because the rate set by the sinoatrial node is depressed or blocked, or when the ventricle assumes control because the rate set by the sinus or atrioventricular nodes is depressed or blocked.

eschar /es´kär/ [Gk *eschara* scab], a scab or dry crust resulting from a thermal or chemical burn, infection, or excoriating skin disease. **–escharotic,** *adj.*

escharotomy /es´kärot´əmē/, a surgical incision into necrotic tissue resulting from a severe burn. It is sometimes necessary to prevent edema from building up sufficient interstitial pressure to impair capillary filling and cause ischemia.

Escherichia coli /eshiri´kē-ə kō´lī/ [Theodor Escherich, German physician, b. 1857; Gk *kolon* colon], a species of coliform bacteria of the family Enterobacteriaceae, normally present in the intestines and common in water, milk, and soil. It is the most frequent cause of urinary tract infection and is a serious pathogen in wounds.

escutcheon /eskuch'ən/ [L *scutum* shield], the shieldlike pattern of distribution of pubic hair.

eserine, eserine sulfate. See **physostigmine.**

Esmarch's bandage /es'märks/ [Johann F. A. von Esmarch, German surgeon, b. 1823], a broad, flat, elastic bandage wrapped around an elevated limb to force blood out of the limb. It is used before certain surgical procedures to create a blood-free field.

ESO, abbreviation for **electric spinal orthosis.**

esophageal atresia /əsof'əjē'əl, es'ofā'jē·əl/ [Gk *oisophagos* gullet], an abnormal esophagus that ends in a blind pouch or narrows to a thin cord and thus fails to provide a continuous passage to the stomach.

esophageal cancer, a malignant neoplastic disease of the esophagus. Risk factors associated with the disease are heavy consumption of alcohol, smoking, betel-nut chewing, Plummer-Vinson syndrome, hiatus hernia, and achalasia. Esophageal cancer does not often cause any symptoms in the early stages but in later stages causes painful dysphagia, anorexia, weight loss, regurgitation, cervical adenopathy, and, in some cases, a persistent cough. Left vocal cord paralysis and hemoptysis indicate an advanced state of the disease.

esophageal dysfunction, any disturbance, impairment, or abnormality that interferes with the normal functioning of the esophagus, such as dysphagia, esophagitis, or sphincter incompetence. The condition is one of the primary symptoms of scleroderma.

esophageal lead, 1. an electrocardiographic conductor in which the exploring electrode is placed within the lumen of the esophagus. It is used to identify cardiac arrhythmias. **2.** *informal;* a tracing produced by such a lead on an electrocardiograph.

esophageal obturator airway, an emergency airway device that consists of a large tube that is inserted into the mouth through an airtight face mask. Because of the design, air passes only into the trachea.

esophageal speech [Gk *oisophagos* gullet; AS *spaec*], alaryngeal sounds made by forcing air in and out of the esophagus, causing it to vibrate. It may be produced by a number of methods.

esophageal varices, a complex of longitudinal, tortuous veins at the lower end of the esophagus, enlarged and swollen as the result of portal hypertension.

esophageal web, a thin membrane that may develop across the lumen of the esophagus, usually near the level of the cricoid cartilage, and associated with iron-deficiency anemia.

esophagectomy /esof'əjek'təmē/ [Gk *oisophagos* + *ektome* excision], a surgical procedure in which all or part of the esophagus is removed, as may be required to treat severe, recurrent, bleeding esophageal varices.

esophagitis /esof'əjī'tis/ [Gk *oisophagos* + *itis*], inflammation of the mucosal lining of the esophagus, caused by infection, irritation from a nasogastric tube, or backflow of gastric juice from the stomach.

esophagogastroscopy /esof'əgōgastros'kəpē/ [Gk *oisophagos* + *gaster* stomach, *skopein* to watch] the examination of the esophagus and stomach using an endoscope.

esophagogastrostomy [Gk *oisophagos* gullet, *gaster* stomach, *stoma* mouth], the surgical creation of a passage between the esophagus and the stomach.

esophagojejunostomy /esof'əgōjijj'-ōōnos'təmē/ [Gk *oisophagos*; L *jejunum* empty, *stoma* mouth], the surgical creation of a direct passage from the esophagus to the jejunum, bypassing the stomach. The procedure is used after total gastrectomy.

esophagoscopy /esof'əgos'kəpē/ [Gk *oisophagos* + *skopein* to look], examination of the esophagus with an endoscope.

esophagospasm /esof'əgōspaz'əm/ [Gk *oisophagos* + *spasmos*], spasmodic contractions of the walls of the esophagus.

esophagus /esof'əgəs/ [Gk *oisophagos*], the muscular canal, about 24 cm long, extending from the pharynx to the stomach. It is the narrowest part of the digestive tube and is most constricted at its commencement and at the point where it passes through the diaphragm. It is composed of a fibrous coat, a muscular coat, and a submucous coat and is lined with mucous membrane. **–esophageal,** *adj.*

esophoria /es'əfôr'ē·ə/ [Gk *eso* inward, *pherein* to bear], deviation of the visual axis of one eye toward that of the other eye in the absence of visual stimuli for fusion. **–esophoric,** *adj.*

esotropia /es'ətrō'pē·ə/ [Gk *eso* + *tropos* turning], a kind of strabismus characterized by an inward deviation of one eye relative to the other eye. **–esotropic,** *adj.*

ESP, abbreviation for **extrasensory perception.**

espundia /espun'dē·ə/ [Sp, cancerous ulcer], a cutaneous form of American leishmaniasis. The primary lesion often disappears spontaneously followed by mucocutaneous lesions that destroy the mucosal surface of the nose, pharynx, and larynx.

ESR, abbreviation for **erythrocyte sedimentation rate.**

essential amino acid [L *essentia* quality], an organic compound not synthesized in the body that is essential for nitrogen equilibrium in adults and optimal growth in infants and children. Adults require isoleucine, leucine, lysine, methionine, phenylalanine, threonine, tryptophan, and valine. Infants need these eight amino acids plus arginine and histidine. Cysteine and tyrosine, limited substitutes respectively for methionine and phenylalanine, are considered quasi-essential.

essential fatty acid (EFA), a polyunsaturated acid, as linoleic, linolenic, and arachidonic, essential in the diet for the proper growth, maintenance, and functioning of the body. A deficiency of essential fatty acids causes changes in cell structure and enzyme function resulting in decreased growth and other disorders. Symptoms include brittle and lusterless hair, nail problems, dandruff, allergic conditions, and dermatoses, especially eczema in infants.

essential fever, any fever of unknown origin.

essential hypertension, an elevated systemic arterial pressure for which no cause can be found and which is often the only significant clinical finding. Elevated blood pressure is always considered a risk, and individuals with elevated pressures are at risk for cardiovascular disease.

essential nutrient, the carbohydrates, proteins, fats, minerals, and vitamins necessary for growth, normal function, and body maintenance.

essential pruritis [L *essentia* quality, *prurire* to itch], localized or general pruritis that begins without any previous skin disorder.

essential tachycardia [L *essentia*; Gk *tachys* fast + *kardia* heart], a heart rhythm with a consistently excessive rate despite the absence of an organic cause for the abnormality.

essential thrombocythemia. See **thrombocytosis.**

essential tremor, an involuntary fine shaking of the hand, the head, and the face, especially during routine movements of the body. The cause is believed to involve the central nervous system. Essential tremor is aggravated by activity and emotion.

essential vertigo [L *essentia* + *vertigo* diz-ziness], a form of vertigo for which no organic cause has been found.

EST, abbreviation for **electric shock therapy.**

established name, the name assigned to a drug by the U.S. Adopted Names Council. The established name, generally shorter than the chemical name, is the name by which the drug is known to health practitioners.

ester /es'tər/ [Gk *aither* air; Ger *Saure* acid], a class of chemical compounds formed by the bonding of an alcohol and one or more organic acids. Fats are esters, formed by the bonding of fatty acids with the alcohol glycerol.

esterase, /es'tərās/ any enzyme that splits esters.

ester-compound local anesthetic, any one of four potent local anesthetics slightly different in chemical structure from the amide group of local anesthetics. Kinds of ester-compound local anesthetics are **chloroprocaine, cocaine hydrochloride,** and **procaine hydrochloride.**

esterified estrogen /ester'ifīd/, an ester of natural estrogen prescribed in the treatment of menstrual irregularities, contraception, and menopausal symptoms.

esthetics, [Gk *aisthetikos* sensitivity], a branch of philosophy dealing with the forms and psychologic effects of beauty. In medicine, esthetics may be applied to dental reconstruction and plastic surgery.

estradiol /es'trɑdī'ôl/, the most potent naturally occurring human estrogen, also found in hog ovaries and in the urine of pregnant mares.

estramustine phosphate sodium /es'trɑmus'tēn/, an antineoplastic agent prescribed for metastatic or progressive carcinoma of the prostate.

estrangement [L *extraneus* not belonging], a psychologic effect caused by the required separation of a mother from her newborn child when the infant is ill, premature, or has a congenital defect, thereby diverting the mother from establishment of a normal relationship with her child.

estriol /es'trē·ôl/, a relatively weak, naturally occurring human estrogen found in high concentrations in urine.

estrogen /es'trojən/ [Gk *oistros* gadfly, *genein* to produce], one of a group of hormonal steroid compounds that promote the development of female secondary sex characteristics. Human estrogen is elaborated in the ovaries, adrenal cortices, testes, and fetoplacental unit. During the menstrual cycle estrogen renders the female genital tract suitable for fertilization, implantation, and nutrition of the early embryo. Kinds of estrogen are **conjugated**

estrogen, esterified estrogen, estradiol, estriol, and **estrone.** —**estrogenic,** *adj.*

estrone /es'trōn/, a relatively potent estrogen. It is prescribed in the treatment of menstrual cycle irregularities, prostatic cancer, and menopausal vasomotor symptoms, and to prevent pregnancy.

estropipate /es'trəpip'āt/, an estrogen prescribed in the treatment of vasomotor symptoms of menopause, atrophic vaginitis, kraurosis vulvae, female hypogonadism, female castration, and primary ovarian failure.

estrus /es'trəs/, the cyclic period of sexual activity in mammals other than primates.

estrus cycle [Gk *oistros* gadfly, *kyklos* circle], the periodic changes in the female body that occur under the influence of sex hormones.

ESWL, abbreviation for **extracorporeal shock-wave lithotripsy.**

eta /ē'tə, ā'tə/, the seventh letter of the Greek alphabet.

état criblé /ātä'krēblā'/ [Fr, sievelike state], a condition or state of multiple sievelike perforations in swollen Peyer's patches of the intestine. It is a frequently fatal complication of untreated typhoid fever.

ethacrynate sodium. See **ethacrynic acid.**

ethacrynic acid /eth'əkrin'ik/, a potent diuretic prescribed to relieve the effects of severe edema and hypertension.

ethambutol hydrochloride /eth'əmbyōō'təl/, a tuberculostatic antibiotic prescribed in the treatment of pulmonary tuberculosis.

ethanoic acid. See **acetic acid.**

ethanol, /eth'ənol/ ethyl alcohol.

ethaverine hydrochloride /eth'aver'ēn/, a smooth muscle relaxant prescribed to relieve spasm of the GI or genitourinary tract, arterial vasospasm, and cerebral insufficiency.

ethchlorvynol /ethklôr'vənôl/, a sedative and hypnotic prescribed in the treatment of insomnia.

ethene. See **ethylene.**

ether /ē'thər/ [Gk *aither* air], a nonhalogenated, volatile liquid used as a general anesthetic. Because it provides excellent analgesia and profound muscle relaxation, adjuncts to anesthesia, such as narcotic analgesics and neuromuscular blocking agents, are often unnecessary. It has an irritating, pungent odor, is highly flammable and explosive, and frequently causes postoperative nausea and vomiting. —**ethereal,** *adj.*

ethics /eth'iks/ [Gk *ethikos* moral duty], the science or study of moral values or principles, including ideals of autonomy, beneficence, and justice.

ethinamate /ethin'əmāt/, a sedative prescribed in the treatment of insomnia.

ethinyl estradiol /eth'inil/, an estrogen prescribed in the treatment of postmenopausal breast cancer, menstrual cycle irregularities and prostatic cancer, and hypogonadism, for contraception, and to relieve menopausal vasomotor symptoms.

ethionamide /eth'ē·ənam'īd/, a tuberculostatic antibacterial prescribed for tuberculosis.

ethmoid /eth'moid/ [Gk, *ethmos,* sieve, *eidos,* form], 1. pertaining to the ethmoid bone. 2. something with a large number of sievelike openings.

ethmoidal air cell /ethmoi'dəl/ [Gk *ethmos* sieve, *eidos* form], one of the numerous, small thin-walled cavities in the ethmoid bone of the skull, rimmed by the frontal maxilla, lacrimal, sphenoidal, and palatine bones.

ethmoid bone, the very light and spongy bone at the base of the cranium, forming most of the walls of the superior part of the nasal cavity.

ethnic group, a population of individuals organized around an assumption of common cultural origin.

ethnocentrism /eth'nōsen'trizm/ [Gk *ethnos* nation, *kentron* center], 1. a belief in the inherent superiority of the "race" or group to which one belongs. 2. a proclivity to consider other ethnic groups in terms of one's own racial origins.

ethoheptazine citrate, /eth'ōhep'təzēn/ a nonnarcotic analgesic prescribed to relieve mild to moderate pain.

ethology /ethol'əjē/ [Gk *ethos* character, *logos* science], 1. (in zoology) the scientific study of the behavioral patterns of animals, specifically in their native habitat. 2. (in psychology) the empiric study of human behavior, primarily social customs, manners, and mores. —**ethologic, ethological,** *adj.,* **ethologist,** *n.*

ethopropazine hydrochloride /eth'ōprō'-pəzēn/, a phenothiazine anticholinergic agent prescribed in the treatment of extrapyramidal parkinsonism and other nervous system disorders.

ethosuximide, /eth'ōsuk'simīd/ an anticonvulsant prescribed in the treatment of petit mal epilepsy.

ethotoin /eth'ōtō'in/, an anticonvulsant prescribed in the treatment of grand mal and psychomotor seizures.

ethyl alcohol. See **alcohol.**

ethyl aminobenzoate. See **benzocaine.**

ethyl chloride, a topical anesthetic for short operations. It is prescribed in the treatment of skin irritations and in minor skin surgery. It is highly flammable.

ethylene /eth′ələn/ [Gk *aither* air, *hyle* stuff], a colorless, flammable gas that is lighter than air and has a slightly sweet odor and taste. It was previously used as a general anesthetic, being slightly more potent than nitrous oxide.

ethylenediamine /eth′əlēndi·am′ēn/, a clear, thick liquid having the odor of ammonia. It is used as a solvent, an emulsifier, and a stabilizer with aminophylline injections.

ethylene dibromide (EDB), a volatile liquid used as an insecticide and gasoline additive. It has been found to be a cause of cancer in animals.

ethylene dichloride poisoning, the toxic effects of exposure to ethylene dichloride, a hydrocarbon solvent, diluent, and fumigant, and one of the most abundant of all chlorinated organic chemicals. It is an eye, ear, nose, throat, and skin irritant. Inhalation or ingestion can lead to serious illness or death.

ethylene glycol poisoning, the toxic reaction to ingestion of ethylene glycol or diethylene glycol, chemicals used in automobile antifreeze preparations. Symptoms in mild cases may resemble those of alcohol intoxication but without the breath odor of alcoholic beverages. There also may be vomiting, carpopedal spasm, lumbar pain, renal failure, respiratory distress, convulsions, and coma.

ethylene oxide, a gas used to sterilize surgical instruments and other supplies.

ethylestrenol, an anabolic steroid.

ethylnorepinephrine hydrochloride /eth′ilnôrep′inef′rin/, a bronchodilator prescribed in the treatment of bronchial asthma.

ethyl oxide, a colorless highly volatile liquid solvent similar to diethyl ether. It is widely used in various pharmaceutical processes.

ethynodiol diacetate /eth′inōdī′ôl/, a synthetic progestin derivative.

ethynodiol diacetate and ethinyl estradiol, an oral contraceptive.

ethynodiol diacetate and mestranol, an oral contraceptive.

etidronate disodium /etid′rənāt/, a regulator of calcium metabolism. It is prescribed in the treatment of Paget's disease, for heterotopic ossification caused by injury to the spinal cord, and after total hip replacement.

etiology /ē′tē·ol′əjē/ [Gk *aitia* cause, *logos* science] **1.** the study of all factors that may be involved in the development of a disease, including susceptibility of the patient and the nature of the disease. **2.** the cause of a disease. –**etiologic,** *adj.*

etomidate /etom′idāt/, a hypnotic and short-acting, investigational nonbarbiturate intravenous induction agent for general anesthesia.

etretinate /etret′ināt/, a synthetic derivative of vitamin A used as an oral drug to treat psoriasis. It is prescribed for severe recalcitrant psoriasis, including generalized pustular and erythrodermic psoriasis.

etymology [Gk *etymos* base; L *logos* words], the study of the origin and development of words.

Eu, symbol for the chemical element **europium.**

eubiotics /yōō′bī·ot′iks/ [Gk *eu* well, *bios* life], the science of healthy living.

eucalyptol /yōō′kəlip′tol/, a substance with an aromatic odor obtained from the volatile oil of *Eucalyptus* and used in nasal emollients.

eucaryon. See **eukaryon.**

eucaryosis. See **eukaryosis.**

eucatropine hydrochloride /yōōkat′rəpin/, an ophthalmic anticholinergic prescribed for dilating the pupil in an ophthalmoscopic examination of the eye.

eucholia /yōōkō′lyə/ [Gk *eu* good, *chole* bile], the normal state of the bile as to the quantity secreted and the condition of the constituents.

euchromatin /yōōkrō′mətin/ [Gk *eu* + *chroma* color], that portion of chromosome material that is active in gene expression during cell division. It stains most deeply during mitosis. –**euchromatic,** *adj.*

euchromosome. See **autosome.**

eugamy /yōō′gəmē/ [Gk *eu* + *gamos* marriage], the union of those gametes that contain the same haploid number of chromosomes. –**eugamic,** *adj.*

eugenics /yōōjen′iks/ [Gk *eu* + *genein* to produce], the study of methods for controlling the characteristics of future human populations through selective breeding.

euglobulin /yōōglob′yəlin/ [Gk *eu* + L *globulus* small sphere], a "true" globulin (a protein insoluble in distilled water). This is one of a number of different properties used to classify proteins.

eugnathic anomaly /yōōnath′ik/ [Gk *eu* + *gnathos* jaw; *anomalia* irregularity], (in dentistry) an abnormality of the teeth and their alveolar supports.

eukaryocyte /yōōker′ē·ōsīt′/ [Gk *eu* + *karyon* nut, *kytos* cell], a cell with a true nucleus, found in all higher organisms and in some microorganisms, as amebae, plasmodia, and trypanosomes. Also spelled **eucaryocyte.** –**eukaryotic,** *adj.*

eukaryon /yōōker′ē·on/ [Gk *eu* good,

karyon nut] **1.** a nucleus that is highly complex, organized, and surrounded by a nuclear membrane, usually characteristic of higher organisms. **2.** an organism containing such a nucleus. Also spelled **eucaryon.**

eukaryosis /yoōker'i·ō'sis/ [Gk *eu* + *karyon* nut, *osis* condition], the state of having a highly complex, organized nucleus containing organelles surrounded by a nuclear membrane.

eukaryote /yoōker'ē·ot/ [Gk *eu* + *karyon* nut], an organism having cells that contain a true nucleus. Also spelled **eucaryote. –eukaryotic, eucaryotic,** *adj.*

eunuch /yoō'nək/ [Gk *eune* couch, *echein* to guard], a male whose testicles have been destroyed or removed. If this occurs before puberty, secondary sex characteristics fail to develop.

eunuchoidism /yoō'nəkoidiz'əm/, deficiency of the function of male hormone or of its formation by the testes. The deficiency leads to sterility and to abnormal tallness, small testes, and deficient development of secondary sexual characteristics, libido, and potency.

euphoretic /yoō'fəret'ik/ [Gk *eu* + *pherein* to bear] **1.** (of a substance or event) tending to produce a condition of euphoria. **2.** a substance tending to produce euphoria, as LSD, mescaline, marijuana, and other hallucinogenic drugs.

euphoria /yoōfôr'ē·ə/ [Gk *eu* + *pherein* to bear] **1.** a feeling or state of well-being or elation. **2.** an exaggerated or abnormal sense of physical and emotional well-being not based on reality or truth, disproportionate to its cause, and inappropriate to the situation.

euploid /yoō'ploid/ [Gk *eu* + *ploos* multiple], **1.** of or pertaining to an individual, organism, strain, or cell with a chromosome number that is an exact multiple of the normal, basic haploid number characteristic of the species, as diploid, triploid, tetraploid, or polyploid. **2.** such an individual, organism, strain, or cell.

euploidy /yoō'ploidē/, the state or condition of having a variation in chromosome number that is an exact multiple of the characteristic haploid number.

eupnea /yoōp·nē'ə/ [Gk *eu* + *pnein* to breathe], normal breathing.

European blastomycosis. See **cryptococcosis.**

European typhus. See **epidemic typhus.**

europium (Eu) /yoōrō'pē·əm/ [Europe], a rare-earth, metallic element. Its atomic number is 63; its atomic weight is 151.96.

eustachian tube /yoōstā'shən/ [Bartolomeo Eustachio, Italian anatomist, b. 1520; L *tubus*], a tube lined with mucous membrane that joins the nasopharynx and the tympanic cavity, allowing equalization of the air pressure in the inner ear with atmospheric pressure.

eustress /yoō'stres/, **1.** a positive form of stress. **2.** a balance between selfishness and altruism through which an individual develops the drive and energy to care for others.

euthanasia /yoō'thənā'zhə/ [Gk *eu* + *thanatos* death], deliberately bringing about the death of a person who is suffering from an incurable disease or condition, actively, such as by administering a lethal drug, or passively, by allowing the person to die by withholding treatment.

euthenics /yoōthen'iks/ [Gk *eu* + *tithenai* to place], the science that deals with improvement of the human species through the control of environmental factors, as pollution, malnutrition, disease, and drug abuse.

euthymism /yoōthī'mizm/ [Gk *eu* + *thymos* thyme flowers], the characteristic of normal mood responses.

euthyroid /yoōthī'roid/ [Gk *eu* + *thyreos* oblong shield], pertaining to a normal thyroid gland.

evacuant /ivak'yoō·ənt/ [L *evacuare* to empty], any medicine or other agent that causes an organ to discharge its contents, as an emetic or laxative.

evacuate [L *evacuare* to empty], **1.** to discharge or to remove a substance from a cavity, space, organ, or tract of the body. **2.** a substance discharged or removed from the body. **–evacuation,** *n.*

evagination /ēvaj'inā'shən/, the turning inside-out or protrusion of a body part or organ.

evaluating [L *ex* away, *valare* to be strong], (in five-step nursing process) a category of nursing behavior in which a determination is made and recorded regarding the extent to which the established goals of care have been met. To make this judgment, the nurse estimates the degree of success in meeting the goals, evaluates the implementation of nursing measures, investigates the client's compliance with therapy, and records the client's response to therapy. The nurse evaluates effects of the measures used, the need for change in goals of care, the accuracy of the implementation of nursing measures, and the need for change in the client's environment or in the equipment or procedures used.

evaporated milk, homogenized whole milk from which 50% to 60% of the water content has been evaporated. It is fortified with vitamin D, canned, and sterilized.

evaporation [L *ex* + *vapor* steam], the change of a substance from a solid or liquid state to a gaseous state. The process of evaporation is hastened by an increase in temperature and a decrease in atmospheric pressure. —**evaporate,** *v.*

eventration /ē'vəntrā'shən/, the protrusion of the intestines from the abdomen.

event-related potential (ERP) [L *evenire* to happen; *relatus* carry back; *potentia* power], a type of brain wave that is associated with a response to a specific stimulus, such as a particular wave pattern observed when a patient hears a clicking sound.

eversion /ivur'zhən/, a turning outward or inside-out.

evisceration /ivis'ərā'shən/ [L *ex* + *viscera* entrails], **1.** the removal of the viscera from the abdominal cavity; disembowelment. **2.** the removal of the contents from an organ or an organ from its cavity. **3.** the protrusion of an internal organ through a wound or surgical incision, especially in the abdominal wall. —**eviscerate,** *v.*

evocation /ev'ōkā'shən/ [L *evocare* to call forth], (in embryology) a specific morphogenetic change within a developing embryo that occurs as a result of the action of a single evocator.

evocator /ev'ōkā'tər/ [L *evocare* to call forth], a specific chemical substance or hormone that is emitted from the organizer part of the embryonic tissue and acts as a morphogenetic stimulus in the developing embryo.

evoked potential (EP) [L *evocare* to call forth; *potentia* power], an electrical response in the brainstem or cerebral cortex that is elicited by a specific stimulus. The stimulus may affect the visual, auditory, or somatosensory pathways, producing a characteristic brain wave pattern. Kinds of evoked potentials include **brainstem auditory evoked potential, somatosensory evoked potential,** and **visual evoked potential.**

evoked response audiometry, a method of testing hearing ability at the level of the brainstem and auditory cortex.

evolution [L *evolvere* to roll forth], **1.** a gradual, orderly, and continuous process of change and development from one condition or state to another. **2.** (in genetics) the theory of the origin and propagation of all plant and animal species, including humans, and their development from lower to more complex forms through the natural selection of variants produced through genetic mutations, hybridization, and inbreeding. Kinds of evolution are **convergent, determinant, emergent, organic,**

orthogenic, and **saltatory evolution.** —**evolutionist,** *n.*

evolution of infarction the normal healing process after a myocardial infarction, as shown on successive electrocardiograms.

evulsed tooth. See **avulsed tooth.**

Ewing's sarcoma /yōō'ingz/ [James Ewing, American pathologist, b. 1866], a malignant tumor developing from bone marrow, usually in long bones or the pelvis. It is characterized by pain, swelling, fever, and leukocytosis.

exacerbation /igzas'ərbā'shən/ [L *exacerbare* to provoke], an increase in the seriousness of a disease or disorder as marked by greater intensity in the signs or symptoms of the patient being treated.

exanthema /ig'zanthē'mə/ [Gk, eruption], a skin eruption or rash that may have specific diagnostic features of an infectious disease. Chickenpox, measles, roseola infantum, and rubella are usually characterized by a particular type of exanthema. —**exanthematous,** *adj.*

exanthem subitum. See **roseola infantum.**

excessive sweat [L *excedere* to go out; AS *swaeaten*], perspiration greater than normal for the ambient environment. It is usually a sign of septic fever, pulmonary tuberculosis, hyperthyroidism, chronic renal disease, or malaria. Abnormal sweating of the hands and feet is often a sign of nervous irritability or other emotional stress.

excess mortality [L *excedere* to go out; *mortalis* mortal], a premature death or one that occurs before the average life expectancy for a person of a particular demographic category.

exchange transfusion in the newborn [L *ex* + *cambire* to change], the introduction of whole blood in exchange for 75% to 85% of an infant's circulating blood that is repeatedly withdrawn in small amounts and replaced with equal amounts of donor blood. The procedure is performed to improve the oxygen-carrying capacity of the blood in the treatment of erythroblastosis neonatorum by removing Rh and ABO antibodies, sensitized erythrocytes producing hemolysis, and accumulated bilirubin.

excise /iksīz'/ [L *ex* + *caedere* to cut], to remove completely, as in the surgical excision of the palatine tonsils.

excision [L *ex* + *caedere* to cut], **1.** the process of excising or amputating. **2.** (in molecular genetics) the process by which a genetic element is removed from a strand of DNA.

excitability [L *excitare* to arouse], the property of a cell that enables it to react to irritation or stimulation, such as the reaction of a nerve or myocardial cell to an adequate stimulus.

excitant /eksī′tənt/, a drug or other agent that will arouse the central nervous system or other body system in a particular manner.

excitation, a state of mental or physical excitement; nerve or muscle acting on impulse.

excitatory amino acids, amino acids that affect the central nervous system and may in some cases act as neurotoxins. Examples include glutamate and aspartate.

excited state [L *excitare* to rouse + *status*], in nuclear physics, an energy level of a system that is higher than the ground state. The system will decay to the ground state and emit the energy difference, usually in the form of photons.

excitement, (in psychiatry) a pathologic state marked by emotional intensity, impulsive behavior, anticipation, and arousal. Excitement in schizophrenic patients tends to result from blocked communications and hostile feelings between the patients and the hospital staff.

exciting eye, (in sympathetic ophthalmia) the eye that is primarily affected by an injury or infection in a bilateral disorder.

excoriation /ekskôr′ē-ā′shən/ [L *excoriare* to flay], an injury to the surface of the skin or other part of the body caused by scratching or abrasion.

excreta /ekskrē′tə/ [L *excernere* to separate], any waste matter discharged from the body.

excrete /ekskrēt′/ [L *excernere* to separate], to evacuate a waste substance from the body.

excretion, the process of eliminating, shedding, or getting rid of substances by body organs or tissues, as part of a natural metabolic activity. Excretion usually begins at the cellular level.

excretion urography [L *excernere*; Gk *ouron* urine + *graphein* to record], a radiographic examination in which an opaque medium is introduced and its pathways recorded as it passes through the urinary tract.

excretory /eks′krətôr′ē/ [L *excernere* to separate], relating to the process of excretion, often used in combination with a term to identify an object or procedure associated with excretion, as in **excretory urography.**

excretory duct, a duct that is conductive but not secretory.

excretory urography. See **intravenous pyelography.**

excursion [L *ex* out, *currere* to run], a departure or deviation from a direct or normal course.

executive physical, a physical examination including extensive laboratory, x-ray, and other tests that is provided periodically to management level personnel at employer expense. Such examinations may be detailed, expensive, and overly complete.

exercise [L *exercere* to make strong], **1.** the performance of any physical activity for the purpose of conditioning the body, improving health, or maintaining fitness or as a means of therapy for correcting a deformity or restoring the organs and bodily functions to a state of health. **2.** any action, skill, or maneuver that exerts the muscles and is performed repeatedly to develop or strengthen the body or any of its parts. **3.** to use a muscle or part of the body repetitively to maintain or develop its strength. Kinds of exercise are **active assisted, active, active resistance, aerobic, anaerobic, corrective, isometric, isotonic, muscle-setting, passive, progressive resistance, range of motion,** and **underwater exercise.**

exercise electrocardiogram (exercise ECG), a stress test that is important in the diagnosis of coronary artery disease. An exercise electrocardiogram is recorded as a person walks on a treadmill or pedals a stationary bicycle for a given length of time at a specific rate of speed.

exercise-induced asthma, a form of asthma that produces symptoms after strenuous exercise. The effect may be acute but is reversible.

exercise prescription [L *exercere, prae + scribere* to write], an individualized schedule for physical fitness exercises.

exercise tolerance, the level of physical exertion an individual may be able to perform before reaching a state of exhaustion. Exercise-tolerance tests are commonly performed on a treadmill under the supervision of a health professional who can stop the test when signs of distress are observed.

exertional headache [L *exserere* to stretch out; AS *heafod, acan* headache], an acute headache that occurs during strenuous exercise. It usually recedes when the level of effort is reduced or by taking an analgesic medication, or both.

exfoliation /eksfō′lē-ā′shən/ [L *ex + folium* leaf], peeling and sloughing off of tissue cells. This is a normal process that may be exaggerated in certain skin diseases or after a severe sunburn. **–exfoliative,** *adj.*

exfoliative cytology /eksfō′lē-ətiv/, the microscopic examination of desquamated cells for diagnostic purposes. The cells are obtained from lesions, sputum, secretions, urine, or other material.

exfoliative dermatitis, any inflammatory skin disorder in which there is excessive peeling or shedding of skin.

exhalation. See **expiration.**

exhale /eks·hāl'/ [L *exhalare* to breathe out], to breathe out or to let out with the breath. **–exhalation,** *n.*

exhaustion [L *exhaurire* to drain away], a state of extreme loss of physical or mental abilities caused by fatigue or illness.

exhaustion delirium, a delirium that may result from prolonged physical or emotional stress, fatigue, or shock associated with severe metabolic or nutritional problems.

exhaustion psychosis [L *exhaurire* to drain out; Gk *psyche* mind, *osis* condition], an abnormal mental condition attributed to physical exhaustion. The main symptom, a delirious state, may develop in some explorers, mountain climbers, persons lost in the wilderness, and some terminally ill patients.

exhibitionism [L *exhibere* to hold out], **1.** the flaunting of oneself or one's abilities to attract attention. **2.** (in psychiatry) a psychosexual disorder occurring in men in which the repetitive act of exposing the genitals to unsuspecting women is a means of achieving sexual excitement and gratification. **–exhibitionist,** *n.*

eximer laser /ek'simĭr/, a small laser designed to break up organic molecules, such as cholesterol deposits, without producing intense heat.

existential humanistic psychotherapy, See **humanistic existential therapy.**

existential psychiatry [L *exsistere* to spring forth; Gk *psyche* mind, *iatreia* medical care], a school of psychiatry based on the philosophy of existentialism that emphasizes an analytic, holistic approach in which mental disorders are viewed as deviations within the total structure of an individual's existence rather than as caused by any biologically or culturally related factors.

existential therapy, a kind of psychotherapy that emphasizes the development of a sense of self-direction through choice, awareness, and acceptance of individual responsibility.

exit block [L *exire* to depart; Fr *bloc*], (in cardiology) the failure of an expected impulse to emerge from its focus of origin and cause a contraction.

exit dose, (in radiotherapy) the amount of radiation at the side of the body opposite the surface to which the beam is directed.

exocoelom. See **extraembryonic coelom.**

exocrine /ek'səkrin/ [Gk *exo* outside, *krinein* to secrete], of or pertaining to the process of secreting outwardly through a duct to the surface of an organ or tissue or into a vessel.

exocrine gland, any one of the two kinds of multicellular glands that open on the surface of the skin through ducts in the epithelium, as the sweat glands and the sebaceous glands.

exogenous /igzoj'ənəs/ [Gk *exo* + *genein* to produce] **1.** growing outside the body. **2.** originating outside the body or an organ of the body or produced from external causes, such as a disease caused by a bacterial or viral agent foreign to the body. **–exogenic,** *adj.*

exogenous depression. See **reactive depression.**

exogenous hemochromatosis [Gk *exo* + *genein, haima* blood, *chroma* color, *osis* condition], a condition of bronzed pigmentation of the skin due to accumulation of an iron pigment from excessive intake of iron-rich foods or blood transfusions.

exogenous hypertriglyceridemia. See **hyperlipidemia type I.**

exogenous infection [Gk *exo* + *genein*; L *inficere* to stain], an infection that develops from bacteria normally outside the body that have gained access into the body.

exogenous obesity, obesity caused by a caloric intake greater than needed to meet the metabolic needs of the body.

exogenous uric acid [Gk *exo* + *genein, ouron* urine; L *acidus*], the accumulation of uric acid in the body produced by the metabolism of purine-rich foods.

exon /ek'son/ [Gk *exo* + *genein* to produce], (in molecular genetics) the part of a DNA molecule that produces the code for the final messenger RNA.

exonuclease /ek'sōnoo'klē·ās/ [Gk *exo* + *nucleus* nut; *ase* enzyme], (in molecular genetics) a nuclease that digests DNA or RNA from the ends of the strands.

exophoria /ek'səfôr'ē·ə/ [Gk *exo* + *pherein* to bear], deviation of the visual axis of one eye away from that of the other eye, occurring in the absence of visual stimuli for fusion. **–exophoric,** *adj.*

exophthalmia /ek'softhal'mē·ə/ [Gk *exo* + *ophthalmos* eye], an abnormal condition characterized by a marked protrusion of the eyeballs (**exophthalmos, exophthalmus**), usually resulting from the increased volume of the orbital contents caused by a tumor; swelling associated with cerebral, intraocular, or intraorbital edema or hemorrhage; paralysis of or trauma to the extraocular muscles; or cavernous sinus thrombosis. It may also be caused by endocrine disorders, such as hyperthyroidism and Graves' disease. **–exophthalmic,** *adj.*

exophthalmic goiter /ek´softhal´mik/, exophthalmos occurring in association with goiter, as in Graves' disease.

exophthalmometer /ek´softhalmom´ətər/ [Gk *exo* + *ophthalmos* eye, *metron* measure], an instrument used for measuring the degree of forward displacement of the eye in exophthalmos.

exophthalmos. See **exophthalmia.**

exophthalmos-macroglossia-gigantism syndrome. See **EMG syndrome.**

exophthalmus. See **exophthalmia.**

exophytic /ek´səfit´ik/ [Gk *exo* + *phyton* plant], of, or pertaining to the tendency to grow outward, such as an exophytic tumor that grows on the surface or exterior portion of an organ or structure.

exophytic carcinoma, a malignant, epithelial neoplasm that resembles a papilloma or wart.

exoskeletal prosthesis /ek´səskel´ətəl/ [Gk *exo* + *skeletos* dried up; *prosthesis* addition], a prosthetic device in which support is provided by an outside structure.

exoskeleton /ek´səskel´ətən/ [Gk *exo* + *skeletos* dried up], the hard outer covering of many invertebrates, such as crustaceans, which lacks the bony internal structures of vertebrates.

exostosis /ek´səstō´sis/ [Gk *exo* + *osteon* bone], an abnormal, benign growth on the surface of a bone. **–exostosed, exostotic,** *adj.*

exostosis cartilaginea [Gk *ex* out, *osteon* bone; L *cartilago* cartilage], an outgrowth of cartilage at the ends of long bones.

exoteric /ek´səter´ik/ [Gk *exoterikos* external], pertaining to something outside the organism.

exotoxin /ek´sətok´sin/ [Gk *exo* + *toxikon* poison], a toxin that is secreted or excreted by a living microorganism.

exotropia /ek´sətrō´pē·ə/ [Gk *exo* + *tropos* turning], strabismus characterized by the outward deviation of one eye relative to the other. **–exotropic,** *adj.*

expanded role [L *expandere* to spread out; OFr *rolle* an assumed character], the role of a nurse beyond the traditional limits of nursing practice legislation.

expectant treatment [L *exspectare* to wait for; *tractare* to handle], applying therapeutic measures to relieve symptoms as they arise in the course of a disease rather than treating the cause of the illness itself.

expectation [L *exspectare* to wait for], (in nursing) **1.** anticipation by the staff of a patient's behavior based on a knowledge and understanding of the person's abilities and problems. **2.** anticipation of the performance of the nursing staff, as role expectation.

expectation of life. See **life expectancy.**

expected date of delivery (EDD), the predicted date of a pregnant woman's delivery. Pregnancy lasts approximately 266 days or 38 weeks from the day of fertilization but is considered clinically to last 280 days, or 40 weeks, or 10 lunar months, or 9 1/3 calendar months from the first day of the last menstrual period (LMP).

expectorant /ekspek´tərənt/ [Gk *ex* out, *pectus* breast], **1.** of or pertaining to a substance that promotes the ejection of mucus or other exudates from the lung, bronchi, and trachea. **2.** an agent that promotes expectoration by reducing the viscosity of pulmonary secretions or by decreasing the tenacity with which exudates adhere to the lower respiratory tract. **–expectorate,** *v.*

expectoration /ekspek´tərā´shen/, the ejection of mucus, sputum, or fluids from the trachea and lungs by coughing or spitting.

experience rating [L *experientia* testing; *rata*], a rating system used by an insurance company to set the premium to be paid by the insured, based on the risk to the insurance company of providing the insurance.

experimental design [L *experimentum; designare* to mark out], (in research) a study design used to test cause-and-effect relationships between variables. The classic experimental design specifies an experimental group and a control group. Subsequent experimental designs have used more groups and more measurements over longer periods of time.

experimental embryology, the study and analysis through experimental techniques of the factors, mechanisms, and relationships that determine and influence prenatal development.

experimental epidemiology, a stage of epidemiologic investigation that uses an experimental model for studies to confirm a causal relationship suggested by observational studies.

experimental group. See **group.**

experimental medicine, a branch of the practice of medicine in which new drugs or treatments are evaluated for safety and efficacy in a clinical laboratory setting by using animals or, in certain cases, human subjects.

experimental physiology, a branch of the study of physiology in which the functions of various body systems are evaluated in a clinical laboratory setting by using animals or, in some cases, human subjects.

experimental psychology, the study of

mental processes and phenomena by observation in a controlled environment using various tests, manipulations, and experiments.

experimental variable. See **independent variable.**

expertise [L *experiri* to try], pertaining to special skills or knowledge acquired by a person through education, training, or experience.

expert witness [L *experiri* to try; AS *witnes* knowledge], a person who has special knowledge of a subject about which a court requests testimony.

expiration /ik'spirā'shən/ [L *expirare* to breathe out], **1.** breathing out, normally a passive process, depending on the elastic qualities of lung tissue and the thorax. **2.** termination or death. **–expire,** *v.*

expiratory /ikspī'rətôrē/, pertaining to the expiration of air from the lungs.

expiratory center [L *expirare*; Gk *kentron* center], one of several regions of the medulla responsible for the control of respiration. It is a subregion specifically involved in carrying out the activity of expiration.

expiratory dyspnea, a feeling of discomfort or distress in breathing because of bronchospasms of the bronchioles.

expiratory phase, the portion of the respiratory cycle that involves exhalation. The expiratory phase may be passive or active.

expiratory reserve volume (ERV), the maximum volume of gas that can be expired from the resting expiratory level.

expiratory retard, (in respiratory care) a mode of mechanical ventilation that mimics the prolonged expiratory phase and pursed-lip breathing of emphysema. The method adds some resistance to expiration.

expire /ikspī'ər/ [L *expirare* exhale], **1.** to breathe out. **2.** to die.

expired gas (E), any gas exhaled from the lungs.

exploratory [L *explorare* to search out], pertaining to exploration, as in exploratory surgery.

exploratory operation [L *explorare*; *operari* to work], surgical intervention to find the cause of a disorder by opening a body cavity or organ and examining the interior.

explosive personality [L *ex* out, *plaudere* to clap], behavior characterized by episodes of uncontrolled rage and physical abusiveness in reaction to relatively minor stressors.

explosive speech, abnormal speech characterized by slow, jerky articulation interspersed with the sudden loud enunciation of words, often seen in brain disorders.

exponent /ikspō'nənt/, a superscript on the number 10 used to indicate very large or very small numbers in medical or scientific reports, as in the example 10^6 representing 1,000,000. Exponents also are indicated by prefixes, such as mega and micro.

exposed pulp [L *exponere* to lay out; *pulpa* flesh], dental pulp that becomes exposed to the external environment and potential bacterial infection. Causes include fracture of the crown through trauma or loss of a tooth crown or penetration of the dentin during restorative preparation.

exposure [L *exponere* to lay out], (in radiotherapy) a measure of the ionization of air produced by a beam of radiation. Exposure is defined in coulomb per kilogram of air.

exposure angle, the angle of the arc described by the movement of the x-ray tube and film during tomography.

exposure switch, a control switch that is designed to interrupt the power automatically when pressure by the operator's hand or foot is released. The purpose is to prevent accidental continuing exposure of the patient to radiation.

exposure unit, any of the conventional or SI units used to measure radiation exposure. They include roentgen (R), rad, rem, curie (Ci), gray (Gy), sievert (Sv), and becquerel (Bq).

expression [L *exprimere* to make clear], **1.** the indication of a physical or emotional state through facial appearance or vocal intonation. **2.** the act of pressing or squeezing to expel something, such as milk from the breast after pregnancy or the fetus from the uterus by exerting pressure on the abdominal wall. **3.** (in genetics) the detectable effect or appearance in the phenotype of a particular trait or condition. **–express,** *v.*

expressive aphasia. See **motor aphasia.**

expressivity /eks'presiv'itē/ [L *exprimere* to make clear], (in genetics) the variability with which basic patterns of inheritance are modified, both in degree and in variety, by the effect of a given gene in people of the same genotype.

expulsive stage of labor [L *expellere* to drive out; *stare* stand; *labor* work], the second stage of labor, during which the mother's uterine contractions are accompanied by a bearing-down reflex. It begins after full dilatation of the cervix and continues to the complete delivery of the infant.

exsanguinate /eksang'gwināt/ [L *ex* + *sanguis,* blood], to drain away or deprive an organ of blood.

exsanguination /eksang'gwinā'shən/, a loss of blood.

exsiccant. See **desiccant.**

exsiccate. See **desiccate.**

extended arm. See **reacher.**

extended care facility [L *extendere* to stretch], an institution devoted to providing medical, nursing, or custodial care for an individual over a prolonged time, such as during the course of a chronic disease or during the rehabilitation phase after an acute illness. Kinds of extended care facilities are **intermediate care facility** and **skilled nursing facility.**

extended family, a family group consisting of the biologic parents, their children, the grandparents, and other family members. The extended family is the basic family group in many societies.

extended insulin-zinc suspension, a long-acting insulin that is slowly absorbed and slow to act.

extension [L *extendere* to stretch], a movement allowed by certain joints of the skeleton that increases the angle between two adjoining bones, such as extending the leg, which increases the angle between the femur and the tibia.

extensor /iksten'sər/ [L *extendere*], any muscle that extends a body part, as the **extensor indicis,** which extends the index finger.

extensor carpi radialis brevis [L *extendere* + Gk *karpos* wrist; L *radius* ray, *brevis* short], one of the muscles of the posterior forearm. It functions to extend the hand.

extensor carpi radialis longus, one of the seven superficial muscles of the posterior forearm. It serves to extend and flex the hand radially.

extensor carpi ulnaris, one of the muscles of the lateral forearm. It functions to extend and adduct the hand.

extensor digiti minimi, an extensor muscle of the posterior forearm. It functions to extend the little finger.

extensor digitorum, the principal muscle of the medial digits of the posterior forearm. It functions to extend the phalanges and, by continued action, the wrist.

extensor digitorum longus, a penniform muscle located at the lateral part of the anterior leg. It extends the proximal phalanges of the four small toes and dorsally flexes and pronates the foot.

extensor retinaculum of ankle, either of two thick layers of fascia holding tendons in the ankle. The inferior extensor retinaculum of the ankle is a Y-shaped band of fascia passing medially from the lateral side of the upper surface of the calcaneum and dividing into two bands, one going to the medial malleolus and the other to the plantar aponeurosis. The superior extensor retinaculum consists of thick fascia attached to the lower ends of the tibia and fibula and extending over the tendons of the extensor muscles.

extensor retinaculum of the hand. See **retinaculum extensorum manus.**

extensor retinaculum of wrist, a broad thickening of deep fascia over the back of the wrist, over the extensor tendons.

extensor thrust, a spinal-level reflex present in a human in the first 2 months of life. It is an exaggeration of the positive support reflex and consists of an uncontrolled extension of a flexed leg when the sole of the foot is stimulated.

extern /eks'turn/ [L *externus* outward], a medical or dental student who lives outside the institution but provides medical or dental care to patients as an extracurricular activity under the professional supervision of hospital staff members.

external [L *externus* outward], **1.** being on the outside or exterior of the body or an organ. **2.** acting from the outside, such as an external influence or exogenous factor. **3.** pertaining to the outward or visible appearance.

external abdominal region. See **lateral region.**

external absorption, the taking up of substances through the mucous membranes or the skin.

external acoustic meatus, the canal of the external ear, comprised of bone and cartilage, extending from the auricle to the tympanic membrane.

external aperture of aqueduct of vestibule, an external opening for the small canal extending from the vestibule of the inner ear, located on the internal surface of the petrous part of the temporal bone lateral to the opening for the internal acoustic passage.

external aperture of canaliculus of cochlea, an external opening of the cochlear channel on the margin of the jugular opening in the temporal bone.

external aperture of tympanic canaliculus, the lower opening of the tympanic channel on the inferior surface of the petrous part of the temporal bone.

external auditory canal. See **external acoustic meatus.**

external carotid artery, one of a pair of arteries with eight major temporal or maxillary branches, rising from the common carotid arteries and supplying various parts and tissues of the head and neck.

external carotid plexus, a network of nerves around the external carotid artery, formed by the external carotid nerves from the superior cervical ganglion and supplying sympathetic fibers associated with branches of the external carotid artery.

external cervical os, an external opening of the uterus that leads into the cavity of the cervix.

external conjugate, the distance measured with obstetric calipers from the depression below the lowest lumbar vertebra posteriorly to the upper border of the symphysis anteriorly.

external counterpulsation, (in cardiology) a noninvasive technique for providing counterpulsation by encasing the legs of a patient in a rigid case housing a water-filled bladder. The legs are pressurized by the bladder during diastole to produce counterpulsation.

external cuneiform bone. See **lateral cuneiform bone.**

external ear, the outer structure of the ear, consisting of the auricle and the external acoustic meatus.

external fertilization, the union of male and female gametes outside of the bodies from which they originated, such as occurs in fish and frogs.

external fistula, an abnormal passage between an internal organ or structure and the cutaneous surface of the body.

external fixation, a method of holding together the fragments of a fractured bone by employing transfixing metal pins through the fragments and a compression device attached to the pins outside the skin surface.

external iliac artery, a division of the common iliac artery descending into the thigh and becoming the femoral artery.

external iliac node, a node in one of the seven groups of parietal nodes serving the lymphatic system in the abdomen and the pelvis.

external iliac vein, one of a pair of veins in the lower body that joins the internal iliac vein to form the two common iliac veins.

external jugular vein, one of a pair of large vessels in the neck that receives most of the blood from the exterior of the cranium and the deep tissues of the face. It runs perpendicularly down the neck and joins the subclavian vein lateral or ventral to the scalenus anterior.

external malleolus [L externus outward, malleolus little hammer], a rounded bony prominence on either side of the ankle joint.

external oblique muscle. See **obliquus externus abdominis.**

external pacemaker [L externus, passus step; ME maken to make], **1.** a device used to stimulate the heart beat electrically by the discharge of impulses through the chest wall, as used in emergency care of significant bradyarrhythmias. **2.** a cardiac pacemaker in which the impulse generator is outside the chest but connected with the heart by wires that pass under the skin.

external perimysium. See **epimysium.**

external pterygoid muscle. See **pterygoideus lateralis.**

external radiation therapy (ERT), the therapeutic application of ionizing radiation from an external beam of a kilovoltage x-ray machine, a megavoltage cobalt 60 machine, or a supervoltage linear accelerator, cyclotron, or betatron.

external rotation, turning outwardly or away from the midline of the body, such as when a leg is externally rotated with the toes turned outward or away from the body's midline.

external secretion. See **exocrine glands.**

external shunt, a device for the passage of a body fluid from one compartment of the body to another, consisting of a tube or catheter or a series of such containers that passes over the surface of the body from one compartment or cavity to another.

external version, an obstetric procedure in which a fetus is turned, usually from a breech to a vertex presentation, by external manipulation of the fetus through the wall of the abdomen.

exteroceptive /ek′stərōsep′tiv/ [L externus outside, recipere to receive], pertaining to stimuli that originate from outside of the body or to the sensory receptors that they activate.

exteroceptor /ek′stərōsep′tər/ [L externus outside, recipere to receive], any sensory nerve ending, as those located in the skin, mucous membranes, or sense organs, that responds to stimuli originating from outside of the body, such as touch, pressure, or sound.

extirpation /ek′stərpā′shən/ [L extirpare to root out], the total removal of a diseased organ or body part.

extraarticular /ek′strə·ärtik′yələr/ [L extra outside, articulare to divide into joints], pertaining to the area outside a joint or within the joint but not involving the joint structures.

extra beat, an extra systole; an extra heart contraction.

extracapsular /ek′strəkaps′yələr/ [L extra + capsula little box], pertaining to something outside a capsule, such as the articulare capsule of the knee joint.

extracapsular dendrite [L extra + capsula; Gk dendron tree], pertaining to dendrites of some autonomic nerves that penetrate the boundary of the capsule and extend some distance from the cell body.

extracapsular fracture [L *extra* + *capsula* little box], any fracture that occurs near a joint but does not directly involve the joint capsule. This type of fracture is extremely common in the hip.

extracellular [L *extra* + *cella* storeroom], occurring outside a cell or cell tissue or in cavities or spaces between cell layers or groups of cells.

extracellular fluid (ECF), the portion of the body fluid comprising the interstitial fluid and blood plasma. The adult body contains about 11.2 L of interstitial fluid, constituting about 16% of body weight, and about 2.8 L of plasma, constituting about 4% of body weight.

extracoronal retainer /ek'strəkôr'ənəl/ [L *extra* + *corona* crown; *retinere* to hold] **1.** a kind of dental retainer that incorporates a cast restoration lying largely external to the coronal portion of a tooth and complements the contour of the tooth crown. **2.** a direct clasp-type retainer that engages an abutment tooth on its external surface, used for the retention and stabilization of a removable partial denture. **3.** a manufactured direct retainer, the protruding portion of which is attached to the external surface of a cast crown on an abutment tooth.

extracorporeal /ek'strəkôrpôr'ē·əl/ [L *extra* + *corpus* body], something that is outside the body, such as extracorporeal circulation in which venous blood is diverted outside the body to a heart-lung machine and returned to the body through a femoral or other artery.

extracorporeal membrane oxygenator (ECMO), a device that oxygenates the blood of a patient outside the body and returns the blood to the patient's circulatory system. The technique may be used to support an impaired respiratory system.

extracorporeal oxygenation, the use of an artificial membrane outside the body by which to provide for oxygenation in a patient with severe lung disease.

extracorporeal shock-wave lithotriptor (ESWL) [L *extra* + *corpus*, body; Fr *choc*; AS *wafian*; Gk *lithos* stone, *tribein* to wear away], an apparatus that uses vibrations of powerful sound waves to break up calculi in the urinary tract.

extracranial [L *extra*; Gk *kranion* cranium], pertaining to something outside the skull.

extract [L *ex* out, *trahere* to draw], **1.** a substance, usually a biologically active ingredient of a plant or animal tissue, prepared by the use of solvents or evaporation to separate the substance from the original material. **2.** to remove a tooth from the oral cavity by means of elevators or forceps or both. **–extraction,** *n.*

extractor /ikstrak'tər/, a medical instrument, such as a forceps, used to remove a foreign body, tissue sample, or medical device that had been placed in a body cavity.

extradural /ek'trəd͞oͅo͞r'əl/ [L *extra* + *dura* hard], outside the dura mater.

extradural anesthesia, anesthetic nerve block achieved by the injection of a local anesthetic solution into the space in the spinal canal outside the dura mater of the spinal cord.

extradural hemorrhage, a hemorrhage of an area surrounding but outside of the dura of the brain or spinal cord.

extraembryonic blastoderm /ek'strə·em'brē·on'ik/ [L *extra* + Gk *en* in, *bryein* to grow], the area of the blastoderm outside the embryo that gives rise to the membranes that surround the embryo during gestation.

extraembryonic coelom, a cavity external to the developing embryo that forms between the mesoderm of the chorion and that covering the amniotic cavity and yolk sac.

extraembryonic mesoderm [L *extra*; Gk *en* + *bryein* to grow, *mesos* middle, *derma* skin], any mesoderm development in the uterus that is not involved with the embryo itself. Included are mesoderm in the amnion, chorion, and yolk sac.

extramammary Paget's disease /ek'strəmam'ərē/ [L *extra* + *mamma* breast; James Paget; L *dis*; Fr *aise* ease], a gradually spreading red, scaly, and crusted lesion resembling that of Paget's disease, but not occurring on the breast. A common area is the vulva. The lesions give rise to carcinoma.

extramedullary /ek'strəmed'yələr'ē/ [L *extra* + *medulla* marrow], pertaining to something outside the medulla, particularly the medulla oblongata.

extramedullary myeloma [L *extra* + *medulla* marrow], a plasma cell tumor that occurs outside of the bone marrow, usually affecting the visceral organs or the nasopharyngeal and oral mucosa.

extramedullary myelopoiesis, the formation and development of myeloid tissue outside of the bone marrow.

extraocular /ek'strə·ok'y͞ool͞ər/ [L *extra* + *oculus* eye], outside the eye.

extraocular muscle palsy, an abnormal condition characterized by paralysis of the extrinsic muscles of the eye, such as the superior, inferior, medial, and lateral rectus muscles, and the superior and the inferior oblique muscles.

extraoral anchorage [L *extra* + *oralis*

mouth; *ancora* hook], an orthodontic anchorage outside the mouth, typically linking dental attachments to a wire bow or to hooks extending between the lips and attached by elastic to a cap, a neck strap, or another extraoral device.

extraoral orthodontic appliance /ek′strə-·ôr′əl/, a device secured to a portion of the face, the neck, or the back of the head to deliver traction force to the teeth or jaws for changing the relative postitions of dentitions.

extraperitoneal /ek′strəper′itənē′əl/ [L *extra* + Gk *peri* near, around, *teinein* to stretch], occurring or located outside the peritoneal cavity.

extraperitoneal cesarean section, a method for surgically delivering a baby through an incision in the lower uterine segment without entering the peritoneal cavity. The uterus is approached through the paravesicle space.

extrapsychic conflict [L *extra* + Gk *psyche* mind; L *confligere* to strike together], an emotional conflict usually occurring when one's inner needs and desires do not coincide with the restrictions of the environment or society.

extrapyramidal /ek′strəpiram′ədəl/ [L *extra* + Gk *pyramis* pyramid], **1.** of or pertaining to the tissues and structures outside the cerebrospinal pyramidal tracts of the brain that are associated with movement of the body, excluding motor neurons, the motor cortex, and the corticospinal and corticobulbar tracts. **2.** of or pertaining to the function of these tissues and structures.

extrapyramidal disease, any of a large group of conditions characterized by involuntary movement, changes in muscle tone, and abnormal posture, as in tardive dyskinesia, chorea, athetosis, and Parkinson's disease.

extrapyramidal side effects, side effects caused by drugs that block dopamine receptor sites in the extrapyramidal system tract.

extrapyramidal system, the part of the nervous system that includes the basal ganglia, substantia nigra, subthalamic nucleus, part of the midbrain, and the motor neurons of the spine.

extrapyramidal tracts, the tracts of motor nerves from the brain to the anterior horns of the spinal cord, except for the fibers of the pyramidal tracts. Within the brain, extrapyramidal tracts comprise various relays of motoneurons between motor areas of the cerebral cortex, the basal ganglia, the thalamus, the cerebellum, and the brainstem. The extrapyramidal tracts are functional rather than anatomic units.

extrarenal uremia /ek′strərē′nəl/ [L *extra*

+ *ren* kidney; Gk *ouron* urine + *haima* blood], uremia that may be involved with kidney failure, although the cause is outside the kidney, as in alkalosis from excessive alkali ingestion or severe vomiting.

extrasensory [L *extra* + *sentire* to feel], pertaining to awareness of events that cannot be observed by any of the five basic senses. They include telepathy, clairvoyance, and psychokinesis.

extrasensory perception (ESP) [L *extra* + *sentire* to feel; *percipere* to perceive], alleged awareness or knowledge acquired without using the physical senses.

extrasystole /ek′strəsis′təlē/ [L *extra* + Gk *systole* contraction], cardiac contraction that is abnormal in timing or in origin of impulse with respect to the fundamental rhythm of the heart.

extrauterine /ek′strəyoo̅′tərin/ [L *extra* + *uterus* womb], occurring or located outside the uterus, as an ectopic pregnancy.

extravasation /ikstrav′əsā′shən/ [L *extra* + *vas* vessel], a passage or escape into the tissues, usually of blood, serum, or lymph. **–extravasate,** *v.*

extravascular fluid [L *extra* + *vasculum* small vessel, *fluere* to flow], fluids in the body that are outside the blood vessels. Examples include lymph and cerebrospinal fluid.

extraventricular hydrocephalus. See **hydrocephalus.**

extraversion. See **extroversion.**

extremity [L *extremitas*], an arm or a leg. The arm may be identified as an upper extremity and the leg as a lower extremity.

extrinsic /ikstrin′sik/ [L *extrinsecus* on the outside], pertaining to anything external or originating outside a structure or organism, including parts of an organ that are not wholly contained within it, as an extrinsic muscle.

extrinsic allergic alveolitis. See **hypersensitivity pneumonitis.**

extrinsic allergic pneumonia. See **diffuse hypersensitivity pneumonia.**

extrinsic asthma. See **allergic asthma.**

extrinsic factor. See **cyanocobalamin.**

extrinsic muscles (em), **1.** muscles that are outside the organ they control, as the extraocular muscles that control eye movements. **2.** muscles that link a limb to the trunk of the body.

extroversion [L *extra* + *vertere* to turn], **1.** the tendency to direct one's interests and energies toward external values or things outside the self. **2.** the state of being totally or primarily concerned with what is outside the self.

extrovert, 1. a person whose interests are directed away from the self and concerned primarily with external reality and the physical environment rather than with inner feelings and thoughts. **2.** a person characterized by extroversion.

extroverted personality [L *extra* + *vertere* to turn, *personalis* of a person], a persona that is directed to a greater degree toward the outer world of people and events rather than the subjective inner world experience.

extrusion reflex /ekstrōō′zhən/ [L *extrudere* to push out; *reflectere* to bend backward], a normal response in infants to force the tongue outward when touched or depressed. The reflex begins to disappear by about 3 or 4 months of age.

extubation /eks′t(y)ōōbā′shən/ [L *ex* out, *tuba* tube], the process of withdrawing a tube from an orifice or cavity of the body. **–extubate,** *v.*

exuberant callus. See **heterotopic ossification.**

exudate /eks′yōōdāt/ [L *exsudare* to sweat out], fluid, cells, or other substances that have been slowly exuded, or discharged, from cells or blood vessels through small pores or breaks in cell membranes.

exudation /eks′yədā′shən/ [L *exsudare* the discharge of fluid, pus, or serum. The exudate may or may not contain fibrous or coagulated material.

exudative /igzōō′dətiv/, relating to the exudation or oozing of fluid and other materials from cells and tissues, usually as a result of inflammation or injury.

exudative angina. See **croup.**

exudative enteropathy, diarrhea seen in diseases characterized by inflammation or destruction of intestinal mucosa.

exudative inflammation [L *exudare* to sweat out, *inflammare* to set afire], an inflammation of a serous or raw cavity in which fluid is being released from the inflamed surface.

eye [AS *eage*], one of a pair of organs of sight, contained in a bony orbit at the front of the skull, embedded in orbital fat and innervated by one of a pair of optic nerves from the forebrain. Two internal cavities are separated by the crystalline lens. The cavity anterior to the lens is divided by the iris into two chambers, both filled with aqueous humor. The posterior chamber is larger than the anterior chamber and contains the jellylike vitreous body. The outside tunic of the bulb consists of the transparent cornea anteriorly and the opaque sclera posteriorly. The internal tunic of nervous tissue is the retina. Light waves passing through the lens strike a layer of rods and cones in the retina creating impulses that are transmitted by the optic nerve to the brain.

eye bank [AS *éage*; It *banca* bench], a facility for collecting and storing corneas of eyes for transplantation to recipients.

eyebrow [AS *eage* + *bru*], **1.** the supraorbital arch of the frontal bone that separates the orbit of the eye from the forehead. **2.** the arch of hairs growing along the ridge formed by the supraorbital arch of the frontal bone.

eyecup, a small vessel, or cup, that is shaped to fit over the eyeball and used to bathe the exposed surface of the organ.

eye deviation [AS *éage*; L *deviare*, to turn aside], pertaining to the movement of the two eyes in which their visual axes are not parallel. Manifest deviation is the amount in degrees that the visual axis of one eye deviates from that of the other in cases of squint, when both eyes are open.

eye dominance, an unconscious preference to use one eye rather than the other for certain purposes, such as sighting a rifle or looking through a telescope.

eyedrops, a liquid medicine that is administered by allowing it to fall in drops onto the conjunctival surface.

eye glasses, transparent devices held in metal or plastic frames in front of the eyes to correct refractive errors or to protect the eyes from harmful electromagnetic waves or flying objects.

eyeground, the fundus of the eye.

eyelash [AS *eage* + ME *lasche*], one of many cilia growing in double or triple rows along the border of the eyelids in front of a row of ciliary glands that are in front of a row of meibomian glands.

eyelid [AS *eage* + *hlid*], a movable fold of thin skin over the eye, with eyelashes and ciliary and meibomian glands along its margin. The orbicularis oculi muscle and the oculomotor nerve control the opening and closing of the eyelid.

eye memory. See **visual memory.**

F

f, **1.** symbol for *breaths per unit time.* **2.** symbol for *respiratory frequency.*

F, **1.** abbreviation for **Fahrenheit. 2.** abbreviation for **farad. 3.** symbol for the chemical element **fluorine. 4.** abbreviation for **frequency.**

F₁, (in genetics) the symbol for the first filial generation; the heterozygous offspring produced by the mating of two unrelated individuals.

F₂, (in genetics) the symbol for the second filial generation; the offspring produced by mating two members of the F₁ generation.

FA, **1.** abbreviation for **fatty acid. 2.** abbreviation for **femoral artery. 3.** abbreviation for **folic acid.**

FAAN, abbreviation for **Fellow of the American Academy of Nursing.**

Fabere's test /fā′bārāz/, a test for pain or dysfunction in the hip and sacroiliac joints through overpressure applied at the knee during flexion, abduction, and external rotation of the hip.

fabrication, a psychologic reaction in which false statements are contrived to mask memory defects.

Fabry's disease, Fabry's syndrome. See **angiokeratoma corporis diffusum.**

FAC, an anticancer drug combination of fluorouracil, doxorubicin, and cyclophosphamide.

FACCP, abbreviation for *Fellow of the American College of Chest Physicians.*

FACD, abbreviation for *Fellow of the American College of Dentists.*

face [L *facies*], **1.** the front of the head from the chin to the brow, including the skin and muscles and structures of the forehead, eyes, nose, mouth, cheeks, and jaw. **2.** the visage. **3.** to direct the face toward something.– **facial,** *adj.*

face-bow [L *facies* + AS *boga*], a device resembling a caliper, used for measuring the relationship of the maxillae to the temporomandibular joints required for the fabrication of denture casts.

face lift, a plastic surgery procedure in which wrinkles and other signs of aging skin are eliminated.

face presentation [L *facies* face, *praesentare* to show], an obstetric presentation in which the chin of the fetus is the point of direction.

facet /fas′it/ [Fr *facette* little face], **1.** (in dentistry) a flattened, highly polished wear pattern on a tooth. **2.** a small, smooth-surfaced process for articulation.

facial angle [L *facies; angulus* a corner], an anthropomorphic expression of the degree of protrusion of the lower face.

facial artery, one of a pair of tortuous arteries that arise from the external carotid arteries, divide into four cervical and five facial branches, and supply various organs and tissues in the head.

facial diplegia, a rare neuromuscular condition characterized by bilateral paralysis of various muscles of the face.

facial hemiplegia, paralysis of the muscles of one side of the face, with the rest of the body not being affected.

facial muscle, one of five groups of facial muscles. They include the muscles of the scalp, the extrinsic muscles of the ear, the muscles of the nose, the muscles of the eyelid, and the muscles of the mouth.

facial nerve, either of a pair of mixed sensory and motor cranial nerves that arises from the brainstem at the base of the pons and divides just in front of the ear into its six branches, innervating the scalp, forehead, eyelids, muscles of facial expression, cheeks, and jaw.

facial palsy [L *facies* face; Gk *paralyein* to be palsied], a loss of motor nerve function in the facial muscles.

facial paralysis, an abnormal condition characterized by the partial or the total loss of the functions of the facial muscles or the loss of sensation in the face.

facial perception, the ability to judge the distance and direction of objects through the sensation felt in the skin of the face. The phenomenon is commonly experienced by those who are blind.

facial tic [L *facies;* Fr *tic* twitching], any repetitive spasmodic and involuntary contraction of groups of facial muscles.

facial vein, one of a pair of superficial veins that drain deoxygenated blood from the superficial structures of the face.

facial vision. See **facial perception.**

facies /fā′shē·ēs/, *pl.* **facies** /fā′shē·ēs/ [L, face], **1.** the face. **2.** the surface of any body structure, part, or organ. **3.** facial expression or appearance.

facilitation /fəsil'itā'shən/ [L *facilitas* easiness] **1.** the enhancement or reinforcement of any action or function so that it is carried out with increased ease. **2.** (in neurology) the phenomenon whereby two or more afferent impulses that individually are not strong enough to elicit a response in a neuron can collectively produce a reflex discharge greater than the sum of the separate responses. **3.** (in neurology) the process of lowering the threshold action potential of a neuron by the repeated passage of an impulse along the same pathway.

FACOG, abbreviation for *Fellow of the American College of Obstetricians and Gynecologists.*

FACP, abbreviation for *Fellow of the American College of Physicians.*

FACS, abbreviation for *Fellow of the American College of Surgeons.*

FACSM, abbreviation for *Fellow of the American College of Sports Medicine.*

factitial /fakti'shəl/ [L *facticius* artificial], artificial or self-induced, such as a factitial dermatitis.

factitial dermatitis, a skin rash caused by the patient, usually for secondary gain or as a manifestation of psychiatric illness.

factitious disorders /faktish'əs/, conditions marked by disease symptoms caused by deliberate efforts of a person to gain attention. Such attempts to gain attention may be repeated, even when the individual is aware of the hazards involved.

factor I. See **fibrinogen.**

factor II. See **prothrombin.**

factor III. See **thromboplastin.**

factor IV, a designation for calcium as an element in the process of the coagulation of blood.

factor V, an unstable procoagulant that occurs in normal plasma but is deficient in the blood of parahemophiliacs. It is needed to convert prothrombin rapidly to thrombin.

factor VI, a hypothetic chemical agent that some suggest is derived from proaccelerin, or factor V, in the process of blood coagulation.

factor VII, a blood procoagulant present in the blood plasma and synthesized in the liver in the presence of vitamin K.

factor VIII, a coagulation factor present in normal plasma but deficient in the blood of persons with hemophilia A.

factor IX, a coagulation factor present in normal plasma but deficient in the blood of persons with hemophilia B.

factor IX complex, a hemostatic containing factors II, VII, IX, and X. It is pre-

scribed in the treatment of hemophilia B. It is a vitamin K-dependent protein synthesized in the liver.

factor X, a coagulation factor that occurs in normal plasma but is deficient in some inherited defects in coagulation.

factor XI, a coagulation factor present in normal plasma. Deficiency results in hemophilia C.

factor XII, a coagulation factor present in normal plasma. It triggers the formation of bradykinin and associated enzymatic reactions.

factor XIII, a coagulation factor present in normal plasma that acts with calcium to produce an insoluble fibrin clot.

factor-searching study, (in nursing research) a study design that produces a qualitative, narrative description including categories or classifications of phenomena.

facultative /fak'əltā'tiv/ [L *facultus* capability], not obligatory; having the ability to adapt to more than one condition, as a facultative **anaerobe.**

facultative aerobe, an organism able to grow under anaerobic conditions but that develops most rapidly in an aerobic environment.

facultative anaerobe, an organism able to grow under aerobic conditions but that develops most rapidly in an anaerobic environment.

facultative parasite. See **parasite.**

faculty [L *facultus* capability], **1.** any normal physiologic function or natural ability of a living organism, such as the digestive faculty or the ability to perceive and distinguish sensory stimuli. **2.** an ability to do something specific, such as learn languages or remember names. **3.** any mental ability or power, such as memory or thought. **4.** a department in an institution of learning or the people who teach in a department of such an institution.

FAD, abbreviation for *fetal activity determination.*

Faget's sign /fazhāz'/ [Jean C. Faget, American physician, b. 1818], a falling pulse rate associated with a constant temperature, or a constant pulse associated with a rising temperature.

fagicladosporic acid /faj'iklad'ōspôr'ik/, a toxin produced by *Cladosporium epiphyllum,* a member of a genus of fungi that cause "black spot" in stored meat, tinea negra, and black degeneration of the brain.

Fahrenheit (F) /fer'ənhīt/ [Daniel G. Fahrenheit, German physicist, b. 1686], a scale for the measurement of temperature in which the boiling point of water is

212° and the freezing point of water is 32° at sea level.

failed forceps, an attempted mid-forceps obstetric procedure that is abandoned because there is a greater degree of resistance to rotation or traction than anticipated.

failure to thrive [L *fallere* to deceive; ME *thriven* to grasp], the abnormal retardation of the growth and development of an infant resulting from conditions that interfere with normal metabolism, appetite, and activity.

faint, *nontechnical.* [OFr *faindre* to feign] **1.** to lose consciousness, as in a syncopal attack. **2.** a syncopal attack.

faith healing [L *fidere* to trust; AS *hoelen* to make whole], alleged healing through the power to cause a cure or recovery from an illness or injury without the aid of conventional medical treatment because the healer is believed to have been given that power by a supernatural force.

falciform body. See **sporozoite.**

falciform ligament /fal'sifôrm/, a triangular or sickle-shaped ligament of the body.

falciparum malaria /falsip'ərəm/ [L *falx* sickle, *forma* form; It, bad air], the most severe form of malaria, caused by the protozoan *Plasmodium falciparum,* characterized by extremely grave systemic symptoms, mental confusion, enlarged spleen, edema, GI symptoms, and anemia.

fallectomy /fəlek'təmē/, the surgical removal of one or both of the fallopian tubes.

fallopian canal /fəlō'pē·ən/ [Gabriele Fallopius, Italian anatomist, b. 1523; L, *canalis*], a passageway for the facial nerve through the petrous bone.

fallopian tube [Gabriele Fallopio, Italian anatomist, b. 1523], one of a pair of ducts opening at one end into the uterus and at the other end into the peritoneal cavity, over the ovary. Each tube serves as the passage through which an ovum is carried to the uterus and through which spermatozoa move out toward the ovary.

Fallot's syndrome. See **tetralogy of Fallot.**

fallout [AS *feallan* to fall, *ut*], the deposition of radioactive debris after a nuclear explosion.

false ankylosis [L *fallere* to deceive; Gk *ankylosis* joint stiffness], a type of joint immobility resulting from abnormal inflexibility of body parts outside the joint.

false anorexia. See **pseudoanorexia.**

false diverticulum [L *fallere, diverticulare* to turn aside], a protrusion of mucous membrane through a muscular coat defect of a hollow organ.

false imprisonment [L *falsus* deceptive; ME *imprisonen*], (in law) the intentional, unjustified, nonconsensual detention or confinement of a person for any length of time.

false joint [L *fallere, jungere* to join], a joint that develops at the site of a former fracture.

false labor. See **Braxton Hicks contractions.**

false negative, an incorrect result of a diagnostic test or procedure that falsely indicates the absence of a finding, condition, or disease.

false-negative rate [L *fallere, negare* to deny, *ratum* calculate], the rate of occurrence of negative test results in subjects known to have the disease or behavior for which the individual is being tested.

false neuroma, 1. a neoplasm that does not contain nerve elements. **2.** a cystic neuroma.

false nucleolus. See **karyosome.**

false pelvis, the part of the pelvis superior to a plane passing through the linea terminalis.

false personification, (in psychiatry) the labeling and prejudgment of others without validating impressions.

false positive, a test result that wrongly indicates the presence of a disease or other condition the test is designed to reveal.

false-positive rate [L *fallere, positivus, ratum* calculate], the rate of occurrence of positive test results in tests of individuals known to be free of a disease or disorder for which the individual is being tested.

false pregnancy. See **pseudocyesis.**

false rib. See **rib.**

false suture, an immovable fibrous joint in which rough articulating surfaces form the connection between certain bones of the skull. Two kinds of false sutures are **sutura plana** and **sutura squamosa.**

false transactions, transactions in which communication is stopped or distorted by one individual relating from a different ego state than was expected.

false twins. See **dizygotic twins.**

false vertebrae, the vertebral segments that form the sacrum and the coccyx.

false vocal cord, either of two thick folds of mucous membrane in the larynx separating the ventricle from the vestibule.

falx /falks, fôlks/, *pl.* **falces** /fal'sēz, fôl'sēz/ [L, sickle], **1.** a sickle-shaped structure. **2.** sickle-shaped.

falx cerebelli /falks ser'əbel'ī/, a small sickle-shaped process of the dura mater attached to the occipital bone above and projecting into the posterior cerebellar notch between the two cerebellar hemispheres.

falx cerebri /falks ser'əbrī/, a sickle-shaped fold of dura mater membrane extending into and following along the longitudinal fissure of the two hemispheres of the cerebrum.

falx inguinalis, transverse and internal oblique muscles.

falx ligamentosa, the broad ligament of the liver.

FAM, an anticancer drug combination of fluorouracil, **doxorubicin,** and **mitomycin.**

familial [L *familia* household], pertaining to a characteristic, condition, or disease that is present in some families and not others or that occurs in more family members than would be expected by chance.

familial cretinism, a rare genetic disorder caused by an inborn error of metabolism resulting from an enzyme deficiency that interferes with thyroid hormone biosynthesis. Clinical manifestations include lethargy, stunted growth, and mental retardation.

familial histiocytic reticulosis [L *familia;* Gk *histion* web, *kytos* cell; L *reticulum* little net; Gk *osis* condition], a hereditary disease, transmitted as an autosomal recessive trait, characterized by anemia, granulocytopenia, and thrombocytopenia. Phagocytosis of blood cells and infiltration of bone marrow by histocytes commonly results in death in childhood.

familial hypercholesterolemia, an inherited disorder transmitted as a dominant trait and characterized by a high level of serum cholesterol, tendinous xanthomas, and early evidence of atherosclerosis, especially of the coronary arteries. Affected individuals at 50 years of age have three to 10 times greater risk of ischemic heart disease than the general population. In Type IIA familial hypercholesterolemia, only **low-density lipoprotein (LDL)** is elevated, whereas in Type IIB, LDL and **very low-density lipoprotein (VLDL)** are increased.

familial hyperglyceridemia. See hyperlipidemia type I.

familial iminoglycinuria. See iminoglycinuria.

familial juvenile nephronophthisis. See medullary cystic disease.

familial lipoprotein lipase deficiency. See hyperchylomicronemia.

familial osteochondrodystrophy. See Morquio's disease.

familial periodic paralyis [L *familia;* Gk *peri* near, *hodos* way, *paralysein* to be palsied], a rare inherited disorder in which clients suffer attacks of general flaccid paralysis following attacks of hypokalemia or potassium depletion. The attacks may follow administration of glucose and are relieved by the administration of potassium salts.

familial polyposis, an abnormal condition characterized by multiple polyps in the colon and rectum. The disease, which has high malignancy potential, is inherited. A kind of familial polyposis is **Gardner's syndrome.**

familial spinal muscular atrophy. See Werdnig-Hoffmann disease.

familial tremor. See essential tremor.

family [L *familia* household], **1.** a group of people related by heredity, such as parents, children, and siblings. The term sometimes is broadened to include persons related by marriage or those living in the same household, who are emotionally attached, interact regularly, and share concerns for the growth and development of the family and its individual members. **2.** a group of persons having a common surname, such as the Anderson family. **3.** a category of animals or plants situated on a taxonomic scale between order and genus. Humans are members of the genus *Homo sapiens,* which is a part of the hominid family which, in turn, is a division of the primate order of mammals. **–familial,** *adj.*

family APGAR, a family therapy rating system in which APGAR is an acronym formed by the first letters of five words, adaptability, partnership, growth, affection, and resolve. Each family member indicates a degree of satisfaction in each of the five categories on a scale of 0 to 2. The system is used most frequently in studies of families with a geriatric member.

family care leave, absence from a job that is permitted for an employee to care for a family member who is ill, disabled, or pregnant. The U.S. Family and Medical Leave Act of 1993 provides 12 weeks unpaid leave per year from a job for the birth or adoption of a child, for the care of a seriously ill child, spouse, or parent, or for a serious illness afflicting the employee. The law applies only to companies with 50 or more employees. Employers must guarantee that a worker can return to the same or a comparable job.

family-centered care, primary health care that includes an assessment and implementation of actions needed to maintain or improve the health of the family unit and its members.

family-centered maternity care, a system for the delivery of safe, high-quality health care adapted to the physical and psychosocial needs of the patient, the patient's family, and the newly born offspring.

family-centered nursing care, nursing

care directed toward improving the potential health of a family or any of its members.

family counseling, a program of providing information and professional guidance to members of a family concerning specific health matters, such as care of a severely retarded child.

family disorganization, a breakdown of a family system. It may be associated with parental overburdening or loss of support systems for family members. Family disorganization can contribute to the loss of social controls that families usually impose on their members.

family dynamics, the forces at work within the family that result in particular behaviors or symptoms.

family functions, processes by which the family operates as a whole, including communication and manipulation of the environment for problem solving.

family health, (in a health history) an account of the health of the members of the immediate family. Hereditary and familial diseases are especially noted. The age and health of each person, the ages at death, and the causes of death are charted.

family history, an essential portion of a patient's medical history in which the patient is asked about the health of the other members of the family in a series of specific questions to discover any diseases to which the patient may be particularly vulnerable.

family medicine, the branch of medicine that is concerned with the diagnosis and treatment of health problems in people of either sex and any age. Practitioners of family medicine are often called family practice physicians, family physicians, or, formerly, general practitioners.

family myths, myths that are constructed to deny the reality of family situations.

family nurse practitioner (FNP), a nurse practitioner possessing skills necessary for the detection and management of acute self-limiting conditions and management of chronic stable conditions.

family of origin, the family into which a person is born.

family of procreation, the family a person forms through marriage and/or having children.

family physician, **1.** a medical practitioner of the specialty of family medicine. **2.** a general practitioner. **3.** a family practice physician.

family planning. See **contraception.**

family practice [L *familia;* Gk *praktikos* ready for action], a medical specialty that combines the knowledge derived from several branches of medicine, including

internal medicine, pediatrics, surgery, psychiatry, and obstetrics and gynecology, and establishes a medical discipline of client management, counseling, and problem solving while at the same time serving as a personal physician coordinating total health care delivery to all members of a family, regardless of the sex or age of the patient.

family practice physician, a practitioner of family medicine, usually one who has completed a residency program in the specialty.

family processes, altered, a NANDA-accepted nursing diagnosis of a situational or developmental change or crisis within the family network. Defining characteristics include the inability of the family system to meet the needs of its members; the inability to communicate adequately; the parents' disrespect for each other's views on child-rearing practices; family rigidity in function and roles; the inability to accept or receive help, to adapt to change, or to deal with traumatic experience; disrespect for individuality and autonomy; failure to accomplish developmental tasks; ineffective decision-making processes; and inappropriate or poorly communicated family rules or rituals.

family structure, the composition and membership of the family and the organization and patterning of relationships among individual family members. In planning health care for a family, an awareness of that family's structure may be important.

family therapy, (in psychiatry) a therapy modality that focuses treatment on the process between family members that supports and perpetuates symptoms; a way of conceptualizing human relationship problems that focuses on the context in which an emotional problem is generated.

famine fever. See **relapsing fever.**

famotidine /famot′idēn/, an oral and parenteral antiulcer drug prescribed for the short-term treatment of active duodenal ulcer, maintenance therapy for duodenal ulcer after healing, and for pathologic hypersecretory conditions such as Zollinger-Ellison syndrome.

fan beam, a geometric pattern that results from collimating a spatially extended x-ray beam with a long, narrow slit.

FANCAP, *U.S.;* a mnemonic device that stands for fluids, aeration, nutrition, communication, activity, and pain. A variant is FANCAS, in which case the *S* stands for stimulation.

Fanconi's anemia /faukō′nēs/ [Guido Fanconi, Swiss pediatrician, b. 1892], a rare, usually congenital disorder, characterized by aplastic anemia in childhood or early adult life, bone abnormalities, chromatin breaks, and developmental anomalies.

Fanconi's syndrome, a group of disorders including renal tubular dysfunction, glycosuria, phosphaturia, and bicarbonate wasting. The condition is often marked by osteomalacia, acidosis, and hypokalemia. Idiopathic Fanconi's syndrome is inherited and usually appears in early middle age. Acquired Fanconi's syndrome is usually the result of toxicity, including the ingestion of outdated tetracycline.

fango /făn′gō/ [It, mud], mud taken from thermal springs at Battaglia, Italy, and used to treat gout and other rheumatic diseases.

fan lateral projection, a technique for making an x-ray image of the hand without superimposition of the phalanges. The patient places the fingers about a sponge wedge designed so that each finger will appear separately, in a fanlike pattern, on the x-ray film.

fantasy [Gk *phantasia* imagination] **1.** the unrestrained free play of the imagination; fancy. **2.** a mental image, usually distorted or grotesque in nature, often the result of the action of drugs or a disease of the central nervous system. **3.** the mental process of transforming undesirable experiences into imagined events.

FAOTA, abbreviation for *Fellow of the American Occupational Therapy Association.*

FAPTA, abbreviation for *Fellow of the American Physical Therapy Association.*

farad (F) /fer′əd/ [Michael Faraday, English scientist, b. 1791], a unit of capacitance that increases the potential difference between the plates of a capacitor by 1 volt with a charge of 1 coulomb.

Faraday cage /fer′ədā/, (in nuclear magnetic resonance imaging) a wire-mesh cage that surrounds the NMR scanner to shield it from stray radio frequency waves, which can distort the results of NMR imaging.

Farber test, a microscopic examination of newborn meconium for lanugo and squamous cells. The absence of hair or skin cells is suggestive of intestinal obstruction or atresia and requires further evaluation.

Far Eastern hemorrhagic fever, a form of epidemic hemorrhagic fever, indigenous to Asia, that is transmitted by a virus carried by an Asian rodent. The infection is characterized by chills, fever, headache, abdominal pain, nausea, vomiting, anorexia, and extreme thirst.

far field. See **Fraunhofer zone.**

farmer's lung [L *firmare* to make firm], a

respiratory disorder caused by the inhalation of actinomycetes or other organic dusts from moldy hay. It is a form of **hypersensitivity pneumonitis.**

far point [ME *farr*; L *punctus* pricked], **1.** the farthest distance from the eye that an object can be seen clearly when eye is at rest and accommodation is fully relaxed. **2.** the point at which the visual axes of the two eyes meet when at rest.

farsightedness. See **hyperopia.**

FAS, abbreviation for **fetal alcohol syndrome.**

fascia /fash′ē-ə/, *pl.* **fasciae** [L, band], the fibrous connective tissue of the body that may be separated from other specifically organized structures, such as the tendons, the aponeuroses, and the ligaments. Kinds of fasciae are **deep fascia, subcutaneous fascia,** and **subserous fascia; –fascial,** *adj.*

fascia bulbi, a thin membranous socket that envelops the eyeball from the optic nerve to the ciliary region and allows the eyeball to move freely.

fascial cleft /fash′ē-əl/ [L *fascia* + ME *clift*], a place of cleavage between two contiguous fascial surfaces, such as the deep fasciae and the subcutaneous fasciae.

fascial compartment, a part of the body that is walled off by fascial membranes, usually containing a muscle or group of muscles or an organ.

fascial membrane lamination, a pad of connective tissue that contains fat and an occasional blood vessel or a lymph node.

fascia thoracolumbalis, the extensive subdivision of the vertebral fascia that sheaths the sacrospinalis muscle.

fascicle. See **fasciculus.**

fascicular neuroma /fəsik′yələr/, a neoplasm composed of myelinated nerve fibers.

fasciculation /fasik′yōōlā′shən/ [L *fasciculus* little bundle, *atio* process], a localized, uncoordinated, uncontrollable twitching of a single muscle group innervated by a single motor nerve fiber or filament that may be palpated and seen under the skin. Fasciculation of the heart muscle is known as **fibrillation. –fascicular,** *adj.,* **fasciculate,** *v.*

fasciculus /fəsik′yələs/, *pl.* **fasciculi** [L, little bundle], a small bundle of muscle, tendon, or nerve fibers. **–fascicular,** *adj.*

fasciitis /fas′ē-ī′tis/ **1.** an inflammation of the connective tissue, which may be caused by streptococcal or other types of infection, an injury, or an autoimmune reaction. **2.** an abnormal, benign growth (*Pseudosarcomatous fasciitis*) resembling a tumor that develops in the subcutaneous oral tissues, usually in the cheek.

fascioliasis /fas′ē·ōlī′əsis/ [L *fasciola* little band; Gk *osis* condition], infection with the liver fluke *Fasciola hepatica,* characterized by epigastric pain, fever, jaundice, eosinophilia, urticaria, and diarrhea, with fibrosis of the liver a consequence of prolonged infection.

fasciolopsiasis /fas′ē·ōlopsī′əsis/ [L *fasciola* little band; Gk *opsis* appearance, *osis* condition], an intestinal infection, prevalent in the Far East, characterized by abdominal pain, diarrhea, constipation, eosinophilia, ascites, and, sometimes, edema; caused by the fluke *Fasciolopsis buski.*

Fasciolopsis buski /fas′ē·əlop′sis bus′kē/, a species of flukes that is an important intestinal parasite endemic in the Orient and tropics.

fascioscapulohumeral muscular dystrophy /fas′ē·ōskap′yŏōlōhy ōō′mərəl/ [L *fasciculus* little bundle, *scapula* shoulderblade, *humerus* shoulder], an abnormal congenital condition and one of the main types of muscular dystrophy. It is characterized by progressive symmetric wasting of the skeletal muscles, especially the muscles of the face, the shoulders, and the upper arms, without any associated neural or sensory disorders.

fasciotomy /fas′ē·ot′əmē/, a surgical incision into an area of fascia.

FASRT, abbreviation for *Fellow of the American Society of Radiologic Technologists.*

fast [AS *faest* firm], **1.** resistant to change, especially to the action of a specific drug or chemical, as a staining agent. **2.** to abstain from all or certain foods.

fast-acting insulin, one of a group of insulin preparations in which the onset of action is rapid, approximately 1 hour. Kinds of fast-acting insulins include **regular insulin (injection)** and **prompt insulin zinc suspension.**

fastigium /fastij′ē·əm/ [L, ridge] **1.** the highest point in the course of a fever, or the most symptomatic point in the course of an illness. **2.** the angle at the top of the roof of the fourth ventricle in the brain.

fasting [AS *foestan* to observe], the act of abstaining from food for a specific period of time, usually for therapeutic or religious purposes.

fast-twitch (FT) fiber, a muscle fiber that can develop high tension rapidly.

fat [AS *faett*], **1.** a substance composed of lipids or fatty acids and occurring in various forms or consistencies ranging from oil to tallow. **2.** a type of body tissue composed of cells containing stored fat (depot fat). Stored fat is usually identified as white fat, which is found in large cellular vesicles, or brown fat, which consists of lipid droplets. Stored fat contains more than twice as many calories per gram as sugars and serves as a source of quickly mobilized body energy.

fatal [L *fatum* what has been spoken], leading inevitably to death.

fat cell lipoma. See **hibernoma.**

fat embolism, a serious circulatory condition characterized by the blocking of an artery by an embolus of fat that entered the circulatory system after the fracture of a long bone or, less commonly, after traumatic injury to adipose tissue or to a fatty liver. Fat embolism usually occurs suddenly 12 to 36 hours after the injury and is characterized by severe chest pain, pallor, dyspnea, tachycardia, delirium, prostration, and, in some cases, coma.

FA test. See **fluorescent antibody test.**

father complex [L *pater; complecti* to embrace], *nontechnical;* a repressed desire for an incestuous relationship with one's father.

father fixation, an arrest in psychosexual development characterized by an abnormally persistent, close, and often paralyzing emotional attachment to one's father.

fatigability, a tendency to become tired or exhausted quickly or easily. Fatigability may occur in certain types of cells that undergo periods of excessive activity.

fatigue [L *fatigare* to tire], **1.** a state of exhaustion or a loss of strength or endurance, as may follow strenuous physical activity. **2.** loss of ability of tissues to respond to stimuli that normally evoke muscular contraction or other activity. **3.** an emotional state associated with extreme or extended exposure to psychic pressure, as in battle or combat fatigue. **4.** a NANDA-accepted nursing diagnosis of an overwhelming sense of exhaustion and decreased capacity for physical and mental work regardless of adequate sleep. Defining characteristics include verbalization of fatigue or lack of energy and inability to maintain usual routines, an increase in physical complaints, impaired ability to concentrate, and decreased libido.

fatigue fever, a benign episode of fever and muscle pain after overexertion. The symptoms are caused by an accumulation of the metabolic waste products of muscle contractions.

fatigue fracture, any fracture that results from excessive physical activity and not from any specific injury, as commonly occurs in the metatarsal bones of runners.

fatigue state [L *fatigare, status* condition], the state of lowest energy of a system.

fat metabolism, the biochemical process by which fats are broken down and elaborated by the cells of the body. Fats provide more food energy than carbohydrates; the catabolism of 1 g of fat provides 9 kcal of heat as compared with 4.1 kcal yielded in the catabolism of 1 g of carbohydrate. Before the final reactions in fat catabolism can occur, fats must be hydrolyzed into fatty acids and glycerol. The body synthesizes fats from fatty acids and glycerol or from compounds derived from excess glucose or from amino acids. The body can synthesize only saturated fatty acids. Essential unsaturated fatty acids can be supplied only by the diet. Certain hormones, such as insulin, growth hormone, adrenocorticotropic hormone, and the glucocorticoids, control fat metabolism.

fat necrosis [AS *faett;* Gk *nekros* dead, *osis* condition], a condition caused by trauma or infection in which neutral tissue fats are broken down into fatty acids and glycerol. Fat necrosis occurs most commonly in the breasts and subcutaneous areas. It also may develop in the abdominal cavity following an attack of pancreatitis causing a release of enzymes from the pancreas.

fat pad, a mass of closely packed fat cells surrounded by fibrous tissue septa. Fat pads may be generously supplied with capillaries and nerve endings. Intraarticular fat pads are also covered by a layer of synovial cells.

fatty acid [AS *faett* + L *acidus* sour], any of several organic acids produced by the hydrolysis of neutral fats. Essential fatty acids are unsaturated molecules that cannot be produced by the body and must therefore be included in the diet. Kinds of essential fatty acids are **arachidonic** and **linoleic.**

fatty alcohol, a hydroxide of a hydrocarbon from the paraffin series.

fatty ascites. See **chylous ascites.**

fatty cirrhosis. See **cirrhosis.**

fatty cirrhosis [AS *faett;* Gk *kirrhos* yellow, *osis* condition], a form of cirrhosis that develops over a long period of poor nutrition resulting in fatty infiltration of the liver.

fatty degeneration [AS *faett;* L *degenerare* to deviate], the abnormal deposition of fat within cells or the fatty tissue invasion of organs.

fatty infiltration, a normal phase of breast development, characterized by accumulation of increased amounts of fat around the parenchymal breast tissue.

fatty infiltration of heart [AS *faett;* L *in* + *filtrare;* AS *heorte*], an accumulation of large amounts of fat within the cells of the heart. The heart muscle may be marked by irregular streaks of pale areas of fatty infiltration. It is sometimes associated with severe and prolonged anemia.

fatty liver, an accumulation of triglycerides in the liver. The causes include alcoholic cirrhosis, IV administration of drugs such as tetracycline and corticosteroids, and exposure to toxic substances, such as carbon tetrachloride and yellow phosphorus.

fatty stool [AS *faett, stol* seat], a stool containing an abnormally large amount of fat, as indicated by a stool that floats on water.

fatty tissue [AS *faett;* OFr *tissu*], loose connective tissue with many cells containing fat droplets.

fauces /fô′sēz/ [L *faux* throat], the opening of the mouth into the pharynx. The anterior pillars of the fauces form the glossopalatine arch, and the posterior pillars form the pharyngopalatine arch.

faucial isthmus /fô′shəl/, an aperture between the pharynx and the mouth.

faulty restoration [L *fallere* to deceive; *restaurare* to renew], any dental restoration that contains flaws, such as overhanging or incomplete tooth fillings, incorrect anatomy of occlusal and marginal ridge areas, and faulty clasps.

favism /fā′vizəm/ [It *fava* bean], an acute hemolytic anemia caused by ingestion of the beans or inhalation of the pollen from the *Vicia faba* (fava) plant. Symptoms include dizziness, headache, vomiting, fever, jaundice, eosinophilia, and often diarrhea.

favus /fā′vəs/ [L, honeycomb], a fungal infection of the scalp caused by *Trichophyton* fungi. Favus is characterized by thick, yellow crusts with suppuration, a distinct "mousy" odor, permanent scars, and alopecia.

FCAP, abbreviation for *Fellow of the College of American Pathologists.*

Fc fragment, a part of a molecule of an antibody after it has been split by a proteolytic enzyme. The Fc portion is sometimes identified as the crystallizable fragment.

FDA, abbreviation for **Food and Drug Administration.**

Fe, symbol for the chemical element **iron.**

fear [ME *fer* danger], a NANDA-accepted nursing diagnosis of a feeling of dread related to an identifiable source that the client is able to validate. Defining characteristics may be subjective or objective. Subjective characteristics include increased tension, apprehension, impulsiveness, terror, panic, and decreased self-assurance. Objective characteristics are increased alertness and concentration on the source of fear; a wide-eyed, aggressive attack mode of behavior or withdrawal from the source of fear; and cardiovascular excitation, superficial vasoconstriction, and pupil dilatation.

fear-tension-pain syndrome, a concept formulated by Grantly Dick-Read, MD, to explain the pain commonly expected and reported in childbirth. The concept proposes that mistaken cultural attitudes induce anxiety before labor and cause fear in labor. He advocated education, exercise, and warm emotional and physical support in labor to counteract the syndrome, coining the term "natural childbirth" for a delivery in which the woman participates in the natural experience.

febrifuge. See **antipyretic.**

febrile /fē′bril, feb′ril/ [L *febris* fever], pertaining to or characterized by an elevated body temperature, such as a febrile reaction to an infectious agent. **–febrility,** *n.*

febrile delirium [L *febris, delirare* to rave], a symptom of disordered central nervous system functions, with excitement, restlessness, and disorientation, accompanying some acute fevers.

febrile seizure, a seizure associated with a febrile illness. Treatment depends on the age of the patient and the number of seizures. Generalized recurrent febrile seizures in children may be treated as grand mal epilepsy.

febrile state [L *febris, status* condition], a significant increase in body temperature accompanied by increased pulse and respiration rates, anorexia, constipation, insomnia, headache, pains, and irritability.

fecal fistula [L *faex* dregs; *fistula* pipe], an abnormal passage from the colon to the external surface of the body, discharging feces.

fecal impaction /fē′kəl/, an accumulation of hardened or inspissated feces in the rectum or sigmoid colon that the individual is unable to move. Diarrhea may be a sign of fecal impaction since only liquid material is able to pass the obstruction. Persons who are dehydrated, nutritionally depleted, on long periods of bedrest, receiving constipating medications, or undergoing barium x-ray studies are at risk of developing fecal impaction.

fecalith /fē′kəlith/ [L *faex* + Gk *lithos* stone], a hard, impacted mass of feces in the colon.

fecal softener, a drug that lowers the surface tension of the fecal mass, allowing the intestinal fluids to penetrate and soften the stool.

feces /fē′sēz/ [L *faex* dregs], waste or excrement from the digestive tract that is formed in the intestine and expelled through the rectum. Feces consist of water, food residue, bacteria, and secretions of the intestines and liver. **–fecal,** *adj.*

fecundation /fē′kəndā′shən, fek′-/ [L *fecundare* to make fruitful], impregnation or fertilization; the act of fertilizing. **–fecundate,** *v.*

fecundity /fikun′ditē/, the ability to produce offspring, especially in large numbers and rapidly; fertility. **–fecund,** *adj.*

Federal Register, a document published by the U.S. government each working day to inform the public of executive regulations, presidential orders, hearings and meetings schedules of the Food and Drug Administration, the Environmental Protection Agency, and other government bureaus that regulate matters of health and safety.

Federal Tort Claims Act, a statute passed in 1946 that allows the federal government to be sued for the wrongful action or negligence of its employees.

Federal Trade Commission (FTC), an agency in the executive branch of the federal government created to promote trade and to prevent practices that restrain free enterprise and competition, including in the area of health care.

Federation Licensing Examination (FLEX), the standardized licensing examination for state licensure of physicians. Developed by the Federation of State Medical Boards of the United States, the examination is based on National Board of Medical Examiners' test materials.

Fede's disease. See **Riga-Fede disease.**

feeblemindedness. See **mental retardation.**

feedback [AS *faedan, baec*], (in communication theory) information produced by a receiver and perceived by a sender that informs the sender about the receiver's reaction to the message.

feeding [AS *faedan*], the act or process of taking or giving food or nourishment. Kinds of feeding include **breastfeeding** and **forced feeding.**

fee-for-service [AS *feoh* property; L *servitum* slavery], **1.** a charge made for a professional activity, as for a physical examination, the fitting of a contraceptive diaphragm, or the monitoring of a person's blood pressure. **2.** a system for the payment of professional services in which the practitioner is paid for the particular service rendered, rather than receiving a salary.

Feer's disease. See **acrodynia.**

fee screen system, a method of establishing payment for physician services based on the usual, customary, or reasonable charge according to a regional evaluation.

feet. See **foot.**

Fehling's solution /fā′lingz/ [Hermann C. von Fehling, German chemist, b. 1812], a solution containing cupric sulfate with sodium hydroxide and potassium sodium tartrate, used for testing for the presence of glucose and other reducing substances in the urine.

Feingold diet /fīn′gōld/, a diet developed by American pediatrician Benjamin Feingold for treating hyperactive children. The diet excludes foods manufactured with synthetic colorings, flavorings, and preservatives and limits the intake of fruits and vegetables that contain salicylates.

Feldenkrais therapy /fel′dənkrīs′/, (in psychiatry) a therapy based on establishment of a good self-image through awareness and correction of body movements.

feldspar /feld′spär/ [Ger *feld* field, *spath* spar], a crystalline mineral of aluminum silicate with potassium, sodium, barium, and calcium. It is an important component of dental porcelain.

fellatio /fəlā′shō/, oral stimulation of the male genitalia.

Fellow of the American Academy of Nursing (FAAN), a member of the American Academy of Nursing.

fellowship [AS *feolaga* partnership], a grant given to a person for study or training or to allow payment for work on a special project, but not for study toward a degree.

felon [L *fel* venom], a suppurative abscess on the distal phalanx of a finger.

felonious assault. See assault, felony.

felony, (in criminal law) a crime declared by statute to be more serious than a misdemeanor and deserving of a more severe penalty.

Felty's syndrome /fel′tēz/ [Augustus R. Felty, American physician, b. 1895], hypersplenism occurring with adult rheumatoid arthritis, characterized by splenomegaly, leukopenia, and frequent infections.

female [L *femella* young woman], **1.** of or pertaining to the human sex that becomes pregnant and bears children; feminine. **2.** a female person.

female catheterization, a procedure for removing urine by means of a urinary catheter introduced through the urinary meatus and urethra into the bladder. The procedure is performed to relieve distention if voluntary micturition is not possible (as after trauma or surgery), as a preparation for and during anesthesia, if a specimen of urine from the bladder is required, or if medication is to be instilled into the bladder. A straight catheter or a retention catheter with a balloon may be used.

female reproductive system assessment, an evaluation of a patient's genital tract and breasts and an investigation of past and present disorders that may be factors in the individual's current gynecologic condition.

female sexual dysfunction, impaired or inadequate ability of a woman to engage in or enjoy satisfactory sexual intercourse and orgasm. Causes include anxiety, fear, negative emotions associated with sexual arousal and intercourse, and interpersonal problems. Treatment is focused on eliminating physical problems and sexual anxieties and on enhancing erotic sensitivities.

female sterility [L *femella* little woman, *sterilis* barren], a condition of being an infertile woman because of congenital defects in the reproductive system, such as failure of the uterus to develop normally, or disease, injury, or corrective surgery affecting functioning of the ovaries, fallopian tubes, uterus, cervix, or vagina.

feminist therapy, a consciousness-raising therapy that focuses on the presence of sexism and sex role stereotyping in society.

feminization [L *femina* woman], **1.** the normal development or induction of female sex characteristics. **2.** the induction of female sex characteristics in a genotypic male. Testicular feminization may be caused by the inability of target tissues to respond to endogenous or administered androgen.

feminizing adrenal tumor, a rare neoplasm of the adrenal cortex, characterized in males by gynecomastia, hypertension, diffuse pigmentation, a high level of estrogen in urine, and loss of potency.

femoral /fem′ərəl/ [L *femur* thigh], of or pertaining to the femur or the thigh.

femoral artery, an extension of the external iliac artery into the lower limb, starting just distal to the inguinal ligament and ending at the junction of the middle and lower thirds of the thigh.

femoral condyle, one of a pair of large flared prominences on the distal end of the femur.

femoral epiphysis, a secondary bone-forming center of the femur, separated from the main part of the bone by cartilage during the period of bone immaturity.

femoral hernia, a hernia in which a loop of intestine descends through the femoral canal into the groin.

femoral nerve, the largest of the seven branches from the lumbar plexus and the main nerve of the anterior part of the thigh.

femoral pulse, the pulse of the femoral artery, palpated in the groin.

femoral reflex [L *femur* thigh, *reflectere* to bend back], a reflex that results in extension of the knee and plantar flexion of the foot when the skin is stimulated on the upper anterior third of the thigh.

femoral torsion, an extreme lateral or a medial twisting rotation of the femur on its longitudinal axis, as may occur because of the action of the gluteal muscles.

femoral vein, a large vein in the thigh originating in the popliteal vein and accompanying the femoral artery in the proximal two thirds of the thigh. Its distal portion lies lateral to the artery; its proximal portion deeper to the artery. Below the inguinal ligament it is joined by the deep femoral vein. Near its termination it is joined by the great saphenous vein.

femur /fē'mər/, *pl.* **femora, femurs** [L, thigh], the thigh bone, which extends from the pelvis to the knee. It is largely cylindric and is the longest and strongest bone in the body.

fenestra /fines'trə/, *pl.* **fenestrae** [L, window], an aperture, especially in a bandage or cast, that is often cut out to relieve pressure or to administer regular skin care.

fenestrated /fen'əstrā'tid/ [L, *fenestra*, window], pertaining to a membrane or other object that has numerous small holes or openings.

fenestrated drape, a drape with a round or slitlike opening in the center.

fenestration /fen'əstrā'shən/ [L *fenestra* window], **1.** a surgical procedure in which an opening is created in order to gain access to the cavity within an organ or a bone. **2.** an opening created surgically in a bone or organ of the body. **–fenestrate,** *v.*

fenfluramine hydrochloride /fenflŏŏr'əmēn/, a sympathomimetic anorectic agent prescribed to decrease the appetite in exogenous obesity.

fenoprofen calcium /fē'nəprō'fən/, a nonsteroidal antiinflammatory agent and analgesic prescribed in the treatment of arthritis and other painful inflammatory conditions.

fenoterol /fen'ōter'ol/, a beta-adrenergic drug used in respiratory therapy.

fentanyl /fen'tanil/, a potent narcotic analgesic, used most commonly with the sedative and antipsychotic drug droperidol as an adjunct in anesthesia.

fentanyl citrate, a narcotic analgesic prescribed as an adjunct to general anesthesia, as a preoperative and postoperative analgesic, and as a component in neuroleptanesthesia and analgesia.

Ferguson's reflex, a contraction of the uterus after the cervix is stimulated. The reflex is an important function of labor.

fermentation [L *fermentare* to cause to rise], a chemical change that is brought about in a substance by the action of an enzyme or microorganism, especially the anaerobic conversion of foodstuffs to certain products. Kinds of fermentation are **acetic, alcoholic, ammoniacal, amylic, butyric, caseous, dextran, diastatic, lactic acid, propionic, storing,** and **viscous fermentation.**

fermentative dyspepsia /fərmen'tətiv/, an abnormal condition characterized by impaired digestion associated with the fermentation of digested food.

fermium (Fm) /fur'mē·əm/ [Enrico Fermi, Italian physicist, b. 1901], a synthetic transuranic metallic element. Its atomic number is 100; its atomic weight is 257.

ferning test /fur'ning/ [AS *faern* fern; L *testum* crucible], a technique used to determine the presence of estrogen in the uterine cervical mucus. It is often used as a test for ovulation; high levels of estrogen cause the cervical mucus to dry on a slide in a fernlike pattern.

ferric /fer'ik/, pertaining to a compound of iron in which the metal is trivalent, such as ferric chloride.

ferritin /fer'itin/ [L *ferrum* iron], an iron compound formed in the intestine and stored in the liver, spleen, and bone marrow for eventual incorporation into hemoglobin molecules. Serum ferritin levels are used as an indicator of the body's iron stores.

ferromagnetic /fer'ōmagnat'ik/, pertaining to substances, such as iron, that are strongly affected by magnetism.

ferrous sulfate /fer'əs/, a hematinic agent prescribed in the treatment of iron deficiency anemia.

fertile [L *fertilis* fruitful], **1.** capable of reproducing or bearing offspring. **2.** of a gamete, capable of inducing fertilization or being fertilized. **3.** prolific; fruitful; not sterile. **–fertility,** *n.,* **fertilize,** *v.*

fertile eunuch syndrome, a hypogonadotropic hormonal disorder occurring only in males in which the quantity of testosterone and follicle-stimulating hormone is inadequate for the induction of spermatogenesis and the development of secondary sexual characteristics.

fertile period, the time in the menstrual cycle during which fertilization may occur. Spermatozoa can survive for 48 to 72 hours; the ovum lives for 24 hours. Thus, the fertile period begins 2 to 3 days before ovulation and lasts for 2 to 3 days afterward.

fertility, the ability to reproduce.

fertility factor. See F factor.

fertility rate, the number of live births per 1,000 women aged 15 through 44.

fertilization [L *fertilis* fruitful], the union of male and female gametes to form a zygote from which the embryo develops. The process takes place in the fallopian tube of the female when a spermatozoon, carried in the seminal fluid discharged during coitus, comes in contact with and penetrates the ovum. Kinds of fertilization include **cross-fertilization, external fertilization,** and **internal fertilization.**

fertilization age. See **fetal age.**

fertilization membrane, a viscous membrane surrounding the fertilized ovum that prevents the penetration of additional spermatozoa.

fertilizin /fərtil'izin/, a glycoprotein found on the plasma membrane of the ovum in various species.

festinating gait [L *festinare* to hasten], a manner of walking in which the speed of the person increases in an unconscious effort to "catch up" with a displaced center of gravity. It is a common characteristic of Parkinson's disease.

festoon [Fr *feston* scallop], a carving in the base material of a denture that simulates the contours of the natural gingival tissues.

fetal abortion /fē'təl/ [L *fetus*], termination of pregnancy after the twentieth week of gestation but before the fetus has developed enough to live outside of the uterus.

fetal advocate, a person who regards the health and well-being of the fetus as a matter of top priority.

fetal age, the age of the conceptus computed from the time elapsed since fertilization.

fetal alcohol syndrome (FAS) [L *fetus*; Ar *alkohl* essence; Gk *syn* together, *dromos* course], a set of congenital psychologic, behavioral, cognitive, and physical abnormalities that tend to appear in infants whose mothers consumed alcoholic beverages during pregnancy. It is characterized by typical craniofacial and limb defects, cardiovascular defects, intrauterine growth retardation, and retarded development. The most serious cases have involved infants born to mothers who were chronic alcoholics and drank heavily during pregnancy. Women who drank less reportedly gave birth to infants with less serious malformations, or **fetal alcohol effects (FAE),** but it is not known if there is a lower limit to alcohol consumption during pregnancy or if there is a particular period in embryonic life when the offspring is most vulnerable to effects of alcohol.

fetal alveoli, the terminal pulmonary sacs of a fetus, which are filled with fluid before birth.

fetal asphyxia, a condition of hypoxemia, hypercapnia, and respiratory and metabolic acidosis that may occur in the uterus.

fetal attitude, the relationship of the fetal parts to each other in which the fetal head is not flexed and the chin on chest is as usual but is held straight up.

fetal bradycardia, an abnormally slow fetal heart rate, usually below 100 beats per minute.

fetal circulation, the pathway of blood circulation in the fetus. Oxygenated blood from the placenta travels through the umbilical vein to the liver and the ductus venosus, which carries it to the inferior vena cava and right atrium. The blood enters the right atrium at a pressure sufficient to direct the flow across the atrium and through the foramen ovale into the left atrium; thus, oxygenated blood is available for circulation through the left ventricle to the head and upper extremities. The blood is returned to the placenta through the umbilical arteries.

fetal death, the intrauterine death of a fetus, or the death of a fetus weighing at least 500 g or after 20 or more weeks of gestation.

fetal distress, a compromised condition of the fetus, usually discovered during labor, characterized by a markedly abnormal rate or rhythm of myocardial contraction.

fetal dose, the estimated amount of radiation received by a fetus during an x-ray examination of a pregnant woman.

fetal heart rate (FHR), the number of heartbeats in the fetus occurring in a given unit of time. The FHR varies in cycles of fetal rest and activity and is affected by many factors, including maternal fever, uterine contractions, maternal-fetal hypotension, and many drugs. The normal FHR is more than 100 beats per minute and less than 160 beats per minute.

fetal heart sound [L *fotus*; AS *heorte*; L *sonus* sound], the beats of the fetal heart as detected by auscultation or by electronic fetal monitoring. The embryonic heart begins beating at about 14 days of intrauterine life.

fetal heart tones (fht), the pulsations of the fetal heart heard through the maternal abdomen in pregnancy.

fetal hemoglobin, hemoglobin F, the major hemoglobin present in the blood of a fetus and neonate.

fetal hydantoin syndrome (FHS), a complex of birth defects associated with prenatal maternal ingestion of hydantoin derivatives. Symptoms of FHS include microcephaly, hypoplasia or absence of nails on the fingers or toes, abnormal facies, mental and physical retardation, and cardiac defects.

fetal hydrops. See **hydrops fetalis.**

fetal lie, the relationship of the long axis of the fetus to the long axis of the mother.

fetal lipoma. See **hibernoma.**

fetal membranes, the structures that protect, support, and nourish the embryo and fetus, including the yolk sac, allantois, amnion, chorion, placenta, and umbilical cord.

fetal monitor. See **electronic fetal monitor.**

fetal mortality, the number of fetal deaths per 1,000 births, or per live births.

fetal movements [L, *fotus, movere,* to move], muscular movements produced by the fetus *in utero* beginning around the fifth month of life. The early fetal movements can be felt by the mother.

fetal placenta [L, *fotus, placenta,* flat cake], the portion of the placenta that is formed from the shaggy chorion frondosum, the villi of which invade the decidua basalis.

fetal position, the relationship of the part of the fetus that presents in the pelvis to four quadrants of the maternal pelvis identified by initial L (left), R (right), A (anterior), and P (posterior). The presenting part is also identified by initial O (occiput), M (mentum), and S (sacrum). If a fetus presents with the occiput directed to the posterior aspect of the mother's right side, the fetal position is right occiput posterior (ROP).

fetal presentation, the part of the fetus that first appears in the pelvis. Cephalic presentations include vertex, brow, and chin; breech presentations include frank breech, complete breech, and single or double footling breech.

fetal rest. See **embryonic rest.**

fetal rickets. See **achondroplasia.**

fetal rotation [L *fotus, rotare* to rotate], the turning of the head of the fetus as it begins the descent through the birth canal. The fetal head may be rotated by hand or with forceps if needed to guide the body in a proper position for delivery.

fetal stage, (in embryology) the interval of time from the end of the embryonic stage, at the end of the seventh week of gestation, to birth, 38 to 42 weeks after the first day of the last menstrual period.

fetal tachycardia, a fetal heart rate that continues at 160 or more beats per minute for more than 10 minutes.

feticide. See **embryoctony.**

fetid /fet'id, fē'tid/ [L *fetere* to stink], pertaining to something that has a foul or putrid odor.

fetish [Fr *fetiche* artificial], **1.** any object or idea given unreasonable or excessive attention or reverence. **2.** (in psychology) any inanimate object or any part of the body not of a sexual nature that arouses erotic feelings or fixation. **–fetishism,** *n.*

fetishist /fet'ishist/, a person who believes in or receives erotic gratification from fetishes.

fetochorionic /fē'tōkôr'ē·on'ik/ [L *fetus* + Gk *chorion* a skin], of or pertaining to the fetus and the chorion.

fetofetal transfusion. See **parabiotic syndrome.**

fetography /fētog'rəfē/ [L *fetus* + Gk *graphein* to record], roentgenography of the fetus in utero.

fetology /fētol'əjē/ [L *fetus* + Gk *logos* science], the branch of medicine that is concerned with the fetus in utero, including the diagnosis of abnormalities, congenital anomalies, the prevention of teratogenic influences, and the treatment of certain disorders.

fetometry /fētom'ətrē/ [L *fetus* + Gk *metron measure*], the measurement of the size of the fetus, especially the diameter of the head and circumference of the trunk. A kind of fetometry is **roentgen fetometry.**

fetoplacental /fēto'pləsen'təl/ [L *fetus* + *placenta* flat cake], of or pertaining to the fetus and the placenta.

fetoprotein /fēto'prō'tēn/ [L *fetus* + Gk *proteios* first rank], an antigen that occurs naturally in fetuses and occasionally in adults as the result of certain diseases. An increased amount of **alpha fetoprotein** in the fetus is diagnostic for neural tube defects. Leukemia, hepatoma, sarcoma, and other neoplasms are associated with **beta-fetoprotein** in the blood of adults.

fetor hepaticus [L, stench; *hepar* liver], foul-smelling breath associated with severe liver disease.

fetoscope /fē'təskōp'/ [L *fetus* + Gk *skopein* to look], a stethoscope for auscultating the fetal heartbeat through the mother's abdomen.

fetoscopy /fētos'kəpē/, a procedure in which a fetus may be directly observed in utero, using a fetoscope introduced through a small incision in the abdomen under local anesthesia.

fetotoxic /fēto'tok'sik/ [L *fetus* + Gk *toxikon* poison], pertaining to anything that is poisonous to a fetus.

fetus /fē'təs/ [L, fruitful], the unborn offspring of a viviparous animal after it has attained the particular form of the species; more specifically, the human child in utero after the embryonic period and the beginning of the development of the major structural features, usually from the eighth week after fertilization until birth. Kinds of fetuses include **acardius, anideus, lithopedion, mummified fetus, parasitic**

fetus, and **sirenomelia.** **–fetal, foetal,** *adj.*

fetus acardiacus, fetus acardius. See **acardius.**

fetus amorphus, a shapeless conceptus in which there are no formed or recognizable parts.

fetus anideus. See **anideus.**

fetus in fetu /fē′təs infē′tōo/, a fetal anomaly in which a small, imperfectly formed twin, incapable of independent existence, is contained within the body of the normal twin, the autosite.

fetus papyraceus, a twin fetus that has died in utero early in development and has been pressed flat against the uterine wall by the living fetus.

fetus sanguinolentis /sang′gwinəlen′tis/, a darkly colored, partly macerated fetus that has died in utero.

FEV, abbreviation for **forced expiratory volume.**

fever [L *febris*], an abnormal elevation of the temperature of the body above 37° C (98.6° F) because of disease. Fever results from an imbalance between the elimination and the production of heat. Exercise, anxiety, and dehydration may increase the temperature of healthy people. Infection, neurologic disease, malignancy, pernicious anemia, thromboembolic disease, paroxysmal tachycardia, congestive heart failure, crushing injury, severe trauma, and many drugs may cause the development of fever. Fever has no recognized function in conditions other than infection. It increases metabolic activity by 7% per degree Celsius, requiring a greater intake of food. Kinds of hyperthermia include **habitual fever, intermittent fever,** and **relapsing fever.**

fever blister, a cold sore caused by herpesvirus 1 or 2.

fever of unknown origin (FUO), a fever of at least 101° F (38.3° C) that persists for at least 3 weeks without discovery of the cause despite at least 1 week of intensive study.

fever therapy. See **artificial fever.**

fever treatment, the care and management of a person with an elevated temperature.

F factor, (in bacterial genetics) an episome present in conjugating male bacteria but absent in females.

^{18}F-FDG, symbol for [^{18}F]-2-fluoro-2-deoxy-D-glucose, a sugar analog used in positron emission tomography to determine the local cerebral metabolic rate of glucose as a measure of neural activity in the brain.

FHR, abbreviation for **fetal heart rate.**

FHS, abbreviation for **fetal hydantoin syndrome.**

fht, abbreviation for **fetal heart tones.**

fiber diet [L *fibra*; Gk *diata* way of living], a diet that contains an abundance of fibrous material that resists digestion. Fibrous foods are found mainly in vegetables, fruits, and cereals. They add bulk to the diet and reportedly reduce the risk of bowel cancer.

fiberoptic bronchoscopy [L *fibra* + Gk *optikos* sight], the visual examination of the tracheobronchial tree through a fiberoptic bronchoscope.

fiberoptic duodenoscope, an instrument for visualizing the interior of the duodenum, consisting of an eyepiece, a flexible tube incorporating bundles of coated glass or plastic fibers with special optic properties, and a terminal light.

fiberoptics, the technical process by which an internal organ or cavity can be viewed, using glass or plastic fibers to transmit light through a specially designed tube and reflect a magnified image. **–fiberoptic,** *adj.*

fiberscope [L *fibra* + Gk *skopein* to look], a flexible fiberoptic instrument designed for the examination of particular organs and cavities of the body, as in bronchoscopy, endoscopy, and gastroscopy.

fibril /fī′bril/ [L *fibrilla* small fiber], a small filamentous structure that often is a component of a cell, as in a mitotic spindle.

fibrillation /fī′brilā′shən/ [L *fibrilla* small fiber, *atio* process], involuntary recurrent contraction of a single muscle fiber or of an isolated bundle of nerve fibers. Fibrillation is usually described by the part that is contracting abnormally, such as atrial fibrillation or ventricular fibrillation.

fibrillin /fibri′lin/ [L, *fibrilla,* small fiber], a major component of elastin-associated microfibrils linked to Marfan syndrome by immunohistochemical studies. Fibrillin is also associated with a disease similar to Marfan syndrome, **congenital contractural arachnodactyly.**

fibrin /fī′brin/ [L *fibra* fiber], a stringy, insoluble protein that is a product of the action of thrombin on fibrinogen in the clotting process. It is responsible for the semisolid character of a blood clot.

fibrinase. See **factor XIII.**

fibrinogen /fibrin′əjən/ [L *fibra* fiber; Gk *genein* to produce], a plasma protein essential to the blood clotting process that is converted into fibrin by thrombin in the presence of calcium ions.

fibrinogenic. See **fibrogenous; fibrinogenous.**

fibrinogenopenia /fĭbrōjen'ōpē'nē·ə/ [L *fibra* + Gk *genein* to produce, *penes* poor], a condition in which there is a deficiency of fibrinogen in the blood.

fibrinogenous /fĭbrinōj'ənəs/ [L *fibra* + Gk *genein* to produce], pertaining to the characteristics or properties of fibrinogen, or the production of fibrin.

fibrinokinase /fĭ'brinōkī'nās/ [L *fibra* + Gk *kinesis* motion], a non-water-soluble enzyme in animal tissue that activates plasminogen.

fibrinolysin /fĭ'brinol'isin/ [L *fibra* + Gk *lysein* to loosen], a proteolytic enzyme that dissolves fibrin.

fibrinolysis /fĭ'brinol'isis/, the continual process of fibrin decomposition by fibrinolysin that is the normal mechanism for the removal of small fibrin clots. –**fibrinolytic,** *adj.*

fibrinopeptide /fĭ'brinōpep'tīd/ [L *fibra* + Gk *peptein* to digest], a product of the action of thrombin on fibrinogen.

fibrinous pericarditis [L *fibra;* Gk *peri* near, *kardia* heart, *itis* inflammation], a condition in which a lymph exudate accumulates on the pericardium and coagulates. The coagulated exudate may acquire a thick buttery appearance.

fibrin-stabilizing factor. See **factor XIII.**

fibroadenoma /fĭ'brō·ad'inō'mə/, *pl.* **fibroadenomas, fibroadenomata** [L *fibra* + Gk *aden* gland, *oma*], a benign tumor composed of dense epithelial and fibroblastic tissue.

fibroangioma. See **angiofibroma.**

fibroareolar tissue. See **areolar tissue.**

fibroblast /fĭ'brəblast'/ [L *fibra* + Gk *blastos* germ], a flat, elongated undifferentiated cell in the connective tissue that gives rise to various precursor cells, such as the chondroblast, collagenoblast, and osteoblast, that form the fibrous, binding, and supporting tissue of the body. –**fibroblastic,** *adj.*

fibroblastoma, /fĭ'brōblastō'mə/ *pl.* **fibroblastomas, fibroblastomata** [L *fibra* + Gk *blastos* germ, *oma*], a tumor derived from a fibroblast, now differentiated as a fibroma or a fibrosarcoma.

fibrocarcinoma. See **scirrhous carcinoma.**

fibrocartilage [L *fibra* + *cartilago*], cartilage that consists of a dense matrix of white collagenous fibers. –**fibrocartilaginous,** *adj.*

fibrocartilaginous joint. See **symphysis.**

fibrocystic disease [L *fibra* + Gk *kystis* bag], **1.** (of the breast) the presence of single or multiple cysts in the breasts. The cysts are benign and fairly common, yet must be considered potentially malignant and observed carefully for growth or change. **2.** See **cystic fibrosis.**

fibrocyte. See **fibroblast.**

fibroelastic tissue. See **fibrous tissue.**

fibroepithelial papilloma /fĭ'brō·ep'ithē'lē·əl/ [L *fibra* + Gk *epi* above, *thele* nipple; L *papilla* nipple; Gk *oma* tumor], a benign epithelial tumor containing extensive fibrous tissue.

fibroepithelioma /fĭ'brō·ep'ithē'lē·ō'mə/, *pl.* **fibroepitheliomas, fibroepitheliomata** [L *fibra* + Gk *epi* above, *thele* nipple, *oma* tumor], a neoplasm consisting of fibrous and epithelial components. A kind of fibroepithelioma is **premalignant fibroepithelioma.**

fibroid /fĭ'broid/ [L *fibra* + Gk *eidos* form], **1.** having fibers. **2.** *informal;* a fibroma or myoma, particularly of the uterus.

fibroidectomy /fĭ'broidek'təmē/ [L *fibra* + Gk *eidos* + *ektome* cutting out], the surgical removal of a fibrous tumor, such as a uterine fibromyoma.

fibroid tumor. See **fibroma.**

fibrolipoma /fĭ'brōlipō'mə/, a fibrous tumor that also contains fatty material.

fibroma /fĭbrō'mə/, *pl.* **fibromas, fibromata** [L *fibra* + Gk *oma* tumor], a benign neoplasm consisting largely of fibrous or fully developed connective tissue.

fibroma cavernosum, a tumor containing large vascular spaces, an excessive amount of fibrous tissue, and blood or lymph vessels.

fibroma cutis, a fibrous tumor of the skin.

fibroma durum. See **hard fibroma.**

fibroma molle. See **soft fibroma.**

fibroma mucinosum, a fibrous tumor in which there is mucoid material with degeneration.

fibroma myxomatodes. See **myxofibroma.**

fibroma of breast [L *fibra* + Gk *oma* tumor; AS *braest*], a connective tissue tumor of the breast. It is usually benign and painless.

fibroma pendulum, a pendulous fibrous tumor of the skin.

fibroma sarcomatosum. See **fibrosarcoma.**

fibroma thecocellulare xanthomatodes. See **theca cell tumor.**

fibromatosis /fĭ'brōmatō'sis/ [L *fibra* + Gk *oma* tumor, *osis* condition], a gingival enlargement believed to be hereditary, manifesting in the permanent dentition and characterized by a firm hyperplastic tissue that covers the surfaces of the teeth.

fibromyoma uteri. See **leiomyoma uteri.**

fibromyomectomy /fī'brōmī'ōmek'təmē/, a surgical procedure for removal of a uterine fibroma or other type of fibromyoma.

fibromyositis /fī'brōmī'əsī'tis/ [L *fibra* + Gk *mys* muscle, *itis* inflammation], any one of a large number of disorders in which the common element is stiffness and joint or muscle pain, accompanied by localized inflammation of the muscle tissues and of the fibrous connective tissues. Kinds of fibromyositis include **lumbago, pleurodynia,** and **torticollis.**

fibropapilloma. See **fibroepithelial papilloma.**

fibrosarcoma /fī'brōsärkō'mə/ *pl.* **fibrosarcomas, fibrosarcomata** [L *fibra* + Gk *sarx* flesh, *oma* tumor], a sarcoma that contains connective tissue. It develops suddenly from small nodules on the skin.

fibrosing alveolitis /fī'brōsing/ [L *fibra* + *alviolus* small hollow; Gk *itis* inflammation], a severe form of alveolitis characterized by dyspnea and hypoxia, occurring in advanced rheumatoid arthritis and other autoimmune diseases.

fibrosis /fībrō'sis/ [L *fibra* + Gk *osis* condition], **1.** a proliferation of fibrous connective tissue. **2.** an abnormal condition in which fibrous connective tissue spreads over or replaces normal smooth muscle or other normal organ tissue. Fibrosis is most common in the heart, lung, peritoneum, and kidney.

fibrosis of the lungs [L *fibra* + Gk *osis;* AS *lungen*], the formation of scar tissue in the connective tissue of the lungs as a sequel to any inflammation or irritation caused by tuberculosis, bronchopneumonia, or a pneumoconiosis. Localized fibrosis may be complicated by infarction, abscess, or bronchiectasis.

fibrositis /fī'brəsī'tis/, an inflammation of fibrous connective tissue, usually characterized by a poorly defined set of symptoms, including pain and stiffness of the neck, shoulder, and trunk.

fibrous /fī'brəs/ [L *fibra* fiber], consisting mainly of fibers or fiber-containing materials, such as fibrous connective tissue.

fibrous capsule, **1.** the external layer of an articular capsule. It surrounds the articulation of two adjoining bones. **2.** the external, tough membranous envelope surrounding some visceral organs, such as the liver.

fibrous dysplasia, an abnormal condition characterized by the fibrous displacement of the osseous tissue within the bones affected. The distinct kinds of fibrous dysplasia are monostotic fibrous dysplasia, polyostotic fibrous dysplasia, and polyostotic fibrous dysplasia with associated endocrine disorders. The initial signs may be a limp, a pain, or a fracture on the affected side. Pathologic fractures are frequently associated with this process, and angulation deformities may follow.

fibrous goiter, an enlargement of the thyroid gland, characterized by hyperplasia of the capsule and connective tissue.

fibrous gold. See **gold foil.**

fibrous histiocytoma. See **dermatofibroma.**

fibrous joint, any one of many immovable joints, such as those of the skull segments, in which a fibrous tissue or a hyaline cartilage connects the bones.

fibrous thyroiditis, a disorder characterized by slowly progressive fibrosis of an enlarged thyroid with replacement of normal thyroid tissue by dense fibrous tissue. Symptoms include a choking sensation, dyspnea, dysphagia, and hypothyroidism, but in some patients the gland functions normally.

fibrous tissue, the fibrous connective tissue of the body, consisting of closely woven elastic fibers and fluid-filled areolae.

fibula /fib'yo͞olə/ [L, buckle], one of the two bones of the lower leg, lateral to and smaller than the tibia. In proportion to its length, it is the most slender of the long bones and presents three borders and three surfaces for attaching various muscles.

fibular /fib'yələr/ [L, *fibula,* clasp], pertaining to the fibula.

Fick principle [Adolf E. Fick, German physiologist, b. 1829], a method for making indirect measurements, based on the law of conservation of mass. It is used specifically to determine cardiac output, in which the amount of oxygen uptake of each unit of blood as it passes through the lungs is equal to the oxygen concentration difference between arterial and mixed venous blood.

Fick's law [Adolf E. Fick], **1.** (in chemistry and physics) an observed law stating that the rate at which one substance diffuses through another is directly proportional to the concentration gradient of the diffusing substance. **2.** (in medicine) an observed law stating that the rate of diffusion across a membrane is directly proportional to the concentration gradient of the substance on the two sides of the membrane and inversely related to the thickness of the membrane.

fictive kin /fik'tiv/, people who are regarded as being part of a family even though they are not related.

FID, abbreviation for **free-induction decay.**

field [AS *feld*], a defined space, area, or

distance. The field of vision represents the total area that can be seen with one fixed eye. The binocular field is the area that can be seen with both eyes.

field fever, a form of leptospirosis affecting primarily agricultural workers. It is characterized by fever, abdominal pain, diarrhea, vomiting, stupor, and conjunctivitis.

field of vision [AS *feld*; L *visio* seeing], the area of space in which objects are visible at the same time when the eye is fixed and the face is turned so as to exclude the limiting effects of the orbital margins and nose.

fiery serpent [AS *fyre*; L *serpere* to creep], an informal term for *Dracunculus medinesis*.

fièvre boutonneuse. See **African tick typhus.**

fifth disease. See **erythema infectiosum.**

fifth nerve. See **trigeminal nerve.**

fight-or-flight. See **flight-or-fight reaction.**

FIGLU, abbreviation for **formiminoglutamic acid.**

figure 4 test. See **Fabere's test.**

figure-ground relationship [L *figura* form; AS *grund*; L *relatus* carry back], a perceptual field that is divided into a figure, which is the object of focus, and a diffuse background.

figure-of-eight bandage, a bandage with successive laps crossing over and around each other like the figure eight.

figure-of-eight suture [L *sutura*], a suture that begins at the deepest layer on each side of a wound, then crosses over to pass through the superficial layers on the opposite side before being tied.

filament /fil'əmənt/ [L *filare* to spin], a fine threadlike fiber. Filaments are found in most tissues and cells of the body and serve various morphologic or physiologic functions.

filamentous, /fil'əmen'təs/ [L *filamentum* thread], pertaining to something that is threadlike or capable of being drawn out into a threadlike structure.

filariasis /fil'ərī'əsis/ [L *filum* thread; Gk *osis* condition], a disease caused by the presence of filariae or microfilariae in the tissues of the body. Filarial worms are round, long, and threadlike and tend to infest the lymph glands and channels after entering the body as microscopic larvae through the bite of an insect.

filariform /filer'ifôrm/, pertaining to a structure or organism that is threadlike.

file, a collection of related data or information kept as a unit.

filial generation /fil'ē·əl/ [L *filius* son; *generare* to beget], the offspring produced from a given mating or cross in a genetic sequence.

filiform bougie /fil'ifôrm/ [L *filum* thread, *forma* form; Fr *bougie* candle], an extremely thin bougie for passage through a narrow stricture, such as a sinus tract.

filiform catheter, a catheter with a slender, threadlike tip that allows the wider portion of the instrument to be passed through canals that are constricted or irregular.

filiform papilla. See **papilla.**

filling factor [AS *fyllan* filling; L *factor* a maker], a measure of the geometric relationship of a radiofrequency coil used in NMR imaging and the body.

filling pressure, the pressure in the left ventricle at the end of diastole.

film [AS *filmen* membrane], **1.** a thin sheet or layer of any material, such as a coating of oil on a metal part. **2.** (in photography and radiography) a thin, flexible, transparent sheet of cellulose acetate or similar material coated with a light-sensitive emulsion, used to record images.

film badge, a photographic film packet, sensitive to ionizing radiation, used for estimating the exposure of personnel working with x-rays and other radioactive sources.

film development, the processing of photographic or x-ray films to make manifest the latent image resulting from exposure of the chemically treated gelatin emulsion to a pattern of electromagnetic radiation.

film fault, a defect in a photograph or radiograph, usually caused by a chemical, physical, or electric error in its production.

film on teeth, a collection of mucinous deposits adhering to the teeth, which contains microorganisms, desquamated tissue elements, blood cellular elements, and other debris.

film screen mammography, a breast x-ray technique in which a special single-emulsion film and high-detail intensifying screens are used.

filter [Fr *filtrer* to strain], **1.** a device or material through which a gas or liquid is passed to separate out unwanted matter. **2.** (in radiology) a device added to x-ray equipment to selectively remove low-energy x-rays that have no chance of getting to the film.

filtered back projection, a mathematical technique used in NMR imaging and computed tomography to create images from a set of multiple projection profiles.

filtration [Fr *filtrer* to strain], the addition of sheets of metal into a beam of x-rays, altering the energy spectrum and thus the imaging characteristics and penetrating ability of the radiation. Filtration is generally provided by aluminum or copper at low to medium energies, and by tin, copper, and aluminum for higher energy beams.

filum /fī′ləm/, a threadlike structure.

fimbria /fim′frē·ə/ [L, fringe], any structure that forms a border or edge or that resembles a fringe. Kinds of fimbria are **fimbria hippocampi, ovarica,** and **tubae.**

fimbriae tubae /fim′bri·ī/, the branched, fingerlike projections at the distal end of each of the fallopian tubes.

fimbria hippocampi, a band of efferent fibers formed by the alveus hippocampi that is continuous with the posterior pillar of the fornix.

fimbrial tubal pregnancy, a kind of tubal pregnancy in which implantation occurs in the fimbriated distal end of one of the fallopian tubes.

fimbria ovarica, the longest of the fimbriae tubae. It extends from the infundibulum to the ovary.

fimbriated [L *fimbria* fringe], pertaining to or resembling the fimbria or fringelike structure of the ovaries or the nerve fibers along the border of the hippocampus.

finastride /fin′əstrīd, finas′trīd/, a drug used to treat prostatic hypertrophy by reversing the progressive enlargement of the gland.

fine motor skills [Fr *fin* thin; L *movere;* ONorse *skilja* to cut apart], the use of precise coordinated movements in such activities as writing, buttoning, cutting, tracing, or visual tracking.

fineness [Fr *fin* thin], (in dentistry) a means of grading alloys relative to gold content. The fineness of an alloy is designated in parts per thousand of pure gold.

fine tremor [Fr *fin;* L *tremor* to tremble], a tremor that occurs after a voluntary movement or one that develops as a result of fatigue in the corresponding muscle group.

finger [AS *fingar*], any of the digits of the hand. The fingers of the hand are composed of a metacarpal bone and three bony phalanges. Some anatomists regard the thumb as a finger.

finger agnosia, a neurologic disorder in which a patient is unable to distinguish between stimuli applied to two different fingers without visual clues.

finger goniometer [AS *finger;* Gk *gonia* angle, *metron* meter], an instrument for measuring the angle of a finger joint, or of an arm or leg.

finger-nose test [AS *finger, nosu;* L *testum* crucible], a test of the coordination of the arms. The patient is asked to bring the tip of the index finger quickly to the nose, first with the eyes open, then with the eyes closed. An inability to accurately perform the test may be an indication of cerebellar disease.

finger percussion. See **percussion.**

finger stick, the act of puncturing the tip of the finger to obtain a small sample of capillary blood.

Finnish bath. See **Russian bath.**

Fio₂, the percentage of inspired oxygen a patient is receiving, usually expressed as a fraction.

fire damp. See **damp.**

fireman's cramp. See **heat cramp.**

first aid [AS *fyrst;* Fr *aider* to help], the immediate care that is given to an injured or ill person before treatment by medically trained personnel. Attention is directed first to the most critical problems: evaluation of the patency of the airway, the presence of bleeding, and the adequacy of cardiac function.

first cuneiform. See **medial cuneiform bone.**

first dentition. See **deciduous dentition.**

first-dollar coverage, an insurance plan under which the third-party payer assumes liability for covered services as soon as the first dollar of expense for such services is incurred, without requiring the insured to pay a deductible.

first filial generation. See **F₁.**

first-generation scanner, an early type of computed tomography device.

first intention. See **intention.**

first metacarpal bone, the metacarpal bone of the thumb.

first nerve. See **olfactory nerve.**

first-order change, a change within a system that itself remains unchanged.

first-order kinetics, a chemical reaction in which the rate of decrease in the number of molecules of a substrate is proportional to the concentration of substrate molecules remaining. The rate of metabolism of most drugs follows the rule of first-order kinetics and is independent of the dose.

first rib, the highest rib of the thoracic cage. It moves about the axis of its neck, raising and lowering the sternum.

first stage of labor [ME *fyrst;* OFr *estage;* L *labor* work], a period of 8 to 12 hours marked by the onset of regular contractions of the uterus with full dilation of the cervix and the appearance of a bit of blood-tinged mucus. Danger signs of the first stage include abnormal bleeding, abnormal fetal heart rate, and abnormal presentation and position of the fetus.

first-state cementoma. See **periapical fibroma.**

Fishberg concentration test, a test of the ability of the kidneys to concentrate urine,

413

developed by American physician Arthur M. Fishberg. The test involves measuring the specific gravity of morning urine samples following overnight deprivation of fluid intake.

fish poisoning, toxic effects caused by ingestion of fish containing substances that may produce symptoms ranging from nausea and vomiting to respiratory paralysis. Scrombroid poisoning usually results from a histamine-like toxin produced by bacterial activity in mackerel, tuna, or bonito. Tetraodon poisoning is caused by a toxin in puffer fish.

fish skin disease. See **ichthyosis.**

fish tapeworm infection [AS *fisc* fish], an infection caused by the tapeworm *Diphyllobothrium latum* that is transmitted to humans when they eat contaminated raw or undercooked freshwater fish.

fission /fish'ən/ [L *fissio* splitting], **1.** the act or process of splitting or breaking up into parts. **2.** a type of asexual reproduction common in bacteria, protozoa, and other lower forms of life in which the cell divides into two or more equal components, each of which eventually develops into a complete organism. Kinds of fission are **binary fission** and **multiple fission. 3.** (in physics) the splitting of the nucleus of an atom and subsequent release of energy.

fissiparous /fisip'ərəs/, reproduced by fission.

fissural angioma /fish'ərəl/ [L *fissura* cleft, a tumor composed of a cluster of dilated blood vessels found in an embryonal fissure, especially on a lip, the face, or the neck.

fissure /fish'ər/ [L *fissura* cleft], **1.** a cleft or a groove on the surface of an organ, often marking division of the organ into parts, such as the lobes of the lung. **2.** a cracklike lesion of the skin, such as an anal fissure. **3.** a lineal fault on a bony surface occurring during the development of a part, such as a fissure in the enamel of a tooth. **—fissured,** *adj.*

fissured tongue /fish'ərd/ [L *fissura* cleft; AS *tunge*], a tongue with deep surface furrows that may radiate outward. The condition may be inherited as an autosomal dominant trait.

fissure fracture, any fracture in which a crack extends into the cortex of the bone but not through the entire bone.

fissure-in-ano /fish'ərinā'nō/, a painful linear ulcer at the margin of the anus.

fissure of Bichat. See **transverse fissure.**

fissure of Rolando. See **central sulcus.**

fissure of Sylvius. See **lateral cerebral sulcus.**

fistula /fis'chŏŏlə, -chələ/, *pl.* **fistulas, fistulae** [L, pipe], an abnormal passage from an internal organ to the body surface or between two internal organs. **—fistulous, fistular, fistulate,** *adj.*

fistula in ano. See **anal fistula.**

fistulectomy /fis'chəlek'təmē/ [L *fistula* pipe; Gk *ektome* cutting out], the surgical removal of a fistula.

fit, 1. *nontechnical;* a paroxysm or seizure. **2.** the sudden onset of an episode of symptoms, as a fit of coughing. **3.** the manner in which one surface is aligned to another, such as the fit of a denture to the gingiva and jaw.

Fitzgerald factor, a high molecular weight kinogen that may be required for the interaction of factors XII and XI in the coagulation process.

Fitzgerald treatment. See **zone therapy.**

five-day fever, *informal;* trench fever.

five-step nursing process, a nursing process comprising five broad categories of nursing behaviors: assessing, analyzing, planning, implementing, and evaluating.

fixating eye [L *figere* to fasten; AS *eage*], (in strabismus) the normal eye that can be focused.

fixation [L *figere* to fasten, *atio* process], (in psychoanalysis) an arrest at a particular stage of psychosexual development, such as anal fixation. **—fixate,** *v.,* **fixated,** *adj.*

fixation muscle, a muscle that acts to hold a part of the body in appropriate position.

fixative [L *figere* to fasten], **1.** any substance used to bind, glue, or stabilize. **2.** any substance used to preserve gross or histologic specimens of tissue for later examination.

fixed anions, anions that are not part of the body's buffer anions.

fixed bridgework, a dental device incorporating artificial teeth permanently attached in the upper or the lower jaw.

fixed cations, cations that are not part of the body's metabolic buffering system.

fixed-combination drug [L *figere* to fasten; *combinare* to combine; Fr *drogue*], any of a group of multiple-ingredient preparations that provides concomitant administration of specific amounts of two or more drugs.

fixed coupling, a precise distance between a normal and ectopic beat that is duplicated each time the ectopic beat occurs.

fixed delusion [L figere, deludere to deceive], a deluison that is consistent and unaltered.

fixed dressing, a dressing usually made of gauze impregnated with a hardening agent, such as plaster of paris, sodium silicate, starch, or dextrin, applied to support or immobilize a part of the body.

fixed-drug eruption, well-defined red to purple lesions that appear at the same sites on the skin and mucous membranes each time a particular drug is used.

fixed fulcrum, a tomographic fulcrum that remains at a fixed height.

fixed idea, 1. a persistent, obsessional thought or notion. **2.** in certain mental disorders, especially obsessive-compulsive neurosis, a delusional idea that dominates mental activity and persists despite contrary evidence.

fixed interval (FI) reinforcement, (in psychiatry) a specific lapse of time required for reinforcement.

fixed macrophage [L *figere*; Gk, *makros* large, *pagein* to eat], nonmotile mononuclear phagocytes in the liver sinuses, spleen, lymph glands, and other tissues.

fixed orthodontic appliance, a prosthetic device cemented to the teeth or attached by adhesive material, for changing the relative positions of dentitions.

fixed-performance oxygen delivery system. See **high-flow oxygen delivery system.**

fixed phagocyte. See **phagocyte.**

fixed pupil [L *figere, pupilla* little girl], an abnormal condition in which the pupils fail to dilate or contract when stimulated. The cause is commonly adhesions that bind the iris to the lens capsule, or because of interference with the nerve supply of the iris in acute glaucoma.

fixed rate pacemaker [L *figere, ratum* calculate, *passus* step; ME *maken*], an artificial cardiac pacemaker that delivers impulses to the cardiac muscle at a preset rate regardless of the heart's independent activity.

fixed ratio (FR) reinforcement, (in psychiatry) reinforcement given after a specific number of responses have occurred.

fixed torticollis [L *figere, tortus* twisted, *collum* neck], a condition in which neck muscles on one side are so short that the head is held continuously in the same position.

fixed vertebrae. See **false vertebrae.**

fixer, a chemical product used in processing photographic or x-ray film. Applied after the developing phase, it neutralizes any developer remaining on the film, removes undeveloped silver halides, and hardens the emulsion.

flaccid /flak′sid/ [L *flaccus* flabby], weak, soft, and flabby; lacking normal muscle tone, such as flaccid muscles. **–flaccidity, flaccidness,** *n.*

flaccid bladder, a form of neurogenic bladder caused by interruption of the reflex arc associated with the voiding reflex in the spinal cord.

flaccid paralysis, an abnormal condition characterized by the weakening or the loss of muscle tone.

flagella /fləjel′ə/ [L *flagellum* whip], hairlike projections that extend from some unicellular organisms and aid in their movement.

flagellant /flaj′ələnt/, a person who receives sexual gratification from the practice of flagellation.

flagellate /flaj′əlāt′, -lit/ [L *flagellum* whip], a microorganism that propels itself by waving whiplike filaments or cilia behind its body, such as *Trypanosoma, Leishmania, Trichomonas,* and *Giardia.*

flagellation, 1. the act of whipping, beating, or flogging. **2.** a type of massage administered by tapping the body with the fingers. **3.** a type of sexual deviation in which a person is erotically gratified by being whipped or by whipping another. **4.** the arrangement of flagella on an organism; exflagellation.

flail chest /flāl/ [ME *fleyl* whip; AS *cest* box], a thorax in which multiple rib fractures cause instability in part of the chest wall and paradoxical breathing, with the lung underlying the injured area contracting on inspiration and bulging on expiration.

flame photometry [L *flagrare* to burn; Gk *phos* light, *metron* measure], measurement of the wavelength of light rays emitted by excited metallic electrons exposed to the heat energy of a flame, used to identify characteristics in clinical specimens of body fluids.

flange /flanj/, **1.** the part of a denture base that extends from the cervical ends of the teeth to the border of the denture. **2.** a prosthesis with a lateral vertical extension designed to direct a resected mandible into centric occlusion.

flank, the posterior portion of the body between the ribs and the ilium.

flapping tremor. See **asterixis.**

flare /fler/, **1.** a red blush on the skin at the periphery of an urticarial lesion seen in immediate hypersensitivity reactions. **2.** an expanding skin flush, spreading from an infective lesion or extending from the principal site of a reaction to an irritant. **3.** the sudden intensification of a disease.

flaring of nostrils, a widening of the nostrils during inspiration, a sign of air hunger or respiratory distress.

flashback, a phenomenon experienced by persons who have taken hallucinogenic drugs and unexpectedly reexperience the drug effects.

flask closure [L *vasculum* small vessel; *claudere* to close], (in dentistry) the joining of two halves of a flask that encloses and forms a denture base.

flat affect, the affect of a patient who does not communicate feelings in verbal or nonverbal responses to events.

Flatau-Schilder disease. See **Schilder's disease.**

flat bone [AS *flet* floor], any of the bones that provide structural contours of the skeleton. Examples include ribs and bones of the skull.

flat electroencephalogram, a graphic chart on which no tracings were recorded during electroencephalography, indicating a lack of brain-wave activity.

flatfoot. See **pes planus.**

flat spring contraceptive diaphragm, a kind of contraceptive diaphragm in which the flexible metal spring that forms the rim is a thin, light, flat band made of stainless steel.

flatulence /flach'ələns/ [L *flatus* a blowing], the presence of an excessive amount of air or gas in the stomach and intestinal tract, causing distension of the organs and in some cases mild to moderate pain.

flatulent /flach'ələnt/, pertaining to gas or air in the digestive tract.

flatus /flā'təs/ [L, a blowing], air or gas in the intestine that is passed through the rectum.

flat wart. See **verruca plana.**

flavone /flā'vōn/ [L *flavus* yellow], a colorless, crystalline, flavonoid derivative and component of bioflavonoid that increases capillary resistance.

flavoxate hydrochloride /flavok'sāt/, a smooth muscle relaxant prescribed for spastic conditions of the urinary tract.

fl. dr., abbreviation for **fluid dram.**

flea [AS], a wingless, bloodsucking insect of the order Siphonaptera, some species of which transmit arboviruses to humans by acting as host or vector to the organism.

flea bite, a small puncture wound produced by a blood-sucking flea. Certain species of fleas transmit plague, murine typhus, and probably tularemia.

flea bites, *informal.* Erythema toxicum neonatorum.

flea-borne typhus. See **murine typhus.**

flecainide acetate /flekā'nīd/, an oral antiarrhythmic drug prescribed for the treatment of ventricular dysrhythmias.

Fleet Enema, trademark for a manufactured enema formula containing 16 gm sodium biphosphate and 6 gm sodium phosphate per 100 ml solution, made available in disposable plastic pouches fitted with prelubricated rectal tubes.

Fleischner method /flīsh'nər/, a technique for producing lordotic x-ray projec-

tions of the lungs. The patient is placed in P-A projection position while leaning backward from the waist to a nearly 45-degree posterior inclination.

Fletcher factor, a prekallikrein blood coagulation substance that interacts with both factor XII and Fitzgerald factor, activating both and accelerating thrombin formation.

FLEX, abbreviation for **Federation Licensing Examination.**

flexibilitas cerea. See **cerea flexibilitas.**

flexion /flek'shən/ [L *flectere* to bend], **1.** a movement allowed by certain joints of the skeleton that decreases the angle between two adjoining bones, such as bending the elbow. **2.** (in obstetrics) a resistance to the descent of the fetus through the birth canal that causes the neck to flex so the chin approaches the chest.

flexion jacket, a corset designed to provide spinal immobility.

flexor /flek'sər/ [L, bender], a muscle that flexes a joint.

flexor carpi radialis [L *flexor* bender], a slender, superficial muscle of the forearm that lies on the ulnar side of the pronator teres. It functions to flex and to help abduct the hand.

flexor carpi ulnaris, a superficial muscle lying along the ulnar side of the forearm. It functions to flex and adduct the hand.

flexor digitorum superficialis, the largest superficial muscle of the forearm, lying on the ulnar side under the palmaris longus. The muscle flexes the second phalanx of each finger and, by continued action, the hand.

flexor retinaculum of ankle [L *flexor, retinaculum* halter, AS *ancleow*], an overgrowth of fascia from the medial malleolus to the calcaneum, passing over the long flexor tendons and blood vessels and nerves of the posterior tibia.

flexor retinaculum of the hand. See **retinaculum flexorum manus.**

flexor retinaculum of wrist [L *flexor, retinaculum;* AS *wrist*], a strong ligament across the front of the hollow of the carpus and over the flexor tendons of the fingers and median nerve.

flexor withdrawal reflex, a common cutaneous reflex consisting of a widespread contraction of physiologic flexor muscles and relaxation of physiologic extensor muscles. It is characterized by abrupt withdrawal of a body part in response to painful or injurious stimuli.

flextime [L *flectere* to bend; AS *tima*], a system of staffing that allows the individualization of work schedules.

flexure /flek'shər/, a normal bend or

curve in a body part, such as the dorsal flexure of the spine.

flight into health [AS *fleogan* to fly], an abnormal but common reaction to an unpleasant physical sensation or symptom in which the person denies the reality of the feeling or observation, insisting that there is nothing wrong.

flight of ideas, (in psychiatry) a continuous stream of talk in which the patient switches rapidly from one topic to another, each subject being incoherent and not related to the preceding one.

flight-or-fight reaction [AS *fleogan* to fly; *feohtan* to fight; L *reagere* to act again], **1.** (in physiology) the reaction of the body to stress, in which the sympathetic nervous system and the adrenal medulla act to increase the cardiac output, dilate the pupils of the eyes, increase the rate of the heartbeat, constrict the blood vessels of the skin, increase the glucose and fatty acids in the circulation, and induce an alert, aroused mental state. **2.** (in psychiatry) a person's reaction to stress by either fleeing from a situation or remaining and attempting to deal with it.

flight to illness, the effort of the patient to convince the therapist that he or she is too ill to terminate therapy and that continued support is needed.

flip angle, in NMR imaging, the amount of rotation of the macroscopic magnetization vector produced by a radiofrequency pulse with respect to the direction of the static magnetic field.

floater [AS *flotian* to float], one or more spots that appear to drift in front of the eye, caused by a shadow cast on the retina by vitreous debris. Most floaters are benign and represent remnants of a network of blood vessels that existed prenatally in the vitreous cavity. The sudden onset of several floaters may indicate serious disease. The technical term for floaters is **muscae volitantes.**

floating head [AS *flotian* to float; *heafod*], unengaged fetal head.

floating kidney, a kidney that is not securely fixed in the usual anatomic location because of congenital malplacement or traumatic injury.

floating patella [AS *flotian*; L *patella* small pan], a patella that has been forced away from the femoral condyle by an effusion into the knee joint.

float nurse, a nurse who is available for assignment to duty on an ad hoc basis, usually to assist in times of unusually heavy work loads or to assume the duties of absent nursing personnel.

flocculant /flok′yo͞olənt/, an agent or substance that causes flocculation.

flocculation test /flok′yo͞olā′shən/ [L *floccus* flock of wool, a serologic test in which a positive result depends on the degree of flocculent precipitation produced in the material being tested. Many tests for syphilis are flocculation tests.

flocculent /flok′yo͞olənt/ [L *floccus* flock of wool], clumped or tufted, such as a cloud, or covered with a woolly, fuzzy surface. **–flocculate,** *v.,* **flocculation, floccule,** *n.*

flood fever. See **typhus.**

flooding [AS *flod*], a technique used in behavior therapy for the reduction of anxiety associated with various phobias. Exposure to a stimulus that usually provokes anxiety desensitizes a person to that stimulus.

floppy infant syndrome [ME *flappe* slap; L *infans* speechless], a general term for juvenile spinal muscular atrophies, including Werdnig-Hoffmann disease and Wohlfart-Kugelberg-Welander disease.

flora /flôr′ə/, microorganisms that live on or within a body to compete with disease-producing microorganisms and provide a natural immunity against certain infections.

florid /flôr′id/ [L *floridus* flower], in human skin complexion or wound appearance, a bright red color.

flossing, the mechanical cleansing of tooth surfaces with stringlike waxed or unwaxed dental floss.

flotation device [Fr *flotter* to float], a foam mattress with a gel-like pad located in its center, designed to protect bony prominences and distribute pressure more evenly against the skin's surface.

flotation therapy, a state of semiweightlessness produced by various types of hospital equipment and used in the treatment and prevention of decubitus ulcers.

flowmeter. See **rotameter.**

flow sheet, (in a patient record) a graphic summary of several changing factors, especially the patient's vital signs or weight and the treatments and medications given. In labor, the flow sheet displays the progress of labor.

flow transducer, a spirometer that calculates volume by dividing flow by time.

flow-volume curve, a graphic representation of the instantaneous volumetric flow rates achieved during a forced expiratory vital capacity maneuver. It may be a maximum expiratory flow-volume curve (MEFV) or a partial expiratory flow-volume (PEFV) curve.

flow-volume loop, a pulmonary function test system in which the patient breathes into an electronic spirometer and performs a forced inspiratory and expiratory vital capacity maneuver. The data are displayed graphically as a loop whose shape indicates lung volume and other data through the complete respiratory cycle.

floxuridine /floksy o͞or′ədēn/, an antineoplastic agent prescribed in the treatment of malignant neoplastic disease of the brain, breast, liver, and gallbladder.

fl. oz., abbreviation for **fluid ounce.**

flu /flo͞o/, *informal.* **1.** influenza. **2.** any viral infection, especially of the respiratory or intestinal system.

fluctuant /fluk′cho͞o·ənt/, pertaining to a wavelike motion that is detected when a structure containing a liquid is palpated.

fluctuation /fluk′cho͞o-ā′shən/ [L *fluctuare* to wave], **1.** a wavelike motion of fluid in a body cavity after succussion. **2.** a variation in a fixed value or mass.

flucytosine /flo͞osī′təsēn/, an antifungal prescribed in the treatment of certain serious fungal infections.

fluent aphasia [L *fluere* to flow; Gk *a* not, *phasis* speech], forms of aphasia in which the patient says words easily although the words may be unintelligible or not be related to a particular stimulus. Types of fluent aphasia include **Wernicke's aphasia** and **conduction aphasia.**

fluid [L *fluere* to flow], **1.** a substance, as a liquid or gas, that is able to flow and to adjust its shape to that of a container because it is composed of molecules that are able to change positions with respect to each other without separating from the total mass. **2.** a body fluid, either intracellular or extracellular, that is involved in the transport of electrolytes and other vital chemicals to, through, and from tissue cells.

fluid balance, a state of equilibrium in which the amount of fluid consumed equals the amount lost in urine, feces, perspiration, and exhaled water vapor.

fluid dram (fl. dr.), a unit of liquid measure equal to 3.696 milliliters (ml), 60 minims, or ⅛th of a fluid ounce.

fluidic ventilator, a ventilator that applies the Coanda effect to the movement of the flow of air or gases.

fluid ounce (fl. oz.), a measure of liquid volume in the apothecaries' system, which is equal to 8 fluid drams or 29.57 ml.

fluid retention, a failure to excrete excess fluid from the body. Causes may include renal, cardiovascular, or metabolic disorders.

fluid therapy, the regulation of water balance in patients with impaired renal, cardiovascular, or metabolic function by carefully measuring fluid intake against daily losses.

fluid volume deficit, 1. a NANDA-accepted nursing diagnosis of a failure of the body's homeostatic mechanisms that regulate the retention and excretion of body fluids. Defining characteristics include dilute urine, increased output of urine, a sudden loss of body weight, hypotension, increased pulse rate, decreased turgor, increased body temperature, hemoconcentration, weakness, and thirst. **2.** a NANDA-accepted nursing diagnosis of the active loss of excessive amounts of body fluid. Defining characteristics include decreased output of urine, high specific gravity of the urine, output of urine that is greater than the intake of fluid, a sudden loss of weight, hemoconcentration, increased serum levels of sodium, increased thirst, alteration in mental state, dryness of skin and mucous membranes, elevated temperature, and an increased pulse rate.

fluid volume deficit, high risk for, a NANDA-accepted nursing diagnosis of a state in which an individual experiences vascular, cellular, or intracellular dehydration. Defining characteristics include increased fluid output, urinary frequency, thirst, and any alteration in fluid intake.

fluid volume excess, a NANDA-accepted nursing diagnosis of a compromised regulatory mechanism of the homeostatic mechanisms that regulate the retention and excretion of body fluids, or of an excess fluid or sodium intake. Defining characteristics include edema, effusion, weight gain, shortness of breath, third heart sound, pulmonary congestion, changes in respiratory pattern, abnormal breath sounds, decreased hemoglobin and hematocrit, blood pressure changes, an alteration in electrolyte balance, restlessness, anxiety, and other changes in mental status.

fluke /flo͞ok/, a parasitic flatworm of the class Trematoda, including the genus *Schistosoma.*

fluocinolone acetonide /flo͞o′ōsin′əlōn/, a topical glucocorticoid prescribed as an antiinflammatory agent.

fluocinonide /flo͞o′ōsin′ənīd/, a synthetic corticosteroid prescribed to reduce inflammation.

fluorescence /flo͞ores′əns/ [L *flux* a discharge], the emission of light of one wavelength (usually ultraviolet) when exposed to light of a different, usually shorter, wavelength. **–fluoresce,** *v.,* **fluorescent,** *adj.*

fluorescent antibody test (FA test), a test in which a fluorescent dye is used to stain an antibody for identification of clinical specimens. Fluorescent dyes make the dyed organisms glow visibly when examined under a fluorescent microscope. Kinds of fluorescent antibody tests include the **FTA-ABS test.**

fluorescent microscopy, examination with a fluorescent microscope equipped with a source of ultraviolet light rays, used to study specimens that have been stained with fluorescent dye.

Fluorescent Treponemal Antibody Absorption Test (FTA-ABS test), a serologic test for syphilis.

fluoridation /flôr'idā'shən/ [L *fluere* to flow], the process of adding fluoride, especially to a public water supply, to reduce tooth decay.

fluoride /flŏŏr'id/, a salt of hydrofluoric acid introduced into drinking water and applied directly to the teeth to prevent tooth decay.

fluoride dental treatment [L *fluere, dens* tooth; Fr *traitment*], the direct oral application of fluoride compounds to reduce dental caries.

fluoride poisoning [L *fluere, potio* drink], the toxic effects of contact with compounds of fluorine, an intensely poisonous pale yellow gas. Sodium fluoroacetate is a powerful rodent poison whereas methyl fluoroacetate is regarded as too toxic to use as a pesticide. The fluoroacetate compounds inhibit enzymes of the citric-acid cycle. Inhalation of hydrogen fluoride can lead to bronchospasm, laryngospasm, and pulmonary edema.

fluorine (F) /flŏŏr'ēn/ [L *fluere* to flow], an element of the halogen family and the most reactive of the nonmetals. Its atomic number is 9; its atomic weight is 19. Small amounts of sodium fluoride are added to the water supply of many communities to harden tooth enamel and decrease dental caries. Excessive amounts of fluoride can mottle tooth enamel and cause osteosclerosis. Acute fluoride poisoning and death can result from the accidental ingestion of insecticides and rodenticides containing fluoride salts.

fluorination /flŏŏr'inā'shən/, the addition of a fluorine group to a compound, such as those commonly found in topical corticosteroids.

fluoroacetic acid /flŏŏr'ō·asē'tik, -aset'ik/, a colorless, water-soluble, highly toxic compound that blocks the Krebs' citric acid cycle, causing convulsions and ventricular fibrillation. It is derived from a South African tree and is used in some potent pesticides.

fluorocarbons /flŏŏr'ōkär'bəns/ [L *fluere, carbo* coal], hydrocarbons that contain fluorine. Fluorocarbons are generally colorless, nonflammable gases, but some are liquids at room temperature. The com-

pounds can produce mild upper respiratory tract irritation; excessive exposure has been cited as a cause of central nervous system depression.

fluorometry /flŏŏrom'ətrē/ [L *fluere* + Gk *metron* measure], measurement of fluorescence emitted by compounds when exposed to ultraviolet or other intense radiant energy. Fluorometry is used to measure urinary estrogens, triglycerides, catecholamines, and other substances. **–fluorometric,** *adj.*

fluoroscope /flŏŏr'əskōp'/ [L *fluere* + Gk *skopein* to look], a device used for the immediate projection of an x-ray image on a fluorescent screen for visual examination. **–fluoroscopic,** *adj.*

fluoroscopic compression device /flŏŏr'əskop'ik/, any of several objects that can be placed on a specific area of the patient's abdomen to compress the exterior surface during fluoroscopy of the digestive tract.

fluoroscopy /flŏŏros'kəpē/, a technique in radiology for visually examining a part of the body or the function of an organ using a fluoroscope.

fluorosis /flŏŏrō'sis/ [L *fluere* + Gk *osis* condition], the condition that results from excessive, prolonged ingestion of fluorine. Severe chronic fluorine poisoning will lead to osteosclerosis and other pathologic bone and joint changes in adults.

fluorouracil /flŏŏr'ōyŏŏr'əsil/, an antineoplastic prescribed in the treatment of malignant neoplastic disease of the skin and internal organs.

fluoxymesterone /flōōok'simes'tərōn/, an androgenic and anabolic steroid prescribed in the treatment of testosterone deficiency, breast cancer in females, and delayed puberty in males.

fluphenazine hydrochloride /flōōfen'əzēn/, a phenothiazine tranquilizer prescribed in the treatment of psychotic disorders.

flurandrenolide /flōō'rəndren'əlīd/, a topical glucocorticoid prescribed as an antiinflammatory agent.

flurandrenolone. See **flurandrenolide.**

flurazepam hydrochloride /flōōraz'əpam/, a benzodiazepine minor tranquilizer prescribed in the treatment of insomnia.

flush [ME *fluschen*], 1. a blush or sudden reddening of the face and neck. 2. a sudden, subjective feeling of heat. 3. a prolonged reddening of the face such as may be seen with fever, certain drugs, or hyperthyroidism. 4. a sudden, rapid flow of water or other liquid.

flush device, a device for the accurate

transmission of a pressure wave from a catheter to a transducer in an IV line.

flutter, a rapid vibration or pulsation that may interfere with normal function.

flutter-fibrillation [AS *fleotan* to move quickly; L *fibrilla* small fiber], a type of atrial fibrillation in which the irregular fibrillatory line resembles atrial flutter.

flux gain /fluks/, (in radiology) the ratio between the number of light photons at the output phosphor of an image-intensifier tube and the number at the input phosphor.

fly [AS *flyge*], a two-winged insect of the order Diptera, some species of which transmit arboviruses to humans.

fly bites, bites that may be caused by species of deer, horse, or sand flies. Such bites produce a small painful wound with swelling because of substances in the insect's saliva that are injected beneath the surface of the skin.

Fm, symbol for the chemical element **fermium.**

FMET, abbreviation for **formylmethionine.**

FMG, abbreviation for **foreign medical graduate.**

FMR-1, the symbol for a gene associated with a mental retardation disorder of the **fragile X chromosome** disease. The normal function of the gene has not been determined.

FNP, abbreviation for **family nurse practitioner.**

foam bath [AS *fam, baeth*], a bath taken in water containing a saporin substance that covers the surface of the liquid and through which air or oxygen is blown to form the foam.

focal [L *focus,* hearth], pertaining to a focus.

focal illumination. See **illumination.**

focal lesion [L *focus* fireplace, *laesio* hurting], an infection, tumor, or injury that develops at a restricted or circumscribed area of tissue.

focal motor seizure. See **motor seizure.**

focal plane, the plane of tissue that is in focus on a tomogram.

focal point [L *focus, punctus* pricked], a point at which rays of light meet when deflected, either by reflection or refraction.

focal seizure [L *focus;* OFr *seisir*], a transitory disturbance in motor, sensory, or autonomic function resulting from abnormal neuronal discharges in a localized part of the brain, most frequently motor or sensory areas adjacent to the central sulcus. Focal motor seizures commonly begin as spasmodic movements in the hand, face, or foot and may spread progressively to other muscles to end in a generalized convulsion. Focal seizures may be caused by localized anoxia or a small lesion in the brain.

focal spot, the area on the cathode of an x-ray tube or the target of an accelerator that is struck by electrons and from which the resulting x-rays are emitted. The shape and size of a focal spot influence the resolution of a diagnostic image.

focal symptom [L *focus;* Gk *symptoma* that which happens], a bodily function disturbance focused on a specific body system or part.

focal zone, (in ultrasonography) the distance along the beam axis of a focused transducer assembly, from the point where the beam area first becomes equal to 4 times the focal area to the point beyond the focal surface where the beam area again becomes equal to 4 times the focal area.

focus [L, fireplace], a specific location, as the site of an infection or the point at which an electrochemical impulse originates. **–focal,** *adj.*

focused activity, a therapeutic technique of actively focusing the patient toward adaptive coping abilities and away from maladaptive ones.

focused grid, (in radiography) an x-ray grid that has lead foils placed at an angle so that they all point toward a focus at a specific distance.

foetus. See **fetus.**

fogged film fault [Dan *spray;* AS *filmen* membrane; L *fallere* to deceive], a defect in a photograph or radiograph, which appears as a foggy image or image area.

fogging [ME *fogge*], a method of determining refractive error, particularly in cases of astigmatism, by placing excessively convex or concave lenses before the eyes. The patient is made artificially myopic by means of plus spheres in order to relax all accommodation.

fog nebulizer /fog neb′yəlī′zər/, (in respiratory care) a device that humidifies by producing large volumes of particles.

foil assistant. See **foil holder.**

foil carrier. See **foil passer.**

foil holder [L *folium* leaf; AS *haldan*], an instrument used for holding a foil pellet in place for various dental restorations.

foil passer, a pointed or forked instrument for carrying pellets of gold foil through an annealing flame or from the annealing tray to a prepared tooth cavity.

foil pellet, a loosely rolled piece of gold foil, used for making various dental restorations, as a permanent tooth cavity filling or tooth crown.

folacin. See **folic acid.**

folate /fō′lāt/, **1.** a salt of folic acid. **2.** any of a group of substances found in some foods and in mammalian cells that act as coenzymes and promote the chemical transfer of single carbon units from one molecule to another.

folate deficiency. See **folic acid.**

Foley catheter /fō'lē/ [Frederick E. B. Foley, American physician, b. 1891], a rubber catheter with a balloon tip to be filled with air or a sterile liquid after it has been placed in the bladder. This kind of catheter is used when continuous drainage of the bladder is desired, as in surgery.

folic acid /fō'lik, fol'ik/, a yellow, crystalline, water-soluble vitamin of the B complex group essential for cell growth and reproduction. It functions as a coenzyme with vitamins B_{12} and C in the breakdown and utilization of proteins and in the formation of nucleic acids and heme in hemoglobin. It also increases the appetite and stimulates the production of hydrochloric acid in the digestive tract.

folic acid deficiency anemia, a form of anemia caused by a lack of folic acid in the diet.

folie /fōlē'/ [Fr, madness], a mental disorder; any of a variety of psychopathologic reactions.

folie à deux. See **shared paranoid disorder.**

folie circulaire. See **bipolar disorder.**

folie du doute /dYd ᴏᴏt'/ [Fr, madness of doubts], an extreme obsessive-compulsive reaction characterized by persistent doubting, vacillation, repetition of behavior, and pathologic indecisiveness.

folie du pourquoi /dYpᴏᴏrkwô·ä'/ [Fr, madness of why], a psychopathologic condition characterized by the persistent tendency to ask questions, usually concerning unrelated topics.

folie gemellaire /zhemeler'/ [Fr, madness in twins], a psychotic condition occurring simultaneously in twins, sometimes in those not living together or closely associated at the time.

folie musculaire /mYskYler'/, severe chorea.

folie raisonnante /rezônäNt'/ [Fr, madness with reason], a delusional form of any psychosis marked by an apparent logical thought process but lacking common sense.

folinic acid /fōlin'ik/, an active form of folic acid.

folk illnesses, health disorders that are attributed to nonscientific causes.

follicle /fol'ikəl/ [L *folliculus* small bag], a pouchlike depression, such as the dental follicles that enclose the teeth before eruption or the hair follicles within the epidermis. **–follicular,** *adj.*

follicle-stimulating hormone (FSH), a

gonadotropin, secreted by the anterior pituitary gland, that stimulates the growth and maturation of graafian follicles in the ovary and promotes spermatogenesis in the male.

follicle-stimulating hormone releasing factor (FSH-RF) [L *folliculus, stimulare* to incite; Gk *horaein* to set in motion; ME *relesen;* L *facere* to do], the gonadotropin-releasing hormone.

follicular adenocarcinoma /fōlik'yələr/, a neoplasm characterized by a follicular arrangement of cells that are usually derived from the thyroid gland. It is not especially malignant, but it has a greater tendency to metastasize.

follicular cyst, an odontogenic cyst that arises from the epithelium of a tooth bud and dental lamina. The kinds of follicular cysts are dentigerous, primordial, and multilocular.

follicular goiter, an enlargement of the thyroid gland characterized by proliferation of the follicles and epithelial tissue.

follicular phase, the first part of the menstrual cycle, when ovarian follicles grow to prepare for ovulation.

follicular tonsillitis [L *folliculus, tonsilla;* Gk *itis* inflammation], an inflammation of the tonsils accompanied by a purulent infection of the tonsillar crypts.

follicular vulvitis [L *folliculus, vulva* a wrapper; Gk *itis* inflammation], an inflammation of the skin follicles of the vulva.

folliculitis /fōlik'yᴏᴏli'tis/, inflammation of hair follicles, as in sycosis barbae.

folliculoma. See **granulosa cell tumor.**

folliculosis /fōlik'yᴏᴏlō'sis/, a condition characterized by the development of a large number of lymph follicles, which may or may not be associated with an infection.

fomentation /fō'mentä'shən/ [L *fomentare* to apply a poultice], **1.** a topical treatment of pain or inflammation with a warm, moist application. **2.** a substance or poultice that is used as a warm, moist application.

fomite /fō'mīt/ [L *fomes* tinder], nonliving material, such as bed linens, which may convey pathogenic organisms.

Fone's method /fōnz/, a toothbrushing technique that employs large, sweeping, scrubbing circles over occluded teeth, with the toothbrush held at right angles to the tooth surfaces.

fontanel /fon'tənel/ [Fr *fontaine* fountain], a space covered by tough membranes between the bones of an infant's cranium. Also spelled **fontanelle.**

fonticulus /fontik'yələs/ [L, little fountain], fontanel or fontanelle.

food [AS *foda*], **1.** any substance, usually of plant or animal origin, consisting of carbohydrates, proteins, fats, and such supplementary elements as minerals and vitamins, that is ingested or otherwise taken into the body and assimilated to provide energy and to promote the growth, repair, and maintenance essential for sustaining life. **2.** nourishment in solid form as contrasted with liquid form. **3.** a particular kind of solid nourishment, such as breakfast food or snack food.

food additives, substances that are added to foods to prevent spoilage, improve appearance, enhance flavor, or increase nutritional value. Most food additives must be approved by the FDA after tests to determine if they could be a cause of cancer, birth defects, or other health problems.

food allergy, a hypersensitive state resulting from the ingestion of a specific food antigen. Symptoms of sensitivity to specific foods can include allergic rhinitis, bronchial asthma, urticaria, angioneurotic edema, dermatitis, pruritus, headache, labyrinthitis and conjunctivitis, nausea, vomiting, diarrhea, pylorospasm, colic, spastic constipation, mucous colitis, and perianal eczema. Food allergens are predominantly protein in nature.

Food and Drug Administration (FDA), a federal agency responsible for the enforcement of federal regulations regarding the manufacture and distribution of food, drugs, and cosmetics as protection against the sale of impure or dangerous substances.

food and drug interactions, adverse health effects of certain combinations of foods and medications. A thiazide diuretic may be a cause of depletion of potassium from body tissues, a vitamin C deficiency may reduce activity of drug-metabolizing enzymes, and isoniazid can interfere with the function of pyridoxine. Monoamine oxidase inhibitors may react with tyramine in certain cheeses, wines, and pickled seafood to produce a life-threatening hypertensive crisis.

food chain [ME *fode, chaine*], an ecological sequence in which the various organisms within a community subsist upon a species lower in the sequence, as man eats the bird that eats the fish that eats the worm, and so on. Each level within the chain has a purpose and destruction of any one member in the chain affects the rest of the chain negatively.

food contaminants, substances that make food unfit for human consumption. Examples include bacteria, toxic chemicals, carcinogens, teratogens, and radioactive materials. Also regarded as contaminants are basically harmless substances, such as water, that may be added to food to increase its weight.

food exchange list, a grouping of foods in which the carbohydrate, fat, and protein values are equal for the items listed. For example, starchy vegetables are listed as bread exchanges; fish and cheese are meat exchanges.

food poisoning, any of a large group of toxic processes resulting from the ingestion of a food contaminated by toxic substances or by bacteria containing toxins. Kinds of food poisoning include **bacterial food poisoning, ciguatera poisoning, Minamata disease, mushroom poisoning,** and **shellfish poisoning.**

food pyramid, a diagrammatic representation of human nutritional needs devised by the U.S. Department of Agriculture in 1992. It replaced the "four food groups" pie chart used since the 1950s. The USDA "Food Guide Pyramid" features a relatively wide base of 6 to 11 servings daily of grains and cereals beneath a layer representing 5 to 9 servings daily of fruits and vegetables. A third tapering level represents 4 to 6 daily servings of meats and dairy products. At the peak of the pyramid are fats and sweets, to be eaten sparingly.

food service administrator, a member of a hospital staff who is responsible for the planning and management of the food service system of the facility.

food service department, the department of a hospital or similar health facility that is responsible for food preparation and services to patients and personnel.

foot [AS *fot*], the distal extremity of the leg, consisting of the tarsus, the metatarsus, and the phalanges.

foot-and-mouth disease, an acute, extremely contagious, rhinovirus infection of cloven-hooved animals. Horses are immune. Uncommonly, the virus is transmitted to humans by direct contact with infected animals or their secretions or with contaminated milk. Symptoms and signs in humans include headache, fever, malaise, and vesicles on tongue, oral mucous membranes, hands, and feet.

footboard, a board or open box placed at the foot of a patient's bed and at a level above the top of the mattress, so as to prevent the weight of the top sheet and blankets from resting on the feet. Its purpose is to help the bedfast patient retain normal posture and prevent footdrop.

footdrop [AS *fot, dropa*], an abnormal neuromuscular condition of the lower leg and foot, characterized by an inability to dorsiflex, or evert, the foot because of damage to the common peroneal nerve.

footling breech [AS *fot;* ME *brech*], an intrauterine position of the fetus in which one or both feet are folded under the buttocks at the inlet of the maternal pelvis, one foot presenting in a single footling breech, both feet in a double footling breech.

foot-pound, a unit for the measurement of work or energy. One foot-pound is the amount of work required to move 1 pound a distance of 1 foot in the same direction as that of the applied force.

foramen /fôrā′mən/, *pl.* **foramina** [L, hole], an opening or aperture in a membranous structure or bone, such as the apical dental foramen and the carotid foramen.

foramen magnum, a passage in the occipital bone through which the spinal cord enters the spinal column.

foramen of Monro /monrō′/, a passage between the lateral and third ventricles of the brain.

foramen ovale /ōvā′lē, ōvä′lä/, **1.** an opening in the septum between the right and the left atria in the fetal heart. This opening provides a bypass for blood that would otherwise flow to the fetal lungs. **2.** an oval foramen situated laterally to the foramen rotundum of the sphenoid bone.

foramen rotundum, one of a pair of rounded apertures in the greater wings of the sphenoid bone.

foramen spinosum, a small opening near the posterior angle of the greater wing of the sphenoid bone.

Forbes-Albright syndrome /fôrbsôl′brīt/ [A. P. Forbes; Fuller Albright, American physician, b. 1900], an endocrine disease characterized by amenorrhea, prolactinemia, and galactorrhea, caused by an adenoma of the anterior pituitary.

Forbes' disease. See **Cori's disease.**

forbidden clone theory [AS *forbeodan;* Gk *klon* a cutting; *theoria* speculation], a theory, associated with autoimmunity, that certain clone cells that can react against the body persist after birth and can be activated by a viral infection or by some metabolic change.

force [L *fortis* strong], **1.** energy applied in such a way that it initiates motion, changes the speed or direction of motion, or alters the size or shape of an object. **2.** a push or pull defined as mass times acceleration.

forced expiratory flow (FEF), the average volumetric flow rate during any stated volume interval while a forced expired vital capacity is performed. It is usually expressed as a percentage of vital capacity.

forced expiratory volume (FEV), the volume of air that can be forcibly expelled in a fixed time period after full inspiration.

forced expired vital capacity (FEVC), a pulmonary function test of the maximal volume of gas that can be forcefully and rapidly exhaled starting from the position of full inspiration.

forced feeding, the administration of food by force, such as nasal feeding, to persons who cannot or will not eat.

forced-inhalation abdominal breathing, a respiratory therapy technique in which the patient is trained to inhale through the nose with an effort that is forceful enough to lift small sandbag weights placed on the abdomen.

forceps, /fôr′seps/ *pl.* **forceps** [L, pair of tongs], a pair of any of a large variety and number of surgical instruments, all of which have two handles or sides, each attached to a blade, and used to grasp, handle, compress, pull, or join tissue, equipment, or supplies.

forceps delivery, an obstetric operation in which instruments are used to deliver a baby. It is performed to overcome dystocia, to quickly deliver a baby experiencing fetal distress, or, most often, to shorten normal labor. Kinds of forceps delivery are **high forceps, low forceps,** and **mid forceps.**

forceps rotation, an obstetric operation in which forceps are used to turn a baby's head that is arrested in transverse or posterior position in the birth canal. Kinds of forceps rotation are **Kielland rotation** and **Scanzoni rotation.**

forceps tenaculum. See **tenaculum.**

forcible inspiration [L *fortis* strong, *inspirare*], breathing that is assisted by a mechanical ventilator that forces air into the lungs during inspiration but allows a return to ambient pressure as the patient exhales passively.

Fordyce-Fox disease /fôr′disfoks′/, an apocrine gland disorder producing symptoms similar to those of miliaria.

Fordyce's disease, the presence of enlarged oil glands in the mucosal membranes of the lips, cheeks, gums, and genitalia. It is a common condition and may be symptomless.

forearm, the portion of the upper extremity between the elbow and the wrist. It contains two long bones, the radius and ulna.

forebrain. See **prosencephalon.**

forefinger, the first, or index, finger.

forefoot, the portion of the foot that includes the metatarsus and toes.

foregut /fôr′gut/ [AS *fore* in front, *guttas*], the cephalic portion of the embryonic alimentary canal.

foreign body [Fr *forain* alien; AS *bodig*],

any object or substance found in the body in an organ or tissue in which it does not belong under normal circumstances, such as a particle of dust in the eye.

foreign body granuloma [OFr *forain;* AS *bodig;* L *granulum* little grain; Gk *oma* tumor], a chronic inflammatory mass of tissue that accumulates around foreign bodies such as gravel, splinters, or bits of sutures.

foreign body in ear [OFr *forain;* AS *bodig, eare*], anything found in the ear that is not normally there.

foreign body in esophagus [OFr *forain;* AS *bodig;* Gk *oisophagos* gullet], anything found in the esophagus that is not normally a part of the tissue.

foreign body in eye [OFr *forain;* AS *bodig, éage*], anything found in the eye that is not a normal part of the tissue.

foreign body in larynx [OFr *forain;* AS *bodig;* Gk *larynx*], anything found in the larynx tissues that is not normally present.

foreign body in throat [OFr *forain;* AS *bodig, throte*], anything found in throat tissue that is not normally present. A common foreign body in the throat is a posteriorly displaced tongue.

foreign body obstruction, a disturbance in normal function or a pathologic condition caused by an object lodged in a body orifice, passage, or organ. Most cases occur in children who suddenly inhale or swallow a foreign object or insert it in a body opening.

foreign medical graduate (FMG), a physician trained in and graduated from a medical school outside the United States and Canada. United States citizens graduated from medical schools outside the United States and Canada are also classified as FMGs.

forensic /fôren'sik/ [L *forensis* public forum], pertaining to courts of law.

forensic dentistry, the branch of dentistry that deals with the legal aspects of professional dental practices and treatment.

forensic medicine [L *forum* market place, *medicinus* physician], a branch of medicine that deals with the legal aspects of health care.

forensic psychiatry [L *forum;* Gk *psyche* mind + *iatreia* treament], a branch of psychiatry concerned with the application of psychiatry to law, including criminal responsibility, guardianship, and competence to stand trial.

foreplay, sexual activities, such as kissing and fondling, that precede coitus.

foreshortened image, a distortion in x-ray imaging caused by inclination of an object or improper alignment of the x-ray tube, resulting in an image that is smaller than the object itself.

foreskin [AS *fore* + *skinn*], a loose fold of skin that covers the end of the penis or clitoris. Its removal constitutes circumcision.

forest yaws [L *foris* outside; Afr *yaw* strawberry], a cutaneous form of American leishmaniasis caused by *Leishmania guyanensis.* The disease is chronic, with multiple deep skin ulcers that occasionally spread to the nasal mucosa.

forewaters [AS *fore* + *waeter*], the amniotic fluid between the presenting part and the intact membranes.

forked tongue [L *furca;* AS *tunge*], a tongue divided by a longitudinal fissure.

formaldehyde /formal'dəhīd/, a toxic, colorless, foul-smelling gas that is soluble in water and used in that form as a disinfectant, fixative, or preservative.

formalin /fôr'məlin/, a clear solution of formaldehyde in water. A 37% solution is used for fixing and preserving biological specimens for pathologic and histologic examination.

formation, a cluster of people or objects that occupies and therefore defines a quantum of space.

formative evaluation, judgments made about effectiveness of nursing interventions as they are implemented.

forme fruste /fôrm' frῙst', fôrm' frōōst'/ *pl.* **formes frustes, 1.** an incomplete or atypical form of a disease or a disease that is spontaneously arrested before it has run its usual course. **2.** (in genetics) an inherited disorder in which there is minimal expression of an abnormal trait.

formic acid /fôr'mik/, a colorless, pungent liquid found in nature in nettles, in ants, and in other insects.

formiminoglutamic acid (FIGLU) /fôrm-im'inōglōōtam'ik/, a compound formed in the metabolism of histidine, occurring in urine in elevated levels in folic acid deficiency.

formol. See **formaldehyde.**

formula /fôr'm(y)ələ/, [L *forma* pattern], a simplified statement, generally using numerals and other symbols, expressing the constituents of a chemical compound, a method for preparing a substance, or a procedure for achieving a desired value or result. **–formulaic,** *adj.*

formulary [L *forma* pattern], a listing of drugs intended to include a large enough range of drugs and sufficient information about them to enable health practitioners to prescribe treatment that is medically appropriate. Hospitals maintain formularies that list all drugs commonly stocked in the hospital pharmacy.

formulation [L *forma* pattern], **1.** a pharmacologic substance prepared according to a formula. **2.** a systematic and precise statement of a problem, a theory, or a method of analysis in research.

formylmethionine (FMET) /fôr′milməthī′ənēn/, (in molecular genetics) the first amino acid in a protein sequence.

fornication [L *fornix* arch], (in law) sexual intercourse between two people who are not married to each other. The specific legal definition varies from one jurisdiction to another.

fornix /fôr′niks/, *pl.* fornices /fôr′nisēz/ [L, arch], an archlike structure or space, such as the fornix cerebri, the superior or inferior conjunctival fornices, or the vaginal fornices.

fornix cerebri /fôr′niks ser′əbrī/, an archlike body of nerve fibers that lies beneath the corpus callosum of the cranium and serves as the efferent pathway from the hipppocampus.

fornix vaginae. See **vaginal fornix.**

forskolin (FSK), an activator of adenylate cyclase. FSK interacts directly with ion channels, increasing glutamine responses and amplitude and decay time of sponateous excitatory postsynaptic currents.

Fort Bragg fever. See **pretibial fever.**

fortified milk [L *fortis* strong; AS *milc*], pasteurized milk enriched with one or more nutrients, usually vitamin D, which has been standardized at 400 International Units per quart (fortified vitamin D milk).

forward-leaning posture, a respiratory therapy technique that is intended to reduce or eliminate accessory muscle activity in ambulatory patients with breathing difficulty. It involves walking in a slightly stooped, foward-leaning posture.

fossa /fos′ə/, *pl.* fossae [L, ditch], a hollow or depression, especially on the surface of the end of a bone, such as the olecranon fossa or the coronoid fossa.

Foster bed, a special bed used in the care and treatment of severely injured patients, especially those with spinal injuries. It consists of two Bradford frames mounted on a castered base and secured with locking bars to the head and foot assemblies. The assembly at each end is attached to a rotary-bearing mechanism, permitting horizontal turning of the patient without moving the spine.

foulage. See **pétrissage.**

foundation [L *fundamentum*], **1.** a charitable organization usually established to allocate private funds to worthy projects or to provide other services. **2.** (in dentistry) any device or material added to a remaining tooth structure to enhance the stability

and retention of an overlying cast restoration.

fourchette /f̄oorshet′/ [Fr, fork], a tense band of mucous membranes at the posterior angle of the vagina connecting the posterior ends of the labia minora.

four-handed dentistry, a technique of chairside operating in which four hands simultaneously perform tasks directly associated with dental work being accomplished in the oral cavity of a patient.

Fourier transform (FT) /f̄ooryā′/ [Jean B. J. Fourier, French mathematician, b. 1768; L *transformare* to change form], (in medical physics) a mathematical procedure that separates the frequency components of a signal from its amplitudes as a function of time, or vice versa.

Fourier transform imaging, (in medical physics) NMR imaging techniques in which at least one dimension is phase encoded by applying variable gradient pulses along that dimension before "reading out" the NMR signal with a gradient magnetic field perpendicular to the variable gradient. The Fourier transform is then used to reconstruct an image from the set of encoded NMR signals.

four-poster cast, a cast to immobilize the cervical vertebrae. It contains four vertical posts or poles on the anterior and posterior lateral sides of the head and is placed over the shoulders. The head is supported under the chin and occiput, and the posts prevent movement.

four-tailed bandage, a narrow piece of cloth with two ties on each end for wrapping a joint, such as an elbow or knee, or a prominence, such as the nose or chin.

fourth-generation scanner, a computed tomography machine in which the x-ray source rotates but the detector assembly does not.

fourth nerve. See **trochlear nerve.**

fourth stage of labor [ME *feower* four; OFr *estage;* L *labor* work], a postpartum period of about four hours following the third stage, or delivery of the placenta. Some complications, especially hemorrhage, occur at this time, requiring careful observation of the mother.

fourth ventricle [ME *feower* four; L *ventriculum* belly], a cavity with a diamond-shaped floor in the hindbrain, communicating below with the central canal of the spinal cord and above with the cerebral aqueduct of the midbrain. At the bottom of the ventricle are surfaces of the pons and medulla.

fovea capitis [L *fovea* pit], **1.** a depression on the proximal surface of the head of the radius where it meets the capitulum of the humerus. **2.** a fovea on the head of the femur, where the ligamentum teres is attached.

fovea centralis /fō'vē·ə/, an area at the center of the retina where cone cells are concentrated and there are no rod cells.

foxglove, a common name for a plant that is a source of digitalis, *Digitalis purpura.*

Fowler's position [George R. Fowler, American surgeon, b. 1848], the posture assumed by the patient when the head of the bed is raised 18 or 20 inches and the individual's knees are elevated.

Fox's knife. See **Goldman-Fox knife.**

Fr, symbol for the chemical element **francium.**

fractional anesthesia. See **continuous anesthesia.**

fractional dilatation and curettage, a diagnostic technique in which each section of the uterus is examined and curetted to obtain specimens of the endometrium from all parts of the uterus.

fractionation /frak'shənā'shən/ [L *frangere* to break], **1.** (in neurology) a mechanism within the neural arch of the vertebrae whereby only a portion of the efferent nerves innervating a muscle reacts to a stimulus, even when the reflex requirement is maximal, so that there is a reserve of neurons to respond to additional stimuli. **2.** (in chemistry) the separation of a substance into its basic constituents, by using such procedures as fractional distillation or crystallization. **3.** (in bacteriology) the process of isolating a pure culture by successive culturing of a small portion of a colony of bacteria. **4.** (in histology) the process of isolating the different components of living cells by centrifugation. **5.** (in radiology) the process of administering a dose of radiation in smaller units over a period of time to minimize tissue damage rather than in a single large dose.

fraction of inspired oxygen (Fio₂), the proportion of oxygen in the air that is inspired.

fracture /frak'chər/ [L *fractura* break], a traumatic injury to a bone in which the continuity of the tissue of the bone is broken. A fracture is classified by the bone involved, the part of that bone, and the nature of the break, such as a comminuted fracture of the head of the tibia. Kinds of fracture include **butterfly, comminuted, complete, compression, displaced, impacted, incomplete, segmental, spiral,** and **undisplaced fracture.**

fracture-dislocation, a fracture involving the bony structures of any joint, with associated dislocation of the same joint.

fracture of clavicle [L *fractura, clavicula* little key], a break in the long bone of the shoulder girdle. It is usually accompanied by pain, swelling, and a protuberance and depression over the site of the injury. The patient usually supports the injured arm at the elbow. Treatment usually involves application of a clavicle strap or a figure-of-eight wrap.

fracture of olecranon [L *fractura;* Gk *olekranon* point of the elbow], a fracture of the bony prominence of the ulna at the elbow joint. Different types of olecranon fractures may occur, depending upon the articular surfaces involved and possible displacement of the radius. The triceps, which normally extends the elbow, may become spastic as a result of the injury.

fracture of patella [L *fractura, patella* small pan], a break in the sesamoid knee cap. The fracture often occurs in automobile accidents in which the knee strikes the dashboard. The damage is complicated by the reflex bracing of the quadriceps femoris muscle that pulls the fragments apart. Treatment includes suturing the bone fragments and confining the patient in a lower body cast.

fracture of radius [L *fractura, ray*] a fracture and dislocation of the lower end of the radius, usually with backward and radial displacement of the wrist and hand. The fracture commonly occurs when a falling person extends the arm and hand in an effort to cushion the impact.

fracture of skull [L *fractura;* AS *skulle* bowl], a break in the structure of one or more of the cranial bones. A fracture of bones in the vault of the skull is usually a compound fracture and complicated by possible damage to brain tissue, particularly if shards of cranial bones are driven into the brain by the force of the trauma.

fragile X syndrome, a reproductive disorder characterized by a nearly broken X chromosome, which has a tip hanging by a flimsy thread. It is the most common inherited cause of mental retardation. Tests for the broken chromosome are effective only about 75% of the time. Some healthy individuals may possess fragile X chromosomes without exhibiting symptoms and may transmit the condition to children or grandchildren.

fragilitas ossium. See **osteogenesis imperfecta.**

fragmented fracture [L *frangere* to break; *fractura* break], a fracture that results in multiple bone fragments.

frail elderly, an older person (usually over the age of 75) who is afflicted with physical or mental disabilities that may interfere with the ability to independently perform activities of daily living.

frambesia. See **yaws.**

frame of reference [AS *framian* to help; L

referre to carry back], the personal guidelines of an individual, such as the person's social status, cultural norms, and concepts.

Franceschetti's syndrome /fran'ches-ket'ēz/ [Adolphe Franceschetti, Swiss ophthalmologist, b. 1896], a complete form of mandibulofacial dysostosis.

franchise dentistry /fran'chīz/ [Fr, exemption; L *dens* tooth], the practice of dentistry under a trade name, which has been purchased from another dentist or dental practice.

francium (Fr) /fran'sē-əm/ [France], a metallic element of the alkali metal group and formed from the decay of actinium. Its atomic number is 87; its atomic weight is 223.

frank [L *francus* forthright], obvious or clinically evident, such as the unequivocal presence of a condition or a disease.

Frank biopsy guide, a device consisting of a long needle containing a hooked wire used to obtain biopsy samples of breast tissue.

frank breech [L *francus* + ME *brec*], an intrauterine position of the fetus in which the buttocks present at the maternal pelvic inlet, the legs are straight up in front of the body, and the feet are at the shoulders.

Frankfort horizontal plane [Frankfurt-am-Main Congress of German Anthropologists Agreement, 1882], (in dentistry) a craniometric plane determined by the inferior borders of the bony orbits and the upper margin of the auditory meatus, passing through the two orbitales and the two tragions.

Frankfort-mandibular incisor angle (FMTA), (in dentistry) the precumbency of the mandibular incisor tooth to the Frankfort horizontal plane.

Frank-Starling relationship [Otto Frank, German physiologist, b. 1865; Ernest H. Starling, English physiologist, b. 1866], an index for determining cardiac output, based on the length of the myocardial fibers at the onset of contraction. The force exerted per beat of the heart is directly proportional to the length or degree of stretch of the myocardial fiber.

fraternal twins. See **dizygotic twins.**

fraud [L *fraudare* to cheat], (in law) the act of intentionally misleading or deceiving another person by any means so as to cause him legal injury, usually the loss of something valuable or the surrender of a legal right.

Fraunhofer zone /froun'hōfər/, (in ultrasonography) the zone farthest from the transducer face.

FRC, abbreviation for **functional residual capacity.**

freckle [ME *freken*], a brown or tan macule on the skin, usually resulting from exposure to sunlight. There is an inherited tendency to freckling.

Fredet-Ramstedt's operation. See **pyloromyotomy.**

free-air chamber [AS *freo* free; Gk *aer* air; L *camera* vault], a device used as a primary standard for calibrating x-ray exposure. It is used in national calibration laboratories throughout the world.

free association, 1. the spontaneous, consciously unrestricted association of ideas, feelings, or mental images. **2.** spontaneous verbalization of thoughts and emotions entering the consciousness during psychoanalysis.

freebasing, a chemical process used to increase the stimulating effect of cocaine.

free clinic, a clinic or health program, usually located in a neighborhood setting, that provides health care for ambulatory patients at nominal or no cost.

free fatty acid (FFA) [AS *freo, faett;* L *acidus* sour], nonesterified fatty acids, released by the hydrolysis of triglycerides within adipose tissue. Free fatty acids can be used as an immediate source of energy by many organs and can be converted by the liver into ketone bodies.

free-floating anxiety, a generalized, persistent, pervasive fear that is not attributable to any specific object, event, or source.

free-form foot orthosis, an orthosis that is molded directly to a patient's foot.

free gingiva, the unattached coronal portion of the gingiva that encircles a tooth and forms a gingival sulcus.

free gingival groove, a shallow line or depression on the gingival surface at the junction of the free and attached gingivae.

free graft [AS *freo;* Gk *graphein* stylus], a graft completely removed from its original site and replaced at a new site in a single one-stage operation.

free-induction decay (FID), (in nuclear magnetic resonance imaging), a signal emitted by a tissue after a radio frequency (RF) pulse has excited the nuclear spins of the tissue at resonance. The decaying oscillation back to the normal state is the signal from which an NMR image is made.

free macrophage [AS *freo;* Gk *makros* large, *phagein* to eat], a motile macrophage derived from a monocyte. It responds to chemotactic stimuli and migrates from blood vessels to tissue spaces.

free nerve ending, a receptor nerve ending that is not enclosed in a capsule.

free phagocyte. See **phagocyte.**

free radical, a compound with an extra

electron or proton. It is unstable and reacts readily with other molecules.

free-radical theory of aging, a concept of aging based on the premise that the main causative factor is an imbalance between the production and elimination of free chemical radicals in the body tissues.

free thyroxine, the amount of the unbound, active thyroid hormone, thyroxine (T_4), circulating in the blood, measured by special laboratory procedures.

free thyroxine index, the amount of unbound, physiologically active thyroxine (T_4) in serum, determined by direct assay or, more frequently, calculated on the basis of an in vitro uptake test.

freeway space [AS *freo, wegan;* L *spatiaum*], the interocclusal distance or separation between the occlusal surfaces of the teeth when the mandible is in its rest position.

freezing point [ME, *fresen,* to be cold; L, *punctus,* pricked], the temperature at which a substance changes from a liquid to a solid state. The freezing point for water is 32° on the **Fahrenheit** scale and 0° on the **Celsius** scale.

Freiberg's infarction [Albert H. Freiberg, American surgeon, b. 1868; L *infarcire* to stuff], an abnormal orthopedic condition characterized by osteochondritis or aseptic necrosis of bone tissue, most commonly affecting the head of the second metatarsal.

Frei test /frī/ [William S. Frei, German dermatologist, b. 1885], a test performed to confirm a diagnosis of lymphogranuloma venereum.

Frejka splint /frā′kə/, a corrective device consisting of a pillow that is belted between the legs of a baby born with dislocated hips to maintain abduction and articulation of the head of the femur with the acetabulum.

fremitus /frem′itəs/ [L, a growling], a tremulous vibration of the chest wall that can be auscultated or palpated during physical examination. Kinds of fremitus include **bronchial, coarse, tactile,** and **vocal fremitus.**

frenectomy /frənek′təmē/ [L *fraenum* bridle; Gk *ektome* excision], a surgical procedure for excising a frenum or frenulum, such as the excision of the lingual frenum from its attachment into the mucoperiosteal covering of the alveolar process to correct ankyloglossia.

Frenkel exercises, a system of slow repetitious exercises of increasing difficulty developed to treat ataxia in multiple sclerosis and similar disorders.

frenotomy /frənot′əmē/ [L *fraenum* + Gk *temnein* to cut], a surgical procedure for

repairing a defective frenum, such as the cutting or lengthening of the lingual frenum to correct ankyloglossia.

frenulum linguae. See **lingual frenum.**

frenulum of tongue /fren′yələm/ [L *fraenum;* AS *tunge*], a longitudinal fold of mucous membrane connecting the floor of the mouth to the underside of the tongue in midline. A congenital defect causes an abnormal shortness of the frenulum, resulting in tongue-tie, which can be surgically corrected.

frenum /frē′nəm/, *pl.* **frenums, frena** [L *fraenum* bridle], a restraining portion or structure.

frequency [L *frequens* frequent], **1.** the number of repetitions of any phenomenon within a fixed period of time, such as the number of heart beats per minute. **2.** (in biometry) the proportion of the number of persons having a discrete characteristic to the total number of persons being studied. **3.** (in electronics) the number of cycles of a periodic quantity that occur in a period of 1 second. Electromagnetic frequencies are expressed in hertz (Hz).

fresh frozen plasma, an unconcentrated form of blood plasma containing all of the clotting factors except platelets. It can be used to supplement RBCs when whole blood is not available for exchange transfusion or to correct a bleeding problem of unknown etiology.

Fresnel zone /freznel′/, (in ultrasonography) the region nearest the transducer face.

Freud, Sigmund /froid/ [Austrian neurologist, b. 1856], founder of a complex integrated theory of psychologic causes of mental disorders, some, such as hysteria, with physical symptoms. Among tenets of Freudian theory: human beings are motivated by a pleasure principle; receive internal stimulation from a sex instinct and a death instinct; have personality structures that can be divided into ego, superego, and id; and have unconscious, preconscious, and conscious levels of mental activity.

freudian /froi′dē·ən/ [Sigmund Freud], **1.** pertaining to the theories and doctrines of Freud, which stress the formative years of childhood as the basis for later psychoneurotic disorders, primarily through the unconscious repression of instinctual drives and sexual desires, and his system of psychoanalysis for treating such disturbances. **2.** pertaining to the school of psychiatry based on Freud's teachings. **3.** pertaining to one who adheres to Freud's school of psychiatry.

freudian fixation, an arrest in psychosexual development characterized by a firm emotional attachment to another per-

F

son or object. Some kinds of freudian fixation are **father fixation** and **mother fixation.**

freudianism /froi'dē-əniz'əm/, the school of psychiatry based on the psychoanalytic theories and psychotherapeutic methods of treating psychoneurotic disorders developed by Sigmund Freud and his followers.

friable /frī'əbəl/ [L *friare* to crumble], pertaining to something that is easily shattered, crumbled, or pulverized.

Fricke dosimeter, a chemical radiation dosimeter that uses the change of concentration of ferric ions in a solution subject to irradiation to quantify the amount of dose delivered to the sample.

friction [L *fricare* to rub], **1.** the act of rubbing one object against another. **2.** a type of massage in which deeper tissues are stroked or rubbed, usually through strong circular movements of the hand.

frictional force, the force component parallel to the surfaces at the point of contact between two objects. It may be increased or decreased by such factors as moisture on a surface.

friction burn, tissue injury caused by abrasion of the skin.

friction rub, a dry, grating sound heard with a stethoscope during auscultation. It is a normal finding when heard over the liver and splenic areas.

Friedländer's bacillus /frēd'lendərz/ [Carl Friedländer, German pathologist, b. 1847], a bacterium of the species *Klebsiella pneumonia,* which is associated with infection of the respiratory tract, especially lobar pneumonia.

Friedländer's disease, a severe arterial inflammation. There may be swelling and overgrowth of tissue cells lining the blood vessel, leading to complete obstruction of the artery.

Friedländer's pneumonia [Carl Friedländer; Gk *pneumon* lung], a form of bronchopneumonia with a high mortality rate, particularly among older patients. The pneumonic patches tend to become confluent and those who survive may experience pulmonary abscesses and necrosis.

Friedman curve /frēd'mən/ [Emanuel A. Friedman, American obstetrician, b. 1926], a graph depicting the progress of labor, used to facilitate detection of dysfunctional labor.

Friedman's test [Maurice H. Friedman, American physiologist, b. 1903], a modification of the Aschheim-Zondek pregnancy test. A sample of urine from a woman is injected into a mature, unmated female rabbit. If, days later, the rabbit ovaries contain fresh corpora lutea or hemor-

rhaging corpora, the test is positive as a sign that the woman is pregnant.

Friedreich's ataxia /frēd'rīshs/ [Nickolaus Friedreich, German physician, b. 1825], an abnormal condition characterized by muscular weakness, loss of muscular control, weakness of the lower extremities, and an abnormal gait. The primary pathologic feature of the disease is pronounced sclerosis of the posterior columns of the spinal cord with possible involvement of the spinocerebellar tracts and the corticospinal tracts.

Friedreich's sign [Nikolaus Friedreich, German physician, b. 1825; L, *signum,* sign], the diastolic collapse of the jugular veins in adherent pericardium.

Fried's rule, a method of estimating the dose of medicine for a child by multiplying the adult dose by the child's age in months and dividing the product by 150.

frigid [L *frigidus* cold], **1.** lacking warmth of feeling; unemotional; unimaginative; without passion or ardor and stiff or formal in manner. **2.** a woman who is unresponsive to sexual advances or stimuli, abnormally indifferent or averse to sexual intercourse, or unable to have an orgasm during sexual intercourse. –**frigidity,** *n.*

fringe field, (in magnetic resonance imaging) the part of a magnetic field that extends away from the confines of the magnet and cannot be used for imaging. It may affect nearby equipment and personnel.

frit /frit, frē/ [Fr, fried], a partially or wholly fused porcelain from which dental porcelain powders are made.

Fröhlich's syndrome. See **adiposogenital dystrophy.**

frôlement /frôlmäN'/ [Fr, brushing], **1.** the rustling type of sound often heard on auscultating the chest in diseases of the pericardium. **2.** a kind of massage that uses a light brushing stroke with the hand.

frontal bone [L *frons* forehead], a single cranial bone that forms the front of the skull, from above the orbits, posteriorly to a junction with the parietal bones at the coronal suture.

frontal lobe, the largest of five lobes constituting each of the two cerebral hemispheres. It lies beneath the frontal bone, occupies part of the lateral, the medial, and the inferior surfaces of each hemisphere, and extends posteriorly to the central sulcus and inferiorly to the lateral fissure. Research indicates that the right frontal and the right temporal lobes are associated with the nonverbal, specialized activities of the right cerebral hemisphere and that the left frontal and the left temporal lobes are associated with the verbal activities of the left cerebral hemisphere.

frontal lobe syndrome, behavioral and personality changes observed after a neoplastic or traumatic frontal lobe lesion. The patient may become sociopathic, boastful, hypomanic, uninhibited, exhibitionistic, and subject to outbursts of irritability or violence. The person may also become depressed, apathetic, lacking in initiative, negligent about personal appearance, and inclined to perseverate.

frontal plane, any one of the vertical planes passing through the body from the head to the feet, perpendicular to the sagittal planes, dividing the body into front and back portions.

frontal pole [L *frons, polus*], the anterior extremity of the frontal lobe of the cerebrum.

frontal section [L *frons, sectio* a cutting], a section of the head or other body part cut into anterior and posterior portions.

frontal sinus, one of a pair of small cavities in the frontal bone of the skull that communicates into the nasal cavity. Each sinus opens into the anterior part of the middle meatus through the frontonasal duct.

frontal vein, one of a pair of superficial veins of the face, arising in the plexus of the forehead.

frontocortical aphasia. See **motor aphasia.**

frostbite [AS *frost, bitan*], traumatic effect of extreme cold on skin and subcutaneous tissues that is first recognized by distinct pallor of exposed skin surfaces, particularly the nose, ears, fingers, and toes. Vasoconstriction and damage to blood vessels impair local circulation and result in anoxia, edema, vesiculation, and necrosis. Gentle warming is appropriate first aid treatment.

frostnip. See **frostbite.**

frottage /frôtäzh′/ [Fr, rubbing], sexual gratification obtained by rubbing (especially one's genital area) against the clothing of another person, as can occur in a crowd.

frotteur /frôtœr′/ [Fr], a person who obtains sexual gratification by the practice of frottage.

frozen section [ME *fresen;* L *sectio*], a histologic section of tissue that has been frozen by exposure to dry ice.

frozen section method [AS *freosan* to freeze; L *sectio* a cutting; Gk *meta* order, *hodos* path], (in surgical pathology) a method used in preparing a selected portion of tissue for pathologic examination. The tissue is moistened and is rapidly frozen and cut by a microtome in a cryostat.

FRSC, abbreviation for *Fellow of the Royal Society of Canada.*

fructokinase /fruk′tōkī′nās/, an enzyme that catalyzes the transfer of a phosphate group from adenosine triphosphate to D-fructose.

fructose /fruk′tōs, frōōk′-/, a yellowish-to-white, crystalline, water-soluble levorotatory ketose monosaccharide that is sweeter than sucrose and found in honey, several fruits, and combined in many disaccharides and polysaccharides.

fructose intolerance [L *fructus* fruit, *in* + *tolerare* to bear], an inherited disorder marked by an absence of enzymes needed to metabolize fructose. Symptoms include sweating, tremors, confusion, and digestive distress, with vomiting, and failure of infants to grow. The condition is transmitted as an autosomal dominant trait.

fructosemia /frōōk′tōsē′mē·ə/ [L *fructus* fruit; Gk *haima* blood], the presence of fructose in the blood.

fructosuria /frōōk′tōsōōr′ē·ə/, presence of the sugar fructose in the urine.

fruit sugar. See **fructose.**

frustration, a feeling that results from an interference with one's ability to attain a desired goal or satisfaction.

FSH, abbreviation for **follicle-stimulating hormone.**

FSH-RF, abbreviation for **follicle-stimulating hormone releasing factor.**

FT, abbreviation for *fast-twitch.*

FTA-ABS test. See **Fluorescent Treponemal Antibody Absorption Test.**

FTC, abbreviation for **Federal Trade Commission.**

fuchsin bodies. See **Russell's bodies.**

fugue /fyōōg/ [L *fuga* running away], a state of dissociative reaction characterized by amnesia and physical flight from an intolerable situation. During the episode, the person appears normal and acts as though consciously aware of what may be very complex activities and behavior, but after the episode, the person has no recollection of the actions or behavior.

fulcrum /fŏōl′krəm, ful′-/ [L *fulcire* to support] **1.** the stable point or the position on which a lever, such as the ulna or the femur, turns. Numerous common movements of the body, such as raising the arm and walking, are combinations of lever actions involving fulcrums. **2.** (in radiology) an imaginary pivot point about which the x-ray tube and film move.

fulfillment [AS *fullfyllan* to make full], a perception of harmony in life that results when an individual has found meaning and leads a purposeful life.

fulgurate /ful′gyərāt/ [L *fulgur* lightning], **1.** pertaining to sudden, intense, sharp pain. **2.** the use of a movable electrode to destroy superficial tissue.

fulguration. See **electrodesiccation.**

full-arch wire, a wire that is attached to the teeth and extends from the molar region of one side of a dental arch to the other.

full bath [AS *fol; baeth*], a bath in which the patient's body is immersed in water up to the neck.

full denture [ME *full*; L *dens* tooth], a removable dental prosthetic that replaces all of the natural teeth in the maxillary and/or mandibular arch. The denture is usually made of acrylic resin and completely supported by the mouth tissues.

full diet. See **regular diet.**

full-liquid diet, a diet consisting of only liquids and foods that liquefy at body temperature. The diet is prescribed after surgery, in some acute infections of short duration, in the treatment of acute GI disorders, and for patients too ill to chew.

full-lung tomography, a technique of producing general tomographic surveys of both lungs to detect possible occult nodules of metastases.

full pulse [ME *full*; L *pulsare* to beat], a large volume pulse with a low pulse pressure.

full term [ME *full*; Gk *terma* limit], pertaining to the normal period of human gestation, between 38 and 41 weeks.

full weight-bearing (FWB) [ME *full*; AS *gewiht*; ME *beren*], in radiology, a view that shows the response to stresses of a natural posture. Full weight-bearing views of the foot are useful in studying flatfoot or cave foot.

fulminant hepatitis, a rare and frequently fatal form of acute hepatitis in which there is rapid deterioration in the condition of the patient, with hepatic encephalopathy, necrosis of the hepatic parenchyma, blood coagulation disorders, renal failure, and coma. The prognosis for adults is generally unfavorable.

fulminating /ful′minā′ting/ [L *fulminare* lightening flash], (of a disease or condition) rapid, sudden, severe, as an infection, fever, or hemorrhage. Also **fulminant.** –**fulminate,** *v.*

fumagillin, fumigacin. See **helvolic acid.**

function /fungk′shən/ [L *functio* performance], 1. an act, process, or series of processes that serve a purpose. 2. to perform an activity or to work properly and normally.

functional, 1. pertaining to a function. 2. affecting the functions but not the structure of an organism or organ system.

functional analysis, (in psychiatry) a type of therapy that traces the sequence of events involved in producing and maintaining undesirable behavior.

functional antagonism, (in pharmacology) a situation in which two agonists interact with different receptors and produce opposing effects.

functional bowel syndrome. See **irritable bowel syndrome.**

functional contracture. See **hypertonic contracture.**

functional differentiation, (in embryology) the specialization or diversification as a result of the particular function of a cell or tissue.

functional disease, 1. a disease that affects function or performance. 2. a condition marked by signs or symptoms of an organic disease or disorder although careful examination fails to reveal any evidence of structural or physiologic abnormalities. Headache, impotence, certain heart murmurs, and constipation may be symptoms of functional disease.

functional dyspepsia, an abnormal condition characterized by impaired digestion caused by an atonic or a neurologic problem.

functional imaging, (in nuclear medicine) a diagnostic procedure in which a sequence of radiographic or scintillation camera images of the distribution of an administered radioactive tracer delineates one or more physiologic processes in the body.

functional impotence. See **impotence.**

functional murmur, a heart murmur caused by an alteration of function without structural heart disease or damage, as in a murmur related to anemia rather than an organic heart disorder.

functional nursing, a centralized system of nursing care that is task and activity oriented, using auxiliary health workers trained in a variety of skills.

functional occlusal harmony, an occlusal relationship of opposing teeth in all functional ranges and movements that provides the maximum masticatory efficiency without pathogenic force on the supporting oral structures.

functional overlay, an emotional aspect of an organic disease. It is characterized by symptoms that continue long after clinical signs of the disease have ended.

functional pathology [L *functio* performance; Gk *pathos* disease, *logos* science], a study of the functional changes resulting from structural alterations in tissues.

functional position of the hand, a position for splinting the hand, including the wrist and fingers. The thumb is abducted and in opposition and alignment with the pads of the fingers.

functional progression, a rehabilitative sequence for a musculoskeletal or similar injury. It usually progresses from immobilization for primary healing to endurance and strengthening activities.

functional psychosis, a severe emotional disorder characterized by personality derangement and the loss of ability to function in reality, but without evidence that the disorder is related to the physical processes of the brain.

functional residual capacity, the volume of gas in the lungs at the end of a normal expiration. The functional residual capacity is equal to the residual volume plus the expiratory reserve volume.

functional splint [L *functio* performance; ME *splent*], a splint that allows or assists a patient's movements.

fundal height /fun′dəl/ [L *fundus* bottom; AS *heightho*], the height of the fundus, measured in centimeters from the top of the symphysis pubis to the highest point in the midline at the top of the uterus.

fundal placenta [L *fundus, placenta* flat cake], a placenta that is attached to the fundus of the uterus.

fundamentals of nursing, the basic principles and practices of nursing as taught in educational programs for nurses. The emphasis of this phase of training is the acquisition by the student of the basic skills of nursing.

fundoplication /fun′dəplikā′shən/ [L *fundus, plicare* to fold], a surgical procedure involving making tucks in the fundus of the stomach around the lower end of the esophagus.

fundoscopy, /fundos′kəpē/ [L *fundus*; Gk *skopein* to view], an examination of the ocular fundus with an ophthalmoscope.

fundus /fun′dəs/, *pl.* *fundi* /fun′dī/ [L, bottom], the base or the deepest part of an organ; the portion farthest from the mouth of an organ, such as the fundus of the uterus or the fundus of an eye.

funduscope. See **ophthalmoscope.**

funduscopy /fundus′kəpē/ [L *fundus* + Gk *skopein* to look], the examination and study of the fundus of the eye by means of an ophthalmoscope. –**fundoscopic, funduscopic,** *adj.*

fundus microscopy, examination of the base of the interior of the eye using an instrument that combines an ophthalmoscope and a lens with high magnifying power for observing minute structures in the cornea and iris.

fungal infection [L *fungus* mushroom; *inficere* to stain], any inflammatory condition caused by a fungus. Most fungal infections are superficial and mild, though persistent and difficult to eradicate. Some kinds of fungal infections are **aspergillosis, blastomycosis, candidiasis, coccidioidomycosis,** and **histoplasmosis.**

fungal septicemia [L *fungus*; Gk *septikos* putrid, *haima* blood], a form of blood poisoning in which the causative agent is a fungus.

fungemia /funjē′mē·ə/ [L *fungus* + Gk *haima* blood], the presence of fungi in the blood.

fungi [L *fungus*], the plural of fungus, a general term for a eukaryotic, thallus forming organism that requires an external carbon source. Fungi lack both chlorophyll and chemolithotrophic systems. They may be saprophytes or parasites and reproduce by spore production. They may invade living organisms, including humans, as well as nonliving organic substances.

fungicide /fun′jisīd/, a drug that kills fungi.

fungiform /fun′jifôrm/, shaped like a mushroom.

fungiform papilla. See **papilla.**

fungistatic /fun′jēstat′ik/, having an inhibiting effect on the growth of fungi.

fungus /fung′gəs/, *pl.* fungi /fun′jī/ [L, mushroom], a simple parasitic plant that, lacking chlorophyll, is unable to make its own food and is dependent on other life forms. A simple fungus reproduces by budding; multicellular fungi reproduce by spore formation. –**fungal, fungous,** *adj.*

funic presentation /fy$\overline{oo}$′nik s$\overline{oo}$′fəl/ [L *funis, praesentare* to show], in obstetrics, the appearance of the umbilical cord before the main presenting part of the fetus.

funic souffle [L *funis* cord; Fr *souffle* breath], a soft, muffled blowing sound produced by blood rushing through the umbilical vessels and synchronous with the fetal heart sound.

funiculitis /fənik′y$\overline{oo}$lī′tis/, any abnormal inflammatory condition of a cordlike structure of the body, such as the spinal cord or spermatic cord.

funiculus /fənik′yələs/ [L, little cord], a division of the white matter of the spinal cord, consisting of fasciculi or fiber tracts.

funiculus umbilicalis. See **umbilical cord.**

funis /fy$\overline{oo}$′nis, f$\overline{oo}$′nis/, a cordlike structure.

funis presentation, See **funic presentation.**

funnel chest [L *fundere* to pour], a skeletal abnormality of the chest characterized by a depressed sternum. The deformity may not interfere with breathing, but surgical correction is often recommended for cosmetic reasons.

funnel feeding, a technique in which liq-

432

funny bone   **FWB**

uids may be given orally to a patient who cannot move the lips or masticate. A rubber tube attached to a funnel is placed in the mouth, usually at one corner, and a liquid is poured slowly through the funnel and tube into the mouth near the back of the tongue.

funny bone, a popular name for a point at the lower end of the humerus where the ulnar nerve is near the surface and subject to external pressure, resulting in a tingling sensation.

FUO, abbreviation for **fever of unknown origin.**

furazolidone /fŏo'rəzol'idōn/, an antiinfective and antiprotozoal prescribed for certain bacterial or protozoal infections of the GI tract.

furcation /fərkā'shən/ [L *furca* fork], the region of division of the root portion of a tooth.

furfuraceous desquamation /fur'fərā'sē·əs/ [L *furfur* bran, *desquamare* to scale off], the shedding of epidermis in large scales.

furosemide /fŏorōsəmīd/, a diuretic prescribed in the treatment of hypertension, renal failure, and edema.

furred tongue [ME *furre* sheath; AS *tunge*], a tongue, the surface of which is coated by a white to brown accumulation of desquamated epithelial cells, bacteria, mycelia, and other debris. It is a common occurrence in some fevers.

furrow /fur'ō/ [AS *furh*], a groove, such as the atrioventricular furrow that separates the atria from the ventricles of the heart.

furuncle /fyŏŏr'ungkəl/ [L *furunculus* a boil], a localized, suppurative staphylococcal skin infection originating in a gland or hair follicle, characterized by pain, redness, and swelling. Necrosis deep in the center of the inflamed area forms a core of dead tissue that will be spontaneously extruded, eventually resorbed, or surgically removed. **–furunculous,** *adj.*

furunculosis /fyŏŏrung'kyŏŏlō'sis/, an acute skin disease characterized by boils or successive crops of boils that are caused by staphylococci or streptococci.

fusiform /fyŏŏ'sifôrm/ [L *fusus* spindle, *forma* form], a structure that is tapered at both ends.

fusiform aneurysm, a localized dilatation of an artery in which the entire circumference of the vessel is distended.

fusiform gyrus [L *fusus* spindle, *forma* form; Gk *gyros* turn], a convolution of the cerebral hemispheres that lies below the collateral fissures and joins the occipital and temporal lobes.

fusimotor /fyŏŏ'zimō'tər/ [L *fusus* + *motare* to move about], pertaining to the motor nerve fibers, or gamma efferent fibers, that innervate the intrafusal fibers of the muscle spindle.

fusion /fyŏŏ'zhən/ [L *fusio* outpouring], **1.** the bringing together into a single entity, as in optic fusion. **2.** the act of uniting two or more bones of a joint. **3.** the surgical joining together of two or more vertebrae, performed to stabilize a segment of the spinal column after severe trauma, a herniated disk, or degenerative disease. **4.** (in psychiatry) the tendency of two people experiencing an intense emotion to unite.

fusion beat, (in electrocardiography) a P wave or QRS complex resulting from the concurrent activation of the atria or the ventricles by two stimuli in the same chamber.

fusospirochetal disease /fyŏŏ'zōspī'rōkē'təl/ [L *fusus* spindle; Gk *speira* coil, *chaite* hair], any infection characterized by ulcerative lesions in which both a fusiform bacillus and a spirochete are found, such as trench mouth or Vincent's angina.

FVIII, symbol for **recombinant blood factor VIII,** a large glycoprotein containing more than 2,300 amino acids, 24 cysteine residues, and 25 potential glycosylation sites. The factor is used to treat bloodclotting disorders, such as **hemophilia A,** in which the factor is deficient or missing.

f waves, (in cardiology) waves that represent fibrillation or flutter.

F wave, a wave form recorded in electroneuromyographic and nerve conduction tests. It appears on supramaximal stimulation of a motor nerve and is caused by antidromic transmission of a stimulus. The F wave is used in studies of motor nerve function in the arms and legs.

FWB, abbreviation for **full weightbearing.**

g, abbreviation for **gram.**

Ga, symbol for the chemical element **gallium.**

GA, abbreviation for **general anesthesia.**

GABA, abbreviation for **gamma-aminobutyric acid.**

GABHS, abbreviation for **group A beta-hemolytic streptococcal (skin disease).**

gadolinium (Gd) /gad′əlin′ē·əm/ [Johan Gadolin, Finnish chemist, b. 1760], a rare earth metallic element. Its atomic number is 64; its atomic weight is 157.25.

gag [ME *gaggen* to strangle], **1.** a dental device for holding the jaws open during oral surgery or dental restoration. **2.** to retch or attempt to vomit.

gag reflex [ME *gaggen;* L *reflectere* to bend backward], a normal neural reflex elicited by touching the soft palate or posterior pharynx, the response being elevation of the palate, retraction of the tongue, and contraction of the pharyngeal muscles.

gait [ONor *geta* a way], the manner or style of walking, including rhythm, cadence, and speed.

gait determinant, one of a number of the kinetic anatomic factors that govern the locomotion of an individual in the process of walking. Authorities have defined pelvic rotation, pelvic tilt, knee and hip flexion, knee and ankle interaction, and lateral pelvic displacement as the main determinants of gait.

gait disorder, an abnormality in the manner or style of walking, usually as a result of neuromuscular, arthritic, or other body changes.

galactocele /gəlak′təsēl′/, a cyst or hydrocele caused by blockage of a mammary gland milk duct.

galactokinase /gəlak′tōkī′nās/ [Gk *gala* milk, *kinesis* movement, Fr *diastase* enzyme], an enzyme that functions in the metabolism of glycogen.

galactokinase deficiency, an inherited disorder of carbohydrate metabolism in which the enzyme galactokinase is deficient or absent. As a result, dietary galactose is not metabolized, galactose accumulates in the blood, and cataracts may develop.

galactophorous duct /gəlak′tōmôr′fəs/ [Gk *gala* + *pherein* to bear; L *ducere* to

lead], a passage for milk in the lobes of the breast.

galactorrhea /gəlak′tərē′ə/ [Gk *gala* + *rhoia* flowing], lactation not associated with childbirth or nursing. The condition is sometimes a symptom of a pituitary gland tumor.

galactose /gəlak′tōs/ [Gk *gala* + *glykys* sweet], a simple sugar found in the dextrorotatory form in lactose (milk sugar), nerve cell membranes, sugar beets, gums, and seaweed and, in the levorotatory form, in flaxseed mucilage.

galactosemia /gəlak′tōsē′mē·ə/ [Gk *gala* + *glykys* sweet, *haima* blood], an inherited, autosomal recessive disorder of galactose metabolism, characterized by a deficiency of the enzyme galactose-1-phosphate uridyl transferase. Shortly after birth, an intolerance to milk is evident. Hepatosplenomegaly, cataracts, and mental retardation develop.

galactosuria /gəlak′tōsŏŏr′ē·ə/, the presence of galactose in the urine.

galactosyl ceramide lipidosis /gəlak′təsil/ [Gk *gala* + *glykys* sweet; L *cera* wax, *lipos* fat, *osis* condition], a rare, fatal, inherited disorder of lipid metabolism, present at birth. Infants become paralyzed, blind, deaf, and increasingly retarded, and eventually die of bulbar paralysis.

galacturia /gal′əktŏŏr′ē·ə/ [Gk *gala* + *ouron* urine], a condition in which the urine has a milky color because of the abnormal presence of galactose, a monosaccharide, in the urine.

Galant reflex /gəlant′/, a normal response in the neonate to move the hips toward the stimulated side when the back is stroked along the spinal cord.

galea aponeurotica. See **epicranial aponeurosis.**

Galeazzi's fracture /gal′ē·at′sēz/ [Riccardo Galeazzi, Italian surgeon, b. 1866], a fracture of the distal radius accompanied by dislocation of the radioulnar joint.

Galen's bandage /gā′lənz/ [Claudius Galen, Greek physician, b. 130 AD], a bandage for the head, consisting of a strip of cloth with each end divided into three pieces.

gall. See **bile.**

gallbladder /gôl′blad′ər/ [ME *gal;* AS

blaedre], a pear-shaped excretory sac lodged in a fossa on the visceral surface of the right lobe of the liver. It serves as a reservoir for bile. About 8 cm long and 2.5 cm wide at its thickest part, it holds about 32 ml of bile. During digestion of fats, the gallbladder contracts, ejecting bile through the common bile duct into the duodenum.

gallbladder carcinoma, a malignant neoplasm of the bile reservoir, characterized by anorexia, nausea, vomiting, weight loss, progressively severe right upper quadrant pain, and, eventually, jaundice. Tumors of the gallbladder are predominantly adenocarcinomas and are often associated with biliary calculi.

gallium (Ga) /gal′ē·əm/ [L *Gallia* Gaul], a metallic element. Its atomic number is 31; its atomic weight is 69.72. Because of its high boiling point (1983° C; 3602° F), it is used in high-temperature thermometers. Radioisotopes of gallium are used in total body scanning procedures.

gallop /gal′əp/ [Fr *galop*], a pathologic third or fourth heart sound, which at certain heart rates sometimes mimics the gait of a horse.

gallop rhythm [Fr *galop;* Gk *rhythmos*], a cadence resembling that of a galloping horse produced by an abnormal third or fourth heart sound.

gallstone. See **biliary calculus.**

galvanic /galvan′ik/ [Luigi Galvani, Italian physician, b. 1737], pertaining to or involving electricity.

galvanic cautery, galvanocautery. See **electrocautery.**

galvanic electric stimulation [Luigi Galvani], the use of a high-voltage electric stimulator to treat muscle spasms, edema of acute injury, myofascial pain, and certain other disorders.

galvanic skin response (GSR) [Luigi Galvani; AS *scinn;* L *respondere* to reply], a reaction to certain stimuli as indicated by a change in the electrical resistance of the skin. The effect is related to unconscious activity of the sweat glands and may result from pleasant as well as unpleasant stimuli. The GSR is used in some polygraph examinations.

galvanometer /gal′vənom′ətər/ [Luigi Galvani], a device that indicates or measures electrical current by its effects on a needle or coil in a magnetic field. Galvanometers are used in certain diagnostic instruments, such as electrocardiographs.

Gambian trypanosomiasis /gam′bē·ən/, a usually chronic form of African trypanosomiasis, caused by the parasite *Trypanosoma brucei gambiense.*

game knee [ME *gamen;* AS *cneow*], a common term for any injury or condition that interferes with normal function of the knee joint.

gamete /gam′ēt/ [Gk, marriage partner], **1.** a mature male or female germ cell that is capable of functioning in fertilization or conjugation and contains the haploid number of chromosomes of the somatic cell. **2.** the ovum or spermatozoon. **–gametic,** *adj.*

gamete intrafallopian transfer (GIFT), a human fertilization technique in which male and female gametes are injected through a laparoscope into the fimbriated ends of the fallopian tubes.

gametic /gəmat′ik/ [Gk *gametes*/husband, *gamete*/wife], pertaining to a reproductive cell such as a spermatozoon or ovum.

gametic chromosome, any of the chromosomes contained in the haploid cell, specifically the spermatozoon or ovum, as contrasted to those in the diploid, or somatic cell.

gametocide /gəmē′tōsīd/ [Gk *gamete* + L *caedere* to kill], any agent that is destructive to gametes or gametocytes, specifically to the malarial gametocytes. **–gametocidal,** *adj.*

gametocyte /gəmē′tōsīt/ [Gk *gamete* + *kytos* cell], (in genetics) any cell capable of dividing into or in the process of developing into a gamete, specifically an oocyte or spermatocyte.

gametogenesis /gam′itōjen′əsis/ [Gk *gamete* + *genein* to produce], the origin and maturation of gametes, which occurs through the process of meiosis. **–gametogenic, gametogenous,** *adj.*

gametophyte /gəmē′tōfīt/ [Gk *gamete* + *phyton* plant], a cell in the reproductive stage when the nuclei are in a haploid condition.

gamma, Γ, γ, the third letter of the Greek alphabet, and symbol for photon, heavy-chain immunoglobulins, third in a series of certain chemical groups, and source of *G,* the seventh letter of the English alphabet.

gamma-aminobutyric acid (GABA), an amino acid with neurotransmitter activity found in the brain and also in the heart, lungs, kidneys, and certain plants.

gamma-benzene hexachloride. See **lindane.**

gamma camera [Gk *gamma* + L *camera* vault], a device that uses the emission of light from a crystal struck by gamma rays to produce an image of the distribution of radioactive material in a body organ. The light is detected by an array of light-sensitive electronic tubes and is converted to electric signals for further processing.

gamma efferent fiber [Gk *gamma* + L *efferre* to carry out; *fibra* fiber], any of the motor nerve fibers that transmit impulses from the central nervous system to the intrafusal fibers of the muscle spindle.

gamma globulin. See **immune gamma globulin.**

gamma-glutamyl transpeptidase, an enzyme that appears in the serum of patients with several types of liver or gallbladder disorders, including drug hepatotoxicity and biliary tract obstruction.

gamma radiation [Gk *gamma* + L *radiare* to emit rays], a very high-frequency electromagnetic emission of photons from certain radioactive elements in the course of nuclear transition or from nuclear reactions. Gamma radiation is more penetrating than alpha radiation and beta radiation but has less ionizing power and is not deflected in electric and magnetic fields. The wavelengths of gamma rays emitted by radioactive substances are characteristic of the radioisotopes involved and range from about 4×10^{-10} to 5×10^{-13}m. The depth to which gamma rays penetrate depends on their wavelengths and energy. Gamma radiation and other forms of radiation can injure, distort, or destroy body cells and tissue, especially cell nuclei, but controlled radiation is used in the diagnosis and treatment of various diseases. Gamma radiation can penetrate thousands of meters of air and several centimeters of soft tissue and bone.

gamma ray, an electromagnetic radiation of short wavelength emitted by the nucleus of an atom during a nuclear reaction. Composed of high-energy photons, gamma rays lack mass and an electric charge and travel at the speed of light.

gammopathy /gamop'əthē/, an abnormal condition characterized by the presence of markedly increased levels of gamma globulin in the blood. **Monoclonal gammopathy** is commonly associated with an electrophoretic pattern showing one sharp, homogenous electrophoretic band in the gamma globulin region. This reflects the presence of excessive amounts of one type of immunoglobulin secreted by a single clone of B cells. **Polyclonal gammopathy** reflects the presence of a diffuse hypergammaglobulinemia in which all immunoglobulin classes are proportionally increased.

gamogenesis /gam'ōjen'əsis/ [Gk *gamos* marriage, *genein* tp produce], sexual reproduction through the fusion of gametes. –**gamogenetic,** *adj.*

gamone /gam'ōn/ [Gk *gamos* marriage], a chemical substance secreted by the ova and spermatozoa that supposedly attracts the gametes of the opposite sex to facilitate union. Kinds of gamones are **androgamone** and **gynogamone.**

gampsodactyly. See **pes cavus.**

ganciclovir /gansik'lōvir/, an acrylic nucleoside structurally related to acyclovir. It is used to prevent cytomegalovirus disease after allogenic bone marrow transplantation and in persons with AIDS.

ganglion /gang'glē·on/, *pl.* **ganglia** [Gk, knot], **1.** a knot, or knotlike mass. **2.** one of the nerve cells, chiefly collected in groups outside the central nervous system. The two types of ganglia in the body are the sensory ganglia on the dorsal roots of spinal nerves and on the sensory roots of the trigeminal, facial, glossopharyngeal, and vagus nerves and the autonomic ganglia of the sympathetic and parasympathetic systems.

ganglionar neuroma /gang·glē'ənər/ [Gk *ganglion* + *neuron* nerve, *oma* tumor], a tumor composed of a solid mass of ganglia and nerve fibers. It is usually found in abdominal tissues and occurs most commonly in children.

ganglionic blockade /gang'glē·on'ik/, the blocking of nerve impulses at synapses of autonomic ganglia, usually by the administration of ganglionic blocking agents.

ganglionic blocking agent, any one of a group of drugs prescribed to produce controlled hypotension, as required in certain surgical procedures or in emergency management of hypertensive crisis. The drugs act by occupying receptor sites on sympathetic and parasympathetic nerve endings of autonomic ganglia.

ganglionic crest. See **neural crest.**

ganglionic glioma [Gk *ganglion* + *glia* glue, *oma* tumor], a tumor composed of glial cells and ganglion cells that are nearly mature.

ganglionic neuroma. See **ganglionar neuroma.**

ganglionic ridge. See **neural crest.**

ganglionitis /gang'glē·ənī'tis/, an inflammation of a nerve or lymph ganglion.

ganglioside /gang'glē·əsīd'/, a glycolipid found in the brain and other nervous system tissues. Accumulation of gangliosides because of an inborn error of metabolism results in gangliosidosis or Tay-Sachs disease.

gangliosidosis type I. See **Tay-Sachs disease.**

gangliosidosis type II. See **Sandhoff's disease.**

gangrene /gang'grēn/ [Gk *gangraina* a gnawing sore], necrosis or death of tissue, usually the result of ischemia (loss of blood supply), bacterial invasion, and subsequent putrefaction. **Dry gangrene** is a late complication of diabetes mellitus that is already complicated by arteriosclerosis in which the affected extremity becomes

G

cold, dry, and shriveled and eventually turns black. **Moist gangrene** may follow a crushing injury or an obstruction of blood flow by an embolism, tight bandages, or tourniquet. **–gangrenous,** *adj.*

gangrenous appendicitis /gang'grənəs/ [Gk, *gaggraina,* a consuming sore, L, *appendere,* to hang upon, Gk, *itis,* inflammation], a condition in which the appendix becomes gangrenous because obstruction of its lumen blocks the flow of blood to that body part.

gangrenous necrosis. See **necrosis.**

gangrenous stomatitis. See **noma.**

gangrenous vulvitis [Gk *gangraina;* L *vulva* wrapper; Gk *itis* inflammation], the death of tissues in the area of the vulva caused by a severe infection resulting in the sloughing of cells.

ganja. See **cannabis.**

gantry assembly /gan'trē/, (in computed tomography) a subsystem consisting of the x-ray tube, the detector array, the high-voltage generator, the patient support and positioning couch, and the mechanical support for each.

gap [OE *gapa* a hole], (in molecular genetics) a short, missing segment in one strand of double-stranded DNA.

gap phenomenon, (in cardiology) a condition in which a premature stimulus encounters a block where an earlier or later stimulus could be conducted.

Gardner, Mary Sewell (1871–1961), an American public health nurse who wrote the classic *Public Health Nurse.* She was instrumental in the development of the National Organization for Public Health Nursing and of public health nursing in the American Red Cross.

Gardner-Diamond syndrome, a condition resulting from autoerythrocyte sensitization, marked by large, painful, transient ecchymoses that appear without apparent cause but often accompany emotional upsets, various collagen disorders, and abnormalities of protein metabolism.

Gardnerella vaginalis /gärd'nərel'ə/, [Herman L. Gardner, twentieth-century American bacteriologist; L, *vagina,* sheath], a genus of rod-shaped gram-negative bacteria normally found in the female genital tract. The bacteria, formerly identified as *haemophilus vaginalis,* may also be a cause of bacterial vaginitis.

Gardnerella vaginalis **vaginitis** [Herman Gardner, L, *vagina,* sheath, Gk, *itis,* inflammation], an infection of the female genital tract by bacteria of the *Gardnerella vaginalis* strain, often in combination with various anaerobic bacteria. It is assumed that the infection is sexually transmitted. The bacteria are also found in normal women without symptoms. The infection often produces a gray or yellow discharge that has a "fishy" odor that increases after washing the genitalia with alkaline soaps.

Gardner's syndrome [Eldon J. Gardner, American geneticist, b. 1909], familial polyposis of the large bowel, with fibrous dysplasia of the skull, extra teeth, osteomas, fibromas, and epidermal cysts.

Gardner-Wells tongs, braces that are attached to the skull of patients immobilized with cervical injuries.

gargle [Fr. *gargouille* drainpipe], **1.** to hold and agitate a liquid at the back of the throat by tilting the head backward and forcing air through the solution. **2.** a solution used to rinse the mouth and oropharynx.

gargoylism. See **Hurler's syndrome.**

Gartner's duct [Hermann T. Gartner, Danish anatomist, b. 1785], one of two vestigial, closed ducts, each one parallel to a uterine tube.

gas [Gk, chaos], an aeriform fluid possessing complete molecular mobility and the property of indefinite expansion. A gas has no definite shape and its volume is determined by temperature and pressure.

gas bacillus [Gk *chaos;* L *bacillum* small rod], any of several species of bacillus that produce a gas as a byproduct of their metabolism. Examples include *E. coli,* which ferments lactose and glucose, and the Clostridial species, which produce gas gangrene.

gas chromatography, the separation and analysis of different substances according to their different affinities for a standard absorbent. In the process a gaseous mixture of the substances is passed through a glass cylinder containing the absorbent, which may be dampened with a nonvolatile liquid solvent for one or more of the gaseous components.

gas distention. See **flatulence.**

gas embolism, an occlusion of one or more small blood vessels, especially in the muscles, tendons, and joints, caused by expanding bubbles of gases. Gas emboli can rupture tissue and blood vessels, causing decompression sickness and death. This phenomenon commonly affects deep-sea divers who rise too quickly to the surface without adequate decompression.

gaseous /gas'ē·əs, gash'əs/ [Gk, chaos], pertaining to or resembling gas.

gas exchange, impaired, a NANDA-accepted nursing diagnosis of a condition in which the individual experiences a decreased passage of oxygen and/or carbon dioxide between the alveoli of the lungs and the vascular system. Defining characteristics include confusion, restlessness, irritability, somnolence, hypercapnea, and hypoxia.

gas gangrene, necrosis accompanied by gas bubbles in soft tissue after surgery or trauma. It is caused by anaerobic organisms, such as various species of *Clostridium*. Symptoms include pain, swelling, and tenderness of the wound area, moderate fever, tachycardia, and hypotension. A characteristic finding is toxic delirium. If untreated, gas gangrene is rapidly fatal.

gasoline poisoning. See **petroleum distillate poisoning.**

gas pains. See **flatulence.**

gas-scavenging system, the equipment and procedures used to eliminate anesthetic gases that escape into the atmosphere of the operating room.

gas sterilization, [Gk *chaos;* L *sterilis* barren] the use of a gas such as ethylene oxide, C_2H_4O, used to sterilize medical equipment.

gas therapy, the use of medical gases in respiratory therapy. Kinds of gas therapy include **carbon dioxide therapy, controlled oxygen therapy, helium therapy,** and **hyperbaric oxygenation.**

gastrectasia /gas′trektā′zhə/ [Gk *gaster* stomach, *ektasis* stretching], an abnormal dilatation of the stomach. It may be accompanied by pain, vomiting, rapid pulse, and falling body temperature. Causes can include overeating, obstruction of the pyloric valve, or a hernia.

gastrectomy /gastrek′əmē/, surgical excision of all or, more commonly, part of the stomach, performed to remove a chronic peptic ulcer, to stop hemorrhage in a perforating ulcer, or to remove a malignancy. Preoperatively, a GI series is done and a nasogastric tube is introduced. Under general anesthesia, one half to two thirds of the stomach is removed, including the ulcer and a large area of acid-secreting mucosa.

gastric /gas′trik/ [Gk *gaster* stomach], of or pertaining to the stomach.

gastric analysis, examination of the contents of the stomach, primarily to determine the quantity of acid present and incidentally to ascertain the presence of blood, bile, bacteria, and abnormal cells.

gastric antacid. See **antacid.**

gastric atrophy. See **atrophic gastritis.**

gastric cancer, a malignancy of the stomach with symptoms of vague epigastric discomfort, anorexia, weight loss, and unexplained iron deficiency anemia. Many cases are asymptomatic in the early stages, and metastatic enlargement of the left supraclavicular lymph node may be the first manifestation of a stomach lesion.

gastric dyspepsia, pain or discomfort localized in the stomach.

gastric digestion [Gk, *gaster,* stomach, L, *digere,* to separate], digestion by gastric juice in the stomach.

gastric emesis [Gk, *gaster,* stomach, *emesis,* vomiting], vomiting associated with a stomach disorder, such as stomach cancer, stomach ulcer, or severe gastritis.

gastric fistula, an abnormal passage into the stomach, communicating most frequently with an opening on the external surface of the abdomen. A gastric fistula may be created surgically to provide tube feeding for patients with severe esophageal disorders.

gastric glands, glands in the stomach mucosa that secrete hydrochloric acid, mucin, and pepsinogen.

gastric inhibitory polypeptide (GIP), a gastrointestinal hormone found in the mucosa of the small intestine. Release of the hormone, mediated by the presence of glucose or fatty acids in the duodenum, results in the release of insulin by the pancreas and inhibition of gastric acid secretion.

gastric intubation, a procedure in which a Levin tube or other small-caliber catheter is passed through the nose into the esophagus and stomach for the introduction into the stomach of liquid formulas to provide nutrition for unconscious patients or for premature or sick newborn infants. Medication or a contrast medium may be instilled for treatment or for radiologic examination.

gastric juice, digestive secretions of the gastric glands in the stomach, consisting chiefly of pepsin, hydrochloric acid, rennin, lipase, and mucin. The pH is strongly acid (0.9 to 1.5).

gastric lavage, the washing out of the stomach with sterile water or a saline solution.

gastric motility, the spontaneous peristaltic movements of the stomach that aid in digestion, moving food through the stomach and out through the pyloric sphincter into the duodenum.

gastric mucin [Gk *gaster* stomach; L *mucus*], a viscous secretion of glycoproteins produced from the mucous membrane lining of swine stomachs and formerly used in the treatment of peptic ulcers.

gastric node, a node in one of three groups of lymph glands associated with the abdominal and pelvic viscera supplied by branches of the celiac artery.

gastric partitioning, a surgical procedure in which a portion of the stomach is closed, reducing its capacity. It is used in the treatment of certain cases of obesity.

gastric resection [Gk *gaster;* L *re* + *secare* to cut], the surgical removal of part or all of the stomach, usually performed in the treatment of stomach cancer or peptic ulcer.

gastric ulcer, a circumscribed erosion of the mucosal layer of the stomach that may penetrate the muscle layer and perforate the stomach wall. It tends to recur with stress and is characterized by episodes of burning epigastric pain, belching, and nausea, especially when the stomach is empty or after eating certain foods. Characteristically, antacid medication or milk quickly relieves the pain.

gastrin /gas'trin/ [Gk *gaster* stomach], a polypeptide hormone, secreted by the pylorus, that stimulates the flow of gastric juice and contributes to the stimulus causing bile and pancreatic enzymes secretion.

gastrinoma /gas'trinō'mə/, a tumor found usually in the pancreas but sometimes in the duodenum.

gastritis /gastrī'tis/, an inflammation of the lining of the stomach that occurs in two forms. **Acute gastritis** may be caused by severe burns, major surgery, aspirin or other antiinflammatory agents, corticosteroids, drugs, food allergens, or by the presence of viral, bacterial, or chemical toxins. The symptoms—anorexia, nausea, vomiting, and discomfort after eating—usually abate after the causative agent has been removed. **Chronic gastritis** is usually a sign of underlying disease, such as peptic ulcer, stomach cancer, Zollinger-Ellison syndrome, or pernicious anemia. Kinds of gastritis include **antral, atrophic, hemorrhagic,** and **hypertrophic gastritis.**

gastrocamera /gas'trōkam'ərə/, a small camera that can be lowered into the stomach through the esophagus and retrieved after recording images of the stomach lining.

gastrocnemius /gas'troknē'mē·əs/ [Gk *gastroknemia* calf of the leg], the most superficial muscle in the posterior part of the leg. It arises by a lateral head and a medial head and forms the greater part of the calf.

gastrocnemius gait /gas'trōknē'mē'əs/, an abnormal gait associated with a weakness of the gastrocnemius. It is characterized by the dropping of the pelvis on the affected side at the last moment of the stance phase in the walking cycle, accompanied by the lagging or the slowness of forward pelvic movement.

gastrocnemius test, a test of the function of the gastrocnemius muscle by ankle plantar flexion while the patient is in a prone position. The examiner places fingers for palpation on the posterior of the calf while the patient pulls the heel upward.

gastrocoele. See **archenteron.**

gastrocolic omentum. See **greater omentum.**

gastrocolic reflex /gas'trōkol'ik/ [Gk *gaster* + *kolon* colon; L *reflectere* to bend backward], a mass peristaltic movement of the colon that often occurs when food enters the stomach.

gastrodidymus /gas'trōdid'iməs/ [Gk *gaster* + *didymos* twin], conjoined, equally developed twins united at the abdominal region.

gastrodisciasis /gas'trōdiskī'əsis/ [Gk *gaster* + *diskos* disk, *eidos* form, *osis* condition], an infection of trematodes of the genus *Gastrodiscoides,* which are digestive tract parasites.

gastrodisk. See **embryonic disk.**

gastroduodenal /gas'trōd o͞o'ədēnal/ [Gk *gaster* + L *duodeni* 12 fingers wide], pertaining to the stomach and duodenum.

gastroduodenitis /gas'trōd o͞o'ədenī'tis/ [Gk *gaster* + L *duodeni* + Gk *itis* inflammation], inflammation of the stomach and duodenum.

gastroenteritis /gas'trō·en'tərī'tis/ [Gk *gaster* + *enteron* intestine, *itis* inflammation], inflammation of the stomach and intestines accompanying numerous GI disorders. Symptoms are anorexia, nausea, vomiting, abdominal discomfort, and diarrhea. The condition may be attributed to bacterial enterotoxins, bacterial or viral invasion, chemical toxins, or miscellaneous conditions, such as lactose intolerance.

gastroenterologist /gas'trō·en'tərol'əjist/, a physician who specializes in gastroenterology.

gastroenterology /gas'trō·en'tərol'əjē/ [Gk *gaster* + *enteron* intestine, *logos* science], the study of diseases affecting the GI tract, including the stomach, intestines, gallbladder, and bile duct.

gastroenterostomy /gas'trō·en'təros'təmē/ [Gk *gaster* + *enteron* intestine, *stoma* mouth], surgical formation of an artificial opening between the stomach and the small intestine, usually at the jejunum. The operation is performed with a gastrectomy, to route food from the remainder of the stomach into the small intestine, or by itself, for perforating ulcer of the duodenum.

gastroesophageal /gas'trō·isof'əjē'əl/ [Gk *gaster* + *oisophagos* gullet], of or pertaining to the stomach and the esophagus.

gastroesophageal hemorrhage. See **Mallory-Weiss syndrome.**

gastroesophageal reflux, a backflow of contents of the stomach into the esophagus that is often the result of incompetence of the lower esophageal sphincter. Gastric juices are acid and therefore produce burning pain in the esophagus.

gastrogavage. See **gastrostomy feeding.**

gastrohepatic omentum. See **lesser omentum.**

gastrointestinal (GI) /gas′trō· intes′tinəl/ [Gk *gaster* + L *intestinum* intestine], of or pertaining to the organs of the GI tract, from mouth to anus.

gastrointestinal allergy, an immediate reaction of hypersensitivity after the ingestion of certain foods or drugs. GI allergy differs from food allergy, which can affect organ systems other than the digestive system. Characteristic symptoms include itching and swelling of the mouth and oral passages, nausea, vomiting, diarrhea (sometimes containing blood), severe abdominal pain, and, if severe, anaphylactic shock.

gastrointestinal bleeding, any bleeding from the GI tract. The most common underlying conditions are peptic ulcer, esophageal varices, diverticulitis, ulcerative colitis, and carcinoma of the stomach and colon. Vomiting of bright red blood or the passage of coffee-ground vomitus indicates upper GI bleeding, usually from the esophagus, stomach, or upper duodenum.

gastrointestinal gas. See **flatulence.**

gastrointestinal infection, any infection of the digestive tract caused by bacteria, viruses, parasites, or toxins. All may have common clinical features of nausea, vomiting, diarrhea, and anorexia.

gastrointestinal obstruction, any obstruction of the passage of intestinal contents, caused by mechanical blockage or failure of motility. Blockage may be caused by adhesions resulting from surgery or inflammatory bowel disease, an incarcerated hernia, fecal impaction, tumor, intussusception, or volvulus. Failure of motility may follow anesthesia, abdominal surgery, or occlusion of any of the mesenteric arteries to the gut. Symptoms generally include vomiting, abdominal pain, and increasing abdominal distention.

gastrointestinal system assessment, an evaluation of the patient's digestive system and symptoms. Discussion of symptoms is encouraged, and information is elicited concerning any changes in eating, bowel habits, the color, character, and frequency of stools and urine, the use of laxatives or enemas, and the occurrence of fatigue, hemorrhoids, and edema of the extremities. Diagnostic aids include a complete blood count, stool examination, prothrombin time, and determinations of levels of alkaline phosphatase, serum and urine bilirubin, serum glutamic oxaloacetic transaminase (SGOT), serum glutamic pyruvic transaminase (SGPT), lactic acid dehydrogenase (LDH), blood urea nitrogen, and serum lipase, cholinesterase, calcium, albumin, and glucose. Additional laboratory studies for the evaluation are the total protein level, a serum electrolyte profile, serum carotene, delta-xylose tolerance, galactose tolerance, hippuric acid, and bromosulphalein tests, the albumin-globulin ratio, serum flocculation and thymol turbidity tests, urobilinogen level, the polyvinylpyrrolidone (PVP) test for protein loss, Sulkowitch's test for calcium in urine, and Schilling's test for GI absorption of vitamin B_{12}.

gastrointestinal tract. See **digestive tract.**

gastromalacia /gas′trōmälä′shə/ [Gk *gaster* + *malakia* softness], an abnormal softening of the walls of the stomach.

gastromegaly /gas′trōmeg′əlē/ [Gk *gaster* + *megas* large], an abnormal enlargement of the stomach or abdomen.

gastroplasty /gas′trōplas′tē/ [Gk *gaster* + *plassein* to mold], any surgery performed to reshape or repair any stomach defect or deformity.

gastropore. See **blastopore.**

gastroschisis /gastros′kəsis/ [Gk *gaster* + *schisis* division], a congenital defect characterized by incomplete closure of the abdominal wall with protrusion of the viscera.

gastroscope /gas′trōskōp′/ [Gk *gaster* + *skopein* to look], a fiberoptic instrument for examining the interior of the stomach. **–gastroscopy,** *n.,* **gastroscopic,** *adj.*

gastroscopy /gastros′kəpē/, the visual inspection of the interior of the stomach by means of a gastroscope inserted through the esophagus. **—gastroscopic,** *adj.*

gastrostomy /gastros′təmē/ [Gk *gaster* + *stoma* mouth], surgical creation of an artificial opening into the stomach through the abdominal wall, performed to feed a patient who has cancer of the esophagus or tracheoesophageal fistula, or one who is expected to be unconscious for a prolonged period.

gastrostomy feeding, the introduction of a nutrient solution through a tube that has been surgically inserted into the stomach through the abdominal wall.

gastrothoracopagus /gas′trōthôr′əkop′- əgəs/ [Gk *gaster* + *thorax* chest, *pagos* fixture], conjoined twins that are united at the thorax and abdomen.

gastrula /gas′trŏŏlə/ [Gk *gaster* stomach], the early embryonic stage formed by the invagination of the blastula. The cup-shaped gastrula consists of an outer layer of ectoderm and an inner layer of mesenterm that subsequently differentiates into the mesoderm and endoderm.

gastrulation /gas′trəlā′shən/ [Gk *gaster* stomach], the development of the gastrula in lower animals and the formation of the three germ layers in the embryo of humans and higher animals.

gatch bed /gach/ [William D. Gatch, American surgeon, b. 1879; AS *bedd*], a bed that has an adjustable joint, allowing the knees to be flexed and the legs supported.

gate theory of pain. See **pain mechanism.**

gating, (in magnetic resonance imaging) organizing the data so that information used to construct an image comes from the same point in the cycle of a repeating motion, such as a heartbeat.

gating mechanism, (in cardiology) the increasing duration of an action potential from the AV node to a point in the distal Purkinje system, beyond which it again decreases.

Gaucher's disease /gôshāz′/ [Phillipe C. E. Gaucher, French physician, b. 1854], a rare, familial disorder of fat metabolism, caused by an enzyme deficiency, characterized by widespread reticulum cell hyperplasia in the liver, spleen, lymph nodes, and bone marrow.

gauntlet bandage /gônt′lit/ [Fr *gantlet* small glove; *bande* strip], a glovelike bandage covering the hand and the fingers.

gauss /gôs, gous/ [J. K. F. Gauss, German physicist, b. 1777], a unit of magnetic field strength. It is equal to 1/10,000 of a tesla.

gauze /gôz/ [Fr *gaze* veiled], a transparent fabric of open weave and differing degrees of fineness, most often cotton muslin, used in surgical procedures and for bandages and dressings. It may be sterilized and permeated by an antiseptic or lotion. Kinds of gauze include **absorbable, absorbent,** and **petrolatum gauze.**

gauze sponge [Ar *Gaza*; Gk *spoggia*], a piece of folded gauze used during surgery to wipe up bleeding surfaces and thereby helping to locate any sources of blood loss.

gavage /gäväzh′/ [Fr *gaver* to gorge], the process of feeding a patient through a nasogastric tube.

gavage feeding of the newborn, a procedure in which a tube passed through the nose or mouth into the stomach is used to feed a newborn infant with weak sucking, uncoordinated sucking and swallowing, respiratory distress, tachypnea, or repeated apneic spells.

gay [Fr *gai* merry], **1.** any person who is homosexual. **2.** of or pertaining to homosexuality.

Gay-Lussac's law /gā′ləsaks′/ [Joseph L. Gay-Lussac, French scientist, b. 1778; L *legu* a rule], (in physics) a law stating that the volume of a specific mass of a gas will increase as the temperature is increased if the pressure remains constant.

Gay Nurses' Alliance (GNA), a national organization of homosexual nurses.

gaze /gāz/ [ME *gazen* to stare], a fixed stare or state of looking in one direction. A person with normal vision has six basic positions of gaze, each determined by control of different combinations of contractions of extraocular muscles.

gaze palsy, a partial or complete inability to move the eyes to all directions of gaze. A gaze palsy is often named for the absent direction of gaze, such as a right lateral gaze palsy.

GBIA. See **Guthrie bacterial inhibition assay test.**

g.c., *informal;* abbreviation for **gonococcus.**

Gd, symbol for the chemical element **gadolinium.**

GDM, abbreviation for **gestational diabetes mellitus.**

Ge, symbol for the chemical element **germanium.**

gegenhalten /gā′gənhäl′tən/ [Ger, counterpressure], the involuntary resistance to passive movement of the extremities. The effect may be psychogenic in origin or a sign of dementia or cerebral deterioration.

Geiger-Müller (GM) counter /gī′gərmil′ər/ [Hans Geiger, German physicist, b. 1882; Walther Müller, German physicist; Fr *conter* to tell], an electronic device that indicates the level of radioactivity of any substance by counting the number of subatomic particles, as electrons, emitted by a substance. It cannot identify the type or energy of a particle.

gel /jel/ [L *gelare* to congeal], a colloid that is firm even though it contains a large amount of liquid, used in many medicines as a demulcent, a vehicle for other drugs, an antacid, or an astringent, depending on the drug from which it is derived.

gelatin buildup, an x-ray film artifact that may appear as a sharp area of either increased or reduced density.

gelatin film, absorbable, a hemostatic used to attain hemostasis during surgery, particularly neurologic, thoracic, and ophthalmic procedures.

gelatiniform carcinoma. See **mucinous carcinoma.**

gelatinous /jəlat′ənəs/ [L *gelare* to congeal], pertaining to or resembling a viscous, jellylike substance.

gelatinous carcinoma, a former term for **mucinous carcinoma.**

gelatin sponge, an absorbable local hemostatic prescribed to control bleeding in various surgical procedures and in the treatment of decubitus ulcers to promote healing and hemostasis.

gel diffusion. See **immunodiffusion.**

Gellhorn pessary. See **pessary.**

gemellary /jem′əler′ē/ [L *gemellus* twin], of or pertaining to twins.

gemellipara /jem′əlip′ərə/ [L *gemellus* + *parare* to give birth], a woman who has given birth to twins.

gemellology /jem′əlol′əjē/ [L *gemellus* + Gk *logos* science], the study of twins and the phenomenon of twinning.

gemellus /jəmel′əs/, either of a pair of small muscles arising from the ischium. They rotate the thigh laterally.

gemellus test, a test of the function of the gemellus in hip external rotation while the patient is seated with the knees flexed. The examiner places one hand on the lateral aspect of the knee to prevent flexion or abduction of the hip while the patient rotates the thigh outward by moving the foot medially.

gemfibrozil, an antihyperlipidemic agent prescribed for hyperlipidemia.

gemistocyte /jemis′təsīt/, an astrocyte with an eccentric nucleus and swollen cytoplasm, as seen in areas of nervous tissue affected by edema or infarction.

gemma /jem′ə/, *pl.* **gemmae** [L, bud] **1.** a budlike projection produced by lower forms of life during the budding process of asexual reproduction. **2.** any budlike or bulblike structure, such as a taste bud or end bulb. **–gemmaceous,** *adj.*

gemmate /jem′āt/ [L *gemma* + *atus* function] **1.** having buds or gemmae. **2.** to reproduce by budding.

gemmation /jemā′shən/ [L *gemmare* to produce buds], the process of cell reproduction by budding.

gemmiferous /jemif′ərəs/ [L *gemma* + *fer* bearing], having buds or gemmae; gemmiparous.

gemmiform /jem′ifôrm′/, resembling a bud or gemma.

gemmipara /jemip′ərə/ [L *gemma* + *parare* to give birth], an animal that produces gemmae or reproduces by budding, such as the hydra. **–gemmiparous,** *adj.*

gemmulation. See **gemmation.**

gemmule /jem′yōōl/ [L *gemmula* small bud] **1.** the small, asexual reproductive structure produced by the parent during budding that eventually develops into an independent organism. **2.** (according to the early theory of pangenesis) any of the submicroscopic particles containing hereditary elements that are produced by each somatic cell of the parent, and are transmitted through the bloodstream to the gametes.

gender /jen′dər/ [L *genus* kind], **1.** the classification of the sex of a person into male, female, or intersexual. **2.** the particular sex of a person.

gender identity, the sense or awareness of knowing to which sex one belongs.

gender identity disorder, a condition characterized by a persistent feeling of discomfort or inappropriateness concerning one's anatomic sex.

gender role, the expression of a person's gender identity; the image that a person presents to both himself or herself and others demonstrating maleness or femaleness.

gender testing [L *genus* + *testum* crucible], a procedure for validating the sex of an individual by examining a tissue sample, usually obtained from oral mucous membrane cells for the presence of a Y chromosome.

gene /jēn/ [Gk *genein* to produce], the biologic unit of genetic material and inheritance. It is considered to be a particular nucleic acid sequence within a DNA molecule that occupies a precise locus on a chromosome and is capable of self-replication by coding for a specific polypeptide chain. Kinds of genes include **complementary, dominant, lethal, mutant, operator, pleiotropic, recessive, regulator, structural, subletha, supplementary,** and **wild-type gene.**

gene amplification [Gk *genein*; L *amplus* large], a gene duplicating process in which RNA molecules are transcribed many times in certain cells in response to defined signals or environmental stresses.

gene library, (in molecular genetics) a collection of all of the genetic information of a specific species, obtained from cloned fragments.

gene pool [Gk *genein*; AS *pol*] the total number of genetic traits within a person or species population. In a population that reproduces by random sexual selection, the distribution of genetic traits follows a normal bell curve.

gene probe, a molecular biology device for locating a particular gene on a chromosome. It involves pairing with a short known segment of DNA or RNA with a matching sequence of bases on a chromosome.

general adaptation syndrome (GAS) [L *genus* kind; L *adaptare* to fit; Gk *syn* together, *dromos* course], the defense response of the body or the psyche to injury

G

or prolonged stress, as described by Hans Selye (1907–1982). It consists of an initial stage of shock or alarm reaction, followed by a phase of increasing resistance or adaptation, using the various defense mechanisms of the body or mind, and culminating in either a state of adjustment and healing or of exhaustion and disintegration.

general anesthesia, the absence of sensation and consciousness as induced by various anesthetic agents, given primarily by inhalation or intravenous injection. Four kinds of nerve blocks attained by general anesthesia are sensory, voluntary motor, reflex motor, and mental. There are several levels of mental block: calmness, sedation, hypnosis, narcosis, and complete, potentially lethal depression of all vital regulatory functions of the medulla in the brain.

generalization [L *genus* kind; Gk *izein* to cause], the process of reducing or bringing under a general rule or statement, such as classifying items under general categories.

generalized anaphylaxis, a severe reagin-mediated reaction to an allergen characterized by itching, edema, wheezing respirations, apprehension, cyanosis, dyspnea, pupillary dilatation, a rapid, weak pulse, and falling blood pressure that may rapidly result in shock and death. Systemic anaphylaxis, the most extreme form of hypersensitivity, may be caused by insect stings, proteins in animal sera, food, or certain drugs; parenterally administered penicillin and contrast media containing iodide are frequent causes of anaphylactic shock.

generalized peritonitis [L *genus;* Gk *peri* near, *tenein* to stretch, *itis* inflammation], a bacterial infection of the peritoneum secondary to an infection in another organ, as when an appendix ruptures or an ulcer perforates the gastric wall. The symptoms are usually acute and severe.

generally recognized as effective (GRAE), one of the statutory criteria that must be met by a drug before it can be approved as a "new drug." To be recognized as effective, the drug must be, according to the Act, considered safe and effective by "experts qualified by scientific training and experience."

general paresis [L *genus* kind; Gk, paralysis], an organic mental disorder resulting from chronic syphilitic infection, characterized by degeneration of the cortical neurons; progressive dementia, tremor, and speech disturbances; muscular weakness; and, ultimately, generalized paralysis.

general practitioner (GP) [L *genus* kind;

Gk *praktikos* qualified for action], a family practice physician.

general relaxation [L *genus, relaxare* to ease], a slackening of strain or tension of the entire body, but particularly of the muscles.

general symptom [L *genus;* Gk *symptoma* that which happens], a symptom that affects the entire body rather than a specific organ or location.

generation [L *generare* to beget], **1.** the act or process of reproduction; procreation. **2.** a group of contemporary individuals, animals, or plants that are the same number of life cycles from a common ancestor. **3.** the period of time between the birth of one individual or organism and the birth of its offspring. Kinds of generation include **alternate, asexual, filial, parental, sexual,** and **spontaneous generation.**

generative [L *generare* to beget], pertaining to activity that generates new physical or mental growth, such as creative problem solving.

generic /jənər'ik/ [L *genus* kind], **1.** of or pertaining to a genus. **2.** of or pertaining to a substance, product, or drug that is not protected by trademark. **3.** of or pertaining to the name of a kind of drug that is also the description of the drug, such as penicillin or tetracycline.

generic equivalent, a drug product sold under its generic name, identical in chemical composition to one or more others sold under a trademark but not, necessarily, equivalent in therapeutic effect.

generic name, the official, established nonproprietary name assigned to a drug. A given drug is licensed under its generic name, but it is usually marketed under a trademark chosen by the manufacturer.

generic nursing program, a program to prepare people with no previous professional nursing experience for entry into the field of nursing. The term is now usually used to distinguish baccalaureate programs from master's programs or practitioner programs.

genesis /jen'əsis/ [Gk, origin], **1.** the origin, generation, or developmental evolution of anything. **2.** the act of producing or procreating.

gene splicing, (in molecular genetics) the process by which a segment of DNA is attached to or inserted in a strand of DNA from another source.

gene therapy a procedure that involves injection of "healthy genes" into the bloodstream of a patient to cure or treat a hereditary disease or similar illness. Blood is withdrawn from the patient and the white cells are separated and cultured in a laboratory, then inserted into modified viruses. Normal genes from a volunteer are inserted into the viruses, which, in turn, transfer the normal gene into the chromosomes of the patient's white cells. The white cells containing the normal genes are finally injected into the patient's bloodstream.

genetic /jənet′ik/ [Gk *genesis* origin] **1.** pertaining to reproduction, birth, or origin. **2.** pertaining to genetics or heredity. **3.** pertaining to or produced by a gene; inherited.

genetic affinity, relationship by direct descent.

genetically significant dose (GSD), an arbitrary measure of the estimated annual gonadal radiation received by the population gene pool. In the United States the estimated GSD is 20 mrad. The figure is not intended to suggest possible genetic effects from exposure to that level of radiation.

genetic code, the information carried by the DNA molecules that determines the specific amino acids and their arrangement in the polypeptide chain of each protein synthesized by the cell. Any change in the code results in the incorrect arrangement of the amino acids in the protein, causing a mutation.

genetic colonization, the process by which a parasite introduces into its host genetic information that induces the host to synthesize products solely for the use of the parasite.

genetic counseling, the process of determining the occurrence or risk of occurrence of a genetic disorder within a family and of providing appropriate information and advice about the courses of action that are available, whether care of a child already affected, prenatal diagnosis, termination of a pregnancy, sterilization, or artificial insemination is involved.

genetic death, **1.** the failure of an organism to survive as a result of its genetic makeup. **2.** the removal of a gene or genotype from the gene pool of a population or a given familial descent because of sterility, failure of the individual or organism to reproduce, or death before sexual maturity.

genetic disorder. See **inherited disorder.**

genetic drift, the chance fluctuations in gene frequencies within a population. The smaller the population, the greater the tendency for variation within each generation, so that eventually small, isolated inbreeding groups become genetically quite different from the ancestors from which they derived.

genetic engineering, the process of producing recombinant DNA so that the geno-

type and phenotype of organisms can be altered and controlled. Enzymes are used to break the DNA molecule into fragments so that genes from another organism can be inserted and the nucleotides rearranged in any desired sequence.

genetic equilibrium, the state within a population at which the frequency of genes and genotypes does not change from generation to generation.

genetic homeostasis, the maintenance of genetic variability within a population through adaptation to varied or changing environments and conditions of life as a result of shifts or resistance to shifts in gene frequencies.

genetic immunity. See **natural immunity.**

genetic isolate, a group of plants, animals, cr individuals that is genetically separated by geographic, racial, social, cultural, or any other barriers that prevent them from interbreeding with those outside of the group.

geneticist, one who specializes in the study or application of genetics.

genetic load, the average number of accumulated detrimental genes per individual within a population, including those caused by mutation and selection within a recent generation and those inherited from ancestors.

genetic map, the graphic representation of the linear arrangement of genes on a chromosome and the relative distance between them, as expressed in map or morgan units.

genetic marker, any specific gene that produces a readily recognizable genetic trait that can be used in family and population studies or in linkage analysis.

genetic polymorphism, the recurrence within a population of two or more discontinuous genetic variants of a specific trait in such proportions that they cannot be maintained simply by mutation, such as the sickle cell trait, the Rh factor, and the blood groups.

genetic population. See **deme.**

genetics, **1.** the science that studies the principles and mechanics of heredity, specifically the means by which traits are passed from parents to offspring and the causes of the similarities and differences between related organisms. **2.** the total genetic makeup of a particular individual, family, group, or condition. Kinds of genetics are **clinical, molecular,** and **population genetics.**

genetic screening, the process of investigating a specific population of persons for the purpose of detecting the presence of disease, either incipient or overt, such as the generalized screening of all newborn infants for phenylketonuria.

gene transfer [Gk *genein;* L *transferre* to bring across], a type of gene therapy in which a gene is transplanted from a donor organism into a recipient organism.

Genga's bandage. See **Theden's bandage.**

geniculate neuralgia /jənik'yəlāt/ [L *geniculum*] little knee; Gk *neuron* nerve, *algos* pain], a severe, debilitating, inflammatory condition of the geniculate ganglion of the facial nerve, characterized by pain, loss of the sense of taste, facial paralysis, and a decrease in salivation and lacrimation.

geniculate zoster. See **herpes zoster.**

geniohyoideus /jē'nē-ō·hī·oi'dē·əs/ [Gk *genion* chin, *hyoides* Y-shaped], one of the four suprahyoid muscles, arising from the symphysis menti of the lower jaw and inserting into the body of the hyoid bone. A narrow muscle, it is innervated by a branch of the first cervical nerve, and it acts to draw the hyoid bone and the tongue forward.

genital herpes. See **herpes genitalis, herpes simplex.**

genitalia. See **genitals.**

genital reflex. See **sexual reflex.**

genitals /jen'itəlz/ [L *genitalis*], the sex, or reproductive, organs. In the female they include the vulva, mons veneris, labia majora, labia minora, clitoris, vagina, uterus, fallopian tubes, and ovaries. The male genitals include the penis, scrotum, testicles, epididymis, vas deferens, prostate gland, seminal vesicles, and Cowper's glands. –**genital,** *adj.*

genital stage [L *genitalis* + Fr *stage* trial period], (in psychoanalysis) the final period in psychosexual development, beginning with adolescence and continuing through the adult years when the genitals are the predominant source of pleasurable stimulation.

genital wart [L *genitalis;* AS *wearte*], a small, soft, moist, pink or red swelling that becomes pedunculated. The growth may be solitary or there may be a cauliflowerlike group in the same area of the prepuce or vulva. It is caused by a human papilloma virus (HPV) and is contagious. Atypical genital warts should be biopsied as possible carcinomas because they are associated with cervical cancer. No therapy has been shown to eradicate HPV.

genitourinary (GU) /jen'itō·yoo'riner'ē/ [L *genitalis* + Gk *ouron* urine], referring to the genital and urinary systems of the body, either the organ structures or functions or both.

genitourinary system. See **urogenital system.**

genogram /jē'nōgram/, a diagram that depicts family relationships over at least three generations.

genome /jē'nōm/ [Gk *genein* to produce], the complete set of genes in the chromosomes of each cell of a particular organism.

genontopia. See **senopia.**

genotype /jē'nōtīp'/ [Gk *genos* birth, *typos* mark], **1.** the complete genetic constitution of an organism or group, as determined by the particular combination and location of the genes on the chromosomes. **2.** the alleles situated at one or more sites on homologous chromosomes. The genetic information carried by a pair of alleles determines a specific characteristic or trait. **3.** a group or class of organisms having the same genetic makeup; the type species of a genus. –**genotypic,** *adj.*

gentamicin sulfate /jen'təmī'sin/, an aminoglycoside antibiotic prescribed to relieve the effects of severe infections caused by organisms sensitive to gentamicin.

gentian violet /jen'shən/, an antibacterial antiinfective, antifungal, and anthelmintic. It is prescribed in the treatment of pinworms, superficial infections of the skin, and vaginal infections.

gentiotannic acid /jen'shē·ətan'ik/, a form of tannic acid once used as an astringent and in the treatment of burns but no longer recommended because the compound is hepatotoxic.

genu /jē'noo/ [L, knee], the knee or any angular structure resembling the flexed knee.

genupectoral position /jē'noopek'tərəl/ [L *genu* + *pectus* breast; *positio*], knee-chest position. To assume the genupectoral position, the person kneels so that the weight of the body is supported by the knees and chest, with the abdomen raised.

genu recurvatum [L *genu, recurvare* to bend back], a backward deformity, hyperextension, at the knee joint.

genus /jē'nəs/, *pl. genera* /jen'ərə/ [L, kind], a subdivision of a family of animals or plants. A genus usually is composed of several closely related species, but the genus *Homo sapiens* has only one species, humans.

genu valgum [L, knee; *valgus* bowlegged], a deformity in which the legs are curved inward so that the knees are close together, knocking as the person walks, with the ankles widely separated.

genu varum [L, knee; *varus* bent outwards], a deformity in which one or both legs are bent outward at the knee.

geographic tongue [Gk *ge* earth, *graphein* to record; AS *tunge*], an inflammatory disorder on the dorsal surface of the tongue characterized by numerous and continually changing areas of loss and regrowth of the filiform papillae.

geometric mean. See **mean.**

geotrichosis /jē'ōtrikō'sis/ [Gk *ge* earth, *thrix* hair, *osis* condition], an abnormal condition associated with the fungus *Geotrichum candidum,* which may cause oral, bronchial, pharyngeal, and intestinal disorders. Geotrichosis has been associated with allergic asthmatic reactions similar to allergic aspergillosis and a type of intestinal disorder characterized by abdominal pain, diarrhea, and rectal bleeding.

geriatric day care [Gk *geras* old age; AS *daeg;* L *garrire* chatter], an ambulatory health care facility for elderly people. It usually offers a broad range of professional and community services to maximize functional independence for the patients.

geriatrician /jer'ē-ətrish'ən/, a medical specialist in the field of geriatrics.

geriatric nurse practitioner, a registered nurse with additional education and training through a master's degree program in nursing or a nondegree certificate program that prepares the nurse to deliver primary health care to elderly adults.

geriatrics /jer'ē·at'riks/, the branch of medicine dealing with the physiology of aging and the diagnosis and treatment of diseases affecting the aged.

germ /jurm/ [L *germen* sprout], **1.** any microorganism, especially one that is pathogenic. **2.** a unit of living matter able to develop into a self-sufficient organism, such as a seed, spore, or egg. **3.** (in embryology) the first stage in development, such as a spermatozoon or other germ cell.

germanium (Ge) /jərmā'nē-əm/ [Germany], a metallic element with some nonmetallic properties. Its atomic number is 32; its atomic weight is 72.59.

German measles. See **rubella.**

germ cell, 1. a sexual reproductive cell in any stage of development, from the primordial embryonic form to the mature gamete. **2.** an ovum or spermatozoon or any of their preceding forms. **3.** any cell undergoing gametogenesis.

germ disk. See **embryonic disk.**

germicide /jur'misīd/ [L *germen* sprout, *caedere* to kill], a drug that kills pathogenic microorganisms.

germinal /jur'minəl/ [L *germen* sprout], pertaining to or characteristic of a germ cell or to the early stages of development.

germinal center [L *germen* sprout; Gk *ken-*

tron center], an antigen-localizing primary follicle with lymphoid tissue. It reacts to antigens, enlarging and becoming filled with lymphoblasts and macrophages at the center of a ring of small lymphocytes.

germinal disk. See **embryonic disk.**

germinal epithelium, 1. the epithelial layer covering the genital ridge from which the gonads are derived in early embryonic development. **2.** the epithelial covering of the ovary, formerly thought to be the site of the formation of the oogonia.

germinal infection, an infection transmitted to a child by the ovum or sperm of a parent.

germinal membrane. See **blastoderm.**

germinal nucleus. See **pronucleus.**

germinal pole. See **animal pole.**

germinal spot, the nucleolus of a mature oocyte, before fertilization.

germinal stage, (in embryology) the interval of time from fertilization to implantation during which the ovum undergoes cell division several times, travels to the uterus, and, in the form of a blastocyst, begins to implant itself in the endometrium.

germinal vesicle, the nucleus of a mature oocyte before fertilization. Much larger than the nucleus of other cells, it initiates the completion of meiotic division after fertilization.

germination /jur'minā'shən/ [L *germinare* to germinate] **1.** the initial growth and development of an organism from the time of fertilization to the formation of the embryo. **2.** the sprouting of a spore or the seed of a plant. –**germinate,** *v.*

germ layer, one of the three primordial cell layers formed during gastrulation in the early stages of embryonic development from which the entire range of body tissue is derived.

germ nucleus. See **pronucleus.**

germ plasm, 1. the protoplasm of the germ cells containing the basic reproductive and hereditary material; the sum total of the DNA in a particular cell or organism. **2.** *nontechnical;* germ cells in any stage of development together with the tissues from which they originated.

germ-plasm theory. See **weismannism.**

germ theory [L *germen;* Gk *theoria* speculation], the concept that all infectious and contagious diseases are caused by living microorganisms.

Gerontologic Society of America (GSA), an organization of scientific and academic professionals interested in studies in the nature of the aging process and in the clinical manifestations of disease in the aging organism. GSA members participate with the International Association of Gerontology in periodic seminars at which worldwide research papers on longevity are presented.

gerontology /jer′əntol′əjē/ [Gk *geras* old age, *logos* science], the study of all aspects of the aging process, including the clinical, psychologic, economic, and sociologic problems encountered by the elderly and their consequences for both the individual and society.

gerontoxon. See **arcus senilis.**

geropsychiatry /jer′ōsīkī′ətrē/ [Gk *geras* old age, *psyche* mind], the study and treatment of mental illness in elderly persons.

Gerstmann-Straussler syndrome. See **human prion disease.**

Gesell Developmental Assessment, an evaluation program that provides information on gross motor, fine motor, language, personal-social, and cognitive development.

Gestalt /gəshtält′/, *pl.* Gestalts, Gestalten /gəshtäl′tən/ [Ger, form], a single physical, psychologic, or symbolic configuration, pattern, or experience consisting of a number of elements that has an effect as a whole different from that of the sum of its parts.

Gestalt psychology, a school of psychology, originating in Germany, that maintains that a psychologic phenomenon is perceived as a total configuration or pattern, rising from the relationships among its constituent elements, rather than as discrete elements possessing attributes of their own.

Gestalt therapy, a form of psychotherapy that stresses the unity of self-awareness, behavior, and experience.

gestant anomaly. See **odontoma.**

gestate /jes′tāt/ [L *gestare* to bear], **1.** to carry a developing fetus in the womb. **2.** to grow and develop slowly toward maturity, such as a fetus in the womb.

gestation /jestā′shən/ [L *gestare* to bear], in viviparous animals, the period of time from the fertilization of the ovum until birth. In humans the average duration is 266 days or approximately 280 days from the onset of the last menstrual period.

gestational age [L *gestare* + *aetas* time of life], the age of a fetus or a newborn, usually expressed in weeks dating from the first day of the mother's last menstrual period.

gestational assessment [L *gestare* + *assidere* to sit beside], calculating the fetal age of the offspring, based upon such factors as the menstrual history of the mother, the date that fetal heart sounds are first detected, and evaluation of ultrasound data. The information is important in planning emergency care in the event of premature birth signs.

gestational diabetes mellitus (GDM), a disorder characterized by an impaired ability to metabolize carbohydrate, usually caused by a deficiency of insulin, occurring in pregnancy and disappearing after delivery but, in some cases, returning years later.

gestational psychosis [L *gestare;* Gk *psyche* mind, *osis* condition], any mental disorder that can be attributed to a pregnancy.

gestation period [L *gestare;* Gk *peri* near, *hodos,* way], the time span between conception and labor in humans. The period is approximately 40 weeks.

Getman visuomotor theory, a concept that visual perception is based on developmental sequences of physiologic actions in children. The sequence of eight stages begins with innate response systems and advances to cognitive integration of perceptions, abstractions, and higher symbolic activity.

GFR abbreviation for **glomerular filtration rate.**

GH, abbreviation for **growth hormone.**

ghost cells [AS *gast;* L *cella* storeroom], red blood cells that have lost their hemoglobin so that only the cell membranes are observed in microscopic examinations of urine samples. The hemoglobin is destroyed by the presence of urine.

GHRF, abbreviation for **growth hormone releasing factor.**

GI, abbreviation for **gastrointestinal.**

giant cell [L *gigant* huge; *cella* storeroom], an abnormally large tissue cell. It often contains more than one nucleus and may appear as a merger of several normal cells.

giant cell arteritis. See **temporal arteritis.**

giant cell carcinoma, a malignant epithelial neoplasm characteristically containing numerous very large anaplastic cells.

giant cell interstitial pneumonia. See **interstitial pneumonia.**

giant cell myeloma, a bone tumor of multinucleated giant cells that resembles osteoclasts scattered in a matrix of spindle cells.

giant cell sarcoma. See **giant cell myeloma, osteoblastic sarcoma.**

giant cell thyroiditis. See **de Quervain's thyroiditis.**

giant cell tumor of bone. See **giant cell myeloma.**

giant chromosome, any of the excessively large chromosomes found in insects and the lower animals, specifically the lampbrush chromosome and polytene chromosome.

giant follicular lymphoma, a nodular, well-differentiated, lymphocytic, malignant lymphoma in which many nodules distort the normal structure of a lymph node.

giant hypertrophic gastritis, a rare disease characterized by large folds of nodular gastric rugae that may cover the wall of the stomach, causing anorexia, nausea, vomiting, and abdominal distress.

Giardia /jē·är′dē·ə/ [Alfred Giard, French biologist, b. 1846], a common genus of the flagellate protozoans. Many species of *Giardia* normally inhabit the digestive tract causing inflammation in association with other factors that produce rapid proliferation of the organism.

giardiasis /jē·ärdī′əsis/ [Alfred Giard; Gk *osis* condition], an inflammatory, intestinal condition caused by overgrowth of the protozoon *Giardia lamblia.* The source of infection is usually untreated water contaminated with *G. lamblia* cysts.

gibbus /gib′əs, jib′əs/ [L, hump], **1.** a hump, swelling, or enlargement on a body surface, usually confined to one side. **2.** a convex spinal curvature that may occur after the collapse of a vertebral body as may result from a fracture or tuberculosis of the spine.

Gibraltar fever. See **brucellosis.**

Gibson's murmur, a heart murmur that is heard continuously throughout the cardiac cycle. It waxes at the end of systole and wanes near the end of diastole and is often described as a "machinery-like" murmur.

Gibson walking splint, a kind of Thomas splint that allows a patient to be ambulatory.

Giemsa's stain /gē·em′zəz/ [Gustav Giemsa, German chemist, b. 1867; Fr *teindre* to dye], an azure dye used as a stain in the microscopic examination of the blood for certain protozoan parasites, viral inclusion bodies, and rickettsia, and, more routinely, in the preparation of a smear for a differential white cell count.

GIFT, abbreviation for **gamete intrafallopian transfer.**

gigantic acid, an antibiotic substance derived from *Aspergillus giganteus,* a species of mold.

gigantism /jigan′tizəm/ [L *gigas* giant], an abnormal condition characterized by excessive size and stature, caused most frequently by hypersecretion of growth hormone (GH) and occurring to a lesser degree in hypogonadism and in certain genetic disorders.

giggle incontinence [Du *giggelen;* L *incon-*

tinentia inability to retain], urinary incontinence when intraabdominal pressure is increased by giggling or laughing.

Gilbert's syndrome [Nicolas A. Gilbert, French physician, b. 1858], a benign, hereditary condition characterized by hyperbilirubinemia and jaundice. No treatment is required.

Gilchrist's disease. See **blastomycosis.**

Gilles de la Tourette's syndrome /zhēl′-dələtŏŏrets′/ [George Gilles de la Tourette, French neurologist, b. 1857], an abnormal condition characterized by facial grimaces, tics, and involuntary arm and shoulder movements. In adolescence, the condition worsens; the child may grunt, snort, and shout involuntarily. Coprolalia often develops.

Gillies' operation /gil′ēz/ [Harold D. Gillies, English surgeon, b. 1882], a surgical procedure for reducing fractures of the zygoma and zygomatic arch by making an incision in the temporal hairline.

gingiva /jinji′və/, *pl. gingivae* [L, gum], the gum of the mouth, a mucous membrane with supporting fibrous tissue that overlies the crowns of unerupted teeth and encircles the necks of those that have erupted. **–gingival,** *adj.*

gingival blanching /jinji′vəl/ [L *gingiva;* Fr *blanchir* to whiten], the lightening of gingival color, usually temporary, caused by the stretching of gingival tissue with decreased blood supply.

gingival blood supply, the vascular supply to the gingivae, arising from blood vessels that pass on the gingival side of the outer periosteum of bone and anastomose with blood vessels of the periodontal membrane and intraalveolar blood vessels.

gingival cavity, a cavity that occurs in the gingival third of the clinical crown of the tooth.

gingival color, the color of healthy or diseased gingival tissues. It varies with the thickness and degree of keratinization of the epithelium, blood supply, pigmentation, and alterations produced by gingival diseases.

gingival consistency, the combination of visual and tactile characteristics of healthy gingival tissue.

gingival corium, the most stable connective tissue of the gingiva, lying between the periosteum and the lamina propria mucosae.

gingival crater, a depression in the gingival tissue, especially in the area of the former apex of interdental papilla.

gingival crevice, a normal fissure between the free gingiva and the tooth enamel.

gingival discoloration, a change in the

normal coloration of the gingivae, associated with inflammation, reduced blood supply, abnormal pigmentation, and other problems.

gingival festoon, the distinct rounding and enlargement of the margins of the gingival tissue found in early gingival involvement.

gingival hormonal enlargement, the enlargement of the gingivae associated with hormonal imbalance during pregnancy, puberty, and hormone therapy.

gingival hyperplasia, overgrowth of the soft tissue of the gums, often seen in patients treated with phenytoin for epileptic seizures.

gingival line [L *gingiva* gum, *linea*], the scalloped line formed by the free gingival margin at the neck of the teeth.

gingival massage, the massage of gingival tissues for cleansing purposes, improving tissue tone and blood circulation, and for keratinization of the surface epithelium.

gingival mat, the gingival connective tissue composed of coarse, broad collagen fibers that attach the gingivae to the teeth and hold the free gingivae in close approximation to the teeth.

gingival papilla. See **papilla.**

gingival physiology, the function of the gingivae as supportive and protective investments of the teeth and subjacent tissues.

gingival position, the level of the gingival margin in relation to the teeth.

gingival shrinkage, the reduction in the size of gingival tissue, especially as the result of therapeutic elimination of subgingival deposits and curettement of the soft tissue wall of the gingival pocket.

gingival stippling, a series of small depressions in the surface of healthy gingivae, producing an appearance that varies from that of smooth, undulated velvet to that of an orange peel.

gingival sulcus, any of the normal spaces between the free gingivae and the teeth.

gingivectomy /jin′jīvek′təmē/ [L *gingiva* + Gk *ektome* excision], surgical removal of infected and diseased gingival tissue, performed to arrest the development of pyorrhea.

gingivitis /jin′jivī′tis/ [L *gingiva* + Gk *itis* inflammation], a condition in which the gums are red, swollen, and bleeding.

gingivoplasty /jin′jivōplas′tē/ [L *gingiva* + Gk *plassein* to shape], the surgical contouring of the gingival tissues to maintain healthy gingival tissue.

gingivostomatitis /jin′jivōstō′mətit′tis/ [L *gingiva* + Gk *stoma* mouth, *itis* inflammation], multiple, painful ulcers on the gums and mucous membranes of the mouth, the result of a herpesvirus infection.

ginglymus joint. See **hinge joint.**

ginseng /gin′seng/, a folk remedy prepared from the root of any species of the genus *Panax*. It is used by some Asian populations as a heart tonic, aphrodisiac, and stimulant.

Giordano-Giovannetti diet /jôrdä′nōjō′-vənet′ē/, a low-protein, low-fat, high-carbohydrate diet with controlled potassium and sodium intake, used in chronic renal insufficiency and liver failure. Protein is given only in the form of essential amino acids so that the body will use excess blood urea nitrogen to synthesize the nonessential amino acids for the production of tissue protein.

gipoma /gipō′mə/, a pancreatic tumor that causes changes in secretion of gastric inhibitory polypeptide (GIP).

girdle /gur′dəl/, any curved or circular structure, such as the hipline formed by the bones and related tissues of the pelvis.

girdle pad, a pad that fits over the iliac crests and sacrum to protect the hip area in contact sports.

girdle sensation. See **zonesthesia.**

glabella /gləbel′ə/ [L *glabrum* bald], a flat triangular area of bone between the two superciliary ridges of the forehead. It is sometimes used as a baseline for cephalometric measurements.

glabrous skin /glā′brəs/ [L *glaber* smooth; AS *scinn*], smooth, hairless skin.

glacial acetic acid, a clear, colorless liquid or crystalline substance (CH_3COOH) with a pungent odor. It is obtained by the destructive distillation of wood or from acetylene and water or by the oxidation of ethyl alcohol. Glacial acetic acid is a strong caustic and is potentially flammable with a low flash point.

gland [L *glans* acorn], any one of many organs in the body, comprising specialized cells that secrete or excrete materials not related to their ordinary metabolism. Some glands lubricate; others, such as the pituitary gland, produce hormones; hematopoietic glands take part in the production of blood. –**glandular,** *adj.*

glanders [OFr *glandres* neck gland swelling], an infection caused by the bacillus *Pseudomonas mallei*, transmitted to humans from horses and other domestic animals. It is characterized by purulent inflammation of the mucous membranes and the development of skin nodules that ulcerate.

gland of Montgomery. See **areolar gland.**

glands of Zeiss. See **ciliary gland.**

glandular carcinoma. See **adenocarcinoma.**

glandular epithelium /glan'dyəl/ [L *glandula;* Gk *epi* above, *thele* nipple], epithelium that contains glandular cells.

glandular fever. See **infectious mononucleosis.**

glandular tissue [L, *glandula,* small gland, OFr, *tissu],* a group of epithelial secreting cells composing a definitive glandular organ, such as the thyroid.

glandula vestibularis major. See **Bartholin's gland.**

glans /glanz/, *pl.* **glandes** /glan'dēz/ [L, acorn], **1.** a general term for a small, rounded mass, or glandlike body. **2.** erectile tissue, as on the ends of the clitoris and the penis.

glans of clitoris [L *glans;* Gk *kleitoris*], the erectile tissue at the end of the clitoris, continuous with the intermediate part of the vaginal vestibular bulbs. It comprises two corpora cavernosa enclosed in a dense, fibrous membrane and connected to the pubis and ischium.

glans penis [L], the conical tip of the penis that covers the end of the corpora cavernosa penis and the corpus spongiosum like a cap. The urethral orifice is normally located at the center of the distal tip of the glans penis.

Glanzmann's disease. See **thrombasthenia.**

Glasgow Coma Scale, a quick, practical, and standardized system for assessing the degree of conscious impairment in the critically ill and for predicting the duration and ultimate outcome of coma, primarily in patients with head injuries. The system involves three determinants: eye opening, verbal response, and motor response, all of which are evaluated independently according to a rank order that indicates the level of consciousness and degree of dysfunction.

glass factor. See **factor XII.**

glaucoma /glôkō'mə, glou-/ [Gk, cataract], an abnormal condition of elevated pressure within an eye because of obstruction of the outflow of aqueous humor. **Acute (angle-closure, closed-angle,** or **narrow-angle) glaucoma** occurs if the pupil in an eye with a narrow angle between the iris and cornea dilates markedly, causing the folded iris to block the exit of aqueous humor from the anterior chamber. Acute glaucoma is accompanied by extreme ocular pain, blurred vision, a red eye, and a dilated pupil. Nausea and vomiting may occur. If untreated, acute glaucoma results in complete and permanent blindness within 2 to 5 days. **Chronic (open-angle** or **wide-angle) glaucoma** is much more common, often bilateral; it develops slowly and is genetically determined. The obstruction is believed to be within the canal of Schlemm. Chronic glaucoma may produce no symptoms except for gradual loss of peripheral vision over a period of years. Sometimes headaches, blurred vision, and dull pain in the eye are present. Cupping of the optic discs may be noted on ophthalmoscopic examination. Halos around lights and central blindness are late manifestations. Both types have elevated intraocular pressure by tonometry. **–glaucomatous,** *adj.*

glaucomatocyclitic crisis /glôkom'ətōsiklit'ik/, a recurrent rise in intraocular pressure in one eye, resembling acute angle-closure glaucoma.

glenohumeral /glē'nōhyo͞o'mərəl/ [Gk *glene* joint socket + L *humerus* shoulder], pertaining to the glenoid cavity and the humerus at the shoulder joint.

glenohumeral joint, the shoulder joint, formed by the glenoid cavity of the scapula and the head of the humerus.

glenohumeral ligaments, three thickened bands of connective tissue attached proximally to the anterior margin of the glenoid cavity and labrum and distally to the lesser tuberosity and neck of the humerus.

glenoid cavity /glē'noid/ [Gk *glene* + *eidos* form; L *cavum*], a shallow depression with which the head of the humerus articulates. Also called **glenoid fossa.**

glia. See **neuroglia.**

glia cells /glī'ə, glē'ə/ [Gk *glia* glue; L *cella* storeroom], neural cells that have a connective tissue supporting function in the central nervous system. Examples include astrocytes and oligodendroglial cells of ectodermal origin and microglial cells of mesodermal origin.

gliadin /glī'ədin/ [Gk *glia* glue], a protein substance that is obtained from wheat and rye. Its solubility in diluted alcohol distinguishes gliadin from another grain protein, glutenin.

gliding [AS *glidan* to glide], **1.** a smooth, continuous movement. **2.** the simplest of the four basic movements allowed by various joints of the skeleton. It is common to all movable joints and allows one surface to move smoothly over an adjacent surface, regardless of shape.

gliding joint, a synovial joint in which articulation of contiguous bones allows only gliding movements, as in the wrist and the ankle.

gliding zone, an articular cartilage surface area immediately adjacent to a joint space.

glioblastoma. See **spongioblastoma.**

glioblastoma multiforme /glī′ōblastō′mə mul′tifôr′mē/ [Gk *glia* glue, *blastos* germ, *oma* tumor; L *multus* many *forma* form], a malignant, rapidly growing, pulpy or cystic tumor of the cerebrum or, occasionally, of the spinal cord. The lesion spreads with pseudopod-like projections.

glioma /glī·ō′mə/, *pl. gliomas, gliomata* [Gk *glia* + *oma* tumor], any of the largest group of primary tumors of the brain, composed of malignant glial cells. Kinds of gliomas are **astrocytoma, ependymoma, glioblastoma multiforme,** medulloblastoma, and **oligodendroglioma.**

glioma multiforme. See **gliobastoma multiforme.**

glioma retinae. See **retinoblastoma.**

glioma sarcomatosum. See **gliosarcoma.**

glioneuroma /glī′ōnŏŏrō′mə/, *pl. glioneuromas, glioneuromata* [Gk *glia* + *neuron* nerve, *oma* tumor], a neoplasm composed of nerve cells and elements of their supporting connective tissue.

gliosarcoma /glī′ōsärkō′mə/, *pl. gliosarcomas, gliosarcomata* [Gk *glia* + *sarx* flesh, *oma* tumor], a tumor composed of spindle-shaped cells in the delicate supporting connective tissue of nerve cells.

gliosarcoma retinae. See **retinoblastoma.**

glipizide /glip′izīd/, an oral antidiabetic drug prescribed as an adjunct to diet and exercise in lowering blood glucose levels of patients with non-insulin-dependent diabetes.

Glisson's capsule /glis′ənz/ [Francis Glisson, English physician, b. 1597; L *capsula* little box], the fibrous tissue sheath around lobules of the liver that carries branches of the hepatic artery, portal vein, and bile duct.

glitter cells [ME *gliteren* to shine], white blood cells in whose cytoplasm movement of granules is observed. They are seen in urine samples in cases of pyelonephritis.

Gln, abbreviation for **glutamine.**

global aphasia [L *globus* ball; Gk *a* + *phasis* speech], a loss of ability to use any form of written or spoken language. The condition involves both sensory and motor nerve tracts. Communication is attempted through primitive gestures or the use of automatic words and phrases.

globin /glō′bin/ [L *globus* ball], any of a group of globulin protein molecules. They become bound by the iron in heme molecules to form hemoglobin or myoglobin.

globoid leukodystrophy. See **galactosyl ceramide lipidosis.**

globule /glob′yŏŏl/ [L *globulus* small sphere], a small spheric mass. Kinds of globules are **dentin, Dobie's, Marchi's, Margagni's, milk,** and **myelin globule.**

globulin /glob′yŏŏlin/, one of a broad category of simple proteins classified by solubility, electrophoretic mobility, and size.

globulinuria /glō′binŏŏ′rē·ə/ [L *globulus* + Gk *ouron* urine], the presence of globulin class proteins in the urine.

globus hystericus /glō′bus/ [L, small sphere; Gk *hystera* womb], a transitory sensation of a lump in the throat, often accompanying emotional conflict or acute anxiety.

globus pallidus /glō′bus pal′idəs/ [L, small sphere; pale], the smaller and more medial part of the lentiform nucleus of the brain, separated from the putamen by the lateral medullary lamina.

glomangioma /glōman′jē·ō′mə/, *pl. glomangiomas, glomangiomata* [L *glomus* ball of thread; Gk *aggeion* vessel, *oma*], a benign tumor that develops from a cluster of blood cells in the skin.

glomerular /glōmer′yŏŏlar/ [L *glomerulus* small ball], of or pertaining to a glomerulus, especially a renal glomerulus.

glomerular capsule. See **Bowman's capsule.**

glomerular disease, any of a group of diseases in which the glomerulus of the kidney is affected.

glomerular filtration, the renal process whereby fluid in the blood is filtered across the capillaries of the glomerulus and into the urinary space of Bowman's capsule.

glomerular filtration rate (GFR), [L *glomerulus;* Fr *filtre;* L *ratus*], a kidney function test in which results can be determined from the amount of ultrafiltrate formed by plasma flowing through the glomeruli of the kidney. It may be calculated from insulin and creatinine clearance, serum creatinine, and blood urea nitrogen (BUN). Normal values average around 170 L/day for men and 150 L/day for women, with variations due to differences in age, muscle mass, and other factors.

glomerulonephritis /glōmer′yŏŏlōnəfrī′tis/ [L *glomerulus* small ball; Gk *nephros* kidney, *itis*], an inflammation of the glomerulus of the kidney, characterized by proteinuria, hematuria, decreased urine production, and edema. Kinds of glomerulonephritis are **acute, chronic,** and **subacute glomerulonephritis.**

glomerulosclerosis /glōmer′yŏŏlōsklərō′sis/ [L *glomerulus* + Gk *sklerosis* a hardening, *osis* condition], a severe kidney disease in which glomerular function of blood filtration is lost as fibrous scar tissue replaces the glomeruli. The disease commonly follows an infection or arteriosclerosis.

glomerulus /glōmer'yo͞olǝs/, *pl.* **glomeruli** [L, small ball] **1.** a tuft or cluster. **2.** a structure composed of blood vessels or nerve fibers, such as a renal glomerulus.

glomus /glō'mǝs/, *pl.* **glomera** /glom'ǝrǝ/ [L, ball of thread], a small group of arterioles connecting directly to veins and having a rich nerve supply.

glossectomy /glosek'tǝmē/ [Gk *glossa* tongue, *ektome* cutting out], the surgical removal of all or a part of the tongue.

glossitis /glosī'tis/ [Gk *glossa* tongue, *itis*], inflammation of the tongue. Acute glossitis, characterized by swelling, intense pain that may be referred to the ears, salivation, fever, and enlarged regional lymph nodes, may develop during an infectious disease or after a burn, bite, or other injury.

glossitis parasitica. See **parasitic glossitis.**

glossitis rhomboidea mediana. See **median rhomboid glossitis.**

glossodynia /glos'ōdin'ē-ǝ/ [Gk *glossa* + *odyne* pain], pain in the tongue, caused by acute or chronic inflammation, an abscess, or an ulcer.

glossodynia exfoliativa [Gk *glossa, odyne* + L *ex* without, *folium* leaf], a form of chronic glossitis, characterized by pain and sensitivity to spicy foods without any evidence of a pathologic condition.

glossoepiglottic /glos'ō-ep'iglot'ik/, pertaining to the epiglottis and the tongue.

glossohyal /glos'ōhī'ǝl/ [Gk *glossa* + *hyoeides* Y-shaped], of or pertaining to the tongue and the horseshoe-shaped hyoid bone at the base of the tongue immediately above the thyroid cartilage.

glossolalia /glos'ōlā'lyǝ/ [Gk *glossa* + *lalein* to babble], speech in an unknown "language," as "speaking in tongues" during a state of religious ecstasy.

glossoncus /glosong'kǝs/ [Gk *glossa* + *onkos* swelling], a local swelling or general enlargement of the tongue.

glossopathy /glosop'ǝthē/ [Gk *glossa* + *pathos* disease], a pathologic condition of the tongue, such as acute inflammation caused by a burn, bite, injury, or infectious disease; enlargement resulting from congenital lymphangioma; or a disorder produced by mycotic infection, a malignant lesion, or a congenital anomaly.

glossopexy /glos'ǝpek'sē/ [Gk *glossa* + *pexis* fixation], an adhesion of the tongue to the lip.

glossopharyngeal /glos'ōfǝrin'jē-ǝl/ [Gk *glossa* + *pharynx* throat], of or pertaining to the tongue and pharynx.

glossopharyngeal nerve, either of a pair of cranial nerves essential to the sense of taste, for sensation in some viscera, and for secretion from certain glands.

glossopharyngeal neuralgia, a disorder of unknown origin characterized by recurrent attacks of severe pain in the back of the pharynx, the tonsils, the base of the tongue, and the middle ear.

glossophytia /glos'ǝfit'ē-ǝ/ [Gk *glossa* + *phyton* plant], a condition of the tongue characterized by a blackish patch on which filiform papillae are greatly elongated and thickened like bristly hairs.

glossoplasty /glos'ōplas'tē/ [Gk *glossa* + *plassein* to mold], a surgical procedure or plastic operation on the tongue performed to correct a congenital anomaly, repair an injury, or restore a measure of function after excision of a malignant lesion.

glossoptosis /glos'optō'sis/ [Gk *glossa* + *ptosis* falling], the retraction or downward displacement of the tongue.

glossopyrosis /glos'ōpīrō'sis/ [Gk *glossa* + *pyr* fire, *osis* condition], a burning sensation in the tongue caused by chronic inflammation, by exposure to extremely hot or spicy food, or by psychogenic glossitis.

glossorrhaphy /glosôr'ǝfē/ [Gk *glossa* + *rhaphe* seam], the surgical suturing of a wound in the tongue.

glossotrichia /glos'ǝtrik'ē-ǝ/ [Gk *glossa* + *thrix* hair], a condition of the tongue characterized by a hairlike appearance of the papillae.

glossy skin [ONorse *glosa* smooth and shiny; AS *scinn*], a shiny skin that is usually secondary to neuritis and may be associated with other integumentary disorders, including alopecia, skin fissuring, and ulceration. It usually begins as an erythematous area on an extremity.

glottis, *pl.* **glottises, glottides** [Gk, opening to larynx], **1.** a slitlike opening between the true vocal cords (plica vocalis). **2.** the phonation apparatus of the larynx, composed of the true vocal cords and the opening between them (rima glottidis). **–glottal, glottic,** *adj.*

glow curve, (in thermoluminescence dosimetry) the graphic representation of the emitted light intensity that increases with the increasing phosphor temperature.

Glu, abbreviation for **glutamic acid.**

glucagon /gloo'kǝgon/ [Gk *glykys* sweet, *agaein* to lead], a hormone, produced by alpha cells in the islets of Langerhans, that stimulates the conversion of glycogen to glucose in the liver. Secretion of glucagon is stimulated by hypoglycemia and by the growth hormone of the anterior pituitary.

glucagonoma syndrome /gloo'kəgonō'-mə/ [Gk *glykys, agaein* + *oma* tumor], a disease associated with a glucagon-secreting tumor of the islet cells of the pancreas, characterized by hyperglycemia, stomatitis, anemia, weight loss, and a characteristic rash.

glucocorticoid /gloo'kōkôr'təkoid/ [Gk *glykys* + L *cortex* bark; Gk *eidos* form], an adrenocortical steroid hormone that increases glyconeogenesis, exerts an antiinflammatory effect, and influences many body functions. The most important of the three glucocorticoids is cortisol (hydrocortisone); corticosterone is less active, and cortisone is inactive until converted to cortisol. Glucocorticoids promote the release of amino acids from muscle, mobilize fatty acids from fat stores, and increase the ability of skeletal muscles to maintain contractions and avoid fatigue.

gluconeogenesis /gloo'kōjen'əsis/, the formation of glycogen from fatty acids and proteins rather than carbohydrates.

glucosan /gloo'kəsan/ [Gk *glykys* sweet], any of a large group of anhydrous polysaccharides that on hydrolysis yield a hexose, primarily anhydrides of glucose. The glucosans include cellulose, glycogen, starch, and the dextrins.

glucose /gloo'kōs/ [Gk *glykys* sweet], a simple sugar found in certain foods, especially fruits, and a major source of energy occurring in human and animal body fluids.

glucose 1-phosphate, an intermediate compound in carbohydrate metabolism.

glucose 6-phosphate, an intermediate compound in carbohydrate metabolism.

glucose-6-phosphate dehydrogenase (G-6-PD) deficiency, an inherited disorder characterized by red cells partially or completely deficient in glucose-6-phosphate dehydrogenase, a critical enzyme in aerobic glycolysis. The disorder is associated with episodes of acute hemolysis under conditions of stress or in response to certain chemicals or drugs.

glucose tolerance test, a test of the body's ability to metabolize carbohydrates by administering a standard dose of glucose and measuring the blood and urine for glucose at regular intervals thereafter.

glucosuria /gloo'kōsŏor'ē·ə/ [Gk *glykys* + *ouron* urine], abnormal presence of glucose in the urine resulting from the ingestion of large amounts of carbohydrate or from a disease, such as nephrosis or diabetes mellitus. **–glucosuric,** *adj.*

glucosyl cerebroside lipidosis. See **Gaucher's disease.**

glue sniffing [Gk *gloios;* ME *sniffen*], the practice of inhaling the vapors of toluene, a volatile organic compound used as a solvent in certain glues.

glutamate /gloo'təmāt/, a salt of glutamic acid.

glutamic acid (Glu) /glootam'ik/ [L *gluten* glue, *amine* ammonia; *acidus* sour], a nonessential amino acid occurring widely in a number of proteins. Preparations of glutamic acid are used as aids for digestion.

glutamicacidemia /glootam'ikas'idē'-mē·ə/, an inherited disorder of amino acid metabolism resulting in an excessive level of glutamic acid.

glutamic acid hydrochloride, a gastric acidifier prescribed for hypoacidity.

glutamic-oxaloacetic transaminase. See **aspartate aminotransferase.**

glutamic-pyruvic transaminase. See **alanine aminotransferase.**

glutamine (Gln) /gloo'təmēn/ [L *gluten* + *amine* ammonia], a nonessential amino acid found in many proteins in the body. It functions as an amino donor for many reactions and it is also a nontoxic transport for ammonia.

glutargin /glootär'gin/, arginine glutamate.

glutathione /gloo'təthī'ōn/ [L *gluten* + Gk *theione* sulfur], an enzyme whose deficiency is commonly associated with hemolytic anemia.

gluteal /gloo'tē·əl/ [Gk *gloutos* buttocks], pertaining to the buttocks or to the muscles that form the buttocks.

gluteal gait. See **Trendelenburg gait.**

gluteal tuberosity, a ridge on the lateral posterior surface of the thigh bone to which is attached the gluteus maximus.

gluten /gloo'tən/ [L, glue], the insoluble protein constituent of wheat and other grains.

gluten enteropathy. See **celiac disease.**

glutethimide /glooteth'əmīd/, a sedative prescribed in the treatment of anxiety and insomnia.

gluteus /glootē'əs/, any of the three muscles that form the buttocks. The **gluteus maximus** acts to extend the thigh. The **gluteus medius** acts to abduct and rotate the thigh. The **gluteus minimus** acts to abduct the thigh.

Gly, abbreviation for **glycine.**

glyburide /glī'bərīd/, an oral antidiabetic drug prescribed as an adjunct to diet and exercise in lowering blood glucose levels of patients with non-insulin-dependent diabetes.

glycerin /glis'ərin/ [Gk *glykeros* sweet], a sweet, colorless, oily fluid that is a pharmaceutic preparation of glycerol. Also spelled glycerine.

glycerol /glis'ərôl/ [Gk *glykeros* sweet],

an alcohol that is a component of fats. Glycerol is soluble in ethyl alcohol and water.

glycerol kinase, an enzyme in the liver and kidneys that catalyzes the transfer of a phosphate group from adenosine triphosphate to form adenosine diphosphate and L-glycerol-3-phosphate.

glyceryl alcohol. See **glycerin.**

glyceryl guaiacolate. See **guaifenesin.**

glyceryl triacetate. See **triacetin.**

glycine (Gly) /glī′sin/ [Gk *glykeros* + L *amine* ammonia], a nonessential amino acid occurring widely as a component of animal and plant proteins.

glycobiarsol /glī′kōbī′ərsol/, an antiamebic containing arsenic and bismuth, formerly used to treat intestinal amebiasis.

glycogen /glī′kəjən/ [Gk *glykys* sweet, *genein* to produce], a polysaccharide that is the major carbohydrate stored in animal cells. It is formed from glucose and stored chiefly in the liver and, to a lesser extent, in muscle cells.

glycogenesis /glī′kōjen′əsis/, the synthesis of glycogen from glucose.

glycogenolysis /glī′kōjenol′isis/ [Gk *glykys, genein* + *lysis* loosening], the breakdown of glycogen to glucose.

glycogenosis. See **glycogen storage disease.**

glycogen storage disease [Gk *glykys, genein* + L *instaurare* to renew; *dis* opposite of; Fr *aise* ease], any of a group of inherited disorders of glycogen metabolism.

glycogen storage disease, type I. See **von Gierke's disease.**

glycogen storage disease, type Ib, a form of glycogen storage disease in which excessive amounts of glycogen are deposited in the liver and leukocytes. Additional symptoms include neutropenia and recurrent GI infections.

glycogen storage disease, type II. See **Pompe's disease.**

glycogen storage disease, type III. See **Cori's disease.**

glycogen storage disease, type IV. See **Andersen's disease.**

glycogen storage disease, type V. See **McArdle's disease.**

glycogen storage disease, type VI. See **Hers' disease.**

glycolic acid /glīkol′ik/ [Gk *glykys* + L *acidus* sour], a substance in bile, formed by glycine and cholic acid, that aids in digestion and absorption of fats.

glycolipid /glī′kōlip′id/ [Gk *glykys* + *lipos* fat], a compound that consists of a lipid and a carbohydrate, usually galactose, found primarily in the tissue of the nervous system.

glycolysis /glīkol′isis/ [Gk *glykys* + *lysis* loosening], a series of enzymatically catalyzed reactions by which glucose and other sugars are broken down to yield lactic acid or pyruvic acid, releasing energy in the form of adenosine triphosphate. **Aerobic glycolysis** yields pyruvic acid in the presence of adequate oxygen. **Anaerobic glycolysis** yields lactic acid.

glycoprotein /glī′kōprō′tēn/ [Gk *glykys* + *proteios* first rank], any of the large group of conjugated proteins in which the nonprotein substance is a carbohydrate. These include the mucins, the mucoids, and the chondroproteins.

glycopyrrolate /glī′kōpir′əlāt/, an anticholinergic prescribed as an adjunct to ulcer therapy.

glycoside /glī′kəsīd/ [Gk *glykys* sweet], any of several carbohydrates that yield a sugar and a nonsugar on hydrolysis. The plant *Digitalis purpurea* yields a glycoside used in the treatment of heart disease.

glycosphingolipids /glī′kōsfing′gōlip′ids/, compounds formed from carbohydrates and ceramide, a fatty substance, found in tissues of the central nervous system and also in erythrocytes.

glycosuria /glī′kōsŏŏr′ē·ə/ [Gk *glykys* + *ouron* urine], abnormal presence of a sugar, especially glucose, in the urine. It is a finding most routinely associated with diabetes mellitus. **–glycosuric,** *adj.*

glycosuric acid /glī′kōsŏŏr′ik/ [Gk *glykys* + *ouron* urine; L *acidus* sour], a compound that is an intermediate product of the metabolism of tyrosine. It forms a melanin-like staining substance in the urine of people who have alkaptonuria.

glycosylated hemoglobin (GHb/Hb A_{1c}) /glīkō′silā′tid/, a hemoglobin A molecule with a glucose group on the N-terminal valine amino acid unit of the beta chain. The glycosylated hemoglobin concentration represents the average blood glucose level over the previous several weeks.

glycyl alcohol. See **glycerin.**

gm, abbreviation for **gram.** The abbreviation *g* is preferred.

GMENAC, abbreviation for **Graduate Medical Education National Advisory Committee.**

GMP, abbreviation for **guanosine monophosphate.**

GNA, abbreviation for **Gay Nurses' Alliance.**

gnathic /nath′ik/ [L *gnathos* jaw], of or pertaining to the jaw or cheek.

gnathion /nā′thē·on/ [L *gnathos* jaw], the lowest point in the lower border of the mandible in the median plane. It is a common reference point in the diagnosis and orthodontic treatment of various kinds of malocclusion.

gnathodynamometer /nā'thōdī'nəmom'-ətər/ [Gk *gnathos* + *dynamis* force, *metron* measure], an instrument used for measuring the biting pressure of the jaws of an individual.

gnathodynia /nā'thōdin'ē·ə/ [Gk *gnathos* + *odyne* pain], a pain in the jaw, such as that commonly associated with an impacted wisdom tooth.

gnathology /nāthol'əjē/ [Gk *gnathos* + *logos* science], a field of dental or medical study that deals with the entire masticatory apparatus, including its anatomy, histology, morphology, physiology, pathology, and therapeutics.

gnathoschisis. See **cleft palate.**

gnathostatic cast /nā'thōstat'ik/ [Gk *gnathos* + *statike* weighing; ME *casten*], a cast of the teeth trimmed so that its occlusal plane is in its normal oral attitude when the cast is set on a plane surface.

gnathostatics /nā'thōstat'iks/ [Gk *gnathos* + *statike* weighing], a technique of orthodontic diagnosis based on an analysis of the relationships between the teeth and certain reference points on the skull.

GnRH, abbreviation for **gonadotropin-releasing hormone.**

goal [ME *gol* limit], the purpose toward which an endeavor is directed, such as the outcome of diagnostic, therapeutic, and educational management of a patient's health problem.

goblet cell [ME *gobelet* small bowl], one of the many specialized cells that secrete mucus and form glands of the epithelium of the stomach, the intestine, and parts of the respiratory tract.

goiter [L *guttur* throat], a hypertrophic thyroid gland, usually evident as a pronounced swelling in the neck. The enlargement may be associated with hyperthyroidism, hypothyroidism, or normal levels of thyroid function. The goiter may be cystic or fibrous, containing nodules or an increased number of follicles. See specific goiters. **–goitrous,** *adj.*

gold (Au) [AS *geolu* yellow], a yellowish, soft metallic element that occurs naturally as a free metal and as the telluride $AuAgTe_4$. Its atomic number is 79; its atomic weight is 197. Gold salts, in which gold is attached to sulfur, are often used in the treatment, or chrysotherapy, of patients with rheumatoid arthritis but cause serious toxicity in about 10% of patients and some toxicity in 25% to 50%.

gold 198, a radioactive gold antineoplastic prescribed for cancer of the prostate, cervix, and bladder and for the reduction of fluid accumulation secondary to a cancer.

Goldblatt kidney, an abnormal kidney in which constriction of a renal artery leads to ischemia and the release of renin, a pressor substance associated with hypertension.

gold compound, a drug containing gold salts, usually administered with other drugs in the treatment of rheumatoid arthritis. Gold is potentially toxic and is administered only under the supervision of a specialist in chrysotherapy.

gold file, (in dentistry) an instrument designed for removing surplus gold from gold restorations. It may be designed and used as either a pull-cut or push-cut file.

gold foil, (in dentistry) pure gold that has been rolled and beaten into a very thin sheet. It is commonly compacted into a retentive tooth cavity form, using gold's property of cold welding.

gold inlay, an intracoronal cast restoration of gold alloy.

gold knife, an instrument that may be contraangled, with a blade or cutting edge, used for trimming excess metal and for developing contour in foil restorations.

Goldman-Fox knife, a dental surgical instrument with a sharp cutting edge, designed for the incision and contouring of gingival tissue.

gold sodium thiomalate, an antirheumatic prescribed for rheumatoid arthritis.

gold therapy. See **chrysotherapy.**

golfer's elbow, a popular term for medial epicondylitis associated with repeated use of the wrist flexors.

Golgi apparatus /gôl'jē/ [Camillo Golgi, Italian anatomist, b. 1844; L *ad* towards, *prepare* to prepare], one of many small membranous structures found in most cells, composed of various elements associated with the formation of carbohydrate side chains of glycoproteins, mucopolysaccharides, and other substances.

Golgi-Mazzoni corpuscles /gôl'jēmatsō'nē/ [Camillo Golgi; Vittori Mazzoni, Italian physician, b. 1823], a number of thin capsules enveloping terminal nerve fibrils in the subcutaneous tissue of the fingers.

Golgi's cells [Camillo Golgi; L *cella* storeroom], **1. Golgi type I neurons,** nerve cells having long axons that leave the local neuropil area of the parent cell body, traverse the white matter, and project to the rest of the nervous system. **2. Golgi type II neurons,** nerve cells with short trajectory axons, like stellate cells of the cerebral and cerebellar cortex. They generally do not enter white matter but remain within the local neuropil in the cerebral and cerebellar cortices and the retina.

Golgi tendon organ, a sensory nerve ending that is sensitive to both tension and excessive passive stretch of a skeletal muscle.

gomphosis /gomfō'sis/, *pl.* **gomphoses** [Gk *gomphos* bolt], an articulation by the insertion of a conic process into a socket, such as the insertion of a root of a tooth into an alveolus of the mandible or the maxilla.

gonad /gō'nad/ [Gk *gone* seed], a gamete-producing gland, such as an ovary or a testis. **–gonadal,** *adj.*

gonadal dysgenesis /gō'nədəl/, a general designation for a variety of conditions involving anomalies in the development of the gonads, such as Turner's syndrome, hermaphroditism, and gonadal aplasia.

gonadal dose, a measure of the dose of radiation received by the gonads as a result of an x-ray examination. It may vary from less than 1 mrad for a dental or chest radiograph to 225 mrad for a lumbar spine radiograph and 800 mrad for a fetus during pelvimetry.

gonadal shield, a specially designed contact or shadow shield used to protect the gonadal area of a patient from the primary radiation beam during x-ray procedures. It is generally used for all patients who are potentially reproductive, including all patients under the age of 40 and also older males.

gonadotropin /gō'nədōtrop'in/ [Gk *gone* + *trophe* nourishment], a hormonal substance that stimulates the function of the testes and the ovaries. The gonadotropic follicle stimulating hormone and luteinizing hormone are produced and secreted by the anterior pituitary gland. In early pregnancy, chorionic gonadotropin is produced by the placenta. **–gonadotropic, gonadotrophic,** *adj.*

gonadotropin-releasing   hormone (GnRH) [Gk, *gone,* seed, *trope,* a turn, ME, *relesen,* Gk, *hormaein,* to set in motion], a decapeptide hypophysiotropic hormone secreted by the hypothalamus. It stimulates the release of gonadotropin hormone by the anteriorpituitary gland. It also stimulates the release of the **luteinizing hormone (LH)** and **follicle-stimulating hormone (FSH)** by the anterior pituitary.

gonial angle. See **angle of mandible.**

goniometer /gon'ē·om'ətər/, an instrument used to measure angles, particularly range of motion angles of a joint.

goniometry /gon'ē·om'ətrē/ [Gk *gonia* angle, *metron* measure], a system of testing for various labyrinthine diseases that affect the sense of balance. **–goniometric,** *adj.*

gonioscope /gō'nē·əskōp'/ [Gk *gonia* + *skopein* to look], an ophthalmoscope used to examine the angle of the anterior chamber of the eye and for demonstrating ocular motility and rotation.

goniotomy /gō'nē·ot'əmē/, an eye operation performed to remove any obstruction to the flow of aqueous humor in the front chamber of the eye. The procedure is commonly done in cases of glaucoma.

gonoblast. See **germ cell.**

gonococcal /gon'əkok'əl/ [Gk *gone* seed, *kokkos* berry], pertaining to or resembling gonococcus.

gonococcal pyomyositis [Gk *gone* + *kokkos; pyon* pus, *mys* muscle, *itis* inflammation], an acute inflammatory condition of a muscle caused by infection with a *Neisseria gonorrhoeae,* characterized by abscess formation and pain. It is differentiated from sarcoma by the discovery of the gonococcal diplococci within the abscess.

gonococcal salpingitis [Gk *gone* + *kokkos, salpigx* tube, *itis*], an inflammation of the fallopian tubes caused by a gonoccal infection.

gonococcal urethritis [Gk *gone* + *kokkos, ourethra* urethra, *itis*], an inflammation of the urethra caused by a gonococcal infection.

gonococcus /gon'əkok'əs/, *pl.* gonococci /gon'əkok'sī/ [Gk *gone* + *kokkos* berry], a gram-negative, intracellular diplococcus of the species *Neisseria gonorrhoeae,* the cause of gonorrhea.

gonocyte. See **germ cell.**

gonorrhea /gon'ərē'ə/ [Gk *gone* + *rhoia* flow], a common sexually transmitted disease most often affecting the genitourinary tract and, occasionally, the pharynx, conjunctiva, or rectum. Infection results from contact with an infected person or by contact with secretions containing the causative organism *Neisseria gonorrhoeae.* Urethritis, dysuria, purulent, greenish yellow urethral or vaginal discharge, red or edematous urethral meatus, and itching, burning, or pain around the vaginal or urethral orifice are characteristic. The vagina may be massively swollen and red, and the lower abdomen may be tense and very tender. As the infection spreads, which is more common in women than in men, nausea, vomiting, fever, and tachycardia may occur as salpingitis, oophoritis, or peritonitis develops. Gonococcal ophthalmia involves infection of the conjunctiva and may lead to scarring and blindness. **–gonorrheal, gonorrheic,** *adj.*

gonorrheal arthritis /gon'ərē'əl/ [Gk *gone* + *kokkos, arthron* joint, *itis*], a blood-borne gonococcal infection of the joints. It may affect one or several joints, occur as a chronic or acute form, and often leads to joint fusion. Infection may result in pus formation in an affected joint.

gonorrheal conjunctivitis, a severe, destructive form of purulent conjunctivitis caused by the gonococcus *Neisseria gonorrhoeae.* Newborn infants receive routine prophylaxis of a topical instillation of 1% solution of silver nitrate or an antibiotic ointment, which has largely eradicated the infection in infants.

gonorrheal proctitis [Gk *gone* seed + *rhoia* flow, *proktos* anus + *itis*], an inflammation of the rectum caused by an infection of gonorrhea.

Gonyaulax catanella /gon'ē·ô'laks/, a species of planktonic protozoa that produce a toxin ingested by shellfish along the coasts of North America, resulting in seafood poisoning.

Goodell's sign /gŏodelz'/ [William Goodell, American gynecologist, b. 1829], softening of the uterine cervix, a probable sign of pregnancy.

Goodpasture's syndrome /gŏod'pas·chər/ [Ernest W. Goodpasture, American pathologist, b. 1886], a chronic, relapsing pulmonary hemosiderosis, usually associated with glomerulonephritis and characterized by a cough with hemoptysis, dyspnea, anemia, and progressive renal failure.

Goodrich, Annie Warburton (1866–1954), an American nursing educator. In 1923 she became dean of the newly formed Yale School of Nursing at Yale University, bringing to nursing the same university rank as other professions.

Good Samaritan legislation [good Samaritan, from New Testament parable; L *lex* law, *lator* proposer], laws enacted in some states to protect physicians, dentists, and some other health professionals from liability in rendering emergency medical or dental aid, unless there is proven willful wrong or gross negligence.

gooseflesh. See **pilomotor reflex.**

Gordon's elementary body [Mervyn H. Gordon, English physician, b. 1872], a particle found in tissues containing eosinophils; once thought to be the viral cause of Hodgkin's disease.

Gordon's reflex [Alfred Gordon, American neurologist, b. 1874] **1.** an abnormal variation of Babinski's reflex, elicited by compressing the calf muscles, characterized by extension of the great toe and fanning of the other toes. It is evidence of disease of the pyramidal tract. **2.** an abnormal reflex, elicited by compressing the forearm muscles, characterized by flexion of the fingers or of the thumb and index finger. It is seen in diseases of the pyramidal tract.

Gosselin's fracture /gôslaNz'/ [Leon A. Gosselin, French surgeon, b. 1815], a V-shaped fracture of the distal tibia, extending to the ankle.

GOT, abbreviation for **glutamic-oxaloacetic transaminase.**

goundou /gōōn'dōō/ [West African], a condition characterized by bony exostoses of the nasal and maxillary bones, usually occurring as a late sequela of yaws in people in Africa and Latin America.

gout [L *gutta* drop-by-drop], a disease associated with an inborn error of uric acid metabolism that increases production or interferes with excretion of uric acid. Excess uric acid is converted to sodium urate crystals that precipitate from the blood and become deposited in joints and other tissues. The condition can result in exceedingly painful swelling of a joint, accompanied by chills and fever. The disorder is disabling and, if untreated, can progress to the development of tophi and destructive joint changes.

gouty /gou'tē/ [L *gutta*, drop], pertaining to or resembling the condition of gout.

gouty arthritis. See **gout.**

Gowers' muscular dystrophy. See **distal muscular dystrophy.**

GP, abbreviation for **general practitioner.**

gp160, code for a glycoprotein that provides an outer coat for the HIV (human immunodeficiency virus). The outer coat, in turn, is composed of gp120, which protrudes from the virus surface, and gp41, which is embedded in the envelope coat.

GPT, abbreviation for **glutamic-pyruvic transaminase.**

gr, abbreviation for **grain.**

graafian follicle /graf'ē·ən, gräf'ē·ən/ [Reijnier de Graaf, Dutch physician, b. 1641; L *folliculus* small bag], a mature ovarian vesicle, measuring about 10 to 12 mm in diameter, that ruptures during ovulation to release the ovum. Many primary ovarian follicles, each containing an immature ovum about 35 μ in diameter, are imbedded near the surface of the ovary. Under the influence of the follicle-stimulating hormone from the adenohypophysis, one ovarian follicle ripens into a graafian follicle during the proliferative phase of each menstrual cycle. The cavity of the follicle collapses when the ovum is released, and the remaining follicular cells greatly enlarge to become the corpus luteum.

gracile /gras'il/, long, slender, and graceful.

gracilis /gras'ilis/, the most superficial of the five medial femoral muscles. It functions to adduct the thigh and flex the leg and to assist in the medial rotation of the leg after it is flexed.

gradation of activity /grədā'shən/, therapeutic activities that are appropriately paced and modified to demand maximal capacities at any point in progression or regression of the patient's condition.

graded exercise test (GXT), a test given a cardiac patient during rehabilitation to assess prognosis and quantify maximal functional capacity.

gradient /grā'dē·ənt/ [L *gradus* step], **1.** the rate of increase or decrease of a measurable phenomenon, such as temperature or pressure. **2.** a visual representation of the rate of change of a measurable phenomenon; a curve.

gradient magnetic field, a magnetic field that changes in strength in a certain given direction. Such fields are used in NMR imaging to select a region for imaging and also to encode the location of NMR signals received from the object being imaged.

graduated bath [L *gradus* step; AS *baeth*], a bath in which the temperature of the water is slowly reduced.

graduated resistance exercise. See **progressive resistance exercise.**

graduate medical education, formal medical education pursued after receipt of an MD or other professional degree in the medical sciences.

Graduate Medical Education National Advisory Committee (GMENAC), a committee established by the Secretary of the U.S. Department of Health and Human Services (HHS) to study the personnel issues in medicine.

graduate nurse (GN) [L *gradus* step, *nutrix* nurse], a nurse who is a graduate of an accredited school of nursing.

Graduate Record Examination (GRE), an examination administered to graduates of institutions of higher learning. The scores are used as criteria for admission to masters and doctoral programs in many institutions and areas of specialization.

GRAE, abbreviation for **generally recognized as effective.**

graft [Gk *graphion* stylus], a tissue or an organ taken from a site or a person and inserted into a new site or person, performed to repair a defect in structure. The graft may be temporary, such as an emergency skin transplant for extensive burns, or permanent, with the grafted tissue growing to become a part of the body. Skin, bone, cartilage, blood vessel, nerve, muscle, cornea, and whole organs, such as the kidney or the heart, may be grafted.

graft-versus-host reaction, a rejection response of certain grafts, especially bone marrow. It involves an incompatibility resulting from a deficiency in the immune response of some patients and is commonly associated with inadequate immunosuppressive therapy. Characteristic signs may include skin lesions with edema, erythema, ulceration, scaling, and loss of hair.

Graham's law /grā'əm/, the law stating that the rate of diffusion of a gas through a liquid (or the alveolar-capillary membrane) is directly proportional to its solubility coefficient and inversely proportional to the square root of its density.

grain (gr) [L *granum* seed], the smallest unit of mass in avoirdupois, troy, and apothecaries' weights, being the same in all and equal to 4.79891 mg. The troy and apothecaries' ounces contain 480 grains; the avoirdupois ounce contains 437.5 grains.

gram (g, gm) [L *gramma* small weight], a unit of mass in the metric system equal to 1/1,000 of a kilogram, 15.432 grains, and 0.0353 ounce avoirdupois. The preferred abbreviation is *g*.

gram calorie. See **calorie.**

gram-equivalent weight (gEq), an equivalent weight of a substance calculated as the gram mass that contains, replaces, or reacts with (directly or indirectly) the Avogadro number of hydrogen atoms.

gram-molecular weight (gmW), an amount in grams equal to the molecular weight of a substance, or the sum of all the atomic weights in its molecular formula.

gram-negative [Hans C. J. Gram, Danish physician, b. 1853; L *negare* to say no], having the pink color of the counterstain used in Gram's method of staining microorganisms. This property is a primary method of characterizing organisms in microbiology.

gram-positive [Hans C. J. Gram; L *positivus*], retaining the violet color of the stain used in Gram's method of staining microorganisms. This property is a primary method of characterizing organisms in microbiology.

Gram's stain [Hans C. J. Gram], the method of staining microorganisms using a violet stain, followed by an iodine solution, decolorizing with an alcohol or acetone solution, and counterstaining with safranin. The retention of either the violet color of the stain or the pink color of the counterstain serves as a primary means of identifying and classifying bacteria.

grandiose /L *grandis* great/, pertaining to something or somebody imposing, impressive, magnificent, or also pompous and showy.

grand mal seizure /gräN·mäl'/ [Fr, great; illness; *saisir* to seize], an epileptic seizure characterized by a generalized involuntary muscular contraction and cessation of respiration followed by tonic and clonic spasms of the muscles. Breathing resumes with noisy respirations. The teeth may be clenched, the tongue bitten, and control of the bladder lost. As this phase of the seizure passes, the person may fall into a deep sleep for 1 hour or more. Usually, the person has no recall of the seizure on awakening. A sensory warning, or aura, usually precedes each grand mal seizure.

grand multipara /grand/ [L *grandis* great, *multus* many, *parere* to give birth], a woman who has carried six or more pregnancies to a viable stage.

grand rounds [Fr, great; L *rotundus* wheel], a formal conference in which one usually expert person presents a lecture concerning a clinical issue intended to be educational for the listeners. In some settings grand rounds may be formal teaching rounds conducted by an expert at the bedsides of selected patients.

grant [ME *granten* to believe a request], an award given to an institution, a project, or an individual usually consisting of a sum of money. A grant is given by a granting agency, the federal government, a foundation, private enterprise, or institution to provide financial support for research, service, or training.

granular /gran'yələr/ [L *granulum* little grain], **1.** macroscopically looking or feeling like sand. **2.** microscopically appearing to have a few or many particles within or on its surface, such as a stained granular leucocyte. –**granularity,** *n*.

granular cast [L *granulum;* ONorse *kasta*], a mass of pathologic debris composed of cells filled with protein and fatty granules.

granular conjunctivitis. See **trachoma.**

granular endoplasmic reticulum. See **endoplasmic reticulum.**

granularity. See **granular.**

granulation tissue /gran'yəlā'shən/ [L *granulum* little grain], any soft, pink, fleshy projections that form during the healing process in a wound not healing by first intention, consisting of many capillaries surrounded by fibrous collagen.

granule /gran'yōol/ [L *granulum*], a particle, grain, or other small dry mass capable of free movement. Unlike powders, granules are usually free-flowing because of small surface forces involved.

granulitis /gran'yəli'tis/ [L *granulum;* Gk *itis* inflammation], acute miliary tuberculosis.

granulocyte /gran'yōōləsīt'/ [L *granulum* + Gk *kytos* cell], one of a group of leukocytes characterized by the presence of cytoplasmic granules. Kinds of granulocytes are **basophil, eosinophil,** and **neutrophil.**

granulocyte transfusion, the use of specially prepared leukocytes for the treatment of severe granulocytopenia and prophylactically for the prevention of serious infection in patients with leukemia or those receiving cancer chemotherapy.

granulocytic leukemia. See **acute myelocytic leukemia, chronic myelocytic leukemia.**

granulocytic sarcoma. See **chloroma.**

granulocytopenia /gran'yōōlōsī'tōpē'nē·ə/ [L *granulum* + Gk *kytos* cell, *penia* poverty], an abnormal condition of the blood, characterized by a decrease in the total number of granulocytes. –**granulocytopenic,** *adj*.

granulocytosis /gran'yōōlōsītō'sis/ [L *granulum* + Gk *kytos* cell, *osis* condition], an abnormal condition of the blood, characterized by an increase in the total number of granulocytes.

granuloma /gran'yōōlō'mə/, *pl.* **granulomas, granulomata** [L *granulum* + Gk *oma* tumor], a mass of nodular granulation tissue resulting from inflammation, injury, or infection. It is composed of capillary buds and growing fibroblasts.

granuloma annulare, a self-limited, chronic skin disease of unknown cause, consisting of reddish papules and nodules arranged in a ring and most commonly seen on the distal portions of the extremities in children.

granuloma gluteale infantum, a skin condition of the neonate characterized by large, elevated bluish or brownish red nodules on the buttocks, often occurring as a secondary reaction to the application of strong steroid salves over a period of time.

granuloma inguinale, a sexually transmitted disease characterized by ulcers of the skin and subcutaneous tissues of the groin and genitalia. It is caused by infection with *Calymmatobacterium granulomatis*, a small gram-negative, rod-shaped bacillus.

granulomatosis /gran'yōōlōmətō'sis/ [L *granulum* + Gk *oma* tumor, *osis* condition], a condition or disease characterized by the development of granulomas, such as **berylliosis, pulmonary**

Wegener's granulomatosis, or **Wegener's granulomatosis.**

granulomatous /gran′yəlom′ətəs/ [L, *granulum,* little grain], pertaining to or resembling granulomas.

granulomatous lipophagia [L *granulum* + Gk *lipos* fat, *phagein* to eat], a disease in which enlarged intestinal and mesenteric lymph spaces become filled with fats and fatty acids.

granulomatous thyroiditis. See de Quervain's thyroiditis.

granulosa cell carcinoma. See granulosa cell tumor.

granulosa cell tumor /gran′yŏolō′sə/ [L *granulum* little grain], a fleshy ovarian tumor with yellow streaks that originates in cells of the primordial membrana granulosa and may grow extremely large.

granulosa-theca cell tumor, an ovarian tumor composed of either granulosa (follicular) cells or theca cells or both.

granulosis /gran′yŏolō′sis/, any disorder characterized by an accumulation of granules in an area of body tissue.

graphing /graf′ing/, the organization of data consisting of two or more variables along horizontal and vertical axes of a graph to show relationships between specific quantities or other specific factors.

GRAS, abbreviation for *generally recognized as safe.*

grasp reflex [ME *graspen* grab; L *reflectere* to bend backward], a pathologic reflex induced by stroking the palm or sole with the result that the fingers or toes flex in a grasping motion. In young infants the tonic grasp reflex is normal.

grass. See cannabis.

grass-line ligature [AS *graes;* L *linea* thread; *ligare* to bind], a fine cord composed of the fibers of a grass-cloth plant, used in orthodontics for minor adjustments or movement of the teeth.

Graves' disease /grāvz/ [Robert J. Graves, Irish physician, b. 1796], a disorder characterized by pronounced hyperthyroidism usually associated with an enlarged thyroid gland and exophthalmos. The origin is unknown, but the disease is familial and may be autoimmune; antibodies to thyroglobulin or to thyroid microsomes are found in more than 60% of patients with the disorder. Typical signs are nervousness, a fine tremor of the hands, weight loss, fatigue, breathlessness, palpitations, heat intolerance, increased metabolic rate, and GI motility. There may be an enlarged thymus, generalized hyperplasia of the lymph nodes, blurred or double vision, localized edema, atrial arrhythmias, and osteoporosis. In patients with inadequately controlled Graves' disease, in-

fection or stress may precipitate a life-threatening thyroid storm.

gravid /grav′id/ [L *gravida* pregnant], pregnant; carrying fertilized eggs or a fetus. **–gravidity, gravidness,** *n.*

gravida /grav′idə/, a woman who is pregnant. The patient may be identified more specifically as **gravida I,** if pregnant for the first time, **gravida II,** if pregnant a second time.

gravida I or 1. See primigravida.

gravida II or 2. See secundigravida.

gravidarum chloasma /grav′ider′əm, grä′vidär′ōōm/ [L *gravidus* pregnant; Gk *chloazein* to be green], a pigmentary change in the skin that occurs in some women during pregnancy. It usually occurs as patches of yellow, brown, or black discoloration.

gravidity, gravidness. See gravid.

gravidum gingivitis /grav′idəm/ [L *gravidus, gingiva* gums, *itis* inflammation], a type of gum inflammation that is associated with plaque formation during pregnancy. It may be associated with hormonal changes.

gravid uterus, a pregnant uterus.

gravity /grav′itē/ [L *gravis* heavy], the heaviness or weight of an object resulting from the universal effect of the attraction between any body of matter and any planetary body.

gravity-eliminated plane, a supported position or plane in which the effect of gravity is absorbed or neutralized. In evaluation of muscle strength, certain tests are conducted in the gravity-eliminated plane.

gray (Gy), the absorption of one joule per kilogram by material exposed to ionizing radiation. One gray equals 100 rad.

gray baby syndrome. See gray syndrome.

gray hepatization. See hepatization.

gray matter. See gray substance.

gray scale, (in ultrasonography) a property of the display in which intensity information is recorded as changes in the brightness of the display.

gray scale display, (in ultrasonography) a signal-processing method of selectively amplifying and displaying the level echoes from soft tissues at the expense of the larger echoes.

gray substance [AS *graeg;* L *substantia*], the gray tissue that makes up the inner core of the spinal column, arranged in two large lateral masses connected across the midline by a narrow commissure. The gray substance splays outward, forming the posterior and anterior horns of the spinal cord. The horns consist primarily of cell bodies of interneurons and cell bodies of motorneurons. Nuclei in the gray matter of the spinal cord function as centers for all spinal reflexes.

gray syndrome, a toxic condition in neonates, especially premature infants, caused by a reaction to chloramphenicol. The name of the condition comes from a characteristic ashen-gray cyanosis, which is accompanied by abdominal distention, hypothermia, vomiting, respiratory distress, and vascular collapse. The condition is fatal if the drug is continued.

GRE, abbreviation for **Graduate Record Examination.**

great auricular nerve [AS, large; L *auricula* little ear, *nervus* nerve], one of a pair of cutaneous branches of the cervical plexus, arising from the second and the third cranial nerves. It winds around the border of the sternocleidomastoideus.

great calorie. See **calorie.**

great cardiac vein, one of the five tributaries of the coronary sinus, beginning at the apex of the heart and ascending along the anterior interventricular sulcus to the base of the ventricles. The great cardiac vein drains the blood through its tributaries from the capillaries of the myocardium.

greater multangular. See **trapezium.**

greater omentum [AS *great* large; L *omentum* entrails], a filmy, transparent extension of the peritoneum, draping the transverse colon and coils of the small intestine. It is attached along the greater curvature of the stomach and the first part of the duodenum, and between its two layers contains blood vessels and fat pads.

greater sciatic foramen [ME *grete;* Gk *ischiadikos* hip joint; L *foraminis* a hole], an opening between the hip bone, sacrum, and sacrotuberous ligament.

greater sciatic notch [ME *grete* large; Gk *ischiadikos* hip joint; OFr *enochier* notch], a notch on the posterior border of the hip bone between the posterior inferior iliac spine and the spine of the ischium.

greater trochanter, a large projection of the femur, to which are attached various muscles, including the gluteus medius, gluteus maximus, and obturator internus.

greater vestibular gland. See **Bartholin's gland.**

great saphenous vein, one of a pair of the longest veins in the body, containing 10 to 20 valves along its course through the leg and the thigh before ending in the femoral vein. It begins in the medial marginal vein of the dorsum of the foot.

great vessels, the large arteries and veins entering and leaving the heart. They include the aorta, the pulmonary arteries and veins, and the superior and inferior venae cavae.

green cancer. See **chloroma.**

Greenfield's disease, a disorder of the white matter of the brain tissue, characterized by an accumulation of sphingolipid in both parenchymal and supportive tissues and a diffuse loss of myelination.

Greenough microscope. See **stereoscopic microscope.**

green soap [AS *grene;* L *sapo*], a soft soap made from vegetable oils with sodium or potassium hydroxide with concentrations adjusted to retain the glycerol. The soap actually may be any color, depending upon the ingredient oils added.

green soap tincture [AS *grene;* L *sapo* soap, *tinctura* dyeing], an alcoholic solution of green soap with lavender oil added.

greenstick fracture [AS *grene, stician*], an incomplete fracture in which the bone is bent but fractured only on the outer arc of the bend. Children are particularly likely to have greenstick fractures.

Grenz rays [Ger *Grenze* boundary; L *radius* emit rays], low-energy x-rays used for treatment of skin conditions.

Greulich-Pyle method /groi'lishpīl/, grōō'lik-/, a technique for evaluating the bone age of children, using a single frontal radiograph of the left hand and wrist.

Grey Turner's sign, bruising of the skin of the loin in acute hemorrhagic pancreatitis.

grid [ME *gredire* a grate], (in radiology) a device used to absorb scattered radiation produced during an x-ray examination. A grid selectively absorbs radiation that is not heading along straight lines from the x-ray source to the film. A **linear grid** is a simple x-ray grid consisting of parallel lead strips.

grid cutoff, (in radiology) an undesirable absorption of primary-beam x-rays by the grid so that useful x-rays are literally cut off from the film.

grief [L *gravis* heavy], a nearly universal pattern of physical and emotional responses to bereavement, separation, or loss. The physical components are similar to those of fear, hunger, rage, and pain.

grief reaction, a complex of somatic and psychologic symptoms associated with some extreme sorrow or loss, specifically the death of a loved one. Somatic symptoms include feelings of tightness in the throat and chest with choking and shortness of breath, abdominal distress, lack of muscular power, and extreme tiredness and lethargy. Psychologic reactions involve a generalized awareness of mental anguish and discomfort accompanied by feelings of guilt, anger, hostility, extreme restlessness, inability to concentrate, and the lack of capacity to initiate and maintain organized patterns of activities.

grieving, anticipatory, a NANDA-accepted nursing diagnosis of grieving before an actual loss, as contrasted with grief in response to an actual loss. Defining characteristics include the potential loss of something or someone important; expressions of distress, denial of potential loss, anger, guilt, or sorrow, and changes in eating habits, sleep patterns, activity level, libido, and patterns of communication.

grieving, dysfunctional, a NANDA-accepted nursing diagnosis of an absence or a lack of resolution of a grieving response. Defining characteristics include expressions of distress or a denial of the loss; grief, anger, sadness, and weeping; changes in patterns and habits of sleeping, eating, and dreaming; and alterations in libido and activity levels.

griffe des orteils. See **pes cavus.**

grinder's asthma /grīn′dərz/ [ME *grinden* to crush; Gk, panting], a condition characterized by asthmatic symptoms caused by inhalation of fine particles produced by industrial grinding processes.

grinder's disease. See **silicosis.**

grinding-in, a clinical corrective grinding of one or more natural or artificial teeth to improve centric and eccentric occlusions.

grip and pinch strength, the measurable ability to exert pressure with the hand and fingers. A patient forcefully squeezes grip or pinch dynamometers, which may express results in either pounds or kilograms of pressure.

gripes /grīps/ [AS *gripan* to grasp], severe and usually spasmodic pain in the abdominal region caused by an intestinal disorder.

grippe. See **influenza.**

gripping. See **gripes.**

griseofulvin /gris′ē-ōful′vin/, an antifungal prescribed in the treatment of certain infections of the skin, hair, and nails.

Griswald brace, an orthosis for the control of vertebral body compression fractures. It is designed with two anterior forces with each equal to one half the posterior force to extend the spine.

grocer's itch [AS *gican* itch], a parasitic dermatitis caused by contact with mites found in grain, cheese, or dried foods. *Glyciphagus domesticus.*

groin [ME *grynde*], each of two areas where the abdomen joins the thighs.

Grönblad-Strandberg syndrome /grön′-bladstrand′bårg/ [Ester E. Grönblad, Swedish ophthalmologist, b. 1898; James V. Strandberg, twentieth-century Swedish dermatologist], an autosomal recessive disorder of connective tissue characterized by premature aging and breakdown of the skin, gray or brown streaks on the retina, and hemorrhagic arterial degeneration, including retinal bleeding that causes loss of vision. Angina pectoris and hypertension are common; weak pulse, episodic claudication, and fatigue with exertion may affect the extremities.

groove [AS *grafan* to dig], a shallow, linear depression in various structures throughout the body, as those that form channels for nerves along the bones, those in bones for the insertion of muscles, and those between certain areas of the brain.

gross [L *grossus* large], **1.** macroscopic, such as *gross pathology,* from the study of tissue changes without magnification by a microscope. **2.** large or obese.

gross anatomy, the study of the organs or parts of the body large enough to be seen with the naked eye.

Grossman principle, (in tomography) the principle that when the fulcrum or axis of rotation remains at a fixed height, the focal place level is changed by raising or lowering the table top through this fixed point to the desired height.

gross motor skills [Fr *gros* big; L *movere;* ONorse *skilja* to cut apart], the use of large muscle groups that coordinate body movements required for normal living, such as walking, running, jumping, throwing, and balance.

gross sensory testing, an evaluation procedure that usually precedes motor evaluation of a patient and includes assessment of passive motion sense in the shoulder, elbow, wrist, and fingers and ability to localize touch stimuli to specific fingers.

gross visual skills, the general ability of a person to track a large, bright object side-to-side or up-to-down without jerkiness, nystagmus, or convergence and to discriminate among various basic shapes and colors.

ground [AS *grund*], **1.** (in electricity) a connection between the electric circuit and the ground, which becomes a part of the circuit. **2.** (in psychology) the background of a visual field that can enhance or inhibit the ability of a patient to focus on an object.

ground itch, pruritic papules, urticarial, vesiculo-pustular lesions secondary to penetration of the skin by hookworm larvae, prevalent in tropic and subtropic climates.

ground substance. See **matrix.**

group [Fr *groupe* cluster], (in research) any set of items or groups of people under study. An **experimental group** is studied to determine the effect of an event, a substance, or a technique. A **control group** serves as a standard or reference for comparison with an experimental group. It is similar to the experimental group in number and is identical in specified characteristics, such as sex, age, or other factors.

group A beta-hemolytic streptococcal (GABHS) skin disease, a bacterial skin infection that affects mainly meat packers. The source of the bacteria is believed to be freshly butchered meat.

group dynamics [Fr *groupe;* Gk *dynamis* force], the interactions and relationships that take place within groups as well as between the groups and the rest of society. It includes interdependence of group members, collective problem solving and decision making, and group conformity.

group function, (in dentistry) the simultaneous contacting of opposing teeth in a segment or a group.

group therapy, the application of psychotherapeutic techniques within a small group of emotionally disturbed persons who, usually under the leadership of a psychotherapist, discuss their problems in an attempt to promote individual psychologic growth and favorable personality change. A kind of group therapy is **psychodrama.**

growing fracture [AS *growan;* L *fractura* to break], a fracture, usually linear, in which consecutive x-ray images show a gradual separation of the fracture edges as the pressure of soft tissues force the edges apart.

growing pains, 1. rheumatism-like pains that occur in the muscles and joints of children or adolescents as a result of fatigue, emotional problems, postural defects, and other causes that are not related to growth and that may be symptoms of various disorders. **2.** emotional and psychologic problems experienced during adolescence.

growth [AS *growan* to grow], **1.** an increase in the size of an organism or any of its parts, as measured in increments of weight, volume, or linear dimensions, that occurs as a result of hyperplasia or hypertrophy. **2.** the normal progressive anatomic, physiologic, psychologic, intellectual, social, and cultural development from infancy to adulthood as a result of the gradual and normal processes of accretion and assimilation. In childhood, growth is categorized according to the approximate age at which distinctive physical changes usually appear and at which specific developmental tasks are achieved. **3.** any abnormal localized increase of the size or number of cells, as in a tumor or neoplasm. **4.** a proliferation of cells, specifically a bacterial culture or mold.

growth and development, altered, a NANDA-accepted nursing diagnosis of a condition in which an individual demonstrates deviations in norms from his or her age group. Defining characteristics include delay or difficulty in performing skills typical of the age group, altered physical growth, inability to perform self-care or self-control activities appropriate for the age, flat affect, listlessness, and decreased responses.

growth failure, a lack of normal physical and psychologic development as a result of genetic, nutritional, pathologic, or psychosocial factors.

growth hormone (GH), a single-chain peptide secreted by the anterior pituitary gland in response to growth hormone releasing factor (GHRF) from the hypothalamus. Growth hormone promotes protein synthesis in all cells, increases fat mobilization and use of fatty acids for energy, and decreases use of carbohydrate. A deficiency of GH causes dwarfism; an excess results in gigantism or acromegaly.

growth hormone release inhibiting hormone. See **somatostatin.**

growth hormone releasing factor (GHRF), somatotropin-releasing factor released by the hypothalamus.

Grünfelder's reflex /grYn'feldərz, grēn'-/, an involuntary dorsal flexion of the great toe with a fanlike spreading of the other toes, caused by continued pressure on the posterior lateral fontanel.

grunting [ME *grunten*], abnormal, short audible gruntlike breaks in exhalation that often accompany severe chest pain. The grunt occurs because the glottis briefly stops the flow of air, halting the movement of the lungs and their surrounding or supporting structures.

GSA, abbreviation for **Gerontologic Society of America.**

G-6-PD deficiency, abbreviation for **glucose-6-phosphate dehydrogenase deficiency.**

GSR, abbreviation for **galvanic skin response.**

gt., abbreviation for the Latin, *gutta,* a drop.

GTP, abbreviation for **guanosine triphosphate.**

gtt., abbreviation for the Latin, *guttae,* drops.

G tube. See **stomach tube.**

GU, abbreviation for **genitourinary.**

guaiac /gwī'ak/, a wood resin, commonly used as a reagent in laboratory tests for the presence of occult blood.

guaiacol poisoning. See **phenol poisoning.**

guaiac test, a test, using guaiac as a reagent, performed on feces and urine for detecting occult blood in the intestinal and urinary tracts.

guaifenesin /gwi'əfen'əsin/, glyceryl guaiacolate, a white to slightly gray powder with a bitter taste and faint odor, widely used as an expectorant.

guanabenz acetate /gwan'əbenz/, an antihypertensive agent prescribed for hypertension.

guanadrel sulfate /gwan'ədril/, an antihypertensive agent prescribed in the treatment of hypertension in patients not responding to a thiazide-type diuretic.

guanase. See **guanine deaminase.**

guanethidine sulfate /gwaneth'idēn/, an antihypertensive prescribed in the treatment of moderate and severe hypertension.

guanine /gwan'ēn/, a major purine base found in nucleotides and a fundamental constituent of DNA and RNA. In free or uncombined form it occurs in trace amounts in most cells, usually as a product of the enzymatic hydrolysis of nucleic acids and nucleotides.

guanine deaminase, an enzyme that catalyzes the hydrolysis of guanine to xanthine and ammonia.

guanine deaminase assay, the measurement of an enzyme in the blood that commonly increases in patients with hepatitis and other types of liver disease and mononucleosis.

guanosine /gwan'ōsēn/, a compound derived from a nucleic acid, composed of guanine and a sugar, D-ribose. It is a major molecular component of DNA and RNA.

guanosine monophosphate (GMP), a nucleotide that plays an important role in various metabolic reactions and in the formation of RNA from DNA templates.

guanosine triphosphate (GTP), a high-energy nucleotide, similar to adenosine triphosphate, that functions in various metabolic reactions, such as the activation of fatty acids and the formation of the peptide bond in protein synthesis.

guaranine /gwərä'nin/, caffeine.

guardian ad litem /ad lī'təm/, (in law) a person who is appointed by a court to prosecute or defend a suit for an infant or an incapacitated person. A guardian ad litem is sometimes appointed when a person's life is in imminent danger and that person refuses treatment.

guardianship, a legal instrument that places the care and property of an individual in the hands of another person. Implementation of the law varies in different cases and jurisdictions. Some courts have held as legally incompetent mental patients who have jobs and live independently.

Gubbay test of motor proficiency, a screening test for the identification of developmental dyspraxia.

Guedel's signs /gōō'dəlz/ [Arthur E. Guedel, American anesthesiologist, b. 1883], a system for describing the stages and planes of anesthesia during an operative procedure. **Stage I** (amnesia and analgesia) begins with the administration of an anesthetic and continues to the loss of consciousness. **Stage II** (delirium or excitement) begins with the loss of consciousness and includes the onset of total anesthesia. **Stage III** (surgical anesthesia) begins with establishment of a regular pattern of breathing and total loss of consciousness and includes the period during which signs of respiratory or cardiovascular failure first appear. This stage is divided into four planes: At *plane 1* all movements cease and respiration is regular and "automatic." At *plane 2* the eyeballs become fixed centrally, conjunctivae lose their luster, and intercostal muscle activity diminishes. At *plane 3* intercostal paralysis occurs, and respiration becomes solely diaphragmatic. At *plane 4* deep anesthesia is achieved, with the cessation of spontaneous respiration and the absence of sensation. **Stage IV** (premortem) signals danger. This stage is characterized by pupils that are maximally dilated and skin that is cold and ashen. Blood pressure is extremely low, often unmeasurable, and the brachial pulse is feeble or entirely absent. Cardiac arrest is imminent.

Guérin's fracture /gāraNz'/ [Alphonse F.M. Guérin, French surgeon, b. 1816], a fracture of the maxilla.

guided imagery, a therapeutic technique in which a patient is encouraged to concentrate on an image that helps relieve pain or discomfort.

guide dog [ME *guiden* to guard; OE *docga*], a dog trained to aid in the mobility of a blind person. Guide dogs are usually recruited from certain compatible breeds and tested at the age of 13 weeks. If qualified, the dog is then specially trained in private hands for one year and retested. Most dogs selected for training pass the final test. Guide dogs also may be trained to serve as "ears" for deaf persons.

guide plane [ME *guiden* to guard; L *planum* level ground], **1.** a part of an orthodontic appliance that has an established inclined plane for changing the occlusal relation of the maxillary and mandibular teeth and for permitting their movement to normal positions. **2.** a plane that is developed on the occlusal sufaces of occlusion rims for positioning the mandible in centric relation. **3.** two or more vertically parallel surfaces of abutment teeth shaped to direct the path of placement and removal of a partial denture.

guide-shoe marks, an x-ray image artifact caused by pressure of the guide shoes, curved metal lips that guide x-ray film in automatic developing systems.

guidewire /gīd'wī-ər/ [ME *guiden* + AS *wir*], a device used to position an intravenous catheter.

Guillain-Barré syndrome /gēyaN'bärā'/ [Georges Guillain, French neurologist, b. 1876; Jean A. Barré, French neurologist, b. 1880], an idiopathic, peripheral polyneuritis occurring between 1 and 3 weeks after a mild episode of fever associated with a viral infection or with immunization. Symmetric pain and weakness affect the extremities, and paralysis may develop. The neuritis may spread, ascending to the trunk and involving the face, arms, and thoracic muscles.

guilt [AS *gylt* delinquency], a feeling caused by tension between the ego and superego when one falls below the standards set for oneself.

guilty, (in criminal law) a verdict by the court, finding that to a moral certainty it is beyond reasonable doubt that the defendant committed the crime and is responsible for the offense as charged.

Guinea worm infection. See **dracunculiasis.**

gullet. See **esophagus.**

gum, 1. a sticky excretion from certain plants. **2.** See **gingiva.**

gumboil [AS *goma, byl*], an abscess of the gingiva and periosteum resulting from injury, infection, or dental decay. The gum is characteristically red, swollen, and tender.

gum camphor. See **camphor.**

gum line [L *gummi, linea*], the line formed by the gingival margin at the neck of the tooth.

gumma /gum'ə/, *pl.* **gummas, gummata** [L *gummi* gum] **1.** a granuloma, characteristic of tertiary syphilis, varying from 1 mm to 1 cm in diameter. It is usually encapsulated and contains a central necrotic mass surrounded by inflammatory and fibrotic zones of tissue. **2.** a soft granulomatous lesion sometimes occurring with tuberculosis.

Gunning's splint [Thomas B. Gunning, American dentist, b. 1813; D *splinte* split], a maxillomandibular splint used for supporting the maxilla and the mandible in surgery of the jaws.

gunshot fracture [ME *gunne;* AS *sceotan* to shoot; L *fractura* break], a fracture caused by a bullet or similar missile.

Gunson method, (in radiology) a method of x-ray examination of the pharynx and upper esophagus during the swallowing act.

Gunther's disease /gun'thərz/ [Hans Gunther, German physician, b. 1884], a rare congenital disorder of porphyrin metabolism that is associated with sunlight-induced skin lesions.

gurgling rale [Fr *gargouiller* to gargle; *rale* rattle], an abnormal coarse sound heard during auscultation, especially over large cavities or over a trachea nearly filled with secretions.

gurry /gur'ē/, *slang.* the detritus incident to physical trauma or surgery, including body fluids, secretions, and tissue.

Gurvich radiation. See **mitogenetic radiation.**

gustation /gustā'shən/ [L *gustare* to taste], the sense and act of tasting foods, beverages, or other substances.

gustatory /gus'tətôr'ē/ [L *gustare* to taste], pertaining to the act or sense of taste or the organs of taste.

gustatory hallucination [L *gustare, alucinari* wandering mind], a false taste sensation either of food or beverage on the mucous membrane lining the empty mouth.

gustatory organ. See **taste bud.**

gustatory papilla [L *gustare, papilla* nipple], any of the small tissue elevations in the mouth that contain sense organs of taste such as the circumvallate papilla of the tongue.

gut [AS *guttas*], **1.** intestine. **2.** *informal.* digestive tract. **3.** suture material manufactured from the intestines of sheep.

Guthrie test /guth'rē/, a screening for phenylketonuria used to detect the abnormal presence of phenylalanine metabolites in the blood. A small amount of blood is obtained and placed in a medium with a strain of *Bacillus subtilis,* a bacterium that cannot grow without phenylalanine.

gutta (gt) /gut'ə/ [L, drop], one drop, or about one minim, of a medication, as eye drops or ear drops.

guttae (gtt) [L, drop], the plural of **gutta** and pertaining to more than one drop, as in **guttae pro auribus,** or ear drops, or **guttae ophthalmicae,** or eye drops.

gutta-percha /gut'əpur'chə/ [Malay *getah-percha* latex sap], the coagulated, rubbery sap of various tropical trees, used for temporarily sealing the dressings of prepared tooth cavities.

gutta-percha point, any of the fine, tapered cylinders of gutta-percha that may be used to fill a root canal.

guttate psoriasis /gut'āt/ [L *gutta* drop; Gk, itch], an acute form of psoriasis consisting of teardrop-shaped, red, scaly patches measuring 3 to 10 mm all over the body.

guttural /gut'ərəl/ [L *guttur* throat], pertaining to or belonging to the throat, including low-pitched, raspy voice quality.

Guyon tunnel, a fibroosseous tunnel formed in part by the pisohamate ligament of the hand. It contains the ulnar artery and nerve, and may be the site of a compression injury.

gyn, *informal.* **1.** abbreviation for **gynecologist. 2.** abbreviation for **gynecology.**

gynandrous /gīnan'drəs, jī-/ [Gk *gyne* woman, *aner* man], describing a man or a woman who has some of the physical characteristics usually attributed to the other sex, as a female pseudohermaphrodite. **–gynandry,** *n.*

gynecography /gī'nə-, jin'əkog'rəfē/, the radiologic examination of the female pelvic organs by means of intraperitoneal gas insufflation.

gynecoid pelvis /gī'nəkoid, jin'əkoid/ [Gk *gyne* + *eidos* form; L *pelvis* basin], a type of pelvis characteristic of the normal female and associated with the smallest incidence of fetopelvic disproportion.

gynecologic examination /gī'nə-, jin'əkəloj'ik/, pelvic examination.

gynecologic operative procedures [Gk *gynaikos* of a woman; L *operari* to work, *procedere* to proceed], surgical intervention upon the female reproductive system. Gynecologic and obstetric problems account for one fifth of all female visits to physicians; many require surgical correction. Essential postoperative care demands that the patient be kept warm and quiet. Because of the risk of shock or hemorrhage, the patient should be closely monitored at frequent intervals during the first few hours. Fluids can be given when tolerated. Urine should be collected and measured periodically. Use of elastic stockings and suitable exercises are recommended to reduce the risk of thrombophlebitis.

gynecologist /gī'nəkol'əjist, jī'-, jin'-/, a physician who specializes in gynecology.

gynecology /gī'nəkol'əjē, jī'-, jin'-/ [Gk *gyne* + *logos* science], a branch of medicine concerned with the health care of women, including their sexual and reproductive function and the diseases of their reproductive organs, except diseases of the breast that require surgery. **–gynecologic, gynecological,** *adj.*

gynecomastia /gī'nəkōmas'tē·ə, jī'-, jin'-/ [Gk *gyne* + *mastos* breast], an abnormal enlargement of one or both breasts in men. The condition is usually temporary and benign. It may be caused by hormonal imbalance, tumor of the testis or pituitary, medication with estrogens or steroidal compounds, or failure of the liver to inactivate circulating estrogen, as in alcoholic cirrhosis.

gynephobia /gī'nəfō'bē·ə, jī'-, jin'-/ [Gk *gyne* + *phobos* fear], an anxiety disorder characterized by a morbid fear of women or by a morbid aversion to the society of women.

gynogamone /gī'nōgam'ōn/ [Gk *gyne* + *gamos* marriage], a gamone secreted by the female gamete.

gypsum /jip'səm/, a mineral composed mainly of crushed calcium sulfate hemihydrate. It is used in making plaster of paris surgical casts and impressions for dentures. Gypsum dust has an irritant action on the mucous membranes of the respiratory tract and the conjunctiva.

gyrase /jī'rās/, an enzyme that enables certain DNA molecules to twist themselves into coils in order to replicate.

gyri cerebri /jī'rī/ [Gk *gyro* circle; L *cerebrum* brain], the convolutions of the outer surface of the cerebral hemisphere, separated from each other by sulci.

gyrus /jī'rəs/, *pl.* **gyri** /jī'rī/ [Gk *gyro* circle], one of the tortuous convolutions of the surface of the brain caused by infolding of the cortex.

h, 1. abbreviation for *haustus,* the Latin word for a draught of medicine. 2. abbreviation for **height.** 4. abbreviation for *horizontal.* 5. abbreviation for **hyperopia.** 3. symbol for *hora,* the Latin word for hour.

H, symbol for the element **hydrogen.**

^{2}H, symbol for **deuterium.**

^{3}H, symbol for **tritium.**

[H$^+$], symbol for hydrogen ion concentration.

H$_2$, abbreviation for a subtype of histamine receptor released in the stomach.

Ha, symbol for the chemical element *hahnium* (element 105).

HaAg, abbreviation for *hepatitis A antigen.*

Haas method, a technique for producing x-ray images of the interior of the skull by having the patient rest the head with the forehead and nose on the table so that the beam enters the skull near the base of the occipital bone and emerges 1 inch above the nasion.

habeas corpus /hā′bē·əs kôr′pəs/, a right retained by all psychiatric patients that provides for the release of an individual who claims to be deprived of liberty and detained illegally. A hearing for this determination takes place in a court of law, and the patient's sanity is at issue.

habilitation /həbil′itā′shən/, the process of supplying a person with the means to develop maximum independence in activities of daily living through training or treatment.

habit [L *habitus* condition], 1. a customary or particular practice, manner, or mode of behavior. 2. an involuntary pattern of behavior or thought. 3. *archaic.* appearance or physique, as pyknic habit. 4. the habitual use of drugs or narcotics.

habitat /hab′itat/ [L *habitare* to dwell], a natural environment where a species of a plant or animal, including humans, may live and grow normally.

habit spasm, an involuntary twitching or tic usually involving a small muscle group of the face, neck, or shoulders and resulting in movements such as spasmodic blinking or rapid jerking of the head to the side.

habit tic [L *habitus*; Fr *tic*], a brief recurrent movement of a muscle group, such as a blink, grimace, or sudden head turning, that is of a psychogenic rather than organic cause.

habit training, the process of teaching a child how to adjust to the demands of the external world by forming certain habits, primarily those related to eating, sleeping, elimination, and dress.

habitual abortion /həbich′ōō·əl/ [L *habituare* to become used to], spontaneous termination of three successive pregnancies before the twentieth week of gestation.

habitual dislocation [L *habitus* + *dis, locare* to place], a dislocation that recurs repeatedly after reduction.

habitual hyperthermia, a condition of unknown cause occurring in young females, characterized by body temperatures of 99° F to 100.5° F regularly or intermittently for years, associated with fatigue, malaise, vague aches and pains, insomnia, bowel disturbances, and headaches.

habituation /həbich′ōō·ā′shən/ [L *habituare* to become used to], 1. an acquired tolerance from repeated exposure to a particular stimulus. 2. a decline and eventual elimination of a conditioned response by repetition of the conditioned stimulus. 3. psychologic and emotional dependence on a drug, tobacco, or alcohol resulting from the repeated use of the substance but without the addictive, physiologic need to increase dosage.

habitus /hab′itəs/, describing a person's appearance or physique, as an athletic habitus.

hacking cough [AS *haeccan, cohettan*], a short, weak repeating cough, often caused by irritation of the larynx by a postnasal drip.

Haeckel's law. See **recapitulation theory.**

Haemophilus /hēmof′iləs/ [Gk *haima* blood, *philein* to love], a genus of gramnegative pathogenic bacteria, frequently found in the respiratory tract of humans and other animals. *Haemophilus influenzae,* which causes influenza and one form of meningitis, is an example.

Haemophilus influenzae, a small, gramnegative, nonmotile, parasitic bacterium that occurs in two forms, encapsulated and nonencapsulated, and in six types, a, b, c, d, e, and f. Almost all infections are caused by encapsulated type b organisms.

hafnium (Hf) /haf′nē·əm/ [Hafnia, original name of Copenhagen, Denmark], a hard, brittle, silver-gray metallic element of the first transition group. Its atomic number is 72; its atomic weight is 178.49.

Hagedorn needle /hä′gedôrn/ [Hans C. Hagedorn, Danish physician, b. 1888], a flat surgical needle with a cutting edge near its point and a very large eye at the other end.

Hageman factor. See **factor XII.**

Haglund's deformity, a foot disorder characterized by an enlarged posterior-superior lateral aspect of the calcaneus, often associated with an inverted subtalar joint. It is a common cause of posterior Achilles bursitis.

hair [AS *haer*], a filament of keratin consisting of a root and a shaft formed in a specialized follicle in the epidermis. There are three stages of hair development: **anagen,** the active growing stage; **catagen,** a short interlude between the growth and resting phases; and **telogen,** the resting (club) stage before shedding. Scalp hair grows at an average rate of 1 mm every 3 days, body and eyebrow hair at a much slower rate.

hair analysis [AS *haer*; Gk, a loosening], chemical analysis of a hair sample to find possible evidence of exposure to a toxic substance. Molecules of lead compounds and other chemicals are absorbed and stored in hair shafts. Hair analysis is also used to determine possible causes of malnutrition. Samples for analysis are taken from areas close to the scalp to eliminate chances that toxic chemicals found in the hair may have been absorbed from air pollutants.

hair follicle [AS *haer*; L *folliculus* a small bag], a tiny tube of epidermal cells originating in the corium layer of the skin and containing the root of a hair shaft.

hairline fracture [AS *haer*; L *linea, fractura*], a minor fracture that appears on x-ray film as a thin line between two segments of a bone. The segments remain in alignment and the fracture may not extend completely through the bone. A fatigue hairline fracture may develop without causing injury or in the absence of trauma.

hair matrix carcinoma. See **basal cell carcinoma.**

hair pulling. See **trichotillomania.**

hairy-cell leukemia [AS *haer*; L *cella* storeroom; Gk *leukos* white, *haima* blood], an uncommon neoplasm of blood-forming tissues, characterized by pancytopenia, a

massively enlarged spleen, and the presence in blood and bone marrow of reticulum cells with many fine projections on their surface. The disease usually appears in the fifth decade with an insidious onset and a variable course marked by anemia, thrombocytopenia, and spontaneous bruising.

hairy leukoplakia, a form of leukoplakia characterized by a white plaque that is markedly folded in appearance or smooth and is often found on one or both lateral borders of the tongue. It is associated with severe immunodeficiency, occurs in HIV-infected patients, and is believed to result from the Epstein-Barr virus.

hairy nevus [AS *haer*; L *naevus* birthmark], a mole, usually pigmented, with hairs growing from it.

hairy tongue, a dark, pigmented overgrowth of the filiform papillae of the tongue that is a benign and frequent side effect of some antibiotics.

halcinonide /həlsin′ənīd/, a glucocorticoid prescribed topically as an antiinflammatory agent.

half-life (t½) [AS *haelf, lif*], **1.** the time required for a radioactive substance to lose 50% of its activity through decay. Each radionuclide has a unique half-life. **2.** the amount of time required to reduce a drug level to one half of its initial value.

half-normal saline, (in respiratory therapy) a solution of 0.45% NaCl used for mucosal hydration. As the fluid tends to evaporate, the saline concentration increases, achieving nearly normal saline concentration in the respiratory tract.

half-sibling, one of two or more children who have at least one parent in common; a half brother or half sister.

half-value layer, the amount of material required to attenuate a beam of radiation to one half of its original level.

halfway house, a specialized treatment facility, usually for psychiatric patients who no longer require complete hospitalization but who need some care and time to adjust to living independently.

halisteresis /həlis′tərē′sis/ [Gk *hals* salt, *steresis* absence of], a theoretic process of bone resorption in which bone salts may be removed by humoral mechanisms and returned to body tissue fluids, leaving behind a decalcified bone matrix.

halitosis /hal′itō′sis/[L *halitus* breath; Gk *osis* condition], offensive breath resulting from poor oral hygiene, dental or oral infections, the ingestion of certain foods, use of tobacco, or some systemic diseases, such as the odor of acetone in diabetes and ammonia in liver disease.

Hallervorden-Spatz disease /hol'ərfôr'- dənshpots'/ [Julius Hallervorden, German neurologist, b. 1882; H. Spatz, German neurologist, b. 1888], a progressive neurologic disease of children, with symptoms of parkinsonism. It is characterized by rigidity, athetosis, and dementia.

hallex. See **hallux**.

Hallpike caloric test /hôl'pīk/, a method for evaluating the function of the vestibule of the ear in patients with vertigo or hearing loss. Irrigation of the ears with cool and warm water or air mimics the stimulus of turning in the vestibular apparatus, causing nystagmus.

hallucination /həloo̅'sinā'shən/ [L *alucinari* to dream], a sensory perception that does not result from an external stimulus. It can occur in any of the senses and is classified accordingly as auditory, gustatory, olfactory, tactile, or visual. Kinds of hallucinations are **hypnagogic, lilliputian,** and **stump hallucination.** –**hallucinate,** *v.*

hallucinogen /həloo̅'sənəjen', hal'əsin'- əjən, hal'yəsin'əjən/ [L *alucinari* + Gk *genein* to produce], a substance that causes excitation of the central nervous system, characterized by hallucination, mood change, anxiety, sensory distortion, delusion, depersonalization, increased pulse, temperature, and blood pressure, and dilatation of the pupils. Kinds of hallucinogens are **lysergide, mescaline, peyote, phencyclidine hydrochloride,** and **psilocybin.**

hallucinogenesis /həloo̅'sinäjen'əsis/ [L *alucinari* a wandering mind; Gk *genein* to produce], a cause or source of hallucinations.

hallucinosis /haloo̅'sinō'sis/[L *alucinari* + Gk *osis* condition], a pathologic mental state in which awareness consists primarily or exclusively of hallucinations. A kind of hallucinosis is **alcoholic hallucinosis.**

hallux /hal'əks/, *pl.* **halluces** /hal'yoo̅sēz/ [L *hallex* large toe], the great toe.

hallux rigidus, a painful deformity of the great toe, limiting motion at the metatarsophalangeal joint.

hallux valgus, a deformity in which the great toe is angulated away from the midline of the body toward the other toes; in some cases the great toe rides over or under the other toes.

halo cast /hā'lō/ [Gk *halos* circular floor; AS *kasta*], an orthopedic device used to help immobilize the neck and head. It incorporates the trunk, usually with shoulder straps, and an apparatus by means of an outrigger within the cast to secure pins to a band around the skull.

halo effect, the beneficial effect of an interview or other encounter, as may occur in the course of a research project or a health care visit. It is the result of indefinable interpersonal factors present in the interaction.

halogen /hal'ōjən/ [Gk *hals* salt, *genein* to produce], any member of the group VII elements in the periodic table: fluorine, chlorine, bromine, iodine, and astatine. They are found in sea water as the corresponding halide ion.

halogenated hydrocarbon /həloj'ənā'tid/ [Gk *hals* salt, *genein* to produce; *hydor* water; L *carbo* coal], a volatile liquid used for general anesthesia, administered in combination with nitrous oxide, oxygen, or both. Nausea, vomiting, laryngospasm, and pharyngeal irritation are less severe and frequent when this anesthesia is used. Kinds of halogenated hydrocarbons are **enflurane, halothane, isoflurane, methoxyflurane,** and **trichloroethylene.**

haloperidol /hal'ōper'ədôl/, a butyrophenone tranquilizer prescribed in the treatment of psychotic disorders and in the control of Gilles de la Tourette's syndrome.

haloprogin /hā'lōprō'jin/, an antibacterial and antifungal prescribed in the treatment of susceptible fungal infections, including athlete's foot.

halothane /hal'əthān/, an inhalation anesthetic prescribed for induction and maintenance of general anesthesia.

halothane-related hepatitis, an adverse reaction of some patients to inhalation of halothane, a general anesthetic. The reaction is characterized by hepatitis and a severe fever that develops several days after exposure to the anesthetic.

Halsted's forceps /hal'stedz/ [William S. Halsted, American surgeon, b. 1852], **1.** a small, pointed hemostatic forceps. **2.** a forceps with slender jaws for grasping arteries and other blood vessels.

hamamelis water. See **witch hazel.**

hamate bone /ham'āt/[L *hamatus* hooked], a carpal bone that rests on the fourth and fifth metacarpal bones and projects a hooklike process, the hamulus, from its palmar surface.

Hamman's disease [Louis Virgil Hamman, American physician, b. 1877; L, *dis,* apart; Fr, *aise,* ease], progressive interstitial fibrosis of both lungs, causing right ventricular failure and ventilatory failure.

Hamman-Rich syndrome. See **interstitial pneumonia.**

hammer finger [AS *hamer, finger*], a permanently flexed terminal phalanx resulting from an injury to the extensor tendon.

hammertoe /ham'ərtō/ [AS *hamer, ta*], a foot digit permanently flexed at the mid phalangeal joint, resulting in a clawlike appearance. The anomaly may be present in more than one digit but is most common in the second toe.

hamstring muscle [AS *hamm, streng*], any one of three muscles at the back of the thigh; medially, the semimembranosus and the semitendinosus and laterally, the biceps femoris.

hamstring reflex, a normal deep tendon reflex elicited by tapping one of the hamstring tendons behind the knee, resulting in contraction of the tendon and flexion of the knee.

hamstring tendon, one of the three tendons from the three hamstring muscles in the back of the thigh.

hamular notch. See **pterygomaxillary notch.**

hand [AS], the part of the upper limb distal to the forearm. It is the most flexible part of the skeleton and has a total of 27 bones, 8 forming the carpus, 5 forming the metacarpus, and 14 comprising the phalangeal section.

handblock [AS *hand* + Fr *bloc*], a device made of a wood block several inches high with a firm handle that can be gripped by a disabled patient to provide a certain amount of body support in minor ambulatory activities, such as getting into or out of a bed.

hand condenser, (in dentistry) an instrument for compacting amalgams or gold foil using force applied by the operator.

handedness [AS *hand* + *ness* condition], voluntary or involuntary preference for use of either the left or right hand. The preference is related to cerebral dominance, with left-handedness corresponding to dominance of the right side of the brain and vice versa.

hand-foot-and-mouth disease, a Coxsackie viral infection characterized by the appearance of painful ulcers and vesicles on the mucous membranes of the mouth and on the hands and feet. The disease is highly contagious and affects mainly children.

hand-foot syndrome. See **sickle cell crisis.**

handicapped [E *hand in cap* a game with forfeits], referring to a person who has a congenital or acquired mental or physical defect that interferes with normal functioning of the body system or the ability to be self-sufficient in modern society.

handpiece, a device for holding rotary instruments in a dental engine or condensing points in mechanic condensing units.

hanging drop preparation [ME *hangen* to hang; AS *dropa* to fall; L *praeparer* to make ready], a technique used for the examination and identification of certain microorganisms, such as spirochetes or trichomonads. A specimen suspected of containing the microorganism is diluted with a sterile isotonic solution. A drop of this fluid mixture is placed on a glass cover slip, which is then inverted carefully and placed over the slide so that the drop is hanging from the slip into the concavity in the special slide.

hangman's fracture, a fracture of the posterior elements of the cervical vertebrae with dislocation of C2 or C3.

hangnail [AS *angnaegl* troublesome nail], a piece of partially disconnected epidermis of the cuticle or nail fold. Tearing the skin fragment causes a red, painful, easily infected sore.

hangover, a popular term for a group of symptoms, including nausea, thirst, fatigue, headache, and irritability, resulting from the use of alcohol and certain drugs.

Hanot's disease /hanōz′/ [Victor C. Hanot, French physician, b. 1844], primary biliary cirrhosis.

Hansen's bacillus [Gerard Henrik Armauer Hansen, Norwegian physician, b. 1841; L, *bacillum*, a small rod], the acid-fast *Mycobacterium leprae* that is the cause of leprosy.

Hansen's disease. See **leprosy.**

HA-1A, a genetically engineered antibody used in the treatment of certain blood infections. The HA-1A antibody attacks the bacterial toxin rather than the bacterium directly. It is relatively free of side effects.

haploid /hap′loid/ [Gk *haploos* single, *eidos* form], having only one complete set of nonhomologous chromosomes.

haploid nucleus [Gk *haploos* single, *eidos* form; L *nucleus* nut], a nucleus possessing only half the normal somatic number of chromosomes. It may occur in a germ cell after reduction division and before fertilization.

hapten /hap′tən/[Gk *haptein* to grasp], a nonproteinaceous substance that acts as an antigen by combining with particular bonding sites on an antibody. Unlike a true antigen, it does not induce the formation of antibodies.

haptics /hap′tiks/ [Gk *haptos* touch sensitive], the science concerned with studying the sense of touch. **–haptic,** *adj.*

haptoglobin /hap′tōglō′bin/ [Gk *haptein* to grasp; L *globus* ball], a plasma protein whose only known function is to bind free hemoglobin.

hard chancre [AS *heard;* Fr *canker*], a syphilitic chancre, or primary lesion that develops at the site of a syphilis infection. The lesion begins as a small red papule that gradually hardens and erodes into an extremely contagious ulcer. A secretion exuded by the sore contains *Treponema pallidum,* the organism that is the etiologic agent of syphilis in humans.

hard contact lens [AS *heard;* L *contingere* to touch, *lentil*], a polymethylmethacrylate, or rigid gas-permeable, contact lens that retains its form without support, in contrast with a soft contact lens that easily yields to pressure.

hard data, information about a patient that is obtained by observation and measurement, including laboratory data, as opposed to information collected by interviewing the patient.

hardening of the arteries, arteriosclerosis.

hard fibroma, a neoplasm composed of fibrous tissue in which there are few cells.

hardness of x-rays, the relative penetrating power of x-rays. In general, the shorter the wavelength, the harder the radiation.

hard palate [AS *heard* hard; L *palatum*], the bony portion of the roof of the mouth, continuous posteriorly with the soft palate and bounded anteriorly and laterally by the alveolar arches and the gums.

hard radiation. See **hardness of x-rays.**

hard water [AS *heard, waeter*], water that contains certain cations, particularly calcium and magnesium, that precipitate with soap solutions. The term is generally applied to tap water and the degree of hardness will vary with the source and previous treatment.

Hardy-Weinberg equilibrium principle /här′dēwīn′bərg/ [G. H. Hardy, English mathmatician; Wilhelm Weinberg, German physician, b. 1862; L *aequilibris* equal weight; *principium* a beginning], a mathematical relationship between the frequency of genes and the resulting genotypes in populations.

harelip. See **cleft lip.**

hare's eye. See **lagophthalmos.**

harlequin color /här′lək(w)in/ [It *arlecchino* goblin; L *color* hue], a transient flushing of the skin on the lower side of the body with pallor of the upward side.

harlequin fetus, an infant whose skin at birth is completely covered with thick, horny scales that resemble armor and are divided by deep red fissures.

Harris tube [Franklin Harris, American surgeon, b. 1895], a tube used for gastric and intestinal decompression. It is a mercury-weighted, single-lumen tube that is passed through the nose and carried through the alimentary tract by gravity. The location of the tube is followed by fluoroscopy.

Hartmann's curet [Arthur Hartmann, German physician, b. 1849], a curet used for the removal of adenoids.

Hartnup disease [Hartnup, family name of first patients diagnosed in England, 1956], a recessive genetic metabolic disorder characterized by pellagra-like skin lesions, transient cerebellar ataxia, and hyperaminoaciduria, caused by defects in intestinal absorption and renal reabsorption of neutral amino acids.

Harvard pump, a small pump that can be adjusted to deliver small amounts of medication in solution through an intravenous infusion set.

harvest fever. See **leptospirosis.**

harvest mite. See **chigger.**

Hashimoto's disease /hä′shimō′tōz/ [Hakaru Hashimoto, Japanese surgeon, b. 1881], an autoimmune thyroid disorder, characterized by the production of antibodies in response to thyroid antigens and the replacement of normal thyroid structures with lymphocytes and lymphoid germinal centers. The thyroid, typically enlarged, pale yellow, and lumpy on the surface, shows dense lymphocytic infiltration, and the remaining thyroid tissue frequently contains small empty follicles. The goiter is usually asymptomatic, but occasionally patients complain of dysphagia and a feeling of local pressure. The thymus is usually enlarged, and regional lymph nodes often show hyperplasia.

hashish. See **cannabis.**

HAV, abbreviation for *hepatitis A virus.*

Haverhill fever /hā′vəril/ [Haverhill, Massachusetts, disorder first diagnosed, 1925], a febrile disease, caused by infection with *Streptobacillus moniliformis,* transmitted by the bite of a rat. The spirochete-like bacterium is normally present in rat saliva. Characteristically the wound from the bite heals, but within 10 days fever, chills, vomiting, headache, muscle and joint pain, and a rash appear.

haversian canal /havur′shən/ [Clopton Havers, English physician, b. 1650], one of the many tiny longitudinal canals in bone tissue, averaging about 0.05 mm in diameter. Each contains blood vessels, connective tissue, nerve filaments, and, occasionally, lymphatic vessels.

haversian canaliculus /havur′shən kan′əlik′yələs/, any one of the many tiny passages radiating from the lacunae of bone tissue to larger haversian canals.

haversian glands [Clopton Havers; L *glans* acorn], extrasynovial fat pads that may project into the joint space.

haversian lamella [Clopton Havers; L *lamella* a small plate], one of a series of lamellae (circular layers) arranged around the central haversian canal of an osteon, or cylindrical unit of bone structure.

haversian system, a circular district of bone tissue, consisting of concentric lamellae in the bone around a central blood vessel canal.

Hawthorne effect /hô'thôrn/, a general, unintentional, but usually beneficial effect on a person, a group of people, or the function of the system being studied. It is the effect of an encounter, as with an investigator or health care provider, or of a change in a program or facility, as by painting an office or changing the lighting system.

hay fever [AS *heawan* to hew; L *febris* fever], *informal;* an acute seasonal allergic rhinitis stimulated by tree, grass, or weed pollens.

Hayflick limits [Leonard Hayflick, American scientist, b. 1928; L, *limes,* border], a concept that the life span of living organisms is limited by the number of times that somatic cells will subdivide. On the basis of human cells in cultures, where divisions occur about 50 times, it is estimated the average human life span is limited to around 115 years.

hazard [Fr *hasard* chance], a condition or phenomenon that increases the probability of a loss arising from some danger that may result in injury or illness. **–hazardous,** *adj.*

Hb, abbreviation for **hemoglobin.**

HB, abbreviation for **hepatitis B.**

Hb A, abbreviation for **hemoglobin A.**

Hb A$_2$, abbreviation for **hemoglobin A$_2$.**

HB Ag, abbreviation for *hepatitis B antigen.*

Hb C, abbreviation for **hemoglobin C.**

HBE, abbreviation for **His bundle electrocardiogram.**

Hb F, abbreviation for **hemoglobin F.**

HBIG, abbreviation for **hepatitis B immune globulin.**

Hb S, abbreviation for **hemoglobin S.**

HBsAG, abbreviation for **hepatitis B surface antigen.**

Hb S-C, abbreviation for **hemoglobin S-C.**

HBV, an abbreviation for *hepatitis B virus.*

HCG, abbreviation for **human chorionic gonadotropin.**

HCG radioreceptor assay, a urine test to detect pregnancy or missed abortion, performed by measuring human chorionic gonadotropin, a chemical found only in the urine of pregnant women or in tumors that produce HCG.

HCl, abbreviation for **hydrochloric acid.**

H deflection, (in cardiology) an indication on an electrocardiogram of His bundle activation.

HDL, abbreviation for **high-density lipoprotein.**

He, symbol for the chemical element **helium.**

head [AS *heafd*], the topmost part of the body, containing the brain, special sense organs, mouth, nose, and related structures. Most of the tissues are enclosed within the skull, composed of 22 bones.

headache [AS *heafd* + *acan* to hurt], a pain in the head from any cause. Kinds of headaches include **functional, migraine, organic, sinus,** and **tension headache.**

head and neck cancer, any malignant neoplasms of the upper aerodigestive tract, facial features, and structures in the neck, presenting as masses, ulcerations, or flat lesions that usually produce early symptoms. Tumors of the oral cavity, lips, and tongue characteristically begin as a swelling or nonhealing ulcer. Nasal and paranasal sinus malignancies, most often epidermoid cancers, cause a bloody discharge, obstruction in breathing, and facial and dental pain. Nasopharyngeal tumors, predominantly squamous cell and undifferentiated carcinomas, are associated with nasal obstruction, serous otitis media, hearing loss, lymphadenopathy, and cranial nerve involvement. Oropharyngeal and tonsillar neoplasms, usually squamous cell carcinomas and less frequently lymphomas, produce dysphagia, pain, dyspnea, and trismus. Most hypopharyngeal and laryngeal tumors are carcinomas that cause hoarseness, dysphagia, dyspnea, cough, and cervical adenopathy. Salivary gland carcinomas occur most frequently in the parotid gland and may cause facial palsy. Cancer of the mandible, including extremely painful osteosarcoma and, often, painless giant cell tumor, Ewing's sarcoma, and ameloblastoma, may erode through the gingiva, producing an intraoral ulcer, and may cause pathologic fractures. Ear neoplasms involve the auricle in most cases and are most commonly squamous cell carcinomas that cause pain, deafness, and facial nerve paralysis.

head bobbing, a sign of respiratory distress in an infant. Because neck extensor muscles are not strong enough to stabilize the head, accessory muscle use produces head bobbing.

head box, a clear plastic chamber that fits over a patient's head with an adjustable seal around the neck for mechanical ventilation. Humidified gas enters the chamber and excess gas is released through an outlet valve. The device may help prevent the need for intubation.

head, eye, ear, nose, and throat (HEENT), a specialty in medicine concerned with the anatomy, physiology, and pathology of the head, eyes, ears, nose, and throat and with the diagnosis and treatment of disorders of those structures.

head injury, any traumatic damage to the head resulting from penetration of the skull or from too rapid inertial acceleration or deceleration of the brain within the skull. Blood vessels, nerves, and meninges are torn; bleeding, infection, edema, and ischemia may result.

head kidney. See **pronephros.**

head nurse, the clinical and administrative leader of the nurses working in a given geographic division of an institution, usually a floor, ward, or unit.

head process, a strand of cells that extends forward from the primitive node in the early stages of embryonic development in vertebrates. It is the precursor of the notochord.

head traction [AS *heafod*; L *trahere* to draw], traction that is applied to the head in the treatment of cervical vertebrae injuries.

Heaf test /hēf/ [Frederick R. G. Heaf, English physician, b. 1894], a tuberculin skin test using a multiple-puncture technique.

healing [AS *haelan* to cure], the act or process in which the normal structural and functional characteristics of health are restored to diseased, dysfunctional, or damaged tissues, organs, or systems of the body.

health [AS *haelth*], a condition of physical, mental, and social well-being and the absence of disease or other abnormal condition. It is not a static condition; constant change and adaptation to stress result in homeostasis.

health assessment, an evaluation of the health status of an individual by performing a physical examination after obtaining a health history. Various laboratory tests may also be ordered to confirm a clinical impression or to screen for dysfunction.

health behavior, an action taken by a person to maintain, attain, or regain good health and to prevent illness. Health behavior reflects a person's health beliefs. Some common health behaviors are exercising regularly, eating a balanced diet, and obtaining necessary inoculations.

Health Belief Model, a conceptual framework that describes a person's health behavior as an expression of health beliefs.

health care consumer, any actual or potential recipient of health care, as a patient in a hospital, a client in a community mental health center, or a member of a prepaid

health maintenance organization (HMO).

health care industry, the complex of preventive, remedial, and therapeutic services provided by hospitals and other institutions, nurses, doctors, dentists, government agencies, voluntary agencies, noninstitutional care facilities, pharmaceutic and medical equipment manufacturers, and health insurance companies.

health care proxy [AS, *haelth;* ME, *caru,* sorrow; L, *procuratio,* a deputy], a person designated to make health care decisions for a patient who has become incapacitated.

health care system, the complete network of agencies, facilities, and all providers of health care in a specified geographic area.

health certificate, a statement signed by a health care provider that attests to the state of health of a person.

health consumer. See **health care consumer.**

health culture, a system that attempts to explain and treat sickness and to maintain health. It may be a popular or folk system, or it may be a technical or scientific one.

health economics, a social system that studies the supply and demand of health care resources and the impact of health services on a population.

health education, an educational program directed to the general public that attempts to improve, maintain, and safeguard the health of the community.

health hazard [AS *haelth;* OFr *hasard*], a danger to health resulting from exposure to environmental pollutants, such as asbestos or ionizing radiation, or to a life-style influence, such as cigarette smoking or chemical abuse.

health history, (in nursing and medicine) a collection of information obtained from the patient and from other sources concerning the patient's physical status and psychologic, social, and sexual functions. The history provides a data base on which a plan for management of the diagnosis, treatment, care, and follow-up of the patient may be made. Kinds of history include **complete health history, episodic health history,** and **interval health history.**

health maintenance, a program or procedure planned to prevent illness, to maintain maximal function, and to promote health.

health maintenance, altered, a NANDA-accepted nursing diagnosis of the condition in which the patient is unable to identify, manage, or seek help to maintain health. Defining characteristics include a demonstrated lack of knowledge regarding basic health practices or the inability to take responsibility for meeting those needs, the inability to adapt to internal or external environmental change, a lack of financial or other resources or support systems, a history of the lack of health-seeking behavior, or an increased interest in improving health behavior.

Health Maintenance Organization (HMO), a type of group health care practice that provides basic and supplemental health maintenance and treatment services to voluntary enrollees who prepay a fixed periodic fee that is set without regard to the amount or kind of services received. Some of the first HMOs, Kaiser-Permanente among them, have demonstrated that high-quality medical care can often be provided at less expense by such a system than by other health care systems. In addition to diagnostic and treatment services, including hospitalization and surgery, an HMO often offers supplemental services, such as dental, mental, and eye care, and prescription drugs. Federal financial support for the establishment of HMOs was provided under Title XIII of the 1973 U.S. Public Health Service Act.

health physicist, a health scientist who directs research, training, and management of programs in which patients and health professionals are exposed to potential hazards associated with the use of diagnostic and therapeutic equipment, such as radioactive materials.

health physics, the study of the effects of ionizing radiation on the body and the methods for protecting people from the undesirable effects of the radiation.

health policy, 1. a statement of a decision regarding a goal in health care and a plan for achieving that goal. **2.** a field of study and practice in which the priorities and values underlying health resource allocation are determined.

health professional, any person who has completed a course of study in a field of health, such as a registered nurse, physical therapist, or physician. The person is usually licensed by a government agency or certified by a professional organization.

health-related services, services of a health facility other than medical care that may contribute directly or indirectly to the physical or mental health and well-being of patients, as personal or social services.

health resources, all materials, personnel, facilities, funds, and anything else that can be used for providing health care and services.

health risk, a disease precursor associated with a higher than average morbidity or mortality.

health risk appraisal, a process of gathering, analyzing, and comparing an individual's prognostic characteristics of health with a standard age group.

health screening, a program designed to evaluate the health status and potential of an individual. Health screening may include taking a personal and family health history and performing a physical examination or tests, laboratory tests, or radiologic examination.

health seeking behaviors, a NANDA-accepted nursing diagnosis of a state in which a client in stable health is actively seeking ways to alter personal health habits and the environment in order to move toward optimal health. Defining characteristics include an expressed or observed desire to seek a higher level of wellness, unfamiliarity with wellness community resources, lack of knowledge in health promotion behaviors, desire for increased control of health practice, and concern about environmental conditions or health status.

health service area, a geographic region designated under the National Health Planning and Resources Development Act of 1974, covering such factors as geography, political boundaries, population, and health resources, for the effective planning and development of health services.

health supervision, health teaching, counseling, or monitoring the status of the patient's health other than physical care.

health systems agency (HSA), an agency established under the terms of the National Health Planning and Resources Development Act of 1974 to provide networks of health planning and resource development services in each of several health service areas established by the Act.

health systems plan, a plan in which the long-range health goals of a health services area are specified. Health systems plans are prepared by health systems agencies.

hearing [AS *hieran*], the special sense that enables sound to be perceived. It is the major function of the ear.

hearing aid, an electronic device that amplifies sound for persons with impaired hearing. The device consists of a microphone, a battery power supply, an amplifier, and a receiver.

hearing impairment, a loss of hearing that adversely affects an individual's ability to communicate through the sense of audition alone.

hearing loss, an inability to perceive the normal range of sounds audible to an in-

H

dividual with normal hearing. **Conductive hearing** is a result of damage to the outer middle ear whereas **sensorineural hearing loss** results from damage to the inner ear or auditory nerve.

heart [AS *heorte*], the muscular, cone-shaped organ, about the size of a clenched fist, that pumps blood throughout the body and beats normally about 70 times per minute by coordinated nerve impulses and muscular contractions. Enclosed in pericardium, the heart rests on the diaphragm between the lower borders of the lungs, occupying the middle of the mediastinum. It is covered ventrally by the sternum and the adjoining parts of the third to the sixth costal cartilages. The layers of the heart, starting from the outside, are the epicardium, the myocardium, and the endocardium. The epicardium includes the visceral pericardium and a layer of fibroelastic connective tissue. The myocardium is composed of layers and bundles of cardiac muscle laced by blood vessels. The endocardium is continuous with the endothelial lining of the blood vessels. The chambers of the heart include two ventricles with thick muscular walls, making up the bulk of the organ, and two atria with thin muscular walls. A septum separates the ventricles and extends between the atria, dividing the heart into the right and the left sides. The left side of the heart pumps oxygenated blood from the pulmonary veins into the aorta and on to all parts of the body. The right side of the heart pumps deoxygenated blood, received through the venae cavae, into the pulmonary arteries.

heart block, an interference with the normal conduction of electric impulses that control activity of the heart muscle. Heart block usually is further defined as to the location of the block and the type.

heartburn, a painful burning sensation in the esophagus just below the sternum. Heartburn is usually caused by the reflux of gastric contents into the esophagus but may be caused by gastric hyperacidity or peptic ulcer.

heart disease risk factors [AS *heorte* heart; L *dis*; Fr *aise* ease, *risquer* chance of injury; L *facere* to make], hereditary lifestyle and environmental influences that increase one's chances of developing heart disease. Examples include cigarette smoking, high blood pressure, obesity, foods that contribute exogenous fats, and hereditary factors.

heart failure, a condition in which the heart cannot pump enough blood to meet the metabolic requirements of body tissues. Many of the symptoms associated with heart failure are caused by the dysfunction of organs other than the heart, especially the lungs, kidneys, and liver. Ventricular dysfunction is usually the basic disorder in congestive heart failure and often triggers compensatory mechanisms that preserve cardiac output but produce symptoms and signs, such as dyspnea, orthopnea, rales, and edema. Most kinds of heart disease initially affect the left side of the heart, and clinicians commonly divide associated heart failure into left-sided heart failure and right-sided heart failure.

heart-lung machine, an apparatus consisting of a pump and an oxygenator that takes over the functions of the heart and lungs, especially during cardiac surgery. The blood is shunted from the venous system through an oxygenator and returned to the arterial circulation.

heart massage. See **cardiac massage.**

heart murmur. See **cardiac murmur.**

heart rate, the pulse, calculated by counting the number of QRS complexes or contractions of the cardiac ventricles per unit of time. Tachycardia is a heart rate of more than 100 beats per minute; bradycardia is a heart rate of fewer than 60 beats per minute.

heart scan, a radiographic scan of the heart, performed after injecting a radioactive material into a vein, used for determining the size, shape, and location of the heart, for diagnosing pericarditis, and for viewing the chambers of the heart.

heart sound, a normal noise produced within the heart during the cardiac cycle that can be heard over the precordium and may reveal abnormalities in cardiac structure or function. Cardiac auscultation is performed systematically from apex to base of the heart or from base to apex, using a stethoscope to listen initially with the diaphragm and then with the bell of the instrument. The first heart sound (S_1), a dull, prolonged *lub*, occurs with the closure of the mitral and tricuspid valves and marks the onset of ventricular systole. The second heart sound (S_2), a short, sharp *dup*, occurs with the closing of the aortic and pulmonic valves at the beginning of ventricular diastole.

heart surgery, any surgical procedure involving the heart, performed to correct acquired or congenital defects, to replace diseased valves, to open or bypass blocked vessels, or to graft a prosthesis or a transplant in place. Two major types of heart surgery are performed, closed and open. The closed technique is done through a small incision, without using the heart-lung machine. In the open technique the heart chambers are open and fully visible, and blood is detoured around the surgical field by the heart-lung machine. Hypothermia may also be used to reduce the metabolic rate and the need of the tissues for oxygen. Kinds of heart surgery include **Blalock-Taussig procedure, coronary bypass,** and **endarterectomy.**

heart transplantation [AS *hoerte;* L *transplantare*], the surgical removal of a donor heart and transfer of the organ to a recipient. The procedure usually involves removal of a heart from a healthy individual who may have died in an accident or from another cause unrelated to heart disease and using it to replace a severely diseased heart of another person. Most recipients survive for more than one year with a transplanted heart and nearly three fourths of the recipients are able to return to work. Total ischemic time for a heart transplant is less than 6 hours between donor and recipient. The heart is transplanted with anastomoses of the aorta, pulmonary artery, and pulmonary vein while venous return is provided by an anastomosis between the recipient's right atrium and that of the transplanted organ.

heart valve, one of the four structures within the heart that control the flow of blood by opening and closing with each heartbeat. The valves include two semilunar valves, the aortic and pulmonary, the mitral valve, and the tricuspid valve. The valves permit the flow of blood in only one direction.

heat cramp [AS *haetu; crammian* to fill], any cramp in the arm, leg, or abdomen caused by depletion in the body of both water and salt because of heat exhaustion. It usually occurs after vigorous physical exertion in an extremely hot environment or under other conditions that cause profuse sweating and depletion of body fluids and electrolytes.

heated nebulization, a method of inhalation therapy using a heating device with a nebulizer that produces a spray with a higher water content than that of a cold atomizer. The mist may be administered through a mask or in a tent.

heat exhaustion, an abnormal condition characterized by weakness, vertigo, nausea, muscle cramps, and loss of consciousness, caused by depletion of body fluid and electrolytes resulting from exposure to intense heat or the inability to acclimatize to heat. Body temperature is near normal; blood pressure may drop but usually returns to normal as the person is placed in a recumbent position; the skin is cool, damp, and pale.

heat hyperpyrexia, a severe and sometimes fatal condition resulting from the failure of the temperature-regulating capacity of the body, caused by prolonged exposure to the sun or to high temperatures. Reduction or cessation of sweating is an early symptom. Body temperature of 105° F or higher, tachycardia, hot and dry skin, headache, confusion, unconsciousness, and convulsions may occur.

heat labile. See **thermolabile.**

heat prostration See **heat exhaustion.**

heat rash, a finely papular or vesicular inflammation of the skin resulting from prolonged exposure to heat and high humidity.

heatstroke. See **heat hyperpyrexia.**

heaves /hēvz/ [AS *hebban* to lift], **1.** a chronic pulmonary disease of horses, similar to human pulmonary emphysema, characterized by wheezing, coughing, and dyspnea on exertion. **2.** *informal.* vomiting and retching.

heavy chain disease [AS *heafig;* L *catena* chain; *dis* opposite of; Fr *aise* ease], a plasma cell disorder characterized by a proliferation of immunoglobulin heavy chains. Effects tend to vary according to the predominant type of heavy chain. For example, most gamma heavy chain disease patients are elderly men who have symptoms resembling those of malignant lymphoma. Mu heavy chain disease presents symptoms of chronic lymphocytic leukemia.

heavy function, (in dentistry) an increase in the functional activities of the teeth.

heavy hydrogen. See **deuterium.**

heavy metal, a metallic element with a specific gravity five or more times that of water. The heavy metals are antimony, arsenic, bismuth, cadmium, cerium, chromium, cobalt, copper, gallium, gold, iron, lead, manganese, mercury, nickel, platinum, silver, tellurium, thallium, tin, uranium, vanadium, and zinc.

heavy metal poisoning, poisoning caused by the ingestion, inhalation, or absorption of various toxic heavy metals. Kinds of heavy metal poisoning include **antimony, arsenic, cadmium, lead,** and **mercury poisoning.**

heavy vaginal bleeding. See **vaginal bleeding.**

hebephrenia, hebephrenic schizophrenia. See **disorganized schizophrenia.**

Heberden's node /hē'bərdənz/ [William Heberden, English physician, b. 1710; L *nodus* knot], an abnormal cartilaginous or bony enlargement of a distal interphalangeal joint of a finger, usually occurring in degenerative diseases of the joints.

hebetude /heb'itŏŏd'/ [L *hebeo* to be blunt], a state of dullness or lethargy, characteristic of some forms of schizophrenia.

heboid paranoia. See **paranoid schizophrenia.**

heel [AS *hela*], the posterior part of the foot, formed by the largest tarsal bone, the calcaneus.

heel cup, a plastic device designed to help relieve pain of a heel spur or contusion by pushing the fat pad of the heel under the calcaneus to increase the cushioning effect.

heel-knee test [AS *hela* + *cneow* knee; L *testum* crucible], a method of assessing coordination of movements of the extremities. In the test the patient, lying prone, is asked to touch the knee of one leg with the heel of the other.

heel lift, a form of foot orthosis, usually made of sheets of cork, to correct a dysfunction that may be the result of anatomic limb length differences or decreased flexibility.

heel puncture [AS *hela*; L *punctura*], a method of obtaining a blood sample from a newborn or premature infant by a puncture in the lateral or medial areas of the plantar surface of the heel. Care must be exercised to avoid puncturing the posterior curvature of the heel and to make the puncture as shallow as feasible.

heel-shin test [AS *hela* + *scinu* shin; L *testum* crucible], a method of assessing coordination of movements of the extremities. In the test the patient, lying prone, is asked to pass the heel of one leg slowly down the shin of the other leg from the knee to the ankle.

HEENT, abbreviation for **head, eye, ear, nose, and throat.**

Hegar's sign /hā′gärz/ [Alfred Hegar, German gynecologist, b. 1830; L *signum* sign], a softening of the isthmus of the uterine cervix early in gestation. It is a probable sign of pregnancy.

height [AS *hiehtho*], the vertical measurement of a structure, organ, or other object from bottom to top, when it is placed or projected in an upright position.

height of contour, the greatest convexity of a tooth surface, viewed from a predetermined position.

Heimlich maneuver /hīm′lik, hīm′lish/ [Harry J. Heimlich, American surgeon, b. 1920; Fr *manoeuvre* action], an emergency procedure for dislodging a bolus of food or other obstruction from the trachea to prevent asphyxiation. The choking person is grasped from behind by the rescuer whose fist, thumb side in, is placed just below the victim's sternum with the other hand placed firmly over the fist. The rescuer then pulls the fist firmly and abruptly into the epigastrium forcing the obstruction up the trachea. If repeated attempts do not free the airway, an emergency tracheotomy may be necessary.

Heimlich sign [H.J. Heimlich, American physician, b. 1920; L, *signum*], a universal distress signal that a person is choking and unable to speak, made by grasping the throat with a thumb and index finger, thereby attracting the attention of others nearby.

Heinz bodies /hīnts/ [Robert Heinz, German pathologist, b. 1865], irregularly shaped bits of altered hemoglobin found in the red blood cells of persons who are hypersensitive to certain chemicals, as aniline, phenylhydrazine, and primaquine.

Helen, Sister (Helen Bowden), a nurse who received her education in England and became the first director of the newly formed Bellevue Hospital Training School for Nurses in New York, in 1873. Although she had not trained under Florence Nightingale, she set up the Bellevue school along Nightingale's principles.

Heliodorus' bandage. See **T bandage.**

helium (He) /hē′lē·əm/ [Gk *helios* sun], a colorless, odorless, gaseous element; the second lightest element after hydrogen. Its atomic number is 2; its atomic weight is 4. Helium is one of the rare or inert gases and does not usually combine with other elements. Most of the commercial helium in the world comes from natural gas reservoirs in Texas and Louisiana where it is recovered after natural gas has been liquefied. It is produced in nature by the decay of radioactive elements and is produced in the sun from hydrogen. It occurs in the atmosphere in the ratio of five parts per million. Helium is used industrially in arc welding, refining, and other processes. Because of its lightness and lack of flammability it is also used to lift airships and balloons. The main physiologic and medical uses of helium are in respiratory therapy and testing, the prevention of nitrogen narcosis and decompression sickness in hyperbaric environments, and in pulmonary function testing to calculate the diffusing and residual capacities of the lungs.

helium therapy, the use of helium gas mixtures to treat patients with airway obstruction. Because of its low density, helium can negotiate an obstruction more easily.

helix /hē′liks/ [Gk, coil], a coiled, spiral-like formation characteristic of many organic molecules, such as deoxyribonucleic acid (DNA).

Heller's test, a laboratory test for proteinuria in which urine is layered upon nitric acid. Appearance of a ring of precipitated protein at the junction of the fluids is a positive sign.

Hellin's law, a generalized formula for calculating the ratio of multiple births in any population, stating that if twin births occur at the rate of 1:N, then the rate of triplet births is approximately $1:N^2$, quadruplets $1:N^3$, quintuplets $1:N^4$, and so on, with the exponent of N being one less than the number in the multiple set. The constant N varies with population, although it was originally set at 89.

helmet cells, fragmented red blood cells that have been "scooped out" so they resemble helmets. They are found in patients with carcinomatosis, hemolytic anemia, and thrombotic thrombocytopenic purpura. Helmet cells are also seen in blood samples of persons with prosthetic heart valves.

helminth /hel'minth/[Gk *helmins* worm], a worm, especially one of the pathogenic parasites of the division Metazoa fluke, including flukes, tapeworms, and roundworms.

helminthemesis /hel'minthem'əsis/ [Gk *helmins* + *emesis* vomiting], the vomiting of intestinal worms.

helminthiasis /hel'minthī'əsis/[Gk *helmins* + *osis* condition], a parasitic infestation of the body by helminths that may be cutaneous, visceral, or intestinal. Ascariasis, bilharziasis, filariasis, hookworm, and trichinosis are common forms of the disease.

helminthic /helmin'thik/ [Gk *helmins*], pertaining to worms.

helper T cell. See **T cell, T4 cell.**

helper virus, a virus that is necessary in a phenotypically mixed infection to mediate the replication of a defective virus. Viruses that mature by budding through the cell membrane require the coding of a helper virus.

helplessness, a feeling of a loss of control, usually after repeated failures, with the result that one is unable to make autonomous choices.

Helsinki accords /helsing'kē/, a declaration signed by the representatives of 35 member nations of the Conference on Security and Cooperation in Europe in Helsinki, Finland, on August 1, 1975. The declared goals are the right to self-determination of all people and respect for the fundamental freedoms, including thought, conscience, and religion or belief, without regard to race, language, sex, or religion. The Helsinki accords grew from the precedent set by the judgments at the trials of the Nuremberg tribunals—that crimes against humanity are offenses subject to criminal prosecution. The principle and the practice of informed consent in health care grew from this precedent.

helvolic acid /helvol'ik/, an antibiotic, derived from the mold *Aspergillus fumigatus,* formerly used as an amebicide.

hemacytometer /hē'məsītom'ətər/ [Gk *haima* blood, *kytos* cell, *metron* measure], an apparatus for counting the number of cells in a known volume of blood or other fluid.

hemadsorption /hē'madsôrp'shən, hem'-/ [Gk *haima* blood; L *ad* to, *sorbere* to swallow], a process in which a substance or an agent, as certain viruses and bacilli, adheres to the surface of an erythrocyte.

hemagglutination /hē'məgloo'tinā'shən, hem'-/ [Gk *haima* + L *agglutinare* to glue], the coagulation of erythrocytes.

hemagglutinin [Gk *haima* + L *agglutinare*], a type of antibody that agglutinates red blood cells. It is classified according to the source of cells agglutinated as **autologous** (from the same organism), **homologous** (from an organism of the same species), and **heterologous** (from an organism of a different species).

hemangioblastoma /hēman'jē·ōblastō'mə/, *pl.* **hemangioblastomas, hemangioblastomata** [Gk *haima* + *aggeion* small vessel, *blastos* germ, *oma* tumor], a brain tumor composed of a proliferation of capillaries and of disorganized clusters of capillary cells or angioblasts.

hemangioendothelioma /hēman'jē·ō·en'dōthē'lē·ō'mə/, *pl.* **hemangioendotheliomas, hemangioendotheliomata** [Gk *haima* + *endon* inside, *thele* nipple, *oma* tumor], **1.** a tumor, consisting of endothelial cells, that grows around an artery or a vein. It rarely becomes malignant. **2.** malignant hemangioendothelioma.

hemangiofibroma /hēman'jē·ōfībrō'mə/ [Gk *haima* + L *fibra* fiber; Gk *oma* tumor], a tumor that has the characteristics of both a hemangioma and a fibroma.

hemangioma /hēman'jē·ō'mə/, *pl.* **hemangiomas, hemangiomata** [Gk *haima* + *aggeion* small vessel, *oma*], a benign tumor consisting of a mass of blood vessels. Types of hemangiomas include **capillary hemangioma, cavernous hemangioma,** and **nevus flammeus.**

hemangioma simplex. See **capillary hemangioma.**

hemangiosarcoma. See **angiosarcoma.**

hemapoiesis /hem'əpō·ē'sis/ [Gk *haima* + *poiein* to make], the formation of blood cells.

hemarthros /hem'är'thrəs/ [Gk *haima* + *arthron* joint], the extravasation of blood into a joint.

hemarthrosis. See **hemarthros.**

hematemesis /hē'mətem'əsis, hem'-/ [Gk *haima* + *emesis* vomiting], vomiting of bright red blood, indicating rapid upper GI bleeding, commonly associated with esophageal varices or peptic ulcer.

hematinuria /hem′ətinŏŏr′ē-ə/ [Gk *haima* + *ouron* urine], a dark-colored urine due to the presence of hematin or hemoglobin.

hematocele /hem′ətōsēl′/, a cystlike accumulation of blood within the tunica vaginalis of the scrotum. It is usually caused by injury.

hematochezia /hem′ətōkē′zhə/ [Gk *haima* + *chezo* feces], the passage of red blood through the rectum. The cause is usually bleeding in the colon or rectum, but it can result from the loss of blood higher in the digestive tract, depending on the transit time. Cancer, colitis, and ulcers are among causes of hematochezia.

hematocrit /himat′ōkrit/ [Gk *haima* + *krinein* to separate], a measure of the packed cell volume of red cells, expressed as a percentage of the total blood volume. The normal range is between 43% and 49% in men, and between 37% and 43% in women.

hematocyte /hem′ətōsīt′/ [Gk *haima* + *kytos* cell], a blood cell, particularly a red blood cell.

hematocytoblast /hem′ətōsī′təblast′/ [Gk *haima* + *kytos* + *blastos* germ], a large nucleated reticuloendothelial cell found in bone marrow. It is believed to be a common precursor of various blood elements.

hematogenesis /hem.ətōjen′əsis/ [Gk *haima* + *genein* to produce], pertaining to the formation of blood cells or an increase in the production of blood elements.

hematogenic shock [Gk *haima* + *genein* to produce; Fr *choc*], a condition of shock caused by the loss of blood or plasma.

hematogenous /hēmətoj′ənəs/ [Gk *haima* + *genein* to produce], originating or transported in the blood.

hematogenous pigment [Gk *haima* + *genein* to produce; L *pingere* to paint], pertaining to the red color of erythrocytes that is caused by the presence of hemoglobin.

hematogenous tuberculosis, a form of tuberculosis that is blood-borne.

hematologic death syndrome, a group of clinical signs and symptoms of radiation damage to the blood cells. The condition is characterized by nausea, vomiting, fever, diarrhea, infections, anemia, leukopenia, and hemorrhage. It can result from exposure to a dose of 200 to 1,000 rad. The mean survival time for a person with hematologic death syndrome is estimated at between 10 and 60 days.

hematologic effect, (in radiology) the response of blood cells to radiation exposure. In general, all types of blood cells are destroyed by radiation and the degree of cell depletion increases with increasing dose.

hematologist /hē′mətol′əjist, hem′-/, a medical specialist in the field of hematology.

hematology /hē′mətol′əjē, hem′-/ [Gk *haima* + *logos* science], scientific medical study of blood and blood-forming tissues. **–hematologic, hematological,** *adj.*

hematolysis [Gk *haima* + *lysein* to loosen], the release of hemoglobin from red blood cells by the breakdown of erythrocytes or by osmosis.

hematoma /hē′mətō′mə, hem′-/, *pl.* **hematomas, hematomata** [Gk *haima* + *oma* tumor], a collection of extravasated blood trapped in the tissues of the skin or in an organ, resulting from trauma or incomplete hemostasis after surgery. Initially, there is frank bleeding into the space; if the space is limited, pressure slows and eventually stops the flow of blood. The blood clots, serum collects, the clot hardens, and the mass becomes palpable to the examiner and is often painful to the patient.

hematomyelia /hē′mətōmē′lē-ə/ [Gk *haima* + *meylos* marrow], the appearance of frank blood in the fluid of the spinal cord.

hematopericardium [Gk *haima* + *peri* near, *kardia* heart], a seepage of blood into the pericardium.

hematoperitoneum /hē′mətōper′itanē′əm/ [Gk *haima* + *peri* + *tenein* to stretch], the effusion of blood into the peritoneal cavity.

hematopoiesis /hē′mətōpō·ē′sis, hem′-/ [Gk *haima* + *poiein* to make], the normal formation and development of blood cells in the bone marrow. In severe anemia and other hematologic disorders, cells may be produced in organs outside the marrow (extramedullary hematopoiesis). **–hematopoietic,** *adj.*

hematopoietic syndrome /hē′mətōpō·et′ik/, a group of clinical features associated with effects of radiation on the blood and lymph tissues. It is characterized by vomiting, destruction of the bone marrow, and atrophy of the spleen and lymph nodes.

hematopoietic system [Gk *haima* + *poiein* to make; L *systema*], the system of body organs and tissues involved in the formation and functioning of blood elements. It includes the bone marrow and spleen.

hematospermia /hē′mətōspur′mē′ə/, the presence of blood in the semen. Causes may include vascular congestion, an infection involving seminal vesicles, coitus interruptus, sexual abstinence, or frequent coitus.

hematothorax [Gk *haima* + *thorax* chest],

a seepage of blood into the peritoneal cavity, often due to the presence of a neoplasm.

hematoxylin-eosin /hē′mətok′silin/ [*Haematoxylon campechianum* logwood; Gk *eos* dawn], a stain commonly used to treat tissue sections on microscope slides.

hematuria /hē′mətŏŏr′ē·ə, hem′-/ [Gk *haima* + *ouron* urine], abnormal presence of blood in the urine. Hematuria is symptomatic of many renal diseases and disorders of the genitourinary system. **–hematuric,** *adj.*

heme /hēm/ [Gk *haima* blood], the pigmented, iron-containing, nonprotein portion of the hemoglobin molecule. There are four heme groups in a hemoglobin molecule, each consisting of a cyclic structure of four pyrrole residues, called protoporphyrin, and an atom of iron in the center.

hemeralopia /hem′ərəlō′pē·ə/ [Gk *hemera* day, *alaos* blind, *ops* eye], an abnormal visual condition in which bright light causes blurring of vision. **–hemeralopic,** *adj.*

hemiacephalus /hem′ē·āsef′ələs/ [Gk *hemi* half, *a, kephale* not head], a grossly malformed fetus in which the brain and most of the cranium are lacking.

hemiachromatosia /hem′ē·ak′rōmətō′zhə/, a state of being color blind in only one half of the visual field.

hemiamblyopia /hem′ē·am′blē·ō′pē·ə/ [Gk *hemi* + *amblys* dull, *ops* eye], blindness in half of the normal visual field.

hemianalgesia /hem′ē·an′əljē′sē·ə/ [Gk *hemi* + *a, algos* not pain], a loss of feeling or sensitivity to pain affecting half of the body or one side of the body.

hemianesthesia /hem′ē·an′esthē′zhə/ [Gk *hemi* + *anaisthesia* absence of feeling], a loss of feeling on one side of the body.

hemianopia [Gk *hemi* + *a, opsis* not vision], defective vision or blindness in one half of the visual field.

hemiarthroplasty /hem′ē·är′thrəplas′tē/, a surgical procedure for repair of an injured or diseased hip joint. It involves replacement of the head of the femur with a prosthesis.

hemiarthrosis /hem′ē·ärthrō′sis/ [Gk *hemi* + *arthron* joint, *osis* condition], a false articulation between two bones.

hemiataxia /hem′ē·ətak′sē·ə/, a loss of muscle control affecting one side of the body, usually as a result of a stroke or cerebellar injury.

hemiazygous vein /hem′ē·əzī′gəs/ [Gk *hemi* + *a, zygon* not yoke], one of the tributaries of the azygous vein of the thorax.

hemiballismus. See **ballismus.**

hemicellulose /hem′əsel′yŏŏlōs/ [Gk *hemi* + L *cellula* little cell], any of a group of polysaccharides that constitute the chief part of the skeletal substances of the cell walls of plants and resemble cellulose but are more soluble and more easily extracted and decomposed.

hemicephalia /hem′ēsefā′lyə/ [Gk *hemi* + *kephale* head], a congenital anomaly characterized by the absence of one side of the cerebrum, caused by severe arrest of brain development in the fetus.

hemicephalus /hem′ēsef′ələs/ [Gk *hemi* + *kephale* head], a grossly malformed fetus with congenital absence of one half of the cerebrum.

hemicrania /hem′ēkrā′nē·ə/ [Gk *hemi* + *kranion* skull], **1.** a headache, usually migraine, that affects only one side of the head. **2.** a congenital anomaly characterized by the absence of one half of the skull in the fetus; incomplete anencephaly.

hemicraniectomy /hem′ēkran′ē·ek′təmē/ [Gk *hemi* + *kranion* skull, *ektome* cutting out], a surgical procedure in which part or all of one half of the skull is excised and reflected as a preliminary step to certain types of brain operations.

hemidiaphragm /hem′ēdī′əfram/, either the left or right functional half of the diaphragm. Although the structure is a single anatomic unit, it is divided by the union of its central tendon and the pericardium. Each hemidiaphragm can function independently of the other.

hemiectromelia /hem′ē·ek′trōmē′lyə/ [Gk *hemi* + *ektosis* miscarriage, *melos* limb], a congenital anomaly characterized by the incomplete development of the limbs on one side of the body. **–hemiectromelus,** *n.*

hemignathia /hem′ēnā′thē·ə/ [Gk *hemi* + *gnathos* jaw], **1.** a congenital anomaly characterized by incomplete development of the lower jaw on one side of the face. **2.** a condition of having only one jaw. **–hemignathus,** *n.*

hemihyperplasia /hem′ēhī′pərplā′zhə/ [Gk *hemi* + *hyper* above, *plassein* to form], overdevelopment or excessive growth of one half of a specific organ or part or all of the organs and parts on one side of the body.

hemihypertonia /hem′ēhīpərtō′nē·ə/ [Gk *hemi* + *hyper* excessive, *tonikos* stretching], a condition in which there is exaggerated tension in the muscles on one side of the body, causing tonic contraction. In one form of the disorder, tonic spasms may occur occasionally in different muscle groups on one side of the body.

hemihypertrophy /hem′ēhīpur′trəfē/ [Gk *hemi* + *hyper* + *trophe* nourishment], an abnormal enlargement or overgrowth of half of the body or half of a body part.

hemihypoplasia /hem′ēhī′pōplā′zhə/ [Gk *hemi* + *hypo* under, *plassein* to form], partial or incomplete development of one half of a specific organ or part or all of the organs and parts on one side of the body.

hemikaryon /hem′ēker′ē·on/ [Gk *hemi* + *karyon* nut], a cell nucleus that contains the haploid number of chromosomes, or one half of the diploid number, as that of the gametes. –**hemikaryotic,** *adj.*

hemimelia /hem′ēmē′lyə/ [Gk *hemi* + *melos*], a developmental anomaly characterized by the absence or gross shortening of the lower portion of one or more of the limbs.

hemiopia /hem′ē·ō′pē·ə/ [Gk *hemi* + *ops* eye], a condition involving only one eye or half the visual field.

hemipagus /hemip′əgəs/ [Gk *hemi* + *pagos* fixture], conjoined symmetric twins who are united at the thorax.

hemiparesis /hemipərē′sis/ [Gk *hemi* + *paralyein* to be paralyzed], muscular weakness of one half of the body.

hemiparesthesia /hemiper′esthē′zhə/ [Gk *hemi* + *para* beside, *aisthesis* sensation], a numbness or other abnormal or impaired sensation that is experienced on only one side of the body.

hemiplegia /hem′iplē′jə/ [Gk *hemi* + *plege* stroke], paralysis of one side of the body. Kinds of hemiplegia are **cerebral, facial, infantile,** and **spastic hemiplegia.** –**hemiplegic,** *adj.*

hemiplegic gait [Gk *hemi* + *plege;* O Norse *gata* a way], a manner of walking in which an affected limb moves in a semicircle with each step.

hemisection [Gk *hemi* + L *sectare* to cut], half of a body or other object when divided along a longitudinal plane, producing two lateral halves.

hemisomus /hem′isō′məs/ [Gk *hemi* + *soma* body], a fetus or individual in which one side of the body is malformed, defective, or absent.

hemisphere [Gk *hemi* + *sphaira* sphere], **1.** one half of a sphere or globe. **2.** the lateral half of the cerebrum or of the cerebellum. –**hemispherical,** *adj.*

hemiteras /hem′ēter′əs/, *pl.* **hemiterata** [Gk *hemi* + *teras* monster], any individual with a congenital malformation that is not so severe or disabling as to be classified as a monstrous or teratic condition. –**hemiteratic,** *adj.*

hemivertebra /hem′ēvur′təbrə/, an abnormal condition characterized by the congenital failure of a vertebra to develop completely, possibly caused by the com-

plete failure of the growth center of one vertebral body. Usually one half of the vertebra involved is completely or partially developed and the other half is absent.

hemizygote /hem′ēzī′gōt/ [Gk *hemi* + *zygon* yoke], an individual, organism, or cell that has only one of a pair of genes for a specific characteristic. –**hemizygosity,** *n.,* **hemizygous, hemizygotic,** *adj.*

hemoagglutination /hē′mō·əglōō′tinā′shən/ [Gk *haima* blood; L *agglutinare* to glue], the coagulation of red blood cells.

hemoagglutinin /hē′mō·əglōō′tinin/, an agglutinin that coagulates red blood cells.

hemoblastic leukemia. See **stem cell leukemia.**

hemochromatosis /hē′mōkrō′mətō′sis, hem′-/ [Gk *haima* blood, *chroma* color, *osis* condition], a rare disease of iron metabolism, characterized pathologically by excess iron deposits throughout the body.

hemoclip, a malleable metal clip used to ligate small blood vessels during surgery. Hemoclips also may be used to mark the location of body structures for radiographic procedures.

hemoconcentration [Gk *haima* + L *cum* together with, *centrum* center], an increase in the number of red blood cells resulting either from a decrease in plasma volume or increased production of erythrocytes.

hemocyanin /hē′mōsī′ənin/, an oxygen-carrying protein molecule present in certain lower animals, particularly arthropods and mollusks.

hemocytoblastic leukemia. See **stem cell leukemia.**

hemocytology /hē′mōsītol′əjē/ [Gk *haima* blood, *kytos* cell, *logos* science], the study of the components of blood.

hemodiafiltration /hē′mōdī′əfiltrā′shən/, a technique similar to hemofiltration, used to treat uremia by convective transport of the solute rather than diffusion.

hemodialysis /hē′mōdī·al′isis, hem′-/ [Gk *haima* + *dia* apart, *lysis* loosening], a procedure in which impurities or wastes are removed from the blood, used in treating renal insufficiency and various toxic conditions. The patient's blood is shunted from the body through a machine for diffusion and ultrafiltration and then returned to the patient's circulation. Hemodialysis requires access to the patient's bloodstream, a mechanism for the transport of the blood to and from the dialyzer, and a dialyzer. Access may be achieved by an external shunt or an arteriovenous fistula. The external shunt is constructed by inserting two cannulas through the skin into a large vein and a large artery. An arteriovenous fistula is created by the anastomosis of a large vein to an artery. Dialysis takes from 3 to 8 hours and may be necessary daily in acute situations, or 2 or 3 times a week in chronic renal failure.

hemodialysis technician, a registered nurse who has received special training in the operation of hemodialysis equipment and treatment of patients with kidney disorders.

hemodialyzer. See **dialyzer.**

hemodilution /hē′mōdilŏŏ′shən/ [Gk *haima* + L *diluare* to wash away], a condition in which the concentration of erythrocytes or other blood elements is lowered.

hemodynamics /hē′mōdīnam′iks/ [Gk *haima* + *dynamis* force], the study of the physical aspects of blood circulation, including cardiac function and peripheral vascular physiology.

hemofiltration /hē′mōfiltrā′shən/, a type of hemodialysis in which there is convective transport of the solute through ultrafiltration across the membrane.

hemoglobin (Hb) /hē′məglō′bən/ [Gk *haima* + L *globus* ball], a complex protein-iron compound in the blood that carries oxygen to the cells from the lungs and carbon dioxide away from the cells to the lungs. Each erythrocyte contains 200 to 300 molecules of hemoglobin, each molecule of hemoglobin contains several molecules of heme, and each molecule of heme can carry one molecule of oxygen. A hemoglobin molecule contains four globin polypeptide chains, designated in adults as the alpha (α), beta (β), gamma (γ), and delta (δ) chains. More than 100 hemoglobins with different electrophoretic mobilities and characteristics have been identified and classified, such as S, C, D, and O. New hemoglobins are named for the laboratory, town, or hospital where they are discovered.

hemoglobin A (Hb A), a normal hemoglobin.

hemoglobin A$_2$ (Hb A$_2$), a normal hemoglobin that occurs in small amounts in adults, characterized by the substitution of delta (δ) chains for beta (β) chains.

hemoglobin C, an abnormal type of hemoglobin characterized by the substitution of lysine for glutamic acid at position 6 of the beta (β) chain of the hemoglobin molecule.

hemoglobin C (Hb C) disease, a genetic blood disorder characterized by a moderate, chronic hemolytic anemia and associated with the presence of hemoglobin C, an abnormal form of the red cell pigment.

hemoglobin E disease [Gk *haima* + L *globus,* ball; *E*; Gk *dis* not; Fr *aise* ease], a mild form of anemia caused by a genetic abnormality of the hemoglobin molecule. Worldwide, it is the third most common form of hemoglobin disorder, affecting primarily persons from Southeast Asia and black populations.

hemoglobin electrophoresis, a test to identify various abnormal hemoglobins in the blood, including certain genetic disorders, such as sickle cell anemia.

hemoglobinemia /hē′mōglō′binē′mē·ə, hem′-/, presence of free hemoglobin in the blood plasma.

hemoglobin F (Hb F), the normal hemoglobin of the fetus, most of which is broken down in the first days after birth and replaced by hemoglobin A. It has an increased capacity to carry oxygen and is present in increased amounts in some pathologic conditions.

hemoglobin M disease [Gk *haima* + L *globus* ball; *M*; Gk *dis* not; Fr *aise* ease], a type of anemia in which part of the hemoglobin contains iron in the Fe^{+++} state and is unable to combine with oxygen. The patient may experience cyanosis but is able to function because part of the hemoglobin is normal.

hemoglobinometer /hē′məglō′bən·om′ə-tər/ [Gk *haima* + L *globus* ball; Gk *metron* measure], any of several types of instruments designed to measure the percent of hemoglobin in a blood sample. Some use colorimetric techniques of comparing the color of the blood sample with a standard red color.

hemoglobinopathy /hē′mōglō′binop′əthē, hem′-/ [Gk *haima* + L *globus* ball; Gk *pathos* disease], any of a group of inherited disorders characterized by variation of the structure of the hemoglobin molecule. Kinds of hemoglobinopathies include **hemoglobin C disease, hemoglobin S-C disease,** and **sickle cell anemia.**

hemoglobin oxygen saturation, a quantitative measure of volume of oxygen per volume of blood, depending on the grams of hemoglobin per deciliter of blood.

hemoglobin saturation, the amount of oxygen combined with hemoglobin in proportion to the amount of oxygen the hemoglobin is capable of carrying.

hemoglobin S (Hb S), an abnormal type of hemoglobin, characterized by the substitution of the amino acid valine for glutamic acid in the beta (β) chain of the hemoglobin molecule.

hemoglobin S-C (Hb S-C) disease, a genetic blood disorder in which two different abnormal alleles, one for hemoglobin S and one for hemoglobin C, are inherited.

hemoglobinuria /hē′mōglō′binŏŏr′-ē·ə/ [Gk *haima* + L *globus* ball; Gk *ouron* urine], an abnormal presence in the urine of hemoglobin that is unattached to red blood cells. Kinds of hemoglobinuria include **cold**, **march**, and **nocturnal hemoglobinuria.**

hemoglobinuric, pertaining to the presence of hemoglobin in the urine.

hemoglobin variant, any type of hemoglobin other than hemoglobin A. All variants are characterized by an alteration in the sequence of amino acids in the polypeptide chains of globin contained in the hemoglobin molecule. These variations are genetically determined.

hemoglobin$_{Yakima}$, an abnormal hemoglobin in which histadine replaces aspartic acid at position 99 in the beta (β) chain.

hemogram /hē'məgram/ [Gk *haima* + *gramma* record], a written or graphic record of a differential blood count that emphasizes the size, shape, special characteristics, and numbers of the solid components of the blood.

hemolysin /himol'əsin/ [Gk *haima* + *lysis* loosening], any one of the numerous substances that lyse or dissolve red blood cells. Hemolysins are produced by strains of many kinds of bacteria, including some of the staphylococci and streptococci. They are also contained in venoms and in certain vegetables.

hemolysis /himol'isis/ [Gk *haima* + *lysis* loosening], the breakdown of red blood cells and the release of hemoglobin. It occurs normally at the end of the life span of a red cell, but it may occur under a variety of other circumstances, including certain antigen-antibody reactions, metabolic abnormalities, and mechanical trauma, as in cardiac prosthesis, or exposure to snake venoms. **–hemolytic,** *adj.*

hemolytic anemia /hē'mōlit'ik/ [Gk *haima, lysis* + *a, haima* not blood], a disorder characterized by the premature destruction of red blood cells. Anemia may be minimal or absent, reflecting the ability of the bone marrow to increase production of red blood cells.

hemolytic jaundice, a yellowish discoloration of the skin caused by a breakdown of red blood cells, resulting in excess production of bilirubin.

hemolytic uremia syndrome, a rare kidney disorder marked by renal failure, microangiopathic hemolytic anemia, and platelet deficiency.

hemoperfusion /hē'mōpərfyōō'zhən/, the perfusion of blood through a sorbent device, such as activated charcoal or resin beads, rather than through dialysis equipment. Hemoperfusion may be used in treating uremia, liver failure, and certain forms of drug toxicity.

hemopericardium /hē'mōper'ikär'dē·əm/- [Gk *haima* + *peri* around, *kardia* heart], an accumulation of blood within the pericardial sac surrounding the heart.

hemoperitoneum /hē'mətōper'itōnē'əm/ [Gk *haima* + *peri* around, *tenein* to stretch], the presence of extravasated blood in the peritoneal cavity.

hemophil /hē'mōfil/ [Gk *haima* + *philein* to love], bacteria of the genus *Haemophilus* that thrive in culture media containing blood.

hemophilia /hē'mōfē'lyə, hem'-/ [Gk *haima* + *philein* to love], a group of hereditary bleeding disorders in which there is a deficiency of one of the factors necessary for coagulation of the blood. The two most common forms of the disorder are **hemophilia A** and **hemophilia B**. Greater than usual loss of blood during dental procedures, epistaxis, hematoma, and hemarthrosis are common problems in hemophilia. Severe internal hemorrhage and hematuria are less common. **–hemophiliac,** *n.,* **hemophilic,** *adj.*

hemophilia A, a hereditary blood disorder, transmitted as an X-linked recessive trait, caused by a deficiency of coagulation factor VIII. Hemophilia A is considered the classic type of hemophilia.

hemophilia B, a hereditary blood disorder, transmitted as an X-linked recessive trait, caused by a deficiency of factor IX.

hemophilia C, a hereditary blood disorder, transmitted as an X-linked recessive trait, caused by a deficiency of factor XI.

hemopneumopericardium /hē'mōnōō'- mōper'ikär'dē·əm/ [Gk *haima* + *pneuma* air, *kardia* heart], an accumulation of both blood and air in the pericardium.

hemopneumothorax /hē'mōnōō'mōthô'- aks/ [Gk *haima* + *pneuma* + *thorax* chest], an accumulation of both air and blood in the pleural cavity.

hemopoietic /hē'mōpō·et'ik, hem'-/ [Gk *haima* + *poiein* to make], related to the process of formation and development of the various types of blood cells.

hemoptysis /himop'tisis/ [Gk *haima* + *ptyein* to spit], coughing up of blood from the respiratory tract. Blood-streaked sputum often occurs in minor upper respiratory infections or in bronchitis. More profuse bleeding may indicate *Aspergillus* infection, lung abcess, tuberculosis, or bronchogenic carcinoma.

hemorheology /hē'mōrē·ol'əjē/ [Gk *haima* + *rhoia* flow, *logos* science], the study of the effects of blood flow on the cellular components of blood and walls of blood vessels.

hemorrhage /hem'ərij/ [Gk *haima* + *rhegnynei* to break forth], a loss of a large amount of blood in a short period of time, either externally or internally. Hemorrhage may be arterial, venous, or capillary. Symptoms of massive hemorrhage are related to hypovolemic shock: rapid, thready pulse; thirst; cold, clammy skin; sighing respirations; dizziness; syncope; pallor; apprehension; restlessness; and hypotension. If bleeding is contained within a cavity or joint, pain will develop as the capsule or cavity is stretched by the rapidly expanding volume of blood. **–hemorrhagic,** *adj.*

hemorrhagic diathesis, an inherited predisposition to any one of a number of abnormalities characterized by excessive bleeding.

hemorrhagic disease of newborn, a bleeding disorder of neonates that is usually caused by a deficiency of vitamin K.

hemorrhagic familial angiomatosis. See **Osler-Weber-Rendu syndrome.**

hemorrhagic fever, a group of viral aerosol infections, characterized by fever, chills, headache, malaise, and respiratory or GI symptoms, followed by capillary hemorrhages, and, in severe infection, oliguria, kidney failure, hypotension, and, possibly, death. Many forms of the disease occur in specific geographic areas.

hemorrhagic gastritis, a form of acute gastritis usually caused by a toxic agent, such as alcohol, aspirin or other drugs, or bacterial toxins that irritate the lining of the stomach. If bleeding is significant, vasoconstrictors and ice water lavage of the stomach may be necessary.

hemorrhagic infarct [Gk *haima* + *rhegnynei* to gush; L *infarcire* to stuff], an infarct that has accumulated so much blood that it has a red color.

hemorrhagic jaundice [Gk *haima* + *rhegnynei;* Fr *jaune* yellow], a form of jaundice that occurs in Weil's syndrome, or other forms of leptospirosis in which there is capillary injury and anemia.

hemorrhagic lung. See **congestive atelectasis.**

hemorrhagic measles [Gk *haima* + *rhegnynei;* ME *masalas*], a severe form of measles characterized by bleeding into the skin and mucous membranes.

hemorrhagic pericarditis, an inflammation of the pericardium with a bloody effusion. The condition is frequently caused by tuberculosis or a tumor.

hemorrhagic plague [Gk *haima* + *rhegnynei;* L *plaga* stroke], a severe form of bubonic plague in which there is bleeding under the skin.

hemorrhagic pleurisy, an inflammation

of the pleura in which there in an effusion of blood into the tissues.

hemorrhagic purpura, a form of purpura associated with thrombocytopenia and prolonged bleeding time.

hemorrhagic scurvy. See **infantile scurvy.**

hemorrhagic shock, a state of physical collapse and prostration associated with the sudden and rapid loss of significant amounts of blood. Severe traumatic injuries often cause such blood losses, which, in turn, produce low blood pressure in affected individuals.

hemorrhagic urticaria [Gk *haima* + *rhegnynei;* L *urtica* nettle], a skin eruption in which there is bleeding in the wheals, usually as a complication of another disease, such as nephritis. In some cases, the bleeding occurs first and the wheals become superimposed.

hemorrhoid /hem'əroid/ [Gk *haima* + *rhoia* flow], a varicosity in the lower rectum or anus caused by congestion in the veins of the hemorrhoidal plexus. Internal hemorrhoids originate above the internal sphincter of the anus. If they become large enough to protude from the anus, they become constricted and painful. Small internal hemorrhoids may bleed with defecation. External hemorrhoids appear outside the anal sphincter. They are usually not painful, and bleeding does not occur unless a hemorrhoidal vein ruptures or thromboses. **–hemorrhoidal,** *adj.*

hemorrhoidectomy /hem'əroidek'təmē/, a surgical procedure for excision of a hemorrhoid.

hemosalpinx /hē'mōsal'pinks/ [Gk *haima* + *salpigx* tube], a collection of blood in a fallopian tube.

hemosiderin /hē'mōsid'ərin/ [Gk *haima* + *sideros* iron], an iron-rich pigment that is a product of red cell hemolysis. Iron is often stored in this form.

hemosiderosis /hē'mōsid'ərō'sis, hem'-/ [Gk *haima* + *sideros* iron, *osis* condition], an increased deposition of iron in a variety of tissues, usually in the form of hemosiderin, and usually without tissue damage.

hemostasis /himos'təsis, hē'məstā'sis/ [Gk *haima* + *stasis,* halting], the termination of bleeding by mechanical or chemical means or by the complex coagulation process of the body, consisting of vasoconstriction, platelet aggregation, and thrombin and fibrin synthesis.

hemostat. See **Halsted's forceps.**

hemostatic /hē'mōstat'ik/ [Gk *haima* + *stasis* halting], of or pertaining to a procedure, device, or substance that arrests the flow of blood. Direct pressure, tourniquets, and surgical clamps are mechanical hemostatic measures. Cold applications are hemostatic and include the use of an ice bag on the abdomen to halt uterine bleeding and irrigation of the stomach with an iced solution to check gastric bleeding. Gelatin sponges, solutions of thrombin, and microfibrillar collagen, which causes the aggregation of platelets and the formation of clots, are used to arrest bleeding in surgical procedures.

hemostatic forceps. See **artery forceps.**

hemothorax /hē'mōthôr'aks, hem'-/ [Gk *haima* + *thorax* chest], an accumulation of blood and fluid in the pleural cavity, between the parietal and visceral pleura, usually the result of trauma. Hemothorax may also be caused by the rupture of small blood vessels as a result of inflammation.

hemotroph /hē'mətrof/, the total nutritive substances supplied to the embryo from the maternal circulation after the development of the placenta. **–hemotrophic,** *adj.*

Henderson-Hasselbalch equation [Lawrence J. Henderson, American biochemist, b. 1878; Karl A. Hasselbalch, Danish biochemist, b. 1874], the relationship between pH, the pK_a of a buffer system, and the ratio of the conjugate base and a weak acid.

Henderson, Virginia, a nursing theorist who introduced a holistic approach to nursing in 1966. It is based on the concepts that the body and mind are inseparable, no two individuals are alike, and the role of nursing is independent of the functions of the physician.

Henle's fissure /hen'lēz/ [Friedrich G. J. Henle, German anatomist, b. 1809], one of many patches of connective tissue between the muscle fibers of the heart.

Henle's loop, a U-shaped portion of the renal tubule.

Henoch-Schönlein purpura /hen'ôkhshœn'līn/ [Eduard H. Henoch, German physician, b. 1820; Johannes L. Schönlein, German physician, b. 1793], a self-limited hypersensitivity vasculitis, chiefly of children, characterized by purpuric skin lesions that appear predominantly on the lower abdomen, buttocks, and legs, and usually associated with pain in the knees and ankles. Other joint involvement, GI bleeding, and hematuria are also common findings.

Henry's law [William Henry, English chemist, b. 1774], (in physics) a law stating that the solubility of a gas in a liquid is proportional to the pressure of the gas if the temperature is constant and if the gas does not chemically react with the liquid.

Henschen method, (in radiology) a technique for positioning a patient's head in a true lateral position to produce an x-ray image of the mastoid and petrous portions of the head.

Hensen's knot, Hensen's node. See **primitive node.**

hen worker's lung. See **pigeon breeder's lung.**

heparin /hep'ərin/ [Gk *hepar* liver], a naturally occurring mucopolysaccharide that acts in the body as an antithrombin factor to prevent intravascular clotting. It is produced by basophils and mast cells.

heparin lock flush solution (USP) [Gk *hepar* + OE *loc;* ME *fluschen;* L *solutus* dissolved], a special sterile solution of heparin sodium, saline solution, and benzyl alcohol that is intended for use in maintaining patency in intravenous equipment; not for use in anticoagulant therapy.

heparin rebound, the phenomenon of reactivation of heparin effect occurring from 5 minutes to 5 hours after neutralization with protamine sulfate.

heparin sodium, an anticoagulant prescribed in the treatment and prophylaxis of a variety of thromboembolic disorders.

hepatectomy /hep'ətek'təmē/ [Gk *hepar* + *ektome* cutting out], a surgical procedure to remove a portion of the liver.

hepatic /hepat'ik/ [Gk *hepar* liver], of or pertaining to the liver.

hepatic adenoma, a rapidly growing liver tumor that may become very large and may rupture, causing a lethal internal hemorrhage.

hepatic amebiasis, a disorder characterized by enlargement and tenderness of the liver that often occurs in association with amebic dysentery.

hepatic coma, a neuropsychiatric manifestation of extensive liver damage caused by chronic or acute liver disease. Either endogenous or exogenous waste toxic to the brain is not neutralized in the liver or substances required for cerebral function are not synthesized in the liver. The condition is characterized by variable consciousness, lethargy, stupor, and coma; a tremor of the hands, personality change, memory loss, hyperreflexia, and hyperventilation. Respiratory alkalosis, mania convulsions, and death may occur.

hepatic cord, a mass of cells, arranged in irregular radiating columns and plates, spreading outward from the central vein of the hepatic lobule.

hepatic encephalopathy, a type of brain damage caused by liver disease and consequent ammonia intoxication.

hepatic fistula, an abnormal passage from the liver to another organ or body structure.

hepatic lobes [Gk *hepar* + *lobos* lobes], the large divisions of the liver, including a caudate, quadrate, left, and right divisions.

hepatic node, a node in one of three groups of lymph glands associated with the abdominal and the pelvic viscera supplied by branches of the celiac artery.

hepatic porphyria. See **porphyria.**

hepatic siderosis [Gk *hepar* + *sideros* iron, *osis* condition], a chronic disease in which hemosiderin, an iron-containing pigment, accumulates in the liver and causes a bronze skin pigmentation.

hepatic vein catheterization, the introduction of a long, fine catheter into a hepatic venule for the purpose of recording intrahepatic venous pressure. The catheter is inserted through a vein in the arm.

hepatic veins [Gk *hepar;* L *vena*], the three main veins, the right, middle, and left, that drain the blood of the liver into the inferior vena cava.

hepatin. See **glycogen.**

hepatitis /hep'əti'tis/ [Gk *hepar* + *itis* inflammation], an inflammatory condition of the liver, characterized by jaundice, hepatomegaly, anorexia, abdominal and gastric discomfort, abnormal liver function, clay-colored stools, and dark urine. The condition may be caused by bacterial or viral infection, parasitic infestation, alcohol, drugs, toxins, or transfusion of incompatible blood. Severe hepatitis may lead to cirrhosis and chronic liver dysfunction.

hepatitis A, a form of infectious viral hepatitis caused by the hepatitis A virus (HAV), characterized by slow onset of signs and symptoms. The virus may be spread by direct contact or through fecal-contaminated food or water.

hepatitis B, a form of viral hepatitis caused by the hepatitis B virus (HBV), characterized by rapid onset of acute symptoms and signs. The virus is transmitted in contaminated serum in blood transfusion or by the use of contaminated needles and instruments.

hepatitis B immune globulin (HBIG), a passive immunizing agent prescribed for postexposure prophylaxis against infection by the hepatitis B virus.

hepatitis B surface antigen. See **Australia antigen.**

hepatitis B vaccine, a vaccine prepared from the blood plasma of asymptomatic human carriers of hepatitis B virus or by recombinant DNA techniques. A series of three doses is recommended to achieve immunity.

hepatitis B vaccine (recombinant), a genetically engineered vaccine produced in yeast cells by recombinant DNA technology. The vaccine stimulates immunity against subtypes of the hepatitis B virus. Immunization requires 3 vaccinations by intramuscular injection over a period of 3 months.

hepatitis C (non-A, non-B hepatitis HCV), a type of hepatitis transmitted largely by blood transfusion or percutaneous inoculation as with intravenous drug users sharing needles. The disease progresses to chronic hepatitis in up to 50% of the patients acutely infected. Diagnosis is made through identification of antibodies of HCV.

hepatitis D (delta hepatitis, HDV), a form of hepatitis that occurs only in patients infected with hepatitis B. HDV relies on HBV replication and cannot replicate independently. The disease usually develops into a chronic state. Diagnosis is made by detecting serum antibodies to HDV. It is transmitted sexually and through needle sharing. The only treatment is prevention of HBV.

hepatitis E (epidemic non-A, non-B hepatitis, HEV), a self-limited type of hepatitis that may occur following natural disasters. It is transmitted by fecal-contaminated water or food. No serologic test is currently available.

hepatization /hep'ətizā'shən/ [Gk *hepatizein* like the liver], transformation of lung tissue into a solid mass resembling the liver. In early pneumococcal pneumonia consolidation and effusion of red blood cells in the alveoli produce **red hepatization.** In later stages of pneumococcal pneumonia, when white blood cells fill the alveoli, the consolidation becomes **gray hepatization,** or **yellow hepatization** when infiltrated by fat deposits.

hepatoblastoma /hep'ətōblastō'mə/, a form of liver cancer that tends to occur in children. Hepatoblastoma also may be associated with precocious puberty.

hepatocarcinoma, hepatocellular carcinoma. See **malignant hepatoma.**

hepatocele [Gk *hepar* liver, *kele* hernia], a hernia of a portion of the liver through the diaphragm or the abdominal wall.

hepatocholangitis /hep'ətōkō'lanjī'tis/, an inflammation of both the liver and the bile ducts.

hepatocyte /hep'ətōsīt/ [Gk *hepar* + *kytos* cell], a parenchymal liver cell that performs all the functions ascribed to the liver.

hepatoduodenal ligament /hep'ətōdoo̅'ə-dē'nəl, -doo̅·od'inəl/ [Gk *hepar* + L *duodeni* twelve fingers], the portion of the lesser omentum between the liver and the duodenum, containing the hepatic artery, the common bile duct, the portal vein, lymphatics, and the hepatic plexus of nerves.

hepatogastric ligament /hep′ətōgas′trik/ [Gk *hepar* + *gaster* stomach], the portion of the lesser omentum between the liver and the stomach.

hepatogenous jaundice /hep′ətoj′ənəs/ [Gk *hepar* + *genein* to produce; Fr *jaune* yellow], a type of jaundice caused by a condition of the liver.

hepatojugular /hep′ətōjug′yoŏōlər/ [Gk *hepar* + L, *jugulum* neck], pertaining to the liver and the jugular vein.

hepatojugular reflux [Gk *hepar* + L *jugulum* neck], an increase in jugular venous pressure when pressure is applied for 30 to 60 seconds over the abdomen, suggestive of right-sided heart failure.

hepatolenticular degeneration /həpat′ōlentik′yoŏōlər/ [Gk *hepar* + L *lens* lentil], an abnormal condition associated with defective copper metabolism, characterized by decreased serum ceruloplasmin and copper levels and increased secretion of urinary copper. Individuals with this condition develop tissue deposits of copper associated with hepatic cirrhosis, deep marginal pigmentation of the cornea, and extensive degeneration of the central nervous system.

hepatoma /hep′ətō′mə/, pl. **hepatomas, hepatomata** [Gk *hepar* + *oma* tumor], a primary malignant tumor of the liver characterized by hepatomegaly, pain, hypoglycemia, weight loss, anorexia, ascites, and the presence of alpha-fetoprotein in the plasma.

hepatomegaly /hep′ətōmeg′əlē/ [Gk *hepar* + *megas* large], abnormal enlargement of the liver that is usually a sign of liver disease. Hepatomegaly may be caused by hepatitis or other infection, fatty infiltration, as in alcoholism, biliary obstruction, or malignancy.

hepatopancreatic ampulla /hep′ətōpan′-krē·at′ik/ [Gk *hepar* + *pan* all, *kreas* flesh], the dilatation formed by the junction of the pancreatic and bile ducts as they open into the lumen of the duodenum.

hepatorenal /hep′ətōrēnəl/ [Gk *hepar* + L *ren* kidney], pertaining to the liver and the kidneys.

hepatorenal syndrome, a type of kidney failure in which there is a gradual loss of function but no sign of tissue damage.

hepatosplenomegaly /hep′ətōsplē′nōmeg′-əlē/ [Gk *hepar* + *splen* + *megas* large], enlargement of the spleen and liver.

hepatotoxic /hep′ətōtok′sik/, potentially destructive of liver cells.

hepatotoxicity /hep′ətōtoksis′itē/ [Gk *hepar* + *toxikon* poison, the tendency of an agent, usually a drug or alcohol, to have a destructive effect on the liver.

heptachlor poisoning /hep′təklôr′/ [Gk *hepar* seven; *chloros* green; L *potio* drink], a form of chlorinated organic insecticide poisoning.

heptaploid. See polyploid.

herald patch. See pityriasis rosea.

herb bath /(h)urb/ [L *herba* grass; AS *baeth*], a medicinal bath taken in water containing a decoction of aromatic herbs.

herbicide poisoning /hur′bisīd/ [L *herba* + *caedere* to kill], a poisoning caused by the ingestion, inhalation, or absorption of a substance intended for use as a weed killer or defoliant. Many of the commonly used agricultural herbicides can produce symptoms ranging from skin irritation to hypotension, liver and kidney damage, and coma or convulsions.

herbivorous /hərbiv′ərəs/ [L *herba* + *vorare* to devour], pertaining to feeding on plants or to animals that subsist mostly or entirely on plants.

herd immunity [ME *heord,* group; L, *immunis,* free from], the level of disease resistance of a community or population.

herd instinct [ME *heord;* L *instinctus* impulse], the basic need of social animals, including humans, for the companionship of peers and a tendency to find compatibility with the behavioral standards of others in the group.

hereditability [L *hereditas* inheritance], the degree to which a given trait is controlled by inheritance.

hereditary [L *hereditas* inheritance], pertaining to a characteristic, condition, or disease transmitted from parent to offspring; inborn; inherited.

hereditary ataxia, one of a group of inherited degenerative diseases of the spinal cord, cerebellum, and, often, other parts of the nervous system, characterized by tremor, spasm, wasting of muscle, skeletal change, and sensory disturbances resulting in impaired motor activity. Kinds of hereditary ataxia include **ataxia telangiectasia** and **Friedreich's ataxia.**

hereditary brown enamel. See amelogenesis imperfecta.

hereditary deforming chondroplasia. See diaphyseal aclasis.

hereditary disorder. See inherited disorder.

hereditary elliptocytosis. See elliptocytosis.

hereditary enamel hypoplasia. See amelogenesis imperfecta.

hereditary essential tremor. See essential tremor.

hereditary hemorrhagic telangiectasia. See Osler-Weber-Rendu disease.

hereditary hyperuricemia. See **Lesch-Nyhan syndrome.**

hereditary multiple exostoses, a rare, familial, dyschondroplastic disease in which bony protuberances form on the shafts of the long bones and eventually develop into caps of cartilage covering the ends of the bones.

hereditary opalescent dentin. See **dentinogenesis imperfecta.**

hereditary oral disease, any abnormal condition characterized by genetic defects of oral and paraoral structures, such as deformed dentition, ankyloglossia, hereditary gingivofibromatosis, or cleft palate.

hereditary protoporphyria. See **porphyria.**

hereditary spherocytosis. See **spherocytic anemia.**

hereditary tyrosinemia. See **tyrosinemia.**

heredity [L *hereditas* inheritance], **1.** the process by which particular traits or conditions are genetically transmitted from parents to offspring, resulting in resemblance of individuals related by descent. **2.** the total genetic constitution of an individual; the sum of the qualities inherited from ancestors and the potentialities of transmitting these qualities to offspring.

Hering-Breuer reflexes /her'ing broi'ər/ [Karl E. K. Hering, Austrian physiologist, b. 1834; Joseph Breuer, Austrian psychiatrist, b. 1842], inhibitory and excitatory impulses that maintain the rhythm of respiration and prevent the overdistension of alveoli.

hermaphroditism /hərmaf'rədītiz'əm/ [Gk *Hermaphrodites* son of Hermes and Aphrodite], a rare condition in which both testicular and ovarian tissue exist in the same person, the testicular tissue containing seminiferous tubules or spermatozoa and the ovarian tissue containing follicles or corpora albicantia.

hermetic /hərmet'ik/ [L, *Hermes*], from use in alchemy, pertaining to completely sealing a container so as to make it airtight.

hernia /hur'nē·ə/ [L, rupture], protrusion of an organ through an abnormal opening in the muscle wall of the cavity that surrounds it. A hernia may be congenital, may result from the failure of certain structures to close after birth, or may be acquired later in life because of obesity, muscular weakness, surgery, or illness. Kinds of hernia include **abdominal, diaphragmatic, femoral, hiatus, inguinal,** and **umbilical hernia.** –**hernial,** *adj.*

hernial sac /hur'nē·əl/ [L *hernia;* Gk *sakkos* sack], a pouch of peritoneum into which organs or other tissues pass to form a hernia.

herniated /hur'nē·ā'tid/, a tear or abnormal bulge of an organ or organ part through a retaining tissue.

herniated disk, a rupture of the fibrocartilage surrounding an intervertebral disk, releasing the nucleus pulposus that cushions the vertebrae above and below. The condition most frequently occurs in the lumbar region.

herniated intervertebral disk. See **herniated disk.**

herniation /hur'nē·ā'shən/, a protrusion of a body organ or portion of an organ through an abnormal opening in a membrane, muscle, or other tissue.

herniorrhaphy /hur'nē·ôr'əfē/, the surgical repair of a hernia.

herniotomy /hur'nē·ot'əmē/ [L *hernia;* Gk *tenein* to cut], a surgical procedure to reduce a hernia.

heroin /her'ō·in/ [Ger, originally a trademark for diacetylmorphine], a morphine-like drug with no currently acceptable medical use in the United States. Heroin is included in Schedule I of the Comprehensive Drug Abuse Prevention and Control Act of 1970. As covered in this legislation, it may not be obtained by prescription but only for research and instructional use or for chemical analysis by application to the Drug Enforcement Administration of the Department of Justice. Heroin, like other opium alkaloids, can produce analgesia, respiratory depression, GI spasm, and physical dependence. It produces its major effects on the central nervous system (CNS) and the bowel and alters the endocrine and autonomic nervous systems.

herpangina /hur'panjī'nə/ [Gk *herpein* to creep; L *angina* quinsy], a viral infection, usually of young children, characterized by sore throat, headache, anorexia, and pain in the abdomen, neck, and extremities. Febrile convulsions and vomiting may occur in infants. Papules or vesicles may form in the pharynx and on the tongue, the palate, or the tonsils. The lesions evolve into shallow ulcers that heal spontaneously. The cause is often infection by a strain of coxsackievirus.

herpes genitalis /hur'pēz jen'ital'is/ [Gk *herpein* to creep; L *genitalis* genitalia], an infection caused by Type 2 herpes simplex virus (HSV2), usually transmitted by sexual contact, that causes painful vesicular eruptions on the skin and mucous membranes of the genitalia of males and females. When acquired during pregnancy, HSV2 may be transmitted through the placenta to the fetus and to the newborn by direct contact with infected tissue during birth. In the male, herpes genitalis infections may resemble penile ulcers. A small group of vesicular lesions surrounded by erythematous tissue may occur on the glans or prepuce. The lesions erupt into superficial ulcers that often heal in 5 to 7 days, although they also may become the sites of secondary infections. The lesions are painful and are often associated with a burning sensation, urinary dysfunction, fever, malaise, and swelling of the lymph nodes in the inguinal area. The female patient may exhibit the same or similar systemic effects, and members of both sexes may complain of painful sexual intercourse. In the female, herpes genitalis lesions are likely to appear as multiple superficial eruptions on the surfaces of the cervix, vagina, or perineum. There may be a discharge from the cervix. Vaginal lesions may appear as mucous patches with grayish ulcerations. Laboratory tests from smears of fluid taken from the base of lesions show a positive Tzanck reaction with multiple nucleated giant cells that distinguishes HSV2 infections from other venereal diseases. HSV2 tends to recur.

herpes gestationis [Gk *herpein;* L *gestare* to bear], a generalized, pruritic, vesicular or bullous rash appearing in the second or third trimester of pregnancy and disappearing several weeks postpartum.

herpes labialis. See **herpes simplex.**

herpes menstrualis [Gk *herpein* to creep; L *menstruare*], a form of herpes simplex that tends to erupt during menstrual periods.

herpes simplex [Gk *herpein;* L *simplex* uncomplicated], infection caused by a herpes simplex virus (HSV), which has an affinity for the skin and nervous system and usually produces small, transient, irritating, and sometimes painful fluid-filled blisters on the skin and mucous membranes. HSV1 (oral herpes, herpes labialis) infections tend to occur in the facial area, particularly around the mouth and nose; HSV2 (herpes genitalis) infections are usually limited to the genital region. The initial symptoms of a herpes simplex infection usually include burning, tingling, or itching sensations about the edges of the lips or nose within 1 week or 2 after contact with an infected person. Several hours later, small red papules develop in the irritated area, followed by the eruption of small vesicles, or fever blisters, filled with fluid. Several small vesicles may merge to form a larger blister. The vesicles generally are associated with itching, pain, or similar discomfort. Other effects often include a mild fever and enlargement of the lymph nodes in the neck. Within 1 week after the onset of symptoms, thin yellow crusts form on the vesicles as healing begins.

herpesvirus /hur′pēzvī′rəs/ [Gk *herpein* + L *virus* poison], any of seven related viruses including herpes simplex viruses 1 and 2, varicella-zoster virus, Epstein-Barr virus, and cytomegalovirus, HHV6 and HHV7.

herpesvirus hominis. See **herpes simplex.**

herpes zoster /hur′pēz zos′tər/ [Gk *herpein; zoster* girdle], an acute infection caused by reactivation of the latent varicella-zoster virus (VZV), affecting mainly adults and characterized by the development of painful vesicular skin eruptions that follow the underlying route of cranial or spinal nerves inflamed by the virus. Distribution of the pain and vesicular eruptions is usually unilateral, although both sides of the body may be involved. Any sensory nerve may be affected, but the virus in most cases tends to invade the posterior root ganglia associated with thoracic and trigeminal nerves. The pain, which may be constant or intermittent, superficial or deep, usually precedes other effects and may mimic other disorders, such as appendicitis or pleurisy. Early symptoms may include GI disturbances, malaise, fever, and headache. The vesicles usually evolve from small red macules along the path of a nerve, and the skin of the area is hypersensitive. All the lesions may appear within a period of hours, but they most often develop gradually over a period of several days. The macules vesiculate and, after about 3 days, become turbid with cellular debris. Usually, at the end of the first week, the vesicles develop crusts. The symptoms may persist for 3 to 5 weeks, but in most cases they diminish after 2 weeks.

herpes zoster ophthalmicus, a form of herpes zoster, causing pain and skin eruptions along the ophthalmic branch of the fifth cranial nerve. The infection frequently leads to corneal ulceration or other ocular complications.

herpes zoster oticus, a herpes zoster infection of the eighth cervical nerve ganglia and geniculate ganglion, causing severe pain in the external ear structures and pain or paralysis along the facial nerve. The disease may also result in hearing loss and vertigo.

herpes zoster virus. See **chickenpox.**

herpetic keratitis /hərpet′ik/ [Gk *herpein* to creep, *keras* horn, *itis*], an inflammation of the cornea caused by a herpes virus.

herpetic neuralgia [Gk *herpein, neuron*

nerve, *algos* pain], a form of neuralgia with intractable pain that develops at the site of a previous eruption of herpes zoster.

herpetic stomatitis [Gk *herpein, stoma* mouth, *itis*], a form of inflammation of the mouth caused by a herpes virus infection.

herpetiform /hɜrpet'ifôrm'/ [Gk *herpein* + L *forma* form], having clusters of vesicles; resembling the skin lesions of some herpesvirus infections.

Hers' disease /herz, hurz/ [H. G. Hers, twentieth-century French pathologist; L *dis* opposite of; Fr *aise* ease], an uncommon metabolic disorder of glycogen storage, characterized by hepatomegaly and an accumulation of abnormally large amounts of glycogen in the liver as a result of its inability to break down glycogen. There is no known treatment.

hertz (Hz) /hurts, herts/ [Heinrich R. Hertz, German physicist, b. 1857], a unit of measurement of wave frequency equal to one cycle per second (cps).

Herxheimer's reaction /herks'hī'mərz/, an increase in symptoms after administration of a drug. The reaction was originally discovered in penicillin treatment of syphilis, but has been found to occur with other diseases as well.

Herzog taping protocol, a procedure for immobilizing and balancing a foot with tape after a musculoskeletal injury.

Heschl's gyrus /hesh'əl/ [Richard Ladislaus Heschl, Austrian pathologist, b. 1824; Gk *gyros* turn], any of several small gyri running transversely on the upper surface of the temporal operculum of the insula of the cortex.

hesperidin /hesper'idin/, a crystalline flavone glycoside found in bioflavonoid and occurring in most citrus fruits, especially in the spongy casing of oranges and lemons.

hetastarch /het'əstärch/, a plasma volume extender prescribed as an adjunct in shock and leukophoresis.

heterauxesis. See allometric growth.

heteroallele /het'ərō·əlēl'/ [Gk *heteros* different, *alleolon* of one another], one of a set of genes located at a specific locus on homologous chromosomes that differs from the other of the pair, resulting in a mutation. **–heteroallelic,** *adj.*

heteroblastic /het'ərōblas'tik/ [Gk *heteros* + *blastos* germ], developing from different germ layers or kinds of tissue rather than from a single type.

heterocephalus /het'ərōsef'ələs/ [Gk *heteros* + *kephale* head], a malformed fetus that has two heads of unequal size. **–heterocephalous, heterocephalic,** *adj.*

heterochromatin /het'ərōkrō'mətin/ [Gk *heteros* + *chroma* color], that portion of chromosome material that is inactive in gene expression but may function in controlling metabolic activities, transcription, and cell division.

heterochromatinization, the transformation of genetically active euchromatin into genetically inactive heterochromatin; the inactivation of one of the X chromosomes in the mammalian female during the early stages of embryogenesis.

heterochromosome /het'ərōkrō'məsōm/, a sex chromosome. **–heterochromosomal,** *adj.*

heterodidymus /het'ərōdid'iməs/ [Gk *heteros* + *didymos* twin], a conjoined twin fetus in which the parasitic elements consist of a head, neck, and thorax attached to the thoracic wall of the autosite.

heteroduplex /het'ərōd͞o͞o'pleks/ [Gk *heteros* + L *duoplicare* to double], (in molecular genetics) a DNA molecule in which the two strands are derived from different individuals, with the result that some pairs or blocks of base pairs may not match.

heteroeroticism /het'ərō·irot'isiz'əm/ [Gk *heteros* + *eros* love], sexual feeling or activity directed toward another individual.

heterogamete /het'ərōgam'ēt/ [Gk *heteros* + *gamete* spouse], a gamete that differs considerably in size and structure from the one with which it unites, specifically denoting those of higher organisms as opposed to those of lower plants and animals.

heterogamy /het'ərog'əmē/ [Gk *heteros* + *gamos* marriage], **1.** sexual reproduction in which there is fusion of dissimilar gametes, usually differing in size and structure. **2.** reproduction by the alternation of sexual and asexual generations; heterogenesis. **–heterogamous,** *adj.*

heterogeneous /het'əroj'ənəs/ [Gk *heteros* + *genos* kind], **1.** consisting of dissimilar elements or parts; unlike; incongruous. **2.** not having a uniform quality throughout. **–heterogeneity,** *adj.*

heterogenesis /het'ərōjen'əsis/ [Gk *heteros* + *genein* to produce], **1.** reproduction that differs in successive generations, as the alternation of sexual with asexual reproduction, so that offspring have characteristics different from those of the parents. **2.** asexual generation. **3.** abiogenesis. **–heterogenetic, heterogenic,** *adj.*

heterogenous /het'əroj'ənəs/ [Gk *heteros* + *genos* kind], derived or developed from another source or from two different sources.

heterogenous vaccine [Gk *heteros* + *genein* to produce; L *vaccinus* cow], a vaccine made from a source other than the patient's own tissues.

heterogeny. See **heterogenesis.**

heterograft. See **xenograft.**

heteroinfection /het′ərō·infek′shən/ [Gk *heteros* + L *inficere* to stain], an infection from a microorganism originating outside the body.

heterologous. See **xenogeneic.**

heterologous anaphylaxis /het′ərol′əgəs/ [Gk *heteros* + *logos* relation, *ana* again, *phylaxis* protection], a form of passive anaphylaxis involving the transfer of serum between two animals of the same species.

heterologous insemination. See **artificial insemination-donor.**

heterologous tumor [Gk *heteros* + *logos* relation], a neoplasm consisting of tissue different from that of its site.

heterologous twins. See **dizygotic twins.**

heterometropia /het′ərōmətrō′pē·ə/ [Gk *heteros* + *metron* measure, *ops* eye], a generally mild visual disorder in which one eye refracts differently than the other, resulting in slightly different images being perceived by the right and left eyes.

heteronymous /het′əron′iməs/ [Gk *heteros* + *onyma* name], **1.** having different names; the opposite of synonymous. **2.** an optical phenomenon in which two images are produced by one object.

heterophil(e) /het′ərofil′/ [Gk *heteros* + *philein* to love], a condition of affinity for something unusual or abnormal, as an antibody that reacts to an antigen other than the one it is expected to challenge.

heterophil antibody test, a test for the presence of heterophil antibodies in the serum of patients suspected of having infectious mononucleosis, based on an agglutination reaction between heterophil antibodies in a person's serum and heterophil antigen.

heterophilic leukocyte [Gk *heteros* + *philein, leukos* white, *kytos* cell], a neutrophil of certain animal species that takes an acid stain.

heteroplastic transplantation [Gk *heteros* + *plassein* to mold; L *transplantare*], the transfer of tissue from one animal to another of a different species.

heteroploid /het′ərəploid′/ [Gk *heteros* + *ploos* times, *eidos* form], **1.** of or pertaining to an individual, organism, strain, or cell that has a variation in the number of whole chromosomes characteristic for the somatic cell of the species. **2.** such an individual, organism, strain, or cell.

heteroploidy /het′ərəploi′dē/, the state or condition of having an abnormal number of chromosomes, either more or less than

that characteristic of the somatic cell of the species.

heteropolymer /het′ərəpol′imir/ [Gk *heteros* + *polys* many, *meros* part], a compound formed from subunits that are not all the same, as a protein composed of various amino acid subunits.

heterosexual /het′ərōsek′shəl/ [Gk *heteros* + L *sexus* male or female], **1.** a person whose sexual desire or preference is for people of the opposite sex. **2.** of or pertaining to sexual desire or preference for people of the opposite sex. **–heterosexuality,** *n.*

heterosexual panic, an acute attack of anxiety resulting in the frantic pursuit of heterosexual activity in response to unconscious or latent homosexual impulses.

heterosis /het′ərō′sis/ [Gk *heteros* + *osis* condition], the superiority of first generation hybrid plants and animals in respect to one or more traits when compared with either of the parent strains or with corresponding inbred strains.

heterotopic ossification /het′ərōtop′ik/ [Gk *heteros* + *topos* place], a nonmalignant overgrowth of bone, frequently occurring after a fracture, that is sometimes confused with certain bone tumors when visualized on x-ray film.

heterotopic transplantation [Gk *heteros* + *topos* place; L *transplantare*], the transfer of tissue from one part of a body of a donor to another area of the body of a recipient.

heterotransplant /het′ərōtrans′plant/ [Gk *hetero* + L *transplantare*], the transfer of tissue from one animal to another of a different species.

heterotypic /het′ərōtip′ik/ [Gk *heteros* + *typos* pattern], pertaining to or characteristic of a type differing from the usual or the normal, specifically regarding the first meiotic division of germ cells in gametogenesis as distinguished from the second or mitotic division.

heterotypic chromosomes, any unmatched pair of chromosomes, specifically the sex chromosomes.

heterotypic mitosis, the division of bivalent chromosomes, as occurs in the first meiotic division of germ cells in gametogenesis; a reduction division.

heterozygosis /het′ərōzīgō′sis/ [Gk *heteros* + *zygosis* joining], **1.** the formation of a zygote by the union of two gametes that have dissimilar pairs of genes. **2.** the production of hybrids through crossbreeding. **–heterozygotic,** *adj.*

heterozygote /het′ərōzī′gōt/ [Gk *heteros* + *zygotos* yoked], an organism whose somatic cells have two different allelomorphic genes on the same locus of each pair of chromosomes. It can produce two different types of gametes.

heterozygote detection, the use of amniocentesis and other techniques to identify potential inherited X-linked recessive disorders, such as **Hunter's syndrome** or Duchenne's muscular dystrophy.

heterozygous /het'ərəzī'gəs/ [Gk *heteros* + *zygotos* yoked], having two different genes at corresponding loci on homologous chromosomes. An individual who is heterozygous for a particular characteristic has inherited a gene for that characteristic from one parent and the alternative gene from the other parent.

heuristic /hyo͞oris'tik/ [Gk *heuriskein* to discover] **1.** serving to stimulate interest for further investigation. **2.** a teaching method in which the student is encouraged to learn through independent research and investigation. **3.** a method of argument that postulates what is to be proved.

hexachlorophene /hek'səklôr'əfēn/, a topical antiinfective and detergent used as an antiseptic scrub and as a disinfectant for inanimate objects.

hexafluorenium bromide /hek'səflo͞orē'nē·əm/, an inhibitor of acetylcholinesterase. It is used as an adjunct to anesthesia to prolong the skeletal muscle relaxation caused by succinylcholine.

hexamethonium /hek'səməthō'nē·əm/, a cholinergic blocking agent used to control bleeding and in the treatment of peptic ulcers and hypertension.

hexamethylenamine. See **methenamine.**

hexamethylmelamine /hek'səmeth'ilmel'-əmēn/, an experimental antineoplastic that has been used to treat bronchogenic, cervical, and ovarian carcinomas.

hexanoic acid. See **caproic acid.**

hexaploid. See **polyploid.**

hexenmilch. See **witch's milk.**

hexocyclium methylsulfate /hek'səsi'-klē·əm/, an anticholinergic prescribed as an adjunct to ulcer therapy.

hexokinase /hek'səkī'nās/ [Gk *hex* six, *glykys* sweet, *kinein* to move, *ase* enzyme], an enzyme that catalyzes the transfer of a phosphate group from adenosine triphosphate to D-glucose.

hexose /hek'sōs/ [Gk *hex* six, *glykys* sweet], a monosaccharide that contains six carbon atoms in the molecule. Glucose and fructose are the principal hexoses found in nature.

hexylcaine hydrochloride /hek'silkān/, a local anesthetic for use on intact mucous membranes of the respiratory, upper GI, and urinary tracts.

hexylresorcinol, /hek'ilrəsôr'sənol/ a topical skin anesthetic that is also admin-

istered for the treatment of certain types of worm infestations.

Hf, symbol for the chemical element **hafnium.**

Hg, symbol for the chemical element **mercury.**

HGF, an abbreviation for **human growth factor; hyperglycemic-glycogenolytic factor.**

HHS, abbreviation for **Department of Health and Human Services.**

hiatus /hī·ā'təs/ [L, gap], a usually normal opening in a membrane or other body tissue. **–hiatal,** *adj.*

hiatus aorticus [L *hiare* to yawn; Gk *ae-rein* to raise], an opening in the diaphragm for the aorta and thoracic duct.

hiatus esophagus [L *hiare;* Gk *oisophagos* gullet], the opening in the diaphragm for the esophagus.

hiatus hernia, protrusion of a portion of the stomach upward through the diaphragm. The major difficulty in symptomatic patients is gastroesophageal reflux, the backflow of the acid contents of the stomach into the esophagus.

Hib disease, an infection caused by *Haemophilus influenzae* type b (Hib), which affects mainly children in the first 5 years of life. It is a leading cause of bacterial meningitis as well as pneumonia, joint or bone infections, and throat inflammations.

hibakusha /hē'bäko͞o'shä/ [Jap], persons who have been exposed to atomic bomb explosions. In 1985, some 370,000 hibakusha still lived in Hiroshima and Nagasaki, more than 40 years after the World War II atomic bomb attacks. Their average age was over 60.

hibernoma /hī'bərnō'mə/, *pl.* **hibernomas, hibernomata** [L *hibernus* winter; Gk *oma* tumor], a benign tumor, usually on the hips or the back, composed of fat cells that are partly or entirely of fetal origin.

hiccup, a characteristic sound that is produced by the involuntary contraction of the diaphragm, followed by rapid closure of the glottis. Hiccups have a variety of causes, including indigestion, rapid eating, certain types of surgery, and epidemic encephalitis. Also spelled **hiccough.**

hickory stick fracture. See **greenstick fracture.**

hidradenitis. See **hydradenitis.**

hidrosis /hidrō'sis, hī-/ [Gk *hidros* sweat], sweat production and secretion. **–hidrotic,** *adj.*

high-altitude edema [ME *heigh;* L *altitudo;* Gk *oidema* swelling], a form of pulmonary edema that occurs in persons who move rapidly into altitudes. Fluid accumulates in the lungs as atmospheric pressure decreases.

high blood pressure. See **hypertension.**

high-calorie diet, a diet that provides 1,000 or more calories a day beyond what is ordinarily recommended. It may be prescribed for nursing mothers, patients with severe weight loss caused by illness, or persons with abnormally high metabolic rates or energy requirements.

high-density lipoprotein (HDL) [AS *heah* top; L *densus* thick; Gk *lipos* fat, *proteios* first rank], a plasma protein containing about 50% protein (apoprotein) with cholesterol and triglycerides. It may serve to stabilize very low-density lipoprotein and is involved in transporting cholesterol and other lipids from the plasma to the tissues.

high enema [ME *heigh;* Gk *einienai* to send in], an enema that is inserted into the colon through a long catheter.

high-energy phosphate compound, a chemical compound containing a high-energy bond between phosphoric acid residues and certain organic substances. When the bond is hydrolyzed, a large amount of energy is released.

highest intercostal vein [AS *heah* top; L *inter* between, *costa* rib, *vena* vein], one of a pair of veins that drain the blood from the upper two or three intercostal spaces.

high-flow oxygen delivery system, respiratory care equipment that supplies inspired gases at a preset oxygen concentration.

high forceps, an obstetric operation in which forceps are used to deliver a baby whose head is not engaged in the birth canal. The procedure is considered hazardous and is generally condemned.

high-Fowler's position [AS *heah* top; George R. Fowler, American surgeon, b. 1848], placement of the patient in a semisitting position by raising the head of the bed more than 20 inches.

high-frequency hearing loss [ME *heigh;* L *frequens;* AS *déaf*], a loss of ability to hear high-frequency sounds. It is most commonly associated with aging or noise exposure. Hearing loss may begin in early adulthood with a loss of hearing to frequencies in the range of 18 to 20 kHz. Around the age of 60, loss of hearing may begin to affect lower frequencies, in the range of 4 to 8 kHz. Hearing loss due to noise exposure is greatest at 4kHz.

high-frequency ventilation (HFV), a technique for providing ventilatory support to patients by operating at a breathing rate of 60 breaths per minute or more. **High-frequency jet ventilation (HFJV)** is a type using a high-pressure gas source that has a respiratory rate of 100 to 400 cycles per minute. **High-frequency oscillation (HFO)** is a form that forces small impulses of gas in and out of the airway at frequencies of 400 to 4,000 per minute.

high labial arch, a labial arch wire adapted to lie gingival to the anterior tooth crowns, having auxiliary springs that extend downward in contact with the teeth to be moved.

high-level wellness, a concept of optimal health that emphasizes the integration of body, mind, and environment to maximize the function of an individual.

high-potassium diet, a diet that contains foods rich in potassium, including all leafy green vegetables, brussels sprouts, citrus fruits, bananas, dates, raisins, legumes, meats, and whole grains. It is indicated for conditions resulting in the loss of extracellular fluid.

high-protein diet, a diet that contains large amounts of protein, consisting largely of meats, fish, milk, legumes, and nuts. It may be indicated in protein depletion from any cause.

high-residue diet [ME *heigh* + L *residuum* remaining; Gk *diaita* life-style], a diet that contains a greater than usual proportion of substances the digestive tract will not metabolize and absorb, such as fiber and other cellulose products.

high-risk infant, any neonate, regardless of birth weight, size, or gestational age, who, because of preconceptual, prenatal, natal, or postnatal conditions or circumstances that interfere with the normal birth process or impede adjustment to extrauterine growth and development, has a greater than average chance of morbidity or mortality, especially within the first 28 days of life.

high-speed handpiece, a rotary or vibratory cutting instrument that operates at high speeds, powered by a conventional dental engine and propelled by gears, a belt drive, or turbine.

high-vitamin diet, a dietary regimen that includes a variety of foods that contain therapeutic amounts of all of the vitamins necessary for the metabolic processes of the body. It is often ordered in combination with other therapeutic diets containing larger than usual amounts of protein or calories, especially when treating severe or chronic infection, malnutrition, or vitamin deficiency.

hilar /hī'lär/ [L *hilum* a little thing], pertaining to a hilum.

Hill-Burton Act, a 1946 amendment to the U.S. Public Health Service Act authorizing grants to states for surveying their hospital and public health center needs and for the planning and construction of additional facilities.

Hill-Burton programs, a cluster of programs created by legislation included in the National Health Planning and Resources Development Act of 1974. The programs allow federal monetary assistance for modernization of health facilities, construction of outpatient health centers, construction of inpatient facilities in underserved areas, and the conversion of existing health care facilities for the provision of new health services.

hilum /hī'ləm/, *pl.* **hili** [L *hilum* a trifle], a depression or pit at that part of an organ where vessels and nerves enter.

hindbrain [ME *hind;* AS *bragen*], the division in the brain of an embryo that eventually becomes the pons, the medulla oblongata, and the cerebellum.

hindgut [ME *hind;* AS *guttas*], the caudal portion of the embryonic alimentary canal.

hind kidney. See **metanephros.**

hinge axis, the joint where the mandible meets the skull and the point of rotation of the mandible.

hinge axis-orbital plane, a craniofacial plane that is usually determined by marking three points on the face of the patient. Two of the points, one on each side of the face, are located on the hinge axis. The third point is located on the face at the level of the orbital rim just beneath the eye.

hinged knee, an appliance designed to protect and support the knee during activity. It consists of an elastic sleeve with bars hinged at the axis of the knee joint and stabilized with straps.

hinge joint [AS *hangian* to hang; ME *jointe* a connection], a synovial joint providing a connection in which articular surfaces are closely molded together in a manner that permits extensive motion in one plane.

hip. See **coxa.**

hip bath. See **sitz bath.**

hipbone. See **innominate bone.**

hip joint. See **coxal articulation.**

hip-joint disease [AS *hype;* L *jungere* to join], any abnormal condition of the hip joint, such as **Perthes' disease** or congenital dislocation of the hip.

Hippel's disease, von Hippel-Lindau disease [Eugen von Hippel, German ophthalmologist, b. 1867; Arvid Lindau, Swedish pathologist, b. 1892], a familial disease involving the retina and first described by Hippel. It is characterized by hemangioblastomas of the cerebellar hemispheres, angiomatosis of the retina, and cysts of the kidneys and pancreas.

hippocampal /hip'ōkam'pəl/ [Gk *hippokampos* seahorse], pertaining to the hippocampus, an elongated, curved eleva-

tion projecting into the temporal horn of the lateral ventricle of the brain.

hippocampal commissure [Gk *hippokampos;* L *commissura* a joint], a thin, triangular layer of transverse fibers that connects the medial edges of the posterior pillars of the fornix.

hippocampal fissure, a fissure reaching from the posterior aspect of the corpus callosum to the tip of the temporal lobe.

hippocampal formation [Gk *hippokampos;* L *formatio*], a part of the rhinencephalon, including the dentate gyrus, longitudinal striae, and hippocampus.

hippocampal gyrus [Gk *hippokampos, gyros* turn], a convolution on the medial side of the temporal lobe of the cerebral cortex.

hippocampus /hip'ōkam'pəs/, *pl.* **hippocampi** [Gk *hippokampos* seahorse], a curved convoluted elevation of the floor of the inferior horn of the lateral ventricle of the brain.

hippocampus minor. See **calcar avis.**

Hippocrates /hipok'rətēz/, a Greek physician born about 460 BC on the island of Cos, a center for the worship of Æsculapius. Called the "Father of Medicine," Hippocrates introduced a scientific approach to healing.

Hippocrates' bandage. See **capeline bandage.**

Hippocratic oath /hip'əkrat'ik/, an oath, attributed to Hippocrates, that serves as an ethical guide for the medical profession. It is traditionally incorporated into the graduation ceremonies of medical colleges.

hippuric acid [Gk *hippos* horse, *ouron* urine; L *acidus* sour], a detoxication product in the urine of some animals. It has been used as a medication in the treatment of arthritic diseases.

hip replacement [AS *hype*], replacement of the hip joint with an artificial ball and socket joint, performed to relieve a chronically painful and stiff hip in advanced osteoarthritis, an improperly healed fracture, or degeneration of the joint. Antibiotic therapy is begun preoperatively, and the patient is taught to walk with crutches. The femoral head, neck, and part of the shaft are removed, and the contours of the socket are smoothed. A prosthesis of a durable, hard metal alloy or stainless steel is shaped to resemble a femur and head of a femur and is attached to the femur with screws or an acrylic cement; a metal or a plastic acetabulum is implanted.

Hirschberg's reflex /hursh'bəwrgz/, a diagnostic test for pyramidal tract disease. The test result is regarded as positive if inversion of the foot occurs when the sole is stroked at the base of the great toe.

Hirschfeld-Dunlop file, a kind of periodontal file, used with a pull stroke to remove tooth calculus. Various models with different angulations are available for different tooth surfaces.

Hirschfeld's method [Isador Hirschfeld, American dentist, b. 1881], a toothbrushing technique in which the bristles are placed against the axial surfaces of the teeth at a slight incisal or occlusal angle and in contact with the teeth and gingivae, then vigorously rotated in very small circles.

Hirschsprung's disease /hirsh′sproͦongz/ [Harald Hirschsprung, Danish physician, b. 1831], the congenital absence of autonomic ganglia in the smooth muscle wall of the colon, resulting in poor or absent peristalsis in the involved segment of colon, accumulation of feces, and dilatation of the bowel (megacolon). Symptoms include intermittent vomiting, diarrhea, and constipation. The abdomen may become distended to several times its normal size.

hirsutism /hur′sootiz′əm/ [L hirsutus shaggy], excessive body hair in a masculine distribution as a result of heredity, hormonal dysfunction, porphyria, or medication. Treatment of the specific cause will usually stop growth of more hair. **–hirsute,** adj., **hirsuteness,** n.

hirsutoid papilloma of the penis /hur′sootoid/ [L hirsutus shaggy; Gk eidos form], a condition characterized by clusters of small, white papules on the coronal edge of the glans penis.

His. See **histidine.**

His bundle. See **bundle of His.**

His bundle electrogram (HBE) [Wilhelm His, Jr., German physician, b. 1863], (in cardiology) a direct recording of the electric activity in the bundle of His.

His-Purkinje system /his′pərkin′jē/ [Wilhelm His, Jr.; Johannes E. Purkinje, Czechoslovakian physiologist, b. 1787], the conduction system in the cardiac tissues from the bundle of His to the distal Purkinje fibers.

histamine /his′təmēn, -min/ [Gk histos tissue; L amine ammonia], a compound, found in all cells, produced by the breakdown of histidine. It is released in allergic, inflammatory reactions and causes dilatation of capillaries, decreased blood pressure, increased secretion of gastric juice, and constriction of smooth muscles of the bronchi and uterus.

histamine headache, a headache associated with the release of histamine from the body tissues and marked by symptoms of dilated carotid arteries, fluid accumulation under the eyes, tearing or lacrimation, and rhinorrhea (runny nose).

histamine-proved achlorhydria [Gk histos + amine, a not, chlorhydria hydrochloric acid], the absence of normal hydrochloric acid production by cells in the lining of the stomach as demonstrated by the **histamine test.**

histamine test [Gk histos + amine; L testum crucible], a test for achylia gastrica, or the lack of hydrochloric acid in the stomach. The stomach is emptied and washed out before subcutaneous injection of 0.1% histamine to stimulate gastric acid secretion. The stomach is aspirated continuously. If no acid is produced, it is considered evidence that the stomach is not producing hydrochloric acid.

histidine (His) /his′tidēn/ [Gk histos tissue], a basic amino acid found in many proteins and a precursor of histamine. It is an essential amino acid in infants.

histidinemia /his′tidinē′mē·ə/, an inherited metabolic disorder affecting the amino acid histidine. The condition leads to retardation and nervous system disorders.

histiocyte. See **macrophage.**

histiocytic leukemia. See **monocytic leukemia.**

histiocytic malignant lymphoma /his′tē-ōsit′ik/ [Gk histos + kytos cell], a lymphoid neoplasm containing undifferentiated primitive cells or differentiated reticulum cells.

histiotypic growth /his′tē·ōtip′ik/ [Gk histos + typos mark], the uncontrolled proliferation of cells, as occurs in bacterial cultures and molds.

histocompatibility /his′tōkəmpat′ibil′itē/ [Gk histos + L compatibilis agreeing], the compatibility of the antigens of donor and recipient of transplanted tissue.

histocompatibility antigens, a group of genetically determined antigens on the surface of many cells. Histocompatibility antigens are the cause of most graft rejections.

histocompatibility gene, the gene that determines histocompatibility between the donor and recipient of transplanted tissue.

histocompatibility locus, a set of positions on a chromosome occupied by a complex of genes that govern several tissue antigens.

histocyte /his′təsīt/ [Gk histion web, kytos cell], a macrophage of connective tissue that plays a role in the body's immune system.

histogram /his′təgram′/ [Gk histos + gramma record], (in research) a graph showing the values of one or more variables plotted against time or against frequency of occurrence.

histography /histog'rəfē/ [Gk *histos* + *graphein* to record], the process of describing or creating visualizations of tissues and cells. **–histographer,** *n.,* **histographic,** *adj.,* **histographically,** *adv.*

histoid neoplasm [Gk *histos* + *eidos* form; *neos* new, *plassein* to mold], a growth that resembles the tissues in which it originates.

histoincompatible, pertaining to host and donor tissues that have different genotypes and are therefore likely to induce an immune response, leading to rejection of a tissue graft or organ transplant.

histologic [Gk *histos* + *logos* science], pertaining to the study of the anatomy and physiology of tissue cells.

Histologic Technician/Technologist, an allied health professional who works in a clinical laboratory preparing sections of body tissue for examination by a pathologist. This includes preparation of tissue specimens of human and animal origin for diagnostic, research, or teaching purposes. The tissue sections enable the pathologist to diagnose body dysfunction and malignancy. Histotechnicians process sections of body tissue by fixation, dehydration, embedding, sectioning, decalcification, microincineration, mounting, and routine and special staining.

histologist /histol'əjist/, a medical scientist who specializes in the study of histology.

histology /histol'əjē/ [Gk *histos* + *logos* science] **1.** the science dealing with the microscopic identification of cells and tissue. **2.** the structure of organ tissues, including the composition of cells and their organization into various body tissues. **–histologic, histological,** *adj.,* **histologically,** *adv.*

histone /his'tōn/ [Gk *histos* tissue], any of a group of strongly basic, low molecular weight proteins that are soluble in water, insoluble in dilute ammonia, and combine with nucleic acid to form nucleoproteins. They are found in the cell nucleus.

histopathology /his'tōpəthol'əjē/ [Gk *histos* + *pathos* disease, *logos* science], the study of diseases involving the tissue cells.

histoplasma agglutinin /his'tōplaz'mə/ [Gk *histos* + *plasma* a formation], an agglutinin associated with fungal lung infections.

Histoplasma capsulatum, [Gk *histos, plasma* + L *capsula* little box], a dimorphic fungal organism that is a single budding yeast at body temperature and a mold at room temperature. It is the causative organism in histoplasmosis.

histoplasmosis /his'tōplazmō'sis/ [Gk *histos, plasma* + *osis* condition], an infection caused by inhalation of spores of the fungus *Histoplasma capsulatum.* **Primary histoplasmosis** is characterized by fever, malaise, cough, and lymphadenopathy. Spontaneous recovery is usual; small calcifications remain in the lungs and affected lymph glands. **Progressive histoplasmosis,** the sometimes fatal, disseminated form of the infection, is characterized by ulcerating sores in the mouth and nose, enlargement of the spleen, liver, and lymph nodes, and severe and extensive infiltration of the lungs.

history [L *historia* inquiry], **1.** a record of past events. **2.** a systematic account of the medical and psychosocial occurrences in a patient's life and of factors in family, ancestors, and environment that may have a bearing on the patient's condition.

history of present illness, an account obtained during the interview with the patient of the onset, duration, and character of the present illness, as well as of any acts or factors that aggravate or ameliorate the symptoms.

histotoxin /his'tōtok'sin/ [Gk *histos* + *toxikon* poison], any substance that is poisonous to the body tissues. It is usually generated from within the body rather than being introduced externally. **–histotoxic,** *adj.*

histotroph, histotrophe, histotrophic nutrition. See **embryotroph.**

histrionic /his'trē·on'ik/ [L *histrio* actor], pertaining to exaggerated facial expressions, speech, or body movements, as used on the stage.

histrionic paralysis [L *histrio;* Gk *paralysein*], a condition, such as **Bell's palsy,** in which paralysis of facial muscles result in a histrionic effect.

histrionic personality [L *histrio; persona* role played], a personality characterized by behavioral patterns and attitudes that are overreactive, emotionally unstable, overly dramatic, and self-centered, exhibited as a means of attracting attention, consciously or unconsciously.

histrionic personality disorder, a disorder characterized by dramatic, reactive, and intensely exaggerated behavior, which is typically self-centered and results in severe disturbance in interpersonal relationships that can lead to psychosomatic disorders, depression, alcoholism, and drug dependency.

His-Werner disease [Wilhelm His, Jr., German physician, b. 1863; Heinrich Werner, German physician, b. 1874], trench fever, an acute louse-borne infection that affected soldiers, mainly in World War I.

HIV, abbreviation for **human immuno-deficiency virus.**

hives. See **urticaria.**

HLA, abbreviation for **human leukocyte antigen.**

HLA-A, abbreviation for *human leukocyte antigen A.*

HLA-B, abbreviation for *human leukocyte antigen B.*

HLA complex, human leukocyte group A, the major human histocompatibility complex that enables the immune system to differentiate tissues or proteins between "self" and "nonself." It consists of groups of loci on the short arm of chromosome 6. They are identified by numbers and letters, such as HLA-B27. HLA-A, -B, and -C are cell surface antigens that occur on the surface of all nucleated cells and and platelets and are important in tissue transplants. If donor and recipient HLA antigens do not match, the non-self antigens are recognized and destroyed by killer T cells.

HLA-D, abbreviation for *human leukocyte antigen D.*

HLH, abbreviation for *human luteinizing hormone.*

HMD, abbreviation for **hyaline membrane disease.**

HMG-CoA reductase, a rate-controlling enzyme of cholesterol synthesis.

HMO, abbreviation for **Health Maintenance Organization.**

Ho, symbol for the chemical element **holmium.**

H₂O, symbol for **water.**

Hô, symbol for **null hypothesis.**

Hodgkin's disease /hoj'kinz/ [Thomas Hodgkin, English physician, b. 1798], a malignant disorder characterized by painless, progressive enlargement of lymphoid tissue, usually first evident in cervical lymph nodes; splenomegaly; and the presence of Reed-Sternberg cells, large, atypical macrophages with multiple or hyperlobulated nuclei and prominent nucleoli. Symptoms include anorexia, weight loss, generalized pruritus, low-grade fever, night sweats, anemia, and leukocytosis. Total lymphoid radiotherapy, using a covering mantle to protect other organs, is the treatment of choice for early stages of the disease; combination chemotherapy is the treatment for advanced disease.

Hodgson's disease /hoj'sənz/ [Joseph Hodgson, English physician, b. 1788], an aneurysmal dilatation of the aorta.

Hoffmann's atrophy. See **Werdnig-Hoffmann disease.**

Hoffmann's reflex [Johann Hoffmann, German neurologist, b. 1857], an abnormal reflex elicited by sudden, forceful flicking of the nail of the index, middle, or ring finger, resulting in flexion of the thumb and of the middle and distal phalanges of one of the other fingers.

holandric /holan'drik/ [Gk *holos* whole, *aner* man] **1.** designating genes located on the nonhomologous portion of the Y chromosome. **2.** of or pertaining to traits or conditions transmitted only through the paternal line.

holandric inheritance, the acquisition or expression of traits or conditions only through the paternal line, transmitted by genes carried on the nonhomologous portion of the Y chromosome.

hold-relax, a technique of proprioceptive neuromuscular facilitation used in treating hypertonicity or motor dysfunction. It is often applied when there is muscle tightness on one side of a joint and when immobility is the result of pain.

holism /hō'lizəm/ [Gk *holos* whole], a philosophic concept in which an entity is seen as more than the sum of its parts. Also spelled **wholism.**

holistic /hōlis'tik/ [Gk *holos*], of or pertaining to the whole; considering all factors, as holistic medicine. Also **wholistic.**

holistic counseling, an alternative form of psychotherapy that focuses on the whole person (mind, body, and spirit) and health.

holistic health care, a system of comprehensive or total patient care that considers the physical, emotional, social, economic, and spiritual needs of the person, the response to the illness, and the impact of the illness on the person's ability to meet self-care needs.

Hollenback condenser. See **pneumatic condenser.**

Holliday-Segar formula, a method of estimating the daily caloric needs of the average hospital patient under conditions of bed rest, based on the body weight in kilograms of the patient.

hollow cathode lamp [ME *holg;* Gk *kata* down, *hodos* way; *lampas*], a lamp consisting of a metal cathode and an inert gas. It emits a line spectrum of specific wavelengths related to the metal of the cathode.

holmium (Ho) /hōl'mē·əm/ [L *Holmia* Stockholm, Sweden], a rare earth metallic element. Its atomic number is 67; its atomic weight is 164.93.

holoacardius /hol'ō·ākär'dē·əs/ [Gk *holos* + *kardia* heart], a separate, grossly defective monozygotic twin fetus in which the heart is absent and the circulation in utero is accomplished totally by the heart of the viable twin through a vascular shunt.

holoacardius acephalus, a grossly defective separate twin fetus that lacks a heart, a head, and most of the upper portion of the body.

holoacardius acormus, a grossly defective, separate twin fetus in which the trunk is malformed and little more than the head is recognizable.

holoacardius amorphus, a malformed separate twin fetus in which there are no recognizable or formed parts.

holoarthritis /hol′ō·ärthrī′tis/, a form of arthritis that involves all or most of the joints.

holoblastic /hol′əblas′tik/ [Gk *holos* icpl *blastos* germ], of or pertaining to an ovum that contains little or no yolk and undergoes total cleavage.

holocephalic /hō′lōsifal′ik/ [Gk *holos* + *kephale* head], a malformed fetus in which several parts are deficient although the head is complete.

holocrine /hol′əkrēn/ [Gk *holos* + *krinein* to secrete], pertaining to a gland whose only function is to secrete or whose secretion consists of disintegrated cells of the gland itself

holocrine secretion, a secretion that consists of disintegrated or altered cells of the gland itself, as in the example of sebaceous glands.

holodiastolic. See **pandiastolic.**

holoenzyme /hol′ō·en′zīm/ [Gk *holos* + *en* in, *zymos* ferment], a complete enzyme-cofactor complex that gives full catalytic activity.

holographic reconstruction, a method of producing three-dimensional images with diagnostic ultrasound equipment.

hologynic /hol′ōjin′ik/ [Gk *holos* + *gyne* female] **1.** designating genes located on attached X chromosomes. **2.** of or pertaining to traits or conditions transmitted only through the maternal line.

hologynic inheritance, the acquisition or expression of traits or conditions only through the maternal line, transmitted by genes located on attached X chromosomes. The phenomenon is not known to occur in humans.

holoprosencephaly /hol′ōpros′ensef′əlē/ [Gk *holos* + *pro* before, *enkephalos* brain], a congenital defect characterized by multiple midline facial defects, including cyclopia in severe cases. **–holoprosencephalic, holoprosencephalous,** *adj.*

holorachischisis. See **complete rachischisis.**

holosystolic. See **pansystolic.**

Holter monitor [L *monere* to remind], a device for making prolonged electrocardiograph recordings on a portable tape recorder while the patient conducts normal

daily activities. The patient may also keep an activity diary for the purpose of comparing daily events with ECG tracings.

Holtzman inkblot technique, a modification of the Rorschach test in which many more pictures of inkblots are used, the subject is permitted only one response to each design, and the scoring is predominantly objective rather than subjective.

Homan's sign [John Homan, American surgeon, b. 1877; L *signum* mark], pain in the calf with dorsiflexion of the foot, indicating thrombophlebitis or thrombosis.

home assessment [ME *h/m;* L *assidire* to sit beside], an examination of the living area of a physically challenged person for the purposes of making recommendations about elimination of safety hazards and suggesting architectural or other modifications that would lead to independent functioning of the patient.

home care [AS *ham* village; L *garrire* to chatter], a health service provided in the patient's place of residence for the purpose of promoting, maintaining, or restoring health or minimizing the effects of illness and disability. Service may include medical, dental, and nursing care, speech and physical therapy, homemaking services, or the provision of transportation.

home health agency, an organization that provides health care in the home. Medicare certification for a home health agency is dependent on the providing of skilled nursing services and of at least one additional therapeutic service.

home maintenance management, impaired, a NANDA-accepted nursing diagnosis of a situation in which a person is unable to maintain a safe, healthy home environment without help. Defining characteristics include difficulty in maintaining the home in a comfortable condition, such as having unwashed or unavailable cooking utensils, clothes, or linens, or the presence of accumulations of dirt, food, waste, and refuse, and repeated infections and infestations resulting from a lack of hygiene; a need for help from the outside in maintaining the home, with exhausted or distressed family or household members; and the existence of debt or a financial crisis.

homeodynamics /hō′mē·ədinam′iks/ [Gk *homoios* similar, *dynamis* force], the constantly changing interrelatedness of body components while maintaining an overall equilibrium.

homeopathic [Gk *homoios* + *pathos* disease], pertaining to the medical practice of **homeopathy,** a system based on a concept that the cure of a disease is effected by drugs "proved" to be capable of producing similar symptoms of the disease in a healthy person. The patient is then treated with minute doses of the "proved" drug. The concept of *similia similibus curenter* (like cures like) was first advanced by Hippocrates around 400 BC.

Homeopathic Pharmacopoeia of the United States, one of the three official drug compendia specified in the Federal Food, Drug, and Cosmetic Act.

homeopathist /hō′mē·op′əthist/, a physician who practices **homeopathy.**

homeopathy /hō′mē·op′əthē/ [Gk *homoios* + *pathos* disease], a system of therapeutics based on the theory that "like cures like." The theory was advanced in the late eighteenth century by Dr. Samuel Hahnemann, who believed that a large amount of a particular drug may cause symptoms of a disease and moderate dosage may reduce those symptoms; thus, some disease symptoms could be treated by very small doses of medicine. –**homeopathic,** *adj.*

homeostasis /hō′mē·əstā′sis/ [Gk *homoios* + *stasis* standing still], a relative constancy in the internal environment of the body, naturally maintained by adaptive responses that promote healthy survival. Various sensing, feedback, and control mechanisms function to effect this steady state. Some of the functions controlled by homeostatic mechanisms are the heartbeat, hematopoiesis, blood pressure, body temperature, electrolytic balance, respiration, and glandular secretion. –**homeostatic,** *adj.*

homeotypic /hō′mē·ōtip′ik/ [Gk *homoios* + *typos* mark], pertaining to or characteristic of the regular or usual type, specifically applied to the second meiotic division of germ cells in gametogenesis as distinguished from the first meiotic division. Also **homeotypical.**

homeotypic mitosis, the equational division of chromosomes, as occurs in the second meiotic division of germ cells in gametogenesis.

Home's silver precipitation method, (in dentistry) a technique for depositing silver in enamel and dentin by the application of ammoniac silver nitrate solution and its reduction with formalin or eugenol.

homicide [L *homo* man, *caedere* to kill], the death of one human being caused by another human. Homicide is usually intentional and often violent.

hominal physiology [L *hominis* human; Gk *physis* nature, *logos* science], the study of the specific physical and chemical processes involved in the normal functioning of humans; human physiology.

hominid /hom′inid/ [L *homo* man; Gk *ei-*

dos form], pertaining to the primate family, *Hominidae,* which includes humans.

homiothermal. See **warm-blooded.**

homiothermic /hom′ē·əthur′mik/ [Gk *homos* same, *therme* heat], pertaining to the ability of warm-blooded animals to maintain a relatively stable internal temperature regardless of the temperature of the environment. This ability is not fully developed in newborn humans.

homoblastic /hō′mōblas′tik/ [Gk *homos* + *blastos* germ], developing from the same germ layer or a single type of tissue.

homochronous inheritance /hōmok′rənəs/ [Gk *homos* + *chronos* time], the appearance of traits or conditions in the offspring at the same age as they appeared in the parents.

homocystinuria /hō′mōsis′tinŏŏr′ē·ə/ [Gk *homos* + (cystine); Gk *ouron* urine], a rare biochemical abnormality characterized by the abnormal presence of homocystine, an amino acid, in the blood and urine, caused by any of several enzyme deficiencies in the metabolic pathway of methionine to cystine. –**homocystinuric,** *adj.*

homogenate /hōmoj′ənit/, a tissue that is or has been made homogenous.

homogeneous /hōmoj′ənəs/ [Gk *homos* + *genos* kind], **1.** consisting of similar elements or parts. **2.** having a uniform quality throughout. –**homogeneity,** *adj.*

homogenesis /hō′mōjen′əsis/ [Gk *homos* + *genesis* origin], reproduction by the same process in succeeding generations so that offspring are similar to the parents.

homogenetic /hō′mōjenet′ik/, **1.** of or pertaining to homogenesis. **2.** homogenous.

homogenized /hōmoj′ənīzd/ [Gk *homos* + *genein* to produce], the state of having undergone homogenization, or making something the same texture or consistency throughout.

homogenized milk [Gk *homos* + *genos* kind], pasteurized milk that has been mechanically treated to reduce and emulsify the fat globules so that the cream cannot separate and the protein is more digestible.

homogenous /hōmoj′ənəs/ [Gk *homos* + *genos* kind] **1.** homogeneous. **2.** having a likeness in form or structure because of a common ancestral origin. –**homoplasty.**

homogentisic acid. See **glycosuric acid.**

homogeny /hōmoj′ənē/ [Gk *homos* + *genos* kind] **1.** homogenesis. **2.** a likeness in structure or form because of a common ancestral origin.

homograft. See **allograft.**

homolateral /hō′mōlat′ərəl/, pertaining to the same side of the body.

homolateral limb synkinesis, a condition of hemiplegia in which there appears to be a mutual dependency between the affected upper and lower limbs. Efforts at flexion of an upper extremity cause flexion of the lower extremity.

homolog /hom'əlog/ [Gk *homologos* same relation] **1.** any organ corresponding in function, origin, and structure to another organ, as the flippers of a seal that correspond to human hands. **2.** (in chemistry) one of a series of compounds, each formed by an added common element; for example, CO, carbon monoxide, is followed by CO_2, carbon dioxide, with the addition of an oxygen atom. Also spelled **homologue.** **–homologous,** *adj.*

homologous anaphylaxis /hōmol'əgəs/ [Gk *homos* same, *logos* relation, *ana* back, *phylaxis* protection], a form of passive anaphylaxis in which serum from an animal of the same species is transferred.

homologous chromosomes [Gk *homologos* same relation; *chroma* color, *soma* body], any two chromosomes in the diploid complement of the somatic cell that are identical in size, shape, and gene loci. In humans there are 22 pairs of homologous chromosomes and one pair of sex chromosomes.

homologous disease. See **graft-versus-host reaction.**

homologous graft, a tissue removed from a donor for transplanting to a recipient of the same species.

homologous insemination. See **artificial insemination—husband.**

homologous organs, body parts of different species that are structural equivalents, like the arms of humans and the forelegs of dogs and cats.

homologous tumor, a neoplasm made up of cells resembling those of the tissue in which it is growing.

homonymous /hōmon'iməs/ [Gk *homos* same, *onyma* name], having the same name or sound.

homonymous diplopia, a type of diplopia in which the image seen by the right eye is to the right of the image seen by the left eye.

homonymous hemianopia [Gk *homos* + *onyma* name], blindness or defective vision in the right or left halves of the visual fields of both eyes.

homophobia /hō'mōfō'bē·ə/ [Gk *homos* + *phobos* fear], the fear of or prejudice against homosexuals.

homoplastic transplantation [Gk *homos* + *plassein* to mold; L *transplantare*], the homologous transplantation of tissue from one human to another or from one animal to another of the same species.

homoplasty /hō'məplas'tē/ [Gk *homos* + *plassein* to mold], having a likeness in form or structure acquired through similar environmental conditions or parallel evolution rather than because of common ancestral origin. **–homoplastic,** *adj.*

homopolymer /hō'mōpol'imir/ [Gk *homos* + *poly* many, *meros* part], a compound formed from subunits that are the same, as a carbohydrate composed of a series of glucose units.

Homo sapiens /hō'mō sā'pē·əns, hō'mō sä'pē·ens/ [L *homo* human, *sapere* to know or taste], the scientific term for the genus and species idenifying humans.

homosexual /hō'mōsek'shəl/ [Gk *homos* + L *sexus* male or female], **1.** of, pertaining to, or denoting the same sex. **2.** a person who is sexually attracted to members of the same sex.

homosexual panic, an acute attack of anxiety based on unconscious conflicts concerning gender identity and a fear of being homosexual.

homosexual sexual intercourse [Gk *homos* same; L *sexus* male or female, *intercursus* interposition], sexual activity between members of the same sex ranging from feelings and fantasies to kissing and genital, oral, or anal contact.

homothermal. See **warm-blooded.**

homovanillic acid /hō'mōvənil'ik/, an acid that is produced by normal metabolism of dopamine and may be elevated in the urine in association with tumors of the adrenal gland.

homozygosis /hō'mōzīgō'sis/ [Gk *homos* + *zygon* yoke] **1.** the formation of a zygote by the union of two gametes that have one or more pairs of identical genes. **2.** the production of purebred organisms or strains through the process of inbreeding.

homozygote /hō'mōzī'gōt/ [Gk *homos* + *zygon* yoke], an organism whose somatic cells have identical genes on the same locus on one of the chromosome pairs.

homozygous /hō'məzī'gəs/ [Gk *homos* + *zygon* yoke], having two identical genes at corresponding loci on homologous chromosomes.

homunculus /hōmung'kyələs/, *pl.* **homunculi** [L, little man], **1.** a dwarf in which all the body parts are proportionally developed and in which there is no deformity or abnormality. **2.** (in early embryologic theories of development) a minute and complete human being contained in each of the germ cells that after fertilization grows from the microscopic to normal size. **3.** a small anatomic model of the human form; a manikin. **4.** (in psychiatry) a little man created by the imagination who possesses magical powers.

hook grasp, a type of prehension in which an object is grasped with the fingers alone.

hookworm [AS *hok, wyrm*], nontechnical. a nematode of the genera *Ancylostoma, Necator,* or *Uncinaria*. Most hookworm infections in the western hemisphere are caused by the species *Necator americanus.*

hookworm disease [AS *hok, wyrm*], a roundworm infestation that may involve either of two serious intestinal parasites of humans, *Ancylostoma duodenale* or *Necator americanus.* Both forms of the disease are characterized by abdominal pain and iron-deficiency anemia. The worms enter the human body as larvae by penetrating the skin, traveling to the lungs via the circulatory system, and ascending the respiratory tract, where they are swallowed. In the intestinal tract, the hookworms attach their mouths to the mucosa and subsist on the blood of the host.

hopelessness [AS *hopian* to hope, *laes* less, *ness* condition], a NANDA-accepted nursing diagnosis of a state in which an individual sees limited or no alternatives or personal choices available and is unable to mobilize energy on his or her own behalf. Defining characteristics include passivity, decreased verbalization, decreased affect, verbal cues with a despondent content, lack of initiative, decreased response to stimuli, decreased appetite, increased sleep, and lack of involvement in care or passivity in allowing care.

hordeolum /hôrdē´ələm/ [L *hordeum* barley], a furuncle of the margin of the eyelid originating in the sebaceous gland of an eyelash. Also called **sty.**

horizon [Gk *horizein* to encircle], a specific stage of human embryonic development based on the appearance and ultimate formation of certain anatomic characteristics. The classification comprises 23 stages, each lasting 2 to 3 days, beginning with the fertilization of the ovum.

horizontal angulation [Gk *horizein* to encircle; L *angularis* angle], (in dentistry) the measured angle within the occlusal plane at which the primary x-ray beam is directed, relative to a reference in the vertical or sagittal plane.

horizontal fissure of the right lung, a cleft that marks the separation of the upper and middle lobes of the right lung.

horizontal plane [Gk *horizein;* L *planum* level ground], **1.** any plane of the erect body parallel to the horizon, dividing the body into upper and lower parts. **2.** a plane passing through a tooth at right angles to its long axis.

horizontal pursuit, a visual screening test in which the patient is asked to follow with both eyes a target moving in a horizontal plane while the examiner observes accuracy of alignment and other factors.

horizontal resorption, a pattern of bone reduction in marginal periodontitis whereby the marginal crest of the alveolar bone between adjacent teeth remains level and the bases of the periodontal pockets are supracrestal.

horizontal transmission, the spread of an infectious agent from one person or group to another, usually through contact with contaminated material, such as sputum or feces.

hormic psychology /hôr´mic/ [Gk *hormaien* to begin action], (in psychology) the school that stresses the purposive, goal-oriented nature of human behavior.

hormone [Gk *hormaien* to begin action], a complex chemical substance produced in one part or organ of the body that initiates or regulates the activity of an organ or a group of cells in another part of the body. Hormones secreted by the endocrine glands are carried through the bloodstream to the target organ. **–hormonal,** *adj.*

hormone therapy, the treatment of diseases with hormones obtained from endocrine glands or substances that simulate hormonal effects.

horn, a projection or protuberance on a body structure. An example is the iliac horn.

Horner's syndrome [Johann F. Horner, Swiss ophthalmologist, b. 1831], a neurologic condition characterized by miotic pupils, ptosis, and facial anhidrosis, resulting from a lesion in the spinal cord, with damage to a cervical nerve.

horny layer. See **stratum corneum.**

horripilation. See **pilomotor reflex.**

horse serum [AS *hors;* L *serum* whey], immune serum, especially tetanus antitoxin, prepared from the blood of a horse. Because many people are sensitive to horse serum, a skin test for sensitivity is usually performed before immunization.

horseshoe fistula [AS *hors, scoh* shoe], an abnormal, semicircular passage in the perianal area with both openings on the surface of the skin.

horseshoe kidney, a relatively common congenital anomaly characterized by an isthmus of parenchymal tissue connecting the two kidneys at the lower poles.

Hortega cells. See **microglia.**

Horton's arteritis. See **temporal arteritis.**

Horton's headache. See **migrainous cranial neuralgia.**

Horton's histamine cephalalgia. See histamine headache.

hospice /hos'pis/ [L *hospes* host], a system of family-centered care designed to assist the chronically ill person to be comfortable and to maintain a satisfactory lifestyle through the terminal phases of dying.

hospital [L *hospitium* guesthouse], a health-care facility that provides inpatient beds, continuous nursing services, and an organized medical staff. Diagnosis and treatment are provided to both surgical and medical patients for a variety of diseases and disorders.

hospital-acquired infection. See nosocomial infection.

hospitalism, the physical or mental effects of hospitalization or institutionalization on patients, especially infants and children in whom the condition is characterized by social regression, personality disorders, and stunted growth.

Hospital Survey and Construction Act. See Hill-Burton Act.

host [L *hospes*], **1.** an organism in which another, usually parasitic, organism is nourished and harbored. A **primary** or **definitive host** is one in which the adult parasite lives and reproduces. A **secondary,** or **intermediate host** is one in which the parasite exists in its nonsexual, larval stage. A **reservoir host** is a primary animal host for organisms that are sometimes parasitic in humans and from which humans may become infected. **2.** the recipient of a transplanted organ or tissue.

host defense mechanisms, a group of body protective systems, including physical barriers and the immune response, that normally guard against infective organisms.

hostility [L *hostilis* of the enemy], the tendency of an organism to threaten harm to another or to itself. The hostility may be expressed passively and actively.

hot bath [AS *hat, baeth*], a bath in which the temperature of the water is gradually raised to about 106° F.

hot compress [AS *hat*; L *comprimere* to press together], a heated pad of damp, thickly folded cloth applied to an area to reduce pain or inflammation.

hot flash, a transient sensation of warmth experienced by some women during or after menopause. Hot flashes result from autonomic vasomotor disturbances that accompany changes in the neurohormonal activity of the ovaries, hypothalamus, and pituitary.

hot line, a means of contacting a trained counselor or specific agency for help with a particular problem, as a rape hot line or a battered child hot line. The person needing help calls a telephone number and speaks to a counselor who remains anonymous.

hot spot, (in molecular genetics) a site in a gene sequence at which mutations occur with an unusually high frequency.

Hounsfield unit /hounz'fēld/, (in computed tomography) the numeric information contained in each pixel. It is used to represent the density of tissue.

hour glass uterus [Gk *hora*; AS *glaes*;], a uterus in which a segment of circular muscle fibers contract during labor, causing constriction ring dystocia.

housekeeping department, a unit of a hospital staff responsible for cleaning the hospital premises and furnishings, including control of pathogenic organisms.

housemaid's knee [AS *hus, maeden; cneow* knee], a chronic inflammation of the bursa in front of the kneecap, characterized by redness and swelling. It is caused by prolonged and repetitive pressure of the knee on a hard surface.

house organ, a publication designed for distribution to the employees or members of an institution or business.

house physician [AS *hus*; Gk *physikos* natural], a physician on call and immediately available in a hospital or other health care facility.

house staff, the interns and residents who are employed at a hospital while receiving additional training after graduation from medical college.

house surgeon, a surgeon on call and immediately available on the premises of a hospital.

housewives' eczema [AS *hus, wif*; Gk *ekzein* to boil over], *nontechnical.* contact dermatitis of the hands caused and exacerbated by their frequent immersion in water and by the use of soaps and detergents.

Houston's valves. See plicae transversales recti.

Howell-Jolly bodies /hou'əljol'ē/, spheric and granular inclusions in the erythrocytes observed on microscopic examination of stained blood smears.

HPG, abbreviation for *human pituitary gonadotropin.*

HPL, abbreviation for **human placental lactogen.**

HPV, 1. abbreviation for **human papilloma virus. 2.** abbreviation for **human parvovirus.**

hr, abbreviation for **hour.**

HRIG, abbreviation for *human rabies immune globulin vaccine.*

hs, h.s., abbreviation for the Latin *hora somni,* or at bedtime.

HSA, abbreviation for **health systems agency.**

HSV, abbreviation for *herpes simplex virus.*

HSV1, abbreviation for *herpes simplex type 1.* See **herpes simplex.**

ht, abbreviation for **height.**

Hubbard tank [Carl P. Hubbard, American engineer, b. 1857; Port *tanque*], a tank containing warm water in which patients perform underwater exercise. The water provides buoyancy and heat for the benefit of weakened or painful muscles, or joints with limited active range of motion.

huffing, a type of forced expiration with an open glottis to replace coughing when pain limits normal coughing.

Huhner test /hoo′nər/, a test for male fertility in which a semen sample is examined for spermatozoa activity.

Huhn's gland, an anterior lingual gland imbedded in tissues on the inferior surface and near the apex and midline of the tongue.

human bite [L *humanus;* AS *bitan*], a wound caused by the piercing of skin by human teeth. Bacteria are usually present, and serious infection often follows.

human chorionic gonadotropin (HCG). See **chorionic gonadotropin.**

human chorionic somatomammotropin (HCS), a hormone produced by the syncytiotrophoblast during pregnancy. It regulates carbohydrate and protein metabolism of the mother.

human diploid cell rabies vaccine (HDCV), an inactivated rabies virus vaccine prepared from rabies virus grown in human diploid cell cultures. Active immunization with HDCV begins on the day of exposure, followed by four or five additional injections. Passive immunization with **human rabies immune globulin (RIG)** may be given concurrently with HDCV.

human ecology, the study of interrelationships between individuals and their environments, as well as among individuals within the environment.

human immunodeficiency virus (HIV) /h(y)oo′mən im′yoonōdifish′ənsē/ [L *humanus, immunis* free from, *de* from, *facere* to make, *virus* poison], a type of retrovirus that causes AIDS. Retroviruses produce the enzyme reverse transcriptase that allows transcription of the viral genome onto the DNA of the host cell. It is transmitted through contact with an infected individual's blood, semen, cervical secretions, cerebrospinal fluid, or synovial fluid. HIV infects T-helper cells of the immune system and results in infection with a long incubation period, averaging 10

years. With the immune system destroyed, **AIDS** develops as opportunistic infections, such as **Kaposi's sarcoma, pneumocystis carinii pneumonia, candidiasis,** and **tuberculosis,** that attack organ systems throughout the body. Aside from the initial antibody tests that establish the diagnosis for HIV infection, the most important laboratory test for monitoring the infection is the CD4 lymphocyte test. It determines the percentage of T lymphocytes that are CD4 positive; CD4 counts of greater than 500 per cubic mm are considered most likely to respond to treatment with alpha-interferon and/or zidovudine. A significant drop in the CD4 count is a signal for therapeutic intervention with antiretroviral therapy. Vaccines based on gp120 and gp160 HIV coat glycoproteins, to boost the immune system of persons already infected with HIV, are being investigated.

human insulin, a biosynthetic product manufactured from two forms of *Escherichia coli* using recombinant DNA technology. The advantages of human insulin are in eliminating allergic reactions that occur with the use of animal insulins.

human investigations committee, a committee established in a hospital, school, or university to review applications for research involving human subjects, to protect the rights of the people to be studied.

humanistic existential therapy, a kind of psychotherapy that promotes self-awareness and personal growth by stressing current reality and by analyzing and altering specific patterns of response to help realize the potential of a person. Kinds of humanistic existential psychotherapy are **client-oriented, existential,** and **Gestalt therapy.**

humanistic nursing model, a conceptual framework in which the nurse-patient relationship is analyzed as a human-to-human event rather than a nurse-to-patient interaction.

humanistic psychology, a branch of psychology that emphasizes a person's struggle to develop and maintain an integrated, harmonious personality as the primary motivational force in human behavior.

human leukocyte antigen (HLA), any one of four significant genetic markers identified as specific loci on chromosome 6. They are HLA-A, HLA-B, HLA-C, and HLA-D. Each locus has several genetically determined alleles; each of these is associated with certain diseases or conditions.

human liver fluke. See **liver fluke.**

human natural killer cells, lymphocytes that are able to lyse tumor and virally infected cells as part of the body's natural defense against malignancy and invasion by pathogens.

human papilloma virus (HPV), a virus that is the cause of common warts of the hands and feet, as well as lesions of the mucous membranes. The virus can be transmitted through sexual contact and is frequently found in women with cancer of the cervix.

human parvovirus (HPV), a small, single-stranded DNA virion that has been associated with several diseases, including erythema infectiosum and aplastic crises of chronic hemolytic anemias.

human placental lactogen (HPL), a placental hormone that may be deficient in certain abnormalities of pregnancy.

human prion diseases [L *humanus; Proteinaceous Infection Particle*], a group of neurodegenerative diseases that are unique in having both infectious and genetic etiologies. Examples include **Creutzfeldt-Jakob disease (CJD)** and **Gerstmann-Straussler syndrome.** A homozygous prion protein genotype predisposes in the diseases.

human protein C, an anticoagulant, produced by genetically engineered bacteria, that inactivates coagulation cofactors 5 and 8c and mediates clot lysis by tissue plasminogen activator (t-PA).

human rhinovirus 14, the common cold virus. It has a complex protein coat containing "sticky sites" that help attach the virus to cell receptors in the upper respiratory system. More than 100 strains of the virus are known, making it difficult to devise a vaccine that would protect against all variations.

human subjects investigation committee. See **human investigations committee.**

human synthetic growth hormone. See **Humatrope.**

Humatrope, a trademark for a brand of human synthetic growth hormone produced with recombinant DNA techniques. It is a polypeptide hormone with 191 amino acids in the same sequence as **somatotropin,** the human growth hormone produced by the pituitary gland.

humectant /hyōōmek′tənt/, a substance that promotes retention of moisture.

humeral. See **humerus.**

humeral articulation. See **shoulder joint.**

humerus /hyōō′mərəs/, *pl. humeri* [L, shoulder], the largest bone of the upper arm, comprising a body, a head, and a condyle. The nearly hemispheric head articulates with the glenoid cavity of the scapula. The condyle at the distal end has several depressions into which articulate the radius and ulna.   **–humeral,** *adj.*

humidification [L *humiditas* moist; *facere* to make], the process of increasing the relative humidity of the atmosphere around a patient through the use of aerosol generators or steam inhalators that exert an antitussive effect. Humidification acts by decreasing the viscosity of bronchial secretions.

humidifier, a machine designed to adjust the amount of moisture in the atmosphere of a room or respiratory device.

humidity [L *humidus* moist], pertaining to the level of moisture in the atmosphere, the amount varying with the temperature. The percentage is usually represented in terms of **relative humidity,** with 100% being the point of air saturation or the level at which the air can absorb no additional water.

humor /hyōō′mər/ [L *humor* moisture], any body fluid such as blood or lymph. The term is often used in referring to the **aqueous humor** or the **vitreous humor** of the eye.

humoral immunity /hyōō′mərəl/ [L *humor* liquid; *immunis* freedom], one of the two forms of immunity that respond to antigens such as bacteria and foreign tissue. Humoral immunity is the result of circulating antibodies carried in the immunoglobulins IgA, IgB, and IgM.

humoral response, one of a broad category of hypersensitivity reactions. Humoral responses are mediated by B cell lymphocytes and occur in type I, type II, and type III hypersensitivity reactions.

hung-up reflex, a deep tendon reflex in which, after a stimulus is given and the reflex action takes place, there is a slow return of the limb to its neutral position.

Hunner's ulcer. See **interstitial cystitis.**

Hunter's canal. See **adductor canal.**

Hunter's syndrome [Charles Hunter, twentieth-century English physician; Gk *syn* together, *dromos* course], a hereditary defect in mucopolysaccharide metabolism affecting only males, characterized by dwarfism, kyphosis, gargoylism, and mental retardation.

Huntington's chorea [George S. Huntington, American physician, b. 1851; Gk *choreia* dance], a rare, abnormal hereditary condition characterized by chronic, progressive chorea and mental deterioration that terminates in dementia. An individual afflicted with the condition usually shows the first signs in the fourth decade of life and dies about 15 years later.

Hunt's tremor. See **cerebellar tremor.**

Hurler's syndrome [Gertrude Hurler, German physician, b. 1920], a type of mucopolysaccharidosis, transmitted as an autosomal-recessive trait, that results in severe mental retardation. Facial characteristics include a low forehead and enlargement of the head. Corneal clouding is common, and the neck is short. Marked kyphosis is apparent at the dorsolumbar level, and the hands and the fingers are short and broad.

Hürthle cell adenoma /hirt′lə, hōōrth′lē/ [Karl W. Hürthle, German histologist, b. 1860], a benign tumor of the thyroid gland composed of large cells with granular eosinophilic cytoplasm (Hürthle cells).

Hürthle cell carcinoma, a malignant neoplasm of the thyroid gland composed of Hürthle cells.

Hürthle cell tumor, a neoplasm of the thyroid gland composed of large cells with granular eosinophilic cytoplasm (Hürthle cells); it may be benign **(Hürthle cell adenoma)** or malignant **(Hürthle cell carcinoma).**

husband-coached childbirth. See **Bradley method.**

Hutchinson's disease. See **angioma serpiginosum.**

Hutchinson's freckle [Jonathan Hutchinson, English surgeon, b. 1828], a tan patch on the skin that grows slowly, becoming mottled, dark, thick, and nodular. The lesion is usually seen on one side of the face of an elderly person.

Hutchinson's teeth [Jonathan Hutchinson], a characteristic of congenital syphilis in which the permanent incisor teeth are peg-shaped, widely spaced, and notched at the end with a centrally placed crescent-shaped deformity.

Hutchinson's triad [Jonathan Hutchinson], the interstitial keratitis, notched teeth, and deafness characteristic of congenital syphilis.

Hutchison-type neuroblastoma [Robert G. Hutchison, English physician, b. 1871; Gk typos mark], a neuroblastoma that has metastasized to the cranium.

HVA, abbreviation for **homovanillic acid.**

HV interval (HBE), (in cardiology) the conduction time through the His-Purkinje system, measured from the earliest onset of the His potential to the onset of ventricular activation.

hyaline /hī′əlin/ [Gk hyalos glass], pertaining to substances that are clear or glasslike.

hyaline bodies [Gk hyalos; AS bodig], **1.** the residue of colloidal degeneration found in some cells. **2.** globules of neurosecretory material found in the posterior lobe of the pituitary. **3.** deposits of ho-

mogenous eosinophilic material found in renal tubular epithelium and representing excess protein molecules that cannot be metabolized or transported.

hyaline cartilage [Gk hyalos; L cartilago], the gristly, elastic connective tissue comprised of specialized cells in a translucent, pearly-blue matrix. Hyaline cartilage thinly covers the articulating ends of bones, connects the ribs to the sternum, and supports the nose, trachea, and part of the larynx.

hyaline cast, a transparent cast composed of mucoprotein.

hyaline membrane [Gk, hyalos, glass; L, membrana], a fibrous covering of acinar epithelium in premature infants caused by a lack of pulmonary surfactant associated with prematurity and low-birth-weight delivery.

hyaline membrane disease. See **acute respiratory distress syndrome of the newborn.**

hyaline thrombus, a translucent, colorless mass consisting of hemolyzed erythrocytes.

hyalinization /hī′əlin′īzā′shən/ [Gk hyalos glass], the development of glassy homogenous material within a cell.

hyalinuria /hī′əlinōōr′ē·ə/ [Gk hyalos + ouron urine], the presence of hyaline casts of protein in the acid pH of urine.

hyaloid /hī′əloid/ [Gk hyalos + eidos form], pertaining to or resembling hyaline.

hyaloid artery [Gk hyalos + eidos form], an embryonic blood vessel that branches to supply the vitreous body of the eye. It persists in the adult as a narrow passage through the vitreous body from the optic disc to the posterior surface of the crystalline lens.

hyaloid membrane [Gk hyalos; L membrana], a surface layer of the vitreous body of the eye, at the interface between the primary and secondary vitreous and at the boundaries of the hyaloid canal.

hyaloplasm /hī′əlōplaz′əm/ [Gk hyalos + plasma formation], the portion of the cytoplasm that is clear and more fluid, as opposed to the granular and reticular part.

hyaluronic acid /hī′əlyōōron′ik/, a mucopolysaccharide formed by the polymerization of acetylglucosamine and glucuronic acid. Known as the cement substance of tissues, it forms a gel in intercellular spaces.

hyaluronidase /hī′əlyōōron′ədās/, an enzyme that hydrolyzes hyaluronic acid. It is prescribed to increase the absorption and dispersion of other parenteral drugs, for hypodermoclysis, and for improving resorption of radiopaque agents.

hybrid /hī′brid/ [L *hybrida* offspring], **1.** an offspring produced from mating plants or animals from different species, varieties, or genotypes. **2.** of or pertaining to such a plant or animal.

hybridization, 1. the process of producing hybrids by crossbreeding. **2.** (in molecular genetics) the process of combining single-stranded nucleic acids whose base composition is identical but whose base sequence is different to form stable double-stranded duplex molecules.

hybridoma /hī′bridō′mə/, a hybrid cell formed by the fusion of a myeloma cell and an antibody-producing cell. Hybridomas are used in the production of monoclonal antibodies.

hybrid subtraction, a two step subtraction method for producing digitalized x-ray images that uses at least four images.

hybrid vigor. See **heterosis.**

hydantoin /hīdan′tō·in/, any one of a group of anticonvulsant medications, chemically and pharmacologically similar to the barbiturates, that act to limit seizure activity and reduce the spread of the abnormal electric excitation from the focus of the seizure.

hydatid /hī′dətid/ [Gk *hydatis* water drop], a cyst or cystlike structure that usually is filled with fluid, especially the cyst formed around the developing scolex of the dog tapeworm *Echinococcus granulosus.* –**hydatidiform,** *adj.*

hydatid cyst, a cyst in the liver that contains larvae of the tapeworm *Echinococcus granulosus.* Patients are generally asymptomatic, except for hepatomegaly and a dull ache over the right upper quadrant of the abdomen.

hydatid disease. See **echinococcosis.**

hydatid mole, an intrauterine neoplastic mass of grapelike enlarged chorionic villi. Characteristic signs of the condition are extreme nausea, uterine bleeding, anemia, hyperthyroidism, an unusually large uterus for the length of pregnancy, absence of fetal heart sounds, edema, and high blood pressure.

hydatidosis /hī′dətidō′sis/ [Gk *hydatis* + *osis* condition], infestation with the tapeworm *Echinococcus granulosus.*

hydatiform /hīdat′ifôrm/ [Gk *hydatis* + L *forma*], having the appearance or form of a **hydatid.**

hydradenitis /hī′dradənī′tis/ [Gk *hydos* water, *aden* gland, *itis* inflammation], an infection or inflammation of the sweat glands. Also spelled **hidradenitis.**

hydralazine /hīdral′əzēn/, an antihypertensive prescribed in the treatment of hypertension.

hydralazine hydrochloride, a vasodilator prescribed in the treatment of high blood pressure.

hydramnios /hīdram′nē·əs/ [Gk *hydos* + *amnos* lamb's caul], an abnormal condition of pregnancy characterized by an excess of amniotic fluid. It is associated with maternal disorders, including toxemia of pregnancy and diabetes mellitus.

hydranencephaly /hī′drənsef′əlē/, a neurologic disorder in which the cerebral hemispheres are lacking although the cerebellum, brainstem, and other central nervous system tissues may be normal. The newborn with hydranencephaly may show normal neurologic functions but fails to develop.

hydrargyrism. See **mercury poisoning.**

hydrate /hī′drāt/ [Gk *hydor* water], **1.** a combination of a substance with one or more water molecules. **2.** a molecular association of a substance with water.

hydration /hīdrā′shən/, a chemical process in which water is taken up without disrupting the rest of the molecule.

hydremic ascites /hīdrem′ik/ [Gk *hydor* + *haima* blood; *askos* bag], an abnormal accumulation of fluid within the peritoneal cavity accompanied by hemodilution, as in protein calorie malnutrition.

hydroa /hīdrō′ə/ [Gk *hydor* + *oon* egg], an unusual vesicular and bullous skin condition of childhood that recurs each summer after exposure to sunlight, sometimes accompanied by itching and lichenification.

hydrobilirubin /hī′drōbil′ir$\overline{oo}$′bin/ [Gk *hydor* + L *bilis* bile, *ruber* red], a reddish brown bile pigment produced by the reduction of bilirubin.

hydrocarbon /hī′ [Gk *hydor* + L *carbo* coal], any one of a large group of organic compounds, the molecules of which are composed of hydrogen and carbon, many of which are derived from petroleum.

hydrocele /hī′drōsēl′/ [Gk *hydor* + *kele* hernia], an accumulation of fluid in any saclike cavity or duct, specifically in the tunica vaginalis testis or along the spermatic cord. The condition is caused by inflammation of the epididymis or testis or by lymphatic or venous obstruction in the cord.

hydrocephalus /hī′drōset′ələs/ [Gk *hydor* + *kephale* head], a pathologic condition characterized by an abnormal accumulation of cerebrospinal fluid, usually under increased pressure, within the cranial vault and subsequent dilatation of the ventricles. Interference with the normal flow of cerebrospinal fluid may be caused by increased secretion of the fluid, obstruction within the ventricular system (noncommunicating or intraventricular hydrocephalus), or defective reabsorption from the cerebral subarachnoid space (communicating or extraventricular hydrocephalus), resulting from developmental anomalies, infection, trauma, or brain tumors. **–hydrocephalic,** *adj., n.*

hydrochloric acid /hi′drōklôr′ik/ [Gk *hydor* + *chloros* green], a compound consisting of hydrogen and chlorine. Hydrochloric acid is secreted in the stomach and is a major component of gastric juice.

hydrochlorothiazide /hi′drōklôr′ōthī′-əzīd/, a diuretic and antihypertensive prescribed in the treatment of hypertension and edema.

hydrocholeretics /hi′drōkō′lərет′iks [Gk *hydor* + *chloe* bile, *eresis* removal], drugs that stimulate the production of bile with a low specific gravity, or with a minimal proportion of solid constituents.

hydrocodone bitartrate /hi′drōkō′dōn/, a narcotic antitussive prescribed in the treatment of cough.

hydrocortisone, hydrocortisone acetate, hydrocortisone cyclopentylpropionate, hydrocortisone sodium succinate. See **cortisol.**

hydrocortisone valerate /hi′drōkôr′tisōn/, a topical corticosteroid used as an antiinflammatory agent.

hydroflumethiazide /hi′drōflōōmethī′-əzīd/, a diuretic and antihypertensive prescribed in the treatment of hypertension and edema.

hydrogen (H) /hī′drəjən/ [Gk *hydor* + *genein* to produce], a gaseous, univalent element. Its atomic number is 1; its atomic weight is 1.008. It is the simplest and the lightest of the elements and is normally a colorless, odorless, highly inflammable diatomic gas. It occurs in pure form only sparsely in the earth and the atmosphere but is plentiful in the sun and in many other stars. Hydrogen is a component of numerous compounds, many of them produced by the body. As a component of water, hydrogen is crucial in the metabolic interaction of acids, bases, and salts within the body and in the fluid balance necessary for the body to survive.

hydrogenase /hī′drōjənās′/, an enzyme that catalyzes reduction of molecules by combining them with molecular hydrogen.

hydrogenation. See **reduction.**

hydrogen bonding, the attractive force of compounds in which a hydrogen atom covalently linked to an electronegative element, as oxygen, nitrogen, or sulfur, has a large degree of positive character relative to the electronegative atom, thereby causing the compound to possess a large dipole.

hydrogen ion [H⁺], a positively charged hydrogen atom nucleus.

hydrogen ion concentration of blood, a measure of blood pH and its effect on the ability of the hemoglobin molecule to hold oxygen.

hydrogen peroxide, a topical antiinfective prescribed to cleanse open wounds, as a mouthwash, and to aid in the removal of cerumen in the external ear.

hydrokinetics [Gk *hydor* + *kinesis* motion], the study of movement of fluids.

hydrolase /hi′drōlās/, an enzyme that cleaves ester bonds by the addition of water.

hydrolysis /hīdrol′isis/ [Gk *hydor* + *lysis* loosening], the chemical alteration or decomposition of a compound with water.

hydrolytic, pertaining to or having the ability to produce hydrolysis.

hydrolyze /hi′drōlīz/, **1.** to cause or bring about hydrolysis. **2.** to cause a substance to split into component parts by the addition of water.

hydrometer /hīdrom′ətər/ [Gk *hydor* + *metron* measure], a device that determines the specific gravity or density of a liquid by a comparison of its weight with that of an equal volume of water. A calibrated, hollow glass device is placed in the liquid being examined, and the depth to which the device settles in the liquid is noted.

hydromorphone hydrochloride /hī′drōmôr′fōn/, a narcotic analgesic used to treat moderate to severe pain.

hydronephrosis /hī′drōnefrō′sis/ [Gk *hydor* + *nephros* kidney, *osis* condition], distention of the pelvis and calyces of the kidney by urine that cannot flow past an obstruction in a ureter. Ureteral obstruction may be caused by a tumor, a calculus lodged in the ureter, inflammation of the prostate gland, or edema caused by a urinary tract infection. The person may experience pain in the flank and, in some cases, hematuria, pyuria, and hyperpyrexia. **–hydronephrotic,** *adj.*

hydropenia /hī′drōpēn′ē·ə/, lack of water in the body tissues.

hydrophilic /hī′drōfil′ik/ [Gk *hydor* + *philein* to love], pertaining to the property of attracting water molecules, possessed by polar radicals or ions.

hydrophobia /hī′drōfō′bē·ə/ [Gk *hydor* + *phobos* fear], **1.** *nontechnical.* rabies. **2.** a morbid, extreme fear of water.

hydrophobic [Gk *hydor* + *phobos* fear], pertaining to the property of repelling water molecules or side chains that are more soluble in organic solvents.

hydrophthalmos. See **congenital glaucoma.**

hydrops /hī′drops/ [Gk, dropsy], an abnormal accumulation of clear, watery fluid in a body tissue or cavity, such as a joint, the abdomen, the middle ear, or the gallbladder.

hydrops endolymphatic. See **endolymphatic hydrops.**

hydrops fetalis, massive edema in the fetus or newborn, usually in association with severe erythroblastosis fetalis. Severe anemia and effusions of the pericardial, pleural, and peritoneal spaces also occur.

hydrops gravidarum [Gk *hydor* + L *gravidus* pregnant], edema caused by pregnancy.

hydrops tubae profluens. See **inermittent hydrosalpinx.**

hydroquinone /hī′drōkwin′ōn/, a dermatologic bleaching agent prescribed to reduce pigmentation of the skin in certain skin conditions in which an excess of melanin causes hyperpigmentation.

hydrosalpinx /hī′drōsal′pingks/ [Gk *hydor* + *salpinx* tube], an abnormal condition of the fallopian tube in which the tube is cystically enlarged and filled with clear fluid, the end result of an infection that has previously occluded the tube at both ends.

hydrosis /hī′drō′sis/, pertaining to the production of sweat.

hydrostatic /hī′drōstat′ik/ [Gk *hydor* + *statos* standing], pertaining to fluids at rest or in equilibrium and the pressure they exert.

hydrostatic pressure, the pressure exerted by a liquid.

hydrostatic dosimetry, the weighing of a person under water to determine lean-to-fat body weight.

hydrotherapy /hī′drōther′əpē/ [Gk *hydor* + *therapeia* treatment], the use of water in the treatment of various mental and physical disorders. Hydrotherapy may include continuous tub baths, wet sheet packs, or shower sprays.

hydrothorax /hī′drōthôr′aks/ [Gk *hydor* + *thorax* chest], a noninflammatory accumulation of serous fluid in one or both pleural cavities.

hydrotropism /hī′drōtrō′pizəm/ [Gk *hydor* + *trope* turning], the tendency of a cell or organism to turn or move in a certain direction under the influence of a water stimulus.

hydrous /hī′drəs/ [Gk *hydor* water], pertaining to a substance or object that contains water or is moist.

hydrous wool fat. See **lanolin.**

hydroxide /hīdrok′sīd/, an ionic compound that contains the OH^- ion.

hydroxyamphetamine hydrobromide /hīdrok′sē-əmfet′əmēn/, an adrenergic and mydriatic prescribed for dilatation of the pupil for ophthalmoscopy and as a diagnostic aid in Horner's syndrome.

hydroxyandrosterone /hīdrok′sē-andos′-tərōn/ [Gk *hydor* + *andros* male, *stereos* solid], a sex hormone that is secreted by the testes and adrenal glands. Its normal accumulation in the urine of men after 24-hour collection is 0.1 to 8 mg; in women, 0 to 0.5 mg.

hydroxyapatite /hīdrok′sē-ap′ətīt/, an inorganic compound composed of calcium, phosphate, and hydroxide. It is found in the bones and teeth in a crystallized latticelike form that gives these structures rigidity.

hydroxybenzene. See **carbolic acid.**

hydroxychloroquine sulfate /hīdrok′sē-klôr′əkwīn/, an antiprotozoal, antirheumatic drug that is also a suppressant of lupus erythematosus and of polymorphous light eruption. It is prescribed in the treatment of malaria and for the suppression of acute paroxysmal attacks of the disease, in the treatment of extraintestinal, usually hepatic, amebiasis, and in the reduction of symptoms of lupus erythematosus and rheumatoid arthritis.

17-hydroxycorticosteroid /hīdrok′sēkôr′-tikos′təroid/, any of the hormones, such as cortisol, secreted by adrenal glands, measured in the urine in a test for determining adrenal function and diagnosing hypoadrenalism or hyperadrenalism.

11-hydroxyetiocholanolone /hīdrok′sē-ē′-tē-ōkolan′əlōn., a sex hormone secreted by the testes and adrenal glands.

5-hydroxyindoleacetic acid /hīdrok′sē-in′dōlē-əset′ik/, an acid produced by serotonin metabolism, measured in the blood and urine to aid in the diagnosis of certain kinds of tumors. It commonly rises above normal levels in whole blood in association with asthma, diarrhea, rapid heartbeat, and other symptoms and is elevated in the urine of patients with carcinoid syndrome.

hydroxyl (OH) /hīdrok′sil/, a radical compound containing an oxygen atom and a hydrogen atom.

hydroxyprogesterone caproate /hīdrok′-sēprōjes′tərōn/, a progestational steroid prescribed in the treatment of advanced adenocarcinoma of the uterine corpus, amenorrhea, and abnormal uterine bleeding caused by hormonal imbalance in the absence of organic disease.

hydroxyproline /hīdrok′sēprō′lēn/, an amino acid that is elevated in the urine in diseases of the bone and certain genetic disorders, such as Marfan's syndrome.

5-hydroxytryptamine. See **serotonin.**

hydroxyurea /hīdrok′siyŏŏrē′ə/, an antineoplastic prescribed in the treatment of a variety of neoplasms.

H

hydroxyzine hydrochloride /hīdrok′sə-zēn/, a minor tranquilizer prescribed to relieve anxiety, nervous tension, hyperkinesis, and motion sickness.

hygiene [Gk *Hygieia* the goddess of health], the principles and science of the preservation of health and prevention of disease.

hygienist, one who practices the principles and laws of **hygiene.**

hygrometer /hīgrom′ətər/, [Gk *hygros* moist, *metron* measure], an instrument that directly measures relative humidity of the atmosphere or the proportion of water in a specific gas or gas mixture, without extracting the moisture.

hygroscopic humidifier, a humidifying device attached to the tubing circuit of a mechanical ventilator or anesthesia gas machine to maintain a constant rate of humidity in the patient's trachea.

hymen /hī′mən/ [Gk, membrane], a fold of mucous membrane, skin, and fibrous tissue at the introitus of the vagina. It may be absent, small, thin and pliant, or, rarely, tough and dense, completely occluding the introitus.

hymenal /hī′mənəl/ [Gk *hymen* membrane], pertaining or belonging to the hymen.

hymenal tag, normal, redundant hymenal tissue protruding from the floor of the vagina during the first weeks after birth.

hymenectomy /hī′mənek′təmē/ [Gk *hymen* + *ektome* cutting out], the surgical excision of a membrane, particularly the hymen.

Hymenolepis /hī′minol′əpis/ [Gk *hymen* + *lepis* rind], a genus of intestinal tapeworms infesting humans. Heavy infestation may cause abdominal pain, bloody stools, and disorders of the nervous system. Contaminated food spreads the disease.

hymenotomy /hī′mənot′əmē/ [Gk *hymen* + *temnein* to cut], the surgical incision of the hymen.

hyoglossal. See **glossohyal.**

hyoglossus /hī′ōglos′əs/, a depressor muscle of the tongue arising from the hyoid bone.

hyoid /hī′oid/ [Gk *hyoeides* upsilon, U-shaped], the hyoid bone or pertaining to it.

hyoid arch [Gk *hyoeides;* L *arcus* bow], the second pharyngeal or branchial arch. It is present in typical form in the embryo but the skeletal elements develop into the stapes and styloid process of the temporal bone of the adult.

hyoid bone /hī′oid/ [Gk *hyoeides;* AS *ban* bone], a single U-shaped bone suspended from the styloid processes of the temporal bones. The bone attaches to various muscles, as the hypoglossus and the sternohyoideus.

hyoscine hydrobromide. See **scopolamine hydrobromide.**

hyoscyamine /hī′əsī′əmēn/, an anticholinergic prescribed in the treatment of hypermotility of the GI and the lower urinary tracts.

hypalgesia /hī′paljē′zē-ə/ [Gk *hypo* below, *algesis* pain], the perception of a painful stimulus to a degree that varies significantly from a normal perception of the same stimulus.

hyperacidity [Gk *hyper* excess; L *acidus* sour], an excessive amount of acidity, as in the stomach.

hyperactive child syndrome [Gk *hyper* + L *agere* to do; AS *cild;* Gk *syn* together, *dromos* course], a childhood mental disorder with onset before age 7 and involving inattention, impulsivity, and hyperactivity.

hyperactivity [Gk *hyper* + L *activus* active], any abnormally increased activity involving either the entire organism or a particular organ, as the heart or thyroid.

hyperacuity /hī′pərakyo͞o′itē/ [Gk *hyper* + *akouien* to hear], excessive sensitivity to sounds.

hyperadenosis /hī′pərad′ənō′sis/ [Gk *hyper* + *aden* gland, *osis* condition], a condition characterized by enlarged glands.

hyperadrenalism. See **Cushing's disease.**

hyperadrenocorticism. See **Cushing's syndrome.**

hyperaldosteronism. See **aldosteronism.**

hyperalimentation /hī′pəral′iməntā′shən/ [Gk *hyper* + L *alimentum* nourishment], overfeeding or the ingestion or administration of a greater than optimal amount of nutrients in excess of the demands of the appetite.

hyperammonemia /hī′pəram′ōnē′mē-ə/ [Gk *hyper* + (ammonia), *haima* blood], abnormally high levels of ammonia in the blood. Untreated, the condition leads to asterixis, vomiting, lethargy, coma, and death.

hyperbaric chamber /hī′pərbər′′ik/ [Gk *hyper* + *baros* weight, *kamara* arched roof], an airtight chamber containing an oxygen atmosphere under high pressure. A patient may be placed in the chamber for the treatment of certain infections, tumors, and cardiovascular diseases in which atmospheric oxygen pressures up to three times normal may have therapeutic value.

hyperbaric oxygenation [Gk *hyper* + *baros* weight; *oxys* sharp, *genein* to produce], the administration of oxygen at greater than normal atmospheric pressure. The procedure is performed in specially designed chambers that permit the delivery of 100% oxygen at atmospheric pressure that is three times normal. The technique is employed to overcome the natural limit of oxygen solubility in blood. Hyperbaric oxygenation has been used to treat carbon monoxide poisoning, air embolism, smoke inhalation, acute cyanide poisoning, decompression sickness, Clostridial myonecrosis, and certain cases of blood loss or anemia in which increased oxygen transport may compensate in part for the hemoglobin deficiency.

hyperbaric oxygen therapy. See **hyperbaric oxygenation.**

hyperbaric solution, a type of spinal anesthetic that has a specific gravity greater than the cerebrospinal fluid so it will settle into the lowest parts of the spinal canal.

hyperbarism /hī′pərber′izəm/, any disorder resulting from exposure to increased ambient pressure, usually from sudden exposure to or a significant increase in pressure.

hyperbasemia /hī′pərbase′mē·ə/, elevated arterial bicarbonate concentration that is caused by metabolic or nonrespiratory factors.

hyperbetalipoproteinemia /hī′pərbā′-təlip′ōprō′tēnē′mē·ə/ [Gk hyper + beta second letter of Greek alphabet, lipos fat, proteios first rank, haima blood], type II hyperlipoproteinemia, a genetic disorder of lipid metabolism, in which there are abnormally high levels of serum cholesterol, and xanthomas appear on the tendons of the heels, knees, and fingers.

hyperbilirubinemia /hī′pərbil′ir oo′binē′-mē·ə/ [Gk hyper + L bilis bile, ruber red; Gk haima blood], greater than normal amounts of the bile pigment bilirubin in the blood, often characterized by jaundice, anorexia, and malaise. Hyperbilirubinemia is most often associated with liver disease or biliary obstruction, but it also occurs when there is excessive destruction of red blood cells.

hyperbilirubinemia of the newborn, an excess of bilirubin in the blood of the neonate, resulting from hepatic dysfunction. It is usually caused by a deficiency of an enzyme, resulting from physiologic immaturity, or increased hemolysis, especially from blood group incompatibility, which, in severe cases, can lead to kernicterus.

hypercalcemia /hī′pərkalsē′mē·ə/ [Gk hyper + L calx lime; Gk haima blood], greater-than-normal amounts of calcium in the blood, most often resulting from excessive bone resorption and release of cal-

cium, as occurs in hyperparathyroidism, metastatic tumors of bone, Paget's disease, and osteoporosis. Clinically, patients with hypercalcemia are confused and have anorexia, abdominal pain, and muscle pain and weakness. **–hypercalcemic,** adj.

hypercalcemic nephropathy /hī′pərkalsē′-mik/ [Gk hyper + L calx + haima; Gk nephros kidney, pathos disease], a progressive disorder of kidney function caused by excessive calcium in the blood. The calcium causes cumulative functional and histologic abnormalities, leading to a decreased glomerular filtration rate and kidney failure.

hypercalciuria /hī′pərkal′sēyoōr′ē·ə/ [Gk hyper + L calx + Gk ouron urine], the presence of abnormally great amounts of calcium in the urine, resulting from conditions such as sarcoid, hyperparathyroidism, or certain types of arthritis, characterized by augmented bone resorption. Concentrated amounts of calcium in the urinary tract may form kidney stones. **–hypercalciuric,** adj.

hypercapnia /hī′pərkap′nē·ə/ [Gk hyper + kapnos vapor], greater than normal amounts of carbon dioxide in the blood.

hypercapnic acidosis /hī′pərkap′nik/ [Gk hyper + kapnos; L acidus sour, osis condition], an excessive acidity in body fluids caused by an increase in carbon dioxide tension in the blood. The condition may be secondary to pulmonary insufficiency; as carbon dioxide accumulates in the blood its acidity increases.

hypercarbia /hī′pərkär′bē·ə/ [Gk hyper + carbo coal], an abnormally high concentration of carbon dioxide in the blood.

hyperchloremia /hi′pərklôr′ē′mē·ə/ [Gk hyper + chloros green, haima blood], an excessive level of chloride in the blood.

hyperchlorhydria /hi′pərklôrid′rē·ə/ [Gk hyper, chloros + hydor water], the excessive secretion of hydrochloric acid by cells lining the stomach.

hypercholesterolemia /hi′pərkōles′tərōl-ēmē·ə/ [Gk hyper + chole bile, stereos solid, haima blood], a condition in which greater-than-normal amounts of cholesterol are present in the blood. High levels of cholesterol and other lipids may lead to the development of atherosclerosis.

hypercholesterolemic **xanthomatosis.** See **familial hypercholesterolemia.**

hyperchromia /hi′pərkrō·mə·ə/ [Gk hyper + chroma color], an increase of hemoglobin in the erythrocytes.

hyperchromic [Gk hyper + chroma color], having a greater density of color or pigment.

hyperchylomicronemia /hi′pərkī′lōmī′-krōnē′mē·ə/ [Gk hyper + chylos juice, *mikros* small, *haima* blood], type I hyperlipoproteinemia, a rare congenital deficiency of an enzyme essential to fat metabolism. Fat accumulates in the blood as chylomicrons. The condition affects children and young adults, who develop xanthomas (fatty deposits) in the skin, hepatomegaly, and abdominal pain.

hypercoagulability /hi´pərkō·ag´yələbil´itē/ [Gk *hyper* + L *coagulare* to curdle, *habilis* able], a tendency of the blood to coagulate more rapidly than is normal.

hyperdactyly. See **polydactyly.**

hyperdiploid. See **hyperploid.**

hyperdynamic syndrome [Gk *hyper* + *dynamis* force], a cluster of symptoms that signal the onset of septic shock, often including a shaking chill, rapid rise in temperature, flushing of the skin, galloping pulse, and alternating rise and fall of the blood pressure. This is a medical emergency that requires expert medical support in a hospital.

hyperemesis gravidarum /hi´pərem´isis/ [Gk *hyper* + *emesis* vomiting; L *gravida* pregnant], an abnormal condition of pregnancy characterized by protracted vomiting, weight loss, and fluid and electrolyte imbalance. If the condition is severe and intractable, brain damage, liver and kidney failure, and death may result. Dehydration results in dry mucous membranes, decreased skin elasticity, a rapid pulse, and falling blood pressure. The volume of urine excreted falls. The hematocrit is elevated because of hemoconcentration. Loss of electrolytes in vomitus leads to metabolic acidosis with hypokalemia, hypochloremia, and hyponatremia. Severe potassium deficit alters myocardial function. Forceful vomiting may cause retinal hemorrhages that impair vision and gastroesophageal tears that bleed and result in hematemesis or melena.

hyperemia /hi´pərē´mē·ə/ [Gk *hyper* + *haima* blood], increased blood in part of the body, caused by increased blood flow, as in the inflammatory response, local relaxation of arterioles, or obstruction of the outflow of blood from an area. Skin overlying a hyperemic area usually becomes reddened and warm. **–hyperemic,** *adj.*

hyperesthesia /hi´pəresthē´zhə/, an extreme sensitivity of one of the body's sense organs, such as pain or touch receptors in the skin.

hyperextension [Gk *hyper* + L *extendere* to stretch out], (of a joint) a position of maximum extension.

hyperextension bed, a bed used in pediatric orthopedics to maintain any correction achieved by suspension of a body part and to increase the range of motion of the hips after an operative muscle release procedure.

hyperextension suspension, an orthopedic procedure used in the postoperative positioning of hip muscles. The procedure uses traction equipment, including metal frames, ropes, and pulleys to relieve the weight of the lower limbs and to position properly the muscles of the hip, without applying traction to the lower limbs involved.

hyperflexia [Gk *hyper* + L *flectere* to bend], the forcible overflexion or bending of a limb.

hyperfunction [Gk *hyper* + L *functio* performance], increased function of any organ or system.

hypergenesis /hi´pərjen´əsis/ [Gk *hyper* + *genesis* origin], excessive growth or overdevelopment. The condition may involve the entire body, as in gigantism, or any particular part or it may result in the formation of extra parts, as the development of additional fingers or toes. **–hypergenetic,** *adj.*

hypergenetic teratism [Gk *hyper, genesis* + *teras* monster], a congenital anomaly in which there is excessive growth of a part or organ or the entire body, as in gigantism.

hypergenitalism, the presence of abnormally large external genitalia. The condition is usually associated with precocious puberty.

hyperglobulinemia /hi´pərglob´yəlinē´mē·ə/ [Gk *hyper* + L *globulus* small globe, *haima* blood], an excess of globulin in the blood.

hyperglycemia /hi´pərglīsē´mē·ə/ [Gk *hyper* + *glykys* sweet, *haima* blood], a greater than normal amount of glucose in the blood. Most frequently associated with diabetes mellitus, the condition may occur in newborns, after the administration of glucocorticoid hormones, and with an excess infusion of intravenous solutions containing glucose.

hyperglycemic-glycogenolytic factor. See **glucagon.**

hyperglycemic-hyperosmolar nonketotic coma [Gk *hyper, glykys* + *hyper, osmos* impulse; L *non* not, (ketone); Gk, *deep* sleep], a diabetic coma in which the level of ketone bodies is normal; caused by hyperosmolarity of extracellular fluid and resulting in dehydration of intracellular fluid, often a consequence of overtreatment with hyperosmolar solutions.

hyperglyceridemia /hi´pərglī´səridē´mē·ə/, an excess of glycerides, particularly triglycerides, in the blood.

hypergonadism /hi´pərgō´nədiz´əm/ [Gk

hyper + gone seed], excessive activity of the ovaries or testes.

hyperhidrosis /hī'pərhidrō'sis, -hidrō'sis/ [Gk *hyper + hidros* perspiration], excessive perspiration, often caused by heat, hyperthyroidism, strong emotion, menopause, or infection.

hyperimmune [Gk *hyper* + L *immunis* freedom], a characteristic associated with an unusual abundance of antibodies, producing a greater-than-normal immunity.

hyperinsulinism /hi'pərin'səliniz'əm/ [Gk *hyper* + L *insula* island], an excessive amount of insulin in the body, as may occur when a greater than required dose is administered.

hyperirritability [Gk *hyper* + L *irritare* to tease], a condition of excessive excitability, sensitivity, or exaggerated response to a stimulus.

hyperkalemia /hī'pərkəlē'mē·ə/ [Gk *hyper* + L *kalium* potassium; Gk *haima* blood], greater than normal amounts of potassium in the blood. This condition is seen frequently in acute renal failure. Early signs are nausea, diarrhea, and muscle weakness.

hyperkalemic periodic paralysis. See **adynamia episodica hereditaria.**

hyperkeratinization /hi'pərker'ətinīzā'-shən/ [Gk *hyper* + *keras* horn], an abnormal horny thickening of the epithelium of the palms and soles.

hyperkeratosis /hī'pərker'ətō'sis/ [Gk *hyper* + *keras* + *osis* condition], overgrowth of the cornified epithelial layer of the skin.

hyperkinesis. See **attention deficit disorder.**

hyperlipemia /hi'pərlipē'mē·ə/, an excessive level of blood fats, usually caused by a lipoprotein lipase deficiency or a defect in the conversion of low-density lipoproteins (LDL) to high-density lipoproteins (HDL).

hyperlipidemia /hi'pərlip'idē'mē·ə/ [Gk *hyper* + *lipos* fat, *haima* blood], an excess of lipids in the plasma, including glycolipids, lipoproteins, and phospholipids.

hyperlipidemia type I, a condition of elevated lipid levels in the blood, characterized by an increase in both cholesterol and triglycerides, and caused by the presence of chylomicrons. It is inherited as an autosomal recessive trait with a low risk of atherosclerosis.

hyperlipidemia type IIA, hyperlipidemia type IIB. See **familial hypercholesterolemia.**

hyperlipidemia type III. See **broad beta disease.**

hyperlipidemia type IV, a relatively common form of hyperlipoproteinemia characterized by a slight elevation in cholesterol levels, a moderate elevation of triglycerides, and an elevation of the normal triglyceride carrier protein VLDL. It is sometimes familial and is associated with an increased risk factor for coronary atherosclerosis.

hyperlipidemia type V, a condition of elevated blood lipids, characterized by slightly increased cholesterol, greatly increased triglycerides, elevation of the triglyceride carrier protein VLDL, and chylomicrons. It is a genetically heterogenous disorder.

hyperlipoproteinemia /hī'pərlip'ōprō'-tēnē'mē·ə/ [Gk *hyper* + *lipos* fat, *proteios* first rank, *haima* blood], any of a large group of inherited and acquired disorders of lipoprotein metabolism characterized by greater than normal amounts of certain protein-bound lipids and other fatty substances in the blood.

hypermagnesemia /hī'pərmag'nisē'mē·ə/ [Gk *hyper* + *magnesia* magnesium, *haima* blood], a greater than normal amount of magnesium in the plasma, found in people with kidney failure and in those who use a large quantity of drugs containing magnesium, such as antacids. Toxic levels of magnesium cause cardiac arrhythmias and depression of deep tendon reflexes and respiration.

hypermature cataract [Gk *hyper* + L *maturare* to make ripe; Gk *katarrhaktes* portcullis], an opaque lens that has lost water and has become reduced in size and soft.

hypermenorrhea. See **menorrhagia.**

hypermetria /hī'pərmē'trē·ə/ [Gk *hyper* + *metron* measure], an abnormal condition, a form of dysmetria, characterized by a dysfunction of the power to control the range of muscular action, resulting in movements that overreach the intended goal of the affected individual.

hypermetropia, hypermetropy, See **hyperopia.**

hypermobility [Gk *hyper* + L *mobilis* movable], a form of joint laxity characterized by an abnormally wide range of movement of the joints. The condition is seen in children and may be associated with **Marfan's syndrome** or degenerative joint diseases.

hypermorph /hī'pərmôrf'/ [Gk *hyper* + *morphe* form] **1.** a person whose arms and legs are disproportionately long in relation to the trunk, and whose sitting height is disproportionate to the standing height. **2.** (in genetics) a mutant gene that shows an increased activity in the expression of a trait.

hypermotility, an excessive movement of the involuntary muscles, particularly in the gastrointestinal tract.

hypernatremia /hī′pərnatrē′mē·ə/ [Gk *hyper* + L *natrium* sodium], a greater than normal concentration of sodium in the blood, caused by excessive loss of water and electrolytes resulting from polyuria, diarrhea, excessive sweating, or inadequate water intake. People with hypernatremia may become mentally confused, have seizures, and lapse into coma. Care must be taken to restore water balance slowly, because further electrolyte imbalances may occur.

hyperopia /hī′pərō′pē·ə/ [Gk *hyper* + *ops* eye], farsightedness, a condition resulting from an error of refraction in which rays of light entering the eye are brought into focus behind the retina.

hyperorchidism /hī′pərôr′kidiz′əm/ [Gk *hyper* + *orchis* testis], excessive endocrine activity of the testes.

hyperornithinemia /hī′pərôr′nithinē′mē·ə/, a metabolic disorder involving the amino acid ornithine, which tends to accumulate in the tissues, causing seizures and retardation.

hyperosmia /hī′pəroz′mē·ə/, an abnormally increased sensitivity to odors.

hyperosmolarity [Gk *hyper* + *osmos* impulse], a state or condition of abnormally increased osmolarity. **–hyperosmolar,** *adj.*

hyperosmotic /hī′pərozmot′ik/, pertaining to an increased concentration of osmotically active components.

hyperostosis [Gk *hyper* + *osteon* bone, *osis* condition], an overgrowth of bone. It may occur as a bone swelling or an osteoma, or involve adjacent cartilage.

hyperoxaluria /hī′pərok′səlŏŏr′ē·ə/, an excessive level of oxalic acid or oxalates, primarily calcium oxalate, in the urine. An excess of oxalates may lead to the formation of renal calculi.

hyperoxemia /hī′pəroksē′mē·ə/ [Gk *hyper* + *oxys* sharp *haima* blood], increased oxygen content of the blood.

hyperoxia /hī′pərok′sē·ə/, a condition of abnormally high oxygen tension in the blood.

hyperoxygenation [Gk *hyper* + *oxys* sharp, *genein* to produce], the use of high concentrations of inspired oxygen before and after endotracheal aspiration.

hyperparathyroidism /hī′pərpər′əthī′roidiz′əm/ [Gk *hyper* + *para* beside, *thyreos* shield, *eidos* form], an abnormal endocrine condition characterized by hyperactivity of any of the four parathyroid glands with excessive secretion of parathyroid hormone (PTH) that results in increased resorption of calcium from the skeletal system and increased absorption of calcium by the kidneys and GI system. The condition may be primary, originating in one or more of the parathyroid glands, or secondary, resulting from an abnormal hypocalcemia-producing condition in another part of the body causing a compensatory hyperactivity of the parathyroid glands.

hyperperistalis /hī′pərperistal′is/ [Gk *hyper* + *peristellein* to clasp], a state of excessive motility of the waves of alternate contractions and relaxations that propel contents forward through the digestive tract.

hyperphenylalaninemia /hī′pərfen′ilal′-əninē′mē·ə/ [Gk *hyper* + (phenylalanine), *haima* blood], an abnormally high concentration of phenylalanine in the blood. This symptom may be the result of one of several defects in the metabolic process of breaking down phenylalanine.

hyperphoria /hī′pərfôr′ē·ə/ [Gk *hyper* + *pherein* to bear], the tendency of an eye to deviate upward.

hyperpigmentation [Gk *hyper* + L *pigmentum* paint], unusual darkening of the skin. Causes include heredity, drugs, exposure to the sun, and adrenal insufficiency.

hyperpituitarism [Gk *hyper* + L *pituita* phlegm], overactivity of the anterior lobe of the pituitary gland, leading to such conditions as **acromegaly** and **Cushing's disease.**

hyperplasia /hī′pərplā′zhə/ [Gk *hyper* + *plassein* to mold], an increase in the number of cells of a body part.

hyperplastic gingivitis [Gk *hyper* + *plassein* to mold; L *gingiva* gum; Gk *itis* inflammation], a condition of enlarged and inflamed gingival tissue, resulting from an increase in the number of cells, usually as a result of dental plaque accumulation.

hyperploid /hī′pərploid/·[Gk *hyper* + *eidos* form] **1.** of or pertaining to an individual, organism, strain, or cell that has one or more chromosomes in excess of the basic haploid number or of an exact multiple of the haploid number characteristic of the species. **2.** such an individual, organism, strain, or cell.

hyperploidy /hī′pərploi′dē/, any increase in chromosome number that involves individual chromosomes rather than entire sets, resulting in more than the normal haploid number characteristic of the species, as in Down's syndrome.

hyperpnea /hī′pərpnē′ə/ [Gk *hyper* + *pnoe* blowing], a deep, rapid, or labored respiration. It occurs normally with exercise, and abnormally with pain, fever, hysteria, or any condition in which the supply of oxygen is inadequate, as cardiac disease and respiratory disease. **–hyperpneic, hyperpnoic,** *adj.*

hyperprolactinemia /hī′pərprōlak′tinē′-mē·ə/ [Gk *hyper* + L *pro* before, *lac* milk; Gk *haima* blood], an excessive amount of prolactin in the blood. The condition is caused by a hypothalamic-pituitary dysfunction. In women it is usually associated with gynecomastia, galactorrhea, and secondary amenorrhea; in men it may be a factor in decreased libido and impotence.

hyperproteinemia /hī′pərprō′tēnē′mē·ə/ [Gk *hyper* + *proteios* first rank, *haima* blood], an abnormally high level of protein elements in the blood.

hyperptyalism. See **ptyalism.**

hyperpyrexia /hī′pərpīrek′sē·ə/ [Gk *hyper* + *pyressein* to be feverish], an extremely elevated temperature sometimes occurring in acute infectious diseases, especially in young children. Malignant hyperpyrexia, characterized by a rapid rise in temperature, tachycardia, tachypnea, sweating, rigidity, and blotchy cyanosis, occasionally occurs in patients undergoing general anesthesia. **–hyperpyretic,** *adj.*

hyperreactivity [Gk *hyper* + L *re* again, *activus* active], an abnormal condition in which responses to stimuli are exaggerated.

hyperreflection, a compulsion to devote excessive attention to oneself.

hyperreflexia /hī′pər·riflek′sē·ə/ [Gk *hyper* + L *reflectere* to bend backward], a neurologic condition characterized by increased reflex reactions.

hypersensitivity [Gk *hyper* + L *sentire* to feel], an abnormal condition characterized by an excessive reaction to a particular stimulus. **–hypersensitive,** *adj.*

hypersensitivity pneumonitis, an inflammatory form of interstitial pneumonia that results from an immunologic reaction in a hypersensitive person. The reaction may be provoked by a variety of inhaled organic dusts, often those containing fungal spores. A wide variety of symptoms may occur, including asthma, fever, chills, malaise, and muscle aches, which usually develop 4 to 6 hours after exposure. Kinds of hypersensitivity pneumonitis include **bagassosis, cork worker's lung,** and **farmer's lung.**

hypersensitivity reaction, an inappropriate and excessive response of the immune system to a sensitizing antigen. The antigenic stimulant is an allergen. Hypersensitivity reactions are classified by the components of the immune system involved in their mediation. Humoral reactions, medi-

ated by the circulating B lymphocytes, are immediate and include three types: anaphylactic hypersensitivity, cytotoxic hypersensitivity, and immune system hypersensitivity. Cellular reactions, mediated by the T lymphocytes, are delayed, cell-mediated hypersensitivity reactions.

hypersensitization, a state of increased reactivity or sensitivity to a stimulus.

hypersomnia /hī′pərsom′nē·ə/ [Gk *hyper* + L *somnus* sleep], **1.** sleep of excessive depth or abnormal duration, usually caused by psychologic rather than physical factors and characterized by a state of confusion on awakening. **2.** extreme drowsiness, often associated with lethargy. **3.** a condition characterized by periods of deep, long sleep.

hyperspadias. See **epispadias.**

hypersplenism /hī′pərsplē′nizəm/ [Gk *hyper* + *splen* spleen], a syndrome consisting of splenomegaly and a deficiency of one or more types of blood cells. The numerous causes of this syndrome include lymphomas, hemolytic anemias, malaria, tuberculosis, and various connective tissue and inflammatory diseases. Patients complain of abdominal pain on the left side and often experience fullness after eating very little, because the greatly enlarged spleen is pressing against the stomach.

hypersthenic /hī′pərsthen′ik/, **1.** pertaining to a condition of excessive strength or tonicity of the body or a body part. **2.** pertaining to a body type characterized by massive proportions.

hypertelorism /hī′pərtel′əriz′əm/ [Gk *hyper* + *tele* far, *horizo* separate], a developmental defect characterized by an abnormally wide space between two organs or parts. A kind of hypertelorism is **ocular hypertelorism.**

hypertension /hī′pərten′shən/ [Gk *hyper* + L *tendere* to stretch], a common, often asymptomatic disorder characterized by elevated blood pressure persistently exceeding 140/90 mm Hg. Essential hypertension, the most frequent kind, has no single identifiable cause, but the risk of the disorder is increased by obesity, a high sodium level in serum, hypercholesterolemia, and a family history of high blood pressure. Known causes of hypertension include adrenal disorders, such as aldosteronism, Cushing's syndrome, and pheochromocytoma, thyrotoxicosis, toxemia of pregnancy, and chronic glomerulonephritis. Persons with mild or moderate hypertension may be asymptomatic or may experience suboccipital headaches, especially on rising, tinnitus, lightheadedness, easy fatigability, and palpitations. Malignant hypertension, characterized by a diastolic pressure higher than 120 mm Hg, severe headaches, blurred vision, and confusion, may result in fatal uremia, myocardial infarction, congestive heart failure, or a cerebrovascular accident. Kinds of hypertension are **essential, malignant,** and **secondary hypertension.**

hypertensive, /hī′pərten′siv/ [Gk *hyper* + L *tendere* to stretch], pertaining to high blood pressure, its cause or effects.

hypertensive crisis, a sudden severe increase in blood pressure to a level exceeding 200/120 mm Hg, occurring most frequently in untreated hypertension and in patients who have stopped taking prescribed antihypertensive medication. Characteristic signs include severe headache, vertigo, diplopia, tinnitus, nosebleed, twitching muscles, tachycardia or other cardiac arrhythmia, distended neck veins, narrowed pulse pressure, nausea, and vomiting. The patient may be confused, irritable, or stuporous, and the condition may lead to convulsions, coma, myocardial infarction, renal failure, cardiac arrest, or stroke.

hypertensive encephalopathy [Gk *hyper* + L *tendere*; Gk *enkephalos* brain, *pathos* disease], a set of symptoms, including headache, convulsions, and coma, associated with glomerulonephritis.

hypertensive retinopathy, a condition in which retinal changes occur in association with arterial hypertension. The changes may include blood vessel alterations, hemorrhages, exudates, and retinal edema.

hypertetraploid. See **hyperploid.**

hyperthermia /hī′pərthur′mē-ə/ [Gk *hyper* + *therme* heat], **1.** a much higher than normal body temperature induced therapeutically or iatrogenically. **2.** *nontechnical.* malignant hyperthermia. **3.** a NANDA-accepted nursing diagnosis of a state in which an individual's body temperature is elevated above his or her normal range. Defining characteristics include the increase in body temperature, flushed skin, skin warm to the touch, increased respiratory rate, tachycardia, and seizures or convulsions.

hyperthyroidism /hī′pərthī′roidiz′əm/ [Gk *hyper* + *thyreos* shield, *eidos* form], a condition characterized by hyperactivity of the thyroid gland. The gland is usually enlarged, secreting greater than normal amounts of thyroid hormones, and the metabolic processes of the body are accelerated. Nervousness, exophthalmos, tremor, constant hunger, weight loss, fatigue, heat intolerance, palpitations, and diarrhea may develop.

hypertonia /hī′pərtō′nē-ə/, **1.** abnormally increased muscle tone or strength.

The condition is sometimes associated with genetic disorders. **2.** a condition of excessive pressure, as in the intraocular pressure of glaucoma.

hypertonic /hī′pərton′ik/ [Gk *hyper* + *tonos* stretching], (of a solution) having a greater concentration of solute than another solution, hence exerting more osmotic pressure than that solution, such as a hypertonic saline solution that contains more salt than is found in intracellular and extracellular fluid.

hypertonic bladder, a condition of hypertonicity in the detrusor muscle of the bladder, usually because of an irritant, such as a calculus.

hypertonic contracture, prolonged muscle contraction as a result of continuous nerve stimulation in spastic paralysis.

hypertonicity /hī′pərtənis′itē/, **1.** in ophthalmology, a state of increased intraocular pressure. **2.** condition of excessive tension of the arteries or muscles.

hypertonic saline, a saline solution that contains 1% to 15% sodium chloride (compared with normal saline at 0.9%). It is used as a bronchial lavage to stimulate sputum production and to promote coughing.

hypertonic solution, a solution that increases the degree of osmotic pressure on a semipermeable membrane.

hypertrichosis. See **hirsutism.**

hypertriglyceridemia. See **hyperchylomicronemia.**

hypertriploid. See **hyperploid.**

hypertrophic /hī′pərtrof′ik/ [Gk *hyper* + *trophe* nourishment], pertaining to an increase in cell size.

hypertrophic angioma. See **hemangioendothelioma.**

hypertrophic cardiomyopathy, an abnormality in the structure and function of heart muscle characterized by gross hypertrophy of the interventricular septum and left ventricular free wall. Ventricular outflow obstruction results in impaired diastolic filling and reduced cardiac output. Signs and symptoms, such as fatigue and syncope, are often associated with exercise when the demand for increased cardiac output cannot be met.

hypertrophic catarrh [Gk *hyper* + *trophe* + *kata* down, *rhoia* flow], a chronic condition characterized by inflammation and discharge from a mucous membrane, accompanied by the thickening of the mucosal and submucosal tissue.

hypertrophic gastritis, an inflammatory condition of the stomach characterized by epigastric pain, nausea, vomiting, and distention. It is differentiated from other forms of gastritis by the presence of prominent rugae (folds), enlarged glands, and nodules on the wall of the stomach. This condition often occurs with peptic ulcer, Zollinger-Ellison syndrome, or gastric hypersecretion.

hypertrophic gingivitis. See **gingivitis.**

hypertrophic obstructive cardiomyopathy. See **idiopathic hypertrophic subaortic stenosis.**

hypertrophic scarring, scarring caused by excessive formation of new tissue in the healing of a wound. It has the appearance of a hard, tumorlike keloid.

hypertrophy /hīpur′trəfē/ [Gk *hyper* + *trophe* nourishment], an increase in the size of an organ caused by an increase in the size of the cells rather than the number of cells. Kinds of hypertrophy include **adaptive, compensatory, Marie's, physiologic,** and **unilateral hypertrophy.** –**hypertrophic,** *adj.*

hypertrophy of the heart [Gk *hyper* + *trophe;* AS *heorte*], an increase in the size of the heart secondary to enlargement of the heart muscle, but without an increase in the size of the heart chambers.

hyperuricemia. See **gout.**

hyperventilation [Gk *hyper* + *ventilare* to wave], a pulmonary ventilation rate that is greater than that metabolically necessary for the exchange of respiratory gases. It is the result of an increased frequency of breathing, an increased tidal volume, or a combination of both, and causes excessive intake of oxygen and the blowing off of carbon dioxide. Hypocapnia and respiratory alkalosis then occur, leading to chest pain, dizziness, faintness, numbness of the fingers and toes, and psychomotor impairment.

hyperviscosity /hī′pərviskos′itē/ [Gk *hyper* + L *viscosus* sticky], pertaining to an extremely viscous or thick fluid.

hypervitaminosis /hī′pərvī′təminō′sis/, an abnormal condition resulting from excessive intake of toxic amounts of one or more vitamins, especially over a long period of time. Serious effects may result from overdoses of vitamins A, D, E, or K, but rarely with the water-soluble B and C vitamins.

hypervolemia /hī′pərvōlē′mē·ə/ [Gk *hyper* + L *volumen* paper roll; Gk *haima* blood], an increase in the amount of extracellular fluid, particularly in the volume of circulating blood or its components.

hypesthesia /hī′pəristhē′zhə/ [Gk *hypo* under, *aisthesis* feeling], an abnormal weakness of sensation in response to stimulation of the sensory nerves. Touch, pain, heat, and cold are poorly perceived. –**hypesthetic,** *adj.*

hypha /hī′fə/, *pl.* **hyphae** [Gk *hyphe* web],

the threadlike structure of the mycelium in a fungus.

hyphema /hīfē′mə/ [Gk *hypo* under *haima* blood], a hemorrhage into the anterior chamber of the eye, usually caused by a blunt or percussive injury. Glaucoma may result from recurrent bleeding.

hypnagogic hallucination /hip′nəgoj′ik/ [Gk *hypnos* sleep, *agogos* leading], one that occurs in the period between wakefulness and sleep.

hypnagogue /hip′nəgog/ [Gk *hypnos* + *agogos* leading], an agent or substance that tends to induce sleep or the feeling of dreamy sleepiness, as occurs before falling asleep. –**hypnagogic,** *adj.*

hypnoanalysis /hip′nə·anal′isis/ [Gk *hypnos* + *analyein* to loosen], the use of hypnosis as an adjunct to other techniques in psychoanalysis.

hypnosis /hipnō′sis/ [Gk *hypnos* sleep], a passive, trancelike state that resembles normal sleep during which perception and memory are altered, resulting in increased responsiveness to suggestion. Susceptibility to hypnosis varies from person to person. Hypnosis is used in some forms of psychotherapy, in behavior modification programs, or in medicine to reduce pain and promote relaxation.

hypnotherapy [Gk *hypnos* + *therapeia* treatment], the use of hypnosis as an adjunct to other techniques in psychotherapy.

hypnotics /hipnot′iks/ [Gk *hypnos* sleep], a class of drugs often used as sedatives.

hypnotic sleep [Gk *hypnos;* ME *slep*], sleep induced by hypnosis or by administration of hypnotic medicines.

hypnotic suggestion [Gk *hypnos;* L *suggerere* to suggest], a suggestion implanted in the mind of a person under hypnosis.

hypnotic trance, an artificially induced sleeplike state, as in hypnosis.

hypnotism [Gk *hypnos* sleep], the study or practice of inducing hypnosis.

hypnotist, one who practices hypnotism.

hypnotize, 1. to put into a state of hypnosis. **2.** to fascinate, entrance, or control through personal charm.

hypoacidity /hī′pō·əsid′itē/, a deficiency of acid.

hypoactivity [Gk *hypo* under; L *activus* active], any abnormally diminished activity of the body or its organs, as decreased cardiac output, thyroid secretion, or peristalsis.

hypoacusis /hī′pō·əkoo̅′sis/ [Gk *hypo* + *akouein* to hear], a reduced sensitivity to sounds; it could be conductive or sensorineural in nature.

hypoadrenalism. See **Addison's disease.**

hypoalbuminemia /hī′pō·alb oo′minē′-mē·ə/, a condition of abnormally low levels of albumin in the blood.

hypoalimentation /hī′pō·al′iməntā′shən/ [Gk *hypo* + L *alimentum* nourishment], a condition of insufficient or inadequate nourishment.

hypoallergenic /hī′pō·al′ərjen′ik/ [Gk *hypo* + *allos* other, *ergein* to work], pertaining to a lowered potential for producing an allergic reaction.

hypobarism /hī′pōber′izəm/, air pressure that is significantly less than the sea level normal of 760 mm Hg.

hypobasemia /hī′pōbasē′mē·ə/, reduced arterial bicarbonate concentration that is caused by metabolic or nonrespiratory factors.

hypobetalipoproteinemia /hī′pōbā′təlip′ō-prō′tēnē′mē·ə/ [Gk *hypo* + *beta* second letter of Greek alphabet, *lipos* fat, *proteios* first rank, *haima* blood], an inherited disorder in which there are less than normal amounts of beta-lipoprotein in the serum.

hypocalcemia /hī′pōkalsē′mē·ə/ [Gk *hypo* + L *calx* lime; Gk *haima* blood], a deficiency of calcium in the serum that may be caused by hypoparathyroidism, vitamin D deficiency, kidney failure, acute pancreatitis, or inadequate plasma magnesium and protein. Mild hypocalcemia is asymptomatic. Severe hypocalcemia is characterized by cardiac arrhythmias and tetany with hyperparesthesia of the hands, feet, lips, and tongue. –**hypocalcemic**, *adj.*

hypocalcemic tetany [Gk *hypo* + *calx* + *haima* blood, *tetanos* convulsive tension], a disease caused by an abnormally low level of calcium in the blood. It is characterized by hyperexcitability of the neuromuscular system. A common cause is a deficiency of parathyroid secretion.

hypocalciuria /hī′pōkal′s oōr′ē·ə/ [Gk *hypo* + L *calx* + Gk *ouron* urine], a diminished level of calcium in the urine.

hypocapnia /hī′pōkap′nē·ə/, an abnormally low arterial carbon dioxide level.

hypochloremia /hī′pōklôrē′mē·ə/ [Gk *hypo* + *chloros* green, *haima* blood], a decrease in the chloride level in the blood serum. The condition may occur as a result of prolonged gastric suctioning.

hypochloremic alkalosis /hi′pōklôrē′mik/, a metabolic alkalosis resulting from increased blood bicarbonate secondary to loss of chloride from the body.

hypochlorhydria /hī′pōklôrid′rē′ə/ [Gk *hypo* + *chloros* green, *hydor* water], a deficiency of hydrochloric acid in the stomach's gastric juice.

hypochlorite poisoning /hī′pōklôr′īt/, toxic effects of ingestion or skin contact with household or commercial bleaches or similar chlorinated products. Symptoms include pain and inflammation of the mouth and digestive tract, vomiting, and breathing difficulty.

hypochlorous acid /hī′pōklôr′əs/ [Gk *hypo* + *chloros* green; L *acidus* sour], a greenish yellow liquid derived from an aqueous solution of lime.

hypochondria, hypochondriac neurosis. See **hypochondriasis**.

hypochondriac [Gk *hypo* + *chondros* cartilage], **1.** pertaining to the region of the upper abdomen beneath the lower ribs. **2.** a person who is so preoccupied with health matters that this state of mind becomes a disability.

hypochondriac region [Gk *hypo* + *chondros*; L *regio* direction], the part of the abdomen in the upper zone on both sides of the epigastric region and beneath the cartilages of the lower ribs.

hypochondriasis /hī′pōkəndrī′əsis/ [Gk *hypo* + *chondros* + *osis* condition], **1.** a chronic, abnormal concern about the health of the body. **2.** a disorder characterized by extreme anxiety, depression, and an unrealistic interpretation of real or imagined physical symptoms as indications of a serious illness or disease despite rational medical evidence that no disorder is present. –**hypochondriac** /hī′pōkon′-drē·ak/, *adj., n.,* **hypochondriacal,** *adj.*

hypochondrium. See **hypochondriac region**.

hypochondroplasia /hī′pōkon′drōplā′zhə/, an inherited form of dwarfism that resembles a mild form of achondroplasia.

hypochromic /hī′pōkrō′mik/ [Gk *hypo* + *chroma* color], having less than normal color, usually describing a red blood cell and characterizing anemias associated with decreased synthesis of hemoglobin.

hypochromic anemia, any of a large group of anemias characterized by a decreased concentration of hemoglobin in the red blood cells.

hypocycloidal motion /hī′pōsī′loidəl/, (in computed tomography) a circular pattern of movement of the x-ray tube and film that results in blurring of structures outside the focal plane and elimination of ghost images.

hypocytic leukemia. See **aleukemic leukemia**.

hypodermatoclysis. See **hypodermoclysis**.

hypodermic [Gk *hypo* + *derma* skin], of or pertaining to the area below the skin, as a hypodermic injection.

hypodermic implantation [Gk *hypo* + *derma;* L *implantare* to set into], the introduction of a solid medicine under the skin, usually on the chest or abdominal wall, to ensure local action or slow absorption.

hypodermic needle, a short, thin, hollow needle that attaches to a syringe for injecting a drug or medication under the skin or into vessels and for withdrawing a fluid, such as blood, for examination.

hypodermic syringe [Gk *hypo* + *derma, syrigx* tube], an instrument designed to direct fluid under the skin into subcutaneous tissue through a fine hollow needle.

hypodermoclysis /hī′pōdərmok′lisis/ [Gk *hypo* + *derma* skin, *klysis* flushing out], the injection of an isotonic or hypotonic solution into subcutaneous tissue to supply the patient with a continuous and large amount of fluid, electrolytes, and nutrients. The procedure is used to replace the loss or inadequate intake of water and salt during illness or surgery or after shock or hemorrhage and is performed only when the patient is unable to take fluids intravenously, orally, or rectally. The rate of absorption into the circulatory system is increased with the addition to the solution of the enzyme hyaluronidase.

hypodiploid. See **hypoploid.**

hypoesthesia. See **hypesthesia.**

hypofibrinogenemia /hī′pōfibrinōjənē′mē·ə/ [Gk *hypo* + L *fibra* fiber; Gk *genein* to produce, *haima* blood], a deficiency of fibrinogen, a blood clotting factor, in the blood. The condition may occur as a complication of abruptio placentae.

hypofunction [Gk *hypo* + L *functio* performance], a diminished or inadequate level of activity on the part of an organ system or its parts.

hypogammaglobulinemia /hī′pōgam′əglō′byəlinē′mē·ə/ [Gk *hypo* + *gamma* third letter in Greek alphabet; L *globus* small sphere; Gk *haima* blood], a less than normal concentration of gamma globulin in the blood, usually the result of increased protein catabolism or the loss of protein in the urine, as in nephrosis.

hypogastric [Gk *hypo* + *gaster* stomach], pertaining to the hypogastrium, or the lower abdominal region below the umbilical region and between the right and left iliac regions.

hypogastric artery. See **internal iliac artery.**

hypogastrium. See **pubic region.**

hypogenitalism /hī′pōjen′itəliz′əm/ [Gk *hypo* + L *genitalis* fruitful], a condition of retarded sexual development caused by a defect in male or female hormonal production in the testis or ovary.

hypogeusia /hī′pōgō̄̄o͞o′zē·ə/, reduced taste.

hypoglossal /hī′pōglos′əl/ [Gk *hypo* +

glossa tongue], pertaining to nerves or other structures under the tongue.

hypoglossal nerve, either of a pair of cranial nerves essential for swallowing and for moving the tongue.

hypoglossus /hī′pōglos′əs/, **1.** a muscle that retracts and pulls down the side of the tongue. **2.** the hypoglossal nerve.

hypoglycemia /hī′pōglīsē′mē·ə/ [Gk *hypo* + *glykys* sweet, *haima* blood], a less than normal amount of glucose in the blood, usually caused by administration of too much insulin, excessive secretion of insulin by the islet cells of the pancreas, or dietary deficiency. The condition may result in weakness, headache, hunger, visual disturbances, ataxia, anxiety, personality changes, and, if untreated, delirium, coma, and death. –**hypoglycemic,** *adj.*

hypoglycemic agent /hī′pōglīsē′mik/, any of a large heterogeneous group of drugs prescribed to decrease the amount of glucose circulating in the blood. Hypoglycemic agents include insulin, the sulfonylureas, and the biguanides. Insulin in its various forms is given parenterally and acts by increasing the use of carbohydrates and the metabolism of fats and protein. The sulfonylureas act by stimulating the release of endogenous insulin from the pancreas. The biguanides act by potentiating the action of endogenous insulin, augmenting the use of glucose by the peripheral cells of the body.

hypoglycemic coma, a loss of consciousness that results from abnormally low blood sugar levels.

hypogonadism /hī′pōgō′nədiz′əm/, a deficiency in the secretory activity of the ovary or testis. The condition may be primary, caused by a gonadal dysfunction involving the Leydig cells in the male, or secondary to a hypothalamic-pituitary disorder.

hypoinsulinism /hī′pō·in′səliniz′əm/ [Gk *hypo* under + L *insula* island (of Langerhans)], a deficiency of insulin secretion by cells of the pancreas and associated signs and symptoms of diabetes.

hypokalemia /hī′pōkəlē′mē·ə/ [Gk *hypo* + L *kalium* potassium; Gk *haima* blood], a condition in which an inadequate amount of potassium, the major intracellular cation, is found in the circulating bloodstream. Hypokalemia is characterized by abnormal ECG, weakness, and flaccid paralysis and may be caused by starvation, treatment of diabetic acidosis, adrenal tumor, or diuretic therapy.

hypokalemic [Gk *hypo* + L *kalium* potassium; Gk *haima* blood], a condition of low potassium blood levels.

hypokalemic alkalosis, a pathologic condition resulting from the accumulation of base or the loss of acid from the body, associated with a low level of serum potassium.

hypokalemic periodic paralysis, a state of recurring attacks of muscular weakness associated with low blood levels of potassium.

hypokinesia /hī'pōkinē'zhə/, a condition of abnormally diminished motor activity.

hypokinetic /hī'pōkinet'ik/ [Gk *hypo* + *kinesis* movement], a condition of diminished power of movement or motor function. It may or may not be accompanied by a mild form of paralysis.

hypolipemia. See **hypolipoproteinemia.**

hypolipoproteinemia /hī'pōlip'ōprō'tēnē'mē·ə/ [Gk *hypo* + *lipos* fat, *proteios* first rank, *haima* blood], a group of defects of lipoprotein metabolism that result in varying complexes of signs. Primary, or hereditary, hypolipoproteinemia factors include abnormal transport of triglycerides in the blood, low levels of high-density lipoproteins, high levels of low-density lipoproteins, and abnormal deposition of lipids in the body. Kinds of hypolipoproteinemias are **abetalipoproteinemia, hypobetalipoproteinemia, lecithin-cholesterol acyltransferase deficiency,** and **Tangier disease.**

hypomagnesemia /hī'pōmag'nisē'mē·ə/, an abnormally low concentration of magnesium in the blood plasma, resulting in nausea, vomiting, muscle weakness, tremors, tetany, and lethargy. Mild hypomagnesemia is usually the result of inadequate absorption of magnesium in the kidney or intestine. A more severe form is associated with malabsorption syndrome, protein malnutrition, and parathyroid disease.

hypomania /hī'pōmā'nē·ə/ [Gk *hypo* + *mania* madness], a psychopathologic state characterized by optimism, excitability, a marked hyperactivity and talkativeness, heightened sexual interest, quick anger and irritability, and a decreased need for sleep. **–hypomaniac,** *n., *hypomanic, adj.*

hypometria /hī'pōmē'trē·ə/ [Gk *hypo* + *metron* measure], an abnormal condition, a form of dysmetria, characterized by a dysfunction of the power to control the range of muscular action, resulting in movements that fall short of the intended goals of the affected individual.

hypomobility /hī'pōmōbil'itē/, a lack of normal movement of a joint or body part, as may result from an articular surface dysfunction or from disease or injury affecting a bone or muscle.

hypomorph /hī'pōmôrf/ [Gk *hypo* + *morphe* form], **1.** a person whose legs are disproportionately short in relation to the trunk and whose sitting height is greater in proportion than the person's standing height. **2.** (in genetics) a mutant allele that has a reduced effect on the expression of a trait but at a level too low to result in abnormal development.

hypomotility /hī'pōmōtil'itē/ [Gk *hypo* + L *motare* to move frequently], a state of diminished motility or loss of power to move about.

hyponatremia /hī'pōnatrē'mē·ə/ [Gk *hypo* + L *natrium* sodium; Gk *haima* blood], a less than normal concentration of sodium in the blood, caused by inadequate excretion of water or by excessive water in the circulating bloodstream. In a severe case the person may develop water intoxication with confusion and lethargy, leading to muscle excitability, convulsions, and coma.

hypoosmolarity /hī'pō·os'mōler'itē/ [Gk *hypo* + *osmos* impulse], a state or condition of abnormally reduced osmolarity.

hypoparathyroidism /hī'pōper'əthī'-roidiz'-əm/ [Gk *hypo* + *para* beside, *thyreos* shield, *eidos* form], a condition of diminished parathyroid function, which can be caused by primary parathyroid dysfunction or by elevated serum calcium levels.

hypoperistalsis /hī'pōper'istal'sis/ [Gk *hypo* + *peristellein* to clasp], a state of abnormally slow motility of waves of alternate contraction and relaxation that impel contents forward through the digestive tract.

hypopharyngeal /hī'pōfərin'jē·ə/ [Gk *hypo* + *pharynx* throat], **1.** of, pertaining to, or involving the hypopharynx. **2.** situated below the pharynx.

hypopharynx, the inferior portion of the pharynx, between the epiglottis and the larynx. It is a critical dividing point in separating solids and fluids from air entering the region.

hypophonia [Gk *hypo* + *phone* voice], a weak or whispered voice.

hypophoria, a type of strabismus in which the patient may not show signs of ocular muscle imbalance until the affected eye is covered, resulting in a downward deviation.

hypophosphatasia /hī'pōfos'fatā'zhə/ [Gk *hypo* + *phosphoros* lightbearing], congenital absence of alkaline phosphatase, an enzyme essential to the calcification of bone tissue.

hypophosphatemic rickets /hī'pōfos'fatē'-mik/, a rare familial disorder in which there is impaired resorption of phosphate in the kidneys and poor absorption of calcium in the small intestine, resulting in osteomalacia, retarded growth, skeletal deformities, and pain.

hypophosphaturia /hī′pōfos′fətŏŏr′ē·ə/ [Gk hypo + phosphoros bringer of light, ouron urine], a deficiency in the normal level of phosphates in the urine.

hypophyseal cachexia. See **panhypopituitarism.**

hypophyseal dwarf. See **pituitary dwarf.**

hypophyseal hormones /hī′pōfizē′əl, hī′po′fiz′ē-əl/, hormones that are associated with body growth and exercise effects, such as luteinizing hormone, growth hormone, and antidiuretic hormone.

hypophysectomy /hīpof′əsek′təmē/ [Gk hypo + phyein to grow, ektome excision], surgical removal of the pituitary gland. It may be performed to slow the growth and spread of endocrine-dependent malignant tumors of the breast, ovary, or prostate gland; to halt deterioration of the retina in diabetes; or to excise a pituitary tumor. −**hypophysectomize,** v.

hypophysis /hīpof′isis/ [Gk, hypo, under, phyein, to grow], the pituitary body (gland). The anterior lobe is sometimes identified as the **adenohypophysis** and the posterior lobe as the **neurohypophysis.** −**hypophyseal,** adj.

hypophysis cerebri. See **pituitary gland.**

hypopigmentation /hī′pōpig′məntā′shən/ [Gk hypo + L pigmentum paint], unusual lack of skin color, seen in albinism or vitiligo.

hypopituitarism /hī′pōpityŏŏ′iteriz′əm/ [Gk hypo + L pituita phlegm], an abnormal condition caused by diminished activity of the pituitary gland and marked by excessive deposits of fat and persistence or acquisition of adolescent characteristics.

hypoplasia /hī′pōplā′zhə/ [Gk hypo + plassein to mold], incomplete or underdeveloped organ or tissue, usually the result of a decrease in the number of cells. Kinds of hypoplasia are **cartilage-hair hypoplasia** and **enamel hypoplasia.** −**hypoplastic,** adj.

hypoplasia of the mesenchyme. See **osteogenesis imperfecta.**

hypoplastic anemia, a broad category of anemias characterized by decreased production of red blood cells.

hypoplastic dwarf. See **primordial dwarf.**

hypoploid /hī′pəploid/ [Gk hypo + eidos form], **1.** also **hypoploidic.** Of or pertaining to an individual, organism, strain, or cell that has fewer than the normal haploid number or an exact multiple of the haploid number of chromosomes charac-

teristic of the species. **2.** such an individual, organism, strain, or cell.

hypoploidy /hī′pōploi′dē/, any decrease in chromosome number that involves individual chromosomes rather than entire sets, resulting in fewer than the normal haploid number characteristic of the species, as in Turner's syndrome.

hypopnea /hī′pōp′nē·ə, hī′pōnē′ə/ [Gk hypo + pnoe breath], shallow or slow respiration. In well-conditioned athletes it is normal and is accompanied by a slow pulse; otherwise, it is characteristic of damage to the brainstem, in which case it is accompanied by a rapid, weak pulse and is a grave sign.

hypopotassemia /hī′pōpot′əse′mē·ə [Gk hypo + Dutch potasschen potash; Gk haima blood], a deficiency of potassium in the blood.

hypoproliferative anemias /hī′pōprolif-′ərətic′/, a group of anemias caused by inadequate production of erythrocytes. The condition is associated with protein deficiencies, renal disease, and myxedema.

hypoproteinemia /hī′pōprō′tēnē′mē·ə/ [Gk hypo + proteios first rank, haima blood], a disorder characterized by a decrease in the amount of protein in the blood to an abnormally low level, accompanied by edema, nausea, vomiting, diarrhea, and abdominal pain.

hypoprothrombinemia /hī′pōprōthrom-′binē′mē·ə/ [Gk hypo + L pro before; Gk thrombos lump, haima blood], an abnormal reduction in the amount of prothrombin (factor II) in the circulating blood, characterized by poor clot formation, longer bleeding time, and possible hemorrhage.

hypoptyalism /hī′pōtī′əliz′əm/ [Gk hypo + ptyalon spittle], a condition in which there is a decrease in the amount of saliva secreted by the salivary glands.

hypopyon /hīpō′pē·on/ [Gk hypo + pyon pus], an accumulation of pus in the anterior chamber of an eye, appearing as a gray fluid between the cornea and the iris. It may occur as a complication of conjunctivitis, herpetic keratitis, or corneal ulcer.

hyporeflexia /hīpōriflek′sē·ə/ [Gk hypo + L reflectere to bend backward], a neurologic condition characterized by weakened reflex reactions.

hyposalivation /hīpōsal′ivā′shən/ [Gk hypo + L saliva spittle], a decreased flow of saliva that may be associated with dehydration, radiation therapy of the salivary gland regions, anxiety, the use of drugs such as atropine and antihistamines, vitamin deficiency, various forms of parotitis,

H

or various syndromes such as Plummer-Vinson syndrome.

hyposensitization. See **immunotherapy.**

hypospadias /hī′pəspā′dē-əs/ [Gk *hypo* + *spadon* a split], a congenital defect in which the urinary meatus is on the underside of the penis. Incontinence does not occur because the sphincters are not defective.

hypostatic /hīpōstat′ik/ [Gk *hypo* + *stasis* standing still], pertaining to an accumulation of deposits of substances or congestion in a body area, resulting from a lack of activity.

hypostatic lung collapse [Gk *hypo* + *stasis;* AS *lungen;* L *collabi* to fall together], a lung disorder in which the settling or pooling of fluids or suspended solids results in congestion because of the effects of gravity in a dependent part.

hypostatic pneumonia, a type of pneumonia associated with elderly or debilitated persons who remain in the same position for long periods. Gravity tends to accelerate fluid congestion in one area of the lungs, increasing the susceptibility to infection.

hyposthenic /hī′pōsthen′ik/, 1. pertaining to a lack of strength or muscle tone. 2. pertaining to a body type characterized by a slender build.

hypotelorism /hī′pōtel′ə riz′əm/ [Gk *hypo* + *tele* far, *horizo* separate], a developmental defect characterized by an abnormally decreased distance between two organs or parts. A kind of hypotelorism is **ocular hypotelorism.**

hypotension [Gk *hypo* + L *tendere* to stretch], an abnormal condition in which the blood pressure is not adequate for normal perfusion and oxygenation of the tissues. An expanded intravascular space, a decreased intravascular volume, or a diminished cardiac thrust may be the cause.

hypotensive, pertaining to a condition of abnormally low blood pressure.

hypotensive anesthesia. See **deliberate hypotension.**

hypotetraploid. See **hypoploid.**

hypothalamic amenorrhea /hīpōthal-am′ik/ [Gk *hypo* + *thalamos* chamber], cessation of menses caused by disorders that inhibit the hypothalamus from initiating the cycle of neurohormonal interactions of the brain, pituitary, and ovary necessary for ovulation and subsequent menstruation.

hypothalamic hormones, a group of hormones secreted by the hypothalamus, including vasopressin, oxytocin, and the thyrotropin-releasing and gonadotropin-releasing hormones.

hypothalamic obesity [Gk *hypo* +

thalamos; L *obesitas* fatness], obesity that is caused by damage or a functional disturbance involving the hypothalamus.

hypothalamic-pituitary-adrenal axis, the combined system of neuroendocrine units that regulate the body's hormonal activities.

hypothalamus /hī′pōthal′əməs/ [Gk *hypo* + *thalamos* chamber], a portion of the diencephalon of the brain, forming the floor and part of the lateral wall of the third ventricle. It activates, controls, and integrates the peripheral autonomic nervous system, endocrine processes, and many somatic functions, such as body temperature, sleep, and appetite. **–hypothalamic,** *adj.*

hypothenar /hīpoth′ənär, hī′pōthē′när/ [Gk *hypo* + *thenar* palm], an eminence or fleshy elevation on the ulnar side of the palm of the hand.

hypothermal /hī′pōthur′məl/ [Gk *hypo* + *therme* heat], 1. pertaining to a condition in which the body temperature is significantly below normal or has been reduced markedly for surgical or therpeutic purposes. 2. pertaining to temperatures that are tepid to slightly warm.

hypothermia /hī′pōthur′mē-ə/ [Gk *hypo* + *therme* heat], 1. an abnormal and dangerous condition in which the temperature of the body is below 95° F (35° C), usually caused by prolonged exposure to cold. Respiration is shallow and slow, and the heart rate is faint and slow. The person is very pale and may appear to be dead. People who are very old or very young, people who have cardiovascular problems, and people who are hungry, tired, or under the influence of alcohol are most susceptible to hypothermia. Treatment includes slowly warming the person. Hospitalization is necessary for evaluating and treating any metabolic abnormalities that may result from hypothermia. 2. the deliberate and controlled reduction of body temperature with cooling mattresses or ice in preparation for some surgical procedures. 3. a NANDA-accepted nursing diagnosis of the state in which an individual's body temperature is reduced below his or her normal range but not below 96° F (rectal) or 97.5° F (rectal newborn). Defining characteristics include mild shivering, cool skin, moderate pallor, slow capillary refill, tachycardia, cyanotic nail beds, hypertension, and piloerection.

hypothermia blanket, a covering used to conserve heat in the body of a patient suffering from hypothermia.

hypothermia therapy, the reduction of a patient's body temperature to counteract high prolonged fever caused by an infectious or neurologic disease, or, less frequently, as an adjunct to anesthesia in heart or brain surgery. Hypothermia may be produced by placing crushed ice around the patient, by immersing the body in ice water, by autotransfusing blood after it is circulated through coils submerged in a refrigerant, or, most commonly, by applying cooling blankets or vinyl pads containing coils through which cold water and alcohol are circulated by a pump.

hypothesis /hīpoth'isis/ [Gk, groundwork], (in research) a statement derived from a theory that predicts the relationship among variables representing concepts, constructs, or events. Kinds of hypotheses include **causal, null,** and **predictive hypothesis.**

hypothrombinemia /hī'pōthrom'binē'mē·ə, a deficiency of the clotting factor thrombin in the blood.

hypothyroid /hī'pōthī'roid/ [Gk hypo + thyreos shield, eidos form], pertaining to or resembling a condition of thyroid deficiency.

hypothyroid dwarf. See **cretin dwarf.**

hypothyroidism /hī'pōthī'roidiz'əm/ [Gk hypo + thyreos + eidos form], a condition characterized by decreased activity of the thyroid gland. It is caused by surgical removal of all or part of the gland, overdosage with antithyroid medication, decreased effect of thyroid releasing hormone secreted by the hypothalamus, decreased secretion of thyroid stimulating hormone by the pituitary gland, or by atrophy of the thyroid gland itself. Weight gain, sluggishness, dryness of the skin, constipation, arthritis, and slowing of the metabolic processes of the body may occur. Untreated, hypothyroidism leads to myxedema, coma, and death.

hypotonia /hī'pōtō'nē·ə/ [Gk hypo + tonos stretching], a condition of diminished tone or tension that may involve any body structure.

hypotonic /hī'pōton'ik/ [Gk hypo + tonikos a stretching], (of a solution) having a smaller concentration of solute than another solution, hence exerting less osmotic pressure than that solution, as a hypotonic saline solution that contains less salt than is found in intracellular or extracellular fluid. Cells expand in a hypotonic solution.

hypotonic saline, a saline solution that is less than isotonic in strength.

hypotriploid. See **hypoploid.**

hypoventilation [Gk hypo + L ventilare to wave], an abnormal condition of the respiratory system, characterized by cyanosis, clubbing of the fingers, polycythemia, increased carbon dioxide arterial tension, Cheyne-Stokes breathing, and generalized decreased respiratory function. Hypoventilation may be caused by uneven distribution of inspired air (as in bronchitis), obesity, neuromuscular or skeletal disease affecting the thorax, decreased response of the respiratory center to carbon dioxide, and reduced functional lung tissue, as in atelectasis, emphysema, and pleural effusion. The result of hypoventilation is hypoxia, hypercapnia, pulmonary hypertension with cor pulmonale, and respiratory acidosis.

hypovitaminosis. See **avitaminosis.**

hypovolemia /hī'pōvōlē'mē·ə/ [Gk hypo + L volumen paper roll; Gk haima blood], an abnormally low circulating blood volume.

hypovolemic shock /hī'pōvōlē'mik/, a state of physical collapse and prostration caused by massive blood loss, circulatory dysfunction, and inadequate tissue perfusion. The common signs include low blood pressure, feeble pulse, clammy skin, tachycardia, rapid breathing, and reduced urinary output. The associated blood losses may stem from GI bleeding, internal hemorrhage, external hemorrhage, or excessive reduction of intravascular plasma volume and body fluids. Disorders that may cause hypovolemic shock are dehydration from excessive perspiration, severe diarrhea, protracted vomiting, intestinal obstruction, peritonitis, acute pancreatitis, and severe burns, which deplete body fluids.

hypoxemia /hī'poksē'mē·ə/ [Gk hypo + oxys sharp, genein to produce, haima blood], an abnormal deficiency of oxygen in the arterial blood. Symptoms of acute hypoxemia are cyanosis, restlessness, stupor, coma, Cheyne-Stokes breathing, apnea, increased blood pressure, tachycardia, and an initial increase in cardiac output that later falls, resulting in hypotension and ventricular fibrillation or asystole. Chronic hypoxemia stimulates red blood cell production by the bone marrow, leading to secondary polycythemia.

hypoxia /hīpok'sē·ə/ [Gk hypo + oxys sharp, genein to produce], an inadequate, reduced tension of cellular oxygen, characterized by cyanosis, tachycardia, hypertension, peripheral vasoconstriction, dizziness, and mental confusion. The tissues most sensitive to hypoxia are the brain, heart, pulmonary vessels, and liver.

hypoxic drive /hīpok'sik/, the low arterial oxygen pressure stimulus to respiration that is mediated through the carotid bodies.

hypsibrachycephaly /hips'ibrakisef'əlē/ [Gk hypsi high, brachys short, kephale

head], the condition of having a skull that is high with a broad forehead. –hypsibrachycephalic, *adj., n.*

hypsicephaly See **oxycephaly.**

hysterectomy /his'tərek'təmē/ [Gk *hystera* womb, *ektome* excision], surgical removal of the uterus, performed to remove fibroid tumors of the uterus or to treat chronic pelvic inflammatory disease, severe recurrent endometrial hyperplasia, uterine hemorrhage, and precancerous and cancerous conditions of the uterus. Types of hysterectomy include **total hysterectomy,** in which the uterus and cervix are removed, and **radical hysterectomy,** in which ovaries, oviducts, lymph nodes and lymph channels are removed with the uterus and cervix. Menstruation ceases after either type is performed. One or both ovaries and oviducts may be removed at the same time. A kind of hysterectomy is **cesarean hysterectomy. –hysterectomize,** *v.*

hysteresis /his'tərē'sis/ [Gk *hysterein* to be late] **1.** a lagging or retardation of one of two associated phenomena, or a failure to act in unison. **2.** the influence of the previous condition or treatment of the body on its subsequent response to a given force.

hysteria /histir'ē·ə/ [Gk *hystera* womb], **1.** a general state of tension or excitement in a person or a group, characterized by unmanageable fear and temporary loss of control over the emotions. **2.** *obsolete.* a psychoneurosis, now commonly called **hysteric neurosis.**

hysteric /hister'ik/ [Gk *hystera,* womb], pertaining to or resembling hysteria. Also called **hysterical.**

hysterical aphonia [Gk *hystera; a* not, *phone* voice], an inability to produce vocal sounds, usually psychogenic in nature.

hysterical tremor [Gk *hystera;* L *tremere* to tremble], **1.** a fine tremor in one extremity or generalized that may be an expression of fear, anxiety, or hysteria. **2.** a coarse irregular tremor that increases with voluntary movements. **3.** a tremor that is transient and is caused by exposure to drugs or toxic substances rather than an organic disorder.

hysteric amaurosis [Gk *hystera* + *amauroein* to darken, monocular or, more rarely, binocular blindness occurring after an emotional shock and lasting for hours, days, or months.

hysteric ataxia [Gk *hystera; ataxia* lack of order], a loss of control over voluntary movements in walking or standing although the involved muscles function normally when the patient is lying or sitting down.

hysteric chorea [Gk *hystera; choreia* dance], a condition in which a patient shows choreiform movements, usually associated with the person's occupation, although the actions are the result of hysteria rather than true chorea.

hysteric paralysis [Gk *hystera; paralyein* to be palsied], a loss of movement or muscular weakness that is caused by hysteria rather than an identifiable organic defect.

hysteritis /his'tərī'tis/, an inflammation of the uterus.

hysterogram /his'tərōgram'/ [Gk *hystera* + *gramma* record], the radiographic record of a uterus made after the injection of a contrast medium into the uterine cavity.

hysterography /his'tərog'rəfē/ [Gk *hystera* + *graphein* to record], the use of x-ray film and other instruments to make a medical assessment of the condition of the uterus.

hysterolaparotomy /his'tərōlap'ərot'əmē/ [Gk *hystera* + *lapara* loin, *temnein* to cut], abdominal hysterectomy or hysterotomy.

hystero-oophorectomy /his'tərō·ō'əfərek'-təmē/ [Gk *hystera* + *oophoron* ovary, *ektome* cutting out], the surgical removal of both the uterus and the ovaries.

hysteropathy /his'tərop'əthē/, any disease of the uterus.

hysterosalpingogram /his'tərōsalping'-gōgram'/ [Gk *hystera* + *salpinx* tube, *gramma* record], an x-ray film of the uterus and the fallopian tubes using gas or a radiopaque substance introduced through the cervix to allow visualization of the cavity of the uterus and the passageway of the tubes.

hysterosalpingography /his'tərōsal'-ping·gog'rəfē/, a method of producing x-ray images of the uterus and fallopian tubes as part of the diagnosis of abnormalities in the reproductive tract of a nonpregnant woman.

hysterosalpingo-oophorectomy /his'tərō-salping'gō·ō'əfərek'təmē/ [Gk *hystera* + *salpinx* tube; *oophoron* ovary, *ektome* excision], surgical removal of one or both ovaries and oviducts along with the uterus, performed commonly to treat malignant neoplastic disease of the reproductive tract and chronic endometriosis. To avoid the severe symptoms of sudden menopause, a portion of one ovary is left, unless a malignancy is present.

hysteroscopy /his'təros'kepē/ [Gk *hystera* + *skopein* to look], direct visual inspection of the cervical canal and uterine cavity through a hysteroscope, performed to examine the endometrium, to secure a specimen for biopsy, to remove an intra-uterine device, or to excise cervical polyps. **–hysteroscope,** *n.,* **hysteroscopic,** *adj.*

hysterospasm /his'tərōspaz'əm/ [Gk *hystera* + *spasmos*], a spasmodic contraction of the uterus.

hysterotome /his'tərotōm'/ [Gk *hystera* + *temnein* to cut], a surgical knife used for certain procedures involving the uterus.

hysterotomy /his'tərot'əmē/ [Gk *hystera* + *temnein* to cut], surgical incision of the uterus, performed as a method of abortion in a pregnancy beyond the first trimester of gestation in which a saline-injection abortion was incomplete, or in which a tubal sterilization is to be done with the abortion.

hysterovagino-enterocele /his'tərōvaj'-inō·en'tərōsēl'/ [Gk *hystera* + L *vagina* sheath; Gk *enteron* bowel, *kele* hernia], a hernia involving the uterus, vagina, and intestines.

Hz, abbreviation for **hertz.**

HZV, abbreviation for **herpes zoster virus.**

H

I

I, 1. symbol for **inspired gas.** 2. symbol for **iodine.**

¹³¹I, symbol for radioactive iodine, atomic weight 131.

¹³²I, symbol for radioactive iodine, atomic weight 132.

IABP, abbreviation for **intraaortic balloon pump.**

IADR, abbreviation for **International Association for Dental Research.**

I and O, abbreviation for *intake and output.*

iatrogenic /ī′atrōjen′ik, yat-/ [Gk *iatros* physician, *genein* to produce], caused by treatment or diagnostic procedures. **–iatrogenesis,** *n.*

iatrogeny [Gk *iatros* physician + *genein* to produce], pertaining to disorders traced to fears instilled in patients by remarks or questions of examining physicians.

iatrology, the science of medicine.

I band [ME *band* flat strip], an isotropic band of striated muscle fiber that appears dark in polarized light but light when stained.

IBC, abbreviation for *iron-binding capacity.*

ibuprofen /ībyo͞o′prəfin/, a nonsteroidal antiinflammatory agent prescribed in the treatment of rheumatoid and osteoarthritis conditions.

IBW, abbreviation for *ideal body weight.*

IC, abbreviation for **inspiratory capacity.**

ICD, abbreviation for *International Classification of Diseases.*

ICDA, abbreviation for *International Classification of Disease Adapted for Use in the United States.*

Iceland disease, a group of symptoms associated with effects of a viral infection of the nervous system, including muscular pain and weakness, depression, and sensory changes.

ice pack [ME *is* + *pakke*], a container of crushed ice used to reduce tissue temperatures, relieve pain, soothe inflamed tissues, or control bleeding.

ICF, abbreviation for **intermediate care facility.**

ICF/MR, abbreviation for *intermediate care facility for the mentally retarded.*

ichthammol /ik′thəmôl/, a topical antiin-

fective used for treating certain skin diseases.

ichthyoid /ik′thē·oid/ [Gk *ichthys* fish, *eidos* form], pertaining to objects or structures that are fish-shaped.

ichthyosis /ik′thē·ō′sis/ [Gk *ichthys* fish, *osis* condition], any of several inherited dermatologic conditions in which the skin is dry, hyperkeratotic, and fissured, resembling fish scales. It usually appears at or shortly after birth and may be part of one of several rare syndromes. **–ichthyotic,** *adj.*

ichthyosis congenita, ichthyosis fetalis. See **lamellar exfoliation of the newborn.**

ichthyosis fetus. See **harlequin fetus.**

ichthyosis vulgaris [Gk *ichthys, osis;* L *vulgaris* common], a hereditary skin disorder characterized by large, dry, dark scales that cover the face, neck, scalp, ears, back, and extensor surfaces but not the flexor surfaces of the body.

ICN, abbreviation for **International Council of Nurses.**

ICP, abbreviation for **intracranial pressure.**

ICS, abbreviation for **International Congress of Surgeons.**

ICSH, abbreviation for **interstitial cell-stimulating hormone.**

ictal /ik′təl/ [L *ictus* a stroke], pertaining to a sudden, acute onset, as convulsions of an epileptic seizure.

icteric /ikter′ik/ [Gk *ikteros* jaundice], pertaining to or resembling jaundice.

icterus. See **jaundice.**

icterus gravis neonatorum /ik″tərəs/ [Gk *ikteros* jaundice; L *gravis* weight, *neonatus* newborn], a hemolytic jaundice of the newborn caused by incompatibility between the mother's serum and the red corpuscles of the infant.

icterus index [Gk *ikteros;* L *index* pointer], a liver function test in which the blood serum is compared in intensity of color with that of potassium dichromate. When an excessive amount of bilirubin is present and jaundice becomes apparent, the index is higher; subnormal values are associated with various anemias.

icterus neonatorum, a jaundice condition in a newborn infant.

ictus /ik′təs/, *pl.* **ictuses, ictus** [L, stroke],

1. a seizure. **2.** a cerebrovascular accident. **–ictal, ictic,** *adj.*

ICU, abbreviation for **intensive care unit.**

id [L, it], **1.** (in psychoanalysis) the part of the psyche functioning in the unconscious that is the source of instinctive energy, impulses, and drives. **2.** the true unconscious.

ID, abbreviation for **infectious disease.**

IDDM, abbreviation for **insulin-dependent diabetes mellitus.**

idea [Gk, form], any thought, concept, intention, or impression that exists in the mind as a result of awareness, understanding, or other mental activity. Kinds of ideas include **autochthonous, compulsive, dominant,** and **fixed.**

ideal gas law [Gk *idea* form, *chaos* gas; AS *lagu* law], a rule that PV = nRT, with the product of pressure (P) and volume (V) equal to the product of the number of moles of gas (n), temperature (T), and a gas constant (R).

idealized image, a self-concept of a person with a compulsive craving for perfection and admiration. It results in high unrealistic and unattainable goals.

idea of influence, an obsessive delusion, often seen in paranoid disorders, that external forces or persons are controlling one's thoughts, actions, and feelings.

idea of persecution, an obsessive delusion, often seen in paranoid disorders, that one is being threatened, discriminated against, or mistreated by other persons or by external forces.

idea of reference, an obsessive delusion that the statements or actions of others refer to oneself, usually taken to be depreciatory, often seen in paranoid disorders.

ideational apraxia [Gk *idea* form; *a, prassein* not to do], a condition in which the conceptual process is lost, often because of a lesion in the parietal lobe. The individual is unable to formulate a plan of movement and does not know the proper use of an object because of a lack of perception of its purpose. There is no loss of motor movement.

idée fixe. See **fixed idea.**

identical twins. See **monozygotic twins.**

identification [L *idem* the same, *facere* to make], an unconscious defense mechanism by which a person patterns his or her personality on that of another person, assuming the person's qualities, characteristics, and actions. Kinds of identification are **competitive** and **positive identification.**

identity, a component of self-concept characterized by one's persisting consciousness of being oneself, separate and distinct from others. **Identity confusion** refers to an altered self-concept in which one does not maintain a clear consciousness of a consistent and continuous self. **Identity diffusion** is a lack of clarity and consistency in one's perception of the self, resulting in a high degree of anxiety.

identity crisis [L *idem* the same; Gk *krisis* turning point], a period of disorientation concerning an individual's sense of self and role in society, occurring most frequently in the transition from one stage of life to the next. Identity crises are most common during adolescence, when a sudden increase in the strength of internal drives combined with greater peer pressure and adult expectations of more mature behavior often results in conflicts.

ideology [Gk *idea*], a scheme of ideas or systematic organization of ideas associated with doctrine and philosophy.

ideomotor apraxia /ī·dē·ə·mō′tər/ [Gk *idea* + L *motare* to move about; Gk *a, prassein* not to do], the inability to translate an idea into motion, resulting from some interference with the transmission of the appropriate impulses from the brain to the motor centers. There is no loss of the ability to perform an action automatically, but the action cannot be performed on request.

ideophobia /ī′dē·ōfō′bē·ə/ [Gk *idea* + *phobos* fear], an anxiety disorder characterized by the irrational fear or distrust of ideas or reason.

idiogram /id′ē·əgram′/, a diagram or graphic representation of a karyotype, showing the number, relative sizes, and morphology of the chromosomes of a species, individual, or cell.

idiojunctional rhythm /id′ē·ōjungk′shənəl/ [Gk *idios* own; L *jungere* to join; Gk *rhythmos*], a heart rhythm emanating from the AV junction but without retrograde conduction to the atria.

idiomere. See **chromomere.**

idiopathic /id′ē·ōpath′ik/ [Gk *idios* + *pathos* disease], without a known cause.

idiopathic disease, a disease that develops without an apparent or known cause, although it may have a recognizable pattern of signs and symptoms and may be curable.

idiopathic gangrene [Gk *idios* + *pathos* disease, *gaggraina*], a gangrenous condition of unknown etiology.

idiopathic hypertrophic subaortic stenosis, a cardiomyopathic disorder, usually involving the left ventricle of the heart, that obstructs emptying.

idiopathic multiple pigmented hemorrhagic sarcoma. See **Kaposi's sarcoma.**

idiopathic nephrotic syndrome [Gk *idios*

+ *pathos; nephros* kidney, *syn* together, *dromos* course], a kidney disease of unknown origin, characterized by hematuria, albuminuria, edema, and blood pressure, and changes in the glomeruli capillaries.

idiopathic neuralgia [Gk *idios* + *pathos; neuron* nerve, *algos* pain], a form of neuralgia that occurs without any identifiable structural nerve lesion.

idiopathic pericarditis [Gk *idios* + *pathos; peri* near, *kardia* heart, *itis*], an inflammation of the pericardium that occurs without a known etiology.

idiopathic pulmonary fibrosis [Gk *idios* + *pathos;* L *pulmoneous* lungs, *fibra* fiber], fibrosis of the lungs that may follow an earlier inflammation or disease, such as tuberculosis or pneumoconiosis.

idiopathic respiratory distress syndrome. See **hyaline membrane disease.**

idiopathic scoliosis, an abnormal condition characterized by a lateral curvature of the spine. It is the most common type of scoliosis. The main factors in diagnosing idiopathic scoliosis are the degree, balance, and rotational component of the curvature. The rotational component may contribute to rib cage deformities and impingement on the pulmonary and the cardiac systems. Neurologic deficits are commonly associated with severe curvature and vary according to the extent to which the curvature has impinged on the spinal cord. Some signs of such impingement are reflex, sensation, and motor alterations of the lower extremities.

idiopathic steatorrhea [Gk *idios* + *pathos; stear* fat, *rhoia* flow], a condition of excess fat in the stools, particularly as in celiac disease in adults.

idiopathic tetanus [Gk *idios* + *pathos; tetanos* convulsive tension], a tetanus infection of unknown etiology.

idiopathic thrombocytopenic purpura (ITP), bleeding into the skin and other organs caused by a deficiency of platelets. **Acute ITP** is a disease of children that may follow a viral infection, lasts a few weeks to a few months, and usually has no residual effects. **Chronic ITP** is more common in adolescents and adults, begins more insidiously, and lasts longer. Antibodies to platelets are found in patients with ITP.

idiopathy /id′ē·op′əthē/, any primary disease that arises without an apparent cause. –**idiopathic,** *adj.*

idiosyncrasy /id′ē·ōsin′krəsē/ [Gk *idios* + *synkrasis* mixing together], **1.** a physical or behavioral characteristic or manner that is unique to an individual or to a group. **2.** an individual's unique hyper-

sensitivity to a particular drug, food, or other substance. –**idiosyncratic,** *adj.*

idiosyncracy to a drug [Gk *idios* + *synkrasis* mixing together; Fr *drogue*], an individual sensitivity to effects of a drug due to inherited or other bodily constitution factors. In some cases, a drug may have indiosyncratic effects that are contrary to the expected results.

idiot savant /idē·ō′ savänt′/, *pl. idiot savants, idiots savants,* an individual with severe mental retardation who is nonetheless capable of performing certain unusual mental feats, primarily those involving music, puzzle-solving, or the manipulation of numbers.

idiotype /id′ē·ətīp′/ [Gk *idios* + *typos* mark], the portion of an immunoglobulin molecule conferring unique character; most often including its binding site.

idioventricular /id′ē·əventrik′yələr/ [Gk *idios* + L *ventriculum* belly], originating in a ventricle.

idioventricular rhythm, a slow heart rhythm caused by a repeated discharge of impulses from a focus within a ventricle. The condition occurs in heart block and sinus arrest.

IDL (intermediate-density lipoprotein), a lipid-protein complex with a density between VLDL (very-low-density lipoprotein) and LDL (low-density lipoprotein). In a type III hyperlipoproteinemic person the IDL concentration in the blood is found to be elevated.

IDM, abbreviation for *infant of a diabetic mother.*

idoxuridine /ī′doksy·ōōr′ədēn/, an ophthalmic antiviral prescribed for herpes simplex keratitis.

id reaction, the autosensitization resulting from a fungal infection that causes pruritus and vesicular lesions. These secondary lesions, caused by circulating antigens, are usually distant from the primary fungal infection.

I:E ratio, (in respiratory therapy) the duration of inspiration to expiration. A range of 1:1.5 to 1:2 for an adult is considered acceptable for mechanical ventilation. Ratio increases to 1:1 or 2:1 or higher may cause hemodynamic complications.

Ig, abbreviation for **immunoglobulin.**

IgA, abbreviation for **immunoglobulin A.**

IgA deficiency, a selective lack of immunoglobulin A, the most common type of immunoglobulin deficiency. Immunoglobulin A is a major protein antibody in the saliva and the mucous membranes of the intestines and the bronchi. It protects against bacterial and viral infections. A deficiency of immunoglobulin A is associated with heredity and with autoimmune abnormalities. The IgA deficiency is common in patients with rheumatoid arthritis and in patients with systemic lupus erythematosus. Common symptoms are respiratory allergies associated with chronic sinopulmonary infection.

IgD, abbreviation for **immunoglobulin D.**

IgE, abbreviation for **immunoglobulin E.**

IgG, abbreviation for **immunoglobulin G.**

IgM, abbreviation for **immunoglobulin M.**

IGT, abbreviation for **impaired glucose tolerance.**

IH, an abbreviation for **infectious hepatitis.**

Ikwa fever. See **trench fever.**

ILD, abbreviation for **interstitial lung disease;** *interstitial lung disorders.*

Ile, abbreviation for **isoleucine.**

ileac /il′ē·ak/ [L *ilia intestines*], pertaining to the ileum.

ileal bypass /il′ē·əl/ [L *ilia* intestines; AS *bi* near; Fr *passer*], a surgical procedure for treating obesity by anastomosing the upper portion of the small intestine to a part closer to the end of the small intestine, thereby bypassing much of the length of the ileum that normally absorbs nutrients.

ileal conduit, a method of urinary diversion through intestinal tract tissue. Ureters are implanted in a section of dissected ileum that is then sewed to an ostomy in the abdominal wall, where a collecting device is attached.

ileitis /il′ē·ī′tis/ [L *ileum* intestine; Gk *itis*], inflammation of the ileum.

ileo-anal anastomosis /il′ē·ō·ā′nəl/, a surgical procedure in which the colon and rectum are removed but the anus is left intact along with the anal sphincter. An anastomosis is formed between the lower end of the small intestine and the anus.

ileocecal /il′ē·ōsē′kəl/ [L *ilia* intestines, *caecus* blind], pertaining to both the ileum and the cecum and the region where they are joined.

ileocecal valve, the valve between the ileum of the small intestine and the cecum of the large intestine. The valve consists of two flaps that project into the lumen of the large intestine, just above the vermiform appendix.

ileocecostomy. See **cecoileostomy.**

ileocolic node /il′ē·ōkol′ik/ [L *ileum* + Gk *kolon* colon; L *nodus* knot], a node in one of three groups of superior mesenteric lymph glands, forming a chain around the ileocolic (mesenteric) artery.

ileocystoplasty /il′ē·ōsis′təplas′tē/ [L *ileum* + Gk *kystis* bag, *plassein* to mold], a surgical procedure in which the bladder is reconstructed using a segment of the ileum for the bladder wall.

ileocystostomy /il′ē·ōsistos′təmē/ [L *ileum* + Gk *kystis* + *stoma* mouth], a surgical procedure to form a passage to direct urine through the abdominal wall using a segment of small intestine as a tube from the bladder.

ileostomate /il′ē·os′təmāt/, a person who has undergone an ileostomy.

ileostomy /il′ē·os′təmē/ [L *ileum* + Gk *stoma* mouth, *temnein* to cut], surgical formation of an opening of the ileum onto the surface of the abdomen, through which fecal matter is emptied. The operation is performed in advanced or recurrent ulcerative colitis, Crohn's disease, or cancer of the large bowel. Intestinal antibiotics are given to decrease the bacterial count. A nasogastric or intestinal tube is passed. The diseased portion of the large bowel is removed in a permanent ileostomy; occasionally, the distal and proximal segments of bowel may be reconnected after ulcerated areas have healed. A loop of the proximal ileum is then brought out onto the abdomen and sutured in place, and a stoma is formed. Postoperatively, the patient wears a temporary disposable bag to collect the semiliquid fecal matter, which begins to drain once peristalsis is restored and the tube is removed.

ileum /il′ē·əm/, *pl.* ilea [L, intestine], the distal portion of the small intestine, extending from the jejunum to the cecum. It ends in the right iliac fossa, opening into the medial side of the large intestine. **–ileac, ileal,** *adj.*

ileus /il′ē·əs/ [L; Gk *eilein* to twist], an obstruction of the intestines, such as an adynamic ileus caused by immobility of the bowel, or a mechanic ileus in which the intestine is blocked by mechanical means.

iliac circumflex node /il′ē·ak/ [L *ilium* flank; *circum* around, *flectere* to bend; *nodus* knot], a node in one of the seven clusters of parietal lymph nodes of the abdomen. This node is one of a group found along the course of the deep iliac circumflex vessels.

iliac crest, the upper elevated margins of the ilium.

iliac fascia, the portion of the endoabdominal fascia that is attached with the iliacus to the crest of the ilium and passes under the inguinal ligament into the thigh.

iliac region. See **inguinal region.**

iliacus /ilī′əkəs/ [L *ilium* flank], a flat, triangular muscle that covers the inner curved surface of the iliac fossa. It acts to flex and laterally rotate the thigh.

iliofemoral /il'ē·ō·fem'ərəl/, of or pertaining to the ilium and femur.

iliofemoral ligament [L *ilium* + *femur* thigh, *ligamentum*], a triangular band of connective tissue attached by its apex to the anterior inferior spine of the ilium and acetabular margin and by its base to the interotrochanteric line of the femur.

ilioinguinal /il'ē·ō·ing'gwinəl/ [L *ilium* + *inguen* groin], of or pertaining to the hip and inguinal regions.

iliolumbar ligament /il'ē·ōlum'bər/ [L *ilium* + *lumbus* loin; *ligare* to bind], one of a pair of ligaments forming part of the connection between the vertebral column and the pelvis. Each iliolumbar ligament attaches to a transverse process of the fifth lumbar vertebra and passes to the base of the sacrum.

iliopectineal line /il'ē·ōpek'tērəl/ [L *ilium* + *pectus* breast; *linea*], a bony ridge on the inner surface of the ilium and pubic bones that divides the true and false pelvises.

iliopsoas /il'ē·ōsō'əs/ [L *ilium* + Gk *psoa* loin muscle], one of the pair of muscle complexes that flexes the thigh and the lumbar vertebral column.

iliopsoas abscess [L *ilium* flank], an abscess, possibly tuberculous in origin, that spreads from the thoracic or lumbar spine to the upper leg muscles.

iliotibial band /il'ē·ōtib'ē·əl/ [L *ilium* flank, *tibia* shinbone], a layer of connective tissue that extends from the iliac crest to the knee and links the gluteus maximus to the tibia.

ilium /il'ē·əm/, *pl.* *ilia* [L, flank], one of the three bones that make up the innominate bone. The ilium forms part of the acetabulum and provides attachment for several muscles, including the obturator internus, the gluteals, the iliacus, and the sartorius. —**iliac,** *adj.*

illegitimate [L *in* + *legitimatus* not lawful], 1. not authorized by law. 2. born out of wedlock. 3. abnormal.

illicit [L *illicitus* unlawful], pertaining to an act that is unlawful or otherwise not permitted.

illness [ME, unhealthy condition], an abnormal process in which aspects of the social, physical, emotional, or intellectual condition and function of a person are diminished or impaired, compared with that person's previous condition.

illness behavior, the manner in which individuals monitor the structure and functions of their own bodies, interpret symptoms, take remedial action, and make use of health care facilities.

illness experience, the process of being ill, comprising five stages: phase I, experiencing a symptom; phase II, assuming a sick role; phase III, making contact for health care; phase IV, being dependent (a patient); and phase V, recovering or being rehabilitated. Each stage is characterized by certain decisions, behaviors, and end points.

illness prevention, a system of health education programs and activities directed toward protecting patients from real or potential health threats, minimizing risk factors, and promoting healthy behavior.

illumination [L *illuminare* to make light], the lighting up of a part of the body or of an object under a microscope for the purpose of examination. —**illuminate,** *v.*

illusion [L *illudere* to mock], a false interpretation of an external sensory stimulus, usually visual or auditory, such as a mirage in the desert or voices on the wind.

IL-6, abbreviation for *interleukin-6,* an antiviral compound also used in the treatment of some types of cancer.

IM, abbreviation for **intramuscular.**

IMA, abbreviation for **Industrial Medical Association.**

image [L *imago* likeness], 1. a representation or visual reproduction of the likeness of someone or something, such as a painting, photograph, or sculpture. 2. an optic representation of an object, such as that produced by refraction or reflection. 3. a person or thing that closely resembles another; semblance. 4. a mental picture, representation, idea, or concept of an objective reality. 5. (in psychology) a mental representation of something previously perceived and subsequently modified by other experiences. Kinds of images include **body, eidetic, memory, mental, motor,** and **tactile image.**

image acquistion time, the time required to carry out an NMR imaging procedure comprising only the data acquisition time.

image foreshortening, (in radiology) an x-ray image distortion caused by improper positioning of the object or the x-ray tube. It results in an image that is smaller than the object itself.

image format, (in computed tomography) the manner in which an image is stored, such as on a floppy disk, magnetic tape, or film.

image intensifier, an electronic device used to produce a fluoroscopic image with a low-radiation exposure. A beam of x-rays is converted into a pattern of electrons. The electrons are accelerated and concentrated onto a small fluorescent screen.

image matrix, (in radiology) an arrangement of columns or rows of imaginary cells, or pixels, forming a digital image.

imagery [L *imago*], (in psychiatry) the formation of mental concepts, figures, or ideas; any product of the imagination. In mentally disturbed persons these images are often bizarre and delusional.

imagination [L *imaginare* picture to oneself, **1.** the ability to form, or the act or process of forming mental images or conscious concepts of things that are not immediately available to the senses. **2.** (in psychology) the ability to reproduce images or ideas stored in the memory by the stimulation or suggestion of associated ideas.

imaging [L *imago*], the formation of a mental picture or representation of someone or something using the imagination.

imago /imā′gō/ [L, likeness], (in analytic psychology) an unconscious, usually idealized mental image of a significant individual, such as one's mother, in a person's early, formative years.

imbalance [L *im* not, *bilanx* having two scales], **1.** lack of balance between opposing muscle groups. **2.** an abnormal balance of fluid and electrolytes in the body tissues. **3.** an unequal distribution of subjects in a population group. **4.** a person with mental abilities that are remarkable in one area but deficient in others, as an idiot savant.

imbricate /im′brikāt/ [L *imbrex* roofing tile], to build a surface with overlapping layers of material. Surgeons may imbricate with layers of tissue when closing a wound or other opening in a body part. **–imbrication,** *n.*

iminoglycinuria /im′inōglī′sinŏŏr′ē·əl/, a benign familial condition characterized by the abnormal urinary excretion of the amino acids glycine, proline, and hydroxyproline.

imipenem-cilastatin sodium /im′ipē′-nəmsil′əstat′in/, a broad spectrum parenteral antibiotic. It is prescribed for the treatment of infections caused by susceptible organisms in the lower respiratory or urinary tracts, skin, abdomen, reproductive organs, bones, or joints. It is also used in the treatment of endocarditis and septicema.

imipramine hydrochloride /imip′rəmēn/, a tricyclic antidepressant with a slow onset of action. It is prescribed in the treatment of mental depression.

immature baby [L *im* not, *maturare* to make ripe], a term sometimes applied to an infant weighing less than 1,134 g (2.5 lb) and who is considerably underdeveloped at birth.

immature cataract [L *in* + *maturus* ripe; Gk *katarrhaktes*], a cataract at an early stage of development when the lens absorbs fluid and increases in swelling; only part of the lens is opaque.

immature erythrocyte [L *in* + *maturus;* Gk *erythros* red, *kytos* cell], any of the intermediate blood cells between the hemocytoblasts and non-nucleated red blood cells. They may be found in the blood circulation after birth of the fetus.

immediate auscultation [L *im* + *medius* middle; *auscultare* to listen], a method of examining a patient by placing an ear or stethoscope on the skin directly over the body part being studied.

immediate automatism a state in which a person acts spontaneously and automatically with no recollection of the behavior.

immediate denture, a removable artificial denture that is placed in the mouth immediately after removal of the natural teeth in order to maintain normal appearance and ability to masticate food. The immediate denture may be full or partial.

immediate hypersensitivity, an allergic reaction that occurs within minutes after exposure to an allergen.

immediate percussion. See **percussion.**

immediate postoperative fit prosthesis (IPOF), a temporary or preparatory prosthesis, such as a pylon.

immediate posttraumatic automatism, a posttraumatic state in which a person acts spontaneously and automatically without having any recollection of the behavior.

immersion /imur′zhən/ [L *im* + *mergere* to dip], the placing of a body or an object into water or other liquid so that it is completely covered by the liquid. **–immerse,** *v.*

immersion foot, an abnormal condition of the feet characterized by damage to the muscles, nerves, skin and blood vessels, caused by prolonged exposure to dampness or by prolonged immersion in cold water.

imminent abortion. See **inevitable abortion.**

immiscible /imis′əbəl/ [L *im* + *miscere* to mix], not capable of being mixed, such as oil and water.

immotile cilia syndrome /imō′til/ [L *im* + *motilis* movable, *cilia* eyelashes; Gk *syn* together, *dromos* course], a condition in which the hairlike processes of epithelial and other cells fail to function normally. As a result, the patient has difficulty in removing dust and other airborne debris from the respiratory system.

immune /imyŏŏn′/ [L *immunis* free from], a state of being protected against infective or allergic diseases by a system of antibody molecules and related resistance factors.

immune body. See **antibody.**

immune complex hypersensitivity [L *immunis* free; *complexus* embrace; Gk *hyper* excess; L *sentire* to feel], an IgG or IgM complement dependent, immediate acting humoral hypersensitivity to certain soluble antigens. It is seen in serum sickness, Arthus reaction, and glomerulonephritis.

immune cytolysis, cell destruction mediated by a particular antibody in conjunction with complement.

immune gamma globulin, passive immunizing agents obtained from pooled human plasma. It is prescribed for immunization against measles, poliomyelitis, chickenpox, serum hepatitis following transfusion, hepatitis A, agammaglobulinemia, and hypogammaglobulinemia.

immune globulin. See **immune gamma globulin.**

immune human globulin, a sterile solution of globulins that is used as a passive immunizing agent and derived from adult human blood.

immune proteins [L *immunis;* Gk *proteios* first rank], proteins in the form of antibodies or antitoxins that contribute to the immunity of a host.

immune reaction [L *immunis;* re + *agere* to act], a local reaction to an antigen, as may occur following a vaccination.

immune response, a defense function of the body that produces antibodies to destroy invading antigens and malignancies. Important components of the immune system and response are immunoglobulins, lymphocytes, phagocytes, complement, properdin, the migratory inhibitory factor, and interferon. The kinds of immune response are humoral immune response, involving B lymphocytes or B cells, and cell-mediated immune response, involving T lymphocytes or T cells. The B cells and the T cells derive from the hemopoietic stem cells. The receptor sites on the surface membranes of the B cells are the combining sites of immunoglobulin molecules, identified by letter names, M, G, A, E, and D. Immunoglobulin M, the antibody that immature B cells synthesize and incorporate in their cytoplasmic membranes, is the predominant antibody produced. The T cells develop in the thymus gland and proliferate with antigen receptors on their surface membranes. The T cells assist in the antigen-antibody reaction of the B cells and control the cell-mediated response. The cell-mediated response is also effective against fungi, viruses, and tumors and is the major reaction in the rejection of organ transplants.

immune serum. See **antiserum.**

immune serum globulin. See **chickenpox, immune human globulin, immunoglobulin antibody.**

immune system, a biochemical complex that protects the body against pathogenic organisms and other foreign bodies. The system incorporates the humoral immune response, which produces antibodies to react with specific antigens, and the cell-mediated response, which uses T cells to mobilize tissue macrophages in the presence of a foreign body.

immunity /imy$\overline{oo}$'nitē/ [L *immunis* free], **1.** (in civil law) exemption from a duty or an obligation generally required by law, as an exemption from taxation, exemption from penalty for wrongdoing, or protection against liability. **2.** the quality of being insusceptible to or unaffected by a particular disease or condition. Kinds of immunity are **active immunity** and **passive immunity.** –**immune,** *adj.*

immunization [L *immunis* free], a process by which resistance to an infectious disease is induced or augmented.

immunoassay /im'yənō·as'ā/ [L *immunis* + Fr *essayer* to try], a competitive-binding assay in which the binding protein is an antibody.

immunocompetence, the ability of an immune system to mobilize and deploy its antibodies and other responses to stimulation by an antigen.

immunocompromised [L *immunis* + *compromittere* to promise mutually], an immune response that has been weakened by a disease or immunosuppressive agent.

immunodeficiency disease, any of a group of health conditions caused by a defect in the immune system and generally characterized by susceptibility to infections and chronic diseases. The diseases are sometimes classified as B cell (antibody) deficiencies, T cell (cellular deficiencies), combined T and B cell deficiencies, defects of cell movement, and defects of microbicidal activity.

immunodeficient [L *immunis* + *de* from, *facere* to make], pertaining to an abnormal condition of the immune system in which cellular or humoral immunity is inadequate and resistance to infection is decreased. Kinds of immunodeficient conditions are **hypogammaglobulinemia** and **lymphoid aplasia.**

immunodiagnosis. See **serologic diagnosis.**

immunodiagnostic [L *immunis* + Gk *dia* through, *gnosis* knowledge], pertaining to or characterizing a diagnosis based on an antigen-antibody reaction.

immunodiffusion [L *immunis* + *diffundere*

to spread], a technique for the identification and quantification of any of the immunoglobulins. It is based on the presence of a visible precipitate that results from an antigen-antibody combination under certain circumstances. **Gel diffusion** is a technique that involves evaluation of the precipitin reaction in a clear gel. **Electro-immunodiffusion** is a gel diffusion to which an electric field is applied, accelerating the reaction. **Double gel diffusion** is a technique that permits identification of antibodies in mixed specimens. In an agar plate, each antigen-antibody combination forms a separate line; observation of the location, shape, and thickness of a line permits identification and quantification of the antibody.

immunoelectrodiffusion. See **immunodiffusion.**

immunoelectrophoresis /im′yənō·ilek′trō-fôrē′sis/ [L *immunis* + Gk *elektron* amber, *pherein* to bear], a technique that combines electrophoresis and immunodiffusion to separate and allow identification of complex proteins. The proteins in the test serum are spread out in agar and separated by electrophoresis. **–immunoelectrophoretic,** adj.

immunofluorescence /im′yənōflŏŏres′əns/ [L *immunis* + *fluere* to flow], a technique used for the rapid identification of an antigen by exposing it to known antibodies tagged with the fluorescent dye fluorescein and observing the characteristic antigen-antibody reaction of precipitation. **–immunofluorescent,** adj.

immunofluorescence test. See **fluorescent antibody test.**

immunofluorescent microscopy. See **fluorescent microscopy, immunofluorescence.**

immunogen /imyŏŏ′nəjən/ [L *immunis* + Gk *genein* to produce], any agent or substance capable of provoking an immune response or producing immunity. **–immunogenic,** adj.

immunoglobulin /im′yənōglob′yəlin/ [L *immunis* + *globus* small sphere], any of five structurally and antigenically distinct antibodies present in the serum and external secretions of the body. Kinds of immunoglobulins are **IgA, IgD, IgE, IgG,** and **IgM.**

immunoglobulin A (IgA), one of the five classes of humoral antibodies produced by the body and one of the most prevalent. It is found in all secretions of the body and is the major antibody in the mucous membrane lining the intestines and in the bronchi, saliva, and tears. IgA combines with a protein in the mucosa and defends body surfaces against invading microorganisms.

immunoglobulin D (IgD), one of the five classes of humoral antibodies produced by the body. It is a specialized protein found in small amounts in serum tissue. It increases in quantity during allergic reactions to milk, insulin, penicillin, and various toxins.

immunoglobulin E (IgE), one of the five classes of humoral antibodies produced by the body. It is concentrated in the lung, the skin, and the cells of mucous membranes. It reacts with certain antigens to release certain chemical mediators that cause Type I hypersensitivity reactions characterized by wheal and flare.

immunoglobulin G (IgG), one of the five classes of humoral antibodies produced by the body. It is a specialized protein synthesized by the body in response to invasions by bacteria, fungi, and viruses.

immunoglobulin M (IgM), one of the five classes of humoral antibodies produced by the body and the largest in molecular structure. It is the first immunoglobulin the body produces when challenged by antigens and is found in circulating fluids. It is the dominant antibody in ABO incompatibilities.

immunohematology /im′yənōhem′-ət ol′əjē/ [L *immunis* + Gk *haima* blood, *logos* science], the study of antigen-antibody reactions and their effects on blood.

immunologic disease /im′yənōloj′ik/ [L *immunis* + Gk *logos* science; L *dis;* Fr *aise* ease], the signs and symptoms of reactions of antibodies to antigens, as in anaphylaxis.

immunologic surveillance [L *immunis* + Gk *logos;* Fr *surveiller* to watch over], a theory contending that the immune system destroys tumor cells, which are constantly arising during the life of the individual.

immunologic tests [L *immunis* + *testum* crucible], tests based on the principles of antigen-antibody reactions.

immunologic theory of aging, a concept based on the premise that normal cells are unrecognized as such, thereby triggering immune reactions within the individual's own body.

immunologist /im′yənol′əjyist/, a specialist in immunology.

immunology /im′yənol′əjē/ [L *immunis* + Gk *logos* science], the study of the reaction of tissues of the immune system of the body to antigenic stimulation.

immunomodulator /im′yənomod′yəlā′tər/ [L *immunis* + *modulus* little measure], a substance that acts to alter the immune response by augmenting or reducing the ability of the immune system to produce specifically modified serum antibodies.

Corticosteroids, cytotoxic agents, thymosin, and the immunoglobulins are among the immunomodulating substances. **–immunomodulation,** n.

immunopotency /im′yənopō′tənsē/ [L *immunis* + *potentia* power], the ability of an antigen to elicit an immune response.

immunoselection [L *immunis* + *seligere* to select], **1.** the survival of certain cells because they lack surface antigens that would otherwise make them vulnerable to attack and destruction by antibodies of an immune system. **2.** the chance of survival of a fetus because its genotype is compatible with that of the mother's immune system.

immunosuppression [L *immunis* + *supprimere* to press down] **1.** the administration of agents that significantly interfere with the ability of the immune system to respond to antigenic stimulation by inhibiting cellular and humoral immunity. Immunosuppression may be deliberate, such as in preparation for transplantation to prevent rejection by the host of the donor tissue, or incidental, such as often results from chemotherapy for the treatment of cancer. **2.** an abnormal condition of the immune system characterized by markedly inhibited ability to respond to antigenic stimuli. **–immunosuppressed,** adj.

immunosuppressive, 1. of or pertaining to a substance or procedure that lessens or prevents an immune response. **2.** an immunosuppressive agent, such as immunosuppressive drugs used to prevent homograft rejection.

immunosurveillance [L *immunis* + Fr *surveiller* to watch over], the continuous detection and protection activity of the immune system in guarding against the presence of "nonself," or foreign proteins in the body tissues.

immunotherapy [L *immunis* + Gk *therapeia* treatment], a special treatment of allergic responses that administers increasingly large doses of the offending allergens to gradually develop immunity. Immunotherapy is based on the premise that low doses of the offending allergen will bind with IgG to prevent an allergic reaction by damping the action of IgE by fostering the synthesis of the blocking IgG antibody. **–immunotherapeutic,** adj.

immunotoxin (IT) /im′yənōtok′sin/, a plant or animal toxin that is attached to a monoclonal antibody and used to destroy a specific target cell.

impacted [L *impingere* to drive against], tightly or firmly wedged in a limited amount of space. **–impact,** v., **impaction,** n.

impacted fracture, a bone break in which the adjacent fragmented ends of the fractured bone are wedged together.

impacted tooth, a tooth so positioned against another tooth, bone, or soft tissue that its complete and normal eruption is impossible or unlikely. It may be further described according to its position as buccoangular, distoangular, or vertical.

impaction /impak′shən/, **1.** an obstacle or malposition that prevents a tooth from erupting. **2.** the presence of a large or hard fecal mass in the rectum or colon.

impaired glucose tolerance (IGT) [L *impejorare* to make worse; Gk *glykys* sweet; L *tolerare* to endure], a condition in which fasting plasma glucose levels are higher than normal but lower than those diagnostic of diabetes mellitus.

impairment [L *impejorare* to make worse], any disorder in structure or function resulting from anatomic, physiologic, or psychologic abnormalities that interfere with normal activities.

impedance /impē′dəns/ [L *impedire* to entangle], a form of electric resistance observed in an alternating current that is analagous to the classic electric resistance that occurs in a direct current circuit.

impedance audiometry. See **audiometry.**

impedance plethysmography, a technique for detecting blood vessel occlusion that determines volumetric changes in the limb by measuring changes in its girth as indicated by changes in the electric impedance of mercury-containing Silastic tubes in a pressure cuff.

imperative conception [L *imperare* to command], a thought or impression that appears spontaneously in the mind and cannot be eliminated, such as an obsession.

imperative idea. See **compulsive idea.**

imperforate /impur′fərit/ [L *im* not, *perforare* to pierce], lacking a normal opening in a body organ or passageway. An infant may be born with an imperforate anus.

imperforate anus, any of several congenital, developmental malformations of the anorectal portion of the GI tract. The most common form is anal agenesis, in which the rectal pouch ends blindly above the surface of the perineum. Other forms include anal stenosis, in which the anal aperture is small, and anal membrane atresia, in which the anal membrane covers the aperture, creating an obstruction.

imperforate hymen [L *im* + *perforare* to pierce through; Gk, *hymen*, membrane], a hymen that completely encloses the external orifice of the vagina.

impermeable /impur′mē·əbəl/ [L *im* not, *permeare* to pass through], (of a tissue, membrane, or film) preventing the passage of a substance through it.

impetigo /im′pətī′gō/ [L *impetus* an attack], a streptococcal, a staphylococcal, or a combined infection of the skin beginning as focal erythema and progressing to pruritic vesicles, erosions, and honey-colored crusts. Lesions usually form on the face and spread locally. The disorder is highly contagious by contact with the discharge from the lesions. **–impetiginous** /im′petij′inəs/, *adj.*

impetigo contagiosa [L *impetus* attack, *contingere* to touch], an acute, contagious, superficial infection of the skin. It is characterized by vesicles that rupture, leaving a purulent exudate that dries into golden crusts.

impetigo herpetiformis [L *impetus;* Gk *herpein* to creep; L *forma*], an acute form of impetigo that affects mainly pregnant women, beginning as an eruption in the genitofemoral area and spreading to other areas. The eruptions are usually irregular or circular groups of pustules that tend to coalesce.

implant /im′plant, implant′/ [L *im* within, *plantare* to set], **1.** (in radiotherapy) an encapsulated radioactive substance embedded in tissue for therapy. Examples include iodine 125 implanted in prostate and chest tumors and iridium 192 embedded in head and neck cancers. **2.** (in surgery) material inserted or grafted into an organ or structure of the body. The implant may be of tissue, such as in a blood vessel graft, or of an artificial substance, such as in a hip prosthesis, a cardiac pacemaker, or a container of radioactive material.

implantation [L *implantare* to set into], (in embryology) the process involving the attachment, penetration, and embedding of the blastocyst in the lining of the uterine wall during the early stages of prenatal development. Kinds of implantation include **eccentric, interstitial,** and **superficial implantation.**

implantation dermoid cyst, a tumor derived from embryonal tissues, caused by an injury that forces part of the ectoderm into the body.

implantation endometriosis [L *implantare;* Gk *endon* within, *metra* womb, *osis* condition], ectopic endometrial tissue found throughout the peritoneal cavity.

implant denture, an artificial or partial denture that consists of a subperiosteally or intraperiosteally implanted framework in contact with alveolar bone.

implanted imfusion port, a self-sealing silicone septum encased in a metal or plastic case with an attached silicone catheter.

implanted suture [L *implantare, sutura*], a suture formed by inserting pins on opposite sides of a wound and bringing the edges of the wound together by winding thread tightly around the pins.

implant restoration, a single-tooth implant crown or multiple-tooth implant crown or bridge that replaces a missing tooth or teeth.

implementation [L *implere* to fill], a deliberate action performed to achieve a goal, such as carrying out a plan in caring for a patient. **–implement,** *v.*

implementation mechanism, the means by which innovations are transferred from the planners to the units of service.

implementing [L *implere* to fill], (in five-step nursing process) a category of nursing behavior in which the actions necessary for accomplishing the health care plan are initiated and completed. Implementing includes the performance or assisting in the performance of the patient's activities of daily living; counseling and teaching the patient or the patient's family; giving care to achieve therapeutic goals and to optimize the achievement of health goals by the patient; supervising and evaluating the work of staff members; and recording and exchanging information relevant to the patient's continued health care.

implied consent [L *implicare* to involve, *consentire* to feel], the granting of permission for health care without a formal agreement between the patient and health care provider. An example is an appointment made with a physician by a patient with a physical complaint; it is implied that by making the appointment the patient gives consent to the physician to make offer a diagnosis and treatment.

implosion [L *im* within, *plaudere* to strike], **1.** a bursting inward. **2.** a psychiatric treatment for people disabled by phobias and anxiety in which the person is desensitized to anxiety-producing stimuli by repeated intense exposure in imagination or reality, until the stimuli are no longer stressful. **–implode,** *v.*

implosive therapy. See **flooding.**

impotence /im′pətəns/ [L *im* not, *potentia* power], **1.** weakness. **2.** inability of the adult male to achieve penile erection or, less commonly, to ejaculate having achieved an erection. **Functional impotence** has a psychologic basis. **Anatomic impotence** results from physically defective genitalia. **Atonic impotence** involves disturbed neuromuscular function. **–impotent,** *adj.*

impregnate /impreg′nāt/ [L *impregnare* to make pregnant], **1.** to inseminate and make pregnant; to fertilize. **2.** to saturate or mix with another substance. **–impregnable,** *adj.,* **impregnation,** *n.*

impression [L *imprimere* to press into], **1.** (in dentistry and prosthetic medicine) a mold of a part of the mouth or other part of the body from which a replacement or prosthesis may be formed. **2.** (in the medical record) the examiner's diagnosis or assessment of a problem, disease, or condition. **3.** a strong sensation or effect on the mind, intellect, or feelings.

impression material [L *imprimere* + *materia* stuff], any material used for making impressions of teeth and oral structures for the purpose of producing dental restorations.

imprinting [Fr *empreindre* to impress], (in ethology) a special type of learning that occurs at critical points during the early stages of development in animals.

imprisonment [Fr *emprisonner* to confine], (in law) the act of confining, detaining, or arresting a person or in any way restraining personal liberty and preventing free exercise of movement.

impulse [L *impellere* to drive], **1.** (in psychology) a sudden, irresistible, often irrational inclination, urge, desire, or action resulting from a particular feeling or mental state. **2.** (in physiology) the electrochemical process involved in neural transmission. **–impulsive,** *adj.*

impulse-conducting system [L *impellere* + *conducere* to conduct; Gk *systema*], the Purkinje fibers within the heart muscle that conduct impulses controlling the contractions of the atria and ventricles.

impulsion /impul'shən/ [L *impellere* to drive], an abnormal, irrational urge to commit an unlawful or socially unacceptable act.

IMV, abbreviation for **intermittent mandatory ventilation.**

In, symbol for the chemical element **indium.**

inactivated measles virus vaccine [L *in, activus;* OE *masala* blister; L *virus* poison; *vaccinus* of a cow], a measles vaccine virus that has been treated so it is no longer capable of replication. It is an alternative to live attenuated measles vaccine, which is contraindicated for some individuals, such as those who are immunocompromised.

inactivation [L *in* not, *activus* active], a reversible denaturation of a protein.

inactivation of complement [L *in, activus, complere* to complete], the loss of activity of the enzymatic proteins in blood achieved by heating the serum to about 55° C. Inactivation of complement is a step in the process of **complement fixation.**

inactive colon [L *in* not, *activus* active; Gk *kolon* colon], hypotonicity of the bowel resulting in decreased contractions and propulsive movements and a delay in the normal 12-hour transit time of luminal contents from cecum to anus. Colonic inactivity may be caused by acquired or congenital megacolon, aging, anticholinergic drugs, depression, faulty habits of elimination, inadequate fluid intake, lack of exercise, a low-residue or starvation diet, neuroendocrine response to surgical stress, prolonged bed rest, or a neurologic disease such as diabetic visceral neuropathy, multiple sclerosis, parkinsonism, and spinal cord lesions. Normal motility of the colon is frequently compromised by the continued use of laxatives.

inadequate personality [L *in* not, *adaequare* to equal; *personalis* of a person], a personality characterized by a lack of physical stamina, emotional immaturity, social instability, poor judgment, reduced motivation, ineptness—especially in interpersonal relationships—and an inability to adapt or react effectively to new or stressful situations.

inanimate /inan'imit/ [L *in* not, *animus* life spirit], not alive; lacking signs of life.

inanition /in'anish'ən/ [L *inanis* empty], **1.** an exhausted condition resulting from lack of food and water or a defect in assimilation; starvation. **2.** a state of lethargy characterized by a loss of vitality or vigor in all aspects of social, moral, and intellectual life.

inanition fever, a temporary, mild, febrile condition of the newborn in the first few days after birth, usually caused by dehydration.

inborn [L *in* within; AS *beran* to bear], innate; acquired or occurring during intrauterine life, with reference to both normally inherited traits and developmental or genetically transmitted anomalies.

inborn error of metabolism, one of many abnormal metabolic conditions caused by an inherited defect of a single enzyme or other protein. People with such diseases generally display a large number of physical signs that are characteristic of the genetic trait. Inborn errors of metabolism may be detected in the fetus in utero by the examination of squamous and blood cells obtained by amniocentesis and fetoscopy. Laboratory tests after birth often show higher than normal levels of particular metabolites in the blood and urine, such as phenylpyruvic acid and phenylalanine in PKU and galactose in galactosemia. Kinds of inborn errors of metabolism include **phenylketonuria, Tay-Sachs disease, Lesch-Nyhan syndrome, galac-**

tosemia, and **glucose-6-phosphate dehydrogenase deficiency.**

inborn reflex. See **unconditioned response.**

inbreeding [L *in* within; AS *bredan* to reproduce], the production of offspring by the mating of closely related individuals, organisms, or plants; self-fertilization is the most extreme form, which normally occurs in certain plants and lower animals. The practice provides a greater chance for recessive genes for both desirable and undesirable traits to become homozygous and to be expressed phenotypically.

incandescent [L *incandescere* to begin to glow], hot to the point of glowing or emitting intense light rays, as in an incandescent light bulb.

incarcerate [L *in* within, *carcerare* confinement], to trap, imprison, or confine, such as a loop of intestine in an inguinal hernia.

incarcerated hernia, a loop of bowel with ends occluded so that solids cannot pass and the hernia will not return to its normal position without manipulation or surgery.

incentive spirometry, spirometric therapy in which the patient is given special encouragement to achieve a maximum inspiratory capacity.

inception [L *incipere* to begin], the origin or beginning of anything.

incest [L *incestum* defiled], sexual intercourse between members of the same family who are so closely related as to be legally prohibited from marrying one another by reason of their consanguinity. –**incestuous,** *adj.*

incidence [L *incidere* to happen], **1.** the number of times an event occurs. **2.** (in epidemiology) the number of new cases in a particular period of time.

incidence rate, the rate of new cases of a disease in a specified population over a defined period of time.

incidental additives [L *incidere* to happen; *additio* something added], food additives caused by the use of pesticides, herbicides, or chemicals involved in food processing.

incident report, a document describing any accident or deviation from policies or orders involving a person on the premises of a health care facility.

incineration [L *incinerare* to burn to ashes], the removal or reduction of waste materials by burning.

incipient [L *incipire* to commence], coming into existence; at an initial stage; beginning to appear, such as a symptom or disease.

incipient dental caries, a dental condi-

tion in which a lesion of tooth decay is initially detectable.

incisal angle /insī′səl/ [L *incidere* to cut into; *angulus* corner], the degree of slope between the axis-orbital plane and the discluding surface of the maxillary incisor teeth.

incisal guide, the part of a dental articulator that maintains the incisal guide angle.

incisal guide pin, a metal rod, attached to the upper member of an articulator, that touches the incisal guide table to maintain the established vertical separation of the upper and lower members of the articulator.

incision /in sizh′ən/ [L *incidere* to cut into], **1.** a cut produced surgically by a sharp instrument, creating an opening into an organ or space in the body. **2.** the act of making an incision.

incisional hernia [L *incidere, hernia* rupture], a herniation through a surgical scar.

incisor /insī′zər/, one of the eight front teeth, four in each dental arch, that first appear as milk teeth during infancy, are replaced by permanent incisors during childhood, and last until old age. The crown of the incisor is chisel-shaped and has a sharp cutting edge. The upper incisors are larger and stronger than the lower and are directed obliquely downward and forward.

incisura /in′sisyōō′rə/ [L *incidere* to cut into], a notch or indentation on an organ or body part.

inclusion [L *in* within, *claudere* to shut], **1.** the act of enclosing or the condition of being enclosed. **2.** a structure within another, such as inclusions in the cytoplasm of the cells.

inclusion bodies, /inklōōzhən/ microscopic objects of various shapes and sizes observed in the nucleus or cytoplasm of blood cells or other tissue cells, depending on the type of disease.

inclusion conjunctivitis, an acute, purulent, conjunctival infection caused by *Chlamydia* organisms. It occurs in two forms: bilateral chemosis, redness, and purulent discharge characterize the infection in infants; the adult variety is unilateral, less severe, less purulent, and associated with preauricular lymphadenopathy.

inclusion dermoid cyst, a tumor derived from embryonal tissues, caused by the inclusion of a foreign tissue when a developmental cleft closes.

inclusiveness principle [L *in* within, *claudere* to shut; *principium* a beginning], a rule that response to various objects in the environment is proportional to the amount of stimulus provided by each object.

inclusive rate, a method of calculating inpatient hospital charges in which a fixed amount covers all services, regardless of the number or intensity of services provided.

incoherent [L *in* not, *cohaere* to hold together], **1.** disordered; without logical connection; disjointed; lacking orderly continuity or relevance. **2.** unable to express one's thoughts or ideas in an orderly, intelligible manner, usually as a result of emotional stress.

incompatibility [L *in* + *compatibilus* agreeing], a state of not being able to exist in harmony, as when transfused blood produces adverse effects because the donor and recipient blood groups are in conflict with each other.

incompatible [L *in* not, *compatibilis* agreement], unable to coexist. A tissue transplant may be rejected because recipient and donor antibody factors are incompatible.

incompetence [L *in,* not *competentia* capable], lack of ability. Body organs that do not function adequately may be described as incompetent. Kinds of incompetence include **aortic, ileocecal,** and **valvular incompetence. –incompetent,** *adj.*

incompetency, a legal status of a person declared to be unable to provide for his or her own needs and protection.

incompetent cervix [L *in* not, *competentia* capable; *cervix* neck], (in obstetrics) a condition characterized by painless dilatation of the cervical os of the uterus before term, without labor or contractions of the uterus. Miscarriage or premature delivery may result.

incomplete abortion [L *in* not, *complere* to fill; *ab* from, *oriri* to be born], termination of pregnancy in which the products of conception are not entirely expelled or removed, often causing hemorrhage that may require surgical evacuation by curettage, oxytocics, and blood replacement.

incomplete dislocation, a partial abnormal separation of the articular surfaces of a joint.

incomplete fistula. See **blind fistula.**

incomplete fracture, a bone break in which the crack in the osseous tissue does not completely traverse the width of the affected bone but may angle off in one or more directions.

incomplete hernia [L *in* + *complere; hernia* rupture], a hernia that has not yet protruded through a weak spot or opening.

incongruent communication, a communication pattern in which the sender gives conflicting messages on verbal and nonverbal levels and the listener does not know which message to accept.

incontinence /inkon′tinəns/ [L *incontinentia* inability to retain], the inability to control urination or defecation. Urinary incontinence may be caused by cerebral clouding in the aged, infection, lesions in the brain or spinal cord, damage to peripheral nerves of the bladder, or injury to the sphincter or perineal structures, sometimes occurring in childbirth. Stress incontinence precipitated by coughing, straining, or heavy lifting occurs more often in women than in men. Fecal incontinence may result from relaxation of the anal sphincter or by central nervous system or spinal cord disorders and may be treated by a program of bowel training. **–incontinent,** *adj.*

incontinence, bowel, a NANDA-accepted nursing diagnosis of a change in normal bowel habits characterized by involuntary passage of stool.

incontinence, functional, a NANDA-accepted nursing diagnosis of an involuntary, unpredictable passage of urine. Defining characteristics include the urge to void or bladder contractions sufficiently strong to result in loss of urine before reaching an appropriate receptacle.

incontinence, reflex, a NANDA-accepted nursing diagnosis of an involuntary loss of urine occuring at somewhat predictable intervals when a specific bladder volume is reached. Defining characteristics include no awareness of bladder filling; no urge to void or feelings of bladder fullness; or uninhibited bladder contractions or spasms at regular intervals.

incontinence, stress, a NANDA-accepted nursing diagnosis of a loss of urine of less than 50 ml occurring with increased abdominal pressure. Defining characteristics include reported or observed dribbling with increased abdominal pressure, urinary urgency, or urinary frequency (more often than every 2 hours).

incontinence, total, a NANDA-accepted nursing diagnosis of a continuous and unpredictable loss of urine. Defining characteristics include a constant flow of urine occurring at unpredictable times without distention or uninhibited bladder contractions or spasms, unsuccessful incontinence refractory treatments, nocturia, lack of perineal or bladder awareness, and unawareness of incontinence.

incontinence, urge, a NANDA-accepted nursing diagnosis of an involuntary passage of urine occurring soon after a strong sense of urgency to void. Defining characteristics include urinary urgency, frequency (voiding more often than every 2 hours), bladder contractions or spasms, nocturia (urination more than two times per night), voiding in small amounts (less than 100 ml) or in large amounts (500 ml), and an inability to reach a toilet on time.

increment [L *incresere* to grow], **1.** an increase or gain. **2.** the act of growing or increasing. **3.** the amount of an increase or gain in intrauterine pressure as uterine contractions begin in labor. **–incremental,** *adj.*

incrustation, hardened exudate, scale, or scab.

incubation period /in'kyəbā'shən/ [L *incubare* to lie on; Gk *peri* around, *hodos* way] **1.** the time between exposure to a pathogenic organism and the onset of symptoms of a disease. **2.** the time required to induce the development of an embryo in an egg or to induce the development and replication of tissue cells or microorganisms in culture media. **3.** the time allowed for a chemical reaction or process to proceed.

incubator, an apparatus used to provide a controlled environment, especially a particular temperature.

incudectomy /in'kyo͞odek'təmē/ [L *incus* anvil, *ektome* incision], surgical removal of the incus, performed to treat conductive deafness resulting from necrosis of the tip of the incus. The defective incus is excised and replaced with a bone chip graft so that sound vibrations are again transmitted.

incus /ing'kəs/, *pl.* incudes /ink o͞o'dēz/ [L, anvil], one of the three ossicles in the middle ear, resembling an anvil. It communicates sound vibrations from the malleus to the stapes.

IND, abbreviation for **investigational new drug.**

indandione derivative /indan'dē·ōn/, one of a small group of oral anticoagulants designed for long-term therapeutic use in patients who cannot tolerate other oral anticoagulants.

indentation [L *in* within, *dens* tooth], a notch, pit, or depression in the surface of an object, such as toothmarks on the tongue or skin. **–indent,** *v.*

independence [L *in* not, *de* from, *pendere* to hang], **1.** the state or quality of being independent; autonomy; free from the influence, guidance, or control of a person or a group. **2.** a lack of requirement or reliance on another for physical existence or emotional needs. **–independent,** *adj.*

independent assortment [L *in* not, *dependere* to hang from; *ad* towards, *sortiri* to cast lots], (in genetics) a basic principle stating that the members of a pair of genes are randomly distributed in the gametes, independent of the distribution of other pairs of genes.

independent living centers, rehabilitation facilities in which disabled persons can receive special education and training in the performance of all or most activities of daily living with a particular handicap.

independent practice, (in nursing) the practice of certain aspects of professional nursing that are encompassed by applicable licensure and law and require no supervision or direction from others. Nurses in independent practice may have an office in which they see patients and charge fees for service. In all nursing settings, state practice acts define certain aspects of nursing practice that are independent and may define those that must be done only under supervision or direction of another individual, usually a physician.

independent practice association (IPA), a prepaid health service system in which office-based physicians contract for the care of patients on a prenegotiated fee-for-service basis.

independent variable, (in research) a variable that is controlled by the researcher and evaluated by its measurable effect on the dependent variable or variables.

indeterminate cleavage /in'ditur'minit/ [L *in* not *determinare* to fix limits; AS *cleofan* to split], mitotic division of the fertilized ovum into blastomeres that have similar developmental potential and, if isolated, can give rise to a complete individual embryo.

index astigmatism [L *indicare* to indicate, *a, stigma* point], an astigmatism caused by unequal refractive indices in different parts of the lens.

index case [L, pointer], (in epidemiology) the first case of a disease as contrasted with the appearance of subsequent cases.

Index Medicus, an index published monthly by the National Library of Medicine, which lists articles from the medical literature from throughout the world by subject and by author.

index myopia, a kind of nearsightedness caused by a variation in the index of refraction of the media of the eye.

Indian Health Service, a bureau within the Department of Health and Human Services for providing public health and medical services to Native Americans in the United States.

Indian tick fever. See **Marseilles fever.**

indican /in'dikən/ [Gk *indikon* indigo], a substance (potassium indoxyl sulfate) produced in the intestine by the decomposition of tryptophan, absorbed by the intestinal wall, and excreted in the urine.

indication [L *indicare* to make known], a reason to prescribe a medication or perform a treatment, as a bacterial infection may be an indication for the prescription of a specific antibiotic or as appendicitis is an indication for appendectomy. **–indicate,** *v.*

indicator, a tape, paper, tablet, or any other substance that is used to test for a particular reaction because it changes in a predictable visible way. Some kinds of indicators are **autoclave indicator, dipsticks,** and **litmus paper.**

indigence /in′dijəns/ [L *indigere* to want], a condition of having insufficient income to pay for adequate medical care without depriving oneself or one's dependents of food, clothing, shelter, or other living essentials.

indigenous /indij′ənəs/ [L *indigena* a native], native to or occurring naturally in a specified area or environment, as certain species of bacteria in the human digestive tract.

indigestible [L *in* not, *digerere* to separate], a descriptive term for a food substance that cannot be broken down by the digestive tract and converted into an absorbable nutrient.

indigestion. See **dyspepsia.**

indirect anaphylaxis [L *in* not, *directus* straight; Gk *ana* again, *phylaxis* protection], an exaggerated reaction of hypersensitivity to a person's own antigen that occurs because the antigen has been altered in some way.

indirect calorimetry, the measurement of the amount of heat generated in an oxidation reaction by determining the intake or consumption of oxygen or by measuring the amount of carbon dioxide or the amount of nitrogen released and translating these quantities into a heat equivalent.

indirect division. See **mitosis.**

indirect laryngoscopy [L *in, directus* not straight; Gk *larynx, skopein* to view], a method of examining the larynx with a mirror.

indirect nursing care functions, liaison nurse activities used to solve problems with a consultee who is responsible for implementing and evaluating any recommended changes.

indirect ophthalmoscope, an ophthalmoscope with a biconvex lens that produces a reversed direct image.

indirect percussion. See **percussion.**

indirect provider reimbursement, a method of payment to an agency for health services delivered by providers, such as nurses.

indirect restorative method, the technique for fabricating a restoration on a cast of the original, such as the indirect construction of an inlay.

indirect retainer, a portion of a removable partial denture that resists movement of a distal extension away from its tissue support by means of lever action opposite the fulcrum line of the direct retention.

indirect transfusion [L *in, directus, transfundere* to pour through], the transfusion of blood to a recipient after the donor blood has been prepared with anticoagulants, defibrinating agents, or other substances, as opposed to transfusing blood directly from donor to recipient.

indirect vision [L *in, directus, visio* seeing], a visual sensation caused by stimulation of the extramacular portion of the retina.

indium (In) [L *indicum* indigo], a silvery metallic element with some nonmetallic chemical properties. Its atomic number is 49; its atomic weight is 114.82.

individual immunity [L *individuus* indivisible; *immunis* free], a form of natural immunity not shared by most other members of the race and species.

individual psychology, a modified system of psychoanalysis, developed by Alfred Adler, that views maladaptive behavior and personality disorders as resulting from a conflict between the desire to dominate and feelings of inferiority.

indoleacetic acid /in′dōləsē′tik, -əset′ik/, a major terminal metabolite of tryptophan that is present in very small amounts in normal urine and excreted in elevated quantities by patients with carcinoid tumors.

indolent [L *in* + *dolere* to suffer pain], pertaining to an organic disorder that is accompanied by little or no pain.

indomethacin /in′dōmeth′əsin/, a nonsteroidal antiinflammatory agent prescribed in the treatment of arthritis and certain other inflammatory conditions.

induce /ind(y)o͞os′/ [L *inducere* to bring in], to cause or stimulate the start of an activity, as an enzyme induces a metabolic activity. **–inducer, induction,** *n.*

induced abortion, an intentional termination of pregnancy before the fetus has developed enough to live if born.

induced fever, a deliberate elevation of body temperature by application of heat or by inoculation with a fever-producing organism in order to kill heat-sensitive pathogens.

induced hypotension. See **deliberate hypotension.**

induced lethargy, a trancelike state produced during hypnosis.

induced mutation [L *inducere; mutare* to change], a mutation that has been produced by treatment with a physical or chemical agent that affects the DNA molecules of a living organism.

induced phagocytosis [L *inducere;* Gk *phagein* to eat, *kytos* cell], the ingestion of microorganisms and other foreign particles by cells of the reticuloendothelial system.

induced trance, a somnambulistic state resulting from a hysteric neurosis or hypnotism.

induced vomiting [L *inducere; vomere* to vomit], vomiting produced by administration of ipecac syrup, soapy water, or handwashing liquid detergent, or by inserting a finger or blunt instrument into the throat. Vomiting may be medically indicated in cases of ingested noncaustic poisons but may also be self-induced by patients afflicted with **bulimia.**

inducer /indoo'sər/, (in molecular genetics) a substance, usually a molecular substrate of a specific enzyme, that combines with and deactivates the active repressor produced by the regulator gene.

induction /induk'shən/ [L *inducere* to bring in], (in embryology) the process of stimulating and determining morphogenetic differentiation in a developing embryo through the action of chemical substances transmitted from one to another of the embryonic parts.

induction of anesthesia, all portions of the anesthetic process that occur before attaining the desired level of anesthesia, including premedication with a sedative, hypnotic, tranquilizer, or curariform adjunct to anesthesia, intubation; administration of oxygen; and administration of the anesthetic.

induction of labor, an obstetric procedure in which labor is initiated artificially by means of amniotomy or the administration of oxytocics. It is performed electively or for fetal or maternal indications. Elective induction is carried out for the convenience of the mother or the obstetrician, often to avert the possibility of delivery outside of the hospital when labor is judged to be imminent and the mother is expected to have an unusually rapid birth.

induction phase, the period of time during which a normal cell becomes transformed into a cancerous cell.

inductive approach, the analysis of data and examination of practice problems within their own context rather than from a predetermined theoretical basis.

inductor /induk'tər/ [L *inducere* to bring in], (in embryology) a tissue or cell that emits a chemical substance that stimulates some morphogenetic effect in the developing embryo.

induration /in'dyərā'shən/ [L *indurare* to make hard], hardening of a tissue, particularly the skin, because of edema, inflammation, or infiltration by a neoplasm. —**indurated,** *adj.*

indurative myocarditis /in'dyərā'tiv/ [L *indurare;* Gk *mys* muscle, *kardia* heart, *itis* inflammation], a form of myocarditis in which the inflammation leads to a hardening of the muscles of the heart walls.

industrial health [Fr *industriel;* ME *helthe*], the health concerns associated with the workplace, such as exposure to asbestos, mining and milling dusts, metal and acid vapors; lighting; and ergonomics.

Industrial Medical Association (IMA), a professional organization whose members are concerned with the identification, prevention, diagnosis, and treatment of disorders associated with technology and industry.

industrial psychology [L *industria* diligence], the application of psychologic principles and techniques to the problems of business and industry, including the selection of personnel, the motivation of workers, and the development of training programs.

indwelling catheter [L *in* within; AS *dwellan* to remain], any catheter designed to be left in place for a prolonged period.

inebriant /inē'brē-ənt/ [L *inebriare* to make drunk], a substance such as ethanol that induces inebriation or intoxication.

inebriate, to make drunk.

inert /inurt'/ [L *iners* idle], **1.** not moving or acting, such as inert matter. **2.** (of a chemical substance) not taking part in a chemical reaction or acting as a catalyst, such as neon or an inert gas. **3.** (of a medical ingredient) not active pharmacologically; serving only as a bulking, binding, or other excipient in a medication.

inert gas, a chemically inactive gaseous element. The inert gases are argon, helium, krypton, neon, radon, and xenon.

inertia /inur'shə/ [L, idleness], **1.** the tendency of a body at rest to remain at rest unless acted on by an outside force, and the tendency of a body in motion to remain at motion in the direction in which it is moving unless acted on by an outside force. **2.** an abnormal condition characterized by a general inactivity or sluggishness, such as colonic inertia or uterine inertia.

inertial impaction, the deposition of large aerosol particles on the walls of an airway conduit. The impaction caused by inertia tends to occur where the airway direction changes.

inevitable abortion [L *inevitablilis* unavoidable], a condition of pregnancy in which spontaneous termination is imminent and cannot be prevented. It is characterized by bleeding, uterine cramping, dilatation of the cervix, and presentation of the conceptus in the cervical os.

in extremis, in the extremity, or at the point of death.

infant [L *infans* unable to speak], **1.** a child who is in the earliest stage of extra-uterine life, a time extending from birth to approximately 12 months of age, when the baby is able to assume an erect posture; some extend the period to 24 months of age. **2.** (in law) a person not of full legal age; a minor. **3.** of or pertaining to infancy; in an early stage of development. **–infantile,** *adj.*

infant botulism, an intoxication from neurotoxins produced by *Clostridium botulinum* that occurs in children less than 6 months of age. The condition is characterized by severe hypotonicity of all muscles, constipation, lethargy, and feeding difficulties, and it may lead to respiratory insufficiency. The botulism neurotoxin is usually found in the GI tract rather than in the blood, indicating that it is probably produced in the gut rather than ingested.

infant death, the death of a live-born infant before 1 year of age.

infant feeder, a device for feeding small or weak infants who cannot suck hard enough to nurse from the breast or to get milk from a bottle. The feeder resembles a bulb syringe with a long soft nipple on the end.

infant feeding. See **bottle feeding, breastfeeding.**

infant feeding pattern, ineffective, a NANDA-accepted nursing diagnosis of a state in which an infant demonstrates an impaired ability to suck or coordinate the suck-swallow response. The defining characteristics are an inability to initiate or sustain an effective suck and inability to coordinate sucking, swallowing, and breathing. Related factors are prematurity, neurologic impairment or delay, oral hypersensitivity, prolonged NPO status, and anatomic abnormalities.

infanticide /infan'tisīd/ [L *infans* unable to speak, *caedere* to kill], **1.** the killing of an infant or young child. **2.** one who takes the life of an infant or young child. **–infanticidal,** *adj.*

infantile /in'fəntīl/ [L *infans* unable to speak], **1.** of, relating to, or characteristic of infants or infancy. **2.** lacking maturity, sophistication, or reasonableness. **3.** affected with infantilism. **4.** being in a very early stage of development.

infantile amnesia, (in psychology) the in-

ability to remember events from early childhood.

infantile arteritis, a disorder in infants and young children characterized by inflammation of many arteries in which atherosclerotic lesions are rarely present.

infantile autism, a disability characterized by abnormal emotional, social, and linguistic development in a child. It may result from organic brain dysfunction, in which case it occurs before 3 years of age, or it may be associated with childhood schizophrenia, in which case the autism occurs later, but before the onset of adolescence. The autistic child remains fixed at one of the consecutive stages through which a normal infant passes as it develops. Treatment includes psychotherapy, often accompanied by play therapy.

infantile celiac disease. See **celiac disease.**

infantile cerebral ataxic paralysis [L *infans* unable to speak; *cerebrum* the brain; Gk *ataxia* lack of order; *paralyein* to be palsied], a form of congenital diplegia. It is characterized by cerebral maldevelopment, ataxia, spasticity of the legs, and possible mental deficiency.

infantile cerebral sphingolipidosis. See **Tay-Sachs disease.**

infantile colic, a descriptive term for a suggested intestinal cause of discomfort in a newborn infant. However, specific causes and mechanisms have not been defined. The typical infantile colic patient eats and gains weight but may also appear excessively hungry. Aerophagia from crying may lead to flatulence and abdominal distention.

infantile cortical hyperostosis, a familial disorder characterized in infants by bony swellings and tenderness in the affected areas. The mandible is most commonly involved.

infantile dwarf, a person whose mental and physical development is greatly retarded as a result of various causes, such as genetic or developmental defects.

infantile eczema. See **atopic dermatitis.**

infantile encephalitis [L *infans*; Gk *enkephalos* brain, *itis* inflammation], any of a group of brain inflammation conditions affecting infants. The cause may be a direct viral infection or a secondary encephalitis that is a complication of measles, chickenpox, rubella, or other diseases.

infantile hemiplegia, paralysis of one side of the body that may occur at birth from a cerebral hemorrhage, in utero from lack of oxygen, or during a febrile illness in infancy.

infantile hydrocele [L *infans*; Gk *hydor*

water, *kele* hernia], an accumulation of fluid in the tunica vaginalis. It may be present at birth or acquired.

infantile paralysis. See **poliomyelitis.**

infantile poliomyelitis. See **acute atrophic paralysis.**

infantile scurvy, a nutritional disease caused by an inadequate dietary supply of vitamin C, most commonly occurring because cow's milk, unfortified with vitamin C, is the principal food in an infant's diet.

infantile spinal muscular atrophy. See **Werdnig-Hoffmann disease.**

infantile spinal paralysis [L *infans, spina;* Gk *paralyein* to be palsied], acute anterior poliomyelitis, a viral infection characterized by nonspecific illnesses, aseptic meningitis, and flaccid weakness of muscle groups.

infantile uterus, a uterus that has failed to attain adult characteristics.

infantilism /infan'tiliz'əm/ [L *infans* unable to speak] **1.** a condition in which various anatomic, physiologic, and psychologic characteristics of childhood persist in the adult. **2.** a condition, usually of psychologic rather than organic origin, characterized by speech and voice patterns in an older child or adult that are typical of very young children.

infant mortality, the statistical rate of infant death during the first year after live birth, expressed as the number of such births per 1,000 live births in a specific geographic area or institution in a given period of time.

infant of addicted mother, a newborn infant showing withdrawal symptoms, usually within the first 24 hours of life, most commonly caused by maternal antepartum dependence on heroin, methadone, diazepam, phenobarbital, or alcohol. Characteristic symptoms include tremors, irritability, hyperactive reflexes, increased muscle tone, twitching, increased mucus production, nasal congestion, respiratory distress, excessive sweating, elevated temperature, vomiting, diarrhea, and dehydration. The infants cry shrilly, sneeze often, frantically suck their fists but feed poorly, and yawn frequently but have difficulty falling asleep. They are usually pale, are often born with nose and knee abrasions, and are subject to convulsions.

infant stimulation [L *infans; stimulare* to incite], the testing of sensory inputs for newborns, usually through the performance of tasks involving coordination and manipulation.

infarct /infärkt'/ [L *infarcire* to stuff], a localized area of necrosis in a tissue, vessel, organ, or part resulting from tissue anoxia caused by an interruption in the blood supply to the area, or, less frequently, by circulatory stasis produced by the occlusion of a vein that ordinarily carries blood away from the area. Kinds of infarct include **anemic, calcareous, cicatrized, hemorrhagic,** and **uric acid infarct.** **–infarcted,** *adj.*

infarct extension, a myocardial infarction that has spread beyond the original area, usually as a result of the death of cells in the ischemic margin of the infarct zone.

infarction /infärk'shən/ [L *infarcire* to stuff], **1.** the development and formation of an infarct. **2.** an infarct. Kinds of infarction include **myocardial infarction** and **pulmonary infarction.**

infect [L *inficere* to taint], to transmit a pathogen that may induce development of an infectious disease in another person.

infected abortion, a spontaneous or induced termination of an immature pregnancy in which the products of conception have become infected, causing fever and requiring antibiotic therapy and evacuation of the uterus.

infection [L *inficere* to taint], **1.** the invasion of the body by pathogenic microorganisms that reproduce and multiply, causing disease by local cellular injury, secretion of a toxin, or antigen-antibody reaction in the host. **2.** a disease caused by the invasion of the body by pathogenic microorganisms. **–infectious,** *adj.*

infection control, the policies and procedures of a hospital or other health facility to minimize the risk of nosocomial or community-acquired infections spreading to patients or members of the staff.

infection control committee, a group of hospital health professionals composed of infection control personnel, with medical, nursing, administrative, and occasionally dietary and housekeeping department representatives, who plan and supervise infection control activities.

infection control nurse, a registered nurse who is assigned responsibility for surveillance and infection prevention and control activities.

infection, high risk for, a NANDA-accepted nursing diagnosis of the state in which an individual is at increased risk for being invaded by pathogenic organisms. Risk factors include inadequate primary defenses, such as broken skin and altered peristalsis; inadequate secondary defenses, such as decreased hemoglobin and immunosuppression; inadequate acquired immunity; tissue destruction and increased environmental exposure; chronic disease; invasive procedures; malnutrition; pharmaceutical agents; trauma; and rupture of amniotic membranes.

infections following splenectomy [L *inficere* to stain; ME *folwen*; Gk *splen, ektome* cutting out], infections that may follow removal of the spleen, an organ that plays a vital role in the body's immune system. The spleen is a major phagocytic organ of the reticuloendothelial network and also serves as an important site of antibody production. Splenectomized patients are particularly prone to certain bacterial infections.

infectious, 1. capable of causing an infection. **2.** caused by an infection.

infectious bulbar paralysis [L *inficere; bulbus* swollen root; Gk *paralyein* to be palsied], a herpesvirus disease of animals that may cause a mild pruritis when transmitted to humans.

infectious disease, any communicable disease, or one that can be transmitted from one human being to another, or from animal to human, by direct or indirect contact.

infectious granuloma [L *inficere; granulum* little grain; Gk *oma* tumor], a lumpy lesion of granuloma tissue that may develop in diseases such as tuberculosis, syphilis, and actinomycosis.

infectious hepatitis. See **hepatitis A.**

infectious isolation [L *inficere;* It *isolare* to detach], the practice of confining to an isolated room or other area a patient with a particularly virulent disease so as to reduce the risk of contact and spread of the disease among hospital personnel.

infectious mononucleosis [L *inficere;* Gk *monos* single; L *nucleus* nut; Gk *osis* condition], an acute herpesvirus infection caused by the Epstein-Barr virus (EBV). It is characterized by fever, sore throat, swollen lymph glands, atypical lymphocytes, splenomegaly, hepatomegaly, abnormal liver function, and bruising. Rupture of the spleen may occur, requiring immediate surgery and blood transfusion.

infectious myringitis, an inflammatory, contagious condition of the eardrum caused by viral or bacterial infection, characterized by the development of painful vesicles on the drum.

infectious nucleic acid, DNA or, more commonly, viral RNA that is able to infect the nucleic acid of a cell and to induce the host to produce viruses.

infectious parotitis. See **mumps.**

infectious polyneuritis. See **Guillain-Barré syndrome.**

infective endocarditis [L *inficere;* Gk *endon* within, *kardia* heart, *itis* inflammation], a bacterial infection of the innermost lining of the heart, usually following

rheumatic fever or another febrile disease. Subacute bacterial endocarditis may lead to vegetation on the heart valves or ulceration of the valve cusps.

infective tubulointerstitial nephritis [L *inficere; tubulus* tubule, *interstitium* space between], an acute inflammation of the kidneys caused by an infection by *Escherichia coli* or other pyogenic pathogen. The condition is characterized by chills, fever, nausea and vomiting, flank pain, dysuria, proteinuria, and hematuria. The kidney may become enlarged, and portions of the renal cortex may be destroyed.

infectivity /in'fektiv'itē/ [L *inficere* to taint], the ability of a pathogen to spread rapidly from one host to another.

inferior [L *inferus* lower], **1.** situated below or lower than a given point of reference, as the feet are inferior to the legs. **2.** of poorer quality or value.

inferior alveolar artery, an artery that descends with the inferior alveolar nerve from the first or mandibular portion of the maxillary artery to the mandibular foramen.

inferior aperture of minor pelvis, an irregular aperture bounded by the coccyx, the sacrotuberous ligaments, part of the ischium, the sides of the pubic arch, and the pubic symphysis.

inferior aperture of thorax, an irregular opening bounded by the twelfth thoracic vertebra, the eleventh and twelfth ribs, and the edge of the costal cartilages as they meet the sternum.

inferior carotid triangle [L *inferus;* Gk *karos* heavy sleep; L *triangulus* three-cornered], a triangular area bounded by the midline of the neck, the superior belly of the omohyoid muscle above, and the sternocleidomastoid muscle behind.

inferior conjunctival fornix, the space in the fold of conjunctiva created by the reflection of the conjunctiva covering the eyeball and the lining of the lower eyelid.

inferior gastric node, a node in one of two groups of gastric lymph glands, lying between the two layers of the lesser omentum along the pyloric half of the greater curvature of the stomach.

inferiority complex, 1. a feeling of fear and resentment resulting from a sense of being physically inadequate, characterized by a variety of abnormal behaviors. **2.** (in psychoanalysis) a complex characterized by striving for unrealistic goals because of an unresolved Oedipus complex. **3.** *informal;* a feeling of being inferior.

inferior maxillary bone. See **mandible.**

inferior mesenteric node, a node in one of the three groups of visceral lymph glands serving the viscera of the abdomen and the pelvis.

inferior mesenteric vein, the vein in the lower body that returns the blood from the rectum, the sigmoid colon, and the descending colon.

inferior olivary nucleus [L *inferus; oliva* olive, *nucleus* nut], a small purse-shaped collection of nerve cells lying posterolateral to the pyramid, just below the level of the pons. It is a source of cerebellar climbing fibers.

inferior orbital fissure, a groove in the inferolateral wall of the orbit that contains the infraorbital and zygomatic nerves and the infraorbital vessels.

inferior phrenic artery, a small, visceral branch of the abdominal aorta, arising from the aorta itself, the renal artery, or the celiac artery.

inferior pole of kidney. See **poles of kidney.**

inferior radioulnar joint. See **distal radioulnar articulation.**

inferior sagittal sinus, one of the six venous channels of the posterior dura mater, draining blood from the brain into the internal jugular vein. It receives deoxygenated blood from several veins from the falx cerebri and, in some individuals, a few veins from the cerebral hemispheres.

inferior subscapular nerve /subskap′-yŏŏlər/, one of two small nerves on opposite sides of the back that supply the distal part of the subscapularis and ends in the teres major.

inferior thyroid vein, one of the few veins that arise in the venous plexus on the thyroid gland and form a plexus ventral to the trachea, under the sternothyroideus muscle. The veins receive the esophageal, the tracheal, and the inferior laryngeal veins.

inferior ulnar collateral artery, one of a pair of branches of the deep brachial arteries carrying blood to the muscles of the forearm.

inferior vena cava, the large vein that returns deoxygenated blood to the heart from parts of the body below the diaphragm. It is formed by the junction of the two common iliac veins at the right of the fifth lumbar vertebra and ascends along the vertebral column, pierces the diaphragm, and opens into the right atrium of the heart.

inferolateral /in′fərōlat′ərəl/ [L *inferus* lower, *latus* side], situated below and to the side.

inferomedial /in′fərōmē′dē·əl/ [L *inferus* lower, *medius* middle], situated below and toward the center.

infertile /infur′təl/ [L *in* not, *fertilis* fruit-

ful], denoting the inability to produce offspring. This condition may be present in one or both sex partners and may be temporary and reversible. The condition is classified as primary, in which pregnancy has never occurred, and secondary, when there have been one or more pregnancies. **–infertility.** *n.*

infest /infest′/, to attack, invade, and subsist on the skin or in the internal organs of a host.

infestation [L *infestare* to attack], the presence of animal parasites in the environment, on the skin, or in the hair of a host.

infiltrate [L *in + filtrare* to strain through], **1.** to perform the process of infiltration. **2.** a substance that seeps through a filter.

infiltration [L *in* within, *filtare* to strain through], the process whereby a fluid passes into the tissues, such as when a local anesthetic is administered.

infirmary [L *infirmus* weak], a hospital, originally a part of a monastery, that provides care for sick or infirm persons, particularly indigent patients.

inflammation [L *inflammare* to set afire], the protective response of the tissues of the body to irritation or injury. Inflammation may be acute or chronic; its cardinal signs are redness (rubor), heat (calor), swelling (tumor), and pain (dolor), accompanied by loss of function. Histamine, kinins, and various other substances mediate the inflammatory process.

inflammation of the liver. See **hepatitis.**

inflammatory [L *inflammare* to set afire], pertaining to or resembling inflammation.

inflammatory bowel disease. See **ulcerative colitis.**

inflammatory dysmenorrhea [L *inflammare;* Gk *dys, men* month, *rhein* to flow], dysmenorrhea that accompanies pelvic infection, fibroids, or endometritis.

inflammatory fracture [L *inflammare; fractura* break], a fracture of bone tissue weakened by inflammation.

inflammatory response, a tissue reaction to injury or an antigen. The response may include pain, swelling, itching, redness, heat, loss of function, or a combination of symptoms.

inflammatory scoliosis [L *inflammare;* Gk *skoliosis* curvature], a form of scoliosis caused by muscle spasms associated with acute inflammation.

inflatable pessary. See **pessary.**

inflatable splint [L *in + flare* to blow; ME *splente*], a tubular device that placed around a patient's extremity and inflated with air to maintain rigidity.

influenza /in′floo·en′zə/ [It, *influence*], a highly contagious infection of the respiratory tract caused by a myxovirus and transmitted by airborne droplet infection. Symptoms include sore throat, cough, fever, muscular pains, and weakness. The onset is usually sudden, with chills, fever, and general malaise. Treatment is symptomatic and usually involves bed rest, aspirin, and drinking of fluids. Fever and constitutional symptoms distinguish influenza from the common cold. Complete recovery in from 3 to 10 days is the rule. Three main strains of influenza virus have been recognized: type A, type B, and type C. New strains of the virus emerge at regular intervals and are named according to their geographic origin. **Asian flu** is a type A influenza.

influenza-virus vaccine, an active immunizing agent prescribed for immunization against influenza.

informal admission, a type of admission to a psychiatric hospital in which there is no formal or written application and the patient is free to leave at any time.

information systems director [L *informationis* idea], a person who directs and administers the data processing facilities of a hospital or other health facility.

informed consent [L *informare* to give form; *consentire* to sense], permission obtained from a patient to perform a specific test or procedure. Informed consent is required before performing most invasive procedures and before admitting a patient to a research study.

infraclavicular fossa /in′frəkləvik′yələr/, a small pocket or indentation just below the clavicle on both sides of the body.

infraction fracture /infrak′shən/ [L *infractio* a breaking; *fractura* break], a pathologic fracture characterized by a small radiolucent line and most commonly associated with a disorder of metabolism.

infranodal block /in′franō′dəl/ [L *infra* below, *nodus* knot; Fr *bloc*], a type of atrioventricular (AV) block in which an impairment of the stimulatory mechanism of the heart causes blockage of the impulse in the bundle of His or in both bundle branches after leaving the AV node. The condition is often the result of arteriosclerosis, degenerative diseases, a defect in the conduction system, or tumor; it is most often seen in older patients. Symptoms include frequent episodes of fainting and a pulse rate of between 20 and 50 beats per minute.

infraorbital /in′frə·ô′bitəl/ [L *infra* below, *orbita* wheeltrack], pertaining to the area beneath the floor of the bony cavity in which the eyeball is located.

infraorbital foramen [L *infra + orbita; foramen* hole or aperture], an opening on the anterior aspect of the maxilla. Through it pass the inferior orbital nerves and blood vessels.

infrapatellar fat pad /in′frəpətel′ər/, an area of palpable soft tissue in front of the joint space on either side of the patellar tendon.

infraradian rhythm /in′frərā′dē·ən/ [L *infra + radians* diverging from center; Gk *rhythmos*], a biorhythm that repeats in patterns greater than 24-hour periods.

infrared radiation /in′frəred′/ [L *infra* + AS *read* red; L *radiare* to emit rays], electromagnetic radiation in which the wavelengths are between 10^{-5} m and 10^{-4} m, or longer than those of visible light waves but shorter than those of radio waves. Infrared radiation striking the body surface is perceived as heat.

infrared therapy, treatment by exposure to various wavelengths of infrared radiation. Infrared treatment is performed to relieve pain and to stimulate circulation of blood.

infrared thermography, measurement of temperature through the detection of infrared radiation emitted from heated tissue.

infraspinous fossa. See **supraspinous fossa.**

infundibular stalk /in′fundib′yələr/ [L *infundibulum* funnel; ME *stalke*], an elongated funnel-shaped structure that connects the diencephalon with the pituitary gland.

infundibulum /in′fundib′yələm/ *pl.* **infundibula** [L, funnel], a funnel-shaped structure or passage, such as the cavity formed by the fimbriae tubae at the distal end of the fallopian tubes.

infusate /infyōō′sāt/, a parenteral fluid infused into a patient over a specific time period.

infusion /infyōō′zhən/ [L *in* within, *fundere* to pour], **1.** the introduction of a substance, such as a fluid, electrolyte, nutrient, or drug, directly into a vein or interstitially by means of gravity flow. **2.** the substance introduced into the body by infusion. **3.** the steeping of a substance, such as an herb, to extract its medicinal properties. **4.** the extract obtained by the steeping process. –**infuse,** *v.*

infusion pump, an apparatus designed to deliver measured amounts of a drug through injection over a period of time. Some kinds of infusion pumps can be implanted surgically.

ingestion [L, *in, gerere,* to carry], the oral taking of substances into the body. It is generally applied to both nutrients and medications.

ingrown hair [L *in* within; AS *growen* to grow; *haer*], a hair that fails to follow the normal follicle channel to the surface, with the free end becoming embedded in the skin.

ingrown toenail, a toenail whose free distal margin grows or is pressed into the skin of the toe, causing an inflammatory reaction.

inguinal /ing'gwinəl/ [L *inguen* groin], of or pertaining to the groin.

inguinal canal, the tubular passage through the lower layers of the abdominal wall that contains the spermatic cord in the male and the round ligament in the female. It is a common site for hernias.

inguinal falx, the inferior terminal portion of the common aponeurosis of the obliquus internus abdominis and the transverse abdominis.

inguinal hernia, a hernia in which a loop of intestine enters the inguinal canal, sometimes filling, in a male, the entire scrotal sac.

inguinal node, one of approximately 18 nodes in the group of lymph glands in the upper femoral triangle of the thigh.

inguinal region, the part of the abdomen surrounding the inguinal canal, in the lower zone on both sides of the pubic region.

inguinal ring, either of the two apertures of the inguinal canal, the internal end opening into the abdominal wall and the external end opening into the aponeurosis of the obliquus externus abdominis above the pubis.

inguinocrural hernia /ing'gwinə'krōō'rəl/ [L *inguen* + *crus* thigh, *hernia* rupture], an inguinal hernia that has turned from the inguinal canal laterally over the groin.

INH. See isoniazid.

inhalant /inhā'lənt/, a substance introduced into the body by inhalation. It may be a medication, such as an aerosol or a volatile chemical.

inhalation administration of medication [L *in* within, *halare* to breathe], the administration of a drug by inhalation of the vapor released from a fragile ampoule packed in a fine mesh that is crushed for immediate administration. The medication is absorbed into the circulation through the mucous membrane of the nasal passages. Vaporized medication is also given by inhalation.

inhalation analgesia, the occasional administration of anesthetic gas during the second stage of labor to reduce pain. Consciousness is retained to allow the woman to follow instructions and to avoid the adverse effects of general anesthesia.

inhalation anesthesia, surgical narcosis achieved by the administration of an anesthetic gas or a volatile anesthetic liquid

via a carrier gas. Administration of an inhalation anesthetic is usually preceded by intravenous or intramuscular administration of a short-acting sedative or hypnotic drug, often a barbiturate. Among the principal inhalation anesthetics are nitrous oxide, cyclopropane, ethylene, halothane, enflurane, fluroxene, methoxyflurane, trichloroethylene, and isoflurane.

inhalation therapy, a treatment in which a substance is introduced into the respiratory tract with inspired air. Oxygen, water, and various drugs may be administered using techniques of inhalation therapy.

inhale [L *in* within, *halare* to breathe], to breathe in or to draw in with the breath. –**inhalation,** *n*.

inhaler, a device for administering medications to be inhaled, such as vapors, fine powders, or volatile substances. An inhaler also may be designed to administer anesthetic gases.

inherent /inhir'ənt/ [L *inhaerere* to cling to], inborn, innate; natural to an environment.

inherent rate, the frequency of impulse formation attributed to a given pacemaker location.

inheritance [L *in* within, *hereditare* to inherit], **1.** the acquisition or expression of traits or conditions by transmission of genetic material from parents to offspring. **2.** the sum total of the genetic qualities or traits transmitted from parents to offspring; the total genetic makeup of the fertilized ovum. Kinds of inheritance include **alternative, amphigenous, autosomal, blending, codominant, complemental, crisscross, cytoplasmic, holandric, hologynic, homochronous, maternal, mendelism, monofactorial, multifactorial, supplemental,** and **x-linked inheritance.** –**inherited,** *adj.* **inherit,** *v.*

inherited disorder, any disease or condition that is genetically determined and involves either a single gene mutation, multifactorial inheritance, or a chromosomal aberration.

inherited trait [L *in* + *hereditare;* Fr *trait* a draft], a distinguishing quality or characteristic that is transmitted genetically from one generation to the next.

inhibin /inhib'in/, a reproductive system hormone that inhibits activity of the follicle-stimulating hormone.

inhibiting gene [L *inhibere* to restrain; Gk *genein* to produce], a gene that prevents the expression of another gene.

inhibiting hormone. See **hormone.**

inhibition /in'hibish'ən/ [L *inhibere* to restrain], **1.** (in psychology) the unconscious restraint of a behavioral process, usually resulting from the social or cultural forces of the environment; the condition inducing such restraint. **2.** (in psychoanalysis) the process in which the superego prevents the conscious expression of an unconscious instinctual drive, thought, or urge. **3.** (in physiology) restraining, checking, or arresting the action of an organ or cell or the reducing of a physiologic activity by an antagonistic stimulation. **4.** (in chemistry) the stopping or slowing down of the rate of a chemical reaction.

inhibition assay, an immunoassay in which an excess of antigens prevents or inhibits the completion of either the initial or indicator phase of the reaction.

inhibition of reflexes [L *inhibere; reflectere* to bend back], **1.** the prevention of a reflex action, requiring a series of biochemical mechanisms to restrict the flow of excitatory impulses at presynaptic and postsynaptic points in the system. **2.** a negative reflex effect that may become established during differential conditioning. The negative conditioned reflex represents an inhibition of a conditioned reflex.

inhibitor /inhib'itər/, a drug or other agent that prevents or restricts a certain action.

inhibitory [L *inhibere* to restrain], tending to stop or slow a process, such as a neuron that suppresses the intensity of a nerve impulse.

inhibitory enzyme [L *inhibere;* Gk *en* within, *zyme* ferment], an enzyme that blocks rather than catalyzes a chemical reaction.

inion /in'ē·on/ [Gk], the most prominent point of the back of the head, where the occipital bone protrudes the farthest.

initial contact stance stage [L *initium* beginning; *contigere* to touch], one of the five stages in the stance phase of walking or gait, specifically associated with the moment when the foot touches the ground or floor, and the leg prepares to accept the weight of the body.

initiation codon /kō'don/ [L *initium* beginning; *caudex* book], (in molecular genetics) the triplet of nucleotides that code for formylmethionine, the first amino acid in protein sequences.

initiator, a cocarcinogenic factor that causes a usually irreversible genetic mutation in a normal cell and primes it for uncontrolled growth. Examples include radiation, aflatoxins, urethane, and nitrosamines.

injectable silicone [L *in* + *jacere* to throw; *silex* silicon], the use of polymeric organic compounds of silicone in plastic surgery. The silicones are injected beneath the skin for cosmetic benefits.

injection /injek'shən/ [L *in* within, *jacere* to throw], **1.** the act of forcing a liquid into the body by means of a syringe. Injections are designated according to the anatomic site involved; the most common are intraarterial, intradermal, intramuscular, intravenous, and subcutaneous. **2.** the substance injected. **3.** redness and swelling observed in the physical examination of a part of the body, caused by dilatation of the blood vessels secondary to an inflammatory or infectious process. **–inject,** *v.*

injection cap, a rubber diaphragm covering a plastic cap. It permits needle insertion into a catheter or vial.

injection technique. See **intradermal injection, intramuscular injection, intrathecal injection, intravenous injection, subcutaneous injection,** and other specific injection techniques.

injunction [L *injungere* to enjoin], a court order that prevents a party from performing a particular act.

injury, high risk for, a NANDA-accepted nursing diagnosis of a potential for injury that may be somatic (internal) or environmental (external). Defining characteristics include (somatic) abnormal sensory function, autoimmune condition, malnutrition, abnormal hematologic condition, broken skin, developmental abnormality, or psychologic dysfunction; (environmental) lack of immunization, pathogenic microorganisms, chemical pollutants, poisons, alcohol, nicotine, food additives, modes of transportation, physical aspects of the community, nosocomial agents, nonavailability of assistance, and various psychologic factors.

inlay splint [L *in* within; AS *lecan* lay], a casting for fixing or supporting one or more approximating teeth.

inlet [L *in* within; ME *leten*], a passage leading into a cavity, such as the pelvic inlet that marks the brim of the pelvic cavity.

inlet contraction. See **contraction.**

in loco parentis /in lō'kō pəren'tis/ [L *in* within; *loco* to place; *parentis* a parent], the assumption by a person or institution of the parental obligations of caring for a child without adoption.

innate /in'āt, ināt'/ [L *innatus* inborn], **1.** existing in or belonging to a person from birth; inborn; hereditary; congenital. **2.** a natural and essential characteristic of something or someone; inherent. **3.** originating in or produced by the intellect or the mind.

innate immunity. See **natural immunity.**

inner cell mass [AS *innera* within; L *cella*

storeroom; *massa* lump], a cluster of cells localized around the animal pole of the blastocyst of placental mammals from which the embryo develops.

inner ear. See **internal ear.**

innervate /in′ərvāt/ [L *in* + *nervus*], pertaining to the nerves or nervous stimuli that supply a body part or organ.

innervation /in′ərvā′shən/ [L *in* witin, *nervus* nerve], the distribution or supply of nerve fibers or nerve impulses to a part of the body.

innervation apraxia. See **motor apraxia.**

innidation. See **nidation.**

innocent [L *innocens* harmless], benign, innocuous, or functional; not malignant, such as an innocent heart murmur.

innocuous [L *innocuus* harmless], pertaining to use of a substance or procedure that would cause no ill effects.

innominate /inom′ināt/ [L *innominatum* nameless], without a name; unnamed. The term is traditionally applied to certain anatomic structures, such as the hipbone.

innominate artery, one of the three arteries that branch from the arch of the aorta.

innominate bone, the hipbone. It consists of the ilium, ischium, and pubis and unites with the sacrum and coccyx to form the pelvis.

innominate vein, a large vein on either side of the neck that is formed by the union of the internal jugular and subclavian veins. The two veins drain blood from the head, neck, and upper extremities and unite to form the superior vena cava.

inoculate /inok′yəlāt/ [L *inoculare* to graft], to introduce a substance (**inoculum**) into the body to produce or to increase immunity to the disease or condition associated with the substance.

inoculum /inok′yo͞oləm/, *pl. inocula* [L *inocuus* harmless], a substance introduced into the body to cause or to increase immunity to a specific disease or condition. It may be a toxin, a live, attenuated, or killed virus or bacterium, or an immune serum.

inoperable [L *in* + *operari* to work], pertaining to a medical condition that would not benefit from surgical intervention or for which the risk would preclude a radical approach.

inorganic [L *in* not; Gk *organikos* natural], (in chemistry) a chemical compound that does not contain carbon.

inorganic acid, a compound containing no carbon that is made up of hydrogen and an electronegative element, such as hydrochloric acid.

inorganic chemistry, the study of the properties and reactions of all chemical el-

ements and compounds other than hydrocarbons.

inorganic dust, dry, finely powdered particles of an inorganic substance, especially dust, which, when inhaled, can cause abnormal conditions of the lungs.

inorganic phosphorus, phosphorus that may be measured in the blood as phosphate ions.

inosine /in′əsēn, -sīn/, a nucleoside, derived from animal tissue, especially intestines, originally used in food processing and flavoring.

inosiplex /inō′sipleks/, a form of inosine that acts as a stimulator of the immune system.

inositol /inō′sətōl, inos′-/, an isomer of glucose that occurs widely in plant and animal cells.

inotropic /in′ōtrop′ik/ [Gk *inos* fiber, *trope* turning], pertaining to the force or energy of muscular contractions, particularly contractions of the heart muscle. An inotropic agent increases myocardial contractility.

inpatient [L *in* within, *patior* to suffer], **1.** a patient who has been admitted to a hospital or other health care facility for at least an overnight stay. **2.** of or pertaining to the treatment or care of such a patient or to a health care facility to which a patient may be admitted for 24-hour care.

inpatient care unit, a unit of a hospital organized for medical and continuous nursing services for a group of inpatients who are usually grouped according to diagnosis or other common characteristics, such as maternity or surgical patients.

input, the information or material that enters a system.

inquest [L *in* + *quaerere* to seek], a legal inquiry into the cause, manner, and circumstances of a sudden, unexpected, or violent death.

insane [L *in* not, *sanus* sound], a legal term for an unsound, diseased, or deranged mind, particularly of a person who is unable to provide adequate self-care and there is a need to protect the patient and the public from each other. In the United States, the precise legal definition varies from state to state.

insanity, [L *in* not, *sanus* sound] *informal.* a severe mental disorder or defect, such as a psychosis, rather than a neurosis. It is used more in legal and social than in medical terminology. When a person is classified as insane, various legal actions can ensue, such as commitment to an institution, appointment of a guardian, or dissolution of a contract.

insatiable /insā′sh(ē)əbəl/ [L *insatiatus* not satisfied], pertaining to an appetite for food or other needs that cannot be satisfied.

insect bite [L *in* within, *secare* to cut], the bite of any parasitic or venomous arthropod such as a louse, flea, mite, tick, or arachnid. Many arthropods inject venom that produces poisoning or severe local reaction, saliva that may contain viruses, or substances that produce mild irritation.

insecticide, a chemical agent that kills insects.

insecticide poisoning. See **chlorinated organic insecticide poisoning.**

insemination /insem'inā'shən/, the injection of semen into the uterine canal. It may involve an artificial process unrelated to sexual intercourse.

insenescence /in'sines'əns/ [L *insenescere* to begin to grow old], **1.** the process of aging. **2.** the state of being chronologically old but retaining the vitality of a person with a younger biological age.

insensible [L *in* not, *sentire* to feel], **1.** pertaining to a person who is unconscious for any reason. **2.** pertaining to a person who is apathetic or deprived of normal sense perceptions.

insensible perspiration [L *in* not, *sentire* to feel; *per* through, *spirare* to breath], a small amount of perspiration continually excreted by the sweat glands in the skin that evaporates before it may be observed.

insertion /insur'shən/ [L *inserere* to introduce], (in anatomy) the place of attachment, such as of a muscle to the bone it moves.

insertion forceps. See **point forceps.**

insertion site, the point in a vein where a needle or catheter is inserted.

in-service education [L *in* within, *servus* a slave; *educare* to rear], a program of instruction or training that is provided by an agency or institution for its employees.

insidious /insid'ē-əs/ [L *insidiosus* cunning], of, pertaining to, or describing a development that is gradual, subtle, or imperceptible.

insight [L *in* within; AS *gesihth* sight], **1.** the capacity of comprehending the true nature of a situation or of penetrating an underlying truth. **2.** an instance of comprehending an underlying truth, primarily through intuitive understanding. **3.** (in psychology) a type of self-understanding encompassing both an intellectual and emotional awareness of the unconscious nature, origin, feelings, and mechanisms of one's attitudes, feelings, and behavior.

insipid /insip'id/ [L *in* + *sapidus* savory], pertaining to something that is dull, tasteless, or lifeless.

in situ /in sī'tōō, sit' ōō/ [L *in* within; *situs* position] **1.** in the natural or usual place.

2. describing a cancer that has not metastasized or invaded neighboring tissues, such as carcinoma in situ.

insoluble [L *in* not, *solubilis* soluble], unable to be dissolved, usually in a specific solvent, such as a substance that is insoluble in water.

insomnia /insom'nē-ə/ [L *in* not, *somnus* sleep], chronic inability to sleep or to remain asleep throughout the night; wakefulness; sleeplessness.

insomniac, 1. a person with insomnia. **2.** pertaining to, causing, or associated with insomnia. **3.** characteristic of or occurring during a period of sleeplessness.

inspiration /in'spirā'shən/ [L *in* within, *spirare* to breathe], the act of drawing air into the lungs in order to exchange oxygen for carbon dioxide, the end product of tissue metabolism. The major muscle of inspiration is the diaphragm, the contraction of which creates a negative pressure in the chest, causing the lungs to expand and air to flow inward. Lungs at maximal inspiration have an average total capacity of 5,500 to 6,000 ml of air.

inspiratory /inspī'rətôr'ē/ [L *in* within, *spirare* to breathe], of or pertaining to inspiration.

inspiratory capacity (IC), the maximum volume of gas that can be inhaled from the resting expiratory level.

inspiratory dyspnea [L *inspirare* to breathe in; Gk *dys* without; *pnoia* breath], a form of breathing difficulty caused by an obstruction in the larynx, trachea, or bronchi. The patient attempts to compensate for this deficiency with prolonged deep inspirations.

inspiratory hold, either of two kinds of modification in an intermittent positive pressure breathing (IPPB) pressure waveform. They are: (1) a pressure hold, in which a preset pressure is reached and held for a designated period, and (2) a volume hold, in which a predetermined volume is delivered and then held for a designated period.

inspiratory reserve volume, the maximum volume of gas that can be inspired from the end-tidal inspiratory level.

inspiratory resistance muscle training, respiratory therapy exercises that require inhalation against some type of resisting force, such as abdominal breathing practice with weights on the abdomen.

inspirometer /in'spirom'ətər/ [L *inspirare;* Gk *metron* measure], an apparatus used to measure the volume, force, and frequency of a patient's inspirations.

inspissate /inspis'āt/ [L *inspissare* to thicken], (of a fluid) to thicken or harden through the absorption or evaporation of the liquid portion, such as milk in an inspissated milk duct. **–inspissation,** *n.*

instillation [L *instillare* to drip], **1.** a procedure in which a fluid is slowly introduced into a cavity or passage of the body and allowed to remain for a specific length of time before being drained or withdrawn. **2.** a solution so introduced. **–instill,** *v.*

instinct [L *instinctus* impulse], an inborn psychologic representation of a need, such as life instincts of hunger, thirst, and sex, and the destructive and aggressive death instincts.

instinctive reflex. See **unconditioned response.**

institutionalism syndrome, a condition characterized by apathy, withdrawal, submissiveness, and a lack of inititiative. The person may resist leaving a hospital, even when the surroundings are barely adequate, because it is familiar and predictable.

institutionalize [L *instituere* to put in place], to place a person in an institution for psychologic or physical treatment or for the protection of the person or society. **–institutionalization,** *n.*, **institutionalized,** *adj.*

institutional licensure [L *instituere* to put in place; *licere* to be permitted], a proposed procedure in which licensure for almost all health professions would be abandoned and the responsibility for assessing professional competence would fall to the health care facility where the health professional is employed.

institutional review board (IRB), a federally approved committee that reviews all research proposals before submission of requests for funding to federal government granting agencies.

instrument [L *nstrumentum* tool], a surgical tool or device designed to perform a specific function, such as cutting, dissecting, grasping, holding, retracting, or suturing. Some kinds of instruments are **clamp, needle holder, retractor,** and **speculum.**

instrumental conditioning. See **operant conditioning.**

instrumental labor, child delivery in which the use of instruments, such as forceps or perforators, is required.

instrumentation, the use of instruments for treatment and diagnosis.

insufficiency [L *in* not, *sufficere* to be adequate], inability to perform a necessary function adequately. Some kinds of insufficiency are **adrenal, aortic, ileocecal, pulmonary,** and **valvular insufficiency.**

insufflate /in'səflāt, insuf'lāt/ [L *insufflare* to blow into], to blow a gas or powder into a tube, cavity, or organ to allow visual examination, to remove an obstruc-

tion, or to apply medication. **–insufflation,** *n.*

insufflator /in'səflā'tər/, an apparatus used to blow air or gas into a body cavity.

insulation, a nonconducting substance that offers a barrier to the passage of heat or electricity.

insulin /in'səlin/ [L *insula* island], **1.** a naturally occurring hormone secreted by the beta cells of the islands of Langerhans in the pancreas in response to increased levels of glucose in the blood. The hormone acts to regulate the metabolism of glucose and the processes necessary for the intermediary metabolism of fats, carbohydrates, and proteins. Insulin lowers blood glucose levels and promotes transport and entry of glucose into the muscle cells and other tissues. **2.** a pharmacologic preparation of the hormone administered in treating diabetes mellitus. The various preparations of insulin available for prescription vary in promptness, intensity, and duration of action. They are termed **rapid-acting, intermediate-acting,** and **long-acting.**

insulin-dependent diabetes mellitus (IDDM), an inability to metabolize carbohydrate caused by an overt insulin deficiency, occurring in children and characterized by polydipsia, polyuria, polyphagia, loss of weight, diminished strength, and marked irritability. Insulin-dependent diabetes mellitus tends to be unstable and brittle, with the patients quite sensitive to insulin and physical activity and liable to develop ketoacidosis. Previously called brittle diabetes, juvenile diabetes, juvenile-onset diabetes, JOD, juvenile-onset-type diabetes, ketosis-prone diabetes.

insulinemia /in'səlinē'mē·ə/ [L, *insula,* island (of Langerhans); Gk, *haima,* blood], an abnormally high level of insulin in the blood.

insulin injection, a fast-acting, regular insulin prescribed in the treatment of diabetes mellitus when the desired action is prompt, intense, and short-acting. Insulin injection is the only form of insulin suitable for intramuscular administration.

insulin injection sites, body tissue areas that offer optimum utilization of subcutaneous injections of insulin. The choice of sites can affect the rate of absorption and peak action times but repeated use of the same injection sites can lead to localized tissue damage, resulting in malabsorption of insulin and misdiagnosis of insulin resistance. These problems are minimized by systematic rotation of injection sites.

insulin kinase, an enzyme, assumed to be present in the liver, that activates insulin.

insulin lipodystrophy [L *insula* + Gk *lipos* fat; *dys* bad, *trophe* nourishment], the loss of local fat deposits in diabetes patients as a complication of repeated insulin injections.

insulinogenic /in'səlin'ōjen'ik/ [L *insula* + Gk *genein* to produce], promoting the production and release of insulin by the islands of Langerhans in the pancreas.

insulinoma /in'səlinō'mə/, *pl.* insulinomas, insulinomata [L *insula* + Gk *oma* tumor], a benign tumor of the insulin-secreting cells of the islands of Langerhans.

insulin pump [L *insula*; ME *pumpe*], a portable battery-powered instrument that delivers a measured amount of insulin through the abdominal wall. It can be programmed to deliver varied doses of insulin according to the body's needs at the time.

insulin reaction, the adverse effects caused by excessive levels of circulating insulin.

insulin resistance, a complication of diabetes mellitus characterized by a need for more than 200 units of insulin per day to control hyperglycemia and ketosis. The cause is associated with insulin binding by high levels of antibody.

insulin shock, hypoglycemic shock caused by an overdose of insulin, a decreased intake of food, or excessive exercise. It is characterized by sweating, trembling, chilliness, nervousness, irritability, hunger, hallucination, numbness, and pallor. Uncorrected, it will progress to convulsions, coma, and death. Treatment requires an immediate dose of glucose.

insulin tolerance test, a test of the body's ability to use insulin, in which insulin is given and blood glucose is measured at regular intervals.

insulintropin /in'səlintrop'in/ [L, *insula,* island], a naturally occurring hormone produced in the intestines when food is ingested. It causes the release of insulin from the pancreas, which, in turn, regulates blood-sugar levels. It has been administered to Type II diabetes patients but it would not be useful in its present form in the treatment of Type I diabetes patients as their pancreases do not secrete insulin.

insuloma. See **insulinoma.**

intake [L *in* within; AS *tacan* to take], **1.** the process in which a person is admitted to a clinic or hospital or is signed in for an office visit. The reason for the visit and various identifying data about the patient are noted. **2.** the amount of food or fluids ingested in a given period.

integral dose /in'təgrəl/ [L *integrare* to make whole; Gk *dosis* giving], (in radiotherapy) the total amount of energy ab-

sorbed by a patient or object during exposure to radiation.

integrating dose meter, (in radiotherapy) an ionization chamber, usually designed to be placed on the patient's skin, with a measuring system for determining the total radiation administered during an exposure.

integration [L *integrare* to make whole], **1.** the act or process of unifying or bringing together. **2.** (in psychology) the organization of all elements of the personality into a coordinated, functional whole that is in harmony with the environment. **–integrate,** *v.*

integration of self, one of the components of high-level wellness. It is characterized by the integration of mind, body, and spirit into one harmoniously functioning unit.

integument /integ'yŏŏmənt/ [L *integumentum* a covering], a covering or skin. **–integumentary,** *adj.*

integumentary system /integ'yəmen'tərē/, the skin and its appendages, hair, nails, and sweat and sebaceous glands.

integumentary system assessment, an evaluation of the general condition of a patient's integument and of factors or abnormalities that may contribute to the presence of a dermatologic disorder. The nurse asks if the patient suffers from itching, pain, rashes, blisters, or boils; if the skin usually is dry, oily, thin, rough, bumpy, or puffy; or if it feels hot or cold, peels, changes in color, or is marked with dark liver (aging) spots. Observations are made of the intactness, turgor, elasticity, temperature, cleanliness, odor, wetness or dryness, and color of the skin. Cyanosis of the lips, circumoral area, or mucous membranes, earlobes, or nailbeds; jaundice of the sclera; pale conjunctivae; the distribution of pigment; and evidence of plethora are noted. Indications of rashes, edema, needle marks, insect bites, scabies, acne, sclerema, decubiti, uremic frost on the beard or eyebrows, or pressure areas over bony prominences are recorded. The nails are examined for brittleness, lines, a convex ram's horn or concave spoon shape, and the condition of surrounding tissue, including clubbing of the fingers and toes. The existence and characteristics of maculae, papules, vesicles, pustules, bullae, hives, warts, moles, ulcers, scars, keloids, petechiae, lipomas, crusts of dried exudate, flakes of dead epidermis, excoriations, blackheads, or a chancre are noted.

intellect [L *intellectus* perception], **1.** the power and ability of the mind for knowing and understanding, as contrasted with feeling or with willing. **2.** a person possessing a great capacity for thought and knowledge. **–intellectual,** *adj., n.*

intellectualization [L *intellectus* + Gk *izein* to cause], (in psychiatry) a defense mechanism in which reasoning is used as a means of blocking a confrontation with an unconscious conflict and the emotional stress associated with it.

intelligence [L *intelligentia* perception], **1.** the potential ability and capacity to acquire, retain, and apply experience, understanding, knowledge, reasoning, and judgment in coping with new experiences and in solving problems. **2.** the manifestation of such ability. **–intelligent,** *adj.*

intelligence quotient (IQ), a numeric expression of a person's intellectual level as measured against the statistical average of his or her age group. On several of the traditional scales it is determined by dividing the mental age, derived through psychologic testing, by the chronologic age and multiplying the result by 100. Average IQ is considered to be 100.

intelligence test, any of a variety of standarized tests designed to determine the mental age of an individual by measuring the relative capacity to absorb information and to solve problems. Two kinds of intelligence tests are **Stanford-Binet and Wechsler-Bellevue scale.**

intemperance [L *in* + *temperare* to moderate], excessive indulgence in eating, drinking, or other lifestyle functions.

intensifying screen [L *intensus* tighten, *facere* to make; ME *screne*], a device consisting of fluorescent material, which is placed in contact with the film in a radiographic cassette. Radiation from a therapeutic process interacts with the fluorescent phosphor, releasing light photons. These expose the film with greater efficiency than would the radiation alone. Thus patient exposure can be reduced.

intensive care [L *intensus* tightened, *garrire* to chatter], constant, complex, detailed health care as provided in various acute life-threatening conditions, such as multiple trauma, severe burns, myocardial infarction, or after certain kinds of surgery.

intensive care unit (ICU), a hospital unit in which patients requiring close monitoring and intensive care are housed for as long as needed. An ICU contains highly technical and sophisticated monitoring devices and equipment, and the staff in the unit is educated to give critical care as needed by the patients.

intention [L *intendere* to aim], a kind of healing process. Healing by **first intention** is the primary union of the edges of a wound, progressing to complete healing without scar formation or granulation;

healing by **second intention** is wound closure in which the edges are separated, granulation tissue develops to fill the gap, and, finally, epithelium grows in over the granulations, producing a scar. Healing by **third intention** is wound closure in which granulation tissue fills the gap between the edges of the wound with epithelium growing over the granulation at a slower rate and producing a larger scar than results from healing from second intention.

intentional additives, substances that are deliberately added in the manufacture of food or pharmaceutic products to improve or maintain flavor, color, texture, or consistency, or to enhance or conserve nutritional value.

intention tremor, fine, rhythmic, purposeless movements that tend to increase during voluntary movements.

interactional model [L *inter* between, *agere* to do], a family therapy model that views the family as a communication system comprising interlocking subsystems. Family dysfunction occurs when the rules governing family interaction become ambiguous. The therapeutic goal is to help the family clarify its rules.

interactionist theory, an aging theory that views age-related changes as resulting from the interaction between the individual characteristics of the person, the circumstances in society, and the history of social interaction patterns of the person.

interaction processes, a component of the theory of effective practice. The processes consist of a series of interactions between a nurse and a patient in a sequence of actions and reactions until the patient and the nurse both understand what is wanted and the desired act is achieved.

interalveolar /in'təralvē'ələr/ [L *inter* + *alveolus* little hollow], pertaining to the area between alveoli.

interarticular /in'tərärtik'yələr/ [L *inter* + *articulus* joint], pertaining to the areas between two joints or between facing surfaces of a joint.

interarticular fibrocartilage, one of four kinds of fibrocartilage, consisting of flattened fibrocartilaginous plates between the articular cartilage of the most active joints, such as the sternoclavicular, wrist, and knee joints.

intercalary /intur'kələr'ē, in'tərkal'ərē/ [L *intercalare* to insert], occurring between two others, such as the absence of the middle part of a bone with the proximal and the distal parts present.

intercalate /intur'kəlāt/ [L *intercalare*], to insert between adjacent surfaces or structures. **–intercalation,** *n.*

intercapillary glomerulosclerosis /in'- tərkap' iler'ē/ [L *inter* + *capillaris* hair-like; *gomerulus* small ball; Gk *sklerosis* a hardening], an abnormal condition characterized by degeneration of the renal glomeruli. It is associated with diabetes and often produces albuminuria, nephrotic edema, hypertension, and renal insufficiency.

intercavernous sinuses /in'tərkav'ərnəs/ [L *inter* + *caverna* cavity; *sinus* curve], the cavities through which the cavernous sinuses of the dura mater communicate.

intercellular [L *inter* + *cella* storeroom], between or among cells.

intercellular bridge, a structure that connects adjacent cells, occurring primarily in the epithelium and other stratified squamous epithelia. It consists of slender strands of cytoplasm that project from the surfaces of adjacent cells.

intercerebral /in'tərser'əbrəl/ [L *inter* + *cerebrum* brain], pertaining to the area between the left and right cerebral hemispheres.

interchange. See **reciprocal translocation.**

interclavicular /in'tərkləvik'yələr/ [L *inter* + *clavicula* little key], pertaining to the area between the clavicles.

interconceptional gynecologic care [L *inter* + *concipere* to take in], health care of a woman during her reproductive years, between pregnancies, and after 6 weeks after delivery. Papanicolaou testing for cervical cancer, breast and pelvic examinations, evaluation of general health, and laboratory determination of glucosuria and proteinuria and of the hematocrit or hemoglobin are common and routine aspects of interconceptional care.

intercondylar fracture /in'tərkon'dilər/ [L *inter* + Gk *kondylos* knuckle], a fracture of the tissue between condyles.

intercostal /in'tərkos'təl/ [L *inter* + *costa* rib], of or pertaining to the space between two ribs.

intercostal bulging, the visible bulging of the soft tissues of the intercostal spaces that occurs when increased expiratory effort is needed to exhale, as in asthma, cystic fibrosis, or obstruction of a respiratory passage by a foreign body.

intercostal muscles, the muscles between adjacent ribs. They are designated as external and internal, and function as secondary ventilatory muscles.

intercostal node, a node in one of three groups of thoracic parietal lymph nodes situated near the dorsal parts of the intercostal spaces and associated with lymphatic vessels that drain the posterolateral area of the chest.

intercostal space, the region between the ribs.

intercourse [L *intercursus* running between], *informal.* sexual intercourse.

intercristal /in'tərkris'təl/ [L *inter* + *crista* ridge], of or pertaining to the space between two crests.

intercurrent disease [L *intercurrere* to run between], a disease that develops in and may alter the course of another disease.

interdental canal [L *inter* + *dens* tooth], any one of the nutrient channels that pass upward to the teeth through the body of the mandible.

interdental gingiva, the soft supporting tissue, consisting of prominent horizontal collagen fibers, that normally fills the space between two approximating teeth.

interdental groove, a linear, vertical depression on the surface of the interdental papillae, which functions as a sluiceway for the egress of food from the interproximal areas.

interdental spillway, a sluiceway formed by the interproximal contours of adjoining teeth and their investing tissues.

interference [L *inter* + *ferire* to strike], the effect of a component on the accuracy of measurement of the desired analyte.

interferent /in'tərfir'ənt/ [L *inter* + *ferire* to strike], any chemical or physical phenomena that can interfere or disrupt a reaction or process.

interferential current therapy /in'- tərfərən'shəl/, a form of electric stimulation therapy using two or three different currents that are passed through a tissue from surface electrodes. Portions of each current are canceled by the other, resulting in a different net current applied to the target tissue.

interferon /in'tərfir'on/ [L *inter* + *ferire* to strike], a natural cellular protein formed when cells are exposed to a virus or other foreign particle of nucleic acid. It induces the production of translation inhibitory protein (TIP) in noninfected cells. TIP blocks translation of viral RNA, thus giving other cells protection against both the original and other viruses. Interferon is species specific.

interferon alfa-2a, recombinant, a parenteral antineoplastic drug administered in the treatment of hair cell leukemia.

interferon alfa-2b, recombinant, a parenteral antineoplastic drug similar to **interferon alfa-2a, recombinant.**

interferon nomenclature, a system recommended by the International Interferon Nomenclature Committee for identifying interferon compounds. For a specific isolated product, "interferon" is the first word of the name. It is followed by a

Greek letter, spelled out, an arabic number, and a lower case letter appended by a dash, as in the example: interferon alfa-2a.

interfibrillar mass of Flemming, interfilar mass. See **hyaloplasm.**

interim rate [L, meanwhile; *ratum* calculate], a method of third-party payment for costs of hospital services in which an amount is paid periodically pending an accounting of actual costs at the end of a designated period.

interiorization /intir′ē·ôrīzā′shən/ [L *interior* inner; Gk *izein* to cause], the merging of reflex and cognitive processes as a response to the environment.

interior mesenteric artery [L, inner; Gk *mesos* middle, *enteron* intestine; *arteria* air pipe], a visceral branch of the abdominal aorta, arising just above the division into the common iliacs and supplying the left half of the transverse colon, all of the descending and iliac colons, and most of the rectum.

interkinesis /in′tərkinē′sis, -kīnē′sis/ [L *inter* + Gk *kinein* to move], the interval between the first and second nuclear divisions in meiosis.

interlace mode /in′tərlās′/, (in radiology) a process whereby a conventional TV camera tube reads off its target assembly so that each of two fields represents repeated adjacent active traces and horizontal retraces of the electron beam across a TV screen.

interleukin-1 (IL-1) /in′tərloo′kin/, a protein with numerous immune system functions, including activation of resting T cells, and endothelial and macrophage cells, mediation of inflammation, and stimulation of synthesis of lymphokines, collagen, and collagenases.

interleukin-2 (IL-2), a protein with various immunologic functions, including the ability to initiate proliferation of activated T cells. IL-2 is used in the laboratory to grow T-cell clones with specific helper, cytotoxic, and suppressor functions.

interleukin-3 (IL-3), an immune response protein that supports the growth of pluripotent bone marrow stem cells and is a growth factor for mast cells.

interleukin-4 (IL-4), an immune response protein that is a growth factor for activated B cells, resting T cells, and mast cells.

interlobular duct /in′tərlob′yələr/ [L *inter* + *lobulus* small lobe], any duct connecting or draining the lobules of a gland.

interlocked twins [L *inter* + AS *loc* a fastening], monozygotic twins so positioned in the uterus that the neck of one becomes entwined with that of the other

during presentation so that vaginal delivery is not possible.

intermediary /in′tərmē′dē·er′ē/ [L *inter* + *mediare* to divide], a Blue Cross plan, private insurance company, or public or private agency selected by health care providers to pay claims under Medicare.

intermediary metabolism [L *inter* + *mediare*; Gk *metabole* change], the metabolic processes involved in the synthesis of cellular components between digestion of food and excretion of waste products.

intermediate-acting insulin [L *inter* + *mediare*; *activus* active], a preparation of the antidiabetic principle of beef pancreas or pork pancreas modified by interaction with zinc under specific chemical conditions and having an intermediate range of action.

intermediate care, a level of medical care for certain chronically ill or disabled individuals in which room and board are provided but skilled nursing care is not.

intermediate care facility, a health facility that provides medical-related services to persons with a variety of physical or emotional conditions requiring institutional facilities but without the degree of care provided by a hospital or skilled nursing facility.

intermediate cell mass. See **nephrotome.**

intermediate cuneiform bone, the smallest of the three cuneiform bones of the foot, located between the medial and the lateral cuneiform bones.

intermediate host, any animal in which the larval or intermediate stages of a parasite develop. Humans are intermediate hosts for malaria parasites.

intermediate mesoderm. See **nephrotome.**

intermenstrual /in′tərmen′stroo·əl/ [L *inter* + *menstruum* menstrual fluid], of or pertaining to the time between menstrual periods.

intermenstrual fever, the normal, slight elevation of temperature that marks ovulation, usually occurring about 14 days before the onset of menses.

intermittent /in′tərmit′ənt/ [L *inter* + *mittere* to send], occurring at intervals; alternating between periods of activity and inactivity, such as rheumatoid arthritis, which is marked by periods of signs and symptoms followed by periods of remission.

intermittent assisted ventilation (IAV), (in respiratory therapy) a system in which an assisted rate is combined with spontaneous breathing.

intermittent claudication. See **claudication.**

intermittent fever, a fever that recurs in cycles of paroxysms and remissions, such as in malaria. Kinds of intermittent fever include **bidoutertian malaria, double quartan malaria, and quartan malaria.**

intermittent hydrosalpinx /in'tərmit'ənt hī'drōsal'pingks/ [L *inter* + *mittere*; Gk *hydor* water, *salpigx* tube], a fluid accumulation in a fallopian tube. The fluid is released periodically through the uterine cavity.

intermittent incontinence [L *inter* + *mittere; incontinentia* inability to retain], urinary incontinence that occurs only when there is pressure on the bladder or during muscular effort.

intermittent mandatory ventilation (IMV), a method of respiratory therapy in which the patient is allowed to breathe independently and then at certain prescribed intervals.

intermittent positive pressure breathing. See **IPPB.**

intermittent positive pressure breathing unit. See **IPPB unit.**

intermittent positive pressure ventilation. See **IPPV.**

intermittent pulse [L *inter* + *mittere; pulsare* to beat], a pulse in which an occasional beat is absent. It tends to occur with second-degree heart block or extrasystole.

intermittent torticollis [L *inter* + *mittere; tortus* twisted; *collum* neck], intermittent spasms of the neck muscles, drawing the head to one side. The powerful contractions usually occur in the sternocleidomastoid muscle.

intermittent tremor [L *inter* + *mittere; tremor* trembling], a rhythmic involuntary shaking that occurs intermittently, or a tremor that occurs after a voluntary movement is attempted.

intern [L *internus* inward], **1.** a physician in the first postgraduate year, learning medical practice under supervision before beginning a residency program. **2.** any immediate postgraduate trainee in a clinical program. **3.** to work as an intern.

internal [L *internus* inward], within or inside. **–internally,** *adv.*

internal aperture of tympanic canaliculus, the upper opening of the tympanic channel in the temporal bone, leading to the tympanum.

internal bleeding [L *internus*; AS *blod*], any hemorrhage from an internal organ or tissue, such as intraperitoneal bleeding into the peritoneal cavity or intestinal bleeding into the bowel.

internal carotid artery, each of two arteries starting at the bifurcation of the common carotid arteries, opposite the cranial border of the thyroid cartilage, through which blood circulates to many structures and organs in the head.

internal carotid plexus, a network of nerves on the internal carotid artery, formed by the internal carotid nerve.

internal cervical os, an internal opening of the uterus that corresponds to the slight constriction or isthmus of that organ about midway in its length.

internal cuneiform bone. See **medial cuneiform bone.**

internal ear, the complex inner structure of the ear, communicating directly with the acoustic nerve, transmitting sound vibrations from the middle ear. It has two parts: the osseous labyrinth and the membranous labyrinth.

internal fertilization, the union of gametes within the body of the female after insemination.

internal fistula, an abnormal passage between two internal organs or structures.

internal fixation, any method of holding together the fragments of a fractured bone without the use of appliances external to the skin. After open reduction of the fracture, smooth or threaded pins, Kirschner wires, screws, plates attached by screws, or medullary nails may be used to stabilize the fragments.

internal iliac artery, a division of the common iliac artery, supplying the walls of the pelvis, the pelvic viscera, the genital organs, and part of the medial thigh.

internal iliac node, a node in one of seven groups of parietal lymph nodes serving the abdomen and the pelvis.

internal iliac vein, one of the pair of veins in the lower body that join the external iliac vein to form the two common iliac veins.

internal injury, any hurt, wound, or damage to the viscera.

internalization [L *internus* + Gk *izein* to cause], the process of adopting within the self, either unconsciously or consciously through learning and socialization, the attitudes, beliefs, values, and standards of another person or, more generally, of the society or group to which one belongs.

internal jugular vein, one of a pair of veins in the neck. Each vein collects blood from one side of the brain, the face, and the neck, and both unite with the subclavian vein to form the brachiocephalic vein.

internal locus of control. See **locus of control.**

internal malleolus [L *internus; malleolus* little hammer], the rounded process of the tibia forming the internal surface of the ankle joint.

internal mammary artery bypass, a surgical procedure to correct a coronary artery obstruction. The internal mammary artery in situ and still attached to the subclavian artery is anastomosed to the coronary artery beyond the obstruction.

internal medicine, the branch of medicine concerned with the study of the physiology and pathology of the internal organs and with the medical diagnosis and treatment of disorders of these organs.

internal oblique muscle. See **obliquus internus abdominis.**

internal os, the internal opening of the cervical canal.

internal podalic version and total breech extraction. See **version and extraction.**

internal pterygoid muscle. See **pterygoideus medialis.**

internal respiratory nerve of Bell. See **phrenic nerve.**

internal rotation, the turning of a limb toward the midline of the body.

internal secretion [L *internus; secernere* to separate], a type of secretion in which substances pass directly from a gland into the bloodstream.

internal standard, an element or compound added in a known amount to yield a signal against which an instrument or an analyte to be measured can be calibrated.

internal strabismus. See **esotropia.**

internal strangulation [L *internus; strangulare* to choke], a state of extreme constriction of an organ, such as a loop of intestine trapped in an opening, resulting in an interruption in the blood supply and ischemia.

internal thoracic artery, one of a pair of arteries that arise from the first portions of the subclavian arteries, supplying the pectoral muscles, the breasts, the pericardium, and the abdominal muscles.

internal thoracic vein, one of a pair of veins that accompanies the internal thoracic artery, receiving tributaries that correspond to those of the artery.

International Association for Dental Research (IADR), an international organization concerned with research in dentistry and the exchange of information regarding such research.

International Classification of Disease Adapted for Use in the United States (ICDA), a classification system adapted by the U.S. Public Health Service from the parent system developed by the World Health Organization. The system is used in categorizing and indexing hospital records. Each disease is listed as belonging to a major section, such as infectious disease or neoplastic disease, and then further coded into major disease categories

and subdivisions. The system is updated every 10 years.

International Classification of Diseases (ICD), an official list of categories of diseases, physical and mental, issued by the World Health Organization (WHO). It is used primarily for statistic purposes in the classification of morbidity and mortality data.

International Commission on Radiation Protection (ICRP), a nongovernmental organization founded in England in 1928 to provide general guidance on the safe use of radiation sources, including appropriate protective measures and codes of practice for medical radiology. The ICRP was reorganized in 1950 to include effects of nuclear energy.

International Congress of Surgeons (ICS), an international professional organization of surgeons.

International Council of Nurses (ICN), the oldest international health organization. It is a federation of nurses' associations from 93 nations and was one of the first health organizations to develop strict policies of nondiscrimination based on nationality, race, creed, color, politics, sex, or social status. The objectives of the ICN include promotion of national associations of nurses, improvement of standards of nursing and competence of nurses, improvement of the status of nurses within their countries, and provision of an authoritative international voice for nurses. The ICN is active in the World Health Organization (WHO), the United Nations Educational, Scientific, and Cultural Organization (UNESCO), and other international organizations.

International Red Cross Society, an international philanthropic organization, based in Geneva, Switzerland, concerned primarily with the humane treatment and welfare of the victims of war and calamity and with the neutrality of hospitals and medical personnel in times of war.

International System of Units (SI), an internationally accepted scientific system of expressing length, mass, and time in basic units (IU) of centimeters, grams, and seconds, replacing the old centimeter-gram-second system (CGS). The SI system also includes as standard measurements, **ampere, kelvin, candela,** and **mole.**

International Unit (IU), a unit of measure in the International System of Units.

internist /intur'nist, in'turnist/ [L *internus* inward], a physician who specializes in internal medicine.

internship, a period of apprenticeship for

a medical school graduate who serves in a hospital for a specified period before beginning a professional practice.

internuncial neuron /in'tərnun'sē·əl/ [L *inter* + *nuntius* messenger], a connecting neuron in a neural pathway, usually serving as a link between two other neurons.

interocclusal record /in'tərəkloo'səl/, a record of the positional relation of opposing teeth or jaws to each other, made on the occlusal surfaces of occlusal rims or teeth with a plastic material that hardens, such as plaster of paris, wax, zinc oxide-eugenol paste, or acrylic resin.

interoceptive /in'tərōsep'tiv/ [L *internus* inward, *capere* to take], pertaining to stimuli originating from within the body regarding the functioning of the internal organs or to the receptors they activate.

interoceptor [L *internus* + *capere* to take], any sensory nerve ending located in cells in the viscera that responds to stimuli originating from within the body regarding the function of the internal organs, such as digestion, excretion, and blood pressure.

interosseous /in'tərōs'ē·əs/ [L *inter* between + *os* bone], pertaining to an area between bones or pertaining to a structure, such as a ligament, connecting two bones.

interparietal fissure. See **intraparietal sulcus.**

interparoxysmal /in'tərper'əksis'məl/ [L *inter* + *paroxysmos* irritation], pertaining to something that happens between paroxysms.

interperiosteal fracture /in'tərper'ē·os'tē·əl/ [L *inter* + Gk *peri* around, *osteon* bone], an incomplete fracture in which the periosteum is not disrupted.

interpersonal [L *inter* + *persona* mask], pertaining to the interactions between individuals.

interpersonal psychiatry, a theory of psychiatry introduced by Sullivan that stresses the nature and quality of relationships with significant others as the most critical factor in personality development.

interpersonal therapy, a kind of psychotherapy that views faulty communications, interactions, and interrelationships as basic factors in maladaptive behavior. A kind of interpersonal therapy is **transactional analysis.**

interphase /in'tərfās'/ [L *inter* + Gk *phasis* phase], the metabolic stage in the cell cycle during which the cell is not dividing, the chromosomes are not individually distinguishable, and such biochemical and physiologic activities as DNA synthesis occur.

interpleural space /in'tərploor'əl/ [L *inter* + Gk *pleura* rib; L *spatium*], the potential space of the mediastinum between the two pleural linings.

interpolated PVC [L *interpolare* to refurbish], a ventricular extrasystole sandwiched between two sinus-conducted beats.

interpolated VPB /intur'pəlā'tid/, a ventricular extrasystole that occurs between two consecutive beats of the dominant heart rhythm.

interpolation /intur'pəlā'shən/, 1. the transfer of tissues, as in plastic surgery or transplants. 2. in statistics, the introduction of an estimated intermediate value of a variable between known values of the variable.

interproximal film. See **bite-wing film.**

interpubic disk /in'tərpyoo'bik/ [L *inter* + *os pubis* pubic bone; Gk *diskos* flat plate], the fibrocartilaginous plate connecting the opposed surfaces of the pubic bones at the pubic symphysis.

interradicular space /in'tər·radik'yələr/ [L *inter* + *radix* root; *spatium*], the area between the roots of a multirooted tooth, normally occupied by a bony septum and the periodontal membrane.

interrogatories /in'tərog'ətōr'ēz/ [L *inter* + *rogare* to ask], (in law) a series of written questions submitted to a witness or other person having information of interest to the court. The answers are transcribed and are sworn to under oath.

interrupted suture [L *interrumpere* to sever; *sutura*], a single suture tied separately, as distinguished from a continuous suture.

intersex /in'tərseks/ [L *inter* + *sexus* male or female], any individual who has anatomic characteristics of both sexes or whose external genitalia are ambiguous or inappropriate for either the normal male or female.

intersexuality [L *inter* + *sexus* male or female], the condition in which an individual has both male and female anatomic characteristics to varying degrees or in which the appearance of the external genitalia is ambiguous or differs from the gonadal or genetic sex. –**intersexual,** *adj.*

interspinal ligament [L *inter* + *spina* spine; *ligare* to bind], one of many thin, narrow membranous ligaments that connect adjoining spinous processes and extend from the root of each process to the apex.

interspinous /in'tərspī'nəs/ [L *inter* + *spina* spine], of or pertaining to the space between any spinous processes.

interstitial /in'tərstish'əl/ [L *inter* + *sistere* to stand], of or pertaining to the space between tissues, as interstitial fluid.

interstitial cell-stimulating hormone (ICSH), the luteinizing hormone that also stimulates the production of testosterone by the Leydig, or interstitial, cells of the testis.

interstitial cystitis, an inflammation of the bladder, believed to be associated with an autoimmune or allergic response. The bladder wall becomes inflamed, ulcerated, and scarred, causing frequent, painful urination. Hematuria often occurs.

interstitial emphysema, a form of emphysema in which air or gas escapes into the interstitial tissues of the lung after a penetrating injury or as the result of a rupture in an alveolar wall. Because the alveoli must be decompressed, there is danger that the pleura will be torn, resulting in a pneumothorax.

interstitial fibroid, a fibrous tumor that develops in the muscular wall of the uterus and tends to grow inward.

interstitial fluid, an extracellular fluid that fills the spaces between most of the cells of the body and provides a substantial portion of the liquid environment of the body. Formed by filtration through the blood capillaries, it is drained away as lymph.

interstitial growth, an increase in size by hyperplasia or hypertrophy within the interior of a part or structure that is already formed.

interstitial hypertrophic neuropathy. See **Dejerine-Sottas disease.**

interstitial implantation, (in embryology) the complete embedding of the blastocyst within the endometrium of the uterine wall.

interstitial inflammation, an inflammation in an area of connective tissues.

interstitial infusion. See **hypodermoclysis.**

interstitial keratitis, an uncommon inflammation within the layers of the cornea, the first symptom of which is a diffuse haziness. Blood vessels may grow into the area and cause permanent opacities. Its causes are syphilis, tuberculosis, leprosy, and vascular hypersensitivity.

interstitial lung disease, a respiratory disorder characterized by a dry, unproductive cough and dyspnea on exertion. X-ray films usually show fibrotic infiltrates in the lung tissue. The fibrosing or scarring of lung tissue is often the result of an immune reaction to an inhaled substance. Interstitial lung disease may also result from infections, uremic pneumonitis, cancers, congenital or inherited disorders, or circulatory impairment.

interstitial mastitis [L *interstitium,* space between; Gk *mastos* breast], an inflammation of the connective tissue between the ducts of the breast.

interstitial myositis. See **myositis.**

interstitial nephritis, inflammation of the interstitial tissue of the kidney, including the tubules. The condition may be acute or chronic. **Acute interstitial nephritis** is an immunologic, adverse reaction to certain drugs, often sulfonamide or methicillin. Acute renal failure, fever, rash, and proteinuria are characteristic of this condition. **Chronic interstitial nephritis** is a syndrome of interstitial inflammation and structural changes, sometimes associated with such conditions as ureteral obstruction, pyelonephritis, exposure of the kidney to a toxin, rejection of a transplant, and certain systemic diseases. Gradually, renal failure, nausea, vomiting, weight loss, fatigue, and anemia develop. Acidosis and hyperkalemia may follow.

interstitial plasma cell pneumonia. See **pneumocystosis.**

interstitial pneumonia, a diffuse, chronic inflammation of the lungs beyond the terminal bronchioles, characterized by fibrosis and collagen formation in the alveolar walls and by the presence of large mononuclear cells in the alveolar spaces. The symptoms of this condition are progressive dyspnea, clubbing of the fingers, cyanosis, and fever. The disease may result from a hypersensitive reaction to drugs. Interstitial pneumonia may also be an autoimmune reaction, since it often accompanies celiac disease, rheumatoid arthritis, Sjögren's syndrome, and systemic sclerosis.

interstitial pregnancy. See **ectopic pregnancy.**

interstitial therapy, radiotherapy in which needles or wires that contain radioactive material are implanted directly into tumor areas.

interstitial tissue, the connective and supporting tissue within and surrounding major functional elements of an organ.

interstitial tubal pregnancy, a kind of tubal pregnancy in which implantation occurs in the proximal, interstitial portion of one of the fallopian tubes.

intertransverse ligament /in'tərtransvurz'/ [L *inter* + *transversus* cross-direction], one of many fibrous bands connecting the transverse processes of vertebrae.

intertrigo /in'tərtrī'gō/ [L *inter* + *terere* to scour], an erythematous irritation of opposing skin surfaces caused by friction. Common sites are the axillae, the folds beneath large or pendulous breasts, and the inner aspects of the thighs. **–intertriginous,** *adj.*

intertrochanteric crest /in'tɔrtrō'-kanter'ik/ [L *inter* + *trochanter* runner; *crista* ridge], one of a pair of ridges along the thigh bones, curving obliquely from the greater to the lesser trochanter.

intertrochanteric fracture, a fracture characterized by a crack in the tissue of the proximal femur between the greater and the lesser trochanters.

intertrochanteric line, a line that runs across the anterior surface of the thigh bone from the greater to the lesser trochanter, winding around the medial surface, and ending in the linea aspera.

intertuberous diameter /in'tɔrtōo'bərəs/ [L *inter* + *tuber* swelling; Gk *dia* across, *metron* measure], the distance between the ischial tuberosities, a factor used in determining the dimensions of the pelvic outlet.

interval [L *intervallum* space between ramparts], a space between things or events, or a break or interruption in an otherwise continuous flow.

interval health history [L *intervallum* space between], a kind of health history that notes the general condition of a client during the period between visits and is not limited to facts relevant to a particular condition. The interval health history provides an ongoing account of a person's health.

intervention [L *inter* + *venire* to come], any act performed to prevent harm from occurring to a patient or to improve the mental, emotional, or physical function of a patient. A physiologic process may be monitored or enhanced; a pathologic process may be arrested or controlled. **Independent intervention** is any health care activity pertaining to certain aspects of professional practice that are encompassed by applicable licensure and law and require no supervision or direction from others. **Interdependent intervention** refers to any health care activity carried out by one health care professional in collaboration with another.

interventricular /in'tɔrventrik'yələr/ [L *inter* + *ventriculum* chamber], located between the ventricles, as the septum of the heart.

interventricular septum, the wall between the ventricles of the heart.

intervertebral /in'tɔrvur'təbrəl/ [L *inter* + *vertebra* back joint], of or pertaining to the space between any two vertebrae, such as the fibrocartilaginous disks.

intervertebral disk, one of the fibrous disks found between adjacent spinal vertebrae, except the axis and the atlas. The disks vary in size, shape, thickness, and number depending on the location in the back and on the particular vertebrae they separate.

intervertebral fibrocartilage. See **intervertebral disk.**

intervertebral foramen, any of the passages between adjacent vertebrae through which the spinal nerves and vessels pass.

intervertebral ganglion [L *inter* + *vertebra*; Gk *gagglion* knot], the ganglionic enlargement of a spinal nerve root between adjacent vertebrae.

interview, a communication with a patient initiated for a specific purpose and focused on a specific content area. A **problem-seeking interview** is an inquiry that focuses on gathering data to identify problems the patient needs to resolve. A **problem-solving interview** focuses on problems that have been identified by the patient or health care professional.

intervillous space /in'tɔrvil'əs/ [L *inter* + *villus* hair; *spatium*], one of many spaces between the chorionic villi of the endometrium of the gravid uterus, beneath the placenta. The intervillous spaces act as small reservoirs for oxygenated maternal blood.

intestinal /intes'tinəl/ [L *intestinum*], pertaining to the intestines.

intestinal absorption [L *intestinum* intestine; *absorbare* to swallow], the passage of the products of digestion from the lumen of the small intestine into the blood and lymphatic vessels in the wall of the gut. The surface area of the intestine is greatly increased by the presence of fingerlike villi, each of which contains capillaries and a lymphatic vessel, or lacteal.

intestinal amebiasis. See **amebic dysentery.**

intestinal angina, chronic vascular insufficiency of the mesentery caused by atherosclerosis and resulting ischemia of the smooth muscle of the small bowel. Abdominal pain or cramping after eating, constipation, melena, malabsorption, and weight loss are characteristic of the condition.

intestinal apoplexy, the sudden occlusion of one of the three principal arteries to the intestine by an embolism or a thrombus. This condition leads rapidly to necrosis of intestinal tissue and is often fatal.

intestinal atresia [L *intestinum*; Gk *a, tresis* boring], a pathologic obstruction of the continuous lumen of the intestinal tract due to a defect in development in utero.

intestinal bypass surgery [L *intestinum*; AS *bi*; Fr *passer*; Gk *cheirourgos*], a surgical procedure to shorten the digestive tract so that less intestinal surface will be available to absorb nutrients from the digested food passing through, or to bypass a blocked or diseased portion of the intestine. The technique usually involves anastomosing the jejunum to the ileum.

intestinal colic [L intestinum; Gk kolikos colonic pain], spasmodic pain in intestinal disorders.

intestinal dyspepsia an abnormal condition characterized by impaired digestion associated with a problem that originated in the intestines.

intestinal fistula, an abnormal passage from the intestine to an external abdominal opening or stoma, usually created surgically for the exit of feces after removal of a malignant or severely ulcerated segment of the bowel.

intestinal flora [L intestinum; flos flowers], the natural bacterial content of the inside of the digestive tract.

intestinal flu, a viral gastroenteritis, usually caused by infection by an enterovirus. It is characterized by abdominal cramps, diarrhea, nausea, and vomiting.

intestinal fluke [L intestinum; AS floc], any internal parasite of the genera Fasciolopsis, Heterophyes, and Metagonimus, in North America and of other genera in the Orient and in tropical countries. They enter the body through the mouth as encysted larvae in aquatic vegetation or freshwater fish. Symptoms of intestinal fluke infestation usually include abdominal pain and obstruction and diarrhea.

intestinal gases [L intestinum], gas in the digestive tract arising from three sources—swallowed air, gas produced by digestive processes, and blood gases diffused into the intestinal lumen. Gases produced in the intestine and diffused from blood are mainly hydrogen, (H_2), most of which is a bacterial fermentation product of ingested carbohydrates, carbon dioxide, (CO_2), and methane, (CH_4).

intestinal glands. See **Lieberkühn's glands.**

intestinal juices, the secretions of glands lining the intestine.

intestinal lymphangiectasia. See **hypoproteinemia.**

intestinal obstruction, any obstruction that results in failure of the contents of the intestine to pass through the lumen of the bowel. The most common cause is a mechanical blockage resulting from adhesions, impacted feces, tumor of the bowel, hernia, intussusception, volvulus, or the strictures of inflammatory bowel disease. Obstruction of the small bowel may cause severe pain, vomiting of fecal matter, dehydration, and eventually a drop in blood pressure. Obstruction of the colon causes less severe pain, marked abdominal distention, and constipation.

intestinal perforation [L intestinum; per-

forare to pierce], the escape of digestive tract contents into the peritoneal cavity due to trauma or a disease condition, such as a ruptured appendix or perforated ulcer. The condition inevitably leads to peritonitis.

intestinal strangulation, the arrest of blood flow to the bowel, resulting in edema, cyanosis, and gangrene of the affected loop of bowel. This condition is usually caused by a hernia, intussusception, or volvulus. Early signs of intestinal strangulation resemble those of intestinal obstruction.

intestinal tonsil, one of a group of lymphatic nodules forming a single layer in the mucous membrane of the ileum opposite the mesenteric attachment.

intestinal tract [L intestinum; tractus], the segments of small and large intestines between the pyloric valve and the rectum.

intestinal tubes [L intestinum; tubus], the alimentary canal or digestive tract.

intestine /intes'tin/ [L intestinum], the portion of the alimentary canal extending from the pyloric opening of the stomach to the anus. It includes the small and large intestines. **–intestinal,** adj.

intima /in'timə/, pl. intimae [L intimus innermost], the innermost layer of a structure, such as the lining membrane of an artery, vein, lymphatic, or organ. **–intimal,** adj.

intimal sclerosis [L intimus inmost; Gk sklerosis hardening], a hardening of the intimal layer of a blood vessel.

intoe. See **metatarsus varus.**

intolerance [L in not, tolerare to bear], a condition characterized by an inability to absorb or metabolize a nutrient or medication. Exposure to the substance may cause an adverse reaction.

intoxicant /intok'sikənt/ [L in within; Gk toxikon poison], any agent that can cause a state of intoxication or poisoning.

intoxication [L in + Gk toxikon poison] **1.** the state of being poisoned by a drug or other toxic substance. **2.** the state of being inebriated because of an excessive consumption of alcohol. **3.** a state of mental or emotional hyperexcitability, usually euphoric.

intraabdominal pressure /in'trə·abdom'inəl/ [L intra within, abdomen belly], the degree of pressure within the abdominal cavity.

intraalveolar pocket. See **periodontal pocket.**

intraaortic balloon pump /in'trə·ā·ôr'tik/ [L intra + aeirein to rise], a counterpulsation device that provides temporary cardiac assist in the management of refractory left ventricular failure, as may follow

myocardial infarction or occur in prein-
farction angina.

intraarterial /in'trə·ärtir'ē·əl/, pertaining
to a structure or action inside an artery.

intraarticular /in'trə·ärtik'yələr/ [L *intra*
+ *articulus* joint], within a joint.

intraarticular fracture, a fracture involving the articular surfaces of a joint.

intraarticular injection, the injection of
a medication into a joint space, usually to
reduce inflammation, such as in bursitis or
fibromyositis.

intraarticular ligament, a ligament that
forms part of the joints between 16 of the
24 ribs, dividing the joints into two cavities, each containing a synovial membrane.

intraatrial /in'trə·ā'trē·əl/ [L *intra* +
atrium entrance hall], within an atrium
in the heart.

intraatrial block, delayed or abnormal
conduction within the atria, identified on
an electrocardiogram by a prolonged and
often notched P wave.

intracanalicular fibroma /in'trəkan'-
əlik'yōōlär/ [L *intra* + *canaliculus* small
channel], a tumor containing glandular
epithelium and fibrous tissue, occurring in
the breast.

intracanicular papilloma /in'trəkənik'-
yōōlər/, a benign warty growth in certain glands, especially the breast.

intracapsular fracture /in'trəkap'sōōlər/
[L *intra* + *capsula* little box], a fracture
within the capsule of a joint.

intracardiac [L *intra* + Gk *kardia* heart],
pertaining to the interior of the heart
chambers.

intracardiac catheter. See **cardiac catheter.**

intracardiac lead /lēd/ [L *intra* + Gk *kardia* heart; AS *laedan* lead], 1. an electrocardiographic conductor in which the
exploring electrode is placed within one of
the cardiac chambers, usually by means of
cardiac catheterization. 2. *informal;* a
tracing produced by such a lead on an
electrocardiograph.

intracartilaginous ossification. See **ossification.**

intracatheter /in'trəkath"atər/ [L *intra* +
Gk *katheter* something lowered], a thin,
flexible plastic catheter introduced and
threaded into a blood vessel to infuse
blood, fluid, or medication.

intracavitary /in'trəkav'itər'ē/ [L *intra* +
cavum cave], pertaining to the space
within a body cavity.

intracavitary therapy, a kind of radiotherapy in which one or more radioactive
sources are placed, usually with the help
of an applicator or holding device, within

a body cavity to irradiate the walls of the
cavity or adjacent tissues.

intracellular [L *intra* + *cella* storeroom],
pertaining to the interior of a cell.

intracellular fluid [L *intra* + *cella; fluere*
to flow], a fluid within cell membranes
throughout most of the body, containing
dissolved solutes that are essential to electrolytic balance and to healthy metabolism.

intracerebral /in'trəser'əbrəl/ [L *intra* +
cerebrum brain], within the tissue of the
brain, inside the bony skull.

intracistronic /in'trəsistron'ik/ [L *intra* +
cis this side, *trans* across], within a cistron.

intracoronal retainer /in'trəkôr'ənəl/ [L
intra + *corona* crown] 1. a retainer in
which the prepared tooth cavity and its
cast restoration lie largely within the body
of the coronal portion of a tooth and within
the contour of the tooth crown, such as an
inlay. 2. a direct retainer used in the construction of removable partial dentures. It
consists of a female portion within the coronal segment of the crown of an abutment
and a fitted male portion attached to the
denture proper.

intracranial /in'trəkrā'nē·əl/ [L *intra* + Gk
kranion skull], within the cranium.

intracranial aneurysm, any aneurysm of
any of the cerebral arteries. Characteristics
of the condition include sudden severe
headache, stiff neck, nausea, vomiting,
and, sometimes, loss of consciousness.
Kinds of intracranial aneurysms include
berry aneurysm, fusiform aneurysm,
and **mycotic aneurysm.**

intracranial   electroencephalography.
See **electroencephalography.**

intracranial hemorrhage [L *intra* + Gk
kranion; haima blood], a hemorrhage
within the cranium.

intracranial pressure, pressure that occurs within the cranium.

intractable /intrak'təbəl/ [L *in* not, *tracta-
bilis* manageable], having no relief, as a
symptom or a disease that remains unrelieved by the therapeutic measures employed.

intractable pain [L *intractabilis* hard to
manage; *poena* penalty], pain that is unrelieved by ordinary medical and surgical
measures. The pain is often chronic, persistent, and psychogenic in nature.

intracutaneous /in'trəkyōōtā'nē·əs/ [L *intra* + *cutis* skin], within the layers of the
skin.

intracystic papilloma /in'trəsis'tik/ [L *intra* + Gk *kystis* bag], a benign epithelial
tumor formed with a cystic adenoma.

intradermal /in'trədur'məl/ [L *intra* + Gk

derma skin], within the tissue of the skin.

intradermal injection, the introduction of a hypodermic needle into the dermis for the purpose of instilling a substance, such as a serum or vaccine.

intradermal test, a procedure used to identify suspected allergens by subcutaneously injecting the patient with small amounts of extracts of the suspected allergens.

intraductal carcinoma [L intra + ductus duct], a frequently large neoplasm occurring most often in the breast.

intradural lipoma [L intra + dura hard], a fatty tumor in or beneath the dura mater of the spine or sacrum that tends to infiltrate the dorsal column and roots of spinal nerves, causing pain and dysfunction.

intraepidermal carcinoma .in'trə·ep'·idur'məl/ [L intra + Gk epi above, derma skin], a neoplasm of squamous epidermal cells that does not proliferate into the basal area and often occurs at many sites simultaneously.

intraepidermal vesicle, a fluid-filled blisterlike cavity within the epidermis.

intraepithelial carcinoma. See carcinoma in situ.

intrafusal muscle /in'trəfyoō'zəl/, the striated muscle tissue within a muscle spindle.

intramembranous ossification. See ossification.

intramenstrual pain /in'trəmen'strr͞oo·əl/ [L intra + menstrualis monthly; poena penalty], pelvic or lower abdominal pain that occurs about midway between menses and may be associated with ovulation.

intramural /in'trəmy͞oo'rəl/ [L intra + murus wall], pertaining to events or structures within the walls of an organ or body part or cavity.

intramuscular [L intra + musculus muscle], pertaining to the interior of muscle tissue.

intramuscular injection, the introduction of a hypodermic needle into a muscle to administer a medication.

intraocular /in'trə·ok'yələr/ [L intra + oculus eye], pertaining to structures or substances within the eyeball.

intraocular pressure, the internal pressure of the eye, regulated by resistance to the flow of aqueous humor through the fine sieve of the trabecular meshwork. Contraction or relaxation of the longitudinal muscles of the ciliary body affects the size of the apertures in the meshwork.

intraoperative [L intra + operari to work], pertaining to the period of time during a surgical procedure.

intraoperative hyperthermia [L intro + operari to work], hyperthermia delivered to internal sites that have been exposed by a surgical procedure.

intraoperative ultrasound, a diagnostic technique that uses a portable ultrasound device to scan the spinal cord during spinal surgery. Intraoperative ultrasound can distinguish between syrinxes, or fluid-filled cysts, and neoplastic growths in nervous system tissue.

intraoral orthodontic appliance /in'trə·ôr'əl/ [L intra + oralis mouth], an orthodontic device placed inside the mouth to correct or alleviate malocclusion.

intraosseous infusion /in'trə·os'ē·əs/, the injection of blood, medications, or fluids into bone marrow rather than into a vein. The technique may be performed in emergency treatment of a child when IV infusion is not feasible.

intraosseous [L intra + os bone], pertaining to the interior of bone.

intraparietal sulcus /in'trəperi'ətəl/ [L intra + paries wall; sulcus groove], an irregular groove on the convex surface of the parietal lobe that marks the division of the inferior and superior parietal lobules.

intrapartal care /in'trəpär'təl/ [L intra + partus birth], care of a pregnant woman from the onset of labor to the completion of the third stage of labor with the expulsion of the placenta.

intrapartal period, the period spanning labor and birth.

intrapartum, /in'trəpär'təm/ pertaining to the period of labor and delivery.

intraperiosteal fracture /in'trəper'ē·os'tē·əl/ [L intra + Gk peri around, osteon bone], a fracture that does not rupture the periosteum.

intrapsychic conflict [L intra + Gk psyche mind], an emotional conflict within oneself.

intrapulmonary /in'trəpul'məner'ē/ [L intra + pulma lung], pertaining to the interior of the lungs.

intrapulmonary shunt [L intra + pulmoneus relating to the lung], (in respiratory therapy) a condition of perfusion without ventilation, expressed as a ratio of QS/QT, with QS reflecting the difference between end capillary oxygen content and mixed venous oxygen content, and QT representing cardiac output. The condition may occur in atelectasis, pneumonia, pulmonary edema, and adult respiratory distress syndrome (ARDS).

intrarenal hemodynamics /in'trərē'nəl [L intra + ren kidney], the pattern of blood flow or distribution in the various parts of the kidney. Normally the renal cortex and outer medulla receive the major portion of renal blood flow.

intraspinal hypodermic [L *intra* + *spina* spine; *hypo* under, *derma* skin], pertaining to the injection of a substance into the spinal canal.

intrathecal /in'trəthē'kəl/ [L *intra* + *theca* sheath], of or pertaining to a structure, process, or substance within a sheath, such as the cerebrospinal fluid within the theca of the spinal canal.

intrathecal injection, the introduction of a hypodermic needle into the subarachnoid space for the purpose of instilling a material for diffusion throughout the spinal fluid.

intrathoracic goiter /in'trəthôras'ik/ [L *intra* + Gk *thorax* chest; L *guttur* throat], an enlargement of the thyroid gland that protrudes into the thoracic cavity.

intrauterine /in'trəyōō'tərin/ [L *intra* + *uterus* womb], pertaining to the inside of the uterus.

intrauterine device (IUD) [L *intra* + *uterus* womb; Fr *devise*], a contraceptive device consisting of a bent strip of radiopaque plastic with a fine monofilament tail that is inserted and left in the uterine cavity for the purpose of altering the physiology of the uterus and fallopian tubes to prevent pregnancy.

intrauterine fracture, a fracture that occurs during fetal life.

intrauterine growth curve, a line on a standardized graph representing the mean weight for gestational age through pregnancy to term.

intrauterine growth retardation, an abnormal process in which the development and maturation of the fetus is impeded or delayed by genetic factors, maternal disease, or fetal malnutrition caused by placental insufficiency.

intravascular /in'trəvas'kyələr/ [L *intra* + *vasculum* little vessel], pertaining to the inside of a blood vessel.

intravascular coagulation test [L *intra* + *vasculum* little vessel], a test for detecting internal coagulation of blood.

intravenous (IV) /in'trəvē'nəs/ [L *intra* + *vena* vein], of or pertaining to the inside of a vein, as of a thrombus or an injection, infusion, or catheter.

intravenous alimentation. See **total parenteral nutrition.**

intravenous bolus, a relatively large dose of medication administered IV in a short period of time, usually within 1 to 30 minutes. The IV bolus is commonly used when administration of a medication is needed quickly, such as in an emergency, when drugs are administered that cannot be diluted, such as many cancer chemo-

therapeutic drugs, and when the therapeutic purpose is to achieve a peak drug level in the bloodstream of the patient.

intravenous catheter [L *intra* + *vena* vein; Gk *katheter* a thing lowered], a catheter that is inserted into a vein to supply medications or nutrients directly into the bloodstream, or for diagnostic purposes such as studying blood pressure.

intravenous cholangiography, (in diagnostic radiology) a procedure for outlining the major bile ducts. A radiopaque contrast material is injected intravenously.

intravenous controller, any one of several devices that automatically delivers IV fluid at a selectable flow rate, usually between 1 and 69 drops per minute. The controller is commonly equipped with a rate selector, drop sensor, drop indicator, and drop alarm. When the infusion does not flow at the prescribed rate, the drop alarm emits a visual and an audible signal.

intravenous DSA (IV-DSA), a form of digital subtraction angiography in which radiopaque dye is injected into a vein, rather than an artery, in order to visualize arteries in the body.

intravenous fat emulsion, a preparation of 10% fat administered intravenously to help maintain the weight of an adult patient or the weight and growth of a younger patient. Such fat emulsions are prepared from refined soybean oil and egg-yolk phospholipids and may contain such major fatty acids as linoleic, oleic, palmitic, and linolenic acids. The IV fat emulsion is isotonic and may be administered into a peripheral vein, but it is not mixed with other solutions employed in parenteral alimentation. Intravenous fat emulsions are often administered when hyperalimentation is not sufficient to maintain adequate treatment of a patient or when the patient needs calories but cannot tolerate the high percentage of dextrose contained in hyperalimentation solutions.

intravenous feeding, the administration of nutrients through a vein or veins.

intravenous infusion, 1. a solution administered intravenously through an infusion set that includes a plastic or glass vacuum bottle or bag containing the solution and tubing connecting the bottle to a catheter or a needle in the patient's vein. 2. the process of administering a solution intravenously.

intravenous infusion filter, any one of numerous devices used in helping to ensure the purity of an IV solution. Intravenous filters strain the IV solution to remove such contaminants as dissolved impurities (detergents, proteins, and polysaccharides), extraneous salts, microorganisms, particles, precipitates, and undissolved drug powders. Any such contaminants may complicate the IV therapy and the recovery of the patient. Some filters are built into the primary IV tubing; others must be attached.

intravenous infusion technique, the calculations for determining the delivery rate of IV fluid for the individual patient and the necessary spiking of the container and priming of the tubing before venipuncture and administration of the fluid.

intravenous injection, a hypodermic injection into a vein for the purpose of instilling a single dose of medication; injecting a contrast medium; or beginning an IV infusion of blood, medication, or a fluid solution, such as saline or dextrose in water.

intravenous medication [L *intra + vena* vein; *medicare* medicine], the delivery of a medication directly into the bloodstream via a vein.

intravenous peristaltic pump, any one of several devices for administering IV fluids by exerting pressure on the IV tubing rather than on the fluid itself. Most peristaltic pumps operate with normal IV tubing and deliver fluid at a selectable drop-per-minute rate. This device typically can infuse between 1 and 99 drops of IV fluid per minute and is equipped with a drop sensor, rate selector, power switch indicator lamp, and drop indicator and alarm. The drop indicator flashes whenever a drop of IV fluid passes the drop sensor.

intravenous piston pump, any one of several devices that accurately control the infusion of IV fluids by piston action. Most IV piston pumps can be operated by battery as well as by electric current, and require special tubing. Some models are portable. Intravenous piston pumps are commonly equipped with controls that allow selectable flow rates and indicators that display flow rates, dose limits, and cumulative fluid volumes.

intravenous pump, a pump designed to regulate the rate of flow of a fluid given intravenously through an intracatheter or a scalp vein needle.

intravenous push. See **intravenous bolus.**

intravenous pyelography (IVP), a technique in radiology for examining the structures and evaluating the function of the urinary system. A contrast medium is injected intravenously, and serial x-ray films are taken as the medium is cleared from the blood by glomerular filtration. The renal calyces, renal pelvis, ureters, and urinary bladder are all visible on the x-ray films.

intravenous syringe pump, any one of several devices that automatically compress a syringe plunger at a controlled rate. Such devices are used with disposable syringes that can deliver blood, medications, or nutrients by IV, arterial, or subcutaneous routes. They are especially useful in treating ambulatory patients.

intravenous team, a group of registered nurses and licensed practical nurses with special training who administer IV therapy under the direction of a physician.

intravenous therapy, the administration of fluids or drugs, or both, into the general circulation through a venipuncture.

intravenous urography. See **intravenous pyelography.**

intraventricular /in′trəventrik′yələr/ [L *intra + ventriculum* belly], of or pertaining to the space within a ventricle.

intraventricular block, the slowed conduction or stoppage of the cardiac excitatory impulse, occurring within the ventricles. The block can occur as a right bundle branch block, a left bundle branch block, or left anterior or posterior fascicular block. The block is identified on an electrocardiogram. Kinds of intraventricular block include **bundle branch block** and **infranodal block.**

intraventricular conduction defect (ICD), a delay in conduction of a ventricular contraction impulse that may occur beyond the Purkinje myocardial gates. It is seen in patients with acute myocardial infarction and is caused by faulty cell-to-cell conduction of the impulse.

intraventricular hydrocephalus. See **hydrocephalus.**

intraventricular pressure [L *intra + ventriculum*], the pressure of the blood within the heart's ventricles; it varies with the phase of the cardiac cycle.

intrinsic /intrin′sik/ [L *intrinsecus* inside], **1.** denoting a natural or inherent part or quality. **2.** originating from or situated within an organ or tissue.

intrinsic asthma, a nonseasonal, nonallergic form of asthma, usually first occurring later in life than allergic asthma, that tends to be chronic and persistent rather than episodic. The precipitating factors include inhalation of irritating pollutants in the atmosphere, such as dust particles, smoke, aerosols, strong cooking odors, paint fumes, and other volatile substances.

intrinsic factor, a substance secreted by the gastric mucosa that is essential for the intestinal absorption of cyanocobalamin. A deficiency of intrinsic factor results in pernicious anemia.

intrinsic muscles, muscles that are entirely within the body part or segment moved by them, as the tongue muscles.

introitus /intrō′itəs/ [L *intro* inside, *ire* to go], an entrance or orifice to a cavity or a hollow tubular structure of the body, such as the vaginal introitus.

introjection /in′trōjek′shən/ [L *intro* + *jacere* to throw], an unconscious mechanism in which an individual incorporates into his own ego structure the qualities of another person.

intromission /in′trōmish′ən/, the insertion of one object into another, such as the introduction of the penis into the vagina.

intron /in′tron/ [L *intra* within, *regionis* region], (in molecular genetics) a sequence of base pairs in DNA that interrupts the continuity of genetic information.

introspection [L *introspicere* to look into], **1.** the act of examining one's own thoughts and emotions by concentrating on the inner self. **2.** a tendency to look inward and view the inner self. –**introspective,** *adj.*

introsusception /in′trōsusep′shən/ [L *intro* + *suscipere* to receive], the telescoping or invagination of one segment of the digestive tract into another segment, usually a lower segment. The result can be obstruction and strangulation of the bowel.

introversion /in′trōvur′zhən/ [L *intro* + *vertere* to turn], **1.** the tendency to direct one's interests, thoughts, and energies inward or toward things concerned only with the self. **2.** the state of being totally or primarily concerned with one's own intrapsychic experience. Also spelled **intraversion.**

introvert [L *intro* + *vertere* to turn], **1.** a person whose interests are directed inward and who is shy, withdrawn, emotionally reserved, and self-absorbed. **2.** to turn inward or to direct one's interests and thoughts toward oneself.

introverted personality [L *intro* + *vertere* to turn; *personalis*], a personality that is preoccupied with inner thoughts and fantasies rather than with the outer world of people and things.

intubate /in′tyo̅o̅bāt/ [L *in* within, *tubus* tube], to catheterize or insert a tube into an organ or body part.

intubation [L *in* + *tubus* + *atio* process], passage of a tube into a body aperture, specifically the insertion of a breathing tube through the mouth or nose or into the trachea to ensure a patent airway for the delivery of an anesthetic gas or oxygen. **Blind intubation** is the insertion of a breathing tube without the use of a laryngoscope. Kinds of intubation are **endotra-**

cheal intubation and **nasogastric intubation.**

intussusception /in′təsəsep′shən/ [L *intus* within, *suscipere* to receive], prolapse of one segment of bowel into the lumen of another segment. This kind of intestinal obstruction may involve segments of the small intestine, the colon, or the terminal ileum and cecum.

inulin /in′yo̅o̅lin/, a fructose-derived substance used as a diagnostic aid in tests of kidney function, specifically glomerular filtration. It is not metabolized or absorbed by the body but is readily filtered through the kidney.

inulin clearance, a test of the rate of filtration of the starch inulin in the glomerulus of the kidney. Inulin is given by mouth, and the glomerular filtration rate can be estimated from the length of time needed for the inulin to appear in the urine.

inunction /inungk′shən/ [L *in* within, *ungere* to smear], **1.** the rubbing of a drug mixed with an oil or fatty substance into the skin, with absorption of the active ingredient. **2.** any compound so applied.

inundation fever. See **scrub typhus.**

in utero /yo̅o̅′tərō/, inside the uterus.

invagination /invaj′ənā′shən/ [L *in* within, *vagina* sheath], **1.** a condition in which one part of a structure telescopes into another part, as the intestine during peristalsis. If the invagination is extensive or involves a tumor or polyps, it may cause an intestinal obstruction. **2.** surgery for repair of a hernia by replacing the contents of the hernial sac in the abdominal cavity. –**invaginate,** *v.*

invariable behavior [L *in* not, *variare* to vary], behavior that results from physiologic response to a stimulus and is not modified by individual experience, such as a reflex.

invasion [L *in* within, *vadere* to go], the process by which malignant cells move into deeper tissue and through the basement membrane and gain access to blood vessels and lymphatic channels.

invasion of privacy, (in law) the violation of another person's right to be left alone and free from unwarranted publicity and intrusion.

invasive [L *in* within, *vadere* to go], characterized by a tendency to spread, infiltrate, and intrude.

invasive carcinoma, a malignant neoplasm composed of epithelial cells that infiltrate and destroy surrounding tissues.

invasive mole. See **chorioadenoma destruens.**

invasive procedure [L *in* + *vadere*; *procedere* to proceed], a diagnostic or therapeutic technique that requires entering a body cavity or interrupting normal body functions. Examples include the Pap test and colonoscopy.

invasive thermometry, measurement of tissue temperature using probes placed directly in the tissue.

inverse anaphylaxis /invurs', in'vurs/, an exaggerated reaction of hypersensitivity induced by an antibody rather than by an antigen.

inverse I:E ratio, an inspiratory/expiratory ratio in which the frequency of inhalations is greater than the rate of exhalations. Such situations occur when there is a need to improve oxygenation.

inverse relationship. See **negative relationship.**

inverse square law, a law stating that the amount of radiation emitted is inversely proportional to the square of the distance between the source and the irradiated surface, such as a person 2 feet from a patient being treated with radium is exposed to four times more radiation than he or she would be exposed to at 4 feet.

inversion /invur'zhən/ [L *invertere* to turn over], **1.** an abnormal condition in which an organ is turned inside out, such as a uterine inversion. **2.** a chromosomal defect in which two or more segments of a chromosome break off and become separated. They rejoin the chromosome in the wrong order.

invert /in'vurt/ [L *invertere* to turn over], **1.** a homosexual. **2.** to turn something upside down or inside out.

invert sugar [L *invertere*; Gk *sakcharon*], a mixture of glucose and fructose produced by the hydrolysis of sucrose. The process results in an inversion of optical rotation from dextrorotation of sucrose to levorotation of the mixture.

investigational device exemption (IDE) [L *investigare* to search for], an agreement through which the federal government permits the testing of new medical devices.

investigational new drug (IND), a drug not yet approved for marketing by the Food and Drug Administration and available only for use in experiments to determine its safety and effectiveness.

invisible differentiation [L *in* not, *visibilis* visible; *differentia* difference], (in embryology) a fixed determination for specialization and diversification that exists in embryonic cells but is not yet visibly apparent.

in vitro /in vē'trō/ [L *in* within; *vitreus* glassware], (of a biologic reaction) occurring in laboratory apparatus.

in vitro fertilization (IVF), a method of fertilizing human ova outside the body by collecting the mature ova and placing them in a dish with a sample of spermatozoa. After the ova are allowed to incubate over a period of 48 to 72 hours, the fertilized ova are injected into the uterus through the cervix. The procedure takes from 2 to 3 days.

in vivo /in vē'vō/ [L *in* within, *vivo* alive], (of a biological reaction) occurring in a living organism.

in vivo tracer study, (in nuclear medicine) a diagnostic procedure in which a series of radiograms of an administered radioactive tracer as it passes through a compartment in the patient's body demonstrates normal or abnormal structures or processes.

involucrum /in'vəloo'krəm/, *pl.* **involucra** [L *involvere* to wrap up], a sheath or coating, such as that encasing a sequestrum of necrotic bone.

involuntary [L *in* not, *voluntas* will], occurring without conscious control or direction.

involuntary muscle. See **smooth muscle.**

involuntary nervous system. See **visceral nervous system.**

involuntary patient, a patient admitted to a psychiatric facility through the commitment process.

involution /in'vəloo'shən/ [L *involvere* to wrap up], **1.** a normal process characterized by a decrease in the size of an organ and a decrease in the size of its cells, such as postpartum involution of the uterus. **2.** (in embryology) a developmental process in which a group of cells grows over the rim at the border of the organ or part and, rolling inward, rejoins the organ or part to form a tube.

involutional melancholia [L, *involvere* + Gk, *melas,* black, *chole* bile] a state of depression occurring during the climacteric.

inward aggression [AS *inweard*], destructive behavior that is directed against oneself.

iodide /ī'ədīd/ [Gk *ioeides* violetlike], any salt of hydroiodic acid. Sodium and potassium iodide are the salts most commonly used in medicine.

iodinated ^{125}**I serum albumin** /ī'ədinā'- tid/, a sterile, buffered isotonic solution containing radioiodinated normal human serum adjusted to provide not more than 1 mCi of radioactivity per milliliter in diagnostic tests of blood volume and cardiac output.

iodine (I) /ī'ədīn/ [Gk *ioeides* violet], a nonmetallic element of the halogen group. Its atomic number is 53; its atomic weight is 126.90. An essential micronutrient or trace element, almost 80% of the iodine present in the body is in the thyroid gland. Iodine deficiency can result in goiter or cretinism. Radioisotopes of iodine are used in radioisotope scanning procedures and in palliative treatment of cancer of the thyroid.

iodine poisoning [Gk *ioeides;* L *potio* drink], toxic effects of ingesting iodine, a potent antiseptic with a low tissue toxicity. Symptoms include burning pain in the mouth and esophagus, abdominal pain, vomiting, diarrhea, shock, nephritis, laryngeal edema, and circulatory collapse. The mucous membranes are stained brown by the iodine.

iodism /ī'ədiz'əm/ [Gk *ioeides* + *ismos* process], a condition produced by excessive amounts of iodine in the body. It is characterized by increased lacrimation and salivation, rhinitis, weakness, and a typical skin eruption.

iodize /ī'ədīz/ [Gk *ioeides* + *izein* to cause], to treat or impregnate with iodine or an iodide. Table salt is iodized to prevent the occurrence of goiter in areas with insufficient iodine in the drinking water or food.

iodized salt [Gk *ioeides;* AS *sealt*], table salt to which potassium or sodium iodide has been added as a preventive measure to protect against goiter, particularly in regions where there is a low iodine content in the soil and drinking water. The iodides are added in a ratio of approximately 100 ppm.

iodochlorhydroxyquin /ī·ō'dōklôrhīdrok'-səkwin/, an antiamebic and topical antiinfective prescribed in the treatment of eczema, athlete's foot, and other fungal infections.

iododerma /ī·ō'dōdur'mə/ [Gk *ioeides* + *derma* skin], a skin rash caused by a hypersensitivity to ingested iodides. The lesions may be acneiform, bullous, or fungating.

iodoform /ī·ō'dəfôrm/ [Gk *ioeides* + (chloroform)], a topical antiinfective used as an antiseptic.

iodophor /ī·ōdəfôr/ [Gk *ioeides* + *phoros* bearer], an antiseptic or disinfectant that combines iodine with another agent, such as a detergent.

iodopsin /ī'ədop'sin/ [Gk *ioeides* + *optikos* vision], a photosensitive chemical in the cones of the retina that reacts in association with other chemicals and plays a part in color vision. Iodopsin is more stable when exposed to bright light than rhodopsin, which is found in the rods of the retina.

iodoquinol /ī'ōdō'kwinol/, an amebicide

prescribed in the treatment of intestinal amebiasis.

ion /ī'ən, ī'on/ [Gk *ienai* to go], an atom or group of atoms that has acquired an electric charge through the gain or loss of an electron or electrons.

ion exchange chromatography, the process of separating and analyzing different substances according to their affinities for chemically stable but very reactive synthetic exchangers, which are composed largely of polystyrene and cellulose. Ion exchange chromatography is often used to separate components of nucleic acids and proteins elaborated by various structures throughout the body.

ionic bonding [Gk *ienai* + ME *band* to bind], a force that holds atoms together by the transfer of a single valance electron, such as from a cation to an anion. Ionic compounds do not form true molecules and in aqueous solution break down into their constituent ions.

ionic dissociation, a phenomenon whereby ions in ionic compounds in an aqueous solution are freed from their mutual bonds and distribute themselves uniformly throughout the solvent.

ionic strength, the sum of the concentrations of all ions in a solution, weighted by the squares of their charges.

ionization /ī'ənīzā'shən/ [Gk *ienai* + *izein* to cause], the process in which a neutral atom or molecule gains or loses electrons and thus acquires a negative or positive electric charge. Ionization can also cause cell death or mutation.

ionization chamber, a small cavity filled with air that has the capability of collecting the ionic charge liberated during irradiation.

ionization constant (K), after establishment of ionic equilibrium, the product of the molar concentration of the ions divided by the molar concentration of the nonionized molecules.

ionize /ī'ənīz/ [Gk *ienai* + *izein* to cause], to separate or change into ions.

ionized calcium, the ionized, unbound, noncomplexed fraction of serum calcium that is biologically active.

ionizing energy, the average energy lost by ionizing radiation in producing an ion pair in a gas.

ionizing radiation, high-energy electromagnetic waves (such as x-rays and gamma rays) and particulate rays (such as alpha particles, beta rays, electrons, neutrons, positrons, protons, and heavy nuclei) that dissociate substances in their paths into ions. High energy x-rays penetrate deeply, most beta particles penetrate only a few millimeters, and alpha particles penetrate only a fraction of a millimeter, but they all produce intense ionization along their tracks.

ionizing radiation injury [Gk *ion* going; L *radiare* to shine; *injuria*], damage or ill effects suffered by exposure to ionizing radiation, including cellular harm resulting from radiation for diagnostic or therapeutic application. The risk of cell death or injury from radiation depends upon the type of tissue cells, the stage of cell division at the time of exposure, the intensity and time span of exposure, and the type of radiation administered.

ion-selective electrode, a potentiometric electrode that develops a potential in the presence of one ion (or class of ions) but not in the presence of a similar concentration of other ions.

iontophoresis /ī·on′tōfôrē′sis/ [Gk *ion* going; *pherein* to carry], the introduction of ions of soluble salts into the tissues by direct current.

iontophoretic pilocarpine test /ī·on′tōfôret′ik/ [Gk *ienai* + *pherein* to carry], a sweat test used in the diagnosis of cystic fibrosis. Pilocarpine iontophoresis is employed to stimulate production of sweat, which is analyzed for concentrations of sodium and chloride electrolytes.

Iowa trumpet, a kind of needle guide used in performing a pudendal block. It consists of a long thin cylinder through which a needle may be passed. A ring is attached to the proximal end of the guide, allowing the operator to hold it securely.

IPA, abbreviation for **independent practice association.**

ipecac /ip′əkak/, an emetic prescribed to cause emesis in certain types of poisoning and drug overdose.

IPOF, abbreviation for **immediate postoperative fit prosthesis.**

IPPB (intermittent positive pressure breathing), a form of assisted or controlled respiration produced by a ventilatory apparatus in which compressed gas is delivered under positive pressure into the person's airways until a preset pressure is reached. Passive exhalation is allowed through a valve.

IPPB unit, a pressure-cycled ventilator for providing a flow of air into the lungs at a predetermined pressure. As the pressure is attained, the flow is stopped, pressure is released, and the patient exhales.

IPPV, abbreviation for **intermittent positive pressure ventilation.**

ipsilateral [L *ipse* same, *latus* side], pertaining to the same side of the body.

IPSP, abbreviation for *inhibitory postsynaptic potential.*

IQ, abbreviation for **intelligence quotient.**

Ir, symbol for the chemical element **iridium.**

IRB, abbreviation for **institutional review board.**

Ir g, abbreviation for *immune response function gene.*

iridectomy /ī′ridek′təmē/ [Gk *iris* + *ektome* excision], surgical removal of part of the iris of the eye, performed most often to restore drainage of the aqueous humor in glaucoma or to remove a foreign body or a malignant tumor.

iridescence /ir′ides′əns/ [L *iridescere* to shine like a rainbow], the property of light interference or ability to break up light waves into colors of the spectrum.

iridium (Ir) /irid′ē·əm/ [Gk *iris* rainbow], a silvery-bluish metallic element. Its atomic number is 77; its atomic weight is 192.2.

iridology /ī′ridol′əjē/ [Gk *iris* rainbow; *logos* science], a science that specializes in relations between disease and the shape, color, and other individual characteristics of the iris.

iridoplegia /ī′ridōplē′jə/ [Gk *iris* + *plege* stroke], a condition of paralysis of the sphincter muscle of the iris or the dilator muscle, or both.

iridotomy /ī′ridot′əmē/ [Gk *iris* + *temnein* to cut], a surgical incision into the iris of the eye, performed to relieve occlusion of the pupil, to enlarge the pupil in cataract extraction, or to treat postoperative glaucoma.

iris /ī′ris/ [Gk, rainbow], a circular, contractile disc suspended in aqueous humor between the cornea and the crystalline lens of the eye and perforated by a circular pupil. The periphery of the iris is continuous with the ciliary body and is connected to the cornea by the pectinate ligament. The iris divides the space between the lens and the cornea into an anterior and a posterior chamber. Dark pigment cells under the translucent tissue of the iris are variously arranged in different people to produce different colored irises. **–iridic,** *adj.*

iritis /īrī′tis/ [Gk *iris* + *itis*], an inflammatory condition of the iris of the eye characterized by pain, lacrimation, photophobia, and, if severe, diminished visual acuity. On ophthalmic examination the eye looks cloudy, the iris bulges, and the pupil is contracted.

iron (Fe) [AS *iren*], a common metallic element essential for the synthesis of hemoglobin. Its atomic number is 26; its atomic weight is 55.85. It is used as a hematinic in the form of its salts and complexes.

iron deficiency anemia, a microcytic, hypochromic anemia caused by inadequate supplies of iron needed to synthesize hemoglobin, characterized by pallor, fatigue, and weakness. Iron deficiency may be the result of an inadequate dietary supply of iron, of poor absorption of iron in the digestive system, or of chronic bleeding.

iron dextran, an injectable hematinic prescribed in the treatment of iron deficiency anemia not responsive to oral iron therapy.

iron lung. See **Drinker respirator.**

iron metabolism, a series of processes involved in the entry of iron into the body through its absorption, its transport and storage throughout the body, its utilization for the formation of hemoglobin and other iron compounds, and its eventual excretion. Iron normally enters the body through the epithelium of the intestinal mucosa, being oxidized from ferrous to ferric iron in the process. Once iron enters the blood, it cycles between the plasma and the reticuloendothelial or erythropoietic system. Plasma iron is delivered to the normoblast for hemoglobin synthesis where it remains for up to 4 months in the hemoglobin molecules of a mature red cell. When red cells deteriorate and break down, the iron is released from the hemoglobin by the reticuloendothelial system to reenter the transport pool for recycling.

iron poisoning [AS *iren;* L *potio* drink], toxic effects of ingesting iron salts, particularly ferrous sulfate and ferrous chloride. Ferrous sulfate tablets, sometimes mistaken for candy, can cause vomiting, collapse, and liver necrosis. Ferrous chloride, a corrosive substance, when taken internally, causes vomiting, diarrhea, and hemorrhages. Iron encephalopathy has occurred from excessive use of iron preparations.

iron-rich food, any nutrient containing a relatively large amount of iron. The best source of dietary iron is liver, with oysters, clams, heart, kidney, lean meat, and tongue as second choices. Leafy green vegetables are the best plant sources.

iron salts poisoning, poisoning caused by overdose of ferric or ferrous salts, characterized by vomiting, bloody diarrhea, cyanosis, and gastric and intestinal pain.

iron saturation, the capacity of iron to saturate transferrin, measured in the blood to detect iron excess or deficiency.

iron transport, the process whereby iron is carried from its entry point into the body, the intestinal mucosa, to the various sites of utilization and storage. Transferrin binds with free iron and shuttles it to storage and utilization sites.

irradiation /irā′dē-ā′shən/ [L *irradiare* to emit rays], exposure to any form of radiant energy like heat, light, or x-ray. Radioactive sources of radiant energy, such as x-rays or isotopes of iodine or cobalt, are used diagnostically to examine internal body structures or to destroy microorganisms or tissue cells that have become cancerous. Infrared or ultraviolet light may be used to produce heat in body tissues to relieve pain and soreness or to treat skin ailments. Ultraviolet light is also used to identify certain bacteria and toxic molds. –**irradiate,** *v.*

irrational [L *irrationalis* contrary to reason], pertaining to events, conditions, or behavior that may be considered unreasonable.

irreducible /ir′əd(y)oo′sibəl/ [L *in* not, *reducere* to bring back], unable to be returned to the normal position or condition, as an irreducible hernia.

irregular pulse [L *in* + *regula* rule, *pulsare* to beat], any pulse that is of irregular force or rhythm.

irreversible [L *irrevertere* to not turn back], describing a situation or condition that cannot be reversed.

irreversible coma. See **brain death.**

irrigate /ir′igāt/ [L *irrigare* to supply water], to flush with a fluid, usually with a slow steady pressure on a syringe plunger. It may be done to cleanse a wound or to clear tubing.

irrigation, the process of washing out a body cavity or wound with a stream of water or other fluid. –**irrigate,** *v.*

irrigator, an apparatus with a flexible tube for flushing or washing out a body cavity.

irritability [L *irritare* to tease], a condition of abnormal excitability or sensitivity.

irritable bladder [L *irritare;* AS *blaedre*], a condition in which there is a nearly constant urge to urinate despite the lack of evidence of a cause, such as inflammation or a kidney stone.

irritable bowel syndrome [L *irritare;* OFr *boel;* Gk *syn* together, *dromos* course], abnormally increased motility of the small and large intestines, generally associated with emotional stress. Most of those affected are young adults, who complain of diarrhea and, occasionally, pain in the lower abdomen. The pain is usually relieved by moving the bowels. Because there is no organic disease present in irritable bowel syndrome, no specific treatment is necessary.

irritant [L *irritare* to tease], an agent that produces inflammation or irritation.

irritant poisons [L *irritare; potio* drink], any of a large number of toxic substances in the environment that can cause pain in the digestive tract, diarrhea, vomiting, abdominal cramps, and urinary tract disorders. Some irritant chemicals are industrial gases, such as ammonia, chlorine, phosgene, sulfur dioxide, hydrogen sulfide, and nitrogen dioxide that may leak into the atmosphere.

irritation fibroma, a localized peripheral, tumorlike enlargement of connective tissue caused by prolonged irritation. It commonly develops on the gingivae or the buccal mucosa.

IRV, abbreviation for **inspiratory reserve volume.**

ischemia /iskē'mē·ə/ [Gk *ischein* to hold back, *haima* blood], decreased blood supply to a body organ or part, often marked by pain and organ dysfunction, as in ischemic heart disease. –**ischemic,** *adj.*

ischemic contracture. See **Volkmann's contracture.**

ischemic heart disease /iskē'mik/, a pathologic condition of the myocardium caused by lack of oxygen reaching the tissue cells.

ischemic lumbago, a pain in the lower back and buttocks caused by vascular insufficiency, as in occlusion of the abdominal aorta.

ischemic pain, the unpleasant, often excruciating sensation associated with ischemia, resulting from peripheral vascular disease, from decreased blood flow caused by constricting orthopedic casts, or from insufficient blood flow caused by surgical trauma or accidental injury. Ischemic pain caused by occlusive arterial disease is often severe and may not be relieved, even with narcotics. The individual with peripheral vascular disease may experience ischemic pain only while exercising because the metabolic demands for oxygen cannot be met by the occluded flow of blood.

ischemic pericarditis [Gk *ischein* to hold back; *haima* blood; *peri* near, *kardia* heart, *itis*], an inflammation of the pericardium caused by interruption of its blood supply during myocardial infarction.

ischial spines /is'kē·əl/ [Gk *ischion* hip joint; L *spina* thorn], two relatively sharp bony projections into the pelvic outlet from the ischial bones that form the lower border of the pelvis.

ischial tuberosity [Gk *ischion;* L *tuber* swelling], a rounded protuberance of the lower part of the ischium. It forms a bony area on which the human body rests when in a sitting position.

ischium /is'kē·əm/, *pl.* **ischia** [L; Gk *is-chion* hip joint], one of the three parts of the hip bone, joining the ilium and the pubis to form the acetabulum. The ischium comprises the dorsal part of the hip bone and is divided into the body of the ischium, which forms two fifths of the acetabulum, and the ramus, which joins the inferior ramus of the pubis.

ISCLT, abbreviation for *International Society of Clinical Laboratory Technologists.*

ISG, abbreviation for **immune serum globulin.**

Ishihara color test /ish'ēhä'rə/ [Shinobu Ishihara, Japanese ophthalmologist, b. 1879], a test of color vision using a series of plates on which are printed round dots in a variety of colors and patterns. People with normal color vision are able to discern specific numbers or patterns on the plates; the inability to pick out a given number or shape is symptomatic of a specific deficiency in color perception.

island fever. See **scrub typhus.**

islands of Langerhans /lang'gərhanz/ [AS *igland* island; Paul Langerhans, German pathologist, b. 1847], clusters of cells within the pancreas that produce insulin, glucagon, and pancreatic polypeptide. They form the endocrine portion of the gland and their hormonal secretions released into the bloodstream are balanced, important regulators of sugar metabolism.

islet cell adenoma. See **insulinoma.**

islet cell antibody /ī'lit/ [OFr *islette* little island], an immunoglobulin that reacts with the cytoplasm of all of the cells of the pancreatic islets. These antibodies occur in most of newly diagnosed insulin-dependent diabetic patients.

islet cell tumor, any tumor of the islands of Langerhans.

islets of Langerhans. See **islands of Langerhans.**

isoagglutination /ī'sō·əgloo'tinā'shən/ [Gk *isos* equal; L *agglutinare* to glue], the clumping of erythrocytes by agglutinins from the blood of another individual of the same species.

isoagglutinin /ī'sō·əgloo'tinin/ [Gk *isos* equal; L *agglutinare* to glue], an antibody that causes agglutination of erythrocytes in other members of the same species that carry an isoagglutinogen on their erythrocytes.

isoagglutinogen /ī'sō·əglootin'əjən/ [Gk *isos* + L *agglutinare* to glue; Gk *genein* to produce], an antigen that causes the agglutination of erythrocytes in others of the same species that carry a corresponding isoagglutinin in their serum.

isoamyl alcohol. See **amyl alcohol.**

isoantibody /ī'sō·an'tibo'ē/ [Gk *isos* + *anti* against; AS *bodig* body], an antibody to isoantigens found in other members of the same species.

isoantigen /ī'sō·an'tijən/ [Gk *isos* + *anti* against; AS *bodig* body; Gk *genein* to produce], a substance that interacts with isoantibodies in other members of the same species.

isobar /ī'səbär/ [Gk *isos* + *baros* weight], **1.** a line connecting points of equal pressure on a graph. **2.** (in nuclear medicine) one of a group of nuclides having the same total number of neutrons and protons in the nucleus but so proportioned as to result in different values of the atomic number.

isobaric /ī'sōbär'ik/ [Gk *isos* equal, *baros* weight], **1.** pertaining to two substances or solutions of the same specific gravity. **2.** pertaining to two isotopes having the same mass number but different atomic numbers.

isobutyl alcohol /ī'sōby ōō'til/ [Gk *isos* + *boutyron* butter, *hyle* matter; AR *alkohl* essence], a clear, colorless liquid that is miscible with ethyl alcohol or ether.

isocapnic /ī'sōkap'nik/, pertaining to a steady level of carbon dioxide in the tissues despite changing levels of ventilation.

isocarboxazid /ī'sōkärbok'səzid/, a monoamine oxidase inhibitor prescribed in the treatment of mental depression.

isochromosome /ī'sōkrō'məsōm/, a chromosome with identical arms on either side of the centromere.

isodose chart /ī'sədōs/ [Gk *isos* + *dosis* giving; *charta* paper], (in radiotherapy) a graphic representation of the distribution of radiation in a medium; lines are drawn through points receiving equal doses.

isoelectric /ī'sō·ilek'trik/ [Gk *isos* + *elektron* amber], pertaining to the electric base line of an electrocardiogram.

isoelectric electroencephalogram. See **flat electroencephalogram.**

isoelectric focusing, the ordering and concentration of substances according to their isoelectric points.

isoelectric period, a period in physiologic activity, such as nerve conduction or muscle contraction, when there is no variation in electrical potential.

isoelectric point, the pH at which a molecule containing many ionizable groups is electrically neutral. The number of positively charged groups equals the number of negatively charged groups.

isoenzyme /ī'sō·en'zīm/ [Gk *isos* + *en* in, *zyme* ferment], a chemically distinct form of an enzyme. The various forms are distinguishable in analysis of blood samples, which aids in the diagnosis of diseases. Isoenzymes that catalyze the same physiologic reaction may also appear in different forms in different animal species. Also called **isozyme.**

isoetharine, isoetharine hydrochloride. See **isoetharine mesylate.**

isoetharine mesylate /ī'sō·eth'ərēn/, a beta-adrenergic bronchodilator prescribed in the treatment of bronchial asthma, bronchitis, and emphysema.

isoexposure lines, (in radiology) imaginary lines representing positions of equal exposure to radiation in the area around fluoroscopic equipment.

isoflows /ī'səflōz/, (in respiratory therapy) a measure of early small airways' dysfunction in a patient made by comparing flow rates between air and helium at fixed points in time.

isoflurophate /ī'sōfl ōō'rōfāt/, a cholinesterase inhibitor prescribed in the treatment of open-angle glaucoma and esotropia.

isofosfamide. See isophosphamide.

isogamete /ī'sōgam'ēt/ [Gk *isos* + *gamete* wife], a reproductive cell of the same size and structure as the one with which it unites. **–isogametic,** *adj.*

isogamy /īsog'əmē/ [Gk *isos* + *gamos* marriage], sexual reproduction in which there is fusion of gametes of the same size and structure, such as in certain algae, fungi, and protozoa. **–isogamous,** *adj.*

isogeneic. See syngeneic.

isogenesis /ī'sōjen'əsis/ [Gk *isos* + *genein* to produce], development from a common origin and according to similar processes. **–isogenetic, isogenic,** *adj.*

isograft /ī'səgraft'/ [Gk *isos* + *graphion* stylus], surgical transplantation of histocompatible tissue obtained from genetically identical individuals, such as between a patient and identical twin.

isohemagglutinin. See isoagglutinin.

isohydric shift [Gk *isos* + *hydor* water; AS *sciftan* to divide], the series of reactions in red blood cells in which CO_2 is taken up and oxygen is released without the production of excess hydrogen ions.

isoimmunization /ī'sō·im'yənīzā'shən/, the development of antibodies against antigens from the same species (isoantigens), such as the development of anti-Rh antibodies in an Rh-negative person.

isokinetic /ī'sōkinet'ik/, pertaining to a concentric or eccentric contraction that occurs at a set speed against a force of maximal resistance produced at all points in the range of motion.

isokinetic exercise [Gk *isos* + *kinesis* motion; L *exercere* to keep at work], a form of exercise in which maximum force is exerted by a muscle at each point through out the range of motion as the muscle contracts. The effort of the patient to resist the movement is measured.

isolate /ī′səlāt/ [It *isolare*, to detach], **1.** to separate a pure chemical substance from contamination by foreign matter. **2.** to derive from any source a pure culture of a microorganism. **3.** to prevent an individual from having contact with the rest of a population.

isolation [L *insula* island], the separation of a seriously ill patient from others to prevent the spread of an infection or to protect the patient from irritating environmental factors.

isolation incubator, an incubator bed regularly maintained for premature or other infants who require special care.

isolation ward [It *isolare* to detach; ME *warden*], a room or section of a hospital in which certain categories of patients, particularly those infected with acute contagious diseases, can be treated with a minimum of contact with the rest of the patients and hospital personnel.

Isolette, a trademark for a self-contained incubator unit that provides a controlled heat, humidity, and oxygen microenvironment for the isolation and care of premature and low birth-weight neonates.

isoleucine (Ile) /ī′sōloo′sēn/ [Gk *isos* + *leukos* white], an amino acid occurring in most dietary proteins that is essential for proper growth in infants and for nitrogen balance in adults.

isologous graft /īsol′əgəs/ [Gk *isos* equal; *logos* relation; *graphion* stylus], a tissue transplant between two individuals who are genetically identical, as identical twins.

isomeric /ī′sōmer′ik/ [Gk *isos* + *meros* part], pertaining to a chemical phenomenon in which two compounds of the same proportion of elements and molecular weight may differ in chemical and physical properties. The difference is due to the arrangement of atoms in the respective molecules, either the connections between the atoms or in the arrangements of the atoms in three-dimensional space.

isomers /ī′səmərz/, molecules that have the same molecular weight and formula but different structures, resulting in different properties.

isomethepotene hydrochloride /ī′sōmethep′tēn/, an antispasmodic and vasoconstrictor drug that is a component in some fixed-combination drugs used to treat migraine.

isometric /ī′səmet′rik/ [Gk *isos* + *metron* measure], maintaining the same length or dimension.

isometric contraction [Gk *isos* + *metron*;

L *contractio* a drawing together], muscular contraction not accompanied by movement of the joint. The muscle is neither lengthened nor shortened but tension changes alone can be measured.

isometric exercise, a form of active exercise that increases muscle tension by applying pressure against stable resistance. This may be accomplished by opposing different muscles in the same individual, such as by making a limb push or pull against an immovable object. There is no joint movement and the length of the muscle remains unchanged.

isometric growth, an increase in size of different organs or parts of an organism at the same rate.

isoniazid /ī′sənī′əzid/, a tuberculostatic antibacterial prescribed in the treatment of tuberculosis caused by mycobacteria sensitive to the drug.

isoosmotic solution /ī′sō-osmot′ik/, a solution with electrolytes that will exert the same osmotic pressure as another solution.

isopentoic acid. See **isovaleric acid.**

isophane insulin suspension /ī′səfān/ [Gk *isos* + *phanein* to show; L *insula* island; *suspendere* to hang up], a modified form of protamine zinc insulin suspension. It is an intermediate-acting insulin that is a stable, commonly prescribed preparation.

isophosphamide /ī′sōfos′fəmīd/, an antineoplastic that is a derivative of cyclophosphamide and is used similarly to cyclophosphamide.

isoprenaline. See **isoproterenol hydrochloride.**

isopropamide iodide /ī′sōprō′pəmīd/, an anticholinergic prescribed as an adjunct to ulcer therapy.

isopropanol. See **isopropyl alcohol.**

isopropylacetic acid. See **isovaleric acid.**

isopropyl alcohol /ī′sōprō′pil/, a clear, colorless, bitter aromatic liquid that is miscible with water, ether, chloroform, and ethyl alcohol.

isopropylaminoacetic acid. See **valine.**

isoproterenol hydrochloride /ī′sōprəter′ənol/, a beta-adrenergic stimulant used as a bronchodilator and as a cardiac stimulant.

isosmotic. See **isotonic.**

isosorbide dinitrate /ī′sōsôr′bīd/, an antianginal agent prescribed as a coronary vasodilator in the treatment of angina pectoris and congestive heart failure.

isotachophoresis /ī′sōtak′ōfôrē′sis/ [Gk *isos* + *tachos* speed, *pherein* to bear], the ordering and concentration of substances of intermediate effective mobilities between an ion of high effective mobility and one of much lower effective mobility, followed by their migration at a uniform velocity.

isothermal /ī'sōthur'məl/ [Gk *isos* + *therme* heat], pertaining to objects or substances having the same temperature.

isotones /ī'sətōnz'/, atoms that have the same number of neutrons but different numbers of protons.

isotonic /ī'səton'ik/ [Gk *isos* + *tonikos* stretching], (of a solution) having the same concentration of solute as another solution, hence exerting the same amount of osmotic pressure as that solution.

isotonic exercise, a form of active exercise in which the muscle contracts and causes movement. Throughout the procedure there is no significant change in the resistance so that the force of the contraction remains constant.

isotonic solution, pertaining to solutions exerting equal osmotic pressures.

isotope /ī'sətōp/ [Gk *isos* + *topos* place], one of two or more forms of a chemical element that have the same number of protons in the atomic nucleus and the same atomic number, but differ in the number of their nuclear neutrons and atomic weights. Carbon (^{12}C) has six nuclear neutrons; its isotope ^{14}C has eight.

isotopic tracer /ī'sətop'ik/ [Gk *isos* + *topos* place; Fr *tracer* to track], an isotope or artificial mixture of isotopes of an element incorporated into a sample to permit observation of the course of the element, alone or in combination, through a chemical, physical, or biologic process.

isotretinoin /ī'sōtrətin'ō-in/, an antiacne agent prescribed for cystic acne.

isovaleric acid /ī'sōvələr'ik/ [Gk *isos* + L *valeriana* herb, *acidus* sour], a fatty acid with a pungent taste and disagreeable odor that is found in valerian and other plant products, as well as in cheese. It also occurs as a metabolite of the amino acid leucine and is found in the sweat of feet and in urine of patients with smallpox, hepatitis, and typhus.

isovolume pressure-flow curve, a curve on a graph describing the relationship of driving pressure to the resulting volumetric flow rate in the airways at any given lung inflation.

isovolumic contraction [Gk *isos* + L *volumen* paper roll; *contractio* drawing together], (in cardiology) an early phase of systole in which the left ventricle is generating enough tension to overcome the resistance of the aortic end-diastolic pressure.

isoxsuprine hydrochloride /īsok'səprēn/, a peripheral vasodilator prescribed for the symptomatic relief of cerebrovascular insufficiency and to improve the circulation in arteriosclerosis, Raynaud's disease, and Buerger's disease.

isthmus /is'məs/, *pl. isthmuses, isthmi* [Gk *isthmos*], a narrow connection between two larger bodies or parts, such as the isthmus of the auditory tube in the ear.

isthmus of thyroid, a part of the thyroid gland, anterior to the trachea, which joins the two lateral lobes of the gland.

IT, abbreviation for **immunotoxin.**

itch [AS *giccan*], **1.** to feel a sensation, usually on the skin, that makes one want to scratch. **2.** a tingling, annoying sensation on an area of the skin that makes one want to scratch it. **3.** the pruritic condition of the skin caused by infestation with the parasitic mite *Sarcoptes scabiei.* **–itchy,** *adj.*

itch mite [AS *giccan, mite*], a tiny eight-legged insect with piercing and sucking mouth parts. At least three genera of itch mites are recognized. They are *Chorioptes, Notoëdres,* and *Sarcoptes.*

ithycyphosis /ith'ēsifō'sis/ [Gk *ithys* straight; *kyphosis* humpback], a backward angular displacement of the spine without lateral displacement.

ITP, abbreviation for **idiopathic thrombocytopenic purpura.**

IU, abbreviation for **International Unit.**

IUCD, abbreviation for *intrauterine contraceptive device.*

IUD, abbreviation for **intrauterine device.**

IV, 1. abbreviation for **intravenous. 2.** *informal.* equipment consisting of a bottle of fluid, infusion set with tubing, and an intracatheter, used in intravenous therapy. **3.** intravenous administration of fluids or medication by injection into a vein.

IVAC pump, a trademark for a portable IV pump that electronically regulates and monitors the flow of fluid.

IVC, abbreviation for **intravenous cholangiography.**

IVCD, abbreviation for **intraventricular conduction defect.**

IVF, abbreviation for **in vitro fertilization.**

ivory bones. See **osteopetrosis.**

IVP, abbreviation for **intravenous pyelography.**

IV push, a technique in which a bolus of medication or a large volume of IV fluid is given rapidly via IV injection or infusion.

IVT, abbreviation for *intravenous transfusion.*

IV-type traction frame, a metal support that holds traction equipment consisting of two metal uprights, one at each end of the bed, which support an overhead metal bar.

ivy poisoning [OE *ifig;* L *potio* drink], a form of contact dermatitis caused by exposure to poison ivy, poison oak, or poison sumac. All are members of the *Rhus* genus of plants that containing an irritating oil. Contact with any part of a Rhus plant can result in severe itching, rashes, and blistering; even the smoke of burning Rhus plants may be toxic.

Ixodes /iksō′dēz/ [Gk, sticky], a genus of parasitic hard-shelled ticks associated with the transmission of a variety of arbovirus infections, such as Rocky Mountain spotted fever.

ixodid /iksod′id, iksō′did/, of or pertaining to hard ticks of the family Ixodidae.

I

J, abbreviation for **joule.**

Jaccoud's dissociated fever /zhäkōōz′/ [Sigismond Jaccoud, French physician, b. 1830], a form of meningitic fever accompanied by a paradoxical slow pulse rate.

jacket [Fr *jaquette*], a supportive or confining therapeutic casing or garment for the torso. Some kinds of jackets are *Minerva jacket* (also called **minerva cast**) and **Sayre's jacket.**

jacket restraint, an orthopedic device used to help immobilize the trunk of a patient in traction and to discourage the patient from sitting up in bed. The jacket restraint is attached to both sides of the bedspring frame by means of buckled webbing straps that are sewn into the side seams of the restraint. The jacket restraint may be used with some kinds of traction.

jackknife position, an anatomic position in which the patient is placed on the back in a semisitting position, with the shoulders elevated and the thighs flexed at right angles to the abdomen. Examination and instrumentation of the male urethra is facilitated by this position.

Jackson crib, a removable orthodontic appliance retained in position by crib-shaped wires.

jacksonian seizure. See **focal seizure.**

Jackson tracheostomy tube, a silver tracheostomy tube with a rubber cuff built onto the tube to prevent accidental migration of the cuff that can result in interference with air flow to the patient.

Jacob's membrane [Arthur Jacob, Irish surgeon, b. 1790; L *membrana* thin skin], the outermost of the nine layers of the retina, composed of rods and cones interacting directly with the optic nerve.

Jacquemier's sign /zhäkmē-āz′/ [Jean M. Jacquemier, French obstetrician, b. 1806], a deepening of the color of the vaginal mucosa just below the urethral orifice. It may sometimes be noted after the fourth week of pregnancy.

jactitation /jak′titā′shən/ [L *jactitare* to toss], twitchings or spasms of muscles or muscle groups, as observed in the restless body movements of a patient with a severe fever.

JADA, abbreviation for *Journal of the American Dental Association.*

jail fever. See **epidemic typhus.**

Jakob-Creutzfeldt disease. See **Creutzfeldt-Jakob disease.**

JAMA /jä′mä, jam′ə, jä′ä′em′ä′/, abbreviation for *Journal of the American Medical Association.*

jamais vu /zhämävY′, -vē′, -vōō′/ [Fr, never seen], the sensation of being a stranger when with a person one knows or when in a familiar place.

Janeway lesion /jān′wā/ [Edward G. Janeway, American physician, b. 1841; L *laedere* to injure], a small erythematous or hemorrhagic macule occurring on the palms or soles, sometimes diagnostic of subacute bacterial endocarditis.

janiceps /jan′əseps/ [L *Janus* two-faced Roman god, *caput* head], a conjoined, twin, grossly malformed fetuses in which the heads are fused, with the faces looking in opposite directions.

Jansen's disease. See **metaphyseal dysostosis.**

Japanese encephalitis, a severe epidemic infection of brain tissue seen in East Asia and the South Pacific, including Australia and New Zealand, characterized by shaking chills, paralysis, and weight loss, and caused by a group of B arboviruses transmitted by mosquitoes.

Japanese flood fever, Japanese river fever. See **scrub typhus.**

JAPHA /jaf′ə, jä′ä′pē′äch′ä′/, abbreviation for *Journal of the American Public Health Association.*

jargon (jar.) [Fr *jargonner* to speak indistinctly], **1.** incoherent speech or gibberish. **2.** a language used by scientists, artists, or others of a professional subculture that is not understood by the general population.

jargon aphasia, a form of speech in which several words are combined in a single word but in a jumbled manner with incorrect accents or words mixed with neologisms. Although outwardly incomprehensible, the speech may be meaningful when analyzed by a psychotherapist.

Jarisch-Herxheimer reaction /jä′risherks′hīmər/ [Adolph Jarisch, Austrian dermatologist, b. 1850; Karl Herxheimer, German dermatologist, b. 1861], a sudden transient fever and exacerbation of skin lesions observed several hours after administration of penicillin or other antibiotics in the treatment of syphilis, leptospirosis, or relapsing fever.

Jarotzky's treatment /jərot'skēz/ [Alexander Jarotsky, Russian physician, b. 1866], therapy for gastric ulcer using a bland diet consisting of egg whites, fresh butter, bread, milk, and noodles.

Jarvik-7 [Robert K. Jarvik, American physician, b. 1946], an artificial heart designed by R. K. Jarvik for use in humans. The Jarvik-7 was an early model that depended on air pressure to drive the ventricles.

jaundice /jôn'dis, jän·dis/ [Fr *jaune* yellow], a yellow discoloration of the skin, mucous membranes, and sclerae of the eyes, caused by greater than normal amounts of bilirubin in the blood. Persons with jaundice may also experience nausea, vomiting, and abdominal pain and may pass dark urine. Jaundice is a symptom of many disorders, including liver diseases, biliary obstruction, and the hemolytic anemias. Newborns commonly develop physiologic jaundice, which disappears after a few days. **–jaundiced**, *adj.*

jaw [AS *ceowan* to chew], a common term used to describe the maxillae and the mandible and the soft tissue that covers these structures.

jaw reflex, an abnormal reflex elicited by tapping the chin with a rubber hammer while the mouth is half open and the jaw muscles are relaxed.

jaw relation, any relation of the mandible to the maxillae.

jaw-winking, an involuntary facial movement phenomenon in which the eyelid droops when the jaw is closed but raises when the jaw is moved. The raising of the eyelid often appears exaggerated.

JCAHO, abbreviation for **Joint Commission on Accreditation of Health Care Organizations.**

J chain, the portion of the IgM molecule possibly holding the structure together, thus "joining chain."

J/deg, abbreviation for *joules per degree.*

Jefferson fracture, a fracture characterized by bursting of the ring of the atlas.

jejunal feeding tube /jij$\overline{oo}$'nəl/, a hollow tube inserted into the jejunum through the abdominal wall for administration of liquified foods.

jejunoileitis. See **Crohn's disease.**

jejunostomy /jij'$\overline{oo}$nos'təmē/, a surgical procedure to create an artificial opening to the jejunum through the abdominal wall. It may be a permanent or a temporary opening.

jejunum /jij$\overline{oo}$'nəm/, *pl.* **jejuna** [L *jejunus*

empty], one of the three portions of the small intestine, connecting proximally with the duodenum and distally with the ileum. The jejunum has a slightly larger diameter, a deeper color, and a thicker wall than the ileum and contains heavy, circular folds that are absent in the lower part of the ileum. **–jejunal**, *adj.*

jellyfish sting [L *gelare* to congeal; AS *fisc; stingan*], a wound caused by skin contact with a jellyfish, a sea animal with a gelatinous body and tentacles containing stinging structures. In most cases a tender, red welt develops on the affected skin. In some cases, severe localized pain and nausea, weakness, excessive lacrimation, nasal discharge, muscle spasm, perspiration, and dyspnea may occur.

Jendrassik's maneuver /yendrä'shiks/ [Ernst Jendrassik, Hungarian physician, b. 1858; Fr *manoeuvre* action], (in neurology) a diagnostic procedure in which the patient hooks the flexed fingers of the two hands together and forcibly tries to pull them apart. While this tension is being exerted, the lower extremity reflexes are tested.

jet humidifier, a humidifier that increases the surface area for exposure of water to gas by breaking the water into small aerosol droplets. A foaming mixture of liquid and gas is produced. Gas issuing from the unit has a maximum amount of water vapor and a minimum of liquid water particles.

jet lag [L *jacere* to throw; Norw *lagga* to fall behind], a condition characterized by fatigue, insomnia, and sluggish body functions caused by disruption of the normal circadian rhythm resulting from air travel across several time zones.

jet nebulizer [L *nebula* mist], a respiratory humidifier that uses the Bernoulli effect to convert a source of liquid into a fine mist of aerosol particles.

Jeune's syndrome /zhœn, zh$\overline{oo}$n/, a form of lethal short-limbed dwarfism characterized by constriction of the upper thorax and, occasionally, polydactylism. It is inherited as an autosomal recessive trait.

jigger. See **chigoe.**

jitters, 1. irregularities in ultrasound echo locations due to mechanical or electronic disturbances. **2.** a very uneasy, nervous feeling.

jkg, abbreviation for *joules per kilogram.*

Jobst garment, a type of pressure wrap applied to control hypertrophic scar formation.

jock itch. See **tinea cruris.**

Jod-Basedow phenomenon /jod'bä'zədō'/, thyrotoxicosis occurring when dietary iodine is given to a patient with endemic goiter in an area of environmental iodine deficiency. It is presumed that iodine deficiency protects some patients with endemic goiter from developing thyrotoxicosis.

jogger's heel [ME *joggen* to shake; AS *hela* heel], a painful condition, common among joggers and distance runners. It is characterized by bruising, bursitis, fasciitis, or calcaneal spurs, caused by repetitive and forceful strikes of the heel on the ground.

Johnson's method, (in dentistry) a technique for filling root canals, in which gutta-percha cones are dissolved in a chloroform-rosin solution in the root canal to form a plastic mass.

joint [L *jungere* to join], any one of the connections between bones. Each is classified according to structure and movability as fibrous, cartilaginous, or synovial. Fibrous joints are immovable, cartilaginous joints slightly movable, and synovial joints freely movable. Typical immovable joints are those connecting most of the bones of the skull with a sutural ligament. Typical slightly movable joints are those connecting the vertebrae and the pubic bones.

joint and several liability, (in law) a condition in which several persons share the liability for a plaintiff's injury and may be found liable individually or as a group.

joint appointment, 1. a faculty appointment to two institutions within a university or system, as to the schools of nursing and medicine of the same university. 2. (in academic nursing) the appointment of a member of the faculty of a university to a clinical service of an associated service institution.

joint audit. See **nursing audit.**

joint capsule [L *jungere* to join; *capsula* little box], a fibrous connective tissue envelope surrounding a joint.

joint chondroma, a cartilaginous mass that develops in the synovial membrane of a joint.

Joint Commission on Accreditation of Health Care Organizations (JCAHO), a private, nongovernmental agency that establishes guidelines for the operation of hospitals and other health care facilities, conducts accreditation programs and surveys, and encourages the attainment of high standards of institutional medical care.

joint conference committee, a hospital organization composed of the governing board, administration, and medical staff representatives whose purpose is to facilitate communication between the groups.

joint fracture, a fracture of the articular surfaces of the bony structures of a joint.

joint instability, an abnormal increase in joint mobility.

joint mouse, a small, movable calculus in or near a joint, usually a knee.

joint planning, the development by two or more health care providers of a strategic plan to serve the health care needs of an area while sharing clinical or administrative services, or the sharing of data, without the sharing of assets.

joint practice, 1. the practice of one or more physicians, nurses, and other health professionals, usually private, who work as a team, sharing responsibility for a group of patients. 2. (in inpatient nursing) the practice of making joint decisions about patient care by committees of the physicians and nurses working on a division.

joint protection, the use of orthotics with therapeutic exercise to prevent damage or deformity of a joint during rehabilitation to restore power and range of motion. An example is a metal ankle-foot orthosis that allows weight-bearing on an extended knee.

Jones criteria, a standardized set of guidelines for the diagnosis of rheumatic fever, as recommended by the American Heart Association.

joule /jōōl/ [James P. Joule, English physicist, b. 1818], a unit of energy or work in the MKS (meter-kilogram-second) system. It is equivalent to 10^7 ergs or 1 watt second.

joystick, a vertical stick or lever that can be manipulated in various directions to control cursor movement on a computer screen or the direction of an electric wheelchair.

J-pouch, a fecal reservoir formed surgically by folding over the lower end of the ileum in an ileo-anal anastomosis.

JRA, abbreviation for **juvenile rheumatoid arthritis.**

Judd method, (in radiology) a technique for positioning a patient for x-ray examination of the atlas and odontoid process.

judgment [L *judicare* to judge], 1. (in law) the final decision of the court regarding the case before it. 2. the reason given by the court for its decision; an opinion. 3. an award, penalty, or other sentence of law given by the court. 4. (in psychiatry) the ability to recognize the relationships of ideas and to form correct conclusions from those data as well as from those acquired from experience.

judgment call, *slang;* a decision based on experience, especially a judgment that resolves a serious problem in which the data are inconclusive or equivocal.

jugular /jug'yələr/ [L, *jugulum,* neck], pertaining to or involving the neck.

jugular foramen [L *jugulum* neck; *foramen* hole], one of a pair of openings between the lateral part of the occipital bone and the petrous part of the temporal bones in the skull.

jugular fossa, a deep depression adjacent to the interior surface of the petrosa of the temporal bone of the skull.

jugular process, a portion of the occipital bone that projects laterally from the squamous part. On its anterior border a deep notch forms the posterior and medial boundary of the jugular foramen.

jugular pulse, a pulsation in the jugular vein caused by waves transmitted from the right side of the heart by the circulating blood.

jugular venous pressure (JVP), blood pressure in the jugular vein, which reflects the volume and pressure of the venous blood in the right side of the heart. With elevated JVP the neck veins may be distended as high as the angle of the jaw.

juice [L *jus* broth], any fluid secreted by the tissues of animals or plants. Kinds of juices include **gastric, intestinal,** and **pancreatic juice.**

jumentous /jo̅o̅men'təs/ [L *jumentum* beast of burden], having a strong animal odor, especially that of a horse. It is used to describe the odor of urine during certain disease conditions.

jumping gene, (in molecular genetics) a unit of genetic information associated with a segment of DNA that can move from one position in the genome to another.

junction [L *jungere* to join], an interface or meeting place for tissues or structures.

junctional bigeminy [L *jungere* to join; *bis* twice, *geminus* twin], a condition in which events occur in pairs, as a bigeminal pulse or nodal extrasystoles, with origination from the junction.

junctional epithelium [L *jungere*; Gk *epi+ thele* nipple], an area of epithelial soft tissue surrounding the abutment post of a tooth.

junctional extrasystole [L *jungere; extra* beyond; Gk *systole* contraction], an extrasystole arising from the atrioventricular junction.

junctional rhythm, the cardiac rhythm originating in the atrioventricular junction.

junctional tachycardia, an automatic heart rhythm of greater than 100 beats/ minute, emanating from the AV junction.

junction lines, (in radiology) vertical lines that appear in the mediastinum on a P-A (posterior-anterior) projection x-ray image.

junction nevus [L *jungere; naevus* birthmark], a hairless, flat or slightly raised, brown skin blemish arising from pigment cells at the epidermal-dermal junction. Malignant change may be signaled by increase in size, hardness or darkening, bleeding, or the appearance of satellite discoloration around the nevus.

junctura cartilaginea. See **cartilaginous joint.**

junctura fibrosa. See **fibrous joint.**

junctura synovialis. See **synovial joint.**

jungian psychology. See **analytic psychology.**

Junin fever. See **Argentine hemorrhagic fever.**

juniper tar /jo̅o̅'nipər/ [L *juniperus;* AS *teoru*], a dark oily liquid obtained by the destructive distillation of the wood of *Juniperus oxycedrus* trees. It is used as an antiseptic stimulant in ointments for skin disorders such as psoriasis and eczema.

junk, *slang.* heroin.

jurisprudence /jo̅o̅'rispro̅o̅'dəns/ [L *juris* law, *prudentia* knowledge], the science and philosophy of law. **Medical jurisprudence** relates to the interfacing of medicine with criminal and civil law.

juvenile [L *juvenus* youthful], **1.** a young person; youth; child; youngster. **2.** of, pertaining to, characteristic of, or suitable for a young person; youthful. **3.** physiologically underdeveloped or immature. **4.** denoting psychologic or intellectual immaturity; childish.

juvenile alveolar rhabdomyosarcoma, a rapidly growing tumor of striated muscle with a grave prognosis, occurring in children and adolescents, chiefly in the extremities.

juvenile angiofibroma. See **nasopharyngeal angiofibroma.**

juvenile delinquency, persistent antisocial, illegal, or criminal behavior by children or adolescents to the degree that it cannot be controlled or corrected by the parents, it endangers others in the community, and it becomes the concern of a law enforcement agency. Such behavioral patterns are characterized by aggressiveness, destructiveness, hostility, and cruelty and occur more frequently in boys than in girls.

juvenile delinquent, a person who performs illegal acts and who has not reached an age at which treatment as an adult can be accorded under the laws of the community having jurisdiction.

juvenile diabetes. See **insulin-dependent diabetes mellitus.**

juvenile glaucoma [L *juvenis* youth; Gk

glaukcos bluish gray], increased intraocular tension in a young adult due to developing structural defects that restrict the outflow of fluid.

juvenile kyphosis. See **Scheuermann's disease.**

juvenile lentigo. See **lentigo.**

juvenile myxedema. See **childhood myxedema.**

juvenile periodontitis, an abnormal condition that may affect the dental alveoli, especially in the anterior and first molar regions of children and adolescents.

juvenile rheumatoid arthritis, a form of rheumatoid arthritis, usually affecting the larger joints of children under 16 years of age. As bone growth in children is dependent on the epiphyseal plates of the distal epiphyses, skeletal development may be impaired if these structures are damaged.

juvenile spinal muscular atrophy, a disorder beginning in childhood in which progressive degeneration of anterior horn and medullary nerve cells leads to skeletal muscle wasting. The condition usually begins in the legs and pelvis.

juvenile xanthogranuloma, a skin disorder characterized by groups of yellow, red, or brown papules or nodules on the extensor surfaces of the arms and legs, and in some cases on the eyeball, meninges, and testes of children.

juxtaarticular /juk′stə-ärtik′yələr/ [L *juxta* adjacent; *articulus* joint], pertaining to a location near a joint.

juxtaglomerular /juk′stəglōmer′ələr/ [L *juxta + glomerulus,* small ball], pertaining to an area between the afferent and efferent arterioles of the kidney glomerulus.

juxtaglomerular cells [L *juxta + glomerulus* small sphere; *cella* storeroom], smooth muscle cells lining the glomerular end of the afferent arterioles in the kidney that are in opposition to the macula densa region of the early distal tubule. These cells synthesize and store renin.

juxtaposition /juk′stəpəzish′ən/, the placement of objects end to end or side by side.

K

K, 1. symbol for *ionization constant.* 2. symbol for **Kelvin scale.** 3. symbol for **kilo,** 1,000, or 10^3. 4. symbol for the element **potassium** (kalium). 5. abbreviation for **kilobyte.** 6. symbol in electronics, 1,024 (2^{10}).

K_m, symbol for *Michaelis-Menten constant.*

ka, abbreviation for *kiloampere.*

Kahn test [Reuben L. Kahn, American bacteriologist, b. 1887] 1. a serologic test for syphilis. The appearance of a white precipitate in a serum sample allowed to stand overnight in a mixture with a sensitized antigen is regarded as a positive reaction. 2. a test for the presence of cancer by measuring the proportion of albumin A in a blood sample.

kainate /kī′nāt/, a non-NMDA (N-methyl-D-aspartate) receptor agonist.

kakke disease. See **beriberi.**

kakosmia. See **cacosmia.**

kala-azar /kä′lə-əzär′/ [Hindi *kala* black; Assamese *azar* fever], a disease caused by the protozoan *Leishmania donovani,* transmitted to humans, particularly to children, by the bite of the sand fly. Kala-azar occurs in Asia, Africa, South and Central American countries, and in the Mediterranean region. The liver and spleen are the main sites of infection; signs and symptoms include anemia, hepatomegaly, splenomegaly, irregular fever, and emaciation.

kalemia /kəlē′mē·ə/, the presence of potassium in the blood.

kaliuresis /kal′iyŏŏrē′sis/, the excretion of potassium in the urine.

kallikrein-kinin system /kalik′rē·in-/, a proposed hormonal system that functions within the kidney, with the enzyme kallikrein in the renal cortex mediating production of bradykinin, which acts as a vasodilator peptide.

Kallmann's syndrome [Franz J. Kallman, American psychiatrist, b. 1897], a condition characterized by the absence of the sense of smell because of agenesis of the olfactory bulbs and by secondary hypogonadism because of the lack of LHRH.

kanamycin /kan′əmī′sin/, an antibacterial substance derived from *Streptomyces kanamyceticus.*

kanamycin sulfate, an aminoglycoside antibiotic prescribed in the treatment of certain severe infections and those resistant to other antibiotics.

Kanner's syndrome. a form of infantile psychosis with an onset in the first 30 months of life. It is characterized by infantile autism. Treatment may include psychotherapy and special education, depending on the intelligence level of the child.

kaodzera. See **Rhodesian trypanosomiasis.**

kaolin /kā′əlin/ [Chin *kao-ling* high ridge], an adsorbent used internally to treat diarrhea, often in combination with pectin.

Kaposi's disease /kap′əsēz/ [Moritz K. Kaposi, Austrian dermatologist, b. 1837], a rare inherited skin disorder that begins in childhood and involves mainly exposed skin areas. Exposure to sunlight results in erythema and vesiculation, followed by increased pigmentation and telangiectasia, skin ulcers, warts, and, malignant epitheliomas.

Kaposi's sarcoma [Moritz J. Kaposi], a malignant, multifocal neoplasm of reticuloendothelial cells that begins as soft, brownish or purple papules on the feet and slowly spreads in the skin, metastasizing to the lymph nodes and viscera. It is occasionally associated with diabetes, malignant lymphoma, AIDS, or other disorders.

Kaposi's varicelliform eruption. See **eczema herpeticum.**

kappa, K, κ, the tenth letter of the Greek alphabet.

karaya powder /kär′äyä/ [Hindi *karayal* resin; L *pulvis* dust], a dried form of *Sterculia urens* or other species of *Sterculia,* used as a bulk cathartic. It reduces the intraluminal rectosigmoid pressure and helps relieve symptoms in patients with irritable bowel disease and diverticular disease of the colon. Externally, it is used as a drying agent for decubitus ulcers.

Kardex. a trademark for a card-filing system that allows quick reference to the particular needs of each patient for certain aspects of nursing care.

Kartagener's syndrome /kärtag′ənərz/, an inherited disorder characterized by bronchiectasis, chronic paranasal sinusitis, and transposed viscera, usually dextrocardia.

karyenchyma. See **karyolymph.**

karyocyte /ker'ē·əsīt'/ [Gk *karyon* nut, *kytos* cell], a normoblast, or developing red blood cell with a nucleus condensed into a homogenous staining body. It is normally found in the red bone marrow.

karyogamy /ker'ē·og'əmē/ [Gk *karyon* + *gamos* marriage], the fusion of cell nuclei, as in conjugation and zygosis. –**karyogenetic,** *adj.*

karyogenesis /ker'ē·ōjen'əsis/ [Gk *karyon* + *genein* to produce], the formation and development of the nucleus of a cell. –**karyogenetic,** *adj.*

karyokinesis /ker'ē·ōkinē'sis, -kīnē'sis/ [Gk *karyon* + *kinesis* motion], the division of the nucleus and equal distribution of nuclear material during mitosis and meiosis. –**karyokinetic,** *adj.*

karyoklasis /ker'ē·ok'ləsis/ [Gk *karyon* + *klasis* breaking], **1.** the disintegration of the cell nucleus or nuclear membrane. **2.** the interruption of mitosis. Also spelled **karyoclasis.** –**karyoklastic, karyoclastic,** *adj.*

karyology /ker'ē·ol'əjē/ [Gk *karyon* + *logos* science], the branch of cytology that concentrates on the study of the cell nucleus, especially the structure and function of the chromosomes. –**karyologic, karyological,** *adj.,* **karyologist,** n.

karyolymph /ker'ē·əlimf'/ [Gk *karyon* + *lympha* water], the clear, usually nonstaining, fluid substance of the nucleus. It consists primarily of proteinaceous, colloidal material in which the nucleolus, chromatin, linin, and various submicroscopic particles are dispersed. –**karyolymphatic,** *adj.*

karyolysis /ker'ē·ol'isis/ [Gk *karyon* + *lysis* loosening], the dissolution of the cell nucleus. It occurs normally, both as a form of necrobiosis and during the generation of new cells through mitosis and meiosis.

karyolytic /ker'ē·əlit'ik/, **1.** of or pertaining to karyolysis. **2.** that which causes the destruction of the cell nucleus.

karyomere /ker'ē·əmir'/ [Gk *karyon* + *meros* part] **1.** a saclike structure containing an unequal portion of the nuclear material after atypical mitosis. **2.** a segment of the chromosome.

karyometry /ker'ē·om'ətrē/, the measurement of the nucleus of a cell. –**karyometric,** *adj.*

karyomit /ker'ē·əmit'/ [Gk *karyon* + *mitos* thread] **1.** a single chromatin fibril of the network within the nucleus of a cell. **2.** a chromosome.

karyomitome /ker'ē·om'itōm/ [Gk *karyon* + *mitos* thread], the fibrillar chromatin network within the nucleus of a cell.

karyomitosis. See **karyokinesis.**

karyomorphism /ker'ē·omôr'fizəm/ [Gk *karyon* + *morphe* form], the shape or form of a cell nucleus, especially that of the leukocyte. –**karyomorphic,** *adj.*

karyon /ker'ē·on/ [Gk, nucleus, nut], the nucleus of a cell. –**karyontic,** *adj.*

karyophage /ker'ē·ōfāj'/ [Gk *karyon* + *phagein* to eat], an intracellular protozoan parasite that destroys the nucleus of the cell it infects. –**karyophagic, karyophagous,** *adj.*

karyoplasm. See **nucleoplasm.**

karyoplasmic ratio. See **nucleocytoplasmic ratio.**

karyopyknosis /ker'ē·ōpiknō'sis/ [Gk *karyon* + *pyknos* thick], the state of a cell in which the nucleus has shrunk and the chromatin has condensed into solid masses. –**karyopyknotic,** *adj.*

karyoreticulum. See **karyomitome.**

karyorrhexis /ker'ē·ərek'sis/ [Gk *karyon* + *rhexis* rupture], the fragmentation of chromatin and distribution of it throughout the cytoplasm as a result of nuclear disintegration. –**karyorrhectic,** *adj.*

karyosome /ker'ē·əsōm'/ [Gk *karyon* + *soma* body], a dense irregular mass of chromatin filaments in the cell nucleus.

karyospherical /ker'ē·ōsfer'ikəl/ [Gk *karyon* + *sphaira* ball], **1.** of or pertaining to a nucleus that is spherical. **2.** such a nucleus.

karyostasis /ker'ē·os'təsis/ [Gk *karyon* + *stasis* standing], the resting stage of the nucleus between cell division. –**karyostatic,** adj.

karyotheca /ker'ē·əthē'kə/ [Gk *karyon* + *theke* sheath], the membrane that encloses a cell nucleus. –**karyothecal,** *adj.*

karyotin. See **chromatin.**

karyotype /ker'ē·ətip'/ [Gk *karyon* + *typos* mark] **1.** the total morphologic characteristics of the somatic chromosome complement of an individual or species, described in terms of number, form, size, and arrangement within the nucleus, as determined by a microphotograph taken during the metaphase stage of mitosis. **2.** a diagrammatic representation of the chromosome complement of an individual or species, arranged in pairs in descending order of size and according to the position of the centromere. –**karyotypic,** *adj.*

Kasabach method /kas'əbak/, (in radiology) a technique for positioning a patient for x-ray examination of the odontoid process.

Kasai operation. See **portoenterostomy.**

Kashin-Bek disease [Nikolai I. Kashin, Russian orthopedist, b. 1825; E.V. Bek; L *dis* + Fr *aise* ease], a form of osteoarthrosis afflicting mainly children living in China, Korea, and eastern Siberia. It is believed to be caused by eating foods made with wheat contaminated by a fungus, *Fusarium sporotrichiella.*

katadidymus /kat′ədid′əməs/ [Gk *kata* down, *didymos* twin], conjoined twins that are united in the lower portion of the body and separated at the top.

katal (K, kat) /kat′al/ [Gk *kata* down], an enzyme unit in moles per second defined by the SI system: 1 K = 6.6 × 10⁹ U.

Kawasaki disease. See **mucocutaneous lymph node syndrome.**

Kayser-Fleischer ring /kī′zərflī′shər/ [Bernhard Kayser, German ophthalmologist, b. 1869; Bruno Fleischer, German ophthalmologist, b. 1874], a gray-green to red-gold pigmented ring at the outer margin of the cornea, pathognomonic of hepatolenticular degeneration, a rare progressive disease caused by a defect in copper metabolism and transmitted as an autosomal recessive trait.

Kazanjian's operation /kasan′jē·ənz/ [Varstad J. Kazanjian, American physician, b. 1879], a surgical procedure for extending the vestibular sulcus to improve prosthetic foundation of edentulous ridges.

kcal, abbreviation for **kilocalorie.**

K cell. See **null cell.**

kCi, abbreviation for *kilocurie.*

ke, abbreviation for **kinetic energy.**

Kedani fever. See **scrub typhus.**

keel, (in prosthetics) a device in a stored-energy foot prosthesis that functions as a cantilever spring, bending the foot upward when weight is applied to the toe.

kefir /kef′ər/ [Russ, fermented milk], a slightly effervescent, acidulous beverage prepared from the milk of cows, sheep, or goats through fermentation by kefir grains, which contain yeasts and lactobacilli.

Kegel exercises. See **pubococcygeus exercises.**

Keith-Flack node. See **sinoatrial node.**

Keith-Wegener-Barker classification system, a method of classifying the degree of hypertension in a patient on the basis of retinal changes. The stages are group 1, identified by constriction of the retinal arterioles; group 2, constriction and sclerosis of the retinal arterioles; group 3, characterized by hemorrhages and exudates in addition to group 2 conditions; and group 4, papilledema of the retinal arterioles.

Kellgren's syndrome /kel′grinz/ [Henry Kellgren, Swedish physician, b. 1827], a form of osteoarthritis affecting the proximal and distal interphalangeal joints, the first metatarsophalangeal and carpometacarpal joints, the knees, and the spine.

Kelly clamp [Howard A. Kelly, American gynecologist, b. 1858; AS *clam* to fasten], a curved hemostat without teeth, used primarily in gynecologic procedures for grasping vascular tissue.

Kelly's pad, a horseshoe-shaped, inflatable rubber drainage pad used in a bed or on the operating table.

keloid /kē′loid/ [Gk *kelis* spot, *eidos* form], an overgrowth of collagenous scar tissue at the site of a wound of the skin. The new tissue is elevated, rounded, and firm, with irregular, clawlike margins. **–keloidal, cheloidal,** *adj.*

keloid acne [Gk *kelis; akme* point], a chronic irritating skin eruption on the nape of the neck that begins as folliculitis and progresses through papulation to a condition of keloid plaques.

keloidosis /kē′loidō′sis/ [Gk *kelis, eidos + osis* condition], habitual or multiple formation of keloids.

keloid scar [Gk *kelis, eidos; eschara* scab], an overgrowth of tissue in a scar at the site of skin injury, particularly a wound or a surgical incision. The amount of tissue growth is excessive for the need to repair the wound and is partially due to an accumulation of collagen at the site.

kelp [ME *culp*], **1.** any of the brown seaweeds species of *Laminaria* found on the Atlantic coast of Europe. **2.** the ashes of *Laminaria* seaweeds burned in a process of extracting iodine and potassium salts.

Kelvin scale (K) [Lord Kelvin (William Thomson), British physicist, b. 1824], an absolute temperature scale calculated in Celsius units from the point at which molecular activity apparently ceases, -273° C. To convert Celsius degrees to Kelvin, add 273.

Kempner rice-fruit diet. See **rice diet.**

Kennedy classification [Edward Kennedy, American dentist, b. 1883], a method of classifying edentulous conditions and partial dentures, based on the position of the spaces of the missing teeth in relation to the remaining teeth.

Kenny treatment. See **Sister Kenny's treatment.**

kenogenesis. See **cenogenesis.**

kenophobia /kē′nōfō′bē·ə/ [Gk *kenos* empty, *phobos* fear], the morbid fear of large and open spaces; agoraphobia.

Kent bundle [Albert F. S. Kent, English physiologist, b. 1863; AS *byndel* to bind], an accessory pathway between atria and ventricles outside of the conduction system and found on both sides of the heart.

Kenya fever. See **Marseilles fever.**

kephir. See **kefir.**

kerasin /ker′əsin/ [L *cera* wax], a cerebroside, found in brain tissue, that consists of a fatty acid, galactose, and sphingosine.

keratectomy /ker′ətek′təmē/ [Gk *keras* horn, *ektome* excision], surgical removal

K

of a portion of the cornea, performed to excise a small, superficial lesion that does not warrant a corneal graft. Corneal epithelium grows rapidly, filling a small surgical area in about 60 hours.

keratic /kərat′ik/ [Gk *keras* horn; L *icus* like], **1.** of or pertaining to keratin. **2.** of or pertaining to the cornea.

keratic precipitate, a group of inflammatory cells deposited on the endothelial surface of the cornea after trauma or inflammation, sometimes obscuring vision.

keratin /ker′ətin/ [Gk *keras* horn], a fibrous, sulfur-containing protein that is the primary component of the epidermis, hair, nails, enamel of the teeth, and horny tissue of animals.

keratinization /ker′ətinīzā′shən/ [Gk *keras* + L *izein* to cause], a process by which epithelial cells exposed to the external environment lose their moisture and are replaced by horny tissue. **–keratinize.** *v.*

keratinocyte /kerat′inōsīt′/ [Gk *keras* + *kytos* cell], an epidermal cell that synthesizes keratin and other proteins and sterols. These cells constitute 95% of the epidermis, being formed as undifferentiated, or basal, cells at the dermal-epidermal junction.

keratitis /ker′ətī′tis/, any inflammation of the cornea. Kinds of keratitis include **dendritic keratitis, interstitial keratitis, keratoconjunctivitis sicca,** and **trachoma. –keratic,** *adj.*

keratoacanthoma /ker′ətō·ak′anthō′mə/, *pl.* **keratoacanthomas, keratoacanthomata** [Gk *keras* + *akantha* thorn, *oma* tumor], a benign, rapidly growing, flesh-colored papule of the skin with a central plug of keratin. The lesion is most common on the face or the back of the hands and arms.

keratoconjunctivitis /ker′ətōkənjungk′-tivī′tis/ [Gk *keras* + L *conjunctivus* connecting; Gk *itis*], inflammation of the cornea and the conjunctiva. Kinds of keratoconjunctivitis include **eczematous conjunctivitis, epidemic keratoconjunctivitis,** and **keratoconjunctivitis sicca.**

keratoconjunctivitis sicca, dryness of the cornea caused by a deficiency of tear secretion in which the corneal surface appears dull and rough, and the eye feels gritty and irritated. The condition may be associated with erythema multiforme, Sjögren's syndrome, trachoma, and vitamin A deficiency.

keratoconus /ker′ətōkō′nəs/ [Gk *keras* + *konos* cone], a noninflammatory protrusion of the central part of the cornea. More common in females, it may cause marked astigmatism.

keratoderma blennorrhagica, the development of hyperkeratotic skin lesions of the palms, soles, and nails. The condition tends to occur in some patients with Reiter's syndrome.

keratohyalin /ker′ətōhī′əlin/ [Gk *keras* + *hyalos* glass], a substance in the granules found in keratinocytes of the epidermis.

keratolysis /ker′ətol′sis/ [Gk *keras* + *lysis* loosening], the loosening and shedding of the outer layer of the skin, which may occur normally by exfoliation or as a congenital condition in which the skin is shed at periodic intervals. **–keratolytic,** *adj.*

keratomalacia /ker′ətōməlā′shə/ [Gk *keras* + *malakia* softness], a condition, characterized by xerosis and ulceration of the cornea, resulting from severe vitamin A deficiency. Early symptoms include night blindness, photophobia, swelling and redness of the eyelids, and drying, roughness, pain, and wrinkling of the conjunctiva. In advanced deficiency, Bitot's spots appear, the cornea becomes dull, lusterless, and hazy, and, without adequate therapy, it eventually softens and perforates, resulting in blindness.

keratomycosis linguae. See **parasitic glossitis.**

keratopathy /ker′ətop′əthē/ [Gk *keras* + *pathos* disease], any noninflammatory disease of the cornea.

keratoplasty /ker′ətōplas′tē/ [Gk *keras* + *plassein* to mold], a procedure in ophthalmologic surgery in which an opaque portion of the cornea is excised.

keratosis /ker′ətō′sis/ [Gk *keras* + *osis* condition], any skin condition in which there is overgrowth and thickening of the cornified epithelium. Kinds of keratosis include **actinic keratosis, keratosis senilis,** and **seborrheic keratosis. –keratotic,** *adj.*

keratosis follicularis, a name of several skin disorders characterized by keratotic papules that coalesce to form brown or black, crusted, wartlike patches.

keratosis seborrheica. See **seborrheic keratosis.**

kerion /kir′ē·on/ [Gk, honeycomb], an inflamed, boggy granuloma that develops as an immune reaction to a superficial fungus infection, generally in association with *Tinea capitis* of the scalp.

Kerley lines /kur′lē/, (in radiology) lines resembling interstitial infiltrate that appear on chest x-ray images and are associated with certain disease conditions, such as congestive heart failure and pleural lymphatic engorgement.

KERMA, abbreviation for *kinetic energy released in the medium,* a quantity that describes the transfer of energy from a photon to a medium as the ratio of energy transferred per unit mass at each point of interaction.

kernicterus /kərnik'tərəs/ [Ger *Kern* kernel; Gk *ikteros* jaundice], an abnormal toxic accumulation of bilirubin in central nervous system tissues caused by hyperbilirubinemia.

Kernig's sign /ker'niks/ [Vladimir M. Kernig, Russian physician, b. 1840], a diagnostic sign for meningitis marked by a loss of the ability of a seated or supine patient to completely extend the leg when the thigh is flexed on the abdomen.

kerosene poisoning [Gk *keros* wax; L *potio* drink], a toxic condition caused by the ingestion of kerosene or the inhalation of its fumes. Symptoms after ingestion include drowsiness, fever, a rapid heartbeat, tremors, and severe pneumonitis if the fluid is aspirated. Vomiting is not induced.

ketamine hydrochloride /ke'təmēn/, a nonbarbiturate general anesthetic administered parenterally to achieve dissociative anesthesia. Ketamine hydrochloride is particularly useful for brief, minor surgical procedures and for the induction of inhalation anesthesia in pediatric, geriatric, and disturbed patients.

ketoacidosis /ke'tō·as'idō'sis/ [Gr *keton* form of acetone; L *acidus* sour, *osis* condition], acidosis accompanied by an accumulation of ketones in the body, resulting from faulty carbohydrate metabolism. It occurs primarily as a complication of diabetes mellitus and is characterized by a fruity odor of acetone on the breath, mental confusion, dyspnea, nausea, vomiting, dehydration, weight loss, and, if untreated, coma. Emergency treatment includes the administration of insulin and IV fluids and the evaluation and correction of electrolyte imbalance. –**ketoacidotic,** *adj.*

ketoaciduria /ke'tō·as'idoor'ē·ə/ [Gr *keton* + L *acidus* sour; Gk *ouron* urine], presence in the urine of excessive amounts of ketone bodies, occurring as a result of uncontrolled diabetes mellitus, starvation, or any other metabolic condition in which fats are rapidly catabolized. –**ketoaciduric,** *adj.*

11-ketoandrosterone /ke'tō-andros'tərōn/, a sex hormone, secreted by the testes and adrenal glands, that may be measured in the urine to assess hormonal and adrenal functions.

ketoconazole /ke'tōkō'nəzōl/, an antifungal agent prescribed for the treatment of candidosis, coccidioidomycosis, histoplasmosis, and other fungal diseases.

11-ketoetiocholanolone /ke'tō-ē'tē-ōkəlan'əlōn/, a sex hormone, secreted by the testes and adrenal glands, that may be measured in the urine to assess hormonal and adrenal functions.

ketogenesis /ke'tōjen'əsis/ [Gr *keton* + Gk *genein* to produce], the formation or production of ketone bodies.

ketogenic diet /ke'tōjen'ik/, a diet that is high in fats and low in carbohydrates.

ketone /ke'tōn/ [Gr *keton* a form of acetone], a general term for an organic chemical compound characterized by having in its structure a carbonyl, or keto, group, CO, attached to two alkyl groups. It is produced by oxidation of secondary alcohols.

ketone alcohol /ke'tōn/ [Gr *keton* + Ar *alkohl* essence], an alcohol containing the ketone group.

ketone bodies, the normal metabolic products, β-hydroxybutyric acid and aminoacetic acid, from which acetone may arise spontaneously. The two acids are products of lipid pyruvate metabolism, via acetyl-CoA in the liver, and are oxidized by the muscles.

ketone group, the chemical carbonyl group with attached hydrocarbons.

ketonemia /ke'tōnē'mē·ə/, the presence of ketones, mainly acetone, in the blood. It is characterized by the fruity breath odor of ketoacidosis.

ketonuria. See **ketoaciduria.**

ketoprofen /ke'tōprō'fən/, a nonsteroidal antiinflammatory drug with analgesic and antipyretic action. It is prescribed for the treatment of rheumatoid and osteoarthritis and related conditions.

ketose /ke'tōs/ [Gr *keton* + *glykys* sweet], the chemical form of a monosaccharide in which the carbonyl group is a ketone.

ketosis /kitō'sis/ [Gr *keton* + *glykys* sweet, *osis* condition], the abnormal accumulation of ketones in the body as a result of a deficiency or inadequate utilization of carbohydrates. Fatty acids are metabolized instead, and the end products, ketones, begin to accumulate. This condition is seen in starvation, occasionally in pregnancy, and, most frequently, in diabetes mellitus. It is characterized by ketonuria, loss of potassium in the urine, and a fruity odor of acetone on the breath. –**ketotic,** *adj.*

ketosis-prone diabetes. See **insulin-dependent diabetes mellitus.**

ketosis-resistant diabetes. See **non-insulin-dependent diabetes mellitus.**

17-ketosteroid /ketō'stəroid/, any of the adrenal cortical hormones, or ketosteroids, that has a ketone group attached to its seventeenth carbon atom, commonly measured in the blood and urine to aid the diagnoses of Addison's disease, Cushing's syndrome, stress, and endocrine problems associated with precocious puberty, femi-

K

nization in men, and excessive hair growth.

ketotic /kētot′ik/, **1.** pertaining to the presence of ketone in the body. **2.** denoting the presence of a carbonyl group in a chemical compound.

keV, an abbreviation for *kiloelectron volts,* an energy unit equivalent to 1,000 electron volts.

Kew Gardens spotted fever. See **rickettsialpox.**

key pinch. See **lateral pinch.**

key points of control, areas of the body that can be handled by a therapist in a specific manner to change an abnormal pattern to reduce spasticity throughout the body and to guide the patient's active movements. The key points are the shoulder and pelvic girdles.

key ridge, the lowest point of the zygomaticomaxillary ridge.

kg, abbreviation for **kilogram.**

kG, abbreviation for *kilogauss.*

kg cal, abbreviation for **kilogram calorie.**

kHz, abbreviation for **kilohertz.**

kidney [ME *kidnere*], one of a pair of bean-shaped urinary organs in the dorsal part of the abdomen, one on each side of the vertebral column, between the level of the twelfth thoracic vertebra, and the third lumbar vertebra. In most individuals the right kidney is more caudal than the left. Each kidney is about 11 cm long, 6 cm wide, and 2.5 cm thick. The kidneys produce and eliminate urine through a complex filtration network and reabsorption system comprising more than 2 million nephrons, composed of glomeruli and renal tubules that filter blood under high pressure, removing urea, salts, and other soluble wastes from blood plasma and returning the purified filtrate to the blood. More than 2,500 pints of blood pass through the kidneys every day.

kidney cancer, a malignant neoplasm of the renal parenchyma or renal pelvis. Factors associated with an increased incidence of disease are exposure to aromatic hydrocarbons or tobacco smoke and the use of drugs containing phenacetin. Characteristic symptoms include hematuria, flank pain, fever, and the detection of a palpable mass.

kidney dialysis. See **hemodialysis.**

kidney disease, any one of a large group of conditions including infectious, inflammatory, obstructive, vascular, and neoplastic disorders of the kidney. Characteristics of kidney disease are hematuria, persistent proteinuria, pyuria, edema, dysuria, and pain in the flank. Specific symptoms vary with the type of disorder. For example: hematuria with severe, colicky pain suggests obstruction by a kidney stone; hematuria without pain may indicate renal carcinoma; proteinuria is generally a sign of disease in the glomerulus, or filtration unit of the kidney; pyuria indicates infectious disease; and edema is characteristic of the nephrotic syndrome.

kidney failure, *informal.* renal failure.

kidney machine. See **artificial kidney, dialyzer.**

kidney stone. See **renal calculus.**

Kielland forceps. See **obstetric forceps.**

Kielland rotation /kē′land/ [Christian Kielland, Norwegian obstetrician, b. 1871], an obstetric operation in which Kielland forceps are used in turning the head of the fetus from an occiput posterior or occiput transverse position to an occiput anterior position.

Kiesselbach's plexus /kē′səlbäkhs′, -bäks′/, a convergence of small, fragile arteries and veins located superficially on the anterosuperior portion of the nasal septum.

killed vaccine [ME *killen*; L *vaccinus* of a cow], a vaccine prepared from dead microorganisms. Killed vaccines are generally used to provide immunization from organisms that are too virulent to be used in the living attenuated state. The immune system reacts to the presence of the pathogen in the same manner whether the organism is live or dead. However, immunity produced by a live, attenuated vaccine, when possible, is usually more effective.

killer cell. See **null cell.**

kilocalorie /kil′əkal′ərē/ [Gk *chilioi* thousand; L *calor* heat], a unit of heat equal to 1,000 small calories (c) or 4,186 joules.

kilogram (kg) /kil′əgram/ [Gk *chiiloi* + Fr *gramme*], a unit for the measurement of mass in the metric system. One kilogram is equal to 1,000 grams or to 2.2046 pounds avoirdupois.

kilogram calorie. See **calorie.**

kilohertz (kHz) /kil′əhurts/ [Gk *chilioi* + *hertz*; Heinrich Rudolf Hertz, German physicist, b. 1857], number of cycles per second, one thousand hertz.

kiloliter (kL) [Gk *chilioi* + Fr *litre*], unit of volume equivalent to 1.057 quarts, one thousand liters.

kilometer (km) [Gk *chilioi* + *metron*], measure equivalent to 39.37 inches, one thousand meters (approx. 0.62 miles).

kilovolt (kV), a unit of electric potential equal to 1,000 volts.

kilovolt peak (kVp), a measure of the maximum electrical potential in kilovolts across an x-ray tube.

Kimmelstiel-Wilson disease. See **intercapillary glomerulosclerosis.**

kinase /kī′nās/ [Gk *kinesis* motion, (ase) enzyme] **1.** an enzyme that catalyzes the transfer of a phosphate group or another high-energy molecular group to an acceptor molecule. **2.** an enzyme that activates a preenzyme (zymogen).

kind firmness, (in psychology) a direct, confident approach to a patient in which rules and regulations are calmly cited in response to infractions and requests.

kinematic face-bow /kin′əmat′ik/, an adjustable caliperlike device, used for precisely locating the axis of rotation of a mandible through the sagittal plane.

kinematics /kin′əmat′iks, kī-′/ [Gk *kinema* motion], (in physiology) the geometry of the motion of the body without regard to the forces acting to produce the motion. The most common types of motions studied in kinematics are flexion, extension, adduction, abduction, internal rotation, and external rotation. Kinematics is especially important in orthopedics and rehabilitation medicine. Also spelled **cinematics.**

kinesia /kīnē′zhə/ [Gk *kinein* to move], any feeling of nausea caused by the sensation of motion, as in sea sickness or car sickness.

kinesic behavior, nonverbal cues of communication that function to achieve and maintain bonds of attachments between people.

kinesics /kinē′siks/ [Gk *kinesis* motion], the study of body position and movement in relation to communication.

kinesiologic electromyography /kinē′-sē·ōloj′ik/, the study of muscle activity involved in body movements.

kinesiology /kīnē′sē·ol′əjē/, [Gk *kinesis* + *logos* science], the scientific study of muscular activity and of the anatomy, physiology, and mechanics of the movement of body parts.

kinesthesia /kin′esthē′zhə/ [Gk *kinein* to move, *aisthesis* feeling], the perception of one's own body parts, weight, and movement.

kinesthetic memory /kin′esthet′ik/, the recollection of movement, weight, resistance, and position of the body or parts of the body.

kinesthetic sense [Gk *kinesis* + L *sentire* to feel], an ability to be aware of muscular movement and position. By providing information through receptors about muscles, tendons, joints, and other body parts, the kinesthetic sense helps control and coordinate such activities as walking and talking.

kinetic analysis /kinet′ik/, analysis in which the change of the monitored parameter with time is related to concentration, such as change of absorbance per minute.

kinetic energy (ke) [Gk *kinesis* + *energeia*], the energy possessed by an object by virtue of its motion. Kinetic energy is expressed by the formula $E = 1/2mv^2$, where m represents the mass of the object and v is its velocity.

kinetic hallucination [Gk *kinesis* + L *allucinari* a wandering mind], a false perception of body movement, as an amputee may feel movement in a missing limb.

kinetic reflex [Gk *kinesis* + L *reflectere* to bend back], a postural response resulting from stimulation of the vestibular apparatus.

kinetics /kinet′iks, kī-/ [Gk *kinesis* + L *icus* like], (in physiology) the study of the forces that produce, arrest, or modify the motions of the body. Newton's laws are applicable to the forces produced by muscles of the body that act on joints. The reaction forces of the muscles contribute to the equilibrium and the motion of the body.

kinetochore. See **centromere.**

kinetotherapeutic bath /kinet′ōthur′-əpyŏŏ′tik/ [Gk *kinesis* + *therapeutike* medical practice; AS *baeth*], a bath in which underwater exercises are performed to strengthen weak or partially paralyzed muscles.

kin group, family members who are related genetically or by marriage.

kinky hair disease [Du *kink* short twist; AS *haer*; L *dis* + Fr *aise* ease], an inherited condition characterized by short, sparse, poorly pigmented hair with shafts that are twisted and broken. Other mental and physical disorders are usually associated with the disease.

kinomere. See **centromere.**

kinship model family group, a family unit comprising the biologic parents and their offspring. It is like a nuclear family but is more closely tied to an extended family.

Kirkland knife [Olin Kirkland, American dentist, b. 1876; AS *cnif*], a surgical knife with a heart-shaped blade, sharp on all edges, used for a primary gingivectomy incision.

Kirklin staging system, a system for determining the prognosis of colon cancer, based on the extent to which the tumor has penetrated the bowel area.

Kirschner's wire /kursh′nərz/ [Martin Kirschner, German surgeon, b. 1879; AS *wir*], a threaded or smooth metallic wire used in internal fixation of fractures or for skeletal traction.

Kite method, (in radiology) a technique for positioning the leg of a patient with congenital clubfoot for x-ray examination.

kiting /kī'ting/, *informal;* the improper and illegal practice of altering a drug prescription to indicate that more of a drug was prescribed than was actually ordered by the physician.

KJ, abbreviation for *knee jerk.*

kL, abbreviation for **kiloliter.**

Klebsiella /kleb'zē·el'ə/ [Theodore A. E. Klebs, German bacteriologist, b. 1834], a genus of diplococcal bacteria that appear as small, plump rods with rounded ends. Several respiratory diseases, including bronchitis, sinusitis, and some forms of pneumonia, are caused by infection by species of *Klebsiella.*

Klebsiella pneumoniae [Theodore Albrecht Edwin Klebs, German bacteriologist, b. 1834; Gk *pneumon* lung], a species of bacteria found in soil, water, cereal grains, and the intestinal tract of humans and other animals. It is associated with several pathologic conditions, including pneumonia.

Klebs-Loeffler bacillus /klebz'lef'lər/ [Theodore A. E. Klebs; Friederich A. J. Loeffler, German bacteriologist, b. 1852; L *bacillum* small rod], *Corynebacterium diphtheriae.*

kleeblattschädel deformity syndrome. See **cloverleaf skull deformity.**

Kleine-Levin syndrome /klīn'ləvēn'/ [Willi Kleine, twentieth-century German psychiatrist; Max Levin, twentieth-century American neurologist], a disorder of unknown cause often associated with psychotic conditions, characterized by episodic somnolence, abnormal hunger, and hyperactivity.

kleptolagnia /klep'tōlag'nē·ə/ [Gk *kleptein* to steal, *lagneia* lust], sexual excitement or gratification produced by stealing.

kleptomania /klep'tōmā'nē·ə/ [Gk *kleptein* + *mania* madness], a neurosis characterized by an abnormal, uncontrollable, and recurrent urge to steal. The objects, taken not for their monetary value, immediate need, or utility but because of a symbolic meaning usually associated with some unconscious emotional conflict, are usually given away, returned surreptitiously, or kept and hidden. **–kleptomaniac,** *n.*

Klinefelter's syndrome /klīn'feltərz/ [Harry F. Klinefelter, American physician, b. 1912], a syndrome of gonadal defects, appearing in males, with an extra X chromosome in at least one cell line. Characteristics are small, firm testes, long legs, gynecomastia, poor social adaptation, subnormal intelligence, chronic pulmonary disease, and varicose veins. The severity of the abnormalities increases with greater numbers of X chromosomes.

Klippel-Feil syndrome [Maurice Klippel, French neurologist, b. 1858; Andre Feil, French neurologist, b. 1884], a condition of short neck and limited neck movements because of congenital fusion of the cervical vertebrae.

Kloehn cervical extraoral orthodontic appliance, a cervical extraoral traction appliance for correcting or improving malocclusion.

Klumpke's palsy /kloomp'kez/, atrophic paralysis of the forearm. It is present at birth and involves the seventh and eighth cervical nerves and the first thoracic nerve. The condition may be accompanied by Horner's syndrome, ptosis, and miosis because of involvement of sympathetic nerves.

km, abbreviation for **kilometer.**

kneading /nē'ding/ [AS *cnedan*], a grasping, rolling, and pressing movement, as is used in massaging the muscles.

knee [AS *cneow*], a joint complex that connects the thigh with the lower leg. It consists of 3 condyloid joints, 12 ligaments, 13 bursae, and the patella.

knee-ankle interaction, one of the five major kinetic determinants of gait, which helps to minimize the displacement of the center of gravity of the body during the walking cycle. The knee and the foot work simultaneously to lower the center of gravity of the body. When the heel of the foot is in contact with the ground, the foot is dorsiflexed and the knee is fully extended so that the associated limb is at its maximum length with the center of gravity at its lower point.

kneecap. See **patella.**

knee-chest position. See **genupectoral position.**

knee-elbow position [AS *cneow, elboga*], a position in which a patient being examined rests on the knees and elbows with the head supported on the hands.

knee-hip flexion, one of the five major kinematic determinants of gait, which allows the passage of body weight over the supporting extremity during the walking cycle. Knee-hip flexion occurs during the stance and the swing phases of the cycle. The knee first locks into extension as the heel of the weight-bearing limb strikes the ground and is unlocked by final flexion and initiation of the swing phase in the walking cycle. Hip flexion is synchronized with these movements, which help to minimize the vertical displacement of the center of gravity of the body in the act of walking.

knee-jerk reflex. See **patellar reflex.**

knee joint, the complex, hinged joint at the knee, regarded as three articulations in one, comprising condyloid joints connecting the femur and the tibia and a partly arthrodial joint connecting the patella and the femur. The knee joint and its ligaments permit flexion, extension, and, in certain positions, medial and lateral rotation. It is a common site for sprain and dislocation.

knee replacement, the surgical insertion of a hinged prosthesis, performed to relieve pain and restore motion to a knee severely affected by osteoarthritis, rheumatoid arthritis, or trauma.

knee sling, a leg support in sling form used under the knee for Russell's traction.

knife needle [AS *cnif; naedl*], a slender surgical knife with a needle point, used in the discission of a cataract and in other ophthalmic procedures, such as goniotomy and goniopuncture.

knock-knee. See **genu valgum.**

Knoop hardness test /nō͞op/, a method of measuring tooth surface hardness by resistance to the penetration of an indenting tool made of diamond.

knot [AS *cnotta*], (in surgery) the interlacing of the ends of a ligature or suture so that they remain in place without slipping or becoming detached. The ends of the suture are passed twice around each other before being pulled taut to make a simple surgeon's knot.

knowledge deficit, a NANDA-accepted nursing diagnosis of a state in which specific information is lacking. Defining characteristics include a statement by the person that the knowledge deficit exists, or that there is a misconception concerning the information, an observed failure to follow through on instructions, the observation of an inadequate performance on a test, a request by the person for information, or the observation of inappropriate or exaggerated behavior.

Kocher's forceps /kō'kərz/ [Emil T. Kocher, Swiss surgeon, b. 1841], a kind of surgical forceps that has notched jaws, interlocking teeth, and thick, curved or straight, powerful handles.

Koch's bacillus /kōks/ [Robert Koch, German bacteriologist, b. 1843; L, *bacillum,* small rod], the *Mycobacterium tuberculosis* microorganism.

Koch's phenomenon [Robert Koch; Gk *phainomenon* anything seen], a tuberculin reaction that occurs when a culture of tubercle bacilli is injected into subjects already infected with the disease. In humans, a positive tuberculin reaction indicates sensitization due to a tuberculosis infection.

Koch's postulates [Robert Koch; L *postulare* to demand], the prerequisites for establishing that a specific microorganism causes a particular disease. The conditions are the following: (1) the microorganism must be observed in all cases of the disease; (2) the microorganism must be isolated and grown in pure culture; (3) microorganisms from the pure culture, when inoculated into a susceptible animal, must reproduce the disease; (4) the microorganism must be observed in and recovered from the experimentally diseased animal.

Koebner phenomenon /kōb'nər/ [Heinrich Koebner, Polish dermatologist, b. 1838; Gk *phainomenon* something observed], the development of isomorphic lesions at the site of an injury occurring in psoriasis, lichen nitidus, lichen planus, and verruca plana.

KOH, chemical symbol for **potassium hydroxide.**

Kohnstamm's phenomenon. See **aftermovement.**

koilonychia /koi'lōnik'ē-ə/ [Gk *koilos* hollow, *onyx* nail], spoon nails; a condition in which nails are thin and concave from side to side.

Kopan's needle /kō'pənz/, a long biopsy needle used to locate the position of a breast tumor on x-ray film.

Koplik's spots /kop'liks/ [Henry Koplik, American pediatrician, b. 1858], small red spots with bluish white centers on the lingual and buccal mucosa, characteristic of measles. The rash of measles usually erupts a day or two after the appearance of Koplik's spots.

Koranyi's sign /kôr'ənyēz/ [Friedrich von Korányi, Hungarian physician, b. 1828; L *signum*], a paravertebral area of dullness found posteriorly on the side opposite a pleural effusion.

Korotkoff sounds /kôrot'kôf/ [Nickolai Korotkoff, Russian physician, b. 1874], sounds heard during the taking of blood pressure using a sphygmomanometer and stethoscope. As air is released from the cuff, pressure on the brachial artery is reduced, and the blood is heard pulsing through the vessel.

Korsakoff's psychosis /kôr'səkôfs/ [Sergei S. Korsakoff, Russian psychiatrist, b. 1854], a form of amnesia often seen in chronic alcoholics, characterized by a loss of short-term memory and an inability to learn new skills. The person is usually disoriented and confabulates to conceal the condition.

kosher [Heb *kasher* fit or proper], pertaining to the preparation and serving of foods according to Jewish dietary laws. Inherently kosher foods include common fruits, vegetables, and cereals, as well as tea and coffee. Foods that are not kosher include pork, birds of prey, and seafood

K

that lacks fins and scales, such as lobster and eels. Some not inherently kosher foods can become kosher if properly processed; they include most domestic poultry and meat products, excluding pork.

Kr, symbol for the element **krypton.**

Krabbe's disease. See **galactosyl ceramide lipidosis.**

Kraske position /kras'kə/ [Paul Kraske, Swiss surgeon, b. 1851], an anatomic position in which the patient is prone, with hips flexed and elevated, head and feet down. The position is used for renal surgery.

kraurosis /krôrō'sis/ [Gk *krauros* dry, *osis* condition], a thickening and shriveling of the skin.

kraurosis vulvae, a skin disease of aged women characterized by dryness, itching, and atrophy of the external genitalia.

Krause's corpuscles [Wilhelm J. F. Krause, German anatomist, b. 1833; L *corpusculum* little body], a number of sensory end organs in the conjunctiva of the eye, mucous membranes of the lips and tongue, epineurium of nerve trunks, the penis, and the clitoris, and the synovial membranes of certain joints. Krause's corpuscles are tiny cylindric oval bodies. They contain a soft, semifluid core in which the axon terminates either in a bulbous extremity or in a coiled mass.

Krebs' citric acid cycle /krebz/ [Hans A. Krebs, English biochemist, b. 1900; Gk *kitron* citron; L *acidus* sour; Gk *kyklos* circle], a sequence of enzymatic reactions involving the metabolism of carbon chains of sugars, fatty acids, and amino acids to yield carbon dioxide, water, and high-energy phosphate bonds. The Krebs' cycle provides a major source of adenosine triphosphate energy and also produces intermediate molecules that are starting points for a number of vital metabolic pathways including amino acid synthesis.

Krebs-Henseleit cycle. See **urea cycle.**

Krukenberg's tumor /krōō'kənbərgz/ [Georg P. H. Krukenberg, German gynecologist, b. 1856], a neoplasm of the ovary that is a metastasis of a GI malignancy, usually stomach cancer.

KS, abbreviation for **Kaposi's sarcoma.**

KUB, abbreviation for *kidney, ureter, and bladder,* a term used in a radiographic examination to determine the location and size of the kidneys.

Kuchendorf method, (in radiology) a technique for positioning a patient for radiography of the patella.

Kufs' disease /kōōfs/ [H. Kufs, German psychiatrist, b. 1871], an adult form of hereditary cerebral sphingolipidosis (amaurotic familial idiocy), characterized by

cerebromacular degeneration, hypertonicity, and progressive spastic paralysis.

Kulchitsky cell carcinoma. See **carcinoid.**

Kulchitsky's cell. See **argentaffin cell.**

Kümmell's disease /kim'əlz/ [Herman Kummell, German surgeon, b. 1852], a set of symptoms that develops after a compression fracture of the vertebrae. They include spinal pain, intercostal neuralgia, kyphosis, and weakness in the legs.

Küntscher nail /kōōn'chər, kin'chər/ [Gerhard Küntscher, German surgeon, b. 1902; AS *naegel*], a stainless steel nail used in orthopedic surgery for the fixation of fractures of the long bones, especially the femur.

Kupffer's cells /kōōp'fərz/ [Karl W. von Kupffer, German anatomist, b. 1829], specialized cells of the reticuloendothelial system lining the sinusoids of the liver. They filter bacteria and other small, foreign proteins out of the blood.

kuru /kōō'rōō/ [New Guinea, trembling], a slow, progressive, fatal viral infection of the central nervous system observed in natives of the New Guinea highlands. Characteristics of kuru are ataxia and decreased coordination progressing to paralysis, dementia, slurring of speech, and visual disturbances. Incidence of the disease has declined with the decline of cannibalism.

Kussmaul breathing /kōōs'moul/ [Adolf Kussmaul, French physician, b. 1822; AS *braeth*], abnormally deep, very rapid sighing respirations characteristic of diabetic acidosis.

Kussmaul's coma [Adolf Kussmaul; Gk *koma* deep sleep], a diabetic coma characterized by acidosis and deep breathing or extreme hypernea.

Kussmaul's sign [Adolf Kussmaul; L *signum* mark], **1.** a paradoxical rise in venous pressure with distention of the jugular veins during inspiration, as seen in constrictive pericarditis or mediastinal tumor. **2.** conditions of convulsions and coma associated with a GI disorder caused by absorption of a toxic substance.

kv, abbreviation for **kilovolt.**

Kveim reaction [Morton A. Kveim, Norwegian physician, b. 1892; L *re* again, *agere* to act], a reaction used in a diagnostic test for sarcoidosis, based on an intradermal injection of antigen derived from a lymph node known to be sarcoid.

kVp, abbreviation for **kilovolt peak.**

kVp test cassette, (in radiology) a cassette containing a copper filter, a series of stepwedges, and an optical attenuator, used to test the accuracy of kVp settings for peak electrical potential across an x-ray tube.

kwashiorkor /kwä′shē·ôr′kôr/ [Afr], a malnutrition disease, primarily of children, caused by severe protein deficiency, usually occurring when the child is weaned from the breast. Characteristics include retarded growth, changes in skin and hair pigmentation, diarrhea, loss of appetite, nervous irritability, edema, anemia, fatty degeneration of the liver, necrosis, dermatoses, and fibrosis, often accompanied by infection and multivitamin deficiencies.

Kyasanur forest disease, an arbovirus infection transmitted by the bite of a tick that is harbored by shrews and other animals in India. Characteristics of the infection include fever, headache, muscle ache, cough, abdominal and eye pain, and photophobia.

kymography /kēmog′rəfē/ [Gk *kyma* wave, *graphein* to record], a technique for graphically recording motions of body organs, as of the heart and the great blood vessels.

kyphos /kī′fəs/ [Gk *kyphos* hunchback], the hump in the thoracic vertebral column that is associated with kyphosis.

kyphoscoliosis /kī′fōskō′lē·ō′sis/ [Gk *kyphos* + *skolios* curved, *osis* condition], an abnormal condition characterized by an anteroposterior curvature and a lateral curvature of the spine. **–kyphoscoliotic,** *adj.*

kyphosis /kīfō′sis/ [Gk *kyphos*], an abnormal condition of the vertebral column, characterized by increased convexity in the curvature of the thoracic spine as viewed from the side. Kyphosis may be caused by rickets or tuberculosis of the spine. **–kyphotic,** *adj.*

K

L, 1. symbol for *kinetic potential.* 2. abbreviation for ***Lactobacillus.*** 3. symbol for *lambert.* 4. abbreviation for *Latin.* 5. symbol for *liter.* 6. abbreviation for **lung.**

La, symbol for the element **lanthanum.**

LA, abbreviation for *left atrium.*

L & A, abbreviation for *reaction of the pupil to light accommodation.*

lab, abbreviation for **laboratory.**

label [ME, band], 1. a substance with a special affinity for an organ, tissue, cell, or microorganism in which it may become deposited and fixed. 2. the process of depositing and fixing a substance in an organ, tissue, cell, or microorganism. 3. an atom or molecule attached to either a ligand or binding protein and capable of generating a signal for monitoring in the binding reaction. 4. the process of attaching a radio isotope to a compound for the purpose of tracing it during a physiologic action in the body.

labeled compound, a chemical substance in which part of the molecules are labeled with a radionuclide so that observations of the radioactivity or isotopic composition make it possible to follow the compound through physical, chemical, or biological processes.

labeling, 1. the providing of information on a drug, food, device, or cosmetic to the purchaser or user. Regulations for labeling are provided by the Food and Drug Administration. 2. the assignment of a word or term to a form of behavior. 3. the act of classifying a patient according to a diagnostic category. Labeling can be misleading because not all cases conform to defined characteristics of standard diagnostic categories.

la belle indifference /läbeleNdifäräNs'/ [Fr, nice indifference], an air of unconcern displayed by some patients toward their physical symptoms. It is believed the physical symptoms may relieve anxiety and result in secondary gains in the form of sympathy or attention.

labetalol hydrochloride /ləbet'əlol/, an antihypertensive drug prescribed for the treatment of hypertension.

labia, *sing.* **labium** [L, lip], 1. the lips; the fleshy, liplike edges of an organ or tissue. 2. the folds of skin at the opening of the vagina.

labial bar /lā'bē·ə/, a major connector that is installed labial or buccal to the dental arch and joins bilateral parts of a mandibular removable partial denture.

labial flange, the part of a denture flange that occupies the labial vestibule of the mouth.

labial glands [L *labium* lip; *glans* acorn], small mucous or serous glands embedded in the lips.

labial notch, a depression in the denture border that accommodates the labial frenum.

labia majora /majôr'ə/, *sing.* **labium majus** /mā'jəs/, two long lips of skin, one on each side of the vaginal orifice outside the labia minora. The embryologic derivations of the labia majora and the scrotum are homologous.

labia minora /minôr'ə/, *sing.* **labium minus** /mē'nəs/, two folds of skin between the labia majora, extending from the clitoris backward on both sides of the vaginal orifice, ending between it and the labia majora.

labile /lā'bil/ [L *labilis* slipping], 1. unstable; characterized by a tendency to change or to be altered or modified. 2. (in psychiatry) characterized by rapidly shifting or changing emotions, as in bipolar disorder and certain types of schizophrenia; emotionally unstable. –**lability,** *n.*

labiodental /lā'bē·ōden'təl/ [L *labium* lip + *dens* tooth], 1. pertaining to the labial surfaces of the 12 anterior teeth. 2. in speech therapy, sounds of speech that require a special coordination of teeth and lips.

labioglossolaryngeal paralysis. See bulbar paralysis.

labiolingual fixed orthodontic appliance /lā'bē·ōling'gwəl/ [L *labium* lip, *lingua* tongue], an orthodontic appliance for correcting or improving malocclusion, characterized by anchorage to the maxillary and mandibular first permanent molars and by labial and lingual arches.

labium. See labia.

labium majus. See labia majora.

labium minus. See labia minora.

labor [L, work], the time and the processes that occur during parturition from the beginning of cervical dilatation to the delivery of the placenta.

labor, abnormal. See **dystocia.**

laboratory (lab) [L *laborare* to labor], **1.** a facility, room, building, or part of a building in which scientific research, experimentation, testing, or other investigative activities are carried out. **2.** of or pertaining to a laboratory.

laboratory core. See **core.**

laboratory diagnosis, a diagnosis arrived at after study of secretions, excretions, or tissue through chemical, microscopic, or bacteriologic means or by biopsy.

laboratory error, any error made by the personnel in a clinical laboratory in the performance of a test, in the interpretation of the data, or in reporting or recording the results.

laboratory medicine, the branch of medicine in which specimens of tissue, fluid, or other body substance are examined outside of the person, usually in the laboratory. Some fields of laboratory medicine are **chemistry, cytology, hematology, histology,** and **pathology.**

laboratory test, a procedure, usually conducted in a laboratory, that is intended to detect, identify, or quantify one or more significant substances, evaluate organ functions, or establish the nature of a condition or disease.

labor coach, a person who assists a woman in labor and delivery by closely attending to her emotional needs and by encouraging her to use properly the breathing patterns, concentration techniques, body positions, and massage techniques that were taught in a program of psychophysical preparation for childbirth. Usually, the coach is the father of the baby or a close friend of the mother.

labored breathing, abnormal respiration characterized by evidence of increased effort, including use of the accessory muscles of respiration of the chest wall, stridor, grunting, or nasal flaring.

labor pains [L *labor* work + *poena* penalty], pain associated with contraction of the uterus in labor.

labyrinth. See **internal ear.**

labyrinthine /lab'ərinthin/ [Gk *labyrinthos* maze], pertaining to or resembling a labyrinth or maze, such as the structure of the inner ear.

labyrinthine reflex. See **kinetic reflex.**

labyrinthine righting, one of the five basic neuromuscular reactions involved in a change of body positions. The change stimulates cells in the semicircular canals of the inner ear causing neck muscle to re-spond by automatically adjusting the head to the new position.

labyrinthitis [Gk *labyrinthos* maze, *itis*], inflammation of the labyrinthine canals of the inner ear, resulting in vertigo.

labyrinthus osseus. See **osseous labyrinth.**

laceration /las'ərā'shən/ [L *lacerare* to tear to pieces], **1.** the act of tearing or lacerating. **2.** a torn, jagged wound. **–lacerate,** *v.,* **lacerated,** *adj.*

laceration of cervix [L *lacerare; cervix* neck], a wound or irregular tear of the cervix uteri during childbirth.

laceration of the perineum [L *lacerare;* Gk *perineos*], a wound or irregular tear of the perineal tissues during childbirth.

lachrymal. See **lacrimal.**

lachrymation. See **lacrimation.**

lacrimal /lak'riməl/ [L *lacrima* tear], of or pertaining to tears.

lacrimal apparatus, a network of structures of the eye that secrete tears and drain them from the surface of the eyeball. These parts include the lacrimal glands, the lacrimal ducts, the lacrimal sacs, and the nasolacrimal ducts.

lacrimal bone, a small, fragile bone of the face, located at the anterior part of the medial wall of the orbit. It unites with the maxilla to form the lacrimal fossa, which contains the lacrimal duct.

lacrimal canaliculi. See **lacrimal duct.**

lacrimal caruncle, the small, reddish, fleshy protuberance that fills the triangular space between the medial margins of the upper and the lower eyelids.

lacrimal ducts, the two channels through which tears pass from the lacrimal lake to the lacrimal sac of each eye.

lacrimal fold [L *lacrima* tear; AS *fealdan*], a valvelike fold of mucous membrane at the lower part of the nasolacrimal duct.

lacrimal gland, one of a pair of glands situated superior and lateral to the eye bulb in the lacrimal fossa. The watery secretion from the gland consists of the tears, slightly alkaline and saline, that moisten the conjunctiva.

lacrimal papilla, the small conic elevation on the medial margin of each eyelid, supporting an apex pierced by the punctum lacrimale through which tears emerge to moisten the conjunctiva.

lacrimal reflex [L *lacrima; reflectere* to bend back], a release of tears in response to stimulation or irritation of the corneal conjunctiva.

lacrimal sac, the dilated end of each of the two nasolacrimal ducts. The lacrimal sacs fill with tears secreted by the lacrimal glands and conveyed through the lacrimal ducts.

lacrimation /lak′rimā′shən/, **1.** the normal continuous secretion of tears by the lacrimal glands. **2.** an excessive amount of tear production, as in crying or weeping.

lactalbumin /lak′təlbyōō′min/ [L *lac* milk, *albus* white], a simple, highly nutritious protein found in milk. It is similar to serum albumin.

lactam /lak′təm/, a cyclic amide created by the elimination of a molecule of water from aminocarboxylic acid.

lactase //lak′tās/ [L *lac* + Fr *diastase* enzyme], an enzyme that catalyzes the hydrolysis of lactose to glucose and galactose.

lactase deficiency, an inherited abnormality in which the amount of the enzyme lactase is deficient, resulting in the inability to digest lactose, except for the bacterial breakdown of lactose in the large intestine.

lactate /lak′tāt/, a salt of lactic acid.

lactate dehydrogenase (LDH), an enzyme that is found in the cytoplasm of almost all body tissues, where its main function is to catalyze the oxidation of L-lactate to pyruvate. It is assayed as a measure of anaerobic carbohydrate metabolism and as one of several serum indicators of myocardial infarction and muscular dystrophies.

lactation /laktā′shən/ [L *lac* milk, *atio* process], the process of the synthesis and secretion of milk from the breasts in the nourishment of an infant or child.

lacteal /lak′tē-əl/, of or pertaining to milk.

lacteal fistula, an abnormal passage opening into a lacteal duct.

lacteal vessel, one of the many central lymphatic capillaries in the villi of the small intestine. It opens into the lymphatic vessels in the submucosa. The capillary is filled with chyle that turns milky white during the absorption of fat.

lactic /lak′tik/ [L *lac* + *icus* like], referring to milk and milk products.

lactic acid, a three-carbon organic acid produced by anaerobic respiration. There are three forms: L-lactic acid in muscle and blood is a product of glucose and glycogen metabolism; D-lactic acid is produced by the fermentation of dextrose by a species of micrococcus; DL-lactic acid is a racemic mixture found in the stomach, in sour milk, and in certain other foods prepared by bacterial fermentation.

lactic acid fermentation, 1. the production of lactic acid from sugars by various bacteria. **2.** the souring of milk.

lactic acidosis, a disorder characterized by an accumulation of lactic acid in the blood, resulting in a lowered pH in muscle

and serum. The condition occurs most commonly in tissue hypoxia.

lactiferous /laktif′ərəs/ [L *lac* + *ferre* to bear], of or pertaining to a structure that produces or conveys milk, such as the tubules of the breasts.

lactiferous duct, one of many channels carrying milk from the lobes of each breast to the nipple.

lactiferous glands [L *lac* + *ferre*; *glans* acorn], glands that secrete or convey milk, such as mammary glands.

lactim. See **lactam.**

lactin. See **lactose.**

Lactobacillus /lak′tobäsi′əs/ [L *lac* + *bacillum* small rod], any one of a group of nonpathogenic, gram-positive, rod-shaped bacteria that produce lactic acid from carbohydrates.

Lactobacillus acidophilus [L *lac* + *bacillum; acidus* sour; Gk *philein* to love], a bacterium found in milk and dairy products, feces of bottlefed babies and some adults, saliva, and carious teeth. The strain is used to manufacture a fermented milk product.

lactogen /lak′təjən/ [L *lac* + Gk *genein* to produce], a drug or other substance that enhances the production and secretion of milk. –**lactogenic,** *adj.*

lactogenic hormone. See **prolactin.**

lacto-ovo-vegetarian /lak′tō-ov′ōvej′-əter′ē-ən/, one whose diet consists primarily of foods of vegetable origin but also includes some animal products, such as eggs (*ovo*), milk and cheese (*lacto*), but no meat, fish, or poultry.

lactose /lak′tōs/ [L *lac* + Gk *glykys* sweet], a disaccharide found in the milk of all mammals. On hydrolysis lactose yields the monosaccharides glucose and galactose.

lactose intolerance, a sensitivity disorder resulting in the inability to digest lactose because of a deficiency of or defect in the enzyme lactase. Symptoms of the disorder are bloating, flatus, nausea, diarrhea, and abdominal cramps.

lactosuria /lak′təsōōr′ē-ə/ [L *lac* + Gk *glykys* sweet, *ouron* urine], the presence of lactose in the urine, a condition that may occur in late pregnancy or during lactation.

lactotherapy [L *lac* + Gk *therapeia* treatment], any treatment that depends upon a diet consisting exclusively or nearly so of milk.

lacto-vegetarian, one whose diet consists of milk and milk products (*lacto*) in addition to foods of vegetable origin but does not include eggs, meat, fish, or poultry.

lactulose /lak′tyəlōs/, a nonabsorbable synthetic disaccharide, 4-0-β-D-galactopyranosyl-D-fructose, $C_{12}H_{22}O_{11}$. It is hydrolyzed in the colon by bacteria.

lacuna /ləkyo͞o′nə/, *pl.* **lacunae** [L, pit], **1.** a small cavity within a structure, especially bony tissue. **2.** a gap, as in the field of vision.

lacunar /ləkyo͞o′nər/ [L. *lacuna,* pit], pertaining to or characterized by the presence of pits, depressions, hollows, or spaces.

lacunar state, a pseudobulbar disorder characterized by the appearance of small, smooth-walled cavities in the brain tissue. The condition usually follows a series of small strokes, particularly in older adults with arterial hypertension and arteriosclerosis.

lacus lacrimalis /lā′kəs lak′rimā′ləs/ [L *lacus* lake; *lacrimalis* tears], a triangular space separating the medial ends of the upper and lower eyelids.

LAD, abbreviation for *left anterior descending.*

LADME /lad′mē/, an abbreviation for the time course of drug distribution, representing the terms *liberation, absorption, distribution, metabolism,* and *elimination.*

Laënnec's catarrh /lā′əneks′/ [Rene T. H. Laënnec, French physician, b. 1781; Gk *kata* down, *rhoia* flow], a form of bronchial asthma characterized by the discharge of small, round, viscous, beadlike bodies of sputum. These bodies, **Laënnec's pearls,** are formed in the bronchioles and appear in the asthmatic person's expectorated bronchial secretions.

Laënnec's cirrhosis [René T. H. Laënnec; Gk *kirrhos* yellow; *osis* condition], a fibrotic form of cirrhosis precipitated by alcohol abuse.

Laetrile /lā′ətril/, a substance composed primarily of amygdalin, a cyanogenic glycoside derived from apricot pits. Laetrile has been offered as a cancer medication despite clinical studies that failed to show benefits from its use.

LAF, abbreviation for **laminar air flow.**

lagophthalmos /lag′əfthal′məs/ [Gk *lagos* hare, *ophthalmos* eye], an abnormal condition in which an eye may not be fully closed because of a neurologic or muscular disorder.

lag phase [Dan *lakke* go slowly; Gk *phasis* appearance], a time span during which bacteria injected into a fresh medium have not begun to multiply although they may enlarge.

laity /lā′itē/ [Gk *laikos* of the people], a nonprofessional segment of the population, as viewed from the perspective of a member of a particular profession. A cler-

gyman may regard a physician as a member of the laity, and vice versa.

LAK, abbreviation for **lymphokine-activated killer cells.**

laked blood /lākt/ [Fr *laque* a deep red color], blood that is clear, red, and homogenous because of hemolysis of the red blood cells, as may occur in poisoning and severe, extensive burns.

La Leche League International /lälech′ā/, an organization that promotes and provides education about breastfeeding.

lallation /lalā′shən/ [L *lallare* to babble] **1.** babbling, repetitive, unintelligible utterances, like the babbling of an infant, and the mumbled speech of schizophrenics, alcoholics, and the severely mentally retarded. **2.** a speech disorder characterized by a defective pronunciation of words containing the sound /l/.

lalophobia /lal′ōfō′bē·ə/ [Gk *lalia* speech, *phobos,* fear], a morbid dread of talking caused by fear and anxiety that one will stammer or stutter.

lamarckism /ləmär′kizəm/ [Jean B. P. de Lamarck, French naturalist, b. 1744; Gk *ismos* practice], the theory postulated that organic evolution results from structural changes in plants and animals that are caused by adaptation to environmental conditions and that these acquired characteristics are transmitted to offspring. –**lamarckian,** *adj., n.*

Lamaze method /lämäz′/, a method of psychophysical preparation for childbirth developed in the 1950s by a French obstetrician, Fernand Lamaze. It requires classes, practice at home, and coaching during labor and delivery, often by a trained coach called a "monitrice." The classes, given during pregnancy, teach the physiology of pregnancy and childbirth, exercises to develop strength in the abdominal muscles and control of isolated muscles of the vagina and perineum, and techniques of breathing and relaxation to promote control and relaxation during labor. The kind and rate of breathing changes with the advancing stages of labor.

lambda /lam′də/, **1.** the eleventh letter of the Greek alphabet. **2.** a posterior fontanel of the skull marking the point where the sagittal and lambdoidal sutures meet.

lambda chain, one of the immunoglobulin light chains.

lambdacism /lam′dəsiz′əm/ [Gk *lambda* + *ismos* practice], a speech disorder characterized by a defective pronunciation of words containing the sound /l/, or by the excessive use of the sound, or by the substitution of the sound /r/ for /l/.

L

lambdoid /lam'doid/, having the shape of the Greek letter lambda.

lambdoidal suture /lamdoi'dəl/, the serrated connection between the occipital bone and the parietal bones of the skull.

lamella /ləmel'ə/, *pl.* **lamellae** [L, small plate] **1.** a thin leaf or plate, as of bone. **2.** a medicated disk, prepared from glycerin and an alkaloid, for insertion under the eyelid, where it dissolves and is absorbed. –**lamellar,** *adj.*

lamellar exfoliation of the newborn [L *lamella* + *ex* without, *folium* leaf; AS *niwe* new, *boren* born], a congenital skin disorder transmitted as an autosomal recessive trait in which a parchmentlike, scaly membrane that covers the infant peels off within 24 hours of birth.

lameness [ME *lama* to break], a condition of being crippled or disabled, particularly because of a foot or leg injury. The term may also applied to a stiff or painful back that makes walking difficult.

lamina /lam'inə/, *pl.* **laminae** [L, plate], any thin, flat layer of membrane or other tissue. It may be structureless or part of a structure, as the laminae of the vertebral arch.

lamina dura, a sheet of compact alveolar bone that lies adjacent to the periodontal membrane.

lamina propria, a layer of connective tissue that lies just under the epithelium of the mucous membrane.

laminar air flow (laf) /lam'inər/ [L *lamina;* Gk *aer;* AS *flowan*], a system of circulating filtered air in parallel flow planes in hospitals or other health care facilities. The system reduces the risk of bacterial contamination or exposure to chemical pollutants in surgical theaters, food preparation areas, hospital pharmacies, and laboratories.

laminaria /lam'iner'ē·ə/ [L *lamina* plate], a type of seaweed that swells on absorption of water.

laminaria tent, a cone of dried seaweed that swells as it absorbs water and therefore is used to dilate the cervix nontraumatically in preparation for induced abortion or induced labor.

laminated thrombus, a thrombus composed of an aggregation of blood platelets, fibrin, clotting factors, and cellular elements, arranged in layers apparently formed at different times.

laminectomy /lam'inek'təmē/ [L *lamina* + Gk *ektome* excision], surgical removal of the bony arches of one or more vertebrae, performed to relieve compression of the spinal cord, as caused by a bone displaced in an injury or as the result of degeneration of a disk, or to reach and remove a displaced intervertebral disk. Spinal fusion may be necessary for stability of the spine if several laminae are removed. –**laminectomize,** *v.*

lampbrush chromosome [Gk *lampas* torch; AS *bryst* bristle], an excessively large type of chromosome found in the oocytes of many lower animals. It has a hairy, brushlike appearance.

lance [L *lancea* spear], to incise a furuncle or an abscess to release accumulated pus.

Lancefield's classification [Rebecca C. Lancefield, American bacteriologist, b. 1895], a serologic classification of streptococci based on their antigenic characteristics. The bacteria are divided into 13 groups by the identification of their pathologic action.

lancet /lan'sit/ [Fr *lancette*], a short pointed blade used to obtain a drop of blood for a capillary sample.

lancinating /lan'sinā'ting/ [L *lancinare* to tear to pieces], sharply cutting or tearing, such as lancinating pain.

Landau reflex /lan'dou/, a normal response of infants when held in a horizontal prone position to maintain a convex arc with the head raised and the legs slightly flexed.

landmark position [AS *land, meark* mark; L *positio*], the correct placement of the hands on the chest in cardiopulmonary resuscitation.

Landouzy-Déjérine muscular dystrophy. See **facioscapulohumeral muscular dystrophy.**

Landsteiner's classification /land'stī'nərz/ [Karl Landsteiner, American pathologist, b. 1868], the classification of blood groups A, B, AB, and O on the basis of the presence or absence of the two agglutinogens A and B on the erythrocytes in human blood.

Langer's line. See **cleavage line.**

Langhans' layer. See **cytotrophoblast.**

language [L *lingua* tongue], a defined set of characters that when used alone or in combinations form a meaningful set of words and symbols.

lanolin /lan'əlin/ [L *lana* wool, *oleum* oil], a fatlike substance from the wool of sheep. It contains about 25% water as a water-in-oil emulsion and is used as an ointment base and an emollient for the skin.

lanthanum (La) /lan'thənəm/ [Gk *lanthanein* to escape notice], a rare earth metallic element. Its atomic number is 57; its atomic weight is 138.91.

lanugo /lanyōō'gō/ [L, down], **1.** the soft, downy hair covering a normal fetus, beginning with the fifth month of life and almost entirely shed by the ninth month.

2. the fine, soft hair covering all parts of the body except palms, soles, and areas where other types of hair are normally found. **–lanuginous,** *adj.*

lanulous /lan′yo͞oləs/ [L *lana* wool, *osus* filled with], downy or covered with short, fine wooly hair, such as the skin of a fetus.

lap, 1. abbreviation for **laparotomy.** **2.** abbreviation for *left atrial pressure.*

laparoenterostomy /lap′ərō·en′təros′təmē/ [Gk *lapara* loin; *enteron* bowel; *stoma* mouth], the surgical installation of a tube through an external opening in the abdomen in order to drain the bowel. A similar procedure may be used to supply nutrients to a patient with an upper digestive tract obstruction.

laparohysterectomy /lap′ərōhis′tərek′-təmē/ [Gk *lapara* + *hystera* womb + *ektome* excision], a hysterectomy performed by making an excision through the abdominal wall.

laparoscope /lap′ərəskōp′/ [Gk *lapara* loin, *skopein* to look], a type of endoscope, consisting of an illuminated tube with an optical system, that is inserted through the abdominal wall for examining the peritoneal cavity. **–laparoscopic,** *adj.,* **laparoscopy,** *n.*

laparoscopic sterilization [Gk *lapara* + *skopein*; L *sterilis* barren], the process of rendering a woman incapable of reproduction by inserting a specialized endoscope through a small incision in the abdominal wall. Sterilization may be performed through the incision with clips to occlude the fallopian tubes or by electrocoagulation and severance.

laparoscopy /lap′əros′kəpē/, the examination of the abdominal cavity with a laparoscope through a small incision in the abdominal wall.

laparotomy (lap) /lap′ərot′əmē/ [Gk *lapara* + *temnein* to cut], any surgical incision into the peritoneal cavity, usually performed under general or regional anesthesia, often on an exploratory basis. Some kinds of laparotomy are **appendectomy, cholecystectomy,** and **colostomy.** **–laparotomize,** *v.*

lap-board [ME *lappa* + *bord* plank], a flat board placed over the lap to serve as a temporary desk or table.

Laplace's law /läpläs′/ [Pierre Simon Marquis de Laplace, French physicist, b. 1749], a principle of physics that the tension on the wall of a sphere is the product of the pressure times the radius of the chamber and the tension is inversely related to the thickness of the wall.

large calorie. See **calorie.**

large-for-gestational age (LGA) infant, an infant whose fetal growth was accelerated and whose size and weight at birth fall above the 90th percentile of appropriate-for-gestational age infants, whether delivered prematurely, at term, or later than term. Factors other than genetic influences that cause accelerated intrauterine growth include maternal diabetes mellitus and Beckwith's syndrome.

large intestine [L *largus* abundant, *intestinum*], the portion of the digestive tract comprising the cecum, appendix, the ascending, transverse, and descending colons, and the rectum.

lariat structure /ler′ē·ət/, a ring of intron segments that have been spliced out of an mRNA molecule by enzymes. Some introns form a long tail attached to the ring, giving the structure the appearance of a microscopic cowboy lariat.

Larmor frequency [Sir Joseph Larmor, Irish physicist, b. 1857], the frequency of the precession of a charged particle when its motion comes under the influence of an applied magnetic field and a central force.

larva /lär′və/ [L, specter], the early immature form of an animal, which undergoes metamorphosis to assume an adult form.

larva migrans. See **cutaneous larva migrans, visceral larva migrans.**

laryngeal cancer /lerin′jē·əl/ [Gk *larynx* + L *cancer* crab], a malignant neoplastic disease characterized by a tumor arising from the epithelium of the structures of the larynx. Chronic alcoholism and heavy use of tobacco increase the risk of developing the cancer. Persistent hoarseness is usually the first sign; advanced lesions may cause a sore throat, dyspnea, dysphagia, and unilateral cervical adenopathy.

laryngeal catheterization, the insertion of a catheter into the larynx for the purpose of removing secretions or introducing gases.

laryngeal polyp [Gk *larynx* + *poly* many + *pous* foot], a polyp on the vocal cords due to vocal abuse or smoking that causes hoarseness.

laryngeal prominence. See **Adam's apple.**

laryngeal reflex [Gk *larynx*; L *reflectere* to bend back], a cough reflex caused by irritation of the fauces and larynx.

laryngeal vertigo [Gk *larynx*; L *vertere* to turn], a short episode of dizziness or unconsciousness following a paroxysmal attack of coughing or laryngeal spasm.

laryngectomy /ler′injek′təmē/ [Gk *larynx* + *ektome* excision], surgical removal of the larynx, performed to treat cancer of the larynx. **–laryngectomize,** *v.*

laryngismus /ler´injiz´məs/ [Gk *laryngismos* whooping], spasm of the larynx.
Laryngismus stridulus, a condition characterized by sudden laryngeal spasm with a crowing sound on inspiration and the development of cyanosis, occurs in inflammation of the larynx, in connection with rickets, and as an independent disease.

laryngitis /ler´inji´tis/ [Gk *larynx* + *itis*], inflammation of the mucous membrane lining the larynx, accompanied by edema of the vocal cords with hoarseness or loss of voice, occurring as an acute disorder caused by a cold, by irritating fumes, by sudden temperature changes, or as a chronic condition resulting from excessive use of the voice, heavy smoking, or exposure to irritating fumes. In acute laryngitis, there may be a cough, and the throat usually feels scratchy and painful.

laryngocele /ləring´gōsēl´/, an abnormal air-containing cavity connected to the laryngeal ventricle. It is caused by an evagination of the mucous membrane of the ventricle and may displace and enlarge the false vocal cord, resulting in hoarseness and airway obstruction. Because a laryngocele is also a potential reservoir of infection, it is usually excised.

laryngography. See **laryngopharyngography.**

laryngol, abbreviation for **laryngology.**

laryngology /ler´ing·gol´əjē/ [Gk *larynx* + *logos* science], a branch of medicine that specializes in the causes and treatments of disorders of the larynx.

laryngopharyngitis /ləring´gōfer´inji´tis/ [Gk *larynx* + *pharynx* throat, *itis*], inflammation of the larynx and pharynx.

laryngopharyngography /lering´gōfer´ingog´rəfē/ [Gk *larynx, pharynx* + *graphein* to record], the radiographic examination of the larynx and the pharynx.

laryngopharynx /lering´gōfer´ingks/ [Gk *larynx* + *pharynx* throat], one of the three regions of the throat, extending from the hyoid bone to the esophagus. —**laryngopharyngeal** /lering´gōferin´jē·əl/, *adj.*

laryngoscope /ləring´gəskōp´/, an endoscope for examining the larynx.

laryngoscopic, pertaining to the use of a laryngoscope.

laryngoscopy [Gk *larynx* + *skopein* to view], the use of a laryngoscope to view the larynx.

laryngospasm /ləring´gōspaz´əm/ [Gk *larynx* + *spasmos* spasm], a spasmodic closure of the larynx.

laryngostasis. See **croup.**

laryngotomy /ler´ing·got´əmē/ [Gk *larynx* + *temnein* to cut], a surgical incision into the larynx through the cricovocal membrane. It is usually an emergency procedure that is performed when a standard tracheotomy cannot be done.

laryngotracheobronchitis (LTB) /lering´gōtrā´kēōbrongkī´tis/ [Gk *larynx* + L *tractus* trachea; Gk *bronchos* windpipe, *itis*], an inflammation of the major respiratory passages, usually causing hoarseness, nonproductive cough, and dyspnea.

larynx /ler´ingks/ [Gk], the organ of voice that is part of the air passage connecting the pharynx with the trachea. The larynx forms the caudal portion of the anterior wall of the pharynx and is lined with mucous membrane that is continuous with that of the pharynx and the trachea. It is composed of three single cartilages and three paired cartilages, connected by ligaments and moved by various muscles. —**laryngeal,** *adj.*

LAS, abbreviation for **lymphadenopathy syndrome.**

laser /lā´zər/, acronym for *light amplification by stimulated emission of radiation,* a source of intense radiation of the visible, ultraviolet, or infrared portions of the spectrum. Lasers are used in surgery to divide or to cause adhesions or to destroy or to fix tissue in place.

laser bronchoscopy, bronchoscopy that is performed with the aid of a carbon dioxide laser beam directed through fiberoptic equipment in the diagnosis and treatment of bronchial disorders.

Lassa fever /lä´sə/ [Lassa, Nigeria; L *febris* fever], a highly contagious disease caused by a virulent arenavirus. It is characterized by fever, pharyngitis, dysphagia, and ecchymoses. Pleural effusion, edema, renal involvement, mental disorientation, confusion, and death from cardiac failure often ensue.

last sacraments [ME *laste;* L *sacramentum* solemn oath], a religious ceremony performed by a member of the clergy in behalf of a person about to die.

latchkey children, minors who are often at home alone because their parents are at work. They carry a key to their home and are more likely to become involved in accidents or antisocial behavior than children who are supervised by adults when not in school.

late dyspituitary eunuchism. See **acromegalic eunuchoidism.**

latency period /lā´tənsē/ [L *latere* to keep out of sight; Gk *peri* + *hodos* way], **1.** the period between contact with a pathogen and development of symptoms. **2.** the period between stimulus and response. **3.** a period between early childhood and puberty when there is little overt interest in the opposite sex.

latency stage [L *latere* to be concealed; Fr

estage stage], (in psychoanalysis) a period in psychosexual development occurring between early childhood and puberty when sexual motivation and expression are repressed or transferred, through sublimation, to the feelings and behavioral patterns expected as typical of the age.

latent /lā′tənt/ [L *latere* to be concealed], dormant; existing as a potential; for example, tuberculosis may be latent for extended periods and become active under certain conditions.

latent carcinoma. See **occult carcinoma.**

latent diabetes. See **impaired glucose tolerance, previous abnormality of glucose tolerance.**

latent energy, the energy contained in an object because of its position in space, internal structure, and stresses imposed on it.

latent heat [L *latere*; AS *haetu*], the heat absorbed by a substance when it changes from a solid to a liquid, or from a liquid to a gas without an accompanying rise in temperature.

latent image, (in radiology), an invisible image produced in the x-ray film emulsion by x-rays or visible light that can be converted to a visible image by development.

latent learning, learning acquired unintentionally. It may remain in the subconscious, or latent, until a need for it arises.

latent malaria, a continuing infection without clinical symptoms due to a balance established between the parasite and the body's immune system.

latent period, (in radiology) an interval of seeming inactivity between the time of exposure to an injurious dose of radiation and the response.

latent phase, the early stage of labor that is characterized by irregular, infrequent, and mild contractions and little or no dilatation of the cervix or descent of the fetus.

latent syphilis, a stage of infection in which no clinical symptoms appear but serologic tests indicate the presence of the syphilis spirochete.

latent tetany, a form of tetany that is elicited only by mechanical or electrical stimulus.

lateral /lat′ərəl/ [L *latus* side], **1.** on the side. **2.** away from the midsagittal plane. **3.** farther from the midsagittal plane. **4.** to the right or left of the midsagittal plane.

lateral abdominal region. See **lateral region.**

lateral aortic node, a lumbar lymph node in any of three clusters of nodes serving the pelvis and abdomen.

lateral aperture of the fourth ventricle, an opening between the end of each lat-

eral recess of the fourth ventricle and the subarachnoid space.

lateral cerebral sulcus, a deep cleft marking the division of the temporal, frontal, and parietal lobes of brain.

lateral condensation method, a technique for filling and sealing tooth root canals. A preselected gutta-percha cone is sealed into the apex of the root; other cones are forced laterally with a spreader until the canal is filled.

lateral cuneiform bone, one of the three cuneiform bones of the foot, located in the center of the front row of tarsal bones.

lateral decentering, (in radiology) an error in positioning of a focused grid, resulting in partial grid cutoff over the entire film. The error may also be a result of improperly positioning the tube head rather than the grid.

lateral geniculate body, one of two elevations of the lateral posterior thalamus receiving visual impulses from the retina via the optic nerves and tracts and relaying the impulses to the calcarine cortex.

lateral humeral epicondylitis, inflammation of the tissue at the lower end of the humerus at the elbow joint, caused by the repetitive flexing of the wrist against resistance. It may result from athletic activity or manual manipulation of tools or other equipment.

lateral incisal guide angle, (in dentistry) the inclination of the incisal guide in the frontal plane.

laterality. See **handedness.**

lateralization /lat′ərəl·īzā′shən/, the tendency for certain processes to be more highly developed on one side of the brain than the other, such as development of spatial and musical thoughts in the right hemisphere and verbal and logical processes in the left hemisphere in most persons.

lateral lobes of thyroid gland [L *latus* side; Gk *lobos*; *thyreos* shield; L *glans* acorn], the left and right lobes of a highly vascular thyroid gland situated in front of the neck. The two conical lobes lying on either side of and attached to the larynx are connected by a narrow isthmus.

lateral nystagmus [L *latus*; Gk *nystagmos* nodding], an involuntary jerky movement in which the eyes move from side to side.

lateral pectoral nerve, one of a pair of branches from the brachial plexus that, with the medial pectoral nerve, supplies the pectoral muscles.

lateral pelvic displacement, one of the five major kinetic determinants of gait. It helps to synchronize the rhythmic movements of walking and is produced by the horizontal shift of the pelvis or by relative hip abduction.

lateral pinch, a grasp in which the thumb is opposed to the middle phalanx of the index finger.

lateral projection, (in radiology) a position of a patient between the x-ray tube and the film cassette so the beam will travel from the left to the right side of the body, or vice versa.

lateral recumbent position, the posture assumed by the patient lying on the left side with the right thigh and knee drawn up.

lateral region, the part of the abdomen in the middle zone on both sides of the umbilical region.

lateral resolution, (in ultrasonography) the resolution of objects in a plane perpendicular to the axis of the beam. It is a measure of the ability of the system to detect closely separated objects such as adjacent blood vessels.

lateral rocking, a sideways rocking of the body used to move the body forward or backward used when normal muscle action is not possible. The technique is used by some disabled patients to move the body to or from the edge of a chair or to a different sitting position on a bed.

lateral rotation, a turning away from the midline of the body.

lateral sinus [L *latus; sinus* hollow], one of the transverse bilateral sinuses of the dura mater that lie along the attached margin of the tentorium cerebelli. They receive the superior sagittal and straight sinuses and drain into the internal jugular veins.

lateral spinal curvature [L *latus; spina* backbone; *curvatura* bend], a bending or abnormal curve of the vertebral column to the right or left side.

lateral umbilical fold, a fold in the peritoneum produced by a slight protrusion of the inferior epigastric artery and the interfoveolar ligament.

lateral ventricle [L *latus; ventriculum*], a cavity in each cerebral hemisphere that communicates with the third ventricle through the interventricular foramen.

late rickets [Gk *rhachis* backbone], a form of rickets in which bone changes caused by a kidney defect result in a vitamin D or calcium deficiency. The disorder tends to affect older children.

latex [L, liquid], an emulsion or fluidlike sap produced in special cells or vessels of certain plants. Latex contains resins, proteins, and other substances and is a source of rubber.

latex fixation test [L *latex* fluid; *figere* to fasten], a serologic test used in the diagnosis of rheumatoid arthritis in which antigen-coated latex particles agglutinate with rheumatoid factors in a slide specimen of serum or synovial fluid.

Lathrop, Rose Hawthorne (1851–1926), a daughter of Nathaniel Hawthorne, who founded the order of sisters called Servants of Relief for Incurable Cancer. The order founded hospitals wherever there was sufficient need and offered quality care to their patients.

latissimus dorsi /latis′iməs dôr·sī/ [L, widest; *dorsum* the back], one of a pair of large triangular muscles on the thoracic and lumbar areas of the back. It extends, adducts, and rotates the arm medially; draws the shoulder back and down; and, with the pectoralis major, draws the body up when climbing.

latitude [L *latitudinis* breadth], the ability of an x-ray imaging system to produce acceptable images over a range of exposures. If a system has wide latitude, it is possible to image parts of the body that vary in thickness or density with only one exposure.

LATS, abbreviation for **long-acting thyroid stimulator.**

LATS-P, abbreviation for *long-acting thyroid stimulator protector.*

lattice formation [OFr *lattis* geometric design], a three-dimensional, cross-linked structure formed by the reaction of multivalent antigens with antibodies.

Lauenstein method, (in radiology) a technique for positioning a patient in order to x-ray the hip joint with emphasis on the relationship of the femur to the acetabulum. The knee of the affected leg is flexed and the thigh is drawn up to a near right angle.

laughing gas, *informal;* nitrous oxide, a side effect of which is laughter or giggling when administered in less than anesthetizing amounts.

Laurence-Moon-Bardet-Biedl syndrome /lôr′ənsm o͞on′bärdā′bē′dəl/ [John Z. Laurence, English ophthalmologist, b. 1830; Robert C. Moon, American ophthalmologist, b. 1844; Georges Bardet, French physician, b. 1885; Artur Biedl, Czechoslovakian physician, b. 1869], an abnormal condition characterized by obesity, hypogenitalism, mental deficiency, polydactylism, and retinitis pigmentosa.

lavage /ləväzh′/ [Fr, washing], **1.** the process of washing out an organ, usually the bladder, bowel, paranasal sinuses, or stomach for therapeutic purposes. **2.** to perform a lavage. Kinds of lavage are **blood lavage, gastric lavage,** and **peritoneal dialysis.**

law [AS *lagu*], **1.** (in a field of study) a

rule, standard, or principle that states a fact or a relationship between factors, such as Dalton's law regarding partial pressures of gas. **2.** a rule, principle, or regulation established and promulgated by a government to protect or to restrict the people affected.

Law method, (in radiology) any of several techniques for positioning a patient for x-ray examination of the facial bones, sinuses, and relationship of the teeth to the jaw bones.

law of definite composition, (in chemistry) a law stating that a given compound is always made of the same elements present in the same proportion.

law of dominance, formerly considered as a separate principle of Mendel's laws of inheritance, but in modern genetics it is incorporated as part of the first Mendelian law, the law of segregation.

law of independent assortment, law of segregation. See **Mendel's laws.**

law of universal gravitation, (in physics) a law stating that the force with which bodies are attracted to each other is directly proportional to the masses of the objects and inversely proportional to the square of the distance by which they are separated.

lawrencium (Lw) /lôren'sē·əm/ [Ernest O. Lawrence, American physicist, b. 1901], a synthetic transuranic metallic element. Its atomic number is 103; its atomic weight is 257.

lax, 1. abbreviation for **laxative. 2.** a condition of relaxation or looseness.

laxative (lax) [L *laxare* to loosen], **1.** of or pertaining to a substance that causes evacuation of the bowel by a mild action. **2.** a laxative agent that promotes bowel evacuation by increasing the bulk of the feces, by softening the stool, or by lubricating the intestinal wall.

lay referral system, an illness referral system through which a person passes from the first recognition of an abnormality to an announcement to the family, to members of the community, then to traditional or culturally recognized healers, and then to the regular medical system that includes nurses and physicians. Depending on the culture and the medical care available, some steps may be omitted.

lazy colon. See **atonia constipation.**

lazy leukocyte syndrome, an immunodeficiency disease of children characterized by recurrent stomatitis, gingivitis, otitis media, and low-grade fever with severe neutropenia.

lb [L, *libra pondo*], symbol for **pound** in weight.

lb ap, abbreviation for *apothecary pound.*

lb avdp, abbreviation for *avoirdupois pound.*

LBBB, abbreviation for *left bundle branch block.*

LBW, abbreviation for *low birth weight.*

lb cal, abbreviation for *pound calorie.*

lbd, abbreviation for *lower back disorder.*

lbf, abbreviation for *pound-force.*

lbf/ft², abbreviation for *pound-force per square foot.*

lbf/in², abbreviation for *pound-force per square inch.*

lbm, abbreviation for **lean body mass.**

lbp, 1. abbreviation for *lower back pain.* **2.** abbreviation for *low blood pressure.*

L-carnitine /elkär'nitēn/, an oral drug prescribed for the treatment of primary systemic carnitine deficiency.

LCAT, abbreviation for *lecithin-cholesterol acetyltransferase.*

LCBF, abbreviation for **local cerebral blood flow.**

LCMRG, abbreviation for **local cerebral metabolic rate of glucose utilization.**

LD, abbreviation for *lethal dose.*

LD50, (in toxicology) the amount of a substance sufficient to kill one half of the population of test subjects.

LDH, abbreviation for **lactate dehydrogenase.**

LDL, abbreviation for **low-density lipoprotein.**

L-dopa. See **levodopa.**

le, abbreviation for *left eye.*

LE, abbreviation for **lupus erythematosus.**

lead (Pb) /led/ [ME *leed*], a common soft, blue-gray metallic element. Its atomic number is 82; its atomic weight is 207.19. In its metallic form, lead is used as a protective shielding against x-rays. Lead is also poisonous, a characteristic that has led to a reduction in the use of lead compounds.

lead /lēd/ [As *laedan* to lead], an electric connection attached to the body to record electric activity, especially of the heart or brain.

lead apron /led/ [AS *led;* Fr *napperon*], a protective shield of lead and rubber that may be worn by a patient, radiologic technician or radiologist, or both, during exposure to x-rays or other diagnostic or therapeutic radiation. It is intended to guard against excessive exposure of the genitalia and other vital body organs to ionizing radiation.

lead encephalopathy /led/ [AS *led;* Gk *enkephalos* brain; *pathos* disease], a condition of brain structure and function as a result of lead poisoning, including exposure to tetraethyl lead. Children are commonly afflicted after eating chips of lead-based

L

paints. The untreated disorder is characterized by delirium, convulsions, mania, cortical blindness, and coma.

lead equivalent /led/, (in radiology) the thickness of lead required to achieve the same shielding effect against radiation, under specified conditions, as that provided by a given material.

leadership [AS *leadan* to lead, *scieppan* to shape], the ability to influence others to the attainment of goals.

lead pipe fracture /led/, a fracture that compresses the bony tissue at the point of impact and creates a linear fracture on the opposite side of the bone involved.

lead poisoning /led/, a toxic condition caused by the ingestion or inhalation of lead or lead compounds. Poisoning also occurs from the ingestion of water from lead pipes, lead salts in certain foods and wines, the use of pewter or earthenware glazed with a lead glaze, and the use of leaded gasoline. Inhalation of lead fumes is common in industry. The acute form of intoxication is characterized by a burning sensation in the mouth and esophagus, colic, constipation, or diarrhea, mental disturbances, and paralysis of the extremities, followed in severe cases by convulsions and muscular collapse. Chronic lead poisoning is characterized by extreme irritability, anorexia, and anemia. Encephalopathy must be anticipated in children with lead poisoning.

lead shielding /led/, the use of aprons and other devices containing lead as protective measures against radiation. A layer of lead 1.0 mm in thickness should attenuate 99% of x-rays of 50 kVp and 94% of x-rays of 100 kVp.

leakage radiation [ONorse *leka* to drip; L *radiare* to emit rays], radiation, exclusive of the primary beam, that is emitted through the housing of equipment used in radiation therapy.

leaky gene. See **hypomorph.**

lean body mass (lbm) [ME, *lenen*, slender; AS, *bodig;* ME, *massa*, lump], the combination of cell solids, extracellular and intracellular water, and mineral mass of the body.

learned helplessness, a behavioral state and personality trait of a person who believes he or she is ineffectual, responses are futile, and control over reinforcers in the environment has been lost.

learning [AS *leornian* to learn], **1.** the act or process of acquiring knowledge or some skill by means of study, practice, or experience. **2.** knowledge, wisdom, or a skill acquired through systematic study or instruction. **3.** (in psychology) the modification of behavior through practice, experience, or training.

learning disability, an abnormal condition often affecting children of normal or above average intelligence, characterized by difficulty in learning such fundamental procedures as reading, writing, and numeric calculation.

learning theory [ME *lernen;* Gk *theoria* speculation], a group of concepts and principles that attempts to explain the learning process. One concept, Guthrie's contiguous conditioning premise, postulates that each response becomes permanently linked with stimuli present at the time so that contiguity rather than reinforcement is a part of the learning process.

leather-bottle stomach. See **linitis plastica.**

Leber's congenital amaurosis /lā′bərz/ [Theodor von Leber, German ophthalmologist, b. 1840; L *congenitus* born with; Gk *amaurorein* to darken], a rare kind of blindness or severely impaired vision caused by a defect transmitted as an autosomal recessive trait and occurring at birth or shortly thereafter. The eyes appear normal externally, but pupillary constriction to light is sluggish or absent and retinal pigment is degenerated.

Leboyer method of delivery /ləboiyā′/, an approach to the delivery of an infant formulated by the French obstetrician Charles Leboyer. It has four aspects: a gentle, controlled delivery in a quiet, dimly lit room; avoidance of pulling on the head; avoidance of overstimulation of the infant's sensorium; and encouragement of maternal-infant bonding. The goal of the method is to minimize the trauma of birth by gently and pleasantly introducing the newborn to life outside the womb.

LE cell, abbreviation for *lupus erythematosus cell,* a neutrophil that has phagocytosed the nucleus of another leukocyte that has already been altered by interacting with the LE factor in the bloodstream.

lecithin /les′ithin/ [Gk *lekithos* yolk], any of a group of phospholipids common in plants and animals. They are essential for the metabolism of fats and are used in the processing of foods, pharmaceutic products, cosmetics, and inks.

lecithin/sphingomyelin ratio, the ratio of two components of amniotic fluid, used for predicting fetal lung maturity. The normal ratio in amniotic fluid is 2:1 or greater.

lectin /lek′tin/, a protein substance occurring in seeds and other parts of certain plants that binds with glycoproteins and glycolipids on the surface of animal cells, causing agglutination.

Lee-Davidsohn test, a heterophil antibody test for infectious mononucleosis using horse red blood cells.

Leeuwenhoekia australiensis [Anton van Leeuwenhoek, Dutch microscopist, b. 1632; Australia], a mite indigenous to New South Wales that burrows into the skin, producing severe irritation.

Lee-White method [Roger I. Lee, American physician, b. 1881; Paul D. White, American physician, b. 1886; Gk *meta* beyond, *hodos* way], a method of determining the length of time required for a clot to form in a test tube of venous blood.

LeFort I fracture. See **Guérin's fracture.**

left atrioventricular valve. See **mitral valve.**

left brachiocephalic vein [ME *left* weak; Gk *brachys* short, *kephale* head], a vessel that starts in the root of the neck at the junction of the internal jugular and the subclavian veins on the left side and runs obliquely across the thorax to join the right brachiocephalic vein and form the superior vena cava.

left common carotid artery, the longer of the two common carotid arteries, springing from the aortic arch and having cervical and thoracic portions.

left coronary artery, one of a pair of branches from the ascending aorta, arising in the left posterior aortic sinus, dividing into the left interventricular artery and the circumflex branch, supplying both ventricles and the left atrium.

left-handedness, a natural tendency by some persons to favor the use of the left hand in performing certain tasks.

left-heart failure, an abnormal cardiac condition characterized by the impairment of the left side of the heart and by elevated pressure and congestion in the pulmonary veins and capillaries. Left-heart failure is usually related to right-heart failure, because both sides of the heart are part of a circuit and the impairment of one side will eventually affect the other.

left hepatic duct, the duct that drains the bile from the left lobe of the liver into the common bile duct.

left innominate vein. See **left brachiocephalic vein.**

left lateral recumbent position, a position in which the patient lies on the left side with the upper knee and thigh drawn upward.

left lymphatic duct. See **thoracic duct.**

left pulmonary artery, the shorter and smaller of two arteries conveying venous blood from the heart to the lungs, rising from the pulmonary trunk, connecting to the left lung.

left subclavian artery, an artery, divided into three parts, that arises from the aortic arch dorsal to the left common carotid at the level of the fourth thoracic vertebra, ascends to the root of the neck, arches laterally to the scalenus anterior, and forms six main branches to supply the vertebral column, spinal cord, ear, and brain.

left ventricle (LV), the thick-walled chamber of the heart that pumps blood through the aorta and the systemic arteries, the capillaries, and back through the veins to the right atrium. It has walls about three times thicker than those of the right ventricle and contains a mitral valve with two flaps that controls the flow of blood from the left atrium.

left ventricular assist device (LVAD), a mechanical pump that temporarily and artificially aids the natural pumping action of the left ventricle.

left ventricular failure, heart failure in which the left ventricle fails to contract forcefully enough to maintain a normal cardiac output and peripheral perfusion. Pulmonary congestion and edema develop from back pressure of accumulated blood in the left ventricle. Signs include breathlessness, pallor, sweating, and peripheral vasoconstriction. The heart is usually enlarged.

legacy [L *legatus* bequest], something that is handed down from the past or is intended to be bestowed on future generations.

legal [L *lex*], actions or conditions that are permitted or authorized by law.

legal blindness [L *legalis* law; ME *blend* sightless], a state of visual acuity in which no better than 20/200 is measured in the better eye with corrective lenses, or a visual field of not more than 20 degrees is obtained.

legal death. See **death.**

leg cylinder cast [ONorse *leggr;* Gk *kylindros;* ONorse *kasta*], an orthopedic device of plaster of paris or fiberglass used to immobilize the leg in treating fractures in the legs from the ankle to the upper thigh.

Legg-Calvé-Perthes disease. See **Perthes disease.**

Legionella pneumonia /lē′jənəl′ə/ [American Legion; Gk, *pneumon* lung], a form of pneumonia caused by a gram-negative bacillus identified as *Legionella pneumophila.* It was discovered after an outbreak of the disease among veterans attending a 1976 convention of the American Legion.

Legionella pneumophila /lē′jənəl′ə nōōmof′əlä/, a small, gram-negative, rod-shaped bacterium that is the causative agent in **Legionnaires' disease.**

L

Legionnaires' disease /lē'jənerz'/ [L *legionarius* member of a legion], an acute bacterial pneumonia caused by infection with *Legionella pneumophila* and characterized by an influenza-like illness followed within a week by high fever, chills, muscle aches, and headache. The symptoms may progress to dry cough, pleurisy, and sometimes diarrhea. Usually the disease is self-limited, but mortality has been 15% to 20% in a few localized epidemics. Contaminated air-conditioning cooling towers and moist soil may be a source of organisms.

legume /leg'yoom/ [L *legumen* pulse], any of the members of the *Fabales* order of dicotyledenous plants, including dried peas, beans, and lentils.

leiomyoblastoma. See **epithelioid leiomyoma.**

leiomyofibroma /lī'ōmī'ōfībrō'mə/, *pl.* **leiomyofibromas, leiomyofibromata** [Gk *leios* smooth, *mys* muscle; L *fibra* fiber; Gk *oma* tumor], a tumor consisting of smooth muscle cells and fibrous connective tissue, commonly occurring in the uterus in middle-aged women.

leiomyoma /lī'ōmī·ō'mə/, *pl.* **leiomyomas, leiomyomata,** a benign smooth muscle tumor most commonly occurring in the stomach, esophagus, or small intestine.

leiomyoma cutis, a neoplasm of the smooth muscles of the skin. The lesion is characterized by many small, tender, red nodules.

leiomyoma uteri, a benign neoplasm of the smooth muscle of the uterus. The tumor is characteristically firm, well circumscribed, round, and gray-white. Multiple tumors of this kind develop most often in the myometrium and occur most frequently in women between 30 and 50 years of age.

leiomyosarcoma /lī'ōmīsärkō'mə/ [Gk *leios* smooth; *mys* muscle; *sarx* flesh; *oma* tumor], a sarcoma that contains large spindle cells of unstriated muscle.

Leishman-Donovan body /lēsh'mandon'-əvən/ [Sir William B. Leishman, English pathologist, b. 1865; Charles Donovan, Scottish physician, b. 1863], the resting stage of an intracellular, nonflagellated protozoan parasite (*Leishmania donovani*) that causes kala-azar, or visceral leishmaniasis as it appears in infected tissue specimens.

Leishmania /lēshmā'nē·ə/ [Sir William B. Leishman], a genus of protozoan parasites. These organisms are transmitted to humans by any of several species of sand flies.

leishmaniasis /lēsh'mənī'əsis/ [Sir William B. Leishman], infection with any species of protozoan of the genus *Leishmania*. The diseases caused by these organisms may be cutaneous or visceral. Kinds of leishmaniasis are **American leishmaniasis, kala-azar,** and **oriental sore.** –**leishmanial,** *adj.*

lemniscal system /lemnis'kəl/ [Gk *lemniskos* fillet; *systema*], a part of the somatosensory network of large diameter myelinated A fibers. It includes the dorsal columns and the neospinothalamic tract extending from the spinal cord to the thalamus and cortex.

lemniscus /lemnis'kəs/ [Gk *lemniskos,* fillet], a band or tract of central nervous system fibers, particularly the ascending axons of secondary sensory neurons leading to the thalamus.

length of stay (LOS), the period of time a patient remains in a hospital or other health care facility as an inpatient.

lens [L, lentil], **1.** a curved transparent piece of plastic or glass that is shaped, molded, or ground to refract light in a specific way, as in eyeglasses, microscopes, or cameras. **2.** *informal.* the crystalline lens of the eye. –**lenticular,** *adj.*

lens capsule, the clear thin elastic capsule that surrounds the lens of the eye.

lens implant, an artifical lens of clear polymethylmethacrylate that is usually implanted at the time of cataract extraction but may also be used for patients with extreme myopia, diplopia, ocular albinism, and certain other abnormalities.

lenticonus /len'tikō'nəs/, an abnormal spherical or conical protrusion on the lens of the eye. It is a congenital defect found in Alport's syndrome.

lenticular nucleus /lentik'yələr/ [L *lentil* lens; *nucleus* nut], a biconvex basal ganglia of the cerebrum, composed of lateral putamen and medial globus pallidus tissue as part of the corpus striatum.

lentiform /len'tiförm/ [L *lens* + *forma*], pertaining to or resembling a lentil shape, such as the lens of the eye.

lentigo /lentī'gō/, *pl.* **lentigines** /lentij'ənēz/ [L, freckle], a tan or brown macule on the skin brought on by sun exposure, usually in a middle-aged or older person. Another variety, called **juvenile lentigo,** is unrelated to sunlight and appears in children 2 to 5 years of age, before the onset of freckles.

lentigo maligna. See **Hutchinson's freckle.**

lentigo maligna melanoma, a neoplasm developing from Hutchinson's freckle on the face or other exposed surfaces of the skin in elderly patients. It is asymptomatic, flat, and tan or brown, with irregular darker spots and frequent hypopigmentation. It is one of the three major clinical types of melanoma.

lentivirus /len'tivī'rəs/, a member of a subfamily of retroviruses that includes the AIDS virus. Lentiviruses are usually slow viruses, with long incubation periods that may delay the onset of symptoms until several years after exposure.

Leopold's maneuver [Christian Gerhard Leopold, German physician, b. 1846], a series of four steps used in palpating the abdomen of a pregnant woman to determine the position and presentation of the fetus.

leper /lep'ər/ [Gk lepis scaly], an outdated term for a person afflicted with Hansen's disease (leprosy).

LE prep, abbreviation for **lupus erythematosus preparation.**

lepromatous leprosy. See **leprosy.**

lepromin test /lepro'min/, a skin sensitivity test used to distinguish between the lepromatous and tuberculoid forms of leprosy. The test consists of intradermal injection of lepromin.

leprosarium /lep'rōser'ē·əm/ [Gk lepra leprosy; sanitarium], a hospital for persons who have Hansen's disease (leprosy).

leprosy /lep'rəsē/ [Gk lepra], a chronic, communicable disease, caused by *Mycobacterium leprae,* that may take either of two forms, depending on the degree of immunity of the host. **Tuberculoid leprosy,** seen in those with high resistance, presents as thickening of cutaneous nerves and anesthetic, saucer-shaped skin lesions. **Lepromatous leprosy,** seen in those with little resistance, involves many systems of the body, with widespread plaques and nodules in the skin, iritis, keratitis, destruction of nasal cartilage and bone, testicular atrophy, peripheral edema, and involvement of the reticuloendothelial system. Blindness may result. –**lepromatous, leprotic, leprous,** adj.

leptocyte. See **target cell.**

leptocytosis /lep'tōsītō'sis/ [Gk leptos thin, kytos cell, osis condition], a hematologic condition in which target cells are present in the blood. Thalassemia, some forms of liver disease, and absence of the spleen are associated with leptocytosis.

leptomeninges /lep'tōminin'jēz/ [Gk leptos + meninx membrane], the arachnoid membrane and the pia mater, two of the three layers covering the spinal cord.

leptonema /lep'tənē'mə/ [Gk leptos + nema thread], the threadlike chromosome formation in the leptotene stage in the first meiotic prophase of gametogenesis before the beginning of synapsis.

Leptospira /lep'tōspī'rə/ [Gk leptos + speira coil], a genus of the family Trepo-

nemataceae, order Spirochaetales, tightly coiled microorganisms having spirals with hooked ends. The spirochete may cause jaundice, skin hemorrhages, fever, and muscular illness.

Leptospira agglutinin, an agglutinin found in the blood of patients with Weil's disease.

leptospirosis /lep'tōspīrō'sis/ [Gk leptos, speira + osis condition], an acute infectious disease caused by several serotypes of the spirochete *Leptospira interrogans,* transmitted in the urine of wild or domestic animals, especially rats and dogs. Human infections arise directly from contact with an infected animal's urine or tissues or indirectly from contact with contaminated water or soil. Clinical symptoms may include jaundice, hemorrhage into the skin, fever, chills, and muscular pain. The most serious form of the disease is called **Weil's disease.**

leptotene /lep'tətēn/ [Gk leptos + tainia ribbon], the initial stage in the first meiotic prophase in gametogenesis in which the chromosomes become visible as single thin filaments.

Leriche's syndrome /lərēshs'/ [Rene Leriche, French surgeon, b. 1879], a vascular disorder marked by gradual occlusion of the terminal aorta; intermittent claudication in the buttocks, thighs, or calves; absence of pulsation in femoral arteries; pallor and coldness of the legs; gangrene of the toes; and, in men, impotence.

lesbian /lez'bē·ən/ [Gk, island of Lesbos, home of Sappho], **1.** a female homosexual. **2.** of or pertaining to the sexual preference or desire of one woman for another. –**lesbianism,** n.

Lesch-Nyhan syndrome /lesh'nī'han/ [Michael Lesch, American pediatrician, b. 1939; William L. Nyhan, Jr., American pediatrician, b. 1926], a hereditary disorder of purine metabolism, characterized by mental retardation, self-mutilation of the fingers and lips by biting, impaired renal function, and abnormal physical development.

lesion /lē'zhən/ [L laesus an injury], **1.** a wound, injury, or pathologic change in body tissue. **2.** any visible, local abnormality of the tissues of the skin, such as a wound, sore, rash, or boil. A lesion may be described as benign, cancerous, gross, occult, or primary.

lesser multangular bone. See **trapezoid bone.**

lesser occipital nerve [AS losian to lose; L occiput back of the head, nervus nerve], one of a pair of cutaneous branches of the cervical plexus, arising from the second cervical nerve, curving around the sternocleidomastoideus, and ascending along the side of the head behind the ear to supply the skin.

lesser omentum [AS *losian* to lose; L *omentum* entrails], a membranous extension of the peritoneum from the peritoneal layers covering the ventral and the dorsal surfaces of the stomach and the first part of the duodenum.

lesser sciatic notch [ME *les;* Gk *ischiadikos* hip joint; OFr *enochier*], a notch on the posterior border of the hip bone. It is smooth, coated with cartilage, and has several ridges corresponding to subdivisions of the obturator internus tendon.

lesser trochanter, one of a pair of conic projections at the base of the neck of the femur, providing insertion of the tendon of psoas major.

let-down, a sensation in the breasts of lactating women that often occurs as the milk flows into the ducts. It may occur when the infant begins to suck or when the mother hears the baby cry or even thinks of nursing the child.

let-down reflex. See **milk ejection reflex.**

lethal [L *letum* death], deadly, capable of causing death.

lethal equivalent [L *letum; aequus* equal, *valere* to be strong], any recessive gene carried in the heterozygous state that, if homozygous, would be lethal and result in the death of the individual or organism.

lethal gene, any gene that produces a phenotypic effect that causes the death of the organism at some stage of development from fertilization of the egg to adulthood. The gene may be dominant, incompletely dominant, or recessive.

lethality, the probability that a person threatening suicide will succeed, based on the method described, the specificity of the plan, and the availability of the means.

lethargic encephalitis. See **epidemic encephalitis.**

lethargy [Gk *lethargos* forgetful], **1.** the state or quality of being indifferent, apathetic, or sluggish. **2.** stupor or coma resulting from disease or hypnosis. Kinds of lethargy include **hysteric, induced,** and **lucid lethargy. –lethargic,** *adj.*

Letterer-Siwe syndrome /let′ərərzē′və/ [Erich Letterer, German pathologist, b. 1895; Sture A. Siwe, Swedish physician, b. 1897], any of a poorly classified group of malignant neoplastic diseases of unknown origin, characterized by histiocytic elements. Anemia, hemorrhage, splenomegaly, lymphadenopathy, and localized tumefactions over bones are usually present.

leucine (Leu) /lōō′sēn/ [Gk *leukos* white], a white, crystalline amino acid essential for optimal growth in infants and nitrogen equilibrium in adults. It cannot be synthesized by the body and is obtained by the hydrolysis of protein during pancreatic digestion.

leucinosis /lōō′sinō′sis/ [Gk *leukos* + *osis* condition], a condition in which the pathways for the degradation of leucine are blocked and large amounts of the amino acid accumulate in body tissue.

leucocyte. See **leukocyte.**

leucovorin. See **folinic acid.**

leucovorin calcium /lōō′kəvôr′in/, an antianemic prescribed in the treatment of an overdose of a folic acid antagonist and certain cases of megaloblastic anemia.

leukapheresis /lōō′kəfarē′sis/ [Gk *leukos* + *aphairesis* removal], a process by which blood is withdrawn from a vein, white blood cells are selectively removed, and the remaining blood is reinfused in the donor.

leukemia /lōōkē′mē·ə/ [Gk *leukos* + *haima* blood], a malignant neoplasm of blood-forming organs characterized by diffuse replacement of bone marrow with proliferating leukocyte precursors; abnormal numbers and forms of immature white cells in circulation; and infiltration of lymph nodes, the spleen, liver, and other sites. The origin of leukemia is not clear, but it may result from exposure to ionizing radiation, benzene, or other chemicals that are toxic to bone marrow. Leukemia is classified according to the predominant proliferating cells, the clinical course, and the duration of the disease. Acute leukemia usually has a sudden onset and rapidly progresses from early signs, such as fatigue, pallor, weight loss, and easy bruising, to fever, hemorrhages, extreme weakness, bone or joint pain, and repeated infections. Chronic leukemia develops slowly, and signs similar to those of the acute forms of the disease may not appear for years. **–leukemic,** *adj.*

leukemia cutis, a condition in which yellow-brown, red, or purple nodular lesions and diffuse infiltrations or large accumulations of leukemic cells develop in the skin.

leukemic reticuloendotheliosis. See **hairy-cell leukemia.**

leukemoid /lōōkē′moid/, resembling leukemia.

leukemoid reaction [Gk *leukos* + *eidos* form; L *re* again, *agere* to act], a clinical syndrome resembling leukemia in which the white blood cell count is elevated in response to an allergy, inflammatory disease, infection, poison, hemorrhage, burn, or other causes of severe physical stress.

leukoblast /lōō′kəblast/ [Gk *leukos* + *blastos* germ], an immature leukocyte, or white blood cell.

leukocyte /lōō′kəsīt/ [Gk *leukos* + *kytos* cell], a white blood cell, one of the formed elements of the circulating blood system. There are five types of leukocytes, classified by the presence or absence of granules in the cytoplasm of the cell. The agranulocytes are lymphocytes and monocytes. The granulocytes are neutrophils, basophils, and eosinophils. **–leukocytic,** *adj.*

leukocyte alkaline phosphatase, an enzyme that is elevated in various diseases, such as cirrhosis and polycythemia, and in certain infections. It may be measured in the blood to detect these disorders.

leukocythemia. See **leukemia.**

leukocytic crystal. See **Charcot-Leyden crystal.**

leukocytopenia. See **leukopenia.**

leukocytosis /lōō′kōsītō′sis/ [Gk *leukos* + *kytos* cell, *osis* condition], an abnormal increase in the number of circulating white blood cells. An increase often accompanies bacterial, but not usually viral, infections. The normal range is 5,000 to 10,000 white cells per cubic millimeter of blood. Kinds of leukocytosis include **basophilia, eosinophilia,** and **neutrophilia.**

leukoderma /lōō′kōdur′mə/ [Gk *leukos* + *derma* skin], localized loss of skin pigment caused by any of a number of specific causes.

leukodystrophy /lōō′kōdis′trəfē/ [Gk *leukos* + *dys, trophe* nourishment], a disease of the white matter of the brain, characterized by demyelination.

leukoerythroblastic anemia /lōō′kō-erith′rōblas′tik/ [Gk *leukos* + *erythros* red, *blastos* germ; *a, haima* not blood], an abnormal condition in which there are large numbers of immature white and red blood cells. It is characteristic of some anemias that occur as a result of the replacement of normal bone marrow with malignant tumor.

leukonychia /lōō′kōnik′ē-ə/ [Gk *leukos* + *onyx* nail], a benign, congenital condition in which white patches appear under the nails. Trauma, infection, and many systemic disorders can cause white spots or streaks on nails. A common cause is the presence of air bubbles under the nails.

leukopenia /lōō′kōpē′nē-ə/ [Gk *leukos* + *penes* poor], an abnormal decrease in the number of white blood cells to fewer than 5,000 cells per cubic millimeter. It may be caused by an adverse drug reaction, radiation poisoning, or other pathologic conditions and may affect one or all kinds of white blood cells. **–leukopenic,** *adj.*

leukopenic leukemia. See **aleukemic leukemia.**

leukophlegmasia. See **phlegmasia alba dolens.**

leukophoresis /lōō′kōfôrē′sis/ [Gk *leukos* + *phoresis* being transmitted], a laboratory procedure in which white blood cells are separated by electrophoresis for identification and evaluation of the types of cells and their proportions.

leukoplakia /lōō′kōplā′kē-ə/ [Gk *leukos* + *plax* plate], a precancerous, slowly developing change in a mucous membrane characterized by thickened, white, firmly attached patches that are slightly raised and sharply circumscribed.

leukoplakic vulvitis /lōō′kōplā′kik/ [Gk *leukos* + *plakos* plate; *vulva* + *itis* inflammation], a condition in which the skin of the vulva becomes thick and white, develops bleeding fissures, and later becomes atrophic. The condition may progress to cancer.

leukopoiesis /lōō′kōpō-ē′sis/ [Gk *leukos* + *poiein* to make], the process by which white blood cells form and develop. Neutrophils, basophils, and eosinophils are produced in myeloid tissue in the bone marrow. Lymphocytes and monocytes are almost all normally derived from hemocytoblasts in lymphoid tissue, but a few develop in the marrow. **–leukopoietic,** *adj.*

leukorrhea /lōō′kərē′ə/ [Gk *leukos* + *rhoia* flow], a white discharge from the vagina. Normally, vaginal discharge occurs in regular variations of amount and consistency during the course of the menstrual cycle. An irritating, pruritic, copious, foul-smelling, green or yellow discharge may indicate vaginal or uterine infection or other pathologic conditions of gynecologic origin. Leukorrhea is the most common reason for women to seek gynecologic care.

leukotomy. See **lobotomy.**

leukotoxin /lōō′kətok′sin/ [Gk *leukos* + *toxikon* poison], a substance that can inactivate or destroy leukocytes. **–leukotoxic,** *adj.*

leukotrienes /lōō′kōtrī′ēnz/, a class of biologically active compounds that occur naturally in leukocytes and that produce allergic and inflammatory reactions. They are thought to play a role in the development of allergic and autoallergic disease, such as asthma and rheumatoid arthritis.

leukovirus /lōō′kōvī′rus/ [Gk *leukos* + L, *virus* poison], any of a group of RNA viruses that cause disease in animals. The diseases include Rous sarcoma and murine leukemia.

leuprolide acetate /loo'prōlīd/, a parenteral antineoplastic drug prescribed for the palliative treatment of advanced prostatic cancer.

levamisole, a new drug used as an anthelmintic agent against a wide variety of nematodes. It has also been used in the treatment of bacterial and viral infections.

levamphetamine /lev'əmfet'əmēn/, an isomer of amphetamine, formerly used as an anorexiant.

levarterenol bitartrate. See norepinephrine bitartrate.

levator /livā'tər/, pl. **levatores** /lev'ətôr'ēz/ [L levare to lift up], **1.** a muscle that raises a structure of the body, as the levator ani raises parts of the pelvic diaphragm. **2.** a surgical instrument used to lift depressed bony fragments in fractures of the skull and other bones.

levator ani, one of a pair of muscles of the pelvic diaphragm that stretches across the bottom of the pelvic cavity like a hammock, supporting the pelvic organs. It functions to support and slightly raise the pelvic floor. The pubococcygeus draws the anus toward the pubis and constricts it.

levator palpebrae superioris, one of the three muscles of the eyelid, also considered a muscle of the eye. It is innervated by the oculomotor nerve, raises the upper eyelid, and is the antagonist of the orbicularis oculi.

levator scapulae, a muscle of the dorsal and lateral aspects of the neck. It acts to raise the scapula and pull it toward the midline.

LeVeen shunt, a tube that is surgically implanted to connect the peritoneal cavity and the superior vena cava to drain an accumulation of fluid in the peritoneal cavity in cirrhosis of the liver, right-sided heart failure, or cancer of the abdomen.

level of activities [OFr livel; L activus], pertaining to the hierarchy of nervous system activity that determines the level responsible for certain functions while also being controlled by another higher level above it, as in the sequence of events in a reflex action.

level of consciousness (LOC), a degree of cognitive function involving arousal mechanisms of the reticular formation of the brain. Impaired LOC may be expressed in obtundation or reduced alertness, stupor, syncope, or unresponsiveness.

level of inquiry [L libella carpenter's level; inquirere to ask about], (in nursing research) one of the levels in a rank-ordered system of classification and organization of the questions to be answered in a research study.

levels of care, a classification of health care service levels by the kind of care given, the number of people served, and the people providing the care. Kinds of health care service levels are **primary health care, secondary health care,** and **tertiary health care.**

levels of consciousness [OFr livel; L conscire to be aware of], the stages of response of the mind to stimuli, varying from unconsciousness through vague awareness to full attention. The usual standard levels include coma, in which the patient does not appear to be aware of the environment; stupor, in which the patient is vaguely aware of the environment; drowsiness, in which the patient responds to stimuli but may be slow to react, and alert wakefulness.

lever /lē'vər, lev'ər/ [L levare to lift up], (in physiology) any one of the numerous bones and associated joints of the body that act together as a lever so that force applied to one end of the bone to lift a weight at another point tends to rotate the bone in the direction opposite from that of the applied force.

Lévi-Lorain dwarf. See pituitary dwarf.

Levin tube /lev'in/ [Abraham L. Levin, American physician, b. 1880], a No. 16 French plastic catheter used in gastric intubation that has a closed, weighted tip and an opening on the side.

levitation [L levitas lightness, atus process], (in psychiatry) a hallucinatory sensation of floating or rising in the air. –**levitate,** v.

levobunolol hydrochloride /lē'vō-bun'əlol/, a topical ophthalmic drug prescribed for the treatment of chronic open-angle glaucoma and ocular hypertension.

levodopa /lē'vōdō'pə/, an antiparkinsonian prescribed in the treatment of Parkinson's disease, juvenile forms of Huntington's disease, and chronic manganese poisoning.

levopropoxyphene napsylate /lē'vōprō-pok'sifēn/, an antitussive prescribed for cough.

levorphanol tartrate /lē'vôrfə'nol/, a narcotic analgesic prescribed for pain and preoperative analgesia.

levothyroxine sodium /lē'vōthī'rəksēn/, a thyroid hormone prescribed in the treatment of hypothyroidism.

levulose. See fructose.

levulosuria. See fructosuria.

lewisite /loo'isīt/ [Winford L. Lewis, American chemist, b. 1878], 2-chlorovinyl arsine; a poisonous blister gas, used in World War I, that causes irritation of the lungs, dyspnea, damage to the tissues of the respiratory tract, tears, and pain.

Leyden-Möbius muscular dystrophy /lī′dən-mē′bē-əs/, a form of limb-girdle muscular dystrophy that begins in the pelvic girdle.

Leydig cells /lī′dig/ [Franz von Leydig, German anatomist, b. 1821], cells of the interstitial tissue of the testes that secrete testosterone.

Leydig cell tumor, a generally benign neoplasm of interstitial cells of a testis that may cause gynecomastia in adults and precocious sexual development if the lesion occurs before puberty.

LF, abbreviation for *low frequency.*

LFA, abbreviation for *left frontoanterior fetal position.*

LFP, abbreviation for *left frontoposterior fetal position.*

LFT, abbreviation for **liver function test.**

LGA, abbreviation for **large-for-gestational age.**

LGV, abbreviation for **lymphogranuloma venereum.**

LH, abbreviation for **luteinizing hormone.**

Lhermitte's sign /ler′mits/ [Jacques J. Lhermitte, French neurologist, b. 1877], sudden, transient, electric-like shocks spreading down the body when the head is flexed forward, occurring chiefly in multiple sclerosis but also in compression disorders of the cervical spinal cord.

LHRH, abbreviation for **luteinizing hormone-releasing hormone.**

Li, symbol for the element **lithium.**

liability [L *ligare* to bind], **1.** something one is obligated to do or an obligation required to be fulfilled by law, usually financial in nature. **2.** the amount of money required to fulfill a financial obligation.

liaison nursing /lē-ō′zən/, an arrangement with clinical specialists in psychiatric nursing whereby nurses and health professionals in other disciplines obtain consultation services in medical-surgical, parent-child, and geriatric settings.

libel [L *libellus* little book], a false accusation written, printed, or typewritten, or presented in a picture or a sign that is made with malicious intent to defame the reputation of a person who is living or the memory of a person who is dead, resulting in public embarrassment, contempt, ridicule, or hatred.

liberation [L *liber* free], the process of drug release from the dosage form.

libidinal development. See **psychosexual development.**

libidinous /libid′inəs/ [L *libidinosus* lustful], **1.** pertaining to or belonging to the libido. **2.** having or characterized by

sexual desire. Also **libidinal.** –**libidinize,** *v.*

libido /libē′dō, libi′dō/, **1.** the psychic energy or instinctual drive associated with sexual desire, pleasure, or creativity. **2.** (in psychoanalysis) the instinctual drives of the id. **3.** lustful desire or striving.

Libman-Sacks endocarditis /lib′mənsaks′/ [Emanuel Libman, American physician, b. 1872; Benjamin Sacks, American physician, b. 1896], an abnormal condition and the most common manifestation of lupus erythematosus, characterized by verrucous lesions that develop near the heart valves but rarely affect valvular action.

lice, *sing.,* **louse** [AS *lus*], any of the small wingless insect order of *Anoplura.* Lice are ectoparasites of birds and mammals and may spend their entire life cycle on a single host, attaching eggs to the hair shafts or feathers. They transfer to humans by direct contact. Three forms that infect humans are the **head louse,** *Pediculus humanus capitis;* the **body louse,** *Pediculus humanus corporis,* and the **crab louse,** *Phthirus pubis.*

licensed practical nurse (LPN) [L *licere* to be allowed; Gk *praktikos* fit for action; L *nutrix* nurse], *U.S.* a person trained in basic nursing techniques and direct patient care who practices under the supervision of a registered nurse. The course of training usually lasts 1 year. In Canada an LPN is called a certified nursing assistant.

licensed psychologist, a person who has earned a PhD in psychology from an accredited graduate school and has completed 2 to 3 years of postgraduate training with special emphasis on the diagnosis and treatment of psychologic disorders.

licensed vocational nurse. See **licensed practical nurse.**

licensure /lī′sənshŏŏr/ [L *licere* to be allowed], the granting of permission by a competent authority (usually a government agency) to an organization or individual to engage in a practice or activity that would otherwise be illegal. Kinds of licensure include the issuing of licenses for general hospitals or nursing homes, for health professionals, as physicians, and for the production or distribution of biologic products.

lichenification /līken′ifikā′shən/ [Gk *leichen* lichen; *facere* to make], thickening and hardening of the skin, often resulting from the irritation caused by repeated scratching of a pruritic lesion. –**lichenified,** *adj.*

lichen nitidus /lī′kən/ [Gk *leichen* + L *nitidus* bright], a rare skin disorder characterized by numerous flat, glistening, pale, discrete papules measuring 2 to 3 mm in diameter.

lichen planus, a nonmalignant, chronic, pruritic skin disease of unknown cause, characterized by small, flat, purplish papules or plaques having fine, gray lines on the surface.

lichen sclerosis et atrophicus, a chronic skin disease characterized by white, flat papules with an erythematous halo and black, hard follicular plugs. In advanced cases, the papules tend to coalesce into large, white patches of thin, pruritic skin.

lichen simplex chronicus, a form of neurodermatitis characterized by a patch of pruritic, confluent papules.

licorice, a dried root of gummy texture from the leguminous plant *Glycyrrhiza glabra*. It has a sweet, astringent taste and is used as a flavoring in medicines, especially in cough syrups and laxatives. It may cause an elevation in blood pressure.

lid. See eyelid.

lidocaine hydrochloride /lī′dəkān/, a local anesthetic agent prescribed as a local anesthetic for topical administration to skin or to mucous membranes. It is used parenterally as an antiarrhythmic agent.

lie [AS *licgan* position], the relationship between the long axis of the fetus and the long axis of the mother. In a longitudinal lie the fetus is lying lengthwise, or vertically, in the uterus, whereas in a transverse lie the fetus is lying crosswise, or horizontally.

Lieberkühn's glands /lē′bərkēnz/ [Johann Nathanael Lieberkühn, German anatomist, b. 1711; L *glans* acorn], tubular glands between the bases of the villi of the small intestine and on the surface of the epithelium of the large intestine.

lie detector [AS *leogan* untruth; L *detegere* to uncover], an electronic device or instrument used to detect lying or anxiety in regard to specific questions. A commonly used lie detector is the polygraph recorder that senses and records pulse, respiratory rate, blood pressure, and perspiration.

lien. See spleen.

lienal vein /lē-ē′nəl/ [L *lien* spleen; *vena*], a large vein of the lower body that unites with the superior mesenteric vein to form the portal vein. It returns blood from the spleen and arises from about six large tributaries that unite to form the single vessel passing from left to right across the superior, dorsal part of the pancreas.

lienography /lē′ənog′rəfē/, the radiographic examination of the spleen after it has been injected with a contrast medium.

life [AS *lif*], the energy that enables organisms to grow, reproduce, absorb and utilize nutrients, evolve, and in some organisms, achieve mobility, express consciousness, and demonstrate a voluntary use of the senses.

life costs [AS *lif*; L *constare* constant], the mortality, morbidity, and suffering associated with a given disease or medical procedure.

life expectancy, the probable number of years a person will live after a given age, as determined by the mortality rate in a specific geographic area. It may be individually qualified by the person's condition or race, sex, age, or other demographic factors.

life extension [AS *lif*; L *extenere* to stretch out], the process of extending the life span of an individual or population by intervention that promotes greater use of preventive medicine and better utilization of established diagnostic and therapeutic facilities.

life island, a plastic bubble enclosing a bed, used to provide a germ-free environment for a patient.

life review, 1. (in psychiatry) a progressive return to consciousness of past experiences. 2. reminiscences that occur in old age as a consequence of the realization of the inevitability of death.

lifesaving measure, any independent, interdependent, or dependent nursing intervention that is implemented when a patient's physical or psychologic status is threatened.

life science, the study of the laws and properties of living matter. Some kinds of life science are **anatomy, bacteriology,** and **biology.**

life space, a term introduced by American psychologist Kurt Lewin to describe simultaneous influences that may affect individual behavior. The totality of the influences make up the life space.

life-style-induced health problems, diseases with natural histories that include conscious exposure to certain health-compromising or risk factors.

life support [AS *lif*; L *supportare* to bring up to], the use of any therapeutic technique or device to maintain life functions.

lifetime reserve [AS *lif, tid* time; L *re* again, *servare* to keep], a lifetime total of days of inpatient hospitalization benefits that may be drawn on by a patient who has exhausted the maximum benefits allowed under Medicare for a single spell of illness.

lift assessment [AS *lyft* loft; L *assidere* to sit beside], the selection of the most appropriate lift method to use when moving a patient, as from the bed to a chair.

ligament /lig′əmənt/ [L *ligare* to bind], 1. one of many predominantly white, shiny, flexible bands of fibrous tissue binding joints together and connecting various bones and cartilages. **2.** a layer of serous membrane with little or no tensile strength, extending from one visceral organ to another, such as the ligaments of the peritoneum. **–ligamentous,** *adj.*

ligamenta flava [L *ligare* + *flavus* yellow], the bands of yellow elastic tissue connecting the laminae of adjacent vertebrae from the axis to the first segment of the sacrum.

ligamental tear [L *ligare* to bind; AS *teran* to destroy], a complete or a partial tear of a ligamentous structure connecting and surrounding the bones of a joint, caused by an injury to the joint, as by a sudden twisting motion or by a forceful blow. Ligamental tears may occur at any joint but are most common in the knees.

ligament of the neck of the rib, one of five ligaments of each costotransverse joint, consisting of short, strong fibers passing from the neck of the rib to the transverse process of the adjacent vertebra.

ligament of the tubercle of the rib, one of the five ligaments of each costotransverse joint, comprising a short, thick fasciculus passing obliquely from the transverse process of a vertebra to the tubercle of the associated rib.

ligamentum. See **ligament.**

ligamentum latum uteri. See **broad ligament.**

ligamentum nuchae /lig'əmen'təm/, the fibrous membrane that reaches from the external occipital protuberance and median nuchal line to the spinous process of the seventh vertebra.

ligand /lig'ənd, lī'gənd/ [L *ligare* to bind], **1.** a molecule, ion, or group bound to the central atom of a chemical compound, such as the oxygen molecule in hemoglobin, which is bound to the central iron atom. **2.** an organic molecule attached to a specific site on a surface or to a tracer element.

ligases /lī'gāsəz/ [L *ligare* + Fr *diastase* enzyme], a group of enzymes that catalyze the formation of a bond between substrate molecules coupled with the breakdown of a pyrophosphate bond in ATP or a similar donor molecule.

ligation /līgā'shən/ [L *ligare* to bind], the procedure of tying off of a blood vessel or duct with a suture or wire ligature. It may be performed to stop or prevent bleeding during surgery, to stop spontaneous or traumatic hemorrhage, or to prevent passage of material through a duct, as in tubal ligation, or to treat varicosities. **–ligate,** *v.*

ligature /lig'əchər/ [L *ligare* to bind], **1.** a suture. **2.** a wire, as used in orthodontia.

ligature needle, a long, thin, curved needle used for passing a suture underneath an artery for ligation of the vessel.

ligature wire [L *ligare;* AS *wir*], a soft, thin wire used in dental procedures, particularly to connect brackets or attachments in orthodontic appliances.

light [AS *leoht*], **1.** electromagnetic radiation of the wavelength and frequency that stimulate visual receptor cells in the retina to produce nerve impulses that are perceived as vision. **2.** electromagnetic radiation with wavelengths shorter than ultraviolet light and longer than infrared light, the range of visible light generally in the range of 400 to 800 nm.

light-adapted eye [AS *leoht;* L *adaptatio;* AS *éage*], an eye that has been exposed to bright light long enough for chemical and physiologic changes to take place, such as bleaching of the rhodopsin or visual purple. The loss of cone sensitivity to light may require increased light intensity to obtain the same degree of visual acuity.

light bath, the exposure of the patient's uncovered skin to the sun or to actinic light rays from an artificial source for therapeutic purposes.

light chain, a subunit of an immunoglobulin molecule composed of a polypeptide chain of about 22,000 daltons, or atomic mass units. An example of a light chain is a Bence Jones protein molecule associated with multiple myeloma.

light chain disease, a type of multiple myeloma in which plasma cell tumors produce only monoclonal light chain proteins. Persons with light chain disease may develop lytic bone lesions, hypercalcemia, impaired kidney function, and amyloidosis.

light diet, a diet suitable for convalescent or bedridden patients taking little or no exercise. It consists of simple, moderate quantities of soft-cooked and easily digested foods, including meats, potatoes, rice, eggs, pasta, some fruits, refined cereals, and breads.

lightening [AS *leoht* light in weight], a subjective sensation reported by many women late in pregnancy as the fetus settles lower in the pelvis, leaving more space in the upper abdomen.

light film fault [AS *leoht* light; *filmen* membrane; L *fallere* to deceive], a defect in a radiograph or developed photographic film that appears as a barely distinct and inadequate image.

light microscope [AS *leoht;* Gk *mikros* small + *skopein,* to view], a microscope that uses visible light to view objects too small for the naked eye to see.

L

light reflex, the mechanism by which the pupil of the eye becomes more or less open in response to direct or consensual pupillary stimulation.

light therapy [AS *leoht;* Gk *therapeia* treatment], exposure of the body to electromagnetic waves of the infrared, ultraviolet, or visible spectrum for therapeutic purposes. In the winter months, light therapy may be used to treat depressive disorders.

light-touch palpations [AS *leoht;* Fr *toucher;* L *palpare* to touch gently], a method of examination by gently depressing the abdomen 1-2 cm in order to outline the size and position of abdominal organs.

light vaginal bleeding. See **vaginal bleeding.**

ligneous /lig'nē·əs/ [L *ligum* wood], woody or resembling wood in texture or other characteristics.

ligneous thyroiditis. See **fibrous thyroiditis.**

lignin /lig'nin/ [L *lignum* wood], a polysaccharide that with cellulose and hemicellulose forms the chief part of the skeletal substances of the cell walls of plants.

lignocaine. See **lidocaine hydrochloride.**

lilliputian hallucination /lil'ipyoo͞o'shən/ [Lilliput, mythic island in Swift's *Gulliver's Travels*], one in which things seem smaller than they actually are.

limb [AS *lim*], **1.** an appendage or extremity of the body, such as an arm or leg. **2.** a branch of an internal organ, such as a loop of a nephron.

limb-girdle muscular dystrophy [AS *lim* limb; *gyrdel*], a form of muscular dystrophy transmitted as an autosomal recessive trait. The characteristic weakness and degeneration of the muscles begins in the shoulder girdle or in the pelvic girdle. The condition is progressive. Kinds of limb-girdle muscular dystrophy are **Erb's muscular dystrophy, Leyden-Möbius muscular dystrophy.**

limbic /lim'bik/ [L *limbus* edge or border], pertaining to something that is marginal or at a junction between structures.

limbic lobe [L *limbus;* Gk *lobos* lobe], the marginal section of the cerebral hemispheres on the medial aspects. It forms a ring of neural tissue around the hypothalamus and some nuclei.

limbic system [L *limus* border], a group of structures within the rhinencephalon of the brain that is associated with various emotions and feelings, such as anger, fear, sexual arousal, pleasure, and sadness. The structures of the limbic system are the cingulate gyrus, the isthmus, the hippocampal gyrus, the uncus, and the hippocampus. The structures connect with various other parts of the brain.

limb kinetic apraxia. See **ideomotor apraxia.**

limb lead [AS *lim* limb; *laeden* lead], in electrocardiography, an electrode that is attached to an arm or a leg.

lime [AS *lim*], **1.** any of several oxides and hydroxides of calcium. **2.** a citrus fruit yielding a juice with a high ascorbic acid content. Lime juice was one of the first effective agents to be used in the treatment of scurvy.

limen. See **threshold stimulus.**

limitation of motion [L *limes* limit], the restriction or reduction to a normal range of motion of a body part caused by disease or injury.

limited fluctuation method of dosing [L *limes* limit; *fluctuare* to wave], a method of drug administration in which the dose is not allowed to rise or fall beyond specified maximum and minimum limits.

limiting charge, the maximum amount that can be charged in the United States for the services of a physician who does not accept the restrictions on fees established by Medicare laws.

limiting resolution, (in computed tomography) the spatial frequency at a modulation transfer function (MTF) equal to 0.1. The absolute object size that can be resolved by a scanner is equal to the reciprocal of the spatial frequency.

limp [ME, not firm], an abnormal pattern of ambulation in which the two phases of gait are markedly asymmetric.

LINAC, abbreviation for **linear accelerator.**

lincomycin hydrochloride /lin'kəmī'sin/, an antibiotic prescribed in the treatment of certain infections.

lindane /lin'dān/, gamma-benzene hexachloride prescribed in the treatment of pediculosis and scabies.

Lindau-von Hippel disease. See **cerebroretinal angiomatosis.**

Lindbergh pump [Charles A. Lindbergh, American technician, b. 1902; ME *pumpe*], a pump used to preserve an organ of the body by perfusing its tissues with oxygen and other essential nutrients, usually during the transport of an organ from a donor to a recipient.

line [L *linea*], **1.** a connection between two points. **2.** a stripe, streak, or narrow ridge, often imaginary, that serves to connect reference points or to separate various parts of the body, as the hairline or nipple line. **3.** a black absorption line in a continuous spectrum passing through a medium. **4.** an accretion line in the enamel of a tooth marking succesive layers of calcification. **5.** a catheter or wire that may be inserted in a vein, as an intravenous line. **6.** the base line of an electrocardiogram when neither positive nor negative potentials are recorded. **7.** line of sight.

linea /lin′ē-ə/ [L, line], a line defining anatomic features, such as the **linea alba** of the abdomen, the **linea albicantes** or **linea nigra** seen on the abdomen during pregnancy, or the **linea vitalis** curving across the palm at the base of the thumb.

linea alba [L *linea* line; *albus* white], the portion of the anterior abdominal aponeurosis in the middle line of the abdomen, representing the fusion of three aponeuroses into a single tendinous band extending from the xiphoid process to the symphysis pubis. It contains the umbilicus.

linea albicantes, lines, white to pink or gray in color, that occur on the abdomen, buttocks, breasts, and thighs and are caused by the stretching of the skin and weakening or rupturing of the underlying elastic tissue.

linea arcuata, the curved tendinous band in the sheath of the rectus abdominis below the umbilicus. It inserts into the linea alba.

linea aspera, the posterior crest of the thigh bone, extending proximally into three ridges to which are attached various muscles, including the gluteus maximus, pectineus, and iliacus.

linea nigra, a dark line appearing longitudinally on the abdomen of a pregnant woman during the latter part of term. It usually extends from the symphysis pubis to the umbilicus.

linear [L *linea* line], pertaining to a line or lines, particularly straight lines.

linear accelerator (LINAC) [L *linea* line; *accelerare* to quicken], an apparatus for accelerating charged subatomic particles used in radiotherapy, physics research, and the production of radionuclides.

linear array, (in radiology) a contiguous sequence of identical discrete detectors used with a fan beam x-ray generator. The detectors read off once for each x-ray pulse. The resulting electronic signal is converted to a digital number and stored in a computer memory.

linear energy transfer (LET), (in radiology) the rate at which energy is transferred from ionizing radiation to soft tissue. It is expressed in terms of kiloelectron volts (keV) per micrometer of track length in soft tissue.

linear flow velocity, the velocity of a particle carried in a moving stream, usually measured in centimeters per second.

linear fracture, a fracture that extends parallel to the long axis of a bone but does not displace the bone tissue.

linear grid. See **grid.**

linearity /lin′ē·er′itē/, (in radiology) the ability to obtain the same exposure for the same milliampere-seconds (mAs), regardless of mA and exposure time used.

linear regression, a statistical procedure in which a straight line is established through a data set that best represents a relationship between two subsets or two methods.

linear scan, (in ultrasonography) the motion of the transducer at a constant speed along a straight line at right angles to the beam.

linear tomography, tomography that produces a blurring pattern with linear, or unidirectional, motion. The pattern is caused by elongation of structures outside the focal plane.

linea semilunaris, the slightly curved line on the ventral abdominal wall. It marks the lateral border of the rectus abdominis and can be seen as a shallow groove when that muscle is tensed.

linea terminalis, a hypothetical line dividing the upper, or false, pelvis from the lower, or true, pelvis.

line compensator, an electrical device that monitors electric power for medical devices, such as x-ray equipment, and makes automatic adjustments for fluctuations in voltage.

line of demarcation [L *linea*; L *de, marcare* to mark], a line that indicates a change in the condition of tissues, such as the boundary between gangrenous and healthy tissues.

line of gravity, an imaginary line that extends from the center of gravity to the base of support.

line pair (lp), (in computed tomography) a factor in determining spatial frequency. It consists of a line, and its adjacent equal width interspace, forming a pair. As line pairs per centimeter increase, the fidelity of the line pair image decreases.

Lineweaver-Burk transformation [Hans Lineweaver, American chemist, b. 1907; Dean Burk, American scientist, b. 1904; L *transformare* to change shape], a method of converting experimental data from studies of enzyme activity so that they can be displayed on a linear plot.

lingua. See **tongue.**

lingual /ling′gwəl/ [L *lingua* tongue], pertaining to or resembling the tongue.

lingual artery, one of a pair of arteries that arises from the external carotid arteries, divides into four branches, and supplies the tongue and surrounding muscles.

L

lingual bar, a major connector that is installed lingual to the dental arch and joins bilateral parts of a mandibular removable partial denture.

lingual bone. See **hyoid bone.**

lingual crib, an orthodontic appliance consisting of a wire frame suspended lingually to the maxillary incisor teeth. It is used for obstructing undesirable thumb and tongue habits that can produce malocclusions.

lingual flange, the part of a mandibular denture that occupies the space adjacent to the residual ridge and next to the mouth.

lingual frenum, a band of tissue that extends from the floor of the mouth to the inferior surface of the tongue.

lingual gingiva, the gum covering the teeth on the surfaces facing the tongue.

lingual goiter, a tumor at the back of the tongue formed by an enlargement of the primordial thyrolingual duct.

lingualis leukoplakia [L *lingua* tongue; Gk *leukos* white + *plax* plate], a chronic inflammatory lesion characterized by smooth, thick, white patches on the surface of the tongue, generally attributed to excessive use of alcohol and tobacco. The lesions may be a precursor of epithelioma.

lingual papilla. See **papilla.**

lingual rest, a metallic extension onto the lingual surface of an anterior tooth to provide support or indirect retention for a removable partial denture.

lingual tonsil, a mass of lymphoid follicles near the root of the tongue.

lingua villosa nigra. See **parasitic glossitis.**

lingula /ling′gyələ/ [L, small tongue], any anatomic structure that resembles a tongue.

lingula of the lung, a tonguelike projection from the costal surface of the upper lobe of the left lung.

liniment /lin′imənt/ [L *linere* to smear], a preparation, usually containing an alcoholic, oily, or soapy vehicle, that is rubbed on the skin as a counterirritant.

linin /lī′nin/ [Gk *linon* flax, thread], the faintly staining threads seen in the nuclei of cells, with granules of chromatin attached to the threads.

linitis /linī′tis/ [Gk *linon* flax, thread, *itis* inflammation], inflammation of cellular tissue of the stomach as in linitis plastica, seen frequently in adenocarcinoma of the stomach.

linitis plastica, a diffuse fibrosis and thickening of the wall of the stomach, resulting in a rigid, inelastic organ. The layer of connective tissue of the stomach becomes fibrotic and thick, and the stomach wall becomes shrunken and rigid. Causes of this condition include infiltrating undifferentiated carcinoma, syphilis, and Crohn's disease.

linkage [Gk *linke* connection], **1.** (in genetics) the location of two or more genes on the same chromosome so that they do not segregate independently during meiosis but tend to be transmitted together as a unit. The closer the loci of the genes, the more likely they are to be inherited as a group and associated with a specific trait. **2.** (in psychology) the association between a stimulus and the response it elicits. **3.** (in chemistry) the bond between two atoms or radicals in a chemical compound.

linkage group, (in genetics) a group of genes located on the same chromosome that tends to be inherited as a unit.

linkage map. See **genetic map.**

linked genes [Me *linke* + Gk *genein* to produce], genes that are located on the same chromosome and whose position is close enough so that they tend to be transmitted as a linkage group.

linker [ME *linke* connection], (in molecular genetics) a small segment of synthetic DNA having a place on its surface that can be ligated to DNA fragments in cloning.

linoleic acid /lin′əlē′ik/ [L *linum* flax, *oleum* oil], a colorless to straw-colored essential fatty acid with two unsaturated bonds, occurring in linseed and safflower oils.

linolenic acid /lin′ōlen′ik/ [L *linum* flax, *oleum* oil], an unsaturated fatty acid essential for normal human nutrition. It occurs in glycerides of linseed and other vegetable oils.

liothyronine sodium /lī′ōthī′rənēn/, a synthetic thyroid hormone prescribed in the treatment of primary hypothyroidism, myxedema, simple goiter, cretinism, and secondary hypothyroidism.

liotrix /lī′ətriks/, a uniform mixture of the thyroid hormones T_3 and T_4. It is prescribed in the treatment of hypothyroid conditions.

lip [AS *lippa*], **1.** either the upper or lower fleshy structure surrounding the opening of the oral cavity. **2.** any rimlike structure bordering a cavity or groove; labium.

LIP, abbreviation for **lymphoid interstitial pneumonia.**

lipase /lī′pās, lip′ās/ [Gk *lipos* + Fr *diastase* enzyme], any of several enzymes, produced by the organs of the digestive system, that catalyze the breakdown of lipids through the hydrolysis of the linkages between fatty acids and glycerol in triglycerides and phospholipids.

lipectomy /lipek′təmē/ [Gk *lipos* + *ektome*

excision], an excision of subcutaneous fat, as from the abdominal wall.

lipedema /lip'ədē'mə/, a condition in which fat deposits accumulate in the lower extremities, from the hips to the ankles, accompanied by symptoms of tenderness in the affected areas.

lipemia /lipē'mē·ə/ [Gk *lipos* + *haima* blood], condition in which increased amounts of lipids are present in the blood, a normal occurrence after eating.

lipid /lip'id, li'pid/ [Gk *lipos* + *eidos* form], any of the free fatty acid fractions in the blood. They are stored in the body and serve as an energy reserve, but are elevated in various diseases, such as atherosclerosis. Kinds of lipids are **cholesterol, fatty acids, neutral fat, phospholipids, phospholipid as phosphorus,** and **triglycerides.**

lipidosis /lip'idō'sis/ [Gk *lipos* + *osis* condition], a general term including several rare familial disorders of fat metabolism. The chief characteristic of these disorders is the accumulation of abnormal levels of certain lipids in the body. Kinds of lipidoses are **Gaucher's disease, Krabbe's disease, Niemann-Pick disease,** and **Tay-Sachs disease.**

lipiduria /lip'idŏŏr'ē·ə/, the presence of lipids in the urine.

lipoatrophic diabetes /lip'ō·atrof'ik/, an inherited disease characterized by insulin-resistant diabetes mellitus, loss of body fat, acanthosis nigricans, and hypertrophied musculature. It is associated with a disorder of the hypothalamus resulting in excessive blood levels of growth hormone and ACTH-releasing hormones.

lipoatrophy /lip'ō·at'rəfē/, a breakdown of subcutaneous fat at the site of an insulin injection. It usually occurs after several injections at the same site.

lipocele. See **adipocele.**

lipochondrodystrophy. See **Hurler's syndrome.**

lipochrome /lip'əkrōm/ [Gk *lipos* + *chroma* color], any of the naturally occurring pigments that contain a lipid, and which give a yellow color to fats, such as carotene.

lipodystrophia progressiva /lip'ōdistrō'fē·ə/ [Gk *lipos* + *dys* bad, *trophe* nourishment; L *progredior* to go forth], an abnormal accumulation of fat around the buttocks and thighs and a progressive, symmetric disappearance of subcutaneous fat from areas above the pelvis and on the face.

lipodystrophy /lip'ōdis'trəfē/ [Gk *lipos* + *dys* bad, *trophe* nourishment], any abnormality in the metabolism or deposition of fats. Kinds of lipodystrophy are **bitro-** chanteric, insulin, and **intestinal lipodystrophy.**

lip of hip fracture, a fracture of the posterior lip of the acetabulum, often associated with displacement of the hip.

lipofuscin /lip'əfus'in/, a class of fatty pigments consisting mostly of oxidized fats that are found in abundance in the cells of adults.

lipogenesis /lip'ōjen'əsis/ [Gk *lipos* + *genein* to produce], the production and accumulation of fat.

lipogranuloma /lip'ōgran'yŏŏlō'mə/, *pl.* **lipogranulomas, lipogranulomata** [Gk *lipos* + L *granulum* little grain; Gk *oma* tumor], a nodule of necrotic, fatty tissue associated with granulomatous inflammation or with a foreign-body reaction around a deposit of injected material containing an oily substance.

lipohypertrophy /lip'ōhīpur'trəfē/, a buildup of subcutaneous fat tissue at the site of an insulin injection.

lipoic acid /lipō'ik/, a bacterial growth factor found in liver and yeast.

lipoid /lip'oid/, any substance that resembles a lipid.

lipolysis /lipol'isis/, the breakdown or destruction of lipids or fats.

lipolytic /lip'ōlit'ik/ [Gk *lipos* + *lysis* loosening], relating to the chemical breakdown of fat.

lipoma /lipō'mə/, *pl.* **lipomas, lipomata** [Gk *lipos* + *oma* tumor], a benign tumor consisting of mature fat cells. –**lipomatous,** *adj.*

lipoma annulare colli, a diffuse, symmetric accumulation of fat around the neck; not a true lipoma.

lipoma arborescens, a fatty tumor of a joint, characterized by a treelike distribution of fat cells.

lipoma capsulare, a benign neoplasm characterized by the abnormal presence of fat cells in the capsule of an organ.

lipoma cavernosum. See **angiolipoma.**

lipoma diffusum renis. See **lipomatous nephritis.**

lipoma dolorosa. See **lipomatosis dolorosa.**

lipoma fibrosum, a fatty tumor containing masses of fibrous tissue.

lipoma myxomatodes. See **lipomyxoma.**

lipoma sarcomatodes. See **liposarcoma.**

lipomatosis /lip'ōmətō'sis/ [Gk *lipos* + *oma* tumor, *osis* condition], a disorder characterized by abnormal tumorlike accumulations of fat in body tissues.

lipomatosis atrophicans. See **lipodystrophia progressiva, lipomatosis.**

lipomatosis dolorosa, a disorder characterized by the abnormal accumulation of painful or tender fat deposits.

L

lipomatosis gigantea, a condition characterized by massive deposits of fat.

lipomatosis renis. See **lipomatous nephritis.**

lipomatous myxoma /lipō′mətəs/, a tumor containing fatty tissue that arises in connective tissue.

lipomatous nephritis, a rare condition in which the renal nephrons are replaced by fatty tissue. Kidney failure may result.

lipometabolism /lipōmetab′əliz′əm/ [Gk *lipos* fat; *metabole* change], the chemical processes involved in building up or breaking down fat molecules.

lipomyoma /lipōmī·ō′mə/ [Gk *lipos* + *mys* muscle, *oma* tumor], a tumor that combines characteristics of a lipoma and myoma.

lipomyxoma /lip′ōmiksō′mə/, *pl.* **lipomyxomas, lipomyxomata** [Gk *lipos* + *myxa* mucus, *oma* tumor], a myxoma that contains fat.

lipophilia /lipōfil′yə/ [Gk *lipos* + *philein* to love], a tendency to attract or absorb fat.

lipoprotein /lip′ōprō′tēn/ [Gk *lipos* + *proteios* first rank], a conjugated protein in which lipids form an integral part of the molecule. They are synthesized primarily in the liver, and are classified according to their composition and density. Kinds of lipoproteins are **chylomicrons, high-density lipoproteins, low-density lipoproteins,** and **very low-density lipoproteins.**

liposarcoma /lip′ōsärkō′mə/, *pl.* **liposarcomas, liposarcomata** [Gk *lipos* + *sarx* flesh, *oma* tumor], a malignant growth of primitive fat cells.

liposis. See **lipomatosis.**

liposoluble [Gk *lipos* + L *solubilis*], fat soluble.

liposome /lip′əsōm/ [Gk *lipos* + *soma* body], a multilayered spherical particle of a lipid in an aqueous medium in a cell.

liposuction, a technique for removing adipose tissue from obese patients with a suction-pump device. It is used primarily to remove or reduce localized areas of fat around the abdomen, breasts, legs, face, and upper arms where the skin is contractile enough to redrape in a normal manner.

liquefaction /lik′wəfak′shən/ [L *liquere* to flow, *facere* to make], the process in which a solid or a gas is made liquid.

liquid [L *liquere* to flow], a state of matter, intermediate between solid and gas, in which the substance flows freely with little application of force and assumes the shape of the vessel in which it is contained.

liquid diet, a diet consisting of foods that can be served in liquid or strained form plus custard, ice cream, pudding, tapioca, and soft-cooked eggs.

liquid glucose, a thick, syrupy, odorless, and colorless or yellowish liquid obtained by the incomplete hydrolysis of starch, primarily consisting of dextrose with dextrins, maltose, and water.

liquor /lik′ər/, any fluid or liquid, such as liquor amnii, the amniotic fluid.

liquor amnii. See **amniotic fluid.**

Lisfranc's fracture /lisfrangks′/ [Jacque Lisfranc, French surgeon, b. 1790], a fracture dislocation of the foot in which one or all of the proximal metatarsals are displaced.

lisping, the defective pronunciation of one or more of the sibilant consonant sounds, usually *s* and *z*.

Lister, Baron Joseph [Scottish surgeon, b. 1827], introduced the use of antiseptic surgery in London hospitals in 1867. Lister operations were performed under a spray of diluted carbolic acid, instruments were dipped in carbolic acid, and wounds were dressed with gauze similarly treated.

Listeria monocytogenes /mon′ōsītoj′inēz/ [Baron Joseph Lister; Gk *mono* single, *kytos* cell, *genein* to produce], a common species of gram-positive, motile bacillus that causes listeriosis.

listeriosis /listir′ē·ō′sis/ [Baron Joseph Lister; Gk *osis* condition], an infectious disease caused by a genus of gram-positive motile bacteria that are nonsporulating. Transmitted by direct contact from infected animals to humans, by inhalation of dust, or by contact with mud, sewage, or soil contaminated with the organism, it is characterized by circulatory collapse, shock, endocarditis, hepatosplenomegaly, and a dark red rash over the trunk and the legs. Fever, bacteremia, malaise, and lethargy are commonly seen.

Liston's forceps [Robert Liston, Scottish surgeon, b. 1794], a kind of bone-cutting forceps.

liter (L) /lē′tər/ [Fr], a unit of volume equivalent to 1.057 quarts and defined as the volume occupied by a mass of one kilogram of water at standard temperature and pressure.

lithiasis /lithī′əsis/ [Gk *lithos* stone, *osis* condition], the formation of calculi in the hollow organs or ducts of the body. Calculi are formed of mineral salts and may irritate, inflame, or obstruct the organ in which they form or lodge. Lithiasis occurs most commonly in the gallbladder, kidney, and lower urinary tract. Lithiasis may be asymptomatic, but more often the condition is extremely painful.

lithium (Li) /lith′ē·əm/ [Gk *lithos* stone], a silvery-white alkali metal occurring in various compounds, such as petalite and spodumene. Its atomic number is 3; its atomic weight is 6.94. Lithium is the lightest known metal. Its salts are used in the treatment of manias.

lithium carbonate, an antimanic agent prescribed in the treatment of manic episodes of manic-depressive disorder.

lithium fluoride (LiF), a compound commonly used for thermoluminescent dosimetry.

lithogenesis /lith′əjen′əsis/ [Gk *lithos* + *genein* to produce], the origin of the formation of a calculus.

lithopedion /lith′əpē′dē·ən/ [Gk *lithos* + *paidion* child], a fetus that has died in utero and has become calcified or ossified.

lithotomy /lithot′əmē/ [Gk *lithos* + *temnein* to cut], the surgical excision of a calculus, especially one from the urinary tract.

lithotomy forceps, a forceps for the extraction of a calculus, usually from the urinary tract.

lithotomy position, the posture assumed by the patient lying supine with the hips and the knees flexed and the thighs abducted and rotated externally.

lithotripsy /lith′ətrip′sē/ [Gk *lithos* + *tribein* to wear away], a procedure for eliminating a kidney stone by crushing or dissolving it in situ.

lithotrite /lith′ətrit/ [Gk *lithos* + L *terere* to rub], an instrument for crushing a stone in the urinary bladder. **–lithotrity,** *n.*

litigant /lit′əgənt/ [L *litigare* to go to law], (in law) a party to a lawsuit.

litigate, (in law) to carry on a suit or to contest.

litigious paranoia [L *litigare* to go to law; Gk *paranous* madness], a form of paranoia in which the person seeks legal proof or justification for systematized delusions.

litmus paper /lit′məs/ [ONorse *litmosi* coloring herb; L *papyrus* paper], absorbent paper coated with litmus, a blue dye, that is used to determine pH. Acid substances or solutions turn blue litmus to red. Alkaline substances or solutions do not cause a color change in blue litmus.

litter [Fr *lit* bed], a stretcher.

Little's disease. See **cerebral palsy.**

Litzmann's obliquity. See **asynclitism.**

live attenuated measles virus vaccine, a vaccine prepared from live strains of measles virus that have been cultured under conditions that cause them to lose their virulence without losing their ability to induce immunity. The vaccine is not recommended for pregnant women or others who may have certain medical conditions that tend to diminish immunity.

live birth [AS *libben* to be alive; ONorse *byrth*], the birth of an infant, irrespective of the duration of gestation, that exhibits any sign of life, such as respiration, heartbeat, umbilical pulsation, or movement of voluntary muscles.

livedo /livē′dō/ [L *liveo* bluish spot], a blue or reddish mottling of the skin, worse in cold weather and probably caused by arteriolar spasm. **Cutis marmorata** is a transient form of livedo.

livedo reticularis, a vasospastic disorder accentuated by exposure to cold and presenting with a characteristic reddish blue mottling with a typical "fishnet" appearance and involving the entire leg and, less often, the arms.

livedo vasculitis. See **segmented hyalinizing vasculitis.**

live measles and mumps virus vaccine, a vaccine prepared from live strains of measles and mumps viruses. The vaccine is commonly combined with live rubella viruses as **MMR vaccine** and administered to normal infants at the age of 15 months.

live oral poliovirus vaccine, a vaccine prepared from three strains (trivalent) of live polioviruses. Primary immunization with the vaccine usually begins at the age of 2 months.

liver [AS *lifer*], the largest gland of the body and one of its most complex organs. More than 500 of its functions have been identified. It is divided into four lobes, contains as many as 100,000 lobules, and is served by two distinct blood supplies. The hepatic artery conveys oxygenated blood to the liver, and the hepatic portal vein conveys nutrient-filled blood from the stomach and the intestines. Some of the major functions performed by the liver are the production of bile by hepatic cells; the secretion of glucose, proteins, vitamins, fats, and most of the other compounds used by the body; the processing of hemoglobin for vital use of its iron content; and the conversion of poisonous ammonia to urea.

liver biopsy, a diagnostic procedure in which a special needle is introduced into the liver under local anesthesia to obtain a specimen for pathologic examination.

liver breath. See **fetor hepaticus.**

liver cancer, a malignant neoplastic disease of the liver, occurring most frequently as a metastasis from another malignancy. Risk factors include hemochromatosis, schistosomiasis, exposure to vinyl chloride or arsenic, and possibly nutritional deficiencies. Alcoholism may be a predisposing factor, but nonalcoholic cirrhosis is a greater risk than alcoholic cirrhosis. Aflatoxins in moldy grain and peanuts appear to be linked to high rates of hepatocellular carcinoma. Characteristics of liver cancer are abdominal bloating, anorexia, weakness, dull upper abdominal pain, ascites, mild jaundice, and a tender enlarged liver; in some cases tumor nodules are palpable on the liver surface.

liver cell carcinoma. See **malignant hepatoma.**

liver disease, any one of a group of disorders of the liver. The most important diseases in this group are cirrhosis, cholestasis, and viral and toxic hepatitis. Characteristics of liver disease are jaundice, anorexia, hepatomegaly, ascites, and impaired consciousness. The exact diagnosis of liver disease is made through a combination of laboratory tests and clinical findings.

liver failure [AS *lifer*; L *fallere* to deceive], a condition in which the liver fails to fulfill its function or is unable to meet the demands made on it. Anorexia, fatigue, and weakness are common symptoms of liver cell failure whereas jaundice indicates a biliary obstruction and fever may accompany viral or alcoholic liver diseases.

liver flap. See **asterixis.**

liver fluke [AS *lifer*; *floc*], a parasitic Trematode with six genera that may infest the liver. The most important species affecting humans in industrialized countries is *Clonorchis sinensis*, which is usually acquired by eating freshwater fish containing the encysted larvae. The larvae are released in the duodenum, enter the common bile duct, and migrate to other bile ducts, the gall bladder, and pancreatic ducts. The liver fluke may survive for many years in the human biliary tree, releasing eggs into the feces. Infestations are most likely to result from ingestion of raw, dried, salted, or pickled freshwater fish and can be prevented by thorough cooking of freshwater fish.

liver function test, a test used to evaluate various functions of the liver—for example, metabolism, storage, filtration, and excretion. Kinds of liver function tests include **alkaline phosphatase, bromsulfalein test, prothrombin time, serum bilirubin,** and **serum glutamic pyruvic transaminase.**

liver scan, a noninvasive technique of visualizing the size, shape, and consistency of the liver by the intravenous injection of a radioactively labeled compound that is readily taken up and trapped in the Kupffer cells of the liver.

liver spot, *nontechnical;* a senile lentigo or actinic keratosis.

liver transplantation, a treatment for end-stage hepatic dysfunction. A donor liver from a previously healthy but brain-dead individual is matched in size and and blood group to the recipient. The transplanted organ may be introduced as an auxiliary liver or a total replacement. The procedure requires five anastomoses and many units of blood. Because of a shortage of child-sized livers, pediatric transplants often are performed with a segment of an adult liver.

livid [L *lividus* bluish], pertaining to an injury that is congested and discolored.

lividity /livid'itē/, a tissue condition of being red or blue because of venous congestion, as in a contusion.

living-in unit [AS *libben* to be alive; L *in* within; *unus* one], a room provided in some hospitals for mothers who want to assume immediate care of their newborn infants under the supervision of nursing personnel.

living will [AS *libben* + *willa* wish], a written agreement between a patient and physician to withhold heroic measures if the patient's condition is found to be irreversible.

livor mortis /lī'vər/, a purple discoloration of the skin in some dependent body areas following death as a result of blood cell destruction.

lizard [L *lacerta*], a scaly skinned reptile with a long body and tail and two pairs of legs. The symptoms of their bites and the recommended treatment are similar to those of the bites from moderately poisonous snakes.

LLD factor. See **cyanocobalamin.**

LLE, abbreviation for *left lower extremity.*

LLQ, abbreviation for *left lower quadrant of abdomen.*

LMA, abbreviation for *left mentoanterior fetal position.*

LMD. See **dextran preparation.**

LMD, abbreviation for *local medical doctor,* used by house staff or others to distinguish a patient's primary physician from university faculty, attending specialist physicians, or house staff.

LMP, 1. abbreviation for *last menstrual period.* **2.** abbreviation for *left mentoposterior fetal position.*

LMT, abbreviation for *left mentotransverse fetal position.*

LOA, abbreviation for *left occipitoanterior fetal position.*

loading response stance stage [AS *lad*

support; L *responsum* reply], one of the five stages of the stance phase of walking or gait, specifically associated with the moment when the leg reacts to and accepts the weight of the body.

loads [AS *lad* support], *slang.* a fixed combination of a sedative hypnotic, glutethimide, and a major narcotic analgesic, codeine. The medications are taken orally by drug abusers for a euphoric effect reported to be similar to that produced by heroin, but longer lasting.

Loa loa /lō'ä lō'ä/, a parasitic worm of western and central Africa that causes loiasis.

lobar bronchus /lō'bär/ [Gk *lobos* lobe; *bronchos* windpipe], a bronchus extending from a primary bronchus to a segmental bronchus into one of the lobes of the right or left lung.

lobar pneumonia, a severe infection of one or more of the five major lobes of the lungs that, if untreated, eventually results in consolidation of lung tissue. The disease is characterized by fever, chills, cough, rusty sputum, rapid shallow breathing, cyanosis, nausea, vomiting, and pleurisy. Complications include lung abscess, atelectasis, empyema, pericarditis, and pleural effusion.

lobe /lōb/ [Gk *lobos*], **1.** a roundish projection of any structure. **2.** a portion of any organ, demarcated by sulci, fissures, or connective tissue, as the lobes of the brain, liver, and lungs. **–lobar, lobular,** *adj.*

lobectomy [Gk *lobos* + *ektome* excision], **1.** excision of the lobe of any organ or gland. **2.** a type of chest surgery in which a lobe of a lung is excised, performed to remove a malignant tumor and to treat uncontrolled bronchiectasis, trauma with hemorrhage, or intractable tuberculosis. Some compensatory emphysema is expected as the remaining lung tissue overexpands to fill the new space. **–lobectomize,** *v.*

lobe of ear [Gk *lobos*; AS *eare*], the lower portion of the auricle, which contains no cartilage.

lobotomy /lōbot'əmē/ [Gk *lobos* + *temnein* to cut], a neurosurgical procedure in which the nerve fibers in the bundle of white matter in the frontal lobe of the brain are severed to interrupt the transmission of various affective responses. Severe intractable depression and pain are among the indications for the operation. It is rarely performed, because it has many unpredictable and undesirable effects.

lobster claw deformity. See **bidactyly.**

lobular carcinoma /lob'yələr/ [Gk *lobos* + *karkinos* crab, *oma* tumor], a neoplasm that often forms a diffuse mass and accounts for a small percentage of breast tumors.

lobule /lob'yōol/, a small lobe, such as the soft, lower, pendulous part of the external ear. **–lobular,** *adj.*

local [L *locus* place], **1.** of or pertaining to a small circumscribed area of the body. **2.** of or pertaining to a treatment or drug applied locally. **3.** *informal;* a local anesthetic.

local adaptation syndrome (LAS), the localized response of a tissue, organ, or system that occurs as a reaction to stress.

local anaphylaxis [L *locus;* Gk *ana, phylaxis*], a condition in which injections of an antigen result in local swellings and localized necrosis of the skin and subcutaneous tissues.

local anesthesia, the direct administration of a local anesthetic agent to tissues to induce the absence of sensation in a small area of the body. Brief surgical or dental procedures are the most common indications for local anesthesia. The anesthetic may be applied topically to the surface of the skin or membrane or injected subcutaneously through an intradermal weal. The principal drawbacks to the use of local anesthesia are the incidence of allergic reactions to certain agents. The advantages include low cost, ease of administration, low toxicity, and safety. A conscious patient can cooperate and does not require respiratory support or intubation.

local anesthetic, a substance used to reduce or eliminate neural sensation, specifically pain, in a limited area of the body. Local anesthetics act by blocking transmission of nerve impulses. More than 100 drugs are available for local anesthesia; they are classified as members of the alcohol-ester or the aminoamide family. Any substance sufficiently potent to induce local anesthesia has potential for causing adverse side effects, ranging from easily reversible dermatitis to lethal anaphylaxis or simultaneous respiratory and cardiac arrest.

local cerebral blood flow (LCBF), (in positron emission tomography) the parametric image of blood flow through the brain. It is expressed in units of milliliters of blood flow per minute.

local cerebral metabolic rate of glucose utilization (LCMRG), (in positron emission tomography) a parametric image of the brain expressed in units of milligrams of glucose utilization per minute per 100 g of brain tissue.

local control, the arrest of cancer growth at the site of origin.

local hypothermia, the heating of a local area of tissue to therapeutic temperatures.

local infection [L *locus; inficere* to stain], an infection involving bacteria that invade the body at a specific point and remain there, multiplying, until eliminated.

localization [L *locus* place], **1.** the designation of a particular site for a lesion or organ function. **2.** the determination of the site of a biologic function. **3.** the assignment of a position to an object detected by radiography.

localization audiometry. See **audiometry.**

localization film [L *locus;* Gk *izein* to cause; AS *filmen* membrane], (in radiotherapy) a diagnostic film taken to confirm a treatment effect or to view the position of an intracavitary or interstitial implant, especially for the purpose of computing the dose delivered.

localized scleroderma. See **morphea.**

localizer image, (in computed tomography) an image used to localize a specific body part.

localizing symptom, local symptom. See **symptom.**

local lesion [L *locus; laesio* hurting], a lesion of the central nervous system characterized by distinctive local symptoms.

local reaction [L *locus; re, agere* to act], a reaction to treatment that occurs at the site at which it was administered.

lochia /lō'kē·ə/ [Gk *lochos* childbirth], the discharge that flows from the vagina after childbirth. During the first 3 or 4 days postpartum the lochia is red **(lochia rubra)** and is made up of blood, endometrial decidua, fetal lanugo, vernix, and sometimes meconium, small shreds of placental tissue, and membranes. After the third day the amount of blood diminishes, the placental site exudes serous material and lymph, and the lochia becomes darker and thinner **(lochia fusca),** and then serous **(lochia serosa)** as evacuation of particulate material is completed. During the second week white blood cells and bacteria appear in large numbers along with fatty, mucinous decidual material, causing the lochia to appear yellow **(lochia flava** or **lochia purulenta).** During the third week and thereafter, as endometrial epithelialization progresses, the amount of lochia decreases markedly and takes on a seromucinous consistency and a gray-white color **(lochia alba).** Cessation of the flow of lochia at about 6 weeks is usual. **—lochial,** *adj.*

locked-in syndrome [ME *loc;* Gk *syn* together, *dromos* course], a paralytic condition in which a person may be conscious and alert but unable to communicate except by eye movements or blinking. Bilateral destruction of the medulla oblongata or pons has rendered the patient unable to speak or move any of the limbs.

locked knee [AS *loc;* cneow], a condition in which the knee cannot be fully extended, often caused by longitudinal splitting of the medial meniscus.

locked twins. See **interlocked twins.**

lock forceps. See **point forceps.**

locking point [AS *loc* lock; L *punctum* puncture], a point on the body at which light pressure can be applied to help a weak or debilitated patient maintain a desired posture or position. A basic locking point is the body's center of gravity, at the level of the second sacral vertebra, where mild pressure can assist a patient in standing or walking erect.

lockjaw, *informal;* tetanus.

locomotion [L *locus* + *motio* movement], movement or the ability to move from one place or position to another.

locomotor [L, *locus; motio*], pertaining to locomotion.

locomotor ataxia. See **tabes dorsalis.**

loculate /lok'yŏŏlāt/ [L *loculus* little place], divided into small spaces or cavities.

loculus /lok'yŏŏləs/ [L, little place], a small chamber, pocket, or cavity, such as the interior of a polyp.

locum tenens /lō'kəm ten'ənz/ [L *locus* place; *tenere* to hold], a temporary substitute for a physician who is away from the practice.

locus, *pl.* **loci** [L, place], a specific place or position, such as the locus of a particular gene on a chromosome.

locus ceruleus [L *locus; ceruleus* heaven], a deeply pigmented group of several thousand neurons in the floor of the fourth ventricle. It is part of a major norepinephrine route of the central nervous system.

locus of control [L *locus;* Fr *contrôle*], a center of responsibility for one's behavior. Individuals with an **internal locus of control** believe they can control events related to their life whereas those with an **external locus of control** tend to believe that real power resides in forces outside themselves and determines their life.

locus of infection, a site in the body where an infection originates.

Löffler's syndrome /lef'lərz/ [Wilhelm Löffler, Swiss physician, b. 1887], a benign, idiopathic disorder marked by episodes of pulmonary eosinophilia, transient opacities in the lungs, anorexia, breathlessness, fever, and weight loss.

logotherapy /log'ōther'əpē/ [Gk *logos* word, *therapeia* treatment], a treatment modality based on the application of humanistic and existential psychology to assist a patient in finding meaning and purpose in life and unique life experiences.

log roll [ME *logge*; L *roto* turn around], a maneuver used to turn a reclining patient from one side to the other or completely over without flexing the spinal column. The arms of the patient are folded across the chest and the legs extended. A draw sheet under the patient is manipulated by attending nursing personnel to facilitate the procedure.

loiasis /lō-ī′əsis/, a form of filariasis caused by the worm *Loa loa*, which may migrate for 10 to 15 years in subcutaneous tissue, producing localized inflammation known as Calabar swellings. The disease is acquired through the bite of an infected African deer fly.

loin [ME *loyn* flank], a part of the body on each side of the spinal column between the false ribs and the hip bones.

lomustine /lōmus′tēn/, an antineoplastic alkylating agent. It is prescribed in the treatment of a variety of malignant neoplastic diseases.

long-acting drug [AS *lang*; L *agere* to do; Fr *drogue* drug], a pharmacologic agent with a prolonged effect because of a formulation resulting in the slow release of the active principle or the continued absorption of small amounts of the dosage of the drug over an extended period.

long-acting insulin, a preparation of the antidiabetic principle of beef pancreas or pork pancreas modified by an interaction with zinc. An injection of the preparation takes effect within 8 hours, reaches a peak of action in 16 to 24 hours, and has a duration of action of more than 36 hours.

long-acting thyroid stimulator (LATS), an immunoglobulin, probably an autoantibody, that exerts a prolonged stimulatory effect on the thyroid gland, causing rapid growth of the gland and excess activity of thyroid function resulting in hyperthyroidism.

long-arm cast [AS *lang* + *earm* arm; O-Norse *kasta*], an orthopedic cast applied to immobilize upper extremities from the hand to the upper arm.

long bones, the bones that contribute to the height or length of an extremity, particularly the bones of the legs and arms.

longevity /lonjev′itē/ [L *longus* long + *aveum* age], the number of years an average person of a particular age can expect to continue living. It is determined by statistical tables based on mortality rates of various population groups.

longitudinal /lon′jətoō′dənəl/ [L *longitudo* length], **1.** a measurement in the direction of the long axis of an object, body, or organ, such as the longitudinal arch of the foot. **2.** a scientific study that is conducted over a long period of time.

longitudinal diffusion, the diffusion of solute molecules in the direction of flow of the mobile phase.

longitudinal dissociation, (in cardiology) the insulation of parallel pathways of impulses from each other, usually in the AV junction.

longitudinal fissure [L *longitudo; fissura* cleft], the largest and deepest groove between the medial surfaces of the cerebral hemispheres.

longitudinal presentation [L *longitudo; praesentare* to show], the normal presentation of a fetus, with the long axis of the infant body parallel to that of the mother.

longitudinal sound waves, pressure waves formed by the oscillation of particles or molecules parallel to the axis of wave propagation. The compression and expansion of such longitudinal waves at high frequencies is the principle on which ultrasonography is based.

long-leg cast, an orthopedic cast applied to immobilize the leg from the toes to the upper thigh.

long-leg cast with walker, an orthopedic cast applied to immobilize the lower extremities from the toes to the upper thigh in treating certain fractures of the leg. This type of cast is the same as the long-leg cast but incorporates a rubber walker, allowing the patient to walk while the leg is encased in the cast.

long-term care (LTC), the provision of medical, social, and personal care services on a recurring or continuing basis to persons with chronic physical or mental disorders.

long-term memory, the ability to recall sensations, events, ideas, and other information for long periods of time without apparent effort.

long thoracic nerve, one of a pair of supraclavicular branches from the roots of the brachial plexus.

long tract signs, neurologic signs, such as clonus, muscle spasticity, or bladder involvement, that usually indicate a lesion in the middle or upper portions of the spinal cord or in the brain.

loop [ME *loupe*], *informal;* intrauterine device.

loop colostomy [ME *loupe;* Gk *kolon* colon, *stoma* mouth], a type of temporary colostomy performed as part of the surgical repair of Hirschsprung's disease. To perform the procedure an intact segment of colon anterior to the repair is brought through an abdominal incision and sutured onto the abdomen. A loop is formed and held in position by placing a piece of glass rod between the segment and the abdomen.

loop diuretic. See **diuretic.**

loop of Henle /hen'lē/ [ME *loupe*; Friedrich G. J. Henle, German anatomist, b. 1809], the U-shaped portion of a renal tubule, consisting of a thin descending limb and a thick ascending limb.

loose association. See **loosening.**

loose fibrous tissue [ME *lous* not fastened], a constrictive, pliable fibrous connective tissue consisting of interwoven elastic and collagenous fibers, interspersed with fluid-filled areolae.

loosening [ME *lous*], (in psychiatry) a disturbance of thinking in which the association of ideas and thought patterns become so vague, diffuse, and unfocused as to lack any logical sequences or relationship to any preceding concepts or themes.

loose-pack joint position, a point in the range of motion at which articulating surfaces are the least congruent and supporting structures are the most lax.

LOP, abbreviation for *left occipitoposterior fetal position.*

loperamide hydrochloride /lōper'əmīd/, an antiperistaltic prescribed in the treatment of diarrhea.

lorazepam /lôrā'zəpam/, a benzodiazepine tranquilizer prescribed as a minor tranquilizer in the treatment of anxiety, nervous tension, and insomnia.

lordoscoliosis /lôr'dōskō'lē·ō'sis/ [Gk *lordos* bent + *skoliosis* curvature], a combination of lordosis and scoliosis.

lordosis /lôrdō'sis/ [Gk *lordos* bent forward, *osis* condition], **1.** the normal curvature of the lumbar and cervical spine, seen as an anterior concavity if the person is observed from the side. **2.** an abnormal, increased degree of curvature of any part of the back.

lordotic pelvis /lôrdot'ik/ [Gk *lordos*; L *pelvis* basin], a pelvis that is inadequate for childbirth because the spinal column bends forward in the lumbar region.

LOS, abbreviation for *length of stay.*

loss of consortium [ME *lossen* to lose; L *consortionis* companionship], (in law) a claim for damages sought in recompense for the loss of conjugal relations, including society, affection, and assistance, and impairment or loss of sexual relations.

LOT, abbreviation for *left occipitotransverse fetal position.*

lotion [L *lotio* a washing], a liquid preparation applied externally to protect the skin or to treat a dermatologic disorder.

Lou Gehrig's disease. See **amyotrophic lateral sclerosis.**

Louis-Bar syndrome. See **ataxia-telangiectasia.**

loupe /lōōp/ [Fr, magnifying glass], a magnifying lens mounted in a frame worn on the head, as used to examine the eyes.

louse. See **lice.**

louse bite, a minute puncture wound produced by a louse that may transmit typhus, trench fever, and relapsing fever. Secondary infection may result from scratching the affected area.

louse-borne typhus. See **epidemic typhus.**

low back pain [ME *low*; AS *baec*; L *poena* penalty], local or referred pain at the base of the spine caused by a sprain, strain, osteoarthritis, ankylosing spondylitis, a neoplasm, or a prolapsed intervertebral disk. Low back pain is a common complaint and is often associated with poor posture, obesity, sagging abdominal muscles, or sitting for prolonged periods of time. Pain may be localized and static; it may be accompanied by muscle weakness or spasms; or it may radiate down the back of one or both legs, as in sciatica. It may be initiated or increased by coughing, sneezing, rising from a seated position, lifting, stretching, bending, or turning. To guard against the pain, the person may decrease the range of motion of the spine. If an intervertebral disk is prolapsed, deep pressure over the interspace generally causes pain, and flexion of the hip elicits sciatic pain when the knee is extended but not when the knee is flexed (Lasègue's sign).

low birth weight (LBW) infant, an infant whose weight at birth is less than 2,500 g, regardless of gestational age. Many low birth weight infants have no problems and develop normally, their smallness being genetic or idiopathic, or the problem that caused their slowed growth being mild or brief.

low blood, *informal;* anemia.

low-calcium diet, a diet that restricts the use of calcium and that eliminates most of the dairy foods, all breads made with milk or dry skimmed milk, and deep-green leafy vegetables. It is prescribed for patients who form renal calculi.

low-caloric diet, a diet that is prescribed to limit the intake of calories, usually to cause a reduction in body weight. Such diets may be designated as 800 calorie, 1,000 calorie, or other specific numbers of calories.

low cervical cesarean section, a method for surgically delivering a baby through a transverse incision in the thin supracervical portion of the lower uterine segment. This incision bleeds less during surgery and heals with a stronger scar than the higher vertical scar of the classic cesarean section.

low-cholesterol diet, a diet that restricts foods containing animal fats and saturated fatty acids, such as egg yolk, cream, butter, milk, muscle and organ meats, and shellfish, and concentrates on poultry, fish, vegetables, fruits, cottage cheese, and polyunsaturated fats.

low-density lipoprotein (LDL), a plasma protein containing relatively more cholesterol and triglycerides than protein. It is derived in part, if not completely, from the intravascular breakdown of the very low-density lipoproteins.

lower extremity suspension [ME *low;* L *extremitas; suspendere* to hang], an orthopedic procedure used in the treatment of bone fractures and in the correction of orthopedic abnormalities of the lower limbs. The procedure uses traction equipment, including metal frames, ropes, and pulleys, to relieve the weight of the lower limb involved rather than to exert traction pull.

lower level discriminator (LLD), (in nuclear medicine) a radiation energy-sensitive device used to discriminate against all radionuclide pulses whose heights are below the accepted level.

lower motor neuron paralysis, an injury to or lesion in the spinal cord that damages the cell bodies or axons, or both, of the lower motor neurons, which are located in the anterior horn cells and the spinal and peripheral nerves. If complete transection of the spinal cord occurs, voluntary muscle control is totally lost. In partial transection function is altered in varying degrees, depending on the areas innervated by the nerves involved.

lower respiratory infection. See **respiratory tract infection.**

lower respiratory tract, a division of the respiratory system that includes the left and the right bronchi and the alveoli where the exchange of oxygen and carbon dioxide occurs during the respiratory cycle. The bronchi divide into smaller bronchioles in the lungs, the bronchioles into alveolar ducts, the ducts into alveolar sacs, and the sacs into alveoli.

low-fat diet [ME *low;* AS *faett;* Gk *diaita* lifestyle], a diet containing limited amounts of fat and consisting chiefly of easily digestible foods of high carbohydrate content. It includes all vegetables, lean meats, fish, fowl, pasta, cereals, and whole wheat or enriched bread. The diet

may be indicated in gallbladder disease and malabsorption syndromes.

low-fat milk, milk containing 1% to 2% fat, making it an intermediate in fat content between whole and skimmed milk.

low-fiber diet. See **Low-residue diet.**

low-flow oxygen delivery system, respiratory care equipment that does not supply all the inspired gases. The patient inhales some room air along with the oxygen being delivered.

low forceps [ME *low;* L *forceps* pair of tongs], an obstetric operation in which forceps are used to deliver a baby whose head is on the pelvic floor. It is commonly required for the delivery of mothers whose expulsive powers have been weakened by analgesia, anesthesia, or fatigue.

low-grade fever, a temperature that is above 98.6° F but lower than 100.4° F for 24 hours.

low-grade infection [ME *lah;* L *gradus* degree, *inficere* to stain], a subacute or chronic infection with mild fever and no pus production.

low-level radiation, radiated energy that is generally nonionizing. Examples include magnetic fields generated by common household electric lines and appliances.

Lown-Ganong-Levine syndrome (LGL) /loun'gənong'ləvēn'/ [Bernard Lown, American physician, b. 1921; William F. Ganong, American physiologist, b. 1924; S. A. Levine, American physician, b. 1891], a disorder of the atrioventricular (AV) conduction system, marked by ventricular preexcitation. Part or all of the AV nodal connection is bypassed by an abnormal AV connection from the atrial muscle to the bundle of His.

low-power field, the low magnification field of vision under a light microscope.

low-protein diet [ME *lah;* Gk *proteios* first rank; *diaita* life-style], a diet proportionally low in protein, usually designed for persons who must restrict their intake of protein because of a metabolic abnormality associated with kidney failure or a liver disease.

low-residue diet, a diet that will leave a minimal residue in the lower intestinal tract after digestion and absorption. It consists of tender meats, poultry, fish, eggs, white bread, pasta, simple desserts, clear soups, tea, and coffee. The diet is prescribed in cases of diverticulosis and diverticulitis, GI irritability or inflammation, and before and after GI surgery.

low-salt diet. See **low-sodium diet.**

low-saturated-fat diet. See **low-cholesterol diet.**

low-sodium diet, a diet that restricts the

L

use of sodium chloride plus other compounds containing sodium, such as baking powder or soda, monosodium glutamate, sodium citrate, sodium propionate, and sodium sulfate. It is indicated in hypertension, edematous states (especially when associated with cardiovascular disease), renal or liver disease, and therapy with corticosteroids. The degree of sodium restriction depends on the severity of the condition.

loxapine /lok'səpēn/, a tranquilizer prescribed in the treatment of schizophrenia.

lozenge. See troche.

lpm, abbreviation for *liters per minute.*

LP, abbreviation for **lumbar puncture.**

LPN, abbreviation for **licensed practical nurse.**

LPO, abbreviation for *left posterior oblique position.*

LPS Act, a California law named for sponsors of the legislation (Lanterman, Petris, and Short) that provides for the protection and treatment of persons judged to be "gravely disabled" and, thus, unable to provide food, clothing, or shelter for themselves. The legislation was designed to safeguard the constitutional rights of persons threatened with involuntary commitment on the basis of a psychiatric diagnosis.

Lr, symbol for the element **lawrencium.**

LSD, abbreviation for *lysergic acid diethylamide.*

L/S ratio, the lecithin/sphingomyelin ratio, used in a test for fetal lung maturity.

LTB, abbreviation for **laryngotracheobronchitis.**

LTC, abbreviation for **long-term care.**

LTH, abbreviation for *leutotropic hormone.*

ʟ-Trp, abbreviation for *ʟ-tryptophan.*

Lu, symbol for the element **lutetium.**

lubb-dupp, in auscultation, an imitation of the two basic sounds heard in the cardiac cycle. *Lubb* represents the first sound, and is made by closure of the mitral and tricuspid valves. It is lower in pitch and lasts slightly longer than the second sound, *dupp,* which is made by closure of the aortic valve.

lubricant [L *lubricans* making slippery], a fluid, ointment, or other agent capable of diminishing friction and making a surface slippery.

lubricating enema [L *lubricans;* Gk *enienai*], an enema used to lubricate the anal canal after surgery for hemorrhoids or to prevent fecal impaction. The enema solution may be made with warm olive oil.

lucid /lōō'sid/ [L *lucidus* clear], clear, rational, and able to be understood.

lucid interval, a period of relative men-

tal clarity between periods of irrationality, especially in organic mental disorders, such as delirium and dementia.

lucidity, pertaining to clarity of mind, perception, or intelligibility.

lucid lethargy, a mental state characterized by a loss of will; hence, an inability to act, even though the person is conscious and intellectual function is normal.

Ludwig's angina /lōōd'vigz/ [Wilhelm F. von Ludwig, German surgeon, b. 1790; L *angina* quinsy], acute streptococcal cellulitis of the floor of the mouth. It is treated with penicillin.

LUE, abbreviation for *left upper extremity.*

Luer-Lok syringe /lōō'ərlok'/, a glass or plastic syringe for injection having a simple metal lock mechanism that securely holds the needle in place.

lues. See syphilis.

luetic aortitis. See syphilitic aortitis.

Lugol's solution [Jean G. A. Lugol, French physician, b. 1786; L *solutus* unbound], an aqueous solution of iodine (5%) and potassium iodide (10%).

Lukes-Collins classification, a system of identifying non-Hodgkin's lymphomas according to B cell, T cell, true, and unclassifiable types. B cell types include lymphocytic, plasmacytic, follicular cell lymphomas, and B cell-derived immunoblastic sarcoma. T cell types include T cell-derived immunoblastic sarcoma and convoluted cell lymphoma. True types are of histiocytic origin.

lukewarm bath [ME *luke;* AS *wearm, baeth*], a bath in which the temperature of the water is between 90° F and 96° F.

lumbago /lumbā'gō/ [L *lumbus* loin], pain in the lumbar region caused by a muscle strain, rheumatoid arthritis, osteoarthritis, or a herniated intravertebral disk. Ischemic lumbago, characterized by pain in the lower back and buttocks, is caused by vascular insufficiency, as in terminal aortic occlusion.

lumbar /lum'bər, lum'bär/ [L *lumbus* loin], of or pertaining to the part of the body between the thorax and the pelvis.

lumbar nerves, the five pairs of spinal nerves rising in the lumbar region. They become increasingly large the more caudal their location and pass laterally and downward under the cover of the psoas major or between its fasciculi.

lumbar node, a node in one of the seven groups of parietal lymph nodes serving the abdomen and the pelvis.

lumbar plexus, a network of nerves formed by the ventral primary divisions of the first three and the greater part of the fourth lumbar nerves. It is located on the inside of the posterior abdominal wall, either dorsal to the psoas muscle and among its fibers and ventral to the transverse processes of the lumbar vertebrae.

lumbar puncture (LP), the introduction of a hollow needle and stylet into the subarachnoid space of the lumbar portion of the spinal canal. With the use of strict aseptic technique, it is performed in various therapeutic and diagnostic procedures. Diagnostic indications include measuring of cerebrospinal fluid (CSF) pressure, obtaining CSF for laboratory analysis, evaluating the canal for the pressure of a tumor, and injecting air, oxygen, or a radiopaque substance for radiographic visualization of the structures of the nervous system of spinal canal and meninges and brain. Therapeutic indications for lumbar puncture include removing blood or pus from the subarachnoid space, injecting sera or drugs, withdrawing CSF to reduce intracranial pressure, introducing a local anesthetic to induce spinal anesthesia, and placing a small amount of the patient's blood in the subarachnoid space to form a clot to patch a rent or hole in the dura to prevent leak of CSF into the epidural space.

lumbar region. See **lateral region.**

lumbar subarachnoid peritoneostomy, a surgical procedure for draining cerebrospinal fluid in hydrocephalus, usually in the newborn. First a lumbar laminectomy is performed, then a polyethylene tube is passed from the subarachnoid space around the flank and into the peritoneum.

lumbar subarachnoid ureterostomy, a surgical procedure for draining excess cerebrospinal fluid through the ureter to the bladder in hydrocephalus, usually in the newborn. A polyethylene tube is passed from the lumbar subarachnoid space through the paraspinal muscles and into a ureter.

lumbar veins, four pairs of veins that collect blood by dorsal tributaries from the loins and by abdominal tributaries from the walls of the abdomen. They end in the inferior vena cava.

lumbar vertebra, one of the five largest segments of the movable part of the vertebral column, distinguished by the absence of a foramen in the transverse process and by vertebral bodies without facets. The body of each lumbar vertebra is flattened or slightly concave superiorly and inferiorly and is deeply constricted ventrally at the sides.

lumbodorsal fascia. See **fascia thoracolumbalis.**

lumbosacral /lum′bōsā′krəl/ [L *lumbus* loin; *sacrum* sacred], pertaining to the lumbar vertebrae and the sacrum.

lumbosacral plexus [L *lumbus* loin, *sacrum* sacred; *plexus* braided], the combination of all the ventral primary divisions of the lumbar, the sacral, and the coccygeal nerves. The lumbar and the sacral plexuses supply the lower limb. The sacral nerves also supply the perineum through the pudendal plexus and the coccygeal area through the coccygeal plexus.

lumbrical /lum′brikəl/ [L *lumbricus* earthworm], resembling a worm.

lumbrical plus deformity, a complication of rheumatoid arthritis in which the lumbricals (muscles in the hands and feet) become contracted, with a resultant action of extension rather than flexion.

lumen /lōō′mən/, *pl.* **lumina, lumens** [L, light], **1.** a cavity or the channel within any organ or structure of the body. **2.** a unit of luminous flux that equals the flux emitted in a unit solid angle by a point source of one candle intensity. **–luminal, luminal,** *adj.*

luminescence /lōō′mines′əns/ [L *lumen* + *escens* beginning], the emission of light by a material after excitation by some stimulus.

luminiferous /lōō′minif′ərəs/ [L *lumen* + *ferre* to bear], pertaining to a medium that will transmit light.

lumpectomy /lumpek′təmē/ [ME *lump* mass; *ektome* excision], surgical excision of a tumor without removal of large amounts of surrounding tissue or adjacent lymph nodes.

lumpy jaw [ME *lump* mass; *ceowan* to chew], *nontechnical.* actinomycosis of cows, caused by infection with *Actinomyces bovis* and not communicable to humans.

lunar month [L *luna* moon; AS *monath* month], a period of 4 weeks or 28 days, approximately the time required for the moon to revolve about the earth.

lunate bone /lōō′nāt/ [L *luna* moon; AS *ban*], the carpal bone in the center of the proximal row of carpal bones between the scaphoid and triangular bones.

Lundh test, a pancreatic function test in which the pancreas is stimulated by oral intake of a formula diet and lipase values are measured in aspirate from the duodenum.

lung [AS *lungen*], one of a pair of light, spongy organs in the thorax, constituting the main component of the respiratory system. The two highly elastic lungs are the main mechanisms in the body for inspiring air from which oxygen is extracted for the arterial blood system and for exhaling carbon dioxide dispersed from the venous system. The lungs are composed of lobes that are smooth and shiny on their surface.

L

The right lung contains three lobes; the left lung two lobes. Each lung is composed of an external serous coat, a subserous layer of areolar tissue, and the parenchyma. The serous coat comprises the thin, visceral pleura. The subserous areolar tissue contains many elastic fibers and invests the entire surface of the organ. The parenchyma is composed of secondary lobules divided into primary lobules, each of which consists of blood vessels, lymphatics, nerves, and an alveolar duct connecting with air spaces.

lung abscess [AS *lungen;* L *abscedere* to go away], a complication of an inflammation and infection of the lung, often caused by aspiration of infected material from the mouth.

lung cancer, a pulmonary malignancy attributable to cigarette smoking in 50% of cases. Other predisposing factors are exposure to acronitrile, arsenic, asbestos, beryllium, chloromethyl ether, chromium, coal products, ionizing radiation, iron oxide, mustard gas, nickel, petroleum, uranium, and vinyl chloride. Lung cancer develops most often in scarred or chronically diseased lungs, and is usually far advanced when detected, because metastases may precede the detection of the primary lesion in the lung. Symptoms of lung cancer include persistent cough, dyspnea, purulent or blood-streaked sputum, chest pain, and repeated attacks of bronchitis or pneumonia. Epidermoid cancers and adenocarcinomas each account for approximately 30% of lung tumors, about 25% are small- or oat cell carcinomas, and 15% are large-cell anaplastic cancers. Epidermoid tumors tend to remain in the thorax, but other lung lesions metastasize widely; oat cell carcinomas usually invade bone marrow, and large-cell cancers frequently metastasize to mediastinal nodes and GI mucosa. Surgery is the most effective treatment, but only one half of the cases are operable at the time of diagnosis.

lung capacities, lung volumes that consist of two or more of the four primary nonoverlapping volumes. Functional residual capacity is the sum of residual volume and expiratory reserve volume. Inspiratory capacity is the sum of the tidal volume and inspiratory reserve volume. Vital capacity is the sum of the expiratory reserve volume, the tidal volume, and the inspiratory reserve volume. Total lung capacity, at the end of maximal inspiration, is the sum of the functional residual capacity and the inspiratory capacity.

lung compliance, a measure of the ease of expansion by the lungs and thorax during respiratory movements. It is deter-

mined by pulmonary volume and elasticity, a high degree of compliance indicating a loss of elastic recoil of the lungs, as in old age or emphysema. Decreased compliance of the lungs occurs in conditions when greater pressure is needed for changes of volume, as in atelectasis, edema, fibrosis, pneumonia, or absence of surfactant.

lung fluke [AS *lungen* lung, *floc*], a parasitic flatworm of the genus and species *Paragonimus westermani* found throughout Africa, Asia, and Latin America, but rarely in North America. It may enter the body as encysted larvae in crabs and crayfish. Symptoms of infestation include peribronchiolar distress and hemoptysis.

lung scan, a radiographic examination of a lung and its function.

lunula /lōōn′yələ/, *pl.* **lunulae** [L *luna* moon], a semilunar structure, such as the crescent-shaped pale area at the base of the nail of a finger or toe.

lupoid. See **lupus.**

lupoid hepatitis. See **hepatitis.**

lupus /lōō′pəs/ [L, wolf], *nontechnical.* lupus erythematosus. **–lupoid,** *adj.*

lupus erythematosus. See **systemic lupus erythematosus.**

lupus erythematosus preparation (LE prep), a laboratory test for lupus erythematosus in which normal neutrophils are incubated with a specimen of the patient's serum resulting in the appearance of large, spherical, phagocytized inclusions within the neutrophils if the patient has lupus erythematosus.

lupus vulgaris, a rare cutaneous form of tuberculosis in which areas of the skin become ulcerated and heal slowly, leaving deeply scarred tissue. The disease is not related to lupus erythematosus.

LUQ, abbreviation for *left upper quadrant of abdomen.*

lusus naturae /lōō′səs/ [L *lusus* sport; *natura* nature], a congenital anomaly; teratism.

luteal /lōō′tē-əl/, of or pertaining to the corpus luteum or its functions or effects.

luteal hormone [L *luteus* yellow; Gk *hormaein* to set in motion], a hormone produced by the **corpus luteum.**

luteal phase. See **secretory phase.**

lutein /lōō′tē-in/ [L *luteus* yellow], a yellow-red, crystalline, carotenoid pigment found in plants with carotenes and chlorophylls and also in animal fats, egg yolk, the corpus luteum, or any lipochrome.

luteinization /lōō′tē-in′īzā′shən/ [L *luteus* yellow], the formation of the corpus luteum from an ovarian follicle that had recently discharged an ovum. The process involves the hypertrophy of the follicular lutein cells and the development of blood vessels and conective tissue at the site.

luteinizing hormone (LH) /loo'te·ini'zing/ [L *luteus* + Gk *izein* to cause; Gk *hormein* to begin activity], a glycoprotein hormone, produced by the anterior pituitary, that stimulates the secretion of sex hormones by the ovary and the testes and is involved in the maturation of spermatozoa and ova. In men, it induces the secretion of testosterone by the interstitial cells of the testes. In females, LH, working together with FSH, stimulates the growing follicle in the ovary to secrete estrogen.

luteinizing hormone-releasing hormone (LHRH), a neurohormone of the hypothalamus that stimulates and regulates the pituitary gland release of the luteinizing hormone (LH).

luteoma /loo'te·o'mə/, pl. **luteomas, luteomata** [L *luteus* + Gk *oma* tumor], **1.** a granulosa or theca cell tumor whose cells resemble those of the corpus luteum. **2.** a unilateral or bilateral nodular hyperplasia of ovarian lutein cells, occasionally developing during the last trimester of pregnancy.

luteotropin. See **prolactin.**

lutetium (Lu) /lootē'shē·əm/ [L *Lutetia* Paris], a rare earth metallic element. Its atomic number is 71; and its atomic weight is 174.97.

luxated joint /luk'sātid/, a condition of complete dislocation, with no contact between articular surfaces of the joint.

LV, abbreviation for **left ventricle.**

LVAD, abbreviation for **left ventricular assist device.**

LVN, abbreviation for **licensed vocational nurse.**

lyases /lē'āsis/ [Gk *lyein* to loosen; Fr *disastase* enzyme], a group of enzymes that reversibly split carbon bonds with carbon, nitrogen, or oxygen without hydrolysis or oxygen reduction reactions.

lycopene /lī'kəpin/ [Gk *lykopersikon* tomato], a red, crystalline, unsaturated hydrocarbon that is the carotenoid pigment in tomatoes and various berries and fruits. It is considered the primary substance from which all natural carotenoid pigments are derived.

lye poisoning /lī/ [AS *leah* lye; L *potio* drink], toxic effects of ingesting caustic soda or sodium hydroxide (NaOH), a powerful alkali. If the chemical has a pH above 11.5, the chemical burn damage to the mouth and throat is usually irreversible. An alkali burn can be more serious than an acid burn because an acid is usually neutralized by the tissues it contacts.

lying-in [AS *licgan* lying; L *in*] **1.** designating the time before, during, and after childbirth. **2.** designating a hospital that provides care for women in childbirth and the puerperium. **3.** the condition of being in confinement, or childbed.

Lyme disease /līm/ an acute, recurrent inflammatory infection, transmitted by a tickborne spirochete, *Borrelia burgdorferi.* The condition was originally described in Lyme, Connecticut. Knees, other large joints, and temporomandibular joints are most commonly involved, with local inflammation and swelling. Chills, fever, headache, malaise, and an expanding annular, erythematous skin eruption often precede the joint manifestations. Occasionally cardiac conduction abnormalities, aseptic meningitis, and Bell's palsy are associated conditions.

lymph /limf/ [L *lympha* water], a thin opalescent fluid originating in many organs and tissues of the body that is circulated through the lymphatic vessels and filtered by the lymph nodes. Lymph enters the bloodstream at the junction of the internal jugular and subclavian veins. It contains chyle, a few erythrocytes, and variable numbers of leukocytes, most of which are lymphocytes. It is otherwise similar to plasma.

lymphadenitis /limfad'inī'tis, lim'fəd-/ [L *lympha* + Gk *aden* gland, *itis* inflammation], an inflammatory condition of the lymph nodes, usually the result of systemic neoplastic disease, bacterial infection, or other inflammatory condition. The nodes may be enlarged, hard, smooth or irregular, red, and may feel hot.

lymphadenopathy /limfad'inop'əthē/, any disorder of the lymph nodes or lymph vessels.

lymphadenopathy syndrome (LAS), a persistent, generalized swelling of the lymph nodes. It is often a part of the AIDS-related complex.

lymphangiectasia /limfan'jē·ektā'zhə/ [L *lympha* + Gk *aggeion* vessel, *ektasis* stretching], dilatation of the smaller lymphatic vessels, characterized by diarrhea, steatorrhea, and protein malabsorption. It usually results from obstruction in the larger vessels.

lymphangiogram /limfan'jē·əgram'/ [L *lympha* + Gk, *aggeion* vessel, *gramma* record], a radiographic visualization of a part of the lymphatic system.

lymphangiography /limfan'jē·og'rafē/ [L *lympha* + Gk *aggeion* vessel, *graphein* to record], the x-ray examination of lymph glands and lymphatic vessels after an injection of contrast medium.

lymphangioma /limfan'jē·o'mə/, pl. **lymphangiomas, lymphangiomata** [L *lym-*

pha + Gk *aggeion* vessel, *oma* tumor], a benign, yellowish tan tumor on the skin, composed of a mass of dilated lymph vessels.

lymphangioma cavernosum, a tumor formed by dilated lymphatic vessels and filled with lymph that is often mixed with coagulated blood.

lymphangioma circumscriptum, a benign skin lesion that develops from superficial hypertrophic lymph vessels.

lymphangioma cysticum. See **cystic lymphangioma.**

lymphangioma simplex, a growth formed by moderately dilated lymph vessels in a circumscribed area, chiefly on the skin.

lymphangiosarcoma /limfan'jē·o'särkō'mə/ [L, *lympha,* water; Gk, *aggeion,* vessel + *sarx,* flesh + *oma,* tumor], a tumor arising from the lymphatic vessels.

lymphangitis /lim'fanjī'tis/ [L *lympha* + Gk *aggeion* vessel, *itis*], an inflammation of one or more lymphatic vessels, usually resulting from an acute streptococcal infection of one of the extremities. It is characterized by fine red streaks extending from the infected area to the axilla or groin, and by fever, chills, headache, and myalgia. The infection may spread to the bloodstream.

lymphatic /limfat'ik/ [L *lympha* + *icus* form] **1.** of or pertaining to the lymphatic system of the body, consisting of a vast network of tubes transporting lymph. **2.** any one of the vessels associated with the lymphatic network.

lymphatic capillary plexus, one of the numerous networks of lymphatic capillaries that collect lymph from the intercellular fluid and constitute the beginning of the lymphatic system. The lymphatic vessels arise from the capillary plexuses, which vary in size and number in different regions and organs of the body.

lymphatic leukemia. See **acute lymphocytic leukemia, chronic lymphocytic leukemia.**

lymphatic nodule. See **malpighian body.**

lymphatic organ [L *lympha* water; Gk *organon* instrument], any body structure composed of lymphatic tissue, such as the thymus, spleen, tonsils, and lymph nodes.

lymphatic system, a vast, complex network of capillaries, thin vessels, valves, ducts, nodes, and organs that helps to protect and maintain the internal fluid environment of the entire body by producing, filtering, and conveying lymph and by producing various blood cells. The lymphatic network also transports fats, proteins, and other substances to the blood system and

restores 60% of the fluid that filters out of the blood capillaries into interstitial spaces during normal metabolism. Small semilunar valves throughout the lymphatic network help to control the flow of lymph and, at the junction with the venous system, prevent venous blood from flowing into the lymphatic vessels. The lymph collected from throughout the body drains into the blood through two ducts situated in the neck. Various body dynamics, such as respiratory pressure changes, muscular contractions, and movements of organs surrounding lymphatic vessels combine to pump the lymph through the lymphatic system. The system also includes specialized lymphatic organs, such as the tonsils, the thymus, and the spleen. Lymph flows into the general circulation through the thoracic duct.

lymphatic vessels [L *lympha; vascellum* little vase], fine transparent valved channels distributed through most tissues. They are often distinguised by their beaded appearance, which is due to an irregular lumen. The collecting branches form two systems, one generally running with the superficial veins and the other below the deep fascia and including the intestinal lacteals. They drain through a thoracic duct and a right lymphatic duct into the venous system near the base of the neck.

lymph cell [L *lympha; cella* storeroom], a mature leukocyte found in the lymphatic tissue of lymph nodes.

lymphedema /lim'fidē'mə/ [L *lympha* + Gk *oidema* swelling], a primary or secondary disorder characterized by the accumulation of lymph in soft tissue and swelling, caused by inflammation, obstruction, or removal of lymph channels. Congenital lymphedema (Milroy's disease) is a hereditary disorder characterized by chronic lymphatic obstruction. Lymphedema praecox occurs in adolescence, chiefly in females, and causes puffiness and swelling of the lower limbs. Secondary lymphedema may follow surgical removal of lymph channels in mastectomy, obstruction of lymph drainage caused by malignant tumors, or the infestation of lymph vessels with adult filarial parasites. **–lymphedematous, lymphedematose,** *adj.*

lymph node [L *lympha* + *nodus* knot], one of the many small oval structures that filter the lymph and fight infection, and in which there are formed lymphocytes, monocytes, and plasma cells. The lymph nodes are of different sizes, some as small as pinheads, others as large as lima beans. Each node is enclosed in a capsule, is composed of a lighter colored cortical portion and a darker medullary portion, and consists of closely packed lymphocytes, reticular connective tissue laced by trabeculae, and three kinds of sinuses: subcapsular, cortical, and medullary. Lymph flows into the node through afferent lymphatic vessels. Most lymph nodes are clustered in (specific) areas, such as the mouth, the neck, the lower arm, the axilla, and the groin.

lymph nodule [L *lympha; nodulus* small knot], any of the small densely packed spherical nodes or aggregations of lymph cells embedded in the reticular meshwork of the lymphatic system, mainly in the tonsils, spleen, and thymus.

lymphoblastic lymphoma, lymphoblastic lymphosarcoma, lymphoblastoma. See **poorly differentiated lymphocytic malignant lymphoma.**

lymphocyte /lim′fəsīt/ [L *lympha* + Gk *kytos* cell], one of two kinds of small, agranulocytic leukocytes, originating from fetal stem cells and developing in the bone marrow. Lymphocytes normally comprise 25% of the total white blood cell count but increase in number in response to infection. They occur in two forms: **B cells** and **T cells.** B cells circulate in an immature form and synthesize antibodies for insertion into their own cytoplasmic membranes. They reproduce mitotically, each of the clones displaying identical antibodies on their surface membranes. When an immature B cell is exposed to a specific antigen, the cell is activated, traveling to the spleen or to the lymph nodes, differentiating, and rapidly producing plasma cells and memory cells. Plasma cells synthesize and secrete copious amounts of antibody. Memory cells do not secrete antibody, but if reexposure to the specific antigen occurs, they develop into antibody-secreting plasma cells. The function of the B cell is to search out, identify, and bind with specific antigens. T cells are lymphocytes that have circulated through the thymus gland and have differentiated to become thymocytes. When exposed to an antigen, they divide rapidly and produce large numbers of new T cells sensitized to that antigen. T cells are often called "killer cells" because they secrete immunologically essential chemical compounds and assist B cells in destroying foreign protein.

lymphocyte transformation, an in vitro immunity test process in which a patient's lymphocytes are placed in a culture with an antigen. The rate of transformation is measured by the uptake of radioactive thymidine by the lymphocytes, indicating protein synthesis.

lymphocytic choriomeningitis /lim′-fasit′ik/ [L *lympha* + Gk *kytos* cell; *cho-*

rion skin, *meninx* membrane, *itis* inflammation], an arenavirus infection of the meninges and the cerebrospinal fluid, caused by the lymphocytic choriomeningitis virus and characterized by fever, headache, and stiff neck.

lymphocytic leukemia. See **acute lymphocytic leukemia, chronic lymphocytic leukemia.**

lymphocytic lymphoma, lymphocytic lymphosarcoma. See **well-differentiated lymphocytic malignant lymphoma.**

lymphocytic thyroiditis. See **Hashimoto's disease.**

lymphocytoma. See **well-differentiated lymphocytic malignant lymphoma.**

lymphocytopenia /lim′fōsī′təpē′nē-ə/ [L *lympha* + Gk *kytos* cell, *penes* poor], a smaller-than-normal number of lymphocytes in the peripheral circulation, occurring as a primary hematologic disorder or in association with nutritional deficiency, malignancy, or infectious mononucleosis.

lymphocytosis /lim′fōsītō′sis/, a proliferation of lymphocytes, as occurs in certain chronic diseases and during convalescence from acute infections.

lymphoderma perniciosa. See **leukemia cutis.**

lymphoepithelioma /lim′fō·ep′ithē′lē-ō′mə/ [L *lympha* + Gk *epi* above, *thele* nipple, *oma* tumor], a poorly differentiated neoplasm developing from the epithelium overlying lymphoid tissue in the nasopharynx.

lymphogenous leukemia. See **acute lymphocytic leukemia, chronic lymphocytic leukemia.**

lymphogranulomatosis /lim′fōgran′yəlō′mətō′sis/ [L *lympha* + *granulum* small grain; Gk *oma* tumor; *osis* condition], an infectious granuloma of the lymphatic system. The term is used to identify several inflammatory granulomata or sarcomata disorders, such as **Hodgkin's disease, sarcoidosis, lymphadenoma,** and **lymphadenoma venereum.**

lymphogranuloma venereum (LGV) [L *lympha* + *granulum* small grain; Gk *oma* tumor; L *Venus* goddess of love], a sexually transmitted disease caused by a strain of the bacterium *Chlamydia trachomatis.* It is characterized by ulcerative genital lesions, marked swelling of the lymph nodes in the groin, headache, fever, and malaise. Ulcerations of the rectal wall occur less commonly.

lymphography. See **lymphangiography.**

lymphoid /lim′foid/ [L *lympha* + Gk *eidos* form], pertaining to lymph or lymphatics.

lymphoid interstitial pneumonia (LIP), a form of pneumonia that involves the

L

lower lobes with extensive alveolar infiltration by mature lymphocytes, plasma cells, and histiocytes. It is associated with AIDS, dysproteinemia, and Sjögren's syndrome.

lymphoid leukemia. See **acute lymphocytic leukemia, chronic lymphocytic leukemia.**

lymphoidocytic leukemia. See **stem cell leukemia.**

lymphoid tissue [L *lympha* + Gk, *eidos* form; OFr *tissu*], tissue that consists of lymphocytes on a framework of reticular cells and fibers, as the tonsils and adenoids.

lymphokine /lim′fōkīn/ [L *lympha* + Gk *kinesis* motion], one of the chemical factors produced and released by T lymphocytes that attract macrophages to the site of infection or inflammation and prepare them for attack. Kinds of lymphokines include **chemotactic factor, lymphotoxin,** and **mitogenic factor.**

lymphokine-activated killer (LAK) cells, nonspecific cytotoxic cells that are generated in the presence of interleukin-2 and in the absence of antigen.

lympholysis /limfol′əsis/ [L *lympha* + Gk *lysein* to loosen], cellular destruction of lymphocytes, especially of certain lymphocytes in the process of an immune response. **–lympholytic,** *adj.*

lymphoma /limfō′mə/, *pl.* **lymphomas, lymphomata** [L *lympha* + Gk *oma* tumor], a neoplasm of lymphoid tissue that is usually malignant but, in rare cases, may be benign. The various lymphomas differ in degree of cellular differentiation and content, but the manifestations are similar in all types. Characteristically, the appearance of a painless, enlarged lymph node or nodes in the neck is followed by weakness, fever, weight loss, and anemia. With widespread involvement of lymphoid tissue, the spleen and liver usually enlarge, and GI disturbances, malabsorption, and bone lesions frequently develop. Kinds of lymphoma include **Burkitt's lymphoma, giant follicular lymphoma, histiocytic malignant lymphoma, Hodgkin's disease, mixed cell malignant lymphoma.** **–lymphomatoid,** *adj.*

lymphoma staging, a system for classifying lymphomas according to the stage of the disease for the purpose of appropriate treatment. Stage I is characterized by the involvement of a single lymph node region or one extralymphatic organ or site and stage II by the involvement of two or more lymph node regions on the same side of the diaphragm or a localized involvement of an extralymphatic organ or site plus one or more node regions on the same side of the diaphragm. In stage III lymph nodes on both sides of the diaphragm are affected, and there may be involvement of the spleen or localized involvement of an extralymphatic organ or site. Stage IV is typified by diffuse or disseminated involvement of one or more extralymphatic organs or sites with or without associated lymph node involvement.

lymphopathia venereum. See **lymphogranuloma venereum.**

lymphopenia. See **lymphocytopenia.**

lymphopoiesis /lim′fōpō·ē′sis/ [L *lympha* + Gk *poien* to make], the formation of lymphocytes. **–lymphopoietic,** *adj.*

lymphoproliferative /lim′fōprōlif′ərativ′/ [L *lympha* + *prolles* offspring; *ferre* to bear], pertaining to the proliferation of lymphoid tissue.

lymphoreticulosis /lim′fōretik′yəlō′sis/ [L *lympha* + *reticulum* little net; Gk *osis* condition], subacute granulomatous inflammation of lymphoid tissue with proliferation of reticuloendothelial cells, occurring most commonly as the result of a cat scratch. The disorder is characterized by the formation of an ulcerated papule at the site of the scratch, and by fever and tender lymphadenopathy, sometimes progressing to suppuration.

lymphosarcoma. See **non-Hodgkin's lymphoma.**

lymphosarcoma cell leukemia /lim′fōsärkō′mə/ [L *lympha* + Gk *sarx* flesh, *oma* tumor], a malignancy of blood-forming tissues characterized by many lymphosarcoma cells in the peripheral circulation that tend to infiltrate surrounding tissues.

lymph sinuses [L *lympha* + *sinus* hollow], continuous small endothelial-lined spaces just below the capsule of the lymph node. The sinuses slow the flow of lymph through the nodes.

Lyon hypothesis /lī′ən/ [Mary L. Lyon, English geneticist, b. 1925], (in genetics) a hypothesis stating that only one of the two X chromosomes in a female is functional, the other having become inactive early in development.

lyonization /lī′ənīzā′shən/ [Mary L. Lyon; Gk *izein* to cause], the process of random inactivation of one of the X chromosomes in the female gamete to compensate for the presence of the double X gene complement.

Lyon's ring, a type of congenital uropathy in females in which submeatal or distal urethral stenosis causes enuresis, dysuria, and recurring infections.

lyophilic /lī′ōfil′ik/ [Gk *lyein* to dissolve; *philein* to love], pertaining to substances having an affinity for, or stable, in solution. Lyophilic substances are used to stabilize colloids.

lypressin /līpres'in/, an antidiuretic and vasoconstrictor prescribed in diabetes insipidus to decrease urinary water loss.

Lys, abbreviation for **lysine**.

lysergide /līsur'jīd/, a psychotomimetic, semisynthetic derivative of ergot that acts at multiple sites in the central nervous system from the cortex to the spinal cord. The drug may cause pupillary dilatation, increased blood pressure, hyperreflexia, tremor, muscle weakness, piloerection, increased body temperature, dizziness, drowsiness, paresthesia, euphoria or dysphoria, and synesthesias; colors may be heard, sounds visualized, and time is felt to pass slowly. Psychologic dependence may develop, and use of lysergide is associated with significant hazards.

Lysholm method, (in radiology) any of several techniques for positioning a patient for x-ray examination of the cranial base, the mastoid and petrous regions of the temporal bone, and the optic foramen and orbital fissure.

lysine (Lys) /lī'sēn, lī'sin/, an essential amino acid needed for proper growth in infants and for maintenance of nitrogen balance in adults.

lysine intolerance, a congenital disorder resulting in the inability to use the essential amino acid lysine because of an enzyme deficiency or defect.

lysinemia /lī'sinē'mē·ə/, a condition caused by an inborn error of metabolism and resulting in the inability to use the essential amino acid lysine because of an enzyme defect or deficiency. It is characterized by muscle weakness and mental retardation.

lysine monohydrochloride, a salt of the amino acid lysine, used as a dietary supplement to increase the use of vegetable proteins, such as corn, rice, and wheat.

lysis /lī'sis/ [Gk *lysein* to loosen] **1.** destruction or dissolution of a cell or molecule through the action of a specific agent. Cell lysis is frequently caused by a lysin. **2.** gradual diminution in the symptoms of a disease.

lysis of adhesions, surgery performed to free adhesions of tissues.

lysogenesis /lī'səjen'əsis/, the formation of lysins, or antibodies that cause partial or complete dissolution of the target cell.

lysosome /lī'səsōm/ [Gk *lysein* + *soma* body], a cytoplasmic, membrane-bound particle that contains hydrolytic enzymes that function in intracellular digestive processes. If the hydrolytic enzymes are released into the cytoplasm, they cause self-digestion of the cell so that lysosomes may play an important role in certain self-destructive diseases characterized by the wasting of tissue, such as muscular dystrophy.

lysozyme /lī'səzīm/ [Gk *lysein* + *en* within, *zyme* ferment], an enzyme with antiseptic actions that destroys some foreign organisms. It is found in granulocytic and monocytic blood cells and is normally present in saliva, sweat, breast milk, and tears.

lytes /līts/, an informal abbreviation of *electrolytes,* especially the levels of potassium, sodium, phosphorus, magnesium, and calcium in the blood, as determined by laboratory testing.

lytic cocktail /lit'ik/, an informal name for an anesthetic compound of chlorpromazine, meperidine, and promethazine that blocks the autonomic nervous system, depresses the circulatory system, and induces neuroplegia.

L

M

m, 1. abbreviation for **meter.** 2. abbreviation for *milli-*.

M, 1. abbreviation for *mega.* 2. abbreviation for **molar.** 3. abbreviation for *metastasis* in the TNM (tumor, node, metastasis) system for staging malignant neoplastic disease.

ma, MA, abbreviations for **milliampere.**

MA, abbreviation for **mental age.**

MA, abbreviation for *Master of Arts* degree.

MAA, abbreviation for *methacrylic acid.*

Maass, Clara (1876-1901), an American nurse who volunteered for military service at the outbreak of the Spanish-American War. After working at Army camps where soldiers were dying of yellow fever, she volunteered to go to Havana to participate in the experiments being done to determine the cause of that disease. She was bitten by a mosquito and died 10 days later of yellow fever. She was one of the first nurses to be inducted into the Hall of Fame of the American Nurses' Association.

mabp, abbreviation for *mean arterial blood pressure.*

MAC, 1. abbreviation for **midupper arm circumference.** 2. abbreviation for **minimum alveolar concentration.**

MAC AWAKE, the concentration of an inhaled anesthetic that allows a patient to respond rationally to questions and verbal instructions.

macerate /mas'ərāt/ [L *macere* to soften], to soften something solid by soaking. **–maceration,** *n.*

maceration /mas'ərā'shən/, the softening and breaking down of skin from prolonged exposure to moisture.

machinery murmur [L *machina; murmur* humming], a continuous murmur heard throughout systole and diastole, with systolic accentuation. It is heard to the left of the sternum in patients with a ductus arteriosus condition.

machismo /mächis'mō/, (in psychology) a concept of the male that includes the culturally desirable traits of courage, as well as the dysfunctional behaviors of heavy drinking, seduction, and abusive spouse behavior.

Machover Draw-A-Person Test. See **Draw-A-Person Test.**

Machupo. See **Bolivian hemorrhagic fever.**

macrencephaly /mak'rənsef'əlē/ [Gk *makros* large, *enkephalos* brain], a congenital anomaly characterized by abnormal largeness of the brain. **–macrencephalic, macroencephalic,** *adj.*

macrobiosis /mak'rōbī·ō'sis/ [Gk *makros* + *bios* life], a long life.

macroblepharia /mak'rōblifer'ē·ə/ [Gk *makros* + *blepharon* eyelid], the condition of having abnormally large eyelids.

macrocephaly /mak'rōsef'əlē/ [Gk *makros* + *kephale* head], a congenital anomaly characterized by abnormal largeness of the head and brain in relation to the rest of the body, resulting in some degree of mental and growth retardation. The head is more than two standard deviations above the average circumference size for age, sex, race, and period of gestation, with excessively wide fontanels; the facial features are usually normal. There is symmetric overgrowth at the head without increased intracranial pressure, as differentiated from hydrocephalus in which the lateral, asymmetric growth of the head is caused by excessive accumulation of cerebrospinal fluid, usually under increased pressure. **–macrocephalic, macrocephalous,** *adj.,* **macrocephalus,** *n.*

macrocyte /mak'rəsīt/ [Gk *makros* + *kytos* cell], an abnormally large, mature erythrocyte. It is most commonly seen in megaloblastic anemia.

macrocytic /mak'rōsit'ik/ [Gk *makros, kytos* + L *icus* form], (of a cell) larger than normal, such as the erythrocytes in macrocytic anemia.

macrocytic anemia, a disorder of the blood characterized by impaired erythropoiesis and the abnormal presence of large, fragile, red blood cells in the circulation.

macrocytosis /mak'rōsītō'sis/ [Gk *makros, kytos* + *osis* condition], an abnormal proliferation of macrocytes in the peripheral blood.

macrodrip /mak'rōdrip/ [Gk *makros* + AS *drypan* to fall in drops], (in intravenous therapy) an apparatus that is used to deliver measured amounts of IV solutions at

630

specific flow rates based on the size of drops of the solution. The size of the drops is controlled by the fixed diameter of a plastic delivery tube. The drops delivered by a macrodrip are larger than those delivered by a microdrip.

macroelement. See **macronutrient.**

macroencephaly. See **macrencephaly.**

macrogamete /mak′rogam″ēt/ [Gk *makros* + *gamete* spouse], a large, nonmotile female gamete of certain thallophytes and sporozoa, specifically the malarial parasite *Plasmodium.*

macrogametocyte /mak′rōgamē′təsīt/ [Gk *makros, gamete* + *kytos* cell], an enlarged merozoite that undergoes meiosis to form the mature female gamete during the sexual phase of the life cycle of certain thallophytes and sporozoa, specifically the malarial parasite *Plasmodium.*

macrogenitosomia /mak′rōjen′itōsō′mē·ə/ [Gk *makros* + L *genitalis* genitalia; Gk *soma* body], a congenital condition in which the genitalia are abnormal because of an excess of androgen during fetal development. It is characterized in boys by enlarged external genitalia and in girls by pseudohermaphroditism.

macroglobulinemia /mak′rōglob′yŏŏlinē′-mē·ə/ [Gk *makros* + L *globulus* small ball; Gk *haima* blood], a form of monoclonal gammopathy in which a large immunoglobulin (IgM) is vastly overproduced by the clones of a plasma B cell in response to an antigenic signal.

macroglossia /mak′rōglos′ē·ə/ [Gk *makros* + *glossa* tongue], a congenital anomaly characterized by excessive size of the tongue, as seen in certain syndromes of congenital defects, including Down syndrome.

macrognathia /mak′rōnā′thē·ə/ [Gk *makros* + *gnathos* jaw], an abnormally large growth of the jaw. **–macrognathic,** *adj.*

macrolide /ma′krōlīd/, any of a group of antibiotics produced by actinomycetes. They include erythromycin and troleandomycin. Macrolides are generally used against gram-positive bacteria and in patients allergic to penicillins.

macromolecule /ma′krōmol′əkyŏŏl/ [Gk *makros* + L *moles* mass], a molecule of colloidal size, such as proteins, nucleic acids, or polysaccharides.

macronucleus /ma′krōnŏŏ′klē·əs/ [Gk *makros* + L *nucleus* nut], **1.** a large nucleus. **2.** (in protozoa) the larger of two nuclei in each cell; it governs cell metabolism and growth as opposed to the micronucleus, which functions in sexual reproduction.

macronutrient /ma′krōnŏŏ′tri·ənt/ [Gk *makros* + L *nutriens* nourishing], a chemical element required in relatively large quantities for the normal physiologic processes of the body.

macrophage /mak′rəfāj/ [Gk *makros* + *phagein* to eat], any phagocytic cell of the reticuloendothelial system including Kupffer cell in the liver, splenocyte in the spleen, and histocyte in the loose connective tissue.

macrophage activating factor (MAF) [Gk *makros* + *phagein* to eat; L *activus* active; *facere* to make], a lymphokine released from a sensitized leukocyte, which induces changes in the appearance and function of macrophages as needed to make them active against certain antigens.

macrophage migration inhibiting factor, a lymphokine produced by leukocytes that immobilizes macrophages after contact with an antigen.

macropsia /makrop′sē·ə/ [Gk *makros* + *opsis* vision], a visual abnormality in which objects appear larger than they actually are.

macroreentry /mak′rōrē·en′trē/ [Gk *makros*+ L *re* again; Fr *entree* entry], (in cardiology) a reentry circuit with anterograde conduction down one of the bundle branches and retrograde conduction up another. It causes ventricular tachycardia with a BBB pattern and a relatively narrow QRS.

macroscopic /mak′rōskop′ik/ [Gk *makros* + *skopein* to view], large enough to be examined with the naked eye.

macroscopic anatomy. See **gross anatomy.**

macrosis /makrō′sis/, an increase in the size or volume of an object.

macrosomia. See **gigantism.**

macula /mak′yələ/, *pl.* **maculae** [L, spot], a small pigmented area or a spot that appears separate or different from the surrounding tissue.

macula albidae [L, spot; *albidare* to make white], small white areas in the serous membranes of the pericardium or in the peritoneum or pleura.

macula cerulea. See **blue spot.**

macula densa [L, spot; *densus* thick], a thickening in the wall of a distal tubule of the kidney nephron at a point where it is in contact with the afferent glomerulus. It may be part of a negative feedback system for sodium.

macula lutea, an oval yellow spot at the center of the retina 2 mm from the optic nerve. It contains a pit, no blood vessels, and the fovea centralis. Central vision occurs when an image is focused directly on the fovea centralis of the macula lutea.

macular degeneration /mak′yələr/ [L

M

macula spot; *degenerare* to deviate], a progressive deterioration of the maculae of the retina and choroid of the eye. The condition is an effect of several diseases, such as **retinitis pigmentosa.**

macular rash [L *macula;* OFr *rasche*], a skin eruption in which the lesions are flat and less than one centimeter in diameter.

macula solaris [L *macula; solaris* sun], freckle.

macule /mak′yo͞ol/ [L *macula* spot], **1.** a small, flat blemish or discoloration that is flush with the skin surface. **2.** a gray scar on the cornea that is visible without magnification. **–macular,** *adj.*

maculopapular rash /mak′yəlōpap′yələr/ [L *macula* + *papula* pimple; OFr *rasche*], a skin eruption with distinctive macules or papules, or both.

maculopathy /mak′yəlop′əthē/ [L *macula* + Gk *pathos* disease], a form of macular degeneration involving primarily the macula lutea.

Madelung's neck. See **lipoma annulare colli.**

mad hatter's disease. See **mercurialism.**

Madura foot /maj′o͞orə/ [Madura, India; AS *fot* foot], a progressive, destructive, tropical fungal infection of the foot, named for a district in India.

MAF, abbreviation for **macrophage activating factor.**

mafenide acetate /maf′ənīd/, a topical antiinfective prescribed in the treatment of burns.

magaldrate /mag′əldrāt/, an antacid prescribed in the treatment of hypersensitivity and stomach upset associated with heartburn, sour stomach, or acid indigestion.

Magendie's law. See **Bell's law.**

magical thinking, (in psychology) a belief that merely thinking about an event in the external world can cause it to occur. It is regarded as a form of regression to an early phase of development.

magic-bullet approach [Gk *magikos* sorcerer; Fr *boulette* small ball; L *ad* toward, *prope* near], **1.** a therapeutic or diagnostic method that makes use of a specific mechanistic connection between a drug and a disease or organ. **2.** (in clinical medicine) the administration of a specific drug to cure or ameliorate a given disease or condition. **3.** (in traditional diagnostic radiology) the administration of a specific dye to facilitate the visualization by x-ray of a given organ. **4.** (in nuclear medicine) the administration of a specific radionuclide tagged to an appropriate carrier to provide a scintillation camera image of a given organ or structure.

magnesemia /mag′nəsē′mē·ə/, the presence of magnesium in the blood.

magnesia magma. See **milk of magnesia.**

magnesium (Mg) /magnē′sē·əm, magnē′-zhəm/ [Magnesia, ancient Greek town], a silver-white mineral element. Its atomic number is 12; its atomic weight is 24.32. Magnesium is the second most abundant cation of the intracellular fluids in the body and is essential for many enzyme activities. It is important to neurochemical transmissions and muscular excitability. Excess magnesium also causes vasodilatation by directly affecting the blood vessels and by ganglionic blockade. Hypomagnesemia can cause changes in cardiac muscles and skeletal muscle and can cause nephrocalcinosis.

magnesium sulfate, a salt of magnesium prescribed parenterally to prevent seizures, especially in preeclampsia, and orally to treat constipation and heartburn and to correct deficiency of magnesium in the body.

magnetic field [Gk *magnesia* (lodestone); AS *feld*], the region around any magnet in which its effects can be detected.

magnetic lines of force [Gk *magnesia* (lodestone); L *linea* line; *fortis* strong], theoretical lines of magnetism that surround a magnet or fill a magnetic field. The presence of the magnetic force along the imaginary lines can be demonstrated by inserting a sensitive material such as iron filings into the lines of magnetic effect.

magnetic moment [L *lapis Magnes* lodestone; *momentum* movement], a measure of the net magnetic field produced by an elementary particle or an atomic nucleus spinning about its own axis. It is the basis for nuclear magnetic resonance imaging.

magnetic resonance (MR), 1. a phenomenon in which the atomic nuclei of certain materials placed in a strong, static magnetic field will absorb radio waves supplied by a transmitter at particular frequencies. **2.** spectra emitted by phosphorus in body tissues as measured and imaged on phosphorus nuclear magnetic resonance instruments.

magnetic resonance imaging (MRI) [L *lapis Magnes* lodestone; *resonare* to sound again; *imago* image], medical imaging that uses nuclear magnetic resonance as its source of energy.

magnetic susceptibility, a measure of the ability of a substance to become magnetized.

magnetization [L *lapis Magnes* lodestone; Gk *izein* to cause], the magnetic polarization of a material produced by a magnetic field (magnetic moment per unit volume).

magnetron /mag'nətron/ [L *lapis Magnes* lodestone, *trum* device], a source of microwave energy used in medical linear accelerators to accelerate electrons to the therapeutic energies.

magnification, (in psychology) cognitive distortion in which the effects of one's behavior are magnified.

magnification factor, (in radiology) the image size divided by the object size.

Mahaim fibers, conductive tracts in cardiac tissue running between the AV node or His bundle and the muscle of the ventricular septum. They conduct early excitation impulses.

Mahoney, Mary Eliza (1845-1926), the first American black nurse. A medal in her name, established after her death, is given to a black nurse in recognition of an outstanding contribution to the profession.

main en griffe. See **clawhand.**

mainstreaming [OE *maegan* might; ME *strem*], the system of educating disabled or mildly mentally retarded children in regular classrooms, but with special assistance as needed. The term is also applied to the return of persons recovering from mental illness to the community.

maintenance dose [Fr *maintenir* to uphold; Gk *dosis* giving], the amount of drug required to keep a desired mean steady-state concentration in the tissues.

Majocchi's granuloma /mäjok'ēz/ [Domenico Majocchi, Italian dermatologist, b. 1849; L *granulum* small grain; Gk *oma* tumor], a rare type of tinea corporis, mainly affecting the lower legs. It is caused by the fungus *Trichophyton,* which infects the hairs of the affected site and raises spongy granulomas.

major affective disorder [L *magnus* great; *affectus* state of mind; *dis* opposite of, *ordo* rank], any of a group of psychotic disorders characterized by severe and inappropriate emotional responses, by prolonged and persistent disturbances of mood and related thought distortions, and by other symptoms associated with either depressed or manic states, such as occurs in bipolar disorder, depression, and involutional melancholia.

major connector, a metal plate or bar, used for joining the components of one side of a removable partial denture to those on the opposite side of the dental arch.

major depressive episode. See **endogenous depression.**

major element. See **macronutrient.**

major histocompatibility complex (MHC) [ME *maiour* great; Gk *histos* tis-sue; L *compatibilis* agreement; *complexus* embrace], a group of proteins on the outer membrane of a cell that helps identify self and nonself (invading) molecules. MHC Class I molecules normally help the immune system discriminate between healthy body cells and those that may be precancerous or infected by viruses. MHC Class II molecules normally recognize foreign proteins. The MHC Class II molecules resemble the gp120 molecules on the outer membranes of HIV viruses, leading confused antibodies to attack the body's own T helper cells. Individuals with Type I diabetes have lower than normal levels of MHC Class I proteins, a susceptibility marker. Their immune systems fail to recognize their own beta cells.

major hysteria [ME *maiour* great; Gk *hystera* womb], an episode of psychogenic illness affecting a large group of individuals at the same time. Examples include the witchcraft trials of the seventeenth century and irrational mass reaction to the 1938 radio show based on H.G. Well's science-fiction novel, "War of the Worlds."

major medical insurance, insurance coverage designed to offset the costs of prolonged or catastrophic illness and injury.

major renal calyx. See **renal calyx.**

major surgery, any surgical procedure that requires general anesthesia or respiratory assistance.

mal /mal, mäl/ [L *malus* bad], an illness or disease, such as grand mal or petit mal.

malabsorption /mal'əbsôrp'shən/ [L *malus* + *absorbere* to swallow], impaired absorption of nutrients from the GI tract. It occurs in celiac disease, sprue, dysentery, diarrhea, and other disorders.

malabsorption syndrome, a complex of symptoms resulting from disorders in the intestinal absorption of nutrients, characterized by anorexia, weight loss, bloating of the abdomen, muscle cramps, bone pain, and steatorrhea. Anemia, weakness, and fatigue occur because iron, folic acid, and vitamin B_{12} are not absorbed in sufficient amounts.

malacia /məlā'shə/ [Gk *malakia* softness], **1.** a morbid softening or a sponginess in any part or any tissue of the body. **2.** a craving for spicy foods, such as mustard, hot peppers, or pickles. **–malacic,** *adj.*

maladaptation /mal'adaptā'shən/ [L *malus* + *adaptatio*], faulty intrapersonal adaptation to stress or change. It may involve a failure to make necessary changes in the desires, values, needs, and attitudes or an inability to make necessary adjustments in the external world.

maladjusted [L *malus* + *adjuxtare* to bring

together], a state in which an individual appears unable to maintain effective relationships needed to fit into the environment, and shows irritability, depression, and other psychogenic influences.

malady /mal′ədē/ [ME *maladie* sick], a disease or illness.

malaise /malāz′/ [Fr, discomfort], a vague feeling of bodily weakness or discomfort, often marking the onset of disease.

malalignment [L *malus* + *ad* to *linea* line], a failure of parts of the body to align normally, such as the teeth in the dental arch.

malar /mā′lər/ [L *mala* cheek], of or pertaining to the cheek or the cheek bone.

malaria /məler′ē-ə/ [L *malus* bad, *aer* air], a serious infectious illness caused by one or more of at least four species of the protozoan genus *Plasmodium,* characterized by chills, fever, anemia, an enlarged spleen, and a tendency to recur. The disease is transmitted from human to human by a bite from an infected *Anopheles* mosquito. Malarial infection can also be spread by blood transfusion from an infected patient or by the use of an infected hypodermic needle. *Plasmodium* parasites penetrate the erythrocytes of the human host, where they mature, reproduce, and burst out periodically. Malarial paroxysms occur at regular intervals, coinciding with the development of a new generation of parasites in the body. –**malarial,** *adj.*

malarial hemoglobinuria. See **blackwater fever.**

malarial parasite, one of four known species of *Plasmodium* that may be injected into the human bloodstream by an anopheline mosquito to begin the cycle of malarial disease.

Malassezia /mal′əsē′zē-əl/ [Louis C. Malassez, French physiologist, b. 1842], a genus of fungi. *M. furfur* causes tinea versicolor (previous name: *Pityrosporum oviculare*). *M. ovalis* is a nonpathogenic organism found in sebaceous areas (previous name: *Pityrosporum ovale*).

malathion poisoning /malā′thē-on, məl′-əthī′on/, a toxic condition caused by the ingestion or absorption through the skin of malathion, an organophosphorus insecticide. Symptoms include vomiting, nausea, abdominal cramps, headache, dizziness, weakness, confusion, convulsions, and respiratory difficulties.

malaxation. See **pétrissage.**

Malayan pit viper venom. See **ancrod.**

mal del pinto. See **pinta.**

mal de mer. See **motion sickness.**

male [L *mas*], **1.** of or pertaining to the sex that produces sperm cells and fertilizes the female to beget children; masculine. **2.** a male person.

male catheterization. the passage of a catheter through the male urethra for the purpose of draining the urinary bladder. The male catheter is approximately 12 inches long, about twice the length of a female urinary catheter, because it must pass through the length of the urethra within the penis. The male patient is placed in a supine position with the legs extended for insertion of the catheter. Sterile technique is important.

male menopause [L *mas* male; *mensis* month; Gk *pauein* to cease], a late middle-age psychogenic condition affecting men who experience anxiety over diminished potency, increased fatigue, thinning and graying hair, and other signs of aging.

male pattern alopecia [L *mas* male; ME *patron;* Gk *alopex* fox mange], a common form of baldness in males, beginning at the front and spreading gradually until a fringe remains around the back and temples. Individual differences are determined by heredity, androgenic stimulation, and aging. A simlar hair loss pattern may develop in women after menopause.

male reproductive system assessment, an evaluation of the condition of the patient's genitalia, reproductive history, and past and present genitourinary infections and disorders.

male sexual dysfunction, impaired or inadequate ability of a man to carry on his sex life to his own satisfaction. Symptoms, often psychologic in origin, include difficulties in starting and maintaining an erection, premature ejaculation, inability to ejaculate, and even loss of desire.

male sterility [L *mas* + *sterilis* barren], the inability of a man to produce sperm. Causes may include environmental factors such as exposure to heat or radiation, undescended testes, varicocele, prolonged fever, endocrine disorders, and abuse of alcohol or marijuana.

malfeasance /malfē′zəns/ [Fr *malfaire* to do evil], performance of an unlawful, wrongful act.

malformation [L *malus* + *forma* shape], an anomalous structure in the body.

malfunction [L *malus* + *functio* performance], the inability to function normally.

Malgaigne's fracture of pelvis /malgā′-nyəz/ [Joseph F. Malgaigne, French surgeon, b. 1806], trauma involving multiple pelvic fractures, including fracture of the wing of the ilium or sacrum and fracture of the ipsilateral pubic rami, with associated upper displacement of the hemipelvis.

malicious prosecution [L *malitia* wickedness; *prosequi* to pursue], (in law) a suit begun in malice and pursued without sufficient cause.

malign [ME *malignen* deceptive], to show ill will, maliciousness, harm.

malignant /məlig'nənt/ [L *malignus* ill-disposed] **1.** tending to become worse and cause death. **2.** (describing a cancer) anaplastic, invasive, and metastatic. **–malignancy,** *n.*

malignant dysentery [L *malignus;* Gk *dys* bad; *enteron* bowel], a potentially fatal form of dysentery in which symptoms are severe.

malignant endocarditis [L *malignus;* Gk *endon* within; *kardia* heart; *itis* inflammation], a bacterial infection of the innermost layer of the heart but affecting primarily the valves after they have already been damaged by rheumatic fever or another disease. The valve cusps may be perforated or ulcerated. The patient usually experiences fever and sweating, emboli, and possible septicemia.

malignant ependymoma. See **ependymoblastoma.**

malignant granuloma [L *malignus; granulum* little grain; *oma* tumor], a malignant lymphoma, such as Hodgkin's disease, or a lymphosarcoma.

malignant hemangioendothelioma. See **hemangiosarcoma.**

malignant hepatoma, a malignant tumor of the liver.

malignant hypertension, the most lethal form of hypertension. It is a fulminating condition, characterized by severely elevated blood pressure, that commonly damages the intima of small vessels, the brain, retina, heart, and kidneys.

malignant hyperthermia (MH), an autosomal dominant trait characterized by often fatal hyperthermia with rigidity of the muscles occurring in affected people exposed to certain anesthetic agents, particularly halothane, succinylcholine, and methoxyflurane.

malignant malnutrition. See **kwashiorkor.**

malignant melanoma. See **melanoma.**

malignant mesenchymoma, a sarcoma that contains mesenchymal elements.

malignant mole. See **melanoma.**

malignant neoplasm, a tumor that tends to grow, invade, and metastasize. It usually has an irregular shape and is composed of poorly differentiated cells. If untreated, it may result in the death of the organism. The degree to which a neoplasm is malignant varies with the kind of tumor and the condition of the patient.

malignant neuroma. See **neurosarcoma.**

malignant pustule. See **anthrax.**

malignant tumor, a neoplasm that characteristically invades surrounding tissue, metastasizes to distant sites, and contains anaplastic cells. A malignant tumor may result in the death of the host if remission or treatment does not intervene.

malingering [Fr *malingre* sickly], a willful and deliberate feigning of the symptoms of a disease or injury to gain some consciously desired end. **–malinger,** *v.,* **malingerer,** *n.*

malleable /mal'ē·əbəl/ [L *malleare* to beat], able to be pressed, hammered, or otherwise forced into a shape without breaking.

malleolus /məlē'ələs/, *pl.* **malleoli** [L, little hammer], a rounded bony process, such as the protuberance on each side of the ankle.

malleolus fibulae. See **external malleolus.**

mallet deformity [ME *maillet* maul], a flexion abnormality of the distal joint of a finger or toe. It may be caused by severe damage such as rupture of the terminal tendon.

mallet finger. See **hammer finger.**

mallet fracture, avulsion fracture of the dorsal base of a distal phalanx of the hand or foot, involving the associated extensor apparatus and causing dropped flexion of the distal segment.

malleus /mal'ē·əs/, *pl.* **mallei** [L, hammer], one of the three ossicles in the middle ear, resembling a hammer with a head, neck, and three processes. It is connected to the tympanic membrane and transmits sound vibrations to the incus.

Mallory bodies /mal'ərē/ [Frank B. Mallory, American pathologist, b. 1862; AS *bodig* body], an eosinophilic cytoplasmic inclusion, alcoholic hyalin, found in the liver cells. It is typically, but not always, associated with acute alcoholic liver injury.

Mallory-Weiss syndrome [G. Kenneth Mallory, American pathologist, b. 1926; Soma Weiss, American physician, b. 1899], a condition characterized by massive bleeding after a tear in the mucous membrane at the junction of the esophagus and the stomach. The laceration is usually caused by protracted vomiting, most commonly in alcoholics or in persons whose pylorus is obstructed.

malnutrition [L *malus + nutrire* to nourish], any disorder concerning nutrition. It may result from an unbalanced, insufficient, or excessive diet or to the impaired absorption, assimilation, or use of foods.

malocclusion /mal'əklo͞o'zhən/ [L *malus + occludere* to shut up], abnormal contact

M

of the teeth of the upper jaw with the teeth of the lower jaw.

malonic acid /məlō′nik/, a white, crystalline, highly toxic substance used as an intermediate compound in the production of barbiturates.

malpighian body /malpig′ē·ən/ [Marcello Malpighi, Italian physician, b. 1628; AS *bodig* body], **1.** the renal corpuscle, which includes a glomerulus with Bowman's capsule. **2.** lymphoid tissue surrounding the arteries of the spleen.

malpighian corpuscle [Marcello Malpighi; L *corpusculum* little body], one of a number of small, round, deep-red bodies in the cortex of the kidney, each communicating with a renal tubule. Malpighian corpuscles average about 0.2 mm in diameter, each composed of two parts: a central glomerulus and a glomerular capsule.

malpractice [L *malus* + Gk *praktikos* performance], (in law) professional negligence that is the proximate cause of injury or harm to a patient, resulting from a lack of professional knowledge, experience, or skill that can be expected in others in the profession or from a failure to exercise reasonable care or judgment in the application of professional knowledge, experience, or skill.

malpresentation [L *malus* + *praesentare* to show], an abnormal position of the fetus in the birth canal.

malrotation /mal′rōtā′shən/, **1.** any abnormal rotation of an organ or body part, such as the vertebral column or a tooth. **2.** a failure of the intestinal tract or other viscera to undergo normal rotation during embryonic development.

Malta fever. See **brucellosis.**

malunion /malyo̅o̅′nyən/ [L *malus* + *unus* one], an imperfect union of previously fragmented bone or other tissue.

mammary /mam′ərē/ [L *mamma* breast], pertaining to or resembling the mammary gland.

mammary duct. See **lactiferous duct.**

mammary gland [L *mamma* breast; *glans* acorn], one of two discoid, hemispheric glands on the chest of mature females, present in rudimentary form in children and in males. Glandular tissue forms a radius of lobes containing alveoli, each lobe having a system of ducts for the passage of milk from the alveoli to the nipple. The periphery is made up mostly of adipose tissue.

mammary papilla. See **nipple.**

mammillary body /mam′iler′ē/ [L *mammilla* nipple; AS *bodig* body], either of the two small round masses of gray matter in the hypothalamus located close to one another in the interpeduncular space.

mammogram /mam′əgram/ [L *mamma* + Gk *gramma* record], an x-ray film of the soft tissues of the breast.

mammography /mamog′rəfē/, radiography of the soft tissues of the breast to allow identification of various benign and malignant neoplastic processes.

mammoplasty /mam′əplas′tē/ [L *mamma* + Gk *plassein* to mold], plastic reshaping of the breasts, performed to reduce or lift enlarged or sagging breasts, to enlarge small breasts, or to reconstruct a breast after removal of a tumor.

mammothermography /mam′ōthərmog′-rəfē/ [L *mamma* + Gk *therme* heat, *graphein* to record], a diagnostic procedure in which thermography is used to examine the breast to detect abnormal growths.

managed care. a health care system in which there is administrative control over a primary health care services in a medical group practice. Redundant facilities and services are eliminated and costs are reduced.

management of therapeutic regimen (individual), ineffective, a NANDA-accepted nursing diagnosis defined as a pattern of regulating and integrating into daily living a program for treatment of illness and the sequelae of illness that is unsatisfactory for meeting specific health goals. Defining characteristics include ineffective choices of daily living, acceleration of illness symptoms, verbalized desire to manage the treatment and difficulty with regulation, and verbalization that the patient would not attempt to reduce risk factors.

mandible /man′dibəl/ [L *mandere* to chew], a large bone constituting the lower jaw. It contains the lower teeth and consists of a horizontal portion, a body, and two perpendicular rami that join the body at almost right angles. The body of the mandible is curved, somewhat resembling a horseshoe, and has two surfaces and two borders. **–mandibular,** *adj.*

mandibular arch /mandib′yələr/ [L *mandere* + *arcus* bow], the first visceral arch from which the lower jaw bone develops.

mandibular canal [L *mandere* + *canalis* channel], (in dentistry) a passage or channel that extends from the mandibular foramen on the medial surface of the ramus of the mandible to the mental foramen. It holds mandibular blood vessels and a portion of the mandibular branch of the trigeminal nerve.

mandibular notch, a depression in the inferior border of the mandible, anterior to the attachments of the masseter muscle, where the external facial muscles cross the lower border of the mandible.

mandibular process [L *mandere* + *processus*], **1.** the upper alveolar part of the mandible. **2.** the projection of the upper posterior part of the ramus of the mandible bearing the condyle.

mandibular ramus [L *mandere* + *ramus* branch], a broad quadrilateral portion of the mandible projecting upward from the posterior end of the body behind the lower teeth. It has two surfaces, four borders, and two processes.

mandibular reflex [L *mandere* + *reflectere* to bend back], a reflex contraction of the masseter muscle after a downward tap on the point of the jaw while the mouth is open.

mandibular sling, the connection between the mandible and the maxilla, formed by the masseter and the pterygoideus at the angle of the mandible.

mandibulofacial dysostosis /mandib'-yəlofā'shəl/ [L *mandere* + *facies* face; Gk *dys* bad, *osteon* bone], an abnormal hereditary condition characterized by antimongoloid slant of the palpebral fissures, colomboma of the lower lid, micrognathia and hypoplasia of the zygomatic arches, and microtia.

mandrel /man'drəl/ [Fr *mandrin* boring tool], a shaft secured in a handpiece or lathe to support an object to be rotated, such as a dental polishing disk or cutting device.

maneuver [Fr *manoeuvre* action], **1.** an adroit or skillful manipulation or procedure. **2.** (in obstetrics) a manipulation of the fetus performed to aid in delivery.

manganese (Mn) /mang'gənēs/ [L a corruption of *maganesium*, a common metallic element found in trace amounts in tissues of the body where it aids in the functions of various enzymes. Its atomic number is 25; its atomic weight is 54.938.

mania /mā'nē·ə/ [Gk, madness], a state characterized by an expansive emotional state, extreme excitement, excessive elation, hyperactivity, agitation, overtalkativeness, flight of ideas, increased psychomotor activity, fleeting attention, and sometimes violent, destructive, and self-destructive behavior. **–maniac,** *n., adj.,* **maniacal,** *adj.*

manic depressive [Gk *mania* madness; L *deprimere* to sink down], a person with or exhibiting the symptoms of bipolar disorder.

manifest deviation. See **eye deviation.**

manipulation [L *manipulare* to work with the hands], the skillful use of the hands in therapeutic or diagnostic procedures, such as palpation, reducing a dislocation,

turning the position of the fetus, or various treatments in physical therapy and osteopathy. A kind of manipulation is **conjoined manipulation.**

mannitol /man'itol/, a poorly metabolized sugar used as an osmotic diuretic and in kidney function tests. It is prescribed to promote diuresis, to decrease intraocular and intracranial pressure, to promote the excretion of poisons and other toxic wastes, and to evaluate renal function.

manometer /mənom'ətər/ [Gk *manos* thin, *metron* measure], a device for measuring the pressure of a fluid, consisting of a tube marked with a scale and containing a relatively incompressible fluid, such as mercury. The level of the fluid in the tube varies with the pressure of the fluid. Kinds of manometers are **aneroid manometer** and **sphygmomanometer.**

Mansonella ozzardi /man'sənel'ə/, a parasitic worm that is indigenous to Latin America and the Caribbean islands. It is a relatively benign nematode that infects humans. The larvae live in the bloodstream and adult worms are found in the visceral mesenteries.

Mantoux test /mantō̄/ [Charles Mantoux, French physician, b. 1877], a tuberculin skin test that consists of intradermal injection of a purified protein derivative of the tubercle bacillus. A hardened, raised red area of 8 to 10 mm, appearing 24 to 72 hours after injection, is a positive reaction.

manual rotation [L *manualis* hand; *rotare* to turn], an obstetric maneuver in which a baby's head is turned by hand from a transverse to an anteroposterior position in the birth canal to facilitate delivery.

manubriosternal articulation /mənō̄'-brē-ōstur'nəl/ [L *manubrium* handle; Gk *sternum* chest; L *articularis* pertaining to joints], the fibrocartilaginous connection between manubrium and the body of the sternum.

manubrium /mənō̄'brē·əm/ [L, handle], the most anterior of the three bones of the sternum, presenting a broad quadrangular shape that narrows caudally at its articulation with the superior end of the body of the sternum. **–manubrial,** *adj.*

manudynamometer /man'ō̄odī'nəmom'-ətər/ [L *manus* hand; Gk *dynamis* force; *metron* measure], a device for measuring the force or extent of thrust.

manus. See **hand.**

many-tailed bandage [AS *manig* many, *taegel* tail; Fr *bande* strip] **1.** a broad, evenly shaped bandage with both ends split into strips of equal size and number. As the bandage is placed on the abdomen, chest, or limb, the ends may be overlapped. **2.** an irregularly shaped bandage with torn or cut ends that are tied together.

MAO, abbreviation for **monoamine oxidase.**

MAOI, abbreviation for **monoamine oxidase inhibitor.**

MAP, 1. abbreviation for *medical aid post.* **2.** abbreviation for **mean arterial pressure.**

map distance. See **map unit.**

maple bark disease [AS *mapul;* ONorse *bark;* L *dis* opposite of; Fr *aise* ease], a hypersensitivity pneumonitis caused by exposure to the mold *Cryptostroma corticale,* found in the bark of maple trees. In the susceptible person the condition may be acute, accompanied by fever, cough, dyspnea, and vomiting, or it may be chronic, characterized by fatigue, weight loss, dyspnea on exertion, and a productive cough.

maple syrup urine disease [AS *mapul;* Ar *sharab;* Gk *ouron* urine], an inherited metabolic disorder in which an enzyme necessary for the breakdown of the amino acids valine, leucine, and isoleucine is lacking. The disease is recognized by the characteristic maple syrup odor of the urine and by hyperreflexia.

mapping [L *mappa* napkin], (in genetics) the process of locating the relative position of genes on a chromosome through the analysis of genetic recombination.

maprotiline hydrochloride /maprō′tilēn/, an antidepressant similar to the tricyclics prescribed for the treatment of mental depression.

map unit [L *mappa* napkin; *unus* one], (in genetics) an arbitrary unit of measure used to designate the distance between genes on a chromosome. It is calculated from the percentage of recombinations that occur between specific genes so that 1% of crossing over represents one unit on a genetic map.

marasmic kwashiorkor /maraz′mik/ [Gk *marasmos* a wasting; Afr], a malnutrition disease, primarily of children, resulting from the deficiency of both calories and protein. The condition is characterized by severe tissue wasting, dehydration, loss of subcutaneous fat, lethargy, and growth retardation.

marasmus /maraz′mas/ [Gk *marasmos* a wasting], a condition of extreme malnutrition and emaciation, occurring chiefly in young children, that is characterized by progressive wasting of subcutaneous tissue and muscle. It results from a lack of adequate calories and proteins and is seen in failure-to-thrive children and in starvation.

marathon encounter group [Marathon,

Greece; L *in* in, *contra* against; Fr *groupe*], an intensive group experience that accelerates self-awareness and promotes personal growth and behavioral change through the continuous interaction of group members for a period ranging from 16 to more than 40 hours.

marble bones. See **osteopetrosis.**

Marburg-Ebola virus disease /mär′bargeb′ələ/, a serious febrile disease characterized by rash and severe GI hemorrhages. This disease may be transmitted to hospital personnel by improper handling of contaminated needles or from hemorrhagic lesions of patients. The diagnosis is made by serologic abnormalities.

march foot [Fr *marcher* to walk; AS *fot*], an abnormal condition of the foot caused by excessive use, such as in a long march. The forefoot is swollen and painful, and one or more of the metatarsal bones may be broken.

march fracture. See **metatarsal stress fracture.**

march hemoglobinuria, a rare, abnormal condition, characterized by the presence of hemoglobin in the urine, that occurs after strenuous physical exertion or prolonged exercise, such as marching or distance running.

Marchiafava-Micheli disease /mär′kyəfä′-vəmikā′lē/ [Ettore Marchiafava, Italian physician, b. 1847; F. Micheli, Italian physician, b. 1872], a rare disorder of unknown origin characterized by episodic hemoglobinuria, occurring usually, but not always, at night.

Marchi's method /mär′kēz/ [Vittoria Marchi, Italian physician, b. 1851], a laboratory staining procedure for demonstrating degenerated nerve fibers.

Marcus Gunn pupil sign [Robert Marcus Gunn, English ophthalmologist, b. 1850], paradoxical dilation of the pupils in an ophthalmologic examination in response to afferent visual stimuli. In a dark room a beam of light is moved from one eye to the other. Normal miosis is caused by the consensual pupil reaction when the normal eye is illuminated; but as the light is moved to the opposite, abnormal eye, the direct reaction to light is weaker than the consensual reaction; hence both pupils dilate.

Marcus Gunn syndrome. See **jaw winking.**

Marfan's syndrome /märfäNz′/ [Bernard-Jean A. Marfan, French pediatrician, b. 1858], an abnormal condition characterized by elongation of the bones, often with associated abnormalities of the eyes and the cardiovascular system. The disease causes major pathologic musculoskeletal disturbances, such as muscular underdevelopment, ligamentous laxity, joint hypermobility, and bone elongation. With Marfan's syndrome pathologic alterations of the cardiovascular system appear to produce fragmentation of the elastic fibers in the media of the aorta, which may lead to aneurysm. Ocular changes associated with the disease include a variety of disorders, including dislocation of the lens. The disease affects men and women equally, elongating the limbs so that most adult patients with the disease are over 6 feet tall. The extremities of individuals with Marfan's syndrome are very long and spiderlike, with greatly extended metacarpals, metatarsals, and phalanges.

marginal gingiva [L *margo* margin; *gingiva* gum], the uppermost of the free gingiva that overlaps the neck and base of the crown of the tooth.

marginal gyrus [L *margo*; Gk *gyros* turn], the superior frontal convolution on the surface of the cerebral hemispheres.

marginal peptic ulcer [L *margo*; Gk *peptein* to digest; L *ulcus* ulcer], an ulcer that develops postoperatively at the surgical anastomosis of the stomach and jejunum.

marginal placenta previa, placenta previa in which the placenta is implanted in the lower uterine segment, with its margin touching or spreading to some degree over the internal os of the uterine cervix. During labor, as the cervix dilates, bleeding may occur from the separation of the edge of the placenta from the uterus beneath it.

marginal rale. See **atelectatic rale.**

marginal ridge, an elevation of enamel that forms the proximal boundary of the occlusal surface of a tooth.

marginal sinus [L *margo* + *sinus* hollow], a sinus that may encircle the placenta.

Marie's hypertrophy [Pierre Marie, French neurologist, b. 1853; Gk *hyper* excess, *trophe* nourishment], chronic enlargement of the joints caused by periostitis.

Marie-Strümpell disease. See **ankylosing spondylitis.**

marijuana. See **cannabis.**

Marin Amat syndrome, an involuntary facial movement phenomenon in which the eyes close when the mouth opens or when the jaws move in mastication. The effect results from a facial nerve paralysis.

marital rape [L *rapere* to seize], forcible sexual intercourse by a man with his wife.

mark [AS *mearc*], any nevus or birthmark.

marker gene. See **genetic marker.**

markers [AS *mearc*], body language movements that serve as indicators and punctuation marks in interpersonal communication.

marrow. See **bone marrow.**

Marseilles fever /märsālz', märsā'/ [Marseilles, France; L *febris* fever], a disease endemic around the Mediterranean, in Africa, in the Crimea, and in India, caused by *Rickettsia conorii* transmitted by the brown dog tick. Symptoms include chills, fever, an ulcer covered with a black crust at the site of the tick bite, and a rash appearing on the second to fourth day.

Marshall-Marchetti operation [Victor F. Marshall, American urologist, b. 1913; Andrew A. Marchetti, American obstetrician, b. 1901], a surgical procedure performed to correct a condition of stress incontinence. The procedure, a vesicourethropexy, involves a retropubic incision and suturing of the urethra, vesicle neck, and bladder to the posterior surface of the pubic bone.

marsupialize /märsoo'pē·əlīz'/ [L *marsupium* pouch; Gk *izein* to cause], to form a pouch surgically to treat a cyst when simple removal would not be effective, such as in a pancreatic or a pilonidal cyst.

Martorell's syndrome. See **Takayasu's arteritis.**

masculine [L *masculinus* male], having the characteristics of a male.

masculinization [L *masculinus* + Gk *izein* to cause], the normal development or induction of male sex characteristics. **–masculinize,** *v.*

MASER /mā'sər/, acronym for *microwave amplification by stimulated emission of radiation.*

MASH, acronym for *mobile army surgical hospital.*

mask [Fr *masque*], **1.** to obscure, as in symptomatic treatment that may mask the development of a disease. **2.** to cover, as does a skin-toned cosmetic that may mask a pigmented nevus. **3.** a cover worn over the nose and mouth to prevent inhalation of toxic or irritating materials, to control delivery of oxygen or anesthetic gas, or (by medical personnel) to shield a patient during aseptic procedures from pathogenic organisms normally exhaled from the respiratory tract.

mask image, (in digital fluoroscopy) an x-ray image made immediately after contrast material has been injected but before it reaches the anatomic site being examined. The initial mask image is then subtracted electronically from a series of additional images. The technique has the effect of enhancing the image of the tissues being studied.

masking, **1.** the covering or concealing

M

of a disorder by a second condition, as when a person begins a weight-loss diet while an undiagnosed wasting disease such as cancer has developed. **2.** the unconscious display of a personality trait that conceals a behavioral aberration.

masking agent, a cosmetic preparation for covering nevi, surgical scars, and other blemishes.

masklike facies [Fr *masque*; L *facies* face], an immobile expressionless face with staring eyes and the mouth slightly open. It is sometimes associated with parkinsonism.

mask of pregnancy. See **chloasma.**

Maslow's hierarchy of need /mas'lōz/ [Abraham H. Maslow, American psychiatrist, b. 1908; Gk *hierarches* position of authority; AS *nied* obligation], (in psychology) a hierarchic categorization of the basic needs of humans. The most basic needs on the scale are the physiologic or biologic, such as the need for air, food, or water. Of second priority are the safety needs, including protection and freedom from fear and anxiety. The subsequent order of needs in the hierarchic progression are the need to belong, to love, and to be loved; the need for self-esteem; and ultimately, the need for self-actualization.

masochism /mas'ōkiz'əm/ [Leopold von Sacher-Masoch, Austrian author, b. 1836], pleasure or gratification derived from receiving physical, mental, or emotional abuse. **–masochistic,** *adj.*

masochist [Leopold von Sacher-Masoch], a person deriving pleasure or gratification from masochistic acts or abuse.

mass [L *massa* a lump], **1.** the physical property of matter that gives it weight and inertia. **2.** (in pharmacology) a mixture from which pills are formed. **3.** an aggregate of cells clumped together such as a tumor.

massage [Fr *masser* to stroke], the manipulation of the soft tissue of the body through stroking, rubbing, kneading, or tapping, to increase circulation, to improve muscle tone, and to relax the patient. The procedure is performed either with the bare hands or through some mechanical means, such as a vibrator. The most common sites for massage are the back, knees, elbows, and heels. Kinds of massage are **cardiac massage, effleurage, flagellation, friction, frôlement, pétrissage, tapotement,** and **vibration.**

masseter /mase'tər/ [Gk, one who chews], the thick, rectangular muscle in the cheek that functions to close the jaw. It is one of the four muscles of mastication.

mass fragment [L *massa* lump; *frangere* to shatter], a degraded portion of a molecule containing one or more charges.

mass hysteria. See **major hysteria.**

mass number (A), the sum of the number of protons and neutrons in the nucleus of an atom or isotope.

mass reflex, an abnormal condition, seen in patients with transection of the spinal cord, characterized by a widespread nerve discharge, resulting in flexor muscle spasms, incontinence of urine and feces, priapism, hypertension, and profuse sweating. A mass reflex may be triggered by scratching or other painful stimulus to the skin, overdistention of the bladder or intestines, cold weather, prolonged sitting, or emotional stress.

mass spectrometer, an analytic instrument for identifying a substance by sorting a stream of charged particles (ions) according to their mass.

mass spectrometry, (in chemistry) a technique for the analysis of a substance in which the constituents are identified and quantified using a mass spectrometer.

mass transfer, the movement of mass from one phase to another.

MAST, abbreviation for **military anti-shock trousers.**

mastalgia /mastal'jə/ [Gk *mastos* breast, *algos* pain], pain in the breast caused by congestion or "caking" during lactation, an infection, fibrocystic disease, especially during or before menstruation, or advanced cancer. The early stages of breast cancer are rarely accompanied by pain. **–mastalgic,** *adj.*

mast cell [Ger *Mast* fattening; L *cella* storeroom], a constituent of connective tissue containing large basophilic granules that bear heparin, serotonin, bradykinin, and histamine.

mast cell leukemia, a malignant neoplasm of leukocytes characterized by many connective tissue mast cells in circulating blood.

mast cell tumor, a connective tissue tumor composed of mast cells. Granules of the cells stain metachromatically with toluidine blue.

mastectomy /mastek'təmē/ [Gk *mastos* breast, *ektome* excision], the surgical removal of one or both breasts, performed to remove a malignant tumor. In a simple mastectomy, only breast tissue is removed. In a radical mastectomy, some of the muscles of the chest are removed with the breast with all lymph nodes in the axilla. In a modified radical mastectomy, the large muscles of the chest that move the arm are preserved. Emotional support and counseling are essential. **–mastectomize,** *v.*

master problem list, a list of a patient's problems that serves as an index to the patient's record. Each problem, the date the problem was first noted, the treatment, and the outcome are added to the master problem list as each becomes known.

master's degree program in nursing, a postgraduate program in a school of nursing, based in a university setting, that grants the degree Master of Science in Nursing to successful candidates. The degree may be awarded for work in maternal-newborn nursing, medical-surgical nursing, pediatric nursing, psychiatric nursing, or in other fields of nursing.

mastery [L *magister* chief], being in command or control of a situation, as in learning accomplishment.

mastication /mas'tikā′shən/ [L *masticare* to chew], chewing, tearing, or grinding food with the teeth while it becomes mixed with saliva.

masticatory system /mas'tikətôr′ē/ [L *masticare* to chew; Gk *systema*], the combination of organs, structures, and nerves involved in chewing. It includes but is not limited to the jaws, the teeth and their supporting structures, the mandibular musculature, the mandible, the maxillae, the temporomandibular joints, the tongue, the lips, the cheeks, the oral mucosa, and cranial nerves.

mastitis /masti′tis/ [Gk *mastos* breast, *itis* inflammation], an inflammatory condition of the breast, usually caused by streptococcal or staphylococcal infection. **Acute mastitis,** most common in the first 2 months of lactation, is characterized by pain, swelling, redness, axillary lymphadenopathy, fever, and malaise. If untreated or inadequately treated, abscesses may form. **Chronic tuberculous mastitis** is rare; when it occurs, it represents extension of tuberculosis from the lungs and ribs beneath the breast.

mastocytosis /mas'təsītō′sis/ [Ger *Mast* fattening; Gk *kytos* cell, *osis* condition], local or systemic overproduction of mast cells, which, in rare instances, may infiltrate skin, spleen, bones, the GI system, and skin.

mastoid /mas′toid/ [Gk *mastos* breast, *eidos* form], **1.** of or pertaining to the mastoid process of the temporal bone. **2.** breast-shaped.

mastoid cells, air cells in the mastoid process of the temporal bone.

mastoidectomy /mas'toidek′təmē/ [Gk *mastos* + *eidos* form, *ektome* excision], surgical excision of a portion of the mastoid part of the temporal bone, performed to treat chronic suppurative otitis media or mastoiditis when systemic antibiotics are ineffective. In a simple mastoidectomy, in-

fected bone cells are removed and the eardrum is incised to drain the middle ear.

mastoid fontanel, a posterolateral fontanel that is usually not palpable.

mastoiditis /mas'toidī′tis/ [Gk *mastos* + *eidos* form, *itis* inflammation], an infection of one of the mastoid bones, usually an extension of a middle ear infection, characterized by earache, fever, headache, and malaise. The infection is difficult to treat, often requiring antibiotics administered intravenously for several days.

mastoid process, the conic projection of the caudal, posterior portion of the temporal bone, serving as the attachment for various muscles, including the sternocleidomastoideus, splenius capitis, and longissimus capitis.

masturbation [L *masturbari* to masturbate], sexual activity in which the penis or clitoris is stimulated, usually to orgasm, by means other than coitus. **–masturbate,** *v,* **masturbatic, masturbatory,** *adj.*

matched group. See **group.**

materia /mətir′ē·ə/, matter or material, such as **materia medica.**

material fact [L *materia* matter; *factum*], (in law) a fact that establishes or refutes an element essential to the complaint, or charge, or to the defense.

materia medica, 1. the study of drugs and other substances used in medicine, their origins, preparation, uses, and effects. **2.** a substance or a drug used in medical treatment.

maternal [L, *maternus,* motherhood], **1.** inherited, derived, or received from a mother. **2.** a motherly behavior. **3.** related through the mother's side of the family, as a maternal grandfather.

maternal and child health (MCH) services, various facilities and programs organized for the purpose of providing medical and social services for mothers and children. Medical services include prenatal, postnatal, family planning care, and pediatric care in infancy.

maternal-child attachment. See **maternal-infant bonding.**

maternal-child separation syndrome. See **separation anxiety.**

maternal death, the death of a woman during the childbearing cycle.

maternal deprivation syndrome [L *mater* mother; *deprivare* to deprive; Gk *syn* together *dromos* course], a condition characterized by developmental retardation that occurs as a result of physical or emotional deprivation. It is seen primarily in infants. Typical symptoms include lack of physical growth, with weight below the third percentile for age and size, malnutrition, pronounced withdrawal, silence, apa-

M

thy, and irritability, and a characteristic posture and body language, featuring unnatural stiffness and rigidity with a slow response reaction to others.

maternal effect. See **maternal inheritance.**

maternal-infant bonding, the complex process of attachment of a mother to her newborn baby. In the first minutes and hours after birth, a sensitive period occurs during which the baby and the mother become intimately involved with each other through behaviors and stimuli that are complementary and that provoke further interactions. The mother touches the baby and holds it en face to achieve eye-to-eye contact. The infant looks back eye to eye. The mother speaks in a quiet, high-pitched voice. The mother and the baby move in turn to the voice and sounds of the other, a process known as entrainment; it can be likened to a dance. The infant's movements constitute a response to the mother's voice, and she is encouraged to continue the process.

maternal inheritance, the transmission of traits or conditions controlled by cytoplasmic factors within the ovum that are not self-replicating and are determined by genes within the nucleus.

maternal mortality, 1. the death of a woman as a result of childbearing. **2.** the number of maternal deaths per 100,000 births.

maternal placenta, the portion of the placenta that develops from the decidua basalis of the uterus and is usually shed along with the fetal elements.

maternity (mat., matern) [L *maternus* motherhood], the character and quality of a mother.

maternity cycle [L *mater* mother; Gk *kyklos* circle], the antepartal, intrapartal, and postpartal periods of pregnancy and the puerperium, from conception to 6 weeks after birth.

maternity nursing, nursing care of women and their families during pregnancy, during parturition, and through the first days of the puerperium.

mat gold [Fr *mat* dull; AS *geolu* yellow], a noncohesive form of pure gold, which is prepared by electrodeposition and may be used in the base of some dental restorations.

mating [MDu *mate* companion], the pairing of individuals of the opposite sex, primarily for purposes of reproduction.

mat. med., abbreviation for **materia medica.**

matrifocal family /mat'rifō'kəl/ [L *mater* mother, *focus* hearth; *familia* household], a family unit composed of a mother and her children. Biologic fathers have a temporary place in the family during the first years of the children's lives, but they maintain a more permanent position in their own original families.

matrix /mā'triks, mat'riks/ [L, womb], **1.** an intercellular substance, **2.** a basic substance from which a specific organ or kind of tissue develops. **3.** a form used in shaping a tooth surface in dental procedures.

matrix retainer, a mechanical device used to secure the ends of a matrix around a tooth and help compact a restoration in a tooth cavity.

matrix unzuis. See **nailed.**

matter [L *materia*], **1.** anything that has mass and occupies space. **2.** any substance not otherwise identified as to its constituents, such as gray matter, pus, or serum exuding from a wound.

maturation [L *maturare* to ripen], **1.** the process or condition of attaining complete development. In humans it is the unfolding of full physical, emotional, and intellectual capacities that enable a person to function at a higher level of competency and adaptability within the environment. **2.** the final stages in the meiotic formation of germ cells in which the number of chromosomes in each cell is reduced to the haploid number characteristic of the species. **3.** suppuration. **–maturate,** *v.*

maturational crisis, a transitional or developmental period within a person's life, such as puberty, when his or her psychologic equilibrium is upset.

mature [L *maturus* ripe], **1.** to become fully developed; to ripen. **2.** fully developed or ripened.

mature cell leukemia. See **polymorphocytic leukemia.**

maturity (mat.) [L *maturus* ripe], **1.** a state of complete growth or development, usually designated as the period of life between adolescence and old age. **2.** the stage at which an organism is capable of reproduction.

maturity-onset diabetes. See **non-insulin-dependent diabetes mellitus.**

max, 1. abbreviation for *maxima.* **2.** abbreviation for *maximum.*

maxilla /maksil'ə/, *pl.* **maxillae** [L *mala* jaw], one of a pair of large bones that form the upper jaw, consisting of a pyramidal body and four processes: the zygomatic, frontal, alveolar, and palatine.

maxillary /mak'səelerē/ [L *maxilla*], pertaining to the upper jaw bone.

maxillary arch [L *maxilla; arcus* bow], the curved bony ridge of the upper jaw bone, in the shape of a horseshoe, including the dentition and supporting structures.

maxillary artery [L *mala* jaw; Gk *arteria* air pipe], either of two larger terminal branches of the external carotid arteries that rise from the neck of the mandible near the parotid gland and divide into three branches, supplying the deep structures of the face.

maxillary fossa. See **canine fossa.**

maxillary process [L *maxilla, processus*], **1.** the alveolar process of the upper jaw that contains the tooth sockets. **2.** the frontal process that extends upward to articulate with the frontal and nasal bones. **3.** the palatine process that helps form the hard palate. **4.** the zygomatic process or anterior surface that articulates with the zygomatic bone.

maxillary sinus, one of the pair of large air cells forming a pyramidal cavity in the body of the maxilla.

maxillary vein, one of a pair of deep veins of the face, accompanying the maxillary artery. Each maxillary vein is a tributary of the internal jugular and the external jugular veins.

maxillofacial /mak′silōfā′shəl/ [L *maxilla* + *facies* face], pertaining to the maxilla and face.

maxillofacial prosthesis, a prosthetic replacement for part, or all, of the upper jaw, nose, or cheek. It is applied when surgical repair alone is inadequate.

maxillofacial surgery. See **oral surgery.**

maxillomandibular fixation /maksil′-ōmandib′yōōlər/ [L *mala* jaw, *mandere* to chew; *figere* to fasten], stabilization of fractures of the face or jaw by temporarily connecting the maxilla and mandible by wires, elastic bands, or metal splints.

maximal breathing capacity (MBC) [L *maximus* greatest; AS *braeth*; L *capacitas*], the amount of gas exchanged per minute with maximal rate and depth of respiration.

maximal diastolic membrane potential, (in cardiology) the greatest degree of negative transmembrane potential achieved by a cell during diastole.

maximal expiratory flow rate (MEFR), the rate of the most rapid flow of gas from the lungs during the expiratory phase of respiration.

maximal midexpiratory flow rate, the average volumetric rate of gas flow during the middle half (in terms of volume) of a forced expiratory vital capacity maneuver.

maximal voluntary ventilation, the maximal volume of gas that a person can ventilate by voluntary effort per unit of time breathing as quickly and deeply as possible.

maximum diastolic potential. See **maximal diastolic membrane potential.**

maximum inspiratory pressure (MIP) [L *maximus* greatest; *inspirare* to breathe in; *premere* to press], the maximum pressure within the alveoli of the lungs that occurs during the inspiratory phase of respiration.

maximum oxygen uptake, the greatest amount of oxygen that can be transported from the lungs to the working muscle tissue.

maximum permissible dose (MPD), the estimated maximum amount of radiation to which a person may be exposed with a minimum risk of experiencing leukemia, cancer, or genetic effects based on data obtained from dose-response models and actual experience accumulated in more than 50 years. The MPD for the general population is 500 mrems per year.

Mayer's reflex /mā′ərz/ [Karl Mayer, Austrian neurologist, b. 1862], a normal reflex elicited by grasping the ring finger and flexing it at the metacarpophalangeal joint of a person whose hand is relaxed with thumb abducted. The normal response is adduction and apposition of the thumb.

Mayo scissors. See **scissors.**

mazindol /mā′zindōl/, an anorectic prescribed to decrease the appetite in the treatment of exogenous obesity.

mb; mbar, abbreviations for millibar.

MB, abbreviation for *Bachelor of Medicine.*

MBC, abbreviation for **maximal breathing capacity.**

MBD, abbreviation for **minimal brain dysfunction.**

mbp, abbreviation for *mean blood pressure.*

mbt, abbreviation for *mean body temperature.*

mc, **1.** abbreviation for *millicycle.* **2.** abbreviation for **millicurie.**

mC, abbreviation for **millicoulomb.**

Mc, abbreviation for *megacycle.*

MC, **1.** abbreviation for *medical certificate.* **2.** abbreviation for *Medical Corps.*

McArdle's disease /məkär′dəlz/ [Brian McArdle, twentieth-century English neurologist], an inherited metabolic disease marked by an absence of myophosphorylase B and abnormally large amounts of glycogen in skeletal muscle. It is milder than other glycogen storage diseases.

MCAT, abbreviation for **Medical College Aptitude Test.**

McBurney's point /makbur′nēz/ [Charles McBurney, American surgeon, b. 1845; L *pungere* to puncture], a site of extreme sensitivity in acute appendicitis, situated in

M

the normal area of the appendix about 2 inches from the right anterior superior spine of the ilium, on a line between that spine and the umbilicus.

McBurney's sign, a reaction of the patient indicating severe pain and extreme tenderness when McBurney's point is palpated. Such a reaction indicates appendicitis.

McCall's festoon, (in dentistry) any one of the enlargements of the gingival margins that may be associated with occlusal trauma.

mcg, abbreviation for **microgram.**

MCh, abbreviation for *Master of Surgery.*

MCH, **1.** abbreviation for *maternal and child health.* **2.** abbreviation for **mean corpuscular hemoglobin.**

MCHC, abbreviation for **mean corpuscular hemoglobin concentration.**

mc hr, abbreviation for *millicurie hour.*

mCi, abbreviation for **millicurie.**

McManus, R. Louise (b. 1885), an American nurse and writer who established the first national testing service for the nursing profession.

McMurray's sign [Thomas P. McMurray, English surgeon, b. 1887], an audible click heard when rotating the tibia on the femur, indicating injury to meniscal structures.

MCP, abbreviation for *metacarpophalangeal joint.*

McShirley's electromallet. See **electromallet condenser.**

MCTD, abbreviation for **mixed connective tissue disease.**

MCV, abbreviation for **mean corpuscular volume.**

Md, symbol for the element **mendelevium.**

MD, abbreviation for *Doctor of Medicine.*

MD, abbreviation for **muscular dystrophy.**

MDA, abbreviation for *Muscular Dystrophy Association.*

MDR, abbreviation for **minimum daily requirement.**

Me, abbreviation for the methyl radical CH_3.

Meals on Wheels, a program designed to deliver hot meals to elderly, physically disabled, or other persons who lack the resources to provide themselves with nutritionally adequate warm meals on a daily basis.

mean [ME *mene* in the middle], occupying a position midway between two extremes of a set of values or data. The **arithmetic mean** is a value that is derived by dividing the total of a set of values by the number of items in the set. The **geometric mean** is a value that is between the first and last of a set of values organized in a geometric progression.

mean arterial pressure (MAP), the arithmetic mean of the blood pressure in the arterial portion of the circulation.

mean corpuscular hemoglobin (MCH), an estimate of the amount of hemoglobin in an average erythrocyte, derived from the ratio between the amount of hemoglobin and the number of erythrocytes present in a specimen.

mean corpuscular hemoglobin concentration (MCHC), an estimation of the concentration of hemoglobin in grams per 100 ml of packed red blood cells, derived from the ratio of the hemoglobin to the hematocrit.

mean corpuscular volume (MCV), an evaluation of the average volume of each red cell, derived from the ratio of the volume of packed red cells (the hematocrit) to the total number of red blood cells.

mean marrow dose (MMD), an arbitrary measure of the estimated average annual somatic radiation received by the population of the United States. The figure is 77 mrad and represents a weighted average for both persons exposed to radiation and persons not exposed during the period. It is expressed in terms of bone marrow because irradiation of that tissue is assumed to be a cause of leukemia.

measles /mē′zəlz/ [ME *meseles* skin spots], an acute, highly contagious viral disease involving the respiratory tract and characterized by a spreading maculopapular cutaneous rash that occurs primarily in young children who have not been immunized. Measles is caused by a paramyxovirus and is transmitted by direct contact with droplets spread from the nose, throat, and mouth of infected persons, usually in the prodromal stage of the disease. Indirect transmission by uninfected persons or by contaminated articles is unusual. An incubation period of 7 to 14 days is followed by the prodromal stage, characterized by fever, malaise, coryza, cough, conjunctivitis, photophobia, anorexia, and the pathognomonic Koplik's spots, which appear 1 to 2 days before onset of the rash. Pharyngitis and inflammation of the laryngeal and tracheobronchial mucosa develop, the temperature may rise to 103° F or 104° F and there is marked granulocytic leukopenia. The papules of the rash first appear as irregular brownish pink spots around the hairline, the ears, and the neck, then spread rapidly, within 24 to 48 hours, to the trunk and extremities, becoming red, maculopapular, and dense, giving a blotchy appearance. Within 3 to 5 days, the fever subsides, and the lesions flatten, turn a brownish color, and begin to fade, causing a fine desquamation, especially over heavily affected areas.

measles and rubella virus vaccine live, an active immunizing agent prescribed for immunization against measles and rubella.

measles immune globulin. See **immune globulin.**

measles, mumps, and rubella virus vaccine live (MMR), an active immunizing agent prescribed for simultaneous immunization against measles, mumps, and rubella.

measurement [L *mensura*], the determination, expressed numerically, of the extent or quantity of a substance, energy, or time.

meatorrhaphy /mē'ətôr'əfē/ [L *meatus* passage; Gk *rhaphe* suture], the suturing of the cut end of the urethra to the glans penis after surgery to enlarge the urethral meatus.

meatoscopy /mē'ətos'kəpē/ [L *meatus* + Gk *skopein* to look], the visual examination of any meatus, especially the urethra, usually performed with the aid of a speculum.

meatus /mē-ā'təs/, *pl.* **meatuses, meatus** [L, passage], an opening or tunnel through any part of the body, as the external acoustic meatus that leads from the external ear to the tympanic membrane. **–meatal,** *adj.*

meatus acusticus externus, the passage from the external ear to the tympanic membrane.

meatus acusticus internus, the internal acoustic meatus, a passageway for the facial, intermediate, and vestibulocochlear nerves, and the labyrinthine artery.

mebendazole /məben'dəzōl/, an anthelmintic prescribed in the treatment of pinworm, whipworm, roundworm, and hookworm infestations.

MEC, abbreviation for *minimum effective concentration,* or the minimum inhibitory concentration for a drug to be active. The drug is effective at any level above this threshold value.

mecamylamine hydrochloride /mek'-əmil'əmēn/, a ganglionic blocking agent prescribed in the management of hypertensive cardiac disease.

mechanical advantage [Gk *mechane* machine; L *abante* superior position], (in physiology) the ratio of the output force developed by the muscles to the input force applied to the body structures that the muscles move.

mechanical condenser, a device that delivers automatically controlled impacts for condensing restorative material in the filling of tooth cavities.

mechanical dead air space, the volume of air that fills the breathing circuits of a mechanical ventilator. The mechanical dead space may be increased if necessary to control hypocapnia and respiratory alkalosis.

mechanical heart-lung, a device connected to the circulatory system to maintain oxygenated blood flow during surgery that requires interruption of normal heart-lung functions.

mechanical restraint [Gk *machane;* L *restringere* to confine], a straitjacket, chair, bed, or other device used to enforce confinement of a patient, as opposed to the use of chemical restraints, such as neuroleptic medications, for the same purpose.

mechanical vector. See **vector.**

mechanism, 1. an instrument or process by which something is done, results, or comes into being. 2. a machine or machine-like system. 3. a stimulus-response system. 4. a habit or drive.

mechanism of labor. See **cardinal movements of labor.**

mechanoreceptor /mek'ənō'risep'tər/ [Gk *mechane* machine; L *recipere* to receive], any sensory nerve ending that responds to mechanical stimuli, such as touch, pressure, sound, and muscular contractions.

mechlorethamine hydrochloride /mek'-lôreth'əmēn/, an antineoplastic alkylating agent prescribed in the treatment of a variety of neoplasms.

Meckel's diverticulum [Johann F. Meckel, German anatomist, b. 1781], an anomalous sac protruding from the wall of the ileum. It is congenital, resulting from the incomplete closure of the yolk stalk.

meclizine hydrochloride /mek'lizēn/, an antihistamine prescribed in the prevention and treatment of motion sickness.

meclofenamate sodium /mek'lōfen'əmāt/, an antiinflammatory agent prescribed in the treatment of rheumatoid arthritis and osteoarthritis.

mecocephaly. See **scaphocephaly.**

meconium /mikō'nē-əm/ [Gk *mekon* poppy], a material that collects in the intestines of a fetus and forms the first stools of a newborn. It has a thick and sticky consistency, is usually greenish to black, and is composed of secretions of the intestinal glands, some amniotic fluid, and intrauterine debris, such as bile pigments, fatty acids, epithelial cells, mucus, lanugo, and blood.

meconium aspiration, the inhalation of meconium by the fetus or newborn, which can block the air passages and result in failure of the lungs to expand or cause other pulmonary dysfunction.

meconium ileus, obstruction of the small intestine in the newborn caused by impaction of thick, dry, tenacious meconium, usually at or near the ileocecal valve. Symptoms include abdominal distention, vomiting, failure to pass meconium within the first 24 to 48 hours after birth, and rapid dehydration with associated electrolyte imbalance.

meconium plug syndrome, obstruction of the large intestine in the newborn caused by thick, rubbery meconium that may fill the entire colon and part of the terminal ileum. Symptoms include failure to pass meconium within the first 24 to 48 hours after birth, abdominal distention, and vomiting if complete intestinal blockage occurs.

MED, 1. abbreviation for *minimal effective dose;* 2. abbreviation for **minimal erythema dose.**

medcard /med´kärd/, (in nursing) a small card listing the name, dose, and schedule of administration of each patient's medications, used in dispensing medication to each patient.

MEDEX /med´eks/, 1. an educational program accredited by the AMA for training military personnel with *medical experience* to become physician's assistants. 2. a physician's assistant who has gained *medical experience* during military service and further training in a physician's assistant program.

medial /mē´dē·əl/ [L *medialis* middle], 1. situated or oriented toward the midline of the body. 2. pertaining to the tunica media, the middle layer of a blood vessel wall.

medial antebrachial cutaneous nerve, a nerve of the arm that arises from the medial cord of the brachial plexus, medial to the axillary artery.

medial arteriosclerosis. See **Mönckeberg's arteriosclerosis.**

medial brachial cutaneous nerve, a nerve of the arm arising from the medial cord of the brachial plexus and distributed to the medial side of the arm.

medial cuneiform bone, the largest of three cuneiform bones of the foot, situated on the medial side of the tarsus, between the scaphoid bone and the first metatarsal.

medial geniculate body, either of the two areas on the posterior dorsal thalamus, relaying auditory impulses from the lateral lemniscus to the auditory cortex.

medialis /mē´dē·ā´lis/ [L *medius* middle], pertaining to the middle or to the median plane.

medial malleolus. See **internal malleolus.**

medial pectoral nerve, a branch of the brachial plexus that, with the lateral pectoral nerve, supplies the pectoral muscles.

medial rotation, a turning toward the midline of the body.

median /mē´dē·ən/ [L *medianus* middle], (in statistics) the number representing the middle value of the scores in a sample. In an odd number of scores arrayed in ascending order, it is the middle score; in an even number of scores so arrayed, it is the average of the two central scores.

median antebrachial vein /an´tēbrā´kē·əl/, one of the superficial veins of the upper limb that drains the venous plexus on the palmar surface of the hand.

median aperture of fourth ventricle, an opening between the lower part of the roof of the fourth ventricle and the subarachnoid space.

median atlantoaxial joint, one of three points of articulation of the atlas and the axis. It allows rotation of the axis and the skull, the extent of rotation limited by the alar ligaments.

median basilic vein, one of the superficial veins of the upper limb, often formed as one of two branches from the median cubital vein. It is commonly used for venipuncture, phlebotomy, or intravenous infusion.

median effective dose (ED$_{50}$), the dose of a drug that may be expected to cause a specific intensity of effect in one half of the patients to whom it is given.

median glossitis. See **median rhomboid glossitis.**

median jaw relation, (in dentistry) any jaw relation that exists when the mandible is in the median sagittal plane.

median lethal dose (MLD, LD$_{50}$), (in radiotherapy) the amount of radiation that kills 50% of the individuals in a large group of animals or organisms within a specified period.

median nerve, one of the terminal branches of the brachial plexus that extends along the radial portions of the forearm and the hand and supplies various muscles and the skin of these parts.

median palatine suture, the line of junction between the horizontal portions of the palatine bones that extends from both sides of the skull to form the posterior part of the hard palate.

median plane, a vertical plane that divides the body into right and left halves and passes approximately through the sagittal suture of the skull.

median rhomboid glossitis, a red, depressed, diamond-shaped area on the dorsum of the tongue, frequently irritated by alcohol, hot drinks, or spicy foods

median sternotomy   a chest surgery technique in which an incision is made from the suprasternal notch to below the xiphoid process. The sternum is then opened with a saw. Closure requires reunion of the sternum with stainless steel sutures.

median toxic dose (TD$_{50}$), the dosage that may be expected to cause a toxic effect in one half of the patients to whom it is given.

mediastinal /mē′dē·əstī′nəl/ [L. *mediastinus,* midway], pertaining to a medium septum or space between two parts.

mediastinitis, an inflammation of the mediastinum.

mediastinoscopy [L *mediastinus* + Gk *skopein* to view], an examination of the mediastinum through an incision in the suprasternum, using an endoscope with light and lenses.

mediastinum /mē′dē·əstī′nəm/, *pl.* **mediastina** [L *mediastinus* lower servant], a portion of the thoracic cavity in the middle of the thorax, between the pleural sacs containing the two lungs. It extends from the sternum to the vertebral column and contains all the thoracic viscera, except the lungs. It is enclosed in a thick extension of the thoracic subserous fascia. **—mediastinal,** *adj.*

mediate /mē′dē·āt/ [L *medio* to divide in the middle], **1.** to cause a change to occur, as in stimulation by a hormone. **2.** to settle a dispute, as in collective bargaining. **3.** situated between two places, things, parts, or terms. **4.** (in psychology) an event that follows one process or event and precedes another; for example, in the process of cognition, perception follows stimulation and precedes thinking. **—mediating,** *adj.,* **mediator,** *n.*

medic [L *medicus* healer], a physician, medical student, medical corpsman, or other medical professional.

Medicaid /med′ikād/, a federally funded, state-operated program of medical assistance to people with low incomes, authorized by Title XIX of the Social Security Act. Under broad federal guidelines the individual states determine benefits, eligibility, rates of payment, and methods of administration.

Medicaid mill, *informal;* a health program or facility that solely or primarily serves persons eligible for Medicaid. Such facilities are found mainly in depressed areas where there are few other health services.

medical assistant [L *medicare* to heal; *as-*

sistere to stand by], a person who, under the direction of a physician, performs various routine administrative and nontechnical clinical tasks in a hospital, clinic, or similar facility.

medical care, the provision by a physician of services related to the maintenance of health, prevention of illness, and treatment of illness or injury.

medical care plan, a long-range program of professional medical guidance designed to meet specific health objectives.

medical center, 1. a health care facility. **2.** a hospital, especially one staffed and equipped to care for many patients and for a large number of kinds of diseases and dysfunctions, using sophisticated technology.

Medical College Aptitude Test (MCAT), an examination taken by persons applying to medical school, the score on this examination being an important criterion for acceptance.

medical consultation, a procedure whereby, on request by one physician, another physician reviews a patient's medical history, examines the patient, and makes recommendations as to care and treatment. The medical consultant often is a specialist with expertise in a particular field of medicine.

medical corpsman /kôr′man/ [L *medicare* to heal; *corpus* body]. **1.** a member of a military medical unit. **2.** a paramedic.

medical decision level, a concentration of analyte at which some medical action is indicated for proper patient care.

medical diagnosis [L *medicare;* Gk *dia* through; *gnosis* knowledge], the determination of the cause of a patient's illness or suffering by the combined use of physical examination and patient interview, laboratory tests, review of the patient's medical records, knowledge of the etiology of observed signs and symptoms, and differential elimination of similar possible causes.

medical diathermy [L *medicare, dia* through, *thereme* heat], the application of high-frequency electrical currents to generate therapeutic heat in diseased tissues.

medical directive, a general term for documents that provide direction on the type of care a person desires.

medical director, a physician who is usually employed by a hospital to serve in a medical and administrative capacity as head of the organized medical staff.

medical engineering, a field of study that involves biomedical engineering and technologic concepts to develop equipment

M

and instruments required in health care delivery.

MedicAlert, a nonprofit U.S. organization that maintains a huge database of information about individuals who are taking one or more medications for a chronic disorder. The database also includes emergency telephone numbers for physicians treating the patients and provides bracelets or pendants to alert paramedics, interns, or other emergency medical personnel of the patient's medical condition and prescription drugs taken by the patient, who may be unconscious or confused after an accident or episode of illness. Medic Alert maintains access to the database for emergency medical personnel through a 24-hour telephone service.

medical ethics [L *medicare;* Gk *ethikos*], the moral conduct and principles that govern members of the medical profession.

medical examiner. See **coroner.**

medical genetics. See **clinical genetics.**

medical history. See **health history.**

medical illustrator, an artist qualified by special training in preparing illustrations of organs, tissues, and medical phenomena in normal and abnormal states.

medical indigency /in'dijen'sē/, the lack of financial reserves adequate to pay for medical care, especially a person or family able to manage other basic living expenses.

medical induction of labor. See **induction of labor.**

medical jurisprudence, the interaction of medicine with civil and criminal law.

medical laboratory technician, a person who, under the supervision of a medical technologist or physician, performs microscopic and bacteriologic tests of human blood, tissue, and fluids for diagnostic and research purposes.

medical model, the traditional approach to the diagnosis and treatment of illness in which the physician focuses on the defect, or dysfunction, within the patient. The medical history and the physical examination and diagnostic tests provide the basis for the identification and treatment of a specific illness.

medical pathology, the study of diseases not easily treated by surgical procedures.

medical record [L *medicare;* ME *recorden* to report], that portion of a patient's health record that is made by physicians and is a written or transcribed history of various illnesses or injuries requiring medical care, innoculations, allergies, treatments and prognosis, and, frequently, health information about the parents, siblings, occupation, and military service. The record may be reviewed by a physician in diagnosing the condition.

medical record administrator, a person who maintains records of patients' medical histories, diagnoses, treatment, and outcome, in a condition that meets medical, administrative, legal, ethical, regulatory, and institutional requirements.

medical record technician, a health professional responsible for maintaining components of health information systems consistent with the medical, administrative, ethical, legal, accreditation, and regulatory requirements of the health care delivery system.

medical secretary, a person who prepares and maintains medical records and performs related secretarial duties.

medical staff, all physicians, dentists, and health professionals responsible for providing health care in a hospital or other health care facility.

medical staff, courtesy, physicians and dentists who meet certain qualifications of the medical staff of a hospital but who admit patients only occasionally or act as consultants. They are ineligible to participate in medical staff activities.

medical staff, honorary, physicians and dentists, usually retired, who are recognized by the hospital medical staff for their noteworthy contributions but who may not admit patients to the hospital or participate in medical staff activities.

medical-surgical nursing, the nursing care of patients whose conditions or disorders are treated pharmacologically or surgically.

medical technologist, a person who, under the direction of a pathologist or other physician or medical scientist, performs specialized chemical, microscopic, and bacteriologic tests of blood, tissue, and fluids. A medical technologist who has successfully completed an examination by the Board of Registry of the American Society of Clinical Pathologists, or a similar professional body, may be designated a certified medical technologist.

medical transcriptionist, a health professional who prepares a written record of patient data that has been dictated by a physician. A **certified medical transcriptionist** is one who has met qualifying standards of the American Association of Medical Transcription.

medical vagotomy. See **pharmacologic vagotomy.**

medical waste, any discarded biological product, such as blood or tissues, removed from operating rooms, morgues, laboratories, or other medical facilities. The term may also be applied to bedding, bandages, syringes, ad similar materials that have been used in treating patients, as well as animal carcasses or body parts used in research.

Medical Women's International Association (MWIA), an international professional organization of women physicians.

medicamentosus /med′ikəmen′təs/ [L *medicamentum* drug], pertaining to a drug, particularly an adverse reaction attributed to a medication.

Medicare /med′iker/, a federally funded national health insurance for certain persons over 65 years of age. The program is administered in two parts. Part A provides basic protection against costs of medical, surgical, and psychiatric hospital care. Part B is a voluntary medical insurance program financed in part from federal funds and in part from premiums contributed by persons enrolled in the program. Medicare enrollment is offered to persons 65 years of age or older who are entitled to receive Social Security or railroad retirement benefits.

medicate [L *medicare* to heal], to treat an illness by the administration of drugs.

medicated bougie [L *medicare* to heal; Fr, candle], a bougie containing a medicated agent.

medicated enema, a medication administered via an enema. It is usually used preoperatively with patients scheduled for bowel surgery.

medicated tub bath, a therapeutic bath in which medication is dispersed in water, usually in the treatment of dermatologic disorders.

medication [L *medicare* to heal], **1.** a drug or other substance that is used as a medicine. **2.** the administration of a medicine.

medication error, any incorrect or wrongful administration of a medication, such as a mistake in dosage or route of administration, a failure to prescribe or administer the correct drug or formulation for a particular disease or condition, the use of outdated drugs, failure to observe the correct time for administration of the drug, or lack of awareness of adverse effects of certain combinations.

medication order, a written order by a physician, dentist, or other designated health professional for a medication to be dispensed by a hospital pharmacy for administration to an inpatient.

medicinal restraint, the use of hypnotics or other sedatives to control a potentially violent patient.

medicinal treatment, therapy of disorders based chiefly on the use of appropriate pharmacologic agents.

medicine [L *medicina* art of healing], **1.** a drug or a remedy for illness. **2.** the art and science of the diagnosis, treatment, and prevention of disease and the maintenance of good health. **3.** the art or technique of treating disease without surgery. Some of the many branches of medicine include **environmental, family, forensic, internal,** and **physical medicine.** –**medical,** *adj.*

medicolegal /med′ikōlē′gəl/ [L *medicina* art of healing, *lex* law], of or pertaining to both medicine and law. Medicolegal considerations, decisions, definitions, and policies provide the framework for informed consent, professional liability, and many other aspects of current practice in the health care field.

meditation [L *meditari* to consider], a state of consciousness in which the individual eliminates environmental stimuli from awareness so the mind can focus on a single thing, producing a state of relaxation and relief from stress.

meditation therapy, a method of achieving relaxation and consciousness expansion by focusing on a mantra, or a key word, sound, or image while eliminating outside stimuli from one's awareness.

Mediterranean anemia. See **thalassemia.**

Mediterranean fever. See **brucellosis.**

medium, *pl.* **media** [L *medius* middle], a substance through which something moves or through which it acts. A **contrast medium** is a substance that has a density different from that of body tissues, permitting visual comparison of structures when used with imaging techniques such as x-ray film. A **culture medium** is a substance that provides a nutritional environment for the growth of microorganisms or cells. A **dispersion medium** is the substance in which a colloid is dispersed. A **refractory medium** is the transparent tissues and fluid of the eye that refract light.

medium-chain triglyceride (MCT), a glycerine ester combined with an acid and distinguished from other triglycerides by having 8 to 10 carbon atoms. MCTs in foods are usually high in calories and easily digested.

MEDLARS /med′lärs/, abbreviation for *Medical Literature Analysis and Retrieval System,* a computerized literature retrieval service of the National Library of Medicine in Bethesda, Maryland. The references are filed in 15 data bases, including MEDLINE, TOXLINE, CHEMLINE, RTECS, CANCERLIT, and EPILEPSYLINE.

MEDLINE /med′līn/, a National Library of Medicine computer data base that covers approximately 600,000 references to biomedical journal articles published currently and in the 2 preceding years. The files duplicate the contents of the *Unabridged Index Medicus*, also published by the National Library of Medicine, which indexes medical reports from 3,000 professional journals in more than 70 countries.

MedRC, abbreviation for *medical reserve corps*.

medroxyprogesterone acetate /medrok'-sēprōjes'tərōn/, a progestin prescribed in the treatment of menstrual disorders caused by hormone imbalance.

MedScD, abbreviation for *Doctor of Medical Science*.

Med Tech, abbreviation for *medical technician*.

medulla /mədul'ə/, *pl.* **medullas, medullae** [L, marrow] **1.** the most internal part of a structure or organ, such as the spinal medulla. **2.** *informal;* medulla oblongata.

medulla oblongata, the most vital part of the entire brain, continuing as the bulbous portion of the spinal cord just above the foramen magnum. The medulla contains the cardiac, the vasomotor, and the respiratory centers of the brain, and medullary injury or disease often proves fatal.

medulla of the kidney, a part of the parenchyma of the kidney, beneath the cortex, including the renal pyramids and columns. It contains few, if any, glomeruli. An inner layer contains the papillae and the outer portion, which extends as far as the arcuate vessels, contains the thick ascending limbs of the loop of Henle.

medullary /med'ələr'ē, mədul'erē, med'-yələr'ē/ [L *medulla* marrow], **1.** of or pertaining to the medulla of the brain. **2.** of or pertaining to the bone marrow. **3.** of or pertaining to the spinal cord and central nervous system.

medullary carcinoma, a soft, malignant neoplasm of the epithelium containing little or no fibrous tissue.

medullary cystic disease, a chronic familial disease of the kidney, characterized by the slow onset of uremia. The disease appears in young children or adolescents, who pass large volumes of dilute urine with greater than normal amounts of sodium.

medullary fold. See **neural fold.**

medullary groove. See **neural groove.**

medullary nerve sheath. See **nerve sheath.**

medullary plate. See **neural plate.**

medullary sponge kidney, a congenital defect of the kidney, leading to cystic dilatation of the collecting tubules. Persons with this defect often develop a kidney stone or an infection of the kidney caused by urinary stasis.

medullary tube. See **neural tube.**

medulla spinalis. See **spinal cord.**

medullated /med'yəlā'tid/ [L *medulla* marrow], enclosed by a marrowlike substance, such as the myelin sheath of a nerve fiber.

medullated neuroma. See **fascicular neuroma.**

medulloblastoma /mədul'ōblastō'mə/ [L *medulla* + Gk *blastos* germ, *oma* tumor], a poorly differentiated malignant neoplasm composed of tightly packed cells of spongioblastic and neuroblastic lineage. The tumor usually arises in the cerebellum.

medulloepithelioma. See **neurocytoma.**

mefenamic acid /mef'ənam'ik/, a nonsteroidal antiinflammatory agent and analgesic prescribed in the treatment of mild to moderate pain.

mefloquine /mef'ləkēn/, an antimalarial that has been shown to be effective in the prophylaxis and treatment of chloroquine-resistant falciparum and vivax malaria.

MEFR, abbreviation for **maximal expiratory flow rate.**

megabladder. See **megalocystis.**

megacaryocyte /meg'əker'ē·əsīt'/ [Gk *megas* large, *karyon* nut, *kytos* cell], an extremely large bone marrow cell having a nucleus with many lobes. Megacaryocytes are essential for the production and proliferation of platelets in the marrow and are normally not present in circulating blood. –**megacaryocytic,** *adj.*

megacolon /meg'əkō'lən/ [Gk *megas* + *kolon* colon], massive, abnormal dilation of the colon that may be congenital, toxic, or acquired. **Congenital megacolon** (Hirschsprung's disease) is caused by the absence of autonomic ganglia in the smooth muscle wall of the colon. **Toxic megacolon** is a grave complication of ulcerative colitis and may result in perforation of the colon, septicemia, and death. **Acquired megacolon** is the result of a chronic refusal to defecate, usually occurring in children who are psychotic or mentally retarded. The colon becomes dilated by an accumulation of impacted feces.

megadose /meg'ədōs/, a dose that is greatly in excess of the amount usually prescribed or recommended.

megaesophagus /meg'ə·isof'əgəs/ [Gk *megas* + *oisophagos* gullet], abnormal dilatation of the lower segments of the esophagus caused by distention resulting from the failure of the cardiac sphincter to relax and allow the passage of food into the stomach.

megahertz (MHz) /meg'əhurts/, a unit of frequency equal to a million cycles per second.

megakaryocytic leukemia /meg'əker'-ē·ōsit'ik/ [Gk *megas* + *karyon*nut, *kytos* cell], a rare malignancy of blood-forming tissue in which megakaryocytes proliferate abnormally in the bone marrow and circulate in the blood in relatively large numbers.

megalencephaly /meg'əlensef'əlē/ [Gk *megas* + *enkephalos* brain], a condition characterized by pathologic parenchymal overgrowth of the brain. In some cases generalized cerebral hyperplasia is associated with mental retardation or a brain disorder. **–megalencephalic, megalencephalous,** *adj.*

megaloblast /meg'əlōblast'/ [Gk *megas* + *blastos* germ], an abnormally large nucleated immature erythrocyte that develops in large numbers in the bone marrow and is plentiful in the circulation in many anemias associated with deficiency of vitamin B_{12}, folic acid, or intrinsic factor. **–megaloblastic,** *adj.*

megaloblastic anemia, a hematologic disorder characterized by the production and peripheral proliferation of immature, large, and dysfunctional erythrocytes. Megaloblasts are usually associated with severe pernicious anemia or folic acid deficiency anemia.

megalocephaly. See **macrocephaly.**

megalocystis /meg'əlōsis'tis/ [Gk *megas* + *kystis* bag], an abnormal condition characterized by an enlarged and thin-walled bladder.

megalomania /meg'əlōmā'nē·ə/ [Gk *megas* + *mania* madness], an abnormal mental state characterized by delusions of grandeur in which one believes oneself to be a person of great importance, power, fame, or wealth.

megaloureter /meg'əlōyōōrē'tər/ [Gk *megas* + *oureter* ureter], an abnormal condition characterized by marked dilation of one or both ureters, resulting from dysfunctional peristaltic action of the smooth muscle in the ureters. Treatment may include surgical resection.

megavitamin therapy, a type of treatment that involves the administration of large doses of certain vitamins and minerals.

megestrol acetate /məjes'trōl/, an antineoplastic progestational agent prescribed to treat endometrial cancer and to palliate advanced endometrial and breast cancer.

meibomian cyst. See **chalazion.**

meibomian gland /mēbō'mē·ən/ [Heinrich Meibom, German physician, b. 1638], one of several sebaceous glands that secrete sebum from their ducts on the posterior margin of each eyelid. The glands are embedded in the tarsal plate of each eyelid.

Meigs' syndrome /megz/ [Joseph V. Meigs, American gynecologist, b. 1892], ascites and hydrothorax associated with a fibroma of the ovaries or other pelvic tumor.

meiocyte /mī'əsīt/ [Gk *meiosis* becoming smaller, *kytos* cell], any cell undergoing meiosis.

meiogenic /mī'əjen'ik/ [Gk *meiosis* + *genein* to produce], producing or causing meiosis.

meiosis /mī·ō'sis/ [Gk, becoming smaller], the division of a sex cell, as it matures, into two, then four gametes, the nucleus of each receiving one half of the number of chromosomes present in the somatic cells of the species. **–meiotic** /mī·ot'ik/, *adj.*

Meissner's corpuscle. See **tactile corpuscle.**

Meissner's plexus /mīs'nərz/ [Georg Meissner, German anatomist, b. 1829; L, *plaited*], small aggregations of gangion cells located in the submucosa of the intestine.

mel ', honey, a mixture of invert sugars and polysaccharides produced from the nectar of flowers by enzymes secreted by the honey bee, *Apis mellifica.*

melancholia /mel'angkō'lē·ə/ [Gk *melas* black, *chole* bile], extreme sadness.

melaniferous /mel'ənif'ərəs/ [Gk *melas* + L *ferre* to bear], pertaining to a black pigment.

melanin /mel'ənin/ [Gk *melas* black], a black or dark brown pigment that occurs naturally in the hair and skin, and in the iris and choroid of the eye.

melanoblast /me'ənōblast'/ [Gk *melas* + *blastos* germ], an epithelial tissue cell containing black granules. It develops into a melanocyte.

melanocyte /mel'ənōsīt', məlen'ōsīt/ [Gk *melas* + *kytos* cell], a body cell capable of producing melanin. Such cells are distributed throughout the basal cell layer of the epidermis and form melanin pigment from tyrosine, an amino acid.

melanocyte-stimulating hormone (MSH), a polypeptide hormone, secreted by the anterior pituitary gland, that controls the intensity of pigmentation in pigmented cells.

melanoderma /mel'ənōdur'mə/ [Gk *melas* + *derma* skin], any abnormal darkening of the skin caused by increased deposits of melanin or by the salts of iron or silver.

melanoma /mel'ənō'mə/ [Gk *melas* + *oma*

M

tumor], any of a group of malignant neoplasms, primarily of the skin, that are composed of melanocytes. Most melanomas develop from a pigmented nevus over a period of several months or years and occur most commonly in fair-skinned people having light-colored eyes. Any black or brown spot having an irregular border, pigment appearing to radiate beyond that border; a red, black, and blue coloration observable on close examination; or a nodular surface is suggestive of melanoma and is usually excised for biopsy. Kinds of melanoma are **amelanotic, benign juvenile, lentigo maligna, nodular, primary cutaneous,** and **superficial spreading melanoma.**

melanosis coli /mel′əno′sis/, an abnormal condition in which the mucous membrane of the colon is pigmented with melanin.

melanotrichia linguae. See **parasitic glossitis.**

melasma. See **chloasma.**

melasma gravidarum /məlaz′mə/, a dark pigment or discoloration that may appear on the skin of pregnant women.

melatonin /mel′ətō′nin/ [Gk *melas* + *tonikos* stretching], the only hormone secreted into the bloodstream by the pineal gland. The hormone appears to inhibit numerous endocrine functions, including the gonadotropic hormones, and to decrease the pigmentation of the skin.

melena /məlē′nə/ [Gk *melaina* black], abnormal, black, tarry stool containing digested blood. It usually results from bleeding in the upper GI tract and is often a sign of peptic ulcer or small bowel disease.

melena neonatorum, the passage of dark tarry stools by a newborn. The cause is usually altered blood pigments associated with hemorrhage. Normal meconium stools are greenish to black.

melioidosis /mel′ē·oidō′sis/ [Gk *melis* glanders, *eidos* form, *osis* condition], an infection that is uncommon in humans and is caused by the gram-negative bacillus *Malleomyces pseudomallei.* **Acute melioidasis** is fulminant and usually characterized by pneumonia, empyema, lung abscess, septicemia, and liver or spleen involvement. **Chronic melioidosis** is associated with osteomyelitis, multiple abscesses of the internal organs, and the development of fistulas from the abscesses. The disease is acquired by direct contact with infected animals.

melphalan /mel′fəlan/, an antineoplastic alkylating agent prescribed in the treatment of malignant neoplastic diseases, including multiple myeloma.

melting point (mp) [AS *meltan;* L *punctus* pricked], a characteristic temperature at which the solid and liquid forms of a substance are in equilibrium. The mp of ice is 32° F, or 0° C.

membrana tectoria /membrä′nə/ [L *membrana* thin skin; *tectorium* a covering] **1.** the broad, strong ligament covering the dens and helping to connect the axis to the occipital bone of the skull. **2.** a spiral membrane projecting from the vestibular lip of the cochlea over the organ of Corti.

membrana tympani. See **tympanic membrane.**

membrane /mem′brān/ [L *membrana* thin skin], a thin layer of tissue that covers a surface, lines a cavity, or divides a space, such as the abdominal membrane that lines the abdominal wall. The principal kinds of membranes are **mucous, serous, synovial,** and **cutaneous membranes. –membranous,** *adj.*

membrane conductance, (in cardiology) the degree of permeability of a cellular membrane to certain ions.

membrane diffusion coefficient, a component of total pulmonary diffusing capacity. It includes qualitative and quantitative characteristics of the functioning alveolar-capillary membrane.

membrane potential, the difference in electrical polarization or charge between two sides of a membrane or a cell wall.

membrane responsiveness, (in cardiology) the relationship between the membrane potential at the time of stimulation and the maximal rate of depolarization of the action potential.

membranous /mem′brənəs/ [L, *membrana*], resembling or consisting of a membrane.

membranous dysmenorrhea [L, *membrana;* Gk, *dys,* bad; *mens,* month; *rhein,* to flow], a form of spasmodic dysmenorrhea in which a cast of the uterine cavity is passed.

membranous labyrinth [L *membrana* + *labyrinthos* a maze], a network of three fluid-filled, membranous, semicircular ducts suspended within the bony semicircular canals of the inner ear, associated with the sense of balance.

membranous pharyngitis [L *membrana;* Gk *pharynx* throat], a diphtheric inflammation of the pharynx with the formation of a false membrane in the throat.

membranous stomatitis. See **pseudomembranous stomatitis.**

memory [L *memoria*], **1.** the mental faculty or power that enables one to retain and to recall, through unconscious associative processes, previously experienced sensations, impressions, ideas, concepts, and all information that has been consciously learned. **2.** the reservoir of all past experiences and knowledge that may be recollected or recalled at will. **3.** the recollection of a past event, ideas, sensations, or previously learned knowledge. Kinds of memory include **affect, antero-grade, kinesthetic, long-term, screen, short-term,** and **visual memory.**

memory cell. See **lymphocyte.**

memory image, a sensation, impression, or sense perception as it is recalled in the memory.

menadiol sodium diphosphate /men'-ədī'ol/, a water-soluble analog of vitamin K.

menadione /men'ədī'ōn/, a synthetic form of vitamin K₃. A water-soluble injectable form of the product is menadiol sodium diphosphate.

menarche /menär'kē/ [L *memsis* month; Gk *archaios* from the beginning], the first menstruation and the commencement of cyclic menstrual function. It usually occurs between 9 and 17 years of age.

menarcheal age /menär'kē·əl/ [L *mensis* + Gk *archaios*; L *aetas* age], the age at which menstruation begins. The normal range is from 9 to 17 years.

mendelevium (Md) /men'dəlē'vē·əm/ [Dimitri I. Mendeleyev, Russian chemist, b. 1834], a synthetic element in the actinide group. Its atomic number is 101. The atomic weight of its most stable isotope is 256. It is the ninth transuranic element.

mendelian genetics. See **Mendel's laws.**

mendelism /men'dəliz'əm/ [Gregor J. Mendel, Austrian geneticist, b. 1822], the concept of inheritance derived from the application of Mendel's laws. **—mendelian,** *adj.*

Mendel's laws [Gregor J. Mendel], the basic principles of inheritance based on breeding experiments of garden peas. These are usually stated as two laws, commonly called the law of segregation and the law of independent assortment. According to the first, each characteristic of a species is represented in the somatic cells by a pair of units, now known as genes, which separate during meiosis so that each gamete receives only one gene for each trait. According to the second law, the members of a gene pair on different chromosomes segregate independently from other pairs during meiosis, so that the gametes show all possible combinations of factors.

Mendelson's syndrome [Curtis L. Mendelson, American obstetrician, b. 1913], a respiratory condition caused by the chemical pneumonia resulting from the aspiration of acid gastric contents into the lungs. It usually occurs when a person vomits

when inebriated, when stuporous from anesthesia, or when unconscious, such as during a seizure.

Ménétrier's disease. See **giant hypertrophic gastritis.**

Ménière's disease /mānē·erz'/ [Prosper Ménière, French physician, b. 1799], a chronic disease of the inner ear characterized by recurrent episodes of vertigo, progressive unilateral nerve deafness, and tinnitus. The cause is unknown although occasionally the condition follows middle ear infection or trauma to the head. There also may be associated nausea, vomiting, and profuse sweating. Attacks last from a few minutes to several hours.

meningeal hydrops. See **pseudotumor cerebri.**

meninges /menin'jēz/, *sing.* **meninx** /mē'ningks, men'-/ [Gk *meninx* membrane], any one of the three membranes that enclose the brain and the spinal cord, comprising the dura mater, the pia mater, and the arachnoid. **—meningeal,** *adj.*

meningioma /menin'jē·ō'mə/, *pl.* **meningiomas, meningiomata** [Gk *meninx* + *oma* tumor], a mesenchymal fibroblastic tumor of the membranes enveloping the brain and spinal cord. The tumors may be nodular, plaquelike, or diffuse lesions that invade the skull, causing bone erosion and compression of brain tissue.

meningism /menin'jizəm/ [Gk *meninx* + *ismos* process], an abnormal condition characterized by irritation of the brain and the spinal cord and by symptoms that mimic those of meningitis. In meningism, however, there is no actual inflammation of the meninges.

meningismus /men'injis'məs/ [Gk, *menigx,* membrane; a condition in which the patient shows signs of meningitis but examination fails to reveal pathologic changes in the meninges. The condition is associated with cases of pneumonia in small children.

meningitis /mən'inji'tis/, *pl.* **meningitides** [Gk *meninx* + *itis* inflammation], any infection or inflammation of the membranes covering the brain and spinal cord. It is usually purulent and involves the fluid in the subarachnoid space. It is characterized by severe headache, vomiting, and pain and stiffness in the neck. The most common causes are bacterial infection with *Streptococcus pneumoniae, Neisseria meningitidis,* or *Haemophilus influenzae.* Aseptic meningitis may be caused by other kinds of bacteria, by chemical irritation, by neoplasm, or by viruses. Many of these diseases are benign and self-limited, such as meningitis caused by strains of coxsackievirus or echovirus. Others are more severe, such as those involving arbovi-

M

ruses, herpesviruses, or poliomyelitis viruses. Yeasts such as *Candida* and fungi such as *Cryptococcus* may cause a severe, often fatal, meningitis. Tuberculous meningitis, invariably fatal if untreated, may result in a variety of neurologic abnormalities even with the best treatment available. A kind of meningitis is **tuberculous meningitis.**

meningocele /mǝning'gōsēl'/ [Gk *meninx* + *kele* hernia], a saclike protrusion of either the cerebral or spinal meninges through a congenital defect in the skull or the vertebral column. It forms a hernial cyst that is filled with cerebrospinal fluid but does not contain neural tissue. The anomaly is designated a cranial meningocele or spinal meningocele, depending on the site of the defect; it can be easily repaired by surgery.

meningococcal polysaccharide vaccine /mǝning'gōkok'ǝl/, either of two active immunizing agents against group A and group C meningococcal organisms. It is prescribed for immunization against meningococcal meningitis.

meningococcemia /mǝning'gōkoksē'mē·ǝ/ [Gk *meninx* + *kokkos* berry, *haima* blood], a disease caused by *Neisseria meningitidis* in the bloodstream. Onset is sudden, with chills, pain in the muscles and joints, headache, petechiae, sore throat, and severe prostration. Tachycardia is present, respirations and pulse rate are increased, and fever is intermittent.

meningococcus /mǝning'gōkok'ǝs/, *pl.* **meningococci** /-kok'sī/ [Gk *meninx* + *kokkos* berry], a bacterium of the genus *Neisseria meningitidis*, a nonmotile, gram-negative diplococcus, frequently found in the nasopharynx of asymptomatic carriers, that may cause septicemia or epidemic cerebrospinal meningitis. **–meningococcal,** *adj.*

meningoencephalitis /mǝnin'gō·ensef'ǝlī'tis/ [Gk *meninx* + *enkephalos* brain, *itis*], an inflammation of both the brain and the meninges, usually caused by a bacterial infection.

meningoencephalocele /mǝning'gō·ensef'ǝlōsēl'/ [Gk *meninx* + *enkephalos* brain, *kele* hernia], a saclike cyst containing brain tissue, cerebrospinal fluid, and meninges that protrudes through a congenital defect in the skull.

meningomyelitis /mǝnin'gōmī'ǝlī'tis/, an inflammation of the spinal cord and its surrounding membranes.

meningomyelocele. See **myelomeningocele.**

meningovascular neurosyphilis /mǝnin'gōvas'kyǝlǝr/, a neurosyphilis inflammation of the supporting and nutrient tissues of the central nervous system.

meniscectomy /men'isek'tǝmē/ [Gk *meniskos* crescent, *ektome* excision], surgical excision of one of the crescent-shaped cartilages of the knee joint, performed when a torn cartilage results in chronic pain and in instability or locking of the joint.

meniscocystosis. See **sickle cell anemia.**

meniscus /menis'kǝs/ *pl. menisci* [Gk *meniskos* crescent], **1.** the interface between a liquid and air. **2.** a lens with both convex and concave aspects. **3.** a curved, fibrous cartilage in the knees and other joints.

Menkes' kinky hair syndrome /men'kēz/ [John H. Menkes, American neurologist, b. 1928; Dutch *kinke* tight twist; AS *haer*], a familial disorder affecting the normal absorption of copper from the intestine, characterized by the growth of sparse, kinky hair. Infants with the syndrome suffer cerebral degeneration, retarded growth, and early death.

menometrorrhagia /men'ōmet'rōrā'jē·ǝ/ [L *mensis* month; Gk *metra* womb, *rhegynein* to burst forth], excessive menstrual and uterine bleeding other than that caused by menstruation.

menopause /men'ǝpôz/ [L *mensis* month; Gk *pausis* to cease], strictly, the cessation of menses, but commonly used to refer to the period of the female climacteric. Menses stop naturally with the decline of cyclic hormonal production and function between 35 and 60 years of age but may stop earlier in life as a result of illness or the surgical removal of the uterus or both ovaries. As the production of ovarian estrogen and pituitary gonadotropins decreases, ovulation and menstruation become less frequent and eventually stop. Fluctuations in the circulating levels of these hormones occur as the levels decline. Hot flashes are the only nearly universal symptom of the menopause. Occasionally, heavy irregular bleeding occurs at this time, usually associated with myomata (fibroids) or other uterine pathologic condition.

menorrhagia /men'ǝrā'jē·ǝ/ [L *mensis* + *rhegynein* to burst forth], abnormally heavy or long menstrual periods. Menorrhagia occurs occasionally during the reproductive years of most women's lives. If the condition becomes chronic, anemia from recurrent excessive blood loss may result. Abnormal bleeding after menopause always warrants investigation to rule out malignancy. **–menorrhagic,** *adj.*

menorrhea /men'ôrē'ǝ/ [L *mensis* + Gk

rhoia flow], the normal discharge of blood and tissue from the uterus.

menostasis /mənos′tasis/ [L *mensis* + Gk *stasis* stand still], an abnormal condition in which the products of menstruation cannot escape the uterus or vagina because of stenosis, an occlusion of the cervix, or the introitus of the vagina. An imperforate hymen is a rare cause of menostasis. –**menostatic,** *adj.*

menotropins /men′ōtrop′inz/ [L *mensis* + Gk *trepein* to turn], a preparation of gonadotropic hormones from the urine of postmenopausal women. It is prescribed with chorionic gonadotropin to induce ovulation.

menoxenia /men′okse′nē·ə/ [L *mensis* + Gk *xenos* strange], any abnormality relating to menstruation.

menses /men′sēz/ [L *mensis* month], the normal flow of blood and decidua that occurs during menstruation. The first day of the flow of the menses is the first day of the menstrual cycle.

menstrual age /men′strōo·əl/ [L *menstrualis* monthly; *aetas* lifetime], the age of an embryo or fetus as calculated from the first day of the last menstrual period.

menstrual colic, a form of dysmenorrhea characterized by abdominal pain during or just before menstruation.

menstrual cramps, low abdominal pain that may range from a colicky feeling to a constant dull ache. The pain may radiate to the lower back and legs. Menstrual cramps are often associated with the beginning of menses.

menstrual cycle, the recurring cycle of change in the endometrium during which the decidual layer of the endometrium is shed, then regrows, proliferates, is maintained for several days, and sheds again at menstruation. The average length of the cycle, from the first day of bleeding of one cycle to the first of another, is 28 days. The duration and character vary greatly among women. Menstrual cycles begin at menarche and end with menopause. The three phases of the cycle are the **proliferative phase, secretory phase,** and **menstrual phase.**

menstrual period [L *menstrualis* monthly; Gk *peri, hodos* way], the periodic discharge of blood and cellular debris from the uterus.

menstrual phase, the final of the three phases of the menstrual cycle in which menstruation occurs. The necrotic mucosa of the endometrium is shed, leaving the stratum basale; bleeding, primarily from the spiral arteries, occurs. The average blood loss is 30 ml. For convenience, the days of the menstrual cycle are counted from the first day of the menstrual phase.

menstrual sponge, a small natural sponge or a piece of a sponge of synthetic material to which a loop of string is attached. It is inserted in the vagina to absorb the menstrual flow and is removed by pulling the string. It may be washed, squeezed dry, and reused as necessary through menstruation.

menstruation /men′strōo·ā′shən/ [L *menstruare* to menstruate], the periodic discharge through the vagina of a bloody secretion containing tissue debris from the shedding of the endometrium from the nonpregnant uterus. The average duration of menstruation is 4 to 5 days, and it recurs at approximately 4-week intervals throughout the reproductive life of nonpregnant women. Kinds of menstruation are **anovular, retrograde,** and **vicarious menstruation. –menstrual,** *adj.,* **menstruate,** *v.*

mental[1] [L *mens* mind], **1.** of, relating to, or characteristic of the mind or psyche. **2.** existing in the mind; performed or accomplished by the mind. **3.** of, relating to, or characterized by a disorder of the mind.

mental[2] [L *mentum* chin], of or pertaining to the chin.

mental age (MA), the age level at which one functions intellectually, as determined by standardized psychologic and intelligence tests and expressed as the age at which that level is average.

mental deficiency. See **mental retardation.**

mental disorder, any disturbance of emotional equilibrium, as manifested in maladaptive behavior and impaired functioning, caused by genetic, physical, chemical, biologic, psychologic, or social and cultural factors.

mental handicap, any mental defect or characteristic resulting from a congenital abnormality, traumatic injury, or disease that impairs normal intellectual functioning and prevents a person from participating normally in activities appropriate for a particular age group.

mental health, a relative state of mind in which a person who is healthy is able to cope with and adjust to the recurrent stresses of everyday living in an acceptable way.

Mental Health Association (MHA), a voluntary, nonprofessional agency dedicated to the improvement of mental health facilities and services in community clinics and hospitals, the recruitment and training of volunteers, and the promotion of mental health legislation. Formerly

M

called the **National Association for Mental Health.**

mental health consultation, any interaction between two or more health care professionals regarding a problem in psychotherapy.

mental health nursing. See **psychiatric nursing.**

mental health service, any one of a group of government, professional, or lay organizations operating at a community, state, national, or international level to aid in the prevention and treatment of mental disorders.

mental hygiene, the study of development of healthy mental and emotional habits, attitudes, and behavior and with the prevention of mental illness.

mental illness. See **mental disorder.**

mental image, any concept or sensation produced in the mind through memory or imagination.

mentality [L *mens* mind], **1.** the functional power and the capacity of the mind. **2.** intellectual character.

mental retardation, a disorder characterized by subaverage general intellectual function with deficits or impairments in the ability to learn and to adapt socially. The cause may be genetic, biologic, psychosocial, or sociocultural.

mental ridge [L *mentum* chin; AS *hrycg*], (in dentistry) a dense elevation that extends from the symphysis to the premolar area on the anterolateral aspect of the body of the mandible.

mental status, the degree of competence shown by a person in intellectual, emotional, psychologic, and personality functioning as measured by psychologic testing with reference to a statistical norm.

mental status examination, a diagnostic procedure for determining the mental status of a person. The trained interviewer poses certain questions in a carefully standardized manner and evaluates the verbal responses and behavioral reactions.

mentation /mentā′shən/ [L *mens* mind, *atus* process], any mental activity, including conscious and unconscious processes.

menthol /men′thol/ [L *mentha* mint], a topical antipruritic with a cooling effect that relieves itching. It is an ingredient in many topical creams and ointments.

mentholated camphor, a mixture of equal parts of camphor and menthol, used as a local counterirritant.

menton /men′ton/ [L *mentum* chin], the most inferior point on the chin in the lateral view. It is a cephalometric landmark.

mentor /men′tər/ [Gk *Mentor* mythic educator], an older, trusted adviser or counselor who offers helpful guidance to younger colleagues.

mentum /men′təm/ [L, chin], **1.** the chin, especially of the fetus. **2.** a fetal reference point in designating the position of the fetus with respect to the maternal pelvis, as left mentum anterior (LMA) indicates the fetal chin is presenting in the left anterior quadrant of the pelvis.

mep, abbreviation for *mean effective pressure.*

mepenzolate bromide /mepen′zəlāt/, an anticholinergic agent prescribed in the treatment of GI hypermotility and as an adjunct in treating peptic ulcer.

meperidine hydrochloride /meper′idēn/, a narcotic analgesic used to treat moderate to severe pain and as preoperative medication to relieve pain and allay anxiety.

mephenesin /mefen′isin/, a curare-like skeletal muscle relaxant sometimes prescribed in the relief of muscle spasm.

mephenytoin /mefen′ətō′in/, an anticonvulsant prescribed for the control of seizures in epilepsy when less toxic medications have not been effective.

mephobarbital /mef′ōbär′bitol/, an anticonvulsant and sedative prescribed in the treatment of anxiety, nervous tension, insomnia, and epilepsy.

meprednisone /mepred′nisōn/, an oral glucocorticoid prescribed in the treatment of a large number of inflammatory conditions.

meprobamate /meprō′bəmāt/, a sedative prescribed in the treatment of anxiety and tension and as a muscle relaxant.

mEq, abbreviation for **milliequivalent.**

mEq/L, abbreviation for **milliequivalent per liter.**

meralgia /miral′jə/ [Gk *meros* thigh, *algos* pain], the presence of pain in the thigh.

meralgia paresthetica /per′esthet′ikə/, a condition characterized by pain, paresthesia, and numbness on the lateral surface of the thigh in the region supplied by the lateral femoral cutaneous nerve. The cause of the condition is ischemia of the nerve caused by its entrapped position in the inguinal ligament.

mercaptopurine /mərkap′təpy$\overline{oo}$′rēn/, an antineoplastic and immunosuppressive prescribed in the treatment of a variety of malignant neoplastic diseases, including acute lymphocytic leukemia.

mercurial /mərky$\overline{oo}$r′ē-əl/, **1.** of or pertaining to mercury, particularly a medicine containing the element mercury. **2.** an adverse effect associated with the administration of a mercurial medication, such as a mercurial tremor caused by mercury poisoning.

mercurial diuretic, any one of several diuretic agents that contain mercury in an organic chemical form. Mercurial diuretics inhibit tubular reabsorption of sodium and chloride and the excretion of potassium but do not produce diuresis in patients who are in metabolic alkalosis. The principal use for the drugs is in treating edema of cardiac origin, ascites associated with cirrhosis, or oliguria in the nephrotic stage of glomerulonephritis.

mercurialism. See **mercury poisoning.**

mercury (Hg) /mur′kyərē/ [L *Mercurius* mythic messenger of the gods], a metallic element. Its atomic number is 80; its atomic weight is 200.6. It is the only common metal that is liquid at room temperature, and it occurs in nature almost entirely in the form of its sulfide, cinnabar. Mercury is produced commercially and is used in dental amalgams, thermometers, barometers, and other measuring instruments. It forms many poisonous compounds. Elemental mercury is only mildly toxic when ingested, because it is poorly absorbed. The vapor of elemental mercury, however, is readily absorbed through the lungs and enters the brain before it is oxidized. The kidneys retain mercury longer than any of the other body tissues.

mercury poisoning, a toxic condition caused by the ingestion or inhalation of mercury or a mercury compound. The chronic form, resulting from inhalation of the vapors or dust of mercurial compounds or from repeated ingestion of very small amounts, is characterized by irritability, excessive saliva, loosened teeth, gum disorders, slurred speech, tremors, and staggering. Symptoms of acute mercury poisoning appear in a few to 30 minutes and include a metallic taste in the mouth, thirst, nausea, vomiting, severe abdominal pain, bloody diarrhea, and renal failure that may result in death.

mercury thermometer, a thermometer in which the expandable indicator is mercury.

mercy killing. See **euthanasia.**

merergasia /mer′ərgā′zhə/ [Gk *meros* part, *ergein* to work], a mild mental incapacity characterized by some emotional instability and some anxiety. –**merergastic,** *adj.*

merethoxylline procaine /mer′əthok′-silēn/, a diuretic.

merisis /mer′isis/ [Gk *merizein* to divide into parts], an increase in size as a result of cell division and the addition of new material rather than of cell expansion.

meroblastic /mer′əblas′tik/ [Gk *meros* + *blastos* germ], pertaining to or characterizing an ovum that contains a large amount of yolk and in which cleavage is restricted to a part of the cytoplasm.

merocrine secretion /mer′əkrin/ [Gk *meros* + *krinein* to separate; L *secernere* to separate], a secretion in which the secreting cell remains intact while producing and releasing a secretory product.

meromelia /mer′əmē′lyə/ [Gk *meros* + *melos* limb], a general designation for the congenital absence of any part of a limb. It is used in reference to such conditions as adactyly, hemimelia, or phocomelia.

merozoite /mer′əzō′īt/ [Gk *meros* + *zoon* animal], an organism produced from segmentation of a schizont during the asexual reproductive phase of the life cycle of a sporozoan, specifically the malarial parasite *Plasmodium.*

merozygote /mer′əzī′gōt/, an incomplete zygote that contains only part of the genetic material of one of the parents. It occurs in bacterial genetics.

Merrifield's knife, a surgical knife with a long, narrow, triangular blade set into a shank, used for gingivectomy incisions.

mesangial IgA nephropathy. See **Berger's disease.**

mesangium /mesan′jē·əm/, a cellular network in the renal glomerulus that helps support the capillary loops.

mescaline /mes′kəlēn, -lin/ [Mex *mezcal*], a psychoactive, poisonous alkaloid derived from a colorless alkaline oil in the flowering heads of the cactus *Lophophora williamsii.* Closely related chemically to epinephrine, mescaline causes heart palpitations, diaphoresis, pupillary dilation, and anxiety. The drug, taken in capsules or dissolved in a drink, produces visual hallucinations.

mescalism /mes′kəliz′əm/ [Mex *mezcal*], a type of chemical dependence on the effects of mescal, an intoxicant spirit obtained from a species of cactus.

mesencephalon /mes′ensef′əlon/ [Gk *mesos* middle, *enkephalos* brain], one of the three parts of the brainstem, lying just below the cerebrum and just above the pons. It consists primarily of white substance with some gray substance around the cerebral aqueduct. A red nucleus lies within the reticular formation of the mesencephalon and contains the terminations of fibers from the cerebellum and the frontal lobe of the cerebral cortex. Deep within the mesencephalon are nuclei of the third and the fourth cranial nerves and the anterior part of the fifth cranial nerve. The mesencephalon also contains nuclei for certain auditory and certain visual reflexes. –**mesencephalic** /mes′ensifal′ik/, *adj.*

mesenchymal chondrosarcoma /meseng'-kəməl/ [Gk *mesos* middle, *enchyma* infusion; *chondros* cartilage, *sarx* flesh, *oma* tumor], a malignant cartilaginous tumor that develops in many sites.

mesenchyme /mes'engkīm/ [Gk *mesos* + *enchyma* infusion], a diffuse network of tissue derived from the embryonic mesoderm. It consists of stellate cells embedded in gelatinous ground substance with reticular fibers.

mesenchymoma /mes'engkimō'mə/ [Gk *mesos* + *enchyma* infusion, ioma tumor], a mixed mesenchymal neoplasm composed of two or more cellular elements not usually associated and fibrous tissue.

mesenteric adenitis. See **adenitis.**

mesenteric node /mes'enter'ik/ [Gk *mesos* + *enteron* intestine; L *nodus* knot], a node in one of three groups of superior mesenteric lymph glands serving parts of the intestine.

mesentery proper /mez'ənter'ē/ [Gk *mesos* + *enteron* intestine; L *propius* more suitable], a broad, fan-shaped fold of peritoneum connecting the jejunum and the ileum with the dorsal wall of the abdomen. The root of the mesentery proper is connected to certain structures ventral to the vertebral column. The intestinal border of the mesentery proper separates to enclose the intestine. The cranial part of the mesentery suspends the small intestine and various nerves and arteries. **—mesenteric,** *adj.*

MESH, an acronym derived from *Medical Subject Headings,* the list of medical terms used by the U.S. National Library of Medicine (NLM) for its computerized system of storage and retrieval of published medical reports.

mesial. See **medial.**

mesiobuccoocclusal /mē'zē-obuk'ō-oklōō'zə/ [Gk *mesos* middle; L *bucca* cheek; L *occludere* to close up], pertaining to the angle formed by the mesial, buccal, and occlusal surfaces of a tooth.

mesiocclusion /mē'zē-oklōō'zhən/ [Gk *mesos* + L *occludere* to close up], an occlusal relationship in which the lower teeth are positioned mesially.

mesiodens /mē'zē-adenz'/ [Gk *mesos* + L *dens* tooth], a supernumerary erupted or unerupted tooth that develops between two maxillary central incisors.

mesiolinguoocclusal /mē'sē-oling'gwō-oklōō'zəl/ [Gk *mesos* + *ligua* tongue; L *occludere* to close up], pertaining to the angle formed by the mesial, lingual, and occlusal surfaces of a tooth.

mesioversion /mē'zē-ōvur'zhən/ [Gk *mesos* + L *vertere* to turn], **1.** a condition in which one or more teeth are closer than normal to the midline. **2.** a condition in which the maxillae or mandible is positioned more anteriorly than normal.

mesmerism /mez'məriz'əm/ [Franz Anton Mesmer, Austrian physician, b. 1734], a practice of hypnotism introduced by Mesmer, who believed health was affected by "celestial magnetic forces." Some patients were reported cured or experienced diminished symptoms by undergoing a "grand crisis," or seizure, while under hypnosis. Mesmer was regarded as a fraud by the medical profession but his work led to serious studies of the health effects of the power of suggestion.

mesocolic node /mes'ōkol'ik/ [Gk *mesos* + *kolon* colon; L *nodus* knot], a node in one of three groups of superior mesenteric lymph glands, proliferating between the layers of the transverse mesocolon, close to the transverse colon.

mesocolopexy /mes'ōkō'ləpek'sē/ [Gk *mesos* + *kolon* colon, *pexis* fixation], suspension or fixation of the mesocolon.

mesoderm /mes'ōdurm/ [Gk *mesos* + *derma* skin], (in embryology) the middle of the three cell layers of the developing embryo. It lies between the ectoderm and the endoderm. Bone, connective tissue, muscle, blood, vascular and lymphatic tissue, and the pleurae of the pericardium and peritoneum are all derived from the mesoderm.

mesoduodenum /mez'ōdōō'ədē'nəm/ [Gk *mesos* + L *duodeni* 12 fingers], a fold of tissue that joins the duodenum to the wall of the abdomen of the fetus. The membrane sometimes persists in later life as the **duodenal mesentery.**

mesogastric /mez'ōgas'trik/ [Gk *mesos* + *gaster* belly], pertaining to the **mesogastrium,** a mesentery of the embryonic stomach.

mesoglia. See **microglia.**

mesomere /mez'əmir/ [Gk *mesos* + *meros* part], a row of mesodermal cells between the mesothelium and epimere of the embryo. It develops into the renal tubules.

mesometritis. See **myometritis.**

mesomorph /mes'əmôrf'/ [Gk *mesos* + *morphe* form], a person whose physique is characterized by a predominance of muscle, bone, and connective tissue, structures that develop from the mesodermal layer of the embryo.

mesonephric duct /mez'ōnef'rik/ [Gk *mesos* + *nephros* kidney; L *ducere* to lead], (in embryology) a duct that, in the male, gives rise to the ducts of the reproductive system (ductus epididymidis, ductus deferens, seminal vesicle, ejaculatory duct). In the female, it persists vestigially as **Gartner's duct.**

mesonephric tubule, any of the embryonic renal tubules comprising the mesonephros. They function as excretory structures during the early embryonic development of humans and other mammals but are later incorporated into the reproductive system. In males the tubules give rise to the efferent and aberrant ductules of the testes, the appendix epididymis, and paradidymis, and in females to the epoophoron, paroophoron, and vesicular appendices. All of the structures are vestigial except the efferent ductules of the testes.

mesonephros /mez'ōnef'rəs/, *pl.* **mesonephroi, mesonephra** [Gk *mesos* + *nephros* kidney], the second type of excretory organ to develop in the vertebrate embryo. It consists of a series of twisting tubules that arise from the nephrogenic cord caudal to the pronephros and that at one end form the glomerulus and at the other connect with the excretory mesonephric duct. –**mesonephric, mesonephroid,** *adj.*

mesoridazine /mez'ərid'əzēn/, a phenothiazine tranquilizer prescribed in the treatment of psychotic disorders, behavioral problems in mental deficiency, and alcoholism.

mesosalpinx /mes'ōsal'pingks/ [Gk *mesos* + *salpinx* tube], the cephalic, free border of the broad ligament in which the uterine tubes lie.

mesothelioma /mes'ōthē'lē·ō'mə/, *pl.* **mesotheliomas, mesotheliomata** [Gk *mesos* + *epi* above, *thele* nipple, *oma* tumor], a rare, malignant tumor of the mesothelium of the pleura or peritoneum, associated with earlier exposure to asbestos.

mesothelium /mes'ōthē'lē·əm/ [Gk *mesos* + *epi* above, *thele* nipple], a layer of cells that lines the body cavities of the embryo and continues as a layer of squamous epithelial cells covering the serous membranes of the adult.

messenger RNA (mRNA) [ME *messangere* message bearer; *RNA* ribonucleic acid], (in molecular genetics) an RNA fraction that transmits information from DNA to the protein-synthesizing ribosomes of cells.

mestranol /mes'trənōl/, an estrogen prescribed in fixed-combination drugs with a progestin as an oral contraceptive.

Met, abbreviation for the amino acid **methionine.**

MET, abbreviation for **metabolic equivalent.**

metabolic /met'əbol'ik/ [Gk *metabole* change], of or pertaining to **metabolism.**

metabolic acidosis, acidosis in which excess acid is added to the body fluids or bicarbonate is lost from them. In starvation and in uncontrolled diabetes mellitus glucose is not present or is not available for oxidation for cellular nutrition. The plasma bicarbonate of the body is used up in neutralizing the ketones that result from the breakdown of body fat for energy that occurs in compensation for the lack of glucose. Metabolic acidosis also occurs when oxidation takes place without adequate oxygen, as in heart failure or shock. Severe diarrhea, renal failure, and lactic acidosis also may result in metabolic acidosis. Hyperkalemia often accompanies the condition.

metabolic alkalosis, an abnormal condition characterized by the significant loss of acid in the body or by increased levels of base bicarbonate. The reduction of acid may be caused by excessive vomiting, insufficient replacement of electrolytes, hyperadrenocorticism, and Cushing's disease. A decrease in base bicarbonate may be caused by various problems, such as the ingestion of excessive bicarbonate of soda and other antacids during the treatment of peptic ulcers, and by the administration of excessive intravenous fluids containing high concentrations of bicarbonate. Severe, untreated metabolic alkalosis can lead to coma and death. Signs and symptoms of metabolic alkalosis may include apnea, headache, lethargy, irritability, nausea, vomiting, and atrial tachycardia.

metabolic balance [Gk *metabole* change; L *bilanx* two scales], an equilibrium between the intake of nutrients and their eventual loss through absorption or excretion. If the intake of a nutrient exceeds its loss, it is called a positive balance while a negative balance indicates that a nutrient is utilized or excreted faster than it is consumed in the diet.

metabolic component, the bicarbonate component of plasma.

metabolic disorder, any pathophysiologic dysfunction that results in a loss of metabolic control of homeostasis in the body.

metabolic equivalent (MET), a unit of measurement of heat production by the body. One MET is equal to 50 kilogram calories (kcal) per hour per square meter of body surface of a resting individual.

metabolic rate, the amount of energy liberated or expended in a given unit of time. Energy is stored in the body in energy-rich phosphate compounds (adenosine triphosphate, adenosine monophosphate, and adenosine diphosphate) and in proteins, fats, and complex carbohydrates.

metabolic respiratory quotient (R), the ratio of production of CO_2 to the corresponding consumption of O_2. The values of R change according to the fuel being

M

burned; the R of fat is lower than that of glucose, whereas the R of protein is between that of glucose and fat.

metabolic waste products [Gk *metabole;* L *vastere* to destroy, *producere* to produce], the products of metabolic activity after oxygen and nutrients have been supplied to a cell. These include mainly water and carbon dioxide, along with sodium chloride, and soluble nitrogenous salts, which are excreted in urine, feces, and exhaled air.

metabolism /mɔtab'ɔliz'ɔm/ [Gk *metabole* change, *ismos* process], the aggregate of all chemical processes that take place in living organisms, resulting in growth, generation of energy, elimination of wastes, and other bodily functions as they relate to the distribution of nutrients in the blood after digestion. Metabolism takes place in two steps: anabolism, the constructive phase, in which smaller molecules (such as amino acids) are converted to larger molecules (such as proteins); and catabolism, the destructive phase, in which larger molecules (such as glycogen) are converted to smaller molecules (such as pyruvic acid). The metabolic rate is customarily expressed (in calories) as the heat liberated in the course of metabolism. **–metabolize,** *v.*

metabolite /mɔtab'ɔlīt/ [Gk *metabole* change], a substance produced by metabolic action or necessary for a metabolic process. An essential metabolite is one required for a vital metabolic process.

metacarpal phalanx /mɔtakär'pɔl/ [Gk *meta* beyond, *karpos* wrist, *phalagx* line of soldiers], pertaining to the hands and fingers, particularly phalanges that articulate with carpal bones.

metacarpophalangeal /mɔtakär'pōfɔlan'-jē·ɔl/, pertaining to the metacarpal bones of the hand and the phalanges of fingers, as in metacarpalphalangeal joints.

metacarpophalangeal joint dislocation [Gk *meta* + *karpos* + *phalagx;* L *jungere* to join; *dis, locare* to place], the dislocation of a finger, usually with damage to tendons and other structures.

metacarpus /met'ɔkär'pɔs/ [Gk *meta* beyond, *karpos* wrist], the middle portion of the hand, consisting of five slender bones numbered from the thumb side, metacarpals I through V. Each metacarpal consists of a body and two extremities. **–metacarpal,** *adj., n.*

metacentric /met'ɔsen'trik/ [Gk *meta* + *kentron* center], pertaining to a chromosome in which the centromere is located near the center so that the arms of the chromatids are of approximately equal length.

metachromasia /mɔtakrōmā'zhē·ɔ/ [Gk *meta* + *chroma* color], a tissue staining phenomenon in which cells being examined acquire a color other than that of the dye used. Cartilage cells, for example, may appear red after being stained with a blue dye. The cause is an interaction between the dye molecules and the acidic radicals of the tissue cells.

metachromatic lipids /mɔtakrōmat'ik/ [Gk *meta* + *chroma;* *lipos* fat], lipid molecules that accumulate in the central nervous system, peripheral nerves, and internal organs of infants who inherit a lipidosis disorder.

metachromatic stain [Gk *meta* + *chroma;* OFr *desteindre* to dye], a basic dye, such as toluidine, that can stain substances a different color than that of the stain.

metachromism, See **meta chromasia.**

metacommunication /mɔtakɔnyōō'-nikā'shɔn/ [Gk *meta* + L *communicare* to inform], communication that indicates how verbal communication should be interpreted. It may support or contradict verbal communication.

metagenesis /met'ɔjen'ɔsis/ [Gk *meta* + *genein* to produce], the regular alternation of sexual with asexual methods of reproduction within the same species. **–metagenetic, metagenic,** *adj.*

metal [Gk *metallon* a mine], any element that conducts heat and electricity, is malleable and ductile, and forms positively charged ions (cations) in solution.

metal fume fever, an occupational disorder caused by the inhalation of fumes of metallic oxides and characterized by symptoms similar to those of influenza.

metallesthesia /met'ɔlesthē'zhɔ/ [Gk *metallon* mine; *aisthesia* perception], an ability to identify a metal through the sense of touch.

metallurgy [Gk *metallon* + *ergein* to work], the theoretical and applied sciences of the nature and uses of metals.

metamorphopsia /met'ɔmôrfop'sē·ɔ/ [Gk *meta* + *morphe* form, *opsis* sight], a defect in vision in which objects are seen as distorted in shape, resulting from disease of the retina or imperfection of the media.

metamorphosis /met'ɔmôr'fɔsis/ [Gk *meta* + *morphe* form], a change in shape or structure, especially a change from one stage of development to another, such as the transition from the larval to the adult stage.

metamyelocyte /met'ɔmī'ɔlōsīt'/ [Gk *meta* + *myelos* marrow, *kytos* cell], a stage in the development of the granulocyte series of leukocytes. It is intermediate between the myelocyte stage and the mature granulocyte.

metanephrine /met'ənef'rin/, one of the two principal urinary metabolites of epinephrine and norepinephrine in the urine, the other being vanillylmandelic acid.

metanephrogenic /met'ənef'rəjen'ik/ [Gk *meta* + *nephros* kidney, *genein* to produce], capable of forming the metanephros, or fetal kidney.

metanephros /met'ənef'rəs/, *pl.* **metanephroi, metanephra** [Gk *meta* + *nephros* kidney], the third, and permanent, excretory organ to develop in the vertebrate embryo. It consists of a complex structure of secretory and collecting tubules that develop into the kidney.

metaphase /met'əfāz/ [Gk *meta* + *phasis* appearance], the second of the four stages of nuclear division in mitosis and in each of the two divisions of meiosis, during which the chromosomes become arranged in the equatorial plane of the spindle to form the equatorial plate, with the centromeres attached to the spindle fibers in preparation for separation.

metaphyseal dysostosis /mətaf'izē'əl, met'əfiz'ē-əl/ [Gk *meta* + *phyein* to grow; *dys* bad, *osteon* bone], an abnormal condition that affects the skeletal system and is characterized by a disturbance of the mineralization of the metaphyseal area of the bones, resulting in dwarfism. Metaphyseal dysostosis is classified as the Gansen type, Schmidt type, Spahar-Hartmann type, or cartilage-hair hypoplasia. The Gansen type is characterized by metaphyseal alterations similar to those of achondroplasia but not involving the skull or the epiphyses of the long bones. The Schmidt type of metaphyseal dysostosis is characterized by developmental changes from the weight-bearing age to approximately 5 years of age. The Spahar-Hartmann type is characterized by skeletal changes and severe genu varum. Cartilage-hair hypoplasia is characterized by severe dwarfism and hair that is sparse, short, and brittle.

metaphyseal dysplasia, an abnormal condition characterized by disordered modeling of the long cylindric bones.

metaphysis /mətaf'əsis/ [Gk *meta* + *phyein* to grow], a region of bone in which diaphysis and epiphysis converge.

metaplasia /met'əplā'zhə/, the conversion of normal tissue cells into an abnormal form in response to chronic stress or injury.

metaproterenol sulfate /met'əprōter'inôl/, a beta-adrenergic bronchodilator prescribed in the treatment of bronchial asthma.

metaraminol bitartrate /met'äram'inol/, an adrenergic vasopressor prescribed in the treatment of hypotension and shock.

metarubricyte [Gk *meta* + L *ruber* red, *kytos* cell], a red blood cell possessing a nucleus. Such cells, usually normoblasts in their final stage, are not normally found in the blood of adults.

metastable solution. See **supersaturate solution.**

metastasis /mətas'təsis/, *pl.* **metastases** /-sēz/ [Gk *meta* + *stasis* standing], **1.** the process by which tumor cells are spread to distant parts of the body. Because malignant tumors have no enclosing capsule, cells may escape and be transported by the lymphatic circulation or the bloodstream to other organs far from the primary tumor. **2.** a tumor that develops in this way. **–metastatic,** *adj.,* **metastasize,** *v.*

metastasizing mole. See **chorioadenoma destruens.**

metastatic abscess /met'astat'ik/ [Gk *meta* + *stasis* standing; L *abscedere* to go away], any secondary abscess that develops at a point distant from an original infection, the infectious particles being transported to other locations in the bloodstream.

metastatic calcification [Gk *meta* + *stasis;* L *calx* lime, *facere* to make], the pathologic process whereby calcium salts accumulate in previously healthy tissues.

metastatic endometriosis [Gk *meta* + *stasis; endon* within, *metra* womb, *osis* condition], extraperitoneal lesions that resemble metastases from a carcinoma.

metastatic ophthalmia. See **sympathetic ophthalmia.**

metastatic survey [Gk *meta* + *stasis;* OFr *surveoir* to examine], a method of monitoring the spread of a cancer by taking a periodic series of x-ray films.

metatarsal /met'ətär'səl/ [Gk *meta* + *tarsos* plate], **1.** of or pertaining to the metatarsus of the foot. **2.** any one of the five bones comprising the metatarsus.

metatarsalgia /met'ətärsal'jə/ [Gk *meta, tarsos* + *algos* pain], a painful condition around the metatarsal bones caused by an abnormality of the foot or recalcification of degenerated heads of metatarsal bones.

metatarsal phalanx [Gk *meta* + *tarsos* sole of foot, *phalanx* line of soldiers], pertaining to the bones of the foot and toes.

metatarsal stress fracture, a break or rupture of a metatarsal bone, resulting from prolonged running or walking. The condition is often difficult to diagnose with x-ray films.

metatarsus /met'ətär'səs/ [Gk *meta* + *tarsos* plate], a part of the foot, consisting of five bones numbered I to V, from the medial side. Each bone has a long, slen-

M

der body, a wedge-shaped proximal end, a convex distal end, and flattened, grooved sides for the attachment of ligaments. Kinds of metatarsus include **metatarsus valgus** and **metatarsus varus.** **–metatarsal,** adj.

metatarsus adductus. See **metatarsus varus.**

metatarsus valgus, a congenital deformity of the foot in which the forepart rotates outward away from the midline of the body and the heel remains straight.

metatarsus varus, a congenital deformity of the foot in which the forepart rotates inward toward the midline of the body and the heel remains straight.

metathalamus /met´əthal´əməs/ [Gk meta + thalamos chamber], one of five parts of the diencephalon. It is composed of a medial geniculate body and a lateral geniculate body on each side. The medial geniculate body acts as a relay station for nerve impulses between the inferior brachium and the auditory cortex. The lateral geniculate body accommodates the terminal ends of the fibers of the optic tract. **–metathalamic,** adj.

metaxalone /metak´səlōu/, a skeletal muscle relaxant prescribed as an adjunct in the treatment of acute skeletal muscle spasm.

metazoa /metazō´ə/ [Gk meta + zoon animal], a category of multicellular animals whose cells have become differentiated into tissues and organs, particularly those possessing a digestive tract.

Metchnikoff's theory /mech´nikofs/ [Elie Metchnikoff, Russian-French biologist, b. 1845; Gk theoria speculation], a theory that living cells ingest microorganisms, as seen in the process of phagocytosis and the ingestion of injurious microbes by leukocytes.

meteorism [Gk meteorizein to hold up], accumulation of gas in the abdomen or the intestine, usually with distention.

meteorotropism /mē´tē·ərətrō´pizəm/ [Gk meteors high in the air, trope turning], a reaction to meteorologic influences shown by various biological occurrences, such as sudden death, attacks of arthritis, and angina. **–meteorotropic,** adj.

meter (m) /mē´tər/ [Gk metron measure], a metric unit of length equal to 39.37 inches.

metered dose inhaler, a device designed to deliver a measured dose of an inhalation drug. It consists usually of a canister of aerosol spray, mist, or fine powder that releases a specific dose each time the canister is pushed against a dispensing valve. It is intended to reduce the risk of overmedication by the person.

methacholine challenge /meth´əkō´lēn/, a method of measuring airway activity by an inhalation challenge test. It consists of inhaling a saline aerosol as a control, followed by increasing concentrations of methacholine chloride, a cholinergic drug. It is used to confirm the diagnosis of asthma when symptoms are present.

methacycline hydrochloride /meth´əsī´klēn/, a tetracycline antibiotic prescribed in the treatment of a variety of infections.

methadone /meth´ədōn/, a synthetic narcotic analgesic prescribed for relief of severe pain, for treatment in detoxification, and in treatment programs for opiate-addicted patients.

methadone hydrochloride, a narcotic analgesic used for anesthesia or as a substitute for heroin, permitting withdrawal without development of acute abstinence syndrome. Methadone does not produce marked euphoria, sedation, or narcosis. It is not given to pregnant women or to patients with liver disease.

methamphetamine hydrochloride /meth´amfet´əmēn/, a central nervous system stimulant prescribed in the treatment of narcolepsy and hyperkinesis and to reduce the appetite in exogenous obesity.

methandriol /methan´drē·ol/, an anabolic hormone used as adjunctive therapy in senile and postmenopausal osteoporosis.

methanol /meth´ənol/, a clear, colorless, toxic, liquid distillate of wood miscible with water, alcohol, and ether. It is widely used as a solvent and in the production of formaldehyde. Ingestion of methanol paralyzes the optic nerve and may cause death.

methanol extractable residue, an immunotherapeutic substance, prepared from a methanol extracted fraction of the bacillus Calmette-Guérin (BCG).

methaqualone /methak´wəlōn/, a sedative-hypnotic prescribed in the treatment of anxiety and insomnia.

metharbital /methär´bitəl/, an anticonvulsant prescribed in the treatment of epilepsy.

methazolamide /meth´əzō´ləmīd/, a carbonic anhydrase inhibitor prescribed in the treatment of glaucoma.

methdilazine /methdil´əzēn/, a phenothiazine antihistamine prescribed to relieve itching.

methemoglobin /met´hēməglō´bin/, a form of hemoglobin in which the iron component has been oxidized from the ferrous to the ferric state. Methemoglobin cannot carry oxygen and so contributes nothing to the oxygen transporting capacity of the blood.

methemoglobinemia, the presence of methemoglobin in the blood.

methemoglobinuria, the presence of methemoglobin in the urine.

methenamine /methē′nəmēn/, a urinary antibacterial prescribed in the treatment of urinary tract infections.

methionine (Met) /methī′ənēn/, an essential amino acid needed for proper growth in infants and for maintenance of nitrogen balance in adults. It is a source for methyl groups and sulfur in the body.

methocarbamol /meth′əkär′bəmol/, a skeletal muscle relaxant prescribed in the treatment of skeletal muscle spasm.

method [Gk *meta* beyond, *hodos* way], a technique or procedure for producing a desired effect, such as a surgical procedure, a laboratory test, or a diagnostic technique.

methodology [Gk *meta, hodos + logos* science], **1.** a system of principles or methods of procedure in any discipline, as education, research, diagnosis, or treatment. **2.** the section of a research proposal in which the methods to be used are described. **–methodologic,** *adj.*

methohexital sodium /meth′ōhek′sitōl/, an intravenous barbiturate prescribed for the induction of anesthesia in short surgical procedures as a supplement to other anesthetics.

methotrexate /meth′ōtrek′sāt/, an antineoplastic antimetabolite prescribed in the treatment of severe psoriasis and a variety of malignant neoplastic diseases.

methoxamine hydrochloride /methok′-səmēn/, an adrenergic that acts as a vasoconstrictor prescribed for use during anesthesia to maintain blood pressure and in the treatment of paroxysmal supraventricular tachycardia.

methoxsalen /methok′sələn/, a pigmentation agent used topically to enhance pigmentation or for repigmentation in vitiligo.

3-methoxy-4-hydroxymandelic acid /methok′sē, hīdrok′sēməndel′ik/, a product of metabolism that may be measured in the urine to determine the levels of the catecholamines (adrenaline and noradrenaline). Increased concentrations of this acid may raise the blood pressure, indicate the presence of tumors, muscular dystrophy, or myasthenia gravis.

methscopolamine bromide /meth′skōpō′-ləmēn/, an anticholinergic prescribed in the treatment of hypermotility of the GI tract and as an adjunct in treating peptic ulcer.

methsuximide /methsuk′simīd/, an anticonvulsant prescribed in the treatment of refractory petit mal epilepsy.

methyclothiazide /məthī′klōthī′əzīd/, a diuretic and antihypertensive prescribed in the treatment of hypertension and edema.

methyl (Me), the chemical radical $-CH_3$.

methyl alcohol. See **methanol.**

methylate [Gk *methy* wine; *hyle* matter], to add a methyl group, $-CH_3$, to a chemical compound.

methylation /meth′ilā′shən/ [Gk *methy* wine; *hyle* matter], **1.** the introduction of a methyl group, $-CH_3$, to a chemical compound. **2.** the addition of methyl alcohol and naptha to ethanol to produce denatured alcohol.

methylbenzethonium chloride /meth′-ilben′zəthō′nē-əm/, a topical antiinfective prescribed for the prevention and treatment of diaper rash and other dermatoses.

methyldopa /meth′ildō′pə/, an antihypertensive prescribed for the reduction of high blood pressure.

methylene blue /meth′əlēn/, a bluish green crystalline substance used as a histologic stain and as a laboratory indicator. It is also used in the treatment of cyanide poisoning and methemoglobinemia.

methylergonovine maleate /meth′-ilərgon′əvēn/, a synthetic ergot alkaloid prescribed as an oxytocic to prevent or to treat postpartum uterine atony, hemorrhage, or subinvolution.

methylphenidate hydrochloride /meth′il-fen′idāt/, a central nervous system stimulant prescribed in the treatment of hyperkinesis in children and in the treatment of narcolepsy in adults.

methylprednisolone /meth′ilprednis′əlōn/, a glucocorticoid prescribed in the treatment of inflammatory conditions, including rheumatic fever and rheumatoid arthritis.

methylrosaniline chloride. See **gentian violet.**

methyl salicylate, a nearly colorless volatile oil with an aromatic flavor prepared from the leaves of *Gaultheria procumbens* or the bark of *Betula lenta* (black birch). It is widely used in liniments as a local irritant and rubefacient.

methyltestosterone /meth′iltəstos′tərōn/, an androgen prescribed in the treatment of testosterone deficiency, osteoporosis, and female breast cancer, and to stimulate growth, weight gain, and red blood cell production.

methyprylon /meth′əprī′lon/, a sedative and hypnotic prescribed in the treatment of insomnia.

methysergide maleate /meth′isur′jīd/, a vasoconstrictor prescribed for relief of migraine headache.

metoclopramide hydrochloride /met′-əklō′prəmīd/, a GI stimulant prescribed to stimulate motility and to increase the tone of gastric contractions of the upper GI tract and as an antiemetic.

M

metocurine iodide /met′əkyoo͞o′rēn/, a potent neuromuscular blocking agent. It is given to produce flaccid paralysis as an adjunct to anesthesia, to reduce muscle spasm in tetanus, and to assist controlled ventilation.

metolazone /mətō′ləzōn/, a diuretic and antihypertensive prescribed for the treatment of edema and high blood pressure.

"me-too" drug, *informal;* a drug product that is similar, identical, or closely related to a drug for which a manufacturer has obtained a new drug application. On the assumption that the new drug has been recognized as safe and effective, clinical trials required of the original manufacturer are not required of the new supplier.

metopic /mətō′pik/, of or pertaining to the forehead.

metoprolol tartrate /metop′rəlol/, an antiadrenergic (beta-receptor) prescribed in the treatment of hypertension.

metralgia /mətral′jə/ [Gk *metra* womb, *algos* pain], tenderness or pain in the uterus.

metric, of or pertaining to a system of measurement that uses the meter as a basis.

metric equivalent [Gk *metron* measure; L *aequus* equal, *valare* to be strong], any value in metric units of measurement that equals the same value in English units, such as 2.54 cm equals 1 inch or 1 L equals 1.0567 quarts.

metric system, a decimal system of measurement based on the meter (39.37 inches) as the unit of length, on the gram (15.432 grains) as the unit of weight or mass, and, as a derived unit, on the liter (0.908 U.S. dry quart or 1.0567 U.S. liquid quart) as the unit of volume.

metritis /mətrī′tis/ [Gk *metra* womb, *itis* inflammation], inflammation of the walls of the uterus.

metrocarcinoma /met′rōkär′sinō′mə/ [Gk *metra* + *karkinos* crab; *oma* tumor], a cancer of the uterus.

metrodynia. See **metralgia.**

metronidazole /met′rənī′dəzōl/, an antimicrobial prescribed in the treatment of amebiasis, trichomonas, and certain bacterial infections.

metronoscope /mətron′əskōp/, **1.** a device that exposes a small amount of reading matter to the eyes for brief preset time periods. It is used in testing and to help increase reading speed. **2.** an apparatus that exercises the eyes rhythmically to improve binocular coordination.

metrorrhagia /met′rōrā′jē-ə/ [Gk *metra* womb, *rhyegnynai* to burst forth], uterine bleeding other than that caused by menstruation. It may be caused by uterine lesions and may be a sign of a urogenital malignancy.

metyrapone /metir′əpōn/, a diagnostic test drug. It is used to test hypothalamico-pituitary function.

metyrosine /mətir′əsēn/, an antihypertensive prescribed in the treatment of pheochromocytoma.

Metzenbaum scissors. See **scissors.**

Meuse fever. See **trench fever.**

mev, MeV, abbreviation for *million electron volts,* the equivalent of 3.82×10^{-14} small calories, or 1.6×10^{-6} ergs.

mevalonate kinase /məval′ənāt/, an enzyme in the liver and in yeast that catalyzes the transfer of a phosphate group from adenosine triphosphate to produce adenosine diphosphate and 5-phosphomevalonate.

Mexican typhus [Gk *typhos* fever], a form of epidemic typhus carried by lice in Mexico.

mexiletine hydrochloride /mek′sile′tin/, an oral antiarrhythmic drug prescribed for the treatment of symptomatic ventricular dysrhythmias.

Meynet's node /mānāz′/, any one of the numerous nodules that may develop within the capsules surrounding joints and in tendons affected by rheumatic diseases, especially in children.

mezlocillin sodium /mezlos′ilin/, a semisynthetic penicillin antibiotic prescribed for lower respiratory tract, intraabdominal, urinary tract, gynecologic, and skin infections and bacterial septicemia caused by susceptible strains of multiple microorganisms.

mF, abbreviation for *millifarad.*

MFCC, abbreviation for *Marriage, Family, and Child Counselor.*

mfd, abbreviation for **microfarad.**

MFD, abbreviation for *minimal fatal dose.*

μg (microgram) [Gk *mikros* small, *gramma* letter], a unit of weight equal to one millionth of a gram.

mg, abbreviation for **milligram.**

Mg, symbol for the element **magnesium.**

MH, 1. abbreviation for **malignant hyperthermia. 2.** abbreviation for **mental health.**

MHA, abbreviation for **Mental Health Association.**

MHC, abbreviation for **major histocompatibility complex.**

MHz, abbreviation for **megahertz.**

MI, abbreviation for **myocardial infarction.**

miasma /mī·az′mə/ [Gk *miainein* defilement], an unwholesome, polluted atmosphere or environment, as a marsh or swamp with rotting organic matter.

MIC, abbreviation for **minimal inhibitory concentration.**

micellar chromatography /mīsel′ər/, a method of monitoring minute quantities of drugs in whole body fluids by using micellar or colloidal compounds to keep proteins in solution. The technique eliminates the need to remove proteins that usually interfere with chromatographic analysis of blood serum, urine, or saliva.

Michaelis-Menten kinetics [Leonor Michaelis, American biochemist, b. 1875; Maud R. Menten, Canadian physician, b. 1879], a method of transforming drug plasma levels into a linear relationship using the parameters of drug concentration and a constant, K_m, which is a measure of enzyme-substrate affinity.

miconazole nitrate /mīkon′əzōl/, an antifungal used topically in the treatment of certain fungal infections of the skin and vagina and parenterally to treat systemic fungal infections.

micrencephalia. See **microcephaly.**

micrencephalon /mī′krənsef′əlon/, an abnormally small brain. **–micrencephalic,** adj., n.

microabscess /mī′krō·ab′ses/, a very small abscess.

microaerophile /mī′krō·er′ōfil/ [Gk mikros small, aer air, philein to love], a microorganism that requires free oxygen for growth but at a lower concentration than that contained in the atmosphere. **–microaerophilic,** adj.

microaerotonometer /mī′krō·er′ətonom′ətər/ [Gk mikros + aer air, tonos tension, metron measure], an instrument for measuring the volume of gases in the blood or other fluids.

microaggregate recipient set /mī′krō·ag′rəgāt/ [Gk mikros + L ad to, gregare to collect; recipere to receive; AS settan], a device composed of plastic components for the intravenous delivery of large volumes of stored whole blood or of packed blood cells.

microampere, one millionth of an ampere.

microaneurysm /mī′krō·an′yəriz′əm/ [Gk mikros + aneurysma widening], a microscopic aneurysm characteristic of thrombotic purpura.

microangiopathy /mī′krō·an′jē·op′əthē/ [Gk mikros + aggerion vessel, pathos disease], a disease of the small blood vessels, such as diabetic microangiopathy, in which the basement membrane of capillaries thickens, or thrombotic microangiopathy, in which thrombi form in the arterioles and the capillaries.

microbe /mī′krōb/, a microorganism. **–microbial,** adj.

microbicide /mīkrō′bisīd/, any drug, chemical, or other agent that can kill microorganisms.

microbiology [Gk mikros + bios life, logos science], the branch of biology concerned with the study of microorganisms, including algae, bacteria, viruses, protozoa, fungi, and rickettsiae.

microbiology technologist, a medical technologist who specializes in the identification of bacteria and other microorganisms found in patient tissues and other specimens.

microblast /mī′krōblast′/ [Gk mikros + blastos germ], a very small immature red blood cell.

microbrachia /mī′krōbrā′kē·ə/ [Gk mikros + brachion arm], a developmental defect characterized by abnormal smallness of the arms. **–microbrachius,** n.

microcentrum. See **centrosome.**

microcephaly /mī′krōsef′əlē/ [Gk mikros + kephale head], a congenital anomaly characterized by abnormal smallness of the head in relation to the rest of the body and by underdevelopment of the brain, resulting in some degree of mental retardation. The head is more than two standard deviations below the average circumference size for age, sex, race, and period of gestation. The facial features are generally normal. **–microcephalic, microcephalous,** adj., **microcephalic, microcephalus,** n.

microcheiria /mī′krōkī′rē·ə/ [Gk mikros + cheir hand], a developmental defect characterized by abnormal smallness of the hands. The condition is usually associated with other congenital malformations or with bone and muscle disorders.

microcirculation, the flow of blood throughout the system of smaller vessels of the body, particularly the capillaries.

microcurie (μCi, μc) /mī′krōkyōōr′ē/ [Gk mikros + curie Marie and Pierre Curie], a unit of radiation equal to one millionth (10^{-6}) of a curie.

microcyte /mī′krəsīt/ [Gk mikros + kytos cell], an abnormally small erythrocyte, often occurring in iron deficiency and other anemias.

microcythemia /mī′krōthē′mē·ə/ [Gk mikros + kytos; haima blood], an excessive amount of microcytes in the blood.

microcytic /mī′krōsit′ik/ [Gk mikros + kytos cell], (of a cell) smaller than normal, such as the erythrocytes in microcytic anemia.

microcytic anemia, a hematologic disorder characterized by abnormally small erythrocytes, usually associated with chronic blood loss or a nutritional anemia.

microcytosis /mī′krōsītō′sis/ [Gk mikros, kytos + osis condition], a hematologic condition characterized by erythrocytes that are smaller than normal. Microcytosis and hypochromatosis are usual in iron deficiency anemia. **–microcytic,** *adj.*

microdactyly /mī′krōdak′təlē/ [Gk *mikros* + *dactylos* finger], a developmental defect characterized by abnormal smallness of the fingers and toes. The condition is usually associated with bone and muscle disorders.

microdrepanocytic /mī′krōdrep′ənōsit′ik/ [Gk *mikros* + *drepane* sickle, *kytos* cell], pertaining to a blood disorder marked by the presence of both microcytes and drepanocytes, such as occurs in sickle cell-thalassemia.

microdrip /mī′krōdrip′/, (in intravenous therapy) an apparatus for delivering relatively small, measured amounts of intravenous solutions at specific flow rates. A microdrip is usually used to deliver small volumes of solution over a long time. With a microdrip, 60 drops deliver 1 ml of solution.

microelement. See **micronutrient.**

microencapsulation /mī′krō·enkap′-syəlā′shən/ [Gk *mikros* + *en* in; L *capsula* little box], a laboratory technique used in the bioassay of hormones in which certain antibodies are encapsulated with a perforated membrane. The antibodies cannot escape through the tiny perforations, but hormones that bind with the antibodies may enter the structure to bind with them.

microencephaly /mī′krō·ensef′əlē/ [Gk *mikros* + *egkephalos* brain], a condition of an infant born with an abnormally small brain.

microfarad (mfd) /mī′krōfer′əd/ [Gk *mikros* + *farad* Michael Faraday], a unit of capacitance that equals one millionth of a farad.

microfiche /mī′krōfēsh′/ [Gk *mikros* + Fr *fiche* peg], a sheet of microfilm that contains several separate photographic reproductions. The sheet is a convenient size for filing and enables large amounts of data to be stored in a relatively small space.

microfilament /mī′krōfil′əmənt/, any of the submicroscopic cellular filaments, such as the tonofibrils, found in the cytoplasm of most cells, that function primarily as a supportive system.

microfilaria /mī′krōfiler′ē·ə/, *pl.* **microfilariae** [Gk *mikros* + L *filum* thread], the prelarval form of any filarial worm.

microfilm, a strip of 16-mm or 35-mm film that contains photographic reproductions of pages of books, documents, or other library or medical records in greatly reduced size. The film is viewed through special machines that enlarge the photographic images.

microfluorometry. See **cytophotometry.**

microgamete /mī′krōgam′ēt/, the small, motile male gamete of certain thallophytes and sporozoa, specifically the malarial parasite *Plasmodium.* It corresponds to the sperm of the higher animals.

microgametocyte /mī′krōgamē′təsīt/ [Gk *mikros* + *gamete* spouse, *kytos* cell], an enlarged merozoite that undergoes meiosis to form the mature male gamete during the sexual phase of the life cycle of certain thallophytes and sporozoa.

microgenitalia /mī′krōjen′itā′lē·ə/, a condition characterized by abnormally small external genitalia.

microglia /mīkrog′lē·ə/ [Gk *mikros* + *glia* glue], small migratory interstitial cells that form part of the central nervous system. They serve as phagocytes that collect waste products of the nerve tissue of the body.

micrognathia /mī′krōnā′thē·ə/ [Gk *mikros* + *gnathos* jaw], underdevelopment of the jaw, especially the mandible. **–micrognathic,** *adj.*

microgram (mg, μg), a unit of measurement of mass equal to one millionth (10^{-6}) of a gram.

microgyria /mī′krōjī′rē·ə/ [Gk *mikros* + *gyros* turn], a developmental defect of the brain in which the convolutions are abnormally small, resulting in structural malformation of the cortex. The condition is usually associated with mental retardation and physical defects.

microgyrus /mī′krōjī′rəs/, *pl.* **microgyri,** an underdeveloped, malformed convolution of the brain.

microhm /mī′krōm/ [Gk *mikros* + *ohm* George Ohm], a unit of electric resistance equal to one millionth of an ohm.

microinvasive carcinoma /mī′krō·invā′-siv/ [Gk *mikros* + L *in* within, *vadere* to go], a squamous epithelial neoplasm that has penetrated the basement membrane, the first stage in invasive cancer.

microlevel interventions, health-generating changes performed at the individual level, such as in conditioning or stimulus control therapies.

microliter (μL), a unit of liquid volume equal to one millionth of a liter.

microlith /mī′krəlith/ [Gk *mikros* + *lithos* stone], a small rounded mass of mineral matter or calcified stone.

micromelic dwarf /mī′krōmē′lik/ [Gk *mikros* + *melos* limb], a dwarf whose limbs are abnormally short.

micrometer, /mīkrom′ətər/, **1.** an instrument used for measuring small angles or distances on objects being observed through a microscope or telescope. **2.** /mī′krōmē′tər/, a unit of measurement, commonly referred to as a *micron*, that is, one thousandth (10^{-3}) of a millimeter.

micromillimeter [Gk *mikros* + L *mille* thousand; Gk *metron*], a nanometer.

micromyeloblastic leukemia /mī′krōmī′-əlōblas′tik/ [Gk *mikros* + *myelos* marrow, *blastos* germ], a malignant neoplasm of blood-forming tissues, characterized by the proliferation of small myeloblasts distinguishable from lymphocytes only by special staining techniques and microscopic examination.

micron (μ, mu) /mī′kron/ [Gk *mikros* small], **1.** a metric unit of length equal to one millionth of a meter; micrometer. **2.** (in physical chemistry) a colloidal particle with a diameter of between 0.2 and 10 microns.

micronucleus /mī′krōnoo′klē·əs/, **1.** a small or minute nucleus. **2.** (in protozoa) the smaller of two nuclei in each cell; it functions in sexual reproduction as opposed to the macronucleus, which governs cell metabolism and growth.

micronutrient /mī′krōnoo′trē·ənt/, an organic compound, such as a vitamin, or a chemical element, such as zinc or iodine, essential only in minute amounts for the normal physiologic processes of the body.

microorganism /mī′krō-ôr′ganiz′əm/ [Gk *mikros* + *organon* instrument], any tiny, usually microscopic entity capable of carrying on living processes. Kinds of microorganisms include **bacteria, fungi, protozoa,** and **viruses.**

micropenis. See **microphallus.**

microphage /mī′krəfāj/ [Gk *mikros* + *phagein* to eat], a neutrophil capable of ingesting small things, such as bacteria. **–microphagic,** *adj.*

microphallus /mī′krōfal′əs/ [Gk *mikros* + *phallos* penis], an abnormally small penis. When observed in the newborn, the nurse examines the child for other signs of ambiguous genitalia.

microphthalmos /mī′krəfthal′məs/ [Gk *mikros* + *ophthalmos* eye], a developmental anomaly characterized by abnormal smallness of one or both eyes. When the condition occurs in the absence of other ocular defects, it is called pure microphthalmos or nanophthalmos. **–microphthalmic,** *adj.*

microplasia. See **dwarfism.**

micropodia /mī′krōpō′dē·ə/ [Gk *mikros* + *pous* foot], a developmental anomaly characterized by abnormal smallness of the feet. The condition is often associated with other congenital malformations or with bone and skeletal disorders.

microprosopus /mī′krōprō′səpəs, -prəsō′-pəs/ [Gk *mikros* + *prosopon* face], a fe-

tus in which the face is abnormally small or underdeveloped.

micropsia /mīkrop′sē·ə/ [Gk *mikros* + *opsis* sight], a condition of vision by which a person perceives objects as smaller than they really are. **–microptic,** *adj.*

microreentry [Gk *mikros* + L *re* again; Fr *entree* entry], (in cardiology) an impulse reentry involving a very small circuit, such as within Purkinje fibers.

microscope [Gk *mikros,* small; *skopein,* to view], an instrument with lenses for viewing very small objects. An electron microscope uses a beam of electrons instead of visible light.

microscopic [Gk *mikros* + *skopein* to look], **1.** of or pertaining to a microscope. **2.** very small; visible only when magnified and illuminated by a microscope.

microscopic anatomy, the study of the microscopic structure of the tissues and cells. Kinds of microscopic anatomy are **cytology** and **histology.**

microscopy /mīkros′kəpē/ [Gk *mikros* + *skopein* to look], a technique for observing minute materials using a microscope. Kinds of microscopy include **darkfield, electron,** and **immunofluorescent microscopy.**

microshock, the passage of current directly into the cardiac tissue.

microsomal enzymes /mī′krōsō′məl/, a group of enzymes associated with a certain particulate fraction of liver homogenate that plays a role in the metabolism of many drugs.

microsomia /mī′krōsō′mē·ə/ [Gk *mikros* + *soma* body], the condition of having an abnormally small and underdeveloped yet otherwise perfectly formed body with normal proportionate relationships of the various parts.

Microsporum /mī′krōspôr′əm/ [Gk *mikros* + *sporos* seed], a genus of dermatophytes of the family Moniliaceae. The type species is *M. audouinii,* which causes epidemic tinea capitis in children.

microstomia /mī′krōstō′mē·ə/ [Gk *mikros* + *stoma* mouth], pertaining to an abnormally small mouth.

microsurgery [Gk *mikros* + *cheirourgos* surgery], surgery that involves microdissection and micromanipulation of tissues.

microthermy /mī′krōthur′mē/ [Gk *mikros* + *therme* heat], a form of therapy in which heat generated by radio wave conversion is used in physical therapy.

microtome /mī′krətōm/ [Gk *mikros* + *temnein* to cut], a device that cuts specimens of tissue prepared in paraffin blocks into extremely thin slices for microscopic study by a surgical pathologist.

M

microtubule, a hollow cylindrical structure that occurs widely within plant and animal cells. They increase in number during cell division and are associated with the movement of DNA material.

microvascular, pertaining to the portion of the circulatory system that is composed of the capillary network.

microvilli /mī′krōvil′ī/ [Gk *mikros* + L *villus* shaggy hair], tiny hairlike processes that extend from the surface of many cells. They are visible with an electron microscope.

microwave interstitial system [Gk *mikros* + AS *wafian* wave], a microwave-generated hyperthermia system that creates a heat field in certain accessible tumors no more than 2 inches beneath the skin. The microwaves produce a temperature of about 109° F to destroy the tumor cells. The treatment can be monitored on a video terminal that shows location of the tumor and heat applicators.

microwaves, electromagnetic radiation in the frequency range of 300 to 2,450 MHz.

microwave thermography, measurement of temperature through the detection of microwave radiation emitted from heated tissue.

micturate, micturition. See **urination.**

micturition reflex /mik′chərish′ən/ [L *micturire* to urinate; *reflectere* to bend backward], a normal reaction to a rise in pressure within the bladder, resulting in contraction of the bladder wall and relaxation of the urethral sphincter. Voluntary inhibition normally prevents incontinence.

micturition syncope [L *micturire*; Gk *syn* together, *koptein* to cut], a temporary loss of consciousness that tends to affect some adult males after arising from a reclining posture to urinate in an upright posture. The effect is due to a brief interruption of blood flow to the brain and is often associated with the use of alcohol, which contributes to vasodilation.

MICU, abbreviation for *medical intensive care unit.*

midarm muscle circumference, an indication of muscle wasting in the upper arm calculated by subtracting the triceps skin fold (TSF) from the midupper arm circumference (MAC) measurement.

midaxillary line /midak′siler′ē/, an imaginary vertical line that passes midway between the anterior and posterior axillary folds.

midazolam hydrochloride /midaz′əlam/, a parenteral central nervous system depressant. It is prescribed for preoperative sedation and impairment of memory of preoperative events, and for conscious sedation before short diagnostic or endoscopic procedures.

midbody, 1. the middle of the body, or the midregion of the trunk. 2. a mass of granules that appears in the middle of the spindle during mitotic anaphase.

midbrain. See **mesencephalon.**

midclavicular line /mid′kləvik′yōōlər/ [AS *midd*; L *clavicula* little key; *linea* line], (in anatomy) an imaginary line that extends downward over the trunk from the midpoint of the clavicle, dividing each side of the anterior chest into two parts.

middle adult [AS *middel*; L *adultus* grown up], an individual in the transitional age span between young adult and elderly.

middle cardiac vein, one of the five tributaries of the coronary sinus that drains blood from the capillary bed of the myocardium. It receives tributaries from both ventricles, and ends in the right extremity of the coronary sinus.

middle costotransverse ligament. See **ligament of the neck of the rib.**

middle cuneiform bone. See **intermediate cuneiform bone.**

middle ear, the tympanic cavity and the auditory ossicles contained in an irregular space in the temporal bone. It is separated from the external ear by the tympanic membrane and from the inner ear by the oval window. The auditory tube carries air from the posterior pharynx into the middle ear.

middle kidney. See **mesonephros.**

middle lobe syndrome, localized atelectasis of the middle lobe of the right lung, characterized by chronic infection, cough, dyspnea, wheezing, and obstructive pneumonitis. Asymptomatic obstruction of the bronchus may occur. The condition is caused by enlargement of the surrounding cuff of lymphatic glands.

middle mediastinum, the widest part of the mediastinum containing the heart, ascending aorta, lower half of the superior vena cava, pulmonary trunk, and phrenic nerves.

middle plate. See **nephrotome.**

middle sacral artery, a small, visceral branch of the abdominal aorta, descending to the fourth and fifth lumbar vertebrae, the sacrum, and the coccyx.

middle suprarenal artery, one of a pair of small, visceral branches of the abdominal aorta, arising opposite the superior mesenteric artery, and supplying the suprarenal gland.

middle temporal artery, one of the branches of the superficial temporal artery on each side of the head.

middle temporal gyrus, the middle of three gyri of the temporal area of the surface of the brain. It runs horizontally and lies between the inferior and superior temporal sulci of the temporal lobe.

middle umbilical fold, the fold of peritoneum over the urachal remnant within the abdomen.

mid forceps [AS *midd;* L *forceps* pair of tongs], an obstetric operation in which forceps are applied to the head of the baby when the head has reached the midplane of the mother's pelvis. An episiotomy is usually performed, and anesthesia is provided. In some cases, such as severe fetal distress, mid forceps may be the most rapid and the safest means of delivery.

midgut [AS *midd, guttas*], the middle portion of the embryonic alimentary canal. It consists of endodermal tissue, is connected to the yolk sac during early prenatal development, and eventually gives rise to some of the small intestine and part of the large intestine.

midlife transition, a period between early adulthood and middle adulthood that occurs between 40 and 45 years of age.

midline [AS *midd;* L *linea* line], an imaginary line that divides the body into right and left halves.

midline episiotomy. See **episiotomy.**

midpelvic contraction. See **contraction.**

midposition, the end-expiratory or end-tidal level or position of the lung-chest system under any given conditions, defining the patient's functional residual capacity.

midsagittal plane. See **median plane.**

midstance /mid′stans/ [AS *midd* + L *stare* to stand], one of the five stages in the stance phase of walking, or gait, directly associated with the period of single-leg support of body weight or the period during which the body advances over the stationary foot.

midsternum /midstur′nəm/ [AS *midd* + Gk *sternon* chest], the body of the breast bone, or sternum.

midstream catch urine specimen [AS *midd, stream;* L *captere* to capture], a urine specimen collected during the middle of a flow of urine, after the urinary opening has been carefully cleaned.

midupper arm circumference (MAC), an indication of upper arm muscle wasting based on measurement of the circumference of the arm at a midpoint between the tip of the acromial process of the scapula and olecranon process of the ulna.

midwife [AS *midd, wif*], **1.** (in traditional use) a (female) person who assists women in childbirth. **2.** (according to the International Confederation of Midwives, World Health Organization, and Federation of International Gynecologists and Obstetricians) a person who, having been regularly admitted to a midwifery educational program fully recognized in the country in which it is located, has successfully completed the prescribed course of studies in midwifery and has acquired the requisite qualifications to be registered and/or legally licensed to practice midwifery. Among the responsibilities of the midwife are supervision of the woman's pregnancy, labor, delivery, and puerperium. The midwife conducts the delivery independently. **3.** a lay midwife. **4.** a nurse midwife or Certified Nurse Midwife.

midwifery [AS, *midd; wif*], the employment of a person who is qualified by special training and experience to assist a woman in childbirth. Generally, a midwife is required to attend an approved school of midwifery and pass an examination.

MIF, abbreviation for *macrophage inhibition factor.*

migraine /mī′grān/ [Gk *hemi* half, *kranion* skull], a recurring vascular headache characterized by a prodromal aura, unilateral onset, and severe pain, photophobia, and autonomic disturbances during the acute phase, which may last for hours or days. The disorder occurs more frequently in women than in men, and a predisposition to migraine may be inherited. The head pain is related to dilatation of extracranial blood vessels, which may be the result of chemical changes that cause spasms of intracranial vessels. An impending attack may be heralded by visual disturbances, such as flashing lights or wavy lines, or by a strange taste or odor, numbness, tingling, vertigo, tinnitus, or a feeling that part of the body is distorted in size or shape. The acute phase may be accompanied by nausea, vomiting, chills, polyuria, sweating, facial edema, irritability, and extreme fatigue.

migrainous cranial neuralgia /mīgrā′nəs/ [Gk *hemi* half, *kranion* skull; L *osus* having], a variant of migraine, characterized by closely spaced episodes of excruciating, throbbing, unilateral headaches often accompanied by dilation of temporal blood vessels, flushing, sweating, lacrimation, nasal congestion or rhinorrhea, ptosis, and facial edema. Repeated episodes usually occur in clusters within a few days or weeks and may be followed by a relatively long remission period. A typical attack begins abruptly without prodromal signs, as a burning sensation in an orbit or temple.

migrating phlebitis [L *migrare* to wander; Gk *phleps* vein + *itis* inflammation], a form of phlebitis characterized by inflammation in one part of a vein and, after remission, in another part of the vein.

migration [L *migrare* to wander], the passage of the ovum from the ovary into a fallopian tube and then into the uterus.

migratory gonorrheal polyarthritis. See **migratory polyarthritis.**

migratory ophthalmia. See **sympathetic ophthalmia.**

migratory polyarthritis, arthritis progressively affecting a number of joints and finally settling in one or more, occurring in patients with gonorrhea and developing a few days to a few weeks after the onset of gonorrheal urethritis. The patient usually has a moderate fever. Large joints are most affected; after the swelling subsides, the overlying skin may peel.

migratory thrombophlebitis, an abnormal condition in which multiple thromboses appear in both superficial and deep veins. It may be associated with malignancy, especially carcinoma of the pancreas, often preceding other evidence of cancer by several months.

Mikulicz's syndrome /mik′yŏŏlich′ēz/ [Johann von Mikulicz-Radecki, Polish surgeon, b. 1850], an abnormal bilateral enlargement of the salivary and lacrimal glands, found in a variety of diseases, including leukemia, tuberculosis, and sarcoidosis.

mild [AS *milde* soft], gentle, subtle, or of low intensity, such as a mild infection.

milia neonatorum /mil′ē·ə/ [L *milium* millet; Gk *neo* new; L *natus* born], a nonpathologic dermatologic condition characterized by minute epidermal cysts consisting of keratinous debris that occur on the face and, occasionally, the trunk of the newborn.

miliaria /mil′ē·er′ē·ə/ [L *milium* millet], minute vesicles and papules, often with surrounding erythema, caused by occlusion of sweat ducts during times of exposure to heat and high humidity.

miliary /mil′ē·er′ē/ [L *milium* millet], describing a condition marked by the appearance of very small lesions the size of millet seeds, such as miliary tuberculosis, which is characterized by tiny tubercules throughout the body.

miliary carcinosis, a condition characterized by the presence of numerous cancerous nodules resembling miliary tubercles.

miliary fever, an inflammatory skin eruption caused by sweat retention. Sweat trapped in the dermis or epidermis causes irritation.

miliary tuberculosis, extensive dissemination by the bloodstream of tubercle bacilli. In children it is associated with high fever, night sweats, and, often, meningitis, pleural effusions, or peritonitis. A similar illness may occur in adults but with a less abrupt onset and, occasionally, with weeks or months of nonspecific symptoms, such as weight loss, weakness, and low-grade fever. Multiple small opacities resembling millet seeds may be evident on chest x-ray films.

milieu /milyœ′, milyŏŏ′/, *pl.* **milieus, milieux** [Fr, middle], the environment, surroundings, or setting. Kinds of milieus are **milieu extérieur** and **milieu intérieur.**

milieu extérieur /eksterē·œr′/, the external or physical surroundings of an organism, including the social environment, especially the home, school, and recreational facilities, that plays a dominant role in personality development.

milieu intérieur /aNterē·œr′/, a basic concept in physiology that multicellular organisms exist in an aqueous internal environment composed of the blood, lymph, and interstitial fluid that bathes all cells and provides a medium for the elementary exchange of nutrients and waste material. All fundamental processes necessary for the maintenance and life of the tissue elements depend on the stability and balance of this environment.

milieu therapy, a type of psychotherapy in which the total environment is used in treating mental and behavioral disorders. It is primarily conducted in a hospital or other institutional setting where the entire facility acts as a therapeutic community.

military antishock trousers (MAST), a garment designed to produce pressure on the lower part of the body, thereby preventing the pooling of blood in the legs and abdomen during aviation maneuvers or weightless experience in space travel. The trousers have also been used in treating postural hypotension and to control internal bleeding.

milium, *pl.* **milia** /mil′ē·ə/ [L, millet], a minute, white cyst of the epidermis caused by obstruction of hair follicles and eccrine sweat glands. One variety is seen in newborn infants and disappears within a few weeks. Another type is found primarily on the faces of middle-aged women.

milk [AS *meoluc*], a liquid secreted by the mammary glands or udders of animals that suckle their young. After breast feeding, people consume the milk of the cow, as well as that of many other animals, including the goat, camel, mare, reindeer, llama, and yak. Milk is a basic food containing carbohydrate (in the form of lactose), protein (mainly casein, with small amounts of lactalbumin, and lactoglobulin), suspended fat, the minerals calcium and phosphorus, the vitamins A, riboflavin, niacin, thiamine, and, when the milk is fortified, vitamin D. It is a valuable nutrient for adults and a nearly complete food for infants.

milk-alkali syndrome, a condition of alkalosis caused by the excessive ingestion of milk, antacid medications containing calcium, or other sources of absorbable alkaline substances. The condition results in hypercalcemia, hypocalciuria, and calcium deposits in the kidneys and other tissues.

milk baby, an infant with iron deficiency anemia caused by ingestion of excessive amounts of milk and the delayed or inadequate addition of iron-rich foods to the diet.

milk bath, a bath taken in milk for cosmetic or emollient reasons.

milk ejection reflex, a normal reflex in a lactating woman elicited by tactile stimulation of the nipple, resulting in release of milk from the glands of the breast.

milker's nodule, a smooth, brownish red papilloma of the fingers or palm that begins as a macule and progresses through a vesicular stage to become a nodule. The disease is acquired from pustular lesions on the udder of a cow infected with poxvirus.

milk fever, *nontechnical.* postpartum fever that begins with the onset of lactation. Maternal oral temperature during the puerperium does not normally exceed 100.4° F; higher elevations usually indicate infection.

milk globule, a spherical droplet of fat in milk that tends to separate out as cream.

milking, a procedure used to express the contents of a duct or tube, to test for tenderness, or to obtain a specimen for study. The examiner compresses the structure with a finger and moves the finger firmly along the duct or tube to its opening.

milk leg. See **phlegmasia alba dolens.**

Milkman's syndrome, a form of osteomalacia characterized by multiple, bilateral, symmetric absorption stripes, indicating pseudofractures in hypocalcified long bones and the pelvis and scapula.

milk of magnesia, a laxative and antacid containing magnesium hydroxide prescribed to relieve constipation and acid indigestion.

milk patch. See **macula albidae.**

milkpox. See **alastrim.**

milk sugar. See **lactose.**

milk therapy, a nutritional treatment used in the therapy of Curling's ulcer in patients who have been severely burned. Cool, homogenized milk is administered in doses of 1 to 2 ounces every hour through a nasogastric tube. After instillation the tube is clamped for 5 minutes and then unclamped. Milk remaining in the stomach is allowed to flow into a basin. As the con-

dition improves, the nasogastric tube is withdrawn, and milk may be continued by mouth.

milk tooth. See **deciduous tooth.**

milky ascites. See **chylous ascites.**

Miller-Abbott tube [Thomas G. Miller, American physician, b. 1886; William O. Abbott, American physician, b. 1902], a long, small-caliber, double-lumen catheter, used in intestinal intubation for decompression. It has several openings on the side of its tip.

milliampere (ma, MA) /mil′ē·am′pir/ [L *mille* thousand; Andre Ampere], a unit of electric current that is one thousandth of an ampere.

milliampere seconds (mAs), the product obtained by multiplying the electric quantity in milliamperes by the time in seconds.

millicoulomb (mC) /mil′ēk oo̅′lom/ [L *mille* thousand; Charles A. de Coulomb], a unit of electric charge that is one thousandth of a coulomb.

millicurie (mCi, mc) /mil′ēk oo̅r′ē/ [L *mille* thousand; Marie and Pierre Curie], a unit of radioactivity that is equal to one thousandth of a curie, or 3.70×10^7 disintegrations per second.

milliequivalent (mEq) [L *mille* + *aequus* equal, *valere* to be strong] **1.** the number of grams of solute dissolved in 1 ml of a normal solution. **2.** one thousandth of a gram equivalent.

milliequivalent per liter (mEq/L), one thousandth of 1 gram of a specific substance dissolved in 1 L of plasma.

milligram (mg) [L *mille* + Fr *gramme* small weight], a metric unit of weight equal to one thousandth (10^{-3}) of a gram.

milliliter (ml) [L *mille* + Fr *litre* a measure], a metric unit of volume that is one thousandth (10^{-3}) of a liter.

millimeter (mm), a metric unit of length equal to one thousandth (10^{-3}) of a meter.

millimole (mmol) [L *mille* + *moles* mass], a unit of metric measurement of mass that is equal to one thousandth (10^{-3}) of a mole.

milliosmol /mil′ē·oz′mōl/, a unit of measure representing the concentration of an ion in a solution, expressed in milligrams per liter divided by atomic weight. **–milliosmolar,** *adj.*

millipede /mil′ipēd′/ [L *mille* + *pedes* going on foot], a many-legged, wormlike arthropod. Certain species squirt irritating fluids that may cause dermatitis.

millirad /mil′ērad/, one thousandth (10^{-3}) of a rad, a unit of measurement of absorbed dose of ionizing radiation.

milliroentgen (mR, mr) /mil′irent′gən,-jən/ [L, *mille,* thousand; William von Roentgen], a unit of radiation that is

M

equal to one thousandth (10^{-3}) of a roentgen.

millisecond (msec) [L *milli* thousand; ME *seconde* small part], one one-thousandth of a second.

millivolt (mV, mv) [L *mille* thousand; Alessandro Volta], a unit of electromotive force equal to one thousandth of a volt.

Milwaukee brace [Milwaukee, Wisconsin; OFr *bracier* to embrace], an orthotic device that helps immobilize the torso and the neck of a patient in the treatment or correction of scoliosis, lordosis, or kyphosis. It is usually constructed of strong but light metal and fiberglass supports lined with rubber to protect against abrasion.

mimic spasm [Gk *mimetikos* imitative; *spasmos* spasm], involuntary, stereotyped movements of a small group of muscles, as of the face. The spasm is usually psychogenic and may be aggravated by stress or anxiety but is generally controllable.

min, abbreviation for **minim.**

Minamata disease /min´əmä´tə/, a severe, degenerative, neurologic disorder caused by the ingestion of grain or of seafood contaminated by soluble mercuric salts. The term is derived from a tragedy involving Japanese who ate seafood from Minamata Bay. Symptoms may not appear for several weeks or months; they include paresthesia of the mouth and extremities, tunnel vision, difficulties with speech, hearing, muscular coordination, and concentration, weakness, emotional instability, and stupor.

mind [AS *gemynd*], **1.** the part of the brain that is the seat of mental activity and that enables one to know, reason, understand, remember, think, feel, and to react and adapt to surroundings and all external and internal stimuli. **2.** the totality of all conscious and unconscious processes of the individual that influence and direct mental and physical behavior. **3.** the faculty of the intellect or understanding in contrast to emotion and will.

mine damp. See **damp.**

mineral [L *minera* mine], **1.** an inorganic substance occurring naturally in the earth's crust, having a characteristic chemical composition and (usually) crystalline structure. **2.** (in nutrition) a mineral usually referred to by the name of a metal, nonmetal, radical, or phosphate rather than by the name of the compound of which it is a part.

mineral deficiency, the inability to use one or more of the mineral elements essential in human nutrition because of a genetic defect, malabsorption dysfunction, or

the lack of that mineral in the diet. Minerals act as catalysts in nerve response, muscle contraction, and the metabolism of nutrients in foods. They also regulate electrolyte balance and hormonal production, and strengthen skeletal structures. See also specific minerals.

mineralization [L *minera* + Gk *izein* to cause], the addition of any mineral to the body.

mineralocorticoid /min´əral˝ōkôr´tikoid/ [L *minera* + *cortex* bark; Gk *eidos* form], a hormone, secreted by the adrenal cortex, that maintains normal blood volume, promotes sodium and water retention, and increases urinary excretion of potassium and hydrogen ions. Aldosterone, the most potent mineralocorticoid in regard to electrolyte balance, and corticosterone, a glucocorticoid and a mineralocorticoid, act on the distal tubules of the kidneys to enhance the reabsorption of sodium into the plasma.

mineral oil, a laxative, stool softener, emollient, and pharmaceutical aid used as a solvent. It is prescribed to prevent constipation, to treat mild constipation, to prepare the bowel for surgery or examination, and as a solvent for various preparations.

mineral soap. See **bentonite.**

miner's cramp. See **heat cramp.**

miner's elbow [L *minera* + AS *elboga*], an inflammation of the olecranon bursa, caused by resting the weight of the body on the elbow, as in some coal mining activities. The condition is sometimes seen in school children who lean on their elbows.

miner's pneumoconiosis. See **anthracosis.**

Minerva cast /minur´və/ [L *Minerva* Roman goddess of wisdom; ONorse *kasta*], an orthopedic cast applied to the trunk and the head, with spaces cut out for the face area and the ears. The section encasing the trunk extends to the sternum and the distal rib border anteriorly and across the distal rib border posteriorly. The cast is used for immobilizing the head and part of the trunk in the treatment of torticollis, cervical and thoracic injuries, and cervical spinal infections. Also called *Minerva jacket.*

minim (min) /min´im/ [L *minimum* smallest], a measurement of volume in the apothecaries' system, originally one drop (of water). Sixty minims equal 1 fluid dram. One minim equals 0.06 ml.

minimal bactericidal concentration. See **minimal inhibitory concentration.**

minimal brain dysfunction. See **attention deficit disorder.**

minimal care unit [L *minimum* smallest],

a unit for the treatment of inpatients who are ambulatory and able to meet many of their own daily living needs but require minimal nursing care.

minimal dose, the smallest dose of a drug or other agent necessary to produce a desired effect. Because of individual variations in drug response, the minimal dose for one person may be either excessive or insufficient for another patient.

minimal erythema dose. See **threshold dose.**

minimal inhibitory concentration (MIC), the lowest concentration of an antibiotic medication in the blood that is effective against an infection, determined by injecting infected venous blood into a culture medium containing various concentrations of a proposed antibiotic.

minimal occlusive volume (MOV), the volume of endotracheal cuff inflation that still permits a minimum airway leak during the inspiratory phase of ventilation.

Mini-Mental State Examination, a brief psychologic test designed to differentiate between dementia, psychosis, and affective disorders. It may include ability to identify common objects such as a pencil and a watch, write a sentence, and demonstrate orientation by identifying the day, month, and year, as well as town and country.

minimization [L minimum smallest; Gk izein to cause], (in psychology) cognitive distortion in which the effects of one's behavior are minimized.

minimum alveolar concentration (MAC), the smallest amount of a gas detected and measured in the alveoli of the lungs.

minimum daily requirement (MDR) [L minimum; OE daeglie; L requirere to seek], the daily human requirements of nutrients, for health and as needed to prevent a deficiency disease. The figures, established by the U.S. Food & Drug Administration, are generally extrapolated from experimental animal studies, and include an added small margin for safety.

minimum lethal dose (MLD) [L minimum, lethum death; Gk dosis giving], the smallest dose of a drug, relative to body weight, that will kill an experimental animal. The MLD may vary with the species of animal tested.

Minnesota Multiphasic Personality Inventory (MMPI), a psychologic test that includes 550 statements for interpretation by the subject, used clinically for evaluating personality and for detecting various disorders, such as depression and schizophrenia.

minocycline hydrochloride /min′əsī′klēn/,

a tetracycline antibiotic active against bacteria, rickettsia, and other organisms. It is prescribed in the treatment of a variety of infections.

minor [L, smaller], (in law) a person not of legal age; a person beneath the age of majority. A kind of minor is an **emancipated minor.**

minor connector, (in dentistry) a device that links the major connector or base of a removable partial denture to other denture units, such as rests and retainers.

minor element. See **micronutrient.**

minor epilepsy. See **petit mal epilepsy.**

minor hysteria, a mild disorder which may be expressed in emotional outbursts, repressed anxieties, or conversion of unconscious conflicts into physical symptoms.

minor renal calyx. See **renal calyx.**

minor surgery, any surgical procedure that does not require general anesthesia or respiratory assistance.

minoxidil /mĭnok′sidil/, a vasodilator prescribed in the treatment of severe refractory hypertension.

minute ventilation /min′it/ [L minitus very small], the total ventilation per minute measured by expired gas collection for a period of 1 to 3 minutes.

miosis /mī·ō′sis/ [Gk meiosis becoming less] **1.** contraction of the sphincter muscle of the iris, causing the pupil to become smaller. **2.** an abnormal condition characterized by excessive constriction of the sphincter muscle of the iris, resulting in very small, pinpoint pupils.

miotic /mē·ot′ik/, **1.** of or pertaining to miosis. **2.** causing constriction of the pupil of the eye. **3.** any substance or pharmaceutic that causes constriction of the pupil of the eye. Such agents are used in the treatment of glaucoma.

MIP, abbreviation for **maximum inspiratory pressure.**

miracidium /mir′əsid′ē·əm/, pl. **miracidia** [Gk meirakidion youthfulness], the ciliated larva of a parasitic trematode that hatches from an egg and can survive only by penetrating and further developing within a host snail, whereupon the larva further develops into a maternal sporocyte that produces more larvae.

mirage /miräzh′/ [L mirari to look at], an optical illusion caused by the refraction of light through air layers of different temperatures, such as the illusionary sheets of water that seem to shimmer over stretches of hot sand and pavement.

mirror image, 1. an image formed by a reflection in a plane mirror. **2.** a kind of reversed asymmetry of characteristics of-

M

ten found in sets of monzygotic twins. **3.** chemical molecules with the same composition but with asymmetrical arrangement of the atoms.

mirror speech [L *mirari* to look at; AS *spaec* speech], abnormal speech characterized by the reversal of the order of syllables in a word.

miscarriage. See **spontaneous abortion.**

miscible /mis'ibəl/ [L *miscere* to mix], able to be mixed or mingled with another substance.

misdemeanor [AS *missan* to miss; ME *demenen* conduct], (in criminal law) an offense that is considered less serious than a felony and carries with it a lesser penalty, usually a fine or imprisonment for less than 1 year.

misfeasance /misfē'zəns/ [AS *missan* to miss; L *facere* to do], an improper performance of a lawful act, especially in a way that might cause damage or injury.

misogamy /misog'əmē/ [Gk *misein* to hate, *gamos* marriage], an aversion to marriage. **–misogamic, misogamous,** *adj.,* **misogamist,** *n.*

misogyny /misoj'inē/ [Gk *misein* + *gyne* women], an aversion to women. **–misogynist,** *n.,* **misogynistic,** *adj.*

misopedia /mis'ōpē'dē·ə/ [Gk *misein* + *pais* children], an aversion to children. **–misopedic,** *adj.,* **misopedist,** *n.*

misophobia. See **mysophobia.**

missed abortion [AS *missan* to miss; L *aboriri* to miscarry], a condition in which a dead, immature embryo or fetus is not expelled from the uterus for 2 or more months. The uterus diminishes in size, and symptoms of pregnancy abate; infection and disorders of the clotting of the mother's blood may follow.

missed period, an unexplained interruption in the menstrual cycle.

missile fracture [L *mittere* to throw], a penetration fracture caused by a projectile, such as a bullet or a piece of shrapnel.

mistura /mistyoo'rə/ [L, mixture], any of a number of mixtures of drugs, usually containing suspensions of insoluble substances intended for internal use. Examples include **mistura kaolini et morphinae,** a mixture of kaolin and morphine, and **mistura cretae pro infantibus,** a mixture of chalk, tragacanth, chloroform water, and other ingredients formulated for the treatment of GI disorders in infants.

mite /mīt/ [AS], a minute arachnid with a flat, almost transparent body and four pairs of legs. Many species of these relatives of ticks and spiders are parasitic, including the chigger and *Sarcoptes scabiei,* which cause localized pruritus and inflammation.

mite typhus. See **scrub typhus.**

mithramycin. See **plicamycin.**

mithridatism. See **tachyphylaxis.**

mitleiden /mit'līdən/ [Ger *mit* with, *leiden* to suffer], psychosomatic symptoms sometimes experienced by expectant fathers.

mitochondrion /mī'tōkon'drē·on/, *pl.* **mitochondria** [Gk *mitos* thread, *chondros* cartilage], a small rodlike, threadlike, or granular organelle within the cytoplasm that functions in cellular metabolism and respiration and occurs in varying numbers in all living cells except bacteria, viruses, blue-green algae, and mature erythrocytes. Mitochondria provide the principal source of cellular energy through oxidative phosphorylation and adenosine triphosphate synthesis. They also contain the enzymes involved with electron transport and the citric and fatty acid cycles. **–mitochondrial,** *adj.*

mitogen /mī'təjən, mit'-/ [Gk *mitos* + *genein* to produce], an agent that triggers mitosis. **–mitogenic,** *adj.*

mitogenesia /mī'tōjənē'zhə/ [Gk *mitos* + *genein* to produce], the production by or formation resulting from mitosis.

mitogenesis /mī'tōjen'əsis/, the induction of mitosis in a cell. **–mitogenetic,** *adj.*

mitogenetic radiation /mī'tōjənet'ik/, the force or specific energy that is supposedly given off by cells undergoing division.

mitogenic factor /mī'tōjen'ik/, a kind of lymphokine that is released from activated T lymphocytes and stimulates the production of normal unsensitized lymphocytes.

mitogenic radiation. See **mitogenetic radiation.**

mitome /mī'tōm/, the reticular network sometimes observed within the cytoplasm and nucleoplasm of fixed cells.

mitomycin /mī'təmī'sin/, an antineoplastic antibiotic prescribed in the treatment of a variety of malignant neoplastic diseases.

mitosis /mītō'sis, mit-/ [Gk *mitos* thread], a type of cell division that occurs in somatic cells and results in the formation of two genetically identical daughter cells containing the diploid number of chromosomes characteristic of the species. Mitosis is the process by which the body produces new cells for both growth and repair of injured tissue. Kinds of mitosis are **heterotypic, homeotypic, multipolar,** and **pathologic mitosis.** **–mitotic,** *adj.*

mitotane /mī'tətān/, an antineoplastic that destroys normal and neoplastic adrenal cortical cells. It is prescribed in the treatment of carcinoma of the adrenal cortex.

mitotic figure /mītot'ik/ [Gk *mitos* + L *figura* form], any chromosome or chromosome aggregation during any of the stages of mitosis.

mitotic index, the number of cells per unit (usually 1,000) undergoing mitosis during a given time. The ratio is used primarily as an estimation of the rate of tissue growth.

mitral /mī′trəl/ [L *mitra* head dress], **1.** of or pertaining to the mitral valve of the heart. **2.** shaped like a miter.

mitral commissurotomy [L *mitra; commissura* joining together; Gk *temnein* to cut], a closed-heart surgical procedure in which the mitral valve is divided at the junction of its cusps for the treatment of mitral stenosis.

mitral gradient, the difference in pressure in the left atrium and left ventricle during diastole.

mitral murmur, a heart murmur caused by a defective mitral valve.

mitral regurgitation, a lesion of the mitral valve that allows the flow of blood from the left ventricle into the left atrium. The condition may result from congenital valve abnormalities, rheumatic fever, mitral valve prolapse, endocardial fibroelastosis, dilation of the left ventricle because of severe anemia, myocarditis, or myocardiopathy. Symptoms include dyspnea, fatigue, intolerance to exercise, and heart palpitations. Congestive heart failure may ultimately occur.

mitral stenosis. See **mitral valve stenosis.**

mitral valve, a bicuspid valve situated between the left atrium and the left ventricle; the only valve with two, rather than three, cusps. The mitral valve allows blood to flow from the left atrium into the left ventricle but prevents blood from flowing back into the atrium. Ventricular contraction in systole forces the blood against the valve, closing the two cusps and ensuring the flow of blood from the ventricle into the the aorta.

mitral valve prolapse (MVP), protrusion of one or both cusps of the mitral valve back into the left atrium during ventricular systole, resulting in incomplete closure of the valve and the backflow of blood. Most patients are asymptomatic, although some may experience chest pain, palpitations, fatigue, or dyspnea. The condition may lead to mitral regurgitation, resulting in enlargement of the left atrium and ventricle.

mitral valve stenosis, an obstructive lesion in the mitral valve of the heart caused by adhesions on the leaflets of the valve, usually the result of recurrent episodes of rheumatic endocarditis. Hypertrophy of the left atrium develops and may be followed by right-sided heart failure and pulmonary edema (cor pulmonale).

mittelschmerz /mit′əlshmerts/ [Ger *mittel* middle, *schmerz* pain], abdominal pain in the region of an ovary during ovulation, which usually occurs midway through the menstrual cycle. Present in many women, mittelschmerz is useful for identifying ovulation, thus pinpointing the fertile period of the cycle.

Mittendorf's dot, an eye anomaly characterized by the presence of a small dense floating opacity behind the posterior lens capsule. It is a remnant of the hyaloid artery that was present in the eye during embryonic development. The object usually does not affect vision.

mixed anesthesia. See **balanced anesthesia.**

mixed cell malignant lymphoma [L *miscere* to mix], a lymphoid neoplasm containing lymphocytes and histiocytes (macrophages).

mixed cell sarcoma, a tumor consisting of two or more cellular elements, excluding fibrous tissue.

mixed connective tissue disease (MCTD), a systemic disease characterized by the combined symptoms of various collagen diseases, such as synovitis, polymyositis, scleroderma, and systemic lupus erythematosus.

mixed culture [L *miscere* to mix; *colere* to cultivate], a laboratory culture that contains two or more different strains of organisms.

mixed dentition, a phase of dentition during which some of the teeth are permanent and some are deciduous.

mixed glioma, a tumor, composed of glial cells, that contains more than one kind of cell, the most common being nonneural cells of ectodermal origin.

mixed infection, an infection by several microorganisms, as in some abscesses, pneumonia, and infections of wounds. Numerous combinations of bacteria, viruses, and fungi may be involved.

mixed leukemia, a malignancy of blood-forming tissues characterized by the proliferation of eosinophilic, neutrophilic, and basophilic granulocytes, in contrast to one predominant cell line.

mixed lymphocyte culture (MLC) reaction, an assay of the function of the T cell lymphocytes, primarily used for histocompatibility testing before grafting.

mixed neoplasm, a tumor or growth involving two germinal layers of tissue.

mixed nerve, a nerve that contains both sensory and motor fibers.

mixed porphyria. See **variegate porphyria.**

M

mixed sleep apnea, a condition marked by signs and symptoms of both central sleep apnea and obstructive sleep apnea. Mixed sleep apnea often begins as central sleep apnea and is followed by development of the obstructive form.

mixed tumor, a growth composed of more than one kind of neoplastic tissue, especially a complex embryonal tumor of local origin.

mixed venous blood, blood that is composed of the venous blood from the heart and all systemic tissues in proportion to their venous returns. In the absence of abnormalities, mixed venous blood is present in the main pulmonary artery.

mixture [L *miscere* to mix], **1.** a substance composed of ingredients that are not chemically combined and do not necessarily occur in a fixed proportion. **2.** (in pharmacology) a liquid containing two or more medications in suspension. The proportions of the ingredients are specific to each mixture.

ml, abbreviation for **milliliter.**

MLC, abbreviation for **mixed lymphocyte culture.**

MLD, abbreviation for **minimum lethal dose.**

mm, abbreviation for **millimeter.**

MMEF, abbreviation for *maximal midexpiratory flow.*

M-mode, abbreviation for *motion mode,* a variation of B-mode ultrasound scanning. It is used in echocardiography.

mmol, abbreviation for **millimole.**

MMPI, abbreviation for **Minnesota Multiphasic Personality Inventory.**

MMR, abbreviation for **measles, mumps, and rubella virus vaccine live.**

MMWR, abbreviation for *Morbidity and Mortality Weekly Report.*

Mn, symbol for the element **manganese.**

mnemonics [Gk *mnemonikos*], a system of memory training by linking a new concept or image with one already established in the memory, as associating the numbers of a combination lock with a birthday or telephone number.

Mo, symbol for the element **molybdenum.**

MOAB, abbreviation for **monoclonal antibody.**

mobile arm support, a forearm support device that enables persons with upper extremity disabilities to fulfill some activities of daily living, such as by helping to position the hand properly for self-feeding. The orthotic device may be mounted on a wheelchair.

mobility [L *mobilis* movable], the velocity a particle or ion attains for a given applied voltage and a relative measure of how quickly an ion may move in an electric field.

mobility, impaired physical, a NANDA-accepted nursing diagnosis of a state in which an individual experiences a limitation of ability for independent physical movement. Defining characteristics include an inability to achieve a functional level of mobility in the environment, a reluctance to move, a limited range of motion of the limbs or extremities, a decrease in the strength or control of the musculoskeletal system, abnormal or impaired ability to coordinate movements, or any of a large number of imposed restrictions on movement, such as medically required bed rest or traction.

Mobitz I heart block /mō′bits/ [Woldemar Mobitz, German physician, b. 1889; AS *hoerte* heart; Fr *bloc* block], second-degree or partial atrioventricular (AV) block in which the PR interval increases progressively until the propagation of an atrial impulse does not occur and the corresponding ventricular beat drops out. After the pause the progressive shortening of the PR interval begins again. Symptoms include fatigue, dizziness, and, in some cases, syncope. Mobitz I heart block is caused by abnormal conduction of the cardiac impulse in the AV node.

Mobitz II heart block, second degree or partial atrioventricular block, characterized by the sudden nonconduction of an atrial impulse and a periodic dropped beat without prior lengthening of the PR interval. This kind of block usually results from impaired conduction in the bundle branches and may be caused by anterior myocardial infarction, myocarditis, drug toxicity, electrolyte disturbances, rheumatoid nodules, and various degenerative diseases. Long-term therapy requires the implantation of a pacemaker.

Möbius' syndrome /mē′bē·əs/ [Paul J. Möbius, German neurologist, b. 1853], a rare developmental disorder characterized by congenital bilateral facial palsy usually associated with oculomotor or other neurologic dysfunctions, speech disorders, and various anomalies of the extremities.

mode [L *modus* measure], a value or term in a set of data that occurs more frequently than other values or terms.

model [L *modulus* small measure], (in nursing research) a symbolic representation of the interrelations exhibited by a phenomenon within a system or a process. The model is presented as a conceptual framework or a theory that explains a phenomenon and allows predictions to be made.

modeling, a technique used in behavior

therapy in which a person learns a desired response by observing it performed.

moderator band /mod′ərā′tər/ [L *moderari* to restrain; AS *bindan* to bind], a thick bundle of muscle in the central part of the right ventricle of the heart.

modification allele. See **modifying gene.**

modified milk [L *modus* measure, *facere* to make], cow's milk in which the protein content has been reduced and the fat content increased to correspond to the composition of breast milk.

modified radical mastectomy, a surgical procedure in which a breast is completely removed with the underlying pectoralis minor and some of the adjacent lymph nodes. The pectoralis major is not excised. The operation is performed in treating early and well-localized malignant neoplasms of the breast.

modifying gene [L *modus* measure; Gk *genein* to produce], a gene that alters or influences the expression function of another gene, including the suppression or reduction of the usual function of the modified gene.

modulation transfer function (MTF) [L *modulus* small measure; L *transferre* to carry; *functio* performance], a quantitative measure of the ability of an imaging system to reproduce patterns that vary in spatial frequency.

Moeller's glossitis /mel′ərz/ [Julius O.L. Moeller, German surgeon, b. 1819], a form of chronic glossitis, characterized by burning or pain in the tongue and an increased sensitivity to hot or spicy foods.

mohel /mō′əl, môhāl′/, an ordained Jewish circumciser.

moiety /moi′itē/ [L *medietas* middle], a part of a molecule that exhibits a particular set of chemical and pharmacologic characteristics.

moist gangrene. See **gangrene.**

moist heat [OFr *moiste* fresh; AS *haetu*], the use of hot water, towels soaked in hot water, or hot water vapors to reduce inflammation and pain, stimulate circulation and/or relieve symptoms as directed by a physician. Hot towels should be wrung out to remove surplus moisture and should not be too hot to be held in the hands of the person applying moist heat.

moist rale [OFr *moiste, rale* rattle], an abnormal breathing sound heard on auscultation when air bubbles through fluid or secretions in the bronchi or trachea.

mol. See **mole²**.

molality /mōlal′itē/ [L *moles* mass], the numbers of moles of solute per kilogram of water or other solvent.

molar /mō′lər/ [L *moles* mass], 1. any one of the 12 molar teeth, six in each den-

tal arch, three located posterior to the premolar teeth. The crown of each molar is nearly cubical, convex on its buccal and lingual surface, and flattened on its surfaces of contact. It is surmounted by four or five cusps separated by cruciate depressions and has a large rounded neck. 2. of or pertaining to the gram molecular weight of a substance.

molarity /mōler′itē/ [L *moles* mass], the number of moles of solute per liter of water or other solvent.

molar pregnancy, pregnancy in which a hydatid mole develops from the trophoblastic tissue of the early embryonic stage of development. The signs of pregnancy are all exaggerated: the uterus grows more rapidly than is normal, morning sickness is often severe and constant, blood pressure is likely to be elevated, and blood levels of chorionic gonadotropins are extremely high.

molar solution, a solution that contains one mole of solute per liter of solution.

molar volume. See **mole volume.**

mold¹, 1. a fungus. 2. a growth of fungi.

mold², a hollow form for casting or shaping an object, as a prosthesis.

molding [ME *moulde* shaping], the natural process by which a baby's head is shaped during labor as it is squeezed into and through the birth passage by the forces of labor. The head often becomes quite elongated, and the bones of the skull may be caused to overlap slightly at the suture lines. Most of the changes caused by molding resolve themselves during the first few days of life.

mole¹ [L, mass], *informal.* 1. a pigmented nevus. 2. (in obstetrics) a hydatidiform mole.

mole² [L *molecula* small mass], the standard unit used to measure the amount of a substance. A mole of a substance is the amount containing the same number of elementary particles (atoms, electrons, ions, molecules, or other particles) as there are atoms in 12 g of carbon 12. –**molar,** *adj.*

molecular biology, the study of biology from the viewpoint of the physical and chemical interactions of molecules involved in life functions.

molecular genetics [L *molecula* small mass; Gk *genesis* origin], the branch of genetics that focuses on the chemical structure and the functions, replication, and mutations of the molecules involved in the transmission of genetic information, such as DNA and RNA.

molecular lesion. See **point lesion.**

molecular pathology, a branch of the science of disease that is concerned with the health effects of specific molecules.

M

molecular weight, the total of the atomic weights of the atoms in a molecule.

molecule [L *molecula* small mass], the smallest unit that exhibits the properties of an element or compound. A molecule is composed of two or more atoms that are chemically combined.

mole percent, a percentage calculation expressed in terms of moles of a substance in a mixture or solution rather than in terms of molecular weight.

mole volume, the volume occupied by one mole of a substance, which may be a solid, liquid, or gas. It is numerically equal to the molecular weight divided by the density.

molindone hydrochloride /mol'indōn/, an antipsychotic agent prescribed in the treatment of schizophrenia.

molluscum /məlus'kəm/ [L *molluscus* soft], any skin disease having soft, rounded masses or nodules.

molluscum contagiosum, a disease of the skin and mucous membranes, caused by a poxvirus. It is characterized by scattered white papules. Palms of the hands and soles of the feet are not affected. The disease most frequently occurs in children and in adults with an impaired immune response. It is transmitted from person to person by direct or indirect contact.

mol. wt., abbreviation for **molecular weight.**

molybdenum (Mo) /məlib'dənəm/ [Gk *molybdos* lead], a grayish metallic element. Its atomic number is 42; its atomic weight is 95.94. Molybdenum is poisonous if ingested in large quantities.

molybdenum 99, the radionuclide that is the parent of technetium 99, and as such is present as a generator in all nuclear medicine departments.

monarthritis /mon'ärthrī'tis/ [Gk *monos* single, *arthron* joint, *itis* inflammation], arthritis affecting only one joint.

monarticular /mon'ärtik'yələr/ [Gk *monos* + L *articulus* joint], pertaining to only one joint.

monaural /monôr'əl/ [Gk *monos* + L *auris* ear], pertaining to one ear.

Mönckeberg's arteriosclerosis /meng'-kəbərgz/ [Johann G. Mönckeberg, German pathologist, b. 1877], a form of arteriosclerosis in which extensive calcium deposits are found in the media of the artery with little obstruction of the lumen.

Monday morning fever. See **byssinosis.**

Monge's disease. See **altitude sickness.**

Mongolian spot [*Mongol* Asian ethnic group; ME *spotte* stain], a benign, bluish black macule occurring over the sacrum and on the buttocks of some new-

borns. It usually disappears during early childhood.

mongolism, mongoloid idiocy. See **Down syndrome.**

Monilia. See *Candida albicans.*

monilial vulvovaginitis, moniliasis. See **candidiasis.**

monitor [L *monere* to warn], **1.** to observe and evaluate a function of the body closely and constantly. **2.** a mechanical device that provides a visual or audible signal or a graphic record of a particular function, such as a cardiac monitor or a fetal monitor.

monitrice /mon'itris'/ [Fr, female instructor], a labor coach, usually a registered nurse, who is specially trained in the Lamaze method of childbirth. The coach provides emotional support and leads the mother through labor and delivery.

mono, abbreviation for **mononucleosis.**

monoamine /mon'ō·am'in/, an amine containing one amine group.

monoamine oxidase (MAO), an enzyme that catalyzes the oxidation of amines.

monoamine oxidase (MAO) inhibitor, any of a chemically heterogeneous group of drugs used primarily in the treatment of depression. These drugs also exert an antianxiety effect, especially anxiety associated with phobia. The effects of the drugs vary greatly from patient to patient, and their specific actions leading to clinical benefits are poorly understood. Among the most common adverse effects are drowsiness, dry mouth, orthostatic hypotension, and constipation. Overdosage may cause tremor, euphoria, or manic behavior. MAO inhibitors interact with many drugs and with foods containing large amounts of the amino acid tyromine.

monobasic acid /mon'ōbā'sik/, an acid with only one replaceable hydrogen atom, such as hydrochloric acid (HCl).

monobenzone /mon'ōben'zōn/, a depigmenting agent prescribed in the treatment of abnormal skin pigmentation, as in disseminated vitiligo. It is not to be used for more trivial conditions, such as freckles.

monoblast /mon'əblast/ [Gk *monos* single, *blastos* germ], an immature monocyte. Increased production of monoblasts in the marrow and by the abnormal presence of these forms in the peripheral circulation are found in certain leukemias. **–monoblastic,** *adj.*

monoblastic leukemia, a malignancy of blood-forming organs, characterized by the proliferation of monoblasts and monocytes.

monocephalus. See **syncephalus.**

monochorial twins /mon'ôr'kē·əl/, **monochorionic twins.** See **monozygotic twins.**

monochrotic pulse /mon'ōkrot'ik/ [Gk *monos* + *krotein* to strike; L *pulsare* to beat], a pulse characterized by a single wave.

monoclonal /mon'əklō'nəl/ [Gk *monos* + *klon* graft], of, pertaining to, or designating a group of identical cells or organisms derived from a single cell.

monoclonal antibody (MOAB) [Gk *monos* + *klon* a twig; Gk *anti;* AS *bodig* body], antibodies produced by a hybridoma or antibody-producing cell source for a specific antigen.

monoclonal gammopathy. See **gammopathy.**

monocomponent insulin /mon'ōkəmpō'nənt/, See **single component insulin.**

monocular diplopia, a condition in which a double image is perceived with one eye. The cause is a disorder in the refracting medium of the eye, such as cataracts, or partial dislocation of the lens. In rare cases, more than two images may be seen with one eye.

monocular strabismus, a squint that is confined to one eye.

monocular vision /monok'yələr/, a condition of seeing with only one eye.

monocyte /mon'əsīt/ [Gk *monos* + *kytos* cell], a large mononuclear leukocyte with an ovoid or kidney-shaped nucleus, containing lacy, linear chromatin material and gray-blue cytoplasm filled with fine, reddish, and azurophilic granules.

monocytic leukemia /mon'əsit'ik/, a malignancy of blood-forming tissues in which the predominant cells are monocytes. The disease has an erratic course characterized by malaise, fatigue, fever, anorexia, weight loss, splenomegaly, bleeding gums, dermal petechiae, anemia, and unresponsiveness to therapy. There are two forms: **Schilling's leukemia,** in which most of the cells are monocytes that probably arise from the reticuloendothelial system, and the more common **Naegeli's leukemia,** in which a large number of the cells resemble myeloblasts.

monocytosis /mon'ōsītō'sis/, an increased proportion of monocytic white blood cells in the circulation.

monodactylism /mon'ōdak'tiliz'əm/ [Gk *monos* + *daktylos* finger or toe], a congenital defect in which the person is born with only one finger on the hand or one toe on the foot.

monoethanolamine /mon'ō·eth'ənol'əmēn/, an amino alcohol formed by the decarboxylation of serine. It is used as a surfactant in pharmaceutical products.

monofactorial inheritance /mon'-ōfaktôr'ē·əl/ [Gk *monos* + L *factare* to make], the acquisition or expression of a trait or condition that depends on the transmission of a single specific gene.

monohybrid /mon'ōhī'brid/ [Gk *monos* + L *hybrida* mixed offspring], pertaining to or describing an individual, organism, or strain that is heterozygous for only one specific trait or that is heterozygous for the single trait or gene locus under consideration.

monohybrid cross, the mating of two individuals, organisms, or strains that have different gene pairs for only one specific trait or in which only one particular characteristic or gene locus is being followed.

monohydric alcohol /mon'ōhī'drik/, an alcohol containing one hydroxyl group.

monomer /mon'əmər/ [Gk *monos* + *meros* part], a molecule that repeats itself to form a polymer, such as the molecules of fibrin monomer that polymerize to form fibrin in the blood-clotting process. **—monomeric,** *adj.*

monomolecular reaction (E[1]), a first-order chemical kinetic reaction in which only one substance is involved in the reaction.

monomphalus /mənom'fələs/ [Gk *monos* + *omphalos* navel], conjoined twins that are united at the umbilicus.

mononeuritis multiplex. See **multiple mononeuropathy.**

mononeuropathy /mon'ōn·ŏŏrop'əthē/ [Gk *monos* + *neuron* nerve, *pathos* disease], any disease or disorder that affects a single nerve trunk. Some common causes of disorders involving single nerve trunks are electric shock, radiation, and fractured bones that may compress or lacerate nerve fibers. Casts and tourniquets that are too tight may also damage a nerve by compression or by ischemia.

mononuclear [Gk *monos* + L *nucleus* nut], pertaining to one nucleus, as a monocyte.

mononuclear cell [Gk *monos* + L *nucleus* nut kernel, *cella* storeroom], a leukocyte, including lymphocytes and monocytes, with a round or oval nucleus.

mononucleosis (mono) /mon'ōnŏŏ'klē·ō'sis/ [Gk *monos* + L *nucleus;* Gk *osis* condition], an abnormal increase in the number of mononuclear leukocytes in the blood.

monooctanoin /mon'ō·ok'tənō'in/, a gallstone-dissolving agent used to dissolve cholesterol gallstones.

monoovular. See **uniovular.**

monophasic /mon'ōfā'sik/, having one phase, part, aspect, or stage.

monoploid /mon'əploid/, haploid.

monopodial symmelia. See **sympus monopus.**

monopus /mon'əpəs/ [Gk *monos* + *pous*

M

foot], a fetus or individual with the congenital absence of a foot or leg.

monorchid /monôr′kid/, a male who has monorchism.

monorchism /mon′ôrkiz′əm/ [Gk *monos* + *orchis* testicle, *ismos* state], a condition in which only one testicle has descended into the scrotum. **–monorchidic,** *adj.*

monosaccharide /mon′ōsak′ərīd/ [Gk *monos* + *sakcharon* sugar], a carbohydrate consisting of a single basic unit with the general formula $C_n(H_2O)_n$, with n ranging from 3 to 8.

monosome /mon′əsōm/ [Gk *monos* + *soma* body] **1.** an unpaired X or Y sex chromosome. **2.** the single, unpaired chromosome in monosomy.

monosomy /mon′əsō′mē/ [Gk *monos* + *soma* body], a chromosomal aberration characterized by the absence of one chromosome from the normal diploid complement. **–monosomic,** *adj.*

monosomy X. See **Turner's syndrome.**

monospecific [Gk *monos* + L *species* form, *facere* to make], an antibody that will react with only one type of antigen.

monosynaptic reflex /mon′ōsinap′tik/ [Gk *monos* + + *synaptein* to join; L *reflectere* to bend back], a reflex requiring only one afferent and one efferent neuron.

monotropy /mənot′rəpē/ [Gk *monos* + *trepein* to turn], a phenomenon in which a mother appears to be able to bond with only one infant at a time. When one twin is taken home from the hospital earlier than the other, the mother often reports that she does not feel that the baby discharged later is hers. The second baby to reach the home is much more likely to fail to thrive or to be neglected or abused. Monotropy may also explain a mother's common tendency to dress twins alike, in effect making them one. **–monotropic,** *adj.*

monounsaturated fatty acid. See **unsaturated fatty acid.**

monovular. See **uniovular.**

monovulatory /mənō′vyələtôr′ē/ [Gk *monos* + L *ovulum* small egg, *orius* characterized by], routinely releasing one ovum during each ovarian cycle.

monozygotic (MZ) /mon′ozīgo′tik/ [Gk *monos* + *zygon* yoke], pertaining to or developed from a single fertilized ovum, or zygote, such as occurs in identical twins. **–monozygosity,** *n.,* **monozygous,** *adj.*

monozygotic twins, two offspring born of the same pregnancy and developed from a single fertilized ovum that splits into equal halves during an early cleavage phase in embryonic development, giving rise to separate fetuses. Such twins are al-

ways of the same sex, have the same genetic constitution, possess identical blood groups, and closely resemble each other in physical, psychologic, and mental characteristics. Monozygotic twins may have single or separate placentas and membranes, depending on the time during development when division occurred.

mons /mons/ [L, mountain], a mound or slight elevation.

Monson curve [George S. Monson, American dentist, b. 1869; L *curvus* a bend], the curve of occlusion in which each tooth cusp and incisal edge conform to a segment of the surface of a sphere 8 inches (20 cm) in diameter, with its center in the region of the glabella.

mons pubis. See **mons veneris.**

monster [L *monstrum*], a fetus that is grossly malformed and usually nonviable. Kinds of monsters include **compound, double,** and **single monster.**

monstrosity, 1. the state or condition of having severe congenital defects. **2.** anything that deviates greatly from the normal; a monster or teras.

mons veneris /mons ven′əris/ [L *mons* mountain; *Venus* goddess of love], a pad of fatty tissue and coarse skin that overlies the symphysis pubis in the woman.

Monteggia's fracture /montej′əz/ [Giovanni B. Monteggia, Italian physician, b. 1762], fracture of the proximal third of the proximal half of the ulna, associated with radial dislocation or rupture of the annular ligament and resulting in the angulation or overriding of ulnar fragments.

Montercaux fracture /mont′ərko′/, a fracture of the neck of the fibula associated with the diastasis of ankle mortise.

Montgomery's gland. See **Montgomery's tubercle.**

Montgomery straps, bands of adhesive tape that are used to secure dressings that must be changed frequently.

Montgomery's tubercle [William F. Montgomery, Irish gynecologist, b. 1797; L *tuber* swelling], one of several sebaceous glands on the areolae of the breasts. The sebaceous material that is secreted from the ducts of the glands to the skin of each areola serves to lubricate and protect the breast from infection and trauma during breast feeding.

Montgomery tapes. See **Montgomery straps.**

mood, a prolonged emotional state that influences one's whole personality and life functioning.

mood-congruent psychotic features [AS *mod* mind; L *congruere* to come together], the characteristics of a psychosis in which the content of hallucinations or delusions is consistent with an elevated, expansive mood or with a depression.

mood disorders, an affective state characterized by any of a variety of periods of depression or depression elation. If mild and occasional, the feelings may be normal. If more severe, they may be a sign of a dysthymic reaction or symptomatic of an affective disorder.

moon face [AS *mona* moon; L *facies* face], a condition characterized by a rounded, puffy face, occurring in people treated with large doses of corticosteroids, such as those with rheumatoid arthritis or acute childhood leukemia.

Moore's fracture [Edward M. Moore, American surgeon, b. 1814], a fracture of the distal radius with associated dislocation of the ulnar head, resulting in the securement of the styloid process under the annular ligaments of the wrist.

MOPP /mop/, an abbreviation for a combination drug regimen used in the treatment of cancer, containing three antineoplastics, Mustargen (mechlorethamine), Oncovin (vincristine sulfate), Matulane (procarbazine hydrochloride), and prednisone (a glucocorticoid). MOPP is prescribed in the treatment of Hodgkin's disease.

morbid [L *morbidus* diseased], pertaining to a pathologic or diseased condition, either physical or mental.

morbid anatomy. See **pathologic anatomy.**

morbidity /môrbid'itē/ [L *morbidus* diseased], **1.** an illness or an abnormal condition or quality. **2.** (in statistics) the rate at which an illness or abnormality occurs, calculated by dividing the entire number of people in a group by the number in that group who are affected with the illness or abnormality. **3.** the rate at which an illness occurs in a particular area or population.

Morbidity and Mortality Weekly Report (MMWR), a weekly epidemiologic report on the incidence of communicable diseases and deaths in 120 urban areas of the United States. It is compiled by the Centers for Disease Control and Prevention in Atlanta, Georgia.

morbidity rate, the number of cases of a particular disease occurring in a single year per a specified population unit, as x cases per 1,000. It also may be calculated on the basis of age groups, sex, occupation, or other population unit.

morbidity statistics, a branch of statistics that is concerned with the disease rate of a population or geographic region.

morbid obesity, an excess of body fat that threatens normal body functions such as respiration.

morbid physiology. See **pathologic physiology.**

morbilli. See **measles.**

morbilliform /môrbil'ifôrm/ [L *morbilli* little disease, *forma* form], describing a skin condition that resembles the erythematous, maculopapular rash of measles.

Morgagni's globule /môrgan'yēz/ [Giovanni B. Morgagni, Italian anatomist, b. 1682], a minute opaque sphere that may form from fluid coagulation between the eye lens and its capsule, especially in cataract.

Morgagni's tubercle [Giovanni B. Morgagni], one of several small, soft nodules on the surface of each of the areola in women. The tubercles are produced by large sebaceous glands just under the surface of the areolae.

morgan /môr'gən/ [Thomas H. Morgan, American biologist, b. 1896], (in genetics) a unit of measure used in mapping the relative distances between genes on a chromosome.

morgue [Fr, mortuary], a unit of a hospital with facilities for the storage and autopsy of dead persons.

moribund /môr'ibund/ [L *moribundus* dying], pertaining to a person near death or in the act of dying.

Morita therapy /môrē'tä/, an alternative therapy that has as its focus the neurotic symptoms of the patient. The goal of the therapy is to enable the patient to live responsibly and constructively, even if the symptoms persist.

morning after pill [AS *morgen; aefter; pilian* to peel], *informal.* A large dose of an estrogen given orally, over a short period of time, to a woman within 24 to 72 hours after sexual intercourse to prevent conception, most commonly in an emergency situation such as rape or incest.

morning dip, a significant decline in respiratory function observed in some asthmatic persons during the early morning hours.

morning sickness. See **nausea and vomiting of pregnancy.**

morning stiffness [OE *morgen; stif*], a period of muscular stiffness after awakening in the morning, a common complaint of patients with arthritis or similar musculoskeletal disorders.

Moro reflex /môr'ō/ [Ernst Moro, German pediatrician, b. 1874], a normal mass reflex in a young infant elicited by a sudden loud noise, such as by striking the table next to the child, resulting in flexion of the legs, an embracing posture of the arms, and usually a brief cry.

morphea /môr'fē·ə/ [Gk *morphe* form], localized scleroderma consisting of

M

patches of yellowish or ivory-colored, rigid, dry, smooth skin.

morphine sulfate /môr'fēn/, a narcotic analgesic prescribed to reduce pain.

morphogenesis /môr'fəjen'əsis/ [Gk *morphe* + *genein* to produce], the development and differentiation of the structures and the form of an organism, specifically the changes that occur in the cells and tissue during embryonic development.

morphogenetic /môr'fōjənet'ik/, (in embryology) of or pertaining to a substance or hormone that acts as an evocator in differentiation.

morphogeny. See **morphogenesis.**

morphology /môrfol'əjē/ [Gk *morphe* + *logos* science], the study of the physical shape and size of a specimen, plant, or animal. **–morphologic,** *adj.*

Morquio's disease /môrkē'ōz/ [Luis Morquio, Uruguayan physician, b. 1867], a familial form of mucopolysaccharidosis that results in abnormal musculoskeletal development in childhood. Dwarfism, hunchback, enlarged sternum, and knock-knees may occur.

mortal, 1. liable to die. **2.** causing death.

mortality [L *mortalis* perishable], **1.** the condition of being subject to death. **2.** the death rate, which reflects the number of deaths per unit of population in any specific region, age group, disease, or other classification, usually expressed as deaths per 1,000, 10,000, or 100,000.

mortar [L *mortarium* wasting], a cup-shaped vessel in which materials are ground or crushed by a pestle in the preparation of drugs.

mortinatality /môr'tinātal'itē/ [L *mors* death; *natus* birth], the stillbirth rate. It is calculated by multiplying the number of stillbirths by 1,000 and dividing by the total number of births per year.

mortise joint /môr'tis/ [ME *mortays* fixed in; *jungere* to join], the *articulatio talocruralis* joint of the ankle.

Morton's disease [Thomas George Morton, American surgeon, b. 1835; L *dis;* Fr *aise* ease], a form of foot neuralgia caused by a falling metatarsal arch and pressure on the digital branches of the lateral plantar nerve.

Morton's foot. See **metatarsalgia.**

Morton's neuralgia. See **Morton's disease.**

Morton's neuroma. See **metatarsalgia.**

Morton's plantar neuralgia [Thomas G. Morton], a severe throbbing pain that affects a nerve branch between the medial and lateral plantar nerves.

Morton's syndrome [Dudley J. Morton, American orthopedist, b. 1884; Gk *syn* together; *dromos* course], a congenital foreshortening of the first metatarsal segment, causing pain and deformity of the forefoot.

Morton's toe. See **metatarsalgia.**

morula /môr'ələ/, *pl.* **morulas, morulae** [L *morulus* blackberry], a solid, spherical mass of cells resulting from the cleavage of the fertilized ovum in the early stages of embryonic development. **–morular,** *adj.*

Morvan's disease, a form of syringomyelia with tissue changes in the extremities, such a paresthesia of the forearms and hands, and progressive painless ulceration of the fingertips.

mosaic /mōzā'ik/ [L *Musa* goddess of the arts] **1.** (in genetics) an individual or organism that developed from a single zygote but that has two or more kinds of genetically different cell populations. Such a condition results from a mutation, crossing-over, or, more commonly in humans, nondisjunction of the chromosomes during early embryogenesis, which causes a variation in the number of chromosomes in the cells. **2.** (in embryology) a fertilized ovum that undergoes determinate cleavage.

mosaic bone, bone tissue appearing to be made up of many tiny pieces cemented together, as seen on microscopic examination of an x-ray film of the affected bone. It is characteristic of Paget's disease of the bone.

mosaic cleavage. See **determinate cleavage.**

mosaic development, a kind of embryonic development occurring in the blastocyst. The fertilized ovum undergoes determinate cleavage, developing according to a precise, unalterable plan in which each blastomere has a characteristic position, limited developmental potency, and is a precursor of a definite part of the embryo.

mosaicism /mōzā'isiz'əm/ [L *Musa* goddess of the arts], (in genetics) a condition in which an individual or an organism that develops from a single zygote has two or more cell populations that differ in genetic constitution.

mosaic wart, a group of contiguous plantar warts.

mosquito bite [L *musca* a fly; AS *bitan* to bite], a bite of a bloodsucking arthropod of the subfamily Culicidae that may result in a systemic allergic reaction in a hypersensitive person, an infection, or, most often, a pruritic wheal.

mosquito forceps, a small hemostatic forceps.

Mössbauer spectrometer /mes'bou·ər, mœs'bou·ər/ [Rudolf L. Mössbauer, German physicist, b. 1929], an instrument that can detect small changes between an atomic nucleus and its environment, such as caused by changes in temperature, pressure, or chemical state.

mother fixation [AS *modor* mother; L *figere* to fasten], an arrest in psychosexual development characterized by an abnormally persistent, close, and often paralyzing emotional attachment to one's mother.

mother yaw. See yaw.

motile /mō´til/ [L *motare* to move often], capable of spontaneous but unconscious or involuntary movement. **–motility,** *n.*

motion sickness [L *motio* movement; AS *seoc* sick; OE *nes* condition], a condition caused by erratic or rhythmic motions in any combination of directions, such as in a boat or a car. Severe cases are characterized by nausea, vomiting, vertigo, and headache; mild cases by headache and general discomfort.

motivation [L *movere* to move], conscious or unconscious needs, interests, rewards, or other incentives that arouse, channel, or maintain a particular behavior.

motivational conflict [L *motus* cause of motion, *alis* relating to; *confluere* to come together], a conflict resulting from the arousal of two or more motives that direct behavior toward incompatible goals. Kinds of motivational conflict include **approach-approach conflict, approach-avoidance conflict,** and **avoidance-avoidance conflict.**

motoneuron /mō´tōn oor´on/ [L *movere* to move; Gk *neuron* nerve], a motor neuron, or a neuron whose axon ends on muscle fibers or other effector organs.

motor [L *motare* to move about], **1.** of or pertaining to motion, the body apparatus involved in movement, or the brain functions that direct purposeful activities. **2.** of or pertaining to a muscle, nerve, or brain center that produces or subserves motion.

motor aphasia, the inability to utter remembered words, caused by a cerebral lesion in the inferior frontal gyrus (Broca's motor speech area) of the left hemisphere in right-handed individuals. The condition most commonly is the result of a stroke. The patient knows what to say but cannot articulate the words.

motor apraxia, the inability to carry out planned movements or to handle small objects, although the proper use of the object is recognized. The condition results from a lesion in the premotor frontal cortex on the opposite side of the affected limb.

motor area, a portion of the cerebral cortex that includes the precentral gyrus and the posterior part of the frontal gyri and that causes the contraction of the voluntary muscles on stimulation with electrodes. Normal voluntary activity requires associations between the motor area and other parts of the cortex; removal of the motor area from one cerebral hemisphere causes paralysis of voluntary muscles, especially of the opposite side of the body.

motor coordination, the coordination of body functions that involve movement, including gross motor, fine motor, and motor planning.

motor depressant, a drug or agent that reduces the normal functioning level of motor neurons, mainly in voluntary muscles.

motor end plate, a broad band of terminal fibers of the motor nerves of the voluntary muscles. Motor nerves derived from the cranial and spinal nerves enter the sheaths of striated muscle fibers, lose their myelin sheaths, and ramify like the roots of a tree. The neurilemma of the nerve fiber merges with the sarcolemma of the muscle, and the axon synapses with the muscle fibers.

motor fiber, one of the fibers in the spinal nerves that transmit impulses to muscle fibers.

motor hallucination [L *motus* mover; *alucinari* wandering mind], the subjective experience of movement when there is no movement.

motor image, a visual concept of one's bodily movements, real or imagined.

motor nerve. See motor neuron.

motor neuron, one of various efferent nerve cells that transmit nerve impulses from the brain or from the spinal cord to muscular or glandular tissue.

motor neuron disease [L *movere* to move; *neuron* nerve; L *dis;* Fr *aise* ease], a progressive disease that tends to affect middle-aged men with degeneration of anterior horn cells, motor cranial nerve nuclei, and pyramidal tracts. An example is **amyotrophic lateral sclerosis (ALS).**

motor neuron paralysis, an injury to the spinal cord that causes damage to the motor neurons and results in various degrees of functional impairment depending on the site of the lesion.

motor nucleus [L *movere, nucleus* nut], the nucleus of a motor nerve or a collection of motor neurons.

motor pathway [L *movere;* AS *paeth*], the route of motor nerve impulses, from the central neuron to a muscle or gland.

motor planning, the ability to plan and execute skilled nonhabitual tasks.

motor point, 1. a point at which a motor nerve enters the muscle it innervates. **2.** a

M

motor praxis. See **motor planning.**

motor root, the proximal end of a motor nerve at its attachment to the spinal cord.

motor seizure, a transitory disturbance in brain function caused by abnormal neuronal discharges that arise initially in a localized motor area of the cerebral cortex. The manifestations depend on the site of the abnormal electric activity, such as tonic contractures of the thumb, caused by excessive discharges in the motor area of the cortex controlling the first digit.

motor sense, the feeling or perception enabling a person to accomplish a purposeful movement, presumably achieved by evoking a sensory engram or memory of the pattern for that specific movement.

motor speech area, the regions of the cerebral hemispheres that are associated with motor control of speech. For right-handed persons the sites are generally located in the left hemisphere. Patients with specific language defects often are found to have lesions in the left hemisphere.

motor tract, an efferent nerve pathway that conveys impulses controlling movement.

motor unit, a functional structure consisting of a motor neuron and the muscle fibers it innervates.

mottle [ME *motley* mixed colors], an effect observed in radiologic imaging when the dose of radiation employed is reduced to a level where individual quantum effects can be seen.

mountain fever, mountain tick fever. See **Colorado tick fever, Rocky Mountain spotted fever.**

mountain sickness. See **altitude sickness.**

mourning [AS *murnan* to mourn], a psychologic process of reaction activated by an individual to assist in overcoming a great personal loss. The process is finally resolved when a new object relationship is established.

mouse-tooth forceps, a kind of dressing forceps that has one or more fine sharp points on the tip of each blade. The tips turn in, and the delicate teeth interlock.

mouth [AS *muth*]. **1.** the nearly oval oral cavity at the anterior end of the digestive tube, bounded anteriorly by the lips and containing the tongue and the teeth. It consists of the vestibule and the mouth cavity proper. The vestibule, situated in front of the teeth, is bounded externally by the lips and the cheeks, internally by the gums and the teeth. The vestibule receives the secretion from the parotid salivary glands and communicates, when the jaws are closed, with the mouth cavity proper by an aperture on each side behind the molar teeth and by narrow clefts between opposing teeth. The mouth is roofed by the hard and the soft palates. The tongue forms the greater part of the floor of the cavity. **2.** an orifice.

mouth guard, a soft plastic intraoral appliance that covers all the occlusal surfaces and the palate. It is worn in contact sports to limit damage to tissues of the oral surfaces.

mouthstick, a device that can be manipulated with the mouth and can be used to type, push buttons, turn pages, or operate power wheelchairs and other equipment for paralyzed patients.

mouth-to-mouth resuscitation, a procedure in artificial resuscitation, performed most often with cardiac massage. The victim's nose is sealed by pinching the nostrils closed, the head is extended, and air is breathed by the rescuer through the mouth into the lungs.

mouth-to-nose resuscitation, a procedure in artificial resuscitation in which the mouth of the victim is covered and held closed and air is breathed through the victim's nose.

MOV, abbreviation for **minimal occlusive volume.**

movement decomposition [L *movere* to go; *de* away, *componere* to assemble], a distortion in voluntary movement in which the movement occurs in a distinct sequence of isolated steps, rather than in a normal, smooth, flowing pattern.

moving grid, (in radiography) an x-ray grid that is continuously moved or oscillated throughout the exposure of a radiographic film.

moxibustion /mok′səbus′chən/ [Jap *moe kusa* burning herb; L *comburere* to burn up], a method of producing analgesia or altering the function of a system of the body by igniting moxa, wormwood, or other combustible, slow-burning substance and holding it as near the point on the skin as possible without causing pain or burning. It is also sometimes used in conjunction with acupuncture.

MPD, abbreviation for **maximum permissible dose.**

MPH, abbreviation for *Master of Public Health.*

MPL + PRED, an anticancer drug combination of melphalan and prednisone.

MPS, abbreviation for **mucopolysaccharidosis.**

MPS I, abbreviation for *mucopolysaccharidosis I.* See **Hurler's syndrome.**

MPS II, abbreviation for *mucopolysaccharidosis II.* See **Hunter's syndrome.**

MPS IV, abbreviation for *mucopolysaccharidosis IV.* See **Morquio's disease.**

MQF, abbreviation for *mobile quarantine facility.*

mr, mR, abbreviation for **milliroentgen.**

mrad, abbreviation for **millirad.**

mrem, abbreviation for *millirem.*

MRI, abbreviation for **magnetic resonance imaging.**

mRNA, abbreviation for **messenger RNA.**

MS, abbreviation for **multiple sclerosis.**

MS, 1. abbreviation for *Master of Science.* **2.** abbreviation for *Master of Surgery.*

msec, abbreviation for **millisecond.**

MSH, abbreviation for **melanocyte-stimulating hormone.**

MSN, abbreviation for *Master of Science in Nursing.*

MT, abbreviation for **medical technologist.**

MTX + MP + CTX, an anticancer drug combination of methotrexate, mercaptopurine, and cyclophosphamide.

mu /moo, myoo/, **1.** μ, Greek letter. **2.** symbol for **micron.**

Much's granules /mooks, mookhs/ [Hans C. Much, German physician, b. 1880], granules and rods, found in tuberculosis sputum, that stain with gram stain but not by the usual methods for acid-fast bacilli.

mucin /myoo'sin/ [L *mucus* slime], a mucopolysaccharide, the chief ingredient in mucus. Mucin is present in most glands that secrete mucus and is the lubricant protecting body surfaces from friction or erosion.

mucinoid /myoo'sinoid/ [L *mucus* + Gk *eidos* form], resembling mucin.

mucinoid adenocarcinoma. See **mucinous carcinoma.**

mucinous carcinoma /myoo'sinəs/, an epithelial neoplasm with a sticky gelatinous consistency caused by the copious mucin secreted by its cells.

mucocutaneous /myoo'kōkyootā'nē-əs/ [L *mucus* + *cutis* skin, *osus* having], of or pertaining to the mucous membrane and the skin.

mucocutaneous leishmaniasis. See **American leishmaniasis.**

mucocutaneous lymph node syndrome (MLNS), an acute, febrile illness, primarily of young children, characterized by inflamed mucous membranes of the mouth, "strawberry tongue," cervical lymphadenopathy, polymorphous rash on the trunk, and edema, erythema, and desquamation of the skin on the extremities. Other commonly associated findings include arthralgia, diarrhea, otitis, pneumonia, photophobia, meningitis, and electrocardiographic changes.

mucoepidermoid carcinoma /myoo'-kō-ep'idur'moid/ [L *mucus* + Gk *epi* above, *derma* skin, *eidos* form], a malignant neoplasm of glandular tissues, especially the ducts of the salivary glands.

mucogingival junction /myoo kōjinjī'vəl/ [L *mucus* + *gingiva* gum; *jungere* to join], the scalloped linear area of the gums that separates the gingivae from the alveolar mucosa.

mucoid /myoo'koid/ [L *mucus* + Gk *eidos* form] **1.** resembling mucus. **2.** a group of glycoproteins, including colloid and ovomucoid, similar to the mucins, the primary difference being in solubility.

mucoid cyst, a cyst formed by an overgrowth of a mucus gland or by the spread of mucus into the interstitial tissues.

mucoid tissue. See **embryonic tissue.**

mucolytic /myoo'kəlit'ik/ [L *mucus* + Gk *lysis* loosening], **1.** exerting a destructive effect on the mucus. **2.** any agent that dissolves or destroys the mucus.

mucomembranous /myoo'kəmem'brənəs/ [L *mucus* + *membrana* thin skin, *osus* having], of or pertaining to a mucous membrane, such as that of the small intestine or the bladder.

mucopolysaccharide /myoo'kōpol'ēsak'-ərīd/ [L *mucus* + Gk *polys* many, *sakcharon* sugar], a polysaccharide containing hexosamine and sometimes occurring with protein, such as mucins.

mucopolysaccharidosis (MPS) /myoo'-kōpol'ēsak'əridō'sis/, *pl.* **mucopolysaccharidoses** [L *mucus* + *polys* many, *sakcharon* sugar, *osis* condition], one of a group of genetic disorders characterized by greater than normal accumulations of mucopolysaccharides in the tissues, with other symptoms specific to each type. The disorders are numbered MPS I through MPS VII, and each type has a specific eponym. In all types there is pronounced skeletal deformity (especially of the face), mental and physical retardation, and decreased life expectancy. Kinds of mucopolysaccharidoses include **Hunter's syndrome (MPS II), Hurler's syndrome (MPS I),** and **Morquio's disease (MPS IV).**

mucoprotein /myoo'kōprō'tēn, -tē-in/ [L *mucus* + Gk *proteios* first rank], a compound, present in all connective and supporting tissue, that contains polysaccharides combined with protein and is relatively resistant to denaturation.

mucopurulent /myoo'kōpyŏor'yələnt/ [L

mucus + *purulentus* pus], characteristic of a combination of mucus and pus.

mucormycosis. See **zygomycosis.**

mucosa /myo͞okō′sə/, *pl.* mucosae, mucous membrane. –**mucosal,** *adj.*

mucositis /myo͞o′kōsī′tis/, any inflammation of a mucous membrane, such as the lining of the mouth and throat.

mucous. See **mucus.**

mucous colitis. See **irritable bowel syndrome.**

mucous membrane /myo͞o′kəs/ [L *mucus* + *membrana* thin skin], any one of four major kinds of thin sheets of tissue that cover or line various parts of the body. Mucous membranes line cavities or canals of the body that open to the outside, such as the linings of the mouth, the digestive tube, the respiratory passages, and the genitourinary tract. It consists of a surface layer of epithelial tissue covering a deeper layer of connective tissue and protects the underlying structure, secretes mucus, and absorbs water, salts, and other solutes.

mucous plug, (in obstetrics) a collection of thick mucus in the uterine cervix that is often expelled at the onset of dilation of the cervix, just before labor begins or in its early hours.

mucous shreds. See **shreds.**

mucous tissue. See **embryonic tissue.**

mucous tumor. See **myxoma.**

mucoviscidosis. See **cystic fibrosis.**

mucus /myo͞o′kəs/ [L, slime], the viscous, slippery secretions of mucous membranes and glands, containing mucin, white blood cells, water, inorganic salts, and exfoliated cells. –**mucoid,** *adj.,* **mucous** /myo͞o′kəs/, *adj.*

mucus trap suction apparatus, a catheter containing a trap to prevent mucus being aspirated into the nasopharynx and trachea of a newborn infant and entering the mouth of the person operating the device.

mud bath, the application of warm mud to the body for therapeutic purposes.

mulibrey nanism /mul′ibrī/, a rare genetic disorder characterized by dwarfism, constrictive pericarditis, muscular hypotonia, anomalies of the skull and face, and characteristic yellow dots in the ocular fundus. The name of the condition is an acronym composed of the first two letters of the anatomic sites of the principal defects: *mu*scle, *li*ver, *br*ain, and *ey*es.

müllerian duct /miler′ē·ən, mYl-/ [Johannes P. Müller, German physiologist, b. 1801], one of a pair of embryonic ducts that become the fallopian tubes, uterus, and vagina in females and that atrophy in males.

Müller's maneuver [Johannes P. Müller], an inspiratory effort against a closed airway or glottis. The effort decreases intrapulmonary and intrathoracic pressures and expands pulmonary gas.

multicentric mitosis. See **multipolar mitosis.**

multidisciplinary health care team, a group of health care workers who are members of different disciplines, each one providing specific services to the patient.

multifactorial [L *multus* many, *facere* to make], of, pertaining to, or characteristic of any condition or disease resulting from the interaction of many factors, specifically the interaction of several genes, usually polygenes, with or without the involvement of environmental factors. Many disorders, such as spina bifida, are considered to be multifactorial.

multifactorial inheritance, the tendency to develop a physical appearance, disease, or condition that is a condition of many genetic and environmental factors, such as stature and blood pressure.

multifocal [L *multus* + *focus* hearth], an action, such as the transmission of an impulse, that arises from more than two foci.

multiform [L *multus* many, *forma*], an organ, tissue, or other object that may appear in more than one shape.

multigenerational model, a model of family therapy that focuses on reciprocal role relationships over a period of time. The family is viewed as an emotional system where patterns of interacting and coping can be passed from one generation to the next and can cause stress to the members on whom they are projected.

multigenerational transmission process, the repetition of relationship patterns, including divorce, suicide, or alcoholism, associated with emotional dysfunction that can be traced through several generations of the same family.

multigravida /mul′tigrav′idə/ [L *multus* + *gravidare* to impregnate], a woman who has been pregnant more than once.

multihospital system, a group of two or more hospitals owned, sponsored, or managed by a central organization.

multiinfarct dementia /mul′ti·infärkt′/ [L *multus* + *infarcire* to stuff; *de* away, *mens* mind], a form of organic brain disease characterized by the rapid deterioration of intellectual functioning, caused by vascular disease. Symptoms include emotional lability, disturbances in memory, abstract thinking, judgment, and impulse control, and focal neurologic impairment, such as gait abnormalities, pseudobulbar palsy, and paresthesia.

multilocular cyst /mul′tilok′yələr/ [L *mul-*

tus + *locilus* little place; Gk *kystis* bag], one of three kinds of follicular cyst, containing many spaces and not associated with a tooth.

multipara /multip′ərə/, *pl.* **multiparae** [L *multus* + *parere* to bear], a woman who has delivered more than one viable infant.

multiparity /mul′tiper′itē/, the status of a mother of more than one child.

multiparous /multip′ərous/, having given birth to more than one child.

multipenniform /mul′tipen′ifôrm/ [L *multus* + *penna* feather, *forma*], (of a bodily structure) having a shape resembling a pattern of many feathers.

multiphasic screening /mul′tifā′sik/ [L *multus* + *phasis* appearance; ME *scren*], a technique of screening populations for diseases in which there is combined use of a battery of screening tests. The technique serves to identify any of several diseases being screened for in a population.

multiple benign cystic epithelioma. See **trichoepithelioma.**

multiple cartilaginous exostoses. See **diaphyseal aclasis.**

multiple enchondromatosis. See **enchondromatosis.**

multiple endocrine adenomatosis. See **adenomatosis.**

multiple factor. See **polygene.**

multiple family therapy [L *multus* + *plica* fold], psychotherapy in which four or five families meet weekly to confront and deal with problems or issues that they have in common.

multiple fission, cell division in which the nucleus first divides into several equal parts followed by the division of the cytoplasm into as many cells as there are nuclei.

multiple fracture, 1. a fracture extending several fracture lines in one bone. **2.** the fracture of several bones at one time or from the same injury.

multiple gene. See **polygene.**

multiple idiopathic hemorrhagic sarcoma. See **Kaposi's sarcoma.**

multiple lipomatosis, a rare, inherited disorder characterized by discrete, localized, subcutaneous deposits of fat in the tissues of the body.

multiple mononeuropathy, an abnormal condition characterized by dysfunction of several individual nerve trunks. It may be caused by various diseases.

multiple myeloma, a malignant neoplasm of the bone marrow. The tumor, composed of plasma cells, destroys osseous tissue, especially in flat bones, causing pain, fractures, and skeletal deformities.

multiple myositis. See **polymyositis.**

multiple neuroma. See **neuromatosis.**

multiple peripheral neuritis, acute or subacute disseminated inflammation or degeneration of symmetrically distributed peripheral nerves, characterized initially by numbness, tingling in the extremities, hot and cold sensations, and slight fever, progressing to pain, weakness, diminished reflexes, and in some cases flaccid paralysis. The disorder may be caused by toxic substances, such as antimony, arsenic, carbon monoxide, copper, lead, mercury, nitrobenzol, organophosphates, and thallium, or various drugs.

multiple personality, an abnormal condition in which the organization of the personality is fragmented. It is characterized by the presence of two or more distinct subpersonalities.

multiple personality disorder, a dissociative disorder characterized by the existence of two or more distinct, clearly differentiated personality structures within the same individual, any of which may dominate at a particular time. The various subpersonalities are usually dramatically different from one another and may or may not be aware of the existence of the others. Transition from one subpersonality to another is usually sudden and associated with psychosocial stress.

multiple plasmacytoma of bone. See **multiple myeloma.**

multiple pregnancy, a pregnancy in which there is more than one fetus in the uterus at the same time.

multiple sclerosis (MS) [L *multus* + *plica* fold; Gk *sklerosis* hardening], a progressive disease characterized by disseminated demyelination of nerve fibers of the brain and spinal cord. The first signs are paresthesias, or abnormal sensations in the extremities or on one side of the face. Other early signs are muscle weakness, vertigo, and visual disturbances, such as nystagmus, diplopia (double vision), and partial blindness. Later in the course of disease there may be extreme emotional lability, ataxia, abnormal reflexes, and difficulty in urinating.

multiple self-healing squamous epithelioma. See **keratoacanthoma.**

multiple transfusion syndrome, a hemorrhagic reaction to massive transfusions of platelet-poor stored blood. Other clotting factors seldom contribute to the condition. Platelet concentrates may be given to correct the deficiency.

multiplicative growth. See **merisis.**

multipolar mitosis /mul′tipō′lər/ [L *multus* + *polus* pole], cell division in which the spindle has three or more poles and results in the formation of a corresponding number of daughter cells.

multisource drug [L *multus* + OFr *sourse* origin], a drug that can be purchased under any of several trademarks from different manufacturers or distributors.

multisynaptic /mul′tisinap′tik/ [L *multus* + Gk *synaptein* to join], pertaining to a nervous process or system of nerve cells requiring a series of synapses.

multivalent /mul′tivā′lənt/ [L *multus* + *valere* to be strong], **1.** (in chemistry) denoting the capacity of an element to combine with three or more univalent atoms. **2.** (in immunology) able to act against more than one strain of organism.

multivalent vaccine, a vaccine prepared from several antigenic types within a species.

mummification /mum′ifikā′shən/ [Per *mum* wax; L *facere* to make], a dried-up state, such as occurs in dry gangrene or a dead fetus in utero.

mummified fetus, a fetus that has died in utero and has shriveled and dried up.

mumps [D *mompen* to sulk], an acute viral disease, characterized by a swelling of the parotid glands, caused by a paramyxovirus. It is most likely to affect children between 5 and 15 years of age, but it may occur at any age. In adulthood the infection may be severe. The incidence of mumps is highest during the late winter and early spring. The mumps paramyxovirus lives in the saliva of the affected individual and is transmitted in droplets or by direct contact. The virus is present in the saliva from 6 days before to 9 days after the onset of the swelling of the parotid gland. The prognosis in mumps is good, but the disease sometimes involves complications, such as arthritis, pancreatitis, myocarditis, oophoritis, and nephritis. About one half of the men with mumps-induced orchitis suffer some atrophy of the testicles, but because the condition is usually unilateral, sterility rarely results. Common symptoms include anorexia, headache, malaise, and low-grade fever, followed by earache, parotid gland swelling, and a temperature of 101° to 104° F (38.3° to 40° C). The patient also experiences pain when drinking acidic liquids or when chewing. The salivary glands may also become swollen.

mumps virus vaccine live, an active immunizing agent prescribed for immunization against mumps.

Munchausen's syndrome /mun′chousənz/ [Baron von Munchausen, legendary eighteenth-century confabulator], an unusual condition characterized by habitual pleas for treatment and hospitalization for a symptomatic but imaginary acute illness. The affected person may logically and convincingly present the symptoms and history of a real disease.

mural /myŏŏ′rəl/ [L *murus* wall], something that is found on or against the wall of a cavity, as a mural thrombus on an interior wall of the heart.

Murchison fever. See **Pel-Ebstein fever.**

muriatic acid /mŏŏ′rē·at′ik/ [L, *muria,* brine; *acidus,* sour], hydrochloric acid.

murine typhus /myŏŏ′rēn/ [L *mus* mouse; Gk *typhos* stupor], an acute arbovirus infection caused by *Rickettsia typhi* and transmitted by the bite of an infected flea. The disease is similar to epidemic typhus but less severe. It is characterized by headache, chills, fever, myalgia, and rash. A dull-red, maculopapular rash, mainly on the trunk, appears about the fifth day and lasts for 4 to 8 days.

murmur [L, a humming], a low-pitched fluttering or humming sound, such as a heart murmur.

muromonab-CD3 /myŏŏ′rəmon′ab/, a parenteral immunosuppressant drug used in the control of acute renal transplant rejection.

Murphy's sign, a test for gallbladder disease in which the patient is asked to inspire while the examiner's fingers are held under the liver border at the bottom of the rib cage. The inspiration causes the gallbladder to descend onto the fingers, producing pain if the gallbladder is inflamed.

muscae volitantes. See **floater.**

muscarine /mus′kərēn/ [L *musca* fly], a choline-related alkaloid present in the poisonous mushroom *Amanita muscaria.* It is similar pharmacologically to acetylcholine, although it is not used in therapeutics.

muscarinic /mus′kərin′ik/ [L *musca* fly], stimulating the postganglionic parasympathetic receptor.

muscle [L *musculus*], a kind of tissue composed of fibers that are able to contract, causing and allowing movement of the parts and organs of the body. Muscle fibers are richly vascular, irritable, conductive, and elastic. There are two basic kinds, striated muscle and smooth muscle. Striated muscle, which comprises all skeletal muscles except for the myocardium, is long and voluntary; it responds very quickly to stimulation and is paralyzed by interruption of its innervation. Smooth muscle, which comprises all visceral muscles, is short and involuntary; it reacts slowly to all stimuli and does not entirely lose its tone if innervation is interrupted. The myocardium is sometimes classified as a third (cardiac) kind of muscle, but it is basically a striated muscle that does not contract as quickly as the striated muscle of the rest of the body, and it is not completely paralyzed if it loses its neural stimuli.

muscle albumin, albumin present in muscle.

muscle biopsy, an examination of surgically removed muscle tissue for diagnosis.

muscle bridge, a band of myocardial tissue over one or more of the large epicardial coronary vessels. It may cause constriction of the artery during systole.

muscle of expression. See **facial muscle.**

muscle reeducation, the use of physical therapeutic exercises to restore muscle tone and strength after an injury or disease.

muscle relaxant, a chemotherapeutic agent that reduces the contractility of muscle fibers. Curare derivatives and succinylcholine compete with acetylcholine and block neural transmission at the myoneural junction. Quinine sulfate reduces muscle tension by increasing the refractory period of muscle fibers and by decreasing the excitability of the motor end plate. Baclofen inhibits monosynaptic and polysynaptic reflexes at the spinal level. Cyclobenzaprine acts primarily in the brainstem. Chlorzoxazone inhibits multisynaptic arcs in the spinal cord and subcortical areas of the brain. The benzodiazepines reduce muscle tension, chiefly by acting on reticular neuronal mechanisms that control muscle tone. Dantrolene apparently achieves its effect by interfering with the release of calcium from the sarcoplasmic reticulum.

muscle-setting exercise, a method of maintaining muscle strength and tonality by alternately contracting and relaxing a skeletal muscle or any group of muscles without moving the associated part of the body.

muscles of respiration, muscles that provide inspiration, partly by increasing the volume of the chest cavity so that air is drawn into the lungs, include the diaphragm and external intercostals. They are aided during forced breathing by the scaleni, levatores costarum, sternocleidomastoideus, greater pectoral, platysma myoides, and superior posterior serratus. Muscles of forced expiration include the external and internal oblique, rectus abdominus and transverse abdominus.

muscle spindle [L *musculus;* AS *spinel*], a specialized proprioceptive sensory organ composed of a bundle of fine striated intrafusal muscle fibers innervated by gamma nerve fibers. Their nuclei are gathered together near the center of each fiber to form a nuclear sac, which is surrounded in turn by sensory, annulospiral nerve endings, all enclosed in a fibrous sheath.

muscle testing, a method of evaluating the contractile unit, including the muscle, tendons, and associated tissues, of a moving part of the body by neurologic or resistance testing. The tests may include range-of-motion ability, isokinetic measurement of muscle strength, and functional tests, such as specific agility drills, as well as other medical tests.

muscle tone, a normal state of balanced muscle tension.

muscular [L *musculus*], **1.** of or pertaining to a muscle. **2.** characteristic of well-developed musculature.

muscular atrophy, a condition of motor unit dysfunction, usually the result of a loss of efferent innervation.

muscular branch of the deep brachial artery, one of several similar branches of the deep brachial artery, supplying certain arm muscles, such as the coracobrachialis, biceps brachii, and brachialis.

muscular dystrophy [L *musculus* + Gk *dys* bad, *trophe* nourishment], a group of genetically transmitted diseases characterized by progressive atrophy of symmetric groups of skeletal muscles without evidence of involvement or degeneration of neural tissue. In all forms of muscular dystrophy there is an insidious loss of strength with increasing disability and deformity, although each type differs in the groups of muscles affected, the age of onset, the rate of progression, and the mode of genetic inheritance. The main types of the disease are pseudohypertrophic (Duchenne) muscular dystrophy, limb-girdle muscular dystrophy, and facioscapulohumeral (Landouzy-Déjérine) muscular dystrophy. Rarer forms include Becker's muscular dystrophy, distal muscular dystrophy, ocular myopathy, and myotonic muscular dystrophy.

muscular incompetence, a failure of a cardiac valve to close properly because of incompetence of the papillary muscles of the heart.

muscular sarcoidosis, sarcoidosis of the skeletal muscles in which there is interstitial inflammation, fibrosis, atrophy, and damage of the muscle fibers as sarcoid tubercles form within and replace normal muscle cells.

muscular system, all of the muscles of the body, including the smooth, cardiac, and striated muscles, considered as an interrelated structural group.

muscular tension [L *musculus* + *tendere* to stretch], strain that results from muscular contractions. Internal tension is caused by crossbridge activity between the

M

actin and myosin filaments within the muscle fiber. The force generated by these contractile elements is transmitted to the bones via tendons and connective tissue. The bones move and produce external tension.

muscular tone [L *musculus;* Gk *tonos* stretching], a normal degree of tension in muscles at rest.

muscular tremor, minute regular involuntary contraction of individual muscle fasciculi. If the tremors are mild and occasional, the cause may be physiologic. Profuse, persistent or recurrent widespread muscular twitching often indicates a motor neuron disorder.

muscular triangle. See **inferior cartoid triangle.**

muscular tumor. See **myoma.**

musculature, the arrangement and condition of the muscles.

musculocutaneous nerve /mus'-kyəlōkōōtā'nē·əs/ [L *musculus* + *cutis* skin, *osus* having], one of the terminal branches of the brachial plexus. It is formed on each side by division of the lateral cord of the plexus into two branches. Various branches and filaments supply different structures, such as the biceps, the brachialis, the humerus, and the skin of the forearm.

musculoskeletal /mus'kyŏōlōskel'ətəl/ [L *musculus* + Gk *skeletos* dried up], of or pertaining to the muscles and the skeleton.

musculoskeletal system, all of the muscles, bones, joints, and related structures, such as the tendons and connective tissue, that function in the movement of the parts and organs of the body.

musculoskeletal system assessment, an evaluation of the condition and functioning of the patient's muscles, joints, and bones and of factors that may contribute to abnormalities in these body structures.

musculospiral nerve. See **radial nerve.**

mush bite, a procedure used in making dental impressions for the construction of full or partial dentures. The patient brings his or her upper and lower jaws together into a block of softened wax, thus supplying a spatial relationship between the maxilla and mandible.

mushroom [ME *mucheron*], the fruiting body of the fungus of the class Basidomycetes, especially edible members of the order Agaricales, known as the field mushrooms or meadow mushrooms. Mushrooms are composed largely of water and are of limited nutritional value. Fungal poisoning is caused by ingestion of mushrooms of the genus *Amanita,* in particular *A. muscaria* and *A. phalloides.*

mushroom poisoning, a toxic condition caused by the ingestion of certain mushrooms, particularly two species of the genus *Amanita.* Muscarine in *Amanita muscaria* produces intoxication in from a few minutes to 2 hours. Symptoms include lacrimation, salivation, sweating, vomiting, labored breathing, abdominal cramps, diarrhea, and, in severe cases, convulsions, coma, and circulatory failure. Atropine is usually administered in treatment. More deadly but slower-acting phalloidine in *A. phalloides* and *A. verna* causes similar symptoms, as well as liver damage, renal failure, and death in 30% to 50% of the cases.

music therapy [Gk *mousike* music; *therapeia* treatment], a form of adjunctive psychotherapy in which music is used as a means of recreation and communication, especially with autistic children, and as a means to elevate the mood of depressed and psychotic patients.

mustard gas, a poisonous gas used in chemical warfare during World War I. It causes corrosive destruction of the skin and mucous membranes, often resulting in permanent respiratory damage and death.

mustard plaster [L *mustum;* Gk *emplastron*], a mustard medication in a fabric base that can be placed close to the skin for a period of time as a counter-irritant in the form of a poultice.

mutacism /myōō'təsiz'əm/, mimmation, or the incorrect use of /m/ sounds.

mutagen /myōō'təjən/ [L *mutare* to change, *genein* to produce], any chemical or physical environmental agent that induces a genetic mutation or increases the mutation rate. **–mutagenic,** *adj.,* **mutagenicity,** *n.*

mutagenesis /myōō'təjen'əsis/, the induction or occurrence of a genetic mutation.

mutant [L *mutare* to change], **1.** any individual or organism with genetic material that has undergone mutation. **2.** relating to or produced by mutation.

mutant gene, any gene that has undergone a change, such as the loss, gain, or exchange of genetic material, that affects the normal transmission and expression of a trait. Kinds of mutant genes are **amorph, antimorph, hypermorph, hypomorph.**

mutase /myōō'tās/, any enzyme that catalyzes the shifting of a chemical group or radical from one position to another within the same molecule or, occasionally, from one molecule to another.

mutation [L *mutare* to change], an unusual change in genetic material occurring spontaneously or by induction. The alteration changes the original expression of the gene. Genes are stable units, but when a mutation occurs, it often is transmitted to future generations. **–mutate,** *v.,* **mutational,** *adj.*

mutism /myo͞o′tizəm/ [L *mutus* dumb], the inability to speak because of a physical defect or emotional problem.

muton /myo͞o′ton/, (in molecular genetics), the smallest DNA segment whose alteration can result in a mutation.

mutually exclusive categories, categories on a research instrument that are sufficiently precise to allow each subject, factor, or variable to be classified in only one category.

mutual support group, a type of group in which members organize to solve their own problems. They are led by the group members themselves who share a common goal and use their own strengths to gain control over their lives.

mv, mV, abbreviation for **millivolt.**

mV̇O₂, symbol for *myocardial oxygen consumption.*

MVV, abbreviation for **maximal voluntary ventilation.**

MWIA, abbreviation for **Medical Women's International Association.**

MX gene, a human gene that helps the body resist viral infections. When exposed to interferon the MX gene inhibits the production of viral protein and nucleic acid necessary for the proliferation of new viral particles.

myalgia /mī·al′jə/ [Gk *mys* muscle, *algos* pain], diffuse muscle pain, usually accompanied by malaise. **–myalgic,** *adj.*

myalgic asthenia /mī·al′jik/ [Gk *mys* + *algos* pain; *a, sthenos* not strength], a condition characterized by a general feeling of fatigue and muscular pain, often resulting from or associated with psychologic stress.

myasthenia /mī′əsthē′nē·ə/ [Gk *mys* + *a, sthenos* not strength], a condition characterized by an abnormal weakness of a muscle or a group of muscles that may be the result of a systemic myoneural disturbance, as in myasthenia gravis, or myasthenia laryngis involving the vocal cord tensor muscles. **–myasthenic,** *adj.*

myasthenia gravis, an abnormal condition characterized by the chronic fatigability and weakness of muscles, especially in the face and throat, as a result of a defect in the conduction of nerve impulses at the myoneural junction. Muscular fatigability in myasthenia gravis is caused by the inability of receptors at the myoneural junction to depolarize because of a deficiency of acetylcholine; hence the diagnosis may be made by administering an anticholinesterase drug and observing improved muscle strength and stamina. The onset of symptoms is usually gradual, with ptosis

of the upper eyelids, diplopia, and weakness of the facial muscles. The weakness may then extend to other muscles innervated by the cranial nerves, particularly the respiratory muscles. Muscular exertion aggravates the symptoms.

myasthenia gravis crisis, acute exacerbation of the muscular weakness characterizing the disease, triggered by infection, surgery, emotional stress, or an overdose or insufficiency of anticholinesterase medication. Typical signs and symptoms include respiratory distress progressing to periods of apnea, extreme fatigue, increased muscular weakness, dysphagia, dysarthria, and fever. The patient may be anxious, restless, irritable, and unable to move the jaws or to raise one or both eyelids.

myasthenic crisis /mī′asthen′ik/, an acute episode of muscular weakness.

mycelium /mīsē′lē·əm/, *pl.* **mycelia** [Gk *mykes* fungus, *helos* nail], a mass of interwoven, branched, threadlike filaments that make up most fungi.

mycetismus /mī′sitiz′məs/, mushroom poisoning.

mycetoma /mī′sətō′mə/ [Gk *mykes* + *oma* tumor], a serious fungal infection involving skin, subcutaneous tissue, fascia, and bone. One kind of mycetoma is **Madura foot.**

mycobacteria /mī′kōbaktir′ē·ə/ [Gk *mykes* + *bakterion* little rod], acid-fast microorganisms belonging to the genus *Mycobacterium.* **–mycobacterial,** *adj.*

mycobacteriosis /mī′kōbak′tirē·ō′sis/ [Gk *mykes, bakterion* + *osis* condition], a tuberculosis-like disease caused by mycobacteria other than *Mycobacterium tuberculosis.*

Mycobacterium /mī′kōbaktir′ē·əm/ [Gk *mykes* + *bakterion* little rod], a genus of rod-shaped, acid-fast bacteria having two significant pathogenic species: *Mycobacterium leprae* causes leprosy; *M. tuberculosis* causes tuberculosis.

mycology /mīkol′əjē/ [Gk *mykes* + *logos* science], the study of fungi and fungoid diseases. **–mycologic, mycological,** *adj.,* **mycologist,** *n.*

mycomyringitis. See **myringomycosis.**

mycophenolic acid /mī′kōfinō′lik/, a bacteriostatic and fungistatic crystalline antibiotic obtained from *Pencillium brevi compactum* and related species.

Mycoplasma /mī′kōplaz′mə/ [Gk *mykes* + *plassein* to mold], a genus of ultramicroscopic organisms lacking rigid cell walls and considered to be the smallest free-living organisms. Some are saprophytes, some are parasites, and many are pathogens.

M

mycoplasma pneumonia, a contagious disease of children and young adults caused by *Mycoplasma pneumoniae*, characterized by a 9- to 12-day incubation period and followed by symptoms of an upper respiratory infection, dry cough, and fever.

mycosis /mīkō'sis/ [Gk *mykes* + *osis* condition], any disease caused by a fungus. Some kinds of mycoses are **athlete's foot, candidiasis,** and **coccidioidomycosis.** –**mycotic,** *adj.*

mycosis fungoides /fung·goi'dēz/, a rare, chronic, lymphomatous skin malignancy resembling eczema or a cutaneous tumor that is followed by microabscesses in the epidermis and lesions simulating those of Hodgkin's disease in lymph nodes and viscera.

mycotic /mīkot'ik/ [Gk *mykes* fungus], pertaining to a disease caused by a fungus.

mycotic aneurysm, a localized dilatation in the wall of a blood vessel caused by the growth of a fungus, usually occurring as a complication of bacterial endocarditis.

mycotoxicosis /mī'kōtok'sikō'sis/ [Gk *mykes* + *toxikon* poison, *osis* condition], a systemic poisoning caused by toxins produced by fungal organisms.

mydriasis /midrī'əsis/ [Gk *mydros,* hot mass] **1.** dilatation of the pupil of the eye caused by contraction of the dilator muscle of the iris, a muscular sheath that radiates outward like the spokes of a wheel from the center of the iris around the pupil. **2.** an abnormal condition characterized by contraction of the dilator muscle, resulting in widely dilated pupils. –**mydriatic,** *adj.*

mydriatic and cycloplegic agent /mid'rē·at'ik/ [Gk *mydros* + *kyklos* circle, *plege* stroke], any one of several ophthalmic pharmaceutic preparations that dilate the pupil and paralyze the ocular muscles of accommodation. Mydriatics stimulate the sympathetic nerve fibers or block parasympathetic nerve fibers of the eye, temporarily paralyzing the iris sphincter muscle. Cycloplegics temporarily paralyze accommodation while relaxing the ciliary muscle. Some drugs may cause both mydriasis and cycloplegia, whereas others are designed to produce a single effect. These drugs are used in diagnostic ophthalmoscopic and refractive examination of the eye.

myelacephalus /mī'aləsef'ələs/ [Gk *myelos* marrow, *a, kephale* not head], a grossly malformed fetus, usually a separate monozygotic twin, whose form and parts are barely recognizable; a slightly differentiated amorphous mass. –**myelacephalous,** *adj.*

myelatelia /mī'əlatē'lē·ə/ [Gk *myelos* + *atelia* unfinished], any developmental defect involving the spinal cord.

myelauxe /mī'əlôk'sē/ [Gk *myelos* + *auxe* increasing], a developmental anomaly characterized by hypertrophy of the spinal cord.

myelencephalon /mī'əlensef'əlon/, the lower part of the embryonic hindbrain from which the medulla oblongata develops.

myelin /mī'əlin/ [Gk *myelos* marrow], a substance constituting the sheaths of various nerve fibers throughout the body. It is largely composed of fat, which gives the fibers a white, creamy color. –**myelinic,** *adj.*

myelinated /mī'əlinā'tid/, (of a nerve) having a myelin sheath.

myelination /mī'əlinā'shən/ [Gk *myelos* + L *atio* process], the process of furnishing or taking on myelin.

myelin globule, a fatlike droplet found in some sputum.

myelinic /mī'əlin'ik/ [Gk *myelos* + L *icus* form of], of or pertaining to myelin.

myelinic neuroma, a neuroma neoplasm composed of myelinated nerve fibers.

myelinization /mī'əlin'īzā'shən/ [Gk *myelos* + *izein* to cause], development of the myelin sheath around a nerve fiber.

myelinolysis /mī'əlinol'isis/ [Gk *myelos* + *lysein* to loosen], a pathologic process that dissolves the myelin sheaths around certain nerve fibers, such as those of the pons in alcoholic and undernourished people who are afflicted with central pontine myelinolysis.

myelin sheath, a segmented, fatty lamination composed of myelin that wraps the axons of many nerves in the body. In myelinated peripheral nerves, the sheaths are composed of Schwann cells. The myelin sheaths around the central nerve fibers are composed of oligodendroglia. Their lipoid content gives these coverings a whitish appearance. Various diseases, such as multiple sclerosis, can destroy these myelin wrappings.

myelitis /mī'əlī'tis/, an abnormal condition characterized by inflammation of the spinal cord with associated motor or sensory dysfunction. Some kinds of myelitis are **acute transverse myelitis, leukomyelitis,** and **poliomyelitis.** –**myelitic,** *adj.*

myeloblast /mī'əlōblast'/ [Gk *myelos* + *blastos* germ], one of the earliest precursors of the granulocytic leukocytes. The cytoplasm appears light blue, scanty, and nongranular when seen in a stained blood smear through a microscope. –**myeloblastic,** *adj.*

myeloblastemia. See **myeloblastosis.**

myeloblastic leukemia /mī'əlōblas'tik/, a

malignant neoplasm of blood-forming tissues, characterized by many myeloblasts in the circulating blood and tissues.

myeloblastomatosis /mī′əlōblas′tōmətō′-sis/ [Gk *myelos, blastos* + *oma* tumor, *osis* condition], abnormal, localized clusters of myeloblasts in the peripheral circulation.

myeloblastosis /mī′əloblastō′sis/ [Gk *myelos, blastos* + *osis* condition], the abnormal presence of myeloblasts in the peripheral circulation.

myelocele /mī′əlōsēl′/ [Gk *myelos* + *kele* hernia], a saclike protrusion of the spinal cord through a congenital defect in the vertebral column.

myeloclast /mī′əlōclast′/ [Gk *myelos* + *klastos* broken], a cell that breaks down the myelin sheaths of nerves of the central nervous system.

myelocyst /mī′əlōsist′/ [Gk *myelos* + *kystis* cyst], any benign cyst that is formed from the rudimentary medullary canals that give rise to the vertebral canal during embryonic development.

myelocystocele /mī′əlōsis′təsēl′/ [Gk *myelos, kystis* + *kele* hernia], a protrusion of a cystic tumor containing spinal cord substance through a defect in the vertebral column.

myelocystomeningocele /mī′əlōsis′-tōməning′gōsēl/ [Gk *myelos, kystis* + *menix* membrane, *kele* hernia], a protrusion of a cystic tumor containing both spinal cord substance and meninges through a defect in the vertebral column.

myelocyte /mī′əlōsīt′/ [Gk *myelos* + *kytos* cell], the first of the maturation stages of the granulocytic leukocytes normally found in the bone marrow. Granules are seen in the cytoplasm. The nuclear material of the myelocyte is denser than that of the myeloblast, but lacks a definable membrane. The cell is flat and contains increasing numbers of granules. —**myelocytic,** *adj.*

myelocythemia /mī′əlōsīthē′mē·ə/ [Gk *myelos, kytos* + *haima* blood], an abnormal presence of myelocytes in the circulating blood, such as in myelocytic leukemia.

myelocytic leukemia /mī′əlōsit′ik/, a disorder characterized by the unregulated and excessive production of myelocytes of the granulocytic series.

myelocytoma /mī′əlōsītō′mə/ [Gk *myelos* + *oma* tumor], a localized cluster of myelocytes in the peripheral vasculature that may occur in myelocytic leukemia.

myelocytosis. See **myelocythemia.**

myelodiastasis /mī′əlōdī·as′təsis/ [Gk *myelos* + *diastasis* separation], disintegration and necrosis of the spinal cord.

myelodysplasia /mī′əlōdisplā′zhə/ [Gk *myelos* + *dys* bad, *plassis* formation], a general designation for the defective development of any part of the spinal cord.

myelofibrosis. See **myeloid metaplasia.**

myelogenesis /mī′əlōjen′əsis/ [Gk *myelos* + *genein* to produce], **1.** the formation and differentiation of the nervous system during prenatal development. **2.** the development of the myelin sheath around the nerve fiber.

myelogenous /mī′əloj′ənəs/, pertaining to the cells produced in bone marrow or to the tissue from which such cells originate. Also **myelogenetic, myelogenic.**

myelogenous leukemia. See **acute myelocytic leukemia, chronic myelocytic leukemia.**

myelogeny /mī′əloj′ənē/ [Gk *myelos* + *genein* to produce], the formation and differentiation of the myelin sheaths of nerve fibers during the prenatal development of the central nervous system.

myelogram /mī′əlōgram′/, **1.** an x-ray film taken after the injection of a radiopaque medium into the subarachnoid space to demonstrate any distortions of the spinal cord, spinal nerve roots, and the subarachnoid space. **2.** a graphic representation of a count of the different kinds of cells in a stained preparation of bone marrow.

myelography /mī′əlog′rəfē/ [Gk *myelos* + *graphein* to record], a radiographic process by which the spinal cord and the spinal subarachnoid space are viewed and photographed after the introduction of a contrast medium, such as air or an absorbable contrast substance. —**myelographic,** *adj.*

myeloid /mī′əloid/ [Gk *myelos* + *eidos* form], **1.** of or pertaining to the bone marrow. **2.** of or pertaining to the spinal cord. **3.** of or pertaining to myelocytic forms that do not necessarily originate in the bone marrow.

myeloid leukemia. See **acute myelocytic leukemia, chronic myelocytic leukemia.**

myeloid metaplasia, a disorder in which bone marrow tissue develops in abnormal sites. The primary form is also called **agnogenic myeloid metaplasia, myelofibrosis.**

myeloidosis /mī′əloidō′sis/ [Gk *myelos* + *eidos* form, *osis* condition], an abnormal condition characterized by general hyperplasia of the myeloid tissue.

myeloma /mī′əlō′mə/ [Gk *myelos* + *oma* tumor], an osteolytic neoplasm consisting of a profusion of cells typical of the bone marrow. It may develop simultaneously in many sites, causing extensive areas of patchy destruction of the bone.

M

Kinds of myeloma are **endothelial, extramedullary, giant cell, multiple,** and **osteogenic myeloma.**

myelomalacia /mī'əlōmələ'shə/ [Gk *myelos* + *malakia* softening], abnormal softening of the spinal cord, caused primarily by inadequate blood supply.

myelomatosis. See **multiple myeloma.**

myelomeningocele /mī'əlōməning'gōsēl/ [Gk *myelos* + *menix* membrane, *kele* hernia], a developmental defect of the central nervous system in which a hernial sac containing a portion of the spinal cord, its meninges, and cerebrospinal fluid protrudes through a congenital cleft in the vertebral column. The condition is caused primarily by the failure of the neural tube to close during embryonic development, although in some instances it may result from the reopening of the tube from an abnormal increase in cerebrospinal fluid pressure.

myelomere /mī'əlōmir'/ [Gk *myelos* + *meros* part], any of the embryonic segments of the brain or spinal cord during prenatal development.

myelomonocytic leukemia. See **monocytic leukemia.**

myelopathic anemia. See **myelophthisic anemia.**

myelopathy /mī'əlop'əthē/, **1.** any disease of the spinal cord. **2.** any disease of the myelopoietic tissues.

myelophthisic anemia /mī'əlofthiz'ik/ [Gk *myelos* + *phthisis* wasting], a disorder characterized by anemia and the appearance of immature granulocytes and nucleated erythroid elements in the peripheral blood.

myelopoiesis /mī'əlōpō·ē'sis/ [Gk *myelos* + *poiein* to form], the formation and development of the bone marrow or the cells that originate from it. A kind of myelopoiesis is **extramedullary myelopoiesis.** –**myelopoietic,** *adj.*

myeloradiculodysplasia /mī'əlōrədik'-yəlōdisplā'zhə/ [Gk *myelos* + L *radiculus* small root; Gk *dys* bad, *plassein* to form], any developmental abnormality of the spinal cord and spinal nerve roots.

myeloschisis /mī'əlos'kəsis/ [Gk *myelos* + *schisis* cleft], a developmental defect characterized by a cleft spinal cord that results from the failure of the neural plate to fuse and form a complete neural tube.

myelosuppression /mī'əlōsəpresh'ən/, the inhibition of the process of production of blood cells and platelets in the bone marrow.

myenteric plexus /mī'enter'ik/ [Gk *mys* muscle, *enteron* bowel; L *plexus* plaited], a group of autonomic nerve fibers and ganglion cells in the muscular coat of the intestine.

myesthesia /mī'esthē'zhə/, perception of any sensation in a muscle, such as touch, direction, proprioception, contraction, relaxation, or extension.

myiasis /mī'yəsis/ [Gk *myia* fly, *osis* condition], infection or infestation of the body by the larvae of flies, usually through a wound or an ulcer, but, rarely, through the intact skin.

myitis. See **myositis.**

mylohyoideus /mī'lōhī·oi'dē·əs/ [Gk *myle* mill, *hyoeides* U-shaped], one of a pair of flat triangular muscles that form the floor of the cavity of the mouth.

myocardial infarction (MI) /mī'ōkär'dē·əl/ [Gk *mys* muscle, *kardia* heart; L *infarcire* to stuff], necrosis of a portion of cardiac muscle caused by an obstruction in a coronary artery from either atherosclerosis or an embolus. The onset of MI is characterized by a crushing, viselike chest pain that may radiate to the left arm, neck, or epigastrium and sometimes simulates the sensation of acute indigestion or a gallbladder attack. The patient usually becomes ashen, clammy, short of breath, faint, and anxious and often feels that death is imminent. Typical signs are tachycardia, a barely perceptible pulse, low blood pressure, an elevated temperature, cardiac arrhythmia, and electrocardiographic evidence of elevation of the ST segment and Q wave. Laboratory studies usually show an increased sedimentation rate, leukocytosis, and elevated serum levels of creatine phosphokinase, lactic dehydrogenase, and glutamic-oxaloacetic transaminase. Potential complications in MI are pulmonary or systemic embolism, pulmonary edema, shock, and cardiac arrest.

myocardiopathy /mī'ōkär'dē·op'əthē/ [Gk *mys* muscle, *kardia* heart, *pathos* disease], any disease of the myocardium.

myocarditis /mī'ōkärdī'tis/ [Gk *mys, kardia* + *itis* inflammation], an inflammatory condition of the myocardium caused by viral, bacterial, or fungal infection, serum sickness, rheumatic fever, or chemical agent, or as a complication of a collagen disease. Myocarditis most frequently occurs in an acute viral form and is self-limited, but it may lead to acute heart failure.

myocardium /mī'ōkär'dē·əm/ [Gk *mys* muscle, *kardia* heart], a thick, contractile, middle layer of uniquely constructed and arranged muscle cells that forms the bulk of the heart wall. The myocardium contains a minimum of other tissue, except for the blood vessels, and is covered interiorly by the endocardium. The contractile tissue of the myocardium is composed of fibers with the characteristic cross-striations of muscular tissue. The fibers, which are about one third as large in diameter as those of skeletal muscle and contain more sarcoplasm, branch frequently and are interconnected to form a network that is continuous except where the bundles and the laminae are attached at their origins and insertions into the fibrous trigone of the heart. Most of the myocardial fibers function to contract the heart. Contraction involves the action of calcium ions and sodium ions and a complex electrochemical process. **–myocardial,** *adj.*

myoclonus /mī′ōklō′nəs/ [Gk *mys* + *klonos* contraction], a spasm of a muscle or a group of muscles. **–myoclonic,** *adj.*

myodiastasis /mī′ōdī·as′təsis/ [Gk *mys* + *diastasis* separation], an abnormal condition in which there is separation of muscle bundles.

myoedema /mī′ō·idē′mə/, *pl.* **myoedemas, myoedemata,** muscle edema.

myofibril /mī′ōfī′bril/ [Gk *mys* + L *fibrilla* small fiber], a slender striated strand of muscle tissue. Myofibrils occur in groups of branching threads running parallel to the cellular long axis.

myogelosis /mī′ōjəlō′sis/ [Gk *mys* + L *gelare* to freeze; Gk *osis*], a condition in which there are hardened areas or nodules within muscles, especially the gluteal muscles.

myogenic /mī′ōjen′ik/ [Gk *mys* + *genesis* origin], pertaining to muscles, particularly cardiac and smooth muscles that do not require nerves to initiate and maintain contractions.

myoglobin /mī′ōglō′bin/ [Gk *mys* + L *globus* ball], a ferrous globin complex consisting of one heme molecule containing one iron molecule attached to a single globin chain. Myoglobin is found in muscle and is responsible for the red color of that tissue and for its ability to store oxygen.

myoglobinuria /mī′ōglō′binŌŌr′ē·ə/ [Gk *mys;* L *globus* + Gk *ouron* urine], the presence of myoglobin, a respiratory pigment of muscle tissue, in the urine.

myokinase. See **adenylate kinase.**

myoma /mī·ō′mə/, *pl.* **myomas, myomata** [Gk *mys* + *oma* tumor], a common, benign fibroid tumor of the uterine muscle. Menorrhagia, backache, constipation, dysmenorrhea, dyspareunia, and other symptoms develop proportionate to the size, location, and rate of growth of the tumor.

myoma previum. See **leiomyoma uteri.**

myoma striocellulare. See **rhabdomyoma.**

myomectomy /mī′ōmek′təmē/, the surgical removal of muscle tissue.

myomere. See **myotome.**

myometritis /mī′ō′ōmətrī′tis/, an inflammation or infection of the myometrium of the uterus.

myometrium /mī′ōmē′trē·əm/, *pl.* **myometria** [Gk *mys* + *metra* womb], the muscular layer of the wall of the uterus. The fibers of the myometrium course around the uterus horizontally, vertically, and diagonally.

myonecrosis /mī′ōnekrō′sis/ [Gk *mys* + *necrosis* death], the death of muscle fibers. **Progressive** or **clostridial myonecrosis** is caused by the anaerobic bacteria of the genus *Clostridium.* Seen in deep wound infections, progressive myonecrosis is accompanied by pain, tenderness, a brown serous exudate, and a rapid accumulation of gas within the tissue of the muscle.

myoneural /mī′ōn ōŌr′əl/ [Gk *mys* + *neuron* nerve], of or pertaining to a muscle and its associated nerve, especially to nerve endings in muscles.

myoneural junction. See **neuromuscular junction.**

myopathy /mī·op′əthē/ [Gk *mys* + *pathos* disease], an abnormal condition of skeletal muscle characterized by muscle weakness, wasting, and histologic changes within muscle tissue, as seen in any of the muscular dystrophies. **–myopathic,** *adj.*

myope /mī′ōp/, an individual who is nearsighted or afflicted with myopia.

myophosphorylase deficiency glycogenosis. See **McArdle's disease.**

myopia /mī-ō′pē·ə/ [Gk *myops* nearsighted], a condition of nearsightedness caused by the elongation of the eyeball or by an error in refraction so that parallel rays are focused in front of the retina. Some kinds of myopia are **chronic, curvature, index,** and **pathologic myopia. –myopic,** *adj.*

myorrhaphy /mī-ôr′əfē/ [Gk *mys* + *rhaphe* suture], suturing of a wound in a muscle.

myorrhexis /mī′ərek′sis/ [Gk *mys* + *rhexis* rupture], a tearing in any muscle. **–myorrhectic,** *adj.*

myosarcoma /mī′ōsärkō′mə/ [Gk *mys* + *sarx* flesh, *oma* tumor], a malignant tumor of muscular tissue.

myosin /mī′əsin/ [Gk *mys* + *in* within], a cardiac and skeletal muscle protein that makes up close to one half of the proteins that occur in muscle tissue. The interaction of myosin and actin is essential for muscle contraction.

myositis /mī′əsī′tis/, inflammation of muscle tissue, usually of the voluntary muscles. Causes of myositis include infection, trauma, and infestation by parasites. Kinds of myositis include **epidemic, interstitial, parenchymatous, polymyositis,** and **traumatic myositis.**

myositis fibrosa, an uncommon inflammation of the muscles, characterized by abnormal formation of connective tissue.

myositis ossificans /əsif′əkanz/, a rare, inherited disease in which muscle tissue is replaced by bone. It begins in childhood, with stiffness in the neck and back and progresses to rigidity of the spine, trunk, and limbs.

myositis purulenta, any bacterial infection of muscle tissue. This condition may result in the formation of an abscess or multiple abscesses.

myositis trichinosa /trik′ənō′sə/, inflammation of the muscles resulting from infection by the parasite *Trichinella spiralis.*

myostasis /mī′ōstā′sis/ [Gk *mys* + *stasis* standing], an abnormal condition of weakened muscle in which there is a relatively fixed length of muscle fibers in the relaxed state. **–myostatic,** *adj.*

myostatic reflex. See **deep tendon reflex.**

myostroma /mī′əstrō′mə/ [Gk *mys* + *stroma* covering], the framework of muscle tissue.

myotenotomy /mī′ōtenot′əmē/ [Gk *mys* + *tenon* tendon, *temnein* to cut], surgical division of the whole or part of a muscle by cutting through its main tendon.

myotherapy, a technique of corrective muscle exercises involving pressure on the fingers and joints to relieve pain or spasms.

myotome /mī′ətōm/ [Gk *mys* + *temnein* to cut] **1.** the muscle plate of an embryonic somite that develops into a voluntary muscle. **2.** a group of muscles innervated by a single spinal segment. **3.** an instrument for cutting or dissecting a muscle.

myotomic muscle /mī′ōtom′ik/, any of the numerous muscles of the trunk of the body, derived from the myotomes and divided into the deep muscles of the back and the thoracoabdominal muscles.

myotomy /mī-ot′əmē/ [Gk *mys* + *temnein* to cut], the cutting of a muscle, performed to gain access to underlying tissues or to relieve constriction in a sphincter, as in severe esophagitis or pyloric stenosis.

myotonia /mī′ətō′nē-ə/ [Gk *mys* + *tonos* tone], any condition in which a muscle or a group of muscles does not readily relax after contracting. **–myotonic,** *adj.*

myotonia atrophica. See **myotonic muscular dystrophy.**

myotonia congenita /konjen′itə/, a rare, mild, and nonprogressive form of myotonic myopathy evident early in life. The only effects of the disorder are hypertrophy and stiffness of the muscles.

myotonic muscular dystrophy /mī′ōton′-ik/, a severe form of muscular dystrophy marked by ptosis, facial weakness, and dysarthria. Weakness of the hands and feet precedes that in the shoulders and hips. Myotonia of the hands is usually present.

myotonic myopathy, any of a group of disorders characterized by increased skeletal muscle tone and decreased relaxation of muscle after contraction. Kinds of myotonic myopathy include **myotonia congenita** and **myotonic muscular dystrophy.**

myringa. See **tympanic membrane.**

myringectomy /mir′injek′təmē/ [L *myringa* eardrum; Gk *ektome* excision], excision of the tympanic membrane.

myringitis /mir′injī′tis/ [L *myringa* + Gk *itis*], inflammation or infection of the tympanic membrane.

myringomycosis /miring′gōmīkō′sis/ [L *myringa* + Gk *mykes* fungus, *osis* condition], a fungal infection of the tympanic membrane.

myringoplasty /miring′gōplas′tē/ [L *myringa* + Gk *plassein* to mold], surgical repair of perforations of the eardrum with a tissue graft, performed to correct hearing loss. The openings in the eardrum are enlarged, and the grafting material is sutured over them.

myringotomy /mir′ing·got′əmē/ [L *myringa* + Gk *temnein* to cut], surgical incision of the eardrum, performed to relieve pressure and release pus from the middle ear. The drum is incised, and cultures are taken; fluid is gently suctioned from the middle ear. Ear drops may be instilled to improve drainage.

mysophobia /mē′sə-/ [Gk *mysos* anything disgusting, *phobos* fear], an anxiety disorder characterized by an overreaction to the slightest uncleanliness, or an irrational fear of dirt, contamination, or defilement. **–mysophobic, misophobic,** *adj.*

myxedema /mik′sədē′mə/ [Gk *myxa* mucus, *oidema* swelling], the most severe form of hypothyroidism. It is characterized by swelling of the hand, face, feet, and periorbital tissues. At this stage, the disease may lead to coma and death.

myxofibroma /mik′sōfibrō′mə/ [Gk *myxa* + L *fibra* fiber; Gk *oma* tumor], a fibrous tumor that contains myxomatous tissue.

myxoid. See **mucoid.**

myxoma /miksō′mə/ [Gk *myxa* + *oma* tumor], a neoplasm of the connective tissue, characteristically composed of stellate cells in a loose mucoid matrix crossed by delicate reticulum fibers. These tumors may grow to enormous size and may occur under the skin, in bones, and in the genitourinary tract and retroperitoneal area. **–myxomatous,** *adj.*

myxoma fibrosum. See **myxofibroma.**

myxoma sarcomatosum. See **myxosarcoma.**

myxopoiesis /mik′sōpō-ē′sis/ [Gk *myxa* + *poiein* to make], the production of mucus.

myxosarcoma /mik′sōsärkō′mə/ [Gk *myxa* + *sarx* flesh, *oma* tumor], a sarcoma that contains some myxomatous tissue.

myxovirus /mik′sōvī′rəs/ [Gk *myxa* + L *virus* poison], any of a group of medium-sized RNA viruses that are further divided into orthomyxoviruses and paramyxoviruses. Some kinds of myxoviruses are the viruses that cause influenza, mumps, and parainfluenza.

MZ, abbreviation for **monozygotic.**

n, 2n, 3n, 4n, symbols for the haploid, diploid, triploid, and tetraploid number of chromosomes in a cell, organism, strain, or individual.

N, 1. symbol for the element **nitrogen. 2.** abbreviation for **normal. 3.** abbreviation for **node** in the TNM system for staging malignant neoplastic disease. **4.** symbol for **Avogadro's number. 5.** symbol for **magnetic flux.**

N/1, symbol for **normal solution.**

nA, abbreviation for *nanoampere.*

Na, chemical symbol for the element **sodium.**

nabothian cyst /nabō'thē-ən/ [Martin Naboth, German physician, b. 1675; Gk *kystis* bag], a cyst formed in a nabothian gland of the uterine cervix. The cyst, which is pearly white and firm, seldom results in adverse or pathologic effects.

nabothian gland [Martin Naboth; L *glans* acorn], one of many small, mucus-secreting glands of the uterine cervix.

NAD, abbreviation for *no appreciable disease.*

NADH, abbreviation for *nicotine adenine dinucleotide, reduced.*

nadir /nā'dər/, the lowest point, such as the blood count after it has been depressed by chemotherapy.

nadolol /nad'ənol/, a beta-adrenergic blocking agent prescribed for long-term management of angina pectoris and for hypertension.

NADPH, abbreviation for *nicotine adenine disphosphonucleotide, reduced.*

Naegeli's leukemia. See **monocytic leukemia.**

nafcillin sodium /nafsil'in/, an antibacterial prescribed in the treatment of infections caused by penicillinase-producing staphylococci.

Naffziger sign /naf'zigər/, a diagnostic sign for sciatica or a herniated nucleus pulposus. Nerve root irritation is produced by external jugular venous compression by the examiner.

Naffziger syndrome, a condition of scalene muscle spasms secondary to intervertebral disk disease, cervical rib, or other disorder. The spasms result in pressure on the major nerve plexus of the arm and the patient experiences pain in the neck, shoulder, arm, and hand.

Nägele's obliquity. See **asynclitism.**

Nägele's rule /nā'gələz/ [Franz K. Nägele, German obstetrician, b. 1778; L *regula* model], a method for calculating the estimated date of delivery based on a mean length of gestation. Three months are subtracted from the first day of the last normal menstrual period, and 1 year plus 7 days are added to that date.

Nager's acrofacial dysostosis /nā'gərz/ [F. R. Nager, twentieth-century Swiss physician; Gk *akron* extremity; L *facies* face; Gk *dys* bad, *osteon* bone, *osis* condition], an abnormal congenital condition characterized by limb deformities, such as radioulnar synostosis, hypoplasia, and the absence of the radius or of the thumbs.

Nahrungs-Einheit-Milch (nem) /nä-'rōōngz īn'hīt milsh, milkh/ [Ger *Nahrung* food; *Einheit* unit; *Milch* milk], a nutritional unit in Pirquet's system of feeding that is equivalent to 1 g of breast milk.

nail [AS *naegel*], **1.** a flattened, elastic structure with a horny texture at the end of a finger or a toe. Each nail is comprised of a root, body, and free edge at the distal extremity. The root fastens the nail to the finger or the toe by fitting into a groove in the skin and is closely molded to the surface of the corium. The nail matrix beneath the body and the root projects longitudinal vascular ridges. The matrix firmly attaches the body of the nail to the underlying connective tissue. The whitish lunula near the root contains irregularly arranged papillae that are less firmly attached to the connective tissue than the rest of the matrix. The cuticle is attached to the surface of the nail just ahead of the root. **2.** any of various metallic nails used in orthopedics to fasten together bones or pieces of bone.

nail bed [AS *naegle*; *bedd* bed], the corium beneath the nail. It appears through the clear nail as a series of longitudinal ridges.

nail fold, a fold of skin supporting the nail at its base.

nail groove [AS *naegle*; Du *groeve*

groove], a shallow depression between the nail bed and the nail wall.

nail matrix. See **nail bed.**

nail plate, the hard portion of the dorsum of the fingers and thumb, a rigid outer covering that extends about 8 mm under the nail fold and arises from the nail bed.

nail plate avulsion, a temporary partial or complete removal of the nail plate without disruption of the underlying matrix cells.

Nalebuff arthrodesis, an arthrodesis of the wrist in which fusion includes the use of a Steinmann pin.

nalidixic acid /nal'idik'sik/, an antibacterial prescribed in the treatment of certain urinary tract infections.

naloxone hydrochloride /nal'əksōn/, a narcotic antagonist prescribed for reversal of narcotic depression, or for acute narcotic intoxication.

naltrexone hydrochloride /naltrek'sōn/, an oral opioid antagonist prescribed to block the effects of opioid analgesics, including heroin, morphine, and methadone in patients recovering from addiction.

Namaqualand hip dysplasia, an autosomal dominant genetic defect found in African children. It is characterized by a growth failure in the femoral epiphysis, resulting in pain and early degenerative arthritis of the hip.

NAMI, abbreviation for **National Alliance for the Mentally Ill.**

NANB, abbreviation for **non-A, non-B hepatitis.**

NANDA, abbreviation for **North American Nursing Diagnosis Association.**

nandrolone decanoate /nan'drəlōn/, an androgen prescribed in the treatment of testosterone deficiency, osteoporosis, and female breast cancer, and to stimulate growth, weight gain, and the production of red cells.

nandrolone phenpropionate, an anabolic steroid with androgenic properties. It is prescribed in the treatment of osteoporosis, in certain anemias, in metastatic breast cancers of women, and for protein-sparing effects in many situations.

nanism /nā'nizəm, nan'-/ [Gk *nanos* dwarf], an abnormal smallness or underdevelopment of the body; dwarfism. Kinds of nanism are **mulibrey, Paltauf's, pituitary, renal, senile,** and **symptomatic nanism.**

nanocephalic dwarf. See **bird-headed dwarf.**

nanocephaly /nā'nōsef'əlē, nan'-/ [Gk *nanos* + *kephale* head], a developmental defect characterized by abnormal smallness of the head. **–nanocephalous,** *adj.,* **nanocephalus,** *n.*

nanocormia /nā'nōkôr'mē·ə/ [Gk *nanos* + *kormos* trunk], abnormal disproportionate smallness of the trunk of the body in comparison to the head and limbs. **–nanocormus,** *n.*

nanocurie (nc, nC) /nā'nəkyŏŏr'ē, nan'-/ [Gk *nanos* dwarf; Marie and Pierre Curie], a unit of radiation equal to one billionth of a curie.

nanogram (ng) /nan'əgram/ [Gk *nanos* + Fr *gramme* small weight], a unit of weight equal to one billionth of a gram.

nanomelia /nā'nōmē'lyə, nan'-/ [Gk *nanos* + *melos* limb], a developmental defect characterized by abnormally small limbs in comparison to the size of the head and trunk. **–nanomelous,** *adj.,* **nanomelus,** *n.*

nanometer (nm) /nan'əmē'tər/ [Gk *nanos* + *metron* measure], a unit of length equal to one billionth of a meter.

nanophthalmos /nā'nofthal'məs, nan'-/ [Gk *nanos* + *ophthalmos* eye], the condition in which one or both eyes are abnormally small, although other ocular defects are not present.

nanosecond (ns) [Gk *nanos* + L *secundus* second], one billionth (10^{-9}) of a second.

nanosomus /nā'nōsō'məs/ [Gk *nanos* + *soma* body], a person of very short stature; a dwarf.

nanukayami /nä'noōkäyä'mē/ [Jap], an acute, infectious disease caused by one of the serotypes of the spirochete *Leptospira* that is indigenous to Japan.

nanus /nā'nəs/, **1.** a dwarf. **2.** a pygmy. **–nanoid,** *adj.*

napalm /nā'päm/, abbreviation for *napthenate palmitate,* a form of jellied gasoline used in warfare.

napalm burn [AS *baernan* burn], a thermal burn caused by contact with flaming **napalm.**

nape [ME], the back of the neck.

naphazoline hydrochloride /nəfaz'əlēn/, an adrenergic vasoconstrictor prescribed in the treatment of nasal congestion and as an ophthalmic vasoconstrictor.

naphthalene poisoning /naf'thəlēn/ [Gk *naptha* flammable liquid; L *potio* drink], a toxic condition caused by the ingestion of naphthalene or paradichlorobenzene that may cause nausea, vomiting, headache, abdominal pain, spasm, and convulsions.

naphthol camphor /naf'thol/, a syrupy mixture of two parts of camphor and one part betanaphthol, used externally as an antiseptic.

naphthol poisoning. See **phenol poisoning.**

napkin ring tumor [ME *nappekin* tablecloth, *hring* band; L *tumor* swelling], a

N

tumor that encircles a tubular structure of the body, usually impairing its function and constricting its lumen to some degree.

NAP-NAP, abbreviation for **National Association of Pediatric Nurse Associates/Practitioners.**

NAPNES, abbreviation for **National Association for Practical Nurse Education and Services.**

napping [ME *nappen* to doze], periods of sleep, usually during the day, which may last from 15 to 60 minutes without attaining the level of deep sleep.

naproxen /naprok'sən/, a nonsteroidal antiinflammatory agent prescribed for the relief of inflammatory symptoms of arthritis.

NAPT, abbreviation for *National Association of Physical Therapists.*

narc, abbreviation for **narcotic.**

narcissism /när'sisiz'əm/ [Gk *Narcissus* mythic youth in love with himself], **1.** an abnormal interest in oneself, especially in one's own body and sexual characteristics; self-love. **2.** (in psychoanalysis) sexual self-interest that is a normal characteristic of the phallic stage of psychosexual development, occurring as the infantile ego acquires a libido.

narcissistic personality, a personality characterized by behavior and attitudes that indicate an abnormal love of the self.

narcissistic personality disorder, a condition characterized by an exaggerated sense of self-importance and uniqueness, an abnormal need for attention and admiration, preoccupation with grandiose fantasies concerning the self, and disturbances in interpersonal relationships, usually involving the exploitation of others and a lack of empathy for them.

narcoanalysis, an interview conducted while the patient is deeply sedated with medication so that inhibitions are reduced and responses will be more truthful.

narcoanesthesia. See **basal anesthesia.**

narcohypnosis /när'kōhipnō'sis/, hypnosis induced with the aid of a narcotic drug, such as sodium amobarbital or sodium pentothal.

narcolepsy /när'kəlep'sē/ [Gk *narke* stupor, *lambanein* to seize], a syndrome characterized by sudden sleep attacks, cataplexy, sleep paralysis, and visual or auditory hallucinations at the onset of sleep. Persons with narcolepsy experience an uncontrollable desire to sleep, sometimes many times in one day. Episodes may last from a few minutes to several hours. Momentary loss of muscle tone occurs during waking hours (cataplexy), or while the person is asleep.

narcoleptic /när'kəlep'tik/, **1.** of or pertaining to a condition or substance that causes an uncontrollable desire for sleep. **2.** a narcoleptic drug. **3.** a person suffering from narcolepsy.

Narcon, abbreviation for *Narcotics Anonymous.*

narcosis /närkō'sis/ [Gk *narkosis* numbness], a state of insensibility or stupor caused by narcotic drugs.

narcotic (narc) [Gk *narkotikos* benumbing], **1.** of or pertaining to a substance that produces insensibility or stupor. **2.** a narcotic drug. Narcotic analgesics, derived from opium or produced synthetically, alter perception of pain; induce euphoria, mood changes, mental clouding, and deep sleep; depress respiration and the cough reflex; constrict the pupils; and cause smooth muscle spasm, decreased peristalsis, emesis, and nausea. Repeated use of narcotics may result in physical and psychologic dependence.

narcotic analgesic. See **analgesic.**

narcotic antagonist, a drug that is used primarily in the treatment of narcotic-induced respiratory depression. The narcotic antagonists nalorphine, levallorphan, and naloxone are usually administered parenterally.

narcotic antitussive. See **antitussive.**

narcotic poisoning [Gk *narke* stupor; L *potio* drink], the toxic effects of a narcotic drug that depresses the brain centers, causing unconsciousness or coma. Narcotic drugs are generally derived from opium but other drugs, including alcohol, can produce similar effects.

nares /ner'ēz/, *sing.* **naris,** the pairs of anterior openings and posterior openings in the nose that allow the passage of air from the nose to the pharynx and the lungs during respiration.

narrow-angle glaucoma. See **glaucoma.**

nasal (nas) [L *nasus* nose], of or pertaining to the nose and the nasal cavity. **—nasally,** *adv.*

nasal airway, a flexible, curved piece of rubber or plastic, with one wide, trumpet-like end and one narrow end that can be inserted through the nose into the pharynx.

nasal cannula, a device for delivering oxygen by way of two small tubes that are inserted into the nares.

nasal cartilage, a flat plate of cartilage in the lower anterior portion of the nasal septum.

nasal cavity, one of a pair of cavities that open on the face through the pear-shaped anterior nasal aperture and communicate with the pharynx.

nasal decongestant, a drug that provides temporary relief of nasal symptoms in acute and chronic rhinitis and sinusitis.

Most are over-the-counter products compounded with a small amount of vasoconstrictor, such as ephedrine or phenylephrine.

nasal drip, a method of slowly infusing liquid into a dehydrated infant by means of a catheter inserted through the nose down the esophagus.

nasal fossa, one of the pair of approximately equal chambers of the nasal cavity that are separated by the nasal septum and open externally through the nostrils and internally into the nasopharynx through the choanae. Each fossa is divided into an olfactory region, consisting of the superior nasal concha and part of the septum, and a respiratory region, constituting the rest of the chamber.

nasal glioma, a neoplasm characterized by the ectopic growth of neural tissue in the nasal cavity.

nasal instillation of medication, the instillation of a medicated solution into the nostrils by drops from a dropper or by an atomized spray from a squeeze bottle. Drops are instilled in each nostril as the patient's neck is hyperextended and the head tilted back over the edge of the bed. Nasal spray is administered to the patient in a sitting position.

nasalis /nāzal'is/ [L *nasus* nose], one of the three muscles of the nose, divided into a transverse part and an alar part. The transverse part serves to depress the cartilaginous portion of the nose and to draw the alar toward the septum. The alar part serves to dilate the nostril.

nasal obstruction, a narrowing of the nasal cavity, thereby reducing the breathing capacity, caused by an irregular septum, nasal polyps, foreign bodies, or enlarged turbinates. Sinusitis is a common complication of the condition.

nasal polyp, a rounded, elongated bit of boggy, dependent mucosa that projects into the nasal cavity.

nasal septum, the partition dividing the nostrils. It is composed of bone and cartilage covered by mucous membrane.

nasal sinus, any one of the numerous cavities in various bones of the skull, lined with ciliated mucous membrane continuous with that of the nasal cavity. The nasal sinuses are divided into frontal sinuses, ethmoidal air cells, sphenoidal sinuses, and maxillary sinus.

nascent /nas'ənt, nā'sənt/ [L *nasci* to be born], **1.** just born; beginning to exist; incipient. **2.** (in chemistry) pertaining to any substance liberated during a chemical reaction, which, because of its uncombined state, is more reactive.

nascent oxygen, oxygen that has just been liberated from a chemical compound.

nasion /nā'zē·on/ [L *nasus* nose], **1.** the anthropometric reference point at the front of the skull where the midsagittal plane intersects a horizontal line tangential to the highest points in the superior palpebral sulci. **2.** the depression at the root of the nose that indicates the junction of the intranasal and the frontonasal sutures.

nasogastric feeding /nā'zōgas'trik/ [L *nasus* nose; Gk *gaster* stomach; AS *faedan* to feed], the process of introducing nutrients in a liquid form directly into the stomach via a nasogastric tube.

nasogastric intubation, the placement of a nasogastric tube through the nose into the stomach to relieve gastric distention by removing gas, gastric secretions, or food; to instil medication, food, or fluids; or to obtain a specimen for laboratory analysis. After surgery and in any condition in which the person is able to digest food but not eat it, the tube may be introduced and left in place for tube feeding until the ability to eat normally is restored.

nasogastric suction, the removal by suction of solids, fluids, or gases from the gastrointestinal tract through a tube inserted into the stomach or intestines via the nasl cavity.

nasogastric tube, any tube passed into the stomach through the nose.

nasojejuneal tube /nā'zōjij oo'nəl/, a mercury-weighted tube inserted through the nose to allow natural peristaltic movement from the pylorus into the jejunum.

nasolabial /nā'zōlā'bē·əl/ [L *nasus* nose; *labium* lip], pertaining to the nose and lip.

nasolabial reflex, a sudden backward movement of the head, arching of the back, and extension and stretching of the limbs that occurs in infants in response to a light touch to the tip of the nose with an upward sweeping motion.

nasolacrimal /nā'zōlak'riməl/ [L *nasus* + *lacrima* tears], of or pertaining to the nasal cavity and associated lacrimal ducts.

nasolacrimal duct, a channel that carries tears from the lacrimal sac to the nasal cavity.

nasolacrimal groove, a groove on the nasal surface of the upper jaw. It is the site of the nasolacrimal duct.

nasomandibular fixation /nā'zōmandib'-yŏŏlər/ [L *nasus* + *mandere* to chew; *figere* to fasten], a type of maxillomandibular fixation to stabilize fractures of the jaw by using maxillomandibular splints connected to a wire through a hole drilled in the anterior nasal spine of the maxillary bone.

nasomental reflex [L *nasus* + *mentum*

chin; *reflectere* to bend back], a reflex elicited by tapping the side of the nose, thereby causing contraction of the lip and wrinkling of the skin of the chin.

nasopharyngeal angiofibroma /nā'-sōfərin'jē·əl/ [L *nasus* + Gk *pharynx* throat], a benign tumor of the nasopharynx, consisting of fibrous connective tissue with many vascular spaces. Typical signs are nasal and eustachian tube obstruction, adenoidal speech, and dysphagia.

nasopharyngeal cancer, a malignant neoplastic disease of the nasopharynx. Depending on the site of a nasopharyngeal tumor, there may be nasal obstruction, otitis media, hearing loss, sensory or motor nerve damage, bony destruction of the skull, or deep cervical lymphadenopathy. Squamous cell and undifferentiated carcinomas are the most common lesions.

nasopharyngeal fibroangioma. See **nasopharyngeal angiofibroma.**

nasopharyngography /nā'zōfer'ingog'-rəfē/ [L *nasus* + Gk *pharynx* throat, *graphein* to record], radiographic imaging and examination of the nasopharynx.

nasopharyngoscopy /nā'zōfer'ing·go·s'kəpē/ [L *nasus* + Gk *pharynx* throat, *skopein* to look], a technique in physical examination in which the nose and throat are visually examined using a laryngoscope, a fiberoptic device, a flashlight, and a dilator for the nares. **–nasopharyngoscopic,** *adj.*

nasopharynx /nā'zōfer'ingks/ [L *nasus* + Gk *pharynx* throat], the uppermost of the three regions of the throat, situated behind the nose and extending from the posterior nares to the level of the soft palate. Swollen or enlarged pharyngeal tonsils can fill the space behind the posterior nares and may completely block the passage of air from the nose into the throat. **–nasopharyngeal,** *adj.*

nasotracheal tube /nā'zōträ'kē·əl/ [L *nasus* + Gk *tracheia* rough artery; L *tubus*], a catheter inserted into the trachea through the nasal cavity and the pharynx. It is commonly used in respiratory therapy.

natal /nā'təl/, **1.** [L *natus*] of or pertaining to birth. **2.** [L *nates*] of or pertaining to the nates, or buttocks.

nates /nā'tēz/, *sing.* **natis** [L, buttocks], the large fleshy protuberances at the lower posterior portion of the torso comprising fat and the gluteal muscles.

National Alliance for the Mentally Ill (NAMI), a national organization for family members of psychotic patients.

National Association for Mental Health. See **Mental Health Association.**

National Association for Practical Nurse Education and Services (NAPNES), a national professional organization concerned with the education of practical nurses and with the services provided by licensed practical nurses.

National Association of Pediatric Nurse Associates/Practitioners (NAP-NAP), a national organization of nurses who are prepared by training or experience to give primary care to pediatric patients. NAP-NAP works in conjunction with the American Academy of Pediatrics.

National Bureau of Standards (NBS), a federal agency in the Department of Commerce that sets accurate measurement standards for commerce, industry, and science in the United States. The NBS compares and coordinates its standards with those of other countries.

National Council Licensure Examination (NCLEX), a comprehensive integrated examination, developed and administered by the National Council of State Boards of Nursing, designed to test basic competency for nursing practice. The NCLEX-RN test plan has three components including nursing behaviors grouped under nursing process categories, the process of decision making that defines nursing's role, and levels of cognitive ability.

National Eye Institute (NEI), a division of the National Institutes of Health. NEI was established in 1968 to support research in the normal functioning of the human eye and visual system, the pathology of visual disorders, and the rehabilitation of the visually handicapped.

National Formulary (NF), a publication containing the official standards for the preparation of various pharmaceutics not listed in the *United States Pharmacopoeia.* It is revised every 5 years.

national health insurance, a government-financed health insurance program providing comprehensive benefits to most or all of the population.

National Health Planning and Resources Development Act of 1974, U.S. congressional legislation (PL 93-641) that established a nationwide network of health systems agencies. The act provides for the coordination and direction of national health policy through state and regional regulatory agencies.

National Health Service Corps (NHSC), a program of the United States Public Health Service (USPHS) in which health care personnel are placed in areas that are underserved. The Corps was established by the Emergency Health Personnel Act of 1970. Nurses, physicians, and dentists

Nat. Inst. Child Health and Hum. Dev. 703

natural law

serve in rural and urban areas, usually as employees of local health care agencies.

National Institute of Child Health and Human Development (NICHHD), a branch of the National Institutes of Health that is concerned with all aspects of the growth, development, and health of the children of the United States.

National Institute of Mental Health (NIMH), a branch of the National Institutes of Health within the Alcohol, Drug Abuse, and Mental Health Administration. It is responsible for federal research and education programs dealing with mental health.

National Institutes of Health (NIH), an agency within the United States Public Health Service made up of several institutions and constituent divisions, including the Bureau of Health Manpower Education, the National Library of Medicine, the National Cancer Institute, and several research institutes and divisions.

National League for Nursing (NLN), an organization concerned with the improvement of nursing education, nursing service, and the provision of health care in the United States. Among its many activities are accreditation of nursing programs at all levels, preadmission and achievement tests for nursing students, and compilation of statistic data on nursing personnel and on trends in health care delivery.

National Male Nurses' Association (NMNA), a national organization that promotes the interests and practice of male nurses.

National Marrow Donor Program (NMDP), a coordinating center for bone marrow transplants, providing links with national and international registries of prospective volunteer donors of HLA-compatible bone tissue.

National Organization of Victims Assistance, a private, nonprofit organization of victims and witness assistance practitioners, criminal justice professionals, and others committed to the recognition of victims' rights.

National Society of Critical Care Nurses of Canada (NSCCN), an organization of Canadian critical care nurses, established originally in 1975 as the Toronto Chapter of the American Association of Critical-Care Nurses. The group became an independent Canadian organization in 1983.

National Student Nurses' Association (NSNA), a national organization of students in the field of nursing. Among its purposes are the improvement of nursing education to improve health care, to aid in the development of the student nurse, and

to encourage optimal achievement in the professional role of the nurse and the health care of people.

natriuresis /nā′trēy ōōrē′sis/ [L *natrium* sodium; Gk *ouresis* urination], the excretion of greater than normal amounts of sodium in the urine, as from the administration of natriuretic diuretic drugs or from various metabolic or endocrine disorders.

natriuretic /nā′trēy ōōret′ik/, **1.** of or pertaining to the process of natriuresis. **2.** a substance that inhibits the resorption of sodium ions from the glomerular filtrate in the kidneys, thus allowing more sodium to be excreted with the urine.

natural antibody [L *natura* nature; Gk *anti*; AS *bodig* body], an antibody that is present in serum in the absence of an apparent specific antigen contact.

natural childbirth [L *natura* nature; AS *cild* child; ME *bwith* birth], labor and parturition accomplished by a mother with little or no medical intervention. Prerequisites include normal gestation, an adequate birth canal, strong maternal motivation, physical and emotional preparation, and constant and intensive support of the mother during labor and birth.

natural dentition, the entire array of natural teeth in the dental arch at any given time, consisting of deciduous or permanent teeth or a mixture of the two.

natural family planning method, any one of several methods of family planning that does not rely on a medication or a device for effectiveness in avoiding pregnancy. Some of the methods are also used to pinpoint the time of ovulation to increase the chance of fertilization when artificial insemination or extraction of an oocyte for in vitro fertilization is to be performed. Kinds of natural family planning include **basal body temperature method, calendar method, ovulation method,** and **symptothermal method of family planning.**

natural immunity, a usually innate and permanent form of immunity to a specific disease. Kinds of natural immunity include **individual immunity, racial immunity,** and **species immunity.**

naturalistic illness, an illness thought to be caused by impersonal factors, such as the Hispanic model of hot and cold forces.

natural killer (NK) cells, effector cells that have the capacity for spontaneous cytotoxicity toward various target cells. These cells are lymphocytes that are capable of binding to and killing virus-infected and tumor cells by a mechanism not yet understood.

natural law, a doctrine that holds there is

N

a natural moral order or natural moral law inherent in the structure of the universe.

naturally acquired immunity. See **acquired immunity.**

natural network, (in psychiatric nursing) a patient's natural contacts in the community, including church and social groups, friends, family, and occupation that support the person's function outside the hospital environment.

natural pacemaker, any cardiac pacing site in the heart tissues.

natural radiation, radioactivity that emanates from the soil and rocks or particles and rays that reach the earth from cosmic sources, as actinic radiation from the sun.

natural selection, the natural evolutionary processes by which those organisms best suited for adaptation to the environment tend to survive and propagate the species, whereas those unfit are eliminated.

nature versus nurture, a name given to a longstanding controversy as to the relative influences of nature versus the environment in the development of personality. Nature is represented by instincts and genetic factors and nurture by social influences.

naturopath /nach′ərōpath′/, a person who practices naturopathy.

naturopathy /nach′ərop′əthē/ [L *natura* + Gk *pathos* disease], a system of therapeutics based on natural foods, light, warmth, massage, fresh air, regular exercise, and the avoidance of medications. Advocates believe that illness can be healed by the natural processes of the body.

Nauheim bath /nou′hīm/ [Nauheim, Germany; AS *baeth* bath], a bath taken in water through which carbon dioxide is bubbled, followed by systematic exercises, used in the treatment of cardiac conditions. The procedure is named after the natural waters of Bad Nauheim, Germany.

nausea /nô′zē·ə, nô′zhə/ [Gk *nausia* seasickness], a sensation often leading to the urge to vomit. Common causes are seasickness and other motion sicknesses, early pregnancy, intense pain, emotional stress, gallbladder disease, food poisoning, and various enteroviruses. –**nauseate,** *v.,* **nauseous,** *adj.*

nausea and vomiting of pregnancy, a common condition of early pregnancy, characterized by recurrent or persistent nausea, often in the morning, that may result in vomiting, weight loss, anorexia, general weakness, and malaise. The causes of the condition are poorly understood. It usually does not begin before the sixth week after the last menstrual period and ends by the twelfth to the fourteenth week of pregnancy.

nauseous /nôshəs, nô′zē·əs/ [Gk. *nausia.* seasickness], pertaining to feelings of nausea or reaction to things that may stimulate nausea.

navel. See **umbilicus.**

navicular /nəvik′yŏŏlər/, boat-shaped; sunken.

navicular bone. See **scaphoid bone.**

navicular pads, tarsal supports for flat feet. They are inserted directly under the arch of the foot.

n.b., abbreviation for the Latin phrase, *nota bene,* note well.

Nb, symbol for the element **niobium.**

NBRC, abbreviation for *National Board for Respiratory Care.*

NBS standard, (in nuclear medicine) a radioactive source standardized, or certified, or both, by the National Bureau of Standards.

nc, nC, abbreviation for **nanocurie.**

N-CAP, abbreviation for **Nurses' Coalition for Action in Politics.**

NCI, abbreviation for the *National Cancer Institute.*

NCLEX abbreviation for **National Council Licensure Examination.**

Nd, abbreviation for the element **neodymium.**

ND, abbreviation for *Doctor of Naturopathy.*

NDA, abbreviation for *National Dental Association.*

NE, abbreviation for **niacin equivalent.**

Ne, symbol for the element **neon.**

Neal-Robertson litter, a modified spine board for transporting trauma patients with spinal injuries.

near-death experience [ME *nere* + *deth; L experientia* trial], the subjective observations of persons who have either been close to clinical death or who may have recovered after having been declared dead. Many claim to have had witnessed similar episodes of passing through a tunnel toward a bright light and encountering persons who had preceded them in death.

near drowning [AS *near* almost; ME *drounen* to drown], a pathologic state in which the victim has survived exposure to circumstances that usually cause drowning. Cardiopulmonary resuscitation is performed immediately; hospitalization is always indicated.

nearest neighbor analysis, (in molecular genetics) a biochemical method used to estimate the frequency with which pairs of bases are located next to one another.

nearsightedness. See **myopia.**

nebula /neb′yələ/, *pl.* **nebulae** [L, cloud],

1. a slight corneal opacity or scar that seldom obstructs vision and that can be seen only by oblique illumination. **2.** a murkiness in the urine. **3.** an oily concoction that is applied with an atomizer.

nebulization /neb′yəlīzā′shən/ [L *nebula* cloud; Gk *izein* to cause], a method of administering a drug by spraying it into the respiratory passages of the patient.

nebulize, to vaporize or disperse a liquid in a fine spray.

nebulizer, a device for producing a fine spray. Intranasal medications are often administered by a nebulizer.

NEC, abbreviation for **necrotizing enterocolitis.**

Necator [L *necare* to kill], a genus of nematode that is an intestinal parasite and causes hookworm disease.

necatoriasis /nek′ətorī′əsis/ [L *necare* to kill; Gk *osis* condition], hookworm disease, specifically that caused by *Necator americanus,* which is the most common North American hookworm. The larvae live in the soil and reach the human digestive tract through contaminated food and water or through the skin of the feet and legs. Symptoms include diarrhea, nausea, abdominal pain, and anemia in the more severe cases.

neck [AS *hnecca*], a constricted section, such as the part of the body that connects the head with the trunk. Other such constrictions are the neck of the humerus and the neck of the femur.

neck dissection, surgical removal of the cervical lymph nodes, performed to prevent the spread of malignant tumors of the head and neck.

neck of femur [AS *hnecca*; L *femur* thigh], the portion of the long bone of the thigh between the head and the greater and lesser trochanters.

neck righting reflex, 1. an involuntary response in newborns in which turning the head to one side while the infant is supine causes rotation of the shoulders and trunk in the same direction. The reflex enables the child to roll over from the supine to prone position. **2.** any tonic reflex associated with the neck that maintains body orientation in relation to the head.

neck ring, a metal ring at the neck of a cervicothoracolumbosacral orthosis. It opens posteriorly for ease in putting on or removing the orthosis and is an attachment for a throat mold and occiput pads.

neck shaft angle, an angle created by the intersection of a line drawn through the femoral shaft and a line through the femoral head and neck.

necrobiosis lipoidica /nek′rōbī·ō′sis li·poi′dikə/ [Gk *nekros* dead, *bios* life; *lipos* fat, *eidos* form], a skin disease characterized by thin, shiny, yellow to red plaques on the shins or forearms. Telangiectases, crusting, and ulceration of these plaques may occur.

necrogenic, necrogenous [Gk *nekros* + *genein* to produce], pertaining to something that originates in dead material.

necrology (necrol) /nekrol′əjē/ [Gk *nekros* + *logos* science], the study of the causes of death, including the compilation and interpretation of mortality statistics.

necrolysis /nekrol′isis/ [Gk *nekros* + *lysis* loosening], disintegration or exfoliation of dead tissue. **–necrolytic,** *adj.*

necrophilia /nek′rōfil′yə/ [Gk *nekros* + *philein* to love], **1.** a morbid liking for being with dead bodies. **2.** a morbid desire to have sexual contact with a dead body, usually of men to perform a sexual act with a dead woman. **–necrophile, necrophiliac,** *n.*

necrophobia [Gk *nekros* + *phobos* fear], a morbid fear of death and dead bodies.

necropsy, necroscopy. See **autopsy.**

necrosis /nekrō′sis/ [Gk *nekros* + *osis* condition], localized tissue death that occurs in groups of cells in response to disease or injury. In **coagulation necrosis,** blood clots block the flow of blood, causing tissue ischemia distal to the clot; in **gangrenous necrosis,** ischemia combined with bacterial action causes putrefaction to set in.

necrotic /nekrot′ik/, pertaining to the death of tissue in response to disease or injury.

necrotizing, causing the death of tissues or organisms.

necrotizing angiitis. See **periarteritis nodosa.**

necrotizing enteritis [Gk *nekros* + *izein* to cause, *enteron* intestine, *itis*], acute inflammation of the small and the large intestine by the bacterium *Clostridium perfringens,* characterized by severe abdominal pain, bloody diarrhea, and vomiting.

necrotizing enterocolitis (NEC), an acute inflammatory bowel disorder that occurs primarily in preterm or low-birthweight neonates. It is characterized by ischemic necrosis of the GI mucosa that may lead to perforation and peritonitis. The cause of the disorder is unknown, although it appears to be a defect in host defenses with infection resulting from normal GI flora rather than from invading organisms.

necrotizing vasculitis, an inflammatory condition of blood vessels, characterized by necrosis, fibrosis, and proliferation of the inner layer of the vascular wall, in some cases resulting in occlusion and infarction. Necrotizing vasculitis may occur in rheumatoid arthritis and is common in systemic lupus erythematosus, periarteritis nodosa, and progressive systemic sclerosis.

needle bath [AS *naedl* needle], a shower in which fine jets of water are sprayed over the body.

needle biopsy, the removal of a segment of living tissue for microscopic examination by inserting a hollow needle through the skin or the external surface of an organ or tumor and rotating it within the underlying cellular layers.

needle filter, a device, usually made of plastic, used for filtering medications that are drawn into a syringe before administration.

needle holder, a surgical forceps used to hold and pass a suturing needle through tissue.

needle-stick injuries, accidental skin punctures resulting from contact with hypodermic needles. The contact may occur accidentally during efforts to inject a patient or as a result of carelessly touching discarded medical waste. Such injuries can be dangerous, particularly if the needle has been used in the treatment of a patient with a severe blood-borne infection, such as AIDS.

NEEP, abbreviation for **negative end-expiratory pressure.**

Neer and Horowitz classification system, a method of classifying proximal humeral fractures in children, based on the degree of separation of the epiphysis from the shaft.

Neer classification system, a method of classifying femoral supracondylar and intercondylar fractures. The system ranges from *type I* for minimal displacement through *type IIA* and *IIB* to *type III* for conjoined supracondylar and shaft fractures. The Neer system is also applied to humeral head and neck fractures.

negative (neg) [L *negare* to deny persistently], **1.** (of a laboratory test) indicating that a substance or a reaction is not present. **2.** (of a sign) indicating on physical examination that a finding is not present, often meaning that there is no pathologic change. **3.** (of a substance) tending to carry or carrying a negative chemical charge.

negative adaptation. See **habituation.**

negative anxiety, (in psychology) an emotional and psychologic condition in which anxiety prevents a person's normal functioning and interrupts the person's ability to perform the usual activities of daily living.

negative catalysis, a decrease in the rate of any chemical reaction caused by a substance that is not part of the process itself and not consumed or affected by the reaction.

negative electrode [L *negare*; Gk *elektron* amber; *hodos* way], a cathode, or the negative pole of an electric current or of a battery or dry cell.

negative end-expiratory pressure (NEEP), a technique used to counterbalance the increase in mean intrathoracic pressure caused by intermittent positive pressure breathing (IPPB) in an effort to return negative intrathoracic pressure for venous return to the right atrium. Generally, the negative pressure is applied to the circuit on exhalation by using a jet or Venturi system and the resulting subatmospheric pressure is applied to the patient's airways.

negative feedback, 1. (in physiology) a decrease in function in response to a stimulus; for example, the secretion of follicle-stimulating hormone decreases even as the amount of circulating estrogen increases. **2.** *informal;* a critical, derogatory, or otherwise negative response from one person to what another person has communicated.

negative identity, the assumption of an identity that is at odds with the accepted values and expectations of society.

negative pathognomonic symptom [L *negare*; Gk *pathos* disease + *gnomen* index, *symptoma* that which happens], any symptom that is not usually found in a specific condition and if present would not be compatible with the diagnosis.

negative pi meson (pion), a form of electromagnetic radiation emitted from a proton linear accelerator.

negative pi meson (pion) radiotherapy, a form of radiotherapy using a negative pi meson (pion) beam emitted by a proton linear accelerator. In the treatment of certain tumors, negative pi meson particles are beamed at the tumor; the atomic nuclei of malignant cells take in the radioactive particles and explode, scattering intensely radioactive subatomic particles through the adjacent malignant tissue.

negative pressure, less than ambient atmospheric pressure, such as in a vacuum, at an altitude above sea level, or in a hypobaric chamber.

negative punishment, a form of behavior modification in which the removal of something after an operant (behavior) decreases the probability of the operant's recurrence.

negative reinforcer, (in psychology) a stimulus that, when presented immediately after occurrence of a particular behavior, will decrease the rate of responding of the behavior.

negative relationship, (in research) an inverse relationship between two variables; as one variable increases, the other decreases.

negativism [L *negare* to deny persistently], a behavioral attitude characterized by opposition, resistance, the refusal to cooperate with even the most reasonable request, and the tendency to act in a contrary manner.

neglect, a condition that occurs when a parent or guardian is unable to or fails to provide minimal physical and emotional care for a child or other dependent person.

negligence [L *negligentia* carelessness], (in law) the commission of an act that a prudent person would not have done or the omission of a duty that a prudent person would have fulfilled, resulting in injury or harm to another person.

negligence per se, (in law) a finding of negligence rendered in judgment of a professional action or inaction in violation of a statute or so at odds with common sense that beyond any doubt no prudent person would have been guilty of it.

Negri bodies /nā′grē/ [Adelchi Negri, Italian physician, b. 1876; AS, *bodig*], an intracytoplasmic inclusion body found in the brain and central nervous system cells of rabies victims.

NEI, abbreviation for **National Eye Institute.**

Neisseria gonorrhoeae /nīser′ē·ə/ [Albert L. S. Neisser, Polish dermatologist, b. 1855; Gk *gone* seed, *rhoia* flow], a gram-negative, nonmotile, diplococcal bacterium usually seen microscopically as flattened pairs within the cytoplasm of neutrophils. It is the causative organism of gonorrhea.

Neisseria meningitidis. See **meningococcus.**

NEJM, abbreviation for *New England Journal of Medicine.*

Nélaton's dislocation /nālätôNz′/ [Auguste Nélaton, French surgeon, b. 1807], a dislocation of the ankle in which the distal ends of the tibia and fibula are separated and the talus is forced upward between the tibia and fibula.

Nelson's syndrome [Donald H. Nelson, American physician, b. 1925], an endocrine disorder that may follow adrenalectomy for Cushing's disease. It is characterized by a marked increase in the secretion of ACTH and MSH by the pituitary gland.

nem, abbreviation for **Nahrungs-Einheit-Milch.**

nematocides /nəmat′əsidz/ [Gk *nema*

thread, *eidos* form; L *caedere* to kill], chemical pesticides that are employed to kill nematode worms.

nematocyst /nem′ətōsist′/ [Gk *nema* + *eidos* form, *kystis* bag], a barbed threadlike process on the surface of coelenterates and attached to a poison sac. The stinger, found on the Portuguese man-of-war and other types of jellyfish, can be ejected into the skin of a human or animal, causing painful and potentially fatal injury.

nematode /nem′ətōd/ [Gk *nema* + *eidos* form], a multicellular, parasitic animal of the phylum Nematoda. All species of roundworms belong to the phylum.

nematodiasis /nem′ətōdī′əsis/, an infestation of nematode worms.

neoantigen /nē′ō·an′tijən/ [Gk *neos* new, *anti* against, *genein* to produce], a new specific antigen that develops in a cell infected by oncogenic virus; it appears after infection by SV40.

neobehaviorism /nē′ōbihā′vē·əiz′əm/ [Gk *neos* + ME *behaven* behavior], a school of psychology based on the general principles of behaviorism but broader and more flexible in concept. It stresses experimental research and laboratory analyses in the study of overt behavior and in various subjective phenomena that cannot be directly observed and measured.

neobehaviorist, a disciple of the school of neobehaviorism.

neoblastic /nē′ōblas′tik/ [Gk *neos* + *blastos* germ], of or pertaining to a new tissue or development within a new tissue.

neocerebellum /nē′ōser′əbe′əm/, those parts of the cerebellum that receive input via the corticopontocerebellar pathway.

neocortex /nē′ōkôr′teks/ [Gk *neos* + L *cortex* bark], the most recently evolved part of the brain. In humans, the neocortex includes all of the cerebral cortex except for the hippocampal and piriform areas.

neodymium (Nd) /nē′ōdin′ē·əm/ [Gk *neos* + *didymos* twin], a rare earth element. Its atomic number is 60; its atomic weight is 144.27.

neoglottis /nē′ōglot′is/, a vibrating structure that replaces the glottis in alaryngeal speech, as after a laryngectomy.

neologism /nē·ol′əjiz′əm/ [Gk *neos* + *logos* word] **1.** a newly coined word or term. **2.** (in psychiatry) a word coined by a psychotic or delirious patient that is meaningful only to the patient.

neomycin sulfate, an aminoglycoside antibiotic prescribed in the treatment of infections of the intestine, in hepatic coma, and, topically, in the treatment of skin infections.

neon (Ne) /nē·on/ [Gk *neos* new], a colorless, odorless gaseous element and one

N

of the inert gases. Its atomic number is 10; its atomic weight is 20.2. Neon has no compounds and occurs in the atmosphere in the ratio of about 18 parts per million.

neonatal /nē′ōnā′təl/ [Gk *neos* + L *natus* born], the period of time covering the first 28 days after birth.

Neonatal Behavior Assessment Scale, a scale for evaluating and assessing an infant's alertness, motor maturity, irritability, consolability, and interaction with people. It is used as a tool for the evaluation of the neurologic condition and the behavior of a newborn infant.

neonatal breathing, respiration in newborn infants that begins when pulmonary fluid in the lungs is expelled by mechanical compression of the thorax during delivery and by resorption from the alveoli into the bloodstream and lymphatics. As air enters the lungs, the chest and lungs recoil to a resting position, but forceful inspirations are necessary to keep the lungs inflated.

neonatal conjunctivitis. See **ophthalmia neonatorum.**

neonatal death, the death of a live-born infant during the first 28 days after birth. Early neonatal death is usually considered to be one that occurs during the first 7 days.

neonatal developmental profile, an evaluation of the developmental status of a newborn infant based on three examinations: a gestational age inventory, a neurologic examination, and a Neonatal Behavior Assessment score.

neonatal hyperbilirubinemia. See **hyperbilirubinemia of the newborn.**

neonatal intensive care unit (NICU), a hospital unit containing a variety of sophisticated mechanic devices and special equipment for the management and care of premature and seriously ill newborn infants.

neonatal jaundice. See **hyperbilirubinemia of the newborn.**

neonatal mortality, the statistic rate of infant death during the first 28 days after live birth, expressed as the number of such deaths per 1,000 live births in a specific geographic area or institution in a given time.

neonatal period, the interval from birth to 28 days of age. It represents the time of the greatest risk to the infant.

neonatal pustular melanosis, a transient skin condition of the neonate characterized by vesicles present at birth that become pustular. The lesions contain neutrophils rather than eosinophils and they disappear within 72 hours.

neonatal thermoregulation, the regulation of the body temperature of a newborn infant, which may be affected by evaporation, conduction, radiation, and convection.

neonatal tyrosinemia. See **tyrosinemia.**

neonatal unit, a unit of a hospital that provides care and treatment of newborn infants through the age of 28 days, and longer if necessary.

neonate /nē′ōnāt/, an infant from birth to 4 weeks of age.

neonatology /nē′ōnātol′əjē/ [Gk *neos* + L *natus* born; Gk *logos* science], the branch of medicine that concentrates on the care of the neonate and specializes in the diagnosis and treatment of the disorders of the newborn infant. **–neonatologic, neonatological,** *adj.,* **neonatologist,** *n.*

neonatorum encephalitis /nē′ōnātôr′əm/ [Gk *neos* + L *natus*; Gk *enkephalos* brain; *itis*], a brain inflammation that develops in the first four weeks of life.

neoplasia /nē′ōplā′zhə/ [Gk *neos* + *plassein* to mold], the new and abnormal development of cells that may be benign or malignant. **–neoplastic,** *adj.*

neoplasm /nē′ōplaz′əm/ [Gk *neos* + *plasma* formation], any abnormal growth of new tissue, benign or malignant. **–neoplastic,** *adj.*

neoplastic fracture, a fracture resulting from weakened bone tissue caused by neoplasm or by a malignant growth.

neoplastic pericarditis, a pericardial inflammation, usually secondary to a malignant tumor within the area.

neoplasty /nē′ōplas′tē/ [Gk *neos* new + *plassein* to mold], a plastic surgery procedure to restore a part or add a new part.

neostigmine bromide /nē′ostig′mēn/, a cholinergic prescribed in the treatment of myasthenia gravis.

neoteny /nē·ot′ənē/ [Gk *neos* new, *teinein* to stretch], the attainment of sexual maturity during the larval stage of development, as in certain amphibians, especially salamanders.

nephelometer /nef′əlom′ətər/ [Gk *nephele* cloud, *metron* measure], a photometric apparatus used to determine the concentration of solids suspended in a liquid or a gas, as may be used to determine the number of bacteria in a specimen.

nephelometry /nef′əlom′ətrē/, a technique of determining the concentration of solids suspended in a liquid or a gas by use of a nephelometer. **–nephelometric, nephelometrical,** *adj.*

nephrectomy /nəfrek′təmē/ [Gk *nephros* kidney, *ektome* excision], the surgical removal of a kidney, performed to remove a tumor, drain an abcess, or treat hydrone-phrosis. **−nephrectomize,** *v.*

nephritic /nəfrit′ik/, pertaining to an in-flammation of the kidney.

nephritic calculus. See **renal calculus.**

nephritic gingivitis [Gk *nephros* + L *icus* like; *gingiva* gum; Gk *itis* inflammation], a kind of stomatitis and gingivitis associated with kidney function failure, accompanied by pain, ammoniac odor, and increased salivation.

nephritis /nəfrī′tis/ // [Gk *nephros* + *itis* inflammation], any one of a large group of diseases of the kidney characterized by inflammation and abnormal function. Kinds of nephritis include **acute nephritis, glomerulonephritis, hereditary nephritis, interstitial nephritis, parenchymatous nephritis,** and **suppurative nephritis.**

nephroangiosclerosis /nef′rō·an′jē·ōskler-ō′sis/ [Gk *nephros* + *aggeion* vessel, *skleros* hard, *osis* condition], necrosis of the renal arterioles, associated with hypertension. Early signs of the condition are head-aches, blurring of vision, and a diastolic blood pressure greater than 120 mm Hg. Examination of the retina reveals hemor-rhages, vascular exudates, and papill-edema. The heart is usually enlarged, especially the left ventricle. Proteins and red blood cells are found in the urine. Heart failure and kidney failure may occur if the disease remains untreated.

nephroblastoma. See **Wilms' tumor.**

nephrocalcinosis /nef′rōkal′sinō′sis/ [Gk *nephros* + L *calx* lime; Gk *osis* condition], an abnormal condition of the kidneys in which deposits of calcium form in the parenchyma at the site of previous inflammation or degenerative change.

nephrogenic /nef′rōjen′ik/ [Gk *nephros* + *genein* to produce], **1.** generating kidney tissue. **2.** originating in the kidney.

nephrogenic ascites, the abnormal presence of fluid in the peritoneal cavity of patients undergoing hemodialysis for renal failure. The cause of this type of ascites is unknown.

nephrogenic cord, either of the paired longitudinal ridges of tissue that lie along the dorsal surface of the coelom in the early developing vertebrate embryo. It gives rise to the structures comprising the embryonic urogenital system.

nephrogenic diabetes insipidus, an ab-normal condition in which the kidneys do not concentrate the urine, resulting in polyuria, polydipsia, and very dilute urine.

nephrogenous /nəfroj′ənəs/, of or per-taining to the formation and development of the kidneys.

nephrohypertrophy /nef′rōhīpur′trəfē/ [Gk *nephros* + *hyper* excessive, *trophe* nourishment], enlargement of the kid-ney.

nephrolith /nef′rəlith/ [Gk *nephros* + *lithos* stone], a calculus formed in a kid-ney. **−nephrolithic,** *adj.*

nephrolithiasis /nef′rōlithī′əsis/, a disor-der characterized by the presence of cal-culi in the kidney.

nephrology /nəfrol′əjē/ [Gk *nephros* + *logos* science], the study of the anatomy, physiology, and pathology of the kidney. **−nephrologic, nephrological,** *adj.*

nephrolytic /nef′rōlit′ik/ [Gk *nephros* + *lysis* loosening], of or pertaining to the de-struction of the structure and function of a kidney.

nephromere. See **nephrotome.**

nephron /nef′ron/ [Gk *nephros* kidney], a structural and functional unit of the kid-ney, resembling a microscopic funnel with a long stem and two convoluted sections. Each kidney contains about 1.25 million nephrons, each consisting of the renal cor-puscle, the loop of Henle, and the renal tu-bules. Each renal corpuscle consists of the glomerulus of renal capillaries enclosed within Bowman's capsule.

nephronophthisis. See **medullary cystic disease.**

nephroparalysis [Gk *nephros* + *paralyein* to be palsied], a paralysis of the kidney resulting in a cessation of functions of that organ.

nephropathy /nefrop′əthē/ [Gk *nephros* + *pathos* disease], any disorder of the kid-ney, including inflammatory, degenerative, and sclerotic conditions.

nephropexy /nef′rəpek′sē/ /nef′rəpek′sē/ [Gk *nephros* + *pexis* fixation], a surgi-cal operation to fixate a floating or ptotic kidney.

nephroptosis /nef′rəptō′sis/ [Gk *nephros* + *ptosis* falling], a downward displace-ment or dropping of a kidney.

nephrorrhaphy /nəfrôr′əfē/ [Gk *nephros* + *rhaphe* suture], an operation that sutures a floating kidney in place.

nephrosclerosis. See **nephroangioscle-rosis.**

nephroscope /nef′rəskōp′/ [Gk *nephros* + *skopein* to look], a fiberoptic instrument that is used specifically for the disintegra-tion and removal of renal calculi. The ne-phroscope is inserted percutaneously, and the calculi are located through use of x-ray films of the renal pelvis. An ultrasonic probe emitting high-frequency sound waves breaks up the calculi, which are re-moved by suction through the scope.

nephrosis. See **nephrotic syndrome.**

nephrostoma /nef′rəstō′mə/, *pl.* **nephros-tomas, nephrostomata** [Gk *nephros* +

stoma mouth], the funnel-shaped ciliated opening of the excretory tubules into the coelom of the early developing vertebrate embryo. **–nephrostomic,** *adj.*

nephrostomy /nəfros'fəmē/, a surgical procedure in which an incision is made on the flank of the patient so that a catheter can be inserted into the kidney pelvis for the purpose of drainage.

nephrotic syndrome [Gk *nephros* + L *icus* like], an abnormal condition of the kidney characterized by proteinuria, hypoalbuminemia, and edema. It occurs in glomerular disease, thrombosis of a renal vein, and as a complication of many systemic diseases, diabetes mellitus, amyloidosis, systemic lupus erythematosus, and multiple myeloma.

nephrotome /nef'rətom/ [Gk *nephros* + *tome* section], a zone of segmented mesodermal tissue in the developing vertebrate embryo. It is the primordial tissue for the urogenital system and gives rise to the nephrogenic cord.

nephrotomography /nef'rətəmog'rəfē/ [Gk *nephros* + *tome* section, *graphein* to record], sectional radiographic examination of the kidneys.

nephrotomy /nəfrot'əmē/ [Gk *nephros* + *temnein* to cut], a surgical procedure in which an incision is made in the kidney.

nephrotoxic [Gk *nephros* + *toxikon* poison], toxic or destructive to a kidney.

nephrotoxin, a toxin with specific destructive properties for the kidneys.

nephroureterolithiasis /nef'rōyoo't-ərōlithī'əsis/, the presence of calculi in the kidneys and ureters.

neptunium (Np) /nept(y)ōo'nē-əm/ [planet Neptune], a transuranic, metallic element. Its atomic number is 93; its atomic weight is 237.

Nernst equation [Hermann W. Nernst, German physicist, b. 1864; L *aequare* to make equal], (in cardiology) an expression of the relationship between the electric potential across a membrane and the concentration ratio between permeable ions on either side of the membrane.

nerve /nurv/ [L *nervus*], one or more bundles of impulse-carrying fibers that connect the brain and the spinal cord with other parts of the body. Nerves transmit afferent impulses from receptor organs toward the brain and the spinal cord and efferent impulses peripherally to the effector organs. Each nerve consists of an epineurium enclosing fasciculi of nerve fibers, each fasciculus surrounded by its own sheath of connective tissue.

nerve accommodation, the ability of nerve tissue to adjust to a constant source and intensity of stimulation so that some change in either intensity or duration of the stimulus is necessary to elicit a response beyond the initial reaction.

nerve block anesthesia. See **conduction anesthesia.**

nerve cable graft, a multistrand free nerve graft, taken from elsewhere in the body, to bridge a large gap in one of the main nerves in the forearm.

nerve compression, a pathologic event that causes harmful pressure on one or more nerve trunks, resulting in nerve damage and muscle weakness or atrophy. Any nerve that passes over a rigid prominence is vulnerable, and the degree of damage depends on the magnitude and the duration of the compressive force.

nerve conduction test, an electrodiagnostic test of the integrity of the peripheral nerves. It involves placing an electric stimulator over a nerve and measuring the time required for an impulse to travel over a measured segment of the nerve. The test is used in the diagnosis of nerve entrapment syndrome and polyneuropathies.

nerve deafness. See **sensorineural hearing loss.**

nerve entrapment, an abnormal condition and type of mononeuropathy, characterized by nerve damage and muscle weakness or atrophy. Nerves that pass over rigid prominences or through narrow bony and fascial canals are particularly prone to entrapment. The common signs of this disorder are pain and muscular weakness. One of the most common types of entrapment is **carpal tunnel syndrome.**

nerve excitability, the readiness of a nerve cell to respond to a stimulus.

nerve fiber, a slender process of a neuron, usually the axon. Each fiber is classified as myelinated or unmyelinated. Myelinated fibers are further designated as A or B fibers; C fibers are unmyelinated. The A fibers are somatic, 1 to 20 μm in diameter, and have a conduction velocity of 5 to 120 meters per second. B fibers are more finely myelinated than A fibers and have a diameter up to 3 μm and a conduction rate of 3 to 15 meters per second. They are both afferent and efferent and are mainly associated with visceral innervation. The unmyelinated C fibers have a diameter of 0.3 to 1.3 μm and a conduction rate of 0.6 to 2 meters per second. They are efferent postganglionic autonomic fibers and afferent fibers that conduct impulses of prolonged, burning pain sensation from the viscera and periphery.

nerve growth factor (NGF), a protein resembling insulin whose hormonelike action affects differentiation, growth, and maintenance of neurons.

nerve impulse. See **impulse.**

nerve plexus [L *nervus* + *plexus* plaited], an interwoven network of nerves, as the lumbar plexus formed by the anterior primary branch of the upper four lumbar nerves.

nerve sheath [L *nervus*; AS *scaeth*], any of several types of coatings or coverings for nerve fibers and nerve tracts. Kinds of nerve sheaths include **endoneurial, medullary, myelin, neurilemma,** and **notochordal.**

nervous breakdown [L *nervus*; AS *brecan* to break, *dune* down], *informal.* any mental condition that markedly interferes with and disrupts normal functioning.

nervous emesis [L *nervus*; Gk *emesis* vomiting], vomiting that is functional and psychogenic. The condition is most common among young women and is regarded as a psychologic representation of a desire to reject something.

nervous prostration [L *nervus* + *prosternere* to throw down], a condition of irritable weakness and depression, which may be psychogenic or the result of a severe prolonged illness or exhausting experience.

nervous system [L *nervus* nerve; Gk *system*], the extensive, intricate network of structures that activates, coordinates, and controls all the functions of the body. It is divided into the central nervous system, composed of the brain and the spinal cord, and the peripheral nervous system, which includes the cranial nerves and the spinal nerves. These morphologic subdivisions combine and communicate to innervate the somatic and the visceral parts of the body with the afferent and the efferent nerve fibers. Afferent fibers carry sensory impulses to the central nervous system; efferent fibers carry motor impulses from the central nervous system to the muscles and other organs. The somatic fibers are associated with the bones, the muscles, and the skin. The visceral fibers are associated with the internal organs, the blood vessels, and the mucous membranes.

nervous tachypnea [L *nervus*; Gk *tachys* rapid + *pnoia* breath], a neurotic symptom characterized by quick, shallow breathing.

nervus abducens. See **abducens nerve.**

nervus accessorius. See **accessory nerve.**

nervus facialis. See **facial nerve.**

nervus glossopharyngeus. See **glossopharyngeal nerve.**

nervus hypoglossus. See **hypoglossal nerve.**

nervus oculomotorius. See **oculomotor nerve.**

nervus olfactorius. See **olfactory nerve.**

nervus opticus. See **optic nerve.**

nervus terminalis. See **terminal nerve.**

nervus trigeminus. See **trigeminal nerve.**

nervus trochlearis. See **trochlear nerve.**

nervus vagus. See **vagus nerve.**

nested nails, in orthopedic surgery, a pair of nails placed side by side in the medullary canal of long bones.

nettle rash [AS *netele* nettle; Fr *rasche* scurf], a fine, urticarial eruption resulting from skin contact with stinging nettle, a common weed with leaves containing histamine.

networking, 1. (in psychiatric nursing) the process of developing a set of agencies and professional personnel that are able to create a system of communication and support for psychiatric patients, usually those newly discharged from inpatient psychiatric facilities. Kinds of networks include **natural network** and **professional network. 2.** a network of supportive contacts or services, such as the Women's Health Network.

Neufeld nail /noi′felt/ [Alonzo J. Neufeld. American surgeon, b. 1906], an orthopedic nail with a V-shaped tip and shank used for fixating an intertrochanteric fracture. The nail is driven into the neck of the femur until it reaches a round metal plate screwed onto the side of the femur.

Neufeld roller traction, a traction device for a fractured femur, consisting of a cast for the calf and thigh hinged at the knee and suspended by a line to the anterior mid-thigh looped around a pulley and to a spring attached to the anterior midleg.

neural /nŏŏr′əl/ [Gk *neuron* nerve], of or pertaining to nerve cells and their processes.

neural canal. See **neurocoele.**

neural crest, the band of ectodermally derived cells that lies along the outer surface of each side of the neural tube in the early stages of embryonic development.

neural ectoderm, the part of the embryonic ectoderm that develops into the neural tube.

neural fold, either of the paired longitudinal elevations resulting from the invagination of the neural plate in the early developing embryo. The folds unite to enclose the neural groove and form the neural tube.

neuralgia /nŏŏral′jə/ [Gk *neuron* + *algos* pain], an abnormal condition characterized by severe stabbing pain, caused by a variety of disorders affecting the nervous system. **–neuralgic,** *adj.*

neuralgic amyotrophy /nŏŏral′jik/, a brachial plexus disorder characterized by sudden pain and muscle weakness in the upper limbs and possible muscular wasting or atrophy. The cause is unknown.

neural groove, the longitudinal depression that occurs between the neural folds during the invagination of the neural plate to form the neural tube in the early stages of embryonic development.

neural impulse. See **impulse.**

neural plate, a thick layer of ectodermal tissue that lies along the central longitudinal axis of the early developing embryo and gives rise to the neural tube and subsequently to the brain, spinal cord, and other tissues of the central nervous system.

neural tube, the longitudinal tube, lying along the central axis of the early developing embryo, that gives rise to the brain, spinal cord, and other neural tissue of the central nervous system.

neural tube defect, any of a group of congenital malformations involving defects in the skull and spinal column that are caused primarily by the failure of the neural tube to close during embryonic development. In some instances, the cleft results from an abnormal increase in cerebrospinal fluid pressure on the closed neural tube during the first trimester of development.

neural tube formation, the various processes and stages involved in the embryonic development of the neural tube, which subsequently differentiates into the brain, the spinal cord, and other neural tissue of the central nervous system.

neurapraxia /nŏŏr′əprak′sē·ə/, the interruption of nerve conduction without loss of continuity of the axon.

neurasthenia /nŏŏr′asthē′nē·ə/ [Gk *neuron + a, sthenos* not strength], **1.** an abnormal condition characterized by nervous exhaustion and a vague functional fatigue that often follows depression. **2.** (in psychiatry) a stage in the recovery from a schizophrenic experience, during which the patient is listless and apparently unable to cope with routine activities and relationships. **–neurasthenic,** *adj.*

neurectomy /nŏŏrek′təmē/ [Gk *neuron + ektome* cutting out], the surgical excision of a nerve segment.

neurenteric canal /nŏŏr′ənter′ik/ [Gk *neuron + enteron* intestine; L *canalis* channel], a tubular passage between the posterior part of the neural tube and the archenteron in the early embryonic development of lower animals.

neurilemma /nŏŏr′əlem′ə/ [Gk *neuron + lemma* sheath], a layer of cells composed of one or more Schwann cells that encloses the segmented myelin sheaths of peripheral nerve fibers. Each myelinated

nerve fiber has a neurilemma cell for each internodal segment between the nodes of Ranvier. The nerve fibers of the brain and the spinal cord are not enclosed by neurilemma. **–neurilemmal, neurilemmatic, neurilemmatous,** *adj.*

neurilemoma. See **schwannoma.**

neurinoma /nŏŏr′inō′mə/, *pl.* **neurinomas, neurinomata** [Gk *neuron + oma* tumor], **1.** a tumor of the nerve sheath. It is usually benign but may undergo malignant change. A kind of neurinoma is **acoustic neurinoma. 2.** a neuroma.

neuritis /nŏŏrī′tis/, *pl.* **neuritides** [Gk *neuron + itis* inflammation], an abnormal condition characterized by inflammation of a nerve. Some of the signs of this condition are neuralgia, hyperthesia, anesthesia, paralysis, muscular atrophy, and defective reflexes.

neuroarthropathy /nŏŏr′ō·ärthrop′əthē/ [Gk *neuron + arthron* joint, *pathos* disease], a condition in which a disease of a joint is secondary to a disease of the nervous system.

neuroblast /nŏŏr′əblast/ [Gk *neuron + blastos* germ], any embryonic cell that develops into a functional neuron; an immature nerve cell. **–neuroblastic,** *adj.*

neuroblastoma /nŏŏr′ōblastō′mə/, *pl.* **neuroblastomas, neuroblastomata** [Gk *neuron + blastos* germ, *oma* tumor], a highly malignant tumor composed of primitive ectodermal cells derived from the neural plate during embryonic life. Symptoms may include an abdominal mass, respiratory distress, and anemia, depending on the site of the primary tumor and metastases, and hormonally active adrenal lesions may cause irritability, flushing, sweating, hypertension, and tachycardia. A kind of neuroblastoma is **Pepper syndrome.**

neurocele. See **neurocoele.**

neurocentral /nŏŏr′ōsen′trəl/ [Gk *neuron + kentron* center], pertaining to the centrum and the developing vertebrae in the early stages of embryology.

neurocentrum /nŏŏr′ōsen′trəm/ [Gk *neuron + L centrum* center], the embryonic mesodermal tissue that subsequently gives rise to the vertebrae.

neuro check /nŏŏr′ō/ [Gk *neuron + ME chek* stop], *nontechnical;* a brief neurologic assessment, usually performed in the triage of patients in an emergency situation or on admission to an emergency service. The level of consciousness is evaluated as alert and oriented, lethargic, stuporous, or comatose.

neurocirculatory asthenia /nŏŏr′ōsur′kyəlätôr′ē/ [Gk *neuron + L circulare* to go around; Gk *a, sthenos* not strength], a psychosomatic disorder characterized by nervous and circulatory irregularities, including dyspnea, palpitation, giddiness, vertigo, tremor, precordial pain, and increased susceptibility to fatigue.

neurocoele /nŏŏr′əsēl/ [Gk *neuron* + *koilos* hollow], a system of cavities in the central nervous system of humans and other vertebrate animals. It consists of the ventricles of the brain and the central canal of the spinal cord.

neurocytoma /nŏŏr′ōsītō′mə/ [Gk *neuron* + *kytos* cell, *oma* tumor], a tumor composed of undifferentiated nerve cells that are usually ganglionic.

neuroderm. See **neuroectoderm.**

neurodermatitis /nŏŏ′rōdur′mətī′tis/ [Gk *neuron* + *derma* skin, *itis* inflammation], a nonspecific, pruritic skin disorder seen in anxious, nervous individuals. Excoriations and lichenification are found on easily accessible, exposed areas of the body such as the forearms and forehead. Sometimes loosely (and incorrectly) applied to **atopic dermatitis.**

neurodevelopmental adaptation, a type of therapy that emphasizes the inhibition/integration of primitive postural patterns and promotes the development of normal postural reactions and achievement of normal tone. The therapy is employed in the treatment of children with cerebral palsy.

neuroectoderm /nŏŏ′ō·ek′tədurm′/ [Gk *neuron* + *ektos* outside, *derma* skin], the part of the embryonic ectoderm that gives rise to the central and peripheral nervous systems, including some glial cells. –**neuroectodermal,** *adj.*

neuroendocrine /nŏŏr′ō·en′dəkrin/ [Gk *neuron* + *endon* within, *krinein* to secrete], pertaining to or resembling the effects produced by endocrine glands strongly linked with the nervous system.

neuroepithelioma /nŏŏr′ō·ep′ithē′lē·ō′mə/ [Gk *neuron* + *epi* upon, *thele* nipple, *oma* tumor], an uncommon neoplasm of neuroepithelium in a sensory nerve.

neurofibroma /nŏŏr′ōfibrō′mə/, *pl.* **neurofibromas, neurofibromata** [Gk *neuron* + L *fibra* fiber; Gk *oma* tumor], a fibrous tumor of nerve tissue resulting from the abnormal proliferation of Schwann cells.

neurofibromatosis /nŏŏr′ōfī′brōmətō′sis/ [Gk *neuron* + *fibra* fiber; Gk *oma* tumor, *osis* condition], a congenital condition characterized by numerous neurofibromas of the nerves and skin, by café-au-lait spots on the skin, and, in some cases, by developmental anomalies of the muscles, bones, and viscera. Many large, pedunculated soft-tissue tumors may develop.

neurogen /nŏŏr′əjən/ [Gk *neuron* + *genein* to produce], a substance within the early

developing embryo that stimulates the primary organizer to initiate the formation of the neural plate, which gives rise to the primary axis of the body.

neurogenesis /nŏŏr′ōjen′əsis/ [Gk *neuron* + *genesis* origin], the development of the tissue of the nervous system. –**neurogenetic,** *adj.*

neurogenic /nŏŏr′ōjen′ik/ [Gk *neuron* + *genesis* origin], **1.** pertaining to the formation of nervous tissue. **2.** the stimulation of nervous energy. **3.** originating in the nervous system.

neurogenic arthropathy, an abnormal condition associated with neural damage, characterized by the gradual and usually painless degeneration of a joint.

neurogenic bladder, dysfunctional urinary bladder caused by a lesion of the nervous system. Treatment is aimed at enabling the bladder to empty completely and regularly, preventing infection, controlling incontinence, and preserving kidney function. Kinds of neurogenic bladder are **spastic bladder, reflex bladder,** and **flaccid bladder.**

neurogenic fracture, a fracture associated with the destruction of the nerve supply to a specific bone.

neurogenic shock, a form of shock that results from peripheral vascular dilation as a result of neurologic injury.

neuroglia /nŏŏrog′lē·ə/ [Gk *neuron* + *glia* glue], the supporting or connective tissue cells of the central nervous system. Kinds of neuroglia include **astrocytes, oligodendroglia,** and **microglia.** –**neuroglial,** *adj.*

neurography /nŏŏrog′rəfē/, the study of the action potentials of the nerves.

neurohumor [Gk *neuron* + L *humor* fluid], one of the chemical substances, formed and transmitted by a neuron, that is essential for the activity of adjacent neurons or nearby organs or muscles. Kinds of neurohumoral substances are **acetylcholine, dopamine, epinephrine, norepinephrine,** and **serotonin.** –**neurohumoral,** *adj.*

neurohypophyseal hormone /nŏŏr′ōhī′pōfiz′ē·əl/ [Gk *neuron* + *hypo* under, *phyein* to grow], a hormone secreted by the posterior pituitary gland. Kinds of neurohypophyseal hormones are **oxytocin** and **vasopressin.**

neurohypophysis /nŏŏr′ōhīpof′isis/ [Gk *neuron* + *hypo* under, *phyein* to grow], the posterior lobe of the pituitary gland that is the source of antidiuretic hormone (ADH) and oxytocin. Nervous stimulation controls the release of both substances into the blood. The neurohypophysis releases ADH when stimulated by the hypothala-

N

mus by an increase in the osmotic pressure of extracellular fluid in the body. The neurohypophysis releases oxytocin under appropriate stimulation from the hypothalamus.

neuroimmunology /nŏŏr'ō·im'yŏŏnol'əjē/ [Gk *neuron* + L *immunis* freedom; Gk *logos* science], the study of relationships between the immune and nervous systems, such as autoimmune activity in neurologic diseases.

neurolemma. See **neurilemma.**

neurolepsis /nŏŏr'ōlep'sis/ [Gk *neuron* + *lepsis* seizure], an altered state of consciousness, as induced by a neuroleptic agent, characterized by quiescence, reduced motor activity, anxiety, and indifference to the surroundings. Sleep may occur, but usually the person can be aroused and can respond to commands.

neurolept. See **neuroleptic.**

neuroleptanalgesia /nŏŏr'ōlept'anəljē'zē·ə/ [Gk *neuron* + *lepsis* seizure, *a, algos* not pain], a form of analgesia achieved by the concurrent administration of a neuroleptic and an analgesic. Anxiety, motor activity, and sensitivity to painful stimuli are reduced; the person is quiet and indifferent to the environment and surroundings. Sleep may or may not occur, but the patient is not unconscious and is able to respond to commands.

neuroleptanesthesia /nŏŏr'ōlept'anəsthē'zhə/ [Gk *neuron* + *lepsis* seizure, *anaisthesia* loss of feeling], a form of anesthesia achieved by the administration of a neuroleptic agent, a narcotic analgesic, and nitrous oxide in oxygen. Induction of anesthesia is slow, but consciousness returns quickly after the inhalation of nitrous oxide is stopped.

neuroleptic /nŏŏr'ōlep'tik/ [Gk *neuron* + *lepsis* seizure], **1.** of or pertaining to neurolepsis. **2.** a drug that causes neurolepsis, such as the butyrophenone derivative, droperidol.

neuroleptic anesthesia [Gk, *neuron*, nerve; *lepsis*, seizure; *anaisthesia*, lack of feeling], a form of anesthesia induced by an injection of a butyrophenone derivative with a narcotic analgesic.

neuroleptic malignant syndrome [Gk *neuron* + *lepsis*; L *malignus* bad disposition; Gk *syn* together, *dromos* course], a complication of psychotherapy with neuroleptic drugs given in therapeutic doses. It is characterized by hypertonicity, pallor, dyskinesia, hyperthermia, incontinence, unstable blood pressure, and pulmonary congestion.

neurolinguistic programming /nŏŏr'ōling·gwi'stik/, a communication approach based on a conceptualization of levels of experience within the person and levels of the self. It involves both verbal and nonverbal messages, sensory experience, awareness or perception through patterns of behavior that can be observed and perceived.

neurologic assessment /nŏŏr'ōloj'ik/ [Gk *neuron* + *logos* science; L *icus* like; *adsidere* to approximate], an evaluation of the patient's neurologic status and symptoms. If alert and oriented, the patient is asked about instances of weakness, numbness, headaches, pain, tremors, nervousness, irritability, or drowsiness. Information is elicited regarding loss of memory, periods of confusion, hallucinations, and episodes of loss of consciousness. The patient's general appearance, facial expression, attention span, responses to verbal and painful stimuli, emotional status, coordination, balance, cognition, and ability to follow commands are noted. If the patient is disoriented, stuporous, or comatose, demonstrated signs of these states are recorded.

neurologic examination, a systematic examination of the nervous system, including an assessment of mental status, of the function of each of the cranial nerves, of sensory and neuromuscular function, of the reflexes, and of proprioception and other cerebellar functions.

neurologist /nŏŏrol'əjist/, a physician who specializes in neurology.

neurology (neurol.) /nŏŏrol'əjē/ [Gk *neuron* + *logos* science], the field of medicine that deals with the nervous system and its disorders. **–neurologic, neurological,** *adj.*

neuroma /nŏŏrō'mə/, *pl.* **neuromas, neuromata** [Gk *neuron* + *oma* tumor], a benign neoplasm composed chiefly of neurons and nerve fibers, usually arising from a nerve tissue. It may be relatively soft or extremely hard and vary in size. Pain radiating from the lesion to the periphery of the affected nerve is usually intermittent but may become continuous and severe.

neuroma cutis, a neoplasm in the skin that contains nerve tissue and that may be extremely sensitive to painful stimuli.

neuroma telangiectodes. See **nevoid neuroma.**

neuromatosis /nŏŏr'ōmətō'sis/ [Gk *neuron* + *oma* tumor, *osis* condition], a neoplastic disease characterized by numerous neuromas.

neuromodulator, a substance that alters transmission of nerve impulses.

neuromotor [Gk *neuron* + L *mover* to move], pertaining to both the nerves and muscles, or to nerve impulses transmitted to muscles.

neuromuscular /nŏŏr'ōmus'kyələr/ [Gk *neuron* + L *musculus* muscle], of or pertaining to the nerves and the muscles.

neuromuscular blockade, the inhibition of a muscular contraction activated by the nervous system, possibly resulting in muscle weakness or paralysis.

neuromuscular blocking agent, a chemical substance that interferes locally with the transmission or reception of impulses from motor nerves to skeletal muscles. Nondepolarizing agents competitively block the transmitter action of acetylcholine at the postjunctional membrane. Depolarizing blocking agents compete with acetylcholine for cholinergic receptors of the motor end plate. Neuromuscular blocking agents are used to induce muscle relaxation in anesthesia, endotracheal intubation, and electroshock therapy and as adjuncts in the treatment of tetanus, encephalitis, and poliomyelitis.

neuromuscular junction, the area of contact between the ends of a large myelinated nerve fiber and a fiber of skeletal muscle.

neuromuscular spindle, any one of a number of small bundles of delicate muscular fibers, enclosed by a capsule, in which sensory nerve fibers terminate. The nerve fibers end as naked axons encircling the intrafusal fibers with flattened expansions or ovoid disks.

neuromyal transmission /nŏŏr'rōmī'əl/ [Gk *neuron* + *mys* muscle; L *transmittere* to transmit], the passage of excitation from a motor neuron to a muscle fiber at the myoneural junction.

neuromyelitis /nŏŏr'ōmī'əlī'tis/ [Gk *neuron* + *myelos* marrow, *itis* inflammation], an abnormal condition characterized by inflammation of the spinal cord and peripheral nerves.

neuron /nŏŏr'on/ [Gk, nerve], the basic nerve cell of the nervous system, containing a nucleus within a cell body and extending one or more processes. Neurons are classified according to the direction in which they conduct impulses and according to the number of processes they extend. Sensory neurons transmit nerve impulses toward the spinal cord and the brain. Motor neurons transmit nerve impulses from the brain and the spinal cord to the muscles and the glandular tissue. Multipolar neurons have one axon and several dendrites, as do most of the neurons in the brain and the spinal cord. Bipolar neurons have only one axon and one dendrite. Unipolar neurons are embryonic structures that originate as bipolar bodies but fuse dendrites and axons into a single fiber that stretches for a short distance

from the cell body before separating again into the two processes. As the carriers of nerve impulses, neurons function according to electrochemical processes involving positively charged sodium and potassium ions and the changing electric potential of the extracellular and the intracellular fluid of the neuron.

neuronal /nŏŏr'ənəl, nŏŏrō'nəl/, pertaining to or resembling a neuron.

neuronitis /nŏŏr'əni'tis/ [Gk *neuron* + *itis* inflammation], an abnormal condition characterized by inflammation of a nerve or a nerve cell, especially the cells and the roots of the spinal nerves.

neuropathic bladder. See **neurogenic bladder.**

neuropathic joint disease [Gk *neuron* + *pathos* disease], a chronic, progressive, degenerative disease of one or more joints, characterized by swelling, instability of the joint, hemorrhage, heat, and atrophic and hypertrophic changes in the bone. The disease is the result of an underlying neurologic disorder, such as tabes dorsalis from syphilis, diabetic neuropathy, leprosy, or congenital absence or depression of pain sensation.

neuropathy /nŏŏrop'əthē/ [Gk *neuron* + *pathos* disease], any abnormal condition characterized by inflammation and degeneration of the peripheral nerves, as that associated with lead poisoning. **–neuropathic,** *adj.*

neuroplasty [Gk *neuron* + *plassein* to mold], plastic surgery to repair a nerve.

neuroplegia /nŏŏr'ōplē'jē·ə/ [Gk *neuron* + *plege* stroke], nerve paralysis caused by disease, injury, or the effect of neuroleptic drugs, administered to achieve **neuroleptanalgesia** or **neuroleptanesthesia.**

neuropore /nŏŏr'opôr/ [Gk *neuron* + *poros* pore], the opening at each end of the neural tube during early embryonic development. Kinds of neuropores are **anterior neuropore** and **posterior neuropore.**

neuropraxia /nŏŏr'ōprak'sē·ə/ [Gk *neuron* + *prassein* to do], a condition in which a nerve remains in place following a severe injury although it no longer transmits impulses.

neurorrhaphy /nŏŏrôr'əfē/ [Gk *neuron* + *rhaphe* suture], a surgical procedure to suture a severed nerve.

neurosarcoma /nŏŏr'ōsärkō'mə/ [Gk *neuron* + *sarx* flesh, *oma* tumor], a malignant neoplasm composed of nerve tissue, connective tissue, and vascular tissue.

neuroscience /nŏŏr'ōsī'əns/ [Gk *neuron* + L *scientia*], the study of neurology and related subjects, including neuroanatomy, neurophysiology, neuropharmacology, and neurosurgery.

neurosis /nŏŏrō'sis/ [Gk *neuron* + *osis* condition], *informal;* an emotional disturbance other than psychosis.

neuroskeleton [Gk *neuron* + *skeletos* dried up], the parts of the skeleton that surround or otherwise protect the nervous system, particularly the skull and vertebrae.

neurosurgery [Gk *neuron* + *cheirourgos* surgeon], any surgery involving the brain, spinal cord, or peripheral nerves. Brain surgery is performed to treat a wound, remove a tumor or foreign body, relieve pressure in intracranial hemorrhage, excise an abscess, treat parkinsonism, or relieve pain. Kinds of brain surgery include craniotomy, lobotomy, and hypophysectomy. Surgery of the spine is performed to correct a defect, remove a tumor, repair a ruptured intervertebral disk, or relieve pain. Kinds of spinal surgery include fusion and laminectomy. Surgery on the peripheral nerves is performed to remove a tumor, relieve pain, or reconnect a severed nerve. One kind of nerve surgery is **sympathectomy.**

neurosyphilis /nŏŏr'ōsif'ilis/ [Gk *neuron* + *syn* together, *philein* to love], infection of the central nervous system by syphilis organisms, which may invade the meninges and cerebrovascular system. **–neurosyphilitic,** *adj.*

neurotendinous /nŏŏr'ōten'dinəs/ [Gk *neuron* + L, *tendo* tendon], pertaining to both nerves and tendons.

neurotendinous spindle [Gk *neuron* + L *tendo;* AS *spinel* spindle], a capsule containing enlarged tendon fibers, found chiefly near the junctions of tendons and muscles.

neurotic [Gk *neuron* + *osis* condition; L *icus* like], **1.** of or pertaining to neurosis or to a neurotic disorder. **2.** pertaining to the nerves. **3.** one who is afflicted with a neurosis. **4.** *informal;* an emotionally unstable person.

neurotic depression. See **dysthemic disorder.**

neurotic disorder, any mental disorder characterized by a symptom or group of symptoms that a person finds distressing, unacceptable, and alien to the personality, such as severe anxiety, obsessional thoughts, and compulsive acts, and that produces psychologic pain or discomfort disproportionate to the reality of the situation.

neurotic personality [Gk *neuron;* L *personalis* of a person], a personality characterized by traits and tendencies that increase the likelihood of a specific neurotic behavior. For example, the orderly, cautious, meticulous person may be prone to development of an obsessive-compulsive disorder.

neurotmesis /nŏŏr'ōtmē'sis/ [Gk *neuron* + *tmesis* cutting apart], a peripheral nerve injury in which the nerve is completely disrupted by laceration or traction.

neurotomy /nŏŏrot'əmē/, the surgical division of a nerve or nerves.

neurotoxic /nŏŏr'ōtok'sik/, having a poisonous effect on nerves and nerve cells, as when ingested lead degenerates peripheral nerves.

neurotoxicity [Gk *neuron* + *toxikon* poison], the ability of a drug or other agent to destroy or damage nervous tissue.

neurotoxin /nŏŏr'ōtok'sin/ [Gk *neuron* + *toxikon* poison], a toxin that acts directly on the tissues of the central nervous system, traveling along the axis cylinders of the motor nerves to the brain. The toxin may be in the venom of snakes, on the spines of a shell or in the flesh of fish or shellfish, or produced by bacteria.

neurotransmitter [Gk *neuron* + L *transmittere* to transmit], any one of numerous chemicals that modify or result in the transmission of nerve impulses between synapses. Neurotransmitters are released from synaptic knobs into synaptic clefts and bridge the gap between presynaptic and postsynaptic neurons. When a nerve impulse reaches a synaptic knob, neurotransmitter molecules squirt into the synaptic cleft and bind to specific receptors. This flow allows an associated diffusion of potassium and sodium ions that causes an action potential. Kinds of neurotransmitters include **acetylcholine chloride, gamma-aminobutyric acid,** and **norepinephrine.**

neurotripsy /nŏŏr'ōtrip'sē/, the surgical crushing of a nerve.

neurotropic viruses [Gk *neuron* + *tropein* to turn; *virus* poison], an unexplained attraction of viruses to nerve tissue. The predilection also applies to certain toxic chemicals.

neurotropism /nŏŏrot'rəpiz'əm/ [Gk *neuron* + *trepein* to turn], **1.** the tendency for certain microrganisms, poisons, and nutrients to be attracted to nervous tissue. **2.** the tendency of basic dyes to be attracted to nervous tissue.

neurula /nŏŏr'ələ/, *pl.* **neurulas, neurulae** [Gk *neuron* nerve], an early embryo during the period of neurulation when the nervous system tissue begins to differentiate.

neurulation /nŏŏrələ'shən/ [Gk *neuron* + L *atus* process], the development of the neural plate and the processes involved with its subsequent closure to form the neural tube during the early stages of embryonic development.

neutral /n(y)ōō′trəl/ [L *neutralis* neuter], the state exactly between two opposing values, qualities, or properties; for example, in electricity a neutral state is one in which there is neither a positive nor a negative charge.

neutralization [L *neutralis* + Gk *izein* to cause], the interaction between an acid and a base that produces a solution that is neither acidic nor basic. The usual products of neutralization are a salt and water.

neutral rotation, the position of a limb that is turned neither toward nor away from the body's midline.

neutral thermal environment, an environment created by any method or apparatus to maintain the normal body temperature to minimize oxygen consumption and caloric expenditure, such as in an incubator for a premature infant.

neutron /n(y)ōō′tron/ [L *neuter* neither; Gk *elektron* amber], (in physics) an elementary particle that is a constituent of the nuclei of all elements except hydrogen. It has no electric charge and is approximately the same size as a proton.

neutron activation analysis, the analysis of elements in a specimen, performed by exposing it to neutron irradiation to convert many elements to a radioactive form in which they can be identified by measuring their emissions of radiation.

neutropenia /nōō′trōpē′nē·ə/ [L *neuter* neither; Gk *penia* poverty], an abnormal decrease in the number of neutrophils in the blood. Neutropenia is associated with acute leukemia, infection, rheumatoid arthritis, vitamin B_{12} deficiency, and chronic splenomegaly.

neutrophil /nōō′trəfil/ [L *neuter* + Gk *philein* to love], a polymorphonuclear granular leukocyte that stains easily with neutral dyes. Neutrophils are the circulating white blood cells essential for phagocytosis and proteolysis in which bacteria, cellular debris, and solid particles are removed and destroyed.

neutrophil alkaline phosphatase. See **leukocyte alkaline phosphatase.**

neutrophilic leukemia. See **polymorphocytic leukemia.**

Neviaser procedure, the surgical transfer of a coracoacromial ligament to the clavicle for acromioclavicular separation.

nevoid amentia. See **Sturge-Weber syndrome.**

nevoid neuroma /nē′void/ [L *naevus* birthmark; Gk *eidos* form], a tumor of nerve tissue that contains numerous small blood vessels.

nevus /nē′vəs/ [L *naevus* birthmark], a pigmented, congenital skin blemish that is usually benign but may become cancerous.

nevus avaneus. See **spider telangiectasia.**

nevus flammeus /flam′ē·əs/, a flat, capillary hemangioma that is present at birth and that varies in color from pale red to deep reddish purple. These lesions are most often seen on the face. The depth of the color depends on whether the superficial, middle, or deep dermal vessels are involved.

nevus vascularis. See **capillary hemangioma.**

newborn [AS *niwe* new, *boren* to bear], **1.** recently born. **2.** a recently born infant; a neonate.

newborn intrapartal care, care of the newborn in the delivery area during the time after birth before the mother and infant are transferred to the postpartum unit. The nasopharynx and mouth may be suctioned to remove excess mucus as the head is born. Depending on the preference and the condition of the mother and the policies of the maternity service, the baby may then be placed on the mother's abdomen and covered with a warm, dry blanket or taken by the nurse to an infant warmer. Apgar scores are assigned at 1 minute of age and at 5 minutes of age; less commonly, another is assigned at 10 minutes of age. The baby is handled gently and quietly; bright lights are often avoided, and maternal contact is encouraged.

new drug, a drug for which the Food and Drug Administration requires premarketing approval. A new drug is generally regarded as one for which safety and effectiveness have not yet been demonstrated for its prescribed use.

New England Journal of Medicine (NEJM), a weekly professional medical journal that publishes findings of medical research and articles about controversial political and ethical issues in the practice of medicine.

Newington orthosis, a bilateral orthosis similar to the **Toronto orthosis** except that flat bars are used and no joints are incorporated.

new growth, a neoplasm or tumor.

Newman, Margaret A., a nursing theorist who contributed to the study of nursing theories and models by defining three approaches to the discovery of nursing theory. They are: "borrowing" of theories from related disciplines, analyzing nursing practice situations in search of conceptual relationships, and creating new conceptual systems from which theories can be derived.

newspaper sign. See **thumb sign.**

newton [Sir Isaac Newton, English scientist, b. 1642], a unit of force in the SI system that would impart an acceleration to one kilogram of mass of one meter per second per second.

new tuberculin [ME *newe*; L *tuber* swelling], an extract of the tubercle bacillus from which all soluble material has been removed and glycerin added.

New World leishmaniasis. See **American leishmaniasis.**

New World typhus. See **murine typhus.**

Nezelof's syndrome /nez′əlofs/ [C. Nezelof, twentieth-century French physician], an abnormal condition characterized by absent T cell function, deficient B cell function, fairly normal immunoglobulin levels, and little or no specific antibody production. Nezelof's syndrome causes progressively severe, recurrent, and eventually fatal infections. Signs that often appear in infants or in children up to 4 years of age include recurrent pneumonia, otitis media, chronic fungal infections, upper respiratory tract infections, diarrhea, and hepatosplenomegaly. The disease may also enlarge the lymph nodes and the tonsils. Involved patients may also develop a tendency toward malignancy. Infection may cause sepsis, which is the usual cause of death. Symptoms that often suggest Nezelof's syndrome also include weight loss and poor eating habits.

nF, abbreviation for *nanofarad*.

NF, abbreviation for *National Formulary*.

NF1, a gene associated with neurofibromatosis. The gene is normally part of a family that helps regulate the timing of cell divisions. It may become defective, leading to neurofibromatosis expression, when an itinerant sequence of a DNA molecule becomes wedged in the NF1 gene. Other genetic disorders are believed to occur in a similar manner, by the dislocation of a "filler" sequence of a DNA molecule in a gene.

ng, abbreviation for **nanogram.**

NGF, abbreviation for **nerve growth factor.**

NG tube, abbreviation for **nasogastric tube.**

NGU, abbreviation for **nongonococcal urethritis.**

NHSC, abbreviation for **National Health Service Corps.**

Ni, symbol for the element **nickel.**

NIA, abbreviation for *National Institute on Aging.*

niacin /nī′əsin/, a white, crystalline, water-soluble vitamin of the B complex group usually occurring in various plant and animal tissues as nicotinamide. It functions as a coenzyme necessary for the breakdown and use of all major nutrients and is essential for a healthy skin, normal functioning of the GI tract, maintenance of the nervous system, and synthesis of the sex hormones. Symptoms of deficiency include muscular weakness, general fatigue, loss of appetite, various skin eruptions, halitosis, stomatitis, insomnia, irritability, nausea, vomiting, recurring headaches, tender gums, tension, and depression. Severe deficiency results in pellagra.

niacinamide /nī′əsin′əmīd/, a B complex vitamin. It is closely related to niacin but has no vasodilating action.

niacin equivalent (NE), an interconversion factor for estimating the contribution of tryptophan in the diet toward meeting the recommended daily allowance of niacin. The convention is to calculate 60 mg of tryptophan as the equivalent of 1 mg of niacin and to regard each as 1 niacin equivalent (NE).

NIB, abbreviation for **National Institute for the Blind.**

NICHHD, abbreviation for **National Institute of Child Health and Human Development.**

Nicholas procedure, a surgical procedure for repairing severe ligamentous injuries to the knee. It involves five procedures: a medial meniscectomy, a medial collateral ligament repair, a vastus medialis advancement, semitendinosus advancement, and a pes anserinus transfer.

nick [ME *nyke* notch], (in molecular genetics) a fissure or split in a single strand of DNA that can be made with the enzyme deoxyribonuclease or with ethidium bromide.

nickel (Ni) [Ger *Kupfer-nickel* false copper], a silvery white metallic element. Its atomic number is 28; its atomic weight is 58.71. Many people are allergic to nickel.

nickel dermatitis, an allergic contact dermatitis caused by the metal, nickel. Exposure comes usually from jewelry, wristwatches, metal clasps, and coins. Sweating increases the degree of rash.

nick translation, a method of labeling DNA in the laboratory by using the enzyme DNA polymerase.

niclosamide /niklō′səmīd/, an anthelmintic prescribed in the treatment of beef tapeworm and fish tapeworm infestations.

Nicola procedure, the surgical transfer of the long head of the biceps tendon through the humeral head for chronic anterior shoulder dislocation.

Nicholas procedure, a surgical procedure for repairing severe ligamentous injuries to the knee.

nicotinamide. See **niacinamide.**

nicotine /nik′ətēn/ [Jean Nicot Villemain, French ambassador to Portugal, b. 1530], a colorless, rapidly acting toxic substance in tobacco that is one of the major contributors to the ill effects of smoking. It is used as an insecticide in agriculture and as a parasiticide in veterinary medicine. Ingestion of large amounts causes salivation, nausea, vomiting, diarrhea, headache, vertigo, slowing of the heartbeat, and, in acute cases, paralysis of respiratory muscles.

nicotine poisoning, poisoning from intake of nicotine. Nicotine poisoning is characterized by stimulation of the central and autonomic nervous systems followed by depression of these systems. In fatal cases, death occurs from respiratory failure.

nicotine polacrilex /pōlak′rileks/, a chewing gum (nicotine resin complex) source of nicotine as an adjunct for smoking cessation.

nicotinic acid. See **niacin.**

nicotinyl alcohol /nik′ətē′nil/, an alcohol used as a vasodilator, in the form of its tartrate salt, in the treatment of peripheral vascular disease, vascular spasm, varicose ulcers, decubital ulcers, chilblains, Ménière's disease, and vertigo.

NICU, abbreviation for **neonatal intensive care unit.**

NID, abbreviation for *National Institute for the Deaf.*

NIDA, abbreviation for *National Institute on Drug Abuse.*

nidation /nīdā′shən/ [L *nidus* nest], the process by which an embryo burrows into the endometrium of the uterus.

NIDDM, abbreviation for **non-insulin-dependent diabetes mellitus.**

nidus /nī′dəs/ [L, nest], a point or origin, focus, or nucleus of a disease process.

Niebauer prosthesis /nē′bou·ər/, a Silastic prosthesis for interphalangeal and thumb joint replacement.

Niemann-Pick disease /nē′monpik′/ [Albert Niemann, German pediatrician, b. 1880; Ludwig Pick, German pediatrician, b. 1868], an inherited disorder of lipid metabolism in which there are accumulations of sphingomyelin in the bone marrow, spleen, and lymph nodes. The disease is characterized by enlargement of liver and spleen, anemia, lymphadenopathy, and progressive mental and physical deterioration.

nifedipine /nifed′ipēn/, a calcium channel blocker prescribed for the treatment of vasospastic and effort-associated angina.

night blindness. See **nyctalopia.**

night guard. See **bite guard.**

Nightingale, Florence (1820-1910), the founder of modern nursing. After limited formal training in nursing she became superintendent in 1853 of a hospital in Lon-

don. Her success in reorganizing the hospital led to a request by the British government to head a mission to the Crimea, where Britain was fighting a war with Russia. She arrived in November, 1854, with 38 nurses to find 5,000 wounded men lacking adequate food and medical supplies. Working many hours on the wards and sending letters to England to obtain money and supplies and to mobilize the government to act, she brought order out of chaos. After her return to England, in 1856, she founded a training school for nurses at St. Thomas' Hospital, whose graduates became matrons of the most important hospitals in Great Britain, thus raising the standards of nursing around the world. Although later bedridden, she carried on her work on the sanitary reform of India, conducted a study of midwifery, helped establish visiting nurse services, and proposed separate institutions for the sick, the insane, the incurable, and children. After Longfellow wrote *Santa Filomena,* she became known as "The Lady with The Lamp." The Nightingale Pledge, named after her, embodies her ideals and has inspired thousands of nurses.

Nightingale ward, a kind of hospital ward, designed by Florence Nightingale, that revolutionized hospital design. The number of beds allowed in a ward of given size was limited to permit the circulation of air and for general cleanliness and the comfort of patients. Three sides of the ward were windowed to admit light and fresh air.

nightingalism /nī′ting·gāl′izəm/, an ideology emphasizing self-sacrifice on the part of a nurse whose primary concern is the welfare of the patient, with minimum personal attention to the needs of the nurse.

nightmare [AS *niht* night, *mara* incubus], a dream occurring during rapid eye movement sleep that arouses feelings of intense, inescapable fear, terror, distress, or extreme anxiety and that usually awakens the sleeper.

night sight. See **hemeralopia.**

night splint, any splint or similar device used only at night.

nightstick fracture, an undisplaced fracture of the ulnar shaft caused by a direct blow.

night sweat [AS *niht, swaetan*], sweating that occurs with a nocturnal fever, as in a wasting disease like pulmonary tuberculosis.

night terrors [AS *niht*; L *terrour*], a form of dissociated sleep, usually in children, in which there may be repeated episodes of abrupt awakening from sleep with signs of

N

panic and anxiety. The subject may have only fragmentary dream images of a threatening nature.

night vision [AS *niht*; L *visio* seeing], a capacity to see dimly lit objects. It stems from a chemophysical phenomenon associated with the retinal rods. The rods contain the highly light-sensitive chemical rhodopsin, or visual purple, which is essential for the conduction of optic impulses in subdued light.

nightwalking [AS *niht*; ME *walken*], a disorder occurring during non-REM sleep in which the subject usually sits up in bed briefly, then gets up and walks around, opening doors, eating, and so on, and eventually returns to bed. The person will have no memory of the event the following day.

nigrities linguae. See **parasitic glossitis.**

NIH, abbreviation for **National Institutes of Health.**

nihilistic delusion /nī′hilis′tik/ [L *nihil* nothing, *icus* form of; *deludere* to deceive], a persistent denial of the existence of particular things or of everything, including oneself, as seen in various forms of schizophrenia.

nikethamide /nīketh′mīd/, a central nervous system stimulant prescribed as an analeptic in the treatment of depression of the central nervous and respiratory systems.

Nikolsky's sign /nikol′skēz/ [Pyotr V. Nikolsky, Polish dermatologist, b. 1855], easy separation of the stratum corneum layer of the epidermis from the basal cell layer by rubbing apparently normal skin areas; found in pemphigus and a few other bullous diseases.

NIMH, abbreviation for **National Institute of Mental Health.**

90-90 traction. See **traction, 90-90.**

ninth cranial nerve. See **glossopharyngeal nerve.**

niobium (Nb) /nī·ō′bē·əm/ [Gk *Niobe* mythic daughter of Tantalus and Amphion], a silver-gray metallic element. Its atomic number is 41; its atomic weight is 92.906.

nipple [D *knibbelen* to nip], a small cylindric, pigmented structure that projects just below the center of each breast. The tip of the nipple has about 20 tiny openings to the lactiferous ducts. The skin of the nipple is surrounded by the lighter pigmented skin of the areola. Stimulation of the nipple in men and women causes the structure to become erect through the contraction of radiating smooth muscle bundles in the surrounding areola.

nipple cancer, an inflammatory malignant neoplasm of the nipple and areola that is usually associated with carcinoma in deeper breast structures. It represents only a small percentage of breast cancers.

nipple discharge, spontaneous exudation of material from the nipple that may be normal, such as colostrum in pregnancy, or that may be a sign of endocrinologic, neoplastic, or infectious disease.

nipple shield, a device to protect the nipples of a lactating woman. The shield is usually made of soft latex and has a tab on one side with which the mother may hold it. The baby nurses from a nipple at the center of the shield. It is most often used to allow sore or cracked nipples to heal while maintaining lactation.

niridazole /nirid′əzōl/, an antischistosomal. In the United States it is available from the Centers for Disease Control and Prevention.

Nirschl procedure /nur′shəl/, a surgical procedure for chronic epicondylitis. It involves excision of a hypercapsular tendon segment of the extensor carpi radialus brevis and decortication of the anterolateral condyle.

nirvanic state /nirvä′nik, nirvan′ik/, (in Zen meditation) a state in which mental processes cease, leading to a radical and lasting alteration of the personality.

NIS, abbreviation for *Nursing Information System.*

Nissl body /nis′əl/ [Franz Nissl, German neurologist, b. 1860], any one of the large granular structures in the cytoplasm of nerve cells that stains with basic dyes and contains ribonucleoprotein.

nit, the egg of a parasitic insect, particularly a louse. It may be found attached to human or animal hair or to clothing fiber.

nitr, 1. abbreviation for **nitrocellulose. 2.** abbreviation for **nitroglycerin.**

nitrazine paper /nī′trazēn/, an absorbent strip of paper that turns specific colors when exposed to solutions of varied acidity or alkalinity.

nitric acid /nī′trik/ [Gk *nitron* soda; L *acidus* sour], a colorless, highly corrosive liquid that may give off suffocating brown fumes of nitrogen dioxide on exposure to air. Commercially prepared nitric acid is a powerful oxidizing agent used in the manufacture of drugs, and, occasionally, as a cauterizing agent for the removal of warts.

nitrite /nī′trīt/ [Gk *nitron* soda], an ester or salt of nitrous acid, used as a vasodilator and antispasmodic. Among the most widely used nitrites in medicine are amyl, ethyl, potassium, and sodium nitrite.

nitritoid reaction /nī′tritoid/, a group of adverse effects, including hypotension, flushing, lightheadedness, and fainting, produced by administration of arsenicals or gold. The reaction is similar to that caused by administration of nitrites.

nitrobenzene poisoning /nī′trōben′zēn/, a toxic condition caused by the absorption into the body of nitrobenzene, a pale yellow, oily liquid used in the manufacture of aniline, shoe dyes, soap, perfume, and artificial flavors. Exposure in industry is usually by inhalation of the fumes or by absorption through the skin. Symptoms of acute poisoning include headache, drowsiness, nausea, ataxia, cyanosis, and, in extreme cases, respiratory failure.

nitrocellulose (nitr), a mixture of nitrate esters of cellulose made by treating cotton with nitric and sulfuric acids. Solutions in a mixture of ether and alcohol are used as "plastic skin" under the name of **collodion.**

nitrofuran /nī′trōfyoo′ran/, one of a group of synthetic antimicrobials used to treat infections caused by protozoa or by certain gram-positive or gram-negative bacteria.

nitrofurantoin /nī′trōfyoo′rəntō′in/, a urinary antibacterial prescribed in the treatment of certain urinary tract infections.

nitrofurazone /nī′trōfyoo′rəzōn/, a topical antibacterial prescribed in the prophylaxis and treatment of infection in second- and third-degree burns and in the treatment of infections of the skin and mucous membranes.

nitrogen (N) /nī′trəjən/ [Gk *nitron* soda, *genein* to produce], a gaseous, nonmetallic element. Its atomic number is 7; its atomic weight is 14.008. Nitrogen constitutes approximately 78% of the atmosphere and is a component of all proteins and a major component of most organic substances. Compounds of nitrogen are essential constituents of all living organisms, the proteins and the nucleic acids being especially basic to all life forms.

nitrogen balance, the relationship between the nitrogen taken into the body, usually as food, and the nitrogen excreted from the body in urine and feces. Positive nitrogen balance, which occurs when the intake of nitrogen is greater than its excretion, implies tissue formation. Negative nitrogen balance indicates wasting or destruction of tissue.

nitrogen cycle, the circulation of nitrogen through natural processes in either of two ways: from the soil to plants and animals that excrete nitrogen products back into the soil and by bacterial fixation of atmospheric nitrogen through plants and animals that decay and release the element back into the atmosphere.

nitrogen fixation, the process by which free nitrogen in the atmosphere is converted by biological or chemical means to ammonia and to other forms usable by plants and animals.

nitrogen mustard. See **mechlorethamine hydrochloride.**

nitrogen narcosis, a condition of depressed central nervous system functions by high partial pressure of nitrogen.

nitrogen washout curve, a graphic curve obtained by plotting the concentration of nitrogen in expired alveolar gas during oxygen breathing as a function of time. As a person begins to inhale pure oxygen after breathing ambient air the nitrogen concentration decreases so that after 4 minutes healthy subjects have a nitrogen concentration in expired alveolar gas of less than 2%.

nitroglycerin (nitr), a coronary vasodilator prescribed for the prevention or relief of angina pectoris. A potent smooth muscle relaxant and vasodilator, nitroglycerin is used in transdermal patches and as an alcohol solution as well as in oral and sublingual tablets as a coronary vasodilator.

nitroglycerin tablets, tablets of glyceryl trinitrate, a volatile ester prepared by the action of nitric and sulfuric acids on glycerol, prescribed for the relief of heart symptoms.

nitromersol, an organic mercurial antiseptic that is not a highly effective germicide, sometimes used for the disinfecting of surgical instruments and as an antiseptic on the skin and mucous membranes.

nitroprusside sodium. See **sodium nitroprusside.**

nitrosamines /nī′trəsam′ēns/, potentially carcinogenic compounds produced by reactions of nitrites with amines or amides normally present in the body. Nitrites are produced by bacteria in saliva, and in the intestine from nitrates normally present in vegetables and in nitrate-treated fish, poultry, and meats.

nitrosourea /nītrō′sōyŏŏrē′ə/, one of a group of alkylating drugs used as an antineoplastic drug in the chemotherapy of brain tumors, multiple myeloma, Hodgkin's disease, adenocarcinomas, hepatomas, chronic leukemias, lymphomas, myelomas, and cancers of the breast and ovaries.

nitrous oxide (N₂O) /nī′trəs/, a gas used as an anesthetic in dentistry, surgery, and childbirth. It provides light anesthesia and is delivered in various concentrations with oxygen. Nitrous oxide alone does not provide deep enough anesthesia for major surgery, for which it is supplemented with other anesthetic agents.

nl, abbreviation for *natural logarithm.*

N

NLN, abbreviation for **National League for Nursing.**

N-m, abbreviation for *newton meter.*

N/m², abbreviation for *newton per square meter.*

NMDP, abbreviation for **National Marrow Donor Program.**

NMR, 1. abbreviation for **nuclear magnetic resonance.** 2. abbreviation for *nuclear magnetic resonance spectroscopy.*

NMR imaging, See **magnetic resonance imaging.**

No, symbol for the element **nobelium.**

N₂O, symbol for **nitrous oxide.**

nobelium (No) /nōbel'ē·əm/ [Alfred Nobel Institute, Stockholm, Sweden], a synthetic, transuranic metallic element. Its atomic number is 102. The atomic weight of its most stable isotope is 259.

noble gas. See **inert gas.**

Nocardia /nōkär'dē·ə/ [Edmund I. E. Nocard, French veterinarian, b. 1850], a genus of gram-positive aerobic bacteria, some species of which are pathogenic, such as *Nocardia asteroides.*

nocardiosis /nōkär'dē·ō'sis/ [Edmund I. E. Nocard; Gk *osis* condition], infection with *Nocardia asteroides,* an aerobic gram-positive species of actinomycetes, characterized by pneumonia, often with cavitation, and by chronic abscesses in the brain and subcutaneous tissues. The organism enters via the respiratory tract and spreads by the bloodstream, especially in Cushing's syndrome.

nociceptive /nō'sēsep'tiv/ [L *nocere* to injure, *capere* to receive], pertaining to a neural receptor for painful stimuli.

nociceptive reflex, a reflex caused by a painful stimulus.

nociceptive stimulus, a painful, sometimes detrimental or injurious, stimulus.

nociceptor /nō'sēsep'tər/, somatic and visceral free nerve endings of thinly myelinated and unmyelinated fibers. They usually react to tissue injury but may also be excited by endogenous chemical substances.

no code [AS *na* not; L *caudex* book], a note written in the patient record and signed by a qualified, usually senior or attending physician, instructing the staff of the institution not to attempt to resuscitate a particular patient in the event of cardiac or respiratory failure.

noct., abbreviation for the Latin, *nocte,* night.

noctambulation. See **somnambulism.**

nocturia /noktŏōr'ē·ə/ [L *nocturnus* by night; Gk *ouron* urine], urination, particularly excessive urination at night. Whereas it may be a symptom of renal dis-

ease, it may occur in the absence of disease in persons who drink excessive amounts of fluids, particularly alcohol or coffee, before bedtime or in people with prostatic disease.

nocturnal [L *nocturnus* by night], 1. pertaining to or occurring during the night. 2. describing an individual or animal that is active at night and sleeps during the day.

nocturnal emission, involuntary emission of semen during sleep, usually in association with an erotic dream.

nocturnal enuresis [L *nocturnus*; Gk *enourein*], involuntary urination while asleep at night.

nocturnal paroxysmal dyspnea, an abnormal condition of the respiratory system, characterized by sudden attacks of shortness of breath, profuse sweating, tachycardia, and wheezing that awaken the person from sleep.

nocturnal penile tumescence (NPT) [L *nocturnus*; *penile,* pertaining to the penis; *tumescere* to begin to swell], a normal condition of penile erection that occurs during sleep throughout most of the lifetime of a male. The occurrence of NPT is important in the diagnosis of impotence because it indicates that impotence may be psychogenic.

nodal event /nō'dəl/, an occurrence that may cause anxiety, such as birth, death, divorce, marriage, or a child leaving home.

nodal rhythm (NR) [L *nodus* knot; Gk *rhythmos*], a cardiac rhythm that occurs when the atrioventricular node gains control of the heart beat, usually because of a defect in the function of the sinoatrial node.

nodal tachycardia [L *nodus*; Gk *tachys* swift, *kardia* heart], a rapid discharge of impulses from an ectopic focus in the area of the atrioventricular node.

node /nōd/ [L *nodus* knot], 1. a small rounded mass. 2. a lymph node.

nodular /nod'yələr/ [L *nodus* knot], (of a structure or mass) small, firm, and knotty.

nodular circumscribed lipomatosis, a condition in which many circumscribed, encapsulated lipomas are distributed around the neck symmetrically, randomly, or like a collar.

nodular cutaneous angiitis, an inflammatory condition of small arteries accompanied by lesions of the skin.

nodular fasciitis, an inflammation of the fascia that results in the formation of nodules.

nodular goiter, an enlarged goiter that contains nodules.

nodular melanoma, a melanoma that is uniformly pigmented, usually bluish black and nodular and sometimes surrounded by an irregular halo of pale, unpigmented skin.

nodule /nod'yo͞ol/ [L *nodulus* small knot], **1.** a small node. **2.** a small nodelike structure.

noise-induced hearing loss, a gradual loss of hearing caused by exposure to loud noise over an extended period. Although an early hearing loss may be temporary, it becomes permanent with increased exposure to noise.

noise pollution, a noise level in an environment that is uncomfortable for the inhabitants.

nok, abbreviation for *next of kin.*

noma /nō'mə/ [Gk *nome* distribution], an acute, necrotizing ulcerative process involving mucous membranes of mouth and genitalia. There is rapid spreading and painless destruction of bone and soft tissue accompanied by a putrid odor.

nomenclature /nō'mənklā'chər, nōmen'-/ [L *nomen* name, *clamare* to call], a consistent, systematic method of naming used in a scientific discipline to denote classifications and to avoid ambiguities in names, such as binomial nomenclature in biology and chemical nomenclature in chemistry.

Nomina Anatomica, the book of official international nomenclature for anatomy as designated by the International Congress of Anatomists.

nominal aphasia /nom'inəl/ [ME *nominalle*; Gk *a, phasis* speech], a type of speech defect in which the patient uses the incorrect names in identifying objects. Minor episodes may be due to anxiety, fatigue, or senility, but severe cases can indicate a focal lesion on the left side of the brain.

nominal damages. See **damages.**

nomogram /nom'əgram, nō'mə-/ [Gk *nomos* law, *gramma* a record], **1.** a graphic representation, by any of various systems, of a numeric relationship. **2.** a graph on which a number of variables is plotted so that the value of a dependent variable can be read on the appropriate line when the values of the other variables are given.

nonabsorbable surgical sutures /non'-absôr'bəbəl/ [L *non* not + *absorbere*; Gk *cheirourgos* surgeon; L *sutura*], sutures of silk, nylon, steel, or other materials that resist absorption. They are used mainly in deep tissues wher it is important for them to remain *in situ.*

nonadherent dressing /non'ədhir'ənt/ [L *non, adhesio* sticking to; OFr *dresser* to arrange], a dressing that usually does not stick to the dried secretions of a wound.

nonadhesive skin traction [L *non* not, *ad-*

hesio sticking to], one of two kinds of skin traction in which the therapeutic pull of traction weights is applied with foam-backed traction straps that do not stick to the skin over the body structure involved. The straps spread the traction pull over a wide area of skin surface, thus decreasing the vulnerability of the patient to skin breakdown.

non-A, non-B (NANB) hepatitis. See **hepatitis C.**

nonbacterial thrombic endocarditis [L *non* + *bakerion* small rod], one of the three main types of endocarditis, characterized by various kinds of lesions that affect the heart valves. Some studies indicate that this disease may be the first step in the development of bacterial endocarditis and that the lesions involved cause peripheral arterial embolisms resulting in death.

noncohesive gold foil /non'kōhē'siv/ [L *non* + *cohaerere* to stick together], a thin sheet of pure gold, used for making dental restorations, such as crowns, that will not cohere at room temperature because of a protective surface coating.

noncommunicating hydrocephalus. See **hydrocephalus.**

noncompetitive inhibition, (in pharmacology) a form of inhibition in which a substance occupies a receptor and cannot be displaced from the receptor by increasing the numbers of other molecules through the principle of mass action.

noncompliance /non'kəmpli'əns/ [L *non* + *complere* to complete], a NANDA-accepted nursing diagnosis of an informed decision on the part of the client not to adhere to a therapeutic suggestion because of a health belief, a cultural or spiritual value, or a problem in the relationship between the provider of the recommendation and the client. Defining characteristics of non-compliance include objective tests that show noncompliance, observation of physical or psychologic signs that demonstrate lack of compliance, or a failure to keep appointments.

non compos mentis /non'kom'pos men'tis/ [L, not of sound mind], a legal term applied to a person declared to be mentally incompetent.

nondirective therapy [L *non* + *digere* to direct], a psychotherapeutic approach in which the psychotherapist refrains from giving advice or interpretation as the client is helped to identify conflicts and to clarify and understand feelings and values.

nondisjunction [L *non* + *disjungere* to disjoint], failure of homologous pairs of chromosomes to separate during the first meiotic division or of the two chromatids of a chromosome to split during anaphase

N

of mitosis or the second meiotic division. The result is an abnormal number of chromosomes in the daughter cells.

nonfat milk.   See **skimmed milk.**

nonfeasance /nonfē′zəns/ [L *non* + *facere* to do],   a failure to perform a task, duty, or undertaking that one has agreed to perform or that one had a legal duty to perform.

nongonococcal urethritis (NGU) /non′-gon′əkok′əl/ [L *non* + Gk *gone* seed, *kokkos* berry],   an infectious condition of the urethra in males that is characterized by mild dysuria and a scanty to moderate amount of penile discharge. The discharge may be white or clear, thin or mucoid, or, less often, purulent. The infection is often caused by the obligate intracellular parasite *Chlamydia trachomatis.* Nearly 50% of all cases of urethritis are nongonococcal.

nonhemolytic jaundice /non′hē′məlit′ik/ [L *non* + Gk *haima* blood, *lysein* to loosen; Fr *jaune* yellow],   a form of jaundice that is caused by a liver disease rather than the destruction of red blood cells.

non-Hodgkin's lymphoma /non′hoj′kənz/,   any kind of malignant lymphoma except Hodgkin's disease.

nonigravida /nō′nigrav′idə/ [L *nonus* nine; *gravida* pregnant],   indicating a woman pregnant for the ninth time.

non-insulin-dependent diabetes mellitus (NIDDM),   a type of diabetes mellitus (type II) in which patients are not insulin-dependent or ketosis prone although they may use insulin for correction of symptomatic or persistent hyperglycemia, and they can develop ketosis under special circumstances, such as infection or stress. About 60% to 90% are obese; in these patients glucose tolerance is often improved by weight loss. Previously called adult-onset diabetes, ketosis-resistant diabetes, maturity-onset diabetes, maturity-onset-type diabetes, MOD, or stable diabetes.

noninvasive [L *non* + *in* into, *vadere* to go],   pertaining to a diagnostic or therapeutic technique that does not require the skin to be broken or a cavity or organ of the body to be entered, such as obtaining a blood pressure reading by auscultation with a stethoscope and sphygmomanometer.

nonionic,   pertaining to compounds without a net negative or positive charge.

nonionizing radiation [L *non* + Gk *ion* going, *izein* to cause],   radiation for which the mechanism of action in tissue does not directly ionize atomic or molecular systems through a single interaction.

nonipara /nōnip′ərə/ [L *nonus* nine, *parere*

to bear],   denoting a woman who has delivered nine offspring.

nonmedullated nerve fiber /non′med′-yəlā′tid/ [L *non* + *medulla* marrow; *nervus*; *fibra*],   a nerve fiber that lacks the fatty myelin insulating sheath. Such fibers form the gray matter of the nervous system, as distinguished from the white matter of medullated fibers.

nonmyelinated   /non′mī′əlinā′tid/   [L *non* + Gk *myelos* marrow],   pertaining to nerve fibers that lack a fatty myelin insulating sheath.

nonossifying fibroma /non′os′ifī′ing/,   a bone anomaly found in children as a sharply circumscribed, eccentrically located lesion in the metaphysis of long bones. A microscopic examination reveals whorl patterns of spindle cells, fibrous tissue, numerous xanthoma cells, and occasional giant cells.

nonosteogenic fibroma /non′ostē·əjen′ik/,   a common bone lesion in which there is degeneration and proliferation of the medullary and cortical tissue, usually near the ends of the diaphyses of the large long bones.

nonparametric test of significance /non′-per′əmet′rik/ [L *non* + Gk *para* beside, *metron* measure],   (in statistics) one of several tests that use a qualitative approach to analyze rank order data and incidence data that cannot be assumed to have a normal distribution. Kinds of nonparametric tests of significance include **chi-square, Spearman's rho.**

nonparous /non′per′əs/,   indicating a woman who has never delivered a child.

nonpenetrating wound,   a wound that does not break the surface of the skin.

nonpolar /non′pō′lər/ [L *non* + *polus* pole],   pertaining to molecules that have a hydrophobic affinity, are "water hating." Nonpolar substances tend to dissolve in nonpolar solvents.

nonproductive cough [L *non* + *producere* to produce],   a sudden, noisy expulsion of air from the lungs that may be caused by irritation or inflammation and does not remove sputum from the respiratory tract. Intratracheal suctioning may be necessary when secretions cause severe respiratory difficulty and coughing is unproductive.

nonproprietary name [L *non* + *proprietas* owner; *nomen* name],   the chemical or generic name of a drug or device, as distinguished from a brand name or trademark. A nonproprietary name may be indicated by the letters, USAN, or United States Adopted Name.

nonprotein nitrogen (NPN) /non′prō′tēn/ [L *non* + Gk *proteios* first rank; *nitron* soda, *genein* to produce],   the nitrogen in the blood that is not a constituent of protein, such as the nitrogen associated with urea, uric acid, creatine, and polypeptides.

nonrapid eye movement (NREM). See **sleep.**

nonreflex bladder. See **flaccid bladder.**

nonreversible inhibitor [L *non* + *revertere* to turn back; *inhibere* to restrain], an effector substance that binds irreversibly to an active site of an enzyme, inhibiting the normal catalytic activity of the enzyme.

nonsecretor /non'səkrē'tər/ [L *non* + *cernere* to separate], a person who does not secrete ABO blood group substances in mucous secretions of the saliva or gastric juice. The condition is genetically determined.

nonseg., abbreviation for *nonsegmented*.

nonsense mutation. See **amber mutation.**

nonsexual generation. See **asexual generation.**

nonshivering thermogenesis, a natural method by which newborns can produce body heat by increasing their metabolic rate.

nonspecific urethritis (NSU) [L *non* + *species* form], inflammation of the urethra not known to be caused by a specific organism. Onset of symptoms is often related to sexual intercourse. The condition is noted by urethral discharge in men and by reddening of the urethral mucosa in women.

nonstress test (NST), an evaluation of the fetal heart rate response to natural contractile activity or to an increase in fetal activity.

nonthrombocytopenic purpura /non'-throm'bōsī'təpē'ik/, a disorder characterized by purplish or reddish skin areas although the condition does not involve a decrease in the number of platelets.

nontoxic, not poisonous.

nontropical sprue [L *non* not; Gk *tropikos* of the solstice; D *sprouw*], a malabsorption syndrome resulting from an inborn inability to digest foods that contain gluten.

nonulcerative blepharitis [L *non* + *ilcus* ulcer; Gk *blepharon* eyelid, *itis* inflammation], a form of blepharitis characterized by greasy scales on the margins of the eyelids around the lashes and hyperemia and thickening of the skin. Nonulcerative blepharitis is often associated with seborrhea of the scalp, eyebrows, and the skin behind the ears.

nonunion, pertaining to a fractured bone that fails to heal properly.

nonverbal communication, the transmission of a message without the use of words. It may involve any or all of the five senses.

nonviable [L *non* + *via* life], pertaining to an individual unable to exist independently after birth.

nonvital pulp [L *non* + *vita* life, *pulpa* flesh], dead dental pulp in which the canal of the tooth has become necrotic because of a disease or trauma that interferes with the blood supply.

Noonan's syndrome /nōō'nənz/ [Jacqueline A. Noonan, American cardiologist, b. 1921], a hypergonadotropic disorder, occurring only in males, characterized by short stature, low-set ears, webbing of the neck, and cubitus valgus. Testicular function may be normal, but fertility is often decreased. The number and morphology of the chromosomes are normal. The cause is unknown.

norepinephrine /nôr'epinef'rin/, an adrenergic hormone that acts to increase blood pressure by vasoconstriction but does not affect cardiac output. It is synthesized naturally by the adrenal medulla and is available also as a drug, levarterenol, given to maintain the blood pressure in acute hypotension secondary to trauma, heart disease, or vascular collapse.

norepinephrine bitartrate, an adrenergic vasoconstrictor prescribed in the treatment of cardiac arrest and in certain acute hypotensive states.

no response (NR), the condition for which the maximum decrease in treated tumor volume is less than 50%.

norethindrone /nôreth'indrōn/, a progestin prescribed in the treatment of abnormal uterine bleeding and endometriosis and is a component in oral contraceptive medications.

norethindrone acetate and ethinyl estradiol, an oral contraceptive also prescribed for endometriosis, and hypermenorrhea.

norfloxacin /nôrflok'səsin/, an oral antibacterial drug prescribed for the treatment of urinary tract infections.

norgestrel /nôrjes'trəl/, a progestin prescribed alone or in combination with estrogen as a contraceptive.

norm [L *norma* rule], 1. a measure of a phenomenon generally accepted as the ideal standard performance against which other measures of the phenomenon may be measured. 2. abbreviation for **normal.**

norma basalis /nôr'mə basā'lis/ [L, rule; Gk *basis* foundation], the inferior surface of the base of the skull with the mandible removed, formed by the palatine bones, the vomer, the pterygoid processes, and parts of the sphenoid and temporal bones.

normal (N) [L *norma* rule], **1.** describing a standard, average, or typical example of a set of objects or values. **2.** describing a chemical solution in which 1 L contains 1 g of a substance or the equivalent in replaceable hydrogen ions. **3.** people in a nondiseased population. **4.** a gaussian distribution.

normal dental function, the correct and healthy action of opposing teeth during mastication.

normal diet. See **regular diet.**

normal dwarf. See **primordial dwarf.**

normal human plasma [L *norma* rule, *humanus*; Gk *plassein* to mold], sterile, disease-free human blood prepared from a pooled donor supply.

normal human serum albumin, an isotonic preparation of pooled human serum albumin for treating hypoproteinemia, hypovolemia, and threatened or existing shock.

normal hydrogen electrode (NHE), a reference electrode that is assigned a value of 0 volts.

normal last shoes, special orthopedic shoes for infants and children constructed with a normal sole, as opposed to a reverse or straight last shoe.

normal phase, a chromatographic mode in which the mobile phase is less polar than the stationary phase.

normal pressure hydrocephalus [L *norma*; *premere* to press; Gk *hydor* water, *kephale* head], a condition in which there is dilatation of the ventricles without an increase in intracranial pressure.

normal saline solution [L *norma*; *sal, solutus* dissolved], a 0.9% w/v sterile solution of sodium chloride in water that is isotonic with blood and injectable intravenously.

normal sinus rhythm [L *norma*; *sinus* hollow; Gk *rhythmos*], the normal heart beat produced when the pacemaker is in the sinoatrial node.

normal solution [L *norma*; *solutus* dissolved], a solution that contains the gram-equivalent weight of a reagent per liter. It is denoted by the symbols N\l or N.

normal strain, a quantity described by the quotient of the change of length of a line and its original length.

normal stress, (in physics) a quantity described by the quotient of distributed force and area when the force is perpendicular to the area.

normal temperature, for a normal person at rest, the oral clinical temperature is given as 98.6° F or 37.0° C but actual "normal" temperatures may range a fraction of a degree or increments of a whole degree higher or lower because of effects of sleep, exercise, eating, sleeping, metabolism, and

the ambient temperature. Rectal temperatures also average a fraction of a degree higher than oral temperatures; axillary readings are lower than oral temperatures.

normoblast /nôr'məblast/ [L *norma* + Gk *blastos* germ], a nucleated cell that is the normal precursor of the adult circulating erythrocyte. After the extrusion of the nucleus of the normoblast, the young erythrocyte becomes known as a reticulocyte. –**normoblastic,** *adj.*

normochromic /nôr'məkrō'mik/ [L *norma* + Gk *chroma* color], pertaining to a blood cell having normal color, usually because it contains an adequate amount of hemoglobin.

normocyte /nôr'məsīt/ [L *norma* + Gk *kytos* cell], an ordinary, normal, adult red blood cell of average size having a diameter of 7 μ. –**normocytic,** *adj.*

normoglycemic /nôr'məglīsē'mik/, pertaining to a normal blood glucose level.

normotensive /nôr'məten'siv/, pertaining to the condition of having normal blood pressure. –**normotension,** *n.*

normoventilation, the alveolar ventilation rate that produces an alveolar carbon dioxide pressure of about 40 torr at any metabolic rate.

normoxia /nôrmok'sē-ə/, an ambient oxygen pressure of about 150 (plus or minus 10) torr, or the partial pressure of oxygen in atmospheric air at sea level.

North American blastomycosis, an infection caused by inhaling the fungus *Blastomyces dermatitidis.* It may resemble bacterial pneumonia. Painless, well-demarcated, verrucous, or ulcerated skin lesions occur on the face and hands. The disease may progress to involve bones and the brain; many viscera are infected in fatal cases.

North American Nursing Diagnosis Association (NANDA), a professional organization of registered nurses created in 1982. The purpose of the organization is "to develop, refine, and promote a taxonomy of nursing diagnostic terminology of general use to the professional."

North Asian tick-borne rickettsiosis, an infection, acquired in the Eastern Hemisphere, caused by *Rickettsia siberica,* transmitted by ticks, and resembling Rocky Mountain spotted fever. Usual findings include a generalized maculopapular rash involving palms and soles, fever, and lymph node enlargement.

North Asian tick typhus. See **Siberian tick typhus.**

Northern blot test, an electrophoretic test for identifying the presence or absence of particular mRNA molecules and nucleic acid hybridization.

nortriptyline hydrochloride /nôrtrip′-tilēn/, a tricyclic antidepressant prescribed in the treatment of mental depression.

Norwegian scabies [Norway; L *scabere* to scratch], a severe infestation of human skin by an itch mite (*Sarcoptes scabiei*). The condition is associated with intense itching, crusting and scaling of the skin, and insect egg burrows that appear as discolored lines in the affected skin areas.

nose [AS *nosu*], the structure that protrudes from the anterior portion of the skull and serves as a passageway for air to and from the lungs. The nose filters the air, warming, moistening, and chemically examining it for impurities that might irritate the mucous lining of the respiratory tract. The nose also contains the organ of smell, and it aids the faculty of speech. The external portion is considerably smaller than the internal portion, which lies over the roof of the mouth. The hollow interior portion is separated into a right and a left cavity by a septum. Each cavity is divided into the superior, middle, and inferior meati by the projection of nasal conchae. The external portion of the nose is perforated by two nostrils and the internal portion by two posterior nares.

nosebleed [AS *nosu* + ME *blod* blood], abnormal hemorrhage from the nose. Emergency responses to nosebleed include seating the patient upright with the head thrust forward to prevent swallowing of blood. Pressure with both thumbs directly under the nostril and above the lips may block the main artery supplying blood to the nose. Alternatively, pressure with both forefingers on each side of the nostril often slows bleeding by blocking the main arteries and their branches. Continued bleeding may require the insertion of cotton or other absorbent material within the nostril and reapplication of pressure. Cold compresses on the nose, lips, and the back of the head may help control hemorrhage. Continued bleeding may require cautery.

NOSIE, abbreviation for **nurses' observation scale for inpatient evaluation.**

nosocomial /nos′əkō′mē-əl/ [Gk *nosokomeian* hospital], of or pertaining to a hospital.

nosocomial infection, an infection acquired during hospitalization, often caused by *Candida albicans, Escherichia coli,* hepatitis viruses, herpes zoster virus, *Pseudomonas,* or *Staphylococcus.*

nosology /nōsol′əjē/ [Gk *nosos* disease, *logos* science], the science of classifying diseases.

nostrils. See **anterior nares.**

notch [Fr *noche*], an indentation or a depression in a bone or other organ, such as the auricular notch or the cardiac notch.

nothing by mouth (NPO), a patient care instruction advising that the patient is prohibited from ingesting food, beverage, or medicine. It is usually posted above the bed of a patient about to undergo surgery or special diagnostic procedures requiring that the digestive tract be empty.

notifiable [L *nota* mark, *facere* to make], pertaining to certain conditions, diseases, and events that must, by law, be reported to a governmental agency, such as birth, death, certain communicable diseases, and certain violations of public health regulations.

notochord /nō′tōkôrd/ [Gk *noton* back, *chorde* cord], an elongated strip of mesodermal tissue that originates from the primitive node and extends along the dorsal surface of the developing embryo beneath the neural tube, forming the primary longitudinal skeletal axis of the body of all chordates. **–notochordal,** *adj.*

notochordal canal /nō′tōkôr′dəl/ [Gk *noton* + *chorde* cord; L *canalis* channel], a tubular passage that extends from the primitive pit into the head process during the early stages of embryonic development in mammals.

notochordal plate. See **head process.**

notogenesis /nō′tōjen′əsis/ [Gk *noton* + *genein* to produce], the formation of the notochord. **–notogenetic,** *adj.*

notomelus /nətom′ələs/ [Gk *noton* + *melos* limb], a congenital malformation in which one or more accessory limbs are attached to the back.

nourish [L *nutrire* to suckle], to furnish or supply the essential foods or nutrients for maintaining life.

nourishment, 1. the act or process of nourishing or being nourished. **2.** any substance that nourishes and supports the life and growth of living organisms.

NOx, abbreviation for **nitrous oxide,** or any mixture of oxides of nitrogen.

noxious /nok′shəs/ [L *noxa* harmful], harmful, injurious, or detrimental to health.

Noyes test /noiz/, an orthopedic knee test performed with the knee extended and the thigh relaxed. There is anterolateral tibial subluxation. The knee is gradually flexed with reduction of the subluxation occurring at about 30 degrees of flexion.

Np, symbol for the element **neptunium.**

NPN, abbreviation for **nonprotein nitrogen.**

npo, abbreviation for the Latin phrase, *non per os* "nothing by mouth."

_n_-propyl alcohol /en′prō′pil/, a clear,

colorless liquid used as a solvent for resins.

NPT, abbreviation for **nocturnal penile tumescence.**

NR, abbreviation for **nodal rhythm**.

NREM, abbreviation for *nonrapid eye movement.*

NSAID, abbreviation for *nonsteroidal antiinflammatory drug.*

NSCCN, abbreviation for **National Society of Critical Care Nurses of Canada.**

n-s/m², abbreviation for *newton second per square meter.*

NSNA, abbreviation for **National Student Nurses' Association.**

NSR, abbreviation for **normal sinus rhythm.**

NSU, abbreviation for **nonspecific urethritis.**

ntp, abbreviation for *normal temperature and pressure.*

nuc, abbreviation for *nuclear.*

nucha /nōō′kə/, *pl.* **nuchae** [Fr *nuque* nape], the nape, or back of the neck. **–nuchal,** *adj.*

nuchal cord /nōō′kəl/ [Fr *nuque* nape; Gk *chorde*], an abnormal but common condition in which the umbilical cord is wrapped around the neck of the fetus in utero or of the baby as it is being born. It is usually possible to slip the loop or loops of cord gently over the child's head.

nuchal ligament, a large midline posterior ligament in the neck from the base of the skull to the seventh cervical vertebra.

nuchal rigidity, a resistance to flexion of the neck, a condition seen in patients with meningitis.

nuchocephalic reflex /nōō′kəsefal′ik/, a test for diffuse cerebral dysfunction, as in senility. When the shoulders are turned to the left or the right, the head fails to turn in the same direction within 1/2 second.

Nuck's canal, Nuck's diverticulum. See **processus vaginalis peritonei.**

nuclear agenesis. See **Möbius' syndrome.**

nuclear family [L *nucleus* nut kernal; *familia* household], a family unit consisting of the biological parents and their offspring. Dissolution of a marriage results in dissolution of the nuclear family.

nuclear fission. See **fission.**

nuclear hyaloplasm. See **karyolymph.**

nuclear isomer, one of two or more nuclides with the same number of neutrons and protons in the nucleus (the same atomic number, or Z, and the same atomic mass, or A) but existing in different energy states.

nuclear magnetic resonance (NMR), See **magnetic resonance (MR).**

nuclear medicine, a medical discipline that uses radioactive isotopes in the diagnosis and treatment of disease.

nuclear medicine technologist, an allied health professional who specializes in the nuclear properties of radioactive and stable nuclides to make diagnostic evaluations of the anatomic or physiologic conditions of the body and to provide therapy with unsealed radioactive sources. Responsibilities include application of a special knowledge of radiation physics and safety regulations to limit radiation exposure; prepare and administer radiopharmaceuticals; use radiation detection devices and other kinds of laboratory equipment that measure the quantity and distribution of radionuclides deposited in a patient specimen, and perform invivo and invitro diagnostic procedures.

nuclear problem, (in psychology) an underlying reason for an individual's reaction to a precipitating event.

nuclear sap. See **karyolymph.**

nuclear scanning, a diagnostic technique that employs an injected or ingested radioactive material and a scanning device for determining the size, shape, location, and function of various body parts.

nuclear spin, an intrinsic form of angular momentum possessed by atomic nuclei containing an odd number of nucleons (protons or neutrons).

nucleic acid /nōōklē′ik/ [L *nucleus* + *acidus* sour], a polymeric compound of high molecular weight composed of nucleotides, each consisting of a purine or pyrimidine base, a ribose or deoxyribose sugar, and a phosphate group. Nucleic acids are involved in energy storage and release and in the determination and transmission of genetic characteristics. Kinds of nucleic acid are **deoxyribonucleic acid** and **ribonucleic acid.**

nucleocapsid /nōō′klē·ōkap′sid/ [L *nucleus* + *capsa* box], a viral enclosure consisting of a capsid or protein coat that encloses nucleic acid.

nucleochylema /nōō′klē·ōkǝlī′mǝ/ [L *nucleus* + Gk *chylos* juice, *haima* blood], the ground substance of the nucleus, as distinguished from that of the cytoplasm.

nucleochyme. See **karyolymph.**

nucleocytoplasmic /nōō′klē·ōsī′tōplas′mik/ [L *nucleus* + Gk *kytos* cell, *plasma* something formed], of or relating to the nucleus and cytoplasm of a cell.

nucleocytoplasmic ratio, the ratio of the volume of a nucleus of a cell to the volume of the cytoplasm. The proportion is usually constant for a specific cell type.

nucleohistone /nōō′klē·ōhis′tōn/ [L *nucleus* + Gk *histos* tissue], a complex nucleoprotein that consists of deoxyribonucleic acid and a histone. It is the basic constituent of the chromatin in the cell nucleus.

nucleolar organizer /nŏŏklē′əlⱥr/ [L *nucleolus* little nut kernel; Gk *organon* instrument, *izein* to cause], a part of the nucleus of the cell, thought to consist of heterochromatin, that is responsible for the formation of the nucleolus.

nucleolus /nŏŏklē′ⱥlⱥs/, *pl.* **nucleoli** [L, little nut kernel], any one of the small, dense structures composed largely of ribonucleic acid and situated within the cytoplasm of cells. Nucleoli are essential in the formation of ribosomes that synthesize cell proteins.

nucleon /n(y)ŏŏ′klē·on/, a collective term applied to protons and neutrons within the nucleus.

nucleophilic /n(y)ŏŏ′klē·ōfil′ik/, a property of some molecules, particularly nucleic acids and proteins, that have electrons that can be shared, and thus form bonds with alkylating agents.

nucleoplasm /nŏŏ′klē·əplaz′əm/ [L *nucleus* + Gk *plasma* something formed], the protoplasm of the nucleus as contrasted with that of the cell. **–nucleoplasmic,** *adj.*

nucleoplasmic ratio. See **nucleocytoplasmic ratio.**

nucleoprotein [L *nucleus* + Gk *proteios* first rank], a molecule in which protein is combined with nucleic acid in a cell nucleus.

nucleoside monophosphate kinase, /nŏŏ′klē·əsīd′/ a liver enzyme that catalyzes the transfer of a phosphate group from adenosine triphosphate, producing adenosine diphosphate and a nucleoside diphosphate.

nucleosome /nŏŏ′klē·əsōm/ [L *nucleus* + Gk *soma* body], any one of the repeating nucleoprotein units consisting of histones forming a complex with deoxyribonucleic acid that appear as the beadlike structures at distinct intervals along the chromosome.

5-nucleotidase /nŏŏ′klē·ot′idās/, a nonlipid enzyme, elevated in some liver disorders and measured in the blood to distinguish between certain liver and bone diseases. The normal accumulations in serum are 0.1 to 6 units.

nucleotide /nŏŏ′klē·ətīd′/, any one of the compounds into which nucleic acid is split by the action of nuclease. A nucleotide consists of a phosphate group, a pentose sugar, and a nitrogenous base.

nucleus /nŏŏ′klē·əs, ny ŏŏ′-/ [L, nut kernel], **1.** the central controlling body within a living cell, usually a spherical unit enclosed in a membrane and containing genetic codes for maintaining life systems of the organism and for issuing commands for growth and reproduction. **2.** a group of nerve cells of the central nervous system having a common function, such as supporting the sense of hearing or smell. **3.** the center of an atom about which electrons rotate. **4.** the central element in an organic chemical compound or class of compounds. **–nuclear,** *adj.*

nucleus pulposus, the central portion of each intervertebral disk, consisting of a pulpy elastic substance that loses some of its resilience with age.

nuclide /nŏŏ′klīd/ [L *nucleus* nut kernel], a species of atom characterized by the constitution of its nucleus, in particular by the number of protons and neutrons. Thus Co-59 and Co-60 are both isotopes of cobalt and are each nuclides.

nudge control, a prosthetic device with a mechanical unit that can be pressed by the chin to lock or unlock one or more joints of the apparatus.

NUG, abbreviation for *necrotizing ulcerative gingivitis.*

Nuhn's gland /noonz/ [Anton Nuhn, German anatomist, b. 1814], an anterior lingual gland in tissues on the inferior surface and near the apex and midline of the tongue.

null cell [L *nullus* not one, *cella* storeroom], a lymphocyte that develops in the bone marrow and lacks the characteristic surface markers of the B and T lymphocytes. Null cells represent a small proportion of the lymphocyte population. Stimulated by the presence of antibody, null cells can attack certain cellular targets directly and are known as **natural killer,** or **NK,** cells.

null hypothesis (H₀), (in research) a hypothesis that predicts that no difference or relationship exists among the variables studied that could not have occurred by chance alone.

nulligravida /nul′igrav′ədə/ a woman who has never been pregnant.

nullipara /nulip′ərə/, *pl.* **nulliparae** [L *nullus* not one, *parere* to bear], a woman who has not been delivered of a viable infant. The designation "para 0" indicates nulliparity. **–nulliparity,** *n.,* **nulliparous,** *adj.*

num, abbreviation for *number.*

numbness [ME *nomen* loss of feeling], a partial or total lack of sensation in a part of the body, resulting from any factor that interrupts the transmission of impulses from the sensory nerve fibers.

nummular dermatitis /num′yələr/ [L *nummulus* piece of money; Gk *derma* skin, *itis* inflammation], a skin disease characterized by coin-shaped, vesicular, or scaling eczema-like lesions on the forearms and the front of the calves.

Nuremberg tribunal [Nuremberg, Germany; L *tribunus* platform for administration of justice], an international tribunal planned and implemented by the United Nations War Crimes Commission to detect, apprehend, try, and punish persons accused of war crimes. The principle and practice of informed consent was reinforced by the precedent set in the trials in which Nazi physicians were declared guilty of crimes against humanity in performing experiments on human beings who were not volunteers and did not consent.

nurse [L *nutrix*], **1.** a person educated and licensed in the practice of nursing; one who is concerned with "the diagnosis and treatment of human responses to actual or potential health problems" (American Nurses' Association). The practice of the nurse includes data collection, diagnosis, planning, treatment, and evaluation within the framework of the nurse's singular concern with the patient's response to the problem rather than to the problem itself. The nurse may be a generalist or a specialist and, as a professional, is ethically and legally accountable for the nursing activites performed and for the actions of others to whom the nurse has delegated responsibility. **2.** to provide nursing care.

nurse anesthetist, a registered nurse qualified by advanced training in an accredited program in the speciality of nurse anesthesia to manage the anesthetic care of the patient in certain surgical situations.

nurse-client interaction, any process in which a nurse and a client exchange or share information, verbally or nonverbally. It is fundamental to communication and is an essential component of the nursing assessment.

nurse-client relationship, a therapeutic relationship between a nurse and a client built on a series of interactions and developing over time. During the first phase, the phase of establishment, the nurse establishes the structure, purpose, timing, and context of the relationship and expresses an interest in discussing this initial structure with the client. During the middle, developmental, phase of the relationship, the nurse and the client get to know each other better and test the structure of the relationship to be able to trust one another. The last phase, termination, ideally occurs when the goals of the relationship have been accomplished, when both the client and

the nurse feel a sense of resolution and satisfaction.

nurse clinician, a nurse who is prepared to identify and diagnose problems of clients by using the expanded knowledge and skills gained by advanced study in a specific area of nursing practice.

nurse coordinator, a registered nurse who coordinates and manages the activities of nursing personnel engaged in specific nursing services, as obstetrics or surgery, for two or more patient care units.

Nurse Corps, the branch within each of the armed services comprised of the nurses within that service, such as the Army Nurse Corps. In each of the armed services, the members of the Nurse Corps have the rank, title, responsibilities, and status of officer.

nurse educator, a registered nurse whose primary area of interest, competence, and professional practice is the education of nurses.

nurse midwife, a registered nurse qualified by advanced training in obstetric and neonatal care and certified by the American College of Nurse Midwives. The nurse midwife manages the perinatal care of women having a normal pregnancy, labor, and childbirth.

nurse practice act, a statute enacted by the legislature of any of the states or by the appropriate officers of the districts or possessions. The act delineates the legal scope of the practice of nursing within the geographic boundaries of the jurisdiction.

nurse practitioner, a nurse who by advanced training and clinical experience in a branch of nursing, as in a master's degree program in nursing, has acquired expert knowledge in the special branch of practice.

nursery diarrhea [L *nutrix* nurse; Gk *dia* through, *rhein* to flow], diarrhea of the newborn. In nurseries, outbreaks of diarrhea caused by *Escherichia coli, Salmonella,* echoviruses, or adenoviruses are potentially life threatening to the infant. Fluid loss is the most serious aspect of the disease, leading to dehydration and electrolyte imbalance.

nurse's aide, a person who is employed to carry out basic nonspecialized tasks in the care of a patient, such as bathing and feeding, making beds, and transporting patients.

Nurses' Coalition for Action in Politics (N-CAP), an organization that works in association with the American Nurses' Association. It raises funds for political contributions to candidates for public office at the state and national levels.

nurses' observation scale for inpatient evaluation (NOSIE), a systematic, objective behavioral rating scale that is applied by nurses to patient behavior.

nurses' registry, an employment agency or listing service for nurses who wish to work in a specific area of nursing, usually for a short period of time or on a per diem basis.

nurses' station, an area in a clinic, unit, or ward in a health care facility that serves as the administrative center for nursing care for a particular group of patients. It is usually centrally located and may be staffed by a ward secretary or clerk who assists with paperwork and telephone and other communication. Before going on duty, nurses usually meet there to receive daily assignments.

nursing, 1. the practice in which a nurse assists "the individual, sick or well, in the performance of those activities contributing to health or its recovery (or to a peaceful death) that he would perform unaided if he had the necessary strength, will or knowledge. And to do this in such a way as to help him gain independence as rapidly as possible." (Virginia Henderson) **2.** "the diagnosis and treatment of human responses to actual or potential health problems," (American Nurses' Association). There are four principal characteristics that further define nursing care: the phenomena that concern nurses; the use of theories to observe the need for nursing intervention and to plan nursing action; the nursing action taken; and an evaluation of the effects of the actions relative to the phenomena. **3.** the professional practice of a nurse. **4.** the process of acting as a nurse, of providing care that encourages and promotes the health of the person being served.

nursing assessment, an identification by a nurse of the needs, preferences, and abilities of a patient. Assessment follows an interview with and observation of a patient by the nurse and considers the symptoms and signs of the condition, the patient's verbal and nonverbal communication, medical and social history, and any other information available. Among the physical aspects assessed are vital signs, skin color and condition, motor and sensory nerve function, nutrition, rest, sleep, activity, elimination, and consciousness.

nursing assistant, *Canada;* a person trained in basic nursing techniques and direct patient care who practices under the supervision of a registered nurse.

nursing audit, a thorough investigation designed to identify, examine, or verify the performance of certain specified aspects of nursing care using established criteria. A **concurrent nursing audit** is performed during ongoing nursing care. A **retrospective nursing audit** is performed after discharge from the care facility, using the patient's record. Often, a nursing audit and a medical audit are performed collaboratively, resulting in a **joint audit.**

nursing bottle caries. See **baby bottle tooth decay.**

nursing care plan, a plan that is based on a nursing assessment and a nursing diagnosis, devised by a nurse. It has four essential components: identification of the nursing care problems and a statement of the nursing approach to solve those problems; the statement of the expected benefit to the patient; the statement of the specific actions by the nurse that reflect the nursing approach and achieve the goals specified; and the evaluation of the patient's response to nursing care and the readjustment of that care as required.

nursing diagnosis, a statement of a health problem or of a potential problem in the client's health status that a nurse is licensed and competent to treat. Four steps are required in the formulation of a nursing diagnosis: A data base is established by collecting information from all available sources, including interviews with the client and the client's family, a review of any existing records of the client's health, observation of the response of the client to any alterations in health status, a physical assessment, and a conference or consultation with others concerned in the care of the client. The second step includes an analysis of the client's responses to the problems, healthy or unhealthy, and a classification of those responses as psychologic, physiologic, spiritual, or sociologic. The third step is the organization of the data so that a tentative diagnostic statement can be made that summarizes the pattern of problems discovered. The last step is the confirmation of the sufficiency and accuracy of the data base by evaluation of the appropriateness of the diagnosis to nursing intervention and by the assurance that, given the same information, most other qualified practitioners would arrive at the same nursing diagnosis. A number of nursing diagnoses have been identified and are listed as accepted by the North American Nursing Diagnosis Association (NANDA), updated and refined at periodic meetings of the group.

nursing differential, an allowance added to payments to hospitals for services rendered Medicare patients in recognition of the cost of providing nursing services to such patients that is greater than the cost to the general patient population.

nursing ethics, the values or moral principles governing relationships between the nurse and patient, the patient's family, other members of the health professions, and the general public.

nursing goal, a general goal of nursing involving activities that are desirable but difficult to measure, such as self-care, good nutrition, and relaxation.

nursing health history, data collected about a patient's level of wellness, changes in life patterns, sociocultural role, and mental and emotional reactions to illness.

nursing home. See **extended care facility.**

nursing intervention, any act by a nurse that implements the nursing care plan or any specific objective of that plan, such as turning a comatose patient to avoid the development of decubitus ulcers.

nursing intervention model, (in nursing research) a conceptual framework used to determine appropriate nursing interventions. The model is a holistic representation of the patient and the health care system. The goal is to learn what nursing interventions would be most effective for the particular problem within the particular health care system.

nursing objective, a specific aim planned by a nurse to decrease a person's stress, or improve the ability to adapt, or both. A nursing objective may be physical, emotional, social, or cultural and may involve the person's family, friends, and other patients.

nursing observation, an objective, holistic evaluation made by a nurse of the various aspects of a patient's condition. It includes the person's general appearance, emotional affect, and nutritional status, habits, and preferences, as well as body temperature, skin condition, and any obvious abnormal processes.

nursing orders, specific instructions for implementing the nursing care plan, including the patient's preferences, timing of activities, details of health education necessary for the particular patient, role of the family, and plans for care after discharge. Nursing orders must be signed by the professional nurse who writes them.

nursing process, the process that serves as an organizational framework for the practice of nursing. It encompasses all of the steps taken by the nurse in caring for a patient: data collection, diagnosis, planning, treatment, and evaluation.

nursing process model, a conceptual framework in which the nurse-patient relationship is the basis of the nursing process. The nursing process is represented as dynamic and interpersonal, the nurse and the patient being affected by each other's behavior and by the environment around them. Each successful two-way communication is termed a "transaction" and can be analyzed to discover the factors that promote transactions.

nursing research, a detailed process in which a systematic study of a problem in the field of nursing is performed. One basic approach requires the following steps: formulation of the problem; review of the literature; development of a theory; formation of a hypothesis or hypotheses; definition of variables; determination of a method for weighting and counting variables; selection of a research design; choice of a population; plan for the analysis of the data; determination of interpretation; and plan for promulgation of the results.

Nursing Research, a bimonthly refereed journal containing papers and other materials concerning nursing research. The goal of the journal is to stimulate research in nursing.

nursing rounds, chart rounds, walking rounds, teaching rounds, or grand rounds that are held specifically for nurses and that focus on nursing care problems.

nursing specialty, a nurse's particular professional field of practice, such as surgical, pediatric, obstetric, or psychiatric nursing.

nursing supervisor, a nurse whose function is the administrative and clinical leadership of the nursing service of a division of a health care facility, such as a nursing supervisor of maternal and infant care nurses.

nursing theorist, a person who develops integrated concepts of nursing functions, objectives, and disciplines, and their relationships to the roles of physicians and other health professionals. Theorists whose models are used in nursing practice include **Dorothea Orem** and **Sr. Callista Roy.**

nursing theory, an organized framework of concepts and purposes designed to guide the practice of nursing.

nursology /nursol′əjē/ [L *nutrix* nurse; Gk *logos* science], a conceptual framework for the study and practice of nursing.

nurture, to feed, rear, foster, or care for, as in the nourishment, care, and training of growing children.

nutation /no͞otā′shən/ [L *nutare* to nod], the act of nodding, especially involuntary nodding as occurs in some neurologic disorders.

nutcracker esophagus. See **symptomatic esophageal peristalsis.**

nutrient /nōō'trē-ənt/ [L *nutriens* nourishing], a substance that provides nourishment and affects the nutritive and metabolic processes of the body.

nutrient artery of the humerus, one of a pair of branches of the deep brachial arteries, arising near the middle of the arm and entering the nutrient canal of the humerus.

nutrient canal. See **interdental canal.**

nutrient enema [L *nutriens*; Gk *enienai* injection], the introduction of saline or glucose into the body via the rectum.

nutriment /nōō'trimənt/ [L *nutrimentum* food that nourishes], any substance that nourishes and aids the growth and the development of the body.

nutrition /n(y)ōōtrish'ən/ [L *nutrire* to nourish], **1.** nourishment. **2.** the sum of the processes involved in the taking in of nutrients and in their assimilation and use for proper body functioning and maintenance of health. **3.** the study of food and drink as related to the growth and maintenance of living organisms.

nutritional [L, *nutrire,* to nourish], pertaining to the quality of food or eating behavior that provides nourishment through assimilation of food to tissues.

nutritional alcoholic cerebellar degeneration. See **alcoholic nutritional cerebellar degeneration.**

nutritional anemia [L *nutrire* to nourish; Gk *a, haima* without blood], a disorder characterized by the inadequate production of hemoglobin or erythrocytes caused by a nutritional deficiency of iron, folic acid, or vitamin B$_{12}$, or other nutritional disorders.

nutritional care, the substances, procedures, and setting involved in ensuring the proper intake and assimilation of nutrients, especially for the hospitalized patient. Patients who are unable to feed themselves are assisted, and abnormal intake of food is recorded and reported. Supplemental nourishment, when indicated, and fluids are offered between meals.

nutrition, altered: less than body requirements, a NANDA-accepted nursing diagnosis of an inability, based on psychologic, biological, or economic factors, to ingest or to digest food or to absorb nutrients in sufficient quantity for the maintenance of normal health. Defining characteristics include loss of weight, reported intake of less food than is recommended, evidence or report of a lack of food, lack of interest in food, aversion to

eating, alteration in the taste of food, feelings of fullness immediately after eating small quantities, abdominal pain with no other explanation, sores in the mouth, diarrhea or steatorrhea, pallor, weakness, and loss of hair.

nutrition, altered: more than body requirements, a NANDA-accepted nursing diagnosis of an excessive intake of food in relation to the metabolic needs of the body. Defining characteristics include overweight (weight gain of 20% greater than the ideal for the height and body build of the client), sedentary activity level, and dysfunctional eating habits, including eating in response to internal cues other than hunger.

nutrition, altered: high risk for more than body requirements, a NANDA-accepted nursing diagnosis of a risk of an intake of nutrients that exceeds metabolic needs. Risk factors include hereditary predisposition; excessive energy intake during late gestational life, early infancy, and adolescence; frequent, closely spaced pregnancies; rapid transition across growth percentiles in infants or children; the use of solid food as a major food source before 5 months of age; the use of food as a reward; an observed increase in the baseline weight at the onset of each pregnancy; and dysfunctional eating patterns.

nutritionist [L *nutrire* to nourish], one who studies and applies the principles and science of nutrition.

Nutting, Mary Adelaide (1858-1947), a Canadian-born American nursing educator and reformer. At Teachers College, Columbia University, she created and developed the Department of Nursing and Health and became the first professor of nursing in the world. With Lavinia Dock, she wrote *History of Nursing,* a classic in nursing literature.

nux vomica /nuks'vom'ikə/ [L *nux* nut; *vomere* to vomit], the dried ripe seeds of a small Asian tree, *Strychnos nux-vomica,* a source of the alkaloids strychnine and brucine. The seeds are powdered and the strychnine content reduced to a little more than 1% by the addition of lactose for use as a bitter tonic and nerve stimulant.

nvm, abbreviation for *nonvolatile matter.*

NVMA, abbreviation for *National Veterinary Medical Association.*

nyctalopia /nik'təlō'pē·ə/ [Gk *nyx* night, *alaos* obscure, *ops* eye], poor vision at night or in dim light resulting from decreased synthesis of rhodopsin, vitamin A deficiency, retinal degeneration, or a congenital defect. **–nyctalopic,** *adj.*

nyctophobia /nik'tō-/ [Gk *nyx + phobos*

N

fear], an anxiety reaction characterized by an obsessive, irrational fear of darkness.

nycturia. See **nocturia.**

nylidrin hydrochloride /nil'idrin/, a peripheral vasodilator prescribed in the treatment of peripheral vascular disease and circulatory disturbances of the inner ear.

nymphomania /nim'fəmā'nē·ə/ [Gk *nymphe* maiden, *mania* madness], a psychosexual disorder of women characterized by an insatiable desire for sexual satisfaction, often resulting from an unconscious conflict concerning personal adequacy.

nymphomaniac, 1. a person with or displaying characteristics of nymphomania. **2.** of, pertaining to, or exhibiting nymphomania. **–nymphomaniacal,** *adj.*

nystagmus /nīstag'məs/ [Gk *nystagmos* nodding], involuntary, rhythmic movements of the eyes; the oscillations may be horizontal, vertical, rotary, or mixed. Jerking nystagmus, characterized by faster movements in one direction than in the opposite direction, may be a sign of barbiturate intoxication or of labyrinthine vestibular, vascular or neurologic disease. Labyrinthine vestibular nystagmus, most frequently rotary, is usually accompanied by vertigo and nausea. Vertical nystagmus is considered pathognomonic of disease of the brainstem's tegmentum, and nystagmus occurring only in the abducting eye is said to be a sign of multiple sclerosis. Seesaw nystagmus, in which one eye moves up and the other down, may be seen in bilateral hemianopia. Pendular nystagmus occurs in albinism, various diseases of the retina and refractive media, and in miners after many years of working in darkness; in miners the eye movements are very rapid, increase on upward gaze, and are often associated with vertigo, head tremor, and photophobia. **–nystagmic,** *adj.*

nystatin /nis'tətin/, an antifungal antibiotic prescribed in the treatment of fungal infections of the GI tract, vagina, and skin.

nystaxis. See **nystagmus.**

O

o, symbol for *ohm.*

O, symbol for the element **oxygen.**

O₂, symbol for *oxygen molecule.*

OASDHI, abbreviation for **Old Age, Survivors, Disability and Health Insurance Program.**

oat cell carcinoma [AS *ate* oat; L *cella* storeroom; Gk *karkinos* crab, *oma* tumor], a malignant, usually bronchogenic epithelial neoplasm consisting of small, tightly packed, round, oval, or spindle-shaped epithelial cells. Tumors produced by these cells do not form bulky masses but usually spread along submucosal lymphatics. One third of all malignant tumors of the lung are of this type.

OAWO, abbreviation for **opening abductory wedge osteotomy.**

ob., abbreviation for the Latin word, *obit,* "died."

OB, *informal.* 1. abbreviation for **obstetrician.** 2. abbreviation for **obstetrics.**

obduction /əbduk′shən/ [L *obductio* a covering], a forensic medical autopsy.

Ober and Barr procedure, a surgical method of treating weak biceps muscles by transfer of the brachioradialis.

Ober procedure, a method for treatment of paralyzed clubfeet by transfer of the posterior tibial tendon to the third cuneiform or metatarsal.

Ober test, an examination for tight tensor fascia lata. The patient lies on one side with the hip and knee flexed on the surface and the opposite hip is extended while the knee is flexed. Inability to place the knee being tested on the table surface indicates a tight fascia lata.

obese /ōbēs′/ [L *obesus* swollen], pertaining to a corpulent or excessively heavy individual. Generally, a person is regarded as medically obese if the body weight is above 20% of desirable body weight for their age, sex, height, and body build. Because the "normal" human body is approximately 25% fat, the proportion may be doubled for a person who is medically defined as obese.

obesity [L *obesitas* fatness], an abnormal increase in the proportion of fat cells, mainly in the viscera and subcutaneous tissues of the body. **Hyperplastic obesity** is caused by an increase in the number of fat cells in the increased adipose tissue mass. **Hypertrophic obesity** results from an increase in the size of the fat cells in the increased adipose tissue mass.

obfuscation /ob′fəskā′shən/ [L *obfuscare* to darken], the act of making something confused, clouded, or obscure.

OBG, abbreviation for *obstetrics and gynecology.*

OB-Gyn, *informal*; abbreviation for *obstetrics and gynecology.*

object, (in psychology) that through which an instinct can achieve its goal.

objective, [L *objectare* to set against], 1. a goal. 2. of or pertaining to a phenomenon or clinical finding that is observed; not subjective.

objective data collection, the process in which data relating to the patient's problem are obtained by an observer through direct physical examination, including observation, palpation, and auscultation, and by laboratory analyses and radiologic and other studies.

objective lens, (in radiology) a lens that accepts light from the output phosphor of an image-intensifier tube and converts it into a parallel beam for recording the image on film.

objective sign [L *objectum* something cast before; *signum* sign], a clinical observation that is based on what can be seen, heard, measured, or otherwise recorded by an examining physician or other health care provider.

objective symptom [L *objectum* something cast before; Gk *symptoma* that which happens], a symptom that is accompanied by signs that tend to confirm the patient's physical complaint and enables the examining physician to deduce the cause.

object permanence, a capacity to perceive that something exists even when it is not seen.

object relations, emotional bonds between one person and another, as contrasted with interest in and love for the self.

obligate /ob′ligit, -gāt/ [L *obligare* to bind], characterized by the ability to survive only in a particular set of environmental conditions, such as an obligate parasite.

obligate aerobe, an organism that cannot grow in the absence of oxygen.

obligate anaerobe, an organism that cannot grow in the presence of oxygen, such as *Clostridium tetani, C. botulinum,* and *C. perfringens.*

obligate parasite. See **parasite.**

oblique /əblēk'/ [L *obliquus* slanted], a slanting direction or any variation from the perpendicular or the horizontal.

oblique bandage, a circular bandage applied spirally in slanting turns, usually to a limb.

oblique fiber, (in dentistry) any one of the collagenous fibers that are bundled together obliquely in the periodontal ligament.

oblique fissure of the lung, 1. the groove marking the division of the lower and middle lobes in the right lung. **2.** the groove marking the division of the upper and the lower lobes in the left lung.

oblique fracture, a fracture that cracks a bone at an oblique angle.

oblique illumination. See **illumination.**

oblique presentation [L *obliquus* slanting, *praesentare* to show], a presentation in which the long axis of the fetus is oblique to the long axis of the mother.

obliquus externus abdominis /əblī'kə/ [L, slanted], one of a pair of muscles that are the largest and the most superficial of the five anterolateral muscles of the abdomen. A broad, thin, four-sided muscle that arises by eight fleshy digitations from the lower eight ribs and inserts in the iliac crest and the linea alba. It acts to compress the contents of the abdomen and assists in micturition, defecation, emesis, parturition, and forced expiration. Both sides acting together serve to flex the vertebral column. One side alone functions to bend the vertebral column laterally and to rotate it, drawing the shoulder of the same side forward.

obliquus internus abdominis, one of a pair of anterolateral muscles of the abdomen, lying under the obliquus externus abdominis in the lateral and ventral part of the abdominal wall. It functions to compress the abdominal contents and assists in micturition, defecation, emesis, parturition, and forced expiration. Both sides acting together serve to flex the vertebral column. One side acting alone acts to bend the vertebral column laterally and rotate it, drawing the shoulder of the opposite side downward.

obliteration [L *obliterare* to efface], the removal or loss of function of a part of the body by surgery, disease, or degeneration.

obliterative phlebitis /əblit'ərətiv'/ [L *obliterare*; Gk *phleps* vein, *itis* inflammation], a form of phlebitis in which the inflammation results in permanent closure of the vessel.

OBS, abbreviation for **organic brain syndrome.**

observation [L *observare* to watch], **1.** the act of watching carefully and attentively. **2.** a report of what is seen or noted, such as a nursing observation.

observation hip, a condition in which a patient experiences a limp, pain, and limited motion of the hip. Causes may include toxic synovitis, infection, or avascular necrosis.

obsession [L *obsidere* to haunt], a persistent thought or idea with which the mind is continually and involuntarily preoccupied and which suggests an irrational act. **–obsessive,** *adj.*

obsessive-compulsive [L *obsidere* to haunt; *compellere* to impel], **1.** characterized by or relating to the tendency to perform repetitive acts or rituals, usually as a means of releasing tension or relieving anxiety. **2.** describing a person who has an obsessive-compulsive disorder.

obstetric anesthesia /əbstet'rik/ [L *obstetrix* midwife; Gk *anaisthesia* absence of feeling], any of various procedures used to provide anesthesia for childbirth. It includes local anesthesia for episiotomy or episiotomy repair, regional anesthesia for labor or delivery, such as by paracervical block or pudendal block, or, for a wider block—epidural, caudal, or saddle block.

obstetric forceps, forceps used to assist delivery of the fetal head. The several styles of forceps are designed to assist in various clinical situations. Kinds of obstetric forceps include **Barton forceps, Elliot forceps, Kielland forceps,** and **Simpson forceps.**

obstetrician /ob'stətrish'ən/, a physician who specializes in obstetrics.

obstetric position. See **lateral recumbent position.**

obstetrics /əbstet'riks/ [L *obstetrix* midwife], the branch of medicine concerned with pregnancy and childbirth, including the study of the physiologic and pathologic function of the female reproductive tract and the care of the mother and fetus throughout pregnancy, childbirth, and the immediate postpartum period. **–obstetric, obstetrical,** *adj.*

obstetrix. See **midwife.**

obstipation /ob'stipā'shən/ [L *obstipare* to press], **1.** a condition of extreme and persistent constipation caused by obstruction in the intestinal or eliminatory system. **2.** a process of blocking. **–obstipant,** *n.,* **obstipate,** *v.*

obstruction [L *obstruere* to build against],

1. something that blocks or clogs. **2.** the act of blocking or preventing passage. **3.** the condition of being obstructed or clogged. **–obstruct,** *v.,* **obstructive,** *adj.*

obstructive airway disease, a classification of respiratory disease characterized by decreased airway size and increased airway secretions. It includes chronic bronchitis, abnormalities of the bronchi, and emphysema.

obstructive anuria [L *obstruere* to build against; Gk *a, ouron* without urine], an abnormal urologic condition characterized by an almost complete absence of urination and caused by an obstruction of the urinary tract.

obstructive biliary cirrhosis [L *ostruere,* to build against; *bilis,* bile; Gk, *kirrhos,* yellow; *osis,* condition], a form of secondary cirrhosis in which a stricture develops in the bile ducts. The condition may develop after cholecystectomy, gallstones, or a tumor.

obstructive constipation, a condition in which feces are retained in the bowel because of a blockage in the lumen.

obstructive jaundice. See **cholestasis.**

obstructive sleep apnea, a form of sleep apnea involving a physical obstruction in the upper airways. The condition is usually marked by recurrent sleep interruptions, and gasping spells on awakening.

obstructive uropathy, any pathologic condition that results in obstruction of the flow of urine. The condition may lead to impairment of kidney function and an increased risk of urinary infection.

obtund /obtund/ [L *obtundere* to blunt] **1.** to deaden pain. **2.** to render insensitive to unpleasant or painful stimuli by reducing the level of consciousness, such as by anesthesia or a strong narcotic analgesic. **–obtundation, obtundity,** *n.,* **obtunded, obtundent,** *adj.*

obtundation /ob'tundā'shən/ [L *obtundere* to blunt, *atus* process], the use of an agent that soothes and reduces irritation or pain by blocking sensibility at some level of the central nervous system, such as in the preoperative use of anesthesia.

obturator /ob'tərā'tər, ob'tyərā'tər/ [L *obturare* to close], **1.** a device used to block a passage or a canal or to fill in a space, such as a prosthesis implanted to bridge the gap in the roof of the mouth in a cleft palate. **2.** *nontechnical;* an obturator muscle or membrane.

obturator dislocation. See **dislocation of hip.**

obturator externus, the flat, triangular muscle covering the outer surface of the anterior wall of the pelvis. It functions to rotate the thigh laterally.

obturator foramen, a large opening on each side of the lower portion of the hip bone, formed posteriorly by the ischium.

obturator internus, a muscle that covers a large area of the inferior aspect of the lesser pelvis, where it surrounds the obturator foramen. It arises from the superior and the inferior rami of the pubis, the ischium, and the obturator membrane and inserts into the greater trochanter of the femur. It functions to rotate the thigh laterally and to extend and abduct the thigh when it is flexed.

obturator membrane, a tough fibrous membrane that covers the obturator foramen of each side of the pelvis.

obturator muscles [L *obturare* to stop up; *musculus*], a pair of thigh muscles, the external and internal obturators. The external obturator flexes and rotates the thigh laterally; the internal obturator abducts and rotates the thigh laterally.

obturator sign [L *obturare, signus* sign], a diagnostic test for appendicitis. The internal rotation of the hip with a resultant tightening of the internal obturator muscle may cause abdominal discomfort in appendicitis.

obv, abbreviation for *obverse.*

OC, abbreviation for **oral contraceptive.**

occ, abbreviation for **occipital.**

occipital /oksip'itəl/ [L *occiput* back of the head], **1.** of or pertaining to the occiput. **2.** situated near the occipital bone, such as the occipital lobe of the brain.

occipital artery, one of a pair of tortuous braces from the external carotid arteries that divides into six branches and supplies parts of the head and scalp.

occipital bone, the cuplike bone at the back of the skull, marked by a large opening, the foramen magnum, that communicates with the vertebral canal. Its inner surface is divided into four fossae. The occipital bone articulates with the two parietal bones, the two temporal bones, the sphenoid, and the atlas.

occipital lobe, one of the five lobes of each cerebral hemisphere, occupying a relatively small pyramidal portion of the occipital pole. The occipital lobe lies beneath the occipital bone and presents medial, lateral, and inferior surfaces.

occipital sinus, the smallest of the cranial sinuses and one of six posterior superior venous channels associated with the dura mater.

occipitoaxial ligament. See **membrane tectoria.**

occipitobregmatic /oksip'itōbregmat'ik/ [L *occiput* + Gk *bregma* front of the head] of or pertaining to the occiput and the bregma.

occipitofrontal /oksip'itōfrun'təl/ [L *occiput* + *frons* forehead], of or pertaining to the occiput and the frontal bone of the skull.

occipitofrontalis /oksip'itōfrəntal'is/, one of a pair of thin, broad muscles covering the top of the skull, consisting of an occipital belly and a frontal belly connected by an extensive aponeurosis. It is the muscle that draws the scalp and raises the eyebrows.

occipitoparietal fissure. See **pariotooccipital sulcus.**

occiput /ok sipet/, *pl.* **occiputs, occipita** /oksip ite/, the back part of the head.

occluded /əkl o͞o'did/ [l *occludere* to shut up], closed, plugged, or obstructed.

occlusal /əkl o͞o'səl/ [L *occludere*], pertaining to a closure, such as the contact between the teeth of the upper and lower jaws.

occlusal adjustment, (in dentistry) the grinding of the occluding surfaces of teeth to improve the occlusion or relationship between opposing tooth surfaces, their supporting structures, the muscles of mastication, and the temporomandibular joints.

occlusal contouring, the modification by grinding of irregularities of occlusal tooth forms, such as uneven marginal ridges, and extruded or malpositioned teeth.

occlusal form, the shape of the occluding surfaces of a tooth, a row of teeth, or any dentition.

occlusal harmony, a combination of healthy and nondisruptive occlusal relationships between the teeth and their supporting structures, the associated neuromuscular mechanisms, and the temporomandibular joints.

occlusal lug. See **occlusal rest.**

occlusal plane [L *occludere, planum* level ground], a plane passing through the occlusal surfaces of the teeth. It represents the mean of the curvature of the occlusal or biting surface.

occlusal radiograph, an intraoral radiograph made with the film placed on the occlusal surfaces of one of the arches.

occlusal recontouring, the reshaping of an occlusal surface of a natural or artificial tooth.

occlusal relationship, the relationship of the mandibular teeth to the maxillary teeth when in a defined occlusal contact position.

occlusal rest, a support placed on the occlusal surface of a posterior tooth.

occlusal rest angle, (in dentistry) the angle formed by the occlusal rest with the upright minor connector.

occlusal spillway, a natural groove that crosses a cusp ridge or a marginal ridge of a tooth.

occlusal surface [L *occludere, superficies* surface], the surfaces of teeth in one arch that makes contact or near contact with the corresponding surfaces of the teeth in the opposing arch.

occlusal trauma, injury to a tooth and surrounding structures caused by malocclusive stresses, including trauma, temporomandibular joint dysfunction, and bruxism.

occlusion /əkl o͞o'zhən/ [L *occludere* to shut up], **1.** (in anatomy) a blockage in a canal, vessel, or passage of the body. **2.** (in dentistry) any contact between the incising or masticating surfaces of the maxillary and mandibular teeth. **–occlude,** *v.,* **occlusive,** *adj.*

occlusion rim, an artificial dental structure with occluding surfaces attached to temporary or permanent denture bases, used for recording the relation of the maxilla to the mandible and for positioning the teeth.

occlusive /əcl o͞o'siv/, pertaining to something that effects an occlusion or closure, such as an occlusive dressing.

occlusive dressing, a dressing that prevents air from reaching a wound or lesion and that retains moisture, heat, body fluids, and medication. It may consist of a sheet of thin plastic affixed with transparent tape.

occlusometer. See **gnathodymamometer.**

occult /əkult'/ [L *occultare* to hide], hidden or difficult to observe directly, such as occult prolapse of the umbilical cord or occult blood.

occult blood, blood that appears from a nonspecific source, with obscure signs and symptoms. It may be detected by means of a chemical test or by microscopic or spectroscopic examination.

occult blood test [L *occultus* hidden; AS *blod*; L *testum* crucible], a test for the presence of microscopic amounts of blood in the feces secondary to bleeding in the digestive tract.

occult carcinoma, a small carcinoma that does not cause overt symptoms. It may remain localized and be discovered only incidentally at autopsy after death resulting from another cause, or it may metastasize and be discovered in the diagnostic study of the resulting metastatic disease.

occult fracture, a fracture that cannot be initially detected by radiographic examination but may be evident radiographically weeks later. It is accompanied by the usual signs of pain and trauma and may produce soft-tissue edema.

occupancy [L *occupare* to seize], the ratio of average daily hospital census to the average number of beds maintained during the reporting period.

occupancy factor (T), the level of occupancy of an area adjacent to a source of radiation, used to determine the amount of shielding required in the walls. T is rated as full, for an office or laboratory next to an x-ray facility; partial, for corridors and restrooms; and occasional, for stairways, elevators, closets, and outside areas.

occupational accident [L *occupare* to employ; *accidere* to happen], an accidental injury to an employee that occurs in the workplace. Occupational accidents account for over 95% of occupational disabilities.

occupational asthma, an abnormal condition of the respiratory system resulting from exposure in the workplace to allergenic or other irritating substances. The condition is most common among persons working with detergents, Western red cedar, cotton, flax, hemp, grain, flour, and stone.

occupational disability, a condition in which a worker is unable to perform the functions required to complete a job satisfactorily because of an occupational disease or an occupational accident.

occupational disease, a disease that results from a particular employment, usually from the effects of long-term exposure to specific substances or of continuous or repetitive physical acts.

occupational health, the ability of a worker to function at an optimum level of well-being at a worksite as reflected in terms of productivity, work attendance, disability compensation claims, and employment longevity.

occupational history, a portion of the health history in which questions are asked about the person's occupation, source of income, effects of the work on worker's health or the worker's health on the job, the duration of the work, and to what degree the occupation satisfies the person.

occupational lung disease, any one of a group of abnormal conditions of the lungs caused by the inhalation of dusts, fumes, gases, or vapors in an environment where a person works.

occupational medicine, a field of preventive medicine concerned with the medical problems and practices relating to occupations and especially to the health of workers in various industries.

occupational neurosis. See **occupational stress.**

occupational performance tasks, activities that can be used to measure the potential ability or actual proficiency in the handling of certain objects and use of skills related to a given occupation.

occupational socialization, the adaptation of an individual to a given set of job-related behaviors, particularly the expected behavior that accompanies a specific job.

occupational stress, a disorder associated with a job or work. The neurosis may be expressed in the form of extreme tension and anxiety, and the development of physical symptoms such as headache or cramps.

occupational therapist (OT), an allied health professional who practices occupational therapy and who must be licensed, registered, certified, or otherwise regulated by law.

occupational therapy, "the use of purposeful activity with individuals who are limited by physical injury or illness, psychosocial dysfunction, developmental or learning disabilities, poverty and cultural differences, or the aging process to maximize independence, prevent disability, and maintain health. The practice encompasses evaluation, treatment, and consultation." (American Occupational Therapy Association.)

occupational therapy aide, a person who, under the supervision of an occupational therapist, performs clerical and related tasks necessary for the implementation of occupational therapy programs.

occupational therapy assistant. See **certified occupational therapy assistant.**

occurrence policy [L *occurere* to run; *politica* pertaining to the state], a professional liability insurance policy that covers the holder during the period an alleged act of malpractice occurred. Occurrence policies are said to have a "long tail" because the statute of limitations on malpractice allegations is unlimited.

ochre mutation. See **amber mutation.**

ochronosis /ō′krənō′sis/ [Gk *ochros* yellow, *osis*] a condition characterized by the deposition of brown-black pigment in connective tissue and cartilage, often caused by alkaptonuria or poisoning with phenol. The urine may be dark-colored.

OCN, abbreviation for *Oncology Certified Nurse.*

ocontic pressure. See **colloid osmotic pressure.**

OCT, abbreviation for **oxytocin challenge test.**

octaploid, octaploidic. See **polyploid.**

octigravida [L *octo* eight; *gravidare* to impregnate], pertaining to a woman who is pregnant for the eighth time.

ocul., abbreviation for the Latin word, *oculis,* "pertaining to the eyes."

ocular /ok'yələr/ [L *oculus* eye], **1.** of or pertaining to the eye. **2.** an eyepiece of an optic instrument.

ocular dysmetria, a visual disorder in which the eyes are unable to fix the gaze on an object or follow a moving object with accuracy.

ocular herpes [L *oculus* eye; Gk *herpein* to creep], a herpes virus infection of the eye.

ocular hypertelorism, a developmental defect involving the frontal region of the cranium, characterized by an abnormally widened bridge of the nose and increased distance between the eyes.

ocular hypotelorism, a developmental defect involving the frontal region of the cranium, characterized by a narrowing of the bridge of the nose and an abnormal decrease in the distance between the eyes, with resulting convergent strabismus.

ocular myopathy, slowly progressive weakness of ocular muscles, characterized by decreased mobility of the eye and drooping of the upper lid. The disorder may be unilateral or bilateral and may be caused by damage to the oculomotor nerve, an intracranial tumor, or a neuromuscular disease.

ocular refraction [L *oculus, refringere* to break apart], pertaining to refraction of the eye.

oculocephalic reflex /ok'yəlō'səfal'ik/ [L *oculus* + Gk *kephale* head; L *reflectere* to bend backward], a test of the integrity of brainstem function. When the patient's head is quickly moved to one side and then the other, the eyes will normally lag behind the head movement and then slowly assume the midline position. Failure of the eyes to either lag properly or revert back to the midline indicates a lesion at the brainstem level.

oculogyric crisis /ok'yəlōj'rik/ [L *oculus* + *gyrare* to turn around], a paroxysm in which the eyes are held in a fixed position, usually up and sideways, for minutes or several hours, often occurring in postencephalitic patients with signs of parkinsonism.

oculomotor /ok'yəlōmō'tər/, pertaining to movements of the eyeballs.

oculomotor nerve [L *oculus* + *motor*], either of a pair of cranial nerves essential for eye movements, supplying certain extrinsic and intrinsic eye muscles.

oculomotor nucleus [L *oculus* + *motor; nucleus* nut], a nucleus of a third cranial nerve arising in the midbrain.

OD, *informal,* abbreviation for **overdose.**

OD, 1. abbreviation for *oculus dexter,* a Latin phrase meaning "right eye." **2.** abbreviation for *Doctor of Optometry.*

OD'd /ōdēd/ *[slang],* overdosed, usually referring to a person who has suffered adverse effects from an excessively large dose of a drug of abuse.

Oddi's sphincter [Ruggero Oddi, Italian surgeon, b. 1864; Gk *sphigkter* binder], a band of circular muscle fibers around the lower part of the common bile duct and pancreatic duct, near the common duct junction of the duodenum.

odontalgia /ō'dontal'jə/ [Gk *odous* tooth, *algos* pain], a toothache.

odontectomy /ō'dontek'təmē/ [Gk *odous* tooth, *ektome* cut out], the extraction of a tooth.

odontiasis /ō'dontī'əsis/, the process of teething.

odontitis /ō'dontī'tis/ [Gk *odous* + *itis* inflammation], abnormal enlargement of a tooth, usually resulting from an inflammation of the odontoblasts (cells responsible for dentine formation) rather than of the mature, or erupted, tooth.

odontoblast /ōdon'təblast'/ [Gk *odous* + *blastos* germ], one of the connective tissue cells of the periphery of the dental pulp that develops into the primary and secondary dentin of a tooth.

odontodynia. See **odontalgia.**

odontodysplasia /ōdon'tōdisplā'zhə/ [Gk *odous* + *dys* bad, *plasis* forming], an abnormality in the development of the teeth, characterized by deficient formation of enamel and dentin.

odontogenesis /ōdon'tōjen'əsis/ [Gk *odous* + *genein* to produce], the origin and formation of developing teeth.

odontogenesis imperfecta. See **dentinogenesis imperfecta.**

odontogenic /ōdon'tōjen'ik/ [Gk *odous* + *genein* to produce], **1.** generating teeth. **2.** developing in tissues that produce teeth.

odontogenic fibroma, a benign neoplasm of the jaw derived from the embryonic part of the tooth germ, dental follicle, or dental papilla or developing later from the periodontal membrane.

odontogenic fibrosarcoma, a malignant neoplasm of the jaw that develops in a mesenchymal component of a tooth or tooth germ.

odontogenic myxoma, a rare tumor of the jaw; it may develop from the mesenchyme of the tooth germ.

odontoid ligament. See **alar ligament.**

odontoid process [Gk *odous* + *eidos* form; L *processus*], the toothlike projection that rises perpendicularly from the upper surface of the body of the second cervical vertebra or axis, which serves as a pivot point for the rotation of the atlas, or first cervical vertebra, enabling the head to turn.

odontoid vertebra. See **axis.**

odontology /o dontol eje/ [Gk *odous* + *logos* science], the scientific study of the anatomy and physiology of the teeth and of the surrounding structures of the oral cavity.

odontoma /ō'dontō'mə/ [Gk *odous* + *oma* tumor], an anomaly of the teeth that resembles a hard tumor, such as dens in dente, enamel pearl, and complex or composite odontoma.

odor [L, a smell], a scent or smell. The sense of smell is activated when airborne molecules stimulate receptors of the first cranial nerve.

odoriferous [L *odor* + *ferre* to bear], pertaining to something that produces a smell, particularly one that is strong or offensive.

odorous [L *odor* smell], pertaining to something that has an odor, smell, or fragrance.

ODTS, abbreviation for **organic dust toxic syndrome.**

odynophagia /od'inōfā'jə/ [Gk *odyne* pain, *phagein* to swallow], a severe sensation of burning, squeezing pain while swallowing, caused by irritation of the mucosa or a muscular disorder of the esophagus, such as gastroesophageal reflux, bacterial or fungal infection, tumor, achalasia, or chemical irritation.

Oedipus complex /ed'ipəs, ē'dipəs/ [Gk *Oedipus* mythic king who slew his father and married his mother], **1.** (in psychoanalysis) a child's desire for a sexual relationship with the parent of the opposite sex, usually with strong negative feelings for the parent of the same sex. **2.** a son's desire for a sexual relationship with his mother.

OEM, abbreviation for *optical electron microscope.*

OER, abbreviation for **oxygen enhancement ratio.**

o/f, symbol for *oxidation/fermentation.*

off-center grid, (in radiology) a focused grid that is perpendicular to the central-axis x-ray beam but shifted laterally, resulting in a cutoff across the entire grid.

off-focus radiation, (in radiology) x-ray artifacts caused by stray electrons that interact at positions on the anode at points other than the focal spot.

off-level grid, (in radiology) a grid that is not perpendicular to the central-axis x-ray beam. The cause is often a malpositioned x-ray tube rather than an improperly positioned grid.

ofloxacin /ōflak'səsin/, an antibiotic of the carboxyfluoroquinolone type.

Ogden classification system, a system of categories for 17 different kinds of epiphyseal fractures.

Ogden plate, a long metal plate with slots designed to accept encircling bands. It is used for fixing long bone fractures associated with preexisting intramedullary devices such as rods or the stem of a prosthesis.

Ogsten line, a line drawn from the adduction tubercle to the intercondylar notch, used as a guide for transection of the condyle in osteotomy for knock-knee.

o.h., abbreviation for the Latin term, *omni hora,* "hourly."

OH, symbol for **hydroxyl.**

OHD, abbreviation for *organic heart disease.*

OHF, abbreviation for **Omsk hemorrhagic fever.**

ohm [Georg S. Ohm, German physicist, b. 1787], a unit of measurement of electric resistance. One ohm is the resistance of a conductor in which an electric potential of 1 V produces a current of 1 ampere.

Ohm's law [Georg S. Ohm,] the principle that the strength or intensity of an unvarying electric current is directly proportional to the electromotive force and inversely proportional to the resistance of the circuit.

oil [L *oleum*], any of a large number of greasy liquid substances not miscible in water. Oil may be fixed or volatile and is derived from animal, vegetable, or mineral matter.

oil retention enema, an enema containing about 200 to 250 ml of an oil-based solution given to soften a fecal mass.

ointment [L *unguentum* a salve], a semisolid, externally applied preparation, usually containing a drug. Various ointments are used as local analgesic, anesthetic, antiinfective, astringent, depigmenting, irritant, and keratolytic agents.

OL, abbreviation for the Latin term, *oculus laevus,* "left eye."

Old Age, Survivors, Disability and Health Insurance Program (OASDHI), a benefit program, administered by the Social Security Administration, that provides cash benefits to workers who are retired or disabled, their dependents, and survivors.

old dislocation, a dislocation in which inflammatory changes have occurred.

old tuberculin [ME, *ald,* L, *tubercule*], the original formula for an extract of the tubercle bacillus used in the treatment of tuberculosis by Koch.

Old World leishmaniasis. See **oriental sore.**

oleandomycin. See **troleandomycin.**

olecranon /olek renon/ [Gk *olekranon* tip of the elbow], a proximal projection of the ulna that forms the point of the elbow and fits into the olecranon fossa of the humerus when the forearm is extended.

olecranon bursa, the bursa of the elbow.

olecranon fossa, the depression in the posterior surface of the humerus that receives the olecranon of the ulna when the forearm is extended.

olecranon process. See **olecranon.**

olefiant gas. See **ethylene.**

olefin /ō′ləfin/ [L *oleum* oil, *facere* to make], any of a group of unsaturated aliphatic hydrocarbons containing one or more double bonds in the carbon chain.

oleic acid /ōlē′ik/ [L *oleum* oil; *acidus* sour], a colorless, liquid, monounsaturated fatty acid occurring in almost all natural fats.

oleovitamin /ō′lē·ovī′təmin/, a preparation of fish-liver oil or edible vegetable oil that contains one or more of the fat-soluble vitamins or their derivatives.

oleovitamin A, an oily preparation, usually fish-liver oil or fish-liver oil diluted with an edible vegetable oil, containing the natural or synthetic form of vitamin A.

oleovitamin D₂. See **calciferol.**

olfaction [L *olfacere* to smell], **1.** the act of smelling. **2.** the sense of smell.

olfactory /olfak′tere/, of or pertaining to the sense of smell. **–olfaction,** *n.*

olfactory anesthesia. See **anosmia.**

olfactory bulb [L *olfactus* sense of smell; *bulbus* swollen root], the area of the forebrain where the olfactory nerves terminate and the olfactory tracts arise.

olfactory center [L *olfactare* to smell at; Gk *kentron*], the part of the brain responsible for the subjective appreciation of odors; a complex group of neurons located near the junction of the temporal and parietal lobes.

olfactory cortex [L *olfactus; cortex* bark], the part of the cerebral cortex including the pyriform lobe and the hippocampus formation that is concerned with the sense of smell.

olfactory foramen, one of several openings in the cribriform plate of the ethmoid bone.

olfactory hallucination, a condition in which an individual has false perceptions of odors, which are usually repugnant or offensive. The hallucinations are sometimes associated with guilt feelings.

olfactory lobe, a structure involved in the sense of smell in lower animals. Vestiges of the tissue are found in the cerebral hemispheres of humans.

olfactory nerve, one of a pair of nerves associated with the sense of smell. The olfactory nerve is cranial nerve I and is composed of numerous fine filaments that ramify in the mucous membrane of the ol-

factory area. The area in which the olfactory nerves arise is situated in the most superior portion of the mucous membrane that covers the superior nasal concha. The olfactory nerves connect with the olfactory bulb and the olfactory tract, which are components of the portion of the brain associated with the sense of smell.

olfactory receptors [L *olfactus; recipere* to receive], bipolar nerve cells located in the nasal epithelium. Axons of the cells become fibers of the olfactory nerve.

oligemia /ol′ijē′mē·ə/ [Gk *oligos* little, *hamia* blood], a condition of hypovolemia or reduced circulating intravascular volume.

oligoclonal banding /ol′igōklō′nəl/, a process by which cerebrospinal fluid IgG is distributed, following electrophoresis, in discrete bands. Approximately 90% of multiple sclerosis patients show oligoclonal banding.

oligodactyly /ol′igōdak′tile/ [Gk *oligos* + *dactylos* finger], a congenital anomaly characterized by the absence of one or more of the fingers or toes. **–oligodactylic,** *adj.*

oligodendroblastoma. See **oligodendroglioma.**

oligodendrocyte /ol′igōden′drəsīt′/ [Gk *oligos* + *dendron* tree, *kytos* cell], a type of neuroglial cell with dendritic projections that coil around axons of neural cells.

oligodendroglia/ol′igōdendrog′lē·ə/, central nervous system cells that produce myelin.

oligodendroglioma /ol′igōden′drōglī·o′-mə/, *pl.* **oligodendrogliomas, olidodendrogliomata** [Gk *oligos* + *dendron* tree, *glia* glue, *oma* tumor], an uncommon brain tumor composed of nonneural ectodermal cells that usually form part of the supporting connective tissue around nerve cells.

oligodontia /ol′igōdon′shə/ [Gk *oligos* + *odous* tooth], a genetically determined dental defect characterized by the development of fewer than the normal number of teeth.

oligogenic /ol′igōjen′ik/ [Gk *oligos* + *genein* to produce], of or pertaining to hereditary characteristics produced by one or only a few genes.

oligohydramnios /ol′igōhidram′nē·əs/ [Gk *oligos* + *hydor* water, *amnion* fetal membrane], an abnormally small amount or absence of amniotic fluid.

oligomeganephronia /ol′igōmeg′ənefro′nē·ə/ [Gk *oligos* + *megas* large, *nephros* kidney], a type of congenital renal hypoplasia associated with chronic renal failure in children. **–oligomeganephronic,** *adj.*

oligomenorrhea /ol′igōmen′ôrē′ə/ [Gk *oli-*

gos + L *mensis* month, *rhoia* flow], abnormally light or infrequent menstruation. **–oligomenorrheic,** *adj.*

oligopnea, oligopnoea. See **bradypnea.**

oligospermia /ol′igōspur′mē·ə/ [Gk *oligos* + *sperma* seed], insufficient spermatozoa in the semen.

oliguria /ol′igyŏŏr′e·ə/ [Gk *oligos* + *ouron* urine], a diminished capacity to form and pass urine, less than 500 ml in every 24 hours, so that the end products of metabolism cannot be excreted efficiently. **–oliguric,** *adj.*

olisthy /ōlis′thē/ [Gk, *olisthanein,* to slip], the slippage of a bone from its normal anatomic site, as in the example of a "slipped disk." **–olisthetic,** *adj.*

olivary body /ol′iver′ē/ [L *oliva* olive; AS *bodig*], an olivary nucleus, part of an aggregate of small densely packed nerve cells, on the medula oblongata.

olivopontocerebellar /ol′ivopon′toser′əbel′ər/ [L *oliva* olive, *pons* bridge, *cerebellum* small brain], of or pertaining to the olivae, the middle peduncles, and the cerebellum.

olivopontocerebellar atrophy (OPCA), a group of hereditary ataxias characterized by mixed clinical features of pure cerebellar ataxia, dementia, parkinson-like symptoms, spasticity, choreoathetosis, retinal degeneration, myelopathy, and peripheral neuropathy.

Ollier's disease. See **endondromatosis.**

Ollier's dyschondroplasia /ol e az/ [Louis X.E.L. Ollier, French surgeon, b. 1830; Gk *dys* bad, *chrondros* cartilage, *plasis* formation], a rare disorder of bone development in which the epiphyseal tissue responsible for growth spreads through the bones, causing abnormal irregular growth and, eventually, deformity. A kind of dyschondroplasia **heredity multiple exostoses.**

o.m. abbreviation for the Latin term, *omni mane,* "every morning."

omalgia /ōmal′jə/ [Gk *omos* shoulder, *algos* pain], pain in the shoulder.

omarthritis /ō′märthrī′tis/, inflammation of the shoulder joint.

ombudsman /om′bədzmən/ [ONorse *umbothsmathr* commission man], a person who investigates and mediates patients' problems and complaints in relation to a hospital's services.

omega, Ω, ω, the twenty-fourth letter of the Greek alphabet.

omental bursa /ōmen′təl/, a cavity in the peritoneum behind the stomach, the lesser omentum, and the lower border of the liver and in front of the pancreas and duodenum.

omentum /ōmen′təm/, *pl.* **omenta, omen-**

tums [L, fat-skin], an extension of the peritoneum that enfolds one of more adjacent organs in the stomach. **–omental,** *adj.*

omicron, O, o, the fifteenth letter of the Greek alphabet.

omission [L *omittere* to neglect], (in law) intentional or unintentional neglect to fulfill a duty required by law.

omnifocal lens /om′nēfō′kəl/ [L *omnis* all + *focus* hearth; *lentil*], an eyeglass lens designed for both near and far vision with the reading portion in a variable curve.

omnipotence, (in psychology) an infantile perception that the outside world is part of the organism, which leads to a primitive feeling of all-powerfulness.

omnivorous [L *omnis* + *vorare* to devour], pertaining to the eating of both plants and animal flesh.

omn. noct. abbreviation for the Latin term, *omni nocte,* "every night."

omn. quad. hor., abbreviation for the Latin term, *omni quadrante hora,* "every quarter of an hour."

omophagia /om′ōfā′jē·ə/[Gk *omos* raw; *phagein* to eat], the eating of raw foods, particularly raw meat or fish.

omphalic /omfal′ik/ [Gk *omphalos* navel], pertaining to the umbilicus.

omphalitis, an inflammation of the umbilical stump, marked by redness, swelling, and purulent exudate in severe cases.

omphaloangiopagus. See **allantoidoangiopagus.**

omphalocele /om′felosel′/ [Gk *omphalos* + *kele* hernia], congenital herniation of intraabdominal viscera through a defect in the abdominal wall around the umbilicus.

omphalodidymus. See **gastrodidymus.**

omphalogenesis /om′falōjen′əsis/ [Gk *omphalos* + *genesis* origin], the formation of the umbilicus or yolk sac during embryonic development. **–omphalogenetic,** *adj.*

omphalomesenteric artery. See **vitelline artery.**

omphalomesenteric circulation. See **vitelline circulation.**

omphalomesenteric duct. See **yolk stalk.**

omphalomesenteric vein. See **vitelline vein.**

omphalopagus. See **monomphalus.**

omphalosite /om′falōsīt′/ [Gk *omphalos* + *sitos* food], the underdeveloped parasitic member of unequal conjoined twins united by the vessels of the umbilical cord.

OMS, abbreviation for **Organisation Mondiale de la Santé.** See **World Health Organization.**

Omsk hemorrhagic fever (OHF) /omsk/, an acute infection, seen in regions of the USSR, caused by an arbovirus transmitted by the bite of an infected tick or by handling infected muskrats. The disease is characterized by fever, headache, epistaxis, GI and uterine bleeding, and other hemorrhagic manifestations.

o.n., abbreviation for the Latin term, *omni nocte,* "every night."

onanism. See **masturbation, withdrawal method.**

onchocerciasis /on' koserki' esis/ [Gk *onkos* swelling, *kerkos* tail, *osis* condition], a form of filariasis common in Central and South America and in Africa, characterized by subcutaneous nodules, pruritic rash, and eye lesions. It is transmitted by the bites of black flies that deposit *Onchocerca volvulus* microfilariae under the skin. The microfilariae migrate to the subcutaneous tissue and eyes, and fibrous nodules develop around the developing adult worms. Hypersensitive reactions to the dying microfilariae include extreme pruritus, a cellulitis-like rash, lichenification, depigmentation, and, rarely, elephantiasis.

oncofetal protein /ong'kōfē'təl/ [Gk *onkos* + L *fetus* pregnant; Gk *proteios* first rank], a protein produced by or associated with a tumor cell, particularly an embryologic tumor.

oncogene /ong'kōjēn/ [Gk *onkos* + *genein* to produce], a potential cancer-inducing gene. Under normal conditions, such genes play a role in the growth and proliferation of cells, but when altered in some way by a cancer-causing agent, they may cause the cell to be transformed into a malignant state.

oncogenesis /ong'kojem'esis/ [Gk *onkos* + *genesis* origin], the process initiating and promoting the development of a neoplasm through the action of biologic, chemical, or physical agents. **–oncogenic** /ong'kojen'ik/, *adj.*

oncogenic virus, a virus that is able to cause the development of a malignant neoplastic disease. Over 100 oncogenic viruses have been identified.

oncologist /ongkol'ejidt/, a physician who specializes in the study and treatment of neoplastic disease, particularly cancer.

oncology /ongkol'eje/ [Gk *onkos* swelling, *logos* science], 1. the branch of medicine concerned with the study of tumors. 2. the study of cancerous malignancies.

Oncology Nursing Society (ONS), an organization of nurses interested or specializing in nursing of the patient with cancer.

oncotic /ongkot'ik/, pertaining to or resulting from the presence of a tumor.

oncotic pressure, the osmotic pressure of a colloid in solution, as when there is a higher concentration of protein in the plasma on one side of a cell membrane than in the neighboring interstitial fluid.

oncotic pressure gradient, the pressure difference between the osmotic pressure of blood and that of tissue fluid or lymph. It is an important force in maintaining balance between blood and surrounding tissues.

oncovirus /ong'kovi'res/ [Gk *onkos* + L *virus* poison], a member of a family of viruses associated with leukemia and sarcoma in animals and, possibly, in humans.

Ondine's curse /ondenz'/ [L *Undine* mythic water nymph; ME *curs* invocation], apnea caused by loss of automatic control of respiration. A defect in the central chemoreceptor responsiveness to carbon dioxide leaves the patient with hypercapnia and hypoxemia, although fully able to breathe voluntarily.

one-and-a-half spica cast, an orthopedic cast used for immobilizing the trunk of the body cranially to the nipple line, one leg caudally as far as the toes, and the other leg caudally as far as the knee.

one-child sterility. See **acquired sterility.**

one-to-one care, a method of organizing nursing services in an inpatient care unit by which one registered nurse assumes responsibility for all nursing care provided one patient for the duration of one shift.

one-to-one relationship, a mutually defined, collaborative goal-directed patient-therapist relationship for the purpose of psychotherapy.

onlay [AS *ana* up, *licagan* to lie], 1. a cast type of metal restoration retained by friction and mechanical forces in a prepared tooth for restoring one or more cusps and adjoining occlusal surfaces of a tooth. 2. an occlusal set portion of a removable partial denture, extended to cover the occlusal surface of a tooth.

onlay graft, a bone graft in which the transplanted tissue is laid directly onto the surface of the recipient bone.

ONS, abbreviation for **Oncology Nursing Society.**

onset of action, the time required after administration of a drug for a response to be observed.

onset of puberty [L *pubertas*], a stage of development when genitalia reach maturity and secondary sex characteristics appear. The onset normally occurs in females between the ages of 11 and 13 with the development of breasts and during the phase of menarche. In males, puberty usually occurs between the ages of 12 and 14 and is characterized by the ejaculation of sperm.

ontogenesis. See **ontogeny.**

ontogenetic /on′tōjənet′ik/, **1.** of, relating to, or acquired during ontogeny. **2.** an association based on visible morphologic characteristics and not necessarily indicative of a natural evolutionary relationship.

ontogeny /ontoj′ene/ [Gk *ontos* being, *genein* to produce], the life history of one organism from a single-celled ovum to the time of birth, including all phases of differentiation and growth.

onychia /onik′e.e/ [Gk *onyx* nail], inflammation of the nail bed.

onychodystrophy [Gk, *onyx,* nail; *dys,* bad; *trophe,* nourishment], a condition of malformed or discolored finger or toe nails.

onychogryphosis /on′ikogrifo′sis/ [Gk *onyn* + *gryphen* to curve, *osis* condition], thickened, curved, clawlike overgrowth of fingernails or toenails.

onycholysis /on′ikol′isis/ [Gk *onyx* + *lysein* to loosen], separation of a nail from its bed, beginning at the free margin, associated with psoriasis, dermatitis of the hand, fungal infection, *Pseudomonas* infection, and many other conditions.

onychomycosis /on′ikomiko′sis/ [Gk *onyx* + *mykes* fungus, *osis* condition], any fungal infection of the nails.

onychosis [Gk *onyx* nail, *osis* condition], a condition of atrophy or dystrophy of the nails, usually caused by a dermatosis such as a fungal infection.

onychotomy, a surgical incision into a nail bed.

oob, abbreviation for *out of bed.*

oobe, abbreviation for *out of body experience.*

ooblast /o′eblast/ [Gk *oon* egg, *blastos* germ], the female germ cell from which the mature ovum is developed.

oocenter See **ovocenter.**

oocyesis /o esi e sis/ [Gk *oon* + *kyesis* pregnancy], an ectopic ovarian pregnancy.

oocyst /o′esist/ [Gk *oon* + *kyesis* bag], a stage in the development of any sporozoan in which after fertilization a zygote is produced that develops about itself an enclosing cyst wall.

oocyte /o′esit/ [Gk *oon* + *kytos* cell], a primordial or incompletely developed ovum.

oocytin /o′esi′tin/, the substance in a spermatozoon that stimulates the formation of the fertilization membrane after penetration of an ovum.

oogamy /o.og′eme/ [Gk *oon* + *gamos* marriage], **1.** sexual reproduction by the fertilization of a large, nonmotile female gamete by a smaller, actively motile male gamete, such as occurs in certain algae and the malarial parasite *Plasmodium.* **2.** heterogamy. **–oogamous,** *adj.*

oogenesis /o′ejen′esis/ [Gk *oon* + *genesis* origin], the process of the growth and maturation of the female gametes, or ova. **–oogenetic,** *adj.*

oogonium /o′ego′ne.em/, *pl.* **oogonia** [Gk *oon* + *gonos* offspring], the precursor cell from which an oocyte develops in the fetus during intrauterine life.

ookinesis /o ekinet′/ [Gk oon + *kinesis* movement], the mitotic phenomena occurring in the nucleus of the egg cell during maturation and fertilization. **–ookinetic,** *adj.*

ookinete /o ekinet′/ [Gk *ook* + *kinen* to move], the motile elongated zygote that is formed by the fertilization of the macrogamete during the sexual reproductive phase of the life cycle of a sporozoan, specifically the malarial parasite *Plasmodium.*

oolemma. See **zona pellucida.**

oophoralgia /ō′əfôral′jə/ [Gk *oophoron* ovary, *algos* pain], pain in an ovary.

oophorectomy /o′eferek′teme/ [Gk *oophoron* ovary, *ektome* excision], the surgical removal of one or both ovaries, performed to remove a cyst or tumor, excise an abscess, treat endometriosis, or, in breast cancer, remove the source of estrogen. In premenopausal women one ovary or a portion of one ovary may be left intact unless a malignancy is present. The operation often accompanies a hysterectomy.

oophoritis /o′eferi′tis/, an inflammatory condition of one or both ovaries, usually occurring with salpingitis.

oophorosalpingectomy /ō′əfôr′əsal′pinjek′təme/ [Gk *oophoron* + *salpinx* tube, *ektome* excision], the surgical removal of one or both ovaries and the corresponding oviducts, performed to remove a cyst or tumor, excise an abscess, or treat the condition of endometriosis. In a bilateral procedure the patient becomes sterile and menopause is induced.

oophorosalpingitis /ō′əfôr′əsal′pinjī′tis/, an inflammation involving both the ovary and the fallopian tube.

ooplasm /o′eplaz′em/ [Gk *oon* + *plasma* something formed], the cytoplasm of the egg, or ovum, including the yolk in lower animals.

oosperm /o′esprum/ [Gk *oon* + *sperma* seed], a fertilized ovum; the cell resulting from the union of the pronuclei of the spermatoon and the ovum after fertilization; a zygote.

ootid /ō′ətid/ [Gk *ootidion* small egg], the mature ovum after penetration by the spermatozoon and completion of the second meiotic division but before the fusion of the pronuclei to form the zygote.

OP, 1. abbreviation for *operative procedure.* **2.** abbreviation for **outpatient.**

O

opacity [L opacitus shadiness], pertaining to an opaque quality of a substance or object, such as cataract opacity.

opaque [L opacus obscure], **1.** of or pertaining to a substance or surface that neither transmits nor allows the passage of light. **2.** neither transparent nor translucent.

OPD, abbreviation for *Outpatient Department.*

open amputation [AS *offan* open; L *amputare* to cut away], a kind of amputation in which a straight, guillotine cut is made without skin flaps. Open amputation is performed if an infection is probable or developing or has been recurrent.

open-angle glaucoma. See **glaucoma.**

open-bite, an abnormal dental condition in which the anterior teeth do not occlude in any mandibular position.

open charting, a system of medical record keeping in which the patient has access to his chart.

open-circuit breathing system, a type of breathing system used in cardiopulmonary therapy in which rebreathing does not occur. Gas is inspired through a breathing branch that is connected to a gas source or open to the ambient atmosphere and then expired into a reservoir or vented back into the atmosphere.

open dislocation, a dislocation in which the skin is broken, formerly called a **compound dislocation.**

open drainage. See **drainage.**

open-drop anesthesia, the oldest and simplest anesthetic technique, although it is not currently used in developed countries. A volatile liquid anesthetic agent is dripped, one drop at time, onto a porous cloth or mask held over the patient's face.

open fracture. See **compound fracture.**

open fracture grading system, a system of five categories of open fractures, ranging from a less than 1 cm clean wound that communicates to the fracture site to an open fracture requiring repair of arteries.

opening abductory wedge osteotomy (OAWO), a procedure for treating a bunion deformity. It involves the use of a bone graft to open the wedge and bring the first metatarsal closer to the second.

opening pressure, the amount of pressure measured in a manometer following insertion of a spinal needle into the subarachnoid space.

opening wedge osteotomy, a bunion deformity treatment with a proximal cut in the metatarsal and reduction of the deformity. It is performed with or without tendon transfers.

open operation, a surgical procedure that provides a full view of the structures or organs involved through membranous or cutaneous incisions.

open pneumothorax [AS *open;* Gk *pneuma* air, *thorax* chest], the presence of air or gas in the chest as a result of an open wound in the chest wall.

open reduction [AS *open;* L *reducere* to lead back], a surgical procedure for reducing a fracture or dislocation by exposing the skeletal parts involved.

open system, a system that interacts with our environment.

open-wedge osteotomy, a straight cut made across a bone, creating angulation, leaving an open wedge-shaped gap.

open wound [AS *open, wund*], a wound that disrupts the integrity of the skin.

operable /op′ərəbəl/ [L *operari* to work], susceptible to surgical intervention, as a disease or injury may be.

operant /op′ərənt/ [L *operari* to work], any act or response occurring without an identifiable stimulus.

operant conditioning, a form of learning used in behavior therapy in which the person undergoing therapy is rewarded for the correct response and punished for the incorrect response.

operant level, the frequency or form of a performance under baseline conditions before any systematic conditioning procedures are introduced.

operating microscope [L *operari* + Gk *mikros* small, *skopein* to look], a binocular microscope used in delicate surgery, especially surgery of the eye or ear. The operating microscope that attaches to a surgeon's head has interchangeable oculars for different magnifications.

operating room (OR), 1. a room in a health care facility in which surgical procedures requiring anesthesia are performed. **2.** *informal;* a suite of rooms or an area in a health care facility in which patients are prepared for surgery, undergo surgical procedures, and recover from the anesthetic procedures required for the surgery.

operation, any surgical procedure, such as appendectomy or a hysterectomy.

operationalization of behavior, (in psychology) the stating of a patient's complaints or problems in specific, observable behavioral terms.

operative cholangiography [L *operari* + Gk *chole* bile, *aggeion* vessel, *graphein* to record], (in diagnostic radiology) a procedure for outlining the major bile ducts. It is performed during surgery by injecting a radiopaque contrast material directly into these ducts.

operative dental surgeon. See **dental surgeon.**

operator gene [L *operari* + Gk *genein* to produce], (in molecular genetics) a genetic unit that regulates the transcription of structural genes in its operon.

operculum /opur'kyoolem/, *pl.* **opercula, operculums** [L , a lid], a lid or covering, such as the mucous plug that blocks the cervix of the gravid uterus. –**opercular,** *adj.*

operon /op'eron/ [L *operari* to work], (in molecular biology) a segment of **DNA** consisting of an operator gene and one or more structural genes with related functions controlled by the operator gene in conjunction with a regulator gene.

ophth, abbreviation for **ophthalmology.**

ophthalmia /ofthal'me.e/ [Gk *ophthalmos* eye], severe inflammation of the conjunctiva or of the deeper parts of the eye. Some kinds of ophthalmia are **ophthalmia neonatorum, sympathetic ophthalmia,** and **trachoma.** –**ophthalmic,** *adj.*

ophthalmia neonatorum /ne'onetor'em/, a purulent conjunctivitis and keratitis of the newborn resulting from exposure of the eyes to chemical, chlamydial, bacterial, or viral agents. Chemical conjunctivitis usually occurs as a result of the instillation of silver nitrate in the eyes of a newborn to prevent a gonococcal infection.

ophthalmic administration of medication /ofthal'mik/, the administration of a drug by instillation of a cream or ointment or by drops of a liquid preparation in the conjunctival sac. The medication is placed in the sac as the patient is instructed to look away from the point of instillation. The dispenser is not allowed to touch the eye, and the medication is not placed directly on the cornea.

ophthalmic herpes zoster. See **herpes zoster ophthalmicus.**

ophthalmic medical technician and technologist, allied health professionals who assist ophthalmologists by collecting data and administering treatment ordered by the ophthalmologist. Ophthalmic medical technologists perform all duties performed by technicians but are expected to do so at a higher level of expertise.

ophthalmic nerve [Gk *ophthalmos* eye; L *nervus* nerve], the first division of the trigeminal nerve (CN V), supplying the eyeball through the nasociliary branch. Branches also innervate the forehead, scalp, lacrimal gland, and dura mater.

ophthalmitis /of'thalmī'tis/, an inflammation of the eye.

ophthalmodynamometer /ofthal'mōdin'əmom'ətər/, an instrument for measuring pressure on the sclera while the fundus is studied with an ophthalmoscope. It may be used to measure blood pressures in the ophthalmic artery.

ophthalmodynia /ofthal'mōdin'ē·ə/ [Gk *ophthalmos* eye; *odyne* pain], pain in the eye.

ophthalmologist /of'thalmol'ejist/, a physician who specializes in ophthalmology.

ophthalmology /of'thalmol'eje/ [Gk *ophthalmos* + *logos* science], the branch of medicine concerned with the study of the physiology, anatomy, and pathology of the eye and the diagnosis and treatment of disorders of the eye. –**ophthalmologic, ophthalmological,** *adj.*

ophthalmoplasty /ofthal'mōplas'tē/ [Gk *ophthalmos* + *plassein* to mold], plastic surgery of the eye or of the area around the eye.

ophthalmoplegia /ofthal'meple'je.e/ [Gk *ophthalmos* + *plege* stroke], an abnormal condition characterized by paralysis of the motor nerves of the eye. Bilateral ophthalmoplegia of rapid onset is associated with acute myasthenia gravis and acute inflammatory cranial polyneuropathy. Ophthalmoplegia is also associated with ocular dystrophy.

ophthalmoscope /of'thalmol'eskop/ Gk *ophthalmos* + *skopein* to look], a device for examining the interior of the eye. It includes a light, a mirror with a single hole through which the examiner may look, and a dial holding several lenses of varying strengths.

ophthalmoscopy /of'thalmos'kepe/, the technique of using an ophthalmoscope to examine the eye.

ophthalmospasm, a sudden involuntary contraction of the eyeball.

opiate /ō'pē·it/ [Gk *opion* poppy sap], **1.** a narcotic drug that contains opium, derivatives of opium, or any of several semisynthetic or synthetic drugs with opiumlike activity. **2.** *informal;* any soporific or narcotic drug. **3.** of or pertaining to a substance that causes sleep or relief of pain.

opiate poisoning, toxic effects of a potent narcotic, including depression of the brain centers, causing unconsciousness. Acute intoxication is characterized by euphoria, flushing, and itching, followed by reduced rate of respiration, hypotension, lowered body temperature, and abnormally slow heart beat. Withdrawal is marked by effects generally the opposite of opiate poisoning, depending upon the size of the dose and the length of the period of dependence.

opiate receptor, any of a group of cells in the brain that bind to opiate drugs, such as morphine. Some along the aqueduct of Sylvius and the center median have been identified as receptors associated with response to pain; others have been found in the striatum.

opinion [L *opinari* to suppose], **1.** (in law) a statement by the court, usually in writing, of the reasoning behind its decision or judgment in a particular case. **2.** a statement prepared for a client by an attorney that represents the attorney's understanding of the law as it pertains to a legal question posed by the client.

opioid /o'pē·oid/, pertaining to natural and synthetic chemicals that have opium-like effects although they are not derived from opium. Examples include endorphins or enkephalins produced by body tissues or synthetic methadone.

opisthorchiasis /o'posthorki'esis/ [Gk *opisthen* behind, *orchis* testicle, *osis* condition], infection with one of the species of *Opisthorchis* liver flukes commonly found in the Philippines, India, Thailand, and Laos.

Opisthorchis sinensis. See ***Clonorchis sinensis.***

opisthotonos /o'pisthot'enes/ [Gk *opisthios* posterior, *tonos straining*], a prolonged severe spasm of the muscles causing the back to arch acutely, the head to bend back on the neck, the heels to bend back on the legs, and the arms and hands to flex rigidly at the joints.

opium [Gk *opion* poppy sap], a milky exudate from the unripe capsules of *Papaver somniferum* and *Papaver album* yielding 9.5% or more of anhydrous morphine. It is a narcotic analgesic, a hypnotic, and an astringent. Opium contains several alkaloids, including codeine, morphine, and papaverine.

opium alkaloid, one of several alkaloids isolated from the milky exudate of the unripe seed pods of *Papaver somniferum,* a species of poppy indigenous to the Near East. Three of the alkaloids, codeine, papaverine, and morphine, are used clinically for the relief of pain. Morphine is the standard against which the analgesic effect of newer drugs for relief of pain is measured. The opium alkaloids have several other effects on the body: coughing is suppressed; the electric activity pattern of the brain resembles that of sleep; the pupils constrict; respiration is depressed; the secretory activity and motility of the GI tract are diminished; and biliary and pancreatic secretions are reduced.

opium tincture, an analgesic and antidiarrheal prescribed in the treatment of intestinal hyperactivity, cramping, and diarrhea.

Oppenheim reflex /op'enhim/ [Herman Oppenheim, German neurologist, b.

1858], a variation of Babinski's reflex, elicited by firmly stroking downward on the anterior and medial surfaces of the tibia, characterized by extension of the great toe and fanning of other toes. It is a sign of pyramidal tract disease.

opportunistic infection [L *opportunus* convenient, *icus* form], **1.** an infection caused by normally nonpathogenic organisms in a host whose resistance has been decreased by such disorders as diabetes mellitus, AIDS, or cancer or by a surgical procedure. Persons with HIV are particularly susceptible to such infections. **2.** an unusual infection with a common pathogen, such as cellulitis, meningitis, or otitis media.

opposition [L *opponere* to oppose], the relation between the thumb and the other digits of the hand for the purpose of grasping objects between the thumb and fingers.

opscan, abbreviation for *optical scanning.*

opsin, a protein that combines with retinal to form rhodopsin, or visual purple, in the rod photoreceptor cells of the retina.

opsonin /op'senin/ [Gk *opsonein* to supply food], an antibody or complement split product that, on attaching to foreign materials, microorganism, or other antigen, enhances phagocytosis of that substance by leukocytes and other macrophages. **–opsonize,** *v.*

opsonization /op'seniza'shen/ [Gk *opsonein* + *izein* to cause], the process by which opsonins render bacteria more susceptible to phagocytosis by leukocytes.

optic [Gk *optikos* sight], of or pertaining to the eyes or to sight. Also **optical.**

optical illusion [Gk *optikos;* L *illudere* to mock], a false visual image derived from a misinterpretation of sensory stimuli caused by either physical or psychologic factors or both. A common optical illusion is the appearance of railroad tracks to merge in the distance.

optical righting reflex [Gk *optikos;* AS *riht;* L *reflectere* to bend back], a reflex that restores normal posture and head position with the help of visual clues.

optic angle. See **visual angle.**

optic atrophy /op'tik/, wasting of the optic disc resulting from degeneration of fibers of the optic nerve and optic tract. Optic atrophy may be caused by a cogential defect, inflammation, occlusion of the central retinal artery or internal carotid artery, alcohol, arsenic, lead, tobacco, or other toxic substances. Degeneration of the disc may accompany arteriosclerosis, diabetes, glaucoma, hydrocephalus, pernicious anemia, and various neurologic disorders.

optic chiasm [Gk *optikos; chiasma* crossed

lines], a place near the thalamus and hypothalamus where portions of each optic nerve cross over.

optic coupling, a method of attaching the crystal window of a scintillator to the window of a photomultiplier tube so there is a minimum loss of light transmitted from the scintillator to the interior of the photomultiplier tube.

optic cup, a two-layered embryonic cavity that develops in early pregnancy. The cells of the optic cup differentiate to form the retina that first develops its layers of rod and cones in the central portion of the cup.

optic density, a number describing the blackening of an x-ray film in any specified location.

optic disc, the small blind spot on the surface of the retina, located about 3 mm to the nasal side of the macula. It is the only part of the retina that is insensitive to light.

optic foramen [Gk *optikos; foramen* hole], an aperture in the root of the lesser wing of the sphenoid bone transmitting the optic nerve.

optic glioma, a tumor composed of glial cells. It develops slowly on the optic nerve or in the optic chiasm, causing loss of vision , and is often accompanied by secondary strabismus, exophthalmos, and ocular paralysis.

optician [Gk *optikos* sight], a person who grinds and fits eyeglasses and contact lenses by prescription. To become an optician, a person must graduate from high school and complete a 4- or 5-year apprenticeship.

optic laser. See **laser.**

optic maser. See **laser.**

optic nerve, either of a pair of cranial nerves consisting mainly of coarse, myelinated fibers that arise in the retinal ganglionic layer, traverse the thalamus, and connect with the visual cortex. At the optic chiasm the fibers from the inner or nasal half of the retina cross to the optic tract of the opposite side. The remaining fibers from the temporal, or outer, half of each retina are uncrossed and pass to the visual cortex on the same side.

optic neuritis, inflammation, degeneration, or demyelinization of an optic nerve caused by a wide variety of diseases. Loss of vision is the cardinal symptom.

optic neuropathy, a disease, generally noninflammatory, of the vision, characterized by dysfunction or destruction of the optic nerve tissues. Causes may include an interruption in the blood supply, compression by a tumor or aneurysm, a nutritional deficiency, or toxic effects of a chemical.

The disorder, which can lead to blindness, usually affects only one eye.

opticokinetic. See **optokinetic.**

optic papilla. See **papilla.**

optic radiation, a system of fibers from the lateral geniculate body of the thalamus that pass through the sublenticular portion of the internal capsule to the striate area.

optic righting, one of the five basic neuromuscular reactions that enable a person to change body positions. It involves a reflex that automatically orients the head to a new optical or visual fixation point, depending on the body position change.

optics [Gk *optikos* sight], **1.** (in physics) a field of study that deals with the electromagnetic radiation of wavelengths shorter than radio waves but longer than x-rays. **2.** (in physiology) a field of study that deals with vision and the process by which the functions of the eye and the brain are integrated in the perception of shape, patterns, movements, spatial relationships, and color.

optic stalk, one of a pair of slender embryonic structures that become the optic nerve.

optic system assessment, an evaluation of the patient's eyes, vision, and current and past disorders or injuries that may be responsible for abnormalities in the individual's optic system.

optic thermometer, a temperature-measuring device in which the properties of transmission and reflection of visible light are temperature dependent, and whose detection can be related to tissue temperature.

optic tract, a flat band of nerve fibers running backward and laterally around each cerebral peduncle from the optic chiasma to the lateral geniculate body.

optokinetic /op′tōkinet′ik/, pertaining to movement of the eyeballs in response to the movement of objects across the visual field as in optokinetic nystagmus.

optometrist /optom′etrist/ [Gk *optikos* sight, *metron* measure], a person who practices optometry. An optometrist is awarded the degree of Doctor of Optometry (OD) after completion of at least 2 years of college, followed by 4 years in an approved college of optometry. A state examination and license are also required.

optometry /optom′etre/ [Gk *optios* sight, *metron* measure], the practice of testing the eyes for visual acuity, prescribing corrective lenses, and recommending eye exercises.

OPV, abbreviation for **oral poliovirus vaccine.**

OR, abbreviation for **operating room.**

oral [L *oralis* mouth], of or pertaining to the mouth.

oral administration of medication, the administration of a tablet, a capsule, an elixir, or solution or other liquid form of medication by mouth. Kinds of oral administration of medication are **buccal administration of medication** and **sublingual administration of medication.**

oral airway, a curved tubular device of rubber, plastic, or metal placed in the oropharynx during general anesthesia to maintain free passage of air and keep the tongue from falling back and obstructing the trachea.

oral and maxillofacial surgeon. See **dental surgeon.**

oral cancer, a malignant neoplasm on the lip or in the mouth, occurring at an average age of 60 with a frequency eight times higher in men than in women. Predisposing factors in the cause of the disease are alcoholism, heavy use of tobacco, poor oral hygiene, ill-fitting dentures, syphilis, Plummer-Vinson syndrome, betel nut chewing, and, in lip cancer, overexposure to sun and wind. Premalignant leukoplakia or erythroplasia or a painless nonhealing ulcer may be the first sign of oral cancer; localized pain usually appears later, but lymph nodes may be involved early in the course. Almost all oral tumors are epidermoid carcinomas; adenocarcinomas occur occasionally, whereas sarcomas and metastatic lesions from other sites are rare.

oral cavity, the cavity of the mouth, including the tongue and teeth.

oral character, (in psychoanalysis) a kind of personality exhibiting patterns of behavior originating in the oral phase of infancy, characterized by optimism, self-confidence, and carefree generosity reflecting the pleasurable aspects of the stage, or pessimism, futility, anxiety, and sadism manifestations of frustrations or conflicts occurring during the period.

oral contraceptive, oral hormone medication for contraception. The two major hormones used are progestogen and a combination of progestogen and estrogen. The hormones act by inhibiting the productivity of gonadotropin-releasing hormone by the hypothalamus, and therefore the pituitary does not secrete gonadotropins to stimulate ovulation. This results in the endometrium of the uterus being thin and the cervical mucus being thick, thus preventing the penetration of sperm.

oral dosage, pertaining to the administration of a medicine by mouth.

oral eroticism, (in psychoanalysis) libidinal fixation at or regression to the oral stage of psychosexual development, often reflected in such personality traits as passivity, insecurity, and oversensitivity.

oral examination, a critical inspection and investigation of the cavity of the mouth for diagnostic purposes.

oral hairy leukoplakia. See **hairy leukoplakia.**

oral herpes. See **herpes simplex.**

oral hygiene, the condition or practice of maintaining the tissues and structures of the mouth. Oral hygiene includes brushing the teeth to remove food particles, bacteria, and plaque; massaging the gums with a toothbrush, dental floss, or water irrigator to stimulate circulation and remove foreign matter; and cleansing of dentures and ensuring their proper fit to prevent irritation.

oral mucous membrane, altered, a NANDA-accepted nursing diagnosis of disruptions in the tissue layers of the oral cavity. Defining characteristics include oral pain or discomfort, coated tongue, xerostomia (dry mouth), stomatitis, oral lesions or ulcers, lack of or decreased salivation, leukoplakia, edema, hyperemia, oral plaque, desquamation, vesicles, hemorrhagic gingivitis, carious teeth, and halitosis.

oral pathology. See **dental pathology.**

oral poliovirus vaccine (OPV), an attenuated preparation of live poliovirus that confers immunity to poliomyelitis.

oral prophylaxis, the science and practice of preventing the onset of diseases of the teeth and adjoining mouth tissues.

oral rehydration solutions (ORS), solutions of electrolytes and glucose used in oral rehydration therapy. The recommended electrolytes include NaCl, KCl, and trisodium citrate.

oral rehydration therapy (ORT), the adjustment of water, glucose, and electrolyte balance in a dehydrated patient by giving fluids with measured amounts of essential ingredients by mouth.

oral sadism, (in psychoanalysis) a sadistic form of oral eroticism, manifested by such behavior as biting, chewing, and other aggressive impulses associated with eating habits.

oral stage, (in psychoanalysis) the initial stage of psychosexual development, occurring in the first 12 to 18 months of life when the feeding experience and other oral activities are the predominant source of pleasurable stimulation.

oral surgeon. See **dental surgeon.**

oral surgery [L *oralis* pertaining to the mouth; Gk *cheirourgos* surgeon], a branch of surgery that is concerned primarily with operations upon the jaws and surrounding soft tissues.

oral temperature, the mean body temperature of a normal person as recorded by a clinical thermometer placed in the mouth. It is usually around 99° F or 37° C, but may vary within a fraction of a degree depending upon the individual and such factors as time of day, sleep or exercise, and whether measured before or after a meal.

orb [L *orbis* circle], describing something spherical or globelike.

orbicular /ôrbik′yələr/ [L *orbiculus* little disk], pertaining to something round.

orbicular bone, a knob on the end of the long process of the incus that articulates with the stapes.

orbicularis ciliaris /orbik′yoolar′is/ [L *orbiculus* little circle; *cilium* eyelash], one of the two zones of the ciliary body of the eye, extending from the ora serrata of the retina to the ciliary processes at the margin of the iris.

orbicularis oculi, the muscular body of the eyelid comprising the palpebra, orbita, and lacrimal muscles. The palpebral muscle functions to close it more energetically, such as in winking.

orbicularis oris, the muscle surrounding the mouth, consisting partly of fibers derived from other facial muscles, such as the buccinator, that are inserted into the lips and partly of fibers proper to the lips. It serves to close and purse the lips.

orbicularis palpebrarum. See **orbicularis oculi.**

orbicularis pupillary reflex, a normal phenomenon elicited by forceful closure of the eyelids or attempting to close them while they are held apart, resulting first in constriction and then dilatation of the pupil.

orbit /ôr′bit/ [L *orbita* wheel rut], one of a pair of bony conical cavities in the skull that accommodate the eyeballs and associated structures, such as the eye muscles, the nerves, and the blood vessels. **–orbital,** *adj.*

orbital aperture, an opening in the cranium to the orbit of the eye.

orbital fat, a semifluid cushion of fat that lines the bony orbit supporting the eye. Traumatic loss of the fat causes a sunken appearance of the eye.

orbital fissure, the space between the floor and lateral wall of the orbit, serving as a conduit for nerves and blood vessels.

orbital hypertelorism. See **ocular hypertelorism.**

orbital hypotelorism. See **ocular hypotelorism.**

orbital pseudotumor, a specific inflammatory reaction of the orbital tissues of the eye, characterized by exophthalmos and edematous congestion of the eyelids.

orbitomeatal line /ôr′bitō·mē·ā′təl/ [L *orbita* wheel rut, *meatus* passage], a positioning line used in radiography that passes through the outer canthus of the eye and the center of the external auditory meatus.

orcheoplasty. See **orchioplasty.**

orchidectomy /ôr′kidek′təmē/ [Gk *orchis* testis, *ektome* excision], a surgical procedure to remove one or both testes. It may be indicated for serious disease or injury to the testis or to control cancer of the prostate by removing a source of androgenic hormones.

orchietomy. See **orchidectomy.**

orchiopexy /ôr′kē·ōpek′sē/ [Gk *orchis* + *pexis* fixation], an operation to mobilize an undescended testis, bring it into the scrotum, and attach it so that it will not retract.

orchioplasty, a surgical procedure involving a testis.

orchis. See **testis.**

orchitis /ôrkī′tis/ [Gk *orchis* + *itis* inflammation], inflammation of one or both of the testes, characterized by swelling and pain, often caused by mumps, syphilis, or tuberculosis, **–orchitic,** *adj.*

orciprenaline sulfate. See **metaproterenol sulfate.**

ordered pairs [L *ordo* a series; *par* equal], pertaining to graph coordinates in which the first number of the pair represents a distance along the x (horizontal) axis and the second number is plotted along the y (vertical) axis.

order of procedure, the sequence in which the required steps are taken to complete an operation, such as the preparation and filling of a tooth.

Orem, Dorthea E., author of the Self-Care Nursing Model, a nursing theory introduced in 1959. The theory describes the role of the nurse in giving assistance to a person experiencing inabilities in self-care. The goal of the system is to meet the patient's self-care demands until the family is capable of providing care. The process is divided into three categories: Universal, which consists of self-care to meet physiologic and psychosocial needs; Developmental, the self-care required when one goes through developmental stages; and Health Deviation, the self-care required when one has a deviation from a healthy status.

orexigenic /ôrek′sijen′ik/ [Gk *orexis* longing, *genein* to produce], a substance that increases or stimulates the appetite.

oreximania /ôrek′simā′nē·ə/ [Gk *orexis* + *mania* madness], a condition characterized by a greatly increased appetite and excessive eating resulting from an unrealistic or exaggerated fear of becoming thin.

orexis /orek´sis/ [Gk, longing],   **1.** desire, appetite. **2.** the aspect of the mind involving feeling and striving as contrasted with the intellectual aspect.

orf [AS],   a viral skin disease acquired from sheep, characterized by painless vesicles that may progress to red, weeping nodules and, finally, to crusting and healing.

organ [Gk *organon* instrument],   a structural part of a system of the body that is comprised of tissues and cells that enable it to perform a particular function, such as the liver, spleen, digestive organs, reproductive organs, or organs of special sense.

organ albumin,   albumin characteristic of a particular organ.

organelle /orgenel´/ [Gk *organon* instrument],   **1.** any one of various particles of living substance bound within most cells, such as the mitochondria, the Golgi complex, the endoplastic reticulum, the lysosomes, and the centrioles. **2.** any one of the tiny organs of protozoa associated with locomotion, metabolism, and other processes.

organic /ôrgan´ik/ [Gk *organikos*],   **1.** any chemical compound containing carbon. **2.** of or pertaining to an organ.

organic brain syndrome. See **organic mental disorder.**

organic chemistry,   the branch of chemistry concerned with the composition, properties, and reactions of chemical compounds containing carbon.

organic disease,   any disease associated with detectable or observable changes in one or more body organs.

organic dust,   dried particles of plants, animals, fungi, or bacteria that are fine enough to be windborne.

organic dust toxic syndrome (ODTS),   any nonallergic, noninfectious respiratory illness caused by inhalation of organic dust from moldy silage, hay, or other agricultural products. Symptoms include shaking chills or sweats, cough or shortness of breath, headache, anorexia, and myalgia.

organic evolution,   the theory that all existing forms of animal and plant life have descended with modification from previous, simpler forms or from a single cell; the origin and perpetuation of species.

organic foods,   foods that have been produced and processed without the use of commercial chemicals, such as fertilizers, pesticides, or synthetic substances that enhance color or flavor.

organic mental disorder (OMD),   a class of disorders characterized by progressive deterioration of the mental processes, caused by permanent brain damage or temporary brain dysfunction.

organic motivation. See **physiologic motivation.**

organic psychosis,   a condition characterized by a loss of contact with reality caused by an alteration in brain tissue function.

organic vertigo,   vertigo that is associated with a CNS disorder, such as cerebellar lesions or in tabes dorsalis.

Organisation Mondiale de la Santé. See **World Health Organization.**

organism [Gk *organon* instrument],   an individual living animal or plant able to carry on life functions through mutually dependent organs or organelles.

organization center [Gk *organon* + *izein* to cause],   a focal point within the developing embryo from which the organism grows and differentiates.

organizer [Gk *organon* + *izein* to cause],   (in embryology) any part of the embryo that induces morphologic differentiation in some other part. Kinds of organizers include **nucleolar organizer, primary organizer.**

organ of Corti [Gk *organon;* Alfonso Corti, Italian anatomist, b. 1822],   the true organ of hearing, a spiral structure within the cochlea containing hair cells that are stimulated by sound vibrations into nerve impulses that are transmitted by the auditory nerve to the brain.

organ of Giraldes. See **paradidymis.**

organ of Golgi. See **neurotendinous spindle.**

organogenesis /ôr´gənōjen´əsis/ [Gk *organon* + *genesis* origin],   (in embryology) the formation and differentiation of organs and organ systems during embryonic development. In humans the period extends from approximately the end of the second week through the eighth week of gestation. **–organogenetic,** *adj.*

organoid /ôr´gənoid/ [Gk *organon* + *eidos* form],   **1.** resembling an organ. **2.** any structure that resembles an organ in appearance or function, specifically an abnormal tumor mass.

organoid neoplasm,   a growth that resembles a body organ.

organoid tumor. See **teratoma.**

organomegaly /ôr´gənōmeg´əlē/ [Gk *organon* + *megas* large],   abnormal enlargement of an organ, particularly organs of the abdominal cavity.

organon. See **organ.**

organophosphates   /ôr´gənōfos´fāts/,   a

class of anticholinesterase chemicals used in certain pesticides and medications. They act by causing irreversible inhibition of cholinesterase.

organotherapy [Gk *organon* + *therapeia* treatment], the treatment of disease by administering animal gland substances. –**organotherapeutic,** *adj.*

organotypic growth /ôr′gənotip′ik/ [Gk *organon* + *typos* mark], the controlled reproduction of cells, such as occurs in the normal growth of tissues and organs.

organ specificity, a substance or activity that is identified with a specific organ, such as enzymes that function in particular organ systems.

organum. See **organ.**

orgasm [Gk *orgein* to be lustful], the sexual climax, a series of strong, involuntary contractions of the muscles of the genitalia experienced as exceedingly pleasurable, set off by sexual excitation of critical intensity. –**orgasmic,** *adj.*

orgasmic maturity, the physiologic maturity of the reproductive system that enables the individual to complete the adult sexual response cycle.

orgasmic platform [Gk *orgein;* Fr *plate-forme* a flat form], congestion of the lower vagina during sexual intercourse.

orient [L *oriens* rising sun], **1.** to make someone aware of new surroundings, including people and their roles, the layout of a facility, and its routines, rules, and services. **2.** to help a person become aware of a situation or simply of reality, such as when a patient recovers from anesthesia. –**orientation,** *n.,* **oriented,** *adj.*

oriental sore [L *oriens* + AS *sar* painful], a dermatologic disease caused by the parasite *Leishmania* tropical, transmitted to humans by the bite of the sand fly, the characterized by ulcerative lesions. Oriental sore causes no systemic symptoms, but the sores are susceptible to secondary infections.

orientation [L *orients* + *itio* process], **1.** (in molecular genetics) the insertion of a fragment of genetic material into a vector so that the placement of the fragment is in the same direction as the genetic map of the vector (the n orientation) of in the opposite direction (the u orientation). **2.** (in psychiatry) the awareness of one's physical environment with regard to time, place, and the identity of other persons.

orifice /ôr′ifis/ [L *orificium* opening], the entrance or the outlet of any cavity in the body. –**orificial,** *adj.*

ori gene /ôr′ē/, (in molecular genetics) the site or region in which DNA replication starts.

origin [L *origo* source], the more fixed end of a muscle attachment.

ornithine /ôr′nithēn/, an amino acid, not a constituent of proteins, that is produced as an important intermediate substance in the urea cycle.

ornithine carbamoyltransferase, an enzyme in the blood that increases in patients with liver and other diseases. Its normal concentrations in serum are 8 to 20 mIU/ml.

ornithine cycle. See **urea cycle.**

Ornithodoros /ôr′nithod′ərəs/ [Gk *ornis* bird, *doros* leather bag], a genus of ticks, some species of which are vectors for the spirochetes of relapsing fevers.

ornithosis. See **psittacosis.**

orofacial, pertaining to the mouth and face.

orphan drug [L *orbus* deprived of parents; ME *drogge*], any pharmaceutical product that may be available to physicians and patients in countries other than the United States but that has not been "adopted" by a domestic pharmaceutical manufacturer or distributor.

orphan virus, a virus that has been isolated and identified although it has not been associated with any particular disease.

oropharynx /ôr′ō fer′ingks/ [L *os* mouth; Gk *pharynx* throat], one of the three anatomic divisions of the pharynx. It extends behind the mouth from the soft palate above to the level of the hyoid bone below and contains the palatine tonsils and the lingual tonsils. –**oropharyngeal,** *adj.*

Oroya fever. See **bartonellosis.**

orphenadrine citrate /ôrfen′ədrēn/, a skeletal muscle relaxant with anticholinergic and antihistaminic activity prescribed in the treatment of severe muscle strain.

orphenadrine hydrochloride, an anticholinergic and antihistaminic agent prescribed in the treatment of parkinsonism.

ORS, abbreviation for **oral rehydration solutions.**

ORT, abbreviation for **oral rehydration therapy.**

ortho, abbreviation for *orthopedic.*

orthoboric acid. See **boric acid.**

orthoclase ceramic feldspar /ôr′thəklās/ [Gk *orthos* straight, *klassis* breaking; *keramikos* pottery], a plentiful clay in the solid crust of the earth, used as a filler and to give body to fused dental porcelain.

orthodontia. See **orthodontics.**

orthodontic appliance /ôr′thədon′tik/ [Gk *orthos* + *odous* tooth], any device used to modify tooth position. Kinds of such appliances are fixed, movable, active, retaining, intraoral, and extraoral.

orthodontic band, a thin metal ring, usually made of stainless steel, fitted over a tooth for securing orthodontic attachments to a tooth.

orthodontics /ôr′thədon′tiks/ [Gk orthos + *odous* tooth], the specialty of dentistry concerned with the diagnosis and treatment of malocclusion and irregularities of the teeth.

orthodontist /ôr′thədon′tist/, a practitioner of the branch of dentistry that is concerned with the diagnosis, prevention, and correction of malocclusion of the teeth.

orthodromic conduction /ôr′thedrom′ik/ [Gk *orthos* + *dromos* course; L *conducere* to connect], the conduction of a neural impulse in the normal direction, from a synaptic junction or a receptor forward along an axon to its termination with depolarization.

orthogenesis /ôr′thejen′esis/ [Gk *orthos* + *genesis* origin], the theory that evolution is controlled by intrinsic factors within the organism and progresses according to a predetermined course rather than in several directions as a result of natural selection and other environmental factors. **–orthogenetic,** *adj.*

orthogenic /ôr′thəjen′ik/ [Gk *orthos* + *genein* to produce], **1.** of or pertaining to orthogenesis; orthogenetic. **2.** of or pertaining to the treatment and rehabilitation of children who are mentally or emotionally disturbed.

orthogenic evolution, change within an animal or plant induced solely by an intrinsic factor, independent of any environmental elements.

orthokinetic cuff /ôr′thəkinet′ik/, an elastic covering for a muscle to provide tactile stimulation that will induce contraction and at the same time restrict contraction of an opposing muscle.

orthokinetics [Gk *orthos* straight, *kinesis* movement], **1.** therapy for hypertrophic osteoarthritis in which an effort is made to change muscular action from one group to another set in order to protect a joint. **2.** therapy for spasticity by using an orthotic device to enable contraction of one muscle while inhibiting its antagonist. **3.** the effect of gravity on the brownian movement as manifested by the movement of particles in the same direction in sedimentation.

orthomyxovirus /ôr′thəmik′sōvī′rəs/ [Gk *orthos* + *mykes* fungus; L *virus* poison], a member of a family of viruses that includes several organisms responsible for human influenza infection.

orthopantogram /ôr′thəpan′təgram/ [Gk *orthos* + *pan* all, *gramma* record], an x-ray film showing a panoramic view of the entire dentition, alveolar bone, and other contiguous structures on a single film, taken extraorally.

orthopedic nurse [Gk *orthos* + *pais* child], a nurse whose primary area of interest, competence, and professional practice is in orthopedic nursing.

orthopedic oxford, a hard leather shoe with a leather or rubber sole, sometimes with a steel shank between the floor of the shoe and the sole, and with firmly constructed sides that support the foot in an upright position. The shoe is constructed uniformly so that assistive devices can be added.

orthopedics /ôr′thəpē′diks/ [Gk *orthos* + *pais* child], a branch of medicine that is concerned with the prevention and correction of disorders of the locomotor system of the body, including the skeleton, muscles, joints, and related tissues.

orthopedic surgery, a branch of medicine that is concerned with the treatment of the musculoskeletal system mainly by manipulative and operative methods.

orthopedic traction, a procedure in which a patient is maintained in a device attached by ropes and pulleys to weights that exert a pulling force on an extremity or body part while counteraction is maintained. Traction is applied most often to reduce and immobilize fractures, but it also is used to overcome muscle spasm, to stretch adhesions, to correct certain deformities, and to help release arthritic contractures.

orthopedist, a specialist in orthopedics.

orthopnea /ôrthop′nē·e/ [Gk *orthos* + *pnoia* breath], an abnormal condition in which a person must sit or stand in order to breathe deeply or comfortably. It occurs in many disorders of the cardiac and respiratory systems, such as asthma, pulmonary edema, emphysema, pneumonia, and angina pectoris. **–orthopneic,** *adj.*

orthopneic position /ôr′thopne′ik/ [Gk *orthos* straight; *pnoia* breath; L *positio*], a body position that enables a patient to breathe comfortably. Usually, it is one in which the patient is sitting up and is bent forward, with the arms supported on a table or chair arms.

orthopod. See **orthopedist.**

orthopsychiatry [Gk *orthos* + *psyche* mind, *iatreia* treatment], the branch of psychiatry that specializes in correcting incipient and borderline mental and behavioral disorders, especially in children, and in developing preventive techniques to promote mental health and emotional growth and development.

orthoptic /ôrthop′tik/ [Gk *orthos* + *ops* eye], **1.** of or pertaining to normal binocular vision. **2.** of or pertaining to a procedure or technique for correcting the visual axes of eyes improperly coordinated for binocular vision.

orthoptic examination, an ophthalmoscopic examination of the binocular function of the yes. A stereoscopic instrument presents a slightly different picture to each eye. The examiner notes the degree to which the pictures are combined by the normal process of fusion. If the person has diplopia, separate pictures are seen.

orthoptic training, a type of therapy for correction of squint or other ocular muscle disorders by the use of eye exercises.

orthoptist /ôrthop′tist/ [Gk *orthos* + *ops* eye], a person qualified by postsecondary training and successful completion of an examination by the American Orthoptist Council, who, under the supervision of an ophthalmologist, tests eye muscles and teaches exercise programs designed to correct eye coordination defect.

orthoscopy /ôrthos′kəpē/, the use of an orthoscope for examining the fundus of the eye.

orthosis /ôrthō′sis/ [Gk *orthos* straight], a force system designed to control, correct, or compensate for a bone deformity, deforming forces, or forces absent from the body. Orthosis often involves the use of special braces. **–orthotic** /orthot′ik,/ *adj., n.*

orthostatic [Gk *ortos* + *statikos* standing], pertaining to an erect or standing position.

orthostatic albuminuria. See **orthostatic proteinuria.**

orthostatic hypotension, abnormally low blood pressure occurring when an individual assumes the standing posture.

orthostatic proteinuria, presence of protein in the urine of some people, especially teenagers, who have been standing. It disappears when they recline and is of no pathologic significance.

orthotics /ôrthot′iks/, the design and application of external appliances to support a paralyzed muscle, promote a specific motion, or correct musculoskeletal deformities.

orthotist /ôrt′thətist/ [Gk *orthos* straight], a person who designs, fabricates, and fits braces or other orthopedic appliances prescribed by physicians. A certified orthotist is one who successfully completed the examination of the American Orthotist and Prosthetic Association.

orthotonos /ôrthot′anəs/ [Gk *orthos* + *tonos* tension], a straight, rigid posture of the body caused by a tetanic spasm, usually resulting from strychnine poisoning or tetanus infection. The neck and all other parts of the body are in a position of extension but not as severely as in opisthotonos.

orthovoltage [Gk *orthos* straight; Court Alessandro Volta], the voltage range of 100 to 350 KeV supplied by some x-ray generators used for radiation therapy.

Ortolani sign /ôr′təlä′nē/, an audible click heard in a test for a congenital dislocated hip. It is noted in infancy when the hip goes into the socket.

Ortolani's test [Marius Ortolani, twentieth-century Italian surgeon; L *testum* crucible], a procedure used to evaluate the stability of the hip joints in newborns and infants. The baby is placed on his or her back, the hips and knees are flexed at right angles and abducted until the lateral aspects of the knees are touching the table. Internal and external rotation are attempted, and symmetry of mobility is evaluated. A click or a popping sensation (Ortolani's sign) may be felt if the joint is unstable.

os /os/. See **bone.**

Os, symbol for the element **osmium.**

OS, abbreviation for *oculus sinister,* a Latin phrase meaning "left eye."

Osborne and Cotterill procedure, a surgical method of correcting a chronic dislocated elbow by the use of capsular reefing, the folding in or overlapping soft tissue by surgical suture to make the structure tighter.

osc, abbreviation for **oscillator.**

os calcis. See **calcaneus.**

os capitatum. See **capitate bone.**

oscillation /os′ilā′shən/ [L *oscillare* to swing], **1.** a back-and-forth motion. **2.** vibration or the effects of a mechanical or electrical vibrator.

oscillator (osc) /os′ilā′tər/ [L *oscillare* to swing], an electric or other device that produces oscillations, vibrations, or fluctuations, such as an alternating electric current generator.

oscilloscope /osil′əskōp′/ [L *oscillare* to swing; Gk *skopein* to look], an instrument that displays a visual representation of electric variations on the fluorescent screen of a cathode ray tube. The graphic representation is produced by a beam of electrons on the screen.

os coxae. See **innominate bone.**

os cubiodeum. See **cuboid bone.**

Osgood osteotomy, a surgical procedure for correction of malrotation of a femur.

Osgood-Schlatter disease /oz′gŏŏdshlat′er/ [Robert B. Osgood, American surgeon, b. 1873; Carl Schlatter, Swiss surgeon, b. 1864], inflammation or partial separation of the tibial tubercle caused by chronic irritation, usually as a result of

O

overuse of the quadriceps muscle. The condition is characterized by swelling and tenderness over the tibial tubercle that increase with exercise or any activity that extends the leg.

OSHA, abbreviation for *Occupational Safety and Health Administration.*

os hamatum. See **hamate bone.**

os hyoideum. See **hyoid bone.**

Osler's disease. See **Osler-Weber-Rendu syndrome, polycythemia.**

Osler's nodes /ōs'lərz/ [Sir William Osler, American-British physician, b. 1849], tender, reddish or purplish subcutaneous nodules of the soft tissue on the ends of fingers or toes, seen in subacute bacterial endocarditis and usually lasting only 1 or 2 days.

Osler-Weber-Rendu syndrome /ōslər web'ərandoo/ [Sir William Osler; Frederick P. Weber, British physician, b. 1863; Henri J.L.M. Rendu, French physician, b. 1844], a vascular anomaly, inherited as an autosomal dominant trait, characterized by hemorrhagic telangiectasia of skin and mucosa. Small red-to-violet lesions are found on the lips, the oral and nasal mucosa, the tongue, and the tips of fingers and toes. The thin, dilated vessels may bleed spontaneously or as a result of only minor trauma, and this condition becomes progressively severe.

os lunatum. See **lunate bone.**

osm, **1.** abbreviation for **osmosis.** **2.** abbreviation for *osmotic.*

os magnum. See **capitate bone.**

osmethesia /os'məthē'zhə/ [Gk *osme* smell, *aisthesis* feeling], the ability to perceive and distinguish odors; the sense of smell.

osmium (Os) /oz'mē·əm/ [Gk *osme* smell], a hard, grayish, pungent-smelling metallic element. Its atomic number is 76; its atomic weight is 190.2.

osmoceptors /oz'mōsep'tərz/ [Gk *osme* + L *recipere* to receive], receptors in the hypothalamus that respond to osmotic pressure, thereby regulating production of the antidiuretic hormone.

osmol. See **osmole.**

osmolal gap /ozmō'ləl/, a difference between the observed and calculated osmolalities in serum analysis. The calculated osmolar values include sodium concentration multiplied by 2, plus glucose and blood urea nitrogen.

osmolality /oz'mōlal'itē/, the osmotic pressure of a solution expressed in osmoles or milliosmoles per kilogram of water.

osmolar /osmō·lər/, of or pertaining to the osmotic characteristics of a solution of one or more molecular substances, ionic substances, or both, expressed in osmoles or milliosmoles.

osmolarity /oz'mōler'itē/, the osmotic pressure of a solution expressed in osmoles or milliosmoles per kilogram of the solution.

osmole /os'mōl/ [Gk *osmos* impulse, *osis* condition + mole (molecule)], the quantity of a substance in solution in the form of molecules, ions, or both (usually expressed in grams) that has the same osmotic pressure as one mole of an ideal nonelectrolyte. Also **osmol.** **−osmolal,** *adj.*

osmology /ozmol'əjē/, **1.** the science of the sense of smell and the production and composition of odors. **2.** the branch of science that is concerned with osmosis.

osmometry /ozmom'ətrē/ [Gk *osmos* impulse, *metron* measure], a field of study that deals with the phenomenon of osmosis and the measurement of osmotic forces. **−osmometric,** *adj.*

Osmone-Clarke procedure, a therapy for talipes valgus. It involves soft tissue release of the medial and lateral foot with peroneous brevis tendon transfer.

osmoreceptor /os'mōrisep'tər/ [Gk *osmos* impulse; L *recipere* to receive], **1.** a neuron in the hypothalamus that is sensitive to the fluid concentration in the blood plasma and regulates the secretion of antidiuretic hormone. **2.** a receptor of smell stimuli.

osmoregulation /os'mōreg'yəlā'shən/ [Gk *osmos* + L *regula* rule], the act of influencing or controlling the speed and extent of osmosis.

osmosis (osm) /ozmō'sis,os-/ [Gk *osmos* impulse, *osis* condition], the movement of a pure solvent, such as water, through a semipermeable membrane from a solution that has a lower solute concentration to one that has a higher solute concentration. Movement across the membrane continues until the concentrations of the solutions equalize. **−osmotic,** *adj.*

osmotic diarrhea /ozmot'ik/, a form of diarrhea associated with water retention in the bowel resulting from an accumulation of nonabsorbable water-soluble solutes. An excessive intake of hexitols, sorbitol, and mannitol (used as sugar substitutes) can result in slow absorption and rapid small intestine motility.

osmotic diuresis, diuresis resulting from the presence of certain nonabsorbable substances in tubules of the kidney, such as mannitol, urea, or glucose.

osmotic fragility, a sensitivity to change in osmotic pressure characteristic of red blood cells. Exposed to a hypotonic concentration of sodium in a solution, red cells take in increasing quantities of water, swell until the capacity of the cell membrane is exceeded, and burst. Exposed to a hypertonic concentration of sodium in a solution, red cells give up intracellular fluid, shrink, and break up.

osmotic pressure, **1.** the pressure exerted on a semipermeable membrane separating a solution from a solvent, the membrane being impermeable to the solutes in the solution and permeable only to the solvent. **2.** the pressure exerted on a semipermeable membrane by a solution containing one or more solutes that cannot penetrate the membrane, which is permeable only by the solvent surrounding it.

osmotic transfection, a method of inserting foreign DNA molecules into cells by putting cells into a dilute solution that causes them to rupture. The alien DNA is added to the fluid and is absorbed into the cell nuclei. The cell membranes quickly repair themselves. The foreign DNA can be detected in the cells as a transfection marker.

os naviculare pedis. See **scaphoid bone.**

osphresis /osfrē′sis/ [Gk, smell], olfaction; the sense of smell.

osseous /os′ē-əs/ [L os bone], bony; consisting of or resembling bone.

osseous labyrinth [L os bone; Gk labyrinthos maze], the bony portion of the internal ear, composed of three cavities: the vestibule, the semicircular canals, and the cochlea, transmitting sound vibrations from the middle ear to the acoustic nerve. All three cavities contain perilymph, in which a membranous labyrinth is suspended.

ossicle /os′ikəl/ [L ossiculum little bone], a small bone, such as the malleus, the incus, or the stapes, ossicles of the inner ear. **–ossicular,** adj.

ossiferous /osif′ərəs/ [L os bone, ferre to bear], pertaining to bony tissue or to the formation of bone.

ossification /os′ifika shən/ [L os + facere to make], the development of bone. **Intramembranous ossification** is that preceded by membrane, such as in the process initially forming the roof and the sides of the skull. **Intracartilaginous ossification** is that preceded by rods of cartilage, such as that forming the bones of the limbs. **–ossify,** v.

ossifying fibroma [L os + facere to make], a slow-growing, benign neoplasm of bone, occurring most often in the jaws, especially the mandible.

ostealgia /os′tē-al′jə/ [Gk osteon + algos pain], any pain that is associated with an abnormal condition within a bone, such as osteomyelitis. **–ostealgic,** adj.

osteanagenesis. See **osteoanagenesis.**

osteitis /os′tē-ī′tis/ [Gk osteon + itis inflammation], an inflammation of bone, caused by infection, degeneration, or trauma. Swelling, tenderness, dull aching pain, and redness in the skin over the affected bone are characteristic of the condition. Some kinds of osteitis are **osteitis deformans** and **osteitis fibrosa cystica.**

osteitis fibrosa cystica. An inflammatory condition in which normal bone is replaced by cysts and fibrous tissue.

osteitis fibrosa disseminata. See **Albright's syndrome.**

ostembryon. See **lithopedion.**

ostemia, an abnormal congestion of blood in a bone.

ostempyesis /os′təmpī-ē′sis/, an accumulation of pus within a bone.

osteo /os′tē-o/, **1.** an abbreviation for **osteopath. 2.** abbreviation for **osteopathy.**

osteoanagenesis /os′tē-ō-an′əjen əsis/ [Gk osteon + ana again, genesis origin], the regeneration or formation of bone tissue.

osteoaneurysm /os′tē-ō-an′yəriz′əm/, an aneurysm within a bone.

osteoarthritis /os′tē-ō arthrī′tis/ [Gk osteon + arthron joint, itis inflammation], a form of arthritis in which one or many joints undergo degenerative changes, including subchondral bony sclerosis, loss of articular cartilage, and proliferation of bone and cartilage in the joint, forming osteophytes. Inflammation of the synovial membrane of the joint is common late in the disease. The most common form of arthritis, its causes may include chemical, mechanical, genetic, metabolic, and endocrine factors. Emotional stress often aggravates the condition. The condition usually begins with pain after exercise or use of the joint. Stiffness, tenderness to the touch, crepitus, and enlargement develop, and deformity, subluxation, and synovial effusion may eventually occur.

osteoarthritis deformans endemica. See **Kashin-Bek disease.**

osteoarthropathy /os′tē-o′arthrop′əthē/ [Gk osteon + arthron joint, pathos disease], a disorder affecting bones and joints.

osteoarthrosis /os′tē-ō-ärthrō′sis/, a condition of chronic arthritis, usually mechanical, without inflammation.

osteoarticular /os′tē-ō-ärtik′yələr/, pertaining to or affecting bones and joints.

osteoarticular graft, a transplant of bone tissue that contains an articular surface.

osteoblast /os′tē-əblast′/ [Gk osteon + bastos germ], a cell that originates in the embryonic mesenchyme and, during the early development of the skeleton, differentiates from a fibroblast to function in the formation of bone tissue. **–osteoblastic,** adj.

osteoblastoma /os′tē·oblastō′me/, *pl.* **osteoblastomas, osteoblastomata,** a small, benign, fairly vascular tumor of poorly formed bone and fibrous tissue. The lesion causes pain, erosion, and resorption of native bone.

osteocachexia /os′tē·ōkəkek′sē·ə/, a chronic disease that results in wasting of the bone, usually due to malnutrition.

osteocarcinoma /os′tē·ōkär′sinō′mə/, cancer of the bone.

osteochondral graft /os′tē·ōkon′drəl/, a transplant of tissue composed of both bone and cartilage.

osteochondritis /os′tē·ōkəndrī′tis/, a disease of the epiphyses, or bone-forming centers of the skeleton, beginning with necrosis and fragmentation of the tissue, and followed by repair and regeneration. Types of the disorder include **osteochondritis deformans juvenilis, osteochondritis ischiopubica, osteochondritis juvenilis,** and **osteochondritis necroticans.**

osteochondritis dissecans [Gk *osteon* bone, *chondros* cartilage; L *dissecare* to cut apart], a joint disorder in which a piece of cartilage and neighboring bone tissue become detached from the articular surface.

osteochondrodystrophy. See **Morquio's disease.**

osteochondrofibroma /os′tē·ōkon′drōfī-brō′mə/, a tumor containing tissues of osteoma, chondroma, and fibroma.

osteochondrolysis. See **osteochondrosis dissecans.**

osteochondroma /os′tē·ōkondrō′mə/ [Gk *osteon* + *chondros* cartilage, *oma* tumor], a benign tumor made of bone and cartilage.

osteochondromatosis /os′tē·ōkon′drōmə-tō′sis/, the transformation of synovial villi into bone and cartilage masses, causing loose bodies in the joints. It usually develops in joints affected by injury or degenerative diseases.

osteochondropathy /os′tē·ōkəndrop′əthē/, a condition affecting both bone and cartilage and characterized by abnormal enchondral ossification.

osteochondrosarcoma /os′tē·ōkon′drō-särkō′mə/, a condition of sarcomatous tumors in the bone and cartilage.

osteochondrosis /os′ti·ōkondrō′sis/ [Gk *osteon* + *chondros* cartilage, *osis* condition], a disease affecting the ossification centers of bone in children, initially characterized by degeneration and necrosis, followed by regeneration and recalcification. Kinds of osteochondrosis include **Legg-Calve-Perthes disease, Osgood-Schlatter disease,** and **Scheuermann's disease.**

osteochondrosis dissecans, the formation of a separate center of bone and cartilage on an epiphyseal surface. The stray fragment may remain in place, be absorbed, or break off and become a loose body.

osteoclasia /os′tē·ōkla′zhə/ [Gk *osteon* + *klasis* breaking], **1.** the destruction and absorption of bony tissue by osteoclasts, such as during growth or the healing of fractures. **2.** the degeneration of bone through disease.

osteoclasis /os′tē·ōk′ləsis/ the intentional surgical fracture of a bone to correct a deformity. **—osteoclastic,** *adj.*

osteoclast /os′tē·əklast′/ [Gk *esteon* + *klasis* breaking], **1.** a large type of multinucleated bone cell that functions in the development and periods of growth or repair, such as the breakdown and resorption of osseous tissue. During bone healing of fractures, or during certain disease processes, osteoclasts excavate passages through the surrounding tissue by enzymatic action. **2.** a surgical instrument used in the fracturing or refracturing of bones for therapeutic purposes, such as correction of a deformity.

osteoclastic /os′tē·əklas′tik/, **1.** pertaining to or of the nature of osteoclasts. **2.** destructive to bone.

osteoclastoma /os′tē·ōklastō′mə/, *pl.* **osteoclastomas, osteoclastomata** [Gk *osteon* + *klasis* breaking, *oma* tumor], a giant cell tumor of the bone, occurring most frequently at the end of a long bone and appearing as a mass surrounded by a thin shell of new, periosteal bone. The lesion may be benign but is more often malignant. It causes local pain, loss of function, and, in some cases, weakness followed by pathologic fracture.

osteoclasty. See **osteoclasis.**

osteocope /os′tē·əkōp/, a painful syphilitic bone disease.

osteocystoma /os′tē·ōsistō′mə/, a cystic tumor in a bone.

osteocyte /os′tē·əsīt′/ [Gk *osteon* + *kytos* cell], a bone cell; a mature osteoblast that has become embedded in the bone matrix. It occupies a small cavity and sends out protoplasmic projections that anastomose with those of other osteoblasts to form a system of minute canals within the bone matrix. **—osteocytic,** *adj.*

osteodensitometer, an apparatus for measuring the density of bone tissue.

osteodiastasis /os′tē·ōdī·as′təsis/, an abnormal separation of bones.

osteodynia /os′tē·ōdin′ē·ə/, bone pain.

osteodystrophy /os′tē·ōdis′trəfē/ [Gk *osteon* + *dys* bad, *trophe* nourishment], any generalized defect in bone development, usually associated with disturbances in calcium and phosphorus metabolism and renal insufficiency, such as in renal osteodystrophy.

osteoenchondroma /os′tē·ō·en·kəndrō′mə/, a benign bone and cartilage tumor within a bone.

osteofibrochondrosarcoma /os′tē-ōfī′brōkon′drōsärkō′mə/, a malignant tumor containing bone, cartilage, and fibrous tissues.

osteofibroma /os′tē-ōfībrō′mə/ [Gk *osteon* + L *fibra* fiber; Gk *oma* tumor], a tumor composed of both bony and fibrous tissues.

osteogenesis /os′tē-ōjen′əsis/ [Gk *osteon* + *genesis* origin], the origin and development of bone tissue. **−osteogenetic, osteogenic,** *adj.*

osteogenesis imperfecta, a genetic disorder involving defective development of the connective tissue. It is inherited as an autosomal dominant trait and is characterized by abnormally brittle and fragile bones that are easily fractured by the slightest trauma. In its most severe form, the disease may be apparent at birth, when it is known as **osteogenesis imperfecta congenita.** The newborn has multiple fractures that have occurred in utero and is usually severely deformed because of imperfect formation and mineralization of bone. If the disease has a later onset, it is called **osteogenesis imperfecta tarda** and usually runs a milder course. Symptoms generally appear when the child begins to walk, but they become less severe with age. There is a broad expressivity of the disease so that the number and extent of pathologic features may range from minimal to severe involvement.

osteogenic, composed of or originating from any tissue involved in the development, growth, or repair of bone. Also **osteogenous** /os′tē·oj′ənəs/.

osteogenic sarcoma. See **osteosarcoma.**

osteogeny. See **osteogenesis.**

osteohalisteresis /os′tē-ōhal′istərē′sis/, a condition of soft bones caused by a loss or deficiency of mineral elements.

osteoid /os′tē-oid/ [Gk *osteon* + *eidos* form], of, pertaining to, or resembling bone.

osteoid osteoma. See **osteoblastoma.**

osteolipochondroma /os′tē-ōlip′okəndrō′mə/, a cartilage tumor with bone and fat elements.

osteolipoma /os′tē-ōlipō′mə/, a fatty tumor containing bone elements.

osteology /os′tē-ol′əjē/ [Gk, *osteon,* bone; *logos,* science], a branch of medicine concerned with the development and diseases of bone tissue.

osteolysis /os′te·ol′isis/ [Gk *osteon* + *ysis* loosening], the degeneration and disso-

lution of bone, caused by disease, infection, or ischemia. The condition commonly affects the terminal bones of the hands and feet, such as in acroosteolysis. **−osteolytic,** *adj.*

osteoma /os′tē·ō′mə/, *pl.* **osteomas, osteomata,** a tumor of bone tissue.

osteomalacia /os′tē·oməlā′ shə/ [Gk *osteon* + *malakia* softening], an abnormal condition of the lamellar bone, characterized by a loss of calcification of the matrix resulting in softening of the bone, accompanied by weakness, fracture, pain, anorexia, and weight loss. The condition is the result of an inadequate amount of phosphorus and calcium available in the blood for mineralization of the bones and may be caused by a diet lacking these minerals or vitamin D, or by a lack of exposure to sunlight.

osteomesopyknosis /os′tē-ōmez′ōpiknō′sis/, a genetic disorder transmitted as an autosomal trait and characterized by osteosclerosis of the axial spine, the pelvis, and the proximal areas of long bones.

osteomyelitis /os′tēo·omī·əlī′tis/ [Gk *osteon* + *myelos* marrow, *itis* inflammation], local or generalized infection of bone and bone marrow, usually caused by bacteria introduced by trauma or surgery, by direct extension from a nearby infection, or via the bloodstream. Staphylococci are the most common causative agents. The long bones in children and the vertebrae in adults are the commonest sites of infection as a result of hematogenous spread. Persistent, severe, and increasing bone pain, tenderness, guarding on movement, regional muscle spasm, and fever suggest this diagnosis. **−osteomyelitic,** *adj.*

osteomyelodysplasia [Gk *osteon* + *myelos* marrow; *dys, plasis* forming], a loss of bone tissue through absorption of minerals. The condition is usually associated with leukopenia, sometimes with fever, and may result from an excess of parathyroid hormone.

osteon /os′tē·on/ [Gk, bone], the basic structural unit of compact bone, consisting of the haversian canal and its concentric rings of 4 to 20 lamellae.

osteonal bone /os′tē-ō′nəl/, a microscopic description of bone tissue seen in mature adults. It is composed of tiny chalky tubes with an arteriole running down the middle and circular laminations of bone concentric with an artery.

osteonecrosis /os′tē-ōnəkrō′sis/ [Gk *osteon* + *nekros* dead, *osis* condition], the destruction and death of bone tissue, such as from ischemia, infection, malignant neoplastic disease, or trauma. **−osteonecrotic,** *adj.*

O

osteopath (osteo) /os'tē-ōpath/, a physician who specializes in osteopathy.

osteopathic scoliosis. See **congenital scoliosis.**

osteopathology, the study of bone diseases.

osteopathy (osteo) /os'tē-op'əthē/ [Gk *osteon* + *pathos* disease], a therapeutic approach to the practice of medicine that uses all the usual forms of medical therapy and diagnosis, including drugs, surgery, and radiation, but that places greater emphasis on the role of the relationship of the organs and the musculoskeletal system than is done in medicine. Osteopathic physicians recognize and correct structural problems using manipulation. The process is important in both the diagnosis and the treatment of health problems. **—osteopathic,** *adj.*

osteopedion. See **lithopedion.**

osteopenia /ostē-ōpē'nē-ə/ [Gk *osteon* + *penes* poverty], a condition of subnormally mineralized bone, usually the result of a failure of the rate of bone matrix synthesis to compensate for the rate of bone lysis.

osteoperiosteal graft /os'tē-ōper'ē-os'tē-əl/, a bone graft that includes the periosteal membrane covering the bone.

osteopetrosis /os'tē-ōpētrō'sis/ [Gk *osteon* + *petra* stone, *osis* condition], an inherited disorder characterized by a generalized increase in bone density, probably caused by faulty bone resorption resulting from a deficiency of osteoclasts. In its most severe form, there is obliteration of the bone marrow cavity, causing severe anemia, marked deformities of the skull, and compression of the cranial nerves, which may result in deafness and blindness and lead to an early death. **—osteopetrotic,** *adj.*

osteophage. See **osteoclast.**

osteophyte /os'tē-əfīt'/, a bony outgrowth, usually found around the joint area.

osteoplast. See **osteoblast.**

osteoplastica /os'tē-ōplas'tikə/, a form of bone inflammation associated with cystic fibrosis.

osteoplasty /o'stē-əplas'tē/ [Gk *osteon* + *plassein* to form], plastic surgery performed on bone tissue.

osteopoikilosis /os'tē-ōpoi'kilō'sis/ [Gk *osteon* + *poikilos* mottled, *osis* condition], an inherited condition of the bones, characterized by multiple areas of dense calcification throughout the osseous tissue, producing a mottled appearance on x-ray examination. **—osteopoikilotic,** *adj.*

osteoporosis /os'tē-ōpərō'sis/ [Gk *osteon* + *poros* passage, *osis* condition], a disorder characterized by abnormal rarefaction of bone, occurring most frequently in postmenopausal women, in sedentary or immobilized individuals, and in patients on long-term steroid therapy. The disorder may cause pain, especially in the lower back, pathologic fractures, loss of stature, and various deformities. Osteoporosis may be idiopathic or secondary to other disorders, such as thyrotoxicosis or the bone demineralization caused by hyperparathyroidism.

osteoporosis of disuse, a thinning of the bone mass that occurs in sedentary persons or patients confined to bed for a long period.

osteoporotic, pertaining to osteoporosis.

osteopsathyrosis. See **osteogenesis imperfecta.**

osteosarcoma /os'tē-ōsärkō'mə/ [Gk *osteon* + *sarx* flesh, *oma*], a malignant bone tumor composed of anaplastic cells derived from mesenchyme.

osteosclerosis /os'tē-ōsklerō'sis/ [Gk *osteon* + *skleros* hard, *osis* condition], an abnormal increase in the density of bone tissue. The condition is commonly associated with ischemia, chronic infection, and tumor formation, and may be caused by faulty bone resorption as a result of some abnormality involving the osteoclasts. **—osteosclerotic,** *adj.*

osteosclerosis fragilis. See **osteopetrosis.**

osteosclerosis fragilis congenita. See **osteopoikilosis.**

osteosynovitis /os'tē-ōsin'ōvī'tis/, an inflammation of the synovial membrane of a joint and the surrounding bone tissue.

osteosynthesis /os'tē-ōsin'thəsis/, the surgical fixation of a bone using any internal mechanical means. It is usually performed in the treatment of fractures.

osteotabes /os'tē-ōtā'bēz/, a condition usually affecting infants in which bone marrow cells are destroyed and the marrow disappears.

osteotelangiectasia /os'tē-ōtelan'jēkətä'-zhə/, a sarcoma of the bone characterized by dilated capillaries.

osteothrombophlebitis /os'tē-ōthrom'-bōfləbī'tis/, an inflammation through intact bone by progressive thrombophlebitis of small venules.

osteothrombosis /os'tē-ōthrəmbō'sis/, a blockage of the blood vessels in the bone tissue.

osteotome /os'tē-ətōm/ [Gk *osteon* + *temnein* to cut], a surgical instrument for cutting through bone.

osteotomy /os'tē-ot'əmē/ [Gk *osteon* + *temnein* to cut], the sawing or cutting of a bone. Kinds of osteotomy include block osteotomy, in which a section of bone is excised, cuneiform osteotomy to remove a bone wedge, and displacement osteotomy, in which a bone is redesigned surgically to alter the alignment or weight-bearing stress areas.

osteotripsy /os'tē-ōtrip'sē/, a method of treating callosities or any percutaneous reduction of a bony prominence.

ostium. See **orifice.**

ostium primum defect, ostium secundum defect. See **atrial septal defect.**

ostomate /os'təmāt/ [L *ostium* mouth], a patient who has undergone an ostomy.

ostomy /os'təmē/ [L *ostium* mouth], *informal.* a surgical procedure in which an opening is made to allow the passage of urine from the bladder or of intestinal contents from the bowel to an incision or stoma surgically created in the wall of the abdomen. An ostomy procedure may be performed to correct an anatomic defect or to relieve an obstruction in or to permit treatment of a severe infection or injury of the urinary or intestinal tract. Each procedure is named for the anatomic location of the ostomy, such as a colostomy, cecostomy, or cystostomy.

ostomy care, the management and support of a patient with a surgical opening created in the bladder, ileum, or colon for the temporary or permanent passage of urine or feces, necessitated by carcinoma, intestinal obstruction, trauma, or severe ulceration distal to the site of the incision. In most cases the opening is covered with a temporary disposable bag in the operating room.

ostomy irrigation, a procedure for cleansing, stimulating, and regulating evacuation of an artificially created orifice. Fluids used in irrigation include tap water and saline or medicated solutions. Loop and double-barrel colostomies require a sequential irrigation of the proximal loop, distal loop, and rectum to prevent the accumulation of discharge.

os trapezium. See **trapezium.**

os trapezoideum. See **trapezoid bone.**

os trigonum /os'trigō'nəm/, a small foot bone just posterior to the talus. It is sometimes confused with a fracture of the posterior tubercle of the talus.

os triquetrum. See **triangular bone.**

OT, abbreviation for **occupational therapist, occupational therapy.**

otalgia /ōtal'jə/, pain in the ear.

OTC, abbreviation for **over the counter.**

Othello syndrome [Othello, character in a Shakespearean tragedy], a psychopathologic condition, characterized by suspicion of a spouse's infidelity and by morbid jealousy. This condition may be accompanied by rage and violence and is frequently associated with paranoia.

otic /ō'tik, ot'ik/ [Gk *ous* ear], of or pertaining to the ear.

otics /ō'tiks, ot'iks/, a group of drugs used locally to treat inflammation of the external ear canal or to remove excess cerumen.

otitic /ōtit'ik/ [Gk *ous* ear], pertaining to otitis, an ear inflammation.

otitic barotrauma. See **barotrauma.**

otitis /ōtī'tis/ [Gk *ous* + *itis* inflammation], inflammation or infection of the ear. Kinds of otitis are **otitis externa** and **otitis media.**

otitis externa, inflammation or infection of the external canal or the auricle of the external ear. Major causes are allergy, bacteria, fungi, viruses, and trauma. Allergy to nickel or chromium in earrings and to chemicals in hair sprays, cosmetics, hearing aids, and medications is common. *Staphylococcus aureus, Pseudomonas aeruginosa,* and *Streptococcus pyogenes* are common bacterial causes. Herpes simplex and herpes zoster viruses are frequently implicated. Eczema, psoriasis, and seborrheic dermatitis also may affect the external ear.

otitis interna. See **labyrinthitis.**

otitis mastoidea, an inflammation of the inner ear associated with a mastoid infection.

otitis media, inflammation or infection of the middle ear, a common affliction of childhood. Acute otitis media is most often caused by *Haemophilus influenzae* or *Streptococcus pneumoniae.* Chronic otitis media is usually caused by gram-negative bacteria, such as *Proteus, Klebsiella,* and *Pseudomonas.* Allergy, *Mycoplasma,* and several viruses also may be causative factors. Otitis media is often preceded by an upper respiratory infection. Organisms gain entry to the middle ear through the eustachian tube. Obstruction of the eustachian tube and accumulation of exudate may increase pressure within the middle ear, forcing infection into the mastoid bone or rupturing the tympanic membrane. Symptoms of acute otitis media include a sense of fullness in the ear, diminished hearing, pain, and fever. Usually only one ear is affected. Squamous epithelium may grow in the middle ear through a rupture in the tympanic membrane, and development of a cholesteatoma and deafness may occur. Pneumococcal otitis media may spread to the meninges.

otitis sclerotica, a sclerosing type of inflammation of the middle ear.

otocephalus /ō'tōsef'ələs/, a fetus with otocephaly.

otocephaly /ō'tōsef'əlē/ [Gk *ous* + keph-

ale head], a congenital malformation characterized by the absence of the lower jaw, defective formation of the mouth, and union or close approximation of the ears on the front of the neck. **–otocephalic, otocephalous,** *adj.*

otodynia. See **otalgia.**

otolaryngologist /ō′tōler′ing·gol′əjist/ [Gk *ous* + *larynx, logos* science], a physician who specializes in the diagnosis and treatment of diseases and injuries of the ears, nose, and throat.

otolaryngology /ō′tōler′ing·gol′əjē/ [Gk *ous* + *larynx, logos* science], a branch of medicine dealing with the diagnosis and treatment of diseases and disorders of the ears, nose, and throat, and adjacent structures of the head and neck.

otolith /ō′təlith/ [Gk *ous* + *lithos* stone], **1.** a calculus in the middle ear. **2.** any of the crystals of calcium carbonate attached to the hair cells of the inner ear as gravity orientation receptors.

otolith righting reflex [Gk *ous* + *lithos* stone], an involuntary response in newborns in which tilting of the body when the infant is in an erect position causes the head to return to the upright position.

otologist /ōtol′əjist/, a physician trained in the diagnosis and treatment of diseases and other disorders of the ear.

otology /ōtol′əjē/ [Gk *ous* + *logos* science], the study of the ear, including the diagnosis and treatment of its diseases and disorders.

otoneuralgia. See **otalgia.**

otoplasty /ō′təplas′tē/ [Gk *ous* + *plassein* to mold], a common procedure in reconstructive plastic surgery in which, for cosmetic reasons, some of the cartilage in the ears is removed to bring the auricle and pinna closer to the head.

otorrhea /ō′tərē′ə/ [Gk *ous* + *rhoia* flow], any discharge from the external ear. Otorrhea may be serous, sanguineous, purulent, or contain cerebrospinal fluid. **–otorrheal, otorrheic, otorrhetic,** *adj.*

otosclerosis /ō′tōsklərō′sis/ [Gk *ous* + *skleros* hard, *osis* condition], a hereditary condition of unknown cause in which irregular ossification in the bony labyrinth of the inner ear, especially of the stapes, occurs, causing tinnitus, then deafness.

otoscope /ō′təskōp′/ [Gk *ous* + *skopein* to look], an instrument used to examine the external ear, the eardrum, and, through the eardrum, the ossicles of the middle ear. It consists of a light, a magnifying lens, and a device for insufflation.

otoscopy /ōtos′kəpē/ [Gk *ous* + *skopein* to view], an inspection of the tympanic membrane and other parts of the outer ear with an otoscope.

otospongiosus. See **otosclerosis.**

ototoxic /ō′tōtok′sik/ [Gk *ous* + *toxikon* poison], (of a substance) having a harmful effect on the eighth cranial nerve or the organs of hearing and balance. Common ototoxic drugs include the aminoglycoside antibiotics, aspirin, furosemide, and quinine.

OTR, abbreviation for *occupational therapist, registered.*

Otto pelvis /ot′ō/, a type of hip dislocation in which there is a gradual central displacement of the femur. The cause is unknown.

OU, abbreviation for *oculus uterque,* a Latin phrase meaning "each eye."

Ouchterlony double diffusion [Orjan T.G. Ouchterlony, Swedish bacteriologist, b. 1914], a form of gel diffusion technique in which antigen and antibody in separate cells are allowed to diffuse toward each other.

ounce (oz) [L *uncia* one twelfth of an amount], a unit of weight equal to $1/16$ of a pound avoirdupois.

outbreeding [AS *ut* out, *bredan* to breed], the production of offspring by the mating of unrelated individuals, organisms, or plants, which can lead to superior hybrid traits or strains.

outcome [AS *ut* + *couman* to come], the condition of a client at the end of therapy or of a disease process, including the degree of wellness and the need for continuing care, medication, support, counseling, or education.

outcome criteria, criteria that focus on observable or measurable results of nursing and other health service activities.

outcome data, data collected to evaluate the capacity of a patient to function at a level described in the outcome statement of a nursing care plan or in standards for patient care.

outcome measure, a measure of the quality of medical care, the standard on which is made the assessment of the expected end result of the intervention employed.

outlet [AS *ut* + *laetan* to permit], an opening through which something can exit, such as the pelvic outlet.

outlet contraction. See **contraction.**

outlet contracture, an abnormally small pelvic outlet. It may be anteroposterior or transverse and is of significance in childbirth because it may impede or prevent the passage of a baby through the birth canal.

outlet forceps. See **low forceps.**

outline form [AS *ut* + *lin* thread], the shape of the cavosurface of a prepared tooth cavity.

outpatient [AS *ut* + L *patientia* endurance], **1.** a patient, not hospitalized, who is being treated in an office, clinic, or other ambulatory care facility. **2.** of or pertaining to a health care facility for patients who are not hospitalized or to the treatment or care of such a patient.

output [AS *ut* + *putian* to put], **1.** the total of any and all measurable liquids lost from the body, including urine, vomitus, diarrhea, and drainage from wounds, from fistulas, and removed by suction equipment. The output is recorded as a means of monitoring a patient's fluid and electrolyte balance. **2.** the end product of a system.

ova and parasites test /ō'və/, a microscopic examination of feces for detecting parasites, such as amebas or worms and their ova, which are indicators of parasitic disorders.

ovale malaria. See **tertian malaria.**

ovalocytes /ō'vəlōsīts'/ [L *ovalis* egg-shaped; Gk *kytos* cell], oblong or oval-shaped red blood cells with pale centers that are found occasionally in patients with hemolytic anemias, certain other anemias, thalassemias, and hereditary elliptocytosis.

ovalocytosis. See **elliptocytosis.**

oval window [L *ovum;* ME *windoge*], an oval-shaped aperture in the wall of the middle ear, leading to the inner ear. The footplate of the stapes vibrates in the oval window, transmitting sound waves to the cochlea.

ovarian /ōver'ē-ən/ [L *ovum* egg], of or pertaining to the ovary.

ovarian artery, a slender branch of the abdominal aorta, arising caudal to the renal arteries, and supplying an ovary.

ovarian cancer. See **ovarian carcinoma.**

ovarian carcinoma, a malignant neoplasm of the ovaries rarely detected in the early stage and usually far advanced when diagnosed. Risk factors of the disease are infertility, nulliparity or low parity, delayed childbearing, repeated spontaneous abortion, endometriosis, Group A blood type, previous irradiation of pelvic organs, and exposure to chemical carcinogens, such as asbestos and talc. After an insidious onset and asymptomatic period the tumor may become evident as a palpable abdominal or pelvic mass accompanied by irregular or excessive menses or postmenopausal bleeding. In advanced cases the patient may have ascites, edema of the legs, and pain in the abdomen and the backs of the legs. Regular yearly pelvic examinations after 40 years of age contribute significantly to early diagnosis and the possibility of curative treatment.

ovarian cyst, a globular sac filled with fluid or semisolid material that develops in or on the ovary. It may be transient and physiologic or pathologic. Kinds of ovarian cysts include **chocolate cyst, corpus luteum cyst,** and **dermoid cyst.**

ovarian follicle [L *ovum, folliculus* small bag], a cavity or recess in an ovary containing a liquid that divides the follicular cells into layers and surrounds an ovum.

ovarian pregnancy, a rare type of ectopic pregnancy in which the conceptus is implanted within the ovary.

ovarian seminoma. See **dysgerminoma.**

ovarian varicocele, a varicose swelling of the veins of the uterine broad ligament.

ovarian vein, one of a pair of veins that emerge from convoluted plexuses in the broad ligament near the ovaries and the uterine tubes. The right ovarian vein opens into the inferior vena cava, the left ovarian vein into the renal vein.

ovariectomy. See **oophorectomy.**

ovary /ō'vərē/ [L *ovum* egg], one of the pair of female gonads found on each side of the lower abdomen, beside the uterus, in a fold of the broad ligament. At ovulation an egg is extruded from a follicle on the surface of the ovary under the stimulation of the gonadotropic hormones, follicle-stimulating hormone (FSH), and luteinizing hormone (LH). The mature ovarian follicle secretes the hormones estrogen and progesterone that regulate the menstrual cycle by a negative feedback system in which an increase in estrogen decreases the secretion of FSH by the pituitary gland and an increase in progesterone decreases the secretion of LH. Each ovary is normally firm and smooth and resembles an almond in size and shape. The ovaries are homologous to the testes.

overbite [AS *ofer* over, *bitan* to bite], vertical overlapping of lower teeth by upper teeth, usually measured perpendicularly to the occlusal plane.

overclosure [AS *ofer* + L *claudere* to close], an abnormal condition in which the mandible rises too far before the teeth make contact, caused by the loss of occlusal vertical dimension.

overcompensation [AS *ofer* + L *compensare* to weigh together], an exaggerated attempt to overcome a real or imagined physical or psychologic deficit. The attempt may be conscious or unconscious.

overdenture [AS *ofer* + L *dens* tooth], a complete or partial removable denture supported by retained roots to provide improved support, stability, and tactile and proprioceptive sensation and to reduce ridge resorption.

overdose (OD), an excessive use of a drug, resulting in adverse reactions ranging from mania or hysteria to coma or death.

O

overdrive suppression [AS *ofer* + *drifan* to drive], the inhibitory effect of a faster cardiac pacemaker on a slower one.

overflow [AS *ofer* + *flowan*], the flooding or excessive discharge of a fluid, such as urine, saliva, or bile.

overflow incontinence [AS *ofer* + *flowan;* L, *incontinentia,* inability to retain], an overflow of urine from a distended paralyzed bladder.

overgrowth [AS *ofer* + ME *growen*], an excessive growth, usually applied to organ or tissue development.

overhang [AS *ofer* + *hangian* to hang], an excess of dental filling material that projects beyond the margin of the associated tooth cavity.

overhydration, an excess of water in the body.

overinclusiveness [AS *ofer* + L *includere* to include], a type of association disorder observed in some schizophrenia patients. The individual is unable to think in a precise manner because of an inability to keep irrelevant elements outside perceptual boundaries.

overjet [AS *ofer* + Fr *jeter* to throw], a horizontal projection of upper teeth beyond the lower teeth, usually measured parallel to the occlusal plane.

overload, 1. a burden greater than the capacity of the system designed to move or process it. **2.** (in physiology) any factor or influence that stresses the body beyond its natural limits and may impair its health.

overoxygenation /ōvərok'sijənā'shən/ [AS *ofer* + Gk *oxys* sharp, *genein* to produce; L *atio* process], an abnormal condition in which the oxygen concentration in the blood and other tissues of the body is greater than normal, and the carbon dioxide concentration is less than normal. The condition is characterized by a fall in blood pressure, decreased vital capacity, fatigue, errors in judgment, paresthesia of the hands and feet, anorexia, nausea and vomiting, and hyperemia.

overriding, the overlapping or telescoping of body parts, as when one fragment of a fractured bone rests on another.

overripe cataract [AS *ofer* + OE *reap*], a cataract in which a completely opaque lens solidifies and shrinks.

over the counter (OTC), (of a drug) available to the consumer without a prescription.

overweight [AS *ofer* + *gewiht* weight], more than normal in body weight after adjustment for height, body build, and age.

oviduct. See **fallopian tube.**

oviferous /ōvif'ərəs/ [L *ovum* egg, *ferre* to bear], bearing or capable of producing ova (egg cells).

oviparous /ōvip'ərəs/ [L *ovum* + *parere* to bring forth], giving birth to young by laying eggs.

ovocenter /ō'vəsen'tər/ [L *ovum* + *centrum* center], the centrosome of a fertilized ovum.

ovoflavin /ō'vəflā'vin/ [L *ovum* + *flavus* yellow], a riboflavin derived from the yolk of eggs.

ovogenesis. See **oogenesis.**

ovoglobulin /ō'vəglob'yo͞olin/ [L *ovum* + *globulus* small sphere], a globulin derived from the white of eggs.

ovogonium. See **oogonium.**

ovoid arch /ō'void/ [L *ovum* + Gk *eidos* form; L *arcus* bow], a dental arch that curves smoothly from the molars on one side to those on the opposite side to form half an oval.

ovo-lacto-vegetarian. See **lacto-vegetarian.**

ovomucin /ō'vəmyo͞o'sin/ [L *ovum* + *mucus* slime], a glycoprotein derived from the white of eggs.

ovomucoid /ō'vəmyo͞o'koid/ [L *ovum* + *mucus* slime; Gk *eidos* form], of or pertaining to a glycoprotein, similar to mucin, derived from the white of eggs.

ovoplasm. See **ooplasm.**

ovotestis /ō'vətes'tis/ [L *ovum* + *testis* testicle], a gonad that contains both ovarian and testicular tissue; a hermaphroditic gonad. **–ovotesticular,** *adj.*

ovovitellin. See **vitellin.**

ovoviviparous /ō'vəvip'ərəs/ [L *ovum* + *vivus* living, *parere* to bring forth], bearing young in eggs that are hatched within the body, such as some reptiles and fish.

ovulation /ov'yəlā'shən/ [L *ovum* + *atio* process], expulsion of an ovum from the ovary on spontaneous rupture of a mature follicle as a result of cyclic ovarian and pituitary endocrine function. It usually occurs on the fourteenth day after the first day of the last menstrual period and often causes brief, sharp lower abdominal pain on the side of the ovulating ovary. **–ovulate,** *v.*

ovulation method of family planning, a natural method of family planning that uses observation of changes in the character and quantity of cervical mucus as a means of determining the time of ovulation during the menstrual cycle. The cyclic changes in gonadotropic hormones, especially estrogen, cause changes in the quantity and character of cervical mucus. In the first days after menstruation, scant thick mucus is secreted by the cervix. These "dry days" are "safe days." The quantity of mucus then increases; it is pearly white and sticky, becoming clearer and less sticky as ovulation approaches; these "wet days" are "unsafe days." During and just after ovulation the mucus is clear, slippery, and elastic; it resembles the uncooked white of an egg. The day on which this sign is most apparent is the "peak day," probably the day before ovulation. The 4 days after the "peak day" are "unsafe": fertilization might occur. Effectiveness of the method in identifying the most fertile days of the cycle is augmented by using the basal body temperature method.

ovulatory [L *ovum*], pertaining to ovulation.

ovum /ō′vəm/, *pl.* **ova** [L, egg], **1.** an egg. **2.** a female germ cell extruded from the ovary at ovulation.

oxacillin sodium /ok′səsil′in/, a penicillinase-resistant penicillin antibiotic prescribed in the treatment of severe infections caused by penicillinase-producing staphylococci.

oxaluric acid /ok′səlŏŏr′ik/, a compound derived from uric acid or from parabonic acid, which occurs in normal urine.

oxamniquine /oksam′nəkwēn/, an antischistosomal prescribed in the treatment of infection caused by *Schistosoma mansoni*.

oxandrolone /oksan′drəlōn/, an androgen prescribed in the treatment of testosterone deficiency, osteoporosis, and female breast cancer and for the stimulation of growth, weight gain, and red blood cell production.

oxazepam /oksā′zəpam/, a minor tranquilizer prescribed to relieve anxiety and nervous tension.

oxidant /ok′sidənt/ [Gk *oxys* sharp], an oxidizing agent.

oxidase [Gk *oxys* sharp], an enzyme that induces biologic oxidation by activating the oxygen in molecules containing the element, such as hydrogen peroxide.

oxidation [Gk *oxys* sharp, *genein* to produce, *atio* process] **1.** any process in which the oxygen content of a compound is increased. **2.** any reaction in which the positive valence of a compound or a radical is increased because of a loss of electrons. **−oxidize,** *v.*

oxidation-reduction reaction, a chemical change in which electrons are removed (oxidation) from an atom or molecule, accompanied by a simultaneous transfer of electrons (reduction) to another.

oxidative phosphorylation, an ATP-generating process in which oxygen serves as the final electron acceptor. The process occurs in mitochondria and is the major source of ATP generation in aerobic organisms.

oxidative water [Gk *oxys* sharp, *genein* to produce, *atus* process], water produced

by the oxidation of molecules of food substances, such as the conversion of glucose to water and carbon dioxide.

oxidize [Gk *oxys*, *genein* to produce, *izein* to cause], (of an element or compound) to combine or cause to combine with oxygen, to remove hydrogen, or to increase the valence of an element through the loss of electrons. **−oxidation,** *n.,* **oxidizing,** *adj.*

oxidizing agent, a compound that readily gives up oxygen and attracts hydrogen from another compound. In chemical reactions an oxidizing agent acts as an acceptor of electrons, thereby increasing the valence of an element.

oxidoreductase /ok′sidō′riduk′tās/, an enzyme that catalyzes a reaction in which one substance is oxidized while another is reduced. An example is alcohol dehydrogenase.

oximeter /oksim′ətər/, any of several devices used to measure oxyhemoglobin in the blood.

oxtriphylline /oks′trəfil′ēn/, a bronchodilator prescribed in the treatment of bronchial asthma, bronchitis, and emphysema.

oxybenzene. See **carbolic acid.**

oxybutynin chloride /ok′sibōō′tinin/, an anticholinergic prescribed in the treatment of neurogenic bladder.

oxycephaly /ok′sisef′əlē/ [Gk *oxys* + *kephale* head], a congenital malformation of the skull in which premature closure of the coronal and sagittal sutures results in accelerated upward growth of the head, giving it a long, narrow appearance with the top pointed or conic in shape.

oxycodone hydrochloride /ok′sidōn/, a narcotic analgesic used to treat moderate to severe pain.

oxygen (O) [Gk *oxys* sharp, *genein* to produce], a tasteless, odorless, colorless gas essential for human respiration. Its atomic weight is 15.9994; its atomic number is 8. In anesthesia, oxygen functions as a carrier gas for the delivery of anesthetic agents to the tissues of the body. In respiratory therapy, oxygen is administered to increase its amount and thus to decrease the amount of other gases circulating in the blood. Overdose of oxygen can cause irreversible toxicity in people with pulmonary abnormalities, especially when complicated by chronic carbon dioxide retention.

oxygenation, the process of combining or treating with oxygen. **−oxygenate,** *v.*

oxygen capacity of blood, the maximum amount of oxygen that can be made to combine chemically with hemoglobin in a unit of blood, excluding physically dissolved oxygen.

O

oxygen concentration in blood, the concentration of oxygen in a blood sample, including both oxygen combined with hemoglobin and oxygen physically dissolved in blood.

oxygen consumption, the amount of oxygen in milliliters per minute required by the body for normal aerobic metabolism; normally about 250 ml/min.

oxygen cost of breathing, the rate at which the respiratory muscles consume oxygen as they ventilate the lungs.

oxygen debt, the quantity of oxygen taken up by the lungs during recovery from a period of exercise or apnea that is in excess of the quantity needed for resting metabolism during the preexercise period.

oxygen enhancement ratio (OER), a measure of tumor sensitivity to the presence or absence of oxygen, expressed as the ratio of radiation dose required to produce a given effect with no oxygen present to the dose required to produce the same effect in one atmosphere of air.

oxygen half-saturation pressure of hemoglobin, the oxygen pressure necessary for 50% saturation of hemoglobin at body temperature and at pH 7.4 or 40 torr carbon dioxide pressure. The value is commonly used as a measure of the affinity between oxygen and hemoglobin.

oxygen hood, a device placed over the head of neonatal patients to deliver high concentrations of oxygen.

oxygen mask, a device used to administer oxygen. It is shaped to fit snugly over the mouth and nose and may be secured in place with a strap or held with the hand.

oxygen radicals [Gk *oxys* sharp; L *radix* root], a substituent group of chemical elements rich in oxygen but incapable of prolonged existence in a free state. Oxygen radicals are used in some types of therapy.

oxygen saturation, the fraction of a total hemoglobin (HB) in the form of HbO_2 at a defined Po_2.

oxygen store, the total quantity of oxygen normally stored in the various body compartments, including the lungs, arterial and venous blood, and tissues.

oxygen tension, the force with which oxygen molecules that are physically dissolved in blood are constantly trying to escape, expressed as partial pressure (Po_2). The tension at any instant is related to the amount of oxygen physically dissolved in plasma; the larger amount carried in chemical combination with hemoglobin serves as a reservoir that releases oxygen molecules to physical solution when the tension decreases and that stores additional molecules of the gas when the tension increases.

oxygen tent, a canopy that encloses the head and neck of a patient and contains a high oxygen tension.

oxygen therapy, any procedure in which oxygen is administered to a patient to relieve hypoxia.

oxygen tolerance, an increased capacity to withstand the toxic effects of hyperoxia as a result of any adaptive change occurring within an organism.

oxygen toxicity, a condition of oxygen overdosage that can result in pathologic tissue changes, such as retrolental fibroplasia or bronchopulmonary dysplasia.

oxygen transport, the process by which oxygen is absorbed in the lungs by the hemoglobin in circulating deoxygenated red cells and carried to the peripheral tissues. This process is made possible by a special characteristic of hemoglobin, that is, the ability to combine with large quantities of oxygen present at a high concentration, such as in the lungs, and to release this oxygen when the concentration is low, such as in the peripheral tissues.

oxygen uptake, the amount of oxygen an organism removes from the environment, including the amount of oxygen that the lungs remove from the ambient atmosphere, the amount that the blood removes from the alveolar gas in the lungs, or the rate at which an organ or tissue removes oxygen from the blood perfusing it.

oxyhemoglobin /ok'sēhē'məglō'bin, -hem'-/ [Gk *oxys* + *genein* to produce, *haima* blood; L *globus* ball], the product of the combining of hemoglobin with oxygen. It is a loosely bound complex that dissociates easily when there is a low concentration of oxygen.

oxyhemoglobin dissociation curve, a graphic expression of the affinity between oxygen and hemoglobin, or the amount of oxygen chemically bound at equilibrium to the hemoglobin in blood as a function of oxygen pressure. To define the curve completely, it should also include the pH, temperature, and carbon dioxide pressure.

oxyhemoglobin saturation, the amount of oxygen actually combined with hemoglobin, expressed as a percentage of the oxygen capacity of that hemoglobin.

oxymetazoline hydrochloride /ok'sēməta-z'əlēn/, a decongestant prescribed in the treatment of nasal congestion.

oxymetholone /ok'sēmeth'əlōn/, an androgen prescribed in the treatment of testosterone deficiency, osteoporosis, and female breast cancer and for the stimulation of growth, weight gain, and red blood cell production.

oxymorphone hydrochloride /ok′sēmôr-′fōn/, a narcotic analgesic prescribed to reduce moderate to severe pain, as a preoperative medication, and to support anesthesia.

oxyopia /ok′sē·ō′pē·ə/ [Gk *oxys* + *opsis* vision], unusual acuteness of vision. A person with normal (20/20) vision when standing 20 feet from the standard Snellen eye chart can read the seventh line of letters, each of which is an eighth of an inch high, while an individual with oxyopia can read smaller letters at that distance.

oxytetracycline /ok′sētet′rəsī′klēn/, a tetracycline antibiotic prescribed in the treatment of bacterial and rickettsial infections.

oxytetracycline calcium, a tetracycline antibiotic.

oxytocic /ok′sitō′sik/ [Gk *oxys* + *tokos* birth], **1.** of or pertaining to a substance that is similar to the hormone oxytocin. **2.** any one of numerous drugs that stimulate the smooth muscle of the uterus to contract. These drugs are often used to initiate labor at term. Oxytocic agents commonly used include oxytocin, certain prostaglandins, and the ergot alkaloids.

oxytocin /ok′sitō′sin/, an oxytocic prescribed to stimulate contractions in inducing or augmenting labor, and to contract the uterus to control postpartum bleeding.

oxytocin challenge test, a stress test for the assessment of intrauterine function of the fetus and the placenta. It is performed to evaluate the ability of the fetus to tolerate continuation of pregnancy or the anticipated stress of labor and delivery. A dilute intravenous infusion of oxytocin is begun, monitored by a meter, or regulated by an infusion pump. The uterine activity is monitored with a tocodynamometer, and the fetal heart rate is monitored with an ultrasonic sensor as the uterus is stimulated to contract by the oxytocin. Decelerations of the fetal heart rate in certain repeating patterns may indicate fetal distress.

oxyuriasis. See **enterobiasis.**

Oxyuris vermicularis. See *Enterobius vermicularis.*

oz, abbreviation for **ounce.**

oz ap, abbreviation for *apothecary ounce,* a unit of weight equal to 31.1035 grams.

ozena /ōzē′nə/ [Gk *ozein* to have an odor], a condition of the nose characterized by atrophy of the nasal chonchae and mucous membranes. Symptoms include crusting of nasal secretions, discharge, and, especially, a very offensive odor.

ozone /ō′zōn/ [Gk *ozein* to have an odor], a form of oxygen characterized by molecules having three atoms. Ozone is formed when oxygen is electrically charged, as might occur in a lightning storm.

ozone shield, the layer of ozone that hangs in the atmosphere from 20 to 40 miles above the surface of the earth and protects the earth from excessive ultraviolet radiation.

ozone sickness, an abnormal condition caused by the inhalation of ozone that may seep into jet aircraft at altitudes over 40,000 feet. It is characterized by headaches, chest pains, itchy eyes, and sleepiness. Exactly why and how ozone causes this condition is not known. It is more prevalent early in the year and occurs more often over the Pacific Ocean.

oz t, abbreviation for *troy ounce,* a unit of weight equal to 31.103 grams.

P, 1. symbol for the element **phosphorus** 2. symbol for **gas partial pressure.** 3. symbol for **after** or **post.**

p17, symbol for a protein that *lines the interior of the HIV virus envelope.*

p24, symbol for a protein that *surrounds the RNA and reverse transcriptase of the HIV virus.*

P₁, 1. (in genetics) symbol for **first parental generation.** 2. symbol for **first pulmonic sound.**

P₂, symbol for **second pulmonic sound.**

P₅₀, the partial pressure of oxygen at which hemoglobin is half saturated with bound oxygen.

pA, symbol for *picoampere.*

Pa, 1. symbol for *pascal.* 2. symbol for the element **protactinium.** 3. symbol for *partial pressure in arterial blood.*

Paco₂, abbreviation for **partial pressure of carbon dioxide in arterial blood.**

Pao₂, symbol for *partial pressure of arterial oxygen.*

PA, 1. abbreviation for **physician's assistant.** 2. abbreviation for **pulmonary artery.** 3. abbreviation for *partial pressure of alveolar oxygen.*

Pao₂ symbol for *partial pressure of arterial oxygen.*

PAo₂, symbol for *partial pressure of alveolar oxygen.*

P-A, p-a, abbreviation for **posteroanterior.**

P&A, 1. abbreviation for *percussion and auscultation* as noted in the patient's chart after physical examination of the chest. 2. abbreviation for *posterior and anterior.*

PABA, abbreviation for **paraaminobenzoic acid,** a topical sunscreen.

pabulum /pab′yələm/ [L, food], any substance that is food or nutrient.

pac, abbreviation for **phenacetin-aspirin-caffeine.**

PAC, abbreviation for *premature atrial contraction.*

PA catheter, an intravenous catheter that is inserted into the pulmonary artery.

PACE II, an interdisciplinary assessment and planning system that focuses on evaluation of the physical health of nursing home patients. It includes checklists of defined (diagnosed) conditions, abnormal laboratory or other findings, risk factors, and other impairments and disabilities.

pacemaker [L *passus* step; AS *macian* to make] 1. the sinoatrial (or sinus) node, specialized nervous tissue located at the junction of the superior vena cava and the right atrium. It originates the contractions of the atria, which force blood into the ventricles. The impulse then passes on to the atrioventricular node, thereby initiating contraction of the ventricles. 2. an electric apparatus used for maintaining a normal sinus rhythm of myocardial contraction by electrically stimulating the heart muscle. A pacemaker may be permanent or temporary. It may emit the stimulus at a constant rate or may fire only on demand, when the heart is not spontaneously contracting at a minimum rate.

pacemaker installation fluoroscopy, the fluoroscopic monitoring of the insertion of an artificial pacemaker, used as an aid for correct installation of the device.

pacer. See **pacemaker.**

pachometer. See **pachymeter.**

pachycephaly /pak′esef′əle/ [Gk *pachys* thick, *kephale* head], an abnormal thickness of the skull, as in acromegaly. –**pachycephalic, pachycephalous,** *adj.*

pachydactyly /pak′edak′tile/ [Gk *pachys* + *daktylos* finger], an abnormal thickening of the fingers or the toes. –**pachydactylic, pachydactylous,** *adj.*

pachyderma alba /pak′idor′mə/ [Gk *pachys* + *derma* skin; L *albus* white], an abnormal state of the buccal mucosa in which the appearance is suggestive of whitened elephant hide.

pachymeter /pakim′ətər/ [Gk *pachys* + *metron* measure], an instrument used to measure thickness, especially of thin structures, such as a membrane or a tissue.

pachynema /pak′ine′mə/ [Gk *pachys* + *nema* thread], the postsynaptic tetradic chromosome formation that occurs in the pachytene stage of the first meiotic prophase of gametogenesis.

pachyonychia congenita /pak′e-ōnik′e-ə/ [Gk *pachys* + *onyx* nail; L *congenitus* born with], a congenital deformity characterized by abnormal thickening and raising of the nails on the fingers and the toes, and hyperkeratosis of the palms and the soles.

pachytene /pak'itēn/ [Gk *pachys* + *tainia* ribbon], the third stage in the first meiotic prophase of gametogenesis in which the paired homologous chromosomes form tetrads. The bivalent pairs become short and thick and intertwine so that four chromatids are visible.

pacifier [L *pacificare* to make peace] **1.** an agent that soothes or comforts. **2.** a nipple-shaped object used by infants and children for sucking.

pacing [L *passus* step], the artificial electrical stimulation of a heart rhythm. Kinds of pacing include **atrial, coupled, endocardial, epicardial, programmed, AV sequential,** and **ventricular.**

pacing wire, an electrode of a pacemaker, a pacing catheter which is usually inserted into the patient's right ventricle.

Pacini's corpuscles /päsē'nēz/ [Filippo Pacini, Italian anatomist, b. 1812; L *corpusculum* little body], a number of special sensory end organs resembling tiny white bulbs, each attached to the end of a single nerve fiber in the subcutaneous, submucous, and subserous connective tissue of many parts of the body, especially the palms, soles, genital organs, joints, and pancreas. They are pressure sensitive and in cross-section resemble an onion.

pack [ME *pakke* bundle], **1.** a treatment in which the entire body or a portion of it is wrapped in wet or dry towels or in ice for various therapeutic purposes, as with cold packs for the reduction of high temperatures and swellings or for inducing hypothermia during certain surgical procedures, especially heart surgery and organ transplants. **2.** a tampon. **3.** the act of applying a dressing or dental cement to a surgical wound. **4.** a surgical dressing to cover a wound or to fill the cavity left from a tooth extraction, especially of a wisdom tooth.

package insert, a leaflet that, by order of the FDA, must be placed inside the package of prescription drugs. In it the manufacturer is required to describe the drug, to state its generic name, and to give the applicable indications, contraindications, warnings, precautions, adverse effects, form, dosage, and administration.

packed cell volume (PCV), a measured quantity of blood to which an anticoagulant has been added and the cells of which have been pressed together by the force of being centrifuged at 2,000 rpm.

packed cells [ME *pakke* bundle; L *cella* storeroom], a preparation of blood cells separated from liquid plasma, often administered in severe anemia to restore ad-

equate levels of hemoglobin and red cells without overloading the vascular system with excess fluids.

packing, 1. material used to fill a wound or cavity. **2.** the act of inserting material into a wound or cavity.

pad [D *paden* a cushion], **1.** a mass of soft material used to cushion shock, prevent wear, or absorb moisture, such as the abdominal pads used to absorb discharges from abdominal wounds. **2.** (in anatomy) a mass of fat that cushions various structures, such as the infrapatellar pad lying below the patella.

p.ae. [L *partes aequales*], symbol for *equal parts.*

paedogenesis. See **pedogenesis.**

Paget's disease /paj'əts/ [Sir James Paget, English surgeon, b. 1814], a common nonmetabolic disease of bone of unknown cause, usually affecting middle-aged and elderly people, characterized by excessive bone destruction and unorganized bone repair. Most cases are asymptomatic or mild; however, bone pain may be the first symptom. Bowed tibias (saber shins), kyphosis, and frequent fractures are caused by the soft abnormal bone in this condition. Enlargement of the head, headaches, and warmth over involved areas caused by increased vascularity are additional features. The x-ray picture of areas of decreased bone density adjacent to sites of increased density is characteristic. Radioactive bone scans help locate regions of active disease. Complications include fractures, kidney stones if the patient is immobilized, heart failure, deafness or blindness caused by pressure from bony overgrowth, and osteosarcoma.

Paget's disease of the nipple. See **nipple cancer.**

pagophagia /pā'gōfā'jē·ə/ [Gk *pagos* frost, *phagein* to eat], an abnormal condition characterized by a craving to eat enormous quantities of ice. It is associated with a lack of nutrient iron. **–pagophagic, pagophagous,** *adj.*

PAHA, abbreviation for **paraaminohippuric acid.**

PAHA sodium clearance test, a test for detecting kidney damage or certain muscle diseases. The test uses the sodium salt of paraaminohippuric acid for determining the rate at which the kidneys remove this salt from the blood and urine.

PAHO, abbreviation for *Pan American Health Organization.*

pain [L *poena* punishment], **1.** an unpleasant sensation caused by noxious stimulation of the sensory nerve endings. It is a cardinal symptom of inflammation and is valuable in the diagnosis of many

P

disorders and conditions. Pain may be mild or severe, chronic, acute, lancinating, burning, dull, or sharp, precisely or poorly localized, or referred. **2.** a NANDA-accepted nursing diagnosis of the presence of severe discomfort or an uncomfortable sensation. Defining characteristics include (1) verbal or nonverbal communication; (2) behavior that is self-protective with an altered time perception, withdrawal from social contact, or impaired thought processes; (3) distraction behavior with moaning, crying, or restlessness; (4) a facial mask with dull and lusterless eyes, a "beaten" look, or grimace; (5) alteration in muscle tone; and (6) autonomic responses, including diaphoresis, changes in blood pressure and pulse rate, pupillary dilation, and an increased or decreased rate of respiration.

pain and suffering, (in law) an element in a claim for damages that allows recovery for the mental and physical pain, suffering, distress, and trauma that an individual has endured as a result of injury.

pain assessment, an evaluation of the factors that alleviate or exacerbate a patient's pain, used as an aid in the diagnosis and the treatment of disease and trauma. Responses to pain vary widely among individuals and depend on many different physical and psychologic factors, such as specific diseases and injuries and the health, pain threshold, fear and anxiety, and cultural background of the individual involved, as well as the way different individuals express their pain experiences. The patient is asked to describe the cause of the pain, (if known), its intensity, location, and duration, the events preceding it, and the pattern usually followed for handling it. Severe pain causes pallor, cold perspiration, piloerection, dilated pupils, and an increase in the pulse and respiratory rate, blood pressure, and muscle tension. When brief intense pain subsides, the pulse rate may be slower and the blood pressure lower than before the pain began. If pain occurs frequently or is prolonged, the pulse rate and blood pressure may not increase markedly.

pain, chronic, a NANDA-accepted nursing diagnosis of pain that continues for more than 6 months in duration. Defining characteristics include a verbal report or observed evidence of pain experienced for more than 6 months, fear of reinjury, altered ability to continue previous activities, anorexia, weight changes, changes in sleep patterns, facial mask, and guarded movements.

pain intervention, the relief of the painful sensations experienced in suffering the physiologic and the psychologic effects of disease and trauma. The most common method of pain intervention is the administration of narcotics, such as morphine, but many authorities believe that the exclusive use of pain-killing drugs without consideration and implementation of psychologic aids is too narrow an approach. There are few patients without a psychogenic overlay on the physical experience of pain. Methods of pain intervention for acute pain are different from those for chronic pain. Acute pain, occurring in the first 24 to 48 hours after surgery, is often difficult to relieve, and narcotics seldom relieve all such pain. The type of pain intervention usually depends on the description of the pain by the individual experiencing it. Mild pain may best be relieved by comfort measures and the distraction afforded by television, visitors, reading, and other passive activities. Moderate pain may be relieved by a combination of comfort measures and drugs. Cognitive dissonance, often employed to dampen moderate pain, encourages the patient to reflect on pleasant experiences and describe them to health care personnel. Intervention to relieve severe pain often includes the administration of narcotics, purposeful interaction between the patient and attending hospital personnel, reduction of environmental stimuli, increased comfort measures, and "waking imagined analgesia," in which the patient is encouraged to concentrate on and become distracted by former pleasant experiences, such as relaxing on a beach surrounded by cool ocean water. In the alleviation of all types of pain, dampening or decreasing stimuli that create pain is the chief goal. Pain often increases in a cold room because the muscles of the patient tend to contract; but the local application of cold, as with an ice pack, often alleviates pain by reducing swelling. Pain intervention seeks to reduce the effects of other factors that compound pain, such as fatigue and anxiety. Coping with pain becomes increasingly difficult as the patient becomes more tired. Sensory restriction may increase pain, because it blocks otherwise effective distraction; overstimulation may cause fatigue and anxiety, thus increasing pain.

pain mechanism, the nerve network that transmits unpleasant sensations and the perceptions of noxious stimuli throughout the body, most commonly in association with physical disease and trauma involving tissue damage. Some theories about the pain mechanism that have evolved are the gate control theory and the pattern theory. The gate control theory states that pain signals reaching the nervous system excite a group of small neurons that form a "pain pool." When the total activity of these neurons reaches a minimum level, a gate opens and allows the signals to proceed to higher brain centers. The areas where the gates operate are considered to be the dorsal horns of the spinal cord and the brainstem. The pattern theory holds that the intensity of a stimulus evokes a specific pattern of nerve impulses that is interpreted by the brain as pain. This perception is the result of the intensity and frequency of stimulation of a nonspecific end organ. Some authorities believe that bradykinin and histamine, two chemical substances elaborated by the body, cause pain.

pain receptor, any one of the many free nerve endings throughout the body that responds to stimuli of various kinds and thereby warns of potentially harmful changes in the environment, such as excessive pressure or temperature. The free nerve endings constituting most of the pain receptors occur chiefly in the epidermis and in the epithelial covering of certain mucous membranes. They also appear in the stratified squamous epithelium of the cornea, in nerve root sheaths and the papillae of hairs, and around the bodies of sudoriferous glands. The terminal ends of pain receptors consist of unmyelinated nerve fibers that often form small knobs between epithelial cells.

paint [Fr *peindre*], **1.** to apply (a medicated solution) to the skin, usually over a wide area. **2.** a medicated solution that is applied in this way. Kinds of paint include **antiseptics, germicides,** and **sporicides.**

pain threshold, the point at which a stimulus, usually one associated with pressure or temperature, activates pain receptors and produces a sensation of pain. Individuals with low pain thresholds experience pain much sooner and faster than individuals with higher pain thresholds.

PAL, abbreviation for *posterior axillary line.*

palatable [L *palatum* palate], pleasant to the taste.

palatal /pal'ətəl/ [L *palatum* palate], **1.** of or pertaining to the palate. **2.** of or pertaining to the lingual surface of a maxillary tooth.

palate /pal'it/ [L *palatum*], the roof of the mouth. It is divided into the hard palate and the soft palate. **–palatal, palatine** /pal'ətīn/, *adj.*

palatine arch /pal'ətin/ [L *palatum; arcus* bow], the vault-shaped muscular structure between the mouth and the nasopharynx.

palatine bone, one of a pair of bones in the skull that form the posterior part of the hard palate, part of the nasal cavity, and the floor of the orbit.

palatine ridge, any one of the four to six transverse elevations on the anterior surface of the hard palate.

palatine suture, one of several thin wavy lines that mark the joining of processes that form the hard palate.

palatine tonsil, one of a pair of almond-shaped masses of lymphoid tissue between the palatoglossal and the palatopharyngeal arches on each side of the fauces (throat).

palatitis, inflammation of the hard palate.

palatoglossal /pal'ətōglos'əl/ [L *palatum* + Gk *glossa* tongue], pertaining to both the palate and the tongue.

palatomaxillary /pal'ətōmak'siler'ē/ [L *palatum* + *maxilla* jaw], of or pertaining to the palate and the maxilla.

palatonasal /pal'ətōnā'zəl/ [L *palatum* + *nasus* nose], of or pertaining to the palate and the nose.

pale infarct [L *pallidus* pallid; *infarcire* to stuff], a wedge of dead tissue, white in color because of the absence of blood, causing obstruction in an artery.

paleogenesis. See **palingenesis.**

paleogenetic /pā'lē-ōjenet'ik/ [Gk *palaios* long ago, *genesis* origin], **1.** a trait or structure of an organism or species that originated in a previous generation. **2.** relating to the development of such a trait or structure.

palilalia /pal'ilā'lyə/ [Gk *palin* again, *lalein* to babble], an abnormal condition characterized by increasingly rapid repetition of the same word or phrase, usually at the end of a sentence.

palindrome /pal'indrōm'/ [Gk *palin* + *dromos* course], (in molecular genetics) a segment of DNA in which identical, or almost identical, sequences of bases run in opposite directions.

palingenesis /pal'injen'əsis/ [Gk *palin* + *genesis* origin] **1.** the regeneration of a lost part. **2.** the hereditary transmission of ancestral structural characteristics. **–palingenetic, palingenic,** *adj.*

palladium (Pd) /pală'dē-əm/ [Gk *Pallas Athena* mythic goddess and protector of Troy], a hard, silvery metallic element. Its atomic number is 46; its atomic weight is 106.4. Highly resistant to tarnish and corrosion, palladium is used in surgical instruments and in dental inlays, bridgework, and orthodontic appliances.

palliate /pal'ē-āt/ [L *palliare* to cloak], to soothe or relieve. **–palliation,** *n.,* **palliative** /pal'i-ətiv/, *adj.*

palliative treatment /pal'ē-ətiv'/ [L *palliare* to cloak; *tractare* to handle], therapy designed to relieve or reduce the intensity of uncomfortable symptoms but not to produce a cure.

pallid /pal′id/ [L *pallidus* pale], lacking color.

pallidum. See **globus pallidus.**

pallium. See **cerebral cortex.**

pallor [L, paleness], an unnatural paleness or absence of color in the skin.

palm [L *palma*], the lower side of the hand, between the wrist and the bases of the fingers, when the hand is held horizontal with the thumb in medial position. –**palmar,** *adj.*

palm and sole system of identification, a method of identifying individuals by the patterns of ridges in the skin of the palms and soles. Like fingerprints, the patterns are helpful in identification of infants, cadavers, and unconscious persons.

palmar aponeurosis [L *palma* + Gk *apo* from, *neuron* nerve], fascia surrounding the muscles of the palm.

palmar crease, a normal groove across the palm.

palmar erythema, an inflammatory redness of the palms.

palmar fascia. See **palmar aponeurosis.**

palmar grasp reflex [L *palma* + ONor *grapa* grab], a flexion of the fingers caused by stimulation of the palm of the hand. The reflex is present at birth and usually disappears by the age of 6 months.

palmaris longus /pəlmer′is/, a long, slender, superficial, fusiform muscle of the forearm. It functions to flex the hand.

palmar metacarpal artery, one of several arteries arising from the deep palmar arch, supplying the fingers.

palmar pinch, a thumbless grasp in which the tips of the other fingers are pressed against the palm.

palmar reflex, a reflex that curls the fingers when the palm is tickled.

palmature /pal′məchər/ [L *palma*], an abnormal condition in which the fingers are webbed.

palm-chin reflex. See **palmomental reflex.**

palmitic acid, a saturated fatty acid that commonly occurs in animal and vegetable fats and oils. It is used in the manufacture of soaps and candles.

palmityl alcohol. See **cetyl alcohol.**

palmomental reflex /pal′məmen′təl/ [L *palma* + *mentum* chin; *reflectere* to bend backward], an abnormal neurologic sign, elicited by scratching the palm at the base of the thumb, characterized by contraction of the muscles of the chin and corner of the mouth on the same side of the body as the stimulus.

palpable /pal′bəbə/ [L *palpare* to touch gently], perceivable by touch.

palpate /pal′pāt/, to use the hands or fingers to examine.

palpation [L *palpare* to touch gently], a technique used in physical examination in which the examiner feels the texture, size, consistency, and location of certain parts of the body with the hands.

palpatory percussion [L *palpare* to touch gently; *percutere* to strike hard], a technique in physical examination in which the vibrations produced by percussion are evaluated by using light pressure of the flat of the examiner's hand.

palpebra. See **eyelid.**

palpebral commissure. See **canthus.**

palpebral conjunctiva. See **conjunctiva.**

palpebral fissure /pal′pəbrəl/ [L *palpebra* eyelid; *fissura* cleft], the opening between the margins of the upper and lower lids.

palpebral gland. See **meibomian gland.**

palpebrae superior, *pl.* **palpebrae superiores,** the upper eyelid, larger and more movable than the lower eyelid and furnished with an elevator muscle.

palpebrate /pal′pəbrāt/, 1. to wink or blink. 2. having eyelids.

palpitate /pal′pitāt/ [L *palpitare* to flutter], to pulsate rapidly, as an unusually fast beating of the heart under various conditions of stress and in patients with certain heart disorders.

palpitation [L *palpitare* to flutter], a pounding or racing of the heart, associated with normal emotional responses or with certain heart disorders.

PALS, abbreviation for **pediatric advanced life support.**

palsy /pôl′zē/ [Gk *para* beyond, *lysis* loosening], an abnormal condition characterized by paralysis.

Paltauf's dwarf. See **pituitary dwarf.**

Paltauf's nanism /päl′toufs/ [Arnold Paltauf, Czechoslovakian physician, b. 1860; Gk *nanos* dwarf], dwarfism associated with excessive production or growth of lymphoid tissue.

PAMP, abbreviation for *pulmonary arterial mean pressure.*

pampiniform /pampin′ifôrm/, having the shape of a tendril.

pampiniform body. See **epoophoron.**

pampiniform plexus [L, *pampinus,* vine tendril; *plexus, plaited*], a network of veins in the spermatic cord that drains the testes into the testicular vein in the lower abdomen.

panacea /pan′əsē′ə/ [Gk *pan* all, *akeia* remedy], 1. a universal remedy. 2. an ancient name for an herb or a liquid potion with healing properties.

panacinar emphysema /panas′ənər/ [Gk *pan* + L *acinus* grape; Gk *en* in, *physema* blowing], a form of emphysema that affects all lung areas by causing dilation and atrophy of the alveoli and by destroying the vascular bed of the lung.

panarteritis /panär′tərī′tis/ [Gk *pan* + *arteria* artery, *itis*], an inflammation that involves all the tissue layers of an artery.

panarthritis /panärthrī′tis/ [Gk *pan* + *arthron* joint], an abnormal condition characterized by the inflammation of many joints of the body. **–panarthritic,** *adj.*

pancake kidney [ME *panne* pan, *kaka* cake; *kidnere*], a congenital anomaly in which the left and right kidneys are fused into a single mass in the pelvis. The fused kidney has two collecting systems and two ureters.

pancarditis /pankärdī′tis/ [Gk *pan* + *kardia* heart, *itis* inflammation], an abnormal condition characterized by inflammation of the entire heart, including the endocardium, myocardium, and pericardium.

Pancoast's syndrome /pan′cōsts/ [Henry K. Pancoast, American radiologist, b. 1875], **1.** a combination of various signs associated with a tumor in the apex of the lung. The signs include neuritic pain in the arm, an x-ray shadow at the apex of the lung, atrophy of the muscles of the arm and hand, and Horner's syndrome. **2.** an abnormal condition caused by osteolysis in the posterior part of one or more ribs, sometimes involving associated vertebrae.

Pancoast's tumor. See **pulmonary sulcus tumor.**

pancolectomy /pankōlek′təmē/ [Gk *pan* + *kolon* colon, *ektome* excision], excision of the entire colon, requiring also an ileostomy.

pancreas /pan′krē·əs/ [Gk *pan* all, *kreas* flesh], a fish-shaped, grayish pink, nodular gland that stretches transversely across the posterior abdominal wall in the epigastric and hypochondriac regions and secretes various substances, such as digestive enzymes, insulin, and glucagon. A compound racemose gland composed of exocrine and endocrine tissue, it contains a main duct that runs the length of the organ, draining smaller ducts and emptying into the duodenum. **–pancreatic,** *adj.*

pancreas scan, an x-ray scan of the pancreas after the intravenous injection of a radioactive contrast medium, used for detecting various abnormalities, such as tumors, cysts, and infections.

pancreatectomy /pan′krē·ətek′təmē/ [Gk *pan, kreas* + *ektome* excision], the surgical removal of all or part of the pancreas, performed to excise a cyst or tumor, treat pancreatitis, or repair trauma.

pancreatic cancer /pan′krē·at′ik/ [Gk *pan, kreas* + L *crab*], a malignant neoplastic disease of the pancreas, characterized by anorexia, flatulence, weakness, dramatic weight loss, epigastric or back pain, jaundice, pruritus, a palpable abdominal mass, the recent onset of diabetes, and clay-colored stools if the pancreatic ducts are obstructed. Insulin-secreting tumors of islet cells cause hypoglycemia, especially in the morning. Nonfunctioning islet cell lesions produce gastrin, causing symptoms of peptic ulcer or in some cases acute diarrhea and hypokalemia, and achlorhydria due to the lesion's elaboration of secretin.

pancreatic diabetes, diabetes mellitus due to a deficiency of insulin production by the islet cells of the pancreas.

pancreatic diverticulum, one of a pair of membranous pouches arising from the embryonic duodenum.

pancreatic dornase, an enzyme from beef pancreas that has been used as a mucolytic for upper respiratory infections and cystic fibrosis.

pancreatic duct, the primary secretory channel of the pancreas.

pancreatic enzyme, any one of the enzymes secreted by the pancreas during digestion. The most important are trypsin, chymotrypsin, steapsin, and amylopsin.

pancreatic hormone, any one of several chemical compounds, secreted by the pancreas, associated with the regulation of cellular metabolism. Major hormones secreted by the pancreas are insulin, glucagon, and pancreatic polypeptide.

pancreatic insufficiency, a condition characterized by the inadequate production and secretion of pancreatic hormones or enzymes, usually occurring secondary to a disease process destructive of pancreatic tissue. Nutritional malabsorption, anorexia, poorly localized upper abdominal or epigastric pain, malaise, and severe weight loss often occur.

pancreatic juice, the fluid secretion of the pancreas, produced by the stimulation of food in the duodenum. The juice is essential in breaking down proteins to their amino acid components, in reducing dietary fats to glycerol and fatty acids, and in converting starch to simple sugars.

pancreaticolienal **(pancreaticosplenic) node** /pan′krē·at′ikōlī·ē′nəl/ [Gk *pan, kreas* + L *lien* spleen; *nodus* knot], one of several masses of lymph tissue that accompany the splenic artery and are related to the posterosuperior border of the pancreas. They receive lymph from the stomach, spleen, duodenum, liver, and pancreas.

pancreatin /pan′krē·atin′/, a concentrate

of pancreatic enzymes from swine or beef cattle. It is prescribed as an aid to digestion to replace endogenous pancreatic enzymes in cystic fibrosis and after pancreatectomy.

pancreatitis /pan'krē·ətī'tis/ [Gk *pan, kreas* + *itis* inflammation], inflammation of the pancreas that may be acute or chronic. **Acute pancreatitis** is generally the result of damage to the biliary tract, as by alcohol, trauma, infectious disease, or certain drugs. It is characterized by severe abdominal pain radiating to the back, fever, anorexia, nausea, and vomiting. There may be jaundice if the common bile duct is obstructed. **Chronic pancreatitis** is generally the result of agents similar to those that cause the acute form. When the etiology is alcohol abuse, there may be calcification and scarring of the smaller pancreatic ducts. Abdominal pain, nausea, and vomiting, as well as steatorrhea and creatorrhea, may be due to the diminished output of pancreatic enzymes.

pancreatoduodenectomy /pan'krē·ā'tō-dōō'ōdənek'təmē/ [Gk *pan, kreas* + L *duoden* twelve each; Gk *ektome* excision], a surgical procedure in which the head of the pancreas and the loop of duodenum that surrounds it are excised.

pancreatography /pan'krē·ə·stog'rəfē/ [Gk *pan, kreas* + *graphein* to record], visualization of the pancreas and its ducts by means of x rays and contrast medium injected into the ducts at surgery, by an endoscope, or by ultrasonography, computed tomography, or radionuclide imaging.

pancreatolith /pankrē·at'əlith/, a stone or calculus in the pancreas.

pancuronium bromide /pankyərō'nē·əm/, a skeletal muscle relaxant prescribed as an adjunct to anesthesia and mechanical ventilation.

pancytopenia /pan'sītəpē'nē·ə/ [Gk *pan* + *kytos* cell, *penia* poverty], a marked reduction in the number of the red blood cells, white blood cells, and platelets. **–pancytopenic,** *adj.*

pandemia /pandē'mē·ə/ [Gk, *pan,* all + *demos,* people], a disease epidemic that affects all or most of a population group.

pandemic /pandem'ik/ [Gk *pan* + *demos* the people], (of a disease) occurring throughout the population.

pandiastolic /pandī'əstol'ik/ [Gk *pan* + *dia* through, *stellein* to set], of or pertaining to the complete diastole.

panencephalitis /pan'ensef'əlī'tis/ [Gk *pan* + *enkephale* brain, *itis*], inflammation of the entire brain. It is characterized by an insidious onset, a progressive course with deterioration of motor and mental functions, and evidence of a viral cause.

Subacute sclerosing panencephalitis is an uncommon childhood disease thought to be caused by a "slow" latent measles virus after recovery from a previous infection. It results in ataxia, myoclonus, atrophy, cortical blindness, and mental deterioration. **Rubella panencephalitis,** a rare disease of adolescents, follows a chronic progressive course marked by motor and mental deterioration. It sometimes resembles juvenile paresis.

panendoscope [Gk *pan* + *endon* within, *skopein* to look], a cystoscope that allows a wide view of the interior of the bladder.

panesthesia /panesthē'zhə/ [Gk *pan* + *aisthesis* feeling], the total sensations experienced by an individual at one time.

pangenesis /panjen'əsis/ [Gk *pan* + *genesis* origin], a darwinian theory that every cell and particle of the parent reproduces itself in the progeny.

panhypopituitarism /panhī'pōpit͞oo'itəriz'əm/ [Gk *pan* + *hypo* under, *pituita* phlegm], generalized insufficiency of pituitary hormones, resulting from damage to or deficiency of the gland. **Prepubertal panhypopituitarism,** a rare disorder usually associated with a suprasellar cyst or craniopharyngioma, is characterized by dwarfism with normal body proportions, subnormal sexual development, and insufficient thyroid and adrenal function. **Postpubertal panhypopituitarism** may be caused by postpartum pituitary necrosis, resulting from thrombosis of pituitary circulation during or after delivery. Characteristic signs of the disorder are failure to lactate, amenorrhea, weakness, cold intolerance, lethargy, and loss of libido and of axillary and pubic hair.

panhysterectomy /pan'histərek'təmē/ [Gk *pan* + *hystera* uterus, *ektome* excision], complete surgical removal of the uterus and cervix.

panic, an intense, sudden, and overwhelming fear or feeling of anxiety that produces terror and immediate physiologic changes resulting in paralyzed immobility or senseless and hysteric behavior.

panic attack [Gk *panikos* of the god Pan; Fr *attaquer*], an episode of acute anxiety that occurs unpredictably with feelings of intense apprehension or terror accompanied by dyspnea, dizziness, sweating, trembling, and chest pain or palpitations. The attack may last several minutes and recur in certain situations.

panic disorder. See **anxiety attack.**

panivorous /paniv'ərəs/ [L *panis* bread, *vorare* to devour], of or pertaining to the practice of subsisting exclusively on bread. **–panivore,** *n.*

panlobular emphysema. See **panacinar emphysema.**

Panner's disease, a rare form of osteochondrosis in which there is abnormal bony growth in the capitulum of the humerus.

panniculitis /pənik'yəlī'tis/ [L *panniculus* piece of cloth; Gk *itis* inflammation], a chronic inflammation of subcutaneous fat in which the skin becomes hardened, particularly over the abdomen and thorax. Small subcutaneous masses of hard tissue are found in the affected areas.

panniculus /pənik'yələs/, *pl.* **panniculi** [L, small garment], a membranous layer, the many sheets of fascia covering various structures in the body.

pannus /pan'əs/ [L, cloth], an abnormal condition of the cornea in which it becomes vascularized and infiltrated with granular tissue just beneath the surface.

panography, a method of tomography that visualizes curved surfaces of the body at any depth. In dentistry this is accomplished by roentgenography of the maxillary and mandibular dental arches and associated structures by using two axes of rotation to record these structures. An intensifying screen cassette with a 5 × 12 inch film rotates on a drum at the same rate as the radiation unit rotates around the patient's head to record the structures.

panophthalmitis /pan'ofthalmī'tis/ [Gk *pan* + *ophthalmos* eye, *itis*], inflammation of the entire eye, usually caused by virulent pyogenic organisms, such as strains of meningococci, pneumococci, streptococci, anthrax bacilli, and clostridia. Initial symptoms are pain, fever, headache, drowsiness, edema, and swelling. As the infection progresses, the iris appears muddy and gray, the aqueous humor becomes turbid, and precipitates form on the posterior surface of the cornea.

panoramic radiograph [Gk, *pan* + *horama* view; L *radiare* to shine; Gk *graphein* to record], a method of tomography for visualization of curved surfaces in the body, such as the upper and lower jaws, on a single film.

panphobia /panfō'bē-ə/ [Gk *pan* + *phobos* fear], an anxiety disorder characterized by irrational and vague fear or apprehension of some pervading or unknown evil; a generalized fear. **–panophobic,** *adj.*

pansystolic /pansistol'ik/, of or pertaining to the entire systole.

pansystolic murmur. See **systolic murmur.**

panthenol /pan'thənôl/, an alcohol converted in the body to pantothenic acid, a vitamin in the B complex group.

panting [Fr *panteler* to gasp], a ventilatory pattern characterized by rapid and shallow breathing with small tidal volume.

pantograph /pan'təgraf'/, **1.** a jointed device for copying a plane figure to any desired scale. **2.** a device that incorporates a pair of facebows fixed to the jaws and is used for inscribing centrically related points and arcs leading to the bows on segments relatable to the three craniofacial planes.

pantomography /pan'təmog'rəfē/ [Gk *pan* + *graphein* to record], panoramic radiography for obtaining radiographs of the maxillary and mandibular dental arches and related structures.

pantothenic acid /pan'təthen'ik/, a member of the B vitamin complex. It is widely distributed in plant and animal tissues and may be an important element in human nutrition.

pantothenyl alcohol. See **panthenol.**

papain /pəpā'ēn/, an enzyme from the fruit of *Carica papaya,* the tropic melon tree. It has been prescribed for enzymatic debridement of wounds and promotion of healing.

Papanicolaou test /pap'ənikəlou'/ [George N. Papanicolaou, American physician, b. 1883], a simple smear method of examining stained exfoliative cells. It is used most commonly to detect cancers of the cervix, but it may be used for tissue specimens from any organ. A smear (**Pap smear**) is often obtained during a routine pelvic examination. The findings are usually reported descriptively and grouped as follows: Class I, only normal cells seen; Class II, atypical cells consistent with inflammation; Class III, mild dysplasia; Class IV, severe dysplasia, suspicious cells; Class V, carcinoma cells seen.

papaverine hydrochloride /papav'ərēn/, a smooth muscle relaxant prescribed in the treatment of cardiovascular or visceral spasms.

paper chromatography [Gk *papyros* papyrus], the separation of a mixture into its components by filtering through a strip of special paper.

paper-doll fetus. See **fetus papyraceus.**

paper radioimmunosorbent test (PRIST), a technique for determining total IgE levels in patients with type I hypersensitivity reactions.

papilla /pəpil'ə/, *pl.* **papillae** [L, nipple], **1.** a small nipple-shaped projection, such as the conoid papillae of the tongue and the papillae of the corium that extend from collagen fibers, the capillary blood vessels, and sometimes the nerves of the dermis. **2.** the optic papilla, a round white disc in the fundus oculi that corresponds to the entrance of the optic nerve.

P

papilla duodeni major. See **hepatopancreatic ampulla.**

papilla of Vater. See **hepatopancreatic ampulla.**

papillary /pap'ələrē/ [L *papilla* nipple], of or pertaining to a papilla.

papillary adenocarcinoma, a malignant neoplasm characterized by small papillae of vascular connective tissue covered by neoplastic epithelium that projects into follicles, glands, or cysts.

papillary adenocystoma lymphomatosum, an unusual tumor, consisting of epithelial and lymphoid tissues, that develops in the area of the parotid and submaxillary glands.

papillary adenoma, a benign epithelial tumor in which the membrane lining the glandular tissue forms papillary processes that project into the alveoli or grow out of the surface of a cavity.

papillary carcinoma, a malignant neoplasm characterized by fingerlike projections.

papillary duct, one of the thousands of straight collecting tubules that descend through the medulla of the kidney and join with others to form the common ducts opening into the renal papillae.

papillary muscle, one of the rounded or conical muscular projections attached to the chordae tendineae in the ventricles of the heart. The papillary muscles help open and close the atrioventricular valves.

papillary tumor. See **papilloma.**

papillate /pap'ilit/, marked by papillae or nipplelike prominences.

papilledema /pap'ilədē'mə/, *pl.* **papilledemas, papilledemata** [L *papilla* + Gk *oidēma* swelling], swelling of the optic disc caused by increased intracranial pressure. The meningeal sheaths that surround the optic nerves from the optic disc are continuous with the meninges of the brain; therefore, increased intracranial pressure is transmitted forward from the brain to the optic disc in the eye to cause the swelling.

papilliform, shaped like a papilla.

papillitis /pap'ili'tis/ [L *papilla* + Gk *itis* inflammation], **1.** inflammation of a papilla, such as the lacrimal papilla. **2.** inflammation of a renal papilla.

papilloma /pap'ilō'mə/ [L *papilla* + Gk *ōma* tumor], a benign epithelial neoplasm characterized by a branching or lobular tumor.

papillomacarcinoma /pap'ilōkär'sinō'mə/ [L *papilla* + Gk *ōma* tumor, *karkinos* crab, *ōma* tumor], a wartlike cancer that grows inward into a cavity or outward from a surface.

papillomatosis /pap'ilōmətō'sis/ [L *papilla* + Gk *ōma* tumor, *osis* abnormal process], an abnormal condition characterized by widespread development of nipplelike growths.

papillomatosis coronae penis. See **hirsutoid papilloma of the penis.**

papillomavirus /pap'ilōməvī'rəs/ [L *papilla* + Gk *ōma* tumor; L *virus* poison], the virus that causes warts in humans.

papilloretinitis /pap'ilōret'inī'tis/ [L *papilla* + *rete* net; Gk *itis* inflammation], inflammatory occlusion of a retinal vein.

papovavirus /pap'əvəvī'rəs/ [(acronym) *pa*pilloma, *po*lyoma, *va*cuolating, *virus*], one of a group of small DNA viruses, some of which may be potentially cancer producing. The human wart is caused by a papovavirus. Kinds of papovaviruses are **papilloma papovavirus, polyoma papovavirus,** and **SV-40 papovavirus.**

pappataci fever. See **phlebotomus fever.**

pappus /pap'əs/ [Gk *pappos* little bird], the first growth of beard, characterized by downy hairs.

Pap smear [George N. Papanicolaou; ME *smere* grease], *(informal).* a specimen of exfoliated, epithelial cells and cervical mucus collected during a pelvic exam for cytologic evaluation according to the Papanicolaou cytologic classification.

Pap test. See **Papanicolaou test.**

papular scaling disease /pap'yələr/ [L *papula* pimple; AS *scealu*], any of a group of skin disorders in which there are discrete, raised, dry, scaly lesions. Some kinds of papular scaling diseases are **lichen planus, pityriasis rosea,** and **psoriasis.**

papulation /pap'yəlā'shən/ [L *papula* pimple, *atus* process], the development of papules.

papule /pap'yōol/ [L *papula* pimple], a small, solid, raised skin lesion less than 1 cm in diameter, such as the lesions of lichen planus and nonpustular acne. **–papular,** *adj.*

papulosquamous /pap'yələskwä'məs/ [L *papula* + *squama* scale], pertaining to a skin eruption that is both papular and scaly.

papulosquamous disease. See **papular scaling disease.**

papyraceous /pap'irā'shəs/ [Gk *papyros* paper], having a paperlike quality.

papyraceous fetus. See **fetus papyraceus.**

Paquelin's cautery /pak'əlinz/ [Claude A. Paquelin, French physician, b. 1836; Gk *kautērion* branding iron], a cauterizing device consisting of a platinum loop through which a heated hydrocarbon is passed.

par, a pair, specifically a pair of cranial

nerves, as the par nonum or the ninth pair.

PAR, abbreviation for **pulmonary arteriolar resistance.**

para [L *parere* to bear], **1.** pertaining to a woman who has produced a viable infant regardless of whether the child was alive or stillborn. The term is used with numerals to indicate the number of pregnancies carried to term or more than 20 weeks, such as para 2, indicating two pregnancies, regardless of the number of offspring produced in a single pregnancy. **2.** (in chemistry). linked to carbon atoms on opposite sides of the benzene ring.

paraaminobenzoic acid (PABA) /per'ə-amē'nōbenzō'ik/, a substance often occurring in association with B complex vitamin, found in cereals, eggs, milk, and meat and present in detectable amounts in blood, urine, spinal fluid, and sweat. It is widely used as a sunscreen.

paraaminohippuric acid /per'ə-amē'nōhipŏŏr'ik/ **(PAHA, PHA),** the *N*-acetic acid of paraaminobenzoic acid. Its sodium salt is used for measuring the effective renal plasma flow and for determining kidney function.

paraaminosalicylic acid /per'ə-amē'nōsal'isil'ik/ **(PAS, PASA),** a bacteriostatic agent prescribed for the treatment of pulmonary and extrapulmonary tuberculosis.

parabiotic syndrome /per'əbī-ot'ik/ [Gk *para* beside, *bios* life; *syn* together, *dromos* course], a blood transfer condition that can occur between identical twin fetuses because of placental vascular anastomoses. One twin may become anemic and the other plethoric.

paracentesis /per'əsentē'sis/ [Gk *para* + *kentesis* puncturing], a procedure in which fluid is withdrawn from a cavity of the body. Paracentesis is most commonly performed to remove excessive accumulations of ascitic fluid from the abdomen.

paracentesis thoracis [Gk *para* + *kentesis; thorax* chest], the aspiration of fluid or air, or both, through a needle inserted into the pleural cavity.

paracentral /per'əsen'trəl/, close to a center or a central part.

paracervical /per'sur'vikəl/ [Gk *para* + L *cervix* neck], adjacent to the cervix.

paracervical block, a form of regional anesthesia in which a local anesthetic is injected into the area on each side of the uterine cervix that contains the plexus of nerves innervating the uterine cervix. Effective anesthesia for active labor is often achieved.

paracetamol. See **acetaminophen.**

parachute reflex, a variation of the **Moro** or **startle reflex,** wherein an infant is tested for motor nerve development by being dropped gently onto a soft surface from a supine position. If the motor nerve development is normal, the infant at 9 months will first extend and then draw in its arms, hands, and fingers on both sides of the body in a protective movement.

paracoccidioidomycosis /per'əkoksid'-ē-oi'dōmīkō'sis/ [Gk *para* + *kokkos* berry, *eidos* form, *mykes* fungus, *osis* abnormal process], a chronic, occasionally fatal, fungal infection caused by *Paracoccidioides brasiliensis,* characterized by ulcers of the oral cavity, larynx, and nose. Other effects include large, draining lymph nodes, cough, dyspnea, weight loss, and skin, genital, and intestinal lesions. The disease is acquired by inhalation of spores of the fungus.

paradichlorobenzene poisoning. See **naphthalene poisoning.**

paradidymal /per'ədid'iməl/ [Gk *para* + *epi* above, *didymos* twin] **1.** pertaining to the paradidymis. **2.** beside the testis.

paradidymis /per'ədid'imis/, *pl.* **paradidymides** /per'ədidim'idēz/ [Gk *para* + *epi* above, *didymos* twin], a rudimentary structure in the male, situated on the spermatic cord of the epididymis, that consists of the vestigial caudal part of the embryonic mesonephric tubules. A similar structure, the paroophoron, is found in the female.

paradigm /per'ədīm, per'ədim/, a pattern that may serve as a model or example.

paradoxic /per'ədok'sik/ [Gk *paradoxos* strange], pertaining to a person, situation, statement, or act that may appear to have inconsistent or contradictory qualities or that may be true but appear absurd or unbelievable.

paradoxical breathing [Gk *paradoxos; AS braeth*], a condition in which a part of the lung deflates during inspiration and inflates during expiration. The condition usually is associated with a chest trauma, such as an open chest wound or rib cage damage.

paradoxical bronchospasm, a constriction of the airways after treatment with a sympathomimetic bronchodilator.

paradoxical incontinence. See **retention with overflow.**

paradoxical intention, a therapeutic technique that encourages a patient to do what he or she fears and, if possible, exaggerate it to the point of humor. It is used in the treatment of phobias.

paradoxical pulse. See **pulsus paradoxus.**

paraffin /per'əfin/ [L, *paraum,* little + *affinis,* related], any of a group of hydrocarbons or hydrocarbon mixtures of the paraffin series as indicated by the formula

$C_nH_{(2n+2)}$. Examples include methane gas and kerosene.

paraffin bath [L *parum* too little, *affinus* related], the application of heat to a specific area of the body through the use of paraffin. The part is quickly immersed in heated liquid wax and then withdrawn so the wax solidifies to form an insulating layer. The procedure is repeated until the layer is 5 to 10 mm thick, and then the entire area is wrapped in an insulating fabric. The technique is effective for heating traumatized or inflamed areas, especially the hands, feet, and wrists, and is used primarily for patients with arthritis and rheumatism.

paraffin method, (in surgical pathology) a method used in preparing a selected portion of tissue for pathologic examination. The tissue is fixed, dehydrated, and infiltrated and then is embedded in paraffin, forming a block that is cut with a microtome into slices.

paraffin section, a histologic section cut from tissue that has been embedded in paraffin wax.

parafollicular C cell /per'əfolik'yəlɔr/, a calcitonin-secreting cell located between follicles.

paraganglion /per'əgang'glē·on/, *pl.* **paraganglia** [Gk *para* + *ganglion* knot], one of the small groups of chromaffin cells associated with the ganglia of a sympathetic nerve trunk and situated outside the adrenal medulla. The paraganglia secrete epinephrine and norepinephrine.

paragonimiasis /per'əgon'imī'əsis/ [Gk *para* + *gonimos* generative, *osis* abnormal process], chronic infection with the lung fluke *Paragonimus westermani*. It is characterized by hemoptysis, bronchitis, and occasionally abdominal masses, pain, and diarrhea, or by cerebral involvement with paralysis, ocular pathologic conditions, and seizures. The disease is acquired by ingesting cysts in infected freshwater crabs or crayfish, the intermediate hosts.

parahypnosis [Gk *para* + *hypnos* sleep], a form of disordered sleep that is observed in hypnosis and narcosis.

parainfluenza virus /per'ə·in'floo·en'zə/ [Gk *para* + It *influenza* influence], a myxovirus with four serotypes, causing respiratory infections in infants and young children and, less commonly, in adults. Type 1 and type 2 parainfluenza viruses may cause laryngotracheobronchitis or croup; type 3 is a cause of croup, tracheobronchitis, bronchiolitis, and bronchopneumonia in children; types 1, 3, and 4 are associated with pharyngitis and the common cold.

parakinesia /per'əkinē'zhə/ [Gk *para* + *ki-nesis* movement], an abnormality of movement due to a nerve disorder in a muscle, such as an irregularity of one of the ocular muscles.

parakinesis. See **telekinesis.**

paraldehyde /peral'dəhīd/, a clear, colorless, strong-smelling liquid obtained by the polymerization of acetaldehyde with a small amount of sulfuric acid. It is used as a solvent and may be administered orally, intravenously, intramuscularly, or rectally to induce hypnotic states or sedation.

parallax /per'əlaks/ [Gk *parallelos* side-by-side], the apparent displacement of an object at different distances from the eyes when viewed together. It is the basis of stereoscopic vision and depth perception.

parallel grid [Gk *parallelos* side-by-side; ME *gredire*], (in radiography) an x-ray grid that has lead strips oriented parallel to each other.

parallelogram condenser [Gk *parallelos* + *gramma* record; L *condensare* to make thick], (in dentistry) an instrument with a face shaped like a rectangle or parallelogram, used for compacting amalgams in filling teeth.

parallel play [Gk *parallelos* + AS *plegan* to play], a form of play among children, primarily toddlers, in which each engages in an independent activity that is similar to but not influenced by or shared with the others.

parallel talk, a form of speech used during children's play therapy in which the clinician verbalizes activities of the child without requiring answers to questions.

Paralympics /per'əlim'piks/, an acronym formed from *paraplegic* and *Olympics;* an international competitive wheelchair sports event, usually held in association with the official quadrennial Olympic Games.

paralysis /pəral'isis/, *pl.* **paralyses** [Gk *paralein* to be paralyzed], the loss of muscle function or sensation, or both. It may be caused by trauma, disease, or poisoning. Paralyses are classified according to cause, muscle tone, distribution, or the part of the body affected. **–paralytic,** *adj.*

paralysis agitans. See **Parkinson's disease.**

paralytic dementia. See **paresis.**

paralytic ileus [Gk *paralyein* to be paralyzed, *eilein* to twist], a decrease in or absence of intestinal peristalsis that may occur after abdominal surgery or peritoneal injury or in connection with severe pyelonephritis, ureteral stone, fractured ribs, myocardial infarction, extensive intestinal ulceration, heavy metal poisoning, porphyria, retroperitoneal hematomas (especially those associated with fractured vertebrae), or any severe metabolic disease. Paralytic ileus is characterized by abdominal tenderness and distention, absence of bowel sounds, lack of flatus, and attacks of nausea and vomiting. There may be fever, decreased urinary output, electrolyte imbalance, dehydration, and respiratory distress.

paralytic incontinence [Gk *paralyein;* L *incontinentia* inability to retain], urinary or fecal incontinence due to loss of or impaired motor nerve control of the sphincter muscles.

paralytic mydriasis, an area of depressed vision on the periphery of the field.

paralytic poliomyelitis, a flaccid paralysis of the limbs resulting from damaged lower motor neurons. Progressive bulbar paralysis with respiratory and vasomotor failure may result when the brainstem nuclei are involved.

paralytic shellfish poisoning. See **shellfish poisoning.**

paralytic stroke, a sudden attack of paralysis caused by disease or injury to the brain or spinal cord.

paralyze /per'əlīz/ [Gk *paralyein* to be paralyzed], **1.** to produce or enter into a state of paralysis. **2.** to cause loss of muscle power.

paramedic [Gk *para* + L *medicina* art of healing], a person who acts as an assistant to a physician or in place of a physician, especially a person in the military, trained in emergency medical procedures. **–paramedical,** *adj.*

paramedical personnel, health care workers other than physicians, dentists, podiatrists, and nurses who have special training in the performance of supportive health care tasks. Paramedical personnel includes, for example, the **emergency medical technician, audiologist,** and **x-ray technologist.**

paramesonephric duct /per'əmēz'ōnef'-rik/ [Gk *para* + *mesos* middle, *nephros* kidney], one of a pair of embryonic ducts that develop into the uterus and uterine tubes.

parameter /pəram'ətər/ [Gk *para* + *metron* measure] **1.** a value or constant used to describe or measure a set of data representing a physiologic function or system. **2.** a statistical value of a population group. **3.** *informal;* limits or boundary.

paramethadione /per'əmeth'ədī'ōn/, an anticonvulsant for the prevention of seizures in petit mal epilepsy.

paramethasone acetate /per'əmeth'əsōn/, a glucocorticoid in the treatment of inflammatory and allergic conditions.

parametric imaging [Gk *para* + *metron* measure; L *imago* image], (in nuclear medicine) a diagnostic procedure in which an image of an administered radioactive tracer is derived according to a mathematical rule, as by the division of one image by another.

parametric statistics, statistics that assume a population has a symmetric, such as gaussian or log normal, distribution.

parametritis /per'əmetrī'tis/ [Gk *para* + *metra* womb, *itis*], an inflammatory condition of the tissue of the structures around the uterus.

parametrium /per'əmē'trē·əm/, *pl.* **parametria** [Gk *para* + *metra* womb], the lateral extension of the uterine subserous connective tissue into the broad ligament.

paramitome. See **hyaloplasm.**

paramnesia /per'amnē'zhə/ [Gk *para* + *amnesia* forgetfulness], **1.** a perversion of memory in which one believes one remembers events and circumstances that never actually occurred. **2.** a condition in which words are remembered and used without the comprehension of their meaning.

paramyxovirus /per'əmik'sōvī'rəs/ [Gk *para* + *myxa* mucus; L *virus* poison], a member of a family of viruses which includes the organisms that cause parainfluenza, mumps, and some respiratory infections.

paranasal /per'ənā'zəl/ [Gk *para* + L *nasus* nose], situated near or alongside the nose, as the **paranasal sinuses.**

paranasal sinus, one of the air cavities in various bones around the nose, as the frontal sinus in the frontal bone lying deep to the medial part of the superciliary ridge and the maxillary sinus within the maxilla between the orbit, the nasal cavity, and the upper teeth.

paraneoplastic syndromes /per'ənē'ə-plas'tik/ [Gk *para* + *neos* new, *plassein* to mold, *syn* together, *dromos* course], indirect effects of a tumor that occur distant to a tumor or metastatic site. They may result from the production of active proteins, polypeptides, or inactive hormones by the tumor.

parangi. See **yaws.**

paranoia /per'ənoi'ə/ [Gk *para* + *nous* mind], (in psychiatry) a disorder characterized by an elaborate overly suspicious system of thinking, with delusions of persecution and grandeur usually centered on one major theme, such as a financial matter, a job situation, or an unfaithful spouse.

paranoiac /per'ənoi'ak/, **1.** a person afflicted with or exhibiting characteristics of paranoia. **2.** of or pertaining to paranoia.

paranoid /per'ənoid/ [Gk *para* + *nous* mind, *eidos* form], **1.** pertaining to or resembling paranoia. **2.** a person afflicted with a paranoid disorder. **3.** *informal;* a person, or pertaining to a person, who is overly suspicious or exhibits persecutory trends or attitudes.

paranoid disorder, any of a large group of mental disorders characterized by an impaired sense of reality and persistent delusions. Kinds of paranoid disorders include **acute paranoid disorder, paranoia,** and **shared paranoid disorder.**

paranoid ideation, an exaggerated, sometimes grandiose, belief or suspicion, usually not of a delusional nature, that one is being harassed, persecuted, or treated unfairly.

paranoid personality, a personality characterized by paranoia.

paranoid personality disorder, a disorder characterized by extreme suspiciousness and distrust of others to the degree that one blames them for one's mistakes and failures and goes to abnormal lengths to validate prejudices, attitudes, or biases.

paranoid reaction, a psychopathologic condition associated with aging and characterized by the gradual formation of delusions, usually of a persecutory nature and often accompanied by related hallucinations.

paranoid schizophrenia, a form of schizophrenia characterized by persistent preoccupation with illogical, absurd, and changeable delusions, usually of a persecutory, grandiose, or jealous nature, accompanied by related hallucinations.

paranoid state, a transitory abnormal mental condition characterized by illogical thought processes and generalized suspicion and distrust, with a tendency toward persecutory ideas or delusions.

paranormal [Gk *para* + L *normalis* rule], pertaining to phenomena that cannot be explained by normal scientific investigation.

paranuclear body. See **centrosome.**

paraoperative. See **perioperative.**

paraparesis /per'əpərē'sis/ [Gk *para* + *paresis* paralysis], a partial paralysis, usually affecting only the lower extremities.

paraperitoneal nephrectomy /per'əper'i-tənē'əl/ [Gk *para* + *peri, tenein* to stretch, *nephros* kidney, *ektome* cutting out], surgery to remove the kidney through an extraperitoneal incision.

parapertussis /per'əpərtus'is/ [Gk *para* + L *per* very, *tussis* cough], an acute bacterial respiratory infection caused by *Bordetella parapertussis,* having symptoms closely resembling those of pertussis. It is usually milder than pertussis, although it can be fatal.

parapharyngeal abscess /per'əfərin'jē-əl/ [Gk *para* + *pharynx* throat; L *abscedere* to go away], a suppurative infection of tissues adjacent to the pharynx, usually a complication of acute pharyngitis or tonsillitis. Infection may spread to the jugular vein, where it may cause thrombophlebitis and septic emboli.

paraphilia /per'əfil'yə/ [Gk *para* + *philein* to love], sexual perversion or deviation; a condition in which the sexual instinct is expressed in ways that are socially prohibited or unacceptable or are biologically undesirable, such as the use of an inanimate object for sexual arousal. Kinds of paraphilia include **exhibitionism, fetishism, pedophilia, transvestism, voyeurism,** and **zoophilia.** –**paraphiliac,** *adj., n.*

paraphimosis /per'əfimō'sis/ [Gk *para* + *phimoein* to muzzle], a condition characterized by an inability to replace the foreskin in its normal position after it has been retracted behind the glans penis. Caused by a narrow or inflamed foreskin, the condition may lead to gangrene. Circumcision may be required.

paraphrasia /per'əfrā'sē-ə/ [Gk *para* + *phrasein* to utter], speech that is incoherent, unintelligible, and apparently incomprehensible. However, the speech may be meaningful when carefully interpreted by a psychotherapist.

paraplasm /per'əplaz'əm/ [Gk *para* + *plassein* to mold], any abnormal growth or malformation. –**paraplasmic,** *adj.*

paraplastic [Gk *para* + *plassein* to mold], **1.** misshapen or malformed. **2.** showing abnormal formative power; of the nature of a paraplasm.

paraplegia /per'əplē'jē-ə/ [Gk *para* + *plege* stroke], an abnormal condition characterized by motor or sensory loss in the lower limbs. Approximately 11,000 spinal cord injuries reported each year in the United States involve paraplegia. Such injuries commonly occur as the result of automobile and motorcycle accidents, sporting accidents, falls, and gunshot wounds. Paraplegia less commonly results from nontraumatic lesions, such as scoliosis, spina bifida, and alcoholism. The signs and symptoms of paraplegia may develop immediately from trauma and include the loss of sensation, motion, and reflexes below the level of the lesion. Depending on the level of the lesion and whether damage to the spinal cord is complete or incomplete, the patient may lose bladder and bowel control and develop sexual dysfunctions. An incomplete spinal cord injury does not usually inhibit circumanal sensation, voluntary toe flexion, or sphincter control. **–paraplegic,** *adj., n.*

paraplegic, pertaining to a person affected by paraplegia or a condition resembling paraplegia.

parapraxia /per′əprak′sē·ə/ [Gk *para* + *praxis* doing], **1.** the abnormal performance of purposive actions, such as one movement occurring in place of another intended movement. **2.** forgetfulness with a tendency to misplace things.

paraprotein /per′əprō′tēn/, any of the incomplete monoclonal immunoglobulins that occur in plasma cell disorders.

parapsoriasis /per′əsərī′əsis/ [Gk *para* + *psorian* to itch], a group of chronic skin diseases resembling psoriasis, characterized by maculopapular, erythematous, scaly eruptions without systemic symptoms. Parapsoriasis is resistant to all treatment.

parapsychology [Gk *para* + *psyche* mind, *logos* science], a branch of psychology concerned with the study of alleged psychic phenomena, such as clairvoyance, extrasensory perception, and telepathy.

paraquat poisoning /per′əkwot′/ [Gk *para* + L *quaterni* four each; *potio* drink], a toxic condition caused by the ingestion of paraquat dichloride, a highly poisonous pesticide. Characteristically, progressive pulmonary fibrosis and damage to the esophagus, kidneys, and liver develop several days after ingestion. Once fibrosis begins, death is inevitable, usually within 3 weeks.

parasacral /per′əsā′krəl/, pertaining to the area around the sacrum.

parasite [Gk *parasitos* guest], an organism living in or on and obtaining nourishment from another organism. A **facultative parasite** may live on a host but is capable of living independently. An **obligate parasite** is one that depends entirely on its host for survival. **–parasitic,** *adj.*

parasitemia /per′əsītē′mē·ə/ [Gk *parasitos* + *haima* blood], the presence of parasites in the blood.

parasitic fetus [Gk *parasitos* + L *icus* like; *fetus* pregnant], the smaller, usually malformed member of conjoined, unequal, or asymmetric twins that is attached to and dependent on the more normal fetus for growth and development.

parasitic fibroma, a pedunculated uterine fibroid deriving part of its blood supply from the omentum.

parasitic glossitis, a mycosis of the tongue, characterized by a black or brown furry patch on the posterior dorsal surface composed of hypertrophied filiform papillae that measure about 1 cm in length and are easily broken.

parasitic hemoptysis [Gk *parasitos*; *haima* blood, *ptyein* to spit], the spitting of bright red blood due to a parasitic infection. The condition usually involves lung flukes *(Paragonimus)* or tapeworms *(Echinococcus).*

parasitism /per′əsitiz′əm/, an infestation or presence of parasites.

parasympathetic [Gk *para* + *sympathein* to feel with], of or pertaining to the craniosacral division of the autonomic nervous system, consisting of the oculomotor, facial, glossopharyngeal, vagus, and pelvic nerves. The actions of the parasympathetic division are mediated by the release of acetylcholine and primarily involve the protection, conservation, and restoration of body resources. Parasympathetic fibers slow the heart, stimulate peristalsis, promote the secretion of lacrimal, salivary, and digestive glands, induce bile and insulin release, dilate peripheral and visceral blood vessels, constrict the pupils, esophagus, and bronchioles, and relax sphincters during micturition and defecation.

parasympathetic ganglion [Gk *para* + *sympathein* to feel with, *ganglion* knot], a cluster of nerve cell bodies of the parasympathetic division of the autonomic nervous system. The nerves are functionally antagonistic to those of the sympathetic division.

parasympathetic nervous system. See **autonomic nervous system.**

parasympatholytic, parasympatholytic drug. See **anticholinergic.**

parasympathomimetic /per′əsim′pəthōmimet′ik/ [Gk *para* + *sympathein* to feel with, *mimesis* imitation], **1.** of or pertaining to a substance producing effects similar to those caused by stimulation of a parasympathetic nerve. **2.** an agent whose effects mimic those resulting from stimulation of parasympathetic nerves, especially the effects produced by acetylcholine.

parasympathomimetic drug. See **cholinergic.**

parasystole [Gk *para* + *systole* contraction], an independent ectopic rhythm whose pacemaker cannot be discharged by impulses of the dominant, usually sinus, rhythm because of an area of depressed conduction surrounding the parasystolic focus. In the classic parasystole, the interectopic intervals are exact multiples of a common denominator reflecting the protected status of the parasystolic focus.

parataxic distortion /per′ətak′sik/ [Gk *para* + *taxis* arrangement], a defense mechanism in which current interpersonal relationships are perceived and judged according to a mode of reference established by an earlier experience.

parataxic mode, a term introduced by H. S. Sullivan to identify a childhood perception of the physical and social environment as being illogical, disjointed, and inconsistent.

parathion poisoning /per′əthī′on/ [Gk *para* + *thio* phosphate, *on*; L *potio* drink], a toxic condition caused by the ingestion, inhalation, or absorption through the skin of the highly toxic organophosphorus insecticide parathion. Symptoms include nausea, vomiting, abdominal cramps, confusion, headache, lack of muscular control, convulsions, and dyspnea.

parathyroidectomy /per′əthī′roidek′təmē/ [Gk *para* + *thyreos* shield, *eidos* form; *ektome* cutting out], the surgical removal of the parathyroid gland.

parathyroid gland /per′əthī′roid/ [Gk *para* + *thyreos* shield, *eidos* form; L *glans* acorn], one of several small structures, usually four, attached to the dorsal surfaces of the lateral lobes of the thyroid gland. The parathyroid glands secrete parathyroid hormone, which helps maintain the level of blood calcium concentration and ensures normal neuromuscular irritability, blood clotting, and cell membrane permeability.

parathyroid hormone (PH), a hormone secreted by the parathyroid glands that acts to maintain a constant concentration of calcium in the extracellular fluid. The hormone regulates absorption of calcium from the GI tract, mobilization of calcium from the bones, deposition of calcium in the bones, and excretion of calcium in the breast milk, feces, sweat, and urine.

parathyroid injection, bovine parathyroid hormone prescribed to regulate blood levels of calcium, especially in the treatment of hypoparathyroidism with tetany.

parathyroid tetany [Gk *para* + *thyreos*; *tetanos* convulsive tension], a form of tetany that is caused by a deficiency of parathyroid secretion.

paratonia. See **gegenhalten.**

paratrooper fracture [Fr *parasol, troupe* company; L *fractura* break], a fracture of the distal tibia and its malleolus, commonly occurring when an individual jumps from an elevated platform and lands feet first on the ground, subjecting the ankles to extreme force.

paratyphoid fever /per′ətī′foid/ [Gk *para* + *typhos* stupor, *eidos* form; L *febris* fever], a bacterial infection, caused by any *Salmonella* species other than *S. typhi*, characterized by symptoms resembling typhoid fever, although somewhat milder.

paraurethral duct /per′əyŏŏrē′thrəl/ [Gk *para* + *ourethra* urethra; L *ducere* to lead], one of two ducts that drain the bulbourethral glands into the vestibule of the vagina.

paravaccinia virus /per′əvaksin′ē·ə/, a member of a subgroup of pox viruses that can infect humans through direct contact with infected livestock. It is related to the smallpox virus and is the cause of pseudocowpox.

paravertebral /per′əvur′təbrəl/ [Gk *para* + L *vertebra* joint], pertaining to the area alongside the spinal column or near a vertebra.

paravertebral block, 1. the blocking of transmission of somatic impulses by the spinal nerves by injecting a local analgesic solution near the point of their emergence. **2.** the blocking of the paravertebral sympathetic chain of nerves anteriolateral to the vertebral bodies.

paraxial /per′ə·ak′sē·əl/, pertaining to an organ or other structure located near the axis of the body.

parchment skin [Fr *parchemin*; AS *scinn*], thin, wrinkled or stretched atrophic skin.

paregoric /per′əgôr′ik/, a camphorated tincture of opium prescribed in the treatment of diarrhea and as an analgesic.

parenchyma /pəreng′kimə/ [Gk *para* + *enchyma* infusion], the tissue of an organ as distinguished from supporting or connective tissue.

parenchymal. See **parenchymatous.**

parenchymal cell /pəreng′kiməl/, any cell that is a functional element of an organ, such as a hepatocyte.

parenchymatous /per′əngkim′ətəs/, pertaining to or resembling the functional tissues of an organ or gland.

parenchymatous neuritis [Gk *para* + *enchyma* infusion; L *osus* like], any inflammation affecting the substance, axons, or myelin of the nerve.

parent [L *parens*], a mother or father; one who bears offspring. **–parental,** *adj.*

parental generation (P₁), the initial cross between two varieties in a genetic sequence; the parents of any individual, organism, or plant belonging to an F₁ generation.

parental grief, the behavioral reactions that characterize the grieving process and result in the resolution of the loss of a child from expected or unexpected death. Parental grieving begins with the discovery of the diagnosis of a life-threatening condition. The immediate reaction is shock and disbelief, followed by acute grief at the anticipation of losing the child. Periods of depression, anger, hope, fear, and anxiety alternate during induction therapy, remission, and maintenance of the disease as parents learn to accept and cope with the situation. In sudden, unexpected death, parents are denied the advantages of anticipatory grief and, because of the lack of time to prepare, usually have extreme feelings of guilt and remorse.

parental leave. See **Family care leave.**

parental role conflict, a NANDA-accepted nursing diagnosis of parental role confusion and conflict in response to crisis. Defining characteristics include an expression by the parent or parents of concerns or feelings of inadequacy to provide for the child's physical and emotional needs during hospitalization or in the home; a demonstrated disruption in caretaking routines; an expression of concerns about changes in parental role, family functioning, family communication, and family health; expressions of concern about perceived loss of control over decisions relating to the child and reluctance to participate in normal caretaking activities; and verbalized or demonstrated feelings of guilt, anger, fear, anxiety, and frustrations about the effect of the child's illness on the family process.

parent-child relationship. See **maternal-infant bonding.**

parent education, any educational experience geared toward the thoughtful conveyance of information enabling the parent to provide quality childrearing.

parent ego state, (in transactional analysis) a part of the self that offers advice like that of one's own parents, containing messages that emphasize what one "ought to" or "should not" do.

parenteral /pəren'tərəl/ [Gk *para* + *enteron* bowel], not in or through the digestive system. **–parenterally,** *adv.*

parenteral absorption, the taking up of substances within the body by structures other than the digestive tract.

parenteral dosage, pertaining to a medication administered by a route that bypasses the GI tract, such as a drug given by injection.

parenteral fluids. See **administration of parenteral fluids.**

parenteral hyperalimentation. See **total parenteral nutrition.**

parenteral nutrition, the administration of nutrients by a route other than through the alimentary canal, such as subcutaneously, intravenously, intramuscularly, or intradermally. The parenteral fluids usually consist of physiologic saline with glucose, amino acids, electrolytes, vitamins, and medications.

parent figure [L *parens* + *figura* form], **1.** a parent or a substitute parent or guardian who cares for a child, providing the physical, social, and emotional requirements necessary for normal growth and development. **2.** a person who symbolically represents an ideal parent, having those attributes believed as necessary for forming the perfect parent-child relationship.

parent image, a conscious and unconscious concept that a child forms concerning the roles and characteristics of the personality of the mother and father.

parenting, altered, a NANDA-accepted nursing diagnosis of changes in ability of nurturing figures to create an environment that promotes the optimum growth and development of another human being. Defining characteristics include an observed lack of actions that demonstrate attachment to the child; inattentiveness to the needs of the child; inappropriate caretaking behavior; a history of abuse or abandonment of the child; constant complaints about the sex or the appearance of the child; verbal self-assessment of inadequacy in the parental role; expressed disgust about the bodily functions of the child; failure to keep health care appointments for the child; inconsistent disciplinary practices; slow growth and development in the child; and an observed need for the parent to receive approval from others.

parenting, altered, high risk for, a NANDA-accepted nursing diagnosis of the possibility of changes in ability of nurturing figures to create an environment that promotes the optimum growth and development of another human being. Risk factors include lack of parental attachment behaviors; inappropriate visual, tactile, or auditory stimulation; negative identification or attachment of meanings to infant or child characteristics; verbalization of disappointment in or resentment toward the infant or child; noncompliance with health appointments; inappropriate caretaking behaviors; inappropriate or inconsistent discipline practices; history of child abuse or abandonment by primary caretaker; and multiple caretakers without consideration for the needs of the child.

Parents Anonymous, a self-help group for parents who have abused their children or who feel that they are prone to maltreat them.

Parents Without Partners, a self-help group for single parents, including those who are separated, divorced, or widowed.

parepididymis. See **paradidymis.**

paresis /pərē'sis, per'isis/ [Gk *paralyein* to be paralyzed], **1.** motor weakness or partial paralysis related in some cases to local neuritis. **2.** a late manifestation of neurosyphilis, characterized by generalized paralysis, tremulous incoordination, transient seizures, Argyll Robertson pupils, and progressive dementia caused by degeneration of cortical neurons. **–paretic,** *adj.*

paresthesia /per´esthē´zhə/ [Gk *para* + *erethizein* to excite], any subjective sensation, experienced as numbness, tingling, or "pins and needles." When experienced in the extremities, it is sometimes identified as acroparesthesia.

paretic /peret´ik/ [Gk, *paresis,* paralysis], pertaining to or resembling partial paralysis.

paretic dementia. See **paresis.**

pareunia. See **coitus.**

pargyline hydrochloride /per´jəlēn/, a monoamine oxidase (MAO) inhibitor used as an antihypertensive. It is prescribed in the treatment of moderate to severe hypertension.

paries /per´ə-ēz/, *pl.* **parietes** /pərī´itēz/, the wall of an organ or cavity in the body.

parietal /pərī´ətəl/ [L *paries* wall], **1.** of or pertaining to the outer wall of a cavity or organ. **2.** of or pertaining to the parietal bone of the skull, or the parietal lobe of the brain.

parietal bone, one of a pair of bones that form the sides of the cranium.

parietal cells, the cells on the periphery of the gastric glands of the stomach. They are located on the basement membrane beneath the chief cells and secrete hydrochloric acid.

parietal lobe, a portion of each cerebral hemisphere that occupies the parts of the lateral and the medial surfaces that are covered by the parietal bone.

parietal lymph node, one of the small oval glands that filter the lymph coursing through the lymphatic vessels in the walls of the thorax or through the lymphatic vessels associated with the larger blood vessels of the abdomen and the pelvis.

parietal pain, a sharp sensation of distress in the parietal pleura, aggravated by respiration and thoracic movements and caused by pneumonia, empyema, pneumothorax, asbestosis, tuberculosis, neoplasm, or the accumulation of fluid resulting from heart, liver, or kidney disease.

parietal pericardium, an outer layer of the serous pericardium that is not in direct contact with the heart muscle.

parietal peritoneum, the portion of the largest serous membrane in the body that lines the abdominal wall.

parietal pleura. See **parietal peritoneum.**

parietooccipital /pərī´ətō-oksip´itəl/ [L *paries* + *occiput* back of the head], of or pertaining to the parietal and the occipital bones or lobes.

parietooccipital sulcus, a groove on each cerebral hemisphere marking the division of the parietal and occipital lobes of the brain.

parietotemporal /pərī´ətotem´pərəl/ [L *paries* + *tempus* temple], pertaining to the temporal and parietal bones of the cranium.

Parinaud's syndrome /per´ənōz/ [Henri Parinaud, French ophthalmologist, b. 1844], a term often used to refer to conjunctivitis that is usually unilateral, follicular, and followed by enlargement of the preauricular lymph nodes and tenderness. The syndrome is frequently caused by infection with a species of the microorganism *Leptothrix.* It may also be associated with other infections, such as tularemia, cat-scratch fever, and lymphogranuloma venereum.

pari passu /per´ē pas´ o͞o/ [L *par* equal, *passus* step], at the same time or in equal proportions.

paritonsillar abscess. See **parapharyngeal abscess.**

parity [L *parere* to give birth], **1.** (in obstetrics) the classification of a woman by the number of live-born children and stillbirths she has delivered at more than 28 weeks of gestation. Commonly, parity is noted with the total number of pregnancies and represented by the letter *P* or the word *para.* A para 4 (P4) gravida 5 (G5) has had four deliveries after 28 weeks and one abortion or miscarriage before 28 weeks. **2.** (in epidemiology) the classification of a woman by the number of live-born children she has delivered.

parkinsonian [James Parkinson, English physician, b. 1755], pertaining to or resembling Parkinson's disease.

parkinsonian facies [Parkinson; L *facies* face], a masklike and immobile facial expression, usually occurring with Parkinson's disease. Infrequent blinking also occurs.

parkinsonian tremor [Parkinson; L *tremor* shaking], a mild resting tremor with slow, regular oscillations of three to six per second, exacerbated by fatigue, cold, or emotions. The tremors usually, but not always, cease during voluntary movement of the affected part and during sleep.

parkinsonism [James Parkinson], a neurologic disorder characterized by tremor, muscle rigidity, hypokinesia, a slow shuffling gait, difficulty in chewing, swallowing, and speaking, caused by various lesions in the extrapyramidal motor system.

Signs and symptoms of parkinsonism resemble those of idiopathic Parkinson's disease and may develop during or after acute encephalitis or in syphilis, malaria, poliomyelitis, and carbon monoxide poisoning. Parkinsonism frequently occurs in patients treated with antipsychotic drugs.

Parkinson's disease [James Parkinson], a slowly progressive, degenerative, neurologic disorder characterized by resting tremor, pill rolling of the fingers, a masklike facies, shuffling gait, forward flexion of the trunk, and muscle rigidity and weakness. It is usually an idiopathic disease of persons over 60 years of age, though it may occur in younger persons, especially after acute encephalitis or carbon monoxide or metallic poisoning. Typical pathologic changes are destruction of neurons in basal ganglia, loss of pigmented cells in the substantia nigra, and depletion of dopamine in the caudate nucleus, putamen, and pallidum. Signs and symptoms of Parkinson's disease, which include drooling, increased appetite, intolerance to heat, oily skin, emotional instability, and defective judgment, are increased by fatigue, excitement, and frustration. Intelligence is rarely impaired.

Parkinson's mask [Parkinson; Fr *masque*], an expressionless face with eyebrows raised, but immobility of the facial muscles.

paromomycin sulfate /per'əmōmī'sin/, an oral antiamebic aminoglycoside antibiotic prescribed in the treatment of intestinal amebiasis.

paronychia /per'ənik'ē·ə/ [Gk *para* + *onyx* nail], an infection of the fold of skin at the margin of a nail. Treatment includes hot compresses or soaks, antibiotics, and, possibly, surgical incision and drainage.

paroophoritis /per'ō·of'ərī'tis/ [Gk *para* + *oon* egg, *pherein* to bear, *itis*], 1. inflammation of the paroophoron. 2. inflammation of the tissues surrounding the ovary.

paroophoron /per'ō·of'əron/ [Gk *para* + *oon* egg, *pherein* to bear], a small vestigial remnant of the mesonephros, consisting of a few rudimentary tubules lying in the broad ligament between the epoophoron and the uterus. A similar vestigial structure, the aberrant ductule, is found in the male.

parosmia /pəroz'mē·ə/ [Gk *para* + *osme* smell], any dysfunction or perversion concerning the sense of smell.

parotid /pərot'id/ [Gk *para* + *ous* ear], near the ear.

parotid duct /pərot'id/ [Gk *para* + *ous* ear; L *ducere* to lead], a tubular canal, about 7 cm long, that extends from the anterior part of the parotid gland to the mouth.

parotidectomy /pərot'idek'təmē/ [Gk *para* + *ous, ektome* cutting out], the surgical removal of the parotid gland.

parotid gland [Gk *para* + *ous* ear; L *glans* acorn], one of the largest pair of salivary glands that lie at the side of the face just below and in front of the external ear. The main part of the gland is superficial, somewhat flattened, and quadrilateral and lies between the ramus of the mandible, the mastoid process, and the sternocleidomastoideus.

parotitis /per'ətī'tis/ [Gk *para* + *ous* ear, *itis* inflammation], inflammation or infection of one or both parotid salivary glands.

parous /per'əs/, having borne one or more viable offspring.

parovarian /per'ō'ver'ē·ən/ [Gk *para* + L *ovum* egg], pertaining to residual tissues in the area near the fallopian tubes and the ovary.

parovarium. See **epoophoron.**

paroxysm /per'əksiz'əm/ [Gk *paroxynein* to stimulate] 1. a marked, usually episodic increase in symptoms. 2. a convulsion, fit, seizure, or spasm. **–paroxysmal,** *adj.*

paroxysmal atrial tachycardia /per'əksis'məl/ [Gk *paroxynein* to stimulate], a period of very rapid heart beats that begins suddenly and ends abruptly.

paroxysmal cold hemoglobinuria (PCH), a rare autoimmune disorder characterized by hemolysis and hematuria, associated with exposure to cold.

paroxysmal cough [Gk *paroxysmos* irritation; AS *cohhetan* cough], a severe attack of coughing as may accompany whooping-cough, bronchiectasis, or a lung injury.

paroxysmal hemoglobinuria, the sudden passage of hemoglobin in urine, occurring after local or general exposure to low temperatures, as in paroxysmal cold hemoglobinuria.

paroxysmal labyrinthine vertigo. See **Ménière's disease.**

paroxysmal nocturnal dyspnea (PND), a disorder characterized by sudden attacks of respiratory distress, usually occurring after several hours of sleep in a reclining position, most commonly caused by pulmonary edema resulting from congestive heart failure. The attacks are often accompanied by coughing, a feeling of suffocation, cold sweat, and tachycardia with a gallop rhythm.

paroxysmal nocturnal hemoglobinuria (PNH), a disorder characterized by intravascular hemolysis and hemoglobinuria. It occurs in irregular episodes of several days' duration, especially at night.

The basic defect in the red blood cell is an unusual sensitivity to lysis by complement or a deficiency or absence of acetylcholinesterase. It is characterized by abdominal pain, back pain, and headache. Its course may be complicated by thrombotic episodes and by iron deficiency, caused by excessive loss of hemoglobin.

paroxysmal nodal tachycardia, a sudden onset and termination of a rapid heart beat due to a quick succession of discharges from an ectopic site in the area of the atrioventricular node.

paroxysmal supraventricular tachycardia, an ectopic rhythm in excess of 100 per minute and usually faster than 170 per minute that begins abruptly with a premature atrial or junctional beat and is supported by an AV nodal reentry mechanism or by an AV reentry mechanism involving an accessory pathway.

paroxysmal ventricular tachycardia, a sudden onset and termination of rapid heart beat due to a quick succession of discharges from an ectopic site in the ventricle.

parrot fever. See psittacosis.

parry fracture. See **Monteggia's fracture.**

pars /pärs/ [L, part], a part, such as the pars abdominalis esophagi.

pars fetalis. See **fetal placenta.**

part [L *pars*], a portion of a larger area, such as the condylar part of the occipital bone.

part. aeq. abbreviation for the Latin phrase, *partes aequales,* "in equal parts."

parthenogenesis /pär′thənōjen′əsis/ [Gk *parthenos* virgin, *genesis* origin], a type of nonsexual reproduction in which an organism develops from an unfertilized ovum, as in many lower animals. **–parthenogenetic, parthenogenic,** *adj.*

partial breech extraction. See **assisted breech.**

partial cleavage, mitotic division of only part of a fertilized ovum into blastomeres, usually the activated cytoplasmic portion surrounding the nucleus; restricted division.

partial crown, a restoration that replaces surfaces of a tooth.

partial denture, a dental prosthesis, either fixed or removable, used to replace one or more missing teeth. Kinds of partial dentures include **articulated, bridge, extension, fixed, fixed cantilever, removable, sectional,** and **unilateral.**

partial dislocation, the partial abnormal separation of the articular surface of a joint.

partial hospitalization program, an organizational entity that provides therapeutic services to patients who use only day or night hospital services or adult day health services, rather than regular inpatient hospitalization services.

partial involution. See **uterine subinvolution.**

partially edentulous arch, a dental arch in which one or more but not all natural teeth are missing.

partial placenta previa, placenta previa in which the placenta is implanted in the lower uterine segment and partially covers the internal os of the uterine cervix. As the cervix dilates in labor, the portion of the placenta that lies over the cervix is separated, causing bleeding from the villous spaces of the uterine wall.

partial pressure, the pressure exerted by any one gas in a mixture of gases or in a liquid, with the pressure directly related to the concentration of that gas and to the total pressure of the mixture. The concentration of oxygen in the atmosphere represents approximately 21% of the total atmospheric pressure, calculated at 760 mm Hg under standard conditions. Therefore, the partial pressure of atmospheric oxygen is about 160 mm Hg (760×0.21).

partial pressure of carbon dioxide, the portion of total blood gas pressure exerted by carbon dioxide. The normal pressures of carbon dioxide in arterial blood are 35 to 45 mm Hg; in venous blood, 40 to 45 mm Hg.

partial response, the condition in which the maximum decrease in treated tumor volume is at least 50% but less than 100%.

partial thromboplastin time (PTT), a test for detecting coagulation defects of the intrinsic system by adding activated partial thromboplastin to a sample of test plasma and to a control sample of normal plasma. The time required for the formation of a clot in test plasma is compared with that in the normal plasma. The normal PTT in plasma is 60 to 85 seconds after the addition to the plasma sample of partial thromboplastin reagent and ionized calcium.

particulate, pertaining to a minute discrete particle or fragment of a substance or material.

parts per million (PPM, ppm), the ratio of the concentration of one substance to the concentration of another, as a unit of solute dissolved in one million units of solvent. It may be further expressed in terms of weight-to-weight, volume-to-volume, or another relationship of units of measure.

parturient /pärt(y)o͞o′rē·ənt/ [L, *parturire,* to have labor pains], pertaining to the act of childbirth.

parturition /pär′tyŏŏrish′ən/ [L *parturire* to desire to bring forth], the process of giving birth.

parulis. See **gumboil.**

PAS, PASA, abbreviation for **paraaminosalicylic acid.**

Pascal's principle /poskul′, paskal′/ [Blaise Pascal, French scientist, b. 1623] /poskulz′/, (in physics) a law stating that a confined liquid transmits pressure applied to it from an external source equally in all directions. Pascal's principle provides the basis for all hydraulic devices.

passive [L *passivus*], pertaining to behavior that subordinates the individual's own interests to the demands of others.

passive-aggressive personality [L *passivus* + *aggressus* combative; *persona* character], a personality characterized by passivity and aggression in which forceful actions or attitudes are expressed in an indirect, nonviolent manner, such as pouting, obstructionism, procrastination, inefficiency, stubbornness, and forgetfulness.

passive-aggressive personality disorder, a disorder characterized by the indirect expression of resistance to occupational or social demands, resulting in persistent, pervasive ineffectiveness, lack of self-confidence, poor interpersonal relationships, and pessimism that can lead, in severe cases, to major depression, alcoholism, or drug dependence.

passive algolagnia. See **masochism.**

passive anaphylaxis. See **antiserum anaphylaxis.**

passive carrier, 1. a healthy person whose body carries the causal organisms of an infectious disease although the person has not contracted the disease and remains symptomless. **2.** a person who carries a gene associated with a hereditary trait although the trait is not expressed in the person.

passive congestion, an excessive amount of blood accumulation in an organ due to increased venous pressure.

passive-dependent personality [L *passivus* + Fr *dependre* to depend; L *persona* character], a personality characterized by helplessness, indecisiveness, and a tendency to cling to and seek support from others.

passive euthanasia. See **euthanasia.**

passive exercise, repetitive movement of a part of the body as a result of an externally applied force or the voluntary effort of the muscles controlling another part of the body.

passive expiration [L *passivus, expirare* to breathe out], normal expiration that occurs without direct muscular effort, as is the case in normal tidal breathing. The air is compressed from the lungs through recoil effect of elastic tissues of the chest and lungs.

passive immunity, a form of acquired immunity resulting from antibodies that are transmitted naturally through the placenta to a fetus or through the colostrum to an infant or artificially by injection of antiserum for treatment or prophylaxis.

passive incontinence, urine overflow that may occur when the bladder (musculus detrusor vesicae) is paralyzed and greatly distended.

passive lingual arch, an orthodontic appliance that may help maintain tooth space and dental arch length when bilateral primary molars are prematurely lost.

passive lung collapse, a condition of dyspnea, cough, and hemoptysis with pigmented cells due to an obstruction in blood flow from the lungs to the heart.

passive motion, involuntary motion caused by an external force, differentiated from active, voluntary muscular effort.

passive movement, the moving of parts of the body by an outside force without voluntary action or resistance by the individual.

passive play, play in which a person does not participate actively. For younger children such activity may include watching and listening to others, observing other children or animals, listening to stories, or looking at pictures.

passive recoil, the normal, quiet act of exhalation caused by the rebound effect of elastic tissue of the lungs, aided by the force of surface tension.

passive sensitization [L *passivus, sentire* to feel], a temporary form of sensitization induced by injecting serum from a sensitized human or animal.

passive smoking, the inhalation by nonsmokers of the smoke from other people's cigarettes, pipes, and cigars.

passive stretching, stretching that involves only noncontractile elements, such as ligaments. An example is during isometric exercises in which there is no range of motion of the body part involved.

passive symptom, a symptom that attracts little or no attention.

passive transfer test. See **Prausnitz-Küstner test.**

passive transport, the movement of small molecules across the membrane of a cell by diffusion. Passive transport is essential to various processes of metabolism, such as the intake of digestive products by the cells lining the intestines.

passive tremor, an involuntary trembling occurring when the person is at rest, one of the signs of Parkinson's disease.

P

passivity [L *passivus*], a mental state of being submissive, dependent, or inactive, as a form of maladaptation.

paste, a topical semisolid formulation containing a pharmacologically active ingredient in a fatty base, a viscous or mucilaginous base, or a mixture of starch and petrolatum.

Pasteur effect [Louis Pasteur], the inhibiting effect of oxygen on carbohydrate fermentation by living cells.

Pasteurella /pas'tərel'ə/ [Louis Pasteur, French bacteriologist, b. 1822], a genus of gram-negative bacilli or coccobacilli, including species pathogenic to humans and domestic animals. *Pasteurella* infections may be transmitted to humans by animal bites.

pasteurization [Louis Pasteur; Gk *izein* to cause], the process of applying heat, usually to milk or cheese, for a specified time to kill or retard the development of pathogenic bacteria. **–pasteurize,** *v.*

pasteurized milk [Louis Pasteur; Gk *izein* to cause; AS *moluc* milk], milk that has been treated by heat to destroy pathogenic bacteria. By law, pasteurization requires a temperature of 145° F to 150° F for not less than 30 minutes, followed by a temperature of 161° F for 15 seconds, followed by immediate cooling.

Pasteur, Louis (1822-1895) /pastŏŏr, pästœr'/, a French chemist who founded the "germ theory" of infection and developed the "pasteurization" process to kill pathogenic organisms in milk. Pasteur also developed several vaccines and pioneered the development of stereochemistry by separating mirror image isomers.

past health [ME *passen* to pass; AS *hoelth* sound body], (in a health history) an overall summary of the person's general health to date, including past injuries, allergies, surgical procedures, immunizations, hospitalizations, and obstetric and psychiatric history.

pastoral counseling department [L *pastor* shepherd], the hospital chaplaincy service.

past pointing [OFr *passer;* L *punctus* pricked], the inability to place a finger on another part of the body accurately, indicating a lack of coordination in voluntary movements.

Patau's syndrome. See **trisomy 13.**

patch [ME *pacche*], a small spot of surface tissue that differs from the surrounding area in color or texture or both and is not elevated above it.

patch test, a skin test for identifying allergens, especially those causing contact dermatitis. The suspected substance (food, pollen, animal fur) is applied to an adhesive patch that is placed on the patient's skin. Another patch, with nothing on it, serves as a control.

patella /pətel'ə/ [L, small dish], a flat, triangular bone at the front of the knee joint, having a pointed apex that attaches to the ligamentum patellae. **–patellar,** *adj.*

patellar bursa /pətel'ər/, any of fluid-filled connective tissue sacs around the kneecap. Kinds of patellar bursae include **infrapatellar, prepatellar,** and **suprapatella.**

patellar ligament [L *patella* + *ligare* to bind], the central portion of the common tendon of the quadriceps femoris. Its superficial fibers are continuous over the front of the patella with those of the tendon of the quadriceps femoris.

patellar reflex, a deep tendon reflex, elicited by a sharp tap on the tendon just distal to the patella, normally characterized by contraction of the quadriceps muscle and extension of the leg at the knee.

patellar tendon bearing-prosthesis (PTB), an ankle-foot orthosis (AFO) that provides prolonged stretch to the posterior leg musculature and may create extension force at the knee joint.

patellar tendon–bearing supracondylar socket (PTB/SC), a patellar tendon–bearing prosthesis with supracondylar (above a condyle) and suprapatellar (above the patella) suspension.

patellar tendon–bearing supracondylar/suprapatellar (PTBSC/SP) socket, a type of patellar-tendon below the knee (BK) bearing prosthesis with a socket that extends in front, medially, and laterally to accommodate both the patella and femoral condyles. The higher socket increases knee stability and a suspension strap is not required.

patellectomy /pat'əlek'təmē/, the surgical removal of the patella.

patency [L *patens* open], a state of being open or exposed.

patent /pā'tənt/ [L *patens* open], open and unblocked, such as a patent airway or a patent anus.

patent ductus arteriosus (PDA), an abnormal opening between the pulmonary artery and the aorta caused by failure of the fetal ductus arteriosus to close after birth. The defect, which is seen primarily in premature infants, allows blood from the aorta to flow into the pulmonary artery and to recirculate through the lungs, causing an increased workload on the left side of the heart and increased pulmonary vascular congestion and resistance.

patent medicine, a nonprescription drug available to the general public without a prescription. The ingredients and contraindications are usually listed on the label or wrapper.

paternal [L *paternus* father], pertaining to fatherhood, characteristic of a father, or related through a father.

paternal engrossment. See **bonding.**

paternity test, a test based upon genetic blood groups and used mainly to exclude the possibility that a particular man could be the father of a specific child. For example, a man with group AB blood could not be the father of a child with group O blood.

Paterson-Kelly syndrome [Donald R. Paterson, Welsh physician, b. 1863; Adam B. Kelly, Scottish physician, b. 1865], a condition of the digestive system associated with iron deficiency anemia, characterized by the development of esophageal webs in the upper esophagus, making swallowing of solids difficult.

Paterson-Parker dosage system [James R. K. Paterson, English radiologist; H. M. Parker, twentieth-century American-English physicist], a radiotherapy system that uses sources of specific relative loadings arranged according to defined rules, which lead to a homogenous dose in the implanted region.

path., abbreviation for **pathologic, pathology.**

pathodontia. See **dental pathology.**

pathogen /path′əjən/ [Gk *pathos* disease, *genein* to produce], any microorganism capable of producing disease. **–pathogenic,** *adj.*

pathogenesis /path′ōjen′əsis/ [Gk *pathos* + *genesis* origin], the source or cause of an illness or abnormal condition.

pathogenicity /path′ōjənis′itē/, pertaining to the ability of a pathogenic agent to produce a disease.

pathogenic occlusion, an abnormal closure of the teeth, capable of producing pathologic changes in the teeth, supporting tissues, and other components of the stomatognathic system.

pathognomonic /pathog′nəmon′ik/ [Gk *pathos* + *gnomon* index], (of a sign or symptom) specific to a disease or condition, such as Koplik's spots on the buccal and lingual mucosa, which are indicative of measles.

pathognomonic symptom. See **symptom.**

pathologic (path.) [Gk *pathos* + *logos* science], pertaining to a condition that is caused by or involves a disease process.

pathologic absorption, the taking up by the blood of an excretory or morbid substance.

pathologic amenorrhea, a stoppage or absence of menstrual discharge from the uterus due to a disease.

pathologic anatomy, (in applied anatomy) the study of the structure and morphology of the tissues and cells of the body as related to disease.

pathologic diagnosis, a diagnosis arrived at by an examination of the substance and function of the tissues of the body, especially of the abnormal developmental changes in the tissues by histologic techniques of tissue examination.

pathologic fracture. See **neoplastic fracture.**

pathologic histology, the specialized study of the effects of disease on minute structures, composition, and function of tissues.

pathologic microorganisms, any microscopic life form, from a virus to nematode, that has the potential to cause disease.

pathologic mitosis, any cell division that is atypical, asymmetric, or multipolar and results in the unequal number of chromosomes in the nuclei of the daughter cells. It is indicative of malignancy.

pathologic myopia, a type of progressive nearsightedness characterized by changes in the fundus of the eye, posterior staphyloma, and deficient corrected acuity.

pathologic physiology, 1. the study of the physical and chemical processes involved in the functioning of diseased tissues. **2.** the study of the modification of the normal functioning processes of an organism caused by disease.

pathologic reflex, any abnormal reflex that is caused by a lesion in or an organic disease of the nervous system.

pathologic retraction ring, a ridge that may form around the uterus at the junction of the upper and lower uterine segments during the prolonged second stage of an obstructed labor.

pathologic sleep, excessive sleep associated with a neurologic disorder, such as encephalitis lethargica, or sleeping sickness.

pathologic triad, the combination of three respiratory disease conditions: bronchospasm, retained secretions, and mucosal edema.

pathologist /pəthol′əjist/, a physician who specializes in the study of disease, usually in a hospital, school of medicine, or research institute or laboratory. A pathologist usually specializes in autopsy or in clinical or surgical pathology.

pathology (path.) /pəthol′əjē/ [Gk *pathos* disease, *logos* science], the study of the characteristics, causes, and effects of disease, as observed in the structure and function of the body. **Cellular pathology** is the study of cellular changes in disease. **Clinical pathology** is the study of disease by the use of laboratory tests and methods. –**pathologic,** *adj.*

pathomimicry. See **Munchausen's syndrome.**

pathophysiology /path″ōfiz′ē·ol′əjē/ [Gk *pathos* disease, *physis* nature, *logos* science], the study of the biological and physical manifestations of disease as they correlate with the underlying abnormalities and physiologic disturbances. –**pathophysiologic,** *adj.*

pathosis, a disease condition.

pathway [AS *paeth, weg*], **1.** a network of neurons that provides a transmission route for nerve impulses from any part of the body to the spinal cord and the cerebral cortex or from the central nervous system to the muscles and organs. **2.** a chain of chemical reactions that produces various compounds in critical sequence, such as the Embden-Meyerhof pathway.

patient [L *pati* to suffer], **1.** a recipient of a health care service. **2.** a health care recipient who is ill or hospitalized. **3.** a client in a health care service.

patient advocate. See **ombudsman.**

patient care committee, a hospital staff organization, composed of medical, nursing, and other health professionals, with the assigned responsibility of monitoring all patient care practices to ensure that predetermined standards are met.

patient compensation fund, a fund usually established by state law and commonly financed by a surcharge on malpractice premiums and used to pay malpractice claims.

patient-controlled analgesia (PCA), a drug-delivery system that dispenses a preset IV dose of a narcotic analgesic into a patient when the patient pushes a switch on an electric cord.

patient day (PD), a unit in a system of accounting used by health care facilities and health care planners. Each day represents a unit of time during which the services of the institution or facility were used by a patient; thus 50 patients in a hospital for 1 day would represent 50 patient days.

patient dumping, the premature discharge of Medicare or indigent patients from hospitals for economic reasons. A 1986 federal rule required hospitals to advise Medicare patients on admission for treatment of their right to challenge what they consider as premature discharge after treatment.

patient interview, a systematic interview of a patient, the purpose of which is to obtain information that can be used to develop an individualized plan for care.

patient mix, 1. the distribution of demographic variables in a patient population, often represented by the percentage of a given race, age, sex, or ethnic derivation. **2.** the distribution of indications for admission in a patient population, such as surgical, maternity, or trauma.

patient plan of care, a plan of care coordinated to include appropriate participation by each member of the health care team.

patient record, a collection of documents that provides a record of each episode in which a patient visited or sought treatment and received care or a referral for care from a health care facility.

patient representative. See **ombudsman.**

patient representative services, hospital services provided by designated staff members relating to the investigation and mediation of patient complaints and the promotion and protection of patient rights.

Patient's Bill of Rights, a list of patient's rights promulgated by the American Hospital Association. It offers some guidance and protection to patients by stating the responsibilities that a hospital and its staff have toward patients and their families during hospitalization, but it is not a legally binding document.

patterning, the method of treatment or act of establishing a system or pattern of stimuli that will evoke a new set or responses. The process is commonly used to retrain persons who have suffered a brain injury that disrupts normal sensory-motor activities.

pattern theory of pain. See **pain mechanism.**

patulous /pat′yələs/ [L *patulus* open], pertaining to something that is open or spread apart.

Paul-Bunnell test [John R. Paul, American physician, b. 1893; Walls W. Bunnell, American physician, b. 1902], a blood test for heterophil antibodies, used for confirming a diagnosis of infectious mononucleosis.

Pautrier microabscess /pôtrēyā′/ [Lucien M. A. Pautrier, French dermatologist, b. 1876; Gk *mikros* small; L *abscedere* to go away], an accumulation of intensely staining mononuclear cells in the epidermis, characterizing malignant lymphoma of the skin, especially mycosis fungoides.

Pauwels' fracture /pou′əlz/ [Friedrich Pauwels, twentieth-century German surgeon; L *fractura* break], a fracture of the proximal femoral neck with varying degrees of angulation.

Pavlov, Ivan Petrovitch (1849-1936), a Russian physiologist who discovered of a pattern of conditioned stimulus-reflex learning, the manner in which the physiology of digestion is controlled by the nervous system, and a theory of the causes and treatment of human neuroses.

pavor /pā′vôr/ [L, quaking], a reaction to a frightening stimulus characterized by excessive terror.

pavor diurnus /dī·ur′nəs/, a sleep disorder occurring in children during daytime sleep in which they cry out in alarm and awaken in fear and panic.

pavor nocturnus /noktur′nəs/, a sleep disorder occurring in children during nighttime sleep that causes them to cry out in alarm and awaken in fear and panic.

Payr's clamp /pī′ərz/ [Erwin Payr, German surgeon, b. 1871; AS *clam* fastener], a heavy clamp used in GI surgery.

Pb, symbol for the element **lead.**

PBI, abbreviation for **protein-bound iodine.**

PBL, abbreviation for *peripheral blood lymphocytes.*

p.c., abbreviation for the Latin phrase, *post cibum,* "after meals."

PC, abbreviation for *private corporation.*

PCB, abbreviation for **polychlorinated biphenyls.**

pcc, abbreviation for *precipitated calcium carbonate.*

PCH, abbreviation for **paroxysmal cold hemoglobinuria.**

Pco₂, symbol for **partial pressure of carbon dioxide.**

PCP, 1. abbreviation for **phencyclidine hydrochloride. 2.** abbreviation for *Pneumocystis carinii pneumonia.*

PCR, abbreviation for **polymerase chain reaction.**

p.d., abbreviation for the Latin phrase, *per diem,* "by the day."

Pd, symbol for the element **palladium.**

PD, 1. abbreviation for **patient day. 2.** abbreviation for *Doctor of Pharmacy.* **3.** abbreviation for *prism diopter.* **4.** abbreviation for *pupil diameter.* **5.** abbreviation for *pupillary distance.* **6.** abbreviation for *pulse duration.*

PDA, abbreviation for **patent ductus arteriosus.**

PDL, abbreviation for **periodontal ligament.**

PDR, abbreviation for *Physicians' Desk Reference.*

PE, abbreviation for **pulmonary embolism.**

peak [ME *pec*], the amount of medication in the blood that represents the highest level during a drug administration cycle.

peak concentration, the maximum amount of a substance or force, such as the highest concentration of a drug measured immediately after the drug has been administered.

peak height velocity, a point in pubescence in which the tempo of growth is the greatest.

peak level, the highest concentration, usually in the blood, that a substance reaches during the time period under consideration, such as the highest blood glucose level attained during a glucose tolerance test.

peak method of dosing, the administration of a drug dosage so that a specified maximum level is reached to produce a desired effect, such as lowering the blood pressure.

peak mucus sign, a lubricative, cloudy to clear white cervical mucus that occurs during periods of high estrogen levels, particularly at the time of ovulation.

pearly penile papules. See **hirsutoid papillomas of the penis.**

pearly tumor. See **cholesteatoma.**

Pearson's product movement correlation [Karl Pearson, English mathematician, b. 1857], (in statistics) a statistical test of the relationship between two variables measured in interval or ratio scales. Correlations computed fall between $+1.00$ and -1.00.

peau d'orange /pō′dôräNzh′/ [Fr, skin of orange], a dimpling of the skin that gives it the appearance of the skin of an orange.

pectin /pek′tin/ [Gk *pektos* congealed], a gelatinous carbohydrate substance found in fruits and succulent vegetables and used as the setting agent for jams and jellies and as an emulsifier and stabilizer in many foods. It also adds to the diet bulk necessary for proper GI functioning.

pectineus /pektin′ē·əs/ [L *pecten* comb], the most anterior of the five medial femoral muscles. It functions to flex and adduct the thigh and to rotate it medially.

pectoral /pek′tərəl/ [L *pectus* breast], pertaining to the thorax or chest.

pectoralis major [L *pectus* breast], a large muscle of the upper chest wall that acts on the shoulder joint to flex, adduct, and medially rotate the arm.

pectoralis minor, a thin, triangular muscle of the upper chest wall beneath the pectoralis major. It functions to rotate the scapula, to draw it down and forward, and to raise the third, fourth, and fifth ribs in forced inspiration.

pectoriloquy /pek′təril′əkwē/, a phenomenon in which voice sounds, including whispers, are transmitted through the pulmonary structures and are clearly audible

P

through a stethoscope. It is often a sign of lung consolidation.

pectus excavatum. See **funnel chest.**

pedagogy /ped′əgoj′ē/ [Gk *pais* child, *agogos* leader], the art and science of teaching children, based on a belief that the purpose of education is the transmittal of knowledge.

pedal [L *pes* foot], pertaining to the foot.

pederosis. See **pedophilia.**

pedes. See **pedal.**

pediatric [Gk *pais* child, *iatreia* treatment], pertaining to preventive and primary health care and treatment of children and the study of childhood diseases.

pediatric advanced life support (PALS), a system of critical care procedures and facilities, such as the intensive care nursery, for the basic and advanced treatment of seriously ill or injured infants and children. It includes the neonatal resuscitation program (NRP) as recommended by the American Academy of Pediatrics and the American Heart Association.

pediatric anesthesia, a subspecialty of anesthesiology dealing with the anesthesia of neonates, infants, and children up to 12 years of age.

pediatric dosage, the determination of the correct amount, frequency, and total number of doses of a medication to be administered to a child or infant. Various formulas have been devised to calculate pediatric dosage from a standard adult dose, although the most reliable method is to use the proportional amount of body surface area to body weight, based on one of the formulas.

pediatric hospitalization, the confinement of a child or infant in a hospital for diagnostic testing or therapeutic treatment.

pediatrician /pē′dē·ətrish′ən/ [Gk *pais* child, *iatreia* treatment], a physician who specializes in pediatrics.

pediatric nurse practitioner (PNP), a nurse practitioner who, by advanced study and clinical practice, such as in a master's degree program or certificate in pediatric nursing, has gained advanced knowledge in the nursing care of infants and children.

pediatric nursing, the branch of nursing concerned with the care of infants and children.

pediatric nutrition, the maintenance of a proper, well-balanced diet, consisting of the essential nutrients and the adequate caloric intake necessary to promote growth and sustain the physiologic requirements at the various stages of development. Nutritional needs vary considerably with age, level of activity, and environmental conditions, and they are directly related to the rate of growth.

pediatrics (peds) /pē′dē·at′triks/, a branch of medicine concerned with the development and care of children. Its specialties are the particular diseases of children and their treatment and prevention. –**pediatric,** *adj.*

pediatric surgery, the special preparation and care of the child undergoing surgical procedures for injuries, deformities, or disease. In addition to the usual fears and emotional trauma of illness and hospitalization, the child is especially concerned about being anesthetized.

pedicle [L *pediculus* little foot], a narrow stalk, stem, or tube of tissue attached to a tumor, skin flap, or organ.

pedicle clamp /ped′ikəl/ [L *pediculus* little foot; ME *clam* fastener], a locking surgical forceps used for compressing blood vessels or pedicles of tumors during surgery.

pedicle flap operation, a mucogingival surgical procedure for relocating or sliding gingival tissue from a donor site to an isolated defect, usually a tooth surface denuded of attached gingiva.

pediculicide /pədik′yōōlisīd′/ [L *pediculus* louse, *caedere* to kill], any of a group of drugs that kill lice.

pediculosis /pədik′yōōlō′sis/ [L *pediculosus* lousy], infestation with bloodsucking lice. **Pediculosis capitis** is infestation of the scalp with lice. **Pediculosis corporis** is infestation of the skin of the body with lice. **Pediculosis palpebrarum** is infestation of the eyelids and eyelashes with lice. **Pediculosis pubis** is infestation of the pubic hair region with lice. Infestation with lice causes intense itching, often resulting in excoriation of the skin and secondary bacterial infection.

pediculous /pədik′yələs/ [L, a little louse], infested with sucking lice.

Pediculus humanus capitis, a species of head lice.

Pediculus humanus corporis, a species of body lice.

Pediculus pubis. See **crab louse.**

pedigree [Fr *pied de grue* crane's foot pattern], **1.** line of descent; lineage; ancestry. **2.** (in genetics) a chart that shows the genetic makeup of a person's ancestors, used in the mendelian analysis of an inherited characteristic or disease in a particular family.

pedodontics /ped′ədon′tiks/ [Gk *pais* child, *odius* tooth], a field of dentistry devoted to the diagnosis and the treatment of dental problems affecting children.

pedogenesis /pē′dōjen′əsis/ [Gk *pais* child, *genesis* origin], the production of offspring by young or larval forms of animals, often by parthenogenesis, as in certain amphibians. **–pedogenetic,** *adj.*

pedophilia /ped′əfil′ē·ə/ [Gk *pais* child, *philein* to love], **1.** an abnormal interest in children. **2.** (in psychiatry) a psychosexual disorder in which the fantasy or act of engaging in sexual activity with prepubertal children is the preferred or exclusive means of achieving sexual excitement and gratification. **–pedophilic,** *adj.*

peds, *informal;* abbreviation for **pediatrics.**

peduncle /pədung′kəl/ [L *pes* foot], a stemlike connecting part, such as the pineal peduncle or a peduncle graft. **–peduncular, pedunculate,** *adj.*

pedunculated [L *pes* foot], pertaining to a structure with a stalk or peduncle.

pedunculus /pədung′kyələs/ [L *pes* foot], a stalk, stem, or any stalklike anatomic structure.

PEEP, abbreviation for **positive end-expiratory pressure.**

Peeping Tom. See **voyeur.**

peer [L *par* equal], a person deemed an equal for the purpose at hand. It is usually an "age mate," or companion or associate on roughly the same level of age or mental endowment.

peer review, an appraisal by professional co-workers of equal status of the way an individual nurse or other health professional conducts practice, education, or research.

PEL, abbreviation for *permissible exposure limits.*

Pel-Ebstein fever /pel′eb′stēn/ [Pieter K. Pel, Dutch physician, b. 1852; Wilhelm Ebstein, German physician, b. 1836], a recurrent fever, occurring in cycles of several days or weeks, characteristic of Hodgkin's disease or malignant lymphoma.

Pelger-Huët anomaly /pel′gərhyoo̅̅′ət/ [Karel Pelger, Dutch physician, b. 1885; G. J. Huët, Dutch physician, b. 1879; Gk *anomalia* irregular], an inherited disorder characterized by granulocytes with unusually coarse nuclear material and dumbbell- or peanut-shaped nuclei.

pellagra /pəlā′grə, pəlag′rə/ [It *pelle* skin, *agra* rough], a disease resulting from a deficiency of niacin or tryptophan or a metabolic defect that interferes with the conversion of the precursor tryptophan to niacin. It is characterized by scaly dermatitis, especially of the skin exposed to the sun, glossitis, inflammation of the mucous membranes, diarrhea, and mental disturbances, including depression, confusion, disorientation, hallucination, and delirium. Kinds of pellagra are **pellagra sine pellagra** and **typhoid pellagra. –pellagrous,** *adj.*

pellagra sine pellagra /sī′nē, sē′nə/, a form of pellagra in which the characteristic dermatitis is not present.

Pellegrini's disease /pel′əgrē′nēz/ [Augusto Pellegrini, Italian surgeon, b. 1877], ossification of the upper part of the medial collateral ligament, sometimes accompanied by bony growth at the internal condyle of the femur. The condition usually follows a leg injury.

pelvic /pel′vik/ [L *pelvis* basin], of or pertaining to the pelvis.

pelvic abscess, a pus-producing lesion in the pelvic peritoneum, usually originating in the rectouterine pouch.

pelvic axis, an imaginary curved line that passes through the centers of the various anteroposterior diameters of the pelvis.

pelvic bone, a combination of the ilium, ischium, and pubis.

pelvic brim, the curved top of the bones of the hip extending from the anterior superior iliac crest in front on one side and around and past the sacrum to the crest on the other side. Below the brim is the pelvis.

pelvic cellulitis, bacterial infection of the parametrium, occurring after childbirth or spontaneous therapeutic abortion. It represents an extension of infection via the blood vessels and lymphatics from a primary wound infection in the external genitalia, perineum, vagina, cervix, or uterus. It is characterized by fever, uterine subinvolution, chills and sweats, and abdominal pain that spreads laterally and, if untreated, by the formation of a large abscess and by signs of peritonitis.

pelvic classification, 1. a process in which the anatomic and spatial relationships of the bones of the pelvis are evaluated, usually to assess the adequacy of the pelvic structures for vaginal delivery. Caldwell-Moloy's system of classification is the one most commonly used. **2.** one of the types in a classification system of the pelvis.

pelvic congestion syndrome, an abnormal gynecologic condition characterized by chronic low back pain, dysuria, dysmenorrhea, vague lower abdominal pain, vaginal discharge, and dyspareunia.

pelvic diameter, 1. at the rim of the pelvis, a line from the lumbosacral angle to the symphysis pubis. **2.** at the pelvic outlet, a line from the tip of the coccyx to the lower border of the symphysis pubis.

pelvic diaphragm, the caudal aspect of the body wall, stretched like a hammock across the pelvic cavity and comprising the levator ani and the coccygeus muscles. It holds the abdominal contents, supports

P

the pelvic viscera, and is pierced by the anal canal, the urethra, and the vagina.

pelvic examination, a diagnostic procedure in which the external and internal genitalia are physically examined using inspection, palpation, percussion, and auscultation. It should be performed regularly throughout a woman's life.

pelvic exenteration /eksen'tərā'shən/, the surgical removal of all reproductive organs and adjacent tissues.

pelvic floor, the soft tissues enclosing the pelvic outlet.

pelvic girdle, a bony ring formed by the hip bones, the sacrum, and the coccyx.

pelvic inferior aperture. See **pelvic outlet.**

pelvic inflammatory disease (PID), any inflammatory condition of the female pelvic organs, especially one caused by bacterial infection. Characteristics of the condition include fever, foul-smelling vaginal discharge, pain in the lower abdomen, abnormal uterine bleeding, pain with coitus, tenderness or pain in the uterus, affected ovary or fallopian tube on bimanual pelvic examination. If an abscess has already developed, a soft, tender, fluid-filled mass may be palpated.

pelvic inlet, (in obstetrics) the inlet to the true pelvis, bounded by the sacral promontory, the horizontal rami of the pubic bones, and the top of the symphysis pubis. Because the infant must pass through the inlet to enter the true pelvis and to be born vaginally, the anteroposterior, transverse, and oblique dimensions of the inlet are important measurements when assessing the pelvis during pregnancy.

pelvic kidney. See **ptotic kidney.**

pelvic minilaparotomy /min'ēlap'ərot'-əmē/, a surgical operation in which the lower abdomen is entered through a small, suprapubic incision, performed most often for tubal sterilization but also for diagnosis and treatment of eccyesis, ovarian cyst, endometriosis, and infertility. It may be performed as an alternative to laparoscopy, often on an outpatient basis.

pelvic outlet, the space surrounded by the bones of the lower portion of the true pelvis. In women, the shape and size of the pelvis vary and are important in childbirth. The shapes are classified by the length of the diameters as compared with each other and by the thickness of the bones.

pelvic pain, pain in the pelvis, as occurs in appendicitis, oophoritis, and endometritis. The character and onset of pelvic pain and any factors that alleviate or aggravate it are significant in making a diagnosis.

pelvic pole, the end of the axis at which the breech of the fetus is located.

pelvic presentation [L *pelvis* basin, *praesentare* to show], a breech presentation.

pelvic rotation, one of the five major kinematic determinants of gait, involving the alternate rotation of the pelvis to the right and the left of the central axis of the body. The usual pelvic rotation occurring at each hip joint in most healthy individuals is approximately 4 degrees to each side of the central axis. Pelvic rotation occurs during the stance phase of gait and involves a medial to lateral circular motion.

pelvic rotunda [L *pelvis* basin, *rotundus* wheel], a part of the ear appearing as a funnel-shaped depression of the tympanum above the fenestra cochlea.

pelvic tilt, one of the five major kinematic determinants of gait that lowers the pelvis on the side of the swinging lower limb during the walking cycle. Through the action of the hip joint the pelvis tilts laterally downward, adducting the lower limb in the stance phase of gait and abducting the opposite extremity in the swing phase of gait. The knee joint of the non–weight-bearing limb flexes during its swing phase to allow the pelvic tilt, which helps minimize the vertical displacement of the center of gravity of the body, thus conserving energy during walking.

pelvic varicocele. See **ovarian varicocele.**

pelvifemoral /pel'vēfem'ərəl/ [L *pelvis* basin, *femur* thigh], of or pertaining to the structures of the hip joint, especially the muscles and the area around the bony pelvis and the head of the femur that make up the pelvic girdle.

pelvifemoral muscular dystrophy. See **Leyden-Moebius muscular dystrophy.**

pelvimeter /pelvim'ətər/ [L *pelvis* basin; Gk *metron* measure], a device for measuring the diameter and capacity of the pelvis.

pelvimetry /pelvim'ətrē/, the act or process of determining the dimensions of the bony birth canal. Kinds of pelvimetry are **clinical pelvimetry** and **x-ray pelvimetry.**

pelvis /pel'viz/, *pl.* **pelves** [L, basin], the lower portion of the trunk of the body, composed of four bones, the two innominate bones laterally and ventrally and the sacrum and coccyx posteriorly. It is divided into the greater or false pelvis and the lesser or true pelvis by an oblique plane passing through the sacrum and the pubic symphysis. The greater pelvis is the expanded portion of the cavity situated cranially and ventral to the pelvic brim. The lesser pelvis is situated distal to the pelvic brim, and its bony walls are more complete than those of the greater pelvis. The inlet and outlet of the pelvis have three important diameters: anteroposterior, oblique, and transverse. **–pelvic,** *adj.*

pemoline /pem′əlēn/, a central nervous system stimulant prescribed in the treatment of minimal brain dysfunction and attention deficit disorder in children.

pemphigoid /pem′figoid/ [Gk *pemphix* bubble, *eidos* form], a bullous disease resembling pemphigus, distinguished by thicker walled bullae arising from erythematous macules or urticarial bases. Oral lesions are uncommon.

pemphigus /pem′figəs, pemfī′gəs/ [Gk *pemphix* bubble], an uncommon, serious disease of the skin and mucous membranes, characterized by thin-walled bullae arising from apparently normal skin or mucous membrane. The bullae rupture easily, leaving raw patches. The person loses weight, becomes weak, and is subject to major infections.

pemphigus vulgaris, a chronic, progressive, often fatal disease, characterized by the formation of bullae on otherwise normal skin.

pendular nystagmus [L *pendulus* hanging down; Gk *nystagmos* nodding], an undulating involuntary movement of the eyeball.

pendulous /pen′dələs/, hanging loose or lacking proper support.

pendulous abdomen, an abnormal condition in which the anterior abdominal wall becomes relaxed and hangs down over the pubic region.

penetrance [L *penetrare* to penetrate], (in genetics) a variable factor that modifies basic patterns of inheritance. It is the regularity with which an inherited trait is manifest in the person who carries the gene. **–penetrant,** *adj.*

penetrate [L *penetrare*], **1.** to enter or pierce a barrier. **2.** pertaining to the degree to which x-rays pass through matter.

penetrating wound, a wound that enters into a body area, organ, or cavity but does not pass through.

penfluridol /penfloo′ridol/, an antipsychotic drug, chemically similar to pimozide.

penicillamine (D-penicillamine) /pen′isil′-əmēn/, a chelating agent. It is prescribed to bind with and remove metals from the blood in the treatment of heavy metal (especially lead) poisoning, in cystinuria, and in Wilson's disease. It is also prescribed as a palliative in the treatment of sclerosis and rheumatoid arthritis when other medications have failed.

penicillic acid /pen′isil′ik/, an antibiotic compound isolated from various species of the fungus *Penicillium*.

penicillin /pen′isil′in/ [L *penicillum* paintbrush], any one of a group of antibiotics derived from cultures of species of the fungus *Penicillium* or produced semisynthetically. Various penicillins administered orally or parenterally for the treatment of bacterial infections exert their antimicrobial action by inhibiting the biosynthesis of cell wall mucopeptides during active multiplication of the organisms.

penicillinase /pen′əsil′ənās/, an enzyme elaborated by certain bacteria, including many strains of staphylococci, that inactivates penicillin and thereby promotes resistance to the antibiotic. A purified preparation of penicillinase is used in the treatment of adverse reactions to penicillin.

penicillinase-producing staphylococci, strains of staphylococcal organisms that elaborate the penicillin-inactivating enzyme penicillinase (beta-lactamase) and thereby resist the bactericidal action of the antibiotic.

penicillinase-resistant antibiotic, an antimicrobial agent that is not rendered inactive by penicillinase. The semisynthetic penicillins resist the action of penicillinase and are used in treating infections caused by staphylococci that elaborate the enzyme.

penicillin G benzathine, a long-acting, depot form of penicillin. It is used in the treatment of group A beta-hemolytic streptococcal pharyngitis, group A beta-hemolytic streptococcal pyoderma, and syphilitic infection occurring outside the central nervous system. It is given by deep intramuscular injection to achieve steady concentrations in the plasma and to slow systemic absorption from the repository in the muscle over a period of 12 hours to several days.

penicillin G potassium, an antibacterial prescribed in the treatment of many infections, including syphilis, rheumatic fever, and glomerulonephritis.

penicillin phenoxymethyl. See **penicillin V.**

penicillin V, an antibacterial prescribed in the treatment of susceptible infections.

penicilliosis /pen′isil′ē·ō′sis/ [L *penicillum* + Gk *osis* condition], pulmonary infection caused by fungi of the genus *Penicillium*.

Penicillium /pen′isil′ē·əm/ [L *penicillum* paintbrush], a genus of fungi, some species of which have been tentatively linked to disease in humans. Penicillin G is obtained from *Penicillium chrysogenum* and *P. notatum*.

penile /pē′nīl/ [L, penis], pertaining to the penis.

penile cancer /pē′nīl/ [L *penis* male sex organ; *cancer* crab], a rare malignancy of the penis occurring in uncircumcised men and associated with genital herpesvirus infection and poor personal hygiene. Leukoplakia or the flat-topped papules of balanitis xerotica obliterans may be premalignant lesions, and the velvety, red, painful papules of Queyrat's erythroplasia are penile squamous cell carcinoma in situ. Cancer of the penis usually presents as a local mass or a bleeding ulcer and metastasizes early in its course.

penile prosthesis [L *penis* + Gk *prosthesis* addition], a device that can be surgically implanted in the penis, some with mechanisms that control production of an erection. Such prostheses are used to treat impotence. Penile implants may consist of inflatable plastic cavernosal cylinders attached to a fluid reservoir and a pump mechanism. The pump forces fluid into the cylinders to produce an erection.

penis /pē′nis/ [L, male sex organ], the external reproductive organ of a man, homologous with the clitoris of a woman. It is attached with ligaments to the front and sides of the pubic arch and is composed of three cylindrical masses of cavernous tissue covered with skin. The corpora cavernosa penis surrounds a median mass called the corpus spongiosum penis, which contains the greater part of the urethra.

penis envy, literally, female envy of the male penis, but generally a female wish for male attributes, position, and advantages. It is believed by some psychologists to be a significant factor in female personality development.

penniform /pen′ifôrm/ [L *penna* feather, *forma* form], of or pertaining to the shape of a feather, especially the patterns of muscular fasciculi that correlate with the range of motion and the power of muscles.

Penrose drain [Charles Bingham Penrose, American surgeon, b. 1862; AS, *draehen*, teardrop], a surgical drain device of gauze surrounded by rubber or other waterproof materials.

pentadactyl /pen′tədak′til/ [Gk *pente* five, *daktylos* fingers or toes], having five fingers per hand and five toes per foot.

pentaerythritol tetranitrate /pen′tə·er·ith′rətol/, a coronary vasodilator prescribed for the relief of angina pectoris.

pentamidine isethionate /pen′tam′idēn/, a parenteral antiprotozoal drug prescribed in the treatment of pneumonia caused by *Pneumoncystis carinii*, particularly in patients who have AIDS.

pentaploid. See **polyploid.**

pentavalent /pəntav′ələnt/ [Gk *pente* five; L *valere* to have worth], **1.** a chemical radical or element that has a valency of five. **2.** a body formed by the association of five chromosomes held together by chiasmata at the first division of meiosis.

pentazocine hydrochloride /pentā′zəsēn/, an analgesic prescribed for the relief of moderate to severe pain.

pentazocine lactate. See **pentazocine hydrochloride.**

pentobarbital /pen′təbär′bitol/, a sedative and hypnotic prescribed as a preoperative sedative, in the treatment of insomnia, and in the control of acute convulsive disorders.

pentose /pen′tōs/ [Gk *penta* five; L *osus* having], a monosaccharide made of carbohydrate molecules, each containing five carbon atoms. It is produced by the body and is elevated after the ingestion of certain fruits, such as plums and cherries, and in certain rare diseases.

pentosuria /pen′tosŏŏr′ē·ə/ [Gk *penta* + L *osus* having; Gk *ouron* urine], a rare condition in which pentose is found in the urine. Essential or idiopathic pentosuria is caused by a genetically transmitted error of metabolism.

pentoxifylline /pentok′sēfil′ēn/, an oral hemorrheologic drug prescribed for the treatment of intermittent claudication associated with chronic occlusive arterial limb disease.

pentylenetetrazol /pen′tilē′nətet′rəzol/, a central nervous system stimulant prescribed as an analeptic to stimulate the respiratory, vagal, and vasomotor centers of the brain, to counter the effects of depressants, and to increase cerebral blood flow, especially in geriatric patients.

Peplau, Hildegard E., one of the pioneers in nursing theory development and a proponent in the 1950s of the concept that nursing is an interpersonal process. Peplau wrote that the nurse-patient relationship occurs in phases during which the nurse functions as a resource person, a counselor, and a surrogate. The four phases of the process were listed as orientation, identification, exploitation, and resolution.

Pepper syndrome [William Pepper, American physician, b. 1874], a neuroblastoma of the adrenal glands that usually metastasizes to the liver.

pep pills, *slang;* amphetamines.

pepsin /pep′sin/ [Gk *pepsis* digestion], an enzyme secreted in the stomach that catalyzes the hydrolysis of protein. Preparations of pepsin obtained from pork and beef stomachs are sometimes used as digestive aids.

pepsinogen /pəpsin′əjən/ [Gk *pepsis* + *genein* to produce], a zymogenic substance secreted by pyloric and gastric chief cells and converted to the enzyme pepsin in an acidic environment, as in the presence of hydrochloric acid produced in the stomach.

pepsinuria /pep′sin o͞or′ē·ə/, the presence of the pepsin enzyme in urine.

peptic [Gk *peptein* to digest], of or pertaining to digestion or to the enzymes and secretions essential to digestion.

peptic ulcer, a sharply circumscribed loss of the mucous membrane of the stomach or duodenum or of any other part of the GI system exposed to gastric juices containing acid and pepsin. Peptic ulcers may be acute or chronic. Acute lesions are almost always multiple and superficial. They may be totally asymptomatic and usually heal without scarring or other sequelae. Chronic ulcers are true ulcers: they are deep, single, persistent, and symptomatic; the muscular coat of the wall of the organ does not regenerate; a scar forms, marking the site, and the mucosa may heal completely. Peptic ulcers are caused by a combination of poorly understood factors, including an excessive secretion of gastric acid, inadequate protection of the mucous membrane, stress, heredity, and the taking of certain drugs, including the corticosteroids, certain antihypertensives, and antiinflammatory medications. Characteristically, ulcers cause a gnawing pain in the epigastrium that does not radiate to the back, is not aggravated by a change in position, and has a temporal pattern that mimics the diurnal rhythm of gastric acidity.

peptidase /pep′tidās/, a protein-splitting enzyme that breaks peptides into amino acids. They occur naturally in plants, yeasts, certain microorganisms, and digestive juices.

peptide /pep′tīd/ [Gk *peptein* to digest], a molecular chain compound composed of two or more amino acids joined by peptide bonds.

peptone /pep′tōn/, a derived protein, which may be produced by hydrolysis of a native protein with an acid or enzyme.

peracephalus /pur′əsef′ələs/, *pl.* **peracephali** [L *per* completely; Gk *a, kephale* not head], a fetus or individual with a malformed head.

per an., abbreviation for the Latin phrase, *per annum,* "yearly."

perceived severity [L *percipere* to perceive; *severus* serious], (in health belief model) a person's perception of the seriousness of the consequences of contracting a disease.

perceived susceptibility, (in health belief model) a person's perception of the likelihood of contracting a disease.

percentage depth dose [L *per* completely,

centum hundred; ME *dep* deep; L *dosis* something given], (in radiotherapy) the amount of radiation delivered at a specified dose, expressed as a percentage of the skin dose.

percentile, the 100th part of a statistical distribution. A percentile rank of 80 indicates that 20% of the total number of cases scored above and 80% scored below in whatever characteristics were being studied.

percent solution, a relationship of a solute to a solvent, expressed in terms of weight of solute per weight of solution. An example of a true percent solution is 5 g of glucose dissolved in 95 g of water, forming 100 g of solution.

percent systole [L *per, centum* + Gk *systole* contraction], an amount of time of each heartbeat that is devoted to the ejection of blood from the ventricle.

percept /pur′sept/ [L *percipere* to perceive], the mental impression of an object that is perceived through the use of the senses.

perception [L *percipere* to perceive], **1.** the conscious recognition and interpretation of sensory stimuli through unconscious associations, especially memory. **2.** the end result or product of the act of perceiving. Kinds of perception include **depth perception, extrasensory perception, facial perception,** and **stereognostic perception.** –**perceptive, perceptual,** *adj.*

perceptivity, the ability to receive sense impressions; perceptiveness.

perceptual constancy [L *percipere* to perceive; *cum* together with, *stare* to stand], in Gestalt psychology, the phenomenon in which an object is seen in the same way under varying circumstances.

perceptual defect, any of a broad group of disorders or dysfunctions of the central nervous system that interfere with the conscious mental recognition of sensory stimuli. Such conditions are caused by lesions at specific sites in the cerebral cortex that may result from any illness or trauma affecting the brain at any age or stage of development.

perceptual deprivation, the absence of or decrease in meaningful groupings of stimuli, which may result from a constant background noise or constant inadequate illumination.

perceptual monotony, a mental state characterized by a lack of variety in the normal pattern of everyday stimuli.

perchloromethane. See **carbon tetrachloride.**

percolation /pur′kalā′shən/ [L *percolare* to strain], **1.** the act of filtering any liquid through a porous medium. **2.** (in pharmacology) the removal of the soluble parts of a crude drug by passing a liquid solvent through it.

per con., abbreviation for the Latin phrase, *per contra,* "the other side."

percuss, to strike the thoracic or abdominal wall, thereby producing sound vibrations that aid in diagnosis.

percussion [L *percutere* to strike hard], a technique in physical examination used to evaluate the size, borders, and consistency of some of the internal organs and to discover the presence and evaluate the amount of fluid in a cavity of the body. **Immediate** or **direct percussion** refers to percussion performed by striking the fingers directly on the body surface; **indirect, mediate,** or **finger percussion** involves striking a finger of one hand on a finger of the other hand as it is placed over the organ. **–percuss,** *v.,* **percussable,** *adj.*

percussor [L, a striker], a small, hammerlike diagnostic tool having a rubber head that is used to tap the body lightly in percussion.

percutaneous /pur'kyo͞otā'nē·əs/ [L *per* + *cutis* skin], performed through the skin, such as a biopsy or the aspiration of fluid from a space below the skin using a needle, catheter, and syringe or the instillation of a fluid in a cavity or space by similar means.

percutaneous absorption, the process of absorption through the skin from topical application.

percutaneous catheter placement, (in arteriography) the technique in which an intracatheter is introduced through the skin into an artery and placed at the site or structure to be studied.

percutaneous nephrolithotomy, a uroradiologic procedure performed to extract stones from within the kidney or proximal ureter by percutaneous surgery after the stones have been visualized radiologically.

percutaneous nephroscope, a thin fiberoptics probe that can be inserted into the kidney through an incision in the skin. The device is equipped with a tool that can be used to grasp and remove small stones.

percutaneous transhepatic cholangiography, a radiographic examination of the structure of the bile ducts. A needle is passed directly into a hepatic duct after which a contrast medium is injected.

percutaneous transluminal coronary angioplasty (PTCA), a technique in the treatment of atherosclerotic coronary heart disease and angina pectoris in which some plaques in the arteries of the heart are flattened against the arterial walls, resulting in improved circulation. The procedure involves threading a catheter through the

vessel to the atherosclerotic plaque and inflating and deflating a small balloon at the tip of the catheter several times, then removing the catheter. The procedure is performed under x-ray or ultrasonic visualization.

per diem rate /pər dē'əm, dī'əm/ [L *per, diem* daily, *ratus* reckoning], an established rate of payment for hospital services determined by dividing the total cost of providing routine inpatient services for a given period by the total number of inpatient days of care during the period.

Perez reflex /pərez', per'ez/ [Bernard Perez, French physician, b. 1836; L *reflectere* to bend backward], the normal response of an infant to cry, flex the limbs, and elevate the head and pelvis when supported in a prone position with a finger pressed along the spine from the sacrum to the neck.

perfectionism [L *perficere* to complete], a subjective state in which a person pursues an impossibly high standard of performance and, in many cases, demands the same standards of others. Failure to attain the goals leads to feelings of defeat and other adverse psychologic consequences.

perfloxacin /pərflok'səsin/, an antibiotic of the carboxyfluoroquinolone type.

perfluorocarbons, a group of chemicals somewhat capable of performing the function of hemoglobin in red blood cells by transporting oxygen through the circulatory system. They can be used for certain blood substitute purposes, regardless of the blood type of the patient.

perforans /pur'fôrənz/ [L *perforare* to pierce], pertaining to nerves, muscles, or other anatomic features that penetrate other structures.

perforate [L *perforare* to pierce], **1.** to pierce, punch, puncture, or otherwise make a hole. **2.** riddled with small holes. **3.** (of the anus) having a normal opening; not imperforate. **–perforation,** *n.*

perforating fracture, an open fracture caused by a projectile, making a small surface wound.

perforating ulcer, 1. an ulcer that penetrates the thickness of a wall or membrane, as a peptic ulcer of the digestive tract. **2.** a deep, painless ulcer, often on the sole of the foot, of a person whose skin is insensitive due to a disease such as diabetes.

perforation [L *perforare*], a hole or opening made through the entire thickness of a membrane or other tissue or material.

perforation of stomach or intestines, a condition in which disease or injury has resulted in a leakage of digestive tract contents into the peritoneal cavity. A common cause is a ruptured appendix or perforating peptic ulcer. Immediate surgical intervention is needed to prevent peritonitis.

perforation of the uterus, an accidental puncture of the uterus, as may occur with a curet or by an intrauterine contraceptive device.

perfusion [L *perfundere* to pour over], **1.** the passage of a fluid through a specific organ or an area of the body. **2.** a therapeutic measure whereby a drug intended for an isolated part of the body is introduced via the bloodstream.

perfusionist, an allied health professional who assists in performing procedures that involve extracorporeal circulation, such as during open-heart surgery, or hypothermia.

perfusion lung scan, a radiographic examination of the lungs and their function, such as that used to aid in the diagnosis of pulmonary embolism.

perfusion rate, the rate of blood flow through the capillaries per unit mass of tissue, expressed in milliliters per minute per 100 g.

perfusion scan. See **lung scan.**

perfusion technologist, a person who, under the supervision of a physician, operates a heart-lung machine used for cardiopulmonary bypass during surgery.

per gene, a segment of nucleic acid that is associated with circadian rhythms of some animal species. A similar DNA sequence occurs in human genes, but it is not known if it affects human circadian rhythms.

perianal /per′i·ā′nəl/ [Gk *peri* near; L *anus*], located around the anus.

perianal abscess /per′ē·ā′nəl/ [Gk *peri* around; L *anus; abscedere* to go away], a focal, purulent, subcutaneous infection in the region of the anus. Treatment includes hot soaks, antibiotics, and possibly incision and drainage.

periaortic /per′i·ā·ôr′tik/ [Gk *peri* + *aerein* to raise], pertaining to the area around the aorta.

periapical /per′i·ap′ikəl/ [Gk *peri* + L *apex* top], of or pertaining to the tissues around the apex of a tooth, including the periodontal membrane and the alveolar bone.

periapical abscess, an infection around the root of a tooth, usually a result of spread from dental caries.

periapical cyst. See **radicular cyst.**

periapical fibroma, a mass of benign connective tissue that may form at the apex of a tooth with normal pulp.

periapical infection, infection surrounding the root of a tooth, often accompanied by toothache.

periapical radiograph, a dental x-ray used to detect changes in the bone support surrounding the roots of the teeth.

periappendicular /per′i·ap′əndik′yələr/ [Gk *peri* + L *appendere* to hang upon], pertaining to the area around the appendix.

periarterial /per′i·ärtir′ē·əl/ [Gk *peri* + *arteria*], pertaining to the area around an artery.

periarteritis /per′i·är′tərī′tis/ [Gk *peri* + *arteria* air pipe, *itis*], an inflammatory condition of the outer coat of one or more arteries and the tissue surrounding the vessel. Kinds of periarteritis are **periarteritis nodosa** and **syphilitic periarteritis.**

periarteritis gummosa. See **syphilitic periarteritis.**

periarteritis nodosa, a progressive, polymorphic disease of the connective tissue that is characterized by numerous large and palpable or visible nodules in clusters along segments of middle-sized arteries, particularly near points of bifurcation. This process causes occlusion of the vessel, resulting in regional ischemia, hemorrhage, necrosis, and pain. The early signs of the disease include tachycardia, fever, weight loss, and pain in the viscera.

periarticular /per′i·ärtik′yələr/ [Gk *peri* + L *articulus* joint], pertaining to the area around a joint.

peribronchiolar /per′ibrong′kē·ō′lər/, pertaining to the area around the bronchioles.

pericardiac /per′ikär′dē·ak/, **1.** pertaining to the pericardium. **2.** pertaining to the area around the heart.

pericardial adhesion /per′ikär′dē·əl/ [Gk *peri* + *kardia* heart; L *adhesio* sticking to], an adhesion of the pericardium to the heart muscle, sometimes restricting action of the heart muscle. In some cases, a previous inflammation or surgery may result in dense fibrous adhesions that obliterate the pericardium. The condition may be general or localized and may involve adhesion between the two layers of pericardium, *internal adhesive pericarditis,* or between one layer and surrounding tissues, *external adhesive pericarditis.*

pericardial artery [Gk *peri* + *kardia* heart; *arteria* air pipe], one of several small vessels branching from the thoracic aorta, supplying the dorsal surface of the pericardium.

pericardial effusion [Gk *peri* + *kardia* heart; L *effundere* to pour out], a collection of blood or other fluid in the pericardium.

pericardial friction rub, the rubbing together of inflamed membranes of the pericardium, as may occur in pericarditis or following a myocardial infarction, producing a sound audible on auscultation.

pericardial rub. See **pericardial friction rub.**

pericardial tamponade. See **cardiac tamponade.**

pericardiocentesis /per′ikär′dē·ōsintē′sis/ [Gk *peri* + *kardia* heart, *kentesis* pricking], a procedure for aspirating fluid from the pericardial space between the serous membranes by surgical puncture.

pericarditis /per′ikärdī′tis/ [Gk *peri* + *kardia* heart, *itis*], an inflammation of the pericardium associated with trauma, malignant neoplastic disease, infection, uremia, myocardial infarction, collagen disease, or idiopathic causes. Two stages are observed. The first stage is characterized by fever, substernal chest pain that radiates to the shoulder or neck, dyspnea, and a dry, nonproductive cough. On examination a rapid and forcible pulse, a pericardial friction rub, and a muffled heartbeat over the apex are noted. The patient becomes increasingly anxious, tired, and orthopneic. During the second stage, a serofibrinous effusion develops within the pericardium, restricting cardiac activity; the heart sounds become muffled, weak, and distant on auscultation. A bulge is visible on the chest over the precordial area. If the effusion is caused by bacterial infection, a high fever, sweat, chills, and prostration also occur.

pericardium /per′ikär′dē·əm/, pl. **pericardia** [Gk *peri* + *kardia* heart], a fibroserous sac that surrounds the heart and the roots of the great vessels. It consists of the serous pericardium and the fibrous pericardium. Between the layers is the pericardial space which contains a few drops of pericardial fluid that lubricates opposing surfaces of the space and allows the heart to move easily during contraction. The fibrous pericardium, which constitutes the outermost sac and is composed of tough, white fibrous tissue lined by the parietal layer of the serous pericardium, fits loosely around the heart and attaches to large blood vessels emerging from the top of the heart but not to the heart itself. **–pericardial,** *adj.*

pericholangitis /per′əkōlanjī′tis/ [Gk *peri* + *chole* bile, *aggeion* vessel, *itis* inflammation], an inflammatory condition of the tissues surrounding the bile ducts in the liver. Pericholangitis is a complication of ulcerative colitis and is characterized by a recurrent fever, chills, jaundice, and possibly portal hypertension.

perichondrial bone /per′ikon′drē·əl/ [Gk *peri* + *chondros* cartilage; AS *ban*], bone that forms in the perichondrium of the cartilaginous template.

pericoronitis /per′ikôr′ənī′tis/, an inflammation of the gingival flap (gum tissue) around the crown of a tooth, usually associated with the eruption of a third molar.

peridural anesthesia. See **epidural anesthesia.**

perifollicular /per′ifolik′yələr/, pertaining to the area around a follicle.

perifolliculitis /per′əfolik′yəlī′tis/ [Gk *peri* + L *folliculus* small bag; Gk *itis*], inflammation of the tissue surrounding a hair follicle.

perikaryon /per′iker′ē·on/ [Gk *peri* + *karyon* nut], the cytoplasm of a cell body exclusive of the nucleus and any processes, specifically the cell body of a neuron. **–perikaryontic,** *adj.*

perilymph /per′ilimf/ [Gk *peri* + L *lympha* water], the clear fluid separating the osseous labyrinth from the membranous labyrinth in the internal ear.

perimeter [Gk *peri* + *metron* measure], **1.** the circumference, outer edge, or periphery of an object. **2.** an instrument for measuring visual fields. **3.** an instrument for measuring the circumference of teeth.

perimetrium /per′imē′trē·əm/ [Gk *peri* + *metra* womb], the serous membrane enveloping the uterus.

perinatal /per′inā′təl/ [Gk *peri* + L *natus* birth], of or pertaining to the time and process of giving birth or being born.

perinatal AIDS, AIDS acquired by infants from their mothers during pregnancy, during delivery, or from ingesting infected breast milk.

perinatal asphyxia. See **asphyxia neonatorum.**

perinatal death, 1. the death of a fetus weighing more than 1,000 g at 28 or more weeks of gestation. **2.** the death of an infant between birth and the end of the neonatal period.

perinatal mortality, the statistical rate of fetal and infant death, including stillbirths, from 28 weeks of gestation to the end of the neonatal period of 4 weeks after birth.

perinatal period, a period extending approximately from the twenty-eighth week of gestation to the twenty-eighth day after birth.

perinatal physiology, the physiology of the process of giving birth or being born.

perinatologist /per′inätol′əjst/, a physician who specializes in the practice of perinatology.

perinatology /per′inätol′əjē/ [Gk *peri* + L *natus* birth; Gk *logos* science], a branch of medicine concerned with the study of the anatomy and physiology of the mother and her unborn and newborn infant and with the diagnosis and treatment of disorders occurring in them during pregnancy, childbirth, and the puerperium. **–perinatologic,** *adj.*

perineal body /per′inē′əl/ [Gk *perineos* perineum; AS *bodig*], a mass of tissue composed of muscle and fascia between the vagina and rectum in females and between the urethra and rectum in the male.

perineal care [Gk *perineos* perineum], a cleansing procedure prescribed for cleansing the perineum after various obstetric and gynecologic procedures. Sterile or clean perineal care may be prescribed.

perineal dislocation. See **dislocation of hip.**

perineal pad, a cushion of soft material used to cover the perineum to absorb the menstrual flow or to protect a wound or incision.

perineorrhaphy /per′inē·ôr′əfē/ [Gk *perineos + rhaphe* suture], a surgical procedure in which an incision, tear, or defect in the perineum is repaired by suturing.

perineotomy /per′inē·ot′əmē/ [Gk *perineos + temnein* to cut], a surgical incision into the perineum.

perinephric abscess /per′inef′rik/ [Gk *peri + nephros* kidney; L *abscedere* to go away], an abscess that develops in the fatty tissue around a kidney. It is usually secondary to an abscess originating earlier in the cortex of the organ.

perineum /per′inē′əm/ [Gk *perineos*], the part of the body situated dorsal to the pubic arch and the arcuate ligaments, ventral to the tip of the coccyx, and lateral to the inferior rami of the pubis and the ischium and the sacrotuberous ligaments. The perineum supports and surrounds the distal portions of the urogenital and GI tracts of the body. **–perineal,** *adj.*

perinodal fibers /per′inō′dəl/ [Gk *peri +* L *nodus* knot], the atrial fibers surrounding the sinoatrial node.

period. See **menses.**

periodic [Gk *peri + hodos* way], (of an event or phenomenon) recurring at regular or irregular intervals. **–periodicity,** *n.*

periodic apnea of the newborn, a normal condition in the full-term newborn infant characterized by an irregular pattern of rapid breathing followed by a brief period of apnea, usually associated with rapid eye movement (REM) sleep.

periodic breathing. See **Cheyne-Stokes respiration.**

periodic deep inspiration, (in respiratory therapy) periodic deep forced inspiration of compressed gas or air in controlled ventilation.

periodic fever, 1. a hereditary illness affecting mainly Sephardic Jews, Armenians, and Arabs with intermittent episodes of fever accompanied by abdominal or pleuritic pain. Age of onset is between 10 and 20 years. Some cases are complicated by symptoms of arthritis, splenomegaly, and renal amyloidosis, which may progress to a fatal kidney disorder. **2.** a common name for **familial Mediterranean fever.**

periodic hyperinflation, a normal phenomenon of an unconscious sighing or deep breathing. Because of the natural need for periodic hyperinflation of the lungs, an artificial sigh is often programed into the mechanism of mechanical ventilators.

periodicity [Gk *periodikos* periodical], the tendency of some events or episodes to repeat at predictable intervals, such as that of filarial worms to appear in cutaneous blood vessels at night but not in daylight hours and types of malaria that cause paroxysms at 24-, 48-, or 72-hour intervals, depending upon the species of pathogen.

periodic table, a systematic arrangement of the chemical elements, devised in 1869 by Dmitri Ivanovich Mendeléeff (Russian chemist, 1834-1907). By arranging the elements in order of their atomic weights, he was able to show relationships, such as valency, that occurred at regular intervals and was able to predict the properties of elements still undiscovered in the nineteenth century.

periodontal /per′ē·ōdon′təl/ [Gk *peri + odous* tooth], of or pertaining to the area around a tooth, such as the peridontium.

periodontal abscess, a localized collection of inflammatory material, including pus, in the periodontal tissue. It is usually classified according to its location in the periodontal pocket, as lateral alveolar, parietal, peridental, or lateral.

periodontal cyst, an epithelium-lined sac that contains fluid, most often occurring at the apex of a pulp-involved tooth. Periodontal cysts that occur lateral to a tooth root are less common.

periodontal disease, disease of the tissues around a tooth, such as an inflammation of the periodontal membrane or periodontal ligament.

periodontal ligament (PDL), the fibrous tissue that attaches the teeth to the alveoli, composed of many bundles of collagenous tissue arranged in groups between which is loose connective tissue interwoven with blood vessels, lymph vessels, and nerves. It invests and supports the teeth.

periodontal pocket, a pathologic increase in the depth of the gingival crevice or sulcus surrounding the tooth at the gingival margin. Kinds of periodontal pockets include **gingival, infrabony, in-**

P

trabony, intraalveolar, relative, simple, subcrestal, suprabony, and **supracrestal.**

periodontal probe, a slender instrument with indentations spaced in millimeters designed for introduction into the gingival sulcus for the purpose of measuring its depth around the tooth.

periodontics [Gk *peri + odous* tooth], a branch of dentistry concerned with the diagnosis, treatment, and prevention of diseases of the periodontium. **–periodontic, periodontal,** *adj.*

periodontist, a dentist who specializes in periodontics.

periodontitis /per'ē-ōdontī'tis/, inflammation of the periodontium, which includes the periodontal ligament, the gingiva, and the alveolar bone.

periodontoclasia [Gk *peri + odous* tooth, *klasis* breaking], the loosening of permanent teeth.

periodontosis /per'idontō'sis/ [Gk *peri + odous* tooth, *osis* condition], a rare disease that affects young people, especially women, and is characterized by idiopathic destruction of the periodontium.

perioperative /per'i·op'ərativ'/ [Gk *peri +* L *operari* to work], pertaining to the time of the surgery.

perioperative nursing [Gk *peri +* L *operari* to work; *nutrix* nurse], nursing care provided surgery patients during the entire inpatient period, from admission to date of discharge.

periorbita /per'i·ôr'bitə/ [Gk *peri +* L *orbita* wheel mark], the periosteum of the orbit of the eye. It is continuous with the dura mater and the sheath of the optic nerve.

periorbital, pertaining to the area surrounding the socket of the eye.

periosteal /per'i·os'tē·əl/ [Gk *peri + osteon* bone], pertaining to the periosteum, the membrane covering the bone.

periosteum /per'i·os'tē·əm/ [Gk *peri + osteon* bone], a fibrous vascular membrane covering the bones, except at their extremities. It consists of an outer layer of collagenous tissue containing a few fat cells and an inner layer of fine elastic fibers. Periosteum is permeated with the nerves and blood vessels that innervate and nourish underlying bone. The membrane is thick and markedly vascular over young bones but thinner and less vascular in later life.

periostitis /per'i·ostī'tis/ [Gk *peri + osteon* bone, *itis*], inflammation of the periosteum. The condition is caused by chronic or acute infection or trauma and is characterized by tenderness and swelling of the affected bone, pain, fever, and chills.

peripatetic /per'ipətet'ik/ [Gk, *peripatein,* to walk about], pertaining to an ambulatory patient.

peripheral [Gk *periphereia* circumference], of or pertaining to the outside, surface, or surrounding area of an organ or other structure.

peripheral acrocyanosis of the newborn, a normal, transient condition of the newborn, characterized by pale cyanotic discoloration of the hands and feet, especially the fingers and toes.

peripheral angiography, the study of the peripheral blood vessels by radiography after an opaque dye has been injected into the circulation.

peripheral arteriovenography, a radiographic examination of the blood vessels in the peripheral parts of the body, such as the arms and legs, after the injection of a contrast medium into these vessels.

peripheral glioma. See **schwannoma.**

peripheral lesion, an injury to any tissues distal to the main organ systems.

peripheral motor neuron, an effector neuron located outside the central nervous system, usually in a ganglion of the sympathetic or parasympathetic nervous system.

peripheral nervous system, the motor and sensory nerves and ganglia outside the brain and spinal cord. The system consists of 12 pairs of cranial nerves, 31 pairs of spinal nerves, and their various branches in body organs. Sensory, or afferent, peripheral nerves transmitting information to the central nervous system and motor, or efferent, peripheral nerves carrying impulses from the brain usually travel together but separate at the cord level into a posterior sensory root and an anterior motor root. Fibers innervating the body wall are designated somatic; those supplying internal organs are termed visceral. Nerves in the sympathetic division cause peripheral vasoconstriction, cardiac acceleration, coronary artery dilation, bronchodilation, and inhibition of peristalsis. Parasympathetic nerves cause peripheral vasodilation, cardiac inhibition, and bronchoconstriction and stimulate peristalsis.

peripheral neuropathy, any functional or organic disorder of the peripheral nervous system. A kind of peripheral neuropathy is **paresthesia.**

peripheral neurovascular dysfunction, high risk for, a NANDA-accepted nursing diagnosis of a state in which an individual is at risk of experiencing a disruption in circulation, sensation, or motion of an extremity. Risk factors include fractures, mechanical compression (e.g., tourniquet, cast, brace, dressing, or restraint), orthopedic surgery, trauma, immobilization, burns, and vascular obstruction.

peripheral odontogenic fibroma, a fibrous connective tissue tumor associated with the gingival margin and believed to originate from the periodontium.

peripheral plasma cell myeloma. See **plasmacytoma.**

peripheral pulse [Gk *periphereia*; L *pulsare* to beat], the series of waves of arterial pressure caused by left ventricle systoles as measured in the limbs.

peripheral resistance, a resistance to the flow of blood that is determined by the tone of the vascular musculature and the diameter of the blood vessels.

peripheral scotoma [Gk *periphereia, skotos* darkness, *oma* tumor], a lost area of the visual field that is located peripherally and does not involve the central region.

peripheral vascular disease, any abnormal condition that affects the blood vessels outside the heart and the lymphatic vessels. Different kinds and degrees of peripheral vascular disease are characterized by a variety of signs and symptoms, such as numbness, pain, pallor, elevated blood pressure, and impaired arterial pulsations. Various causative factors include obesity, cigarette smoking, stress, sedentary occupations, and numerous metabolic disorders. Some kinds of peripheral vascular disease are **arteriosclerosis** and **atherosclerosis.**

peripheral vision, a capacity to see objects that reflect light waves falling on areas of the retina distant from the macula.

periphery, 1. parts or areas near or outside a perimeter or boundary. **2.** the outer body parts, such as the skin or limbs.

perirectal /per′irek′təl/, pertaining to the area around the rectum.

perisinusitis /per′isī′nəsī′tis/, an inflammation of the structures located around a sinus.

peristalsis /per′istal′sis, -stôl′sis/ [Gk *peristellein* to clasp], the coordinated, rhythmic, serial contraction of smooth muscle that forces food through the digestive tract, bile through the bile duct, and urine through the ureters.

peristaltic, pertaining to peristalsis.

peristomal /per′istō′məl, per′istō′məl/, pertaining to the area of skin surrounding a stoma, or surgically created opening in the abdominal wall.

peritoneal abscess /per′itənē′əl/, an abscess in the peritoneal cavity, the result of peritonitis and usually complicated by adhesions.

peritoneal cavity /per′itōnē′əl/ [Gk *peri* + *teinein* to stretch], the potential space between the parietal and the visceral layers of the peritoneum.

peritoneal dialysis, a dialysis procedure performed to correct an imbalance of fluid or of electrolytes in the blood or to remove toxins, drugs, or other wastes normally excreted by the kidney. The peritoneum is used as a diffusible membrane. Under local anesthesia, a many-eyed catheter is sutured in place and is connected to the inflow and outflow tubing with a Y-connector. The dialysate is introduced through the catheter into the peritoneal cavity. The dialysate remains in the peritoneal cavity; by means of osmosis, diffusion, and filtration the needed electrolytes pass to the bloodstream via the vascular peritoneum to the blood vessels of the abdominal cavity, and the waste products pass from the blood vessels through the vascular peritoneum into the dialysate. During outflow, the dialysate is allowed to drain from the peritoneal cavity by gravity.

peritoneal dialysis solution, a solution of electrolytes and other substances that is introduced into the peritoneum to remove toxic substances from the body.

peritoneal endometriosis [Gk *peri* + *teinein* to stretch, *endon* within + *metra* womb], ectopic endometrial tissue found in the pelvic cavity.

peritoneal fluid, a naturally produced fluid in the abdominal cavity that lubricates surfaces, thereby preventing friction between the peritoneal membrane and internal organs.

peritoneoscope. See **laparoscope.**

peritoneoscopy /per′itō′nē·os′kəpē/, the use of an endoscope to inspect the peritoneum through a stab incision in the abdominal wall.

peritoneum /per′itənē′əm/ [Gk *peri* + *teinein* to stretch], an extensive serous membrane that covers the entire abdominal wall of the body and is reflected over the contained viscera. It is divided into the parietal peritoneum and the visceral peritoneum. In men, the peritoneum is a closed membranous sac. The free surface of the peritoneum is smooth mesothelium, lubricated by serous fluid that permits the viscera to glide easily against the abdominal wall and against one another. The mesentery of the peritoneum fans out from the main membrane to suspend the small intestine. Other parts of the peritoneum are the transverse mesocolon, the greater omentum, and the lesser omentum. **–peritoneal,** *adj.*

peritonitis /per′itənī′tis/ [Gk *peri* + *teinein* to stretch, *itis*], an inflammation of the peritoneum produced by bacteria or irritating substances introduced into the abdomi-

P

nal cavity by a penetrating wound or perforation of an organ in the GI tract or the reproductive tract. Peritonitis is caused most commonly by rupture of the vermiform appendix but also occurs after perforations of intestinal diverticula, peptic ulcers, gangrenous gallbladders, gangrenous obstructions of the small bowel, or incarcerated hernias, as well as ruptures of the spleen, liver, ovarian cyst, or fallopian tube, especially in ectopic pregnancy. Characteristic signs and symptoms of peritonitis include abdominal distention, rigidity and pain, rebound tenderness, decreased or absent bowel sounds, nausea, vomiting, and tachycardia. The patient has chills and fever, breathes rapidly and shallowly, is anxious, dehydrated, and unable to defecate, and may vomit fecal material. Leukocytosis, an electrolyte imbalance, and hypovolemia are usually present, and shock and heart failure may ensue.

peritonitis meconium [Gk *peri* + *teinein*, *itis*, inflammation, *mekon* poppy], a condition of peritonitis in a newborn due to rupture of the digestive tract. The inflammation is caused by leakage of meconium, or fetal contents, into the peritoneal cavity.

peritonsillar /per′iton′silər/ [Gk *peri* + L *tonsilla*], pertaining to the area around a tonsil.

peritonsillar abscess [Gk *peri* + L *tonsilla* tonsil; *abscedere* to go away], an infection of tissue between the tonsil and pharynx, usually after acute follicular tonsillitis. The symptoms include dysphagia, pain radiating to the ear, and fever. Redness and swelling of the tonsil and adjacent soft palate are present.

periumbilical /per′i·umbil′ikəl/ [Gk *peri* + *umbilicus* navel], pertaining to the area around the umbilicus.

periungual /per′i·ung′gwəl/ [Gk *peri* + L *unguis* nail], of or pertaining to the area around the fingernails or the toenails.

perivascular goiter /per′ivas′kələr/ [Gk *peri* + L *vasculum* little vessel; *guttur* throat], an enlargement of the thyroid gland surrounding a large blood vessel.

perivascular spaces [Gk, *peri*, near; L, *vasculum*, little vessel; *spatium*, space], spaces that surround blood vessels as they enter the brain. They communicate with the subarachnoid space.

perivertebral [Gk *peri* + *vertebra* joint], pertaining to the area around a vertebra.

perivitelline /per′ivitel′ēn/ [Gk *peri* + L *vitellus* yolk], surrounding the vitellus or yolk mass.

perivitelline space, the space between the ovum and the zona pellucida of mammals into which the polar bodies are released at the time of maturation.

perle /purl, perl/ [Fr. pearl], a soft capsule filled with medicine.

perlèche. See **cheilosis.**

perlingual /pərling′gwəl/, pertaining to the administration of drugs through the tongue, which absorbs substances through its surface.

permanent dentition [L *permanere* to last], the 32 permanent teeth, beginning with the eruption of the first permanent molars at about 6 years of age. The process is completed by 12 or 13 years of age except for the four wisdom teeth, which usually do not erupt until 18 to 25 years of age, or later.

permanent pacemaker, any pacemaker implanted permanently inside the body of a patient.

permanent tooth, one of the set of 32 teeth that appear during and after childhood and usually last until old age. In each jaw they include four incisors, two canines, four premolars, and six molars. They replace the 20 deciduous teeth of infancy. The permanent teeth start to develop in the ninth week of fetal life with the thickening of the epithelium along the line of the future jaw. They erupt first in the lower jaw: the first molars in about the sixth year; the two central incisors about the seventh year; the two lateral incisors about the eighth year; the first premolars about the ninth year; the second premolars about the tenth year; the canines between the eleventh and the twelfth years; the second molars between the twelfth and the thirteenth years; the third molars between the seventeenth and the twenty-fifth years.

permeability /pur′mē·əbil′itē/ [L *permeare* to pass through], the degree to which one substance allows another substance to pass through it. Kinds of permeability include **capillary** and **magnetic.**

permeable [L *permeare* to pass through], a condition of being pervious so that fluids and certain other substances can pass through, such as a permeable membrane.

permethrin /pərmeth′rin/, a topical pediculicide used for the treatment of head lice and nits.

permissible dose [L *permittere* to permit; *dosis* something given], (in radiotherapy) the amount of radiation that may be received by an individual in a specified period of time with the expectation of no significantly harmful results.

pernicious /pərnish′əs/ [L *perniciosus* dangerous], potentially injurious, destructive, or fatal unless treated, such as pernicious anemia.

pernicious anemia [L *pernicosus* destructive; Gk *a, haima* not blood], a progressive, megaloblastic, macrocytic anemia, affecting mainly older people, that results from a lack of intrinsic factor essential for the absorption of cyanocobalamin. The maturation of red blood cells in bone marrow becomes disordered, the posterior and lateral columns of the spinal cord deteriorate, and the white blood cell count is reduced. Extreme weakness, numbness and tingling in the extremities, fever, pallor, anorexia, and loss of weight may occur.

pernicious vomiting [L *perniciosus* dangerous, *vomere* to vomit], a severe, life-threatening episode of vomiting that may occur during pregnancy.

pernio. See **chilblain.**

perobrachius /pē´rōbrā´kē·əs/ [Gk *peros* damaged, *brachion* arm], a fetus or individual with deformed arms.

perochirus /pē´rōkī´rəs/ [Gk *peros* + *cheir* hand], a fetus or individual with malformed hands.

perocormus. See **perosomus.**

perodactylus /pē´rōdak´tiləs/, a fetus or an individual with a deformity of the fingers or the toes, especially the absence of one or more digits.

perodactyly /pē´rō´dak´tilē/ [Gk *peros* + *daktylos* finger], a congenital anomaly characterized by a deformity of the digits, primarily the complete or partial absence of one or more of the fingers or toes.

peromelia /pē´rōmē´lyə/ [Gk *peros* + *melos* limb], a congenital anomaly characterized by the malformation of one or more of the limbs. **–peromelus,** *n.*

peroneal /per´ənē´əl/ [Gk *perone* brooch], of or pertaining to the outer part of the leg, over the fibula and the peroneal nerve.

peroneal muscular atrophy, symmetric weakening or atrophy of the foot and the ankle muscles and by hammertoes. Affected individuals may have high plantar arches and an awkward gait, caused by weak ankle muscles.

peroneus brevis /per´ənē´əs/ [Gk *perone* + L *brevis* short], the smaller of the two lateral muscles of the leg, lying under the peroneus longus. It pronates and plantar flexes the foot.

peroneus longus, the more superficial of the two lateral muscles of the leg. The muscle pronates and plantar flexes the foot.

peronia /pərō´nē·ə/ [Gk *peros* damaged], a congenital malformation or developmental anomaly.

peropus /pərō´pəs/ [Gk *peros* + *pous* foot], a fetus or individual with malformed feet, often in association with some defect of the legs.

per os [L], by mouth.

perosomus /pē´rōsō´məs/ [Gk *peros* + *soma* body], a fetus or individual whose body, especially the trunk, is severely malformed.

perosplanchnia /pē´rōsplangk´nē·ə/ [Gk *peros* + *splanchnon* viscera], a congenital anomaly characterized by the malformation of the viscera.

peroxide. See **hydrogen peroxide.**

perphenazine /pərfen´əzēn/, an antipsychotic prescribed in the treatment of psychotic disorders and in the control of severe nausea and vomiting in adults.

per primam intentionem [L], by first intention.

per pro., abbreviation for the Latin term, *per procurationem,* "on behalf of."

per rectum [L], by rectum.

PERRLA /pur´lə/, abbreviation for *pupils equal, round, react to light, accommodation.* In the process of performing an assessment of the eyes, the size and shape of the pupils, their reaction to light, and their ability to accommodate are evaluated. If all findings are normal, the acronym is noted in the account of the physicial examination.

per se [L], by itself, or of itself.

per secundum intentionem [L], by second intention.

perseveration [L *per* through, *severus* severe], the involuntary and pathologic persistence of an idea or response.

persistent cloaca [L *persistere* to take a stand, *cloaca* sewer], a congenital anomaly in which the intestinal, urinary, and reproductive ducts open into a common cavity resulting from the failure of the urorectal septum to form during prenatal development.

persona /pərsō´nə/, *pl.* **personae** /-nē/ [L, mask], (in analytic psychology) the personality façade or role that a person assumes and presents to the outer world to satisfy the demands of the environment or society or as an expression of some intrapsychic conflict.

personal and social history, (in a health history) an account of the personal and social details of a person's life that serve to identify the person. Place of birth, religion, race, marital status, number of children, military status, occupational history, and place of residence are the usual components of this part of the history.

personal care services, the services performed by health care workers to assist patients in meeting the requirements of daily living.

personal identity disturbance, a NANDA-accepted nursing diagnosis of the inability to distinguish between self and nonself. The defining characteristics of a disturbance in personal identity are to be developed at a later conference.

P

personality [L *personalis* role], **1.** the composite of the behavioral traits and attitudinal characteristics by which one is recognized as an individual. **2.** the pattern of behavior each person evolves, both consciously and unconsciously, as a means of adapting to a particular environment and its cultural, ethnic, national, and provincial standards.

personality disorder, a disruption in relatedness manifested in any of a large group of mental disorders characterized by rigid, inflexible, and maladaptive behavior patterns that impair a person's ability to function in society by severely limiting adaptive potential.

personality test, any of a variety of standardized tests used in the evaluation or assessment of various facets of personality structure, emotional status, and behavioral traits.

personal orientation, 1. a continually evolving process in which a person determines and evaluates the relationships that appear to exist between the person and other people. **2.** the assessment derived by a person regarding those relationships.

personal space, the area surrounding an individual that is perceived as private by the individual, who may regard a movement into the space by another person as intrusive. Personal space boundaries vary somewhat in different cultures, but in general it is regarded as a distance of 1 meter (3 feet) around the individual.

personal unconscious, (in analytic psychology) the thoughts, ideas, emotions, and other mental phenomena acquired and repressed during one's lifetime.

personal zone, an individual protective zone in which the boundaries may contract or expand according to contextual characteristics between distances of about 18 inches to 4 feet.

person year, a statistical measure representing one person at risk of developing a disease during a period of 1 year.

perspiration [L *per* + *spirare* to breath], **1.** the act or process of perspiring; the secretion of fluid by the sweat glands through pores in the skin. **2.** the fluid excreted by the sweat glands. It consists of water containing sodium chloride, phosphate, urea, ammonia, and other waste products. Perspiration serves as a mechanism for excretion and for regulating body temperature. Kinds of perspiration are **insensible perspiration** and **sensible perspiration.**

perspire, to sweat or excrete sweat.

per tertiam intentionem [L], by third intention.

Perthes' disease /per'tās/ [Georg C. Per-

thes, German surgeon, b. 1869], osteochondrosis of the head of the femur in children, characterized initially by epiphyseal necrosis or degeneration followed by regeneration or recalcification.

perturbation /pur'tərbā'shən/ [L *per* + *tubare* to disturb], a cause or a condition of disturbance, disorder, or confusion.

pertussis /pərtus'is/ [L *per* + *tussis* cough], an acute, highly contagious respiratory disease characterized by paroxysmal coughing that ends in a loud whooping inspiration. It occurs primarily in infants and in children less than 4 years of age who have not been immunized. The causative organism, *Bordetella pertussis,* is a small, nonmotile, gram-negative coccobacillus. A similar organism, *B. parapertussis,* causes a less severe form of the disease called parapertussis.

pertussis immune globulin, a passive immunizing agent prescribed for immunization against whooping cough.

pertussis vaccine, an active immunizing agent prescribed for immunization against pertussis when the administration of diphtheria, pertussis, and tetanus vaccine is contraindicated.

per vaginam [L], through the vagina.

pervasive developmental disorder [L *pervadere* to go through], any of certain disorders of infancy and childhood that are characterized by severe impairment of relatedness and behavioral aberrations previously identified as childhood psychoses. The group of disorders includes infantile autism, childhood schizophrenia, and symbiotic psychosis.

perversion [L *pervertere* to turn about], **1.** any deviation from what is considered normal or natural. **2.** the act of causing a change from what is normal or natural. **3.** *informal;* (in psychiatry) any of a number of sexual practices that deviate from what is considered normal adult behavior.

pervert /pur'vərt/ [L *pervertere*], **1.** *informal;* a person whose sexual pleasure is derived from stimuli almost universally regarded as unnatural, such as a fetishist or sadomasochist; a paraphiliac. **2.** one whose sexual behavior deviates from a social or statistical norm but is not necessarily pathologic.

pes /pēz/, *pl.* **pedes** /pē'dēz/ [L, foot], the foot or a footlike structure.

pes cavus, a deformity of the foot characterized by an excessively high arch with hyperextension of the toes at the metatarsophalangeal joints, flexion at the interphalangeal joints, and shortening of the Achilles tendon. The condition may be present at birth or appear later because of contractures or an imbalance of the muscles of the foot, as in neuromuscular diseases such as Friedreich's ataxia or peroneal muscular atrophy.

pes equinus, a foot deformity in which the toes are extremely flexed, walking is done on the outer surface, and the heel does not touch the ground.

pes planus, an abnormal but relatively common condition characterized by the flattening out of the arch of the foot.

pessary /pes'ərē/ [Gk *pessos* oval stone], a device inserted in the vagina to treat uterine prolapse, uterine retroversion, or cervical incompetence. It is employed in the treatment of women whose advanced age or poor general condition precludes procedures required for surgical repair. Pessaries are also used in younger women in evaluating symptomatic uterine retroversion. A **Smith-Hodge pessary** is a rubber- or vinyl-covered wire rectangle that fits between the pubic bone and the posterior vaginal fornix, supporting the uterus and holding the cervix in a posterior position. A **Gellhorn pessary** is an inflexible device made of Lucite in the form of a large collar button. It has a canal through the stem that allows drainage of vaginal secretions. A **doughnut pessary** is a permanently inflated flexible rubber doughnut that is inserted to support the uterus by blocking the canal of the vagina. An **inflatable pessary** is a collapsible rubber doughnut to which is attached a flexible stem containing a rubber valve. The pessary is inserted collapsed, inflated with a bulb similar to that of a sphygmomanometer, and deflated for removal. A **Bee cell pessary** is a soft rubber cube; in each face of the cube is a conical depression that acts as a suction cup when the pessary is in the vagina. A **diaphragm pessary** is a contraceptive diaphragm used for uterovaginal support. A **stem pessary** is a slim curved rod that is fitted into the cervical canal for uterine positioning. It is rarely used today.

pessimism [L *pessimus* worst], the inclination to anticipate the worst possible results from any action or situation or to emphasize unfavorable conditions, even when progress or gain might reasonably be expected. **–pessimist,** *n.*

pesticide poisoning [L *pestis* plague, *caedere* to kill; *potio* drink], a toxic condition caused by the ingestion or inhalation of a substance used for the eradication of pests. Kinds of pesticide poisoning include **malathion poisoning** and **parathion poisoning.**

pestilence, any epidemic of a virulent infectious or contagious disease.

pestis. See bubonic plague.

pes valgus, deviation of the foot outward at the talocalcanean joint.

PET, abbreviation for **positron emission tomography.**

petaling, a process of smoothing the raw or ragged edges of a plaster cast to prevent skin irritation.

petechiae /pētē'kē·ē/, *sing.* **petechia** /-ə/ [It *petecchie* flea-bite], tiny purple or red spots that appear on the skin as a result of minute hemorrhages within the dermal or submucosal layers. **–petechial,** *adj.*

petechial fever /pitē'kē·əl/ [It *petecchie* + L *febris* fever], any febrile illness accompanied by small petechiae on the skin, as seen in the late stage of typhoid fever.

petechial hemorrhage, a small discrete hemorrhage under the skin.

pethidine. See meperidine hydrochloride.

petit mal seizure. See absence seizure.

petit pas gait, a manner of walking with short, mincing steps and shuffling with loss of associated movements. It is seen in cases of parkinsonism as well as in patients with diffuse cerebral disease resulting from multiple small infarcts.

Petren's gait /pet'rənz/, a hesitant form of walking in which a patient takes a few steps, halts, and then continues to take a few more steps. In some cases, the patient must be encouraged to begin the next brief period of walking. The condition is seen in elderly persons and those with paretic disease.

Petri dish /pē'trē, pä'trē/ [Richard Julius Petri, German bacteriologist, b. 1852], a shallow circular glass dish used to hold solid culture media.

petrification, the process of becoming calcified or stonelike.

pétrissage /pā'trisäzh'/ [Fr *petrir* to knead], a technique in massage in which the skin is gently lifted and squeezed. Pétrissage promotes circulation and relaxes the muscles.

petrolatum [L *petra* rock, *oleum* oil], a purified mixture of semisolid hydrocarbons obtained from petroleum and commonly used as an ointment base or skin emollient.

petrolatum gauze /pet'rəlā'təm/, absorbent gauze permeated with white petrolatum.

petroleum distillate poisoning [L *petra, oleum* + *distillare* to drop down; *potio* drink], a toxic condition caused by the ingestion or inhalation of a petroleum distillate, such as fuel oil, lubricating oil, and various solvents. Nausea, vomiting, chest pain, dizziness, and severe depression of the central nervous system characterize the condition. Severe or fatal pneumonitis may occur if the substance is aspirated.

petrosphenoidal fissure /pet′rōsfēnoi′dəl/ [Gk *petros* stone, *sphen* wedge, *eidos* form], a fissure on the floor of the cranial fossa between the posterior edge of the great wing of the sphenoid bone and the petrous part of the temporal bone.

petrous /pet′rəs/ [Gk *petros* stone], resembling a rock or stone.

Peutz-Jeghers syndrome /poits′jeg′ərz/ [J. L. A. Peutz, twentieth-century Dutch physician; Harold J. Jeghers, American physician, b. 1904], an inherited disorder, transmitted as an autosomal dominant trait, characterized by multiple intestinal polyps, and abnormal mucocutaneous pigmentation, usually over the lips and buccal mucosa.

Peyer's patches. See **intestinal tonsil.**

peyote /pā·ō′tē/ [Aztec *peyotl*], **1.** a cactus from which a hallucinogenic drug, mescaline, is derived. **2.** mescaline.

Peyronie's disease /pārōnēz′/ [François de la Peyronie, French physician, b. 1678], a disease of unknown cause resulting in fibrous induration of the corpora cavernosa of the penis. The chief symptom of Peyronie's disease is painful erection.

pF, abbreviation for *picofarad.*

PFT, abbreviation for **pulmonary function test.**

PG, abbreviation for **prostaglandin.**

PGI₂, abbreviation for **prostacyclin.**

PGY, abbreviation for *postgraduate year,* describing medical school graduates during their postgraduate training as interns (PGY-1, first year), residents (PGY-2, 3, 4), or fellows (PGY-4, 5).

pH, abbreviation for *potential hydrogen,* a scale representing the relative acidity (or alkalinity) of a solution, in which a value 7.0 is neutral, below 7.0 is acid, and above 7.0 is alkaline. The numeric pH value is equal to the negative log of the hydrogen ion concentration expressed in moles per liter.

Ph, symbol for **phenyl.**

Ph¹, symbol for **Philadelphia chromosome.**

PH, abbreviation for **parathyroid hormone.**

PHA, 1. abbreviation for **paraaminohippuric acid. 2.** abbreviation for **phytohemagglutinin.**

phacomalacia /fak′ōmälä′shə/ [Gk *phalos* lens, *malkia* softness], an abnormal condition of the eye in which the lens becomes soft because of the presence of a soft cataract.

phacomatosis. See **phakomatosis.**

phage. See **bacteriophage.**

phage typing /fāj/ [Gk *phagein* to eat; *ty-* *pos* mark], the identification of bacteria by testing their vulnerability to bacterial viruses.

phagocyte /fag′əsīt/ [Gk *phagein* + *kytos* cell], a cell that is able to surround, engulf, and digest microorganisms and cellular debris. **Fixed phagocytes,** which do not circulate, include the fixed macrophages and the cells of the reticuloendothelial system. **Free phagocytes,** which circulate in the bloodstream, include the leukocytes and the free macrophages. **–phagocytic,** *adj.*

phagocytize /fag′əsitīz′/, to engulf and destroy bacteria or other foreign materials.

phagocytosis /fag′əsitō′sis/ [Gk *phagein, kytos* + *osis* condition], the process by which certain cells engulf and dispose of microorganisms and cell debris.

phakomatosis /fak′ōmətō′sis/, *pl.* **phakomatoses** [Gk *phako* lens, *oma* tumor, *osis* condition], (in ophthalmology) any of several hereditary syndromes characterized by benign tumorlike nodules of the eye, skin, and brain. The four disorders designated phakomatoses are neurofibromatosis (Recklinghausen's disease), tuberous sclerosis (Bourneville's disease), encephalotrigeminal angiomatosis (Sturge-Weber syndrome), and cerebroretinal angiomatosis (von Hippel-Lindau disease).

phal, abbreviation for **phalanges; phalanx.**

phalanx /fā′langks/, *pl.* **phalanges** /fəlan′jēz/ [Gk, line of soldiers], any one of the 14 tapering bones composing the fingers and toes. They are arranged in three rows at the distal end of the metacarpus and the metatarsus. The fingers each have three phalanges; the thumb has two. The toes each have three phalanges; the great toe has two. **–phalangeal,** *adj.*

phallic /fal′ik/ [Gk *phallos* penis], pertaining to the penis or penis-shaped.

phallic stage [L *phallus* penis; *stare* to stand], (in psychoanalysis) the period in psychosexual development occurring between 3 and 6 years of age when emerging awareness and self-manipulation of the genitals are the predominant source of pleasurable experience.

phallic symbol [Gk *phallos* penis, *symbolon* pledge], in psychoanalysis, any object that resembles a penis.

phalloidine /faloi′din/, a poison present in the mushroom *Amanita phalloides.* Ingestion of phalloidine results in bloody diarrhea, vomiting, severe abdominal pain, kidney failure, and liver damage.

phallus. See **penis.**

phantasm /fan′taz′əm/ [Gk *phantasma* vision], an illusory image, such as an optical illusion of something that does not exist.

phantom [Gk *phantasma* vision], a mass of material similar to human tissue used to investigate the interaction of radiation beams with human beings. Phantom materials can range from water to complex chemical mixtures that faithfully mimic the human body as it would interact with radiation.

phantom images, (in computed tomography) false images that appear but are not actually in the focal plane. They are created by the incomplete blurring or fusion of the blurred margins of some structures characteristic of the type of tomographic motion used.

phantom limb syndrome, a phenomenon common after amputation of a limb in which sensation or discomfort is experienced in the missing limb.

phantom tumor, a swelling resembling a tumor, usually caused by muscle contraction or gaseous distention of the intestines.

phar, abbreviation for **pharmacy; pharmacology; pharmaceutical.**

PharmB, abbreviation for *Bachelor of Pharmacy.*

PharmD, abbreviation for *Doctor of Pharmacy.*

pharmaceutic, pharmaceutical (phar) [Gk *pharmakeuein* to give drugs], **1.** of or pertaining to pharmacy or drugs. **2.** a drug.

pharmaceutical chemistry, the science dealing with the composition and preparation of chemical compounds used in medical diagnoses and therapies.

Pharm Chem, abbreviation for **pharmaceutical chemistry.**

pharmacist [Gk *pharmakeuein*], a person prepared to formulate and dispense drugs or medications through completion of a university program in pharmacy of at least 4 years' duration.

pharmacodynamics /fär′məkōdīnam′iks/ [Gk *pharmakon* drug, *dynamis* power], the study of how a drug acts on a living organism, including the pharmacologic response observed relative to the concentration of the drug at an active site in the organism.

pharmacogenetics /fär′məkōjənet′iks/ [Gk *pharmakon* drug, *genesis* origin], the study of the effect that the genetic factors belonging to a group or to an individual has on the response of the group or the individual to certain drugs.

pharmacokinetics /fär′məkōkinet′iks/ [Gk *pharmakon* + *kinesis* motion], (in pharmacology) the study of the action of drugs within the body, including the routes and mechanisms of absorption and excretion, the rate at which a drug's action begins and the duration of the effect, the biotrans-

formation of the substance in the body, and the effects and routes of excretion of the metabolites of the drug.

pharmacologic agent /fär′məkōloj′ik/, any oral, parenteral, or topical substance used to alleviate symptoms and treat or control a disease process or aid recovery from an injury.

pharmacologic treatment. See **treatment.**

pharmacologic vagotomy, the use of medications to curtail functions of the vagus nerve.

pharmacologist, a specialist in pharmacology.

pharmacology (phar) [Gk *pharmakon* + *logos* science], the study of the preparation, properties, uses, and actions of drugs.

pharmacopeia, pharmacopoeia /fär′məkəpē′ə/ [Gk *pharmakon* + *poiein* to make], **1.** a compendium containing descriptions, recipes, strengths, standards of purity, and dosage forms for selected drugs. **2.** the available stock of drugs in a pharmacy. **3.** the total of all authorized drugs available within the jurisdiction of a given geographic or political area.

pharmacotherapy [Gk, *pharmakon,* drug + *therapeia*], the use of drugs to treat diseases.

pharmacy (phar) [Gk *pharmakon*], **1.** the study of preparing and dispensing drugs. **2.** a place for preparing and dispensing drugs.

pharyngeal aponeurosis /ferin′jē·əl/ [Gk *pharynx* throat; *apo* from, *neuron* sinew], a sheet of connective tissue just beneath the mucosa of the pharynx.

pharyngeal bursa, a blind sac at the base of the pharyngeal tonsil.

pharyngeal reflex. See **gag reflex.**

pharyngeal tonsil, one of two masses of lymphatic tissue situated on the posterior wall of the nasopharynx behind the posterior nares.

pharynges. See **pharynx.**

pharyngitis /fer′injī′tis/ [Gk *pharynx* + *itis*], inflammation or infection of the pharynx, usually causing symptoms of a sore throat. Some causes of pharyngitis are diphtheria, herpes simplex virus, infectious mononucleosis, and streptococcal infection.

pharyngoconjunctival fever /fəring′gōkon′jungktī′vəl/ [Gk *pharnyx* + L *conjunctivus* connecting; *febris* fever], an adenovirus infection characterized by fever, sore throat, and conjunctivitis. Contaminated water in lakes and swimming pools is a common source of infection.

pharyngoscope /fəring′gəskōp′/ [Gk *pharynx* + *skopein* to view], an endoscopic device for examining the lining of the pharynx.

pharyngoscopy /fer'ing·gos'kəpē/, the examination of the throat with a pharyngoscope.

pharyngotonsillitis /fəring'gōton'silī'tis/ [Gk *pharynx* + L *tonsilla;* Gk *itis*], an inflammation involving the pharynx and the tonsils.

pharynx /fer'inks/ [Gk], the throat, a tubular structure that extends from the base of the skull to the esophagus and is situated just in front of the cervical vertebrae. The pharynx serves as a passageway for the respiratory and digestive tracts and changes shape to allow the formation of various vowel sounds. The pharynx is composed of muscle, is lined with mucous membrane, and is divided into the nasopharynx, the oropharynx, and the laryngopharynx. It contains the openings of the right and the left auditory tubes, the openings of the two posterior nares, the fauces, the opening into the larynx, and the opening into the esophagus. **–pharyngeal,** *adj.*

phase /fāz/ [Gk *phasis* appearance], in a periodic function, such as rotational or sinusoidal motion, the position relative to a particular part of the cycle.

phase 0, (in cardiology) the upstroke of the action potential.

phase 1, (in cardiology) the initial rapid repolarization phase of the action potential.

phase 2, (in cardiology) the plateau of the action potential.

phase 3, (in cardiology) the terminal rapid repolarization phase of the action potential.

phase 4, (in cardiology) the period of electric diastole and the last of the four phases of cardiac action potential.

phase microscope, a microscope with a special condenser and objective containing a phase-shifting ring that allows the viewer to see small differences in refraction indexes as differences in image intensity or contrast.

phase of maximum slope, the time of rapid cervical dilatation and rapid fetal descent in the active phase of labor.

phase one study, a clinical trial to assess the risk that might come from administering a new treatment modality. A phase two study evaluates the clinical effectiveness of the new modality, whereas a phase three study compares its effectiveness with the best existing treatment.

phasic /fā'zik/ [Gk *phasis*], **1.** pertaining to a process proceeding in stages or phases. **2.** pertaining to a type of afferent or sensory nerve receptor of the proprioceptive system that responds to rate versus length changes in a muscle spindle.

PhD, abbreviation for *Doctor of Philosophy.*

phenacemide /fənas'əmīd/, an anticonvulsant prescribed in the treatment of severe epilepsy, particularly mixed forms of psychomotor seizures refractory to other drugs.

phenacetin /fənas'itin/, an analgesic.

phenazopyridine hydrochloride /fen'ə-zōpī'ridēn/, a urinary tract analgesic prescribed to reduce the pain of cystitis or other urinary tract infections.

phencyclidine hydrochloride (PCP) /fen-sī'klidēn/, a piperidine derivative administered parenterally to achieve neuroleptic anesthesia. Because of its marked hallucinogenic properties, it is not used therapeutically in the United States. Its reported use as an abused substance has declined in recent years.

phendimetrazine tartrate /fen'dīmet'-rəsēn/, a sympathomimetic amine used as an anorectic agent to decrease the appetite in the treatment of exogenous types of obesity.

phenelzine sulfate /fē'nəlzēn/, a monoamine oxidase (MAO) inhibitor prescribed in the treatment of endogenous and other types of depression.

phenformin /fen'fôrmin/, phenformin hydrochloride, an oral hypoglycemic.

phenic acid. See **carbolic acid.**

pheniramine maleate /fənir'əmēn, -min/, an antihistamine prescribed in the treatment of a variety of hypersensitivity reactions, including rhinitis, skin rash, and pruritus.

phenmetrazine hydrochloride /fənmet'-rəzēn/, a sympathomimetic amine used as an anorectic agent. It is prescribed to reduce the appetite and in the short-term treatment of exogenous obesity.

phenobarbital /fē'nəbär'bital/, a barbiturate anticonvulsant and sedative-hypnotic prescribed in the treatment of a variety of seizure disorders and as a long-acting sedative.

phenobarbital-phenytoin serum levels /fen'itō'in/, the concentration of phenobarbital and phenytoin in the serum, monitored to maintain concentrations sufficient to control seizures but not high enough to cause toxic reactions.

phenocopy /fē'nōkop'ē/ [Gk *phainein* to appear; L *copia* plenty], a phenotypic trait or condition that is induced by environmental factors but closely resembles a phenotype usually produced by a specific genotype. The trait is neither inherited nor transmitted to offspring. Phenocopies may present problems in genetic screening and genetic counseling, so all exogenous factors must be ruled out before any congenital trait or defect is labeled hereditary.

phenol /fē'nol/ [Gk *phainein* to appear; L *oleum* oil] **1.** a highly poisonous, caustic, crystalline chemical derived from coal tar or plant tar or manufactured synthetically. **2.** Any of a large number and variety of chemical products closely related in structure to the alcohols and containing a hydroxyl group attached to a benzene ring.

phenol block, an injection of hydroxybenzene (phenol) into individual nerves, anesthetizing a selected group of those nerves. The technique is sometimes used to control spasticity in specific muscle groups or to block transmission of nerve impulses in conditions such as trigeminal neuralgia.

phenol camphor, an oily mixture of camphor and phenol, used as an antiseptic and toothache remedy.

phenol coefficient, a measure of the disinfectant activity of a given chemical in relation to carbolic acid.

phenolphthalein /fē'nolthal'ē·in, -thā'lēn/, **1.** a laxative that acts by stimulating the motor activity of the lower intestinal tract. **2.** an indicator of hydrogen ion in urine and gastric juice.

phenolphthalein laxative, a purgative that acts on the wall of the bowel. It is prescribed in the treatment of chronic constipation and to prevent straining at the stool for postoperative patients and those afflicted with heart disease or hypertension.

phenol poisoning, corrosive poisoning caused by the ingestion of compounds containing phenol, such as carbolic acid, creosote, cresol, guaiacol, and naphthol. Characteristic of phenol poisoning are burns of the mucous membranes, weakness, pallor, pulmonary edema, convulsion, and respiratory, circulatory, cardiac, and renal failure.

phenolsulfonphthalein /fē'nəlsul'fōnfthal'ē·in/, a dye used for testing the excretory capacity of the kidney tubules.

phenomenon [Gk *phainomenon* something seen], a sign that is often associated with a specific illness or condition and is therefore diagnostically important.

phenothiazine /fē'nōthī'əzēn/, a yellow to green crystalline compound that is a source of dyes and is used in veterinary medicine to treat infestations of threadworms and roundworms.

phenothiazine derivatives, any of a group of drugs that have a three-ring structure in which two benzene rings are linked by a nitrogen and a sulfur. They represent the largest group of antipsychotic compounds in clinical medicine. Of the many phenothiazines and their congeners that are used as adjuncts to general anesthesia, antiemetics, major tranquilizers (antipsychotic agents), and antihistamines, the most widely used are the two prototypes, chlorpromazine and prochlorperazine.

phenotype /fē'nətīp/ [Gk *phainein* to appear; *typos* mark], **1.** the complete observable characteristics of an organism or group, including anatomic, physiologic, biochemical, and behavioral traits, as determined by the interaction of both genetic makeup and environmental factors. **2.** a group of organisms that resemble each other in appearance. **–phenotypic,** *adj.*

phenoxybenzamine hydrochloride /fēnok'sēben'zəmēn/, an antihypertensive prescribed in the control of hypertension and sweating in pheochromocytoma. If tachycardia is excessive, concomitant administration of propranolol may be necessary.

phenoxymethyl penicillin. See **penicillin V.**

phensuximide /fensuk'simīd/, an anticonvulsant prescribed to prevent and treat seizures in petit mal epilepsy.

phentermine hydrochloride /fen'tərmēn/, a sympathomimetic amine used as an anorexic agent. It is prescribed to decrease the appetite in the short-term treatment of exogenous obesity.

phentolamine /fentol'əmēn/, an antiadrenergic administered as the hydrochloride form in tablets and as the mesylate form for injections. It is prescribed to control symptoms of pheochromocytoma before and during surgery and for dermal necrosis and sloughing after extravasation of parenteral norepinephrine.

phenyl (Ph) /fē'nil, fen'il/, a monovalent organic radical, C_6H_5, derived from benzene.

phenylacetic acid /fen'iləsē'tik/, a metabolite of phenylalanine excreted in urine in conjugation with glutamine.

phenylalanine (Phe) /fen'ilal'ənēn/, an essential amino acid necessary for the normal growth and development of infants and children and for normal protein metabolism throughout life.

phenylalaninemia /fen'ilaləninē'mē·ə/, the presence of phenylalanine in the blood.

phenylbutazone /fē'nilbōō'təzōn/, a nonsteroidal antiinflammatory agent prescribed in the treatment of severe symptoms of arthritis, bursitis, and other inflammatory conditions.

phenyl carbinol. See **benzyl alcohol.**

phenylephrine hydrochloride, an alpha-adrenergic agent prescribed to maintain blood pressure used locally as a nasal or ophthalmic vasoconstrictor.

phenylethyl alcohol, a colorless, fragrant liquid with a burning taste, used as a bacteriostatic agent and preservative in medicinal solutions.

phenylic acid, phenylic alcohol. See **carbolic acid.**

phenylketonuria (PKU) /fen'əlkē'-tōnyŏŏr'ē·ə, fē'nəl-/, abnormal presence of phenylketone and other metabolites of phenylalanine in the urine, characteristic of an inborn metabolic disorder caused by the absence or a deficiency of phenylalanine hydroxylase, the enzyme responsible for the conversion of the amino acid phenylalanine into tyrosine. Accumulation of phenylalanine is toxic to brain tissue. Untreated individuals have very fair hair, eczema, a mousy odor to the urine and skin, and progressive mental retardation. –**phenylketonuric,** adj.

phenyl methanol. See **benzyl alcohol.**

phenylpropanolamine hydrochloride /fen'əlprō'pənol'əmēn/, a sympathomimetic amine with vasoconstrictor action prescribed to relieve nasal congestion and related cold symptoms.

phenylpyruvic acid /fen'ilpīrŏŏ'vik/, a product of the metabolism of phenylalanine. The presence of phenylpyruvic acid in the urine is indicative of phenylketonuria.

phenylpyruvic amentia. See **phenylketonuria.**

phenyl salicylate, the salicylic ester of phenol.

phenyltoloxamine citrate /fen'iltəlok'-səmēn, fē'nil-/, an antihistamine usually used in a fixed-combination drug with an analgesic.

phenytoin /fen'ətō'in/, an anticonvulsant prescribed in grand mal and psychomotor seizure disorders and as an antiarrhythmic agent, particularly in digitalis-induced arrhythmias.

pheochromocytoma /fē'ōkrō'mōsītō'mə/, pl. **pheochromocytomas, pheochromocytomata** [Gk phaios dark, chroma color, kytos cell, oma tumor], a vascular tumor of chromaffin tissue of the adrenal medulla or sympathetic paraganglia, characterized by hypersecretion of epinephrine and norepinephrine, causing persistent or intermittent hypertension. Typical signs include headache, palpitation, sweating, nervousness, hyperglycemia, nausea, vomiting, and syncope. There may be weight loss, myocarditis, cardiac arrhythmia, and heart failure. The tumor occurs most frequently in young people, and only a small percentage of the lesions are malignant.

pheresis. See **apheresis.**

pheromone /fer'əmōn'/ [Gk pherein to carry, hormaein to stimulate], a hormonal substance secreted by an organism that elicits a particular response from another individual of the same species, but usually of the opposite sex.

Philadelphia chromosome (Ph¹) [Philadelphia, Pennsylvania], a translocation of the long arm of chromosome 22, often seen in the abnormal myeloblasts, erythroblasts, and megakaryoblasts of patients who have chronic myelocytic leukemia.

philtrum, the vertical groove in the center of the upper lip.

phimosis /fīmō'sis/ [Gk, muzzle], tightness of the prepuce of the penis that prevents the retraction of the foreskin over the glans. The condition is usually congenital but may be the result of infection.

phimosis vaginalis /vaj'inā'lis/, congenital narrowness or closure of the vaginal opening.

phlebectomy /fləbot'əmē/ [Gk phleps vein, ektome cutting out], the surgical removal of a vein or part of a vein.

phlebitis. See **thrombophlebitis.**

phlebogram /fleb'əgram/ [Gk phleps vein, gramma record] **1.** an x-ray film obtained by phlebography. **2.** a graphic representation of the venous pulse, obtained by phlebograph.

phlebograph /fleb'əgraf'/, a device for producing a graphic record of the venous pulse.

phlebography /fləbog'rəfē/ [Gk phleps + graphein to record], **1.** the technique of preparing an x-ray image of veins injected with a radiopaque contrast medium. **2.** the technique of preparing a graphic record of the venous pulse by means of a phlebograph.

phlebostatic axis [Gk phleps + stasis standing still], the approximate location of the right atrium, found by drawing an imaginary line from the fourth intercostal space at the right side of the sternum to an intersection with the midaxillary line.

phlebothrombosis /fleb'ōthrombō'sis/ [Gk phleps + thrombos lump, osis condition], an abnormal venous condition in which a clot forms within a vein, usually caused by hemostasis, hypercoagulability, or occlusion. In contrast to thrombophlebitis, the wall of the vein is not inflamed.

phlebotomist /fləbot'əmist/ [Gk, phleps, vein + ektome], a physician or other individual with special training in the practice of opening veins to remove blood.

phlebotomize /fləbot'əmiz/, to open a vein to remove blood.

phlebotomus fever /fləbot'əməs/ [Gk phleps + tomos cutting; L febris fever], an acute, mild infection caused by one of five distinct arboviruses transmitted to humans by the bite of an infected sandfly, characterized by rapidly developing fever, headache, eye pain, conjunctivitis, myalgia, and occasionally a macular or urticarial rash.

phlebotomy /fləbot'əmē/ [Gk *phleps* + *temnein* to cut], the incision of a vein for the letting of blood, as in collecting blood from a donor. Phlebotomy is the chief treatment for polycythemia vera and may be performed every 6 months, or more frequently if required.

phlegm /flem/ [Gk *phlegma* mucus], thick mucus secreted by the tissues lining the respiratory passages.

phlegmasia alba dolens [Gk *phlegmone* inflammation; L *albus* white; *dolens* painful], thrombophlebitis of the femoral vein, resulting in edema of the leg and pain. It may occur after childbirth or after a severe febrile illness.

phlegmasia cerulea dolens, a severe form of thrombosis of a deep vein, usually the femoral vein.

phlegmatic /flegmat'ik/ [Gk *phlegmatikos* sluggishness], pertaining to a person who is dull, apathetic, or not easily excitable.

phlegmon /fleg'mon/ [Gk *phlegmone* inflammation], an inflammation of connective tissue.

phlegmonous gastritis /fleg'mənəs/ [Gk *phlegmone* + *osis* condition], a rare but severe form of gastritis involving the connective tissue layer of the stomach wall.

phlyctenular keratoconjunctivitis /flikten'yələr/ [Gk *phlyktaina* blister], an inflammatory condition of the cornea, characterized by tiny, ulcerating nodules, seen most often in children as a response to allergens found in tuberculin, gonococci, *Candida albicans,* or various parasites.

phobia /fō'bē-ə/ [Gk *phobos* fear], an anxiety disorder characterized by an obsessive, irrational, and intense fear of a specific object, such as an animal or dirt; of an activity, such as meeting strangers or leaving the familiar setting of the home; or of a physical situation, such as heights and open or closed spaces. Typical manifestations of phobia include faintness, fatigue, palpitations, perspiration, nausea, tremor, and panic. The fear, which is out of proportion to reality, often results from some early painful or unpleasant experience involving the particular object or situation. Some kinds of phobias are **agoraphobia, algophobia, claustrophobia, erythrophobia, gynephobia, laliophobia, mysophobia, nyctophobia, photophobia, xenophobia,** and **zoophobia. –phobic,** *adj.*

phobiac /fō'bē-ak/, a person who exhibits or is afflicted with a phobia.

phobic desensitization [Gk *phobos* fear; L *de, sentire* to feel], a method of resolving an ego dystonic or uncomfortable behavior pattern by reentry into the emotionally upsetting life situation in stages, first in fantasy and again in real life. It is similar to the psychotherapeutic techniques of **flooding** and **implosive therapy.**

phobic disorder, phobic neurosis, phobic reaction. See phobia.

phobic state, a condition characterized by extreme anxiety resulting from the excessive, irrational fear of a particular object, situation, or activity.

phocomelia /fō'kəmē'lyə/ [Gk *phoke* seal, *melos* limb], a developmental anomaly characterized by the absence of the upper portion of one or more of the limbs so that the feet or hands or both are attached to the trunk of the body by short, irregularly shaped stumps, resembling the fins of a seal. **–phocomelic,** *adj.*

phocomelic dwarf /fō'kəmē'lik/, a dwarf in whom the long bones of any or all of the extremities are abnormally short.

phocomelus /fōkom'ələs/, an individual who has phocomelia.

phonation /fōnā'shən/ [Gk *phone* sound; L *atio* process], the production of speech sounds through the vibration of the vocal folds of the larynx.

phonetics, the science of speech sounds used in language.

phonic, of or pertaining to voice, sounds, or speech.

phonocardiogram /fō'nōkär'dē·əgram'/, a graphic recording obtained from a phonocardiograph.

phonocardiograph /fō'nōkär'dē·əgraf'/ [Gk *phone* + *kardia* heart, *graphein* to record], an electroacoustic device that produces graphic heart sound recordings, used in the diagnosis and monitoring of heart disorders. This instrument produces phonocardiograms by using a system of microphones placed on the chest near the base of the heart and another positioned on the chest over the apex of the heart. **–phonocardiographic,** *adj.*

phonocardiography, the recording of heart sounds and murmurs by electromechanical apparatus.

phonology /fōnol'əjē/, the study of speech sounds, particularly the principles governing the way speech sounds are used in a given language.

phonophoresis /fō'nōfərē'sis/, an ultrasound therapeutic technique in which the high-frequency sound waves are used to force topical medicines into subcutaneous tissues.

phonoreceptor [Gk *phone* + L *recipere* to

receive], a device for receiving sound impulses.

phosphatase /fos'fətāz/, an enzyme that acts as a catalyst in chemical reactions involving phosphorus.

phosphate, a salt of phosphoric acid. Phosphates are extremely important in living cells, particularly in the storage and use of energy and the transmission of genetic information.

phosphate-bond energy, the Gibbs energy for hydrolysis of a phosphate compound; a measure of relative phosphorylation power.

phosphatemia /fos'fātē'mē·ə/ [Gk *phosphoros* bringer of light; Gk *haima* blood], a condition of excessive phosphates in the blood.

phosphatide /fos'fətīd/, a phosphatidic acid from which the choline or colamine portion has been removed. It may occur as an intermediate in the biosynthesis of triglycerides and phospholipids.

phosphaturia /fos'fatŏŏr'ē·ə/ [Gk *phosphoros* + *ouron* urine], a condition of excessive phosphates in the urine.

phosphoglycerate kinase /fos'fōglis'ərāt/, an enzyme that catalyzes the reversible transfer of a phosphate group from adenosine triphosphate to D-3-phosphoglycerate, forming D-1,3-diphosphoglycerate.

phospholipid /fos'fōlip'id/ [Gk *phos* light, *pherein* to bear, *lipos* fat], one of a class of compounds, widely distributed in living cells, containing phosphoric acid, fatty acids, and a nitrogenous base. Two kinds of phospholipids are **lecithin** and **sphingomyelin**.

phosphomevalonate kinase /fos'fōməval'-ənāt/, an enzyme that catalyzes the transfer of a phosphate group from adenosine triphosphate to produce adenosine diphosphate and 5-pyrophosphomevalonate.

phosphoresence [Gk *phos* + *pherein* to bear], **1.** a glow of yellow phosphorus caused by slow oxidation. **2.** the emission of visible light without accompanying heat as observed in phosphorus that has been exposed to radiation, continuing after radiation has ceased.

phosphoric acid, a clear, colorless, odorless liquid that is irritating to the skin and eyes and moderately toxic if ingested.

phosphorus (P) [Gk *phos* light, *pherein* to bear], a nonmetallic chemical element occurring extensively in nature as a component of phosphate rock. Its atomic number is 15; its atomic weight is 30.975. Phosphorus is essential for the metabolism of protein, calcium, and glucose. A nutritional deficiency of phosphorus can cause weight loss, anemia, and abnormal growth.

phosphorus poisoning, a toxic condition caused by the ingestion of white or yellow phosphorus, sometimes found in rat poisons, certain fertilizers, and fireworks. Intoxication is characterized initially by nausea, throat and stomach pain, vomiting, diarrhea, and an odor of garlic on the breath.

phosphorylase /fosfôr'ilās/, any of a group of physiologically important enzymes that catalyze reactions between phosphates and glycogen or other starch components, yielding glucose-1-phosphate.

photic /fō'tik/, pertaining to light.

photic epilepsy [Gk *phos* light; *epilepsia* seizure], a condition in which epileptic attacks may be triggered by flickering light.

photoallergic [Gk *photos* light, *allos* other, *ergein* to work], exhibiting a delayed hypersensitivity reaction after exposure to light.

photoallergic contact dermatitis, a papulovesicular, eczematous, or exudative skin reaction occurring 24 to 48 hours after exposure to light in a previously sensitized person. The sensitizing substance concentrates in the skin and requires chemical alteration by light to become an active antigen.

photoallergy, a sensitivity to light as a cause of allergic reactions.

photochemotherapy [Gk *photos* + *chemeia* alchemy, *therapeia* treatment], a kind of chemotherapy in which the effect of the administered drug is enhanced by exposing the patient to light, such as the treatment of psoriasis with oral methoxsalen followed by exposure to ultraviolet light.

photodisintegration, (in radiology) the interaction of a high-energy x-ray photon with the nucleus of a target atom, resulting in the emission of a nucleon or other nuclear fragment.

photoelectron [Gk *phos* + *elektron* amber], any electron that is discharged when light strikes a metal surface.

photokinetic /ˈkinet'ik/ [Gk *phos* + *kinesis* movement], any movement that is stimulated by light rays.

photometer /fōtom'ətər/ [Gk *photos* + *metron* measure], an instrument that measures light intensity.

photomultiplier [Gk *photos* + L *multiplex* many folds], a device used in many radiation detection applications that converts low levels of light into electric pulses.

photon /fō'ton/ [Gk *photos*], the smallest quantity of electromagnetic energy. It has no mass and no charge but travels at the speed of light. Photons may occur in the form of x-rays, gamma rays, or a quantum of light.

photophobia /fō'tō-/ [Gk *photos* + *phobos* fear] **1.** abnormal sensitivity to light, especially by the eyes. The condition is prevalent in albinism and various diseases of the conjunctiva and cornea and may be a symptom of such disorders as measles, psittacosis, encephalitis, Rocky Mountain spotted fever, and Reiter's syndrome. **2.** (in psychiatry) a morbid fear of light with an irrational need to avoid light places. **–photophobic,** *adj.*

phototopic eye. See **light-adapted eye.**

photopic vision, daylight vision, which depends primarily on the function of the retinal cone cells.

photoprotective, protective against the potential adverse effects of ultraviolet light.

photoreaction, any chemical reaction that is stimulated by the influence of light.

photoreceptor, a nerve cell that is receptive to light stimuli.

photorefractive keratectomy, a procedure for the treatment of near-sightedness in which a 30-second exposure to an excimer laser beam shaves a few layers of cells off the surface of the cornea. The laser flattens the cornea to reduce or eliminate myopia.

photoscan /fō'tōskan'/, a radiograph that shows the distribution of a radiopharmaceutical in the body.

photosensitive [Gk *photos* + L *sentire* to feel], pertaining to increased reactivity of skin to sunlight caused by a disorder, such as albinism or porphyria, or more frequently resulting from the use of certain drugs. Relatively brief exposure to sunlight or to an ultraviolet lamp may cause edema, papules, urticaria, or acute burns in individuals with endogenous or acquired photosensitivity.

photosensitivity, any abnormal response to exposure to light, specifically a skin reaction requiring the presence of a sensitizing agent and exposure to sunlight or its equivalent.

photosensitization, the process of rendering an organism sensitive to the effects of light rays.

photosynthesis /fōtōsin'thəsis/ [Gk *photos* + *synthesis* putting together], a process by which green plants containing chlorophyll synthesize chemical substances, chiefly carbohydrates, from atmospheric carbon dioxide and water, using light for energy and liberating oxygen in the process.

phototherapy [Gk *photos* + *therapeia* treatment], the treatment of disorders by the use of light, especially ultraviolet light. Ultraviolet light may be employed in the therapy of acne, decubiti and other indo-lent ulcers, psoriasis, and hyperbilirubinemia. **–phototherapeutic,** *adj.*

phototherapy in the newborn, a treatment for hyperbilirubinemia and jaundice in the newborn that involves the exposure of an infant's bare skin to intense fluorescent light. The blue range of light accelerates the excretion of bilirubin in the skin, decomposing it by photooxidation.

phototoxic [Gk *photos* + *toxikon* poison], characterized by a rapidly developing, nonimmunologic reaction of the skin when it is exposed to a photosensitizing substance and light.

phototoxic contact dermatitis, a rapidly appearing, sunburnlike response of areas of skin that have been exposed to the sun after contact with a photosensitizing substance. Hyperpigmentation may follow the acute reaction. Among known photosensitizing materials are coal tar derivatives, oil of bergamot, and many plants containing furocoumarin, such as cowslip, buttercup, and yarrow.

pH paper. See **nitrazine paper.**

phren /fren/ [Gk, mind], the diaphragm.

phrenetic /frənet'ik/ [Gk *phren*], frenzied, delirious, maniacal.

phrenic /fren'ik/ [Gk *phren* mind], **1.** of or pertaining to the diaphragm. **2.** of or pertaining to the mind.

phrenic nerve, one of a pair of muscular branches of the cervical plexus, arising from the fourth cervical nerve. It contains about half as many sensory as motor fibers and is generally known as the motor nerve to the diaphragm, although the lower thoracic nerves also help to innervate the diaphragm.

Phthirus /thī'rəs/ [Gk *phtheir* louse], a genus of bloodsucking lice that includes the species *Phthirus pubis,* the pubic louse, or crab.

phthisis /tis'is, thī'sis/ [Gk *phthisis* wasting away], any wasting disease involving all or part of the body, such as pulmonary tuberculosis.

phychologist /fēkol'əjist/, a person who specializes in the study of algae.

phycology /fēkol'əjē/ [Gk *phykos* seaweed, *logos* science], the branch of science that is concerned with algae.

phycomycosis /fī'kōmīkō'sis/ [Gk *phykos* + *mykes* fungus, *osis* condition], a fungal infection caused by a species of the order Phycomycetes.

phylactic /filak'tik/ [Gk *phylax* guard], **1.** serving to protect. **2.** something that produces phylaxis.

phylloquinone. See **vitamin K₁.**

phylogenesis. See **phylogeny.**

phylogenetic /fī'lōgənet'ik/ [Gk *phylon* tribe, *genesis* origin], **1.** of, relating to, or acquired during phylogeny. **2.** based on a natural evolutionary relationship, as a system of classification.

phylogeny /fīloj′ənē/ [Gk *phylon* + *genesis*], the development of the structure of a particular race or species as it evolved from simpler forms of life.

phylum /fī′ləm/ [Gk *phylon* tribe], a major classification category of the plant and animal kingdoms, representing one or more classes.

physiatrics /fiz′ē·at′riks/ [Gr *physis* nature, *iatrikos* treatment], the diagnosis and treatment of disease by the use of physical agents such as heat, cold, light, water, electricity, and mechanical devices.

physiatrist /fiz′ē·at′rist/ [Gk *physikos* natural, *iatros* healing], a physician specializing in physical medicine and rehabilitation who has been certified by the American Board of Physical Medicine and Rehabilitation after completing residency and other requirements.

physical abuse [Gk *physikos* natural; L *abuti* to abuse], one or more episodes of aggressive behavior, usually resulting in physical injury with possible damage to internal organs, sense organs, the central nervous system, or the musculoskeletal system of another person.

physical allergy, an allergic response to physical factors, such as cold, heat, light, or trauma. Usually, specific antibodies are found in people having physical allergies. Common characteristics include pruritus, urticaria, and angioedema.

physical assessment, the part of the health assessment representing a synthesis of the information obtained in a physical examination.

physical chemistry, the natural science dealing with the relationship between chemical and physical properties of matter.

physical diagnosis, the diagnostic process accomplished by the study of the physical manifestations of health and illness revealed in the physical examination, as guided by the patient's complete history and supported by various laboratory tests.

physical examination, an investigation of the body to determine its state of health, using any or all of the techniques of inspection, palpation, percussion, auscultation, and smell.

physical fitness, the ability to carry out daily tasks with alertness and vigor, without undue fatigue, and with enough energy reserve to meet emergencies or to enjoy leisure time pursuits.

physical medicine, the use of physical therapy techniques to return physically diseased or injured patients to a useful life.

physical science, the study of the laws and properties of nonliving matter. Some kinds of physical science are **chemistry, geology,** and **physics.**

physical sign, an objective indicator found during physical diagnosis or one detected by palpation, percussion, or auscultation.

physical therapist, a person who is licensed to assist in the examination, testing, and treatment of physically disabled or handicapped people through the use of special exercise, application of heat or cold, use of sonar waves, and other techniques. A physical therapist usually becomes qualified by taking a 4-year college course leading to a BS in physical therapy or a special 12-month certificate course after obtaining a bachelor's degree in a related field.

physical therapy, the treatment of disorders with physical agents and methods, such as massage, manipulation, therapeutic exercises, cold, heat (including shortwave, microwave, and ultrasonic diathermy), hydrotherapy, electric stimulation, and light to assist in rehabilitating patients and in restoring normal function after an illness or injury.

physical therapy aide, a person who, under the supervision of a licensed physical therapist, assists in carrying out patient treatment programs and performing related clerical tasks.

physician [Gk *physikos* natural], a health professional who has earned a degree of Doctor of Medicine (MD) after completing an approved course of study at an approved medical school. Satisfactory completion of National Board Examinations, usually given during both the second and the final years of medical school and after graduation, is also required. An MD usually enters a hospital internship program for 1 year of postgraduate training before beginning practice or further training in a specialty. To practice medicine, an MD is required to obtain a license from the state in which professional services will be performed.

physician extender, a health care provider who is not a physician but who performs medical activities typically performed by a physician.

physician's assistant (PA), a person trained in certain aspects of the practice of medicine to provide assistance to a physician. A physician's assistant is trained by physicians and practices under the direction and supervision and within the legal license of a physician. Training programs vary in length from a few months to 2 years. National certification is available to qualified graduates of approved training programs. The national organization is the American Association of Physician's Assistants (AAPA).

Physician's Desk Reference (PDR), a compendium compiled annually, containing information about drugs, primarily prescription drugs and products used in diagnostic procedures in the United States, supplied by their manufacturers.

physics [Gk *physikos* natural], the study of the laws and properties of matter and energy, particularly as related to motion and force.

physiologic, physiological, [Gk *physis* nature, *logos* science], pertaining to physiology, particularly normal functions as opposed to the pathologic.

physiologic age, the age of the body as determined by its stage of development or deterioration in terms of functional norms for various systems.

physiologic albuminuria [Gk *physis* + *logos* science; L *albus* white; Gk *ouron* urine], the presence of albumin in the urine in the absence of any disease usually associated with the condition.

physiologic incompatibility, a condition in which substances, such as drugs, may have mutually antagonistic effects on the body.

physiologic murmur, a functional murmur produced by an alteration of function without evidence of heart damage or disease.

physiologic salt solution, a normal saline solution, usually consisting of a sterile 0.9% w/v solution of sodium chloride in distilled water. It is isotonic with normal body fluids.

physiologic amenorrhea, an absence of menstruation for normal reasons, such as pregnancy, lactation, menopause, or prepuberty.

physiologic antidote, a drug that has the opposite effect on the body from that caused by a poisonous or toxic substance.

physiologic chemistry. See **biochemistry.**

physiologic contracture [Gk *physikos* + *logos* science; L *contractio* drawing together], a temporary condition in which muscles may contract and shorten for a considerable period. Drugs, extremes of temperature, and local accumulation of lactic acid are causes.

physiologic dead space. See **dead space.**

physiologic dwarf. See **primordial dwarf.**

physiologic flexion, an excessive amount of flexor tone that is normally present at birth because of the existing level of central nervous system maturation and fetal positioning in the uterus.

physiologic hypertrophy, a temporary increase in the size of an organ or part because of normal physiologic functions, as occurs in the walls of the uterus and in the breasts during pregnancy.

physiologic jaundice, a simple jaundice of newborn infants that involves breaking down the excessive number of red blood cells that may be present at birth.

physiologic motivation, a bodily need, such as food or water, that initiates behavior directed toward satisfying the particular need.

physiologic occlusion, **1.** a closure of the teeth that complements and enhances the functions of the masticatory system. **2.** a closure of the teeth that produces no pathologic effects on the stomatognathic system. **3.** an acceptable occlusion in a healthy gnathic system.

physiologic psychology, the study of the interrelationship of physiologic and psychologic processes, especially the effects of a change from normal to abnormal.

physiologic retraction ring, a ridge around the inside of the uterus that forms during the second stage of normal labor at the junction of the thinned lower uterine segment and thickened upper segment as a result of progressive lengthening of the muscle fibers of the lower segment and concomitant shortening of the muscle fibers of the upper segment.

physiologic saline. See **saline solution.**

physiologic third heart sound, a low-pitched extra heart sound heard early in diastole in a healthy child or young adult. The same sound, heard in an older person who has heart disease, is an abnormal finding called a ventricular gallop.

physiologic tremor [Gk *physis* + *logos; L tremor* shaking], any tremor caused by physiologic factors, such as fatigue, fear, or cold.

physiologist [Gk *physis* + *logos* science], a person who specializes in the science of living organisms.

physiology [Gk *physikos* + *logos* science], **1.** the study of the processes and function of the human body. **2.** the study of the physical and chemical processes involved in the functioning of living organisms and their component parts. Kinds of physiology are **comparative, developmental, hominal,** and **pathologic physiology.**

physiopathologic, pertaining to the physiologic approach to disease.

physiotherapy. See **physical therapy.**

physostigmine /fī′sōstig′min/, a cholinergic prescribed in the treatment of some forms of glaucoma and to reverse effects of neuromuscular blocking agents.

physostigmine salicylate, an anticholinergic drug inhibitor. It is prescribed in the treatment of central nervous system effects caused by drugs in clinical or toxic dosages capable of producing anticholinergic poisoning.

phytanic acid storage disease /fītan'ik/, a rare genetic disorder of lipid metabolism in which there are accumulations of phytanic acid in the plasma and tissues. The condition is characterized by ataxia, peripheral neuropathy, retinitis pigmentosa, and abnormalities of the bone and skin.

phytogenesis /fī'tōjen'əsis/ [Gk *phyton* plant, *genein* to produce], the origin and evolution of plant organisms.

phytogenous /fītoj'ənəs/ [Gk *phyton* + *genein*], pertaining to production by plant growth, origin in a plant, or the origin or formation of plant organisms.

phytohemagglutinin (PHA) /fī'tōhem'-əgloo'tinin/ [Gk *phyton* plant, *haima* blood; L *agglutinare* to glue], a hemagglutinin that is derived from a plant, specifically the lectin obtained from the red kidney bean.

phytohemagglutinin test, a test to identify genetic carriers of cystic fibrosis, performed by exposing white blood cells to phytohemagglutinin. A normal reaction involves a noticeable increase of cell protein.

phytolectin, See **phytohemagglutinin.**

phytonadione. See **vitamin K₁.**

PI, 1. (in patient records) abbreviation for *present illness* 2. abbreviation for *International Pharmacopeia.*

pia, abbreviation for **pia mater.**

piaarachnoid [L *pia* tender; Gk *arachne* spider, *eidos* form], pertaining to both the pia mater and arachnoid layers of the meninges covering the brain and spinal cord.

pia mater /pē'ə mā'tər/ [L *pia* tender, *mater* mother], the innermost of the three meninges covering the brain and the spinal cord. It is closely applied to both structures and carries a rich supply of blood vessels, which nourish the nervous tissue. The cranial pia mater covers the surface of the brain and dips deeply into the fissures and the sulci of the cerebral hemispheres. The spinal pia mater is thicker, firmer, and less vascular than the cranial pia mater.

pian. See **yaws.**

pian bois. See **forest yaws.**

pica /pī'kə/ [L, magpie], a craving to eat substances that are not foods, such as dirt, clay, chalk, glue, ice, starch, or hair. The appetite disorder may occur with some nutritional deficiency states, with pregnancy, and in some forms of mental illness.

Pick's disease¹ [Arnold Pick, Czechoslovakian neurologist, b. 1851], a form of presenile dementia occurring in middle age. This disorder affects mainly the frontal and temporal lobes of the brain and characteristically produces neurotic behavior, slow disintegration of intellect, personality, and emotions, and degeneration of cognitive abilities.

Pick's disease² [Friedel Pick, Czech physician, b. 1867], a condition similar to polyserositis, with constrictive inflammation of the mediastinum and pericardium, leading to chronic venous congestion and cirrhosis.

Pick's disease³ [Ludwig Pick, German physician, b. 1868], a rare chronic familial disease involving lipid metabolism, with large cells of the marrow, spleen, and glands filled with sphyngomyelin. Other characteristics include anemia, digestive disorders, enlarged liver, and distended abdomen.

pickwickian syndrome [*Pickwick Papers* by Charles Dickens], an abnormal condition characterized by obesity, decreased pulmonary function, somnolence, and polycythemia.

picogram (pg) /pī'kəgram/, a unit of measure equal to one trillionth of a gram, or 1×10^{-12} gram.

picornavirus /pīkôr'nəvī'rəs/ [It *pico* small, *RNA* ribonucleic acid; L *virus* poison], a member of a group of small RNA viruses that are ether resistant. These viruses cause poliomyelitis, herpangina, and aseptic meningitis, encephalomyocarditis, and foot-and-mouth disease.

picosecond (ps), a unit of measure equal to one trillionth of a second.

picrotoxin /pik'rōtok'sin/ [Gk *pikros* bitter, *toxikon* poison], a central nervous system stimulant obtained from the seeds of *Anamirta cocculus,* formerly used as an antidote for acute barbiturate poisoning.

PID, abbreviation for **pelvic inflammatory disease.**

PIE, abbreviation for **pulmonary infiltrate with eosinophilia,** a hypersensitivity reaction, characterized by infiltration of alveoli with eosinophils and large mononuclear cells, edema, and inflammation of the lungs. Simple pulmonary eosinophilia, in which patchy, migratory infiltrates cause minimal symptoms, is a self-limited reaction that is elicited by helminthic infections and by certain drugs. A more prolonged illness, characterized by fever, night sweats, cough, dyspnea, weight loss, and more severe tissue reaction, occurs in certain drug allergies and bacterial, fungal, and parasitic infections.

piebald /pī'bôld/ [L *pica* magpie; ME

balled smooth], having patches of white hair or skin because of an absence of melanocytes in those nonpigmented areas. It is a hereditary condition.

Piedmont fracture, an oblique fracture of the distal radius, with fragments of bone pulled into the ulna.

Pierre Robin's syndrome [Pierre Robin, French histologist, b. 1867], a complex of congenital anomalies including a small mandible, cleft lip, cleft palate, other craniofacial abnormalities, and defects of the eyes and ears, including glaucoma. Intelligence is usually normal.

piezochemistry /pī-ē′zōkem′istrē/ [Gk *piezein* to press, *chemeia* alchemy], a branch of chemistry concerned with reactions that occur under pressure.

piezoelectric effect [Gk *piezein* to press, *elektron* amber; L *effectus*], **1.** the generation of a voltage across a solid when a mechanical stress is applied. **2.** the dimensional change resulting from the application of a voltage. **3.** (in ultrasound) the conversion of one form of energy into another, such as the conversion of electrical energy into mechanical energy.

pigeon breast [L *pipio* bird; AS *broest* breast], a congenital structural defect characterized by a prominent anterior projection of the xiphoid and the lower part of the sternum and by a lengthening of the costal cartilages. It may cause cardiorespiratory complications. **–pigeon-breasted,** *adj.*

pigeon breeder's lung, a respiratory disorder caused by acquired hypersensitivity to antigens in bird droppings.

pigeon-toed. See **metatarsus varus.**

piggyback port [AS *piken* pick; ME *pakke* pack; L *portus* haven], a special coupling for the primary IV tubing that allows a supplementary, or piggyback, solution to run into the IV system.

pigment [L *pigmentum* paint], **1.** any organic coloring material produced in the body, such as melanin. **2.** any colored, paintlike, medicinal preparation applied to the skin surface. **–pigmentary, pigmented,** *adj.*, **pigmentation,** *n.*

pigmentary retinopathy, a disorder of the retina characterized by deposits of pigment and increasing loss of vision.

pigmented villonodular synovitis, a disease of the joints characterized by fingerlike proliferative growths of synovial tissue, with hemosiderin deposition within the synovial tissue.

pigmy. See **pygmy.**

pil, abbreviation for the Latin, *pilula,* pill, or *pilulae,* pills.

pilar cyst [L *pilus* hair; Gk *kystis* bag], an epidermoid cyst of the scalp. It originates from the middle portion of the epithelium of a hair follicle.

piles. See **hemorrhoids.**

pili. See **pilus.**

piliform /pī′lifôrm/ [L *pilus* hair], the appearance of hair.

pi lines, x-ray film artifacts that occur as a result of dirt or chemical stains on a processing roller.

pill. See **tablet.**

pillion fracture /pil′yən/ [Gael *pillean* couch; L *fractura* break], a T-shaped fracture of the distal end of the femur with displacement of the condyles posterior to the femoral shaft, caused by a severe blow to the knee.

pilocarpine and epinephrine, a fixed-combination drug used in the treatment of glaucoma, containing a cholinergic (pilocarpine hydrochloride) and an adrenergic vasoconstrictor (epinephrine bitartrate).

pilocarpine and physostigmine, a fixed-combination drug used in the treatment of glaucoma, containing a cholinergic (pilocarpine hydrochloride) and a short-acting cholinesterase inhibitor (physostigmine salicylate). Both ingredients reduce intraocular pressure.

pilocarpine hydrochloride, a cholinergic drug derived from the leaves of the jaborandi tree and other species of *Pilocarpus.* It is used mainly as a miotic to contract the pupil in cases of glaucoma. The drug also increases the secretion of salivary, intestinal, and gastric glands when injected, reduces the heartbeat, and constricts the bronchioles.

pilomotor reflex /pī′lōmō′tər/ [L *pilus* hair, *motor* mover; *reflectere* to bend backward], erection of the hairs of the skin in response to a chilly environment, emotional stimulus, or irritation of the skin.

pilonidal [L *pilus* + *nidus* nest], a growth of hair in a cyst or other internal structure.

pilonidal cyst /pī′lənī′dəl/ [L *pilus* + *nidus* nest], a hairy cyst that often develops in the sacral region of the skin. Pilonidal cysts may sometimes be recognized at birth by a depression, sometimes a hairy dimple, in the midline of the back at the sacrococcygeal area.

pilonidal fistula, an abnormal channel containing a tuft of hair, situated most frequently over or close to the tip of the coccyx but also occurring in other regions of the body.

pilonidal sinus [L *pilus* + *nidus; sinus* curve], a cavity or sinus containing hair, such as the axilla or navel. In most instances the hair originated in another area and became lodged in the sinus.

pilosebaceous /pī′lōsibā′shəs/ [L *pilus* +

P

sebum fat], of or pertaining to a hair follicle or its oil gland.

pilus /pē′ləs/, *pl.* **pili** [L, hair], **1.** a hair or hairlike structure. **2.** (in microbiology) a fine, filamentous appendage found on certain bacteria and similar to flagellum except that it is shorter, straighter, and found in greater quantities in the organism.

pimozide /pim′əzīd/, an oral neuroleptic agent prescribed for the suppression of motor and phonic tics associated with Tourette's disorder.

pimple [ME *pinple*], a small papule, pustule, or furuncle.

pin [AS *pinn*], **1.** (in orthopedics) to secure and immobilize fragments of bone with a nail. **2.** See **nail**, def. 2. **3.** (in dentistry) a small metal rod or peg, used as a support in rebuilding a tooth.

pin and tube fixed orthodontic appliance, an orthodontic appliance for correcting and improving malocclusion. It employs a labial arch with vertical posts that insert into tubes attached to bands on the teeth.

pinch, a compression or squeezing of the end of the thumb in opposition to the end of one or more of the fingers.

pinch graft [Fr *pince;* Gk *graphion* stylus], a small, circular deep graft of skin only a few millimeters in diameter. It is cut so that the center is of whole skin but the edges consist of only epidermis.

pinch grip. See **tip pinch.**

pinch meter, a type of dynamometer that measures the strength of a finger pinch.

pindolol /pin′dəlol/, a beta-adrenergic blocker with sympathomimetic activity. It is prescribed in the treatment of hypertension, alone or concomitantly with a diuretic.

pineal [L *pineus* pine cone], **1.** pertaining to the pineal body. **2.** resembling a pine cone.

pineal body /pin′ē-əl/ [L *pineus* pine cone; AS *bodig* body], a cone-shaped structure in the brain, situated between the superior colliculi, the pulvinar, and the splenium of the corpus callosum. Its precise function has not been established.

pinealectomy /pin′ē-əlek′təmē/, the surgical removal of the pineal body.

pineal hyperplasia syndrome, an abnormal condition caused by overgrowth of the pineal body. It is characterized by severe insulin resistance, dry skin, thick nails, hirsutism, early appearance of dentition, and sexual precocity.

pinealoma /pin′ē-əlō′mə/, *pl.* **pinealomas, pinealomata** [L *pineas* + Gk *oma* tumor], a rare neoplasm of the pineal body in the brain, characterized by hydrocephalus, pupillary changes, gait disturbances, headache, nausea, and vomiting.

pineal peduncle [L *pineus; peduncle* small foot], the stalk of the pineal body.

pineal tumor, a neoplasm of the pineal body.

pine tar [L *pinus* pine; AS *teoru* tar], a topical antieczematic and a rubefacient. It is a common ingredient in creams, soaps, and lotions used in the treatment of chronic skin conditions, such as eczema and psoriasis.

pinhole pupil, a very small pupil, which may be congenital; an effect of the use of miotics, or the result of an inflamed iris.

pinhole retention [AS *pinn* pin, *hol* hole; L *retinere* to hold], retention developed by drilling one or more holes, 2 to 3 mm in depth, in suitable areas of a cavity preparation to supplement resistance and retention form.

pinhole test, a test performed in examining a person who has diminished visual acuity to distinguish a refractive error from organic disease. Several pinholes are punched in a card; the patient selects one and looks through it with one eye at a time, without wearing glasses. If visual acuity is improved, the defect is refractive; if not, it is organic. **2.** (in radiology) a test to identify the size of the focal spot of the x-ray tube. Also, a tomography test used to trace the path of the tube movement.

pink disease. See **acrodynia.**

pinkeye. See **conjunctivitis.**

Pinkus' disease. See **lichen nitidus.**

pinna. See **auricle.**

pinocytic /pī′nəsit′ik/ [Gk *pinein* to drink, *kytos* cell], pertaining to a pinocyte, particularly its ability to absorb liquids by phagocytosis in cellular metabolic processes.

pinocytosis /pī′nōsītō′sis/ [Gk *pinein, kytos* + *osis* condition], the process by which extracellular fluid is taken into a cell. The cell membrane develops a saccular indentation filled with extracellular fluid, then closes around it, forming a vesicle or a vacuole of fluid within the cell.

pinprick test, a test of the ability of a person to detect a cutaneous pain sensation and to differentiate such sensations from pressure stimuli. The test is performed with a pin or needle gently applied to the skin where it cannot be observed by the subject.

pinta /pēn′tə/ [Sp, spot], an infection of the skin caused by *Treponema carateum,* a common organism in South America and Central America. The bacterium gains entry into the body through a break in the skin. The primary lesion is a slowly enlarging papule with regional lymph node enlargement, followed in 1 to 12 months by a generalized red to slate-blue macular rash.

pin track infection [AS *pinn;* ME *trak* trace; L *inficere* to taint], an abnormal condition associated with skeletal traction and characterized by infection of superficial, deeper, or soft tissues or by osteomyelitis. These infections may develop at skeletal traction pin sites.

pinworm. See *Enterobius vermicularis.*

PIo₂, the partial pressure of inspired oxygen.

pions /pī′onz/ [Gk *pi* sixteenth letter of Greek alphabet + *meson* nuclear particle], a family of particles that can be created in nuclear reactions. Pions are unstable but can survive long enough to be formed into beams and used in certain types of medical therapy, such as the treatment of brain tumors.

Piper forceps. See **obstetric forceps.**

piperocaine hydrochloride, a local anesthetic for the induction of spinal or caudal anesthesia.

pipette /pīpet′, pipet′/ [Fr, little pipe], **1.** a calibrated, transparent open-ended tube of glass or plastic used for measuring or transferring small quantities of a liquid or gas. **2.** using a pipette to dispense liquid.

piriform /pir′ifôrm/ [L *pirum* pear, *forma* form], pear-shaped.

piriform aperture [L *pirum* + *forma; apertura* opening], the anterior nasal opening in the skull.

piriformis /pir′ifôr′mis/ [L *pirum* + *forma*], a flat, pyramidal muscle lying almost parallel with the posterior margin of the gluteus medius. It functions to rotate the thigh laterally and to abduct and to help extend it.

Pirquet's test /pirkāz′/ [Clemens P. von Pirquet, Austrian physician, b. 1874], a tuberculin skin test that consists of scratching the tuberculin material onto the skin.

pisiform /pī′sifôrm/ [L *pisum* pea + *forma* form], pea-shaped.

pisiform bone /pē′sifôrm′/ [L *pisum* + *forma;* AS *ban* bone], a small, spheroidal carpal bone in the proximal row of carpal bones. It articulates with the triangular bone and is attached to the flexor retinaculum, the flexor carpi ulnaris, and the abductor digiti minimi.

pistol-shot sound, a sharp, slapping sound heard by auscultation over the femoral pulse of a patient with aortic incompetence. It is caused by a large-volume pulse with a sharp rise in pressure.

pit and fissure cavity [AS *pytt;* L *fissura* cleft; *cavum* cavity], a cavity that starts in tiny faults in tooth enamel, usually on occlusal surfaces of molars and premolars.

pitch [ME *picchen*], the quality of a tone or sound dependent on the relative rapidity of the vibrations by which it is produced.

pithing /pith′ing/ [AS *pitha*], the destruction of the central nervous system of an experimental animal in preparation for physiologic research. It is usually done by inserting a blunt probe through a foramen.

pitting [AS *pytt*], **1.** small, punctate indentations in fingernails or toenails, often a result of psoriasis. **2.** an indentation that remains for a short time after pressing edematous skin with a finger. **3.** small, depressed scars in the skin or other organ of the body. **4.** the removal by the spleen of material from within erythrocytes without damage to the cells.

pitting edema [AS *pytt;* Gk *oidema* swelling], an edema characterized by a condition in which a finger pressed into the skin over an accumulation of fluid will result in a temporary depression in the skin. Normally, skin and subcutaneous tissues quickly rebound when the pressure is released.

pituicyte /pit(y)oo̅′isīt/ [L *pituita* phlegm; Gk *kytos* cell], a cell of the neurohypophysis.

pituitarism /pit(y)oo̅′itəriz′əm/ [L *pituita* phlegm], any condition due to a defect or failure of the pituitary gland.

pituitary. See **pituitary gland.**

pituitary adamantinoma. See **craniopharyngioma.**

pituitary cachexia. See **postpubertal panhypopituitarism.**

pituitary dwarf /pitoo̅′iter′ē/ [L *pituita* phlegm; AS *dweorge*], a dwarf whose retarded development is caused by a deficiency of growth hormone resulting from hypofunction of the anterior lobe of the pituitary. The body is properly proportioned, with no facial or skeletal deformities, and there is normal mental and sexual development.

pituitary gland [L *pituita* phlegm], an endocrine gland suspended beneath the brain in the pituitary fossa of the sphenoid bone, supplying numerous hormones that govern many vital processes. It is divided into an anterior adenohypophysis and a smaller posterior neurohypophysis. The adenohypophysis secretes growth hormone (somatotropin), thyrotropic hormone, adrenocorticotropic hormone (ACTH), two gonadotropic hormones, follicle stimulating hormone (FSH), luteinizing hormone (LH), and prolactin, the hormone that promotes milk secretion. The

P

neurohypophysis stores two hormones, oxytocin and vasopressin.

pituitary myxedema [L *piuita;* Gk *myxa* mucus, *oidema* swelling], a type of hypothyroid condition secondary to an anterior pituitary disease.

pituitary nanism, a type of dwarfism associated with hypophyseal infantilism.

pituitary snuff lung, a type of hypersensitivity pneumonitis that sometimes occurs among takers of pituitary snuff. The antigens to which the hypersensitivity reaction occurs are found in serum proteins of cows and pigs and in pituitary tissue. Symptoms of the acute form of the disease include chills, cough, fever, dyspnea, anorexia, nausea, and vomiting.

pituitary stalk, a structure that connects the pituitary gland with the hypothalamus.

pit viper [AS *pytt;* L *vipera* snake], any one of a family of venomous snakes found in the Western Hemisphere and Asia, characterized by a heat-sensitive pit between the eye and nostril on each side of the head and hollow, perforated fangs that are usually folded back in the roof of the mouth. With the exception of coral snakes, all indigenous poisonous snakes in the United States are pit vipers.

pityriasis [Gk *pityron* bran], any of a number of skin diseases that have in common lesions that resemble dandrufflike scales without obvious signs of inflammation.

pityriasis alba /pitərī′əsis/ [Gk *pityron* bran; L *albus* white], a common idiopathic dermatosis characterized by round or oval, finely scaling patches of hypopigmentation, usually on the cheeks.

pityriasis rosea, a self-limited skin disease in which a slightly scaling, pink, macular rash spreads over the trunk and other unexposed areas of the body. A characteristic feature is the **herald patch,** a larger, more scaly lesion that precedes the diffuse rash by several days. The smaller lesions tend to line up with the long axis parallel to normal lines of cleavage of the skin. Mild itching is the only symptom.

Pityrosporum. See *Malassezia.*

pivot joint [Fr, hinge; L *jungere* to join], a synovial joint in which movement is limited to rotation. The proximal radioulnar articulation is a pivot joint.

pivot transfer, the movement of a person from one site to another, such as from a bed to a wheelchair, when there is a loss of control of one side of the body. The person is helped to a position on the strong side of the body with both feet on the floor, heels behind the knees, and knees lower than the hips. The person stands with the weight on the strong leg and pivots on it, lowering the body into the wheelchair.

PJC, abbreviation for *premature junctional complex.*

PK, abbreviation for **psychokinesis.**

pKₐ, the negative logarithm of the ionization constant of an acid. A measure of the strength of an acid.

PKA, abbreviation for **protein kinase.**

PKD, abbreviation for **polycystic kidney disease.**

PK test, abbreviation for **Prausnitz-Küstner test.**

PKU, abbreviation for **phenylketonuria.**

placebo /pləsē′bō/ [L *placere* to please], an inactive substance, such as saline, distilled water, or sugar, or a less than effective dose of a harmless substance, as a water-soluble vitamin prescribed as if it were an effective dose of a needed medication. Placebos are prescribed for patients who cannot be given the medication they request or who, in the judgment of the health care provider, do not need that medication.

placebo effect, a physical or emotional change occurring after a substance is taken or administered that is not the result of any special property of the substance. The change may be beneficial, reflecting the expectations of the patient.

placement [Fr *placer* to find a place], the positioning of a dental prosthesis, such as a removable denture in its planned site on the dental arch.

placement path, the direction of placement and removal of a removable partial denture on its supporting oral structures.

placenta /pləsen′tə/ [L, flat cake], a highly vascular fetal organ through which the fetus absorbs oxygen, nutrients, and other substances and excretes carbon dioxide and other wastes. It begins to form on approximately the eighth day of gestation when the blastocyst touches the wall of the uterus and adheres to it. At term the normal placenta weighs one seventh to one fifth the weight of the infant. The maternal surface is lobulated and divided into cotyledons. It has a dark red, rough, liverlike appearance. The fetal surface is smooth and shiny, covered with the fetal membranes, marked by the large white blood vessels beneath the membranes that fan out from the centrally inserted umbilical cord. The time between the delivery of the infant and the expulsion of the placenta is the third and last stage of labor. **–placental,** *adj.*

placenta abruptio. See **abruptio placentae.**

placenta accreta, a placenta that invades

the uterine muscle, making separation from the muscle difficult.

placenta battledore, a condition in which the umbilical cord is inserted into the margin of the placenta.

placental bruit [L *placenta* flat cake; Fr *bruit* noise], a humming noise, due to fetal circulation, heard in the pregnant uterus. It is synchronized with the mother's pulse.

placental dysfunction. See **placental insufficiency.**

placental dystocia, a prolonged or otherwise difficult delivery of the placenta.

placental hormone, one of the several hormones produced by the placenta, including human placental lactogen, chorionic gonadotropin, estrogen, progesterone, and a thyrotropin-like hormone.

placental infarct, a localized ischemic, hard area on the fetal or maternal side of the placenta.

placental insufficiency, an abnormal condition of pregnancy, manifested clinically by retardation of the rate of fetal and uterine growth. Some of the abnormalities that can result in placental insufficiency are abnormal implantation of the placenta, multiple pregnancy, abnormal attachments of the umbilical cord or anomalies of the cord itself, and abnormalities of the placental membranes.

placental presentation, a complication of childbirth in which the placenta is located in or near the lower uterine segment.

placental scan, a scan of the uterus of a pregnant woman, performed after an intravenous injection of a contrast medium, used for locating the fetus and placenta and for detecting intrauterine bleeding.

placental stage of labor, the third stage of labor when the placenta and membranes are expelled from the uterus, following birth of the child.

placental thrombosis, intravascular coagulation that occurs in the placenta and veins of the uterus.

placental transmission, the transference of a drug or other substance across the placenta.

placenta previa /prē'vē·ə/, a condition of pregnancy in which the placenta is implanted abnormally in the uterus so that it impinges on or covers the internal os of the uterine cervix. It is the most common cause of painless bleeding in the third trimester of pregnancy. Even slight dilatation of the internal os can cause enough local separation of an abnormally implanted placenta to result in bleeding. Kinds of placenta previa are **central placenta previa, marginal placenta previa,** and **partial placenta previa.**

placenta previa partialis, a placenta that partially obstructs the internal cervical os.

placenta souffle [Fr *souffle* puff], a soft blowing or humming sound produced by fetal circulation at the placenta.

placenta succenturiata, an accessory placenta.

Plafon fracture, a fracture that involves the buttress portion of the malleolus of a bone.

plagiocephaly /plā'jē·ōsef'əlē/ [Gk *plagios* askew, *kephale* head], a congenital malformation of the skull in which premature or irregular closure of the coronal or lambdoidal sutures results in asymmetric growth of the head, giving it a twisted, lopsided appearance. **–plagiocephalic, plagiocephalous,** *adj.*

plague /plāg/ [L *plaga* stroke], an infectious disease transmitted by the bite of a flea from a rodent infected with the bacillus *Yersinia pestis*. Plague is primarily an infectious disease of rats: the rat fleas feed on humans only when their preferred rodent hosts, usually rats, have been killed by the plague under epizootic conditions. Kinds of plague include **bubonic plague, pneumonic plague,** and **septicemic plague.**

plague vaccine, an active immunizing agent prepared with killed plague bacilli. It is prescribed for immunization against plague after probable exposure or as protection for travelers in endemic areas, such as Southeast Asia.

plaintiff [ME *plaintif* one who complains], (in law) a person who files a lawsuit initiating a legal action.

planar xanthoma [L *planum* level; Gk *xanthos* yellow, *oma* tumor], a yellow or orange flat macule or slightly raised papule containing foam cells and occurring in clusters in localized areas, such as the eyelids, or widely distributed over the body.

Planck's constant [Max Planck, German physicist, b. 1858], a fundamental physical constant that relates the energy of radiation to its frequency. It is expressed as 6.63×10^{-27} erg-seconds or 6.63×10^{-34} joule-seconds.

plane [L *planum* level], **1.** a flat surface determined by three points in space. **2.** an extension of a longitudinal section through an axis, such as the coronal, the horizontal, and the sagittal planes used to identify the position of various parts of the body in the study of anatomy. **3.** the act of paring or of rubbing away. **4.** a superficial incision in the wall of a cavity or between tissue layers, especially in plastic surgery. **–planar,** *adj.*

planes of anesthesia. See **Guedel's signs.**

P

planigraphic principle, a rule of tomography in which the fulcrum or axis of rotation is raised or lowered to alter the level of the focal plane but the tabletop height remains constant.

plankton /plangk′tən/ [Gk *planktos* wandering], nearly microscopic bits of plant and animal life that swarms in lakes and oceans and provides the basic food for aquatic animals.

planned change, (in psychotherapy) an alteration of the status quo by means of a carefully formulated program that follows four steps: unfreezing the present level, establishing a change relationship, moving to a new level, and freezing at the new level.

planned parenthood, a philosophic framework central to the development of contraceptive methods, contraceptive counseling, and family planning programs and clinics. Advocates hold that it is the right of each woman to decide when to conceive and bear children and that contraceptive and gynecologic care and information should be available to help her become or avoid becoming pregnant.

planning [L *planum*], (in five-step nursing process) a category of nursing behavior in which a strategy is designed for the achievement of the goals of care for an individual patient, as established in assessing and analyzing. Planning includes developing and modifying a care plan for the patient, cooperating with other personnel, and recording relevant information.

plantago seed /plantā′gō/, a bulk-forming laxative derived from *Plantago psyllium* seeds. It is prescribed in the treatment of constipation and nonspecific diarrhea.

plantar /plan′tər/ [L *planta* sole], of or pertaining to the sole of the foot.

plantar aponeurosis, the tough fascia surrounding the muscles of the soles of the feet.

plantar arch, the arterial arch in the sole of the foot, over the metatarsal bone.

plantar flexion [L *planta* + *flectere* to bend], a toe-down motion of the foot at the ankle. It is measured in degrees from the 0-degree position of the foot at rest on the ground in a standing position.

plantar grasp reflex, a reflex characterized by the flexion of the toes when the sole of the foot is stroked gently. It is present in babies at birth but should disappear after 6 weeks.

plantaris /plantā′ris/ [L *planta*], one of three superficial muscles at the back of the leg, between the soleus and the gastrocnemius. It flexes the foot and the leg.

plantar neuroma, a neuroma of the sole of the foot.

plantar reflex, the normal response, elicited by firmly stroking the outer surface of the sole from heel to toes, characterized by flexion of the toes.

plantar wart, a painful verrucous lesion on the sole of the foot, primarily at points of pressure, as over the metatarsal heads and the heel. Caused by the common wart virus, it appears as a soft, central core and is surrounded by a firm, hyperkeratotic ring resembling a callus.

plantigrade /plan′tigrād′/ [L *planta* + *gradi* to walk], of, pertaining to, or characterizing the human gait; walking on the sole of the foot with the heel touching the ground.

plant or animal classification, the system of identification of organisms according to their natural relationships based on such common factors as embryology, structure, or physiologic chemistry. In the system for plants, the descending order of categories is kingdom, division, class, order, genus, species. For animals, the categories are kingdom, phylum, class, order, family, genus, species. Humans are members of a species, *Homo sapiens,* of the genus *Homo,* in a family of hominidae, which are two-legged members of the order of primates, in a class of mammals, within a subphylum of vertebrates in the animal kingdom.

plant toxin, any poisonous substance derived from a plant, such as the ricin of castor-oil seeds.

plaque /plak/ [Fr, plate], **1.** a flat, often raised, patch on the skin or any other organ of the body. **2.** a patch of atherosclerosis. **3.** a thin film on the teeth made up of mucin and colloidal material found in saliva and often secondarily invaded by bacteria.

plasma /plaz′mə/ [Gk, something formed], the watery, straw-colored, fluid portion of the lymph and the blood in which the leukocytes, erythrocytes, and platelets are suspended. Plasma is made up of water, electrolytes, proteins, glucose, fats, bilirubin, and gases. It is essential for carrying the cellular elements of the blood through the circulation, transporting nutrients, maintaining the acid-base balance of the body, and transporting wastes from the tissues.

plasma cell, a lymphoid or lymphocyte-like cell found in the bone marrow, connective tissue, and sometimes the blood. Plasma cells are involved in the immunologic mechanism.

plasma cell leukemia, an unusual neoplasm of blood-forming tissues in which the predominant cells in peripheral blood are plasmacytes. The disease may develop in the course of multiple myeloma or arise independently.

plasma cell myeloma. See **multiple myeloma.**

plasmacytoma /plaz′məsītō′mə/, *pl.* **plasmacytomas, plasmacytomata,** a focal neoplasm containing plasma cells. It may develop in the bone marrow, as in multiple myeloma, or outside the bone marrow, as in certain tumors of the viscera.

plasma exchange therapy, a method of treating certain diseases by removing a portion of plasma from the blood supply of a patient and replacing it with plasma from a disease-free person.

plasma expander, a substance, usually a high molecular weight dextran, that is administered intravenously to increase the oncotic pressure of a patient.

plasma membrane. See **cell membrane.**

plasmapheresis /plaz′məfərē′sis/, the removal of plasma from withdrawn blood by centrifugation, the reconstitution of the cellular elements in an isotonic solution, and the reinfusion of this solution into the donor.

plasma protein, any one of the various proteins, including albumin, fibrinogen, prothrombin, and the gamma globulins, which constitute about 6% to 7% of the blood plasma in the body.

plasma renin activity, the action of the enzyme renin, measured in plasma to aid in the diagnosis of adrenal disease associated with hypertension.

plasma thromboplastin antecedent. See **factor XI.**

plasma thromboplastin component deficiency. See **hemophilia.**

plasmasome. See **plasmosome.**

plasma volume, the total volume of plasma in the body, elevated in diseases of the liver and spleen and in vitamin C deficiency, lowered in Addison's disease, dehydration, and shock.

plasma volume extender, an intravenous solution of dextran, proteins, or other substances used to treat shock due to blood volume loss.

plasmid /plaz′mid/ [Gk *plasma* something formed], (in bacteriology) any type of intracellular inclusion considered to have a genetic function, especially a molecule of DNA separate from the bacterial chromosome that determines traits not essential for the viability of the organism but that in some way changes the organism's ability to adapt.

plasmidotrophoblast. See **syncytiotrophoblast.**

plasmin. See **fibrinolysin.**

plasminogen. See **fibrinogen.**

Plasmodium /plazmō′dē·əm/ [Gk *plasma* + *eidos* form], a genus of protozoa several species of which cause malaria, transmitted to humans by the bite of an infected *Anopheles* mosquito. *Plasmodium falciparum* causes falciparum malaria, the most severe form of the disease; *P. malariae* causes quartan malaria; *P. ovale* causes mild tertian malaria with oval red blood cells; and *P. vivax* causes common tertian malaria.

plasmosome /plaz′məsōm/ [Gk *plasma* + *soma* body], the true nucleolus of a cell as distinguished from the karyosomes in the nucleus.

plaster [Gk *emplastron*], **1.** any composition of a liquid and a powder that hardens when it dries, used in shaping a cast to support a fractured bone as it heals, such as plaster of paris. **2.** a home remedy consisting of a semisolid mixture applied to a part of the body as a counterirritant or for other therapeutic reasons, such as a mustard plaster.

plaster cast, a traditional cast designed to encase and immobilize a part of the body in a circumferentially wrapped plaster of Paris impregnated gauze roll that has been dipped in warm water. Modern casts are often made of materials such as glass fibers or plastic instead of plaster of paris.

plaster of paris [Gk *plassein* to mold; originated in Paris, France], a white powder, calcium sulfate hemihydate, which is mixed with water to make a paste that can be molded to encase a body part.

plasticity /plastis′itē/ [Gk *plassein* to mold], the quality of being plastic or formative.

plastic surgery [Gk *plassein* to mold; *cheirourgos* surgery], the alteration, replacement, or restoration of visible portions of the body, performed to correct a structural or cosmetic defect. In performing corrective plastic surgery, the surgeon may use tissue from the patient or from another person or an inert material that is nonirritating, has a consistency appropriate to the use, and is able to hold its shape and form indefinitely. See also specific procedures.

plate [Fr *plat* flat dish], **1.** a flat structure or layer, such as a thin layer of bone or the frontal plate between the sides of the ethmoid cartilage and the sphenoid bone in the fetus. **2.** a single partitioning unit of a chromatographic system.

platelet /plat′lit/ [Fr, small plate], the smallest of the cells in the blood. Platelets are disk-shaped and contain no hemoglobin. They are essential for the coagulation of blood.

plateletpheresis [Fr *platelet* + Gk *aphairesis* to carry away], the removal of platelets from withdrawn blood, the remainder of the blood being reinfused into the donor.

platinized gold foil [Sp *plata* silver; AS *geolu* gold; L *folium* leaf], a thin sheet rolled or hammered from platinum sandwiched between two sheets of gold, used for making portions of dental restorations requiring greater hardness than that obtained by using other materials, such as copper amalgam.

platinum (Pt) /plat'ənəm/ [Sp *plata* silver], a silvery white, soft metallic element. Its atomic number is 78; its atomic weight is 195.09. Platinum is used in dentistry.

platinum foil, a very thin sheet of rolled pure platinum that has a high fusing point, making it an ideal matrix in various soldering procedures for fabricating orthodontic appliances and dentures.

Platyhelminthes /plat'ihelmin'thēz/ [Gk *platys* flat, *helmins* worm], a phylum of parasitic flatworms that includes the Cestoda subclass of tapeworms and Trematoda class of flukes.

platypelloid pelvis /plat'əpel'oid/ [Gk *platys* wide, *pella* bowl, *eidos* form; L *pelvis* basin], a rare type of pelvis in which the inlet is round like the gynecoid type in the anterior section, but the posterior section is foreshortened by its flat and heavy border. Vaginal delivery is not usually possible in women who have platypelloid pelves.

platysma /plətiz'mə/ [Gk *platys* flat], one of a pair of wide muscles at the side of the neck. It serves to draw down the lower lip and the corner of the mouth. When the platysma fully contracts, the skin over the clavicle is drawn toward the mandible, increasing the diameter of the neck.

play [AS *plegan* sport], any spontaneous or organized activity that provides enjoyment, entertainment, amusement, or diversion. It is essential in childhood for the development of a normal personality and as a means for developing physically, intellectually, and socially. Play provides an outlet for releasing tension and stress. Kinds of play include **active, associative, cooperative, dramatic, parallel, passive, skill,** and **solitary.**

play therapy, a form of psychotherapy in which a child plays in a protected and structured environment with games and toys provided by a therapist, who observes the behavior, affect, and conversation of the child to gain insight into thoughts, feelings, and fantasies.

pleasure principle [Fr *plaisir* pleasure; L *principium*], (in psychoanalysis) the need for immediate gratification of instinctual drives.

pledget /plej'ət/, a small, flat compress made of cotton gauze, or a tuft of cotton wool, lint, or a similar synthetic material, used to wipe the skin, absorb drainage, or clean a small surface.

pleiotropic gene, a gene that produces a complex of unrelated phenotypic effects.

pleiotropy /plī·ot'rəpē/ [Gk *pleion* more, *trepein* to turn], (in genetics) the production by a single gene of a multiple, different, and apparently unrelated manifestation of a particular disorder, such as the cluster of symptoms in Marfan's syndrome, aortic aneurysm, dislocation of the optic lens, skeletal deformities, and arachnodactyly, any or all of which may be present.

plessimeter. See **pleximeter.**

plethora /pleth'ərə/ [Gk *plethore* fullness], a term applied to the beefy red coloration of a newborn. The "boiled lobster" hue of the infant's skin is caused by an unusually high proportion of erythrocytes per volume of blood. –**plethoric,** *adj.*

plethysmogram /pləthiz'məgram'/ [Gk *plethynein* to increase, *gramma* record], a tracing produced by a plethysmograph.

plethysmograph /pləthiz'məgraf'/, an instrument for measuring and recording changes in the sizes and volumes of extremities and organs by measuring changes in their blood volumes. –**plethysmographic,** *adj.,* **plethysmography,** *n.*

plethysmography /pleth'izmog'rəfē/, the measurement of changes in the volume of organs or other body parts, particularly those changes due to blood flow.

pleura /plŏŏr'ə/, *pl.* **pleurae** [Gk, rib], a delicate serous membrane enclosing the lung, composed of a single layer of flattened mesothelial cells resting on a delicate membrane of connective tissue. The pleura divides into the visceral pleura, which covers the lung, dipping into the fissures between the lobes, and the parietal pleura, which lines the chest wall, covers the diaphragm, and reflects over the structures in the mediastinum. –**pleural,** *adj.*

pleural cavity [Gk *pleura* rib; L *cavum* cavity], the cavity within the thorax that contains the lungs. Between the ribs and the lungs are the visceral and parietal pleurae.

pleural effusion, an abnormal accumulation of fluid in the interstitial and air spaces of the lungs, characterized by fever, chest pain, dyspnea, and nonproductive cough. The fluid involved is an exudate or a transudate from inflamed pleural surfaces.

pleural friction rub, a rubbing, grating sound that occurs with pleurisy as one layer of the pleural membrane slides over the other during breathing.

pleural space, the potential space between the visceral and parietal layers of the pleurae. The space contains a small amount of fluid that acts as a lubricant, allowing the pleurae to slide smoothly over each other as the lungs expand and contract with respiration.

pleura pulmonalis [Gk *pleura* rib; L *pulmo* lung], the portion of the pleural membrane that covers the lungs, as distinguished from the parietal layer of pleura that lines the inner aspect of the thoracic cavity.

pleurisy /plŏŏr'əsē/ [Gk *pleura* + *itis* inflammation], inflammation of the parietal pleura of the lungs, characterized by dyspnea and stabbing pain, leading to restriction of ordinary breathing with spasm of the chest on the affected side. A friction rub may be heard on auscultation. Common causes of pleurisy include bronchial carcinoma, lung or chest wall abscess, pneumonia, pulmonary infarction, and tuberculosis.

pleurisy with effusion, pleurisy in which inflammation has progressed to an effusion into the intrapleural space, characterized by fluid with a high specific gravity caused by a high concentration of fibrin and clots.

pleuritic, pertaining to a condition of pleurisy.

pleuritis. See **pleurisy.**

pleurodynia /plŏŏr'ōdin'ē·ə/ [Gk *pleura* + *odyne* pain], acute inflammation of the intercostal muscles and the muscular attachment of the diaphragm to the chest wall. It is characterized by sudden severe pain and tenderness, fever, headache, and anorexia. These symptoms are aggravated by movement and respiration.

pleuropericardial rub [Gk *pleura* + *peri* around, *kardia* heart; ME *rubben* to scrape], an abnormal coarse friction sound heard on auscultation of the lungs during late inspiration and early expiration. It is caused by the visceral and parietal pleural surfaces rubbing against each other.

pleuroperitoneal cavity. See **splanchnocoele.**

pleuropneumonia [Gk *pleura* + *pneumon* lung], **1.** a combination of pleurisy and pneumonia. **2.** an infection of cattle resulting in inflammation of both the pleura and lungs, caused by microorganisms of the *Mycoplasma* group.

pleuropneumonia-like organism (PPLO), a group of filterable organisms of the genus *Mycoplasma* similar to *M. mycoides,* the cause of pleuropneumonia in cattle.

pleurothotonos /plŏŏr'əthot'ənəs/ [Gk *pleurothen* side of the body, *tonos* tension], an involuntary, severe, prolonged contraction of the muscles of one side of the body, resulting in an acute arch to that side. **–pleurothotonic,** *adj.*

plexiform neuroma [L *plexus* braided, *forma* form; Gk *neuron* nerve, *oma* tumor], a neoplasm composed of twisted bundles of nerves.

pleximeter /pleksim'ətər/ [Gk *plessein* to strike, *metron* measure], a mediating device, such as a percussor or finger, used to receive light taps in percussion.

plexor. See **percussor.**

plexus /plek'səs/, *pl.* **plexuses** [L, braided], a network of intersecting nerves and blood vessels or of lymphatic vessels.

plica /plī'kə/, *pl.* **plicae** /plī'sē/ [L *plicare* to fold], a fold of tissue within the body, as the plicae transversales of the rectum and the plicae circulares of the small intestine. **–plical,** *adj.*

plica circularis. See **circular fold.**

plicae transversales recti, semilunar, transverse folds in the rectum that support the weight of feces.

plicamycin /plī'kəmī'sin/, an antineoplastic agent prescribed primarily in the treatment of malignant tumors of the testis. It is also prescribed in the treatment of hypercalcemia and hypercalciuria associated with cancer.

plica semilunaris, the semilunar fold of the conjunctiva that extends laterally from the lacrimal caruncle.

plication /plīkā'shən/ [L *plicare* to fold], any operation that involves folding, shortening, or decreasing the size of a muscle or hollow organ, such as the stomach, by taking in tucks.

plication of stomach [L *plicare;* Gk *stomakhos* gullet], a surgical treatment for obesity in which tucks are created in the wall of the stomach.

plica umbilicalis lateralis. See **lateral umbilical fold.**

plica umbilicalis mediana. See **middle umbilical fold.**

Plimmer's bodies [Henry G. Plimmer, English biologist, b. 1856], small, round, encapsulated bodies found in cancers; once thought to be the causative parasites.

ploidy /ploi'dē/ [Gk *eidos* form], the status of a cell nucleus in regard to the number of complete chromosome sets it contains.

plug [D *plugge* stopper], a mass of tissue cells, mucus, or other matter that blocks a normal opening or passage of the body, such as a cervical plug.

plumbism /plum'izəm [L *plumbum* lead],

a chronic form of lead poisoning caused by absorption of lead or lead salts.

Plummer's disease [Henry S. Plummer, American physician, b. 1874], goiter characterized by a hyperfunctioning nodule or adenoma and thyrotoxicosis.

Plummer-Vinson syndrome /plum'ər-vin'sən/ [Henry S. Plummer; Porter P. Vinson, American physician, b. 1890], a rare disorder associated with severe and chronic iron deficiency anemia, characterized by dysphagia caused by esophageal webs at the level of the cricoid cartilage.

plunging goiter. See **diving goiter.**

pluricentric blastoma. See **blastoma.**

pluripara [L *pluri* plus, *parere* to bear], a woman who has borne several children.

pluripolar mitosis. See **multipolar mitosis.**

plutonium (Pu) /plo͞otoͦ'nē-əm/ [planet *Pluto*], a synthetic transuranic metallic element. Its atomic number is 94; its atomic weight is 242.

pm, abbreviation for *picometer.*

Pm, symbol for the element **promethium.**

PMD, abbreviation for *private medical doctor.*

pmh, abbreviation for *past medical history.*

PMI, abbreviation for **point of maximum impulse.**

PMN, abbreviation for **polymorphonuclear cell.**

PMS, pms, abbreviation for **premenstrual syndrome.**

PMT, abbreviation for *premenstrual tension.*

PND, 1. abbreviation for **paroxysmal nocturnal dyspnea. 2.** abbreviation for **postnasal drip.**

pneopneic reflex [Gk *pnoe* breath; L *reflectere* to bend back], a change in the normal rhythm of breathing when an irritating gas is introduced into the lungs.

pneumatic /noͦomat'ik/ [Gk *pneuma* air], pertaining to air or gas.

pneumatic condenser [Gk *pneuma* air; L *condensare* to thicken], (in dentistry) a pneumatic device to deliver a compacting force to restorative material used in filling tooth cavities.

pneumatic heart driver, a mechanical device that regulates compressed air delivery to an artificial heart, controlling heart rate, percent systole, and delay in systole.

pneumatocele /noͦomat'əsēl'/, a thin-walled cavity in the lung parenchyma caused by partial airway obstruction.

pneumatogram /noͦomat'əgram/ [Gk *pneuma* + *gramma* record], a tracing made by a pneumograph of chest movements during breathing.

pneumobelt /noͦo'mōbelt/, a corset with an inflatable bladder that fits over the abdominal area and is connected to a ventilator that delivers positive pressure at an adjustable rate. It is used to assist in the respiratory rehabilitation of patients with high cervical injuries.

pneumocentesis [Gk *pneumon* lung, *kentesis* pricking], a procedure in which a lung is punctured to drain fluid contents.

pneumococcal /noͦo'mōkok'əl/ [Gk *pneumon* lung, *kokkos* berry], of or pertaining to bacteria of the genus *Pneumococcus.*

pneumococcal meningitis, meningitis caused by pneumococcal infection.

pneumococcal vaccine, an active immunizing agent containing antigens of the 14 types of *Pneumococcus* associated with 80% of the cases of pneumococcal pneumonia. It is prescribed for people over 2 years of age who are at high risk of developing severe pneumococcal pneumonia.

pneumococcus /noͦo'mōkok'əs/, *pl.* **pneumococci** /noͦo'mōkok'sī/ [Gk *pneumon* + *kokkos* berry], a gram-positive diplococcal bacterium of the species *Diplococcus pneumoniae,* the most common cause of bacterial pneumonia.

pneumoconiosis /noͦo'mōkōnē·ō'sis/ [Gk *pneumon* + *konis* dust, *osis* condition], any disease of the lung caused by chronic inhalation of dust, usually mineral dusts of occupational or environmental origin. Some kinds of pneumoconioses are **anthracosis, asbestosis, silicosis.**

pneumoconstriction, an area of collapsed lung tissue that results from mechanical stimulation of an exposed portion of the lung. It is produced by local reflex muscular closure of alveolar ducts and alveoli.

Pneumocystis carinii, a microorganism that causes pneumocystosis, a type of interstitial cell pneumonitis.

pneumocystis pneumonia [Gk *pneuma* air, *kystis* bag; *pneumon* lung], a type of interstitial plasma cell pneumonia in which the alveoli become honeycombed with an acidophilic material. The patients may or may not be febrile but usually are weak, dyspneic, and cyanotic.

pneumocystosis /noͦo'mōsisto'sis/ [Gk *pneumon* + *kystis* bag, *osis* condition], infection with the parasite *Pneumocystis carinii,* usually seen in patients with AIDS, infants, or debilitated or immunosuppressed people, particularly those with lymphomas, and characterized by fever, cough, tachypnea, and frequently cyanosis. The diagnosis is difficult to make and usually requires bronchoscopy and special staining techniques. Mortality nears 100% in untreated patients.

pneumoencephalogram /nōō′mō·ensef′-əlōgram/, a radiograph of the brain made during pneumoencephalography.

pneumoencephalography /nōō′mō·ensef′-əlog′rəfē/ [Gk *pneuma* air, *enkephalos* brain, *graphein* to record], a procedure for the radiographic visualization of the ventricular space, basal cisterns, and subarachnoid space overlying the cerebral hemispheres of the brain. Air, helium, or oxygen is injected into the lumbar subarachnoid space after the intermittent removal of the cerebrospinal fluid by lumbar puncture. **–pneumoencephalographic,** *adj.*

pneumogastric nerve. See **vagus nerve.**

pneumogram. See **pneumatogram.**

pneumograph, a device that records breathing movements by means of an inflated coil around the chest.

pneumohemopericardium. See **hemopneumopericardium.**

pneumohemothorax, an accumulation of air and blood in the pleural cavity.

pneumomediastinum /nōō′mōmē′dē·əstī′-nəm/ [Gk *pneuma* air, *mediastinus* midway], the presence of air or gas in the mediastinal tissues. The condition may result from bronchitis, acute asthma, pertussis, cystic fibrosis, or bronchial rupture from cough or trauma.

pneumonectomy [Gk *pneumon* lung, *ektome* excision], the surgical removal of all or part of a lung.

pneumonia /nōōmō′nē·ə/ [Gk *pneumon* lung], an acute inflammation of the lungs, usually caused by inhaled pneumococci of the species *Diplococcus pneumoniae*. The alveoli and bronchioles of the lungs become plugged with a fibrous exudate. Pneumonia may be caused by other bacteria, as well as by viruses, rickettsiae, and fungi. Characteristic of pneumonia are severe chills, a high fever (which may reach 105° F), headache, cough, and chest pain. Inflammation of the lower lobe of the right lung may produce a pain suggesting appendicitis. An effusion of red blood cells into the alveolar spaces, resulting from histolytic damage by the microorganism, causes a rust-colored sputum that may be a diagnostic sign of pneumococcal infection. As the disease progresses, sputum may become thicker and more purulent, and the person may experience painful attacks of coughing. Respiration usually becomes more difficult, painful, shallow, and rapid. The pulse increases in rapidity, often measuring 120 or more beats a minute. Other signs may include profuse sweating and cyanosis. GI disorders and an outbreak

of herpes simplex about the face may also occur. In children, pneumonia may be accompanied by convulsion. As the alveoli become filled with exudate, the affected area of a lobe becomes increasingly firm and consolidated. A distinctive kind of rale is heard on auscultation. Kinds of pneumonia are **aspiration pneumonia, bronchopneumonia, eosinophilic pneumonia, interstitial pneumonia, lobar pneumonia, mycoplasma pneumonia,** and **viral pneumonia.**

pneumonic plague [Gk *pneumon* lung; L *plaga* stroke], a highly virulent and rapidly fatal form of plague characterized by bronchopneumonia. There are two forms: **primary pneumonic plague** results from involvement of the lungs in the course of bubonic plague; **secondary pneumonic plague** results from the inhalation of infected particles of sputum from a person having pneumonic plague.

pneumonitis /nōō′mənī′tis/, *pl.* **pneumonitides** [Gk *pneumon* + *itis*], inflammation of the lung. Pneumonitis may be caused by a virus or may be a hypersensitivity reaction to chemicals or organic dusts, such as bacteria, bird droppings, or molds. It is usually an interstitial, granulomatous, fibrosing inflammation of the lung, especially of the bronchioles and alveoli. Dry cough is a common symptom. A kind of pneumonitis is **humidifier lung.**

pneumoperitoneum [Gk *pneuma* air, *peri* around, *teinein* to stretch], the presence of air or gas within the peritoneal cavity of the abdomen. It may be spontaneous, as from rupture of a hollow gas-containing organ, or induced for diagnostic or therapeutic purposes.

pneumotachometer, a device that measures the flow of respiratory gases. The pressure gradient is directly related to flow, thus allowing a computer to derive a flow curve measured in liters per minute.

pneumothorax /nōō′mōthôr′aks/ [Gk *pneuma* air, *thorax* chest], a collection of air or gas in the pleural space causing the lung to collapse. Pneumothorax may be the result of an open chest wound that permits the entrance of air, the rupture of an emphysematous vesicle on the surface of the lung, or a severe bout of coughing, or it may occur spontaneously without apparent cause. The onset of pneumothorax is accompanied by a sudden, sharp chest pain, followed by difficult, rapid breathing, cessation of normal chest movements on the affected side, tachycardia, a weak pulse, hypotension, diaphoresis, an elevated temperature, pallor, dizziness, and anxiety.

P

PNF, abbreviation for **proprioceptive neuromuscular facilitation.**

PNH, abbreviation for **paroxysmal nocturnal hemoglobinuria.**

PNP, abbreviation for **pediatric nurse practitioner.**

p.o., an abbreviation for the Latin phrase, *per os,* "by mouth"; a route for administration of medications.

Po, symbol for the element **polonium.**

Po₂, symbol for *partial pressure of oxygen.*

pockmark [AS pocc, meark], a pitted scar on the skin, usually the result of a smallpox pustule at the site.

podalic /pōdal'ik/ [Gk *pous* foot], pertaining to the feet.

podalic version, the shifting of the position of a fetus so as to bring the feet to the outlet during labor.

podiatrist, a health professional who diagnoses and treats disorders of the feet. Podiatrists complete a 4-year postgraduate educational program leading to a degree of Doctor of Podiatric Medicine (DPM).

podiatry /pədī'ətrē/ [Gk *pous* + *iatros* healer], the diagnosis and treatment of diseases and other disorders of the feet.

podophyllotoxin /pō'dōfil'ətok'sin/ [Gk *pous* + *phyllon* leaf, *toxikon* poison], any one of a group of substances derived from the roots of *Podophyllum peltatum,* a common plant species known as mayapple, or American mandrake. A resinous preparation of podophyllotoxin is prescribed in the topical treatment of condyloma acuminatum and other types of warts. Several podophyllotoxin derivatives have been used as purgatives.

podophyllum /pod'əfil'əm/ [Gk *pous* + *phyllon* leaf], the dried rhizome and roots of *Podophyllum peltatum,* from which a caustic resin is derived for use in removing certain warts.

poikilocytosis /poi'kilōsītō'sis/ [Gk *poikilos* variation, *kytos* cell, *osis* condition], an abnormal degree of variation in the shape of the erythrocytes in the blood.

poikiloderma atrophicans vasculare [Gk *poikilos* variation, *derma* skin; *a,* *trophe* not nourishment; L *vasculum* little vessel], an abnormal skin condition characterized by hyperpigmentation or hypopigmentation, telangiectasia, and atrophy of the epidermis.

poikiloderma of Civatte, a common benign, progressive dermatitis characterized by erythematous patches on the face and neck that become dry and scaly. As the condition progresses, pigment is deposited around the hair follicles extending down the lateral aspects of the neck.

poikilothermic. See **cold blooded.**

point [L *punctus* pricked], a small spot or designated area.

point behavior [L *punctus* pricked; AS *bihabban* to behave], the orientation of body parts in a certain direction within a quantum of space.

point forceps, a dental instrument used in filling root canals. It holds the filling cones during their placement.

point lesion, a disruption of single chemical bonds caused by effects of ionizing radiation on a macromolecule.

point mutation, a mutation in which only a single base-pair of DNA is changed.

point of maximum impulse (PMI), the place in the fifth intercostal space of the thorax, just medial to the left midclavicular line, where the apex beat of the heart is observed.

poise [Jean L. M. Poiseuille, French physiologist, b. 1799], a unit of liquid or gas (fluid) viscosity expressed in terms of gm × cm⁻¹ × sec¹. The centipoise, or 1/100th of a poise, is more commonly used.

poison [L *potio* drink], any substance that impairs health or destroys life when ingested, inhaled, or absorbed by the body in relatively small amounts. **–poisonous,** *adj.*

poison control center, one of a nearly worldwide network of facilities that provide information regarding all aspects of poisoning or intoxication, maintain records of their occurrence, and refer patients to treatment centers.

poisoning, 1. the act of administering a toxic substance. **2.** the condition or physical state produced by the ingestion, injection, inhalation, or exposure of a poisonous substance. Identification of the poison and the presentation of a container label are critical to expeditious diagnosis and treatment.

poisoning, high risk for, a NANDA-accepted nursing diagnosis of the accentuated risk of accidental exposure to or ingestion of drugs or dangerous products in doses sufficient to cause poisoning. The risk factors may be internal (individual) or external (environmental). Internal risk factors include reduced vision, lack of safety or drug education, lack of proper precautions, and cognitive or emotional difficulties. External risk factors include medicines or dangerous products stored in unlocked cabinets; availability of illicit drugs contaminated by poisonous additives; flaking paint or plaster in the presence of young children; chemical contamination of food and water; unprotected contact with heavy metals, chemicals, paint, or lacquer; presence of poisonous vegetation; and presence of atmospheric pollutants.

poisoning treatment, the symptomatic and supportive care given a patient who has been exposed to or who has ingested a toxic drug, commercial chemical, or other dangerous substance. In the case of oral poisoning, a primary effort should be directed toward recovery of the toxic substance before it can be absorbed into the body tissues. If vomiting does not occur spontaneously, it should be induced after first identifying the poison, if possible. If the poison is a petroleum distillate, such as kerosene, or a caustic or corrosive substance, vomiting should *not* be induced.

poison ivy, any of several species of climbing vine of the genus *Rhus,* characterized by shiny, three-pointed leaves. It is common in North America and causes severe allergic contact dermatitis in many people. Localized vesicular eruption with itching and burning results.

poison ivy dermatitis, a type of skin eruption caused by exposure to a nonvolatile oil, toxicodendrol, present in the leaves and other plant parts of poison ivy, a member of the *Rhus toxicodendron* genus. Other *Rhus* species producing the same kind of contact dermatitis are poison oak and poison sumac.

poison oak, any of several species of shrub of the genus *Rhus,* common in North America. Skin contact results in allergic dermatitis in many people. The characteristics and the treatment of the condition are similar to those of poison ivy.

poison sumac /soo'mak/, a shrub of the genus *Rhus,* common in North America. Skin contact results in allergic dermatitis in many people. The characteristics and the treatment of the condition are similar to those of poison ivy.

poker spine. See **bamboo spine.**

polar [L *polus* pole], pertaining to molecules that are hydrophilic, or "water-loving." Polar substances tend to dissolve in polar solvents.

polar body, one of the small cells produced during the two meiotic divisions in the maturation process of female gametes, or ova. It is nonfunctional and incapable of being fertilized.

polarity /pōler'itē/ [L *polus*], **1.** the existence or manifestation of opposing qualities, tendencies, or emotions, such as pleasure and pain, love and hate, strength and weakness, dependence and independence, masculinity and femininity. **2.** (in physics) the distinction between a negative and a positive electric charge.

polarity therapy, a technique of massage based on the theory that the body has posi-

tive and negative energy patterns that must be balanced to establish physical harmony.

polarization [L *polus* + Gk *izein* to cause], the concentration within a population or group of members' interests, beliefs, and allegiances around two conflicting positions.

polarization microscope, a microscope that utilizes polarized light for special diagnostic purposes, such as examining crystals of chemicals found in patients with gout and related disorders.

polarized light [L *polus*; AS *leoht*], light that is propagated in such a way that the radiation waves occur in only one direction in the vibration plane and not at random.

polarographic oxygen analyzer, an electrochemical device used to analyze the proportion of oxygen molecules in respiratory care systems. The oxygen is measured in terms of an electron current produced after it acquires electrons from a negative electrode in a hydroxide bath.

pole [L *polus*], **1.** (in biology) an end of an imaginary axis drawn through the symmetrically arranged parts of a cell, organ, ovum, or nucleus. **2.** (in anatomy) the point on a nerve cell at which a dendrite originates. **–polar,** *adj.*

poles of kidney, either end of an axis through the length of a kidney. They are designated as the **upper pole of the kidney (extremitas superior renis)** and the **inferior pole of the kidney (extremitas inferior renis).**

pol gene, a segment of a retrovirus, such as the human T cell leukemia virus (HTLV), that encodes its reverse transcriptase enzyme.

policy [L *politia* the state], a principle or guideline that governs an activity and that employees or members of an institution or organization are expected to follow.

polio. See **poliomyelitis.**

polioencephalitis /pō'lē·ō·ensef'əli'tis/ [Gk *polios* gray, *enkephalos* brain, *itis*], an inflammation of the gray matter of the brain caused by infection of the brain by a poliovirus.

polioencephalomeningomyelitis [Gk *polios* + *egkephalos* brain, *meninx* membrane, *myelos* marrow, *itis*], an inflammation that involves the gray matter of the brain and spinal cord and also the meninges.

polioencephalomyelitis /pō'lē·ō·ensef'-əlōmī'əli'tis/ [Gk *polios, enkephalos* + *myelos* marrow, *itis*], inflammation of the gray matter of the brain and the spinal cord, caused by infection by a poliovirus.

poliomyelitis /pō'lē·ōmī·əli'tis/ [Gk *polios* + *myelos* marrow, *itis*], an infectious

P

disease caused by one of the three polio-viruses. Asymptomatic, mild, and paralytic forms of the disease occur. It is transmitted from person to person through fecal contamination or oropharyngeal secretions. Asymptomatic infection has no clinical features, but it confers immunity. Abortive poliomyelitis lasts only a few hours and is characterized by minor illness with fever, malaise, headache, nausea, vomiting, and slight abdominal discomfort. Nonparalytic poliomyelitis is longer lasting and is marked by meningeal irritation with pain and stiffness in the back and by all the signs of abortive poliomyelitis. Paralytic poliomyelitis begins as abortive poliomyelitis. The symptoms abate, and for several days the person seems well. Malaise, headache, and fever recur; pain, weakness, and paralysis develop. The peak of paralysis is reached within the first week. In spinal poliomyelitis, viral replication occurs in the anterior horn cells of the spine causing inflammation, swelling, and, if severe, destruction of the neurons. The large proximal muscles of the limbs are most often affected. Bulbar poliomyelitis results from viral multiplication in the brainstem. Bulbar and spinal poliomyelitis often occur together.

poliomyelitis vaccine. See **poliovirus vaccine.**

poliosis /pō′lē-ō′sis/ [Gk *polios* + *osis* condition], depigmentation of the hair on the scalp, eyebrows, eyelashes, mustache, beard, or body. The condition may be inherited and generalized or acquired and localized in patches. Acquired localized poliosis often occurs in alopecia areata.

poliovirus [Gk *polios* + L *virus* poison], the causative organism of poliomyelitis. There are three serologically distinct types of this very small RNA virus. Infection or immunization with one type does not protect against the others.

poliovirus vaccine, a vaccine prepared from poliovirus to confer immunity to it. TOPV, the trivalent live oral form of vaccine, is recommended for all children under 18 years of age who have no specific contraindications. The inactivated poliovirus vaccine (IPV) is recommended for infants and children who are immunodeficient and for unvaccinated adults. TOPV is called Sabin vaccine; IPV is called Salk vaccine. IPV is given subcutaneously.

polishing [L *polire* to make smooth], a tendency of patients with right temporal lobe lesions to deny dysphoric affect and minimize socially disapproved behavior while exaggerating other qualities.

political nursing [L *politia* the state; *nutrix* nourishment], the use of knowledge about power processes and strategies to influence the nature and direction of health care and professional nursing.

pollakiuria /pol′əkēyŏōr′ē-ə/ [Gk *pollache* frequent, *ouron* urine], an abnormal condition characterized by unduly frequent passage of urine.

pollen coryza [L, dust; Gk *koryza* runny nose], acute seasonal rhinitis caused by exposure to an allergenic.

pollex, /pol′eks/ [L], the thumb.

pollinosis. See **hay fever.**

pollutant [L *polluere* to defoul], an unwanted substance that occurs in the environment, usually with health-threatening effects. Pollutants may exist in the atmosphere as gases or fine particles that may be irritating to the lungs, eyes, and skin, as dissolved or suspended substances in drinking water, and as carcinogens or mutagens in foods or beverages.

polonium (Po) [Polonia, Poland], a radioactive element that is one of the disintegration products of uranium. Its atomic number is 84; its atomic weight is approximately 210.

polus /pō′ləs/, *pl.* **poli** [L, pole], either of the opposite ends of any axis; the official anatomic designation for the extremity of an organ. **–polar,** *adj.*

polyacrylamide, a polymer of acrylamide and usually some crosslinking derivative.

polyamine /polē-am′ēn/, any compound that contains two or more amine groups, such as spermidine and spermine, which are normally occurring tissue constituents in humans.

polyanionic /pol′ē-an′ī-on′ik/ [Gk *polys* many, *ana* again, *ion* going], pertaining to multiple negative electric charges.

polyarteritis /pol′ē-är′tərī′tis/ [Gk *polys* + *arteria* air pipe, *itis* inflammation], an abnormal inflammatory condition of several arteries.

polyarteritis nodosa, a severe and poorly understood collagen vascular disease in which there is widespread inflammation and necrosis of small and medium-sized arteries and ischemia of the tissues they serve. It is characterized by fever, abdominal pain, weight loss, neuropathy, and, if the kidneys are affected, hypertension, edema, and uremia. Some symptoms may mimic GI or cardiac disorders.

polyarthritis, an inflammation that involves more than one joint. The inflammation may migrate from one joint to another, or there may be simultaneous involvement of two or more joints.

polyarticular [Gk *polys* + *articulus* joint], pertaining to many joints.

polychlorinated biphenyls (PCBs), a group of more than 30 isomers and compounds used in plastics, insulation, and flame retardants and varying in physical form from oily liquids to crystals and resins. All are potentially toxic and carcinogenic.

polychromasia. See **polychromatophilia.**

polychromatic [Gk *polys* + *chroma* color], a light of many colors or wavelengths. The term is usually applied to white light, although it may also refer to a defined portion of the spectrum.

polychromatophil /pol′ēkrōmat′əfəl/, any cell that may be stained by several different dyes.

polychromatophilia /pol′ēkrō′matəfil′ē·ə/ [Gk *polys*, *chroma* + *philein* to love], an abnormal tendency of a cell, particularly an erythrocyte, to be dyed by a variety of laboratory stains.

polyclonal /pol′ēklō′nəl/ [Gk *polys* + *klon* cutting] **1.** of, pertaining to, or designating a group of identical cells or organisms derived from several identical cells. **2.** of, pertaining to, or designating several groups of identical cells or organisms (clones) derived from a single cell.

polyclonal gammopathy. See **gammopathy.**

polycystic [Gk *polys* + *kystis* bag], characterized by the presence of many cysts.

polycystic kidney disease (PKD), an abnormal condition in which the kidneys are enlarged and contain many cysts. There are three forms of the disease. **Childhood polycystic disease (CPD)** is uncommon and may be differentiated from adult or congenital polycystic disease by genetic, morphologic, and clinical facets. Death usually occurs within a few years as the result of portal hypertension and liver and kidney failure. A portacaval shunt may prolong life into the twenties. **Adult polycystic disease (APD)** may be unilateral, bilateral, acquired, or congenital. The condition is characterized by flank pain and high blood pressure. Kidney failure eventually develops, progressing to uremia and death. **Congenital polycystic disease (CPD)** is a rare congenital aplasia of the kidney involving all or only a small segment of one or both kidneys. Severe bilateral aplasia results in death shortly after birth.

polycystic ovary syndrome, an abnormal condition characterized by anovulation, amenorrhea, hirsutism, and infertility. It is caused by an endocrine imbalance with increased levels of testosterone, estrogen, and luteinizing hormone (LH) and decreased secretion of follicle stimulating hormone (FSH). Numerous follicular cysts, 2 to 6 mm in diameter, may develop.

The affected ovary commonly doubles in size and is invested by a smooth, pearly white capsule.

polycythemia /pol′ēsīthē′mē·ə/ [Gk *polys* + *kytos* cell, *haima* blood], an increase in the number of erythrocytes in the blood. It may be primary or secondary to pulmonary disease or heart disease or to prolonged exposure to high altitudes.

polycythemia rubra vera (PV), a condition of unknown etiology characterized by a marked increase in the red blood cell count, packed cell volume, cellular hemoglobin, leukocytes, platelets, and total blood volume. The skin and mucous membranes acquire a maroon or plum color and the patient develops hepatomegaly, splenomegaly, hypertension, and neurologic symptoms. The condition is associated with an F chromosome defect.

polydactyly [Gk *polys* + *daktylos* finger], a congenital anomaly characterized by the presence of more than the normal number of fingers or toes. The condition is usually inherited.

polydipsia /pol′ēdip′sē·ə/ [Gk *polys* + *dipsa* thirst], **1.** excessive thirst characteristic of several different conditions, including diabetes mellitus, in which an excessive concentration of glucose in the blood osmotically increases the excretion of fluid via urination, which leads to hypovolemia and thirst. **2.** *informal;* alcoholism.

polyelectrolyte /pol′ē·ilek′trəlīt/ [Gk *polys* + *elektron* amber, *lytos* soluble], a substance with many charged or potentially charged groups.

polyendocrine deficiency syndromes. See **polyglandular autoimmune syndromes.**

polyesthesia /pol′ē·esthē′zhə/ [Gk *polys* + *aisthesis* feeling], a sensory disorder involving the sense of touch in which a stimulus to one area of the skin is felt at other sites in addition to the one stimulated.

polyestradiol phosphate, an antineoplastic estrogen compound. It is prescribed for cancer of the prostate and postmenopausal breast cancer.

polygene /pol′ējēn′/ [Gk *polys* + *genein* to produce], any of a group of nonallelic genes that individually exert a small effect but together interact in a cumulative manner to produce a particular characteristic within an individual, usually of a quantitative nature, such as size, weight, or skin pigmentation. **–polygenic,** *adj.*

polygenic inheritance. See **multifactorial inheritance.**

polyglandular autoimmune syndromes, disorders of subnormal functioning of

P

more than one endocrine gland. Type I is characterized by the appearance of mucocutaneous candidiasis, often occurring in childhood, and is associated with hypoparathyroidism and adrenal insufficiency. Type I condition occurs in siblings, without involvement of other generations in the family. Type II involves primary adrenal insufficiency and primary thyroid failure occurring in the same patient for unclear reasons. It has been demonstrated that many of these patients have an autoimmune disorder, with formation of antibodies against cellular fractions of many endocrine glands.

polyglucosan [Gk *polys* + *glykys* sweet], a large molecule consisting of many anhydrous polysaccharides.

polyhybrid [Gk *polys* + L *hybrida* offspring of mixed parents], (in genetics) pertaining to or describing an individual, organism, or strain that is heterozygous for more than three specific traits.

polyhybrid cross, (in genetics) the mating of two individuals, organisms, or strains that have different gene pairs that determine more than three specific traits.

polyhydramnios. See **hydramnios.**

polyleptic /pol′ēlep′tik/ [Gk *polys* + *lambanein* to seize], describing any disease or condition marked by numerous remissions and exacerbations.

polyleptic fever, a fever occurring paroxysmally, such as smallpox and relapsing fever.

polymer /pol′imər/ [Gk *polys* + *meros* part], a compound formed by combining or linking a number of monomers, or small molecules. A polymer may be composed of a variety of different monomers or from many units of the same monomer.

polymerase chain reaction (PCR), a process whereby a strand of DNA can be cloned millions of times within a few hours. The process can be used to make prenatal diagnoses of genetic diseases and to identify an individual by analysis of a single tissue cell.

polymerize /pol′əmərīz/ [Gk *polys* + *meros* parts], to convert two or more molecules into a polymer.

polymicrobial [Gk *polys* + *mikros* small, *bios* life], pertaining to a number of species of microbes.

polymicrobic infections, an infection involving more than one species of pathogens.

polymicrogyria. See **microgyria.**

polymorphism /pol′ēmôr′fizəm/ [Gk *polys* + *morphe* form], **1.** the state or quality of existing or occurring in several different forms. **2.** the state or quality of appearing in different forms at different stages of

development. Kinds of polymorphism are **balanced polymorphism** and **genetic polymorphism.** –**polymorphic,** *adj.*

polymorphocytic leukemia /pol′ēmôr′fəsit′ik/ [Gk *polys, morphe* + *kytos* cell; *leukos* white, *haima* blood], a neoplasm of blood-forming tissues in which mature, segmented granulocytes are predominant.

polymorphonuclear /pol′ēmôr′fōnoō′klē·ər/ [Gk *polys, morphe* + L *nucleus* nut], having a nucleus with a number of lobules or segments connected by a fine thread.

polymorphonuclear cell (PMN), a leukocyte with a multilobed nucleus, as a neutrophil.

polymorphonuclear leukocyte, a white blood cell containing a segmented lobular nucleus; an eosinophil, basophil, or neutrophil.

polymorphous /pol′ēmôr′fəs/ [Gk *polys* + *morphe* form], occurring in many varying forms, possibly changing in structure or appearance at different stages.

polymorphous light eruption, a common, recurrent, superficial vascular reaction to sunlight or ultraviolet light in susceptible individuals. Within 1 to 4 days after exposure to the light, small, erythematous papules and vesicles appear on otherwise normal skin, then disappear within 2 weeks.

polymyalgia rheumatica [Gk *polys* + *mys* muscle, *algos* pain; *rheuma* flux], a chronic, episodic, inflammatory disease of the large arteries that usually develops in people over 60 years of age. It primarily affects the muscles and is characterized by pain and stiffness of the back, shoulder, or neck, usually becoming more severe on rising in the morning. There may also be a severe, throbbing cranial headache, as in cranial arteritis, which affects the temporal and occipital arteries.

polymyositis /pol′ēmī′ōsī′tis/ [Gk *polys* + *mys* muscle, *itis*], inflammation of many muscles, usually accompanied by deformity, edema, insomnia, pain, sweating, and tension.

polymyxin, an antibiotic used topically and systemically in the treatment of gram-negative bacterial infections, including meningitis, corneal ulcerations, and otitis media.

polymyxin B sulfate, an antibiotic prescribed for infections caused by microorganisms sensitive to this drug, including urinary tract infections, septicemia, and conjunctivitis.

polyneuralgia [Gk *polys* + *neuron* nerve, *algos* pain], a type of neuralgia that affects several nerves at the same time.

polyneuritic psychosis. See **Korsakoff's psychosis.**

polyneuritis [Gk *polys* + *neuron, itis*], an inflammation involving many nerves.

polyneuropathy [Gk *polys* + *neuron, pathos* disease], a condition in which many peripheral nerves are afflicted with a disorder.

polyoma papovavirus. See **papilloma-carcinoma.**

polyopia /pol′ē·ōpē·ə/ [Gk *polys* + *ops* eye], a defect of sight in which one object is perceived as many images; multiple vision. The condition can occur in one or both eyes.

polyp /pol′ip/ [Gk *polys* + *pous* foot], a small tumorlike growth that projects from a mucous membrane surface.

polypapilloma, multiple papillomas or stalked tumors.

polypeptide /pol′epep′tīd/, a chain of amino acids joined by peptide bonds. A polypeptide has a larger molecular weight than a peptide but a smaller molecular weight than a protein.

polyphagia /pol′ēfā′jē·ə/ [Gk *polys* + *phagein* to eat], eating to the point of gluttony.

polypharmacy, a term applied to the use of a number of different drugs by a patient who may have one or several health problems.

polyploid /pol′əploid/ [Gk *polys* + *plous* times], **1.** of or pertaining to an individual, organism, strain, or cell that has more than the two complete sets of chromosomes normal for the somatic cell. The multiple of the haploid number characteristic of the species is denoted by the appropriate prefix, as in triploid, tetraploid, pentaploid, and so on. **2.** such an individual, organism, strain, or cell.

polypoid [Gk *polys* + *pous* foot, *eidos* form], like a polyp or tumor on a stalk.

polyploid adenocarcinoma. See **papillary adenocarcinoma.**

polyploidy /pol′əploi′dē/, the state or condition of having more than two complete sets of chromosomes.

polyposis [Gk *polys* + *pous* foot, *osis* condition], an abnormal condition characterized by the presence of numerous polyps on a part.

polyposis coli, a condition of multiple polyps in the large intestine.

polyradiculitis /pol′ērədik′yŏŏlī′tis/ [Gk *polys* + L *radicula* rootlet; Gk *itis*], inflammation of many nerve roots, as found in Guillain-Barré syndrome.

polyribosome. See **polysome.**

polysaccharide [Gk *polys* + *sakcharon* sugar], a carbohydrate that contains three or more molecules of simple carbohydrates. Examples of polysaccharides include dextrins, starches, glycogens, and pentose.

polysome /pol′isōm/ [Gk *polys* + *soma* body], (in genetics) a group of ribosomes joined together by a molecule of messenger RNA containing the genetic code.

polysomy /pol′əsō′mē/, the presence of a chromosome in at least triplicate in an otherwise diploid somatic cell as the result of chromosomal nondisjunction during meiotic division in the maturation of gametes. The chromosome may be duplicated three times (trisomy), four times (tetrasomy), or more.

polysynaptic [Gk *polys* + *synaptein* to join], pertaining to nerve cells that end in synapses.

polysyndactyly [Gk *polys* + *syn* together, *daktylos* finger or toe], multiple webbing or fusion between fingers or toes.

polytene chromosome [Gk *polys* + *tainia* band], an excessively large type of chromosome consisting of bundles of unseparated chromonemata filaments.

polythiazide, a diuretic and antihypertensive prescribed in the treatment of hypertension and edema.

polyunsaturated [Gk *polys* + AS *un* not; L *saturare* to fill], pertaining to a chemical compound containing double or triple valency bonds that can be opened to accept more atoms in the molecule, thereby becoming saturated. A polyunsaturated fatty acid is one in which there are two or more links in the chain of carbon atoms that can be opened to accept hydrogen atoms.

polyunsaturated fatty acid. See **unsaturated fatty acid.**

polyuria /pol′ēyŏŏr′ē·ə/ [Gk *polys* + *ouron* urine], the excretion of an abnormally large quantity of urine. Some causes of polyuria are diabetes insipidus, diabetes mellitus, diuretics, excessive fluid intake, and hypercalcemia.

polyvalent antiserum. See **antiserum.**

polyvalent vaccine [Gk *polys* + L *valere* worth; *vaccinus* cow], a vaccine prepared from several different antigenic types of a species.

polyvinyl chloride (PVC), a common synthetic thermoplastic material that releases hydrochloric acid when burned and that may contain carcinogenic vinyl chloride molecules as a contaminant.

POMP /pomp/, an abbreviation for a combination drug regimen used in the treatment of cancer, containing three antineoplastics, Purinethol (mercaptopurine), Oncovin (vincristine sulfate), methotrexate, and prednisone (a glucocorticoid).

Pompe's disease [J. C. Pompe, twentieth-century Dutch physician; L *dis* opposite of; Fr *aise* ease], a form of muscle glycogen storage disease in which there is a generalized accumulation of glycogen, resulting from a deficiency of acid maltase (alpha-1, 4-glucosidase). Children with Pompe's disease appear mentally retarded and hypotonic, seldom living beyond 20 years of age. In adults muscle weakness is progressive, but the disease is not fatal.

pompholyx. See **dyshidrosis.**

POMR, abbreviation for **problem-oriented medical record.**

ponos. See **kala-azar.**

pons /ponz/, *pl.* **pontes** /pon'tēz/ [L, bridge], 1. any slip of tissue connecting two parts of a structure or an organ of the body. 2. a prominence on the ventral surface of the brainstem, between the medulla oblongata and the cerebral peduncles of the midbrain. The pons consists of white matter and a few nuclei and is divided into a ventral portion and a dorsal portion. The dorsal portion comprises the tegmentum, which contains the nucleus of the abducens nerve, the nucleus of the facial nerve, the motor nucleus of the trigeminal nerve, the sensory nuclei of the trigeminal nerve, the nucleus of the cochlear division of the eighth nerve, the superior olive, and the nuclei of the vestibular division of the eighth nerve.

Pontiac fever. See **Legionnaires' disease.**

pontic /pon'tik/ [L *pons* bridge], the suspended member of a fixed partial denture, such as an artificial tooth, usually occupying the space previously occupied by the natural tooth crown.

pontine /pon'tīn/ [L *pons* bridge], pertaining to the pons.

pontine center. See **apneustic center.**

pontine nucleus, nerve cells in the basilar part of the pons where impulses are relayed between the cerebrum and cerebellum.

pooled plasma [AS *pol*; Gk *plasma* something formed], a liquid component of whole blood, collected and pooled to prepare various plasma products or to use directly as a plasma expander when whole blood is unavailable or is contraindicated.

poorly differentiated lymphocytic malignant lymphoma, a lymphoid neoplasm containing many cells resembling lymphoblasts that have a fine nuclear structure and one or more nucleoli.

popliteal /poplit'ē·əl, pop'litē'əl/ [L *poples* ham], pertaining to the area behind the knee.

popliteal artery /pop'litē'əl/ [L *poples* the ham; Gk *arteria* air pipe], a continuation of the femoral artery, extending from the opening in the abductor magnus, passing through the popliteal fossa at the knee, dividing into eight branches, and supplying various muscles of the thigh, leg, and foot.

popliteal node, a node in one of the groups of lymph glands in the leg.

popliteal pulse, the pulse of the popliteal artery, palpated behind the knee of a person lying prone with the knee flexed.

population [L *populus* the people], 1. (in genetics) an interbreeding group of individuals, organisms, or plants characterized by genetic continuity through several generations. 2. a group of individuals collectively occupying a particular geographic locale. 3. any group that is distinguished by a particular trait or situation. 4. any group measured for some variable characteristic from which samples may be taken for statistical purposes.

population at risk, a group of people who share a characteristic that causes each member to be vulnerable to a particular event, such as nonimmunized children who are exposed to poliovirus.

population genetics, a branch of genetics that applies mendelian inheritance to groups and studies the frequency of alleles and genotypes in breeding populations.

porcine /pôr'sīn/ [L *porcinus* pork], obtained from or related to hogs, as porcine insulin.

porcine graft [L *porcinus* pig; Gk *graphion* plant stylus], a temporary biologic heterograft made from the skin of a pig.

poriomania /pôr'ē·ōmā'nē·ə/, a tendency to leave home impulsively or to be a vagabond.

pork tapeworm. See *Taenia solium.*

pork tapeworm infection [L *porcus* sow; AS *taeppe* tape, *wyrm* worm; L *inficere* to taint], an infection of the intestine or other tissues, caused by adult and larval forms of the tapeworm *Taenia solium*. The pork tapeworm is unique in that it can use humans as both intermediate hosts for larvae and definitive hosts for the adult worm. Humans are usually infected with the adult worm after eating contaminated, undercooked pork.

porosis /pərō'sis/ [Gk *poros* passage], a condition of thinning bone tissue, particularly its supporting connective tissue, as in osteoporosis.

porous /pôr'əs/ [Gk *poros* passage], pertaining to something with pores or openings.

porphobilinogen /pôr'fōbilin'əjən/, a chromogen substance that is an intermediate in the biosynthesis of heme and porphyrins. It appears in the urine of persons with porphyria.

porphyria /pôrfir′ē·ə/ [Gk *porphyros* purple], a group of inherited disorders in which there is abnormally increased production of substances called porphyrins. Two major classifications of porphyria are **erythropoietic porphyria,** characterized by the production of large quantities of porphyrins in the blood-forming tissue of the bone marrow, and **hepatic porphyria,** in which large amounts of porphyrins are produced in the liver. Clinical signs common to both classifications of porphyria are photosensitivity, abdominal pain, and neuropathy.

porphyrin /pôr′fərin/ [Gk *porphyros*], any iron- or magnesium-free pyrrole derivative occurring in many plant and animal tissues.

portacaval shunt [L *porta* gateway, *cavum* cavity; ME *shunten*], a shunt created surgically to increase the flow of blood from the portal circulation by carrying it into the vena cava.

porta hepatitis. See **portal fissure.**

portal /pôr′təl/, **1.** an entrance. **2.** pertaining to the porta hepatis, or portal vein.

portal circulation, the pathway of blood flow from the gastrointestinal tract and spleen to the liver via the portal vein and its tributaries.

portal fissure [L *porta* + *fissura* cleft], a fissure on the visceral surface of the liver along which the portal vein, the hepatic artery, and the hepatic ducts pass.

portal hypertension, an increased venous pressure in the portal circulation caused by compression or by occlusion in the portal or hepatic vascular system. It results in splenomegaly, large collateral veins, ascites, and in severe cases systemic hypertension and esophageal varices.

portal of entry, the route by which an infectious agent enters the body.

portal system, the network of veins that drain the blood from the abdominal portion of the digestive tract, the spleen, the pancreas, and the gallbladder and convey blood from these viscera to the liver.

portal systemic encephalopathy. See **hepatic coma.**

portal vein, a vein that ramifies like an artery in the liver and ends in capillary-like sinusoids that convey the blood to the inferior vena cava through the hepatic veins. The tributaries of the portal vein are the lienal vein, the superior mesenteric vein, the coronary vein, the pyloric vein, the cystic vein, and the paraumbilical vein.

portal venous shunt. See **postcaval shunt.**

Porter-Silber reaction [Curt C. Porter, American biochemist, b. 1914; Robert H. Silber, American biochemist, b. 1915], a

reaction, visible as a change in color to yellow, that indicates the amount of adrenal steroids (the 17-hydroxycorticosteroids) excreted per day in the urine. The test is used to evaluate adrenocortical function.

portoenterostomy /pôr′tō·en′təros′təmē/ [L *porta* bowel, *stoma* mouth, *temnein* to cut], a procedure to correct biliary atresia in which the jejunum is anastomosed by a Roux-en-Y loop to the portal fissure region to establish bile flow from the bile ducts to the intestine.

port-wine stain. See **nevus flammeus.**

position [L *positio*], **1.** any one of many postures of the body, such as the anatomic position, lateral recumbent position, or semi-Fowler's position. **2.** (in obstetrics) the relationship of an arbitrarily chosen fetal reference point, such as the occiput, sacrum, chin, or scapula, on the presenting part of the fetus, with respect to its location in the maternal pelvis.

positional behavior, the orientation of the body regions to claim a quantum of space. Positional behavior involves four body regions: head and neck, upper torso, pelvis and thighs, and lower legs and feet.

positive [L *positivus*], **1.** (of a laboratory test) indicating that a substance or a reaction is present. **2.** (of a sign) indicating on physical examination that a finding is present, often meaning that there is pathologic change. **3.** (of a substance) tending to carry or carrying a positive chemical charge.

positive end-expiratory pressure (PEEP), (in respiratory therapy) the addition of positive airway pressure at the end of the exhalation phase. Each successive breath begins from a new baseline. Ventilation is controlled by a flow of air delivered in cycles of constant pressure through the respiratory cycle. PEEP is used for the relief of respiratory distress secondary to prematurity, pancreatitis, shock, pulmonary edema, trauma, surgery, or other conditions in which spontaneous respiratory efforts are inadequate and arterial levels of oxygen are deficient.

positive feedback, 1. (in physiology) an increase in function in response to a stimulus; for example, micturition increases once the flow of urine has started. **2.** *informal;* an encouraging, favorable, or otherwise positive response from one person to what another person has communicated.

positive identification, the unconscious modeling of one's personality on that of another who is admired and esteemed.

positive pressure, 1. a greater than ambient atmospheric pressure. **2.** (in respiratory therapy) any technique in which com-

P

pressed air or gas is delivered to the respiratory passages at greater than ambient pressure.

positive pressure breathing unit. See **IPPB unit.**

positive relationship, (in research) a direct relationship between two variables; as one increases, the other can be expected to increase.

positive signs of pregnancy, three unmistakable signs of pregnancy: fetal heart tones, heard on auscultation; fetal skeleton, seen on x-ray film or ultrasonogram; and fetal parts, felt on palpation.

positron /pos'itron/, a positive electron, or positively charged particle emitted from neutron-deficient radioactive nuclei.

positron emission tomography (PET) [L *positivus* + Gk *elektron* amber; L *emittere* to send out; Gk *tome* section, *graphein* to record], a computerized radiographic technique that employs radioactive substances to examine the metabolic activity of various body structures. In PET studies the patient either inhales or is injected with a biochemical, such as glucose, carrying a radioactive substance that emits positively charged particles, or positrons, that combine with negatively charged electrons normally found in the cells of the body. When the positrons combine with these electrons, gamma rays are emitted. The electronic circuitry and computers of the PET device detect the gamma rays and convert them into color-coded images that indicate the intensity of the metabolic activity of the organ involved.

Posner-Schlossman   syndrome. See **glaucomatocyclitic crisis.**

postcaval shunt [L *post* after; *vena cava*; ME *shunten*], any of several surgical anastomoses of the portal and systemic circulations to relieve symptoms of portal hypertension.

postcentral gyrus [L *post* + Gk, *kentron* center; *gyros* turn], a convolution of the brain immediately posterior to the central sulcus of the cerebrum.

postcoital [L *post* + *coire* to come together], pertaining to the time after sexual intercourse.

postcommissurotomy syndrome [L *post* after, *commissura* a union; Gk *temnein* to cut], a condition of unknown cause occurring within the first few weeks after cardiac valvular surgery, characterized by intermittent episodes of pain and fever, which may last weeks or months and then resolve spontaneously.

postconcussional syndrome [L *post* + *concussio* shake violently], a condition after head trauma, characterized by dizzi-

ness, poor concentration, headache, hypersensitivity, and anxiety.

postdate pregnancy, a pregnancy that lasts more than 42 weeks.

posterior /postir'ē-ər/ [L, behind], 1. of or pertaining to or situated in the back part of a structure, as of the dorsal surface of the human body. 2. the back part of something. 3. toward the back.

posterior Achilles bursitis, a painful heel condition caused by inflammation of the bursa between the Achilles tendon and the calcaneus. It is commonly associated with Haglund's deformity.

posterior asynclitism. See **asynclitism.**

posterior atlantoaxial ligament, one of five ligaments connecting the atlas to the axis.

posterior atlantooccipital membrane, one of a pair of thin, broad fibrous sheets that form part of the atlantooccipital joint between the atlas and the occipital bone.

posterior auricular artery, one of a pair of small branches from the external carotid arteries, dividing into auricular and occipital branches and supplying parts of the ear, scalp, and other structures in the head.

posterior column, the posterior horns of the gray matter in the spinal cord.

posterior common ligament. See **posterior longitudinal ligament.**

posterior costotransverse ligament, one of the five ligaments of each costotransverse joint, comprised of a fibrous band passing from the neck of each rib to the base of the vertebra above.

posterior drawer sign, an orthopedic test in which the patient is positioned with hips at 45 degrees and knees flexed at 90 degrees while the examiner sits on the foot and pushes the tibia backward. Also, with both the hips and knees flexed at 90 degrees, the heels are held together and the knees are observed for comparison of relative posterior sag of the tibia.

posterior fontanel, a small triangular area between the occipital and parietal bones at the junction of the sagittal and lambdoidal sutures.

posterior fossa, a depression on the posterior surface of the humerus, above the trochlea, that lodges the olecranon of the ulna when the elbow is extended.

posterior horn, the horn-shaped projections of gray matter in the posterior region of the spinal cord.

posterior longitudinal ligament, a thick, strong ligament attached to the dorsal surfaces of the vertebral bodies, extending from the occipital bone to the coccyx.

posterior mediastinal node, a node in one of three groups of thoracic visceral nodes, connected to the part of the lymphatic system that serves the esophagus, pericardium, diaphragm, and convex surface of the liver.

posterior mediastinum, the irregularly shaped caudal portion of the mediastinum, parallel with the vertebral column.

posterior nares, a pair of posterior openings in the nasal cavity that connect the nasal cavity with the nasopharynx and allow the inhalation and the exhalation of air.

posterior neuropore, the opening at the caudal end of the embryonic neural tube.

posterior palatal seal area, the area of soft tissues along the junction of the hard and soft palates on which displacement, within the physiologic tolerance of the tissues, can be applied by a denture to aid its retention.

posterior pituitary, posterior pituitary gland. See **neurohypophysis.**

posterior rhizotomy, a surgical procedure for cutting the posterior, or sensory, nerve root for the relief of intractable pain.

posterior tibial artery, one of the divisions of the popliteal artery, starting at the distal border of the popliteus muscle, passing behind the tibia, dividing into eight branches, and supplying various muscles of the lower leg, foot, and toes.

posterior tibialis pulse, the pulse of the posterior tibialis artery palpated on the medial aspect of the ankle, just posterior to the prominence of the ankle bone.

posterior tooth, any of the maxillary and mandibular premolars and molars of the permanent dentition, or of prostheses.

posterior vein of left ventricle, one of the five tributaries of the coronary sinus that drain blood from the capillary bed of the myocardium.

posteroanterior [L *posterus* coming after, *anterior* before], the direction from back to front.

posteroinferior [L *posterus* + *inferior* lower], pertaining to a position that is both lower and behind.

posterolateral [L *posterus* + *latus* side], pertaining to a position behind and to the side.

posterolateral thoracotomy /pos'tərōlat'-ərəl/, a chest surgery technique in which an incision is made in the submammary fold, below the tip of the scapula.

postganglionic [L *post* + Gk, *gagglion* knot], distal to a ganglion.

postganglionic neuron, a neuron that is distal to or beyond a ganglion.

postgastrectomy care [L *post* + Gk *gaster* stomach, *ektome* excision], nursing care after the removal of all or part of the stomach. Drainage of the nasogastric tube normally changes from bright red to dark in the first 24 hours. When bowel sounds re-

appear and a small amount of water given by the ounce is retained, the nasogastric tube is removed. Small, bland meals are offered hourly as tolerated. An increase in temperature or dyspnea indicates a leakage of oral fluids around the anastomosis. The diet is changed slowly to a regular diet, with five or six dry small feedings daily. Fluids are given hourly between meals. The most common complication of gastrectomy is the dumping syndrome, with fullness and discomfort, including vertigo, sweating, palpitation, and nausea occurring 5 to 30 minutes after eating, as food enters the small bowel.

posthepatic cirrhosis. See **cirrhosis.**

posthepatic jaundice [L *post* + Gk *hepar* liver; Fr *jaune* yellow], jaundice caused by obstruction of the bile ducts.

posthumous /pos'chəməs/ [L *post* + *humare* to bury], pertaining to the time after a person's death.

posthypnotic suggestion [L *post* + Gk *hypnos* sleep; L *suggerere* to suggest], an action suggested to a hypnotized person during a trance and carried out upon awakening from the trance. The action is in response to a cue and the subject usually does not know why he or she is performing the act.

postictal /pōst'iktəl/ [L *post* + Gk *ikteros* jaundice], of or pertaining to the period following a convulsion. **–postictus,** *n.*

postinfectious [L *post* + *inficere* to taint], occurring after an infection.

postinfectious encephalitis. See **encephalitis.**

postinfectious glomerulonephritis, the acute form of glomerulonephritis, which may follow 1 to 6 weeks after a streptococcal infection, most often in childhood. Characteristics of the disease are hematuria, oliguria, edema, and proteinuria, especially in the form of granular casts.

postinfectious psychosis, psychotic behavior that follows a serious infection such as pneumonia, scarlet fever, malaria, uremia, or typhoid fever.

postlumbar puncture headache [L *post* + *lumbus* loin; *punctura*; AS *heafod* + *acan*], a headache that occurs within a few hours of a lumbar puncture and usually lasts 1 or 2 days to several weeks. It may be accompanied by nausea and vomiting and improves when the patient lies down.

postmastectomy exercises [L *post* + Gk *mastos* breast, *ektome* excision], exercises essential to the prevention of shortening of the muscles and contracture of the joints following mastectomy. The woman is asked to flex and extend the fingers of the affected arm and to pronate and supinate the forearm immediately on return to her room after recovery from anesthesia and surgery. On the first postoperative day she is asked to squeeze a rubber ball in her hand. Brushing her teeth and hair is encouraged as effective exercises. Other exercises are usually taught, including four that are called climbing the wall, arm swinging, rope pulling, and elbow spreading.

postmature [L *post* + *maturare* to become ripe], **1.** overly developed or matured. **2.** of or pertaining to a postmature infant. **–postmaturity,** *n.*

postmature infant, an infant, born after the end of the forty-second week of gestation, bearing the physical signs of placental insufficiency. Characteristically, the baby has dry, peeling skin, long fingernails and toenails, and folds of skin on the thighs and sometimes on the arms and buttocks. Hypoglycemia and hypokalemia are common. Postmature infants often look as if they have lost weight in utero.

postmenopausal [L *post* + *mensis* month; Gk *pauien* to cease], of or pertaining to the period of life after the menopause.

postmenopausal vaginitis, an inflammation caused by degenerative changes in the vaginal mucosa after menopause.

postmortem [L *post* + *mors* death], **1.** after death. **2.** *informal;* postmortem examination.

postmortem cesarean section, delivery of a fetus by incision into the uterus after death of a pregnant woman.

postmortem delivery, See **postmortem cesarean section.**

postmortem examination, an examination of a body after death by a person trained in pathology.

postmortem graft, the transplanting of a cornea, artery, or other body part from a dead individual to repair a defect in a living body.

postmyocardial infarction syndrome [L *post* + Gk *mys* muscle, *kardia* heart; L *infarcire* to stuff], a condition that may occur days or weeks after an acute myocardial infarction. It is characterized by fever, pericarditis with a friction rub, pleurisy, pleural effusion, and joint pain. It tends to recur and often provokes severe anxiety, depression, and fear that it is another heart attack.

postnasal [L *post* + *nasus* nose], pertaining to the region behind the nose, or the posterior part of the nasal fossae.

postnasal drip (PND) [L *post* + *nasus* nose; AS *dryppan*], a drop-by-drop discharge of nasal mucus into the posterior pharynx, often accompanied by a feeling of obstruction, an unpleasant taste, and fetid breath, caused by rhinitis, chronic sinusitis, or hypersecretion by the nasopharyngeal mucosa.

postnecrotic cirrhosis [L *post* + Gk *nekros* dead; *kirrhos* yellowish, *osis* condition], a nodular form of cirrhosis that may follow hepatitis or other inflammation of the liver.

postoperative [L *post* + *operari* work], of or pertaining to the period of time after surgery. It begins with the patient's emergence from anesthesia and continues through the time required for the acute effects of the anesthetic or surgical procedures to abate.

postoperative atelectasis, a form of atelectasis in which collapse of lung tissue is caused by the depressant effects of anesthetic drugs. Deep breathing and coughing are encouraged at frequent intervals postoperatively to prevent this condition.

postoperative bed, a bed prepared for a patient who is weak or unconscious, as when recovering from anesthesia. The bed is in the flat position. The bottom sheet may be covered with a cotton bath blanket that is tucked tightly beneath the mattress. The top linen is fan-folded to the far side of the bed and not tucked in. This simplifies transferring a patient from a stretcher into the bed.

postoperative care, the management of a patient after surgery. On the patient's discharge from the operating room the surgical drapes, ground plate, and restraints are removed and a sterile dressing is applied to the incision. The patency and connections of all drainage tubes and the flow rate of parenteral infusions are checked. The patient's cleanliness and dryness are given attention, and the gown is changed, avoiding exposing the individual. Four people transfer the patient slowly and cautiously to a recovery room bed, maintaining body alignment and protecting the limbs. When indicated, an oral or nasal airway is inserted or a previously inserted endotracheal tube is suctioned; respiration may be supported with a pulmonator or intermittent positive pressure breathing (IPPB); if respiration remains impaired, the anesthesiologist is notified. The blood pressure, pulse, and respirations are initially reported to the anesthesiologist and are then checked every 15 minutes or as ordered. At similar intervals, the level of consciousness, reflexes, and movements of extremities are observed, and the incision, drainage tubes, and intravenous infusion site are inspected. Nothing is given orally; medication, blood or blood components, oxygen, and IPPB are administered as ordered, and fluid intake and output are measured.

postoperative cholangiography, (in diagnostic radiology) a procedure for outlining the major bile ducts. A radiopaque contrast material is injected into the common bile duct via a T-tube inserted during surgery. It is usually performed after a cholecystectomy to discover any residual calculi.

postoperative ileus [L *post* + *operari* to work; Gk *eilein* to twist], an obstruction to normal intestinal function due to a loss of peristalsis muscular action of the ileus following surgery.

postparalytic [L *post* + Gk *paralyein* to be palsied], pertaining to something that occurred after paralysis.

postpartal care [L *post* + *partus* bringing forth], care of the mother and her newborn baby during the first few days of the puerperium. The physical and physiologic changes of involution in the mother are observed for deviation from the normal. The uterus contracts after delivery, causing bleeding from the site of placental implantation to diminish. It is the size of a softball, with the fundus below the umbilicus. The lochia changes color and consistency during the first few days. Lochia rubra flows for up to 1 week, followed by straw-colored lochia serosa, and finally by clear, sticky lochia alba. The abdominal wall is soft, but muscle tone returns with time and exercise. On the third day the milk usually begins to fill the breasts.

postpartum /pōstpär′təm/, after childbirth. **–post partum,** *adv.*

postpartum blues, an emotional effect of childbirth experienced by mothers, consisting mainly of transient feelings of depression for a period of about 72 hours. If the depression persists for a longer period, it may be due to lack of interest in the infant or a reaction to the physical and mental stress of pregnancy. The condition may require psychotherapy or antidepressant medications.

postpartum depression [L *post* + *partus; deprimere* to press down], an abnormal psychiatric condition that occurs after childbirth, typically from 3 days to 6 weeks post partum. It is characterized by symptoms that range from mild "postpartum blues" to an intense, suicidal, depressive psychosis. Some women at risk for postpartum depression may be identified during the prenatal period by their having made no preparations for the expected baby, by their expressing unrealistic plans for postpartum work or travel, or by their denying the reality of the responsibilities of parenthood.

postpartum hemorrhage, excessive bleeding (a loss of more than 500 ml of blood) following childbirth.

postpartum iliofemoral thrombophlebitis, a condition of thrombophlebitis involving the iliofemoral artery following childbirth.

postpartum pituitary necrosis, a condition of hypopituitarism resulting from hypovolemia and shock in the immediate postpartum period. The patients may not develop lactation, pubic and axillary hair may be lost, and symptoms of hypoglycemia and amenorrhea are experienced.

postpartum psychosis, an episode of psychosis, either depressive or schizophrenic, following childbirth. Because the condition usually tends to develop in the month after childbirth, it is believed that endocrinologic factors are a cause.

postperfusion syndrome [L *post* + *perfundere* to pour over], a cytomegalovirus (CMV) infection, occurring between 2 and 4 weeks after the transfusion of fresh blood containing CMV. It is characterized by prolonged fever, hepatitis, rash, atypical lymphocytosis, and occasionally jaundice.

postpericardiotomy syndrome /pōst′perikär′dē·ot′əmē/ [L *post* + Gk *peri* around, *kardia* heart, *temnein* to cut], a condition that sometimes occurs days or weeks after pericardiotomy, characterized by symptoms of pericarditis, often without any fever. It appears to be an autoimmune response to damaged muscle cells of the myocardium and pericardium.

postpill amenorrhea [L *post* + *pilla* ball; Gk *a* not, *men* month, *rhoia* flow], failure of normal menstrual cycles to resume within 3 months after discontinuation of oral contraception.

postpoliomyelitis muscular atrophy (PPMA) [L *post* + Gk *polios* gray, *myelos* marrow, *itis*], a recurrence of neuromuscular symptoms in persons who had recovered from acute paralytic polio many years earlier. The chief symptom is muscular weakness, and the condition may affect the same muscles as before or muscles that were not damaged in the earlier polio attack.

postpolycythemic myeloid metaplasia [L *post* + Gk *polys* many, *kytos* cell, *haima* blood; *myelos* marrow, *eidos* form; *meta* with, *plassein* to mold], a late development in polycythemia vera, characterized by anemia caused by sclerosis of the bone marrow. The production of red blood cells then occurs only in extramedullary tissue, such as the liver and spleen.

postprandial, after a meal.

postprandial pain [L *post* + *prandium*

lunch; *poena* penalty], pain that occurs after a meal.

postpubertal panhypopituitarism [L *post* + *pubertas* maturation; Gk *pan* all, *hypo* below, *pituita* phlegm], insufficiency of pituitary hormones, caused by postpartum pituitary necrosis resulting from thrombosis of the circulation of the gland during or after delivery. The disorder, characterized initially by weakness, lethargy, failure to lactate, amenorrhea, loss of libido, and intolerance to cold, leads to loss of axillary and pubic hair, bradycardia, hypotension, premature wrinkling of the skin, and atrophy of the thyroid and adrenal glands.

postpuberty [L *post* + *pubertas*], a period of approximately 1 to 2 years after puberty during which skeletal growth slows and the physiologic functions of the reproductive years are established. **–postpuberal, postpubertal, postpubescent,** *adj.*

postrenal anuria [L *post* + *renes* kidney; Gk *a, ouron* not urine], cessation of urine production caused by obstruction in the ureters.

postresection filling. See **retrograde filling.**

postsynaptic /ˈsinapˈtik/ [L *post* + Gk *synaptein* to join], **1.** situated after a synapse. **2.** occurring after a synapse has been crossed.

postterm infant. See **postmature infant.**

posttransfusion syndrome [L *post* + *transfundere* to pour through], a complex of adverse reactions that may accompany or follow IV administration of blood or blood components. Reactions may include hemolytic effects, headache and back pain, allergies to an unknown component in donor blood, circulatory overloading, effects of cold blood that chill the patient's cardiovascular system, and effects of microaggregates in stored blood.

posttrauma response, a NANDA-accepted nursing diagnosis of a sustained painful response to unexpected extraordinary life events. Defining characteristics include reexperience of the traumatic event (flashbacks, intrusive thoughts, repetitive dreams or nightmares, excessive verbalization of the traumatic event, or verbalization of survival guilt or guilt about behavior required by survival), psychic or emotional numbness, and an altered life-style with self-destructiveness, including substance abuse, suicide attempt, or other acting-out behavior, difficulty with interpersonal relationships, development of a phobia regarding the trauma, poor impulse control or irritability, and explosiveness.

posttraumatic [L *post* after; Gk *trauma* wound], pertaining to any emotional, mental, or physiologic consequences following a major illness or injury.

posttraumatic amnesia [L *post* + Gk *trauma* wound], a period of amnesia between a brain injury resulting in memory loss and the point at which the functions concerned with memory are restored.

posttraumatic epilepsy. See **traumatic epilepsy.**

posttraumatic osteoporosis, osteoporosis that develops after an injury or other severe health episode.

posttraumatic spondylitis. See **Kümmell's disease.**

posttraumatic stress disorder (PTSD), an anxiety disorder characterized by an acute emotional response to a traumatic event or situation involving severe environmental stress, such as a natural disaster, airplane crash, serious automobile accident, military combat, and physical torture.

posttraumatic syndrome. See **postconcussional syndrome.**

postulate [L *postulare* to demand], a hypothesis that is offered as true without proof or as a basis for argument or debate.

postural albuminuria. See **orthostatic proteinuria.**

postural background movements [L *ponere* to place], the spontaneous body adjustments, requiring vestibular and proprioceptive integration, that maintain the center of gravity, keep the head and body in alignment, and stabilize body parts.

postural drainage, the use of positioning to drain secretions from specific segments of the bronchi and the lungs into the trachea. Coughing normally expels secretions from the trachea. Positions are selected that promote drainage from the affected parts of the lungs. Pillows and raised sections of the hospital bed are used to support or elevate parts of the body. The procedure is begun with the patient level, and the head is gradually lowered to a full Trendelenburg position. Inhalation through the nose and exhalation through the mouth is encouraged. Simultaneously the nurse may use cupping and vibration over the affected area of the lungs to dislodge and mobilize secretions. The person is then helped to a position conducive to coughing and is asked to breathe deeply at least three times and to cough at least twice.

postural hypotension. See **orthostatic hypotension.**

postural proteinuria. See **orthostatic proteinuria.**

postural reflex [L *ponere* to place; *reflectere* to turn backward], any of several reflexes associated with the maintenance of normal body posture.

postural vertigo. See **cupulolithiasis.**

posture [L *ponere* to place], the position of the body with respect to the surrounding space. A posture is determined and maintained by coordination of the various muscles that move the limbs, by proprioception, and by the sense of balance.

postvaccinal encephalitis [L *post* after, *vaccinus* of a cow; Gk *enkephalos* brain, *itis* inflammation], acute encephalitis following vaccination.

postvaccinal encephalomyelitis [Gk *enkephalos* brain, *myelos* marrow, *itis* inflammation], acute encephalomyelitis following vaccination.

postviral fatigue syndrome [L *post* + *virus* poison; *fatigare* to tire; Gk *syn* together, *dromos* course], a condition of chronic muscle fatigue unrelieved by rest following a viral infection. Other symptoms may include visual and hearing difficulties, low-grade fever, stiff neck, urinary frequency, and insomnia.

potable /pō′təbəl/ [L *potare* to drink], fit for drinking.

potassemia [Du *potasschen;* Gk *haima* blood], an excess of potassium in the blood.

potassium (K) [D *potasschen* potash], an alkali metal element, the seventh most abundant element in the earth's crust. Its atomic number is 19; its atomic weight is 39.1. Potassium salts are necessary to the life of all plants and animals. Potassium in the body constitutes the predominant intracellular cation, helping to regulate neuromuscular excitability and muscle contraction.

potassium chloride (KCl), a white crystalline salt used as a substitute for table salt in the diet of persons with cardiovascular disorders, to administer the potassium ion, and as a constituent of Ringer's solution. It is prescribed in the treatment of hypokalemia resulting from a variety of causes and in treating digitalis intoxication.

potassium hydroxide (KOH), a white, soluble, highly caustic compound. Occasionally used in solution as an escharotic for bites of rabid animals, KOH has many laboratory uses as an alkalinizing agent, including the preparation of clinical specimens for examination for fungi under the microscope.

potassium indoxyl sulfate. See **indican.**

potassium iodide, a bronchodilator prescribed in the treatment of bronchitis, bronchiectasis, asthma, and in various thyroid disorders.

potassium penicillin V. See **penicillin V.**

potassium-sparing diuretic. See **diuretic.**

potency [L *potentia* power], (in embryology) the range of developmental possibilities of which an embryonic cell or part is capable, regardless of whether the stimulus for growth or differentiation is natural, artificial, or experimental.

potent, powerful or strong.

potential [L *potentia*], an expression of the energy involved in transfering a unit of electric charge. The gradient or slope of a potential causes the charge to move.

potential abnormality of glucose tolerance, a classification that includes persons who have never had abnormal glucose tolerance but who have an increased risk of diabetes or impaired glucose tolerance. Factors associated with an increased risk of insulin-dependent diabetes mellitus (IDDM) include circulating islet cell antibodies, being a monozygotic twin or sibling of an IDDM patient, and being the offspring of an IDDM patient.

potential diabetes. See **potential abnormality of glucose tolerance.**

potential difference, the difference in electric potential between two points.

potential energy, the energy contained in a body because of its position in space, internal structure, and stresses imposed on it.

potential life, a criterion used by the Federal Centers for Disease Control to gauge premature death rates. Among younger individuals, it is based on an assumption that the person would have lived to the age of 65 if life had not been interrupted by a particular disease or injury. The leading cause of loss of potential life in young persons is accidents, followed by cancer and heart disease. For older persons, the system is based on years of potential life lost before the age of 85, in which case the cancer and heart disease rank first and second.

potential trauma, (in dentistry) a change in tissue that may occur because of existing malocclusion or dental disharmony.

potentiate /pōten′shē·āt/, to increase the strength or degree of activity of something.

potentiation /pōten′shē·ā′shən/ [L *potentia*], a synergistic action in which the effect of two drugs given simultaneously is greater than the effect of the drugs given separately.

potentiometer /pōten′shē·om′ətər/ [L *potentia* + Gk *metron* measure], a voltage-measuring device.

Potter-Bucky grid [Hollis E. Potter, American radiologist, b. 1880; Gustav Bucky, American radiologist, b. 1880; ME *gredire* grate], (in radiography) an x-ray grid designed on the principle of a moving grid, which oscillates during the exposure of a radiographic film.

Pott's disease. See **tuberculous spondylitis.**

Pott's fracture [Percival Pott, English physician, b. 1714], a fracture of the fibula near the ankle, often accompanied by a break of the malleolus of the tibia or rupture of the internal lateral ligament.

potty chair [AS *pott;* ME *chaire*], a small chair that has an open seat over a removable pot, used for the toilet training of young children.

pouch [OFr *pouche*], any small saclike appendage or pocket, such as Rathke's pouch in the roof of the embryonic roof cavity.

pouch of Douglas. See **cul-de-sac of Douglas.**

poultice /pōl′tis/ [L *puls* porridge], a soft, moist, pulp spread between layers of gauze or cloth and applied hot to a surface to provide heat or counterirritation. A kind of poultice is a **mustard poultice.**

pound [L *pondus* weight], a unit of measure equal to 16 ounces, avoirdupois; 0.45359 kilogram; 7,000 grains.

poverty [L *paupertas*], **1.** a lack of material wealth needed to maintain existence. **2.** pertaining to a poor bodily condition; lean or feeble. **3.** a loss of emotional capacity to feel love or sympathy.

povidone, a polymerized form of vinylpyrrolidone, a white hygroscopic powder easily soluble in water, used as a dispersing and suspending agent in drugs. It has also been used as a blood volume extender, and, in a complex with iodine, as a topical antiseptic.

povidone-iodine /pō′vidōnī′ədīn/, an antiseptic microbicide prescribed for disinfection of wounds, as a preoperative surgical scrub, for vaginal infections, and for antiseptic treatment of burns.

Powassan virus infection [Powassan, Ontario], an uncommon form of encephalitis caused by a tick-borne arbovirus found in eastern Canada and the northern United States.

powder bed [L *pulvis* dust; AS *bedd*], a treatment in which large areas of a patient's body are kept in contact with a powdered medication for a certain length of time. The patient lies supine on the powdered sheet. Powder is shaken over the patient's body. The powdered sheet is then wrapped around the limbs and the trunk from the side to keep the powder in contact with the body.

powdered gold [L *pulvis* + AS *geolu* yellow], a fine granulation of pure gold, produced by atomizing the molten metal or by chemical precipitation. It is used in some dental restorations, such as prepared tooth cavities.

powerlessness [Fr *pouvoir* to have power; AS *loes* limited, *nes* condition], a NANDA-accepted nursing diagnosis of a perceived lack of control over a current health-related situation or problem and the client's perception that any action he or she takes will not affect the outcome of the particular situation. Defining characteristics include the verbal expression of having no control or influence over self-care, the particular situation, or its outcome; apathy; depression over physical deterioration that occurs despite compliance with regimens; nonparticipation in or lack of interest in the mode of care, in decision making regarding regimens, or in monitoring progress; verbal expression of dissatisfaction and frustration regarding the inability to perform previous activities; reluctance to express true feelings, fearing alienation of others; general irritability or passivity; expressions of resentment, anger, guilt, or doubt regarding role performance; and uncertainty about fluctuating energy levels.

power of attorney [Fr *pouvoir* + OFr *atorne* legal agent], a document authorizing one person to take legal actions in behalf of another, who acts as an agent for the grantor.

power stroke, a working stroke with a dental scaling instrument, used for splitting or dislodging calculus from the surface of a tooth or tooth root.

pox [ME *pokkes* pustules], **1.** any of several vesicular or pustular exanthematous diseases. **2.** the pitlike scars of smallpox. **3.** *archaic.* syphilis.

poxvirus /poksvī′rəs/ [ME *pokkes* + L *virus* poison], a member of a family of viruses that includes the organisms that cause molluscum contagiosum, smallpox, and vaccinia.

PPD, abbreviation for **purified protein derivative,** the material used in testing for tuberculin sensitivity.

PPLO, abbreviation for **pleuropneumonia-like organism.**

ppm, abbreviation for **parts per million.**

PPMA, abbreviation for **postpoliomyelitis muscular atrophy.**

PPO, abbreviation for **preferred provider organization.**

PPS, abbreviation for *prospective payment system.*

PPV, abbreviation for *positive pressure ventilation.*

Pr, symbol for the element **praseodymium.**

practical anatomy. See **applied anatomy.**

practical nurse. See **licensed practical nurse (LPN).**

practice guideline, a detailed description of a process of patient care management that will facilitate improvement of maintenance of health status or slow the decline in health status in certain chronic clinical conditions. The purpose of a practice guideline is to assist health care providers to identify preferred treatment by providing linkages among the diagnoses, treatments, and outcomes, and by describing alternatives for each patient.

practice models [Gk *praktikos* course of action], the different patterns in delivery of health care services by means of which health care is made available to diverse groups of people in different settings.

practice setting, the context or environment within which nursing care is given.

practice theory, (in nursing research) a theory that describes, explains, and prescribes nursing practice in general. It serves as the basis for specific items in the curriculum of nursing education and for the development of theories in the administration of nursing and nursing education.

practicing, the second subphase of the separation-individuation phase in Mahler's system of preoedipal development, when the child is able to move away from the mother and return to her.

practicing medicine without a license, (in law) practicing activities defined under state law in the medical practice act without physician supervision, direction, or control.

practitioner [Gk *praktikos* course of action], a person qualified to practice in a special professional field, such as a nurse practitioner.

Prader-Willi syndrome [A. Prader, twentieth-century Swiss physician; H. Willi; Gk *syn* together, *dromos* course], a metabolic condition characterized by congenital hypotonia, hyperphagia, obesity, and mental retardation. The syndrome is associated with a less than normal secretion of gonadotropic hormones by the pituitary gland.

praevia /prē'vē·ə/, **praevius** [L], pertaining to something that occurred at an earlier time or place.

praecox [L, premature], pertaining to something that occurred at at earlier stage of life or development.

pragmatic, pertaining to a belief that ideas are valuable only in terms of their consequences.

pragmatism [Gk *pragma* deed], a philosophy concerned with actual practice and practical results as opposed to theory and speculation.

pralidoxime chloride /pral'ədok'sēm/, a cholinesterase reactivator prescribed as an antidote for organophosphate poisoning and drug overdosage in the treatment of myasthenia gravis.

pramoxine hydrochloride, a local anesthetic for the relief of pain and itching associated with dermatoses, anogenital pruritus, hemorrhoids, anal fissure, and minor burns.

prandial /pran'dē·əl/ [L *prandium* lunch], pertaining to a meal. The term is used in relation to timing, such as postprandial or preprandial. **–prandiality,** *n.*

praseodymium (Pr) /prā'sē·ōdim'ē·əm/ [Gk *prasaios* light green, *didymos* twin], a rare earth metallic element. Its atomic number is 59; its atomic weight is 140.91.

Prausnitz-Küstner (PK) test /prous'nitskist'nər/ [Otto C. W. Prausnitz, Polish bacteriologist, b. 1876; Heinz Küstner, Polish gynecologist, b. 1897], a skin test in which an allergic response is transferred to a nonallergic person who acts as a surrogate to permit identification of the allergen. The test is performed only when skin sensitivity testing cannot be performed directly on the allergic patient.

praxis /prak'sis/ [Gk, action], a concept that deals with actions and overt behavior, or the performance of an action to the exclusion of metaphysical thought.

prazepam /praz'əpam/, an antianxiety agent derived from benzodiazepine. It is prescribed for the treatment of anxiety disorders and for the short-term relief of symptoms of anxiety.

prazosin hydrochloride /prä'zəsin/, an antihypertensive prescribed in the treatment of hypertension and to decrease afterload in congestive heart disease.

preadmission certification, a system whereby physicians are required to obtain advance approval for nonemergency admission of Medicare patients to hospitals. The system is intended to determine whether the patient can be treated as an outpatient or in another, less expensive manner than hospitalization. Emergency admissions require post hoc approval.

preagonal ascites [L *prae* before; Gk *agon* struggle; *askos* bag], a rapid accumulation of fluid within the peritoneal cavity, representing the transudation of serum from the circulatory system.

preanesthetic medication. See **premedication.**

preaortic node /prē'ā·ôr'tik/ [L *prae* + Gk *aerein* to raise; L *nodus* knot], a node in one of the three sets of lumbar lymph nodes that serve various abdominal viscera supplied by the celiac, superior mesenteric, and inferior mesenteric arteries.

precancerous, pertaining to a stage of abnormal tissue growth that is likely to develop into a malignant tumor.

precancerous dermatitis. See **intraepidermal carcinoma.**

precedent [L *praecedere* to go before], a previously adjudged decision that serves as an authority in a similar case.

precentral gyrus, a convolution of the cerebral hemisphere immediately anterior to the central sulcus of the cerebrum in each hemisphere. It is the location of the motor strip that controls voluntary movements of the contralateral side of the body.

preceptorship [L *prae + capere* to take up], the position of teacher or instructor, usually the headmaster or dean of a school.

precession [L *praecedere* to go before], a comparatively slow gyration of the axis of a spinning body, so as to trace out a cone, caused by the application of a torque.

precipitant [L *praecipitare* to throw down], a substance that causes another substance to settle, separate, or deposit from a solution, such as a reagent that causes certain metals to precipitate.

precipitate /prəsip'ität, -it/ [L *praecipitare* to cast down], **1.** to cause a substance to separate or to settle out of solution. **2.** a substance that has separated from or settled out of a solution. **3.** occurring hastily or unexpectedly.

precipitate delivery, childbirth that occurs with such speed or in such a situation that the usual preparations cannot be made.

precipitating factor, an element that causes or contributes to the occurrence of a disorder.

precipitation, a process whereby solid particles are made to settle out of a solution so they can be separated from other dissolved substances.

precipitin /prəsip'itin/ [L *praecipitare + Gk anti* against; AS *bodig* body; Gk *genein* to produce], an antibody that causes formation of an insoluble complex when combined with a specific soluble antigen.

precision rest [L *praecidere* to cut short; AS *rest*], a rigid denture support consisting of two tightly fitting parts, the insert of which rests firmly against the gingival portion of the device.

preclinical, a stage in a disease when a specific diagnosis cannot be made because adequate signs and symptoms have not yet developed.

precocious [L *praecoquere* to mature early], pertaining to the early, often premature, development of physical or mental qualities.

precocious dentition, the abnormal acceleration of the eruption of the deciduous or permanent teeth, usually associated with an endocrine imbalance, such as excess pituitary growth hormone or hyperthyroidism.

precocious puberty, abnormally early development of sexual maturity. It is usually marked by ovulation in girls before the age of 8 and the production of mature sperm in a boy before the age of 10.

precognition, the foreknowledge of events.

preconscious [L *prae* before, *conscire* to be aware] **1.** before the development of self-consciousness and self-awareness. **2.** (in psychiatry) the mental function in which thoughts, ideas, emotions, or memories not in immediate awareness can be brought into the consciousness without encountering any intrapsychic resistance or repression. **3.** the mental phenomena capable of being recalled, although not present in the conscious mind.

precordia [L *prae + cor* heart], pertaining to the front area of the thorax that lies over the heart.

precordial /prēkôr'dē-əl/ [L *prae + cor* heart], of or pertaining to the precordium, which forms the region over the heart and the lower part of the thorax.

precordial lead, an electrocardiographic lead from the chest wall over the heart.

precordial movement, any motion of the anterior wall of the thorax localized in the area over the heart. Kinds of precordial movements include **apical impulse, left ventricular thrust,** and **right ventricular thrust.**

precordial pain, a pain in the chest wall area over the heart.

precordium, the part of the front of the chest wall that overlays the heart and the epigastrium.

precursor [L *prae + currere* to run], a prognostic characteristic or feature of a patient's health data, such as an x-ray or laboratory finding, that is associated with a higher or lower risk of death than the average.

precursor therapy, a type of treatment involving the use of nutrients that may influence neurologic clinical conditions.

predeciduous dentition [L *prae + decidere* to fall off], the epithelial structures found in the mouth of the infant preceding the eruption of the deciduous teeth.

prediabetes. See **potential abnormality of glucose tolerance, previous abnormality of glucose tolerance.**

prediastole, the part of the cardiac cycle between the late systolic phase and the early diastolic phase.

prediastolic murmur, a murmur heard during the cardiac systole.

predicate /pred'ikāt/, (in neurolinguistic programing) the part of a sentence that tells something about the subject. It can refer to direct sensory experience or can be neutral.

predictive hypothesis [L *prae* + *dicere* to say; Gk, foundation], (in research) a hypothesis that predicts the nature of a relationship among the variables to be studied.

predictive validity, validity of a test or a measurement tool that is established by demonstrating its ability to predict the results of an analysis of the same data using another test instrument or measurement tool.

predictor variable. See **independent variable.**

predisposing cause, any condition that enhances the specific cause of a disease, such as being susceptible because of hereditary or life-style factors.

predisposing factor [L *prae* + *disponere* to dispose], any conditioning factor that influences both the type and amount of resources that the individual can elicit to cope with stress. It may be biological, psychologic, or sociocultural in nature.

predisposition, a state of being particularly susceptible.

prednisolone /prednis'əlōn/, a glucocorticoid prescribed as treatment for inflammation of the skin, conjunctiva, and cornea and for immunosuppression.

prednisone /pred'nisōn/, a glucocorticoid prescribed in severe inflammation and immunosuppression.

preeclampsia /prē'iklamp'sē-ə/ [L *prae* + Gk *ek* out, *lampein* to flash], an abnormal condition of pregnancy characterized by the onset of acute hypertension after the twenty-fourth week of gestation. The classic triad of preeclampsia is hypertension, proteinuria, and edema. Mild preeclampsia is diagnosed if one or more of the following signs develop after the twenty-fourth week of gestation: systolic blood pressure of 140 mm Hg or more or a rise of 30 mm or more above the woman's usual systolic blood pressure; diastolic blood pressure of 90 mm Hg or more or a rise of 15 mm or more above the woman's usual diastolic blood pressure; proteinuria; edema. Severe preeclampsia is diagnosed if one or more of the following is present: systolic blood pressure of 160 mm Hg or more or a diastolic blood pressure of 110 mm Hg or more on two occasions 6 hours apart with the woman at bed rest; proteinuria of 5 g or more in 24 hours; oliguria of less than 400 ml in 24 hours; ocular or cerebral vascular disorders; cyanosis or pulmonary edema.

preemie /prē'mē/, abbreviation for **premature infant.**

preexcitation [L *prae* + *excitare* to arouse], activation of part of the ventricular myocardium earlier than would be expected if the activating impulses traveled only down the normal routes or had experienced a normal delay within the AV node. The degree of preexcitation is determined by how fast the impulse traverses the atrial tissue and the accessory pathway or the AV node.

preexisting condition, any injury, disease, or disability that may have occurred at some time in the past and might predispose an individual to limited health in the future.

preferential anosmia [L *praeferens* being preferred; Gk *a, osme* not smell], the inability to smell certain odors. The condition is often caused by psychologic factors concerning either a particular smell or the situation in which the smell occurs.

preferred provider organization (PPO) [L *praeferre* to put before], an organization of physicians, hospitals, and pharmacists whose members discount their health care services to subscriber patients.

preformation [L *prae* + *formatio* formation], an early theory in embryology in which the organism is contained in minute and complete form within the germ cell and after fertilization grows from microscopic to normal size.

preformed water [L *prae* + *forma* form; AS *waeter*], the water that is contained in foods.

prefrontal lobotomy [L *prae* + *frons* forehead; Gk *lobos* lobe, *temnein* to cut], a surgical procedure in which connecting fibers between the prefrontal lobes of the brain and the thalamus are severed. After surgery, patients are often apathetic, docile, and lacking social graces. If only the white fibers are severed, the procedure is called a prefrontal leukotomy.

preg, abbreviation for **pregnancy.**

preganglionic neuron, a neuron whose axon terminates in contact with another nerve cell located in a peripheral ganglion.

pregnancy [L *praegnans* child bearing], the gestational process, comprising the growth and development within a woman of a new individual from conception through the embryonic and fetal periods to birth. Pregnancy lasts approximately 266 days (38 weeks) from the day of fertilization, but it is clinically considered to last 280 days (40 weeks; 10 lunar months; 9⅓ calendar months) from the first day of the last menstrual period. Of the millions of ejaculated sperm cells, thousands reach the female ovum in the outer end of the fallopian tube, but usually only one penetrates the egg for union of the male and female pronuclei and conception. The zygote, genetically a unique entity, begins cell division as it is transported to the uterine cavity where it implants in the uterine wall. Maternal and embryologic elements together form the beginnings of the placenta, which grows into the substance of the uterus. The placenta functions in maternal-fetal exchange of nutrients and waste products. The conceptus is, in some aspects, like a foreign graft or transplant in the mother. Though the mother normally does not activate an immune response, all of her tissues and organs undergo change, many of them profound and some of them permanent.

pregnancy gingivitis, an enlargement or hyperplasia of the gingivae caused by hormonal imbalance during pregnancy.

pregnancy luteoma. See **luteoma.**

pregnancy rate, (in statistics) the ratio of pregnancies per 100 woman-years, calculated as the product of the number of pregnancies in the women observed multiplied by 1,200 (months) divided by the product of the number of women observed multiplied by the number of months observed. For example, if 50 women used one contraceptive method for 12 months and 5 of them became pregnant, the pregnancy rate would be 10 per 100 woman-years.

pregnancy test. See **HCG radioreceptor assay.**

pregnanediol /pregnān'dē·ol/, a crystalline, biologically inactive compound found in the urine of women during pregnancy or the secretory phase of the menstrual cycle.

pregnant [L *praegnans*], being gravid, with child.

prehensile [L *prehendre* to seize], able to grasp.

prehension, the use of the hands and fingers to grasp or pick up objects.

prehospital care, any medical care given an ill or injured patient by a paramedic or other person before the patient reaches the hospital emergency department.

preinvasive carcinoma. See **carcinoma in situ.**

preload [L *prae* + AS *lad*], the initial stretch of myocardial fiber at end diastole. The ventricular end diastolic pressure and volume reflect this parameter.

preload filling pressure, the load on the ventricular muscle fibers at the end of diastole or just prior to contraction. The preload on the heart is estimated by the left ventricular filling pressure. Cardiac performance increases with preload to a point.

premalignant fibroepithelioma [L *prae* +

malignus bad disposition; *fibra* fiber; Gk *epi* above, *thele* nipple, *oma* tumor], an elevated white flesh–colored sessile neoplasm formed of interlacing ribbons of epithelial cells on a hyperplastic mesodermal stroma. The tumor occurs most often on the lower trunk of older people.

premarket approval (PMA), permission given by the federal government to equipment manufacturers to sell their devices to the medical profession.

premature [L *prae* + *maturare* to ripen], **1.** not fully developed or mature. **2.** occurring before the appropriate or usual time. **–prematurity,** *n.*

premature alopecia [L *praematurus* too soon; Gk *alopex* fox mange], acquired baldness in a person who is not old.

premature atrial complex, a cardiac arrhythmia characterized by an atrial depolarization occurring earlier than expected, indicated electrocardiographically as an early P wave. The dysrhythmia may be the result of atrial enlargement or ischemia, or may be caused by stress, caffeine, or nicotine.

premature beat, a heart contraction, usually ectopic, that occurs earlier than expected in the ongoing rhythm pattern.

premature contraction, any contraction of either the ventricle or atrium that occurs early with respect to the dominant rhythm.

premature ejaculation, uncontrollable, untimely ejaculation of semen often caused by anxiety during sexual intercourse.

premature impulse, any impulse that occurs early with respect to a dominant rhythm.

premature infant, any neonate, regardless of birth weight, born before 37 weeks of gestation. Predisposing factors associated with prematurity include multiple pregnancy, toxemia, chronic disease, acute infection, sensitization to blood incompatibility, and any severe trauma that may interfere with normal fetal development. In most instances the cause is unknown. The premature infant usually appears small and scrawny, with a large head in relation to body size, and weighs less than 2,500 g. The skin is bright pink, smooth, shiny, and translucent with the underlying vessels clearly visible. The arms and legs are extended, not flexed, as in the full-term infant. There is little subcutaneous fat, sparse hair, few creases on the soles and palms, and poorly developed ear cartilage. In boys, the scrotum has few rugae and the testes may be undescended; in girls, the labia gape and the clitoris is prominent.

premature labor, labor that occurs earlier

in pregnancy than normal, either before the fetus has reached a weight of 2,000 to 2,500 g or before the thirty-seventh or thirty-eighth week of gestation. No single measure of fetal weight or gestational age is used universally to designate premature birth; local or institutional policy dictates which of several standards is applied.

premature rupture of membranes, the spontaneous rupture of the amniotic sac before the onset of labor.

premature systole, a systole that occurs too early as a result of a discharge of an ectopic focus in the atria, atrioventricular junction, or ventricle.

premature thelarche. See thelarche.

premature ventricular contraction (PVC), a cardiac sinus conducted dysrhythmia characterized by ventricular depolarization occurring earlier than expected, shown on the electrocardiogram as an early, wide QRS complex without a preceding related P wave. They may be caused by stress, acidosis, electrolyte imbalance, hypoxemia, hypercapnia, ventricular enlargement, or a toxic reaction to drugs.

prematurity, pertaining to a happening before the usual or expected time, as a premature birth.

premed, abbreviation for *premedical student.*

premedication [L *prae* + *medicare* to heal], **1.** any sedative, tranquilizer, hypnotic, or anticholinergic medication administered before anesthesia. The choice of drug depends on variables such as the patient's age and physical condition and the specific operative procedure. **2.** the administration of such medications. –**premedicate,** *v.*

premenarchal [L *prae* + *mensis* month; Gk *archaios* from the beginning], pertaining to the period before the start of menstruation.

premenopausal [L *prae* + *mensis* month; Gk *pauein* to cease], of or pertaining to the time of life preceding the menopause.

premenstrual [L *prae* + *menstrualis* monthly], pertaining to a period before the start of menstruation.

premenstrual syndrome (PMS), a syndrome of nervous tension, irritability, weight gain, edema, headache, mastalgia, dysphoria, and lack of coordination occurring during the last few days of the menstrual cycle before the onset of menstruation.

premise [L *prae* + *mittere* to send], a proposition that is laid down as the base of an argument, and which is usually established beforehand.

premolar /prēmō'lər/ [L *prae* + *mola* mill], one of eight teeth, four in each dental arch, located lateral to and posterior to the canine teeth. The premolars appear during childhood and remain until old age. They are smaller and shorter than the canine teeth.

premonition, a sense of an impending event without prior knowledge of it.

premonitory [L *prae* + *monere* to warn], an early symptom or sign of a disease. The term is commonly used to describe minor symptoms that precede a major health problem.

premorbid personality, a personality characterized by early signs or symptoms of a mental disorder. The specific defects may indicate whether the condition will progress toward schizophrenia, a bipolar disorder, or another type of condition.

prenatal [L *prae* + *natus* birth], prior to birth; occurring or existing before birth, referring to both the care of the woman during pregnancy and the growth and development of the fetus.

prenatal care, the health care provided the mother and fetus before childbirth.

prenatal development, the entire process of growth, maturation, differentiation, and development that occurs between conception and birth. On approximately the fourteenth day before the next expected menstrual period, ovulation usually occurs. If the egg is fertilized, it immediately begins the course to fetal maturity and birth. During the first 14 days the fertilized ovum undergoes cell division several times, becoming a morula, and then a blastocyst that is able to implant in the uterine wall. From the beginning of the third to the end of the seventh week of embryonic development, implantation deepens and completes. By the end of the seventh week all essential systems are present. The period of time from the eighth week to birth is called the fetal stage. Between the seventeenth and the twentieth weeks of pregnancy the mother usually first feels the baby move. The fetus looks like a very small baby at this time. At 28 weeks subcutaneous fat begins to develop, fingernails and toenails are present, the eyelids are separate and the eyes may open, scalp hair is well developed, and in males the testes are at the internal inguinal ring or below. In a modern neonatal intensive care unit more than 80% of the babies born at 28 weeks survive. By the thirty-second week, the fetus weighs between 3 and 4 pounds. At 36 weeks the body and the limbs are fuller and more rounded, creases involve the anterior two thirds of the soles, and the skin is thicker and less translucent. As the fetus reaches term, between 38 and

42 weeks, the vernix decreases, and the ear cartilage is developed. At 40 weeks the average fetus weighs 7¼ pounds and is between 19 and 22 inches long. Prenatal development may be adversely affected by several factors. Between 2 and 14 weeks of gestation, ionizing radiation and some drugs may have profound effects on morphologic and functional development. After 14 weeks when all the organs, systems, and parts of the body have formed, any adverse effects are largely functional; major morphologic damage does not occur.

prenatal diagnosis, any of various diagnostic techniques to determine if a developing fetus in the uterus is affected with a genetic disorder or other abnormality. Such procedures as x-ray examination and ultrasound scanning can be used to follow fetal growth and detect structural abnormalities; amniocentesis enables fetal cells to be obtained from the amniotic fluid for culture and biochemical assay to detect metabolic disorders and for chromosomal analysis; fetoscopy enables fetal blood to be withdrawn from a blood vessel of the placenta and examined for disorders such as thalassemia, sickle cell anemia, and Duchenne's muscular dystrophy.

prenatal surgery, any surgical procedure that is performed on a fetus. The technique has been used to correct hydrocephalus and obstructions of the urinary tract.

preoccupation, a state of being self-absorbed or engrossed in one's own thoughts to a degree that hinders effective contact with or relationship to external reality.

pre-op /prē·op′/, abbreviation for *preparation for operation.*

preoperational thought phase [L *prae* + *operari* work; AS *thot;* Gk *phainein* to show], a piagetian phase of child development, during the period of 2 to 7 years of age, when the child focuses on the use of language as a tool to meet his or her needs.

preoperative [L *prae* + *operari* work], of or pertaining to the period of time before a surgical procedure. Commonly, the preoperative period begins with the first preparation of the patient for surgery, as when, 12 hours before scheduled procedure, fluids or food by mouth is forbidden. It ends with the induction of surgical anesthesia in the operating suite.

preoperative care, the preparation and management of a patient before surgery. The patient's nutritional and hygienic state, medical and surgical history, allergies, current medication, physical handicaps, signs of infection, and elimination habits are noted and recorded. The patient's understanding of the operative, preoperative, and postoperative procedures, the patient's ability to verbalize anxieties, and the family's knowledge of the planned surgery are ascertained. The signed informed consent statement, the physician's preoperative orders, and the patient's identification bands, willingness to receive blood if necessary, and understanding of the use of the call bell and the purpose of the bed's side rails are checked. Blood pressure, temperature, pulse, and respiration are recorded, and any abnormalities are reported to the physician. The physician is also informed if the electrocardiogram, chest x-ray study, or laboratory studies show any abnormalities. On completion of the patient's blood typing, the number of matched blood units required to be held for a possible blood transfusion is determined. When ordered, an enema is given, a bowel preparation is completed, a nasogastric tube or indwelling catheter is inserted, and parenteral fluids are administered. Before bedtime the patient showers, using an antibacterial soap; nothing is given orally after midnight unless ordered. After preoperative medication is administered, the side rails of the bed are raised. Before leaving for the operating room with the completed chart, the patient voids, and dentures, contact lenses, and any valuables are removed for safekeeping.

prep, abbreviation for *prepare* or **preparation,** particularly when referring to preparation for surgery.

preparation [L *praeparare* to make ready], **1.** making a site ready for a procedure. such as removing debris from a tooth cavity before filling. **2.** a medication or other treatment made ready for use. **3.** a specimen.

preparatory prosthesis, a temporary artificial limb that is fitted to the stump soon after amputation. It permits ambulation and biomechanical adaptation during the first several weeks after surgery.

prepared cavity [L *praeparare* to make ready; *cavum* cavity], a tooth cavity that has been prepared to receive and retain a restoration.

prepared childbirth. See **natural childbirth.**

prepartum, pertaining to events that occur before child delivery.

prepatellar [L *prae* + *patella* small disk], located in front of the patella.

prepatellar bursa [L *prae* + *patella* small dish; Gk *byrsa* wineskin], a bursa between the tendon of the quadriceps and the lower part of the femur continuous with the cavity of the knee joint.

prepatellar bursitis, an inflammation of the bursa in front of the patella and beneath the skin over the site.

prepayment [L *prae* + *pacere* to pacify], the payment in advance for health care services, by subscribers to a third-party insurance program, such as Blue Cross.

preprandial [L *prae* + *prandium* lunch], before a meal.

prepubertal panhypopituitarism [L *prae* + *pubertas* maturity; Gk *pan* all, *hypo* under, *pituita* phlegm], insufficiency of pituitary hormones, caused by damage to the gland usually associated with a suprasellar cyst or craniopharyngioma, occurring in childhood. The disorder is characterized by dwarfism with normal body proportions, subnormal sexual development, impaired thyroid and adrenal function, and yellow, wrinkled skin.

prepuberty [L *prae* + *pubertas* maturity], the period immediately preceding puberty, lasting approximately 2 years and characterized by preliminary physical changes, such as accelerated growth and appearance of secondary sex characteristics, that lead to sexual maturity. **–prepuberal, prepubertal,** *adj.*

prepubescence /prē′pyo̅o̅bes′əns/, the state of being prepubertal. **–prepubescent,** *adj.*

prepuce /prē′pyo̅o̅s/ [L *praeputium* foreskin], a fold of skin that forms a retractable cover, such as the foreskin of the penis or the fold around the clitoris. **–prepucial, preputial,** *adj.*

prerenal [L *prae* + *ren* kidney], **1.** located in front of the kidney. **2.** occurring before reaching the kidney.

prerenal anuria [L *prae* + *renes* kidneys; Gk *a, ouron* not urine], cessation of urine production caused by the blood pressure in the kidney being too low to maintain glomerular filtration pressure.

prerenal uremia, a condition of kidney failure in which the primary cause may be outside the kidney, as in some severe cases of alkalosis.

presbycardia /prez′bikär′dē·ə/ [Gk *presbys* old man, *kardia* heart], an abnormal cardiac condition, especially affecting elderly individuals and associated with heart failure in the presence of other complications, such as heart disease, fever, anemia, mild hyperthyroidism, and excess fluid administration. Presbycardia may be associated with decreased elasticity of the musculature of the heart and with mild fibrotic changes of the heart valves, but the basis for these changes and the associated pigmentation of the heart is not known.

presbycusis /pres′bēk o̅o̅′sis/ [Gk *presbys* + *akousis* hearing], the normal loss of hearing acuity, speech intelligibility, auditory threshold, and pitch associated with aging.

presbyopia /prez′bi·ō′pē·ə/ [Gk *presbys* + *ops* eye], farsightedness resulting from a loss of elasticity of the lens of the eye. The condition commonly develops with advancing age. **–presbyopic,** *adj.*

preschizophrenic state [L *prae* + Gk *schizein* to split, *phren* mind], a period before psychosis that is evident when the patient deviates from normal behavior but does not demonstrate psychotic symptoms of delusions, hallucinations, or stupor.

prescreen [L *prae* + ME *scren*], **1.** evaluation of a patient or a group of patients to identify those who are at greater risk of developing a particular condition and therefore in particular need of special diagnostic procedures or health care. **2.** *informal;* a rapid, superficial examination of a person who does not appear to be acutely ill. It may include taking a medical history.

prescribe [L *prae* + *scribere* to write], **1.** to write an order for a drug, treatment, or procedure. **2.** to recommend or encourage a course of action.

prescription, an order for medication, therapy, or a therapeutic device given by a properly authorized person to a person properly authorized to dispense or perform the order. A prescription is usually in written form and includes the name and address of the patient, the date, the ℞ symbol (superscription), the medication prescribed (inscription), directions to the pharmacist or other dispenser (subscription), directions to the patient that must appear on the label, the prescriber's signature, and in some instances an identifying number.

prescription drug [L *prae* + *scribere;* Fr *drogue*], a drug that can be dispensed to the public only with a prescription. The designation as a prescription drug is made by the Food and Drug Administration.

prescriptive intervention mode [L *prae-scriptus* prescribed; *intervenire* to come between; *modus* measure], a therapeutic situation in which the health professional tells the patient explicitly how to solve a problem, so that less collaboration between the consultant and patient is needed.

prescriptive theory, a theory that comprises a description of a specific activity, a statement of the goal of the activity, and an analysis of the elements of the activity that together constitute a prescription for reaching the goal.

presence a mode of being available in a situation with the wholeness of one's in-

P

dividual being; a gift of self which can be given freely, invoked or evoked.

presenile [L *prae* before, *senex* aged], pertaining to a condition in which a person manifests signs of aging in early or middle life.

presenile dementia. See **Alzheimer's disease.**

presentation. See **fetal presentation.**

present health [L *praesentare* to show; AS *haelth*], (in a health history) a chronologic, succinct account of any recent changes in the health of the patient and of the circumstances or symptoms that prompted the person to seek health care.

presenting part [L *praesentare* + *pars* part], the part of the fetus that lies closest to the internal os of the cervix.

presenting symptom. See **symptom.**

preservative [L *praeservare* to keep], a chemical or other agent that reduces the rate of decomposition of a substance.

presomite embryo /prēsō'mīt/ [L *prae* + Gk *soma* body, *en* in, *bryein* to grow], an embryo in any stage of development before the appearance of the first pair of somites, which, in humans, usually occurs around 19 to 21 days after fertilization of the ovum.

pressor /pres'ər/ [L *premere* to press], describing a substance that tends to cause a rise in blood pressure.

pressoreceptor /pres'ōrisep'tər/ [L *premere* + *recipere* to receive], a nerve ending that is sensitive to changes in blood pressure.

pressure [L *premere* to press], a force, or stress, applied to a surface by a fluid or an object, usually measured in units of mass per unit of area, as pounds per square inch.

pressure acupuncture, a system of acupuncture involving the application of pressure, as by the tip of a finger, to certain specified points of the body.

pressure area, an oral area that is subject to excessive displacement of soft tissue by a prosthesis.

pressure bandage, a bandage applied to stop bleeding, prevent edema, or provide support for varicose veins.

pressure dressing, a dressing firmly applied to exert pressure, usually on a wound for hemostasis.

pressure edema, 1. edema of the lower extremities caused by pressure of a pregnant uterus against the large veins of the area. 2. edema of the fetal scalp after cephalic presentation.

pressure point, 1. a point over an artery where the pulse may be felt. Pressure on the point may be helpful in stopping the flow of blood from a wound distal to the point. 2. a site that is extremely sensitive to pressure, such as the phrenic pressure point along the phrenic nerve between the sternocleidomastoid and the scalenus anticus on the right side.

pressure-sensitive adhesive, a drug-delivery device that utilizes polymers that are permanently tacky at room temperature and will adhere to the skin when slight pressure is applied.

pressure sore. See **decubitus ulcer.**

pressure support ventilation (PSV), the augmentation of spontaneous breathing effort with a specific amount of positive airway pressure. The patient initiates the inspiratory flow, generating his or her own V_t and frequencies.

pressure ventilator, a ventilator in which gas delivery is limited by a predetermined pressure.

presumptive signs [L *praesumere* to take beforehand; *signum* mark], manifestations that indicate a pregnancy, although they are not necessarily positive. Presumptive signs may include cessation of menses and morning sickness.

preswing stance stage [L *prae* + AS *swingan* to fling; L *stare* to stand; OFr *estage* stage], one of the five stages in the stance phase of walking or gait, involving a brief transitional period of double limb support during which one leg of the body is rapidly relieved of body-bearing weight and prepared for the swing forward.

presymptomatic disease [L *prae* + Gk *symptoma* a happening], an early stage of disease when physiologic changes have begun although no signs or symptoms are observed.

presynaptic [L *prae* + *synaptein* to join], 1. situated near or before a synapse. 2. occurring before a synapse is crossed.

presystole, an interval in the cardiac cycle immediately before systole.

presystolic [L *prae* + Gk *systole* contraction], of or pertaining to the period preceding systole.

presystolic murmur, a heart murmur heard in cases of mitral stenosis. The murmur is heard during the last phase of ventricular diastole.

preterm, 1. pertaining to events preceding a specific date. 2. pertaining to a shorter than normal period of gestation.

preterm birth, any birth that occurs before the thirty-seventh week of gestation.

preterm infant. See **premature infant.**

preterm labor. See **premature labor.**

pretibial /prētib'ē·əl/ [L *prae* + *tibia* shinbone], of or pertaining to the area of the leg in front of the tibia.

pretibial fever, an acute infection caused by *Leptospira autumnalis,* characterized by headache, chills, fever, enlarged spleen, myalgia, low white blood cell count, and a rash on the anterior surface of the legs.

pretrial discovery. See **discovery.**

prevalence /prev′ələns/ [L *praevalentia* a powerful force], (in epidemiology) the number of all new and old cases of a disease or occurrences of an event during a particular period of time.

prevention [L *praevenire* to anticipate], (in nursing care) any action directed toward preventing illness and promoting health to avoid the need for secondary or tertiary health care.

preventive [L *praevenire* to anticipate], tending to slow, stop, or interrupt the course of an illness or to decrease the incidence of a disease.

preventive care, a pattern of nursing and medical care that focuses on the prevention of disease and health maintenance and includes early diagnosis of disease, discovery and identification of people at risk of developing specific problems, counseling, and other intervention to avert a health problem.

preventive dentistry, the science of prevention of disease affecting the teeth.

preventive health care. See **preventive care.**

preventive medicine, the branch of medicine that is concerned with the prevention of disease and methods for increasing the power of the patient and community to resist disease and prolong life.

preventive nursing, a branch of nursing that is concerned with general health promotion, teaching of early recognition and treatment of disease, encouraging lifestyle modification, and prevention of further deterioration of the disabled.

preventive psychiatry, the use of theoretical knowledge and skills to plan and implement programs designed to achieve primary, secondary, and tertiary prevention.

preventive treatment, a procedure, measure, substance, or program designed to prevent a disease from occurring or a mild disorder from becoming more severe. Various diseases are prevented by immunizations with vaccines, antiseptic measures, regular exercise, a prudent diet, adequate rest, and screening programs for the detection of preclinical signs of disorders.

previa. See **placenta previa.**

previllous embryo /prēvil′əs/ [L *prae* + *villus* hairy; Gk *en* in, *bryein* to grow], an embryo of a placental mammal at any stage before the development of the chorionic villi, which in humans begin to form

between the first and second months after fertilization of the ovum.

previous abnormality of glucose tolerance, a classification that includes persons who previously had diabetic hyperglycemia or impaired glucose tolerance but whose fasting plasma glucose levels have returned to normal. Previously called latent diabetes, prediabetes.

previtamin. See **provitamin.**

prevocational evaluation, an evaluation of the abilities and limitations of a patient undergoing rehabilitation from a disabling disorder. The goal is to find eventual employment in a sheltered workshop or in the general community.

prevocational training, a rehabilitation program designed to prepare a patient for the performance of useful, paid work in a sheltered setting or community. It may involve training in basic work skills and counseling as required for a typical employment setting.

priapism /prī′əpiz′əm/ [Gk *priapos* phallus], an abnormal condition of prolonged or constant penile erection, often painful and seldom associated with sexual arousal. It may result from urinary calculi or a lesion within the penis or the central nervous system.

priapitis /prī′əpī′tis/, inflammation of the penis.

priapus. See **penis.**

prickle cell layer. See **stratum spinosum.**

prickly heat. See **miliaria.**

prilocaine hydrochloride /pril′ōkān/, a local anesthetic agent of the amide family, used for nerve block, epidural, and regional anesthesia. It is not used for spinal or topical anesthesia.

prima facie rights /prī′mə fā′shē·ə/, rights on the surface, or face, that may be overridden by stronger conflicting rights or by other values.

primal scream therapy, a form of psychotherapy developed by Arthur Janov that focuses on repressed pain of infancy or childhood. The goal is for the patient to surrender his or her neurotic defenses and "become real."

primaquine phosphate /prī′məkwin/, an antimalarial prescribed in the treatment of malaria and prevention of relapse during recovery from the disease.

primary [L *primus* first], **1.** first in order of time, place, development, or importance. **2.** not derived from any other source or cause, specifically the original condition or set of symptoms in disease processes, as a primary infection or a primary tumor. **3.** (in chemistry) noting the first and most simple compound in a related series, formed by the substitution of one of two or more atoms or of a group in a molecule.

primary abscess, an abscess that develops at the original point of infection by a pus-producing microorganism.

primary amenorrhea. See **amenorrhea.**

primary amputation, amputation performed after severe trauma, after the patient has recovered from shock, and before infection has set in.

primary amyloidosis. See **amyloidosis.**

primary anesthesia, any anesthetic or analgesic given a surgical patient before the administration of chemical agents that produce reversible unconsciousness.

primary apnea, a self-limited condition characterized by an absence of respiration. It may follow a blow to the head and is common immediately after birth in the newborn who breathes spontaneously when the carbon dioxide in the circulation reaches a certain level. Reflexes are present, and the heart is beating, but the skin color may be pale or blue and muscle tone is diminished.

primary atelectasis, failure of the lungs to expand fully at birth, most commonly seen in premature infants or those narcotized by maternal anesthesia. The infant is usually cared for in an incubator in which the temperature and humidity may be closely monitored.

primary atypical pneumonia. See **mycoplasma pneumonia.**

primary biliary cirrhosis, a chronic inflammatory condition of the liver. It is characterized by generalized pruritus, enlargement and hardening of the liver, weight loss, and diarrhea with pale, bulky stools. Petechiae, epistaxis, or hemorrhage resulting from hypoprothrombinemia may also be evident. Jaundice, dark urine, pale stools, and cutaneous xanthosis may occur in the later stages of this disease.

primary bronchus, one of the two main air passages that branch from the trachea and convey air to the lungs as part of the respiratory system. The right primary bronchus is about 2.5 cm long, wider and shorter than the left primary bronchus, and enters the right lung nearly opposite the fifth thoracic vertebra. The left primary bronchus is about 5 cm long, passes under the aortic arch, and courses ventral to the esophagus, the thoracic duct, and the descending aorta before dividing into bronchi for the superior and the anterior lobes of the lung.

primary carcinoma, a neoplasm at its site of origin.

primary care, the first contact in a given episode of illness that leads to a decision regarding a course of action to resolve the health problem.

primary care physician, a physician who usually is the first health professional to examine a patient and who recommends secondary care physicians, medical or surgical specialists with expertise in the patient's specific health problem, if further treatment is needed.

primary constriction. See **centromere.**

primary cutaneous melanoma, the site of origin for melanoma on the skin.

primary degenerative dementia. See **senile psychosis.**

primary dementia, a gradual progressive deterioration of memory, cognition, judgment, abstract thought, and behavior that may develop in a person around age 65.

primary dental caries, dental caries developing in the enamel of a tooth that was previously unaffected.

primary dentition. See **deciduous dentition.**

primary dermatitis, a skin eruption caused by a substance that can produce cell damage on initial contact, as opposed to dermatitis that develops as a sensitivity reaction to an allergen.

primary dysmenorrhea. See **dysmenorrhea.**

primary endometriosis [L *primus*; Gk *endon* within, *metra* womb, *osis* condition], an ingrowth of the muscle walls of the uterus by the mucous membrane lining of the organ.

primary enuresis, involuntary voiding of urine in a child who has not been toilet trained.

primary fissure, a fissure that marks the division of the anterior and posterior lobes of the cerebellum.

primary gain, a benefit, primarily relief from emotional conflict and freedom from anxiety, attained through the use of a defense mechanism or other psychologic process.

primary gangrene, a form of gangrene that occurs without preceding inflammation.

primary health care, a basic level of health care that includes programs directed at the promotion of health, early diagnosis of disease or disability, and prevention of disease. Primary health care is provided in an ambulatory facility to limited numbers of people, often those living in a particular geographic area. In any episode of illness, it is the first patient contact with the health care system.

primary hemorrhage [L *primus* + Gk *haima* blood, *rhegnynei* to gush], a hemorrhage that follows immediately after an injury.

primary host. See **definitive host.**

primary hypertension. See **essential hypertension.**

primary iritis, an inflammation of the iris that results from a source within the body, such as a systemic disease.

primary lesion [L *primus* + *laesio* hurting], a sore or wound that develops at the point of inoculation of the disease, usually applied to a syphilis chancre.

primary nurse, a nurse who is responsible for the planning, implementation, and evaluation of the nursing care of one or more clients 24 hours a day for the duration of the hospital stay.

primary nursing, a system for the distribution of nursing care in which care of one patient is managed for the entire 24-hour day by one nurse who directs and coordinates nurses and other personnel, schedules all tests, procedures, and daily activities for that patient, and cares for that patient personally when on duty. In an acute care situation, the primary care nurse might be responsible for only one patient; in an intermediate care situation, the primary care nurse might be responsible for three or more patients.

primary organizer, the part of the dorsal lip of the blastopore that is self-differentiating and induces the formation of the neural plate that gives rise to the main axis of the embryo.

primary physician, 1. the physician who usually takes care of a patient; the physician who first sees a patient for the care of a given health problem. **2.** a family practice physician or general practitioner.

primary pneumonic plague. See **pneumonic plague.**

primary polycythemia. See **polycythemia vera.**

primary prevention, a program of activities directed toward improvement of the general well-being while also involving specific protection for selected diseases, such as immunization against measles.

primary processes, unconscious processes, originating in the id, that obey different laws from those of the ego. These processes are seen in the dreams of the adult. Much of the distorted thinking of an acutely psychotic person is based on primary process thinking.

primary proximal renal tubular acidosis. See **proximal renal tubular acidosis.**

primary relationships, relationships with intimates, close friends, and family.

primary sensation, a feeling or impression that results directly from a particular stimulus.

primary sequestrum, a piece of dead bone that completely separates from sound bone during the process of necrosis.

primary shock, a state of physical collapse comparable to fainting. It may be the result of slight pain, such as that produced by venipuncture, or may be caused by fright. Primary shock is usually mild, self-limited, and of short duration.

primary sterility [L *primus* + *sterilis* barren], the inability to produce an offspring because of a functional failure of the ovaries or the testes.

primary tooth. See **deciduous tooth.**

primary triad, in Beck's theory of depression, the three major cognitive patterns that force the individual to view self, environment, and future in a negativistic manner.

primary tuberculosis, the childhood form of tuberculosis, most commonly occurring in the lungs, the posterior pharynx, or rarely the skin. Infants lack resistance to the disease, being easily infected and especially vulnerable to rapid and extensive spread of the infection through their bodies.

primate [L *primus* first], a member of the biological order of animals of the chordate class Mammalia. The primate order includes lemurs, monkeys, apes, and humans. Most primates have large brains, stereoscopic vision, and hands and feet developed for grasping.

prime mover [L *primus* + *movere* to move], a muscle that acts directly to produce a desired movement amid other muscles acting simultaneously to produce indirectly the same movement. Most movements of the body require the combined action of numerous muscles.

primidone /prī′məedōn/, an anticonvulsant prescribed in the treatment of seizure disorders, including grand mal, psychomotor, and focal epilepsy-like seizures.

primigravida /prim′igrav′ idəe/ {*primus* + *gravidus* pregnancy}, a woman pregnant for the first time. **–primigravid,** *adj.*

primipara /primip′əerəe/, *pl.* **primiparae** [L *primus* + *parere* to bear], a woman who has given birth to one viable infant, indicated by "para 1" on the patient's chart.

primiparity /prim′iper′itē/ [L *primus* + *parere* to bear], a condition of having borne one child.

primiparous /primip′ərəs/ pertaining to a woman who has borne one child.

primitive [L *primitus* first time], **1.** undeveloped; undifferentiated; rudimentary; showing little or no evolution. **2.** embryonic; formed early in the course of development; existing in an early or simple form.

primitive fold. See **primitive ridge.**

primitive groove, a furrow in the posterior region of the embryonic disk that indicates the cephalocaudal axis resulting from the active involution of cells forming the primitive streak.

primitive gut. See **archenteron.**

primitive line. See **primitive streak.**

primitive node, a knoblike accumulation of cells at the cephalic end of the primitive streak in the early stages of embryonic development in humans and the higher animals.

primitive pit, a minute indentation at the anterior end of the primitive groove in the early developing embryo.

primitive reflex, any reflex normal in an infant or fetus. Its presence in an adult usually indicates serious neurologic disease. Some kinds of primitive reflexes are **grasp reflex, Moro reflex,** and **sucking reflex.**

primitive ridge, a ridge that bounds the primitive groove in the early stages of embryonic development.

primitive streak, a dense area on the central posterior region of the embryonic disk, formed by the morphogenetic movement of a rapidly proliferating mass of cells that spreads between the ectoderm and endoderm, giving rise to the mesoderm layer.

primordial /prīmôr′dē·əl/ [L *primordium* origin] **1.** characteristic of the most undeveloped or primitive state, specifically those cells or tissues that are formed in the early stages of embryonic development. **2.** first or original; primitive.

primordial cyst, a follicular cyst that appears radiographically as a light area in the affected jaw. It develops from a dental enamel organ before the formation of hard tissue.

primordial dwarf, a person of extremely short stature who is otherwise perfectly formed, with the ususal proportions of body parts and normal mental and sexual development.

primordial germ cell, any of the large spheric diploid cells that are formed in the early stages of embryonic development and are precursors of the oogonia and spermatogonia.

primordial image, (in analytic psychology) the archetype or original parent, representing the source of all life.

primordium /prīmôr′dē·əem/, *pl.***primordia** [L, origin], the first recognizable stage in the embryonic development and differentiation of a particular organ, tissue, or structure.

principal [L *principalis* first in rank], first in authority or importance.

principal cell. See **chief cell.**

principle [L *principium* foundation], **1.** a general truth or settled rule of action. **2.** a prime source or element from which anything proceeds. **3.** a law on which others are founded or from which others are derived.

principles of instrumentation, in dentistry the six principles for the use of mirrors and other hand and motor-driven devices: **1.** grasp; **2.** fulcrum; **3.** insertion; **4.** adaptation and angulation; **5.** activation (lateral pressure and working stroke); **6.** rest.

P-R interval, (in electrocardiography) the interval measured from the beginning of the P wave to the beginning of the QRS complex, representing the atrioventricular conduction time.

Prinzmetal's angina [Myron Prinzmetal, American cardiologist, b. 1908], a variation of angina pectoris in that chest pain is experienced at rest, rather than in relation to effort. The pain tends to occur at night, and there is an electrocardiographic S-T segment elevation instead of depression. It is associated with proximal high-grade coronary artery obstructive lesions or coronary spasm or both.

priority [L *prius* previously], action established in order of importance or urgency to the welfare or purposes of the organization, patient, or other person at a given time.

prism, **1.** a solid figure, with a triangular or polygonal cross-section, bounded by parallelograms. **2.** enamel prisms, or calcified rods, surrounded by organic prism cuticle joined together to form tooth enamel. **3.** an adverse prism or verger prism used to test and train ocular muscles.

privacy, a culturally specific concept defining the degree of one's personal responsibility to others in regulating behavior that is regarded as intrusive. Some privacy-regulating mechanisms are physical barriers, such as closed doors, and interpersonal types, such as lowered voices.

privileged communication, a legal term employed in court-related proceedings concerning the right to reveal information that belongs to the person who spoke. Privileged communication may exist between a patient and a health professional only if the law specifically establishes it.

privileges [L *privilegium* private law], authority granted to a physician or dentist by a hospital governing board to provide care in the hospital. Clinical privileges are limited to the individual's professional license, experience, and competence. Emergency privileges may be granted in an emergency situation and without regard to the physician or dentist's regular service assignment or status. Temporary privileges may be granted a physician or dentist to provide health care to patients for a limited period or to a specific patient.

PRL, abbreviation for **prolactin.**

prn, (in prescriptions) abbreviation for *pro re nata,* a Latin phrase meaning "as needed." The times of administration are determined by the needs of the patient.

Pro, abbreviation for the amino acid **proline.**

proaccelerin. See **factor V.**

probability [L *probabilitas*], **1.** a measure of the increased likelihood that something will occur. **2.** a mathematical ratio of the number of times something will occur to the total number of possible occurrences.

probable signs [L *probabalis* credible; *signum* mark], clinical signs that there is a definite likelihood of pregnancy. Examples include enlargement of the abdomen, Goodell's sign, Hegar's sign, Braxton Hicks' sign, and positive hormonal test results.

proband. See **propositus.**

probenecid /prōben'əsid/, a uricosuric and adjunct to antibiotics. It is prescribed in the treatment of gout and as an adjunct prolonging the activity of penicillin or cephalosporins in some infections, such as gonorrhea.

problem [Gk *proballein* to throw forward], any health care condition that requires diagnostic, therapeutic, or educational action. An active problem requires immediate action, whereas an inactive problem is one of the past. A subjective problem is one reported by the patient, whereas one noted by an observer is regarded as an objective problem.

problem-oriented medical record (POMR), a method of recording data about the health status of a patient in a problem-solving system. The POMR preserves the data in an easily accessible way that encourages ongoing assessment and revision of the health care plan by all members of the health care team. The data base consists of all information from a health assessment or physical examination of the patient, and information from various laboratory tests.

problem-solving approach to patient-centered care, (in nursing) a conceptual framework that incorporates the overt physical needs of a patient with covert psychologic, emotional, and social needs. It provides a model for caring for the whole person as an individual, not as an example of a disease or a medical diagnosis. Nursing is defined within this model as a problem-solving process. The patient is viewed as a person who is in an impaired state, less than usually able to perform self-care activities.

probucol /prōbyōō'kəl/ an anticholisteremic prescribed in the treatment of primary hypercholesterolemia in patients who have not responded to diet, weight control, or other therapies.

procainamide hydrochloride /prōkān'-əmīd/, an antiarrhythmic agent prescribed in the treatment of a variety of cardiac arrhythmias, including premature ventricular contractions, ventricular tachycardia, and atrial fibrillation.

procaine hydrochloride /prō'kān/, a local anesthetic of the ester family. Procaine is administered for local anesthesia by infiltration and injection and for caudal, epidural, and other regional anesthetic procedures. It is not used for topical anesthesia.

procarbazine hydrochloride /prōkär'-bəzēn/, an antineoplastic prescribed in the treatment of a variety of neoplasms, including Hodgkin's disease and lymphomas.

procaryocyte. See **prokaryocyte.**

procaryon. See **prokaryon.**

procaryosis. See **prokaryosis.**

Procaryotae /prōker'ē-ō'tē/, (in bacteriology) a kingdom of plants that includes all microorganisms in which the nucleoplasm has no basic protein and is not surrounded by a nuclear membrane. The kingdom has two divisions, Cyanobacteria, which includes the blue-green bacteria, and Bacteria.

procaryote. See **prokaryote.**

procedure, the sequence of steps to be followed in establishing some course of action.

procerus /prəesir'əes/ [L, stretched], one of three muscles of the nose. The procerus functions to draw down the eyebrows and wrinkle the nose.

process [L *processus*], **1.** a series of related events that follow in sequence from a particular state or condition to a conclusion or resolution. **2.** a natural growth that projects from a bone or other part. **3.** to put through a particular series of interdependent steps, as in preparing a chemical compound.

process criteria, criteria identified by the American Nurses' Association Division on Psychiatric and Mental Health Nursing Practice that focus on nursing activities.

process recording, (in nursing education) a system used for teaching nursing students to understand and analyze verbal and nonverbal interaction. The conversation between nurse and patient is written on special forms or in a special format.

processus vaginalis peritonei /prəses'əs/ [L *processus* process; *vagina* sheath; Gk *peri* around, *tenein* to stretch], a diverticulum of the peritoneal membrane that during embryonic development extends through the inguinal canal. In males it descends into the scrotum to form the processus vaginalis testis; in females it is usually completely obliterated.

prochlorperazine, a phenothiazine antipsychotic and antiemetic prescribed in the treatment of psychotic disorders and for the control of nausea and vomiting.

prochlorperazine maleate. See **prochlorperazine.**

prochromosome. See **karyosome.**

procidentia [L *procidere* to fall forward], the prolapse of an organ. The term is usually applied to a prolapsed uterus.

procoagulant, a precursor or other agent that mediates the coagulation of blood. Examples include fibrinogen and prothrombin.

proconvertin. See **factor VII.**

procreation [L *procreare* to create], the entire reproductive process of producing offspring. **–procreate,** *v.*

proctalgia /proktal'jə/ [Gk *proktos* anus,*algos* pain], a neurologic pain in the anus or lower rectum.

proctalgia fugax [Gk *proktos* + *algos* pain; L *fugax* fleeting], periodic pain in the anus, possibly muscular in origin, that follows a pattern and is sometimes relieved by food and drink.

proctitis /proktī'tis/ [Gk *proktos* anus, *itis*], inflammation of the rectum and anus caused by infection, trauma, drugs, allergy, or radiation injury. Acute or chronic, it is accompanied by rectal discomfort and the repeated urge to pass feces with the inability to do so. Pus, blood, or mucus may be present in the stools, and tenesmus may be present.

proctocele. See **rectocele.**

proctocoletomy /prok'tōkəelek'təemē/, a surgical procedure in which the anus, rectum, and colon are removed. The procedure is a common treatment for severe, intractable ulcerative colitis.

proctodeum /prokto'dē·əm/, *pl.* **proctodea** [Gk *proktos* + *hodiaos* a route], an invagination of the ectoderm, behind the urorectal septum of the developing embryo, that forms the anus and anal canal when the cloacal membrane ruptures. **–proctodeal, proctodaeal,** *adj.*

proctodynia /prok *proktos* + *odyne* pain], pain in or around the anus.

proctologist /proktol'əjist/, a physician who specializes in proctology.

proctology /proktol'əejē/, [Gk *proktos* + *logos* science], the branch of medicine concerned with treating disorders of the colon, rectum, and anus.

proctoplasty /prok'təplas'tē/ [Gk *proktos* + *plassein* to mold], a plastic surgery procedure on the anus and rectum.

proctoscope /prok'təskōp'/ [Gk *prostos* + *skopein* to look], an instrument used to examine the rectum and the distal portion of the colon. It consists of a light mounted on a tube or speculum.

proctoscopy /proktos'kəpē/, the examination of the rectum with an endoscope inserted through the anus.

proctosigmoidoscopy /prok'tosig'moidas'- kəpē/ [Gk *proktos* + *sigmoid* + *skopein* to view], the use of a sigmoidoscope to examine the rectum and pelvic colon.

procyclidine hydrochloride /prōsī'- 'klædēn/, an anticholinergic prescribed in the treatment of parkinsonism, and to relieve extrapyramidal dysfunctions and control sialorrhea, which are side effects of other medications.

prodromal labor /Gk *prodromos* running before; L *laborare* to labor], the early period in parturition before uterine contractions become forceful and frequent enough to result in progressive dilatation of the uterine cervix.

prodromal phase, a clear deterioration in function before the active phase of a mental disturbance that is not caused by a disorder in mood or to a psychoactive substance and includes some residual phase symptoms.

prodromal symptom, a symptom that may be the first indication of the onset of a disease.

prodrome /prō'drōm/ [Gk *prodromos* running before], **1.** an early sign of a developing condition or disease. **2.** the earliest phase of a developing condition or disease. **–prodromal,** *adj.*

prodrug, an inactive or partially active drug that is metabolically changed in the body to an active drug.

product evaluation committee, a hospital committee composed of medical, nursing, purchasing, and administrative staff members whose purpose is to evaluate health care–related products and advise on their procurement.

productive cough [L *producere* + AS *cohhetan* to cough], a sudden, noisy expulsion of air from the lungs that effectively removes sputum from the respiratory tract and helps clear the air passages, permitting oxygen to reach the alveoli. Coughing is stimulated by irritation or by inflammation of the respiratory tract caused most frequently by infection. Deep breathing, with contraction of the diaphragm and intercostal muscles and forceful exhalation, promotes productive coughing in patients with respiratory infections.

professional corporation (PC) [L *professio* profession], a corporation formed according to the law of a particular state for the purpose of delivering a professional service. In some states corporations may not practice law, medicine, surgery, or dentistry, whereas in others nurses may form or be partners in a professional corporation.

professional liability, the legal obligation of health care professionals, or their insurers, to compensate patients for injury or suffering caused by acts of omission or commission by the professionals. Professional liability better describes the responsibility of all professionals to their clients than does the concept of malpractice, but the idea of professional liability is central to malpractice.

professional network, (in psychiatric nursing) the network of professional resources available to support the psychiatric outpatient in the community. The network may include a therapist, a hospital day treatment program, social work agency, and other agencies.

professional organization, an organization, whose members share a professional status, created to deal with issues of concern to the professional group or groups involved.

Professional Standards Review Organization (PSRO), an organization formed under Social Security Act Amendments of 1972 to review the services provided under Medicare, Medicaid, and Maternal Child Health programs. Review is conducted by physicians to ascertain the need for the program, to ensure that it is carried out in accord with certain criteria, norms, and standards, and, in institutional situations, in a proper setting.

profibrinolysin, See **fibrinogen.**

profile [L *profilare* to outline], a short sketch, diagram, or summary relating to a person or thing.

profunda /prōfun'də/ [L *profundus* deep], pertaining to structures, mainly blood vessels, that are deeply embedded in tissues.

profuse sweat [L *profundere* to pour out; AS *swaetan*], excessive perspiration.

progenitive [Gk *pro* before, *genein* to produce], capable of producing offspring; reproductive.

progenitor [Gk *pro* + *genein*], **1.** a parent or ancestor. **2.** one who or anything that originates or precedes; precursor.

progeny /proj'ənē/ [L *progenies*], **1.** offspring; an individual or organism resulting from a particular mating. **2.** the descendants of a known or common ancestor.

progeria /prōjē'rē·ə/ [Gk *pro* + *geras* old age], an abnormal congenital condition characterized by premature aging and the appearance in childhood of gray hair and wrinkled skin and by small stature, absence of pubic and facial hair, and the posture and habitus of an aged person. Death usually occurs before 20 years of age.

progestagen. See **progestogen.**

progestational /prō'jestā'shənəl/ [Gk *pro* + L *gestare* to bear], of or pertaining to a drug with effects similar to those of progesterone, the hormone produced by the corpus luteum and adrenal cortex during the luteal phase of the menstrual cycle that prepares the uterus for reception of the fertilized ovum.

progestational agent [L *pro* + *gestare* to bear, *agere, to do*], any chemical having the same action as progesterone produced by the corpus luteum and the placenta.

progestational phase. See **secretory phase.**

progesterone /prəjes'tərōn/, a natural progestational hormone prescribed in the treatment of various menstrual disorders, infertility associated with luteal phase dysfunction, and repeated spontaneous abortion.

progestin /prōjes'tin/, **1.** progesterone. **2.** any of a group of hormones, natural or synthetic, secreted by the corpus luteum, placenta, or adrenal cortex that have a progesterone-like effect on the uterus.

progestogen /prōjes'təjən/, any natural or synthetic progestational hormone.

proglottid /prōglot'id/ [Gk *pro* + *glossa* tongue], a sexual segment of an adult tapeworm, containing both male and female reproductive organs.

prognathism /prog'nəthiz'əm/ [Gk *pro* + *gnathos* jaw], an abnormal facial configuration in which one or both jaws project forward. It is considered real or imaginary, depending on anatomic and developmental factors involved. **–prognathic,** *adj.*

prognosis /prognō'sis/ [Gk *pro* + *gnosis* knowledge], a prediction of the probable outcome of a disease based on the condition of the person and the usual course of the disease as observed in similar situations.

prognostic /prognos'tik/ [Gk *pro* + *gnosis* knowledge], pertaining to signs and symptoms that may indicate the outcome of a disease or injury.

programmable pacemaker [Gk *pro* + *graphein* to write; L *passus* step; ME *maken*], an electronic pacemaker with multiple settings that can be changed following implantation.

P

progravid [L *pro* + *gravid* pregnant], before pregnancy.

progression, a carcinogenic process whereby some cells altered by initiators undergo a second genetic mutation that allows them to grow uncontrollably without the stimulus of promoters. They progress to fully malignant cells.

progressive [L *progredi* to advance], describing the course of a disease or condition in which the characteristic signs and symptoms become more prominent and severe, such as progressive muscular atrophy.

progressive assistive exercise, an exercise designed to progressively improve the strength of a muscle group by gradually increasing resistance against contractions with the assistance of a therapist.

progressive bulbar paralysis, a motor neuron disease characterized by weakness of the laryngeal, pharyngeal, tongue, and facial muscles. The patient experiences progressive dysarthria and dysphagia.

progressive myonecrosis. See **myonecrosis.**

progressive myopia, a condition in which myopia increases at a more rapid rate than normal, often continuing into adulthood.

progressive ophthalmoplegia, a form of ocular muscle paralysis that usually begins with ptosis and gradually involves all of the extraocular muscles.

progressive patient care, a system of care in which patients are placed in units on the basis of their needs for care as determined by the degree of illness rather than in units based on a medical specialty.

progressive relaxation, a technique for combating tension and anxiety by systematically tensing and relaxing muscle groups.

progressive resistance exercise, a method of increasing the strength of a weak or injured muscle by gradually increasing the resistance against which the muscle works, as by using graduated weights over a period of time.

progressive spinal muscular atrophy of infants. See **Werdnig-Hoffmann disease.**

progressive subcortical encephalopathy. See **Schilder's disease.**

progressive supranuclear palsy, a mild form of paralysis involving muscles innervated by the cranial nerves and affecting primarily the face, throat, and tongue.

progressive systemic sclerosis (PSS), the most common form of scleroderma.

progress notes [L *progredi* + *nota* mark], (in the patient record) notes made by a nurse and physician that describe the patient's condition and the treatments given or planned. Progress notes may follow the problem-oriented medical record format. The physician's progress notes usually focus on the medical or therapeutic aspects of the patient's condition and care; the nurse's progress notes, although recording the medical conditions of the patient, usually focus on the objectives stated in the nursing care plan.

proinsulin /prō·in′s(y)əlin/ [L *pro* + *insula* island], a single-chain protein molecule that is a precursor of insulin.

projectile vomiting, expulsive vomiting that is extremely forceful.

projection [L *projectio* thrown forward], **1.** a protuberance; anything that thrusts or juts outward. **2.** the act of perceiving an idea or thought as an objective reality. **3.** (in psychology) an unconscious defense mechanism by which an individual attributes his or her own unacceptable traits, ideas, or impulses to another.

projection reconstruction imaging, the techniques used in NMR imaging to obtain a cross-sectional image of an object. Such an image is computer reconstructed from a series of NMR profiles.

projective test [L *projectio* thrown forward], a kind of diagnostic, psychologic, or personality test that uses unstructured or ambiguous stimuli, such as inkblots, a series of pictures, abstract patterns, or incomplete sentences, to elicit responses that reflect a projection of various aspects of the individual's personality.

prokaryocyte /prōker′ē·əsīt′/ [Gk *protos* first, *karyon* nut, *kytos* cell], a cell without a true nucleus and with nuclear material scattered throughout the cytoplasm.

prokaryon /prōker′ē·on/ [Gk *protos* + *karyon* nut], **1.** nuclear elements that are not bound by a membrane but are spread throughout the cytoplasm. **2.** an organism containing such unbound nuclear elements.

prokaryosis [Gk *protos, karyon* + *osis* condition], the condition of not containing a true nucleus surrounded by a nuclear membrane.

prokaryote /prōker′ē·ōt/ [Gk *protos* + *karyon*], an organism that does not contain a true nucleus surrounded by a nuclear membrane, characteristic of lower forms, such as bacteria, viruses, and blue-green bacteria. Division occurs through simple fission. **–prokaryotic,** *adj.*

prolactin (PRL) /prōlak′tin/ [Gk *pro* before, *lac* milk], a hormone produced and secreted into the bloodstream by the anterior pituitary. Prolactin, acting with estrogen, progesterone, thyroxine, insulin, growth hormone, glucocorticoids, and human placental lactogen, stimulates the development and growth of the mammary glands. After parturition, prolactin together with glucocorticoids is essential for the initiation and maintenance of milk production.

prolapse /prō'laps, prōlaps'/ [L *prolapsus* fall down], the falling, sinking, or sliding of an organ from its normal position or location in the body, such as a prolapsed uterus.

prolapsed cord, an umbilical cord that protrudes beside or ahead of the presenting part of the fetus.

prolapsed hemorrhoid, internal hemorrhoids that protrude through the anal orifice.

prolapse of anus, the protrusion of the mucous membrane of the anus through the external sphincter.

prolapse of rectum, a protrusion of the mucous membrane of the lower portion of the rectum through the anal orifice.

prolapse of uterus, the descent of the uterine cervix into the vagina, partly into the vagina, or outside the vagina.

proliferate [L *prolles* offspring, *ferre* to bear], to grow by multiplication of cells, parts, or organisms.

proliferation [L *proles* offspring, *ferre* to bear], the reproduction or multiplication of similar forms. The term is usually applied to increases of cells or cysts.

proliferative phase, the phase of the menstrual cycle after menstruation. Under the influence of follicle-stimulating hormone from the pituitary, the ovary produces increasing amounts of estrogen, causing the lining of the uterus to become dense and richly vascular.

prolific, highly productive.

proline (Pro), a nonessential amino acid found in many proteins of the body, particularly collagen.

prolonged gestation [L *prolongare* to lengthen, *gestare* to bear], a pregnancy that lasts longer than the usual time span of 41 weeks.

prolonged release [Gk *pro* before, *longus* long], a term applied to a drug that is designed to deliver a dose of a medication over an extended period of time. The most common device for this purpose is a soft, soluble capsule containing minute pellets of the drug for release at different rates in the GI tract, depending on the thickness and nature of the oil, fat, wax, or resin coating on the pellets.

promethazine hydrochloride, a phenothiazine antiemetic, antihistamine, and sedative. It is prescribed in the treatment of motion sickness, nausea, rhinitis, itching, and skin rash.

promethium (Pm) [L *Prometheus* mythic character who brought fire to Earth], a radioactive, rare earth, metallic element. Its atomic number is 61; its atomic weight is 145.

prominence /prom'inəns/ [L *prominentia* sticking out], any elevation or projection of a structural feature.

promontory of the sacrum [L *promontorium* headland], the superior projecting part of the sacrum at its junction with the L5 vertebra.

promoter [L *promovere* to move forward], **1.** (in molecular genetics) a DNA sequence that initiates RNA transcription of the genetic code. **2.** a cocarcinogenic factor that encourages cells altered by initiators to reproduce at a faster than normal rate, increasing the probability of malignant transformation. Examples include DDT, phenobarbital, and some chemicals in cigarette smoke.

prompt insulin zinc suspension [L *promptus* ready], a fast-acting noncrystalline semilente insulin prescribed in the treatment of diabetes mellitus when a prompt, intense, and short-acting response is desired.

promyelocyte /prōmī'ələsīt'/, a large mononuclear blood cell that contains a single, regular, symmetric nucleus and a few undifferentiated cytoplasmic granules. It is intermediate in development between a myeloblast and a myelocyte and is indicative of leukemia.

pronation /prōnā'shən/ [L *pronare* to bend forward] **1.** assumption of a prone position, one in which the ventral surface of the body faces downward. **2.** (of the arm) the rotation of the forearm so that the palm of the hand faces downward and backward. **3.** (of the foot) the lowering of the medial edge of the foot by turning it outward and producing abduction movements in the tarsal and metatarsal joints. **–pronate,** *v.*

pronator reflex /prōnā'tər/ [L *pronare* + *reflectere* to bend backward], a reflex elicited by holding the patient's hand vertically and tapping the distal end of the radius or ulna, resulting in pronation of the forearm.

pronator syndrome, the compression of the median nerve between the two heads of the pronator teres muscle.

pronator teres, a superficial muscle of the forearm, arising from a humeral and an ulnar head. It functions to pronate the hand.

prone [L *pronus* inclined forward],

1. having a tendency or inclination. **2.** (of the body) being in horizontal position when lying face downward.

proneness profile [L *pronus* + *profilare* to outline], a screening process that evaluates the probability of developmental problems occurring in the early years of a child's life. Several of the variables in the proneness profile that appear to be significant in selecting the infants who are at risk are the perinatal health status of the mother and infant, especially complications of pregnancy, delivery, the neonatal period, and the puerperium; characteristics of the mother; characteristics of the infant, including alertness, activity pattern, and responsiveness; and the behaviors of the infant and care giver as they interact.

prone-on-elbows, a body position in which the person rests the upper part of the body on the elbows while lying face down. The position is used as an initial rehabilitation exercise in training a person with a cerebellar dysfunction to achieve ambulation. From prone-on-elbows the person can practice weight shifting through the hips to a quadruped position without the risk of falling from a standing position.

pronephric duct [Gk *pro* before, *nephros* kidney; L *ducere* to lead], one of the paired ducts that connect the tubules of each of the pronephros with the cloaca in the early developing vertebrate embryo.

pronephric tubule, any of the segmentally arranged excretory units of the pronephros in the early developing vertebrate embryo.

pronephros /prōnef'rəs/ *pl.* **pronephroi** [Gk *pro* + *nephros* kidney], the primordial excretory organ in the developing vertebrate embryo. **–pronephric,** *adj.*

prone position [L *pronare* to bend forward, *positio*], a postural position of facing downward while lying flat.

prone posture [L *pronare* + *ponere* to place], a posture assumed of lying flat with the face forward during certain disorders of the spine or viscera.

pronucleus *pl.* **pronuclei** [Gk *pro* + L *nucleus* nut], the nucleus of the ovum or the spermatozoon after fertilization but before the fusion of the chromosomes to form the nucleus of the zygote.

propagation /prop'əgā'shən/ [L *propagare* to generate], the process of increasing or causing to increase.

propantheline bromide, an anticholinergic prescribed as an adjunct in peptic ulcer therapy.

proparacaine hydrochloride /prōper'-əkān/, a rapid-acting, topical anesthetic of the amide family used for ophthalmologic procedures.

properidin system. See **alternative pathway of complement activation.**

prophase /prō'fāz/ [Gk *pro* + *phasis* appearance], the first of four stages of nuclear division in mitosis and in each of the two divisions of meiosis.

prophylactic /prō'filak'tik/ [Gk *prophylax* advance guard] **1.** preventing the spread of disease. **2.** an agent that prevents the spread of disease. **–prophylactically,** *adv.*

prophylactic forceps. See **low forceps.**

prophylactic odontomy, (in dentistry) the surgical removal of harmful pits and fissures in the posterior primary and permanent molars.

prophylactic treatment. See **preventive treatment.**

prophylaxis /prō'filak'sis/ [Gk *prophylax*], prevention of or protection against disease, often involving the use of a biological, chemical, or mechanical agent to destroy or prevent the entry of infectious organisms.

Propionibacterium /prō'pē·on'ebaktir'-ē·əm/ [Gk *pro* + *pion* fat, *bacterion* small rod], a genus of nonmotile, anaerobic, gram-positive bacteria found on the skin of humans, in the intestinal tract of humans and animals, and in dairy products. *P. acnes* is common in acne pustules.

propionicacidemia /prō'pē·n'ikas'idē'-mē·ə/ [Gk *pro* + *pion*; L *acidus* sour; Gk *haima* blood], a rare inherited metabolic defect caused by the failure of the body to metabolize the amino acids threonine, isoleucine, and methionone, characterized by lethargy and mental and physical retardation. Acidosis occurs as a result of the accumulation of propionic acid in the body. **–propionicacidemic,** *adj.*

propionic fermentation [Gk *pro* + *pion*; L *fermentare* to cause to ferment], the production of propionic acid by the action of certain bacteria on sugars or lactic acid.

proportional gas detector, a device for measuring alpha and beta forms of radioactivity.

proportional mortality [L *pro* + *portio* part; *mortalis* subject to death], a statistical method of relating the number of deaths from a particular condition to all deaths within the same population group for the same period.

proposition [L *proponere* to place forward], **1.** a statement of a truth to be demonstrated or an operation to be performed. **2.** to bring forward or offer for consideration, acceptance, or adoption.

propositus /prōpoz'itəs/ [L *proponere* to place forward], a person from whom a genealogic lineage is traced, as is done to discover the pattern of inheritance of a familial disease or a physical trait.

propoxyphene /prōpok'sǝfēn/, a mild centrally acting narcotic analgesic prescribed to relieve mild to moderate pain.

propoxyphene hydrochloride, an analgesic prescribed for the relief of mild to moderate pain.

propranolol hydrochloride, a beta-adrenergic blocking agent prescribed in the treatment of angina pectoris, cardiac arrhythmias, and hypertension.

proprietary [L *proprietarius* a property], **1.** of or pertaining to an institution or other organization that is operated for profit. **2.** of or pertaining to a product, such as a drug or device, that is made for profit.

proprietary hospital, a hospital operated as a profit-making organization. Many proprietary hospitals are owned by physicians who operate the hospital primarily for their own patients but also accept patients from other physicians. Some proprietary hospitals are owned by investor groups or large corporations.

proprietary medicine, any pharmaceutic preparation or medicinal substance that is protected from commercial competition because its ingredients or method of manufacture is kept secret or is protected by trademark or copyright.

proprioception /prō'prēMDRV·ǝsep'shǝn/ [L *proprius* one's own, *capere* to take], sensation pertaining to stimuli originating from within the body regarding spatial position and muscular activity or to the sensory receptors that they activate.

proprioceptive /prōprē·ǝsep'tiv/, pertaining to the sensations of body movements, and awareness of posture, enabling the body to orient itself in space without visual clues.

proprioceptive neuromuscular facilitation (PNF), an activity, such as a therapeutic technique, that helps initiate a proprioceptive response in a person.

proprioceptive receptors, sensory nerve terminals, found in muscles, joints, tendons, and the inner ear, that are sensitive to body and position movement.

proprioceptive reflex /prō'prē·ǝsep'tiv/ [L *proprius* + *capere* to take; *reflectere* to bend backward], any reflex initiated by stimulation of proprioceptive receptors, such as the increase in respiratory rate and volume induced by impulses arising from muscles and joints during exercise.

proprioceptive sensation [L *propius* + *capere; sentire* to feel], the feelings of body movement and position, including motion of the arms and legs, resulting from stimuli received by special sense organs in the muscles, tendons, joints, and the labyrinth of the ear. The stimuli may be produced by changes in muscle tension or stretching and reaction to the pull of gravity on the body.

proprioceptor /prō'prē·ǝsep'tǝr/ [L *proprius* + *capere*], any sensory nerve ending, such as those located in muscles, tendons, joints, and the vestibular apparatus, that responds to stimuli originating from within the body regarding movement and spatial position.

proptosis /proptō'sis/ [L *prop* + *ptosis* falling], bulging, protrusion, or forward displacement of a body organ or area.

propulsion [L *propellere* to drive forward], **1.** the process of pushing forward. **2.** the tendency of some patients, particularly those afflicted with nervous disorders, to push or fall forward while walking as their center of gravity is displaced.

propylene glycol, a colorless viscous liquid used as a solvent in the preparation of certain medications. It also inhibits the growth of fungi and microorganisms and is used commercially as an antifreeze.

propylformic acid. See **butyric acid.**

propylthiouracil /prō'pilthī'ǝyo͞or'ǝsil/, an inhibitor of thyroid hormone biosynthesis. It is prescribed in the treatment of hyperthyroidism, thyrotoxic crisis, and preparation for thyroidectomy.

pro re nata (p.r.n.), a Latin phrase meaning "according to circumstances," or "as the need arises."

proscribe /prōskrīb/, to forbid. **–proscriptive,** *adj.*

prosector [L *prosecare* to cut off], a person who, under the supervision of a pathologist, performs gross dissections and prepares autopsy specimens for pathologic examination.

prosencephalon /pros'ensef'ǝlon/ [Gk *pro* + *enkephalon* brain], the portion of the brain that includes the diencephalon and the telencephalon. **–prosencephalic,** *adj.*

prosopalgia. See **trigeminal neuralgia.**

prosopopilary virilism /pros'ǝpōpī'lǝrē/, a heavy growth of facial hair.

prosopospasm /pros'ǝpōspaz'ǝm/ [Gk *prosopon* face. *spasmos*], a spasm of the facial muscles, as may occur in tetanus.

prosoposternodidymus /pros'ǝpōstur'nǝdid'ǝmǝs/ [Gk *prosopon* face, *sternon* chest, *didymos* twin], a fetal monster consisting of conjoined twins united laterally from the head through the sternum.

prosopothoracopagus /pros'ǝpōthôr'ǝkop'ǝgǝs/ [Gk *prosopon* + *thorax* chest, *pagos* fixed], conjoined symmetric twins who are united laterally in the frontal plane from the thorax through most of the head region.

prospective medicine [L *proscipere* to look forward; *medicina* art of healing], the early identification of pathologic or potentially pathologic processes and the prescription of intervention to stop the processes.

prospective reimbursement, a method of payment to an agency for health care services to be delivered based on predictions of what the agency's costs will be for the coming year.

prospective study, a study designed to determine the relationship between a condition and a characteristic shared by some members of a group. A prospective study may involve many variables or only two; it may seek to demonstrate a relationship that is an association or one that is causal.

prostacyclin (PG₁₂) /pros'təsī'klin/, a prostaglandin. It is a biologically active product of arachidonic acid metabolism in human vascular walls, and is a potent inhibitor of platelet aggregation.

prostaglandin (PG) /pros'təglan'din/ [Gk *prostates* standing before; L *glans* acorn], one of several potent hormonelike unsaturated fatty acids that act in exceedingly low concentrations on local target organs. They are produced in small amounts and have a large array of significant effects. Some of the pharmacologic uses for the prostaglandins are termination of pregnancy and treatment of asthma and gastric hyperacidity.

prostanoic acid /pros'tənō'ik/, a 20-carbon aliphatic acid that is the basic framework for prostaglandin molecules, which differ according to the location of hydroxyl and keto substitutions at various positions along the molecule.

prostate /pros'tāt/ [Gk *prostates* standing before], a gland in men that surrounds the neck of the bladder and the urethra and elaborates a secretion that liquefies coagulated semen. It is a firm structure about the size of a chestnut, composed of muscular and glandular tissue. The ejaculatory ducts pass obliquely through the posterior part of the gland. The prostatic secretion consists of alkaline phosphatase, citric acid, and various proteolytic enzymes.

prostate cancer, a slowly progressive adenocarcinoma of the prostate gland that affects an increasing proportion of American males after the age of 50. It is the third leading cause of cancer deaths with more than 120,000 new cases reported in the United States each year. The cause is unknown, but it is believed to be hormone related. The disease may cause no direct symptoms but can be detected in the course of diagnosing bladder or uretal obstruction or pyuria. The cancer can spread to cause bone pain in the pelvis, ribs, or vertebrae.

prostatectomy /pros'tətek'təmē/ [Gk *prostates* + *ektome* excision], surgical removal of a portion of the prostate gland, as performed for benign prostatic hypertrophy, or the total excision of the gland, as performed for malignancy. Kinds of approaches include transurethral, the most common, in which a resectoscope is inserted and through it shavings of prostatic tissue are cut off at the bladder opening with a loop, suprapubic, and retropubic. The perineal approach is used for biopsy when early cancer is suspected or for the removal of calculi.

prostate-specific antigen (PSA), a protein produced by the prostate gland that may be present at elevated levels in patients with cancer or other diseases of the prostate.

prostatic /prostat'ik/, pertaining to the prostate gland.

prostatic calculus, a solid pathologic concretion formed in the prostate, usually of calcium carbonate and/or calcium phosphate.

prostatic catheter, a catheter that is approximately 16 inches long and has an angled tip. It is used in male catheterization to pass an enlarged prostate gland obstructing the urethra.

prostatic ductule /duk'tyo̅o̅l/ [Gk *prostates* + L *ductulus* little duct], any one of 12 to 20 tiny excretory tubes that convey the alkaline secretion of the prostate gland and open into the floor of the prostatic portion of the urethra.

prostatic hypertrophy. See **prostatomegaly.**

prostatic syncope, a temporary loss of consciousness because of restricted cerebral blood flow that may occur during a prostate examination.

prostatic utricle, the portion of the urethra in men that forms a cul-de-sac about 6 mm long behind the middle lobe of the prostate. It is homologous with the uterus in women.

prostatism /pros'tətiz'əm/ [Gk *prostates* one standing before], an abnormal condition of the prostate gland, particularly an enlargement of the gland resulting in an obstruction to the urinary flow.

prostatitis /pros'tətī'tis/ [Gk *prostates* + *itis* inflammation], acute or chronic inflammation of the prostate gland, usually the result of infection. The patient complains of burning, frequency, and urgency.

prostatomegaly /pros'tətōmeg'əlē/ [Gk *prostates* + *megas* large], the hypertrophy or enlargement of the prostate gland.

prosthesis /prosthē'sis/, *pl.* **prostheses** [Gk,

addition] **1.** an artificial replacement for a missing part of the body, such as an artificial limb or total joint replacement. **2.** a device designed and applied to improve function, such as a hearing aid.

prosthetic heart valve, an artificial heart valve.

prosthetic restoration. See **restoration.**

prosthetics /prosthet′iks/ [Gk *prosthesis* addition], a branch of surgery concerned with the design, construction, and attachment of artificial limbs or other systems to replace function of a missing body part.

prosthetist /pros′thatist/, a person who fabricates and fits artificial limbs and similar devices prescribed by a physician. A certified prosthetist is one who has successfully completed the examination of the American Orthotic and Prosthetic Association.

prosthodontics /pros′thədon′tiks/ [Gk *prosthesis + odous* tooth], a branch of dentistry devoted to the construction of artificial appliances that replace missing teeth or restore parts of the face.

prostration [L *prosternere* to throw down], a condition of extreme exhaustion and inability to exert oneself further, as in heat prostration or nervous prostration. **–prostrate,** *adj.*

protactinium (Pa) [Gk *protos* first, *aktis* ray], a radioactive element. Its atomic number is 91; its atomic weight is 231.

protamine sulfate /prō′təmēn/, a heparin antagonist derived from fish sperm. It is prescribed to diminish or reverse the anticoagulant effect of heparin, particularly in cases of heparin overdosage.

protamine zinc insulin suspension, a long-acting insulin that is absorbed slowly at a steady rate. Some patients can be treated with only one injection daily.

protanopia, a form of color blindness in which the person is unable to distinguish shades of red.

protaxic mode of experience, (in psychology) a type of primitive experience characterized by sensations, feelings, and fragmented images of short duration that are not logically connected.

protease /prō′tē-ās/, an enzyme that is a catalyst in the breakdown of protein.

protection, altered, a NANDA-accepted nursing diagnosis of a state in which an individual experiences a decrease in an ability to guard the self from internal and external threats, such as illness or injury. Defining characteristics include deficient immunity, impaired healing, altered clotting, maladaptive stress response, neurosensory alteration, immobility, disorientation, and pressure sores. Related factors include extremes of age, drug therapies,

treatments such as surgery and radiation, and diseases such as cancer and immune disorders.

protective [L *protegere* to cover], describing an individual who guards another from danger or injury and provides a safe environment.

protective apron, See **lead apron.**

protective isolation, 1. the practice of confining a patient with a virulent infectious disease in a separate area so that contact with other persons can be minimized. **2.** the practice of placing a highly susceptible person, such as an immunodeficient patient, in a separate area where the risk of contact with pathogenic microorganisms can be controlled.

protein /prō′tē-in, prō′tēn/ [Gk *proteios*], any of a large group of naturally occurring, complex, organic nitrogenous compounds. Each is composed of large combinations of amino acids containing the elements carbon, hydrogen, nitrogen, oxygen, usually sulfur, and occasionally phosphorus, iron, iodine, or other essential constituents of living cells. Twenty-two amino acids have been identified as vital for proper growth, development, and maintenance of health. The body can synthesize 14 of these amino acids, called nonessential, whereas the remaining eight must be obtained from dietary sources and are termed essential. Protein is the major source of building material for muscles, blood, skin, hair, nails, and the internal organs. It is necessary for the formation of hormones, enzymes, and antibodies and as a source of heat and energy, and it functions as an essential element in proper elimination of waste materials. Excessive intake of protein may in some conditions result in fluid imbalance.

proteinase /prō′tē-inās′/, a proteolytic enzyme that splits protein molecules at central linkages.

protein-bound iodine (PBI), iodine that is firmly bound to protein in serum, the measurement of which indirectly indicates the concentration of circulating thyroxine (T_4).

protein calorie malnutrition. See **energy protein malnutrition.**

proteinemia /prō′tē-inē′mē-ə/, an excessive level of protein in the blood.

protein hydrolysate injection, a fluid and nutrient replenisher prescribed to correct a negative nitrogen balance and in other clinical situations requiring parenteral nutrition.

protein kinase, a protein that catalyzes the transfer of a phosphate group from adenosine triphosphate to produce a phosphoprotein.

protein metabolism, the processes whereby protein foodstuffs are used by the body to make tissue proteins, together with the processes of breakdown of tissue proteins in the production of energy. Food proteins are first broken down into amino acids, then absorbed into the bloodstream, and finally used in body cells to form new proteins. Amino acids in excess of the body's needs may be converted by liver enzymes into keto acids and urea.

protein sensitization, a reaction that follows parenteral introduction of a foreign protein into the body. Symptoms of varying severity, including serum sickness, occur when the same foreign protein is re-introduced into the body at a later date.

proteinuria /prō'tēnyŏŏr'ē·ə/ [Gk *proteios* + *ouron* urine], the presence in the urine of abnormally large quantities of protein, usually albumin. Persistent proteinuria is usually a sign of renal disease or renal complications of another disease. However, proteinuria can result from heavy exercise or fever.

proteolipid /prō'tē·ōlip'id/ [Gk *proteios lipos* fat], a type of lipoprotein in which lipid material forms more than half the molecule. It is insoluble in water and occurs primarily in the brain.

proteolysis /prō'tē·ol'isis/ [Gk *proteios* + *lysis* loosening], a process in which water added to the peptide bonds of proteins breaks down the protein molecule. Numerous enzymes may catalyze this process.

proteolytic /prō'tē·əlit'ik/, of or pertaining to any substance that promotes the breakdown of protein.

Proteus /prō'tē·əs/ [Gk *Proteus* mythic god who changed shapes], a genus of motile, gram-negative bacilli often associated with nosocomial infections, normally found in feces, water, and soil. *Proteus* may cause urinary tract infections, pyelonephritis, wound infections, diarrhea, bacteremia, and endotoxic shock.

Proteus morgani, a species of bacteria associated with infectious diarrhea in infants.

Proteus mirabilic, a species of bacteria found in putrid meat, abscesses, and fecal material. It is the leading cause of urinary tract infections.

Proteus vulgaris, a species of bacteria that is a frequent cause of urinary tract infections. The bacteria are found in feces, water, and soil.

prothrombin /prōthrom'bin/ [L *pro* before; Gk *thrombos* lump], a plasma protein that is the precursor to thrombin. It is synthesized in the liver if adequate vitamin K is present.

prothrombinemia, the presence of prothrombin in the blood.

prothrombin time (PT), a one-stage test for detecting certain plasma coagulation defects caused by a deficiency of factors V, VII, or X. Thromboplastin and calcium are added to a sample of the patient's plasma and, simultaneously, to a sample from a normal control. The length of time required for clot formation in both samples is observed.

protocol /prō'təkôl/ [Gk *protos* first, *kolla* glued page], a written plan specifying the procedures to be followed in giving a particular examination, in conducting research, or in providing care for a particular condition.

proton /prō'ton/ [Gk *protos* first], a positively charged particle that is a fundamental component of the nucleus of all atoms. The number of protons in the nucleus of an atom equals the atomic number of the element.

proton density, a measure of proton concentration, or the number of atom nuclei per given volume. It is one of the major determinants of magnetic resonance signal strength in hydrogen imaging.

protopathic /prō'təpath'ik/, pertaining to the somatic sensations of fast localized pain, slow poorly localized pain, and temperature.

protoplasm /prō'təplaz'əm/ [Gk *protos* + *plasma* something formed], the living substance of a cell, usually composed of myriad molecules of water, minerals, and organic compounds. –**protoplasmic,** *adj.*

protoplast /prō'təplast/ [Gk *protos* + *plassein* to mold], **1.** (in biology) the protoplasm of a cell without its containing membrane. **2.** a first entity or an original. –**protoplastic,** *adj.*

protoporphyria /prō'tōpôrfir'ē·ə/ [Gk *protos* + *porphyros* purple, *haima* blood], increased levels of protoporphyrin in the blood and feces.

protoporphyrin /prō'tōpôr'firin/ [Gk *protos* + *porphyros*], a kind of porphyrin that combines with iron and protein to form a variety of important organic molecules, including catalase, hemoglobin, and myoglobin.

protostoma. See **blastopore.**

prototaxic mode [Gk *protos* + *taxis* arrangement; *modus* measure], a stage in infancy, according to a Sullivan theory, characterized by a lack of differentiation between the self and the environment.

prototype /prō'tətīp/ [Gk *protos* + *typos* mark], the primary or original form of an object or organism.

protozoa /prō'təzō'ə/, *sing. protozoon* [Gk *protos* + *zoon* animal], single-celled microorganisms of the class Protozoa, the lowest form of animal life. Protozoa are more complex than bacteria, forming a self-contained unit with organelles that carry on such functions as locomotion, nutrition, excretion, respiration, and attachment to other objects or organisms. Approximately 30 protozoa are pathogenic to humans. **–protozoal, protozoan,** adj.

protozoal infection, any disease caused by single-celled organisms of the class Protozoa. Some kinds of protozoal infections are **amebic dysentery, kala-azar, malaria,** and **trichomonas vaginitis.**

protracted dose [L pro before, trahere to draw; dosis something given], (in radiotherapy) a low amount of radiation delivered continuously over a relatively long period.

protriptyline hydrochloride /prōtrip'-tilēn/, a tricyclic antidepressant prescribed in the treatment of endogenous mental depression marked by withdrawal and anergy.

protrusio bulbi. See exophthalmia.

protrusion [L protrudere to push forward], a state or condition of being forward or projecting.

protrusive incisal guide angle, (in dentistry) the inclination of the incisal guide in the sagittal plane.

protuberance /prōt(y)o͞o'bərəns/ [L pro + tuberare to swell], an anatomic landmark that appears as a blunt projection or swelling, such as the chin, buttock, or bulge of the frontal bone above the eyebrow.

proud flesh [AS prud, flaesc], excessive granulation tissue.

provider, a hospital, clinic, or health care professional, or group of health care professionals, who provide a service to patients.

Provincial/Territorial Nurses' Association (PTNA), an association of Canadian nurses organized at the provincial or territorial level. The Canadian Nurses' Association is a federation of the 11 PTNAs.

provirus, a stage of viral replication in which the viral genetic information has been integrated into the genome of the host cell.

provitamin /prōvī'təmin/, a precursor of a vitamin; a substance found in certain foods that in the body may be converted into a vitamin.

provocative diagnosis [L provocare to call forth; Gk dia through, gnosis knowledge], a diagnosis in which the identity and cause of an illness are discovered by inducing an episode of the condition.

prox, abbreviation for **proximal.**

proxemics /proksē'miks/ [L proximus near-

est], the study of spatial distances between people and its effect on interpersonal behavior, especially in relation to density of population, placement of people within an area, and the opportunity for privacy.

proximal /prok'siməl/ [L proximus], nearer to a point of reference, usually the trunk, than other parts of the body. Proximal interphalangeal joints are those closest to the hand.

proximal cavity, a cavity that occurs on the mesial or distal surface of a tooth.

proximal contact [L proximus nearest, contingere to touch], the contact between the distal surface of one tooth with the mesial surface of an adjacent tooth.

proximal contour, the shape or form of the mesial or the distal surface of a tooth.

proximal dental caries, decay that may occur in the mesial or distal surface of a tooth.

proximal radioulnar articulation, the pivot joint between the circumference of the head of the radius and the ring formed by the radial notch of the ulna and the annular ligament. The joint allows the rotary movements of the head of the radius in pronation and supination.

proximal renal tubular acidosis (proximal RTA), an abnormal condition characterized by excessive acid accumulation and bicarbonate excretion. It is caused by the defective reabsorption of bicarbonate in the proximal tubules of the kidney and the resulting flow of excessive bicarbonate into the distal tubules, which normally secrete hydrogen ions. In **primary proximal RTA** the defective reabsorption of bicarbonate is the sole causative factor. In **secondary proximal RTA** the reabsorptive defect is one of several causative factors and may result from tubular cell damage produced by various disorders, such as Fanconi's syndrome.

proximate [L proximus nearest], the nearest to a point of origin or attachment.

proximate cause [L proximare to approach], a legal concept of cause and effect relationships in determining, for example, whether an injury would have resulted from a particular cause.

proximity principle [L proximus + principium origin], a rule that when two or more objects are close to each other they may be seen as a perceptual unit.

proxymetacaine. See **proparacaine hydrochloride.**

PrP, abbreviation for prion protein, a viruslike infectious agent associated with Creutzfeldt-Jakob disease.

prurigo /pro͞orī'gō/ [L, an itch], any of a group of chronic inflammatory conditions of the skin characterized by severe itching and multiple, dome-shaped, small papules capped by tiny vesicles. Later (as a result of repeated scratching), crusting and lichenification may occur. Some causes of prurigo are allergies, drugs, endocrine abnormalities, malignancies, and parasites. A mild form of the disease is called **prurigo mitis,** and a more severe form **prurigo agria** or **prurigo ferox. –pruriginous,** *adj.*

pruritus /pro͞orī′təs/ [L *prurire* to itch], the symptom of itching, an uncomfortable sensation leading to the urge to scratch. Scratching often results in secondary infection. Some causes of pruritus are allergy, infection, jaundice, lymphoma, and skin irritation. **–pruritic,** *adj.*

pruritus ani, a common chronic condition of itching of the skin around the anus. Some causes are candidal infection, contact dermatitis, external hemorrhoids, pinworms, psoriasis, and psychogenic illness.

pruritus vulvae, itching of the female external genitalia. The condition may become chronic and result in lichenification, atrophy, and occasionally malignancy. Some causes of pruritus vulvae are contact dermatitis, lichen sclerosus et atrophicus, psychogenic pruritus, trichomoniasis, and vaginal candidiasis.

Prussian blue [Prussia, Germany; ME *blew*], a chemical reagent used on microsopic preparations. It demonstrates the presence of copper by developing a bright blue color.

ps, abbreviation for **picosecond.**

PSA, 1. abbreviation for **pressure-sensitive adhesive. 2.** abbreviation for **prostate-specific antigen.**

P sac, abbreviation for *pericardial cavity.*

psammoma /samō′mə/, *pl.* **psammomas, psammomata** [Gk *psammos* sand, *oma* tumor], a neoplasm containing small calcified granules (psammoma bodies) that occurs in the meninges, choroid plexus, pineal body, and ovaries.

psammoma body, a round, layered mass of calcareous material occurring in benign and malignant epithelial and connective tissue neoplasms and in some chronically inflamed tissue.

pseudarthritis /so͞o′därthrī′tis/ [Gr, *pseudes,* false + *arthron,* joint + *itis,* inflammation], musculoskeletal pain that does not involve the joints.

pseudesthesia /so͞o′desthē′zhə/ [Gk *pseudes* false, *aisthesis* feeling], a sensation experienced without an external stimulus or a sensation that does not correspond to the causative stimulus, such as phantom limb pain.

pseudoallele /so͞o′dōəlēl′/ [Gk *pseudes + allelon* of one another], (in genetics) one of two or more closely linked genes on a chromosome that appear to function as a single member of an allelic pair but occupy distinct, nearly corresponding loci on homologous chromosomes. **–pseudoallelic,** *adj.,* **pseudoallelism,** *n.*

pseudoankylosis /so͞o′dōang′kilō′sis/ [Gk *pseudes + agkylosis* joint stiffness], fibrous ankylosis, or false ankylosis caused by inflexibility of body structures outside the joint.

pseudoanorexia [Gk *pseudes + a, orexis* not appetite], a condition in which an individual eats secretly while claiming a lack of appetite and inability to eat.

pseudoarthrosis, See **false joint.**

pseudoataxia /so͞o′dōətak′sē·ə/ [Gk *pseudes + ataxia* lack of order], a loss of control over voluntary movements that does not involve an organic lesion.

pseudobulbar paralysis [Gk *pseudes + L bulbus* swollen root; *paralyein* to be palsied], a condition resembling progressive bulbar paralysis, with dysarthria and dysphagia, but weakness of the bulbar muscles is of the upper motor neuron type and the condition may result from multiple bilateral infarcts of the cerebral cortex in some cases.

pseudochylous ascites /so͞o′dōkī′ləs/ [Gk *pseudes + chylos* juice; *askos* bag], the abnormal accumulation in the peritoneal cavity of a milky fluid that resembles chyle.

pseudocoxalgia. See **Perthes' disease.**

pseudocyesis /so͞o′dōsī·ē′sis/ [Gk *pseudes + kyesis* pregnancy], a condition in which a woman believes she is pregnant when she is not. The condition may be psychogenic or caused by a tumor or endocrine dysfunction.

pseudocyst /so͞o′dəsist/ [Gk *pseudes + kystis* bag], a space or cavity containing gas or liquid but without a lining membrane. Pseudocysts commonly occur after pancreatitis when digestive juices break through the normal ducts of the pancreas and collect in spaces lined by fibroblasts and surfaces of adjacent organs.

pseudodementia, affective disorders, particularly depression, that mimic the signs and symptoms of dementia.

pseudoephedrine hydrochloride /so͞o′-dōef′ədrēn/, an adrenergic that acts as a vasoconstrictor and bronchodilator. It is prescribed for the relief of nasal congestion and eustachian tube congestion.

pseudoephedrine sulfate. See **pseudoephedrine hydrochloride.**

pseudofracture [Gk *pseudes + L fractura*], radiologic evidence of a thickened periosteum and new bone formation over what looks like an incomplete fracture.

pseudogene /sōō′dōjēn′/ [Gk *pseudes* + *genein* to produce], (in molecular genetics) a sequence of nucleotides that resembles a gene and may be derived from one but lacks a genetic function.

pseudoglottis. See **neoglottis**.

pseudogout. See **chondrocalcinosis**.

pseudohermaphrodite [Gk *pseudes* + *Hermaphroditos, son of Hermes and Aphrodite*], a congenital condition in which a person has either male or female gonads but external genitalia of the opposite sex, or both.

pseudohermaphroditism, a condition in which a person exhibits the somatic characteristics of both sexes though possessing the physical characteristics of either males (testes) or females (ovaries).

pseudohypertrophic muscular dystrophy. See **Duchenne's muscular dystrophy**.

pseudojaundice [Gk *pseudes* + Fr *jaune* yellow], a yellow discoloration of the skin that is not caused by hyperbilirubinemia. The excessive ingestion of carotene results in a form of pseudojaundice.

pseudomembrane [Gk *pseudes* + L *membrana* thin skin], a membrane consisting of coagulated fibrin, bacteria, and leukocytes that forms in the throats of diphtheria patients.

pseudomembranous colitis, a diarrheal disease frequently found in hospitalized patients who have received antibiotics that caused overgrowth of the anaerobic, spore-forming toxin producing *Clostridium difficile*.

pseudomembranous enterocolitis. See **necrotizing enterocolitis**.

pseudomembranous stomatitis, a severe inflammation of the mouth that produces a membranelike exudate. The inflammation may be caused by a variety of bacteria or by chemical irritants.

pseudomonad /sōōdom′ənad/, a bacterium of the genus *Pseudomonas*.

Pseudomonas /sōōdom′ənas/ [Gk *pseudes* + *monas* unit], a genus of gram-negative bacteria that includes several free-living species of soil and water and some opportunistic pathogens, such as *Pseudomonas aeruginosa,* isolated from wounds, burns, and infections of the urinary tract. Pseudomonas are notable for their fluorescent pigments and their resistance to disinfectants and antibiotics.

Pseudomonas aeruginosa [Gk *pseudes* + *monas* unit], a species of gram-negative nonsporing motile bacilli that may cause various human diseases ranging from purulent meningitis to nosocomial infected wounds.

pseudomutuality [Gk *pseudes* + L *mutuus* reciprocal], (in psychotherapy) an atmosphere maintained by family members in which there is surface harmony and a high degree of agreement with one another, but in which the atmosphere of agreement covers deep and destructive intrapsychic and interpersonal conflicts.

pseudopod /sōō′dəpod/ [Gk *pseudes* + *pous* foot], a temporary protoplasmic limblike process of an amoeba that can be extended to propel itself or to engulf food.

pseudopregnancy. See **pseudocyesis**.

pseudorabies. See **infectious bulbar paralysis**.

pseudorubella. See **roseola infantum**.

pseudosclerema. See **adiponecrosis subcutanea neonatorum**.

pseudostratified /sōō′dōstra′tifīd/ [Gk *pseudes* + *stratum* cover], pertaining to a type of columnar epithelium in which the nuclei of adjacent cells are at different levels.

pseudotumor [Gk *pseudes* + L *tumor* swelling], a false tumor.

pseudotumor cerebri, a condition characterized by increased intracranial pressure, headache, vomiting, and papilledema without neurologic signs, except, occasionally, palsy of the sixth cranial nerve.

pseudoxanthoma elasticum. See **Grönblad-Strandberg syndrome**.

psi, abbreviation for *pounds per square inch*.

psia, abbreviation for *pounds per square inch, absolute*.

psig, abbreviation for *pounds per square inch, gauge*.

psilocin /sī′ləsin/, one of several indole-derived psychomimetic drugs. It is related chemically to psilocybin.

psilocybin /sī′lōsī′bin, -sib′in/, a psychedelic drug and an active ingredient of various Mexican hallucinogenic mushrooms of the genus *Psilocybe mexicana*. It can produce altered states of mood and consciousness and has no accepted medical use in the United States.

psittacosis /sit′əkō′sis/ [Gk *psittakos* parrot], an infectious illness caused by the bacterium *Chlamydia psittaci,* characterized by respiratory, pneumonia-like symptoms and transmitted to humans by infected birds, especially parrots. The clinical manifestations of the disease are extremely variable and resemble a great number of infectious diseases, but fever, cough, anorexia, and severe headache are almost always present.

psm, abbreviation for **presystolic murmur**.

psoas, one of the muscles of the vertebral column.

P

psoas major /sō'əs/ [Gk *psoa* loin], a long muscle originating from the transverse processes of the lumbar vertebrae and the fibrocartilages and sides of the vertebral bodies of the lower thoracic vertebrae and the lumbar vertebrae. It acts to flex and laterally rotate the thigh and to flex and laterally bend the spine.

psoas minor, a long, slender muscle of the pelvis, ventral to the psoas major. It functions to flex the spine.

psoralen-type photosynthesizer, any one chemical compound that contains photosensitizing psoralen and that reacts on exposure to ultraviolet light to increase the melanin in the skin. Naturally occurring psoralen photosynthesizers, such as 5- and 8-methoxypsoralen, are found in buttercups, carrot greens, celery, clover, cockleburs, dill, figs, limes, parsley, and meadow grass. Some psoralen-type photosynthesizers produced as pharmaceutics are used to enhance skin pigmentation or tanning in the treatment of skin diseases, such as psoriasis and vitiligo.

psoriasis /sərī'əsis/ [Gk, itch], a common, chronic, inheritable skin disorder, characterized by circumscribed red patches covered by thick, dry, silvery, adherent scales that are the result of excessive development of epithelial cells. Exacerbations and remissions are typical. Lesions may be anywhere on the body but are more common on extensor surfaces, bony prominences, scalp, ears, genitalia, and the perianal area. An arthritis, particularly of distal small joints, may accompany the skin disease. Subcategories of psoriasis include **guttate psoriasis** and **pustular psoriasis.** –**psoriatic** /sôr'ē·at'ik/, *adj.*

psoriasis universalis, a severe attack of psoriasis in which most or all of the skin is involved.

psoriatic arthritis /sôr'ī·at'ik/, a form of rheumatoid arthritis associated with psoriatic lesions of the skin and nails, particularly at the distal interphalangeal joints of the fingers and toes.

PSRO, abbreviation for **Professional Standards Review Organization.**

PSS, abbreviation for **progressive systemic sclerosis.**

PSSO, abbreviation for *peer specialist second opinion.*

PSV, abbreviation for **pressure support ventilation.**

PSW, abbreviation for **psychiatric social worker**.

psych, abbreviation for **psychology**.

psychalgia. See **psychic pain.**

psyche /sī'kē/ [Gk, mind], **1.** the aspect of one's mental faculty that encompasses the conscious and unconscious processes.
2. the vital mental or spiritual entity of the individual as opposed to the body or soma.
3. (in psychoanalysis) the total components of the id, ego, and superego, including all conscious and unconscious aspects.

psychedelic /sī'kədel'ik/ [Gk *psyche* + *deloun* manifest], **1.** of or describing a mental state characterized by altered sensory perception and hallucination, accompanied by euphoria or fear, usually caused by the deliberate ingestion of drugs or other substances known to produce this effect. **2.** of or describing any drug or substance that causes this state, such as mescaline or psilocybin.

psychiatric disorder. See **mental disorder.**

psychiatric emergency service [Gk *psyche* + *iatreia* healing], a hospital service that provides immediate initial evaluation and treatment to acutely disturbed mental patients on a 24-hour-a-day basis.

psychiatric foster care, a service for discharged psychiatric patients who receive observation and care in an approved foster home.

psychiatric home care, a service whereby a discharged psychiatric patient is provided observation and care in his or her place of residence.

psychiatric hospital, a health care facility providing inpatient and outpatient therapeutic services to patients with behavioral or emotional illnesses.

psychiatric inpatient unit, a hospital ward or similar area used for the treatment of inpatients who require psychiatric care.

psychiatric nurse practitioner, a nurse practitioner who, by advanced study and clinical practice, as in a master's program in psychiatric nursing, has gained expert knowledge in the care and prevention of mental disorders.

psychiatric nursing, the branch of nursing concerned with the prevention and cure of mental disorders and their sequelae.

psychiatric social worker (PSW), a social worker who specializes or works exclusively with the mentally ill.

psychiatrist, a physician with additional medically qualified training and experience in the diagnostic prevention and treatment of mental disorders.

psychiatry [Gk *psyche* + *iatreia* healing], the branch of medical science that deals with the causes, treatment, and prevention of mental, emotional, and behavioral disorders. Some kinds of psychiatry are **community psychiatry, descriptive psychiatry, dynamic psychiatry, existential psychiatry, forensic psychiatry,** and **orthopsychiatry.** –**psychiatric,** *adj.*

psychic [Gk *psyche* mind], a practitioner of the systematic study of parapsychology, a category of psychologic phenomena that cannot be explained by current scientific thinking.

psychic blindness, a somatoform disorder that is manifested by the total or partial loss of vision in eyes that are organically normal. Despite the symptoms claimed, the patient usually reacts to light and avoids objects that might cause injury.

psychic contagion. See **psychic infection.**

psychic energy, body energy that is used for psychologic tasks such as thinking, perceiving, and remembering.

psychic impotence [Gk *psyche* + L *in, potentia* power], a functional disorder of the male who is unable to perform sexual intercourse despite normal genitalia and sexual desire. The term is generally applied to an inability to achieve and maintain an erection, but may be manifested in other forms such as premature ejaculation or the need for certain conditions.

psychic infection /sī′kik/ [Gk *psyche* + L *inficere* to taint], the spread of neurotic or psychic effects or influences on others on a small scale, as in folie á deux, or on a large scale, as in the spread of hysteric or panic reactions in a crowd.

psychic pain, a functional pain which, in the absence of any organic cause, is usually associated with feelings of acute anxiety. In some cases the person may experience hallucinations or obsessions.

psychic suicide, the termination of one's own life without the use of physical means or agents, as by an older person who becomes sufficiently depressed to lose "the will to live."

psychic trauma, an emotional shock or injury or a distressful situation that produces a lasting impression, especially on the subconscious mind. Common causes of psychic trauma are abuse or neglect in childhood, rape, and loss of a loved one.

psychoactive, pertaining to a drug or other agent that affects such normal mental functioning as mood, behavior, or thinking processes. Examples include stimulants, sedatives, or hallucinogens.

psychoanalysis [Gk *psyche* + *analyein* to separate parts], a branch of psychiatry founded by Sigmund Freud devoted to the study of the psychology of human development and behavior. From its systematized method for investigating the processes of the mind evolved a system of psychotherapy based on the concepts of a dynamic unconscious, using such techniques as free association, dream interpretation, and the analysis of defense mechanisms, especially resistance and transference. Through these devices, emotions and behavior are traced to the influence of repressed instinctual drives in the unconscious.

psychoanalyst, a psychotherapist, usually a psychiatrist, who has had special training in psychoanalysis and who applies the techniques of psychoanalytic theory.

psychoanalytic, 1. of or pertaining to psychoanalysis. **2.** using the techniques or principles of psychoanalysis.

psychobiologic resilience, a concept that proposes a recurrent human need to weather periods of stress and change throughout life. The ability to weather each period of disruption and reintegration successfully leaves the person better able to deal with the next change.

psychobiology [Gk *psyche* + *bios* life, *logos* science] **1.** the study of biochemical foundations of thought, mood, emotion, affect, and behavior. **2.** personality development and functioning in terms of the interaction of the body and the mind. **3.** a school of psychiatric thought introduced by Adolf Meyer that stresses total life experience, including biological, emotional, and sociocultural factors in assessing the psychologic makeup or mental status of an individual.

psychocatharsis. See **catharsis.**

psychodiagnosis, the study of a personality through observations of behavior and mannerisms, combined with various tests.

psychodrama, a form of group therapy, originated by J. L. Moreno, in which people act out their emotional problems through improvisational dramatization.

psychodynamics [Gk *psyche* + *dynamis* power], the study of the forces that motivate behavior.

psychogenesis /sī′kōjen′əsis/ [Gk *psyche* + *genesis* origin], **1.** the development of the mind or of a mental function or process. **2.** the development or production of a physical symptom or disease from mental or psychic origins rather than organic factors. **3.** the development of emotional states, either normal or abnormal, from the interaction of conscious and unconscious psychologic forces.

psychogenic /sī′kōjen′ik/ [Gk *psyche* + *genein* to produce], **1.** originating within the mind. **2.** referring to any physical symptom, disease process, or emotional state that is of psychologic rather than physical origin.

psychogenic pain, a functional pain that is not due to any organic cause.

psychogenic pain disorder, a disorder characterized by persistent and severe pain for which there is no apparent organic cause. The condition is often accompanied by other sensory or motor dysfunction, such as paresthesia or muscle spasm.

psychokinesia /sī′kōkinē′zhə, -kīnē′zhə/ [Gk *psyche* + *kinesis* motion], **1.** impulsive, maniacal behavior resulting from deficient or defective inhibitions. **2.** (in parapsychology) psychokinesis.

psychokinesis (PK) /sī′kōkinē′sis, -kīnē-′sis/ [Gk *psyche* + *kinesis* motion], the alleged direct influence of the mind or will on matter that would result in the production of motion in objects without the intervention of the physical senses or a physical force.

psychokinetics /sī′kōkinet′iks, -kīnet′iks/, the study of psychokinesis.

psychologic miscarriage, an absence or deficiency of a mother's love for her infant.

psychologic test [Gk *psyche* + *logos* science; L *testum* crucible], any of a group of standardized tests designed to measure or ascertain characteristics of an individual such as intellectual capacity, motivation, perception, role behavior, values, level of anxiety or depression, coping mechanisms, and general personality integration.

psychologist, a person who specializes in the study of the structure and function of the brain and related mental processes of animals and humans. A clinical psychologist is one who is qualified by graduate degree in psychology and training in clinical psychology and who provides testing and counseling services to patients with mental and emotional disorders.

psychology [Gk *psyche* + *logos* science], **1.** the study of behavior and of the functions and processes of the mind, especially as related to the social and physical environment. **2.** a profession that involves the practical applications of knowledge, skills, and techniques in the understanding of, prevention of, or solution to individual or social problems, especially in regard to the interaction between the individual and the physical and social environment. **3.** the mental, motivational, and behavioral characteristics and attitudes of an individual or group of individuals. Kinds of psychology include **analytic psychology, animal psychology, behaviorism, clinical psychology, cognitive psychology, experimental psychology, humanistic psychology,** and **social psychology. –psychologic, psychological,** *adj.,* **psychologically,** *adv.*

psychometrician [Gk *psyche* + *metron* measure], a specialist who performs quantitative estimation or measurement of personality and intelligence.

psychometrics /sī′kōmet′riks/ [Gk *psyche* + *metron* measure], the development,

administration, or interpretation of psychologic and intelligence tests.

psychomotor [Gk *psyche* + L *motare* to move about], pertaining to or causing voluntary movements usually associated with neural activity.

psychomotor and physical development of infants, a branch of pediatric psychiatry that is concerned with the development of skills requiring coordination of sensory processes and motor activities, including infant reflexes, developmental timetables, emotional and behavioral disorders.

psychomotor development, the progressive attainment by the child of skills that involve both mental and muscular activity, such as the ability of the infant to turn over, sit, or crawl at will and of the toddler to walk, talk, control bladder and bowel functions, and begin solving cognitive problems.

psychomotor domain, the area of observable performance of skills that require some degree of neuromuscular coordination.

psychomotor epilepsy. See **psychomotor seizure.**

psychomotor learning, the acquisition of ability to perform motor skills.

psychomotor retardation, a slowing of motor activity related to a state of severe depression.

psychomotor seizure, a temporary impairment of consciousness, often associated with temporal lobe disease and characterized by psychic symptoms, loss of judgment, automatic behavior, and abnormal acts. No apparent convulsions occur, but there may be loss of consciousness or amnesia for the episode. During the seizure the individual may appear drowsy, intoxicated, or violent; asocial acts or crimes may be committed, but normal activities, such as driving a car, typing, or eating, may continue at an automatic level.

psychoneuroimmunology, a discipline that studies the relationships between psychologic states and the immune response.

psychoneurosis. See **necrosis.**

psychoneurotic. See **neurotic.**

psychoneurotic disorder. See **neurotic disorder.**

psychopath /sī′kōpath/ [Gk *psyche* + *pathos* disease], a person who has an antisocial personality disorder.

psychopathia. See **psychopathy.**

psychopathia sexualis /sī′kōpā′thē·ə sek′-shoo·al′is/ [Gk *psyche* + *pathos* disease; L *sexus* male or female], a mental disease characterized by sexual perversion.

psychopathic /sī′kōpath′ik/, of or pertaining to antisocial behavior.

psychopathic personality. See **antisocial personality.**

psychopathologist, one who specializes in the study and treatment of mental disorders. –**psychopathology,** *n.*

psychopathology, 1. the study of the causes, processes, and manifestations of mental disorders. **2.** the behavioral manifestation of any mental disorder.

psychopathy /sīkop′əthē/, any disease of the mind, congenital or acquired, not necessarily associated with subnormal intelligence.

psychopharmacology [Gk *psyche* + *pharmakon* drug, *logos* science], the scientific study of the effects of drugs on behavior and normal and abnormal mental functions.

psychophylaxis. See **mental hygiene.**

psychophysical preparation for childbirth, a program that prepares women for giving birth by teaching them the physiology of the process, exercises to improve muscle tone and physical stamina, and various techniques of breathing and relaxation to promote control and comfort during labor and delivery. Methods of psychophysical preparation for childbirth include **Bradley method, Lamaze method,** and **Read method.**

psychophysics [Gk *psyche* + *physikos* natural], the branch of psychology concerned with the relationships between physical stimuli and sensory responses.

psychophysiologic [Gk *psyche* + *physikos* natural], having physical symptoms resulting from psychogenic origins; psychosomatic.

psychophysiologic disorder, any of a large group of mental disorders characterized by the dysfunction of an organ or organ system controlled by the autonomic nervous system, such as a peptic ulcer, which may be caused or aggravated by emotional factors.

psychophysiology, 1. the study of physiology as it relates to various aspects of psychologic or behavioral function. **2.** the study of mental activity by physical examination and observation.

psychoprophylactic preparation for childbirth, a system of prenatal education for giving birth using the Lamaze method of natural childbirth.

psychosexual [Gk *psyche* + L *sexus* male or female], of or pertaining to the psychologic and emotional aspects of sex. –**psychosexuality,** *n.*

psychosexual development, (in psychoanalysis) the emergence of the personality through a series of stages from infancy to adulthood. Each stage is relatively fixed in time and characterized by a dominant mode of achieving libidinal pleasure through the interaction of the person's biologic drives and the restraints of the environment.

psychosexual disorder, any condition characterized by abnormal sexual attitudes, desires, or activities resulting from psychologic rather than organic causes.

psychosexual dysfunction, any of a large group of sexual maladjustments or disorders caused by an emotional or psychologic problem.

psychosis /sīkō′sis/, *pl.* **psychoses** [Gk *psyche* + *osis* condition], any major mental disorder of organic or emotional origin characterized by a gross impairment in reality testing, whereby the individual incorrectly evaluates the accuracy of his or her perceptions and thoughts and makes incorrect references about external reality, even in the face of contrary evidence.

psychosocial [Gk *psyche* + L *socialis* partners], pertaining to a combination of psychologic and social factors.

psychosocial assessment, an evaluation of a person's mental health, social status, and functional capacity within the community.

psychosocial development, (in child development) a description devised by Erik Erikson of the normal serial development of trust, autonomy, identity, and intimacy; the development begins in infancy and progresses as the infantile ego interacts with the environment. For the child to reach a new stage, the preceding one must be fully realized.

psychosomatic /sī′kōsəmat′ik/ [Gk *psyche* + *soma* body], **1.** of or pertaining to psychosomatic medicine. **2.** relating to, characterized by, or resulting from the interaction of the mind or psyche and the body. **3.** the expression of an emotional conflict through physical symptoms.

psychosomatic approach, the interdisciplinary or holistic study of physical and mental disease from a biological, psychosocial, and sociocultural point of view.

psychosomatic illness. See **psychophysiologic disorder.**

psychosomatic medicine, the branch of medicine concerned with the interrelationships between mental and emotional reactions and somatic processes, in particular the manner in which intrapsychic conflicts influence physical symptoms.

psychosomatic pain, pain that is due in part to a psychogenic problem.

psychosomatic reaction. See **psychophysiologic disorder.**

psychosomatics. See **psychosomatic medicine.**

psychosomatogenic, pertaining to factors

that cause or lead to the development of psychophysiologic coping measures as learned responses to stressors.

psychosurgery [Gk *psyche + cheirourgos*], surgical interruption of certain nerve pathways in the brain, performed to treat selected cases of chronic, unremitting anxiety, agitation, or obsessional neuroses when the condition is severe and when alternative treatments, such as psychotherapy, drugs, and electroshock, have proven ineffective.

psychosynthesis, a form of psychotherapy that focuses on three levels of the unconscious—lower, middle, and higher. The goal of treatment is the recreation or integration of the personality.

psychotherapeutic drugs, drugs that are prescribed for their effects in relieving symptoms of anxiety, depression, or other mental disorders.

psychotherapeutics [Gk *psyche + therapeia* treatment], the treatment of personality disorders by means of psychotherapy.

psychotherapist, one who practices psychotherapy, including psychiatrists, licensed psychologists, psychiatric nurses, psychiatric social workers, and individuals trained in counseling.

psychotherapy [Gk *psyche + therapeia* treatment], any of a large number of related methods of treating mental and emotional disorders by psychologic techniques rather than by physical means.

psychotic /sīkot′ik/ [Gk *psyche + osis* condition] **1.** of or pertaining to psychosis. **2.** a person exhibiting the characteristics of a psychosis.

psychotic disorder. See **psychosis.**

psychotic insight, a stage in the development of a psychosis that follows an initial experience of confusion, bizarreness, and apprehension. At this point an insight is reached that enables the patient to interpret the external world in terms of a delusional system of thinking. The factors that had previously been confusing become a part of the systematized pattern of the delusion, which, although irrational to an observer, is perceived by the patient as the attainment of exceptionally lucid thinking.

psychotic reaction. See **psychosis.**

psychotomimetic /sīkot′ōmimet′ik/, a drug or other substance whose effects mimic the symptoms of psychosis, such as hallucinations.

psychotropic [Gk *psyche + trepein* to turn], exerting an effect on the mind or modifying mental activity.

psychotropic drugs, drugs that affect the psychic functions, behavior, or experience of a person using them.

psyllium seed. See **plantago seed.**

pt, 1. abbreviation for *pint.* **2.** abbreviation for **patient.**

Pt, symbol for the element **platinum.**

PT, 1. abbreviation for **physical therapist 2.** abbreviation for **physical therapy. 3.** abbreviation for **prothrombin time.**

PTA, abbreviation for **plasma thromboplastin antecedent.**

PTB, abbreviation for **patellar tendon–bearing prosthesis.**

PTB/SC, abbreviation for **patellar tendon–bearing supracondylar socket.**

PTCA, abbreviation for **percutaneous transluminal coronary angioplasty.**

pteroylglutamic acid. See **folic acid.**

pterygium /tərij′ē·əm/ [Gk *pterygion* wing], a thick, triangular bit of pale tissue that extends medially from the nasal border of the cornea to the inner canthus of the eye.

pterygoid /ter′igoid/ [Gk *pteryx* wing, *eidos* form], pertaining to a winglike structure.

pterygoideus lateralis /ter′igoi′dē·əs/ [Gk *pteryx* wing, *eidos* form], one of the four muscles of mastication. It functions to open the jaws, protrude the mandible, and move the mandible from side to side.

pterygoideus medialis, one of the four muscles of mastication. It acts to close the jaws.

pterygoid plexus /tur′igoid/, one of a pair of extensive networks of veins between the temporalis and the pterygoideus lateralis, extending between surrounding structures in the infratemporal fossa.

pterygoid process [Gk *pteryx* wing, *eidos* form; L *processus*], one of the processes of the sphenoid bone.

pterygomandibular /ter′igōmandib′yələr/, pertaining to the pterygoid process and the mandible.

pterygomaxillary, pertaining to the sphenoid bone and the maxilla.

pterygomaxillary notch, a fissure at the junction of the maxilla and the pterygoid process of the sphenoid bone.

PTH, abbreviation for **parathyroid hormone.**

PTNA, abbreviation for **Provincial/Territorial Nurses' Association.**

ptomaine /tō′mān/ [Gk *ptoma* corpse], an imprecise term introduced in the nineteenth century to identify a group of nitrogenous substances found in putrefied proteins.

ptosis /tō′sis/ [Gk, falling], an abnormal condition of one or both upper eyelids in which the eyelid droops because of a congenital or acquired weakness of the levator muscle or paralysis of the third cranial nerve.

ptotic kidney /tō′tik/, a kidney that is abnormally situated in the pelvis, usually over the sacral promontory behind the peritoneum.

PTT. See **partial thromboplastin time.**

ptyalin /tī′əlin/ [Gk *ptyalon* spittle], a starch-digesting enzyme present in saliva.

ptyalism /tī′əliz′əm/ [Gk *ptyalon* spittle], excessive salivation, as sometimes occurs in the early months of pregnancy. It is also a clinical sign of mercury poisoning.

Pu, symbol for the element **plutonium.**

pubarche /pyo̅o̅bär′kē, pyo̅o̅′bärkē/ [L *puber* maturity, *arch* beginning], the onset of puberty, marked by the beginning of the development of secondary sexual characteristics.

puberism. See **onset of puberty.**

puberty [L *pubertas* age of maturity], the period of life at which the ability to reproduce begins. **–pubertal,** *adj.*

puberulic acid /pyo̅o̅ber′yo̅o̅lik/, an antibiotic isolated from the mold *Penicillium puberulum* that prevents the replication of gram-positive bacteria.

pubescent [L *pubescere* to reach puberty], to arrive at the age of puberty.

pubescent uterus, a uterus in which the cervix and body remain of equal length, the premenstrual state, in adult life.

pubic [L *pubis*], pertaining to or involving the region of the pubic symphysis.

pubic bone. See **pubis.**

pubic dislocation. See **dislocation of hip.**

pubic hair, hair of the pubic region.

pubic region [L *pubes* signs of maturity; *regere* to rule], the most inferior part of the abdomen in the lower zone between the right and left inguinal regions and below the umbilical region.

pubic symphysis, the slightly movable interpubic joint of the pelvis, consisting of two pubic bones separated by a disk of fibrocartilage and connected by two ligaments.

pubis /pyo̅o̅′bis/, *pl.* **pubes** [L *pubes*], one of a pair of pubic bones that, with the ischium and the ilium, form the hip bone and join the pubic bone from the opposite side at the pubic symphysis. The internal surface of the pubis is smooth; it forms part of the anterior wall of the pelvis.

public health [L *publicus* the people; AS *haelth*], a field of medicine that deals with the physical and mental health of the community, particularly in such areas as water supply, waste disposal, air pollution, and food safety.

public health nursing, a field of nursing that is concerned with the health needs of the community as a whole. Public health nurses may work with families in the home, in schools, at the workplace, in government agencies, and at major health facilities. A home care nursing service is provided by nurses who have special training in public health and are employed by such voluntary agencies as the Visiting Nurses Association or Visiting Nurse Service.

publish or perish [L *publicare* to make public; *perire* to come to naught], *informal.* a practice followed in many academic institutions in which a contract for employment is renewed at the same or higher rank only if a candidate has demonstrated scholarship and professional status by having had work published in a book or in a reputable professional journal.

pubococcygeal /p(y)o̅o̅′bokoksijē·əl/ [L *pubes* + Gk *kokkyx* cuckoo's beak], pertaining to the pubis and the coccyx.

pubococcygeus exercises /pyo̅o̅′bōkoksij′ē·əs/ [L *pubes* + Gk *kokkyx* cuckoo's beak; L *exercere* to make strong], a regimen of isometric exercises in which a woman executes a series of voluntary contractions of the muscles of her pelvic diaphragm and perineum in an effort to increase the contractility of her vaginal introitus or to improve her retention of urine. The exercise involves the familiar muscular squeezing action that is required to stop the urinary stream while voiding; that action is performed in an intensive, repetitive, and systematic way throughout each day.

pudendal block [L *pudendum* modest; Fr *bloc* lump], a form of regional anesthetic block administered to relieve the discomfort of the expulsive second stage of labor, or for episiotomy. Pudendal block anesthetizes the perineum, vulva, clitoris, labia majora, and the perirectal area without affecting the muscular contractions of the uterus. When the block is properly administered, the risk is minimal.

pudendal canal. See **Alcock's canal.**

pudendal nerve, one of the branches of the pudendal plexus that arises from the second, third, and fourth sacral nerves, passes between the piriformis and coccygeus, and leaves the pelvis through the greater sciatic foramen.

pudendal plexus, a network of motor and sensory nerves formed by the anterior branches of the second, the third, and all of the fourth sacral nerves.

pudendum /pyo̅o̅den′dəm/, *pl.* **pudenda** [L, modest], the external genitalia, especially of women. In a woman it comprises the mons veneris, the labia majora, the labia minora, the vestibule of the vagina, and the vestibular glands. In a man it comprises the penis, scrotum, and testes. **–pudendal,** *adj.*

puericulture /pyōō'ərikul'chər/ [L *pueri* children, *colere* to cultivate], the rearing and training of children. **–puericulturist,** *n.*

puerile /pyōō'əril, -īl/ [L *puerilis* childish], of or pertaining to children or childhood; juvenile. **–puerility,** *n.*

puerilism /pyōō'əriliz'əm/ [L *puerilis* childish], childishness, particularly when manifested in an older adult.

puerpera /pyōō'ərpərə/, a woman who has just given birth or is in labor.

puerperal /pyōō·ur'pərəl/ [L *puerperus* childbirth], **1.** of or pertaining to the period immediately after childbirth. **2.** of or pertaining to a woman (puerpera) who has just given birth to an infant.

puerperal eclampsia [L *puerperus;* Gk *ek* out, *lampein* to flash], a condition of coma and convulsive seizures caused by toxins that develop during pregnancy or labor.

puerperal endometritis. See **puerperal fever.**

puerperal fever, a syndrome associated with systemic bacterial infection and septicemia that occurs after childbirth, usually as a result of unsterile obstetric technique. It is characterized by endometritis, fever, tachycardia, uterine tenderness, and foul lochia; if untreated, prostration, renal failure, bacteremic shock, and death may occur. The causative organism is most often one of the hemolytic streptococci.

puerperal mania, a rare, acute mood disorder that sometimes occurs in women after childbirth, characterized by a severe manic reaction.

puerperal mastitis, a form of acute mastitis in a nursing mother.

puerperal metritis. See **puerperal fever.**

puerperal phlebitis, an inflammation that begins in a uterine veins after childbirth and spreads to other veins, particularly the iliac and femoral veins.

puerperal psychosis. See **postpartum psychosis.**

puerperal sepsis, an infection acquired during the puerperium.

puerperium /pyōō'ərpir'ē·əm/ [L *puerperus*], the time after childbirth, lasting approximately 6 weeks, during which the anatomic and physiologic changes brought about by pregnancy resolve, and a woman adjusts to the new or expanded responsibilities of motherhood and nonpregnant life.

PUFA, abbreviation for **polyunsaturated fatty acid.**

puff [ME *puf*], a short soft blowing sound heard on auscultation.

Pulex /pyōō'leks/ [L, flea], a genus of fleas, some species of which transmit arthropod-borne infections, such as plague and epidemic typhus.

pulmonary /pōōl'məner'ē/ [L *pulmoneus* relating to the lungs], of or pertaining to the lungs or the respiratory system.

pulmonary acid aspiration syndrome. See **Mendelson's syndrome.**

pulmonary alveolar proteinosis, a condition in which the air sacs of the lungs become filled with protein and lipids. The cause is unknown and the disease progresses to respiratory failure.

pulmonary alveolus, one of the numerous terminal air sacs of the lungs in which oxygen and carbon monoxide are exchanged.

pulmonary angiography, the radiographic study of the blood vessels of the lungs after injecting an opaque contrast medium into the pulmonary circulation.

pulmonary anthrax. See **woolsorter's disease.**

pulmonary arteriolar resistance (PAR), pressure loss per unit of blood flow from the pulmonary artery to a pulmonary vein.

pulmonary artery, either the left pulmonary artery supplying the left lung or the right pulmonary artery supplying the right lung. The lobar branches are named according to the lobe they supply, such as apical *(ramus apicalis).*

pulmonary artery catheter, a catheter inserted into a pulmonary artery to measure cardiac output, pulmonary arterial pressure, and capillary wedge pressure.

pulmonary artery wedge pressure, the blood pressure as measured by a transducer when a catheter is wedged into a distal branch of the pulmonary artery. The pressure measured is that of the pulmonary vein and, indirectly, that of the left atrium and the left ventricle during diastole.

pulmonary atresia, a congenital heart defect of the right ventricular outflow tract. In one form there is an intact ventricular septum with an interatrial communication and a persistent patent ductus arteriosus. A more extreme form is the four-defect **tetralogy of Fallot.**

pulmonary atrium, any of the spaces at the end of an alveolar duct into which alveoli open.

pulmonary carcinosis. See **alveolar cell carcinoma.**

pulmonary circulation, the blood flow through a network of vessels between the heart and the lungs for the oxygenation of blood and removal of carbon dioxide.

pulmonary compliance, a measure of the elasticity or expansibility of the lungs.

pulmonary congestion, an excessive accumulation of fluid in the lungs, usually associated with either an inflammation or congestive heart failure.

pulmonary disease, an abnormal condition of the respiratory system, characterized by cough, chest pain, dyspnea, hemoptysis, sputum production, stridor, and wheezing. Less common symptoms may be anxiety, arm and shoulder pain, tenderness in the calf of the leg, erythema nodosum, swelling of the face, headache, hoarseness, pain in the joints, and somnolence. Pulmonary diseases are either obstructive or restrictive. Obstructive respiratory diseases are the result of an obstacle in the airway that impedes the flow of air, especially during expiration. Obstructive diseases are characterized by reduced expiratory flow rates and increased total lung capacities. Restrictive respiratory diseases are caused by conditions that limit lung expansion by an actual reduction of the volume of inspired air, such as fibrothorax, a neuromuscular disorder, kyphosis, scoliosis, spondylitis, or surgical removal of lung tissue. Characteristic features of restrictive respiratory diseases are decreased forced vital capacity and total lung capacity, with increased work of breathing and inefficient exchange of gases.

pulmonary edema, the accumulation of extravascular fluid in lung tissues and alveoli, caused most commonly by congestive heart failure and also occurring in barbiturate and opiate poisoning, diffuse infections, hemorrhagic pancreatitis, renal failure, and after a stroke, skull fracture, near drowning, the inhalation of irritating gases, and the rapid administration of whole blood, plasma, serum albumin, or intravenous fluids. In congestive heart disease serous fluid is pushed back through the pulmonary capillaries into alveoli and quickly enters bronchioles and bronchi. The patient with pulmonary edema breathes rapidly and shallowly with difficulty, is usually restless, apprehensive, hoarse, pale, or cyanotic, and may cough up frothy, pink sputum. The peripheral and neck veins are usually engorged; the blood pressure and heart rate are increased; and the pulse may be full and pounding or weak and thready. There may be edema of the extremities, rales in the lungs, respiratory acidosis, and profuse diaphoresis.

pulmonary embolism (PE), the blockage of a pulmonary artery by foreign matter such as fat, air, tumor tissue, or a thrombus that usually arises from a peripheral vein. Predisposing factors include an alter-ation of blood constituents with increased coagulation, damage to blood vessel walls, and stagnation or immobilization, especially when associated with childbirth, congestive heart failure, polycythemia vera, or surgery. Pulmonary embolism is difficult to distinguish from myocardial infarction and pneumonia. It is characterized by dyspnea, sudden chest pain, shock, and cyanosis.

pulmonary emphysema, a chronic obstructive disease of the lungs, marked by an overdistention of the alveoli.

pulmonary fibrosis. See **fibrosis of the lungs.**

pulmonary function laboratory, an area of a hospital or other health facility used for examination and evaluation of patients' respiratory functions, using electromechanical and other devices.

pulmonary function test (PFT), a procedure for determining the capacity of the lungs to exchange oxygen and carbon dioxide efficiently. There are two general kinds of respiratory function tests. One measures ventilation, or the ability of the bellows action of the chest and lungs to move gas in and out of alveoli; the other kind measures the diffusion of gas across the alveolar capillary membrane and the perfusion of the lungs by blood. Efficient gas exchange in the lungs requires a balanced ventilation-perfusion ratio, with areas receiving ventilation well perfused and areas receiving blood flow capable of ventilation.

pulmonary hypertension, a condition of abnormally high pressure within the pulmonary circulation.

pulmonary infarction (PI), an obstruction in a branch of a pulmonary artery resulting from a thrombus that may have originated in a leg or pelvic vein. After it is released into the venous circulation, the thromboembolus is carried in the bloodstream to one of the lungs, and filtered by the pulmonary vascular system.

pulmonary infiltrate with eosinophilia. See **PIE.**

pulmonary insufficiency, a failure of the pulmonary valve to close properly.

pulmonary oxygen toxicity, a form of oxygen poisoning caused by breathing high partial pressures of oxygen. Pathophysiologic effects include pulmonary capillary endothelial damage and alveolar epithelial cell destruction. Clinical manifestations include cough, substernal pain, nausea, vomiting, and atelectasis.

pulmonary stenosis, an abnormal cardiac condition, generally characterized by concentric hypertrophy of the right ventricle with relatively little increase in diastolic

P

volume. When the ventricular septum is intact, this condition may be caused by valvular stenosis, by infundibular stenosis, or by both; it produces a pressure difference during systole between the right ventricular cavity and the pulmonary artery.

pulmonary sulcus tumor, a destructive, invasive neoplasm that develops at the apex of the lung and infiltrates the ribs, vertebrae, and the brachial plexus.

pulmonary surfactant, a surfactant agent found in the lungs that functions to reduce the surface tension of the fluid on the surface of the cells of the lower respiratory system, enhancing the elasticity of the alveoli and bronchioles and thus the exchange of gases in the lungs.

pulmonary trunk, the short, wide vessel that conveys venous blood from the right ventricle of the heart to the lungs.

pulmonary tuberculosis. See **tuberculosis.**

pulmonary valve, a cardiac structure composed of three semilunar cusps that close during each heartbeat to prevent blood from flowing back into the right ventricle from the pulmonary artery. The cusps are separated by sinuses that resemble tiny buckets when they are closed and filled with blood. These flaps grow from the lining of the pulmonary artery.

pulmonary vascular resistance (PVR), the resistance in the pulmonary vascular bed against which the right ventricle must eject blood.

pulmonary vein, one of a pair of large vessels that return oxygenated blood from each lung to the left atrium of the heart. The right pulmonary veins pass dorsal to the right atrium and the superior vena cava. The left pulmonary veins pass ventral to the descending thoracic aorta.

pulmonary ventilation, the process of inhaling and exhaling air through the lungs.

pulmonary wedge pressure (PWP), the pressure produced by an inflated latex balloon against a pulmonary artery, as part of a procedure used in the diagnosis of congestive heart failure, myocardial infarction, and other conditions. A balloon-tipped catheter is inserted through a subclavian, jugular, or femoral vein to the vena cava and on through the right atrium and ventricle to the pulmonary artery.

pulmonary Wegener's granulomatosis, a rare, fatal disease of young or middle-aged men, characterized by granulomatous lesions of the respiratory tract, focal necrotizing arteritis, and, finally, widespread inflammation of body organs.

pulmonic. See **pulmonary.**

pulmonic stenosis. See **pulmonary stenosis.**

pulp [L *pulpa* flesh], any soft, spongy tissue, such as that contained within the spleen, the pulp chamber of the tooth, or the distal phalanges of the fingers and the toes. **–pulpy,** *adj.*

pulp abscess [L *pulpa* + *abscedere* to go away], a pus-producing abscess that develops in the pulp of a tooth.

pulp canal, the space occupied by the pulp in the radicular portion of the tooth.

pulp cavity, the space in a tooth bounded by the dentin and containing the dental pulp. It is divided into the pulp chamber and the pulp or root canal.

pulpectomy /pulpek'təmē/ [L *pulpa* + Gk *ektome* excision], the surgical removal either complete or partial of the pulp from a tooth.

pulpitis /pulpī'tis/, infection or inflammation of the dental pulp.

pulpless tooth, a tooth in which the dental pulp is necrotic or has been removed.

pulp stone. See **denticle.**

pulsate [L *pulsare* to beat], to throb or vibrate rhythmically, as the expansion and contraction rhythm of the heart.

pulsatile /pul'sətil/ [L *pulsatio* beating], pertaining to an activity characterized by a rhythmic pulsation.

pulsatile assist device (PAD), a flexible valveless balloon conduit contained within a rigid plastic cylinder that is inserted into the arterial circulation to provide pulsatile cardiopulmonary bypass perfusion.

pulsating exophthalmos [L *pulsare* to beat; Gk *ex, ophthalmos* eye], an eye disorder characterized by a bulging, pulsating eyeball. The cause is an arteriovenous aneurysm involving the internal carotid artery and the cavernous sinus of the orbit.

pulse [L *pulsare* to beat], **1.** a rhythmic beating or vibrating movement. **2.** a brief electromagnetic wave. **3.** the regular, recurrent expansion and contraction of an artery produced by waves of pressure caused by the ejection of blood from the left ventricle of the heart as it contracts. The phenomenon is easily detected on superficial arteries, such as the radial and carotid arteries, and corresponds to each beat of the heart. The normal number of pulse beats per minute in the average adult varies from 60 to 80, with fluctuations occurring with exercise, injury, illness, and emotional reactions.

pulse deficit, a condition that exists when the radial pulse is less than the ventricular rate as auscultated at the apex or seen on the electrocardiogram. The condition indicates a lack of peripheral perfusion for some of the heart contractions.

pulse height analyzer, (in radiology) a

device that accepts or rejects electronic pulses according to their amplitude or energy.

pulseless disease. See **Takayasu's arteritis.**

pulse MR, MR techniques that use radio-frequency pulses and Fourier transformation of the MR signal.

pulse point, any one of the sites on the surface of the body where arterial pulsations can be easily palpated. The most commonly used pulse point is over the radial artery at the wrist. Other pulse points are over the temporal artery in front of the ear, over the common carotid artery at the lower level of the thyroid cartilage, and over the facial artery at the lower margin of the jaw.

pulse pressure, the difference between the systolic and diastolic pressures, normally 30 to 40 mm Hg.

pulse rate [L *pulsare* + *reri* to calculate], the number of beats per minute as measured on the radial, carotid, femoral, and pedal arteries. Normally, it is the same rate as the heart beat, but pulses in various body areas may differ slightly.

pulse wave [L *pulsare* + AS *wafian*], a local blood pressure change caused by the passage of blood from the left ventricle into the aorta. It is accompanied by a wave action through the artery.

pulsus alternans /pul′səs ôl′tərnanz/ [L *pulsare* + *alternare* to alternate], a pulse characterized by a regular alternation of weak and strong beats without changes in the length of the cycle.

pulsus magnus. See **full pulse.**

pulsus paradoxus, an abnormal decrease in systolic pressure and pulse wave amplitude during inspiration.

pulsus parvus et tardus [L *pulsare* to beat, *parvus* small, *tardus* slow], a small pulse with low pressure that rises and falls slowly. The condition occurs in aortic stenosis.

pulsus tardus, a pulse with a gradual rise and fall in amplitude.

Pulvule /pul′vyo̅o̅l/ [L *pulvis* dust], a proprietary capsule containing a dose of a drug in powder form.

pumice [L *pumex*], a very finely divided volcanic rock, used in powdered or solid form for smoothing or polishing surfaces.

pump [ME *pumpe*], **1.** an apparatus used to move fluids or gases by suction or by positive pressure, such as an infusion pump or stomach pump. **2.** a physiologic mechanism by which a substance is moved, usually by active transport across a cell membrane, such as a sodium pump. **3.** to move a liquid or gas by suction or positive pressure.

pump lung. See **congestive atelectasis.**

pump oxygenator [ME, *pumpe*; Gk, *oxys*, sharp + *genein*, to produce], a device that pumps oxygenated blood through the body during cardiopulmonary surgery.

punch biopsy [L *pungere* to prick; Gk *bios* life, *opsis* view], the removal of living tissue for microscopic examination, usually bone marrow from the sternum, by means of a punch.

punch forceps, a surgical instrument used to cut out a disk of dense or resistant tissue, such as bone and cartilage. The ends of the blades of the punch forceps are perforated to grip the involved tissue.

punctum lacrimale /pungk′təm/, *pl.* **puncta lacrimalia** [L *punctus* pricked; *lacrima* tear], a tiny aperture in the margin of each eyelid that opens into the lacrimal duct. The puncta release tears that travel through the lacrimal ducts to the conjunctiva.

puncture [L *punctura*], **1.** to prick or pierce a surface, as with a needle or knife. **2.** a wound or opening made by piercing.

puncture of the antrum [L *punctura*; Gk *antron* cave], to pierce a cavity or hollow, as in piercing the wall of the maxillary sinus to drain pus.

puncture wound [L *punctura*; AS *wund*], a traumatic injury caused by the penetration of the skin by a narrow object, such as a knife, nail, or slender fragment of metal, wood, glass, or other material.

punitive damages. See **damages.**

Punnett square [Reginald C. Punnett, twentieth-century English geneticist; OFr *esquarre*], a checkerboard, graphlike diagram, used in charting genetic ratios, that shows all of the possible combinations of male and female gametes when one or more pairs of independent alleles are crossed.

PUO, abbreviation for *pyrexia of unknown origin.*

pupa /pyo̅o̅′pə/ [L, doll], a second stage in the life cycle of certain *(endopterytgote)* insects between a larva and adult. It shows the basic external features of the adult form but without expanded wings.

pupil [L *pupa* doll], a circular opening in the iris of the eye, located slightly to the nasal side of the center of the iris. The pupil lies behind the anterior chamber of the eye and the cornea and in front of the lens. Its diameter changes with contraction and relaxation of the muscular fibers of the iris as the eye responds to changes in light, emotional states, and other kinds of stimulation. The pupil is the window of the eye through which light passes to the lens and the retina. **–pupillary,** *adj.*

pupilla /pyōoil'ə/ [L], the pupil of the eye.

pupillary reflex. See **accommodation reflex, light reflex.**

pupillary skin reflex. See **ciliospinal reflex.**

PUPs, abbreviation for *previously untreated patients,* usually infants participating in clinical trials.

pure dwarf. See **primordial dwarf.**

pure science. See **science.**

pure tone audiometry. See **audiometry.**

pure vegetarian. See **strict vegetarian.**

purgation. See **catharsis.**

purgative /pur'gətiv/ [L *purgare* to purge], a strong medication usually administered by mouth to promote evacuation of the bowel or several bowel movements.

purge [L *purgare*], **1.** to evacuate the bowels, as with a cathartic. **2.** a cathartic. **3.** to make free of an unwanted substance. **–purgative,** *n., adj.*

purified protein derivative (PPD), a dried form of tuberculin used in testing for past or present infection with tubercle bacilli. This product is usually introduced into the skin during such tests.

purine /pyōor'ēn, -in/ [L *purum* pure, *urina* urine], any one of a large group of nitrogenous compounds, produced as end products in the digestion of proteins in the diet, or synthesized in the body. Purines are also present in many medications and other substances, including caffeine, theophylline, and various diuretics, muscle relaxants, and myocardial stimulants.

purine base [L *purus* pure], any of the purine derivates found in animal waste products. They include hypoxanthine, xanthine, and uric acid.

purine-free diet, a diet that excludes foods that are rich sources of purines, end products of digestion of certain proteins. Foods high in purines include particularly organ meats, such as liver, kidney, and sweetbreads, as well as red meats, poultry, and fish. Those items can be replaced by milk, eggs, cheese, and some vegetable sources of protein.

purine-low diet, a diet that excludes some foods rich in purines, such as certain meat products, fish, and poultry, and particularly anchovies, meat extracts, sardines, and organ meats.

Purkinje cells /pərkin'jəs/ [Johannes E. Purkinje, Polish physiologist, b. 1787], large neurons that provide the only output from the cerebellar cortex after the cortex processes sensory and motor impulses from the rest of the nervous system.

Purkinje's fibers, myocardial fibers that are a continuation of the bundle of His and extend into the muscle walls of the ventricles.

Purkinje's network /pərkin'jēz, pur'kinjēz, -jāz/, a complex network of muscle fibers that spread through the right and the left ventricles of the heart and carry the impulses that contract those chambers almost simultaneously.

purposeful activity, activity that depends on consciously planned and directed involvement of the person.

purpura /pur'pyŏorə/ [L, purple], any of several bleeding disorders characterized by hemorrhage into the tissues, particularly beneath the skin or mucous membranes, producing ecchymoses or petechiae. The two major kinds of purpura are **thrombocytopenic purpura** and **nonthrombocytopenic purpura. –purpuric,** *adj.*

purpura rheumatica, a distinctive clinical sign associated with hemorrhages of the skin and other tissues. The lesions are red or purple and do not blanch on pressure. Purpura is either related to a disorder of the blood or an abnormality affecting the blood vessels.

purpura senile, a skin condition affecting older persons and characterized by fragile blood vessel walls which rupture on minimal trauma.

pursed-lip breathing, respiration characterized by deep inspirations followed by prolonged expirations through pursed lips.

purse-string suture [L *sutura*], a continuous suture inserted in a circle about a round wound. The opening is closed by tightly drawing the ends of the suture together.

purulence /pyōor'(y)ələns/ [L *purulentus* pus formation], the condition of producing or discharging pus.

purulent /pyŏor'ŏŏlənt/ [L, containing pus], producing or containing pus.

purulent conjunctivitis [L *purulentus, conjunctivus* connecting; Gk *itis* inmflammation], an inflammation of the conjunctiva caused by suppurative microorganisms, including species of streptococci, gonococci, and pneumococci.

purulent diarrhea [L *purulentus* + Gk *dia, rhein* to flow], diarrhea in which stools contain pus, a sign of a purulent gastrointestinal tract infection.

purulent inflammation [L *purulentus, inflammare* to set afire], an inflammation that is accompanied by the formation of pus.

purulent iritis [L *purulentus* + Gk *iris* rainbow, *itis* inflammation], an inflammation of the iris accompanied by pus formation.

purulent keratitis [L *purulentus* + Gk

keras horn, *itis*], a severe form of keratitis leading to disintegration of the cornea if untreated. The condition commonly begins with a bacterial infection of the lacrimal sac, occurs frequently in elderly patients who have poor nutrition, and spreads into a pus-producing ulcer.

purulent pancreatitis [L *purulentus* + Gk *pan* all, *kreas* flesh, *itis*], inflammation of the pancreas accompanied by pus formation.

purulent rhinitis [L *purulentus* + Gk *rhis* nose, *itis*], an infection of the nasal mucosa that is accompanied by pus formation. The condition is often secondary to a systemic infection, such as measles.

purulent synovitis [L *purulentus* + Gk *syn* together; L *ovum,* egg], an inflammation of the synovial membrane of a joint with pus formation in the cavity.

pus [L, corrupt matter], a creamy, viscous, pale yellow or yellow-green fluid exudate that is the result of liquefaction necrosis. Its main constituent is an abundance of polymorphonuclear leukocytes. Bacterial infection is its most common cause.

pus in urine, the presence of pus in a urine sample, indicating a urinary tract infection anywhere from the kidneys to the urethra. Cloudiness in urine may be due to either pus or chemicals, a difference determined by simple laboratory tests.

pustular psoriasis [L *pustula* blister; Gk *psoriasis* itch], a severe form of psoriasis consisting of bright red patches and sterile pustules all over the body. Crops of lesions lasting 4 to 7 days occur every few days in cycles over weeks or months. Recurrences are inevitable. Fever, leukocytosis, and hypoalbuminemia are associated.

pustule /pus'chool/ [L *pustula*], a small, circumscribed elevation of the skin containing fluid that is usually purulent. –**pustular,** *adj.*

putamen [L, husk], a part of the lentiform nucleus that is lateral to the globus pallidus. It is associated with the corpus striatum and receives connections from the suppressor centers of the cortex.

putrefaction /pyoo'trəfek'shən/ [L *puter* rotten, *facere* to make], the decay of enzymes, especially proteins, that produces foul-smelling compounds, such as ammonia, hydrogen sulfide, and mercaptans. –**putrefactive,** *adj.*

putrefy /pyoo'trəfi/ [L *puter* rotten, *facere* to make], to decay, with the production of foul-smelling substances, especially putrescine and mercaptans associated with the decomposition of animal tissues and proteins.

putrescine /pyoo'tresēn/, a foul-smelling, toxic ptomaine produced by the decomposition of the amino acid ornithine during the decay of animal tissues, bacillus cultures, and fecal bacteria.

putrid /pyoo'trid/, decomposed.

putromaine /pyootrō'mān/, any toxin produced by the decay of food within a living body.

P value, (in research) the statistical probability attached to the occurrence of a given finding by chance alone in comparison with the known distribution of possible findings, considering the kinds of data, the technique of analysis, and the number of observations.

PVB. See **VBP.**

PVC, 1. abbreviation for **polyvinyl chloride. 2.** abbreviation for **premature ventricular contraction.**

PVR, abbreviation for **pulmonary vascular resistance.**

pW, abbreviation for *picowatt.*

PWA, abbreviation for *person with AIDS.*

P wave, the component of the cardiac cycle shown on an electrocardiogram as an inverted U-shaped curve that follows the end of the T wave and precedes the spike of the QRS complex. It represents atrial depolarization.

P′ wave (P prime wave), a P wave that is generated from other than the sinus node; an ectopic P wave.

PWP, abbreviation for **pulmonary wedge pressure.**

pyelogram /pī'əlōgram'/ [Gk *pyekos* pelvis, *gramma* record], an x-ray picture of the kidneys and ureters. An intravenous pyelogram (IVP), taken after the injection of a radiopaque dye, shows the size and location of the kidneys, the outline of the ureters and bladder, the filling of the renal pelves, the patency of the urinary tract, and any cysts or tumors within the kidneys.

pyelography. See **intravenous pyelography.**

pyelolithotomy /pī'əlō'lithot'əmē/, a surgical procedure in which renal calculi are removed from the pelvis of the ureter.

pyelonephritis /pī'əlōnəfrī'tis/ [Gk *pyelos* + *nephros* kidney, *itis* inflammation], a diffuse pyogenic infection of the pelvis and parenchyma of the kidney. **Acute pyelonephritis** is usually the result of an infection that ascends from the lower urinary tract to the kidney. **Chronic pyelonephritis** develops slowly after bacterial infection of the kidney and may progress to renal failure. Most cases are associated with some form of obstruction, such as a stone or a stricture of the ureter.

pyemic embolism [Gk *pyon* pus, *haima*

P

blood, *embolos* plug], an infective embolus producing an abscess.

pygmalionism /pigmā'lē-əniz'əm/ [Gk *Pygmalion* mythic sculptor who fell in love with his statue], a psychosexual abnormality in which the individual directs erotic fantasies toward an object that he or she has created.

pygmy /pig'mē/ [L *pygmaeus* dwarf], an extremely small person whose bodily parts are proportioned accordingly; a primordial dwarf.

pygoamorphus /pī'gō-əmôr'fəs/ [Gk *pyge* buttocks, *a, morphe* not form], asymmetric, conjoined twins in which the parasitic member is represented by an undifferentiated amorphous mass attached to the autosite in the sacral region.

pygodidymus /pī'gōdid'əməs/ [Gk *pyge* + *didymos* twin], **1.** a malformed fetus that has a double pelvis and hips. **2.** conjoined twins that are fused in the cephalothoracic region but separated at the pelvis.

pygomelus /pīgom'ələs/ [Gk *pyge* + *melos* limb], a malformed fetus that has an extra limb or limbs attached to the buttock.

pygopagus /pīgop'əgəs/ [Gk *pyge* + *pegos* fixed], conjoined twins consisting of two fully formed or nearly formed fetuses that are united in the sacral region so that they are back to back.

pyknic /pik'nik/ [Gk *pyknos* thick], describing a body structure characterized by short, round limbs, a full face, a short neck, stockiness, and a tendency toward obesity.

pylon /pī'lon/ [Gk, gate], an artificial lower limb, often a narrow vertical support consisting of a socket with wooden side-supports and a rubber-clad peg end. It may be used as a temporary prosthesis.

pyloric obstruction and dilation [Gk *pyle* gate, *ouros* guard; L *obstruere* to build against, *dilatare* to widen], a reaction of the stomach to pyloric obstruction, which increases the resistance to the expulsion of partly digested food from the stomach. As a result, the stomach may become hypertrophied, then dilated. Excessive consumption of food and beverages contributes to the condition.

pyloric orifice /pīlôr'ik/ [Gk *pyle* gate, *ouros* guard; L *orificium* opening], the opening of the stomach into the duodenum lying to the right of the middle line at the level of the cranial border of the first lumbar vertebra.

pyloric spasm. See **pylorospasm.**

pyloric sphincter, a thickened muscular ring in the stomach, separating the pylorus from the duodenum.

pyloric stenosis, a narrowing of the pyloric sphincter at the outlet of the stomach, causing an obstruction that blocks the flow of food into the small intestine.

pyloric ulcer. See **peptic ulcer.**

pyloric valve. See **pyloric sphincter.**

pyloromyotomy /pīlō'ōmī-ot'əmē/ [Gk *pyle, ouros* + *mys* muscle, *temnein* to cut], the incision of the longitudinal and circular muscle of the pylorus, which leaves the mucosa intact but separates the incised muscle fibers.

pyloroplasty /pīlôr'əplas'tē/ [Gk *pyle, ouros* + *plassein* to mold], a surgical procedure performed to relieve pyloric stenosis.

pylorospasm /pīlôr'əspaz'əm/ [Gk *pyle, ouros* + *spasmos*], a spasm of the pyloric sphincter of the stomach, as occurs in pyloric stenosis.

pylorotomy /pī'lôrot'əmē/ [Gk *pyle* gate, *ouros* guard, *temnein* to cut], a surgical incision of the pylorus, usually performed to remove an obstruction.

pylorus /pīlôr'əs/, *pl.* **pylori, pyloruses** [Gk *pyle* gate, *ouros* guard], a tubular portion of the stomach that angles to the right from the body of the stomach toward the duodenum. **–pyloric,** *adj.*

pyocyst /pī'əsist/ [Gk *pyon* + *kytos* cell], a pus-filled cyst.

pyoderma /pī'ōdur'mə/ [Gk *pyon* pus, *derma* skin], any purulent skin disease, such as impetigo.

pyogenic /pī'əjen'ik/ [Gk *pyon* + *genein* to produce], producing pus.

pyogenic granuloma, a small, nonmalignant mass of excessive granulation tissue, usually found at the site of an injury. Most often a dull red, it contains numerous capillaries, bleeds easily, and is very tender; it may be attached by a narrow stalk.

pyogenic infection, any infection that results in pus production.

pyogenic microroganisms [Gk *pyon* + *genein; mikros* small, *organon* instrument], microorganisms that produce pus. They include species of bacilli, clostridia, gonococci, meningococci, pseudomonads, staphylococci, and streptococci.

pyohemothorax /pī'ōhem'ōthôr'aks/ [Gk *pyon* + *haima* blood, *thorax* chest], an accumulation of blood and pus in the pleural cavity.

pyophylactic [Gk *pyon* + *phylax* protector], providing protection against purulent infection, such as with taking an antibiotic before its onset.

pyorrhea /pī'ərē'ə/ [Gk *pyon* + *rhoia* flow] **1.** a discharge of pus. **2.** a purulent inflammation of the tissues surrounding the teeth. **–pyorrheal,** *adj.*

pyosalpinx /pī'ōsal'pingks/ [Gk *pyon* + *salpinx* tube], an accumulation of pus in a fallopian tube.

pyramid /pir'əmid/ [Gr *pyramis*], a mass of tissue rising to an apex, as the pyramids of the cerebellum and kidneys.

pyramidal /piram'idəl/ [Gk *pyramis*], of or pertaining to the shape of a pyramid.

pyramidal cell, a neuron with a pyramid-shaped cell body in the gray matter of the cerebral cortex.

pyramidalis /piram'idā'lis/, one of a pair of anterolateral muscles of the abdomen, contained in the lower end of the sheath of the rectus abdominis. It functions to tense the linea alba.

pyramidal nucleus, a band of gray matter lying between the olivary nucleus and the midline that projects fibers contralaterally to the vermis of part of the cerebellum.

pyramidal tract, a pathway composed of groups of nerve fibers in the white matter of the spinal cord through which motor impulses are conducted to the anterior horn cells from the opposite side of the brain. These descending fibers regulate the voluntary and reflex activity of the muscles through the anterior horn cells.

pyrantel pamoate /pīran'təl/, an anthelmintic prescribed in the treatment of infestation by roundworms or pinworms.

pyrazinamide /pī'razin'əmīd/, an antimycobacterial prescribed in combination chemotherapy in the treatment of tuberculosis of hospitalized patients who fail to respond to other medications.

pyrectic, pyretic [Gk *pyretos* fever], pertaining to or characterized by fever.

pyrethrin and piperonyl butoxide, a fixed-combination scabicide and pediculicide. It is prescribed in the treatment of infestations of head, body, and pubic lice.

pyretogenic /pī'ratōjen'ik/ [Gk *pyretos* fever, *genein* to produce], inducing, causing, or resulting from a fever.

pyrexia. See **fever.**

pyridostigmine bromide /pir'idōstig'mēn/, a cholinergic prescribed in the treatment of myasthenia gravis and used as an antagonist to nondepolarizing muscle relaxants, such as curare.

pyridoxal phosphate /pir'ədok'səl/, an enzyme in the body that acts with pyridoxamine phosphate and transaminase to catalyze the reversible transfer of an amino group from an alpha-amino acid to an alpha-keto acid, especially alpha-ketoglutaric acid.

pyridoxamine phosphate /pir'ədok'-səmēn/, an enzyme that participates with pyridoxal phosphate and transaminase in the reversible transfer of an amino group from an alpha-amino acid to an alpha-keto acid.

pyridoxine /pir'idok'sēn/, a water-soluble, white, crystalline vitamin that is part of the B complex group, derived from pyridine, and converted in the body to pyridoxal and pyridoxamine for synthesis. It functions as a coenzyme essential for the synthesis and breakdown of amino acids, the conversion of tryptophan to niacin, the breakdown of glycogen to glucose 1-phosphate, the production of antibodies, the formation of heme in hemoglobin, the formation of hormones important in brain function, the proper absorption of vitamin B_{12}, the production of hydrochloric acid and magnesium, and the maintenance of the balance of sodium and potassium, which regulates body fluids and the functioning of the nervous and musculoskeletal systems.

pyridoxine hydrochloride. See **pyridoxine.**

pyriform /pir'ifôrm/ [L *pirum* pear + *forma*], pear shaped.

pyrilamine maleate /piril'əmēn/, an antihistamine prescribed in the treatment of a variety of hypersensitivity reactions, including rhinitis, skin rash, and pruritus.

pyrimethamine /pir'əmeth'əmēn/, an antimalarial prescribed in the treatment of malaria and toxoplasmosis.

pyrimethamine and sulfadoxine, an antimalarial fixed-combination drug prescribed for prophylaxis and attacks of malaria.

pyrimidine /pərim'ədēn/, an organic compound of heterocyclic nitrogen found in nucleic acids and in many drugs, including the antiviral drugs acyclovir, ribavirin, and trifluridine.

pyrogen /pī'rəjən/ [Gk *pyr* fire, *genein* to produce], any substance or agent that tends to cause a rise in body temperature, such as some bacterial toxins. **–pyrogenic,** *adj.*

pyrolagnia /pī'rōlag'nē·ə/ [Gk *pyr* + *lagneia* lust], sexual stimulation or gratification from watching or setting fires.

pyromania /pī'rōmā'nē·ə/ [Gk *pyr* + *mania* madness], an impulse-control neurosis characterized by an uncontrollable urge to set fires.

pyromaniac /pī'rōmā'nē·ak/, **1.** a person with or displaying characteristics of pyromania. **2.** of, pertaining to, or exhibiting pyromania. **–pyromaniacal,** *adj.*

pyrosis. See **heartburn.**

pyrrole /pirōl', pir'ōl/ [Gk *pyrrhos* red], a heterocyclic substance occurring naturally in many compounds in the body. Heme and porphyrin are pyrrole derivatives.

pyruvate kinase /pī'rəvāt/, an enzyme essential for anaerobic glycolysis in red blood cells. It catalyzes the transfer of a phosphate group from adenosine triphosphate to produce adenosine diphosphate.

pyruvate kinase deficiency, a congenital hemolytic disorder transmitted as an autosomal recessive trait. The homozygous condition is characterized by severe chronic hemolysis.

pyruvic acid /pīr o͞o'vik/, a compound formed as an end product of glycolysis, the anaerobic stage of glucose metabolism. Exposed to oxygen and acetylcoenzyme A at the entrance to the Krebs citric acid cycle, the compound is changed to citric acid.

pyuria /pīy o͞or'ē·ə/ [Gk *pyon* pus, *ouron* urine], the presence of white blood cells in the urine, usually a sign of an infection of the urinary tract. Pyuria occurs most often in cystitis, pyelonephritis, urethritis, and tuberculosis of the kidney.

PZI, abbreviation for *protamine zinc insulin.*

Q, **1.** symbol for *blood volume.* **2.** symbol for *quantity.* **3.** symbol for *coulomb.*

Q̇, symbol for rate of *blood flow.*

QA, abbreviation for **quality assurance.**

Q angle, the angle of incidence of the quadriceps muscle relative to the patella. The Q angle determines the tracking of the patella through the trochlea of the femur. As the angle increases, the chance of patellar compression problems increases.

QAP, abbreviation for **quality assurance program.**

q.d., **1.** (in prescriptions) abbreviation for *quaque die* /dē′ā/, a Latin phrase meaning "every day." **2.** abbreviation for *quartile deviation.*

q diem, See **q.d.**

qdrnt, abbreviation for **quadrant.**

Q fever [query; L *febris*], an acute febrile illness, usually respiratory, caused by the rickettsia, *Coxiella burnetii (Rickettsia burnetii).* The disease is spread through contact with infected domestic animals, either by inhaling the rickettsiae from their hides, drinking their contaminated milk, or being bitten by a tick harboring the organism.

q.h., (in prescriptions) abbreviation for *quaque hora,* a Latin phrase meaning "every hour."

q.2h., (in prescriptions) abbreviation for *quaque secunda hora,* a Latin phrase meaning "every 2 hours."

q.3h., (in prescriptions) abbreviation for *quaque tertia hora,* a Latin phrase meaning "every 3 hours."

q.4h., (in prescriptions) abbreviation for *quaque quarta hora,* a Latin phrase meaning "every 4 hours."

q.6h., (in prescriptions) abbreviation for *quaque sex hora,* a Latin phrase meaning "every 6 hours."

q.8h., (in prescriptions) abbreviation for *quaque octa hora,* a Latin phrase meaning "every 8 hours."

q.i.d., (in prescriptions) abbreviation for *quater in die* /dē′ā/, a Latin phrase meaning "four times a day."

q.l., abbreviation for the Latin phrase, *quantum libet,* "as much as one pleases."

qli, abbreviation for *quality of life index.*

QRS complex, a series of wave forms on an electrocardiogram that represent depo-

larization of ventricular muscle cells. The term "QRS complex" is assigned by convention to describe both normal and abnormal ventricular depolarization. The variable morphologies of the QRS complex are described in detail by labeling each deflection above and below the baseline as Q,R, or S wave; uppercase and lowercase letters are used to describe the amplitude of each waveform. In the QRS complex, a Q wave is the negative deflection preceding an R wave; an R wave is the first positive deflection, and an S wave is the negative deflection following an R wave.

QRST complex [L *complexus*], components of an electrocardiogram, consisting of the QRS complex, the S-T segment, the Q-T interval, the T wave, and the U wave. It represents depolarization and repolarization of the ventricles.

QRST interval [L *intervallum* space between ramparts], the electrocardiographic period of ventricular electrical activity.

q.s., (in prescriptions) abbreviation for *quantum sufficit,* a Latin phrase meaning "quantity required."

Q's test. See **Queckenstedt's test.**

qt, abbreviation for **quart.**

Q-T interval, the portion on an electrocardiogram from the beginning of the QRS complex to the end of the T wave, reflecting the length of the refractory period of the heart. A long Q-T interval is associated with the life-threatening ventricular tachycardia known as **torsades de pointes.**

quack. See **charlatan.**

quad, abbreviation for *quadriceps, quadrilateral,* **quadrant, quadriplegia.**

quadrant /kwod′rənt/ [L *quadrans* a fourth part], **1.** one quarter of a circle. **2.** one quarter of an anatomic area formed by the division of the area by imaginary vertical and horizontal bisecting each other.

quadratus labii superioris. See **zygomaticus minor.**

quadriceps femoris /kwod′risəps/ [L *quattuor* four, *caput* head; *femur* thigh], the great extensor muscle of the anterior thigh, composed of the rectus femoris, the vastus lateralis, the vastus medialis, and the vastus intermedius. The muscle functions to extend the leg.

quadriceps reflex. See **patellar reflex.**

quadrigeminal /kwod'rijem'inəl/ [L *qua-drigeminum* fourfold], **1.** in four parts. **2.** a fourfold increase in size or frequency. **3.** having four symmetric parts.

quadrigeminal pulse, a pulse in which a pause occurs after every fourth beat.

quadrilateral socket /kwod'rilat'ərrl/, a four-sided prosthetic socket design for persons with above-the-knee amputations. The posterior brim is designed to fit directly beneath the ischial tuberosity so that the person literally sits on it.

quadripedal extensor reflex. See **Brain's reflex.**

quadriplegia /kwod'rəplē'jē·ə/ [L *quattuor* four; Gk *plege* stroke], an abnormal condition characterized by paralysis of the arms, the legs, and the trunk of the body below the level of an associated injury to the spinal cord. This disorder may be caused by spinal cord injury, especially in the area of the fifth to the seventh vertebrae. Automobile accidents and sporting mishaps are common causes.

quadruped /kwod'rŏoped'/ [L *quattour* four, *pes* foot], **1.** any four-footed animal. **2.** a human whose body weight is supported by both arms as well as both legs.

quadruplet /kwod'rŏoplit, kwodrŏo'plit/ [L *quadruplus* fourfold], any one of four offspring born of the same gestation period during a single pregnancy.

qual anal, abbreviation for **qualitative analysis.**

quale /kwä'lē/, *pl.* **qualia** /kwä'lē·ə/ [L *qualis* what kind of], **1.** the quality of a particular thing. **2.** a quality considered as an independent entity. **3.** (in psychology) a feeling, sensation, or other conscious process that has its unique, particular quality regardless of its external meaning or frame of reference.

qualified /kwol'ifīd/ [L *qualis*], pertaining to a health professional or health facility that is formally recognized by an appropriate agency or organization as meeting certain standards of professional competence.

qualitative /kwol'itā'tiv/ [L *qualis*], of or pertaining to the quality, value, or nature of something.

qualitative analysis [L *qualis* what kind; Gk *analysis* a loosening], **1.** (in chemistry) the study of a sample of material to determine what chemical substances are present. **2.** (in research) analysis and interpretation of data that cannot be analyzed by statistical methods.

qualitative melanin test, a test for detecting melanin in the urine of patients with malignant melanomas.

qualitative test, a test that determines the presence or absence of a substance.

quality /kwol'itē/ [L *qualis*], (in radiotherapy) a descriptive specification of the penetrating ability of the x-ray beam as influenced by kilovoltage and filtration. Kilovoltage produces more penetration. Filtration removes the "softer" wavelengths and "hardens" the beam.

quality assessment measures, formal, systematic, organizational evaluation of overall patterns or programs of care, including clinical, consumer, and systems evaluation.

quality assurance, (in health care) any evaluation of services provided and the results achieved as compared with accepted standards.

quality assurance program, a system of review of selected hospital medical records by medical staff members, performed for the purposes of evaluating the quality and effectiveness of medical care in relation to accepted standards.

quality factor, (in radiotherapy) evaluation of the biologic damage that radiation can produce. In the field of radiation protection, biologically equivalent doses are set equal to one another by multiplying the actual absorbed dose by a number called the quality factor.

quality of life, a measure of the optimum energy or force that endows a person with the power to cope successfully with the full range of challenges encountered in the real world. The term applies to all individuals, regardless of illness or handicap, on the job, at home, or in leisure activities. Quality enrichment methods can include activities that reduce boredom and allow a maximum amount of freedom in choosing and performing various tasks.

quantitative /kwon'titā'tiv/ [L *quantus* how much], capable of being measured.

quantitative analysis, 1. (in chemistry) the determination of the amounts of constituents in a sample of material. Kinds of quantitative analysis include **gravimetric, volumetric,** and **spectrophotometric analysis. 2.** (in research) the use of statistical methods to analyze data.

quantitative inheritance. See **multifactorial inheritance.**

quantitative test, a test that determines the amount of a substance per unit volume or unit weight.

quantum mechanics. See **quantum theory.**

quantum mottle. See **mottle.**

quantum theory /kwon'təm/ [L *quantus* + Gk *theoria* speculation], (in physics) a theory dealing with the interaction of matter and electromagnetic radiation, particularly at the atomic and subatomic levels, according to which radiation consists of small units of energy called quanta.

quarantine /kwor′əutēn′/ [It *quarantina* forty], **1.** isolation of people with communicable disease or of those exposed to communicable disease during the contagious period in an attempt to prevent spread of the illness. **2.** the practice of detaining travelers or vessels coming from places of epidemic disease, originally for 40 days, for the purpose of inspection or disinfection.

quart (qt) /kwôrt/ [L *quartus* one fourth], a unit of volume fluid measure equivalent to one-fourth gallon, two pints, 32 ounces, or 946.24 milliliters. The British Imperial quart is equal to 1.136 liters amd the American quart for dry measure is 1.101 liters.

quartan /kwôr′tən/ [L *quartanus* relating to the fourth], recurring on the fourth day, or at about 72-hour intervals.

quartan malaria, a form of malaria, caused by the protozoan *Plasmodium malariae,* characterized by febrile paroxysms that occur every 72 hours.

quaternary /kwot′əner′ē, kwətur′nərē/ [L *quattuor* four], pertaining to a chemical compound in which four atoms or groups are elements or four substitutions on one atom.

quarternary ammonium derivative, a substance whose chemical structure has four carbon groups attached to a nitrogen atom. It is usually a strong base, highly water soluble but relatively insoluble in lipids.

quartile /kwôr′təl, kwôr′tīl/ [L *quartus* one fourth], one fourth of the distribution of scores. The 1st quartile would be the lowest 25% of scores, the 2nd quartile would represent the 26% to 50% range of scores, and so on.

quartz silicosis. See **silicosis.**

Queckenstedt's test /kwek′ənstets/ [Hans H. G. Queckenstedt, German physician, b. 1876], a test for an obstruction in the spinal canal in which the jugular veins on each side of the neck are compressed alternately. Normally, occlusion of the veins of the neck causes an immediate rise in spinal fluid pressure; if the vertebral canal is blocked, no rise occurs.

Queensland tick typhus, an infection caused by *Rickettsia australis,* occurring in Australia, transmitted by ticks, and resembling mild Rocky Mountain spotted fever.

quellung reaction /kwel′ung/ [Ger *quellung* swelling; L *re* again, *agere* to act], the swelling of the capsule of a bacterium, seen in the laboratory when the organism is exposed to specific antisera. This phenomenon is used to identify the genera, species, or subspecies of the bacteria causing a disease.

Quengle cast /kwen′gəl/, a two-section, hinged orthopedic cast for immobilizing the lower extremities from the foot or ankle to below the knee and the upper thigh to a level just above the knee. The two parts of the cast are connected by special hinges at knee level.

quercetin /kwur′sitin/, a yellow, crystalline, flavonoid pigment found in oak bark, the juice of lemons, asparagus, and other plants. It is used to reduce abnormal capillary fragility.

querulous paranoia /kwer′(y)ələs/ [L *queri* to complain; Gk *para* beside, *nous* mind], a form of paranoia characterized by extreme discontent and habitual complaining, usually about imagined slights by others.

Quervain's disease /kervānz′, kerveNz′/ [Fritz de Quervain, Swiss surgeon, b. 1868; L *dis;* Fr *aise* ease], chronic tenosynovitis of the abductor pollicis longus and extensor pollicis brevis muscles of the thumb.

quick connect [ME *quic* living; L *connectere* to bind], a plastic or similar connecting device that is attached to or implanted in a patient who will be joined to an electromechanical or other apparatus.

quickening /kwik′(ə)ning/ [ME *quic* living], the first feeling by a pregnant woman of movement of her baby in utero, usually occurring between 16 and 20 weeks of gestation.

Quick's test [Armand J. Quick, American physician, b. 1894] **1.** a test for jaundice. The patient is given an oral dose of sodium benzoate, which is conjugated in the liver with glycine to form hippuric acid. The amount of hippuric acid excreted in the urine is inversely proportional to the degree of liver damage. **2.** a test for hemophilia. A solution of thromboplastin is added to oxalated blood plasma and calcium chloride. The amount of time required for formation of a firm clot is inversely proportional to the amount of prothrombin in the plasma.

Quigley traction /kwig′lē/, a type of traction for lateral malleolar and trimalleolar fractures in which a stockinette is placed around the leg and ankle and is attached to an overhead frame, thus suspending the leg by the ankle.

quinacrine hydrochloride /kī′nəkrēn/, an anthelmintic and an antimalarial. It is prescribed in the treatment of giardiasis and cestodiasis and in the treatment and suppression of malaria.

Quincke's disease /kwing'kēz/ [Heinrich I. Quincke, German physician, b. 1842], angioneurotic edema, a potentially fatal chronic condition of subcutaneous edema, abdominal pain, urticaria, and laryngeal edema.

Quincke's pulse [Heinrich I. Quincke], an abnormal alternate blanching and reddening of the skin that may be observed in several ways, as by pressing the front edge of the fingernail and watching the blood in the nail bed recede and return.

quinethazone /kwəneth'əzōn/, a diuretic and antihypertensive prescribed in the treatment of hypertension and edema.

quinidine /kwin'əden, -din/, an antiarrhythmic agent used as a bisulfate, gluconate, polygalacturonate, or sulfate. It is prescribed in the treatment of atrial flutter, atrial fibrillation, premature ventricular contractions, and tachycardias.

quinidine gluconate. See **quinidine**.

quinine /kwī'nīn/ [Sp *quina* bark], a white, bitter crystalline alkaloid, made from cinchona bark, used in antimalarial medications.

quinine dihydrochloride, an antimalarial.

quinine sulfate, an antimalarial with antipyretic, analgesic, and muscle relaxant activity. It is prescribed in the treatment of malaria, particularly malaria caused by *Plasmodium falciparum,* and nocturnal leg cramps.

quinolone /kwin'əlōn/, any of a class of antibiotics that act by interrupting the replication of DNA molecules in bacteria.

quinsy. See **peritonsillar abscess**.

quintan /kwin'tən/ [L *quintanus* relating to the fifth], recurring on the fifth day, or at about 96-hour intervals.

quintana fever. See **trench fever**.

quintessence /kwintes'əns/ [L *quinta essentia* the fifth essence], **1.** a highly concentrated extract of any substance. **2.** a tincture or extract containing the most essential components of plant materials.

quintuplet /kwin'tooplit, kwintoo'plit/ [L *quintuplex* fivefold], any one of five offspring born of the same gestation period during a single pregnancy.

quotid. See **q.d.**

q.v., 1. abbreviation for the Latin phrase, *quantum vis,* "as much as you please." **2.** abbreviation for the Latin phrase, *quod vide,* "which see."

Q wave, the component of the QRS complex shown on an electrocardiogram as a short downward deflection preceding an R wave.

r, 1. abbreviation for *right.* 2. symbol for *resistance ohm.*

R, 1. abbreviation for **metabolic respiratory quotient.** 2. abbreviation for **resolution.** 3. abbreviation for **respiratory exchange ratio** 4. abbreviation for **roentgen.** 5. symbol for **gas constant.**

R$_f$, symbol for a ratio used in paper chromatography and thin-layer chromatography, representing the distance from the origin to the center of the separated zone divided by the distance from the origin to the solvent front. 2. abbreviation for **radiofrequency.**

R$_i$, symbol for *inhibitory receptor* molecule.

R$_s$, symbol for *stimulatory receptor* molecule.

R$_x$, symbol for the Latin, *recipe,* "take."

Ra, symbol for the element **radium.**

RA, 1. abbreviation for **rheumatoid arthritis.** 2. abbreviation for *right atrium.*

rabbit fever. See **tularemia.**

rabbit test. See **Friedman's test.**

rabid /rab′id/ [L *rabidus* raving], pertaining to or suffering from rabies, displaying signs of madness, agitation, delirium, hallucinations, and bizarre behavior.

rabies /rā′bēz/ [L *rabere* to rave], an acute, usually fatal viral disease of the central nervous system of animals. It is transmitted from animals to people by infected blood, tissue, or, most commonly, saliva. The reservoir of the virus is chiefly wild animals, including skunks, bats, foxes, dogs, raccoons, and cats. After introduction into the human body, often by a bite of an infected animal, the virus travels along nerve pathways to the brain and, later, to other organs. An incubation period ranges from 10 days to 1 year and is followed by a prodromal period characterized by fever, malaise, headache, paresthesia, and myalgia. After several days, severe encephalitis, delirium, agonizingly painful muscular spasms, seizures, paralysis, coma, and death ensue. **–rabid** /rab′id/, *adj.*

rabies immune globulin (RIG), a solution of antirabies immune globulin used in conjunction with rabies duck embryo vaccine for possible protection against rabies

in persons suspected of exposure to rabies.

rabies vaccine (DEV), a sterile suspension of killed rabies virus prepared from duck embryo. It is prescribed for immunization and postexposure prophylaxis against rabies.

rabies virus group [L *rabere* to rave, *virus* poison; It *gruppo* knot], the genus of viruses that includes the organism that causes rabies in humans, the *lyssa* virus.

race [It *razza*], a vague, unscientific term for a group of genetically related people who share certain physical characteristics. 2. a distinct ethnic group characterized by traits that are transmitted through their offspring.

racemic /rāse′mik/ [L *racemus* bunch of grapes], pertaining to a compound made up of levorotatory isomers, rendering it optically inactive under polarized light.

racemic epinephrine, a mixture of two isomers of epinephrine. It is a less potent form of epinephrine, with fewer side effects, and is used as an aerosol in the treatment of acute croup.

racemose /ras′əmōs′/ [L *racemus*], like a bunch of grapes. The term is used in describing a structure in which many branches terminate in nodular, cystlike forms, such as pulmonary alveoli.

racemose aneurysm, a pronounced dilatation of lengthened and tortuous blood vessels, some of which may be distended to 20 times their normal size.

rachial [/rā′kē-əl/ Gk *rhachis* backbone], pertaining to the spinal column.

rachiopagus /rā′kē-op′əgəs/ [Gk *rachis* backbone, *pagos* fixed], conjoined symmetric twins that are united back to back along the spinal column.

rachischisis /rəkis′kəsis/ [Gk *rachis* + *schizein* to split], a congenital fissure of one or more vertebrae.

rachischisis totalis. See **complete rachischisis.**

rachitic /rəkit′ik/, 1. of or pertaining to rickets. 2. resembling or suggesting the condition of one afflicted with rickets.

rachitic dwarf, a person whose retarded growth is caused by rickets.

rachitis /rəkī′tis/ [Gk *rachis* + *itis* inflammation] 1. rickets. 2. an inflammatory disease of the vertebral column.

rachitis fetalis annularis, congenital enlargement of the epiphyses of the long bones.

rachitis fetalis micromelia, congenital shortening of the long bones.

racial immunity /rā′shəl/ [It *razza;* L *immunis* freedom], a form of natural immunity shared by most of the members of a genetically related population.

racial unconscious. See **collective unconscious.**

rad /rad/, abbreviation for **radiation absorbed dose;** the basic unit of absorbed dose of ionizing radiation. One rad is equal to the absorption of 100 ergs of radiation energy per gram of matter.

radarkymography /rā′därkĭmog′rəfē/ [radar + Gk *kyma* wave, *graphein* to record], a radar (radio detection and ranging) technique for showing the size and outline of the heart, using a radar tracking device and a fluoroscopic screen to display images produced by electric impulses passed over the chest surface.

Radford nomogram, a mathematical chart device used in respiratory therapy to estimate combined tidal volumes and rates for mechanical ventilation. It is based on three parameters of body weight, sex, and respiratory rate.

radial /rā′dē·əl/ [L *radius* wheel spoke], pertaining to the radius.

radial artery [L *radius* ray], an artery in the forearm, starting at the bifurcation of the brachial artery and passing in 12 branches to the forearm, wrist, and hand.

radial keratotomy, a surgical procedure in which a series of tiny shallow incisions are made on the cornea, causing it to bulge slightly to correct for nearsightedness.

radial nerve, the largest branch of the brachial plexus, arising on each side as a continuation of the posterior cord. It supplies the skin of the arm and forearm and their extensor muscles.

radial nerve palsy, a compression or entrapment neuropathy involving the radial nerve. Symptoms of muscle weakness and sensory loss are due to compression of the radial nerve against the humerus.

radial notch of ulna, the narrow, lateral depression in the coronoid process of the ulna that receives the head of the radius.

radial paralysis, musculospiral paralysis involving muscles supplied by the radial nerve, mainly the wrist and finger extensors.

radial pulse, the pulse of the radial artery palpated at the wrist over the radius. The radial pulse is the one most often taken, because of the ease with which it is palpated.

radial recurrent artery, a branch of the radial artery, arising just distal to the elbow, ascending between the branches of the radial nerve, and supplying several muscles of the arm and the elbow.

radial reflex, a normal reflex elicited by tapping over the distal radius, with the response being flexion of the forearm.

radiant [L *radiare* to shine], pertaining to any object that emits rays or is the center of rays that spread outward.

radiant energy [L *radiare* to emit rays; Gk *energeia*], the energy emitted by electromagnetic radiation, such as radio waves, visible light, x-rays, and gamma rays.

radiate /rā′ē·āt/ [L *radiare* to emit rays], to diverge or spread from a common point.

radiate ligament, a ligament that connects the head of a rib with a vertebra and an associated intervertebral disk.

radiation /rā′dē-āshən/ [L *radiatio*], **1.** the emission of energy, rays, or waves. **2.** (in medicine) the use of a radioactive substance in the diagnosis or treatment of disease.

radiation absorbed dose (rad), a unit of absorbed dose of ionizing radiation. One rad is equal to 0.01 J/kg, or 100 ergs of ionizing radiation per gram of tissue of other substance.

radiation burn, a burn resulting from exposure to radiant energy in the form of sunlight, x-rays, or nuclear emissions or explosion. Ionizing radiation can produce tissue damage directly by striking a vital molecule such as DNA.

radiation caries, tooth decay caused by ionizing radiation of the oral and maxillary structure. Radiation caries is often a side effect of treatment for oral malignancies.

radiation cataract [L *radiare;* Gk *katarrhaktes* portcullis], a cataract caused by excessive exposure of the eye to x-rays or other types of radiation that cause a change in the protein molecules of the lens.

radiation dermatitis [L *radiare;* Gk *derma* skin, *itis*], an acute or chronic inflammation of the skin due to exposure to ionizing radiation, as in cancer radiation therapy. Symptoms, which may not appear until three weeks after exposure, include redness, blistering, and sloughing of the skin. In severe cases the condition can progress to scarring, fibrosis, and atrophy.

radiation detector, a device for converting radiant energy to an observable form, used for detecting the presence and sometimes the amount of radiation.

Radiation Effects Research Foundation (RERF), an organization that studies the long-term effects of survivors of atomic bombings of Hiroshima and Nagasaki during World War II. The RERF is successor to the Atomic Bomb Casualty Commission.

radiation exposure, a measure of the ionization produced in air by x-rays or gamma rays. It is the sum of the electric charges on all ions of one sign that are produced when all electrons liberated by photons in a volume of air are completely stopped, divided by the mass of air in the volume element. The unit of exposure is the roentgen.

radiation hygiene, the art and science of protecting human beings from injury by radiation by seeking to reduce clinical exposure from external radiation through protective barriers of radiation-absorbing material, ensuring safe distances between people and radiation sources, reducing radiation exposure times, or employing combinations of all these measures.

radiation oncologist, a physician with special training in the use of ionizing radiation in the treatment of cancers.

radiation oncology, the treatment of cancer using radiation.

radiation protection, employment of devices, equipment, distance, and barriers to reduce the risk of exposure to ionizing radiation in a health care facility, research center, or industrial site where radiation-emitting devices are used. The risk also varies with the type and intensity of radiation.

radiation sensitivity, a measure of the response of tissue to ionizing radiation.

radiation sickness, an abnormal condition resulting from exposure to ionizing radiation. Moderate exposure may cause headache, nausea, vomiting, anorexia, and diarrhea; long-term exposure may result in sterility, damage to the fetus in pregnant women, leukemia or other forms of cancer, alopecia, and cataracts.

radiation symbol, a universal symbol consisting of a "purple propeller" pattern of three fan-shaped images arranged at positions 120 degrees apart as if radiating from a solid dark circle on a yellow background. The symbol is intended to identify sources or containers of radioactive materials and areas of potential radiation exposure.

radiation syndrome. See **radiation sickness.**

radiation therapy. See **radiotherapy.**

radiation therapy technologist, an allied health professional who administers radiation therapy services to patients, observing patients during treatment, and maintaining records. Duties may include tumor localization, dosimetry, patient follow-up, and patient education.

radical /rad′ikəl/ [L *radix* root], **1.** a group of atoms that acts together and forms a component of a compound. The group tends to remain bound together when a chemical reaction removes it from a compound and attaches it to another. A radical does not exist freely in nature. **2.** pertaining to drastic therapy, such as the surgical removal of an organ, limb, or other part of the body.

radical dissection, the surgical removal of tissue in an extensive area surrounding the operative site. Most often it is performed to identify and excise all tissue that may possibly be malignant to decrease the chance of recurrence.

radical mastectomy, surgical removal of an entire breast, pectoral muscles, axillary lymph nodes, and all fat, fascia, and adjacent tissues. It is performed in the treatment of cancer of the breast. Chemotherapy and radiation therapy may continue after surgery. The woman is told never to allow blood to be drawn from the affected arm; intravenous injection is also to be avoided in that arm.

radical neck dissection, dissection and removal of all lymph nodes and removable tissues under the skin of the neck, performed to prevent the spread of malignant tumors of the head and neck that have a reasonable chance of being controlled.

radical surgery [L *radix* root; Gk *cheirourgos* surgeon], surgery that is usually extensive and complex and intended to correct a severe health threat such as a rapidly growing cancer.

radical therapy, 1. a treatment intended to cure, not palliate. **2.** a definitive, extreme treatment; not conservative, such as radical mastectomy rather than simple or partial mastectomy.

radical vulvectomy. See **vulvectomy.**

radicular /rədik′yələr/ [L *radix* root], pertaining to a root, such as a spinal nerve root.

radicular cyst [L *radicula* small root; Gk *kystis* bag], (in dentistry) a cyst with a wall of fibrous connective tissue and a lining of stratified squamous epithelium that is attached to the apex of the root of a tooth with dead pulp or a defective root canal filling.

radicular retainer, a type of retainer that lies within the body of a tooth, usually in the root portion, such as a dowel crown.

radicular retention, retention developed by placing metal projections into the root canals of pulpless teeth.

radiculitis /rədik′yəlī′tis/, an inflammation involving a spinal nerve root, resulting in pain and hyperesthesia.

R

radiculopathy /rədik′yəlop′əthē/, a disease involving a spinal nerve root.

radioactive /rā′dē-ō/-ak′tiv/ [L *radius* ray, *activus* active], giving off radiation as the result of the disintegration of the nucleus of an atom.

radioactive contamination, the undesirable addition of radioactive material to the body or part of the environment, such as clothing or equipment. Beta radiation contamination of the body of health care personnel is only possible through the ingestion, inhalation, or absorption of the source, as when the skin is contaminated with a beta emitter contained in an absorbable chemical form. Instruments, drapes, surgical gloves, and clothing that come in contact with serous fluids, blood, and urine of patients containing beta or gamma radiation emitters may be contaminated.

radioactive contrast media, a solution or colloid containing material of high atomic number, used for visualizing soft tissue structures.

radioactive decay, the disintegration of the nucleus of an unstable nuclide by the spontaneous emission of charged particles, photons, or both.

radioactive element, an element subject to spontaneous degeneration of its nucleus accompanied by the emission of alpha particles, beta particles, or gamma rays. All elements with atomic numbers greater than 83 are radioactive.

radioactive half-life. See half-life.

radioactive iodine (RAI), a radioactive isotope of iodine, used as a tracer in biology and medicine.

radioactive iodine excretion, the elimination by the body of radioactive iodine (RAI) administered in a test of thyroid function and in the treatment of hyperthyroidism.

radioactive iodine excretion test, a method of evaluating thyroid function by measuring the amount of radioactive iodine (RAI) in urine after the patient is given an oral tracer dose of the radioisotope ^{131}I. After administration of the tracer, a scintillation detector is placed over the patient's neck at 2, 6, and 24 hours to measure the RAI accumulated by the thyroid.

radioactive iodine uptake (RAIU), the absorption and incorporation by the thyroid of radioactive iodine (RAI), administered orally as a tracer dose in a test of thyroid function and as larger doses for the treatment of hyperthyroidism.

radioactive tracer, a molecule to which a radioactive atom, or tag, has been attached so that it can be followed through a physiologic system with radiation detectors.

radioactivity /-aktiv′itē/, the emission of corpuscular alpha or beta or electromagnetic gamma radiations as a consequence of nuclear disintegration.

radioallergosorbent test (RAST) /rā′dē-ō·alur′gōsôr′bənt/ [L *radius* + Gk *allos* other, *ergein* to work; L *absorbere* to swallow], a test in which a radioimmunoassay is used to identify and quantify IgE in serum that has been mixed with any of 45 known allergens. If an atopic allergy to a substance exists, an antigen-antibody reaction occurs with characteristic conjugation and clumping.

radiobiology /-bō·ol′əjē/ [L *radius* + *bios* life, *logos* science], the branch of the natural sciences dealing with the effects of radiation on biological systems. **–radiobiologic, radiobiological,** *adj.*

radiocarpal articulation /-kär′pəl/ [L *radius* + Gk *karpos* wrist], the condyloid joint at the wrist that connects the radius and distal surface of an articular disk with the scaphoid, the lunate, and the triangular bones. The joint involves four ligaments and allows all movements but rotation.

radiochemistry /-kem′istrē/ [L *radius* + Gk *chemiea* alchemy], the branch of chemistry that deals with the properties and behavior of radioactive materials and the use of radionuclides in the study of chemical and biological problems.

radiocurable /-kyōō′rəbəl/, the susceptibility of tumor cells to destruction by ionizing radiation.

radiofrequency (rf) [L *radius* + *frequens*], that portion of the electromagnetic spectrum with frequencies lower than about 10^{10} Hz.

radiofrequency ablation, /-frē′kwənsē/, unmodulated high-frequency alternating current flow that is applied to tissue to cause heat and cell injury for the purpose of destroying troublesome areas and pathways to the heart. The technique has replaced surgical ablation.

radiograph /rā′dē-əgraf′/, an x-ray image.

radiographer /rā′dē-og′rəfər/, an allied health professional who provides patient services using radiographic imaging modalities as directed by a physician. Duties may include processing of film, evaluating radiologic equipment, managing a radiographic quality assurance program, and providing patient education relevant to specific imaging procedures.

radiographic grid /-graf′ik/, a device used to reduce the amount of scatter radiation reaching the radiographic film.

Grids are fabricated using parallel strips of radiopaque materials with alternating strips of radiolucent materials.

radiographic magnification, a radiographic procedure to improve visualization of fine blood vessels and small bony structures. Magnification is achieved by increasing the distance of the object from the radiographic image receptor.

radiography /rā′dē·og′rəfē/ [L *radius* + Gk *graphein* to record], the production of shadow images on photographic emulsion through the action of ionizing radiation. **–radiographic,** *adj.*

radioimmunoassay (RIA) /-im′yənō·as′ā/ [L *radius* + *immunis* freedom; Fr *essayer* to try], a technique in radiology used to determine the concentration of an antigen, antibody, or other protein in the serum.

radioimmunosorbent assay test /-im′-yənōsôr′bənt/ [L *radius, immunis* + *absorbere* to swallow], a test that uses serum immunoglobulin E to detect allergies to various substances, such as certain cosmetics, animal fur, dust, and grasses.

radioiodine /rā′dē·ō·ī′ədin/ [L *radius* + Gk *ioeides* violet], a radioactive isotope of iodine used in radiotherapy. A common form of radioiodine is ^{131}I.

radioisotope /rā′dē·ō·ī′sətōp/ [L *radius* + Gk *isos* equal, *topos* place], a radioactive isotope of an element, used for therapeutic and diagnostic purposes.

radioisotope scan, a two-dimensional representation of the gamma rays emitted by a radioisotope, showing its concentration in a body site, such as the thyroid gland, brain, or kidney.

radiologic anatomy /-loj′ik/ [L *radius* + Gk *logos* science], (in applied anatomy) the study of the structure and morphology of the tissues and organs of the body based on their x-ray visualization.

radiologic technologist, a person who, under the supervision of a physician radiologist, operates radiologic equipment and assists radiologists and other health professionals, and whose competence has been tested and approved by the American Registry of Radiologic Technologists.

radiologist /rā′dē·ol′əjist/, a physician who specializes in radiology. A certified radiologist is one whose competence has been tested and approved by the American Board of Radiology.

radiology /-ol′əjē/ [L *radius* + *logos* science], the branch of medicine concerned with radioactive substances and, using various techniques of visualization, with the diagnosis and treatment of disease using any of the various sources of radiant energy. Three subbranches of radiology are **diagnostic radiology,** which concerns

itself with imaging using external sources of radiation; **nuclear medicine,** which is involved with imaging radioactive materials that are placed into body organs; and **therapeutic radiology,** which is concerned with the treatment of cancer using radiation. **–radiologic, radiological,** *adj.*

radiolucency /loo′sənsē/ [L *radius* + *lucere* to shine], a characteristic of materials of relatively low atomic number that attenuates x-rays passing through them and produces relatively dark images. **–radiolucent,** *adj.*

radionecrosis /-nəkrō′sis/, tissue death caused by radiation.

radionuclide /-noo′klīd/ [L *radius* + *nucleus* nut kernel] **1.** an isotope (or nuclide) that undergoes radioactive decay. **2.** any of the radioactive isotopes of cobalt, iodine, phosphorus, strontium, and other elements, used in nuclear medicine for treatment of tumors and cancers and for nuclear imaging of internal parts of the body.

radionuclide angiocardiography, the radiographic examination of cardiac blood vessels after an intravenous injection of a radiopharmaceutic.

radionuclide imaging, the noninvasive examination of various parts of the body, especially the heart, using a radiopharmaceutic, such as thallium 201, and a detection device, such as a gamma camera, rectilinear scanner, or positron camera.

radionuclide organ imaging. See **nuclear scanning.**

radiopacity /-pas′itē/, the quality of being radiopaque, or having the ability to stop or reduce the passage of x-radiation.

radiopaque /-pāk′/ [L *radius* + *opacus* obscure], not permitting the passage of x-rays or other radiant energy. Bones are relatively radiopaque and therefore show as white areas on an exposed x-ray film. **–radiopacity,** *n.*

radiopaque dye, a chemical substance that does not permit the passage of x-rays. Various radiopaque iodine compounds are used to outline the interior of hollow organs such as heart chambers, blood vessels, respiratory passages, and the biliary tract in x-ray or fluoroscopic pictures.

radiopharmaceutic, radiopharmaceutical /-fär′məsoo′tik/ [L *radius* + Gk *pharmakeuein* to give a drug], a drug that contains radioactive atoms. Kinds of radiopharmaceutics are **diagnostic radiopharmaceutics, research radiopharmaceutics,** and **therapeutic radiopharmaceutics.**

radiopharmacist /-fär′məsist/, a trained professional responsible for the formula-

R

tion and dispensing of prescribed radioactive tracers and for the clinical aspects of radiopharmacy. Some states require that radioactive drugs be dispensed by licensed pharmacists only; others recognize radiopharmaceutical specialists who are not necessarily graduates of a school of pharmacy.

radiopharmacy /-fär′məsē/ [L *radius* + Gk *pharmakeuein* to give a drug], a facility for the preparation and dispensing of radioactive drugs and for the storage of radioactive materials, inventory records, and prescriptions of radioactive substances.

radioprotective drugs /-prətek′tiv/, pharmaceuticals that protect the body against ionizing radiation. An example is Lugol's solution, an aqueous solution of iodine used to supply iodine internally, thereby blocking the uptake of radioactive iodine.

radioresistance /-risis′təns/ [L *radius* + *resistare* to withstand], the relative resistance of cells, tissues, organs, organisms, chemical compounds, or any other substances to the effects of radiation.

radioresistant /risis′tənt/, unchanged by or protected against damage by radioactive emissions such as x-rays, alpha particles, or gamma rays.

radioresponsive /-rispon′siv/, pertaining to the sensitivity of a chemical or tissue to radiation, whether harmful or beneficial.

radiosensitive /-sen′sitiv/ [L *radius* + *sentire* to feel], capable of being changed by or reacting to radioactive emissions such as x-rays, alpha particles, or gamma rays.

radiosensitivity /sen′sitiv′itē/, the relative susceptibility of cells, tissues, organs, organisms, or any other living substances to the effects of radiation. Cells of self-renewing systems, as those in the crypts of the intestine, are the most radiosensitive. Cells that divide regularly but mature between divisions, such as spermatogonia and spermatocytes, are next in radiosusceptibility. Long-lived cells that usually do not undergo mitosis unless there is a suitable stimulus include the less radiosensitive liver, kidney, and thyroid cells. Least sensitive are fixed postmitotic cells that have lost the ability to divide, such as neurons.

radiosensitizers /-sen′sitī′zərs/ [L *radius, sentire* + Gk *izein* to cause], drugs that enhance the killing effect of radiation of cells.

radiotherapy /-ther′əpē/ [Gk *radius* + Gk *therapeia* treatment], the treatment of neoplastic disease by using x-rays or gamma rays, usually from a cobalt source, to deter the proliferation of malignant cells by decreasing the rate of mitosis or impairing DNA synthesis.

radioulnar articulation /-ul′nər/ [L *radius* + *ulna* elbow], the articulation of the radius and the ulna, consisting of a proximal articulation, a distal articulation, and three sets of ligaments.

radium (Ra) /rā′dē·im/ [L *radius* ray], a radioactive metallic element of the alkaline earth group. Its atomic number is 88. Four radium isotopes occur naturally and have different atomic weights: 223, 224, 226, and 228.

radium insertion, the introduction of metallic radium (Ra) into a body area, such as the uterus or cervix, to treat cancer.

radium therapy, the use of radium and its radioactive emissions to treat disease.

radium 226, a radioactive substance used to fill the needles and tubes required for brachytherapy.

radius /rā′dē·əs/, *pl.* **radii** /rā′dē·ī/ [L, ray], one of the bones of the forearm, lying parallel to the ulna. Its proximal end is small and forms a part of the elbow joint. The distal end is large and forms a part of the wrist joint.

radix. See **root.**

radon (Rn) /rā′don/ [L *radiare* to emit rays], a radioactive, inert, gaseous, nonmetallic element. Its atomic number is 86; its atomic weight is 222. Radon, a decay product of radium, is used in radiation cancer therapy.

radon daughters, electrically charged ions that are decay products of radon gas. Radon daughters are regarded as a potential health hazard by the Environmental Protection Agency (EPA) because they tend to adhere to surfaces, such as alveoli of the lungs, where they can cause ionizing radiation damage. Radon is released by rocks, soil, and groundwater.

radon seed, a small sealed tube of glass or gold containing radon, and visible radiographically, for insertion into body tissues in the treatment of malignancies.

radon 222, the radioactive daughter of radium 226 that has been used to fill seeds for permanent implantation into tumors. This material is being replaced by the more manageable radionuclide iodine 125.

RAI, abbreviation for **radioactive iodine.**

RAIU, abbreviation for **radioactive iodine uptake.**

RA latex test, abbreviation for *rheumatoid arthritis latex test.*

rale [Fr, rattle], a common abnormal respiratory sound heard on auscultation of the chest during inspiration, characterized by discontinuous bubbling noises. Fine rales have a crackling sound produced by air entering distal bronchioles or alveoli that contain serous secretions, as in congestive heart failure, pneumonia, or early tuberculosis. Coarse rales originate in the larger bronchi or trachea and have a lower pitch. Kinds of rales are **sibilant rale** and **sonorous rale.**

ramification /ram'ifikē'shən/ [L *ramus* branch, *facere* to make], a branching, distribution.

Ramsay Hunt's syndrome [James Ramsay Hunt, American neurologist, b. 1874], a neurologic condition resulting from invasion of the seventh nerve ganglia and the geniculate ganglion by varicella zoster virus, characterized by severe ear pain, facial nerve paralysis, vertigo, hearing loss, and often mild, generalized encephalitis.

ramus /rā'məs/, *pl.* **rami** [L, branch], a small, branchlike structure extending from a larger one or dividing into two or more parts, such as a branch of a nerve or artery or one of the rami of the pubis. **–ramification,** *n.* **ramify,** *v.*

random controlled trial [ME *randoun* run violently; Fr *contrôle* check, *trier* to grind], a study plan for a proposed new treatment in which subjects are assigned on a random basis to participate either in an experimental group receiving the new treatment or in a control group that does not.

random genetic drift. See **genetic drift.**

randomization, the process of assigning subjects or objects to a control or experimental group on a random basis.

random mating, a pairing on subjects when each individual has an equal chance of mating with those of other genetic backgrounds.

random sampling, a method of sampling for a study in which each individual has the same chance of being selected and the choice of a particular individual does not affect the chances of the others.

random selection, a method of choosing subjects for a research study in which all members of a particular group have an equal chance of being selected.

random voided specimen, a voided urine specimen obtained at any point of a 24-hour period.

range /rānj/ [OFr *ranger* to arrange in a row], the interval between the lowest and the highest values in a series of data.

range of accommodation, the distance between the farthest point that an object can be seen clearly with accommodation fully relaxed and the nearest distance that an object can be seen with full accommodation, measured in inches or centimeters.

range of motion (ROM), the range of movement of a joint, from maximum extension to maximum flexion, as measured in degrees of a circle.

range of motion exercise [Fr *rang* rank; L

motio movement], any body action involving the muscles, the joints, and natural directional movements, such as abduction, extension, flexion, pronation, and rotation.

ranitidine /ranit'idēn/, a histamine H_2-receptor anatgonist prescribed in the treatment of duodenal and gastric ulcers and gastric hypersecretory conditions.

Rankine scale [William J. M. Rankine, Scottish physicist, b. 1820], an absolute temperature scale calculated in degrees Fahrenheit. Absolute zero on the Rankine scale is $-460°$ F, equivalent to $-273°$ C.

ranula /ran'yōōlə/, *pl.* **ranulae** [L *rana* frog], a large mucocele in the floor of the mouth, usually caused by obstruction of the ducts of the sublingual salivary glands and less commonly by obstruction of the ducts of the submandibular salivary glands.

Ranvier's nodes /ränvē-āz', räN-/ [Louis A. Ranvier, French pathologist, b. 1835], constrictions in the medullary substance of a nerve fiber at more or less regular intervals.

rape [L *rapere* to seize], a sexual assault, homosexual or heterosexual, the legal definitions for which vary from state to state. Rape is a crime of violence or one committed under the threat of violence, and its victims are treated for medical and psychologic trauma.

rape counseling, counseling by a trained person provided to a victim of rape. Rape counseling usually begins at the time the crime is first reported, as in an emergency room. Initially, the counselor offers sensitive support for the victim by accepting the victim in a nonprejudicial, noncritical way. Counseling personnel may provide supportive services and advocacy and liaison between the victim and medical, legal, and law enforcement authorities. This involves staying with the victim during medical examination, police or district attorney's questioning, and throughout the criminal justice process.

rape-trauma syndrome, a NANDA-accepted nursing diagnosis of forced, violent sexual penetration against the victim's will and consent. The trauma syndrome includes an acute phase of disorganization and a longer phase of reorganization in the victim's life. Defining characteristics are divided into three subcomponents: **rape trauma, compound reaction,** and **silent reaction. Rape trauma** in the acute phase includes emotional reactions of anger, guilt, and embarrassment, fear of physical violence and death, humiliation, wish for revenge, and multiple physical complaints. The long-term phase includes changes in

R

the usual patterns of daily life, nightmares and phobias, and a need for support from friends and family. The **compound reaction** includes all of the defining characteristics of rape trauma, reliance on alcohol or drugs, or the recurrence of the symptoms of previous conditions. The **silent reaction** sometimes occurs in place of the rape trauma or compound reaction. Defining characteristics of the silent reaction are an abrupt change in the victim's usual sexual relationships, an increase in nightmares, an increasing anxiety during the interview about the rape incident, a marked change in sexual behavior, denial of the rape or refusal to discuss it, and the sudden development of phobic reactions.

raphe /rā′fē/ [Gk rhaphe seam], a line of union of the halves of various symmetric parts, such as the abdominal raphe of the linea alba or the raphe penis, which appears as a narrow, dark streak on the inferior surface.

raphe of tongue [Gk rhaphe; AS tunge], a fibrous wall that forms a line of union between the right and left sides of the tongue.

rapid-acting insulin. See **short-acting insulin.**

rapid eye movement. See **sleep.**

rapid pulse /rap′id/ [L rapidus rush, pulsare to beat], a pulse faster than normal.

rapport /rapôr′/ [Fr, agreement], a sense of mutuality and understanding; harmony, accord, confidence, and respect underlying a relationship between two persons, an essential bond between a therapist and patient in psychotherapy.

rapprochement /räprôshmäN′/ [Fr rapprocher to bring together], (in psychology) the third subphase of the separation-individuation phase of Mahler's system of preoedipal development. This stage is characterized by a rediscovery of mother after the initial separation of the practicing subphase.

raptus /rap′təs/ [L rapere to seize], 1. a state of intense emotional or mental excitement, often characterized by uncontrollable activity or behavior resulting from an irresistible impulse; ecstasy; rapture. 2. any sudden or violent seizure or attack.

rare earth element [L rarus thin; AS earthe; L elementum], a metallic element having an atomic number between 57 and 71, inclusively. These closely related substances are classified in three groups: the cerium metals, the terbium metals, and the yttrium metals.

rare earth screen, a fluorescent material, such as calcium tungstate, used as the basis of x-ray intensifying screens. Rare earths enable lower radiation doses to be used while producing acceptable film densities.

RAS, abbreviation for **reticular activating system.**

rash [OFr rasche scurf], a skin eruption. Kinds of rashes include **butterfly rash, diaper rash, drug rash,** and **heat rash.**

Rashkind procedure /rash′kind/ [William J. Rashkind, American physician, b. 1922; L procedere to go forth], the enlargement of an opening in the cardiac septum between the right and left atria, performed to relieve congestive heart failure in newborns with certain congenital heart defects by improving the oxygenation of the blood.

RAST. See **radioallergosorbent test.**

rat-bite fever [AS raet; bitan to bite], either of two distinct infections transmitted to humans by the bite of a rat or mouse, characterized by fever, headache, malaise, nausea, vomiting, and rash. In the United States the disease is more commonly caused by Streptobacillus moniliformis, and its unique features are rash on palms and soles, painful joints, prompt healing of the wound, and a duration of 2 weeks. Rat-bite fever resulting from infection caused by Streptobacillus moniliformis is also called **Haverhill fever;** infection caused by Spirillum minus is also called **sodoku.**

rate [L ratus to reckon], a numeric ratio, often used in the compilation of data concerning the prevalence and incidence of events, in which the number of actual occurrences appears as the numerator and the number of possible occurrences appears as the denominator. Standard rates are stated in conventional units of population, such as neonatal mortality per 1,000 or maternal mortality per 100,000.

rate-pressure product, the heart rate multiplied by the systolic blood pressure. It is a clinical indicator of myocardial oxygen demand.

Rathke's pouch /rät′kēz/, a depression that forms in the roof of the mouth of an embryo around the fourth week of gestation. The walls of the diverticulum develop into the anterior lobe of the pituitary gland.

Rathke's pouch tumor. See **craniopharyngioma.**

ratio /rā′shō/ [L, a reckoning], the relationship of one quantity to one or more other quantities expressed as a proportion of one to the others, and written either as a fraction (8/3) or linearly (8:3).

rational /rash′ənəl/ [L rationalis reasonable], 1. of or pertaining to a measure, method, or procedure based on reason. 2. of or pertaining to a therapeutic method based on an understanding of the cause and mechanisms of a specific disease and the potential effects of the drugs or procedures used in treating the disorder. **3.** sane; capable of normal reasoning or behavior.

rationale /rash'ənal'/ [L *rationalis*], a system of reasoning or a statement of the reasons used in explaining data or phenomena.

rational emotive therapy (RET), a form of psychotherapy, originated by Albert Ellis, that emphasizes a reorganization of one's cognitive and emotional functions, a redefinition of one's problems, and a change in one's attitudes to develop more effective and suitable patterns of behavior.

rationalization /rash'ənal'īzā'shən/, the most commonly used defense mechanism in which an individual justifies ideas, actions, or feelings with seemingly acceptable reasons or explanations. It is often used to preserve self-respect, reduce guilt feelings, or to obtain social approval or acceptance.

rational treatment. See **treatment.**

ratio solution, the relationship of a solute to a solvent expressed as a proportion, such as 1 : 100, or parts per thousand.

rattle [ME *ratelen*], an abnormal sound heard by auscultation of the lungs in some forms of pulmonary disease. It consists of a coarse vibration caused by the movement of moisture and the separation of the walls of small air passages during respiration.

rattlesnake [ME *ratelen* + AS *snacan* to creep], a poisonous pit viper with a series of loosely connected, horny segments at the end of the tail that make a noise like a rattle when shaken. More than 25 species of rattlesnakes are found in the Americas, including many parts of the United States. They have a hematoxin in their venom, and they are responsible for most of the poisonous snake bites in the United States.

rat typhus. See **murine typhus.**

rauwolfia /rôwol'fē-ə, rou-, rä-/ [Leonhard Rauwolf, sixteenth-century German botanist], the dried roots of *Rauwolfia serpentina* that provide the extracts for hypotensive agents and tranquilizing alkaloid drugs, such as reserpine.

rauwolfia alkaloid, any one of more than 20 alkaloids derived from the root of a climbing shrub, *Rauwolfia serpentina,* indigenous to India and the surrounding area. Formerly used as an antipsychotic agent, it is today confined to the treatment of hypertension.

rauwolfia serpentina, the dried root from *Rauwolfia serpentina,* used as an antihypertensive. It is prescribed in the treatment of mild hypertension and hypertensive emergencies.

raw data, (in magnetic resonance imaging) the information obtained by radio reception of the MR signal as stored by a computer. Specific computer manipulation of these data is required to construct an image from it.

ray [L *radius*], a beam of radiation, such as heat or light, moving away from a source.

Raynaud's phenomenon /rānōz'/ [Maurice Raynaud, French physician, b. 1834], intermittent attacks of ischemia of the extremities of the body, especially the fingers, toes, ears, and nose, caused by exposure to cold or by emotional stimuli. The attacks are characterized by severe blanching of the extremities, followed by cyanosis, then redness; they are usually accompanied by numbness, tingling, burning, and often pain. The condition is called **Raynaud's disease** when there is a history of symptoms for at least 2 years with no progression of symptoms and no evidence of an underlying cause.

Raynaud's sign. See **acrocyanosis.**

Rb, symbol for the element **rubidium.**

RBBB, abbreviation for **right bundle branch block.**

RBC, abbreviation for **red blood cell.**

RBE, abbreviation for **relative biologic effectiveness.**

RCP, abbreviation for **Royal College of Physicians.**

RCPSC, abbreviation for **Royal College of Physicians and Surgeons of Canada.**

RCS, abbreviation for **Royal College of Surgeons.**

RD, abbreviation for *registered dietician.*

RDA, abbreviation for **recommended dietary allowance.**

rdi, abbreviation for *reference daily intake.*

RDS, abbreviation for *respiratory distress syndrome.*

Re, symbol for the element **rhenium.**

reabsorption /rē'əbsôrp'shən/, the process of something being absorbed again, such as the removal of calcium from the bone back into the blood.

reacher /rē'chər/, a pair of extended tongs that can be used by persons with upper extremity disabilities to grasp objects on shelves and similar areas beyond their usual range.

Reach to Recovery [AS *reacan* to reach; ME *recoveren* to get back], a national volunteer organization that offers counseling and support to women who have breast cancer and to their families. Many of the members have had mastectomies themselves.

reaction /rē·ak'shən/ [L *re* again, *agere* to act], a response in opposition to a substance, treatment, or other stimulus, such as an antigen-antibody reaction in immunology, a hypersensitivity reaction in allergy, or an adverse reaction in pharmacology. **−react,** *v.,* **reactive,** *adj.*

reaction formation, a defense mechanism in which a person avoids anxiety through overt behavior and attitudes that are the opposite of repressed impulses and drives and that serve to conceal those unacceptable feelings.

reaction time, the interval between the application of a stimulus and the beginning of a response.

reactivate /rē·ak'tivāt/, to make active again, as in adding fresh serum to restore the potency of an original supply of the serum.

reactive decision /rē·ak'tiv/ [L *re + activus*], (in psychology) a decision made by an individual in response to the influence or goals of others.

reactive depression, an emotional disorder characterized by an acute feeling of despondency, sadness, and depressive dysphoria, which varies in intensity and duration. The condition is caused by an unrealistic and inappropriate reaction to some identifiable external situation or intrapsychic conflict and is relieved when the circumstance is altered or the conflict understood and resolved.

reactive inflammation, an inflammation that develops as a reaction to an antigen.

reactive schizophrenia, a form of schizophrenia caused by environmental factors rather than by organic changes in the brain. The onset of the disease is usually rapid; symptoms are of brief duration, and the affected individual appears well immediately before and after the schizophrenic episode.

reactor /rē·ak'tər/, 1. (in psychology) a family therapist who lets a family in therapy take the lead and then follows in that direction. 2. (in radiology) a cubicle in which radioisotopes are artificially produced.

reading [AS *raedan*], (in molecular genetics) the linear process in which the genetic information contained in a nucleotide sequence is decoded, as in the translation of the messenger RNA directives for the sequence of the amino acids in a polypeptide.

reading disorders, a language disorder in which a one's reading ability is significantly below intellectual capacity. Tests show the problem does not involve mental retardation, chronologic age, or inadequate schooling, but is marked by faulty oral reading, slow reading, and reduced comprehension.

Read method, a method of psychophysical preparation for childbirth designed by Dr. Grantly Dick-Read. It was the first "natural childbirth" program, a term coined by Dr. Read. Basically, Read held that childbirth is a normal, physiologic procedure and that the pain of labor and delivery is of psychologic origin—the fear-tension-pain syndrome. He countered women's fears with education about the physiologic process, encouraged a positive, welcoming attitude, corrected false information, and led tours of the hospital before birth. To decrease tension, he developed a series of breathing exercises for use during the various stages of labor. To foster relaxation and optimal physical function in labor and in recovery after delivery, he incorporated a series of physical exercises to be performed regularly in classes and in practice at home during pregnancy.

readthrough [AS *raedan + thurh* through], (in molecular genetics) transcription of RNA beyond the normal termination sequence in the DNA template, caused by the occasional failure of RNA polymerase to respond to the end-point signal.

reagent /rē·ā'jənt/ [L *re* again, *agere* to act], a chemical substance known to react in a specific way. A reagent is used to detect or synthesize another substance in a chemical reaction.

reagin /rē'ājin/ [L *re + agere*], 1. an antibody associated with human atopy, such as asthma and hay fever. In antigen-antibody reactions it triggers the release of histamine and other mediators that cause atopic symptoms. 2. a nonspecific, nontreponemal antibody-like substance found in the serum of individuals with syphilis. **−reaginic,** *adj.*

reaginic antibody /rē'əgin'ik/, an IgE immunoglobulin that is elevated in hypersensitive individuals.

reagin-mediated disorder, a hypersensitivity reaction, such as hay fever or an allergic response to an insect sting, produced by reaginic antibodies (IgE immunoglobulins), causing degranulation and the release of histamine, bradykinin, serotonin, and other vasoactive amines. An initial sensitizing dose of the antigen induces the formation of specific IgE antibodies, and their attachment to mast cells and basophils results in hypersensitivity to a subsequent challenging dose of the antigen. The abundance of mast cells in the skin, nose, and lungs makes those areas susceptible to IgE-mediated reactions.

reality /rē·al'itē/ [L *res* factual], the culturally constructed world of perception, meaning, and behavior that members of a culture regard as an absolute.

reality orientation, an activity that uses specific approaches to assist confused or disoriented persons toward an awareness of reality, as by emphasizing the hour, day, month, and weather.

reality principle, an awareness of the demands of the environment and the need for an adjustment of behavior to meet those demands, expressed primarily by the renunciation of immediate gratification of instinctual pleasures to obtain long-term and future goals.

reality testing, an ego function that enables one to differentiate between external reality and any inner imaginative world and to behave in a manner that exhibits an awareness of accepted norms and customs. Impairment of reality testing is indicative of a disturbance in ego functioning that may lead to psychosis.

reality therapy, a form of psychotherapy in which the aims are to help define and assess basic values within the framework of a current situation and to evaluate the person's present behavior and future plans in relation to those values.

real time [L *res* factual; AS *tid* tide], an application of computerized equipment that allows data to be processed with relation to ongoing external events, so that the operators can make immediate diagnostic or other decisions based on the current data output. Ultrasound scanning uses real time control systems.

real-time scanning, the scanning or imaging of an entire object, or a cross-sectional slice of the object, at a single moment. To produce such a "snapshot" image, scanning data must be recorded quickly over a very short time rather than by accumulation over a longer period.

reamer [AS *ryman* to make room], **1.** a tool with a straight or spiral cutting edge, used in a rotating motion to enlarge a hole or clear an opening. **2.** (in dentistry) an instrument with a tapered and loosely spiraled metal shaft, used for enlarging and cleaning root canals.

reapproximate /rē'əprok'simāt/ [L *re* again, *approximare* to come near], to rejoin tissues separated by surgery or trauma so that their anatomic relationship is restored. **–reapproximation,** *n.*

reasonable care /rē'zənəbəl/ [L *rationalis*], the degree of skill and knowledge used by a competent health practitioner in treating and caring for the sick and injured.

reasonable person, (in law) a hypothetical person who possesses the qualities that are used as an objective standard on which to judge a defendant's action in a negligence suit.

reasonably prudent person doctrine /rē'zənəblē'/, a concept that a person of ordinary sense will use ordinary care and skill in meeting the health care needs of a patient.

reattachment /rē'ətach'mənt/, **1.** the rejoining of accidentally severed body parts. **2.** the rejoining of periodontal membrane fibers to the cementum of a tooth and the alveolar bone to restore a loosened tooth.

rebase /rēbās'/ [L *re* again, *basis* base], a process of refitting a denture by replacing its base material without changing the occlusal relationships of the teeth.

rebirthing /rēbur'thing/, a form of psychotherapy that focuses on the breath and breathing apparatus. The goal of treatment is to overcome the trauma of the birth-damaged breathing apparatus so the person is able to use the breath as a supportive and creative part of life.

rebound /rē'bound/ [Fr *rebondir* to bounce], **1.** recovery from illness. **2.** a sudden contraction of muscle after a period of relaxation, often seen in conditions in which inhibitory reflexes are lost.

rebound congestion, swelling and congestion of the nasal mucosa that follows the vasodilator effects of decongestant medications.

rebound phenomenon, a renewal of reflex activity after the stimulus that triggered the original action has been removed. It may be indicative of a lesion of the cerebellum.

rebound tenderness, a sign of inflammation of the peritoneum in which pain is elicited by the sudden release of a hand pressing on the abdomen.

rebreathing /rēbrē'thing/ [L *re* + AS *braeth* breath], breathing into a closed system. Exhaled gas mixes with the gas in the closed system, and some of this mixture is then reinhaled. Rebreathing may result in progressively decreasing concentrations of oxygen and progressively increasing concentrations of carbon dioxide.

rebreathing bag, (in anesthesia) a flexible bag attached to a mask. The rebreathing bag may function as a reservoir for anesthetic gases during surgery or for oxygen during resuscitation. It may be squeezed to pump the gas or air into the lungs.

recalcification /rēkal'sifikā'shən/, the replacement of lost calcium salts in the body needed for normal neuromuscular excitability, excitation-coupling contraction in cardiac and smooth muscle stimulus-secretion coupling, maintenance of tight

R

junctions between cells, blood clotting, and compressional strength of bone.

recannulate /rēka'yəlāt/ [L *re* + *cannula* small reed], to make a new opening through an organ or tissue, such as opening a passage through an occluded blood vessel.

recapitulation theory /rē'kəpit'yəlā'shən/ [L *re* + *capitulum* small head], the theory, formulated by German naturalist Ernst Heinrich Haeckel, that an organism during the course of embryonic development passes through stages that resemble the structural form of several ancestral types of the species as it evolved from a lower to a higher form of life. It is summarized by the statement "Ontogeny recapitulates phylogeny."

receiver /risē'vər/ [L *recipere* to receive], (in communication theory) the person or persons to whom a message is sent.

receptive aphasia /risep'tiv/, a form of sensory aphasia marked by impaired comprehension of language.

receptor /risep'tər/ [L *recipere* to receive], **1.** a chemical structure on the surface of a cell that combines with an antigen to produce a discrete immunologic component. **2.** a sensory nerve ending that responds to various kinds of stimulation. **3.** a specific cellular protein that must first bind a hormone before cellular response can be elicited.

receptor site, a location on a cell surface where certain molecules, such as enzymes, neurotransmitters, or viruses, attach to interact with cellular components.

receptor theory of drug action, the concept that certain drugs produce their effects by acting discretely at some specific receptor site on a cell or molecule within the cell or its membrane.

recess /rē'ses, rises'/ [L *recedere* to retreat], a small hollow cavity, such as the epitympanic recess in the tympanic cavity of the inner ear or the retrocecal recess extending as a small pocket behind the cecum.

recessive /rises'iv/ [L *recedere*], of, pertaining to, or describing a gene the effect of which is masked or hidden if there is a dominant gene at the same locus.

recessive gene, the member of a pair of genes that lacks the ability to express itself in the presence of its more dominant allele; it is expressed only in the homozygous state.

recessive trait, a genetically determined characteristic that is expressed only when present in the homozygous state.

recidivism (recid) /risid'iviz'əm/ [L *recidivus* falling back], a tendency by an ill person to relapse or return to a hospital.

recipient /risip'ē·ənt/ [L *recipere* to receive], the person who receives a blood transfusion, tissue graft, or organ.

reciprocal /rəsip'rəkəl/ [L *reciprocare* to move backward], a type of body movement that aids in communication, such as body language that indicates affiliation between people.

reciprocal beat, an atrial or ventricular complex resulting from a return of an impulse to its chamber of origin.

reciprocal changes, the changes seen in ECG leads facing the opposite wall to a myocardial infarction. The changes were formerly thought to be purely electrical but are now considered a sign of more extensive myocardial damage.

reciprocal gene. See **complementary gene.**

reciprocal inhibition, the theory in behavior therapy that if an anxiety-producing stimulus occurs simultaneously with a response that diminishes anxiety, the stimulus may cause less anxiety, as deep chest or abdominal breathing and relaxation of the deep muscles appear to diminish anxiety and pain in childbirth.

reciprocal roentgens, (in radiology) the measure of x-ray film speed, used in the formula speed = 1/number of roentgens needed to produce a density of 1.

reciprocal translocation, the mutual exchange of genetic material between two nonhomologous chromosomes.

reciprocity /res'ipros'itē/, a mutual agreement to exchange privileges, dependence, or relationships, as an agreement between two governing bodies to accept the medical credentials of physicians licensed in either community.

Recklinghausen's canal /rek'linghou'sənz/ [Friedrich D. von Recklinghausen, German pathologist, b. 1833], the small lymph space in the connective tissues of the body.

Recklinghausen's disease. See **neurofibromatosis.**

Recklinghausen's tumor [Friedrich Recklinghausen], a benign tumor derived from smooth muscle, containing connective tissue and epithelial elements, that occurs in the wall of the oviduct or posterior uterine wall.

reclining /riklī'ning/, leaning backward. **−recline,** v.

reclining position. See **jackknife position.**

recluse spider. See **brown spider.**

recombinant /rēkom'binənt/ [L *re* again, *combinare* to combine], **1.** the cell or organism that results from the recombination of genes within the DNA molecule, regardless of whether naturally or artificially induced. **2.** of or pertaining to such an organism or cell.

recombinant DNA, a DNA molecule in which rearrangement of the genes has been artificially induced. Enzymes are used to break isolated DNA molecules into fragments that are then rearranged in the desired sequence. Portions of DNA material from another organism of the same or a different species may also be introduced into the molecule.

recombination /rē′kämbinā′shən/ [L re + combinare], **1.** (in genetics) the formation of new combinations and arrangements of genes within the chromosome as a result of independent assortment of unlinked genes, crossing over of linked genes, or intracistronic crossing over of nucleotides. **2.** a method of measurement of radiation by ionometric techniques in which it is necessary to collect the liberated charges to arrive at a value of total charge per unit mass of air. Recombination of ions will lower the value collected.

recommended dietary allowance (RDA) /rek′əmen′did/ [L re + commendere to commend], the amount of nutrients, particularly kilocalories, protein, vitamins, and minerals, recommended as a necessary part of one's daily food intake to maintain normal health.

recon /rē′kon/ [L re + combinare + Gk ion going], (in molecular genetics) the smallest genetic unit that is capable of recombination, thought to be a triplet of nucleotides.

reconstitution /rē′konstit(y)oo′shən/ [L re + constituere to establish], the continuous repair of tissue damage.

reconstruction time /rē′kənstruk′shən/, (in computed tomography) the period between the end of a scan and the appearance of an image.

record /ricôrd′/, a written form of communication that permanently documents information relevant to the care of a patient.

Recovery /rikuv′əry/, a self-help group that provides support for persons discharged from inpatient psychiatric hospitals.

recovery room (RR) [ME recoveren; AS rum], an area adjoining the operating room to which surgical patients are taken while still under anesthesia, before being returned to their rooms. Vital signs and adequacy of ventilation are carefully observed as the patient recovers consciousness.

recreational drug, any substance with pharmacologic effects that is taken for personal pleasure or satisfaction rather than for medicinal purposes, such as alcohol, barbiturates, cocaine, and caffeine in coffee or cola beverages.

recreational therapy /rē′krē-āshənəl/ [L recreare to renew], a form of adjunctive psychotherapy in which games or other group activities are used as a means of modifying maladaptive behavior, awakening social interests, or improving the ability to communicate in depressed, withdrawn people.

recrudescence /rē′krōodes′əns/ [L re + crudescere to become hard], a return of symptoms of a disease during a period of recovery. **–recrudescent,** adj.

recrudescent hepatitis /-ənt/, a form of acute viral hepatitis marked by a relapse during the period of recovery.

recrudescent typhus. See **Brill-Zinsser disease.**

recruitment /rikroot′mənt/, **1.** the perception of a rapid growth of loudness, commonly seen in sensorineural hearing losses which are cochlear in nature. The impaired ear cannot hear faint sounds, but hears intense sounds as loudly as a normal ear. **2.** in muscle contractions, the ability to recruit additional motor units into action as the need to overcome resistance increases.

rectal abscess /rek′təl/ [L rectus straight, abscedere to go away], an abscess in the perianal area.

rectal alimentation [L rectus, alimentum nourishment], the delivery of nourishment in concentrated form by injection or installation through the rectum.

rectal anesthesia [L rectus straight], general anesthesia achieved by the insertion, injection, or infusion of an anesthetic agent into the rectum; this procedure is performed rarely because of the unpredictability of absorption of the drug into the blood.

rectal cancer. See **colorectal cancer.**

rectal instillation of medication, the instillation of a medicated suppository, cream, or gel into the rectum. Some conditions treated by this method are constipation, pruritus ani, and hemorrhoids. Occasionally, a drug may be given in a medicated enema.

rectal reflex, the normal response (defecation) to the presence of an accumulation of feces in the rectum.

rectal temperature, temperature as measured in the rectum. Rectal temperatures average 0.3° C to 0.4° C or 0.5 F to 0.75° F higher than oral temperatures.

rectal thermometer [L rectus; Gk therme heat, metron measure], a clinical thermometer suitable for measuring body temperature rectally.

R

rectal tube, a flexible tube inserted into the rectum to assist in the relief of flatus.

rectifier /rek'tifī'ər/, an electrical device that converts alternating current (AC) to direct current (DC).

rectilinear scanner /rek'tilin'ē·ər/, a device that generates an image of a body organ by detecting radioactivity within the structure and recording it on film.

rectitis. See **proctitis.**

rectocele /rek'tō-/ [L *rectus* + Gk *koilos* hollow], a protrusion of the rectum and the posterior wall of the vagina into the vagina. The condition occurs after the muscles of the vagina and pelvic floor have been weakened by childbearing, old age, or surgery.

rectosigmoid /-pig'moid/ [L *rectus* + Gk *sigma* S-shaped, *eidos* form], a portion of the anatomy that includes the lower portion of the sigmoid and the upper portion of the rectum.

rectosigmoidoscopy /-sig'moidəs'kəpē/, the examination of the rectum and pelvic colon with a sigmoidoscope.

rectouterine excavation, rectouterine pouch. See **cul-de-sac of Douglas.**

rectovaginal fistula /-vaj'inə/ [L *rectus* + *vagina* sheath], an abnormal passage or opening between the rectum and the vagina.

rectovaginal ligament, one of the four main uterine support ligaments. It helps hold the uterus in position by maintaining traction on the cervix.

rectovesical /-ves'ikəl/ [L *rectus* + *vesica* bladder], pertaining to the rectum and bladder.

rectum /rek'təm/, *pl.* **rectums, recta** [L *rectus*], the portion of the large intestine, about 12 cm long, continuous with the descending sigmoid colon, just proximal to the anal canal. It follows the sacrococcygeal curve and ends in the anal canal. –**rectal,** *adj.*

rectus abdominis /rek'təs/, one of a pair of anterolateral muscles of the abdomen, extending the whole length of the ventral aspect of the abdomen. It functions to flex the vertebral column, tense the anterior abdominal wall, and assist in compressing the abdominal contents.

rectus femoris, a fusiform muscle of the anterior thigh, one of the four parts of the quadriceps femoris. It functions to flex the leg.

rectus muscle [L, straight; *musculus*], a muscle of the body that has a relatively straight form. Some rectus muscles are **rectus abdominis, rectus capitis anterior,** and **rectus capitis lateralis.**

recumbency /rikum'bənsē/, the state of lying down or leaning against something.

recumbent /rikum'bənt/ [L *recumbere* to lie down], lying down or leaning backward. –**recumbency,** *n.*

recuperate /rik(y)oo'pərāt/ [L *recupare* to regain], to recover one's health and strength.

recuperation /rikoo'pərā'shən/, the process of recovering health and strength.

recurrence /rikur'əns/ [L *recurrere* to run back], the reappearance of a sign or symptom of a disease after a period of remission.

recurrent /rikur'ənt/, a disease sign or symptom that returns periodically.

recurrent bandage [L *recurrere* to run back], a bandage that is wrapped several times around itself, usually applied to the head or an amputated stump.

recurrent fever. See **relapsing fever.**

recurvatum /rē'kərvā'təm/ [L *recurvare* to bend back], backward thrust of the knee caused by weakness of the quadriceps or a joint disorder.

red blindness. See **protanopia.**

red blood cell. See **erythrocyte.**

red blood cell count [AS *read, blod;* L *cella* storeroom; Fr *conter* to count], a count of the erythrocytes in a specimen of whole blood, commonly made with an electronic counting device. The normal concentrations of red blood cells in the whole blood of males are 4.6 to 6.2 million/mm³; in females, the concentrations are 4.2 to 5.4 million/mm³.

Red Book of the American Academy of Pediatrics, a book that serves as the standard reference source of immunization procedures for children and adults.

red bug. See **chigger.**

red cell. See **erythrocyte.**

red cell indexes, a series of relationships that characterize the red cell population in terms of size, hemoglobin content, and hemoglobin concentration. The indexes are useful in making differential diagnoses of several kinds of anemia.

red corpuscle. See **erythrocyte.**

Red Cross. See **American Red Cross, International Red Cross Society.**

red fever. See **dengue fever.**

red hepatization. See **hepatization.**

red infarct [AS *read;* L *infarcire* to stuff], a pathologic change that occurs in brain tissue that has been rendered ischemic by lack of blood. Diapedesis of red blood cells occurs into the parenchyma of the brain, producing only infiltration of erythrocytes.

red marrow [AS *read;* AS *mearh* marrow], the red vascular substance consisting of connective tissue and blood vessels containing primitive blood cells, macrophages, megakaryocytes, and fat cells. It is found in the cavities of many bones, including the flat and the short bones, the bodies of the vertebrae, the sternum, the ribs, and the articulating ends of the long bones.

redon /rē′don/, the smallest unit of the DNA molecule capable of recombination; it may be as small as one deoxyribonucleotide pair.

redox, an abbreviation for *reduction-oxidation* (reaction).

red phenol. See **phenolsulfonphthalein.**

red tide. See **shellfish poisoning.**

reduce /rid(y)o͞o′/ [L *reducere* to draw backward], **1.** (in surgery) the restoration of a part to its original position after displacement, as in the reduction of a fractured bone by bringing ends or fragments back into alignment. **2.** to decrease the amount, size, extent, or number of something, as of body weight.

reducible hernia /rid(y)o͞o′səbəl/, a hernia in which the protruding tissues can be manipulated into a normal position.

reducing agent /rid(y)o͞o′sing/, a substance that donates electrons to another substance in a chemical reaction.

reduction /riduk′shən/ [L *reducere*], **1.** the addition of hydrogen to a substance. **2.** the removal of oxygen from a substance. **3.** the decrease in the valence of the electronegative part of a compound. **4.** the addition of one or more electrons to a molecule or atom of a substance. **5.** the correction of a fracture, hernia, or luxation. **6.** the reduction of data, as in converting interval data to an ordinal or nominal scale of measurement.

reduction diet, a diet that is low in calories, used for reduction of body weight. The diet must supply fewer calories than the individual expends each day while supplying all the essential nutrients for maintaining health. A diet of this type may provide 1,200 calories per day from the basic food groups.

reduction division. See **meiosis.**

reductionism /riduk′shəniz′əm/, an approach that tries to explain a form of behavior or an event in terms of a specific category of phenomena, such as biological, psychologic, or cultural, negating the possibility of an interrelation of causal phenomena.

Reed-Sternberg cell [Dorothy M. Reed, American pathologist, b. 1874; Karl Sternberg, Austrian pathologist, b. 1872], one of a number of large, abnormal, multinucleated reticuloendothelial cells in the lymphatic system in Hodgkin's disease. The number and proportion of cells are the basis for the histopathologic classification of Hodgkin's disease.

reefer. See **cannabis.**

reentry /rē·en′trē/ [L *re* again; Fr *entree*], (in cardiology) the reactivation of myocardial tissue for the second or subsequent time by the same impulse. Reentry is one of the most common arrhythmogenic mechanisms.

refereed journal /ref′ərēd′/ [L *referre* to bring back; *diunalis* daily record], a professional or literary journal in which articles or papers are selected for publication by a panel of referees who are experts in the field.

reference electrode /ref′ərəns/ [L *referre* + Gk *elektron* amber, *hodos* way], an electrode that has an established potential and is used as a reference against which other potentials may be measured.

reference group, a group with which a person identifies or wishes to belong.

referential idea. See **idea of reference.**

referential index deletions /refəren′shəl/, a neurolinguistic programing term that pertains to the omission of the specific person being discussed.

referral /rifur′əl/ [L *referre* to bring back], a process whereby a patient or the patient's family is introduced to additional health resources in the community, as in helping a patient find an appropriate community health nurse after discharge from a hospital.

referred pain /rifurd′/ [L *referre* + *poena* punishment], pain felt at a site different from that of an injured or diseased organ or part of the body. In disease of the gallbladder, pain may be felt in the right shoulder or scapular region.

referred sensation, a feeling or impression that occurs at a site other than at which the stimulus is initiated.

refined birth rate /rifīnd′/ [L *re* + *finire* to finish], the ratio of total births to the total female population, considered during a period of 1 year.

refl, abbreviation for *reflexive*.

reflecting /riflik′ting/, a communication technique in which the listener picks up the feeling tone of the patient's message and repeats it back to the patient. It encourages the patient to continue with clarifying comments.

reflection /riflek′shən/ [L *reflectere* to bend backward], **1.** (in cardiology) a form of reentry in which, after encountering delay in one fiber, an impulse enters a parallel fiber and returns retrogradely to its source. **2.** (in ultrasonography) the reentry of acoustic energy where there is a discontinuity in the characteristic acoustic impedance along the propagation path.

reflective layer /riflek′tiv/, (in radiology) a thin layer of magnesium oxide or tita-

R

nium oxide between the phosphor and the base of an intensifying screen. Its function is to intercept and redirect isotropically emitted light from the phosphor to the x-ray film.

reflex /rē′fleks/ [L *reflectere* to bend backward], **1.** a backward or return flow of energy or of an image, as a reflection. **2.** a reflected action, particularly an involuntary action or movement.

reflex action, the involuntary functioning or movement of any organ or part of the body in response to a particular stimulus.

reflex apnea, involuntary cessation of respiration caused by irritating, noxious vapors or gases.

reflex arc, a simple neurologic unit of a sensory neuron that carries a stimulus impulse to the spinal cord where it connects with a motor neuron that carries the reflex impulse back to an appropriate muscle or gland.

reflex bladder. See **spastic bladder.**

reflex center, any part of the nervous system in which reception of afferent impulses results in a discharge of efferent impulses leading to some change in a muscle or gland.

reflex dyspepsia, an abnormal condition characterized by impaired digestion associated with the disease of an organ not directly involved with digestion.

reflex emesis, vomiting or gagging that is induced by touching the mucous membrane of the throat or as a result of other noxious stimuli.

reflex hammer, a percussion mallet with a rubber head used to tap tendons, nerves, or muscles to elicit reflex reactions.

reflex inhibiting pattern (RIP), a conscious set of neuromuscular actions directed toward inhibition of a natural reflex, as in suppressing a sneeze.

reflexology, a system of treating certain disorders by massaging the soles of the feet, using principles similar to those of acupuncture.

reflex sensation. See **referred sensation.**

reflex tachycardia [L *reflectere*; Gk *tachys* fast, *kardia* heart], a rapid heart sinus rhythm caused by a variety of autonomic nervous system effects, such as blood pressure changes, fever, or emotional stress.

reflex vasodilatation [L *reflectere*, *vas* vessel, *dilatare* to spread out], any blood vessel dilatation that results from stimulation of vasodilator nerves or inhibition of vasoconstrictors of the sympathetic nervous system, including epinephrine-type drugs.

reflux /rē′fluks/ [L *refluere* to flow back], an abnormal backward or return flow of a

fluid. Kinds of reflux include **gastroesophageal reflux, hepatojugular reflux,** and **vesicoureteral reflux.**

reflux esophagitis, esophageal irritation and inflammation that results from reflux of the stomach contents into the esophagus.

refracting angle. See **angle of refraction.**

refracting medium. See **medium.**

refraction /rifrak′shən/ [L *refringere* to break up], **1.** the change of direction of energy as it passes from one medium to another of different density. **2.** an examination to determine and to correct refractive errors of the eye. **3.** (in ultrasonography) the phenomenon of bending wave fronts as the acoustic energy propagates from the medium of one acoustic velocity to a second medium of differing acoustic velocity.

refraction of eye, the deflection of light from a straight path through the eye by various ocular tissues, including the cornea, lens, aqueous humor, and vitreous body.

refractive error /rifrak′tiv/, a defect in the ability of the lens of the eye to focus an image accurately, as occurs in nearsightedness and farsightedness.

refractive index, a numeric expression of the refractive power of a medium, as compared with that of air, which has a refractive index value of 1. It is related to the number, charge, and mass of vibrating particles in the material through which light passes.

refractometer /rē′frəktom′ətər/ [L *refringere* + Gk *metron* measure], an instrument for measuring the refractive index of a substance, used primarily for measuring the refractivity of solutions.

refractoriness /rifrak′ōrines/, the property of excitable tissue that determines how closely together two action potentials can occur.

refractory /rifrak′tərē/ [L *refringere*], pertaining to a disorder that is resistant to treatment.

refractory period, the time from phase 0 to the end of phase 3 of the action potential, divided into effective and relative. In pacing terminology, it is the period during which a pulse generator is unresponsive to an input signal of specified amplitude.

reframing /rēfrā′ming/, changing the viewpoint in relation to which a situation is experienced and placing it in a different frame that fits the "facts" of a concrete situation equally well, thereby changing its entire meaning.

Refsum's syndrome /ref′sōōmz/ [Sigvald Refsum, Norwegian physician, b. 1907], a rare, hereditary disorder of lipid metabolism in which phytanic acid cannot be broken down. The syndrome is characterized by ataxia, abnormalities of the bones and skin, peripheral neuropathy, and retinitis pigmentosa.

regimen /rej'imən/ [L, guidance], a strictly regulated therapeutic program, such as a diet or exercise schedule.

regional /rē'jənəl/ [L regio direction], of or pertaining to a geographic area, such as a regional medical facility, or to a part of the body, such as regional anesthesia.

regional anatomy, the study of the structural relationships within the organs and the parts of the body. Kinds of regional anatomy are **surface anatomy** and **cross-sectional anatomy.**

regional anesthesia, anesthesia of an area of the body by injecting a local anesthetic to block a group of sensory nerve fibers. Kinds of regional anesthesia include **brachial plexus anesthesia, caudal anesthesia, epidural anesthesia, intercostal anesthesia, paracervical block, pudendal block,** and **spinal anesthesia.**

regional control, the control of cancer in sites that represent the first stages of spread from the local origin.

regional enteritis. See **Crohn's disease.**

regional hyperthermia, the elevation of temperature over an extended volume of tissue.

regionalization /rē'jənəl'īzā'shən/, (in health care planning) the organization of a system for the delivery of health care within a region to avoid costly duplication of services and to ensure availability of essential services.

regional medical program (RMP), a program of community health planning that includes all the medical resources available in a region that may be mobilized to meet a specific medical objective. The RMP was authorized by the Health, Disease, Cancer and Stroke Amendments passed by the U.S. Congress in 1965.

region of interest (ROI), (in positron emission tomography) an area that circumscribes a desired anatomic location. Image processing systems permit drawing of ROIs on images.

region of recombination, the first stage of amplitude of an electric signal in a gas-filled radiation detector, when the voltage is very low. No electrons are attracted to the central electrode, and ion pairs produced in the chamber will recombine.

register /rej'istər/ [L regerere to bring back], (in computed tomography) a device in the central processing unit (CPU) that stores information for future use.

registered nurse (RN), 1. U.S.; a profes-

sional nurse who has completed a course of study at a state-approved school of nursing and passed the National Council Licensure Examination (NCLEX-RN). A registered nurse may use the initials RN after the signature. 2. Canada; a professional nurse who has completed a course of study at an approved school of nursing and who has taken and passed an examination administered by the Canadian Nurses Association Testing Service, called the Comprehensive Examination for Nurse Registration Licensure.

registered record administrator (RRA), a medical record administrator who has successfully completed the credentialing examination conducted by the American Medical Record Association.

registered respiratory therapist (RRT), an allied health professional who has successfully completed the registry examination of the National Board for Respiratory Care (NBRC). Usually a 2-year or 4-year college affiliation leading to an associate or bachelor's degree is required.

registered technologist (RT), a title awarded by the American Registry of Radiologic Technologists as certification of qualification to act as an x-ray technologist.

registrar /rej'isträr/, an administrative officer whose responsibility is to maintain the records of an institution.

registration, /rej'istrā'shən/ [L, registratio], 1. a learning or memory recording made in the central nervous system of an impression resulting from a stimulus. 2. the recording of vital personal information, such as health data. 3. the recording of professional qualification information relevant to government licensing regulations.

registry /rej'istrē/ [L regerere to bring back], 1. an office or agency in which lists of nurses and records pertaining to nurses seeking employment are maintained. 2. (in epidemiology) a listing service for incidence data pertaining to the occurrence of specific diseases or disorders, such as a tumor registry.

regression /rigresh'ən/ [L regredi to go back], 1. a retreat or backward movement in conditions, signs, or symptoms. 2. a return to an earlier, more primitive form of behavior. 3. a tendency in physical development to become more typical of the population than of the parents. **–regress,** v.

regular diet /reg'yələr/ [L regula rule], a full, well-balanced diet containing all of the essential nutrients needed for optimal growth, repair of the tissues, and normal functioning of the organs.

R

regular insulin, a fast-acting, amorphous, noncrystalline form of insulin prescribed in the treatment of diabetes mellitus when the desired action is prompt, intense, and short-acting.

regulative cleavage. See **indeterminate cleavage.**

regulative development /reg'yəlā'tiv/ [L *regula* rule], a type of embryonic development in which the fertilized ovum undergoes indeterminate cleavage, producing blastomeres that have similar developmental potencies and are each capable of giving rise to a single embryo. Determination of the particular organs and parts of the embryo occurs during later stages of development and is influenced by inductors and intercellular interaction.

regulator gene /reg'yəlā'tər/, (in molecular genetics) a genetic unit that regulates or suppresses the activity of one or more structural genes.

regulatory sequence /reg'yələtôr'ē/ [L *regula* + *sequi* to follow], (in molecular genetics) a series of DNA nucleotides that regulates the expression of a gene.

regurgitant menstruation. See **retrograde menstruation.**

regurgitant murmur /rigur'jitənt/, a heart murmur caused by a defective valve as blood flows backward through the partly closed valve cusps. Kinds of regurgitant murmurs include diastolic, pansystolic, and systolic.

regurgitation /rēgur'jitā'shən/ [L *re* again, *gurgitare* to flood], 1. the backward flow from the normal direction, as the return of swallowed food into the mouth. 2. the backward flow of blood through a defective heart valve, named for the affected valve, as in **aortic regurgitation.**

regurgitation jaundice, jaundice caused by bile pigment entering the blood and lymphatic systems as a result of biliary obstruction.

rehabilitation [L *re* + *habitalas* aptitude], the restoration of an individual or a part to normal or near normal function after a disabling disease, injury, addiction, or incarceration. **–rehabilitate,** *v.*

rehabilitation center, a facility providing therapy and training for rehabilitation. The center may offer occupational therapy, physical therapy, vocational training, and special training, such as speech therapy.

Rehfuss stomach tube /rā'fəs/ [Martin E. Rehfuss, American physician, b.1887], a specially designed gastric tube with a graduated syringe, used for withdrawing specimens of the contents of the stomach for study after a test meal.

rehydration /rē'hīdrā'shən/, restoration of normal water balance in a patient by giving fluids orally or intravenously.

Reid's base line [Robert W. Reid, Scottish anatomist, b. 1851], the base line of the skull, a hypothetic line extending from the infraorbital point to the superior border of the external auditory meatus.

Reifenstein's syndrome /rī'fənstīnz/ [Edward C. Reifenstein, Jr., American physician, b. 1908], male hypogonadism of unknown origin, marked by azoospermia, undescended testes, gynecomastia, testosterone deficiency, and elevated gonadotropin titers.

reimbursement /rē'imburs'mənt/ [L *re* + *im* in; Fr *bourse* purse], a method of payment, usually by a third-party payer, for medical treatment or hospital costs. Cost-based reimbursement covers payment for all allowable costs incurred in the provision of services to patients included in a contract. Prospective reimbursement provides for additional payment by which costs incurred in providing services to patients are based on actual costs determined at the end of a fiscal period.

reinforcement /rē'infôrs'mənt/ [L *re* + Fr *enforcir* to strengthen], (in psychology) a process in which a response is strengthened by the fear of punishment or the anticipation of reward.

reinforcement-extinction, a process of socialization in which one learns to engage in certain behaviors (reinforcement) or to avoid certain behaviors (extinction).

reinforcer /rē'infôr'sər/, (in psychology) a consequence that increases the probability that an operant will recur.

Reiter's syndrome /rī'tərz/ [Hans Reiter, German physician, b. 1862], an arthritic disorder of adult males, believed to result from a myxovirus or *Mycoplasma* infection. The syndrome most often affects the ankles, feet, and sacroiliac joints and is usually associated with conjunctivitis and urethritis. Lesions that become superficial ulcers may form on the palms and the soles. Arthritis usually persists after the conjunctivitis and urethritis subside, but it may become episodic.

reject analysis /rē'jekt/, (in radiology) the study of repeated radiographs to determine the cause for their being discarded.

rejection /rijek'shən/ [L *re* + *jacere* to throw], 1. (in medicine) an immunologic response to organisms or substances that the system recognizes as foreign, including grafts or transplants. 2. (in psychiatry) the act of excluding or denying affection to another person.

rejunctive /rijungk'tiv/, (in contextual psychotherapy) pertaining to a relationship that is characterized by moves toward trustworthy relatedness.

rejuvenation /rējŏŏ′vənā′shən/, the restoration of youthful health and vitality.

relapse /rilaps′/ [L *relabi* to slide back], **1.** to exhibit again the symptoms of a disease from which a patient appears to have recovered. **2.** the recurrence of a disease after apparent recovery.

relapsing, pertaining to the return of disease after a period of apparent recovery.

relapsing fever, any one of several acute infectious diseases, marked by recurrent febrile episodes, caused by various strains of the spirochete *Borrelia*. The disease is transmitted by both lice and ticks and is often seen during wars and famines. The first episode usually starts with a sudden high fever (104° F to 105° F), accompanied by chills, headache, neuromuscular pains, and nausea. A rash may appear over the trunk and extremities, and jaundice is common during the later stages. Each attack lasts 2 or 3 days and culminates in a crisis of high fever, profuse sweating, and a rise in heart and respiratory rate. This is followed by an abrupt drop in temperature and a return to normal blood pressure. People typically relapse after 7 to 10 days of normal temperature and eventually recover completely.

relapsing polychondritis, a rare disease of unknown cause resulting in inflammation and destruction of cartilage with replacement by fibrous tissue. Autoimmunity may be involved in this condition. Most commonly the ears and noses of middle-aged people are affected with episodes of tender swelling, often accompanied by fever, arthralgias, and episcleritis.

relation searching /rilā′shən/ [L *relatio* a carrying back; *circum* round about], (in nursing research) a study design used to discover and describe relationships between variables.

relationship therapy /rilā′shənship′/ [L *relatio* + AS *scieppan* to shape], a therapy that is based on a totality of patient-therapist relationship and encourages the growth of self in the patient.

relative biologic effectiveness (RBE) /rel′ətiv/ [L *relatio*], (in radiotherapy) a measure of the cell-killing ability of a particular radiation compared with a reference radiation. The ratio of cells killed with the test radiation over that of 250 keV radiation is the RBE.

relative centrifugal force (RCF), a method of comparing the force generated by various centrifuges based on the speeds of rotation and distances from the center of rotation.

relative cephalopelvic disproportion. See **cephalopelvic disproportion.**

relative growth, the comparison of the various increases in size of similar organisms, tissues, or structures at different time intervals.

relative humidity, the amount of moisture in the air compared with the maximum the air could contain at the same temperature.

relative refractory period. See **refractory period.**

relative risk, the ratio of the frequency of a certain disorder in groups exposed or not exposed to a particular hereditary or environmental factor.

relative sterility, a condition of infertility in which one or more factors tend to reduce the chances of becoming pregnant.

relative value unit, a comparable service measure used by hospitals to permit comparison of the amounts of resources required to perform various services within a single department or between departments.

relativism /rel′ətiviz′əm/. See **cultural relativism.**

relax /rilaks′/ [L *relaxare* to ease], to reduce tension.

relaxant /rilak′sənt/, a drug or other agent that tends to reduce tension, as a muscle relaxant or bowel relaxant.

relaxation /rē′laksā′shən/ [L *relaxare* to ease], **1.** a reducing of tension, as when a muscle relaxes between contractions. **2.** a lessening of pain. **3.** (in magnetic resonance imaging) the return of excited nuclei to their normal unexcited state by the release of energy.

relaxation oven, (in mammography) a part of the xerographic plate conditioner system used to eliminate ghost images. The plate is heated in the oven so that any residual electrostatic charge on the surface will be removed.

relaxation response, a protective mechanism against stress that brings about decreased heart rate, lower metabolism, and decreased respiratory rate. It is the physiologic opposite of the "fight or flight," or stress, response.

relaxation therapy, treatment in which patients are taught to perform breathing and relaxation exercises and to concentrate on a pleasant situation. An integral part of the Lamaze method of childbirth, relaxation therapy is also used to relieve various kinds of pain and physical manifestations of stress.

relaxation time, (in MRI) the characteristic time it takes for a sample of atoms, whose nuclei have first been aligned along a static magnetic field and then excited to a higher energy (MR) state by a radio-frequency signal, to return to a lower energy equilibrium state.

relaxin /rilak′sin/, a hormone obtained from the corpora lutea of swine and used to relax the pelvic ligaments and dilate the cervix during labor. The medication has also been used to treat dysmenorrhea.

release therapy /rilēs′/ [ME *relesen* to release], a type of pediatric psychotherapy used to treat children with stress and anxiety related to a specific, recent event.

releasing hormone (RH), one of several peptides produced by the hypothalamus and secreted directly into the anterior pituitary via a connecting vein. Each of the releasing hormones stimulates the pituitary to secrete a specific tropic hormone; thus corticotropic releasing hormone stimulates the pituitary to secrete adrenocorticotropic hormone.

releasing stimulus, (in psychology) an action or behavior by one individual that serves as a cue to trigger a response in others. An example is yawning by one person, which results in yawning by others in the group.

reliability /rilī′əbil′itē/ [L *religare* to fasten behind], (in research) the extent to which a test measurement or a device produces the same results with different investigators, observers, or administration of the test over time.

relief area [L *relevare* to lighten], the portion of the tissue surface under prosthesis on which pressures are reduced or eliminated.

relieving factor /rilē′ving/, an agent that alleviates a symptom.

religiosity /rilij′ē·os′itē/ [L *religiosus*], a psychiatric symptom characterized by the demonstration of excessive or affected piety.

reline /rēlīn′/ [L *re* + *linea*], the resurfacing of the tissue side of a denture with new base material.

relocation stress syndrome, a NANDA-accepted nursing diagnosis of physiologic and/or psychosocial disturbances as a result of a transfer from one environment to another. Defining characteristics include a change in environment or location, anxiety, apprehension, increased confusion (elderly population), depression, loneliness, sleep disturbance, gastrointestinal disturbances, and withdrawal. Related factors include past, concurrent, and recent losses, and decreased physical health status.

rem /rem, är′ē′em′/, abbreviation for *roentgen equivalent man*. A dose of ionizing radiation that produces in humans the same effect as one roentgen of x-radiation or gamma radiation.

REM /rem, är′ē′em′/, abbreviation for **rapid eye movement.**

remasking /rēmas′king/, (in digital fluoroscopy) the production of one or more additional mask images if the first is inadequate due to patient motion, noise, or other factors.

remedial /rimē′dē·əl/ [L *remediare* to cure], designed to improve or cure.

reminiscence /rem′inis′ns/ [L *reminisci* to remember], the recollection of past personal experiences and significant events.

reminiscence therapy, a psychotherapeutic technique in which self-esteem and personal satisfaction are restored, particularly in older persons, by encouraging patients to review past experiences of a pleasant nature.

remission /rimish′ən/ [L *remittere* to abate], the partial or complete disappearance of the clinical and subjective characteristics of a chronic or malignant disease. Remission may be spontaneous or the result of therapy.

remittent fever /rimit′ənt/ [L *remittere* + *febris* fever], diurnal variations of an elevated temperature with exacerbations and remissions but never a return to normal.

remnant radiation /rem′nənt/ [L *remanere* to remain], the measurable radiation that passes through an object and can produce an image on radiographic film.

remodeling /rēmod′əling/, the process of changing a body part or area, as in reconstructive surgery.

remote afterloading /rimōt′/ [L *removere* to remove], (in radiotherapy) a technique in which an applicator, such as an acrylic mold of an area to be irradiated, is placed in or on the patient and then loaded from a safe source with a high-activity radioisotope. Remote afterloading is used in the treatment of head, neck, vaginal, and cervical tumors.

remotivation /rē′mōtivā′shən/ [L *re* + *motus* movement], the use of special techniques that stimulate patients to become motivated to learn and interact.

remotivation group, a treatment group that is organized with the purpose of stimulating the interest, awareness, and communication of withdrawn and institutionalized mental patients.

removable lingual arch /rimoo͞o′vəbəl/ [L *removere* to remove], an orthodontic arch wire designed to fit the lingual surface of the teeth and aid orthodontic movement of the dentition involved.

removable orthodontic appliance, a device placed inside the mouth to correct or alleviate malocclusion and designed to be removed or replaced by the patient.

removable rigid dressing, a dressing

similar to a cast used to encase the stump of an amputated limb. It is usually applied to permit the fitting of a temporary prosthesis so that ambulation can begin soon after surgery.

renal /rē′nəl/ [L *ren* kidney], of or pertaining to the kidney.

renal acidosis [L *ren, acidus* sour; Gk *osis* condition], an excessive increase in the H⁺ ions in body fluids because of impaired kidney function. The acidosis can result from excessive loss of bicarbonate or from the inability to excrete phosphoric and sulfuric acid.

renal adenocarcinoma. See **renal cell carcinoma.**

renal angiography, a radiographic examination of the renal artery and associated blood vessels, after the injection of a contrast medium.

renal anuria, cessation of urine production caused by intrinsic renal disease.

renal artery, one of a pair of large, visceral branches of the abdominal aorta that supplies the kidneys, suprarenal glands, and the ureters.

renal biopsy, the removal of kidney tissue for microscopic examination, conducted to establish the diagnosis of a renal disorder and to aid in determining the stage of the disease, the appropriate therapy, and the prognosis. An open biopsy involves an incision, permits better visualization of the kidney, and carries a lower risk of hemorrhage; a closed or percutaneous biopsy, performed by aspirating a specimen of tissue with a needle, requires a shorter period of recovery and is less likely to cause infection.

renal calculus, a concretion occurring in the kidney.

renal calyx, the first unit in the system of ducts in the kidney carrying urine from the renal pyramid of the cortex to the renal pelvis for excretion through the ureters. There are two divisions: the **minor calyx,** with several others, drains into a larger **major calyx,** which in turn joins other major calyces to form the renal pelvis.

renal capsule [L *ren, capsula* little box], a protective connective tissue capsule surrounding to the kidney.

renal cell carcinoma, a malignant neoplasm of the kidney, composed predominantly of large cells with clear cytoplasm that originate in tubular epithelium. The tumor may develop in any part of the kidney, becoming a large mass that may grow into the tributaries of the renal vein. Hematuria and pain are usually present.

renal colic, sharp, severe pain in the lower back over the kidney, radiating forward into the groin. Renal colic usually accompanies forcible dilatation of a ureter followed by spasm as a stone is lodged or passed through it.

renal corpuscle. See **malpighian corpuscle.**

renal cortex, the soft, granular, outer layer of the kidney, containing approximately 1.25 million glomeruli, which remove body wastes in the form of urine.

renal dialysis [L *ren*; Gk *dia* + *lysis* loosening], a process of diffusing blood across a semipermeable membrane to remove substances that a normal kidney would eliminate, including poisons, drugs, urea, uric acid, and creatinine. Renal dialysis may restore electrolytes and acid-base imbalances.

renal diet, a diet prescribed in chronic renal failure and designed to control the intake of protein, potassium, sodium, phosphorus, and fluids, depending on individual conditions. Carbohydrates and fats are the principal sources of energy. Protein is limited; the amount is determined by the patient's condition.

renal dwarf, a dwarf whose retarded growth is caused by renal failure.

renal failure, inability of the kidneys to excrete wastes, concentrate urine, and conserve electrolytes. The condition may be acute or chronic. **Acute renal failure** is characterized by oliguria and by the rapid accumulation of nitrogenous wastes in the blood. It is caused by hemorrhage, trauma, burn, toxic injury to the kidney, acute pyelonephritis or glomerulonephritis, or lower urinary tract obstruction. **Chronic renal failure** may result from many other diseases. The early signs include sluggishness, fatigue, and mental dullness. Later, anuria, convulsions, GI bleeding, malnutrition, and various neuropathies may occur. The skin may turn yellow-brown and become covered with uremic frost. Congestive heart failure and hypertension are frequent complications, the results of hypervolemia.

renal glycosuria [L *ren*; Gk *glykys* sweet, *ouron* urine], a familial condition characterized by lowered renal threshold to sugar. Blood sugar levels may be normal, although sugar is excreted in the urine.

renal hematuria [L *ren*; Gk *haima* blood, *ouron* urine], presence of blood in the urine because of a kidney disorder.

renal hypertension, hypertension resulting from kidney disease, including chronic glomerulonephritis, chronic pyelonephritis, renal carcinoma, and renal calculi. Analgesic abuse and certain drug reactions may also result in renal hypertension. Untreated renal hypertension is likely to result in kidney damage and cardiovascular disease.

renal insufficiency, partial kidney function failure characterized by less than normal urine excretion.

renal nanism, dwarfism associated with infantile renal osteodystrophy.

renal osteodystrophy, a condition resulting from chronic renal failure and characterized by uneven bone growth and demineralization.

renal papilla. See **papilla.**

renal pelvis [L *ren, pelvis* basin], a funnel-shaped dilatation that drains urine from the kidney into the ureter.

renal pyramid, one of the conical masses of tissue that forms the kidney medulla. The base of each pyramid adjoins the kidney's cortex. The pyramids consist of the loops of Henle and the collecting tubules of the nephrons.

renal rickets, a condition characterized by rachitic changes in the skeleton and caused by chronic nephritis.

renal scan, a scan of the kidneys to determine their size, shape, and exact position, used to aid in the diagnosis of a tumor or other abnormalities and performed after the intravenous injection of a radioactive substance.

renal sclerosis, arteriosclerosis or fibrosis of the arterioles of the kidney.

renal transplantation, the surgical transfer of a complete kidney from a donor to a recipient.

renal tubular acidosis (RTA), an abnormal condition associated with persistent dehydration, metabolic acidosis, hypokalemia, hyperchloremia, and nephrocalcinosis. It is caused by the inability of the kidneys to conserve bicarbonate and to adequately acidify the urine. Prolonged RTA can cause hypercalciuria and the formation of kidney stones. Some common signs and symptoms of RTA, especially in children, may include anorexia, vomiting, constipation, retarded growth, polyuria, nephrocalcinosis, and rickets. In children and adults RTA can also cause urinary tract infections and pyelonephritis.

renal tubule, the part of the kidney's nephron that leads from the glomerulus to the collecting tubules. It consists of a looping segment and two convoluted sections. These are reabsorptive canals that secrete, collect, and conduct urine.

Rendu-Osler-Weber syndrome. See **Osler-Weber-Rendu syndrome.**

renin /rē′nin/ [L *ren* kidney], a proteolytic enzyme, produced and stored in the juxtaglomerular apparatus that surrounds each arteriole as it enters a glomerulus. The enzyme affects the blood pressure by catalyzing the change of angiotensinogen to angiotensin.

renin test. See **plasma renin activity.**

rennin /ren′in/ [ME *rennen* to run], a milk-curdling enzyme that occurs in the gastric juices of infants and is also contained in the rennet produced in the stomach of calves and other ruminants. It is an endopeptidase that converts casein to paracasein.

renogram /rē′nəgram′/, a graphic image made by a radiographic scan of the kidneys after injection of a radiopharmaceutic. It represents radioactivity versus time and is used to assess renal function.

Renshaw cells /ren′shô/ [B. Renshaw, American neurologist, b. 1911], small cells that reduce motor neuron discharge through a feedback circuit involving axon collaterals that excite interneurons. The system prevents rapid repeated firing of motor neurons.

reovirus /rē′ōvī′rəs/ [*respiratory enteric orphan* + L *virus*], any one of three ubiquitous, double-stranded RNA viruses found in the respiratory and alimentary tracts in healthy and in sick people. Reoviruses have been implicated in some cases of upper respiratory tract disease and infantile gastroenteritis.

repercussion /rē′pərkush′ən/ [L *repercussio* rebounding], **1.** (in obstetrics) ballottment. **2.** being driven back by a powerful resistance. **3.** the reduction of a swelling or tumor.

repetition compulsion [L *repetere* to repeat], an unconscious need to revert to and repeat earlier situations, patterns of behavior, and acts to experience previously felt emotions or relationships.

replacement /riplās′mənt/ [Fr *replacer* to put in place again], the substitution of a missing part or substance with a similar structure or substance, such as the replacement of an amputated limb with a prosthesis or the replacement of lost blood with donor blood.

replacement therapy, **1.** the use of a medicinal product to replace a natural hormone or enzyme that the body is no longer able to produce in sufficient amounts. **2.** a psychotherapeutic technique of replacing abnormal behavior with healthy, constructive activities.

replacement transfusion, the removal of all or most of a patient's diseased blood and its simultaneous replacement with an equal volume of normal blood.

replication /rep′likā′shən/ [L *replicare* to fold back], **1.** a process of duplicating, reproducing, or copying; literally, a folding back of a part to form a duplicate. **2.** (in research) the exact repetition of an experiment performed to confirm the initial findings. **3.** (in genetics) the duplication of the polynucleotide strands of DNA or the synthesis of DNA. **–replicate,** *v.*

replicator /rep'likā'tər/ [L *replicare*], (in genetics) the segment of the DNA molecule that initiates and controls the replication of the polynucleotide strands.

replicon /rep'ləkon/ [L *replicare*], (in genetics) a replication unit; the segment of the DNA molecule that is undergoing replication.

repolarization /rē'pōlərīzā'shən/ [L *re + polus* pole; Gk *izein* to cause], (in cardiology) the process by which the cell is restored to its resting potential. It encompasses the effective and the relative refractory periods and correlates with the QT interval on the ECG.

report /ripôrt'/ [L *re + portare* to carry], (in nursing) the transfer of information from the nurses on one shift to the nurses on the following shift. Report is given systematically at the time of change of shift.

reportable diseases /ripôr'təbəl/, diseases that must be reported by the physician to public health authorities, given their contagious nature. They include but are not limited to malaria, influenza, poliomyelitis, relapsing fever, typhus, yellow fever, cholera, and bubonic plague.

repositioning /rēpəzish'rning/ [L *reponere* to put back], the restoration of an organ or body part to its natural position, as in repositioning an inverted uterus or changing the position of the jaws.

representative group /rep'rəsen'tətiv/, a group of individuals whose members represent all the various sectors of a community.

repression /ripresh'ən/ [L *reprimere* to press back], **1.** the act of restraining, inhibiting, or suppressing. **2.** (in psychoanalysis) an unconscious defense mechanism whereby unacceptable thoughts, feelings, ideas, impulses, or memories, especially those concerning some traumatic past event, are pushed from the consciousness because of their painful guilt association or disagreeable content and are submerged in the unconscious, where they remain dormant but operant and dynamic. **–repress,** *v.* **repressive,** *adj.*

repressive-inspirational approach /ripres'iv/, a psychotherapeutic approach used in some groups to encourage focus on positive feelings and group strengths.

repressor /ripres'ər/ [L *reprimere* to press back], (in molecular genetics) a protein produced by the regulator gene. It binds to a sequence of nucleotides in the operator gene, which regulates the structural gene.

repressor gene. See **regulator gene.**

reproduction /rē'prəduk'shən/ [L *re + producere* to produce], **1.** the process by which animals and plants give rise to offspring; procreation; the sum total of the cellular and genetic phenomena involved in the transmission of organic life from one organism to successive generations similar to the parents so that the perpetuation of the species is maintained. Kinds of reproduction include **asexual, cytogenic, sexual, somatic,** and **unisexual reproduction. 2.** the creation of a similar structure, situation, or phenomenon; duplication; replication. **3.** (in psychology) the recalling of a former idea, impression, or something previously learned. **–reproductive,** *adj.*

reproductive endocrinology /rē'prəduk'tiv/, the study of the maternal female hormone system, including the activities of the hypothalamus, pituitary, and ovaries from puberty through menopause.

reproductive system, the male and female gonads, associated ducts and glands, and the external genitalia that function in the procreation of offspring. In women these include the ovaries, fallopian tubes, uterus, vagina, clitoris, and vulva. In men these include the testes, epididymis, vas deferens, seminal vesicles, ejaculatory duct, prostate, and penis.

repulsion /ripul'shən/ [L *repellere* to drive away], **1.** the act of repelling, disjoining. **2.** a force that separates two bodies or things. **3.** (in genetics) the situation in linked inheritance in which the alleles of two or more mutant genes are located on homologous chromosomes so that each chromosome of the pair carries one or more mutant and wild-type genes, which are located close enough to be inherited together.

request for proposal (RFP) [L *requaerere* to require; *propronere* to propound], a solicitation by a funding agency for proposals to accomplish a particular goal. The RFP lists the requirements a project must meet to receive funding.

required arch length [L *requaerere* to require], the sum of the mesiodistal widths of all the natural teeth in a dental arch.

RES, abbreviation for **reticuloendothelial system.**

rescinnamine /risin'əmin/, an alkaloid antihypertensive and sedative. It is prescribed in the treatment of mild hypertension involving the cardiovascular or central nervous system, or both.

research /risurch', rē'surch/ [Fr *rechercher* to investigate], the diligent inquiry or examination of data, reports, and observations in a search for facts or principles.

research instrument, a testing device for

measuring a given phenomenon, such as a paper and pencil test, a questionnaire, an interview, or a set of guidelines for observation.

research measurement, an evaluation of the quantity or incidence of a given variable as obtained by using a research instrument.

research radiopharmaceutical, a drug that is labeled with a small quantity of a radioactive tracer to study its biodistribution; it may later be used in a nonradioactive form.

resect /risekt'/ [L *re + secare* to cut], to remove tissue from the body by surgery.

resection /risek'shən/, the cutting out of a significant portion of an organ or structure. Resection of an organ may be partial or complete. One type of resection is a **wedge resection.**

reserpine /res'ərpēn/, an antihypertensive prescribed in the treatment of high blood pressure and certain neuropsychiatric disorders.

reserve /rizurv'/ [L *reservare* to save], a potential capacity to maintain the vital functions of the body in homeostasis by adjusting to increased need, such as cardiac reserve, pulmonary reserve, and alkali reserve.

reserve capacity, the volume of air that can be exhaled with maximum effort after completion of a normal expiration.

reserve cell carcinoma. See **oat cell carcinoma.**

reservoir /rez'ərvwär/ [Fr], a chamber or receptacle for holding or storing a fluid.

reservoir bag, a component of an anesthesia machine in which gas accumulates, forming a reserve supply of gas for use when the quantity of flow is inadequate.

reservoir host, a nonhuman host that serves as a means of sustaining an infectious organism as a potential source of human infection. Wild monkeys are reservoir hosts for the yellow fever virus.

reservoir of infection, a continuous source of infectious disease. People, animals, and plants may be reservoirs of infection.

resident /rez'idənt/ [L *residere* to remain], a physician in one of the postgraduate years of clinical training after the first, or internship, year. The length of residency varies according to the specialty.

resident bacteria, bacteria living in a specific area of the body.

residential care facility /rez'iden'shəl/, a facility that provides custodial care to persons who, because of physical, mental, or emotional disorders, are not able to live independently.

residual /rizij'ōō·əl/ [L *residuum* remain-

der], pertaining to the portion of something that remains after an activity that removes the bulk of the substance.

residual cyst, an odontogenic cyst that remains in the jaw after the removal of a tooth.

residual dental caries, any decayed material left in a prepared tooth cavity.

residual function, the remaining ability to function after a serious illness or injury.

residual ridge, the portion of the dental ridge that remains after the alveolar process has disappeared after extraction of the teeth.

residual urine, urine that remains in the bladder after urination.

residual volume, the amount of gas in the lungs at the end of a maximum expiration.

residue-free diet /rez'id(y)ōō/, a diet free of nondigestible cellulose or fiber, such as found in semisolid bland food.

residue schizophrenia [L *residuum*], a form of schizophrenia in which the essential features include the presence of residual symptoms without evidence of delusions, hallucinations, incoherence, or gross disorganization.

resilience /rizil'yəns/ [L *resilere* to spring back], the ability of a body to return to its original form after being stretched or compressed.

res ipsa loquitur /räs' ip'sə lok'witōōr/, a Latin phrase meaning literally "the thing speaks for itself," a legal concept that is important in many malpractice suits. Classic examples of res ipsa loquitur are a sponge left in the abdomen after surgery or the amputation of the wrong extremity.

resistance /rizis'təns/ [L *resistere* to withstand], **1.** an opposition to a force, such as the resistance offered by the constriction of peripheral vessels to the blood flow in the circulatory system. **2.** the frictional force that opposes the flow of an electric charge, as measured in ohms. **3.** (in respiratory therapy) the process of acting against a force placed on it, pertaining to thoracic resistance, tissue resistance, and airway resistance.

resistance form, the shape given to a prepared tooth cavity to impart strength and durability to the restoration and remaining tooth structure.

resistance to flow, (in respiratory therapy) the pressure differential required to produce a unit flow change.

resistance transfer factor. See **R factor.**

resistance vessels, the blood vessels, including small arteries, arterioles, and metarterioles that form the major portion of the total peripheral resistance to blood flow.

resistive magnet /risis'tiv/, a simple electromagnet in which electricity passing through coils of wire produces a magnetic field.

resocialization /rēsō′shəlīzā′shən/ [L re + socialis partners; Gk izein to cause], the reintegration of a patient into family and community life after critical or long-term hospitalization.

resolution /rez′əlōō′shən/ [L re + solvere to solve], **1.** the ability of an imaging process to distinguish adjacent structures in the object. **2.** the state of having made a firm determination or decision on a course of action. **3.** the ability of a chromatographic system to separate two adjacent peaks.

resolving power /rizol′ving/, **1.** the ability to separate closely migrating substances, as in electrophoresis. **2.** the ability to distinguish closely positioned objects as distinct entities.

resolving time, (in radiology) the minimum time between ionization that can be detected by a Geiger-Müller scintillation device.

resonance /rez′ənəns/ [L resonare to sound again], **1.** an echo or other sound produced by percussion of an organ or cavity of the body during a physical examination. **2.** the process of energy absorption by an object that is tuned to absorb energy of a specific frequency only. Other frequencies do not affect the object. An example is the vibration of a tuning fork, causing other tuning forks of the same frequency to vibrate also. **−resonant,** adj.

resonating /rez′ənā′ting/, pertaining to vibrations or pulsations that are synchronous with a source of sound waves or electromagnetic oscillations.

resorb /risôrb′/ [L resorbere], to absorb again.

resorbent /risôr′bənt/, a material or agent that is used to absorb blood or other substances.

resorcinated camphor /rizôr′sinā′tid/, a mixture of camphor and resorcinol, used for the treatment of pediculosis and itching.

resorcinol /rizôr′sinol/, an antiseptic substance used as a keratolytic agent in the dermatoses.

resorcinol test. See **Boas' test.**

resorption /risôrp′shən/ [L resorbere to swallow again], **1.** the loss of substance or bone by physiologic or pathologic means. **2.** the cementoclastic and dentinoclastic action that may occur on a tooth root.

Res. Phys., abbreviation for Resident Physician.

respiration /res′pirā′shən/ [L respirare to breathe], the process of the molecular exchange of oxygen and carbon dioxide within the body's tissues, from the lungs to cellular oxidation processes. Certain types of breathing patterns commonly referred to as "respiration" are **Biot's respiration, Cheyne-Stokes respiration,** and **Kussmaul's respiration.**

respiration of infants, a rate of breathing that averages 40 to 50 breaths per minute at birth and declines to 15 to 20 breaths per minute at puberty.

respiration rate, the number of inspirations per minute, ranging from a rapid 40 to 50 for newborns, through 20 to 25 for older children, and 15 to 20 for most teenagers and adults. An adult rate of 25 breaths per minute may be regarded as accelerated, whereas a rate of less than 12 breaths per minute is abnormally slow.

respirator /res′pirā′tər/ [L respirare], an apparatus used to modify air for inspiration or to improve pulmonary ventilation.

respiratory /res′pərətôr′ē, rispī′rətôr′ē/ [L respirare], of or pertaining to respiration.

respiratory acidosis, an abnormal condition characterized by increased arterial Pco_2, excess carbonic acid, and increased plasma hydrogen ion concentration. It is caused by reduced alveolar ventilation, or the suppression of respiratory reflexes with narcotics, sedatives, hypnotics, or anesthetics. The hypoventilation associated with this condition inhibits the excretion of carbon dioxide, which consequently combines with water in the body to produce excessive carbonic acid and thus reduces blood pH. Some common signs and symptoms of respiratory acidosis are headache, dyspnea, fine tremors, tachycardia, hypertension, and vasodilatation. Ineffective treatment of acute respiratory acidosis can lead to coma and death.

respiratory alkalosis, an abnormal condition characterized by decreased Pco_2, decreased hydrogen ion concentration, and increased blood pH. It is caused by pulmonary and nonpulmonary problems. Some pulmonary causes are acute asthma, pulmonary vascular disease, and pneumonia. Some nonpulmonary causes are aspirin toxicity, anxiety, fever, metabolic acidosis, inflammation of the central nervous system, gram-negative septicemia, and hepatic failure. The hyperventilation associated with respiratory alkalosis most commonly stems from extreme anxiety. Deep and rapid breathing at rates as high as 40 respirations per minute is a major sign of respiratory alkalosis. Other symptoms are light-headedness, dizziness, peripheral paresthesia, spasms of the hands and the feet, muscle weakness, tetany, and cardiac

R

arrhythmia. Confirming diagnosis is often based on Pco_2 levels below 35 mm Hg, but the measurement of blood pH is critical in differentiating between metabolic acidosis and respiratory alkalosis.

respiratory arrest, the cessation of breathing.

respiratory assessment, an evaluation of the condition and function of a person's respiratory system. Signs of confusion, anxiety, restlessness, flaring nostrils, cyanotic lips, gums, earlobes, or nails, clubbing of extremities, fever, anorexia, and a tendency to sit upright are noted if present. The person's breathing is closely observed for evidence of slow, rapid, irregular, shallow, or Cheyne-Stokes respiration, hyperventilation, a long expiratory phase or periods of apnea, and for retractions in the suprasternal, supraclavicular, substernal, or intercostal areas during breathing. Percussion is performed to evaluate resonance, hyperresonance, tympany, and dull or flat sounds; and rales, rhonchi, wheezing, friction rubs, the transmission of spoken words through the chest wall, and decreased or absent breath sounds are detected by auscultation. Background information pertinent to the evaluation includes allergies, recent exposure to infection, immunizations, exposure to environmental irritants, previous respiratory disorders and operations, preexisting chronic conditions, medication currently taken, the person's smoking habits, and the family history.

respiratory bronchiole. See **bronchiole.**

respiratory burn, tissue damage to the respiratory system resulting from the inhalation of a hot gas or burning particles, as may occur in a fire or explosion.

respiratory care practitioner, a health professional with special training and experience in the treatment and rehabilitation of patients with respiratory disorders. The respiratory care practitioner typically does not diagnose but must be competent with patient assessment skills in a variety of clinical settings.

respiratory center, a group of nerve cells in the pons and medulla of the brain that control the rhythm of breathing in response to changes in levels of oxygen and carbon dioxide in the blood and cerebrospinal fluid. Change in the concentration of oxygen and carbon dioxide or hydrogen ion levels in the arterial circulation and in cerebrospinal fluid activate central and peripheral chemoreceptors; these send impulses to the respiratory center, increasing or decreasing the breathing rate.

respiratory component (OPco₂) the acid component of an acid-base control system that is modified by the respiratory status.

respiratory cycle, an inspiration followed by an expiration.

respiratory depressant, a drug or other agent that diminishes normal breathing functions. Most respiratory depressants, such as alcohol and opiates, act by depressing the central nervous system.

respiratory depression, respiration that is slow, below 12 inspirations per minute, or feeble breathing that fails to provide full ventilation and perfusion of the lungs.

respiratory distress syndrome of the newborn (RDS), an acute lung disease of the newborn, characterized by airless alveoli, inelastic lungs, more than 60 respirations a minute, nasal flaring, intercostal and subcostal retractions, grunting on expiration, and peripheral edema. It is caused by a deficiency of pulmonary surfactant, resulting in overdistended alveoli and, at times, hyaline membrane formation, alveolar hemorrhage, severe right-to-left shunting of blood, increased pulmonary resistance, decreased cardiac output, and severe hypoxemia.

respiratory exchange ratio (R), the ratio of the net expiration of carbon dioxide to the concurrent net inspiration of oxygen, expressed by the formula $V \cdot co_2 / V \cdot o_2$.

respiratory failure, the inability of the cardiac and pulmonary systems to maintain an adequate exchange of oxygen and carbon dioxide in the lungs. Respiratory failure may be hypoxemic or ventilatory. Hypoxemic failure is characterized by hyperventilation and occurs in diseases that affect the alveoli or interstitial tissues of the lobes of the lungs, such as alveolar edema, emphysema, fungal infections, leukemia, lobar pneumonia, lung carcinoma, various pneumoconioses, pulmonary eosinophilia, sarcoidosis, or tuberculosis. Ventilatory failure, characterized by increased arterial tension of carbon dioxide, occurs in acute conditions in which retained pulmonary secretions cause increased airway resistance and decreased lung compliance, as in bronchitis and emphysema.

respiratory insufficiency, a failure of the respiratory system to maintain adequate ventilation and perfusion of the lungs.

respiratory muscles, the muscles that produce volume changes of the thorax during breathing. The inspiratory muscles include the hemidiaphragms, external intercostals, scaleni, sternomastoids, trapezius, pectoralis major, pectoralis minor, subclavius, latissimus dorsi, serratus anterior, and muscles that extend the back. The expiratory muscles are the internal intercostals, abdominals, and the muscles that flex the back.

respiratory quotient (RQ), the body's total exchange of oxygen for carbon dioxide, expressed as the ratio of the volume of carbon dioxide produced to the volume of oxygen consumed per unit of time.

respiratory rate, the normal rate of breathing at rest, about 14 inspirations per minute. The rate may be more rapid in fever, acute pulmonary infection, diffuse pulmonary fibrosis, gas gangrene, left ventricular failure, thyrotoxicosis, and in states of tension. Slower breathing rates may result from head injury, coma, or narcotic overdose.

respiratory rhythm, a regular oscillating cycle of inspiration and expiration, controlled by neuronal impulses transmitted between the muscles of inspiration in the chest and the respiratory centers in the brain.

respiratory syncytial virus (RSV, RS virus), a member of a subgroup of myxoviruses that in tissue culture causes formation of giant cells or syncytia. It is a common cause of epidemics of acute bronchiolitis, bronchopneumonia, and the common cold in young children and sporadic acute bronchitis and mild upper respiratory tract infections in adults. Symptoms of infection with this virus include fever, cough, and severe malaise.

respiratory system. See **respiratory tract.**

respiratory therapist, a graduate of a school approved by the American Medical Association designed to qualify the person for the registry examination of the National Board of Respiratory Care (NBRC).

respiratory therapy (RT), 1. any treatment that maintains or improves the ventilatory function of the respiratory tract. **2.** *informal;* the department in a health care facility that provides respiratory therapy for the patients of the facility.

respiratory therapy technician, a graduate of an AMA-approved school designed to qualify the person for technician certification examination of the National Board for Respiratory Care (NBRC). It usually requires a 1-year hospital-based program combining a special curriculum of basic sciences with supervised clinical experience.

respiratory therapy technician, certified (CRTT), an allied health professional who administers general respiratory care. Duties can include collection and review of clinical data, examination of the patient by inspection, palpation, percussion, and auscultation, and assembling and maintaining equipment used in respiratory care.

respiratory tract, the complex of organs and structures that perform the pulmonary ventilation of the body and the exchange of oxygen and carbon dioxide between the ambient air and the blood circulating through the lungs. It also warms the air passing into the body and assists in the speech function by providing air for the larynx and the vocal cords.

respiratory tract infection, any infectious disease of the upper or lower respiratory tract. **Upper respiratory tract infections** include the common cold, laryngitis, pharyngitis, rhinitis, sinusitis, and tonsillitis. **Lower respiratory tract infections** include bronchitis, bronchiolitis, pneumonia, and tracheitis.

respiratory zone, the terminal air units where gas exchange actually occurs, usually below the seventeenth division of bronchi.

respirometer /res'pirom'ətər/, an instrument used to analyze the quality of a patient's respirations.

respite care /res'pit/ [L *respicere* to look back], **1.** short-term health services to the dependent older adult, either at home or in an institutional setting. **2.** the provision of temporary care for a patient who requires specialized or intensive care or supervision that is normally provided by his or her family at home.

respite time /res'pit/, relief time from responsibilities for the care of a patient.

respondeat superior /respon'dē·at/, a Latin phrase meaning literally "let the master answer," denoting the doctrine that an employer may be held liable for torts committed by employees acting within the scope of their employment.

respondent conditioning. See **classic conditioning.**

responder /rispon'dər/ [L *respondere* to promise in return], a tumor that shrinks in volume by at least 50% as a result of chemotherapy, radiation, or other treatment.

response /rispons'/ [L *responsum* reply], (in psychology) a cost category of negative punishment in which the reinforcer is lost or withdrawn after an operant.

response time, the period between the application of a stimulus and the response of a cell or cells.

rest [AS *restan* to rest], an extension from a prosthesis that affords vertical support for a dental restoration.

rest angle. See **occlusal rest angle.**

rest area, a surface prepared on a tooth or fixed restoration into which the rest fits, providing support for a removable partial denture.

resting cell, a cell that is not undergoing division.

resting membrane potential, the transmembrane voltage that exists when the heart muscle is at rest.

resting potential, the electrical potential across a nerve cell membrane before it is stimulated to release the charge. The resting potential for a neuron is between 50 and 100 millivolts, with the excess of negatively charged ions inside the cell membrane.

resting tremor. See **passive tremor.**

restitution /res'tit(y)o͞o'shən/, the spontaneous turning of the fetal head to the right or left after it has extended through the vulva.

rest jaw relation, (in dentistry) the postural relation of the mandible to the maxillae when the patient is resting comfortably in the upright position.

rest joint position, the position of a joint where the joint surfaces are relatively incongruent and the support structures are relatively lax. The position is used extensively in passive mobilization procedures.

restless legs syndrome [AS *restlaes;* ONorse *leggr*], a benign condition of unknown origin characterized by an irritating sensation of uneasiness, tiredness, and itching deep within the muscles of the leg, especially the lower part of the limb, accompanied by twitching and sometimes pain. The only relief is walking or moving the legs.

restoration /res'tôrā'shən/ [L *restaurare* to restore], any tooth filling, inlay, crown, partial or complete denture, or prosthesis that restores or replaces lost tooth structure, teeth, or oral tissues.

restoration contour, the profile of the surfaces of teeth that have been restored.

restoration of cusps, a reduction and inclusion of tooth cusps within a tooth cavity preparation and their restoration to functional occlusion with an artificial dental material.

restorative /ristôr'ətiv/, pertaining to the power or ability to restore or renew a person to a normal state of health or consciousness.

restraint /ristrānt'/ [L *restringere* to confine], any one of numerous devices used in aiding the immobilization of patients, especially children in traction. Some kinds of restraints are specially designed slings, jackets, or diapers.

restraint in bed, the confinement of a person to bed rest by the use of mechanical, physical, or chemical means, if needed.

restraint of trade, an illegal act that interferes with free competition in a commercial or business transaction so as to restrict the production of a product or the provision of a service, affect the cost of a product or a service, or control the market in any way to the detriment of the consumers or purchasers of the service or product.

restriction endonuclease /en'dōno͞o'-klē·ās/ [L *restringere* + Gk *endon* within; L *nucleus* nut; Fr *diastase* enzyme], (in molecular genetics) an enzyme that cleaves DNA at a specific site. Each of the many different endonucleases acts at a species-specific cleavage site.

restriction fragment, a fragment of viral or cellular nucleic acid produced by cleavage of the DNA molecule by specific endonucleases.

restriction fragment length polymorphism (RFLP), a marker for a DNA segment of a chromosome that is associated with a hereditary disease. RFLPs are used in the detection of sequence variations in human genomic DNA segments.

restrictive cardiomyopathy, a form of heart disease characterized by diastolic noncompliance or poor compliance of the ventricles as in constrictive pericarditis.

restrictive disease, a respiratory disorder characterized by restriction of expansion of the lungs or chest wall, resulting in diminished lung volumes and capacities.

rest seat. See **rest area.**

resuscitation /risus'itā'shən/ [L *resuscitare* to revive], the process of sustaining the vital functions of a person in respiratory or cardiac failure while reviving him or her, using techniques of artificial respiration and cardiac massage, correcting acid-base imbalance, and treating the cause of failure. **–resuscitate,** *v.*

resuscitator /risus'itā'tər/, an apparatus for pumping air into the lungs. It consists of a mask snugly applied over the mouth and nose, a reservoir for air, and a manually or electrically powered pump.

RET, abbreviation for **rational emotive therapy.**

retail dentistry [ME *retailen* to divide into pieces], the practice of fee-for-service dentistry in an exclusively retail environment, such as a shopping center, with the specific intention of attracting the customers of such retail centers and by using the marketing techniques of the retailers involved.

retained placenta [L *retinere* to hold, *placenta* flat cake], the failure of the placenta to be delivered during an appropriate period, usually 30 minutes, following birth of the infant.

retainer [L *retinere* to hold], **1.** the part

of a dental prosthesis that connects an abutment tooth with the suspended portion of a bridge. **2.** an appliance for maintaining teeth and jaw positions gained by orthodontic procedures. **3.** the portion of a fixed prosthesis that attaches a pontic to the abutment teeth. **4.** any clasp, attachment, or device for fixing or stabilizing a dental prosthesis.

retaining orthodontic appliance, an orthodontic device for holding the teeth in place, following orthodontic tooth movement, until the occlusion is stabilized.

retardation /rē'tärdā'shən/ [L *retardare* to check], the slowing down of any mental or physical activity or failure of intellectual abilities to develop normally. Psychomotor retardation may occur in depression and a conditioned response to an unconditioned stimulus may be retarded in appearance.

retarded /ritär'did/, adj/ [L *retarder* to slow down], (of physical, intellectual, social, or emotional development) abnormally slow. **–retard,** *v.,* /ritärd'/ **retardation,** *n.*

retarded dentition, the abnormal delay of the eruption of the deciduous or permanent teeth resulting from malnutrition, malposition of the teeth, a hereditary factor, or a metabolic imbalance, such as hypothyroidism.

retarded depression, the depressive phase of bipolar disorder.

retarded ejaculation, the inability of a male to ejaculate after having achieved an erection. This often accompanies the aging process.

retch [AS *hraecan* to spit], a strong attempt to vomit without bringing up anything.

rete /rē'tē/ [L, net], a network, especially of arteries or veins. **–retial,** *adj.*

rete arteriosum, an anastomotic network of small arteries at a point before they branch into arterioles and capillaries.

retention /riten'shən/ [L *retinere* to hold], **1.** a resistance to movement or displacement. **2.** the ability of the digestive system to hold food and fluid. **3.** the inability to urinate or defecate. **4.** the ability of the mind to remember information acquired from reading, observation, or other processes. **5.** the inherent property of a dental restoration to maintain its position without displacement under axial stress. **6.** a characteristic of proper tooth cavity preparation in which provision is made for preventing vertical displacement of the cavity filling. **7.** a period of treatment during which an individual wears an appliance to maintain teeth in positions to which they have been moved by orthodontic procedures. **–retain,** *v.*

retention enema, a medicinal or nutrient enema specially formulated so it will remain in the bowel without stimulating the nerve endings that would ordinarily result in evacuation.

retention form, the provision made in a prepared tooth cavity to prevent displacement of the restoration.

retention groove, a depression formed by the opposing vertical constrictions in the preparation of a tooth, which improves the retention of a restoration.

retention of urine, an abnormal, involuntary accumulation of urine in the bladder as a result of a loss of muscle tone in the bladder, neurologic dysfunction or damage to the bladder, obstruction of the urethra, or the administration of a narcotic analgesic.

retention pin, a small metal projection that extends from a dental metal casting into the dentin of a tooth to improve the retention of a tooth restoration.

retention procedure, a method established by state laws or mental health codes for committing a person to a psychiatric institution.

retention time (t_a), **1.** (in chromatography) the amount of elapsed time from the injection of a sample into the chromatographic system to the recording of the peak (band) maximum of the component in the chromatogram. **2.** the length of time a compound is retained on a chromatography column.

retention with overflow, a complication of urinary incontinence in which the pressure of retained urine after a voiding results in dribbling.

rete peg. See **epithelial peg.**

reticular /ritik'yələr/ [L *reticulum* little net], (of a tissue or surface) having a netlike pattern or structure of veins.

reticular activating system (RAS), a functional system in the brain essential for wakefulness, attention, concentration, and introspection. A network of nerve fibers in the thalamus, hypothalamus, brainstem, and cerebral cortex contribute to the system.

reticular formation, a small, thick cluster of neurons, nestled within the brainstem, that controls breathing, the heartbeat, the blood pressure, the level of consciousness, and other vital functions of the body. The reticular formation constantly monitors the state of the body through connections with the sensory and the motor tracts.

reticulation film fault /ritik'yəlā'shən/ [L *reticulum + atio* process], a defect in a radiograph or developed photographic film that appears as a network of corruga-

R

tions. It is usually caused by film development with an excessive temperature difference between any two of the darkroom solutions.

reticulin /ritik′yəlin/ [L *reticulum*], an albuminoid substance found in the connective fibers of reticular tissue.

reticulocyte /ritik′yələsīt/ [L *reticulum* + Gk *kytos* cell], an immature erythrocyte characterized by a meshlike pattern of threads and particles at the former site of the nucleus.

reticulocyte count, a count of the number of reticulocytes in a whole blood specimen, used in determining bone marrow activity. The reticulocyte count is lowered in hemolytic diseases; it is elevated after hemorrhage or during recovery from anemia.

reticulocytopenia /ritik′yələsī′təpē′nē·ə/ [L *reticulum* + Gk *kytos* cell, *penia* poverty], a decrease below the normal range of 0.5% to 1.5% in the number of reticulocytes in a blood sample.

reticulocytosis /-sīto′sis/, an increase in the number of reticulocytes in the circulating blood.

reticuloendothelial cells /ritik′yəlō·en′-dōthē′lē·əl/ [L *reticulum* + Gk *endon* within, *thele* nipple], cells lining vascular and lymph vessels capable of phagocytosing bacteria, viruses, and colloidal particles or of forming immune bodies against foreign particles.

reticuloendothelial system (RES) /-en′dothē′lē·əl/, a functional system of the body involved primarily in defense against infection and in disposal of the products of the breakdown of cells. It is made up of macrophages, the Kupffer cells of the liver, and the reticulum cells of the lungs, bone marrow, spleen, and lymph nodes. Disorders of this system include **eosinophilic granuloma, Gaucher's disease, Hand-Schüller-Christian syndrome,** and **Niemann-Pick disease.**

reticuloendotheliosis /ritik′yəlō·en′dōthē′-lē·ō′sis/, an abnormal condition characterized by increased growth and proliferation of the cells of the reticuloendothelial system.

reticulogranular /-gran′yələr/ [L *reticulum* + *granulum* little grain], pertaining to a cloudy appearance of the lungs on a chest radiograph of a patient with respiratory distress syndrome.

reticulosarcoma. See **undifferentiated malignant lymphoma.**

reticulum cell sarcoma. See **histiocytic malignant lymphoma.**

retina /ret′inə/ [L *rete* net], a 10-layered, delicate nervous tissue membrane of the eye, continuous with the optic nerve, that receives images of external objects and transmits visual impulses through the optic nerve to the brain. The retina is soft, semitransparent, and contains rhodopsin, which gives it a purple tint. The retina becomes clouded and opaque if exposed to direct sunlight. The outer surface of the retina is in contact with the choroid, the inner surface with the vitreous body.

retinaculum /ret′inak′yələm/, *pl.* retinacula [L, halter], **1.** a structure that retains an organ or tissue. **2.** an instrument for retracting tissues during surgery.

retinaculum extensorum manus, the thick band of antebrachial fascia that wraps tendons of the extensor muscles of the forearm at the distal ends of the radius and the ulna.

retinaculum flexorum manus, the thick, fibrous band of antebrachial fascia that wraps the carpal canal surrounding the tendons of flexor muscles of the forearm at the distal ends of the radius and the ulna.

retinal /ret′inəl, ret′inal′/ [L *rete*], **1.** an aldehyde precursor of vitamin A produced by the enzymatic dehydration of retinol. **2.** pertaining to the retina.

retinal detachment, a separation of the retina from the choroid in the back of the eye, usually resulting from a hole in the retina that allows the vitreous humor to leak between the choroid and the retina. Severe trauma to the eye, such as a contusion or penetrating wound, may be the proximate cause, but in the great majority of cases retinal detachment is the result of internal changes in the vitreous chamber associated with aging, or, less frequently, with inflammation of the interior of the eye. In most cases retinal detachment develops slowly. The first symptom is often the sudden appearance of a large number of spots floating loosely suspended in front of the affected eye. The person may also notice a curious sensation of flashing lights as the eye is moved. Because the retina does not contain sensory nerves that relay sensations of pain, the condition is painless. Detachment usually begins at the thin peripheral edge of the retina and extends gradually beneath the thicker, more central areas. The person perceives a shadow that begins laterally and grows in size, slowly encroaching on central vision. If the process of detachment is not halted, total blindness of the eye ultimately results. The condition does not spontaneously resolve itself.

retinene /ret′inin/ [L *rete*], either of the two carotenoid pigments found in the rods of the retina that are precursors of vitamin A and are activated by light.

retinitis /ret′inī′tis/ [L *rete* + Gk, *itis* inflammation], an inflammation of the retina.

retinitis pigmentosa [L *rete* + Gk *itis*; L *pigmentum* paint], a group of diseases, often hereditary, characterized by bilateral primary degeneration of the retina, beginning in childhood and progressing to blindness by middle age. Clinical signs include night blindness, reduced visual fields, and pigmentation of the retina, macular degeneration, and eventually total loss of vision.

retinoblastoma /ret′inōblastō′mə/, *pl.* retinoblastomas, retinoblastomata [L *rete* + Gk *blastos* germ, *oma* tumor], a congenital, hereditary neoplasm developing from retinal germ cells. Characteristic signs are diminished vision, strabismus, retinal detachment, and an abnormal pupillary reflex. The rapidly growing tumor may invade the brain and metastasize to distant sites.

retinocerebral angiomatosis. See **cerebroretinal angiomatosis.**

retinochoroiditis /-kôr′oidī′tis/ [L *rete* + Gk *chorion* skin, *itis*], an inflammation of the retina and choroid coat of the eye.

retinodialysis /ret′inōdī·al′isis/ [L *rete* + Gk *dia* through, *lysis* loosening], a separation or tear in the retina in its anterior part, in the area of the ora serrata, just behind the ciliary body.

retinoid [L *rete* + Gk *eidos* form], pertaining to a structure that resembles the retina.

retinol /ret′inôl/ [L *rete*], the cis-trans form of vitamin A. It is found in the retinas of mammals.

retinopathy /ret′inop′əthē/ [L *rete* + Gk *pathos* disease], a noninflammatory eye disorder resulting from changes in the retinal blood vessels.

retinoscope /ret′inəskōp′/ [L *rete* + Gk *skopein* to view], an instrument used in retinoscopy to determine errors of refraction.

retinoscopy /ret′inos′kəpē/, a procedure for examining the eyes for possible errors of refraction. The examiner shines a light into the eyeball and notes the movements of reflex from the fundus. This indicates the types of lenses needed to neutralize the refractive errors.

retirement center /ritī′ə′mənt/ [Fr *retirer* to withdraw; Gk *kentron* center], a facility or organized program that may be affiliated with a hospital to provide social services and activities for senior citizens who generally do not require ongoing health care.

retract /ritrakt′/ [L *retractare* to draw back], to shrink, make shorter, or pull back.

retracted nipple, a nipple drawn inward as the result of cancer, adhesions below the skin surface, or a natural condition present at birth.

retraction /ritrak′shən/ [L *retractare* to draw back], **1.** the displacement of tissues to expose a part or structure of the body. **2.** a distal movement of the teeth. **3.** a distal or retrusive position of the teeth, dental arch, or jaw.

retraction of the chest, the visible sinking-in of the soft tissues of the chest between and around the firmer tissue of the cartilaginous and bony ribs, as occurs with increased inspiratory effort.

retractor /ritrak′tər/ [L *retractare*], an instrument for holding back the edges of tissues and organs to maintain exposure of the underlying anatomic parts, particularly during surgery, such as an army retractor or a double-ended Richardson retractor.

retroanterograde amnesia /-anter′ōgrād/ [L *retro* + *antero* foremost, *gradus* step; Gk *amnesia* forgetfulness], a memory disorder in which current events may be assigned to the past and past events may be regarded as current.

retroaortic node /re′trō·ā·ôr′tik/ [L *retro* backward; Gk *aerein* to raise], a node in one of three sets of lumbar lymph nodes that serve various structures in the abdomen and the pelvis.

retroauricular /-ôrik′yələr/ [L *retro* + *auricula* little ear], pertaining to a location behind the ear.

retrobulbar /-bul′bər/ [L *retro* + *bulbus* swollen root], **1.** pertaining to the area behind the pons. **2.** pertaining to the area behind the eyeball.

retrobulbar neuritis, a form of neuritis that involves the optic nerve or the optic disc.

retrocecal /-sē′kəl/ [L *retro* + *caecus* blind], pertaining to the region behind the cecum.

retroclusion /ret′roklōō′shən/, a method of controlling hemorrhage from an artery by compressing it between tissues on either side. A needle is inserted through the tissues above the bleeding vessel, then turned around and down so it also passes through the tissues beneath the artery.

retroflexion /-flek′shən/ [L *retro* + *flectere* to bend], an abnormal position of an organ in which the organ is tilted back acutely, folded over on itself.

retroflexion of the uterus, a condition in which the body of the uterus is bent backward at an angle with the cervix, whose position usually remains unchanged.

retrognathia /ret′rōnā′thē′ə/ [L *retro* + Gk, *gnathos* jaw], a condition in which either or both jaws recede with respect to

R

the frontal plane of the forehead. According to Angle's Classification of Malocclusion, the facial profile of a person with Class II or distocclusion is retrognathic.

retrognathism /ret′rōnă′this′əm/ [L *retro* + Gk *gnathos* jaw], a facial abnormality in which one or both jaws, usually the mandible, are posterior to their normal facial positions.

retrograde /ret′rəgrād/ [L *retro* + *gradus* step], **1.** moving backward; moving in the opposite direction to that which is considered normal. **2.** degenerating; reverting to an earlier state or worse condition. **3.** catabolic.

retrograde amnesia, the loss of memory for events occurring before a particular time in a person's life, usually before the event that precipitated the amnesia.

retrograde cystoscopy, a radiologic technique for examining the bladder in which a catheter is inserted through the urethra into the bladder. A radiopaque medium is introduced, filling the bladder, and the contour of the bladder is observed, using serial x-ray films or fluoroscopy.

retrograde ejaculation, an ejaculation of semen in a reverse direction, into the urinary bladder. The effect is sometimes the result of prostate surgery or a congenital condition.

retrograde filling, a filling placed in the apical portion of a tooth root to seal the apical portion of the root canal.

retrograde flow, the flow of fluid in a direction other than normal, as in regurgitation.

retrograde infantilism. See **acromegalic eunuchoidism.**

retrograde infection, an infection that spreads along a tubule or duct against the flow of secretions or excretions, as in the urinary and lymphatic systems.

retrograde menstruation, a backflow of menstrual discharge through the uterine cavity and the fallopian tubes into the peritoneal cavity.

retrograde pyelography, a radiologic technique for examining the structures of the collecting system of the kidneys that is especially useful in locating a urinary tract obstruction. A radiopaque contrast medium is injected through a urinary catheter into the ureters and the calyces of the pelves of the kidneys.

retrograde urography. See **retrograde pyelography.**

retrograde Wenckebach, a progressively lengthening conduction of impulses from the ventricles or AV junction to the atria until an impulse fails to reach the atria.

retrogression /-gresh′ən/ [L *retro* + *gradi* to step], a return to a less complex state,

condition, or behavioral adaptation; degeneration; deterioration.

retrolental fibroplasia /-len′təl/ [L *retro* + *lentil* lens; *fibra* fiber; Gk *plassein* to mold], a formation of fibrous tissue behind the lens of the eye, resulting in blindness. The disorder is caused by administration of excessive concentrations of oxygen to premature infants.

retromolar pad /-mō′lər/ [L *retro* + *mola* mill; D *paden* cushion], a mass of soft tissue, usually pear shaped, that marks the distal termination of the mandibular residual ridge.

retromylohyoid space /ret′rōmī′lōhī′oid/ [L *retro* + Gk *myle* mill, *hyoeides* upsilon shaped; L *spatium*], the part of the alveolingual sulcus that is distal to the distal end of the mylohyoid ridge.

retroperitoneal /-per′itənē′əl/ [L *retro* + Gk *peri* around, *teinein* to stretch], of or pertaining to organs closely attached to the abdominal wall and partly covered by peritoneum, rather than suspended by that membrane.

retroperitoneal fibrosis, a chronic inflammatory process, usually of unknown cause, in which fibrous tissue surrounds the large blood vessels in the lower lumbar area. Symptoms include low-back and abdominal pain, weakness, weight loss, fever, and, with urinary tract involvement, frequency of urination, hematuria, polyuria, or anuria.

retroperitoneal lymph node dissection, surgical removal of lymph nodes behind the peritoneum, usually performed in an attempt to eliminate sites of lymphoma or metastases from malignancies originating in pelvic organs or genitalia.

retroperitoneum /-per′itəmē′əum/ [L *retro* + Gk, *peri*, *teinein* to stretch], the space behind the peritoneum.

retropharyngeal abscess /-fərin′jē·əl/ [L *retro* + Gk *pharynx* throat], a collection of pus in the tissues behind the pharynx accompanied by difficulty in swallowing, fever, and pain. Occasionally, the airway becomes obstructed.

retroplacental /-pləsen′təl/, behind the placenta.

retrospective chart audit /-spek′tiv/ [L *retro* + *spicere* to look], a format for an audit developed by the Joint Commission on the Accreditation of Hospitals. The audit involves several steps that outline a procedure for evaluating the effectiveness of the care given at a particular institution and for correcting any deficiencies found by reviewing the patient's records.

retrospective nursing audit. See **nursing audit.**

retrospective study, a study in which a

search is made for a relationship between one (usually current) phenomenon or condition and another that occurred in the past.

retrosternal /-stur′nəl/ [L *retro* + Gk *sternon* chest], behind the sternum.

retrouterine /re′trōyo͞o′tərin/, behind the uterus.

retroversion /-vur′zhən/ [L *retro* + *vertere* to turn], **1.** a common condition in which an organ is tipped backward, usually without flexion or other distortion. Uterine retroversion is measured as first, second, or third degree, depending on the angle of tilt with respect to the vagina. **2.** an abnormal condition in which the teeth or other maxillary and mandibular structures are posterior to their normal positions. **–retrovert,** *v.*

retrovirus /-vī′rəs/ [L *retro* + *virus*], any of a family of RNA viruses containing reverse transcriptase in the virion. During replication the viral DNA becomes integrated into the DNA of the host cell. Retroviruses are enveloped and assemble their capsids in the cytoplasm of the host cell. The HIV, which causes AIDS, is a retrovirus.

retrusion. See **retroversion.**

revascularization /rēvas′kyələr′īzā′shən/ [L *re* + *vasculum* small vessel; Gk *izein* to cause], the restoration by surgical means of blood flow to an organ or a tissue being replaced, as in bypass surgery.

reverberation /rivur′bərā′shən/, the phenomenon of multiple reflections within a closed system.

Reverdin's needle /reverdaNz′/ [Albert Reverdin, Swiss surgeon, b. 1881], a surgical needle with an eye that can be opened and closed with a slide.

reversal film /rivur′səl/, (in radiology) a reverse-tone duplicate of an x-ray image, showing black changed to white and white to black. It is produced by exposing single-emulsion film through a standard x-ray film.

reverse anaphylaxis. See **inverse anaphylaxis.**

reverse Barton's fracture [L *revertere* to turn back; John R. Barton, American surgeon, b. 1794], a fracture of the volar articular surface of the radius with associated displacement of the carpal bones and radius.

reverse bevel. See **contra bevel.**

reverse curve, (in dentistry) a convex curve of occlusion, as viewed in the frontal plane.

reversed bandage, a roller bandage that is reversed on itself with a half twist so that it lies smoothly, conforming to the contour of the extremity.

reversed coarctation. See **Takayasu's arteritis.**

reversed phase, a chromatographic mode in which the mobile phase is more polar than the stationary phase.

reverse isolation, isolation procedures designed to protect a patient from infectious organisms that might be carried by the staff, other patients, or visitors or on droplets in the air or on equipment or materials. Handwashing, gowning, gloving, sterilization or disinfection of materials brought into the area, and other details of housekeeping vary with the reason for the isolation and the usual practices of the hospital.

reverse peristalsis [L *revertere* to turn back; Gk *peristellein* to clasp], peristalsis that propels the contents in a direction opposite to the normal outward direction.

reverse transcriptase (RT), an enzyme that is present in the virion of retroviruses. Reverse transcriptase occurs in leukoviruses and RNA tumor viruses of eukaryotic cells.

reverse Trendelenburg, a position in which the lower extremities are lower than the body and head.

reversible brain syndrome, any of a group of acute brain disorders characterized by a disruption of cognition. The disorder is related to a variety of biological stressors, and recovery is possible.

review of systems (ROS) [Fr *revoir* to see again], (in a health history) a system-by-system review of the functions of the body. The ROS is begun during the initial interview with the patient and completed during the physical examination, as physical findings prompt further questions.

Reye's syndrome /rāz′/ [Ralph D. K. Reye, twentieth-century Australian pathologist], a combination of acute encephalopathy and fatty infiltration of the internal organs that may follow acute viral infections. This syndrome has been associated with influenza B, chickenpox (varicella), the enteroviruses, and the Epstein-Barr virus. It usually affects people under 18 years of age, characteristically causing an exanthematous rash, vomiting, and confusion about 1 week after the onset of a viral illness. In the late stage, there may be extreme disorientation followed by coma, seizures, and respiratory arrest.

rf, 1. abbreviation for **radiofrequency. 2.** abbreviation for **rheumatic fever.**

RF, abbreviation for **rheumatoid factor.**

R factor, an episome in bacteria that is responsible for drug resistance and is transmissible to progeny and to other bacterial cells by conjugation. The portion of the

R

episome involved in replication and transmission is called **resistance transfer factor.**

RFP, abbreviation for **request for proposal.**

RF test. See **latex fixation test.**

Rh, 1. abbreviation for *Rhesus* (blood factor). **2.** symbol for the chemical element **rhodium.**

r/h, 1. abbreviation for **relative humidity. 2.** abbreviation for *roentgens per hour.*

rhabdomyoma /rab'dōmī·ō'mə/, pl. rhabdomyomas, rhabdomyomata [Gk *rhabdos* rod, *mys* muscle, *oma*], a tumor of striated muscle that may occur in the uterus, vagina, pharynx, or tongue, or in the heart as congenital neoplastic infiltration.

rhabdomyosarcoma /rab'dōmī-ōsärkō'mə/, pl. rhabdomyosarcomas, rhabdomyosarcomata [Gk *rhabdos* + *mys* muscle, *sarx* flesh, *oma*], a highly malignant tumor, derived from primitive striated muscle cells, that occurs most frequently in the head and neck and is also found in the genitourinary tract, extremities, body wall, and retroperitoneum. In some cases, the onset is associated with trauma. The initial symptoms depend on the site and indicate local tissue or organ destruction, such as dysphagia, vaginal bleeding, hematuria, or obstruction of the flow of urine.

rhabdovirus /rab'dōvī'rəs/ [Gk *rhabdos* + L *virus* poison], a member of a family of viruses that includes the organism causing rabies.

rhagades /rag'ədēz/ [Gk, chinks], cracks or fissures in skin that has lost its elasticity, especially common around the mouth.

Rh antiserum, a serum that contains Rh antibodies.

rhaphe. See **raphe.**

Rh blood group. See **Rh factor.**

rhd, 1. abbreviation for *radioactive health data.* **2.** abbreviation for **rheumatic heart disease.**

Rh₀(D) immune globulin, a passive immunizing agent prescribed to prevent Rh sensitization after abortion or miscarriage, post partum, or in ectopic pregnancy.

rhenium (Re) /rē'nē·əm/ [L *Rhenus* Rhine], a hard, brittle metallic element. Its atomic number is 75; its atomic weight is 186.2. Rhenium has a high melting point and is used in thermometers for measuring high temperatures.

rheostat /rē'əstat/ [Gk *rheos* current, *statikos* causing to stand], a variable resistance electrical device that can be adjusted to control the strength of a current.

Rhesus factor. See **Rh factor.**

rheumatic /rōomat'ik/ [Gk *rheuma* flux], of or pertaining to rheumatism.

rheumatic aortitis, an inflammatory condition of the aorta, occurring in rheumatic fever and characterized by disseminated focal lesions that may progressively form patches of fibrosis.

rheumatic arteritis, a complication of rheumatic fever characterized by generalized inflammation of arteries and arterioles. Fibrin, mixed with cellular debris, may invade, thicken, and stiffen the vessel wall, and the vessel may be surrounded by hemorrhage and exudate.

rheumatic carditis [Gk *rheumatismos* that which flows, *kardia* heart, *itis*], the pericarditis, myocarditis, and endocarditis that may be associated with acute rheumatic fever.

rheumatic chorea. See **Sydenham's chorea.**

rheumatic endocarditis [Gk *rheumatismos* that which flows, *endon* within, *kardia* heart, *itis*], an inflammation of the endocardium in association with acute rheumatic fever.

rheumatic fever, an inflammatory disease that may develop as a delayed reaction to inadequately treated group A beta-hemolytic streptococcal infection of the upper respiratory tract. The onset of rheumatic fever is usually sudden, often occurring from 1 to 5 symptom-free weeks after recovery from a sore throat or from scarlet fever. Early symptoms usually include fever, joint pains, nose bleeds, abdominal pain, and vomiting. The major manifestations of this disease include migratory polyarthritis affecting numerous joints and carditis, which causes palpitations, chest pain, and, in severe cases, symptoms of cardiac failure. Sydenham's chorea, which may develop, is usually the sole, late sign of rheumatic fever and may initially be manifested as an increased awkwardness and an associated tendency to drop objects. As the chorea progresses, irregular body movements may become extensive, occasionally involving the tongue and the facial muscles, resulting in incapacitation of the affected individual.

rheumatic heart disease, damage to heart muscle and heart valves caused by episodes of rheumatic fever. When a susceptible person acquires a group A beta-hemolytic streptococcal infection, an autoimmune reaction may occur in heart tissue, resulting in permanent deformities of heart valves or chordae tendineae. Involvement of the heart may be evident during acute rheumatic fever, or it may be discovered long after the acute disease has subsided.

rheumatic nodules, aggregations of fibroblasts and lymphoid cells that may accumulate in soft tissues and over bony prominences of patients afflicted with rheumatoid arthritis and rheumatic fever.

rheumatic scoliosis, a form of scoliosis associated with muscle spasms and acute inflammation.

rheumatid /rōō′mətid/, a skin eruption that sometimes occurs with rheumatic disorders.

rheumatism /rōō′mətiz′əm/ [Gk *rheumatismos* that which flows], *nontechnical.* **1.** any of a large number of inflammatory conditions of the bursae, joints, ligaments, or muscles characterized by pain, limitation of movement, and structural degeneration of single or multiple parts of the musculoskeletal system. **2.** the syndrome of pain, limitation of movement, and structural degeneration of elements in the musculoskeletal system as may occur in gout, rheumatoid arthritis, systemic lupus erythematosus, ankylosing spondylitis, and many other diseases. **–rheumatic, rheumatoid,** *adj.*

rheumatoid arteritis /rōō′mətoid/, inflammation of the arterial walls associated with a rheumatic disorder.

rheumatoid arthritis [Gk *rheumatismos* + *eidos* form; *arthron* joint, *itis* inflammation], a chronic, destructive, sometimes deforming collagen disease that has an autoimmune component. Rheumatoid arthritis is characterized by symmetric inflammation of the synovium and increased synovial exudate, leading to thickening of the synovium and swelling of the joint. The course of the disease is variable but is most frequently marked by remissions and exacerbation.

rheumatoid coronary arteritis, an abnormal condition, characterized by a thickening of the tunica intima of the coronary arteries, which may produce coronary insufficiency. Rheumatoid coronary arteritis is a collagen disease that affects the connective tissue by inflammation and fibrinoid degeneration.

rheumatoid factor (RF), antiglobulin antibodies often found in the serum of patients with a clinical diagnosis of rheumatoid arthritis. Rheumatoid factors may also be found in widely divergent diseases such as tuberculosis, parasitic infections, leukemia, and connective tissue disorders.

rheumatologist /rōō′mətol′əjist/, a specialist in rheumatology.

rheumatology /-ol′əjē/ [Gk *rheuma* flux, *logos* science], the study of disorders characterized by inflammation, degeneration, or metabolic derangement of connective tissue and related structures of the body.

Rh factor, an antigenic substance present in the erythrocytes of most people. A person having the factor is Rh+ (Rh positive); a person lacking the factor is Rh− (Rh negative). If an Rh− person receives Rh+ blood, hemolysis and anemia occur. Rh+ infants may be exposed to antibodies to the factor produced in the Rh− mother's blood, resulting in red cell destruction and erythroblastosis fetalis. Transfusion, blood typing, and crossmatching depend on Rh+ and ABO classification. The Rh factor was first identified in the blood of a rhesus (Rh) monkey.

Rh genes [Rh, rhesus; Gk *genein* to produce], a series of allelic genes that account for the various Rh blood groups. The four variations of the Rh+ gene are identified as R^0, R^1, R^2, and R^z, whereas the four types of Rh− gene are designated as r, r′, r″, and r_y.

Rh immune globulin [Rh, rhesus; L *immunis* free from, *globulus*], an immune globulin that is administered to all Rh− mothers after every abortion or delivery unless the infant is Rh− or unless the mother's serum already contains anti-$Rh_0(D)$ reagent.

Rh incompatibility, (in hematology) a lack of compatibility between two groups of blood cells that are antigenically different because of the presence of the Rh factor in one group and its absence in the other.

rhinencephalon /rī′nensef′əlon/, *pl.* rhinencephala [Gk *rhis* nose, *encephalon* brain], a portion of each cerebral hemisphere that contains the limbic system, which is associated with the emotions. **–rhinencephalic,** *adj.*

rhinitis /rīnī′tis/ [Gk *rhis* + *itis* inflammation], inflammation of the mucous membranes of the nose, usually accompanied by swelling of the mucosa and a nasal discharge. Rhinitis may be acute, allergic, atrophic, or vasomotor.

rhinolaryngitis /rī′nōler′injī′tis/ [Gk *rhis* nose, *larynx* throat, *itis*], an inflammation of the mucous membranes of the nose and throat.

rhinopathy /rīnop′əthē/ [Gk *rhis* + *pathos* disease], any disease or malformation of the nose.

rhinophycomycosis /rī′nōfī′kōmīkō′sis/, an infection of the nasal and paranasal sinuses caused by the phycomycete *Entomophthora coronata.* The infection often spreads to surrounding tissues, including the eye and brain.

rhinophyma /rī′nōfī′mə/ [Gk *rhis* + *phyma* tumor], a form of rosacea in which there is sebaceous hyperplasia, redness, prominent vascularity, swelling, and distortion of the skin of the nose.

R

rhinoplasty /rī'nəplas'tē/ [Gk *rhis* + *plassein* to mold], a procedure in plastic surgery in which the structure of the nose is changed. Bone or cartilage may be removed, tissue grafted from another part of the body, or synthetic material implanted to alter the shape. The procedure is most frequently performed for cosmetic reasons.

rhinorrhagia /rī'nôrā'jə/ [Gk *rhis* + *rhegnynein* to gush forth], a profuse nosebleed.

rhinorrhea /rī'nôrē'ə/ [Gk *rhis* + *rhoia* flow] **1.** the free discharge of a thin nasal mucus. **2.** the flow of cerebrospinal fluid from the nose after an injury to the head.

rhinoscope /rī'nəskōp/, an instrument for examining the nasal passages through the anterior nares or through the nasopharynx.

rhinoscopy /rīnos'kəpē/ [Gk *rhis* + *skopein* to look], an examination of the nasal passages to inspect the mucosa and detect inflammation, deformities, or asymmetry, as in deviation of the septum. The nasal passages may be examined anteriorly, by introducing a speculum into the anterior nares, or posteriorly, by introducing a rhinoscope through the nasopharynx. **−rhinoscopic,** *adj.*

rhinosporidiosis /rī'nōspərid'ē·ō'sis/ [Gk *rhis* + *sporo* seed, *osis* condition], an infection caused by the fungus *Rhinosporidium seeberi,* characterized by fleshy red polyps on mucous membranes of nose, conjunctiva, nasopharynx, and soft palate. The disease may be acquired by swimming or bathing in infected water.

rhinotomy /rīnot'əmē/ [Gk *rhis* + *temnein* to cut], a surgical procedure in which an incision is made along one side of the nose, performed to drain accumulated pus from an abscess or a sinus infection.

rhinovirus /rī'nōvī'rəs/ [Gk *rhis* + L *virus* poison], any of about 100 serologically distinct, small RNA viruses that cause about 40% of acute respiratory illnesses. Infection is characterized by dry, scratchy throat, nasal congestion, malaise, and headache. Fever is minimal. Nasal discharge lasts 2 or 3 days. Complete recovery is usual.

rhitidosis /rit'idō'sis/ [Gk *rhytis* wrinkle, *osis* condition], a wrinkling, especially of the cornea.

rhizomelic /rī'zəmel'ik/ [Gk *rhizo* root, *melos* limb], pertaining to the hip and shoulder joints.

rhizotomy /rīzot'əmē/, the surgical resection of the dorsal root of a spinal nerve, performed to relieve pain.

Rh negative. See **Rh factor.**

Rhodesian trypanosomiasis /rōdē'zhən/, an acute form of African trypanosomiasis, caused by the parasite *Trypanosoma brucei rhodesiense.* The disease may progress rapidly, causing encephalitis, coma, and death in only a few weeks.

rhodium (Rh) /rō'dē·əm/ [Gk *rhodon* rose], a grayish white metallic element. Its atomic number is 45; its atomic weight is 102.91.

rhodopsin /rōdop'sin/ [Gk *rhodon* rose, *opsis* vision], the purple-pigmented compound in the rods of the retina, formed by a protein, opsin, and a derivative of vitamin A, retinal. Rhodopsin gives the outer segments of the rods a purple color and adapts the eye to low-density light. The compound breaks down when struck by light, and this chemical change triggers the conduction of nerve impulses.

rhomboid /rom'boid/ [Gk *rhomb* + *eidos* form], resembling the shape of an oblique equilateral parallelogram, as a rhomboid muscle.

rhomboideus major /romboi'dē·əs/ [Gk *rhombos* rhombus, *eidos* form], a muscle of the upper back below and parallel to the rhomboideus minor. It functions to draw the scapula toward the vertebral column while supporting it and drawing it slightly upward.

rhomboideus minor, a muscle of the upper back, above and parallel to the rhomboideus major. It acts to draw the scapula toward the vertebral column while supporting the scapula and drawing it slightly upward.

rhomboid glossitis. See **median rhomboid glossitis.**

rhonchi /rong'kī/, *sing.* **rhonchus** [Gk *rhonchos* snore], abnormal sounds heard on auscultation of an airway obstructed by thick secretions, muscular spasm, neoplasm, or external pressure. The continuous rumbling sounds are more pronounced during expiration, and they characteristically clear on coughing, which gurgles do not.

rhotacism /rō'təsiz'əm/ [Gk *rho* letter R], a speech disorder characterized by a defective pronunciation of words containing the sound /r/, or by the excessive use of the sound /r/, or by the substitution of another sound for /r/.

Rh positive. See **Rh factor.**

r-HuEPO, abbreviation for *recombinant human erythropoietin.*

rhus dermatitis /rŏos/ [Gk *rhous* sumac], a skin rash resulting from contact with a plant of the genus *Rhus,* such as poison ivy, poison oak, or poison sumac.

rhythm /rith'əm/ [Gk *rhythmos*], the relationship of one impulse to neighboring impulses as measured in time, movement, or regularity of action.

rhythmic nystagmus. See **nystagmus.**

rhythm method. See **natural family planning method.**

rhytidoplasty /ritid'ōplas'tē/ [Gk *rhytis* wrinkle, *plassein* to mold], a procedure in reconstructive plastic surgery in which the skin of the face is tightened, wrinkles are removed, and the skin is made to appear firm and smooth.

rhytidosis. See **rhitidosis.**

RIA. See **radioimmunoassay.**

rib [AS, roof], one of the 12 pairs of elastic arches of bone forming a large part of the thoracic skeleton. The first seven ribs on each side are called **true ribs** because they articulate directly with the sternum and the vertebrae. The remaining five ribs are called **false ribs,** the first three attaching ventrally to ribs above; the last two ribs are free at their ventral extremities and are called **floating ribs.**

ribavirin /rī'bəvir'in/, an aerosol antiviral drug prescribed for the treatment of respiratory synctial virus (RSV) infections for the lower respiratory tract in infants and small children.

rib fracture, a break in a bone of the thoracic skeleton caused by a blow or crushing injury or by violent coughing or sneezing. The ribs most commonly broken are the fourth to eighth, and, if the bone is splintered or the fracture is displaced, sharp fragments may pierce the lung, causing hemothorax or pneumothorax. The patient with a fractured rib suffers pain, especially on inspiration, and usually breathes rapidly and shallowly. The site of the break is generally very tender to the touch, and the crackling of bone fragments rubbing together may be heard on auscultation. Breath sounds may be absent, decreased, or accompanied by rales and rhonchi.

riboflavin /rib'ōflā'vin/ [*ribose* + L *flavus* yellow], a yellow crystalline, water-soluble pigment, one of the heat-stable components of the B vitamin complex. It combines with specific flavoproteins and functions as a coenzyme in the oxidative processes of carbohydrates, fats, and proteins. Deficiency of riboflavin produces cheilosis, local inflammation, desquamation, encrustation, glossitis, photophobia, corneal opacities, proliferation of corneal vessels, seborrheic dermatitis about the nose, mouth, forehead, ears, and scrotum, trembling, sluggishness, dizziness, edema, inability to urinate, and vaginal itching.

ribonuclear protein /rī'bōnoō'klē-ər/, a conjugated protein consisting of a protein molecule and nucleic acid.

ribonuclease /-noō'klē-ās/, a class of endonucleases that hydrolyze ribonucleic acids.

ribonucleic acid (RNA) /rī'bōnoōklē'ik/ [*ribose* + L *nucleus* nut; *acidus* sour], a nucleic acid, found in both the nucleus and cytoplasm of cells, that transmits genetic instructions from the nucleus to the cytoplasm. In the cytoplasm, RNA functions in the assembly of proteins.

ribonucleotide /-noō'klē-ətīd/, a class of nucleotides in which the pentose is D-ribose.

ribose /rī'bōs/, a 5-carbon pentose sugar that occurs as a component of ribonucleic acid.

ribosome /rī'bəsōm/ [*ribose* + Gk *soma* body], a cytoplasmic organelle composed of ribonucleic acid and protein that functions in the synthesis of protein. Ribosomes interact with messenger RNA and transfer RNA to join together amino acid units into a polypeptide chain according to the sequence determined by the genetic code.

rib shaking, a procedure in physiotherapy involving constant downward pressure with an intermittent shaking motion of the hands on the rib cage over the area being drained. It is done with the flat part of the palm of the hand over the lung segment being drained.

rib vibration, a procedure in physiotherapy, similar to rib shaking, but done with a downward vibrating pressure with the flat part of the palm during exhalations.

RICE, abbreviation for *rest, ice, compression, elevation,* the treatment for sprains and strains.

rice diet [Gk *oryza* rice, *diaita* life-style], a diet consisting only of rice, fruit, fruit juices, and sugar, supplemented with vitamins and iron. Salt is strictly forbidden. It is prescribed for the treatment of hypertension, chronic renal disease, and obesity.

Richards, Linda (1841-1930), considered to be the first American-trained nurse, having graduated in the first class of the New England Hospital for Women and Children. She is credited with being the first to keep written records on patients, a practice she started when she worked as night superintendent at Bellevue Hospital in New York under Sister Helen.

Richet's aneurysm. See **fusiform aneurysm.**

rickets /rik'əts/ [Gk *rachis* backbone, *itis* inflammation], a condition caused by the deficiency of vitamin D, calcium, and usually phosphorus, seen primarily in infancy and childhood, and characterized by abnormal bone formation. Symptoms include

R

soft pliable bones causing deformities such as bowlegs and knock-knees, nodular enlargements on the ends and sides of the bones, muscle pain, enlarged skull, chest deformities, spinal curvature, enlargement of the liver and spleen, profuse sweating, and general tenderness of the body when touched. Kinds of rickets include **adult rickets, celiac rickets, renal rickets,** and **vitamin D-resistant rickets.**

Rickettsia /riket'sē-ə/ [Howard Taylor Ricketts, American pathologist, b. 1871], a genus of microorganisms that combine aspects of both bacteria and viruses. They can be observed with a light microscope, divide by fission, and may be controlled with antibiotics. They also exist as viruslike intracellular parasites, living in the intestinal tracts of insects, such as lice. Thus, a human infested with lice is also likely to be infected with a form of typhus transmitted by *Rickettsia prowazeki.* Rickettsial diseases have been responsible for many of history's worst epidemics. The various species are distinguished on the basis of similarities in the diseases they cause: The spotted fever group includes Rocky Mountain spotted fever, rickettsialpox, and others; the typhus group includes epidemic typhus, scrub typhus, murine typhus; and a miscellaneous group includes Q fever and trench fever. Rickettsial diseases are uncommon in parts of the world where insect and rodent populations are well controlled. **-rickettsial,** *adj.*

rickettsial disease, an infection caused by a species of *Rickettsia.* Examples include Rocky Mountain spotted fever and typhus.

rickettsialpox /riket'sē-əlpoks'/ [Howard T. Ricketts; ME *pokkes* pustules], a mild, acute infectious disease caused by *Rickettsia akari* and transmitted from mice to humans by mites. It is characterized by an asymptomatic, crusted primary lesion, chills, fever, headache, malaise, myalgia, and a rash resembling chickenpox. About 1 week after onset of symptoms, small, discrete, maculopapular lesions appear on any part of the body.

rickettsiosis /riket'sē-ō'sis/, *pl.* rickettsioses [Howard T. Ricketts; Gk *osis* condition], any of a group of infectious diseases caused by microorganisms of the genus *Rickettsia.* Kinds of rickettsioses include a spotted fever group (**boutonneuse fever, rickettsialpox, Rocky Mountain spotted fever**), a typhus group (**epidemic typhus, murine typhus, scrub typhus**), and a miscellaneous group (**Q fever, trench fever**).

rider's bone [AS *ridan* to ride, *ban* bone], a bony deposit that sometimes develops in

horseback riders on the inner side of the lower end of the tendon of the adductor muscle of the thigh.

rider's sprain [OFr *espreindre* to force out], a sprain of the adductor muscles of the thigh due to horseback riding.

ridge /rij/ [AS *hrycg*], a projection or projecting structure, such as the gastrocnemial ridge on the posterior surface of the femur, giving attachment to the gastrocnemius muscle.

ridge extension, an intraoral surgical operation for deepening the labial, buccal, or lingual sulci.

ridge lap, the part of an artificial tooth that is adjacent to or laps the residual ridge.

Riedel's struma, Riedel's thyroiditis. See **fibrous thyroiditis.**

Rieder's cell leukemia /rē'dərz/ [Hermann Rieder, German physician, b. 1858], a malignant neoplasm of blood-forming tissues, characterized by the presence in blood of large numbers of atypical myeloblasts with immature cytoplasm and relatively mature lobulated, indented nuclei.

RIF, abbreviation for *resistance-inducing factor.*

rifampin /rif'əmpin/, an antibacterial prescribed in the treatment of tuberculosis, in meningococcal prophylaxis, and as an antileprotic.

Rift Valley fever, an arbovirus infection of Egypt and east Africa spread by mosquitoes or by handling infected sheep and cattle. It is characterized by abrupt fever, chills, headache, and generalized aching, followed by epigastric pain, anorexia, loss of taste, and photophobia.

RIG, abbreviation for **rabies immune globulin.**

Riga-Fede disease /rē'gäfā'dā/ [Antonio Riga, Italian physician, b. 1832; Francesco Fede, Italian pediatrician, b. 1832], an ulceration of the lingual frenum in some infants, caused by abrasion of the frenum by natal or neonatal teeth.

right atrial catheter, an indwelling intravenous catheter inserted centrally or peripherally and threaded into the superior vena cava and right atrium.

right atrioventricular valve. See **tricuspid valve.**

right brachiocephalic vein [AS *riht;* Gk *brachion* arm, *kephale* head], a vessel, about 2.5 cm long, that starts in the root of the neck at the junction of the internal jugular and the subclavian veins on the right side and descends vertically from behind the sternal end of the clavicle to join the left brachiocephalic vein and form the superior vena cava.

right bundle branch block, an abnormal

cardiac condition characterized by impaired transmission of an electrical impulse down the right bundle branch of fibers that transmit impulses from the bundle of His to the right ventricle. A right bundle branch block is often associated with right ventricular hypertrophy, especially in individuals under 40 years of age. In older individuals a right bundle branch block is commonly caused by coronary artery disease.

right common carotid artery, the shorter of the two common carotid arteries, arising from the brachiocephalic trunk, passing obliquely from the level of the sternoclavicular articulation to the cranial border of the thyroid cartilage, and dividing into the right carotid arteries.

right coronary artery, one of a pair of branches of the ascending aorta, arising in the right posterior aortic sinus, passing along the right side of the coronary sulcus, dividing into the right interventricular artery and a large marginal branch, supplying both ventricles, the right atrium, and the sinoatrial node.

right coronary vein. See **small cardiac vein.**

right-handedness, a natural tendency to favor the use of the right hand.

right-hand rule, a principle of physics in which the direction of current flow in a wire is related to the position of the imaginary lines of force of the magnetic field about the wire.

right-heart failure, an abnormal cardiac condition characterized by the impairment of the right side of the heart and congestion and elevated pressure in the systemic veins and capillaries. Right-heart failure is often related to left-heart failure because both sides of the heart are part of a circuit and what affects one side will eventually affect the other.

right hepatic duct, the duct that drains bile from the right lobe of the liver into the common bile duct.

righting reflex [AS *riht;* L *refectere* to bend backward], any reflex that tends to return an animal to its normal body position in space when it has been moved from the normal position and that adjusts head to body position or vice versa. The head and trunk are thus kept in alignment.

right interventricular artery. See **dorsal interventricular artery.**

right lymphatic duct, a vessel that conveys lymph from the right upper quadrant of the body into the bloodstream in the neck at the junction of the right internal jugular and the right subclavian veins.

right-to-know laws, laws that require employers to inform workers regarding health effects of materials they must handle, including toxic chemicals and radioactive substances. Under the authority of the U.S. Occupational Safety and Health Act of 1970, the National Institute for Occupational Safety and Health (NIOSH) periodically revises recommendations or limits of exposure to potentially hazardous substances in the workplace. It also recommends appropriate preventive measures designed to reduce or eliminate adverse health effects of these hazards and publishes its recommendations in a variety of public documents.

right-to-left shunt, a venoarterial shunt in which unoxygenated venous blood passes directly into the arterial system, bypassing the lungs as in the tetralogy of Fallot and other conditions.

right pulmonary artery, the longer and slightly larger of the two arteries conveying venous blood from the heart to the lungs, rising from the pulmonary trunk, bending to the right behind the aorta, and dividing into two branches at the root of the right lung.

right-sided failure. See **right-heart failure.**

right subclavian artery, a large artery that arises from the brachiocephalic artery. It has several important branches: the axillary, vertebral thoracic, and internal thoracic arteries and the cervical and costocervical trunks, perfusing the right side of the upper body.

right ventricle, the relatively thin-walled chamber of the heart that pumps blood received from the right atrium into the pulmonary arteries to the lungs for oxygenation. The right ventricle is shorter and rounder than the long, conical left ventricle.

rigidity /rijd′itē/ [L *rigere* to be stiff], a condition of hardness, stiffness, or inflexibility. **−rigid,** *adj.*

rigidus /rij′idəs/ [L, stiff], a deformity characterized by limited motion, especially dorsiflexion of the great toe.

rigor /rig′ər/ [L, stiffness], **1.** a rigid condition of the tissues of the body, as in rigor mortis. **2.** a violent attack of shivering that may be associated with chills and fever.

rigor mortis /môr′tis/, the rigid stiffening of skeletal and cardiac muscle shortly after death.

rim [OE *rima* edge], an outer edge, which may be curved or circular, as on an occluding surface built on a temporary or permanent denture base.

rima glottidis. See **glottis.**

ring chromosome [AS *hring*], a circular chromosome formed by the fusion of the

R

two ends. It is the primary type of chromosome found in bacteria.

Ringer's lactate solution, a fluid and electrolyte replenisher. It is prescribed for correction of extracellular volume and electrolyte depletion.

ring removal from swollen finger, a technique for removing a ring from a swollen finger in which a string is slipped under the ring while moving the ring toward the hand. The string is then wound around the swelling a number of times, after which it is unwound, while gradually easing the ring toward the free end of the finger.

ringworm. See **tinea.**

Rinne tuning fork test /rin′ē/ [Heinrich A. Rinne, German otologist, b. 1819], a method of distinguishing conductive from sensorineural hearing loss. The test is performed with tuning forks of 256, 512, and 1,024 cycles, and while each ear is tested, the other is masked. In sensorial loss the sound is heard longer by air conduction, whereas in conductive hearing loss the sound is heard longer by bone conduction.

Rio Grande fever. See **abortus fever.**

RIP, abbreviation for **reflex inhibiting pattern.**

ripe cataract [OE *ripan*; Gk *katarrhaktes portcullis*], a mature cataract that produces swelling and opacity of the entire lens.

risk-benefit analysis, the consideration as to whether a medical or surgical procedure, particularly a radical approach, is worth the risk to the patient as compared to possible benefits if the procedure is successful.

risk factor [Fr *risque* hazard; L *factor* maker], a factor that causes a person or a group of people to be particularly vulnerable to an unwanted, unpleasant, or unhealthful event, such as immunosuppression, which increases the incidence and severity of infection.

risk management, a function of administration of a hospital or other health facility directed toward identification, evaluation, and correction of potential risks that could lead to injury to patients, staff members, or visitors and in property loss or damage.

risorius /risôr′ē·əs/ [L *ridere* to laugh], one of the 12 muscles of the mouth. Arising in the fascia over the masseter and inserting into the skin at the corner of the mouth. It acts to retract the angle of the mouth, as in a smile.

Risser cast /ris′ər/ [Joseph C. Risser, American surgeon, b. 1892], an orthopedic device for encasing the entire trunk of the body, extending over the cervical area to the chin. In rare cases it extends over the hips to the knees.

risus sardonicus /rē′səs särdon′ikəs/ [L, laughter; Gk *sardonius* mocking], a wry, masklike grin caused by spasm of the facial muscles, as seen in tetanus.

Ritgen maneuver, an obstetric procedure used to control delivery of the head. It involves applying upward pressure from the coccygeal region to extend the head during actual delivery.

ritodrine hydrochloride /rit′ədrēn/, a beta-sympathomimetic agent prescribed in pregnancy management to stop the uterus from contracting in preterm labor.

Ritter's disease [Gottfried Ritter von Rittershain, Czechoslovakian pediatrician, b. 1820], a rare, staphylococcal infection of newborns that begins with red spots about the mouth and chin, gradually spreading over the entire body and followed by generalized exfoliation. Vesicles and yellow crusts may also be present. Ritter's disease is usually fatal unless treated with antibiotics.

river blindness. See **onchocerciasis.**

Rivinus' notch /rēvē′nəs/ [Augustus Q. Rivinus, German anatomist, b. 1652], a deficiency in the tympanic sulcus of the ear that forms an attachment for the flaccid part of the tympanic membrane and the mallear folds.

RLE, abbreviation for *right lower extremity.*

RLL, abbreviation for *right lower lobe of lung.*

r-loop, (in molecular genetics) a distinctive loop formation seen under an electron microscope. It is composed of a single helical strand of DNA, wound with a hybrid strand containing another single strand of DNA with a strand of RNA.

RLQ, abbreviation for *right lower quadrant.*

RMP, abbreviation for *right mentoposterior presentation* of fetal face.

RMSF, abbreviation for **Rocky Mountain spotted fever.**

RMT, abbreviation for *right mentotransverse* fetal position.

Rn, symbol for the element **radon.**

RN, abbreviation for **registered nurse.**

RNA, abbreviation for **ribonucleic acid.**

RNA polymerase, (in molecular genetics) an enzyme that catalyzes the assembly of ribonucleoside triphosphates into RNA, with single-stranded DNA serving as the template.

RNase, abbreviation for **ribonuclease.**

RNA splicing, (in molecular genetics) the process by which base pairs that interrupt the continuity of genetic information in

DNA are removed from the precursors of messenger RNA.

RN, C, abbreviation for *Registered Nurse, Certified.*

RN, CNA, abbreviation for *Registered Nurse, Certified in Nursing Administration.*

RN, CNAA, abbreviation for *Registered Nurse, Certified in Nursing Administration, Advanced.*

RN, CS, abbreviation for *Registered Nurse, Certified Specialist.*

ROA, abbreviation for *right occipitoanterior fetal position.*

Robb, Isabel Hampton (1860-1910), a Canadian-born American nursing educator and writer. She was the first to institute a systematic, step-by-step course for nursing students that integrated clinical experience and classwork and the first educator to arrange for the affiliation of her students at other hospitals for specialized training. She was one of the founders of *The American Journal of Nursing* and the forerunner of the American Nurses' Association.

robertsonian translocation /rob'ərtsō'-nē·ən/, the exchange of entire chromosome arms, with the break occurring at the centromere, usually between two nonhomologous acrocentric chromosomes, to form one large metacentric chromosome and one extremely small chromosome that carries little genetic material and through successive cell divisions may be lost.

rocker knife, a knife that cuts with a rocking motion, designed for patients who have the use of only one hand.

rock fever. See *brucellosis.*

Rocky Mountain spotted fever (RMSF), a serious tick-borne infectious disease occurring throughout the temperate zones of North and South America, caused by *Rickettsia rickettsii* and characterized by chills, fever, severe headache, myalgia, mental confusion, and rash. Erythematous macules first appear on wrists and ankles, spreading rapidly over the extremities, trunk, face, and usually on the palms and soles. Hemorrhagic lesions, constipation, and abdominal distention are also common. Care must be taken not to crush ticks, because infection may be acquired through skin abrasions.

rod [AS *rodd*], **1.** a straight cylindric structure. **2.** one of the tiny cylindric elements arranged perpendicular to the surface of the retina. Rods contain the chemical rhodopsin, which adapts the eye to detect low-intensity light and gives the rods a purple color.

rodenticide poisoning /rōden'tisīd/ [L *rodere* to gnaw, *caedere* to kill; *potio* drink], a toxic condition caused by the ingestion

of a substance intended for the control of rodent populations.

rodent ulcer /rō'dənt/ [L *rodere* to gnaw; *ilcus* ulcer], a slowly developing serpiginous ulceration of a basal cell carcinoma of the skin.

rods and cones [AS *rodd*; Gk *konos*], the light-sensitive cells of the retina. The rods, under the visual purple pigment epithelium, are located mainly around the periphery of the retina. The cones receive color stimuli.

roentgen (R) /rent'gən, ren'jən/ [William K. Roentgen, German physicist, b. 1845], the quantity of x- or gamma radiation that creates 1 electrostatic unit of ions in 1 ml of air at 0° C and 760 mm of pressure. In radiotherapy or radiodiagnosis the roentgen is the unit of the emitted dose.

roentgen fetometry, the use of radiographic techniques to measure the fetus in utero.

Rogers, Martha, author of Rogers' Science of Unitary Man, a nursing theory introduced in 1970. The Rogers theory has strong ties to the general systems theory with elements of a developmental model. It considers four "building blocks": Energy Fields, Universe of Open Systems, Pattern and Organization, and Four Dimensionality.

Rohrer's constants, the constants in an empiric equation for airway resistance. It is expressed as $R = K_1 + K_2V$, where R is resistance, V is instantaneous volumetric flow rate, K_1 is a constant representing gas viscosity and airway geometry, and K_2 is a constant representing gas density and airway geometry.

Rokitansky's disease. See **Budd-Chiari syndrome.**

Rolando's fissure [Luigi Rolando, Italian anatomist, b. 1773; L *fissura* cleft], the central sulcus of the cerebrum.

Rolando's fracture /rōlan'dōz/ [Luigi Rolando], a fracture of the base of the first metacarpal.

role [Fr, character], a socially expected behavior pattern associated with an individual's function in various social groups. Roles provide a means for social participation and a way to test identities for consensual validation by significant others.

role ambiguity. See **role strain.**

role blurring, the tendency for professional roles to overlap and become indistinct.

role change, a situation in which status is retained while role expectations change.

role clarification, gaining the knowledge, information, and cues needed to perform a role.

R

role conflict, the presence of contradictory and often competing role expectations.

role induction interview, a therapeutic technique that provides information to the patient in advance about the ways patients are expected to behave.

role model, a person who inspires others to imitate his or her persona. The role model may be a real person, as a parent, or a symbolic character as depicted in movies or television programs.

role overload, a condition in which there is insufficient time in which to carry out all of the expected role functions.

role overqualification. See **role strain.**

role performance, altered, a NANDA-accepted nursing diagnosis of a disruption in the way one perceives one's role performance. Defining characteristics include a change in self-perception of one's role, denial of the role, a change in others' perception of one's role, conflict in roles, a change in physical capacity to resume one's role, lack of knowledge of role, and change in usual patterns of responsibility.

role playing, a psychotherapeutic technique in which a person acts out a real or simulated situation as a means of understanding intrapsychic conflicts.

role playing therapy. See **psychodrama.**

role reversal act, the act of assuming the role of another person to appreciate how the person feels, perceives, and behaves in relation to himself and others.

role strain, stress associated with expected roles or positions, experienced as frustration. **Role ambiguity** occurs when shared specifications set for an expected role are incomplete or insufficient to tell the involved individual what is desired and how to do it. **Role incongruence** occurs when an individual undergoes role transitions requiring a significant modification in attitudes and values. **Role overqualification** occurs when a role does not require full use of a person's resources.

Rolfing. See **structural integration.**

roll [OFr *rolle*], intrinsic joint movements on an axis parallel to the articulating surface. The axis can remain stationary or move in a plane parallel to the joint surface.

roller bandage, a long, tightly wound strip of material that may vary in width. It is generally applied as a circular bandage.

roller clamp, a device, usually made of plastic, equipped with a small roller that may be rolled counterclockwise to close off primary intravenous tubing or clockwise to open it.

rolling effleurage, a circular rubbing stroke used in massage to promote circulation and muscle relaxation, especially on the shoulder and buttocks. It is performed with the hand flat, the palm and closely held fingers acting as a unit.

ROM, abbreviation for **range of motion.**

Romberg sign /rom'bərg/ [Moritz H. Romberg, German physician, b. 1795; L *signum* mark], an indication of loss of the sense of position in which the patient loses balance when standing erect, feet together, and eyes closed.

rongeur forceps /rônzhur', rôNzhr'/ [Fr *ronger* to gnaw; L *forceps* pair of tongs], a kind of biting forceps that is strong and heavy, used for cutting bone.

R-on-T phenomenon, a cardiac event in which a stimulus causes premature depolarization of cells that have not completed the repolarization process.

room [AS *rum*], any area surrounded by four walls within a building, especially one in which a patient is housed, treated, or cared for.

rooming-in, (in a hospital) a recent practice that allows mothers and new babies to share accommodations, remaining together in the hospital as they would at home rather than being separated.

root /rōōt, rŏŏt/ [AS *rot*], the lowest part of an organ or a structure by which something is firmly attached, such as the anatomic root of the tooth.

root amputation. See **apicoectomy.**

root canal. See **pulp canal.**

root canal file, a small metal hand instrument with tightly spiraled blades, used for cleaning and shaping a root canal.

root canal filling, a material placed in the root canal system of a tooth to seal the space previously occupied by the dental pulp.

root curettage, the débridement and planing of the root surface of a tooth to remove accretions and induce the development of healthy gingival tissues.

root end cyst. See **radicular cyst.**

root furcation, 1. the anatomic area at which the roots of a multirooted tooth divide. 2. abnormal resorption of bone in multirooted teeth, resulting from periodontal disease.

rooting reflex, a normal response in newborns when the cheek is touched or stroked to turn the head toward the stimulated side and begin to suck.

root resection. See **apicoectomy.**

root resorption of teeth, destruction of the cementum, dentin, or bone by cementoclastic or osteoclastic activity. If only the apex is dissolved, it may result in a short, blunted root. When resorption occurs in the middle of the root, it generally results in penetration of the pulp canal.

root retention, a technique that removes the crown of a root canal–treated tooth and retains enough of the root and gingival attachment to support a removable prosthesis.

root submersion, a root retention in which the tooth structure is reduced below the level of the alveolar crest and the soft tissue is allowed to heal over it.

ROP, abbreviation for *right occipitoposterior* fetal position.

Rorschach test /rôr′shäk, rôr′shokh/ [Hermann Rorschach, Swiss psychiatrist, b. 1884], a projective personality assessment test developed by the Swiss psychiatrist Hermann Rorschach. It consists of 10 pictures of inkblots, five in black and white, three in black and red, and two multicolored, to which the subject responds by telling, in as many interpretations as is desired, what images and emotions each design evokes. The test is designed to assess the degree to which intellectual and emotional factors are integrated in the subject's perception of the environment.

ROS, abbreviation for **review of systems.**

rosacea /rōzā′shē-ə/ [L *rosaceus* rosy], a chronic form of acne seen in adults of all ages and associated with telangiectasia, especially of the nose, forehead, and cheeks.

rose fever [L *rosa; febris* fever], a common misnomer for seasonal allergic rhinitis caused by pollen, most frequently of grasses, that is airborne at the time roses are in bloom.

Rosenmüller's organ. See **epoophoron.**

Rosenthal's syndrome. See **hemophilia C.**

roseola /rōzē′ələ/ [L *roseus*], any rose-colored rash.

roseola infantum, a benign, endemic illness of infants and young children, attributed to a parovirus and characterized by abrupt, high sustained or spiking fever, mild pharyngitis, and lymph node enlargement. Febrile convulsions may occur. After 4 or 5 days the fever suddenly drops to normal, and a faint, pink, maculopapular rash appears on the neck, trunk, and thighs. The rash may last a few hours to 2 days.

rose spots [L *rosa* + ME *spotte*], small erythematous macules occurring on the upper abdomen and anterior thorax and lasting 2 or 3 days, characteristic of typhoid and paratyphoid fevers.

rostral /ros′trəl/, beak-shaped. **–rostrum,** *n.*

rostrum /ros′trəm/ [L, beak], a beaklike projection, as the rostrum of the sphenoid bone.

ROT, abbreviation for *right occipitotransverse* fetal position.

rotameter /rotam′ətər/ [L *rota* wheel; Gk *metron* measure], a device operated by a needle valve in an anesthetic gas machine that measures gases by speed of flow, according to their viscosity and density.

rotary nystagmus /rō′tərē/ [L *rotare* to rotate; Gk *nystagmos* nodding], a form of nystagmus in which the eyeball makes rotary motions, around an axis.

rotating tourniquet /rō′tāting/ [L *rotare* to rotate; Fr *tourniquet* garrote], one of four constricting devices used in a rotating order to pool blood in the extremities to relieve congestion in the lungs in the treatment of acute pulmonary edema. Use of the rotating tourinquet has declined in recent years due to the development of vasodilating drugs and diuretics.

rotation /rōtā′shən/ [L *rotare*], **1.** a turning around an axis. **2.** one of the four basic kinds of motion allowed by various joints: the rotation of a bone around its central axis, which may lie in a separate bone, as in the pivot formed by the dens of the axis around which the atlas turns. A bone, such as the humerus, may also rotate around its own longitudinal axis, or the axis of rotation may not be quite parallel to the long axis of the rotating bone, as in movement of the radius on the ulna during pronation and supination of the hand. **3.** (in obstetrics) the turning of the fetal head to descend through the pelvis.

rotator /rō′tātər/, a muscle that rotates on an axis, such as the cervical, thoracic, and lumbar musculi rotatores, which function to extend and rotate the vertebral column toward the opposite side.

rotavirus /rō′təvīrəs/, a double-stranded RNA molecule that appears as a tiny wheel, with a clearly defined outer layer, or rim, and an inner layer of spokes. The organism is a cause of acute gastroenteritis with diarrhea.

Rotokinetic treatment table /rō′tokinet′ik/, a special bed equipped with an automatic turning device that completely immobilizes patients while rotating them from 90 to 270 degrees around a horizontal axis.

Rotor syndrome /rō′tər/, a rare condition of the liver inherited as an autosomal recessive trait. It is similar to Dubin-Johnson syndrome.

rotula. See **troche.**

roughage. See **dietary fiber.**

rouleaux /roolō′/, *sing.* **rouleau** [Fr, cylinder], an aggregation of red cells that may be caused by abnormal proteins, as in multiple myeloma or macroglobulinemia, but is most often a microscopic artifact.

round ligament [L *rotundus* round; *ligare* to bind], **1.** a curved fibrous band that is attached at one end to the fovea of the head of the femur and at the other to the transverse ligament of the acetabulum. **2.** a fibrous cord extending from the umbilicus to the anterior part of the liver. **3.** in the female, a fibromuscular band that extends from the anterior surface of the uterus through the inguinal canal to the labium majus. The structure is homologous to the spermatic cord in the male.

rounds, *informal;* a teaching conference or a meeting in which the clinical problems encountered in the practice of nursing, medicine, or other service are discussed. Kinds of rounds include **grand rounds, nursing rounds, teaching rounds,** and **walking rounds.**

round window, a round opening in the medial wall of the middle ear leading into th cochlea and covered by a secondary tympanic membrane.

roundworm, any worm of the class Nematoda, including *Ancylostoma duodenale, Ascaris lumbricoides, Enterobius vermicularis,* and *Strongyloides stercoralis.*

route of administration [Fr *route* course; L *administrare* to serve], (of a drug) any one of the ways in which a drug may be administered, such as intramuscularly, intranasally, intravenously, orally, rectally, subcutaneously, sublingually, topically, or vaginally.

Roux-en-Y /rōō'enwī, rōō'änēgek'/ [César Roux, Swiss surgeon, b. 1857], an anastomosis of the small intestine in the shape of the letter *Y*. The proximal end of the divided intestine is anastomosed end-to-side to the distal loop and a portion of the distal loop is anastomosed to another part of the digestive tract, such as the esophagus.

Rovsing's sign /rov'singz/ [Nils T. Rovsing, Danish surgeon, b. 1862], an indication of acute appendicitis in which pressure on the left lower quadrant of the abdomen causes pain in the right lower quadrant.

Royal College of Physicians (RCP), a professional organization of physicians in the United Kingdom.

Royal College of Physicians and Surgeons of Canada (RCPSC), a national Canadian organization that recognizes and confers membership on certain qualified physicians and surgeons.

Royal College of Surgeons (RCS), a professional organization of surgeons in the United Kingdom.

Roy, Sister Callista, a nursing theorist who introduced the Adaptation Model of Nursing in 1970 as a conceptual framework for nursing curricula, practice, and research. In the Roy model, the human is

viewed as an adaptive system. Changes occur in the system in response to stimuli. If the change promotes the integrity of the individual, it is an adaptive response. Otherwise, it is a maladaptive response.

RPF, abbreviation for *renal plasma flow.*

rpm, abbreviation for *revolutions per minute.*

RQ, abbreviation for **respiratory quotient.**

RR, abbreviation for **recovery room.**

RRA, abbreviation for **registered record administrator.**

R-R interval, the interval from the peak of one QRS complex to the peak of the next as shown on an electrocardiogram.

rRNA, abbreviation for *ribosomal RNA.*

RRT, abbreviation for **registered respiratory therapist.**

RSV, RS virus, abbreviation for **respiratory syncytial virus.**

RT, abbreviation for **respiratory therapy.**

RT, abbreviation for **registered technologist.**

RTA, abbreviation for **renal tubular acidosis.**

r.t.c., abbreviation for *return to clinic,* noted on the chart, usually followed by a date on which a subsequent appointment has been made for the patient.

Ru, symbol for the element **ruthenium.**

rub, [ME *rubben* to tear out], the movement of one surface moving over another, thereby producing friction, as when pleural membranes produce friction rub.

rubber, *informal;* condom.

rubber-band ligation, a method of treating hemorrhoids by placing a rubber band around the hemorrhoidal portion of the blood vessel, causing it to slough off after time.

rubber dam [ME *rubben* to scrape; AS *demman* to dam up], a thin sheet of latex rubber for isolating one or more teeth during a dental procedure.

rubber dam clamps forceps, (in dentistry) a type of forceps with beaks designed to engage holes in a rubber dam clamp to facilitate its placement.

rubbing alcohol [ME *rubben* to scrape; Ar *alkohl* essence], a disinfectant for skin and instruments. It contains 70% ethyl alcohol by volume, the remainder consisting of water and denaturants, with or without color or perfume. It may cause dryness of the skin. Rubbing alcohol is for external use only and is flammable.

rubefacient /rōō'bəfā'shənt/ [L *ruber* red, *facere* to make], **1.** a substance or agent that increases the reddish coloration of the skin. **2.** increasing the reddish coloration of the skin.

rubella /rōōbel'ə/ [L *rubellus* somewhat

red], a contagious viral disease characterized by fever, symptoms of a mild upper respiratory tract infection, lymph node enlargement, arthralgia, and a diffuse, fine, red, maculopapular rash. The virus is spread by droplet infection, and the incubation time is from 12 to 23 days. The symptoms usually last only 2 or 3 days except for arthralgia, which may persist longer or recur. One attack confers lifelong immunity. If a woman acquires rubella in the first trimester of pregnancy, fetal anomalies may result, including heart defects, cataracts, deafness, and mental retardation. An infant exposed to the virus in utero at any time during gestation may shed the virus for up to 30 months after birth. Complications of postnatal rubella are rare.

rubella and mumps virus vaccine, a suspension containing live attenuated mumps and rubella viruses. It is prescribed for immunization against rubella and mumps.

rubella embryopathy, any congenital abnormality in an infant caused by maternal rubella in the early stages of pregnancy.

rubella panencephalitis. See **panencephalitis.**

rubella titer, [L *ruber* red; Fr *titre* standard], a serologic test to determine a patient's state of immunity against rubella.

rubella virus vaccine, a suspension containing live attenuated rubella virus. It is prescribed for immunization against rubella.

rubeola. See **measles.**

ruber /roo'bər/, the Latin word for red.

rubescent /roobes'ənt/, reddening.

rubidium (Rb) /roobid'ē·əm/ [L *rubidus* reddish], a soft metallic element of the alkali metals group. Its atomic number is 37; its atomic weight is 85.47. Slightly radioactive, it is used in radioisotope scanning.

Rubin's test [Isador C. Rubin, American gynecologist, b. 1883], a test performed in the process of evaluating the cause of infertility by assessing the patency of the fallopian tubes. Carbon dioxide gas (CO_2) is introduced into the tubes under pressure through a cannula inserted into the cervix. The CO_2 is passed through from a syringe connected to a manometer at pressures of up to 200 mm Hg. If the tubes are open, the gas enters the abdominal cavity and the recorded pressure falls below 180 mm Hg.

rubivirus /roo'bēvī'rəs/, a member of the togavirus family, which includes the rubella virus.

rubor /roo'bôr/, redness, especially when accompanying inflammation.

rubricyte /roo'brisīt/ [L *ruber* red; Gk *kytos* cell], a nucleated red blood cell; the

marrow stage in the normal development of an erythrocyte.

ructus. See **eructation.**

rudiment /roo'diment/ [L *rudimentum* beginning], an organ or tissue that is incompletely developed or nonfunctional. **–rudimentary,** *adj.*

Ruffini's corpuscles /roofē'nēz/ [Angelo Ruffini, Italian histologist, b. 1864], a variety of oval nerve endings in the subcutaneous tissue, located principally at the junction of the corium and the subcutaneous tissue.

RU486, a drug that can end a pregnancy when administered as a one-dose pill within the first 6 weeks after conception.

ruga /roo'gə/, *pl.* rugae /roo'jē/ [L, wrinkle], a ridge or fold, such as the rugae of the stomach, in the mucous membrane of an organ.

rugae of vagina, the transverse ridges on the mucous membrane lining the vagina that allow the vagina to stretch during childbirth.

RUL, abbreviation for *right upper lobe* of lung.

rule of bigeminy [L *regula* model; *bis* double, *geminus* twin], (in cardiology) the tendency of a lengthened ventricular cycle to precipitate a ventricular premature beat.

rule of confidentiality, a principle that personal information about others, particularly patients, should not be revealed to persons not authorized to receive such information.

rule of co-occurrence, a mandate that a person use the same level of lexical and syntactic structure when speaking.

rule of nines, a formula for estimating the amount of body surface covered by burns by assigning 9% to the head and each arm, twice 9% (18%) to each leg, and the anterior and posterior trunk, and 1% to the perineum. This is modified in infants and children because of the different body proportions.

rule of three, (in respiratory therapy) an arterial oxygen tension that is three times the value of the inspired oxygen concentration. It is regarded as an empirical guide to a temporarily acceptable minimal oxygenation or expression of clinical observation and has no scientific basis.

ruminant /roo'minənt/ [L *ruminare* to chew again], pertaining to animals that chew their cud and to human infants that may regurgitate and reswallow a meal.

rumination /roo'minā'shən/ [L *ruminare* to chew again], habitual regurgitation of small amounts of undigested food with little force after every feeding, a condition commonly seen in infants. It may be a symptom of overfeeding, of eating too fast, or of swallowing air.

runner's high, a feeling of euphoria experienced by some runners and joggers as they near the end of a run. The feeling of elation is believed to be associated with the body's production of endorphins during physical stress.

rupture /rup'chər/ [L *rumpere* to break], **1.** a tear or break in the continuity or configuration of an organ or body tissue, including those instances when other tissue protrudes through the opening. **2.** to cause a break or tear.

ruptured intervertebral disk. See **herniated disk.**

rupture of membranes, the rupture of the amniotic sac usually at the start of labor.

rupture of uterus in pregnancy, a tear or break in the uterus because of trauma or other causes, possibly accompanied by displacement of fetus and amniotic sac into peritoneal cavity. The patient may experience acute pain because of tissue damage and irritation of peritoneal tissues. Excessive loss of blood may be marked by hypotension, fluid volume deficit, and altered cardiac output.

RUQ, abbreviation for *right upper quadrant.*

Rural Clinics Assistance Act, an act of Congress that permitted the establishment of clinics in certain areas designated rural and underserved and in some inner cities. The clinics are designed to provide primary care through teams of physicians and nurse practitioners.

Russell dwarf [Alexander Russell, twentieth-century Scottish physician; AS *dweorge*], a person affected with **Russell's syndrome,** a congenital disorder in which short stature is associated with various anomalies of the head, face, and skeleton and with varying degrees of mental retardation.

Russell's bodies [William Russell, Scottish physician, b. 1852; AS *bodig* body], the mucoprotein inclusions found in globular plasma cells in cancer and inflammations. The bodies contain surface gamma globulins.

Russell's syndrome. See **Russell dwarf.**

Russell traction [R. Hamilton Russell, twentieth-century Australian surgeon; L *trahere* to pull along], a unilateral or a bilateral orthopedic mechanism that combines suspension and traction to immobilize, position, and align the lower extremities in the treatment of fractured femurs and hip and knee contractures and in the treatment of disease processes of the hip and the knee.

Russian bath, a hot steam bath followed by a cold plunge.

rusty sputum [AS *rust*; L *sputum* spittle], sputum that is reddish, indicative of blood.

ruthenium (Ru) /rōōthē'nē·əm/ [Ruthenia, region of western Ukraine, USSR], a hard, brittle, metallic element. Its atomic number is 44; its atomic weight is 101.07.

rutin /rōō'tin/, a bioflavonoid obtained from buckwheat and used in the treatment of capillary fragility.

RV, abbreviation for **residual volume.**

RVC, abbreviation for *responds to verbal commands.*

R wave. See **QRS complex.**

rxn, RXN, symbols for drug reaction.

s, 1. abbreviation for **steady state. 2.** abbreviation for **sinister** (left).

s̄, s, symbol for the Latin word, *sine*, "without."

S, 1. symbol for **sulfur 2.** symbol for *saturation of hemoglobin.*

S₁, the first heart sound in the cardiac cycle occurring with ventricular systole. It is associated with closure of the mitral and tricuspid valves and is synchronous with the apical pulse.

S₂, the second heart sound in the cardiac cycle. It is associated with closure of the aortic and pulmonary valves just before ventricular diastole.

S₃, the third heart sound in the cardiac cycle. Normally, it is audible only in children and physically active young adults. In older people, it is an abnormal finding and usually indicates myocardial failure.

S₄, the fourth heart sound in the cardiac cycle. It occurs late in diastole on contraction of the atria. Rarely heard in normal subjects, it indicates an abnormally increased resistance to ventricular filling.

S1, S2, . . . , symbols for sacral nerves.

SA, 1. abbreviation for **sinoatrial (S-A node). 2.** abbreviation for **surface area. 3.** abbreviation for **surgeon's assistant.**

Sabin-Feldman dye test /sā'binfeld'mən/ [Albert B. Sabin, American virologist, b. 1906; H. A. Feldman; AS *deag;* L *testum* crucible], a diagnostic test for toxoplasmosis that depends on the presence of specific antibodies that block the uptake of methylene blue dye by the cytoplasm of the *Toxoplasma* organisms.

Sabin Vaccine. See **oral poliovirus vaccine.**

sac [Gk *sakkos* sack] /sak/, a pouch or a baglike organ, such as the abdominal sac of the embryo that develops into the abdominal cavity.

saccade /sakād'/ [Fr *saccader* to jerk], pertaining to something jerky, broken, or abrupt, such as rapid shifts of eye movement or a staccato voice.

saccadic eye movement /sakad'ik/, an extremely fast voluntary movement of the eyes, allowing the eyes to accurately fix on a still object in the visual field as the person moves or the head turns.

saccharide /sak'ərīd'/, any of a large group of carbohydrates, including all sugars and starches. Almost all carbohydrates are saccharides.

saccharin /sak'ərin/ [Gk *sakcharon* sugar] **1.** a white, crystalline, synthetic sweetening agent derived from coal tar. Although it is up to 500 times as sweet as sugar, it has no food value. **2.** having a sweet taste, especially cloyingly sweet.

Saccharomyces /sak'ərōmī'sēz/ [Gk *sakcharon* + *mykes* fungus], a genus of yeast fungi, including brewer's and baker's yeast, as well as some pathogenic fungi, that cause such diseases as bronchitis, moniliasis, and pharyngitis.

saccharomycosis /sak'ərōmīkō'sis/ [Gk *sakcharon, mykes* + *osis* condition], infection with yeast fungi, such as the genera *Candida* or *Cryptococcus.*

saccular aneurysm /sak'yələr/, a localized dilatation of an artery in which only a small area of the vessel is distended, forming a saclike swelling or protrusion.

sacculated /sak'yələ'tid/ [L *sacculus* small sack], a condition of small sacs or pouches or saclike dilatations.

saccule /sak'yōōl/ [L *sacculus*], a small bag or sac, such as the air saccules of the lungs. –**saccular,** *adj.*

sacculus /sak'yōōləs/, *pl.* **sacculi,** a little sac or bag, especially the smaller of the two divisions of the membranous labyrinth of the vestibule, which communicates with the cochlear duct through the ductus reuniens in the inner ear.

Sachs' disease. See **Tay-Sachs disease.**

SA conduction time, the conduction time for an impulse from the sinus node to the atrial musculature, measured from the SA deflection in the SA nodal electrocardiogram to the beginning of the P wave in a bipolar record, or to the beginning of the high right atrial electrogram in a unipolar record.

sacral bone, a composite bone formed by the fusion during maturation of five sacral vertebrae that were separate at birth. The sacrum forms the back of the pelvis.

sacral canal, an extension of the vertebral canal through the sacrum.

sacral foramen, one of several openings between the fused segments of the sacral vertebrae in the sacrum through which the sacral nerves pass.

sacral nerves, the five segmental nerves from the sacral portion of the spinal cord, the first four emerging through the anterior sacral foramina and the fifth from between the sacral foramen and the coccyx.

sacral node, a node in one of the seven groups of parietal lymph nodes of the abdomen and the pelvis, situated within the sacrum.

sacral plexus, a network of motor and sensory nerves formed by the lumbosacral trunk from the fourth and fifth lumbar, and by the first, second, and third sacral nerves. They converge toward the caudal portion of the greater sciatic foramen and unite to become a large, flattened band, most of which continues into the thigh as the sciatic nerve.

sacral vertebra, one of the five segments of the vertebral column that fuse in the adult to form the sacrum. The ventral border of the first sacral vertebra projects into the pelvis. The bodies of the other sacral vertebrae are smaller than that of the first and are flattened and curved ventrally, forming the convex, anterior surface of the sacrum.

sacrococcygeal /sā′krōkoksij′ē-əl/ [L *sacer* + Gk *kokkyx* cuckoo's beak], pertaining to the sacrum and the coccyx.

sacroiliac /sā′krō·il′ē·ak/ [L *sacer* + *ilia* flank], pertaining to the part of the skeletal system that includes the sacrum and the ilium bones of the pelvis.

sacroiliac articulation, an immovable joint in the pelvis formed by the articulation of each side of the sacrum with an iliac bone.

sacroiliac joint, an irregular synovial joint between the sacrum and the ilium on either side.

sacrospinalis /sak′rōspīnal′is/ [L *sacer* + *spina* backbone], a large, fleshy muscle of the back that divides into a lateral iliocostalis column, an intermediate longissimus column, and a medial spinalis column.

sacrum /sā′krəm, sak′rəm/ [L *sacer* sacred], the large, triangular bone at the dorsal part of the pelvis, inserted like a wedge between the two hip bones. The base of the sacrum articulates with the last lumbar vertebra, and its apex articulates with the coccyx. **–sacral,** *adj.*

SAD, abbreviation for **seasonal affective disorder.**

saddle block anesthesia [AS *sadol;* Fr *bloc;* Gk *anaisthesia* lack of feeling], a form of regional nerve block in which the parts of the body anesthetized are those that would touch a saddle, were the patient sitting astride one. It is performed by injecting a local anesthetic into the spinal cavity as the patient sits with the head on the chest, back curved, and legs down.

saddle joint, a synovial joint in which surfaces of contiguous bones are reciprocally concavoconvex. A saddle joint permits no axial rotation but allows flexion, extension, adduction, and abduction.

saddle nose, a sunken nasal bridge caused by injury or disease and resulting in damage to the nasal septum.

sadism /sā′dizəm, sad′izəm/ [Donatien A. F. de Sade, French Marquis, b. 1740], **1.** abnormal pleasure derived from inflicting physical or psychologic pain or abuse on others; cruelty. **2.** (in psychiatry) a psychosexual disorder characterized by the infliction of physical or psychologic pain or humiliation on another person, either a consenting or nonconsenting partner, to achieve sexual excitement or gratification. Kinds of sadism are **anal sadism** and **oral sadism. –sadistic,** *adj.*

sadist /sā′dist/, a person who is afflicted with or practices sadism.

sadomasochism /sā′dōmas′əkiziəm/ [Marquis de Sade; Leopold von Sacher-Masoch, Austrian author, b. 1836], a personality disorder characterized by traits of sadism and masochism.

sadomasochist /sā′dōmas′əkist/ [Comte de Sade; Sacher-Masoch], a person who practices sadomasochism.

safe period. See **natural family planning method.**

safe sex, intimate sexual practices between partners who use condoms or other methods to prevent the exchange of sexually related diseases and who are not promiscuous by having intimate sexual relations with other partners. Although perfect safety is virtually impossible without abstinence, the known risks of infections by HIV viruses or other organisms transmitted through sexual contact can be reduced by safe sex practices.

safety director /sāf′tē/ [Fr *sauver* to save, *directeur* manager], a member of a hospital staff whose activities are related to safety functions, such as fire prevention, environmental safety, and disaster planning activities.

sagittal /saj′ətəl/ [L *sagitta* arrow], (in anatomy) of or pertaining to a suture or an imaginary line extending from the front to the back in the midline of the body or a part of the body.

sagittal axis, a hypothetical line through the mandibular condyle that serves as an axis for rotation movements of the mandible.

sagittal fontanel, a soft area located in

the sagittal suture, halfway between the anterior and posterior fontanels. It may be found in some normal newborns and also some with Down syndrome.

sagittal plane, the anteroposterior plane or the section parallel to the median plane of the body.

sagittal sinus, either of two venous sinuses of the dura mater. The superior venous sinus begins near the crista galli and drains backward to empty into a confluence of sinuses near the occipital area. The inferior venous sinus begins in the lower margin of the cerebral falx and follows the superior venous sinus, emptying into the straight sinus.

sagittal suture, the serrated connection between the two parietal bones of the skull, coursing down the midline from the coronal suture to the upper part of the lambdoidal suture.

SaH, SAH, abbreviation for **subarachnoid hemorrhage.**

SAIN, abbreviation for **Society for Advancement in Nursing.**

Saint Vitus' dance /säntvī'təs/, a motor nerve disorder characterized by irregular, involuntary jerky movements of the limbs and facial muscles. Historically, the condition was once confused with symptoms of a dance mania that reportedly was cured by a pilgrimmage to the shrine of Saint Vitus.

salaam convulsion /säläm'/, a violent muscle spasm of the sternomastoid muscles marked by head bobbing or bowing.

salbutamol. See **albuterol.**

salicylanilide /sal'isilan'ilīd/, a topical antifungal prescribed in the treatment of tinea capitis caused by *Microsporum audouinii.*

salicylate /səlis'əlāt/ [Gk *salix* willow, *hyle* matter], any of several widely prescribed drugs derived from salicylic acid. Salicylates exert analgesic, antipyretic, and antiinflammatory actions. The most important is acetylsalicylic acid, or aspirin. Sodium salicylate has also been used systemically, and it exerts similar effects. Methyl salicylate can be absorbed through the skin in amounts capable of causing systemic toxicity. Another salicylate, salicylic acid, is too irritating to be used systemically and is used topically as a keratolytic agent, for example, for removing warts.

salicylated /səlis'ilā'tid/ [Gk *salix* willow, *hyle* matter], pertaining to a chemical formed as a salt or ester of salicylic acid.

salicylate poisoning, a toxic condition caused by the ingestion of salicylate, most often in aspirin or oil of wintergreen. Intoxication is characterized by rapid breathing, vomiting, headache, irritability, keto-

sis, hypoglycemia, and, in severe cases, convulsions and respiratory failure.

salicylazosulfapyridine /səlisilaz'ōsul'-fəpir'idēn/, See **sulfasalazine.**

salicylic acid /sal'isil'ik/, a keratolytic agent prescribed in the treatment of hyperkeratotic skin conditions and as an adjunct in fungal infections.

salicylism /sal'isil'izəm/ [Gk *salix* willow, *hyle* matter, *ismos* practice], a syndrome of salicylate toxicity.

saline /sā'līn/ [L *sal* salt], **1.** pertaining to a substance that contains a salt of an alkali metal or earth. **2.** pertaining to something that is salty or has the characteristics of common table salt.

saline cathartic [L *sal* salt; Gk *katharsis* cleansing], one of a large group of cathartics administered to achieve prompt, complete evacuation of the bowel. A watery semifluid evacuation usually occurs within 3 to 4 hours.

saline enema, a salt-water enema. Hypertonic saline enemas are used to treat a worm infestation, both by inducing peristalsis and evacuation. A normal saline enema of 1 teaspoonful of salt per 0.5 liter of water is instilled slowly and retained as long as possible to combat shock or replace lost fluids.

saline infusion, the therapeutic introduction of a physiologic salt solution into a vein.

saline irrigation, the washing out of a body cavity or wound with a stream of salt solution, usually an isotonic aqueous solution of sodium chloride.

saline solution, a solution containing sodium chloride. Depending on the use, it may be hypotonic, isotonic, or hypertonic with body fluids.

saliva /səlī'və/ [L, spittle], the clear, viscous fluid secreted by the salivary and mucous glands in the mouth. Saliva contains water, mucin, organic salts, and the digestive enzyme ptyalin. It moistens the oral cavity, to initiate the digestion of starches, and to aid in the chewing and swallowing of food.

salivary /sal'iver'ē/ [L, saliva], of or pertaining to saliva or to the formation of saliva.

salivary duct, any one of the ducts through which saliva passes. Kinds of salivary ducts are **Bartholin's duct, duct of Rivinus, parotid duct,** and **submandibular duct.**

salivary fistula, an abnormal communication from a salivary gland or duct to an opening in the mouth or on the skin of the face or neck.

salivary gland, one of the three pairs of glands secreting into the mouth, thus aiding the digestive process. The salivary glands are the parotid, the submandibular, and the sublingual glands. They are racemose structures consisting of numerous lobes subdivided into smaller lobules connected by dense areolar tissue, vessels, and ducts.

salivary gland cancer, a malignant neoplastic disease of a salivary gland, occurring most frequently in a parotid gland. About 75% of tumors that develop in the salivary glands are benign, characteristically slow-growing, painless, mobile masses that are cystic or rubbery in consistency. The most common malignant neoplasms are mucoepidermoid, adenoid cystic, solid, and squamous cell carcinomas.

salivation /sal′ivā′shən/, the process of saliva secretion by the salivary glands.

salivatory /sal′ivətôr′ē/, stimulation of the production of saliva.

Salk Vaccine. See **poliovirus vaccine.**

sallow /sal′ō/ [ME *salou* dirty-gray], sickly in complexion.

salmon calcitonin. See **calcitonin.**

Salmonella /sal′mənel′ə/ [Daniel E. Salmon, American pathologist, b. 1850], a genus of motile, gram-negative, rod-shaped bacteria that includes species causing typhoid fever, paratyphoid fever, and some forms of gastroenteritis.

Salmonella enteritidis [Daniel E. Salmon; Gk *enteron* intestine], a species of *Salmonella* causing food poisoning and gastroenteritis in humans.

salmonellosis /sal′mənəlō′sis/ [Daniel E. Salmon; Gk *osis* condition], a form of gastroenteritis, caused by ingestion of food contaminated with a species of *Salmonella*, characterized by an incubation period of 6 to 48 hours followed by sudden, colicky abdominal pain, fever, and bloody, watery diarrhea. Nausea and vomiting are common, and abdominal signs may resemble acute appendicitis or cholecystitis. Symptoms usually last from 2 to 5 days, but diarrhea and fever may persist for up to 2 weeks. Dehydration may occur.

salol. See **phenyl salicylate.**

salol camphor /sal′ol/ /sal·l/, a clear, oily mixture of two parts of camphor and three parts of phenyl salicylate, used as a local antiseptic.

Salonica fever. See **trench fever.**

salpingectomy /sal′pinjek′təmē/ [Gk *salpinx* tube, *ektome* excision], surgical removal of one or both fallopian tubes, performed to remove a cyst or tumor, excise an abscess or, if both tubes are removed, as a sterilization procedure.

salpingitis /sal′pinjī′tis/ [Gk *salpinx* + *itis* inflammation], an inflammation or infection of the fallopian tube.

salpingo-oophorectomy /salping′gō-ō′-əfôrek′təmē/, the surgical removal of a fallopian tube and an ovary.

salpingo-oophoritis /-ō′əfôri′tis/, an inflammation of a fallopian tube and associated ovary.

salpingostomy /sal′ping·gos′təmē/ [Gk *salpinx* + *stoma* mouth], the formation of an artificial opening in a fallopian tube, performed to restore patency in a tube whose fimbriated ostium has been closed by infection or by chronic inflammation or to drain an abscess or an accumulation of fluid. A prosthesis may be inserted to maintain the patency of the fallopian tube and to direct the route of the ova to assist fertilization.

salpinx /sal′pingks/, pl. **salpinges** /salpin-′jēz/ [Gk, tube], a tube, such as the *salpinx auditiva* or the *salpinx uterina.* **–salpingian,** adj.

salt /sôlt/ [AS *sealt*], **1.** a compound formed by the chemical reaction of an acid and a base. Salts are usually composed of a metal and a nonmetal and may behave chemically as metals or nonmetals. **2.** sodium chloride (common table salt). **3.** a substance, such as magnesium sulfate (Epsom salt), used as a purgative.

saltation /saltā′shən/ [L *saltare* to dance], (in genetics) a mutation causing a significant difference in appearance between parent and offspring or an abrupt variation in the characteristics of the species. **–saltatorial, saltatoric, saltatory** /sal′tətôr′ē/, adj.

saltatory conduction [L *saltare* + *conducere* to lead together], impulse transmission that skips from node to node.

saltatory evolution, the appearance of a sudden, abrupt change within a species, caused by mutation; the progression of a species by sudden major changes rather than by the gradual accumulation of minor changes.

salt cake, sodium sulfate anhydrous; a technical grade of sodium sulfate used in detergents, dyes, soaps, and other industrial products.

salt depletion, the loss of salt from the body through excessive elimination of body fluids by perspiration, diarrhea, vomiting, or urination, without corresponding replacement.

Salter fracture. See **epiphyseal fracture.**

salt-free diet. See **low-sodium diet.**

saltpeter /sôlt′pē′tər/ [L *sal* salt, *petra* rock], common name for potassium nitrate, KNO_3, used in gunpowder, pickling, and medicines.

salt-poor diet, a diet providing 500 mg or less of sodium chloride daily. To ensure that the maximum intake of salt does not exceed the limit, it is necessary to record the amount of dietary sodium chloride including amounts contained in medications taken by a patient. Note: some "salt-free" diets may contain as much as 1,000 mg of sodium chloride per day.

salvage therapy /sal′vij/ [Fr *sauver* to save; Gk *therapeia* treatment], therapy administered to sites at which previous therapies have failed and the disease has recurred.

salve. See **ointment.**

samarium (Sm) /səmer′ē·əm/ [Colonel Samarski, nineteenth-century Russian mine official], a rare earth, metallic element. Its atomic number is 62; its atomic weight is 150.35.

sample [L *exemplum*], in research, a group or portion of the whole that can be used to demonstrate characteristics of the whole. Kinds of samples include **cluster, convenience, random,** and **stratified.**

sanatorium. See **sanitarium.**

sand bath, the application of warm, dry sand or of damp sand to the body.

sand flea. See **chigoe.**

sandfly fever. See **phlebotomus fever.**

Sandhoff's disease, a variant of Tay-Sachs disease that includes defects in both the enzymes hexosaminidase A and B. It is characterized by a progressively more rapid course and is found in the general population, not restricted as is Tay-Sachs disease.

Sandoz Clinical Assessment-Geriatric, an examination of psychologic function that is administered to elderly persons to assist in the diagnostic process.

sand tumor. See **psammoma.**

sanguine /sang′gwin/ [L *sanguis* blood], pertaining to an abundant and active blood circulation, ruddy complexion, and an attitude full of vitality and confidence.

sanguineous /sang·gwin′ē·əs/ [L *sanguis* blood], pertaining to blood.

sanitarium /san′iter′ē·əm/ [L, *sanare* to restore health], a facility for the treatment of patients suffering from chronic mental or physical diseases, or the recuperation of convalescent patients.

sanitary landfill /san′iterē/ [L *sanitas* health; AS *land, fyllan* to fill], a solid waste disposal site, usually a swamp area, ravine, or canyon where the waste is compacted by heavy machines and covered with earth.

sanitation /san′itā′shən/, the science of maintaining a healthful, disease-free, and hazard-free environment.

sanitize /san′itīz/, to take action needed to clean the environment or a part of it, removing or reducing pathogenic microorganisms and their habitats.

San Joaquin fever /san′wôkēn′/ [San Joaquin Valley, California; L *febris* fever], the primary stage of coccidioidomycosis.

SA node. See **sinoatrial node.**

SaO₂, symbol for the percent of *oxygen saturation of arterial blood.*

saphenous [Gk *saphenes* manifest], pertaining to certain anatomic structures in the leg, such as arteries, veins, or nerves.

saphenous nerve /səfē′nəs/ [Gk *saphenes* manifest; L *nervus* nerve], the largest and longest branch of the femoral nerve, supplying the skin of the medial side of the leg.

saphenous vein. See **great saphenous vein.**

saponaceous /sap′ənā′shəs/ [L *sapo* soap], pertaining to soap.

saponification /sapon′ifikā′shən/ [L *sapo* + *facere* to make], the production of soap.

saponified /sapon′ifīd/, pertaining to a substance chemically hydrolized into soaps or acid salts and glycerol by heating with an alkali.

saponin /sap′ənin/ [L *sapo* soap], a soapy material found in some plants, especially soapwort (Bouncing Bet) and certain lilies. It is used in demulcent medications to provide a sudsy quality.

saprophyte /sap′rəfīt/ [Gk *sapros* rotten, *phyton* plant], an organism that lives on dead organic matter. **–saprophytic,** *adj.*

SAR, abbreviation for **structure-activity relationship.**

saralasin, a competitive antagonist of angiotensin. It is administered by intravenous injection to assess the role of the renin-angiotensin system in the maintenance of blood pressure.

sarcoadenoma /sär′kōad′ənō′mə/ [Gk *sarx* flesh, *aden* gland, *oma* tumor], a mixed tumor containing both glandular and connective tissue characteristics.

sarcocarcinoma /-kär′sinō′mə/ [Gk *sarx* + *karkinos* crab, *oma* tumor], a mixed tumor with characteristics of both sarcomas and carcinomas.

sarcoidosis /sär′koidō′sis/ [Gk *sarx* flesh, *eidos* form, *osis* condition], a chronic disorder of unknown origin characterized by the formation of tubercles of nonnecrotizing epithelioid tissue. Common sites are the lungs, spleen, liver, skin, mucous membranes, and lacrimal and salivary glands, usually with involvement of the lymph glands. The lesions usually disappear over a period of months or years but progress to widespread granulomatous inflammation and fibrosis.

sarcoidosis cordis, a form of sarcoidosis in which granulomatous lesions develop in the myocardium. In severe cases the myo-

S

cardium may be infiltrated with many tumors and cardiac failure may follow.

sarcolemma /-lem′ə/ [Gk *sarx* + *lemma* sheath], a membrane that covers smooth, striated, and cardiac muscle fibers.

sarcoma /särkō′mə/, *pl.* **sarcomas, sarcomata** [Gk *sarx* + *oma* tumor], a malignant neoplasm of the soft tissues arising in fibrous, fatty, muscular, synovial, vascular, or neural tissue, usually first presenting as a painless swelling. The tumor, composed of closely packed cells in a fibrillar or homogeneous matrix, tends to be vascular and is usually highly invasive. Trauma probably does not play a role in the cause, but sarcomas may arise in burn or radiation scars.

sarcoma botryoides /bot′rē·oi′dēz/, a tumor derived from primitive striated muscle cells, occurring most frequently in young children and characterized by a painful, edematous, polypoid grapelike mass in the upper vagina or on the uterine cervix or the neck of the urinary bladder.

sarcomagenesis /särkō′məjen′əsis/ [Gk *sarx, oma* + *genesis* origin], the process of initiating and promoting the development of a sarcoma. –**sarcomagenetic,** *adj.*

sarcomere /sär′kōmir/ [Gk *sarx* + *meros* part], the smallest functional unit of a myofibril. Sarcomeres occur as repeating units along the length of a myofibril, occupying the region between Z disks of the myofibril.

sarcoplasm /sär′kōplaz′əm/ [Gk *sarx* + *plassein* to mold], the semifluid cytoplasm of muscle cells.

sarcoplasmic reticulum /-plas′tik/ [Gk *sarx* + *plassein* to mold; L *reticulum* little net], a network of tubules and sacs in skeletal muscles that plays an important role in muscle contraction and relaxation by releasing and storing calcium ions.

Sarcoptes scabiei /särkop′tēz skā′bē·ī/ [Gk *sarx* + *koptein* to cut; L *scabere* to scratch], the genus of itch mite that causes scabies.

sartorius /särtôr′ē·əs/ [L *sartor* tailor], the longest muscle in the body, extending from the pelvis to the calf of the leg. It acts to flex the thigh and rotate it laterally and to flex the leg and rotate it medially.

satellite cells /sat′əlīt/ [L *satelles* attendant, *cella* storeroom], glial cells that form around damaged nerve cells.

satellite clinic [L *satelles* attendant; Gk *kline* bed], a health care facility usually operated under the auspices of a large institution but situated in a location some distance from the larger health center.

satiety /sətī′ətē/, the satisfied feeling of being full after eating.

saturated /sach′ərā′tid/ [L *saturare* to fill], having absorbed or dissolved the maximum amount of a given substance, such as a solution in which no more of the solute can be dissolved.

saturated calomel electrode (SCE), a reference electrode commonly used in polarography.

saturated fatty acid, any of a number of glyceryl esters of certain organic acids in which all the atoms are joined by single-valence bonds. These fats are chiefly of animal origin and include beef, lamb, pork, veal, whole-milk products, butter, most cheeses, and a few plant fats such as cocoa butter, coconut oil, and palm oil.

saturated hydrocarbon, an organic compound that contains the maximum number of hydrogen atoms so that only single valence bonds exist in the carbon chain, such as in saturated fatty acids.

saturated solution, a solution in which the solvent contains the maximum amount of solute it can take up.

saturation /sach′ərā′shən/ [L, *saturare*, to fill], **1.** a condition in which a solution contains as much solute as can remain dissolved. **2.** a measure of the degree to which oxygen is bound to hemoglobin, expressed as a percentage of the possible limit. **3.** a condition in which all of the valency bonds of a chemical compound have been filled.

saturation index of hemoglobin, a measure of the amount of hemoglobin in a given amount of blood, compared with normal.

Saturday night palsy, a radial nerve paralysis caused by pressure on the arm after falling asleep, usually during an alcoholic binge. A similar type of palsy may result in the legs during alcoholic slumber on a sofa.

satyriasis /sat′irī′əsis/ [Gk *satyros* lecherous, *osis* condition], excessive or uncontrollable sexual desire in the male.

sauna bath /sô′nə/ [Finn *sauna*; AS *baeth*], a bath in which hot vapor is used to induce sweating, followed by rubbing of the body, and ending with a cold shower.

Sayre's jacket /serz/ [Lewis A. Sayre, American surgeon, b. 1820; ME *jaket*], a cast applied for support and immobilization in the treatment of certain abnormalities of the spinal column.

Sb, symbol for the element **antimony.**

SBE, 1. abbreviation for **self-breast examination. 2.** abbreviation for **subacute bacterial endocarditis.**

sc, 1. abbreviation for *sine correctione*, a Latin phrase meaning "without correction." **2.** abbreviation for *subcutaneously.*

Sc, symbol for the element **scandium.**

scab. See **eschar.**

scabicide /skab′isīd/ [L *scabere* to scratch, *caedere* to kill], any one of a large group of drugs that destroy the itch mite, *Sarcoptes scabiei.* These drugs are applied topically in a lotion or cream-based preparation. All are potentially toxic and irritating to the skin. Kinds of scabicides include **crotamiton, lindane.**

scabies /skā′bēz/ [L *scabere* to scratch], a contagious disease caused by *Sarcoptes scabiei,* the itch mite, characterized by intense itching of the skin and excoriation from scratching. The mite, transmitted by close contact with infected humans or domestic animals, burrows into outer layers of the skin where the female lays eggs. Two to 4 months after the first infection, sensitization to the mites and their products begins, resulting in a pruritic papular rash. Secondary bacterial infection may occur.

scabietic /skā′bē-et′ik/, pertaining to scabies.

scald /skôld/ [L *calidus* hot], a burn caused by exposure of the skin to a hot liquid or vapor.

scalded skin syndrome. See **toxic epidermal necrolysis.**

scale [OFr *escale* husk], **1.** a small, thin flake of keratinized epithelium. **2.** to remove encrusted material from the surface of a tooth.

scalene /skā′lēn/ [Gk *skalenos* uneven], pertaining to one of the scalenous muscles.

scalenus /skālē′nəs/ [Gk *skalenos*], one of a group of four muscles arising from the cervical vertebrae with insertions on the first or second rib.

scalenus anticus syndrome. See **Nafziger's syndrome.**

scalp [ME], the skin covering the head, not including the face and ears.

scalpel /ska′pəl/ [L *scalprum* knife], a small pointed knife with a convex edge. Some scalpels use interchangeable blades for specific surgical procedures, such as operating and amputating.

scalp medication, 1. a cream, ointment, lotion, or shampoo used to treat dermatologic conditions of the scalp. **2.** the application of a medication to the scalp.

scalp tourniquet, a bandage applied to the scalp to restrict blood flow during administration of antineoplastic drugs. The tourniquet controls the hair loss that commonly accompanies use of cancer-suppressing drugs.

scalp vein needle, a thin-gauge needle designed for use on the veins of the scalp or other small veins, especially in children.

scamping speech [ONorse *skammr* scant; ME *speche*], abnormal speech in which consonants or whole syllables are left out of words because of the person's inability to shape the sounds.

scandium (Sc) /skan′dē-əm/ [Scandinavia], a grayish metallic element. Its atomic number is 21; its atomic weight is 44.956.

scanning [L *scandere* to climb], a technique for carefully studying an area, organ, or system of the body by recording and displaying an image of the area. A concentration of a radioactive substance that has an affinity for a specific tissue may be administered by IV to enhance the image. –**scan,** *n., v.*

scanning electron microscope (SEM), an instrument similar to an electron microscope in that a beam of electrons instead of visible light is used to scan the surface of a specimen. The image produced is of less magnification than that produced by an electron microscope, but it appears to be three-dimensional and lifelike.

scanning electron microscopy, the technique using a scanning electron microscope on an electrically conducting sample.

scanning speech, abnormal speech characterized by a staccato-like articulation in which the words are clipped and broken because the person pauses between syllables.

scanography /skanog′rəfē/ [L *scandere* to climb; Gk *graphein* to record], a method of producing a radiogram of an internal body organ or structure by using a series of parallel beams that eliminate size distortion.

Scanzoni rotation /skanzō′nē/ [Friedrich W. Scanzoni, German gynecologist, b. 1821; L *rotare* to rotate], an obstetric operation in which forceps having a curved shank are applied to the fetal head while it is still high in the pelvis. The head is displaced upward and rotated to the occiput anterior position.

scapegoating /skāp′gōting/ [ME *escapen* to escape; *goot*], the projection of blame, hostility, or suspicion onto one member of a group by other members to avoid self-confrontation.

scaphocephaly /skaf′ōsef′əlē/ [Gk *skaphe* skiff, *kephale* head], a congenital malformation of the skull in which premature closure of the sagittal suture results in restricted lateral growth of the head, giving it an abnormally long, narrow appearance with a cephalic index of 75 or less. –**scaphocephalic, scaphocephalous,** *adj.*

scaphoid /skaf′oid/ [Gk *skaphe* + *eidos* form], boat-shaped, such as the scaphoid bone of the wrist.

S

scaphoid abdomen, an abdomen with a sunken anterior wall.

scaphoid bone [Gk *skaphe* + *eidos* form; AS *ban*], either of two similar bones of the hand and the foot. The scaphoid bone of the hand is slanted at the radial side of the carpus. The scaphoid bone of the foot is located at the medial side of the tarsus between the talus and cuneiform bones.

scapula /skap'yələ/, one of the pair of large, flat, triangular bones that form the dorsal part of the shoulder girdle.

scapular line /skap'yələr/, an imaginary vertical line drawn through the inferior angle of the scapula.

scapulohumeral /skap'yəlohy͞oo'mərəl/ [L *scapula* + *humerus* shoulder], of or pertaining to the structures of muscles and the area around the scapula and humerus that make up the shoulder girdle.

scapulohumeral muscular dystrophy. See **Erb's muscular dystrophy.**

scapulohumeral reflex, a normal response to tapping the vertebral border of the scapula, resulting in adduction of the arm.

scapus /skā'pəs/ [Gk *skapos* rod], a stem or shaft, such as the scapus penis.

scar. See **cicatrix.**

scarification /sker'ifikā'shən/ [L *scarifare* to scratch], multiple superficial scratches or incisions in the skin, such as those made for the introduction of a vaccine.

scarify /sker'əfi/ [L *scarifare*], to make multiple superficial incisions into the skin; to scratch. Vaccination against smallpox is achieved by scarifying the skin under a drop of vaccine.

scarlatina. See **scarlet fever.**

scarlatiniform /skär'lətē'nifôrm/ [It *scarlattina*; L *forma* form], resembling the rash of **scarlet fever.**

scarlet fever /skär'lit/ [OFr *escarlate*; L *febris* fever], an acute contagious disease of childhood caused by an erythrotoxin-producing strain of group A hemolytic *Streptococcus*. The infection is characterized by sore throat, fever, enlarged lymph nodes in the neck, prostration, and a diffuse bright red rash.

scarlet rash [OFr *escarlate, rasche* scurf], any scarlitini or rosy skin eruption that accompanies an infection, such as scarlet fever or German measles.

scarlet red, an azo dye that has been used to impart color to pharmaceutic preparations.

scatologic /skat'əloj'ik/, pertaining to **scatology.**

scatology /skatol'əjē/ [Gk *skatos* dung, *logos* science], the science of feces.

scattered radiation /skat'ərd/ [ME *scateren* to throw away; L *radiare* to shine],

radiation that travels in a direction other than that of its source energy, such as secondary radiation and stray radiation.

scattergram /skat'ərgram [ME *scateren* + Gk *gramma* record], a graph representing the distribution of two variables in a sample population. One variable is plotted on the vertical axis; the second on the horizontal axis. A scattergram demonstrates the degree or tendency to which the variables occur in association with each other.

scattering [ME *scateren*], (in radiology) an effect produced by the interaction of low-energy x-rays with matter. The incident photon interacts with a target atom, causing it to become excited and release the excess energy as a secondary or scattered photon with a change in direction.

scavenger cell /skav'ənjər/, a phagocytic cell that removes tissue debris and some invading pathogens. It may or may not be mobile.

scavenging system. See **gas scavenging system.**

ScD, abbreviation for *Doctor of Science.*

Schedule I, a category of drugs not considered legitimate for medical use. Among the substances so classified by the Drug Enforcement Agency are mescaline, LSD, heroin, and marijuana. Special licensing procedures must be followed to use Schedule I substances.

Schedule II, a category of drugs considered to have a strong potential for abuse or addiction, but which have legitimate medical use. Among the substances so classified by the Drug Enforcement Agency are morphine, cocaine, pentobarbital, oxycodone, alphaprodine, and methadone.

Schedule III, a category of drugs that have less potential for abuse or addiction than Schedule II or I drugs. Among the substances so classified by the Drug Enforcement Agency are glutethimide and various analgesic compounds containing codeine.

Schedule IV, a category of drugs that have less potential for abuse or addiction than those of Schedules I to III. Among the substances so classified by the Drug Enforcement Agency are chloral hydrate, chlordiazepoxide, meprobamate, and oxazepam.

Schedule V, a category of drugs that have a small potential for abuse or addiction. Among the substances so classified by the Drug Enforcement Agency are many commonly prescribed medications that contain small amounts of codeine or diphenoxylate. The specific drugs in Schedule V vary greatly from state to state.

Schedule of Drugs [L *scheda* sheet of paper; Fr *drogue*], a classification system that categorizes drugs by their potential for abuse. The schedule is divided into five groups: Schedules I to V. All substances in Schedules II to V require a written prescription signed by a physician. Schedule I substances are not approved for medical use. Specific regulations for dispensing these substances vary from state to state and from institution to institution.

schema /skē′mə/, an innate knowledge structure that allows a child to organize in his or her mind ways to behave in his or her environment.

Scheuermann's disease /shoi′ərmonz/ [Holger W. Scheuermann, Danish surgeon, b. 1877], an abnormal skeletal condition characterized by a fixed kyphosis that develops at puberty and is caused by wedge-shaped deformities of one or several vertebrae. The cause of the disease is unknown, but authorities have speculated that it may result from infection, inflammatory processes, aseptic necrosis, disk deterioration, mechanical influences, inadequate circulation during rapid growth, or disturbances of epiphyseal growth resulting from protrusion of the intervertebral disk through deficient or defective cartilaginous plates. The most striking pathologic feature of Scheuermann's disease is the presence of wedge-shaped vertebral bodies, seen on radiographic examination, that create an excessive curvature.

Schick test /shik/ [Bela Schick, Austrian-American physician, b. 1877], a skin test to determine immunity to diphtheria in which diphtheria toxin is injected intradermally. A positive reaction, indicating susceptibility, is marked by redness and swelling at the site of injection.

Schick test control [Bela Schick, Austrian pediatrician, b. 1877; L, *testum*, crucible; Fr, *contrôle*, check], a preparation used in carrying out the Schick test for diphtheria immunization.

Schilder's disease /shil′dərz/ [Paul F. Schilder, American neurologist, b. 1886], a group of progressive, severe, neurologic diseases beginning in childhood. All are characterized by demyelination of the white matter of the brain with muscle spasticity, optic neuritis, aphasia, deafness, adrenal insufficiency, and dementia. Many of the signs resemble those of multiple sclerosis.

Schiller's test /shil′ərz/ [Walter Schiller, American pathologist, b. 1887], a procedure for indicating areas of abnormal epithelium in the vagina or on the cervix of the uterus as a guide in selecting biopsy sites for cancer detection. A potassium iodide or aqueous iodine solution is painted on the vaginal walls and cervix under direct visualization. Normal epithelium contains glycogen and stains a deep brown color; abnormal epithelium, containing no glycogen, will not stain, and nonstaining sites may then be included in tissue biopsies.

Schilling's leukemia. See **monocytic leukemia.**

Schilling test /shil′ing/ [Robert Schilling, American physician, b. 1919], a diagnostic test for pernicious anemia in which vitamin B_{12} tagged with radioactive cobalt is administered orally, and GI absorption is measured by determining the radioactivity of urine samples collected over a 24-hour period.

schindylesis /skin′dilē′sis/ [Gk, splintering], an articulation of certain bones of the skull in which a thin plate of one bone enters a cleft formed by the separation of two layers of another bone.

Schiötz' tonometer /shē·ets′/ [Hjalmar Schiötz, Norwegian ophthalmologist, b. 1850; Gk *tonos* stretching, *metron* measure], a tonometer used to measure intraocular pressure by observing the depth of indentation of the cornea made by the weighted plunger on the device after a topical anesthetic is applied.

Schirmer's test. See **test for lacrimation.**

schistocyte /shis′tōsīts/ [Gk *schistos* cleft, *kytos* cell], an erythrocyte cell fragment characteristic of hemolysis or cell fragmentation associated with severe burns and intravascular coagulation.

Schistosoma /shis′təsō′mə/ [Gk *schistos* cleft, *soma* body], a genus of blood flukes that may cause urinary, GI, or liver disease in humans and that requires freshwater snails as intermediate hosts. *Schistosoma hematobium*, found chiefly in Africa and the Middle East, affects the bladder and pelvic organs, causing painful, frequent urination and hematuria. *S. japonicum*, found in Japan, the Philippines, and Eastern Asia, causes GI ulcerations and fibrosis of the liver. *S. mansoni*, found in Africa, the Middle East, the Caribbean, and tropical America, causes symptoms similar to those caused by *S. japonicum*.

schistosomiasis /shis′təsōmī′əsis/ [Gk *schistos, soma + osis* condition], a parasitic infection caused by a species of fluke of the genus *Schistosoma*, transmitted to humans, the definitive host, by contact with fresh water contaminated by human feces. A single fluke may live in one part of the body, depositing eggs frequently, for up to 20 years. The eggs are irritating to mucous membrane, causing it to thicken

S

and become papillomatous. Symptoms depend on the part of the body infected.

schistosomicide /shis'təsō'məsīd/ [Gk *schistos, soma* + L *caedere* to kill], a drug destructive to schistosomes, blood flukes transmitted by snails to human hosts. –schistosomicidal, *adj.*

schizoaffective disorder /skit'sō·afek'tiv/ [Gk *schizein* to split; L *affectus* state of mind; *dis* opposite of, *ordo* rank], a condition that includes characteristics of schizophrenia and a mood disorder but fails to meet the DSM-III-R criteria for either diagnosis.

schizogenesis /skit'səjen'əsis/ [Gk *schizein* + *genesis* origin], reproduction by fission. –schizogenetic, schizogenic, schizogenous, *adj.*

schizogony /skitsog'ənē/ [Gk *schizein* + *genein* to produce], 1. reproduction by multiple fission. 2. the asexual reproductive stage of sporozoans, specifically the portion of the life cycle of the malarial parasite that occurs in the erythrocytes or liver cells.

schizoid /skit'soid, skiz'oid/ [Gk *schizein* + (*phren* mind), *eidos* form], 1. characteristic of or resembling schizophrenia; schizophrenic. 2. a person, not necessarily a schizophrenic, who exhibits the traits of a schizoid personality.

schizoid personality, a functioning but maladjusted person whose behavior is characterized by extreme shyness, oversensitivity, introversion, seclusiveness, and avoidance of close interpersonal relationships.

schizoid personality disorder, a personality disorder (DSM-III-R) characterized by a defect in the ability to form social relationships, as shown by emotional coldness and aloofness, withdrawn and seclusive behavior, and indifference to praise, criticism, and the feelings of others.

schizont /skit'sont/ [Gk *schizein* + *on* being], the multinucleated cell stage during the sexual reproductive phase in the life cycle of a sporozoan, such as the malarial parasite *Plasmodium*. It is produced by the multiple fission of the trophozoite in a cell of the vertebrate host and subsequently segments into merozoites.

schizonticide /skitson'təsīd/ [Gk *schizein* + *on* being; L *caedere* to kill], a substance that destroys schizonts. –schizonticidal, *adj.*

schizophasia /skit'səfā'zhə, skiz'ə-/ [Gk *schizein* + *phasis* speech], the disordered, incomprehensible speech characteristic of some forms of schizophrenia.

schizophrene /skit'səfrēn', skiz'ə-/ [Gk *schizein* to split, *phren* mind], a person afflicted with schizophrenia.

schizophrenia /skit'səfrē'nē·ə, skiz'ə-/ [Gk *schizein* to split, *phren* mind], any one of a large group of psychotic disorders characterized by gross distortion of reality, disturbances of language and communication, withdrawal from social interaction, and the disorganization and fragmentation of thought, perception, and emotional reaction. Apathy and confusion; delusions and hallucinations; rambling or stylized patterns of speech, such as evasiveness, incoherence, and echolalia; withdrawn, regressive, and bizarre behavior; and emotional lability often occur. No single cause of the disease is known; genetic, biochemical, psychologic, interpersonal, and sociocultural factors are usually involved.

schizophrenic /skit'səfren'ik, skiz'ə-/ 1. of or pertaining to schizophrenia. 2. a person with schizophrenia.

schizophreniform disorder /skit'səfren'ifôrm/ [Gk *schizein, phren* + L *forma* form], a condition exhibiting the same symptoms as schizophrenia but characterized by an acute onset with resolution in 2 weeks to 6 months.

schizophrenogenic /skit'səfren'əjen'ik, skiz'ə-/ [Gk *schizein, phren* + *genein* to produce], tending to cause or produce schizophrenia.

Schizotrypanum cruzi. See Chagas' disease.

schizotypal personality disorder /skit'sōtī'pəl/ [Gk *schizein* + *typos* mark; L *personalis* character; *dis* opposite of, *ordo* rank], a condition characterized by oddities of thought, perception, speech, and behavior that are not severe enough to meet the clinical criteria for schizophrenia. Symptoms include magical thinking, such as belief in clairvoyance and telepathy; ideas of reference; recurrent illusions, such as sensing the presence of a person not actually present; social isolation; peculiar speech patterns, including words used deviantly; and hypersensitivity to criticism.

Schlatter-Osgood disease, Schlatter's disease. See Osgood-Schlatter disease.

Schlemm's canal. See canal of Schlemm.

Schneiderian carcinoma /shnīdir'ē·ən/, an epithelial malignancy of the nasal mucosa and paranasal sinuses.

Schönlein-Henoch purpura. See Henoch-Schönlein purpura.

school nurse practitioner (SNP), a registered nurse who is qualified through satisfactory completion of a nurse practitioner program to serves a nurse practitioner in a school system.

school phobia [AS *scol*; Gk *phobos* fear], an extreme separation anxiety disorder of children, usually in the elementary grades, characterized by a persistent, irrational fear of going to school or being in a school-like atmosphere. Such children are usually oversensitive, shy, timid, nervous, and emotionally immature and have pervasive feelings of inadequacy. They typically try to cope with their fears by becoming overdependent on others, especially the parents.

Schüffner's dots, coarse pink or red granules seen in the red blood cells of patients with tertiary malaria. They are signs of *Plasmodium vivax* or *P. ovale* and are absent in blood cells of patients infected with other types of malaria.

Schultz-Charlton phenomenon [Werner Schultz, German physician, b. 1878; Willy Charlton, German physician, b. 1889], a cutaneous reaction to the intradermal injection of scarlatina antiserum in a person who has a scarlatiniform rash. The rash blanches.

Schultze's mechanism, the delivery of a placenta with the fetal surfaces presenting.

Schwann cells /shwon/ [Friedrich T. Schwann, German anatomist, b. 1810], cells of ectodermal origin that comprise the neurilemma.

schwannoma /shwonō′mə/, *pl.* **schwannomas, schwannomata** [Friedrich Schwann; Gk *oma* tumor], a benign, solitary, encapsulated tumor arising in the neurilemma (Schwann's sheath) of peripheral, cranial, or autonomic nerves.

schwannosis /shwonō′sis/ [Friedrich Schwann; Gk *osis* condition], a condition of overgrowth of the neurilemma or sheath of Schwann.

Schwann's sheath /shwons/. See **neurilemma.**

Schwartz bed. See **hyperextension bed.**

Schwartzman-Sanarelli phenomenon /shvôrts′man san′ərel′ē/ [Gregory Schwartzman, American physician, b. 1896; Guiseppe Sanarelli, Italian physician, b. 1864], a phenomenon induced experimentally in the investigation of the role of coagulation in renal disease. Animals injected twice with a bacterial endotoxin develop massive disseminated intravascular coagulation with thrombosis of the blood vessels in the kidneys.

sciatic /sī·at′ik/ [Gk *ischiadikos* hip joint], near the ischium, such as the sciatic nerve or the sciatic vein.

sciatica /sī·at′ikə/, an inflammation of the sciatic nerve, usually marked by pain and tenderness along the course of the nerve through the thigh and leg. It may result in a wasting of the muscles of the lower leg.

sciatic dislocation. See **dislocation of hip.**

sciatic nerve, a long nerve originating in the sacral plexus and extending through the muscles of the thigh, leg, and foot, with numerous branches.

SCID, abbreviation for **severe combined immunodeficiency disease.**

science /sī′əns/ [L *scientia* knowledge], a systematic attempt to establish theories to explain observed phenomena and the knowledge obtained through these efforts. **Pure science** is concerned with the gathering of information solely for the sake of obtaining new knowledge. **Applied science** is the practical application of scientific theory and laws.

Science of Unitary Human Beings, a conceptual model and theory of nursing proposed by Martha Rogers in 1970. Its four basic concepts focus on the nature and direction of "unitary human development."

scientific method /sī′əntif′ik/, a systematic, ordered approach to the gathering of data and the solving of problems. The basic approach is the statement of the problem followed by the statement of a hypothesis. An experimental method is established to help prove or disprove the hypothesis. The results of the experiment are observed, and conclusions are drawn from observed results.

scientific rationale, a reason, based on supporting scientific evidence, why a particular action is chosen.

scintigram /sin′tigram′/ [L *scintillatio* sparkling; Gk *gramma* record], in nuclear medicine, a recording of the radioactivity emitted by a tracer in an organism or organ system.

scintigraph /sin′tigraf′/, a photographic recording produced by an imaging device showing the distribution and intensity of radioactivity in various tissues and organs after the administration of a radiopharmaceutical.

scintillating scotoma /sin′tilā′ting/, an abnormal area of the visual field that is positive and luminous, sometimes becoming hemianopic and appearing in a migraine aura.

scintillation detector /sin′tilā′shən/ [L *scintillatio* sparkling], **1.** a device that relies on the emission of light or ultraviolet radiation from a crystal subjected to ionizing radiation. The light is detected by a photomultiplier tube and converted to an electric signal that can be processed further. **2.** a device used to measure the amount of radioactivity in an area of the body.

scintiscan /sin′tiscan′/, a photographic display of the distribution of a radiopharmaceutical within the body.

S

scirrhous carcinoma /skir′əs/ [Gk *skirrhos* hard; *karkinos* crab, *oma* tumor], a hard, fibrous, particularly invasive tumor in which the malignant cells occur singly or in small clusters or strands in dense connective tissue.

scissor gait /siz′ər/, a manner of walking cross-legged as observed in spastic paraplegia.

scissor legs, legs that are crossed due to a disorder of the adductor muscles of the thigh or a deformity of the hip.

scissors [L *scindere* to cut], a sharp instrument composed of two opposing cutting blades, held together by a central pin on which the blades pivot. The most common dissecting scissors are the straight **Mayo,** for cutting sutures; the **Snowden-Pencer,** for deep, delicate tissue; the long, curved **Mayo,** for deep, heavy, or tough tissue; the short, curved **Metzenbaum,** for superficial, delicate tissue; and the long, blunt, curved **Metzenbaum,** for deep, delicate tissue.

SCL, abbreviation for **soft contact lens.**

sclera /sklir′ə/ [Gk *skleros* hard], the tough, inelastic, opaque membrane covering the posterior five sixths of the eyeball. It maintains the size and form of the bulb and attaches to muscles that move the bulb. Posteriorly, it is pierced by the optic nerve and, with the transparent cornea, comprises the outermost of three tunics covering the eyeball.

scleredema /sklir′ədē′mə/ [Gk *skleros* + *oidema* swelling], an idiopathic skin disease characterized by nonpitting induration beginning on the face or neck and spreading downward over the body, sparing the hands and feet. There also may be swelling of the tongue, restriction of the movements of the eyes, and pericardial, pleural, and peritoneal effusions.

sclerema neonatorum /sklirē′mə/ [Gk *skleros* + *neos* new; L *natus* birth], a progressive generalized hardening of the skin and subcutaneous tissue of the newborn. It is usually a fatal condition that occurs as a result of severe cold stress in severely ill premature infants.

scleritis /sklirī′tis/, an inflammation of the sclera.

sclerodactyly /sklir′ōdak′tilē/ /skler′ōdak-′tilē/ [Gk *skleros* + *daktylos* finger], a musculoskeletal deformity affecting the hands of persons with scleroderma. The fingers are fixed in a semiflexed position, with tightened skin to the wrist. The fingertips may be ulcerated.

scleroderma /skler′ōdur′mə/ [Gk *skleros* + *derma* skin], a relatively rare autoimmune disease affecting the blood vessels and connective tissue. The disease is characterized by fibrous degeneration of the connective tissue of the skin, lungs, and internal organs, especially the esophagus and kidneys. Scleroderma is most common in middle-aged women. The most common initial complaints are changes in the skin of the face and fingers. Raynaud's phenomenon occurs with a gradual hardening of the skin and swelling of the distal extremities. In the early stages, the disease may be confused with rheumatoid arthritis or Raynaud's disease. As the disease progresses, there is deformity of the joints and pain on movement. Skin changes include edema, then pallor; then the skin becomes firm; finally, it becomes slightly pigmented and fixed to the underlying tissues. At this stage the skin of the face is taut, shiny, and masklike, and the patient may have difficulty in chewing and swallowing.

scleroderma neonatorum. See **sclerema neonatorum.**

scleromalacia perforans /-məlā′shə/ [Gk *skleros* + *malakia* softening; L *perforare* to pierce], a condition of the eyes in which devitalization and sloughing of the sclera occur as a complication of rheumatoid arthritis. The pigmented uvea becomes exposed and glaucoma, cataract formation, and detachment of the retina may result.

sclerose /sklerōz′/ [Gk *skleros*], to harden or to cause hardening. –**sclerotic,** *adj.*

sclerosing hemangioma /sklirō′zing/ [Gk *skleros* + *haima* blood, *aggeion* vessel, *oma* tumor], a solid, encapsulated tumorlike nodule of the skin or a mass of histiocytes, thought to arise from a hemangioma by the proliferation of endothelial and connective tissue cells.

sclerosing keratitis [Gk *skleros* + *keras* horn, *itis*], **1.** a form of corneal inflammation in which nodular infiltrates appear near the margin of the cornea in association with a ring of anterior scleritis. **2.** a form of corneal inflammation characterized by an opaque triangle in the deep layers of the cornea, with the base of the triangle near the sclerosing area.

sclerosing phlebitis [Gk *skleros* + *phleps* vein, *itis*], an inflammation of a vein that has become hardened and obstructed.

sclerosing solution [Gk *skleros* + L *solvere* to dissolve], a liquid containing an irritant that causes inflammation and resulting fibrosis of tissues. It may be used in cauterizing ulcers, arresting hemorrhage, and treating hemangiomas.

sclerosis /sklerō′sis/ [Gk *sklerosis* hardening], a condition characterized by hardening of tissue resulting from any of several causes, including inflammation, the deposit of mineral salts, and infiltration of connective tissue fibers. **–sclerotic,** *adj.*

sclerotherapy /-ther′əpē/ [Gk *skleros* + *therapeia* treatment], the use of sclerosing chemicals to treat varicosities such as hemorrhoids or esophageal varices. The agent produces inflammation and later fibrosis and obliteration of the lumen.

sclerotomal pain distribution /-tō′məl/, the referral of pain from pain-sensitive tissues covering the axial skeleton along a sclerotomal segment.

sclerotome /sklir′ətōm/ [Gk *skleros* + *temnein* to cut], (in embryology) the part of the segmented mesoderm layer in the early developing embryo that originates from the somites and gives rise to the skeletal tissue of the body.

scolex /skō′leks/, *pl.* **scoleces** /skō′ləsēz/ [Gk, worm], the headlike segment or organ of an adult tapeworm that has hooks, grooves, or suckers by which it attaches itself to the wall of the intestine.

scoliometer /skō′lē·om′ətər/ [Gk *skoliosis* curvature], a device for measuring the amount of abnormal curvature in the spine.

scoliosis /skō′lē·ō′sis/ [Gk *skoliosis* curvature], lateral curvature of the spine, a common abnormality of childhood. Causes include congenital malformations of the spine, poliomyelitis, skeletal dysplasias, spastic paralysis, and unequal leg length. Unequal heights of hips or shoulders may be a sign of this condition.

scoliotic pelvis /skō′lē·ot′ik/, an abnormal pelvic area due to the effects of scoliosis bending the sacrum to one side.

scombroid /skom′broid/ [Gk *scombros* mackerel, *eidos* form], pertaining to fish of the spiny-finned percoid *Scombridae* and *Scomberescidae* families, which include skipjack, mackerel, bonito, and tuna.

scombroid poisoning, toxic effects of eating scombroid types of fish that have begun bacterial decomposition after being caught. Scombroid fish contain large amounts of free histidine in the muscle tissue, which gives rise to toxic levels of histamine under conditions of histidine decarboxylation by any of a dozen species of bacteria. Scombroid poisoning is not limited to consumption of fresh fish; the problem may also affect commercially canned tuna. Symptoms, which usually last no more than 24 hours, include nausea, vomiting, diarrhea, epigastric pain, and urticaria. Treatment is symptomatic.

scopolamine /skōpol′əmēn/ [Giovanni A. Scopoli, Italian naturalist, b. 1723], an anticholinergic alkaloid obtained from the leaves and seeds of several solanaceous plants. It is a central nervous system depressant and is used to prevent motion sickness and as an antiemetic, a sedative in obstetrics, and a cycloplegic and mydriatic.

scopolamine hydrobromide, an anticholinergic prescribed in the treatment of nausea and vomiting, as a sedative and preanesthetic medication, and as a cycloplegic and mydriatic medication in ophthalmic procedures.

scopophilia /skō′pəfil′ē·ə, skop′-/ [Gk *skopein* to look, *philein* to love], **1.** sexual pleasure derived from looking at sexually stimulating scenes or at another person's genitals; voyeurism. **2.** a morbid desire to be seen; exhibitionism. **–scopophiliac, scopophilic, scoptophiliac, scoptophilic.** *adj., n.*

scopophobia /skō′pə-/ [Gk *skopein* + *phobos* fear], an anxiety disorder characterized by a morbid fear of being seen or stared at by others. The condition is commonly seen in schizophrenia.

scorbutic gingivitis /skôrbyoo̅′tik/ [Fr *scorbutique* scurvy; L *gingiva* gum; Gk *itis* inflammation], an abnormal condition, characterized by inflamed or bleeding gums and caused by vitamin C deficiency.

scorbutic pose, the characteristic posture of a child with scurvy, with thighs and legs semiflexed and hips rotated outward. The child usually lies motionless without voluntary movements of the extremities because of the pain that accompanies any motion.

scorbutus. See **scurvy.**

scorpion sting /skôr′pē·on/ [Gk *skorpios*; AS *stingan*], a painful wound produced by a scorpion, an arachnid with a hollow stinger in its tail. The stings of many species are only slightly toxic, but some, including *Centruroides sculpturatus* of the southwestern United States, may inflict fatal injury, especially in small children. Initial pain is followed within several hours by numbness, nausea, muscle spasm, dyspnea, and convulsion.

scotoma /skōtō′mə/, *pl.* **scotomas, scotomata** [Gk *skotos* darkness, *oma* tumor], a defect of vision in a defined area in one or both eyes. A common prodromal symptom is a shimmering film appearing as an island in the visual field.

scotopic vision /skōtop′ik/ [Gk *skotos*; L *visio* seeing], the ability of the eye to adjust for vision in darkness or dim light.

scratch test [ME *scratten*; L *testum* crucible], a skin test for identifying an allergen, performed by placing a small quantity of a solution containing a suspected allergen on a lightly scratched area of the skin. If a wheal forms within 15 minutes, allergy to the substance is indicated.

S

screamer's nodule. See **vocal cord nodule.**

screening [ME *scren*], **1.** a preliminary procedure, such as a test or examination, to detect the most characteristic sign or signs of a disorder that may require further investigation. **2.** the examination of a large sample of a population to detect a specific disease or disorder, such as hypertension.

screen memory [ME *scren;* L *memoria*], a consciously tolerable memory that replaces one that is emotionally painful to recall.

screw clamp [OFr *escroe* screw; AS *clam* fastener], a device, usually made of plastic, equipped with a screw that can be manipulated to close and open the primary IV tubing for regulating the flow of intravenous solution.

Scribner shunt [Belding S. Scribner, American physician, b. 1921], a type of arteriovenous bypass, used in hemodialysis, consisting of a special tube connection outside the body.

scripting /skrip'ting/, a technique of family therapy involving the development of new family transactional patterns.

scrotal cancer /skrō'təl/ [L *scrautum* quiver for arrows], an epidermoid malignancy of the scrotum, characterized initially by a small sore that may ulcerate. The lesion occurs most frequently in elderly men who have been exposed to soot, pitch, crude oil, mineral oils, polycyclic hydrocarbons, or arsenic fumes from copper smelting. In the eighteenth century, Sir Percival Pott associated scrotal cancer in chimney sweeps with exposure to soot. It is the first malignancy shown to be caused by an environmental carcinogen.

scrotal raphe, a line of union of the two halves of the scrotum. It is generally more highly pigmented than the surrounding tissue.

scrotal tongue, a nonpathologic condition in which the tongue is deeply furrowed and resembles the surface of the scrotum.

scrotum /skrō'təm/ [L *scrautum* quiver for arrows], the pouch of skin containing the testes and parts of the spermatic cords. It is divided on the surface into two lateral portions by a ridge that continues ventrally to the undersurface of the penis and dorsally along the middle line of the perineum to the anus. The two layers of the scrotum are the skin and the dartos tunic. The skin is very thin, has a brownish color, and is usually wrinkled. It is supplied with sebaceous follicles that secrete a substance with a characteristic odor and has thinly scattered, kinky hairs with roots that are visible through the skin. The dartos tunic is composed of a thin layer of unstriated muscular fibers around the base of the scrotum, continuous with the two layers of the superficial fascia of the groin and the perineum. The tunic projects an internal septum that divides the pouch into two cavities for the testes, extending between the scrotal ridge and the root of the penis. **–scrotal,** *adj.*

scrub. See **surgical scrub.**

scrubbed team members [ME *scrobben* to scrub], the surgeons and physicians, nurses, and technicians who are scrubbed for surgical procedures in a sterile environment.

scrub itch. See **Leeuwenhoekia australiensis.**

scrub nurse, a registered nurse or operating room technician who assists surgeons during operations.

scrub room, a special hospital area where surgeons and surgical teams use disposable sterile brushes and bactericidal soaps to wash and scrub their fingernails, hands, and forearms before performing or assisting in surgical operations.

scrub typhus, an acute, febrile disease of Asia, India, northern Australia, and the western Pacific islands, caused by several strains of the genus *Rickettsia tsutsugamushi* and transmitted from infected rodents to humans by mites. The clinical course is characterized by a necrotic papule or black eschar at the site of the lesion caused by the bite of the small arachnid. Tender, enlarged regional lymph nodes, fever, severe headache, eye pain, muscle aches, and a generalized rash usually occur. In severe cases, the myocardium and the central nervous system may be involved.

scruple /skr̄oo'pəl/ [L *scrupulus* small stone], a measure of weight in the apothecaries' system, equal to 20 grains or 1.296 g.

sculpting /skulp'ting/, a technique of family therapy involving construction of a live family portrait that depicts family alliances and conflicts.

scultetus bandage /skəltē'təs/ [Johann Schultes, German surgeon, b. 1595], a many-tailed bandage with an attached central piece. The tails are overlapped; the last two tied or pinned act to secure the others. A scultetus bandage may be opened or removed without moving the bandaged part of the body.

scurvy /skur'vē/ [Scan *scurfa* scabby], a condition resulting from lack of ascorbic acid in the diet. It is characterized by weakness, anemia, edema, spongy gums, often with ulceration and loosening of the teeth, and tendency to mucocutaneous hemorrhages, and induration of the muscles of the legs.

scut work [L *scutella* kitchen maid; AS *werc*], a derogatory, colloquial term for menial tasks, usually of a nontherapeutic nature, that are a necessary part of the work routine performed by the staff of a health care facility.

SD, abbreviation for **standard deviation.**

SDMS, abbreviation for *Society for Diagnostic Medical Sonographers.*

Se, symbol for the element **selenium.**

SE, abbreviation for **standard error.**

sealed source [ME *seel* mark; Fr *sourdre* to spring], (in radiotherapy) a source of radiant energy in which the radioactive material is permanently encased in a container or bonding material in a manner to prevent leakage.

sealer cement, a compound used in filling a root canal. It is applied as a plastic that solidifies after insertion and fills depressions in the surface of the canal.

seal limbs. See **phocomelia.**

seasickness. See **motion sickness.**

seasonal affective disorder (SAD) /sē′zənəl/, a mood disorder associated with the shorter days and longer nights of autumn and winter. Symptoms include lethargy, depression, and work difficulties. The patients also consume excess amounts of carbohydrates. The symptoms recede in the spring. The condition is associated with the effect of light on melatonin secretion and is treated with exposure to bright light.

seatworm. See *Enterobius vermicularis.*

sea urchin sting /ur′chin/ [AS *sae, herichon* hedgehog], an injury inflicted by any of a variety of sea urchins, in which the skin is punctured and, in some species, venom released. A venomous sting is characterized by pain, muscular weakness, numbness around the mouth, and dyspnea.

seawater bath [AS *sae, waeter*], a bath taken in warm seawater or in saline solution.

sebaceous /sibā′shəs/ [L *sebum* grease], fatty, oily, or greasy, usually referring to the oil-secreting glands of the skin or to their secretions.

sebaceous cyst, a misnomer for epidermoid cyst or pilar cyst.

sebaceous follicle, a sebaceous gland that opens into a hair follicle.

sebaceous gland, one of the many small sacculated organs in the dermis. They are located throughout the body in close association with all types of body hair but are especially abundant in the scalp, face, anus, nose, mouth, and external ear. Each gland consists of a single duct that

emerges from a cluster of oval alveoli. Each alveolus is composed of a transparent basement membrane enclosing epithelial cells. The ducts from most sebaceous glands open into the hair follicles but some open onto the surface of the skin. The sebum secreted by the glands oils the hair and the surrounding skin helps prevent evaporation of sweat and aids in the retention of body heat.

seborrhea /seb′ərē′ik/ /seb′ərē′ə/ [L *sebum* + Gk *rhoia* flow], any of several common skin conditions in which there is an overproduction of sebum resulting in excessive oiliness or dry scales. **–seborrheic** /seb′ərē′ik/, *adj.*

seborrhea capitis, seborrhea of the scalp.

seborrheic blepharitis, a form of seborrheic dermatitis in which the eyelids and the margins are covered with a granular crust.

seborrheic dermatitis, a common, chronic, inflammatory skin disease characterized by dry or moist, greasy scales and yellowish crusts. Common sites are the scalp, eyelids, face, external surfaces of the ears, axillae, breasts, groin, and gluteal folds. In acute stages there may be exudate and infection resulting in secondary furunculosis. In some people seborrheic dermatitis is associated with paralysis agitans, diabetes mellitus, malabsorption disorders, epilepsy, or an allergic reaction to gold or arsenic. Kinds of seborrheic dermatitis include **cradle cap, dandruff,** and **seborrheic blepharitis.**

seborrheic keratosis, a benign, well-circumscribed, slightly raised, tan to black, warty lesion of the skin of the face, neck, chest, or upper back. The macules are loosely covered with a greasy crust that leaves a raw pulpy base when removed. Itching is common.

sebum /sē′bəm/ [L, grease], the oily secretion of the sebaceous glands of the skin, composed of keratin, fat, and cellular debris. Combined with sweat, sebum forms a moist, oily, acidic film that is mildly antibacterial and antifungal and protects the skin against drying.

Seckel's syndrome. See **bird-headed dwarf.**

seclusion /siklo̅o̅′zhən/ [L *secludere* to isolate], (in psychiatric nursing) the isolation of a patient in a special room to decrease stimuli that might be causing or exacerbating the patient's emotional distress.

secobarbital /sek′obär′bital/, a sedative and hypnotic prescribed in the treatment of insomnia, agitation, and as an anticonvulsant and preoperative sedative.

secondary /sek′ənder′ē/ [L *secundus* second], second in importance or in incidence or belonging to the second order of sophistication or development, such as a secondary health care facility or secondary education.

secondary amenorrhea. See **amenorrhea.**

secondary amputation, amputation performed after suppuration has begun following severe trauma.

secondary amyloidosis. See **amyloidosis.**

secondary analysis, the study of a problem using previously compiled data.

secondary apnea, an abnormal condition in which respiration is absent and will not begin again spontaneously. Secondary apnea may result from any event that severely impedes the absorption of oxygen into the bloodstream.

secondary areola, a second ring appearing around the areola of the breast during pregnancy that is more pigmented than the areola before pregnancy.

secondary biliary cirrhosis, an abnormal hepatic condition characterized by obstruction of the bile duct with or without infection.

secondary care, 1. the provision of a specialized medical service by a physician specialist or a hospital on referral by a primary care physician. **2.** the retardation of an existing illness or other pathologic condition.

secondary dementia, dementia resulting from another, concurrent form of psychosis.

secondary dental caries, dental caries developing in a tooth already affected by the condition; often a new cavity forms adjacent to or beneath the restorative filling of an old cavity.

secondary dentition. See **permanent dentition.**

secondary dysmenorrhea. See **dysmenorrhea.**

secondary enuresis, enuresis in an older child who has demonstrated bedtime control for a year or more. It is typically the result of psychologic stress, but it may also be an early sign of an organic disorder, such as diabetes mellitus.

secondary fissure, a fissure between the uvula and the pyramid of the cerebellum.

secondary fracture. See **neoplastic fracture.**

secondary gain, an indirect benefit, usually obtained through an illness or debility. Such gains may include monetary and disability benefits, personal attentions, or escape from unpleasant situations and responsibilities.

secondary gangrene, a form of gangrene in which putrefaction follows the primary

tissue necrosis, resulting in malodorous and toxic products.

secondary gestation, a pregnancy in which the ovum becomes displaced from its original site of implantation but continues development at a different location.

secondary health care, an intermediate level of health care that includes diagnosis and treatment, performed in a hospital having specialized equipment and laboratory facilities.

secondary hemorrhage, a hemorrhage that develops 24 hours or more after the original injury or surgery. It is often due to an infection.

secondary host. See **intermediate host.**

secondary hydrocephalus, hydrocephalus that develops after an injury or infection, such as syphilis or meningitis.

secondary hypertension, elevated blood pressure associated with several primary diseases, such as renal, pulmonary, endocrine, and vascular diseases.

secondary hypertrophic osteoarthropathy. See **clubbing.**

secondary infection, an infection by a microorganism that follows an initial infection by another kind of organism.

secondary iritis, an inflammation of the iris that follows an infection or other disorder in a neighboring part of the eye, such as the cornea.

secondary nutrient, a substance that acts as a stimulant to activate the flora of the GI tract to synthesize other nutrients.

secondary occlusal traumatism, occlusal stress that affects previously weakened periodontal structures.

secondary peritonitis, inflammation of the peritoneum caused by the spread of infection from neighboring tissue.

secondary pneumonia, a condition of pneumonia that develops during the course of another disease, such as diphtheria or tularemia.

secondary polycythemia, a form of polycythemia that develops as a result of another disorder, such as a pulmonary disease.

secondary port, a control device for regulating the flow of a primary and a secondary intravenous solution. It consists of a Y-shaped plastic apparatus that attaches to the primary IV tubing and allows the primary and secondary IV solutions to flow separately or to flow simultaneously.

secondary prevention, a level of preventive medicine that focuses on early diagnosis, use of referral services, and rapid initiation of treatment to stop the progress of disease processes or a handicapping disability.

secondary proximal renal tubular acidosis. See **proximal renal tubular acidosis.**

secondary radiation, radiation that results from the scattering of primary x-rays. Secondary radiation often accounts for fogging of x-ray film.

secondary relationships, relationships with those who provide or accept services, or with acquaintances and friends, as distinguished from family members and intimate friends.

secondary sequestrum, a piece of dead bone that partially separates from sound bone during the process of necrosis but may be pushed back into position.

secondary sex characteristic, any of the external physical characteristics of sexual maturity secondary to hormonal stimulation that develops in the maturing individual.

secondary shock, a state of physical collapse and prostration caused by numerous traumatic and pathologic conditions. It develops over a period of time after severe tissue damage and may merge with primary shock, accompanied by various signs, such as weakness, restlessness, low body temperature, low blood pressure, cold sweat, and reduced urinary output. Blood pressure drops progressively in this state, and death may occur within a relatively short time after onset unless appropriate treatment intervenes. Secondary shock is often associated with heat stroke, crushing injuries, myocardial infarction, poisoning, fulminating infections, burns, and other life-threatening conditions. The pathology of this state reflects changes in the capillaries, which become dilated and engorged with blood.

secondary teeth. See **permanent teeth.**

secondary thrombocytosis. See **thrombocytosis.**

second cranial nerve. See **optic nerve.**

second cuneiform bone. See **intermediate cuneiform bone.**

second filial generation. See F_2.

second intention. See **intention.**

second messenger, a chemical substance inside a cell that carries information along the signal pathway from the internal portion of a membrane-spanning receptor embedded in the cell membrane.

second opinion [L *secundus* + *opinari* to suppose], a patient privilege of requesting an examination and evaluation of a health condition by a second physician to verify or challenge the diagnosis by a first physician.

second-order change, a change that changes the system itself.

second-order kinetics, a chemical reaction in which the rate of the reaction is determined by the concentration of two chemical entities involved.

second sight. See **senopia.**

second stage of labor, the period of childbirth from full dilatation of the cervix to delivery of the fetus.

secrete /sikrēt´/ [L *secernere* to separate], to discharge a substance into a cavity, vessel, or organ or onto the surface of the skin, such as a gland. **–secretion,** *n.*

secretin /sikrē´tin/ [L *secernere*], a digestive hormone that is produced by certain cells lining the duodenum and jejunum when fatty acids of partially digested food enter the intestine from the stomach. It stimulates the pancreas to produce a fluid high in salts but low in enzymes.

secretin test, a test of pancreatic function after stimulation with a hormone, secretin. The test measures the volume and bicarbonate concentration of pancreatic secretions.

secretion /sikrē´shən/ [L *secernere*], **1.** the release of chemical substances manufactured by cells of glandular organs. **2.** a substance released.

secretoinhibitory /sikrē´tō-inhib´itôr´ē/ [L *secernere* + *inhibere* to restrain], pertaining to a function of inhibiting secretion.

secretory /sikrē´tərē/ [L *secernere*], pertaining to or contributing to the function of secretion.

secretory duct [L *secernere*], (of a gland) a small duct that has a secretory function and joins with an excretory duct.

secretory phase, the phase of the menstrual cycle after the release of an ovum from a mature ovarian follicle. The corpus luteum secretes progesterone, which stimulates the development of the glands and arteries of the endometrium, causing it to become thick and spongy. In a negative feedback response to the increased level of progesterone in the blood, the secretion of LH from the pituitary decreases.

secretory piece, a polypeptide chain attached to an IgA molecule. The secretory piece is necessary for secretion of the immunoglobulin molecule into mucosal spaces.

section /sek´shən/ [L *sectio* a cutting], **1.** a cut surface or slice of tissue. **2.** the act of cutting tissue.

sectional arch wire /sek´shənəl/ [L *sectio; arcus* bow; AS *wir*], a wire attached to only a few teeth, usually on one side of a dental arch or in the anterior segment of the arch to cause or guide orthodontic tooth movement.

secundigravida /səkund´dəgrav´idə/ [L *secundus* second, *gravidus* pregnancy], a

S

woman who is pregnant for the second time. **–secundigravid,** *adj.*

secundines /səkun′dīnz/ [L *secundus*], the placenta, umbilical cord, and membranes of afterbirth.

secundipara /sek′əndip′ərə/ [L *secundus + parere* to give birth], a woman who has borne two viable children in separate pregnancies.

sedation /sidā′shən/ [L *sedatio* soothing], an induced state of quiet, calmness, or sleep, as by means of a sedative or hypnotic medication.

sedative /sed′ətiv/ [L *sedatus*], **1.** of or pertaining to a substance, procedure, or measure that has a calming effect. **2.** an agent that decreases functional activity, diminishes irritability, and allays excitement.

sedative bath, the immersion of the body in water for a prolonged period, used especially as a calming procedure for agitated patients.

sedative-hypnotic, a drug that reversibly depresses the activity of the central nervous system, used chiefly to induce sleep and to allay anxiety. Barbiturates and many nonbarbiturate sedative-hypnotics with diverse chemical and pharmacologic properties share the ability to depress the activity of all excitable tissue, but the arousal center in the brainstem is especially sensitive to their effects. Various sedative-hypnotics and minor tranquilizers with similar effects are used in the treatment of insomnia, acute convulsive conditions, and anxiety states, and to facilitate the induction of anesthesia.

sedentary /sed′ənter′ē/ [L *sedentarius* sitting], pertaining to a condition of inaction, such as work or recreation that can be performed in the sitting posture.

sedentary living, a pattern of daily living that requires a minimum amount of physical effort.

sediment /sed′imənt/ [L *sedimentum* settling], a deposit of relatively insoluble material that settles to the bottom of a container of liquid.

sedimentation /sed′iməntā′shən/ [L *sedimentum*], the deposition of insoluble materials to the bottom of a liquid. The process may be accelerated by centrifugation.

sedimentation rate, the speed of settling of red blood cells in a vertical glass column of citrated plasma. It is used to monitor inflammatory or malignant disease and to aid in the detection and diagnosis of occult diseases, such as tuberculosis.

sed. rate, *informal;* erythrocyte sedimentation rate.

segment /seg′mənt/, a component, por-

tion, or part of a structure, as a lobe of the liver or part of the intestine.

segmental bronchus /segmen′təl/ [L *segmentum* piece cut off], a bronchus branching from a lobar bronchus to a bronchiole.

segmental fracture, a bone break in which several large bone fragments separate from the main body of a fractured bone. The ends of such fragments may pierce the skin, as in an open fracture, or may be contained within the skin, as in a closed fracture.

segmental reflex, a reflex that involves a pathway through only a single segment of the spinal cord.

segmental resection, a surgical procedure in which a part of an organ, gland, or other part of the body is excised, such as a segmental resection of a part of an ovary performed to diminish the hormonal secretion of the gland by decreasing the amount of secretory tissue in the gland.

segmentation /seg′məntā′shən/ [L *segmentum + atio* process], **1.** the repetition of structured parts or the process of dividing into segments or similar parts, such as the formation of somites or metameres. **2.** the division of the zygote into blastomeres; cleavage.

segmentation cavity. See **blastocoele.**

segmentation cell. See **blastomere.**

segmentation method, a technique for filling tooth root canals in which a preselected gutta-percha cone is cut into segments and the tip section sealed into the apex of a root. The other sections are usually warmed and condensed against the first piece with a plugger.

segmentation nucleus, the nucleus of the zygote resulting from the fusion of the male and female pronuclei in the fertilized ovum. It is the final stage in fertilization.

segmented hyalinizing vasculitis, a chronic, relapsing inflammatory condition of the blood vessels of the lower legs associated with nodular or purpuric skin lesions that may become ulcerated and leave scars.

segmented neutrophil /segmen′tid/, a neutrophil with a filament between the lobes of its nucleus.

segregation /seg′rəgā′shən/ [L *segregare* to separate], (in genetics) a principle stating that the pairs of chromosomes bearing genes derived from both parents are separated during meiosis. Chance alone determines which gene, maternal or paternal, will travel to which gamete.

seizure /sē′zhər/ [Fr *saisir* to seize], a hyperexcitation of neurons in the brain leading to a sudden, violent, involuntary series of contractions of a group of muscles that may be paroxysmal and episodic, as in a seizure disorder, or transient and acute, as after a head concussion. A seizure may be clonic or tonic, focal, unilateral, or bilateral.

seizure threshold, the amount of stimulus necessary to produce a convulsive seizure. All humans can have seizures if the provocation is sufficient.

selection /silek′shən/ [L *seligere* to choose], **1.** the act or product of choosing. **2.** (in genetics) the process by which various factors or mechanisms determine and modify the reproductive ability of a genotype within a specific population, thus influencing evolutionary change. Kinds of selection are **artificial, natural,** and **sexual selection.**

selective abstraction /silek′tiv/ [L *seligere* to choose], a type of cognitive distortion in which focus on one aspect of an event negates all other aspects.

selective angiography, a graphic procedure that allows selective visualization of the aorta, the major arterial systems, or a particular vessel. It is performed using a percutaneous catheter. A few milliliters of a radiopaque substance are injected when the catheter is in place.

selective grinding, any modification of the occlusal forms of the teeth, produced by corrective grinding at selected places to improve occlusion and tooth function.

selective inattention, the screening out of unwanted stimuli, particularly the part of a message the listener does not want to hear.

selectivity /silektiv′itē/ [L *seligere*], the capacity factor ratios of two substances measured under identical chromatographic conditions.

selectivity coefficient, the degree to which an ion-selective electrode (ISE) responds to a particular ion with respect to a reference ion.

selenium (Se) /silē′nē·əm/ [Gk *selene* moon], a metalloid element of the sulfur group. Its atomic number is 34; its atomic weight is 78.96. Selenium occurs as a trace element in foods, and research continues to determine the most effective daily allowances for different age groups.

selenium sulfide, an antifungal and antiseborrheic prescribed for dandruff and for seborrheic dermatitis of the scalp.

self, *pl.* **selves** /selvz/ [AS], **1.** the total essence or being of a person; the individual. **2.** those affective, cognitive, and spiritual qualities that distinguish one person from another; individuality. **3.** a person's awareness of his or her own being or identity; consciousness; ego.

self-acceptance [AS *self;* L *accipere* to

take], the recognition and acceptance of one's own qualities and limitations.

self-actualization, (in humanistic psychology) the fundamental tendency toward the maximum realization and fulfillment of one's human potential.

self-alien. See **ego-dystonic.**

self-alienation. See **depersonalization.**

self-anesthesia, the self-administered inhalational anesthesia in which whiffs of anesthetic gas are inhaled from a handheld breathing device controlled by the patient.

self-breast examination (SBE), a procedure in which a woman examines her breasts and their accessory structures for evidence of change that could indicate malignant process. The SBE is usually performed 1 week to 10 days after the first day of the menstrual cycle, when the breasts are smallest and cyclic nodularity is least apparent. The techniques are similar to those of the examination of the breast as performed in the health assessment or physical examination.

self-care, **1.** the personal and medical care performed by the patient, usually in collaboration with and after instruction by a medical professional. **2.** the health care by laypeople of their families, friends, and themselves, including identification and evaluation of symptoms, medication, and treatment. **3.** personal care accomplished without technical assistance, such as eating, washing, dressing, using the telephone, attending to one's own elimination, appearance, and hygiene. The goal of rehabilitation medicine is maximal personal self-care.

self-care deficit, bathing/hygiene, a NANDA-accepted nursing diagnosis of an impaired ability to perform or complete bathing and hygiene activities for himself or herself. Defining characteristics include an inability to wash the body or parts of the body, an inability to get or to get to water for bathing, and an inability to regulate water temperature or flow.

self-care deficit, dressing/grooming, a NANDA-accepted nursing diagnosis of an impaired ability to perform or complete dressing and grooming activities for himself or herself. Defining characteristics include an impaired ability to don or to remove necessary items of clothing and an impaired ability to fasten clothing, to obtain or replace articles of clothing, and to maintain a satisfactory appearance.

self-care deficit, feeding, a NANDA-accepted nursing diagnosis of an impaired ability to perform or complete feeding activities for himself or herself. The major defining characteristic is an inability to bring food from a receptacle to the mouth.

S

self-care deficit, toileting, a NANDA-accepted nursing diagnosis of an impaired ability to perform or complete toileting activities for himself or herself. Defining characteristics include an inability to get to the toilet or to the commode, to sit down on or to arise from the toilet or commode, to get the necessary clothing on or off, and to perform the usual toilet hygiene.

self-care theory, a model, used to provide a conceptual framework for nursing care directed toward self-care by the patient to the greatest degree possible. The model requires an assessment of the patient's capability for self-care and need for care.

self-catheterization, a procedure performed by a patient to empty the bladder and prevent it from becoming overdistended with urine. The patient who cannot empty the bladder completely but can retain urine for 2 to 4 hours at a time can be taught self-catheterization if the person is willing to learn and has some manual dexterity and the ability to palpate the bladder.

self-concept, the composite of ideas, feelings, and attitudes that a person has about his or her own identity, worth, capabilities, and limitations.

self-conscious, 1. the state of being aware of oneself as an individual entity that experiences, desires, and acts. **2.** a heightened awareness of oneself and one's actions as reflected by the observations and reactions of others; socially ill at ease. **–self-consciousness,** *n.*

self-confrontation, a technique for behavior modification that depends on a patient's recognition of and dissatisfaction with inconsistencies in his or her own values, beliefs, and behaviors, or between his or her own personal system and that of a significant other.

self-defeating personality disorder a personality characterized by a type of behavior that inhibits the individual from achieving his or her own desires and goals. It is characterized by involvement in situations that continuously lead to failure, rejection, and loss even when other options for involvement are available.

self-destructive behavior, any behavior, direct or indirect, that if uninterrupted, will ultimately lead to the death of the individual.

self-diagnosis, the diagnosis of one's own health problems, usually without direction or assistance from a physician.

self-differentiation, specialization and diversification of a tissue or part resulting solely from intrinsic factors.

self-disclosure, the process by which one person lets his or her inner being,

thoughts, and emotions be known to another. It is important for psychologic growth in individual and group psychotherapy.

self-esteem, the degree of worth and competence one attributes to oneself.

self-esteem, chronic low, a NANDA-accepted nursing diagnosis of a long-standing negative self-evaluation and negative feelings about the self or self-capabilities. Defining characteristics include self-negating verbalization, expression of shame or guilt, evaluation of self as unable to deal with events, rejection of positive feedback, exaggeration of negative feedback, hesitancy to try new situations, frequent lack of success in work or other life events, being overly conforming and dependent on others' opinions, being nonassertive, indecisive, and excessively seeking reassurance.

self-esteem disturbance, a NANDA-accepted nursing diagnosis of a negative self-evaluation and negative feelings about the self or self-capabilities, which may be directly or indirectly expressed. Defining characteristics include self-negating verbalization, expressions of shame or guilt, evaluation of self as unable to deal with events, rationalization or rejection of positive feedback, exaggeration of negative feedback, hesitancy to try new situations, denial of problems obvious to others, projection of blame or responsibility for problems on others, rationalization of personal failures, being hypersensitive to slight or criticism, and showing grandiosity.

self-esteem, situational low, a NANDA-accepted nursing diagnosis of a negative self-evaluation with feelings about the self that develop in response to a loss or change in an individual who previously had a positive self-evaluation. Defining characteristics include an episodic occurrence of negative self-appraisal in response to life events, verbalization of negative feelings about the self, such as helplessness or uselessness, self-negating verbalizations, expression of shame or guilt, evaluation of oneself as unable to handle situations or events, and difficulty in making decisions.

self-fulfilling prophecy, a principle that states that a belief in or the expectation of a particular resolution is a factor that contributes to its fulfillment.

self-help group, a group of people who meet to improve their health through discussion and special activities. Characteristically, self-help groups are not led by a professional.

self-hypnosis [AS *self;* Gk *hypnos* sleep], the process of putting oneself into a trancelike state by autosuggestion such as concentration on a single thought or object. Some subjects are more susceptible than others.

self-ideal, a perception of how one should behave based on personal standards. The standard may be either a carefully constructed image of the kind of person one would like to be or a number of aspirations one would like to achieve.

self-image, the total concept, idea, or mental image one has of oneself and of one's role in society; the person one believes oneself to be.

self-imposed guilt, a restrictive type of guilt of which the individual is aware and from which he or she is unable to break free.

self-insurance, a system whereby hospitals or health professionals may, in lieu of commercial insurance, assume financial responsibility for their liability.

self-limited, (of a disease or condition) tending to end without treatment.

self-limited disease, a disease restricted in duration by its own pattern of characteristics and not by other influences.

self-management approach, a treatment approach in which patients assume responsibility for their behavior, changing their environment, and planning their future.

self-mutilation, high risk for, a NANDA-accepted nursing diagnosis of the state in which an individual is at high risk to perform an act on the self to injure but not kill, and that produces tissue damage and tension relief. Risk factors include being a member of an at-risk group, inability to cope with increased psychologic/physiologic tension in a healthy manner, feelings of rejection, self-hatred, parental emotional deprivation, and a dysfunctional family.

self-other, a concept that characterizes people who believe that sources of power are within the self as opposed to those who believe the source of power is in others.

self-radiolysis, a process in which a compound is damaged by radioactive decay products originating in an atom within the compound.

self-responsibility, a concept of holistic health by which individuals assume responsibility for their own health.

self-retaining catheter, an indwelling urinary catheter that has a double lumen. One channel allows urine to drain from the bladder into a collecting bag; the other channel has a balloon at the bladder end and a diaphragm at the other end. Several centimeters of air or sterile water are injected through the diaphragm to fill the balloon in the bladder and hold the catheter in place.

self-system, the organization of experiences that acts as a protective mechanism against anxiety.

self-theory, a personality theory that uses one's self-concept in integrating the function and organization of the personality.

self-threading pin, a threaded pin screwed into a hole drilled in tooth dentin to improve the retention of a restoration.

self-transcendence, the ability to focus attention on doing something for the sake of others, as opposed to self-actualization in which doing something for oneself is an end goal.

sella turcica /sel′ə tur′sikə/ [L *sella* seat; *turcica* Turkish], a transverse depression crossing the midline on the superior surface of the body of the sphenoid bone and containing the pituitary gland.

SEM. See **scanning electron microscope.**

semantics /siman′tiks/ [Gk *semantikos* significant], the study of language with special concern for the meanings of words or other symbols.

semen /sē′mən/ [L, seed], the thick, whitish secretion of the male reproductive organs discharged from the urethra on ejaculation. It contains various constituents, including spermatozoa in their nutrient plasma and secretions of the prostate, seminal vesicles, and various other glands. **–seminal,** *adj.*

semicircular canal /sem′ēsur′kyələr/ [L *semi* half, *circulare* to go around; *canalis* channel], any of three bony, fluid-filled loops in the osseous labyrinth of the internal ear, associated with the sense of balance.

semicircular duct, one of three ducts that make up the membranous labyrinth of the inner ear.

semicoma. See **coma.**

semicomatose /-kō′mətōs/ [L *semi* + Gk *koma* deep sleep], pertaining to a condition of semicoma, from which a patient can be aroused.

semiconductor /-kənduk′tər/, a solid crystalline substance whose electrical conductivity is intermediate between that of a conductor and an insulator. An **n-type semiconductor** has loosely bound electrons that are relatively free to move about inside the material. A **p-type semiconductor** is one with holes, or positive traps, in which electrons may be bound. The holes may be free to migrate through the material.

semiconscious, an impaired state of consciousness, characterized by obtundation, stupor, or hypersomnia, from which a patient can be aroused only by energetic stimulation.

semi-Fowler's position /-fou′lərz/ [L *semi;* George R. Fowler], placement of the patient in an inclined position, with the upper half of the body raised by elevating the head of the bed.

semilente insulin. See **intermediate-acting insulin.**

semilunar bone. See **lunate bone.**

semilunar valve /-lōō′nər/ [L *semi + luna* moon; *valva* folding door] **1.** a valve with half-moon-shaped cusps, such as the aortic valve and the pulmonary valve. **2.** any one of the cusps constituting such a valve.

semimembranosus /sem′ēmem′brənō′səs/ [L *semi + membrana* membrane], one of three posterior femoral muscles. The tendon of insertion forms one of the two medial hamstrings. The muscle functions to flex the leg, to rotate it medially after flexion, and to extend the thigh.

semimembranous /-mem′brənəs/ [L *semi + membrana*], a muscle or other tissue that is partly membrane or fascia, such as the semimembranous hamstring muscle.

seminal duct /sem′inəl/ [L *semen + ducere* to lead], any duct through which semen passes, such as the vas deferens or the ejaculatory duct.

seminal emission [L *semen + emittere* to send out], a discharge of semen.

seminal fluid. See **semen.**

seminal fluid test, any of several tests of semen to detect abnormalities in a male reproductive system and to determine fertility. Some common factors considered are seminal fluid liquefaction time, spermatic quantity, morphology, motility, volume, and pH.

seminal vesicle, either of the paired, sac-like glandular structures that lie behind the urinary bladder in the male and function as part of the reproductive system. The seminal vesicles produce a fluid that is added to the secretion of the testes and other glands to form the semen.

seminal vesiculitis, inflammation of a seminal vesicle.

seminarcosis. See **twilight sleep.**

semination /sem′inā′shən/, the introduction of semen into the female genital tract.

seminiferous /sem inif′ eres/ [L *semen + ferre* to bear], transporting or producing semen, such as the tubules of the testes.

seminiferous tubules, long threadlike tubes packed in areolar tissue in the lobes of the testes.

seminoma /sem ino me/, *pl.* **seminomas, seminomata** [L *semen + oma* tumor], a malignant tumor of the testis. It is the most common testicular tumor and is believed

to arise from the seminiferous epithelium of the mature or maturing testis.

semipermeable /-pur′mē·əbəl/ [L *semi + permare* to pass through], pertaining to a membrane that allows the passage of some molecules but prevents the passage of others.

semipermeable membrane [L *semi + permeare* to pass through], a membrane barrier to the passage of substances above a specific size, but which allows the movement through the membrane of substances below that size.

semiprone /-prōn′/ [L *semi + pronus* leaning forward], lying on one's side, with the thigh on the upper side flexed against the abdomen, and the arm on the lower side extended back.

semiprone side position. See **Sims' position.**

semirecumbent /-rikum′bənt/, a reclining position.

semisynthetic /-sinthet′ik/ [L *semi + Gk synthesis* putting together], pertaining to a natural substance that has been partially altered by chemical manipulation.

semitendinosus /sem iten dion ses/ [L *semi + tendere* to stretch], one of three posterior femoral muscles of the thigh. It functions to flex the leg and rotate it medially after flexion and to extend the thigh.

semustine /semus ten/, an antineoplastic prescribed in the treatment of Lewis lung carcinoma, brain tumors, malignant melanoma, and Hodgkin's disease.

sender [AS *sendan* to send], (in communication theory) the person by whom a message is encoded and sent.

senescent /sənes′ənt/ [L *senescere* to grow old], aging or growing old. **–senescence** /sənes′əns/, *n.*

Sengstaken-Blakemore tube [Robert W. Sengstaken, American neurosurgeon, b. 1923; Arthur H. Blakemore, American surgeon, b. 1987], a thick catheter having a triple lumen and two balloons, used to produce pressure to arrest hemorrhaging from esophageal varices. Attached to a tube, one balloon is blown up in the stomach and exerts pressure against the upper orifice. Similarly attached, another balloon exerts pressure on the walls of the esophagus. The third tube is used for withdrawing gastric contents.

senile /sē′nīl/ [L *senilis* old man], pertaining to or characteristic of old age or the process of aging, especially the physical or mental deterioration accompanying aging. **–senescent,** *adj.,* **senility,** *n.*

senile angioma. See **cherry angioma.**

senile cataract, a kind of cataract, associated with aging, in which a hard opacity forms in the nucleus of the lens of the eye.

senile delirium, disorientation and mental feebleness associated with extreme age and characterized by restlessness, insomnia, aimless wandering, and, less commonly, hallucination.

senile dementia. See **senile psychosis.**

senile dental caries, tooth decay occurring at an advanced age. Senile dental caries is usually characterized by cavity formation in or around the cementum layer and root surfaces.

senile involution, a pattern of retrograde changes occurring with advancing age and resulting in the progressive shrinking and degeneration of tissues and organs.

senile keratosis. See **actinic keratosis.**

senile memory. See **anterograde memory.**

senile nanism, dwarfism associated with progeria.

senile psychosis, an organic mental disorder of the aged, resulting from the generalized atrophy of the brain with no evidence of cerebrovascular disease. Symptoms include loss of memory, impaired judgment, decreased moral and aesthetic values, inability to think abstractly, periods of confusion, confabulation, and irritability, all of which may range from mild to severe.

senile tremor, a tremor associated with aging.

senile vaginitis, a condition of atrophy of the vagina resulting from the postmenopausal loss of estrogen secretion.

senile wart. See **actinic keratosis.**

senility /sinil′itē/, the general state of reduced mental and physical vigor associated with aging.

senna /sen′ə/ [Ar *sana*], the dried leaflets of pods of *Cassia acutifolia* or *Cassia augustifolia,* used as a cathartic.

senopia /seno pe e/ [L *senex* old man, *posis* vision], an improvement in the near vision of the aged caused by the myopia associated with increasing lenticular nuclear sclerosis.

sensate focus technique /sen′sāt/, a therapeutic program for the treatment of erectile dysfunction in males.

sensation /sensā′shən/ [L *sentire* to feel], **1.** a feeling, impression, or awareness of a bodily state or condition that results from the stimulation of a sensory receptor site and transmission of the nerve impulse along an afferent fiber to the brain. Kinds of sensation include **delayed, epigastric, primary, referred,** and **subjective sensation. 2.** a feeling or an awareness of a mental or emotional state, which may or may not result in response to an external stimulus.

sense [L *sentire*], **1.** the faculty by which stimuli are perceived and conditions outside of and within the body are distinguished and evaluated. The major senses are sight, hearing, smell, taste, touch, and pressure. Other senses include hunger, thirst, pain, temperature, proprioception, spatial, time, and visceral sensations. **2.** the ability to feel; a sensation. **3.** the capacity to understand; normal mental ability. **4.** to perceive through a sense organ.

sensible perspiration /sen′sibəl/ [L *sensibilis* perceptible], loss of fluid from the body through the secretory activity of the sweat glands in a quantity sufficient to be observed.

sensitive /sen′sitiv/ [L *sentire* to feel], **1.** the ability to perceive and transmit a sensation or stimulus. **2.** affected by low concentrations of antimicrobial drugs, said of microorganisms. **3.** abnormally susceptible to a subject, such as a drug or foreign protein.

sensitive volume [L *sentire* + *volumen* paper roll], (in NMR imaging) the region of the object from which an NMR signal will preferentially be acquired because of strong magnetic field inhomogeneity elsewhere.

sensitivity /sen′sitiv′itē/ [L *sentire*], **1.** capacity to feel, transmit, or react to a stimulus. **2.** susceptibility to a substance, such as a drug or an antigen. **–sensitive,** *adj.*

sensitivity test, a laboratory method for testing the effectiveness of antibiotics. It is usually done on organisms known to be potentially resistant to antibiotic therapy in vitro. A report of "resistant" means the antibiotic is not effective in inhibiting the growth of a pathogen, whereas use of an effective antibiotic results in a "sensitive" report.

sensitivity training group, a group that offers members a supportive atmosphere in which to experiment with and alter behavioral patterns and interpersonal reactions.

sensitization /sen′sitizā′shən/ [L *sentire* + Gk *izein* to cause], **1.** an acquired reaction in which specific antibodies develop in response to an antigen. This is deliberately caused in immunization by injecting a disease-causing organism that has been altered in such a way that it is no longer infectious yet remains able to cause the production of antibodies to fight the disease. **2.** a photodynamic method of destroying microorganisms by inserting into a solution substances, such as fluorescing dyes, that absorb visible light and emit energy at wavelengths destructive to the organism. **3.** *nontechnical;* anaphylaxis. **–sensitize,** *v.*

sensitized /sen′sitīzd/, pertaining to tissues that have been made susceptible to antigenic substances.

sensitized vaccine, a vaccine that is prepared by suspending microorganisms in their own homologous immune serum.

sensorimotor /sen′sərēmō′tər/ [L *sentire* to feel + *motor* mover], pertaining to both sensory and motor nerve functions.

sensorimotor phase [L *sentire* + *motor* mover], the developmental phase of childhood, encompassing the period from birth to 2 years of age, according to piagetian psychology.

sensorimotor therapy, therapy that is designed to enhance the integration of reflex phenomena and the emergence of voluntary motor behaviors concerned with posture and locomotion.

sensorineural /sen′sərēnŏŏr′əl/ [L *sentire* + Gk *neuron* nerve], pertaining to sensory nerves.

sensorineural hearing loss [L *sentire* + Gk *neuron* nerve], a form of hearing loss in which sound is conducted normally through the external and middle ear but a defect in the inner ear or auditory nerve results in a hearing loss.

sensorium /sensôr′ē·əm/, (in psychology) the part of the consciousness that includes the special sensory perceptive powers and their central correlation and integration in the brain. A clear sensorium conveys the presence of a reasonably accurate memory together with a correct orientation for time, place, and person.

sensory /sen′sərē/ [L *sentire* to feel], **1.** pertaining to sensation. **2.** pertaining to a part or all of the body's sensory nerve network.

sensory apraxia. See **ideational apraxia.**

sensory area, the regions of the cerebral cortex that receive impulses from sensory nerves, including thalamic, nucleic, and parietal lobes.

sensory-based language, the use of nonverbal behavior in neurolinguistic communication. Examples include puzzled expressions and finger-pointing.

sensory deficit, a defect in the function of one or more of the senses.

sensory deprivation [L *sentire* + ME *depriven* to deprive; L *atio* process], an involuntary loss of physical awareness caused by detachment from external sensory stimuli. Such deprivation often results in psychologic disorders, such as panic, mental confusion, depression, and hallucinations.

sensory end organ [L *sentire; AS ende;* Gk *organon* instrument], any of the specialized nerve endings devoted to detection of specific environmental stimuli, such as smell, sight, hearing, temperature, or touch.

sensory integration, the organization of sensory input for use, a perception of the body or environment, an adaptive response, a learning process, or the development of some neural function.

sensory integrative dysfunction, a disorder or irregularity in brain function that makes sensory integration difficult. Many, but not all, learning disorders stem from sensory integrative dysfunctions.

sensory integrative therapy, therapy that involves sensory stimulation and adaptive responses to it according to a child's neurologic needs. Treatment usually involves full body movements that provide vestibular, proprioceptive, and tactile stimulation. The goal is to improve the brain's ability to process and organize sensations.

sensory nerve, a nerve consisting of afferent fibers that conduct sensory impulses from the periphery of the body to the brain or spinal cord via the dorsal spinal roots.

sensory nucleus of trigeminal nerve, a collection of nerve cells in the pons that serve as the main nucleus for reception of tactile fibers of the trigeminal area.

sensory overload, a condition in which the central nervous system receives much more sound, visual, or other environmental stimuli per time frame than can be processed effectively.

sensory pathway, the route followed by a sensory nerve impulse from an end organ to a reflex center in the brain or spinal cord.

sensory/perceptual alterations (visual, auditory, kinesthetic, gustatory, tactile, olfactory) /pərsep′chŏŏ·əl/, a NANDA-accepted nursing diagnosis of a change in the amount or patterning of incoming stimuli accompanied by a diminished, exaggerated, distorted, or impaired response to such stimuli. Defining characteristics include disorientation, change in the ability to abstract, conceptualize, or solve problems, change in behavior and in sensory acuity, restlessness, irritability, inappropriate response to stimuli, lack of concentration, rapid mood changes, and exaggerated emotional responses, noncompliance, motor incoordination, hallucination, complaints of fatigue, changes in posture and muscular tension, and inappropriate responses.

sensory-perceptual overload, a state in which the volume and intensity of various stimuli overcome the ability of the individual to discriminate among the varying stimuli.

sensory receptor, a specialized nerve ending that, when stimulated, initiates an afferent or sensory nerve impulse.

sensory root, the proximal end of a dorsal afferent nerve as it is attached to the spinal cord.

sensory threshold, the point at which increasing stimuli trigger the start of an afferent nerve impulse. Absolute threshold is the lowest point at which response to a stimulus can be perceived.

sensual /sen′sho͞o·əl/ [L *sensualis*], pertaining to a great interest in sex, food, or other sensory satisfying activities.

sentient /sen′shənt/ [L *sentire* to feel], possessing sensitivity or powers of sensation and perception.

sentinel gland /sen′tinəl/ [Fr *sentinelle*; L *glans* acorn], a node or growth that is associated with the presence of a nearby tumor or ulcer. An example is a supraclavicular node with cancer cells that have metastasized from an undiscovered primary cancer.

sentinel node. See **Virchow's node.**

SEP, abbreviation for **somatosensory evoked potential.**

s-EPO, abbreviation for *serum erythropoietin.*

separation anxiety /sep′ərā′shən/ [L *separare* to separate, *atio* process], fear and apprehension caused by separation from familiar surroundings and significant people. The syndrome occurs commonly in an infant when separated from its mother or from its mothering figure or when it is approached by a stranger.

separation factor. See **selectivity.**

separator /sep′ərā′tər/ [L *separare* to separate], an instrument for wedging teeth apart, used in the examination of proximal tooth surfaces and in finishing proximal restorations.

sepsis /sep sis/ [Gk *sepein* to become putrid], infection, contamination. **–septic,** *adj.*

septal cartilage. See **nasal cartilage.**

septal defect /sep′təl/ [L *saeptum* enclosure; *defectus* failure], an abnormal, usually congenital defect in the wall separating two chambers of the heart. Oxygenated and deoxygenated blood mix, causing a decrease in the amount of oxygen carried in the blood to the peripheral tissues. Kinds of septal defects are **atrial septal defect** and **ventricular septal defect.**

septate /sep′tāt/, pertaining to a structure divided by a septum.

septic /sep′tik/ [Gk, *septikos*, putrid], pertaining to an infection with pyogenic microorganisms.

septic abortion [Gk *sepein* to become putrid], spontaneous or induced termination of a pregnancy in which the life of the mother may be threatened because of the invasion of germs into the endometrium, myometrium, and beyond, requiring immediate and intensive care, massive antibiotic therapy, evacuation of the uterus, and, often, emergency hysterectomy to prevent death from overwhelming infection and septic shock.

septic arthritis, an acute form of arthritis, characterized by bacterial inflammation of a joint caused by the spread of bacteria through the bloodstream from an infection elsewhere in the body or by contamination of a joint during trauma or surgery. The joint is stiff, painful, tender, warm, and swollen.

septicemia [Gk *sepein* + *haima* blood], systemic infection in which pathogens are present in the circulating bloodstream, having spread from an infection in any part of the body. Characteristically, septicemia causes fever, chill, prostration, pain, headache, nausea, or diarrhea. **–septicemic,** *adj.*

septicemic plague /sep′tisē′mik/, a rapidly fatal form of bubonic plague in which septicemia with meningitis occurs before buboes have had time to form.

septic fever, an elevation of body temperature associated with infection by pathogenic microorganisms or in response to a toxin secreted by a microorganism.

septic infarct [Gk *septikos* putrid; L *infarcire* to stuff], an infected segment of dead tissue.

septic shock, a form of shock that occurs in septicemia when endotoxins are released from certain bacteria in the bloodstream. The endotoxins cause decreased vascular resistance, resulting in a drastic fall in the blood pressure. Fever, tachycardia, increased respirations, and confusion or coma may also occur. Septic shock is usually preceded by signs of severe infection, often of the genitourinary or GI system. Kinds of septic shock include **toxic shock syndrome** and **bacteremic shock.**

septic sore throat, a severe throat infection, usually caused by a streptococcus strain, resulting in fever and marked exhaustion.

septostomy /septos′təme/, the creation of an opening in a septum by surgery.

septum /sep tem/, *septa* [L *saeptum* enclosure], a partition, such as the interauricular septum that separates the atria of the heart. **–septal,** *adj.*

septuplet /septup′lit/, any one of seven children born of a single pregnancy.

sequela /sikwē′lə/, *pl.* **sequelae** [L *sequi* to follow], any abnormal condition that follows and is the result of a disease, treatment, or injury, such as paralysis after poliomyelitis.

sequence /sē′kwəns/ [L *sequi* to follow], an order of arrangement of objects or events, such as the sequence of peptides in a protein molecule.

sequential imaging /sikwen′shəl/, (in nuclear medicine) a diagnostic procedure in which a series of closely timed images of the rapidly changing distribution of an administered radioactive tracer is used to determine a physiologic process or precesses within the body.

sequential line imaging, (in NMR imaging) techniques in which the image is built up from successive lines through the object.

sequential multiple analysis (SMA), the biochemical examination of various substances in the blood, such as albumin, alkaline phosphatase, bilirubin, calcium, cholesterol, and others, using a computerized laboratory analyzer that produces a printout showing measured values of the substances tested.

sequential pacing. See **pacing.**

sequential plane imaging, (in MRI) a technique in which the image of an object is built up from successive planes in the object.

sequential point imaging, (in MRI) techniques in which the image is built from successive point positions in the object.

sequester /sikwes′tər/ [L *sequestri* to deposit], to detach, separate, or isolate, such as a patient sequestered to prevent the spread of an infection.

sequestered antigens theory, a theory of autoimmunity, stressing the relationship between antigen exposure, immunogenic cells, and body cells and maintaining that immunologic tolerance depends on a certain degree of contact between immunologic cells and body cells and on a certain degree of antigen exposure.

sequestered edema, edema localized in the tissues surrounding a newly created surgical wound.

sequestration /sēkwestrā′shən/ [L *sequestare* to lay aside], **1.** the isolation of a patient or group of patients. **2.** a method of controlling hemorrhage of the head or trunk by isolating fluid in the arms and legs from the general circulation. **3.** allowing blood from the systemic circulation to perfuse a nonfunctioning part of a lung.

sequestrum /sikwes′trəm/, *pl.* **sequestra** [L, a deposit], a fragment of dead bone that is partially or entirely detached from the surrounding or adjacent healthy bone.

sequestrum forceps, a forceps with small, powerful teeth used for extracting necrotic or sharp fragments of bone from surrounding tissue.

sequoiasis /sikwoi′əsis/ [sequoia (tree) + Gk *osis* condition], a type of hypersensitivity pneumonitis common among workers in sawmills where redwood is processed. The antigens are the fungus *Pullalaria pullulans* and species of the genus *Graphium,* found in moldy redwood sawdust. Characteristics of the acute disease include chills, fever, cough, dyspnea, anorexia, nausea, and vomiting. Symptoms of the chronic disease include productive cough, dyspnea on exertion, fatigue, and weight loss.

Ser, abbreviation for the amino acid **serine.**

serendipity /ser′əndip′itē/ [Serendip, author Horace Walpole's mythic land of pleasant surprises], the act of accidental discovery. A number of important medications have evolved through serendipity, such as the discovery of antidepressant activity in a drug originally developed to treat tuberculosis.

serial /sir′ē-əl/ [L *series* row], pertaining to a succession, arrangement, or order of items.

serial determination [L *series* in a row; *determinare* to limit], a laboratory test that is repeated at stated intervals, as in a series of repeated tests for cardiac enzymes in blood samples taken from a suspected myocardial infarction patient.

serial dilution, a laboratory technique in which a substance, such as blood serum, is decreased in concentration in a series of proportional amounts.

serial extraction, the extraction of selected primary teeth over a period of years, frequently ending with the removal of the first premolar teeth, to relieve crowding of the dental arches during eruption of the lateral incisors, canines, and premolars.

serial section, one of a number of consecutive slices of tissue.

serial speech, overlearned speech involving a series of words, such as counting or reciting days of the week.

series /sir′ēs/, *pl.* **series** / sir′ēs/ [L, in a row], a chain of objects or events arranged in a predictable order, such as the series of stages through which a mature blood cell develops.

serine (Ser) /ser′ēn/, a nonessential amino acid found in many proteins in the body. It is a precursor of the amino acids, glycine, and cysteine.

seroconversion /sir′ōkənvur′zhən/ [L *serum* whey, *conversio* turned about], a change in serologic tests from negative to positive as antibodies develop in reaction to an infection or vaccine.

serodiagnosis /-dī'əgnō'sis/ [L *serum* + Gk *dia* through + *gnosis* knowledge], the use of serologic tests in the diagnosis of disease.

serofibrinous pericarditis /-fī'brinəs/, a form of fibrinous pericarditis marked by a serous exudate.

serologic diagnosis /-loj'ik/ /siroloj'ik/ [L *serum* whey; Gk *dia* through, *gnosis* knowledge], a diagnosis that is made through laboratory examination of antigen-antibody reactions in the serum.

serologic test, any diagnostic test made with serum.

serologist /sirol'əjist/ [L *serum* + Gk *logos* science], a bacteriologist or medical technologist who prepares or supervises the preparation of serums used to diagnose and treat diseases and to immunize people against infectious diseases.

serology /sirol'əjē/ [L *serum* + Gk *logos* science], the branch of laboratory medicine that studies blood serum for evidence of infection by evaluating antigen-antibody reactions in vitro. **–serologic, serological,** *adj.*

seronegative /-neg'ətiv/, a serologic test with negative results.

seropositive /-pos'itiv/, a serologic test with positive results.

seroprevalence /-prev'ələns/, the overall occurrence of a blood-borne disease within a defined population at one point in time. An example is HIV seroprevalence.

serosa /sirō'sə/ [L *serum*], any serous membrane, such as the tunica serosa that lines the walls of body cavities and secretes a watery exudate.

serosanguineous /sir'ōsang·gwin'ē·əs/, (of a discharge) thin and red; composed of serum and blood. Also **serosanguinous** /sir'ōsang'gwinəs/.

serotonin /ser'ətō'nin, sir'-/ [L *serum* + Gk *tonos* tone], a naturally occurring derivative of tryptophan (5-hydroxytryptamine) found in platelets and in cells of the brain and the intestine. It acts as a potent vasoconstrictor and as a neurotransmitter.

serous [L *serum* whey], pertaining to, resembling, or producing serum.

serous fluid /sir'əs/ [L *serum* + *fluere* to flow], a fluid that has the characteristics of serum.

serous membrane, one of the many thin sheets of tissue that line closed cavities of the body, such as the pleura lining the thoracic cavity, the peritoneum lining the abdominal cavity, and the pericardium lining the sac that encloses the heart. Between the visceral layer of serous membrane covering various organs and the parietal layer lining the cavity containing such organs is a potential space moistened by serous fluid. The fluid reduces the friction of the structures covered by the serous membrane, such as the lungs, which move against the thoracic walls in respiration.

serpent ulcer /sur'pənt/ [L *serpens* snake], an ulceration of the skin that heals in one area while extending to another.

Serratia /serā'shə/ [L *serra* saw teeth], a genus of motile, gram-negative bacilli capable of causing infection in humans, including bacteremia, pneumonia, and urinary tract infections. *Serratia* organisms are frequently acquired in hospitals.

serratus anterior /serā'təs/ [L *serra* saw teeth], a thin muscle of the chest wall extending from the ribs under the arm to the scapula. It acts to rotate the scapula and to raise the shoulder, as in full flexion and abduction of the arm.

Sertoli cell /sertō'lē/ [Enrico Sertoli, Italian physiologist, b. 1842], one of the supporting cells of the seminiferous tubules of the testes. The cytoplasm of the cells contain spermatids.

Sertoli-Leydig cell tumor. See **arrhenoblastoma.**

serum /sir'əm/ [L, whey], **1.** any serous fluid that moistens the surfaces of serous membranes. **2.** any clear, watery fluid that has been separated from its more solid elements, such as the exudate from a blister. **3.** the clear, thin, and sticky fluid portion of the blood that remains after coagulation. **4.** a vaccine or toxoid prepared from the serum of a hyperimmune donor for prophylaxis against a particular infection or poison.

serum albumin, a major protein in blood plasma, important in maintaining the oncotic pressure of the blood.

serum bank, a facility for the storage of frozen samples of blood serum. The specimens are used mainly for medical research.

serum C-reactive protein. See **C-reactive protein.**

serum creatinine level, the concentration of creatinine in the serum, used as a diagnostic sign of possible renal impairment.

serum diagnosis. See **serologic diagnosis.**

serum globulin, a protein fraction of blood serum with antibody qualities. The several types of fractions, α, β, and γ, have different specific properties.

serum glutamic oxaloacetic transaminase (SGOT), a catalytic enzyme found in various parts of the body, especially the heart, liver, and muscle tissue. Increased amounts of the enzyme occur in the serum as a result of myocardial infarction, acute liver disease, the actions of certain drugs,

S

and any disease or condition in which cells are seriously damaged.

serum glutamic pyruvic transaminase (SGPT), a catalytic enzyme normally found in high concentration in the liver. Greater than normal amounts in the serum indicate liver damage.

serum hepatitis. See **hepatitis B.**

serum osmolality [L *serum;* Gk *osmos* impulse], pertaining to the osmotic concentration of blood serum, expressed in terms of ions of solute per unit of solution.

serum protein, any of the proteins in blood serum.

serum sickness, an immunologic disorder that may occur 2 to 3 weeks after the administration of an antiserum. It is caused by an antibody reaction to an antigen in the donor serum and is characterized by fever, splenomegaly, swollen lymph nodes, skin rash, and joint pain.

service of process /sur'vis/ [L *servus* a slave; *processus* going forth], (in law) the delivery of a writ, summons, or complaint to a defendant. Once delivered or left with the party for whom it is intended, it is said to have been served.

sesamoid /ses'amoid/ [Gk *sesamon* sesame, *eidos* form], nodular objects having the shape and size of sesame seeds.

sesamoid bone [Gk *sesamon* sesame, *eidos* form], any one of numerous small, round, bony masses embedded in certain tendons that may be subjected to compression and tension. The largest sesamoid bone is the patella, which is embedded in the tendon of the quadriceps femoris at the knee.

sessile /ses'əl/ [L *sessilis* sitting], 1. (in biology) attached by a base rather than by a stalk or a peduncle, such as a leaf that is attached directly to its stem. 2. permanently connected.

set, a predisposition to behave in a certain way.

settlement [AS *setlan* to put in place], (in law) an agreement made between parties to a suit before a judgment is rendered by a court.

setup [AS *settan* to set, *up* on high], 1. an arrangement of teeth on a trial denture base. 2. a laboratory procedure in which teeth are removed from a plaster cast and repositioned in wax, used as a diagnostic procedure, or to produce a mold for a positioner appliance.

seventh cranial nerve. See **facial nerve.**

severe combined immunodeficiency disease (SCID) /sivir'/ [L *servus* slave], an abnormal condition characterized by the complete absence or by the marked deficiency of B cells and T cells with the consequent lack of humoral immunity and cell-mediated immunity. This disease occurs as an X-linked recessive disorder only in males and as an autosomal recessive disorder affecting both males and females. It results in a pronounced susceptibility to infection and is usually fatal. The precise cause of SCID is not known, but research indicates it may be caused by a cytogenic dysfunction of the embryonic stem cells in differentiating B cells and T cells. The affected individual consequently has a very small thymus and little or no protection against infection.

Sever's disease. See **calcaneal epiphysitis.**

sex [L *sexus* male or female], 1. a classification of male or female based on many criteria, among them anatomic and chromosomal characteristics. 2. coitus.

sex chromatin, a densely staining mass within the nucleus of all nondividing cells of normal mammalian females. It represents the facultative heterochromatin of the inactivated X chromosome.

sex chromosome, a chromosome that is responsible for the sex determination of offspring; it carries genes that transmit sex-linked traits and conditions. In humans and other mammals there are two distinct sex chromosomes, the X and the Y chromosomes.

sex chromosome mosaic, an individual or organism whose cells contain variant chromosomal numbers involving the X or Y chromosomes. Such variations are found in most of the syndromes associated with sex chromosome aberrations, primarily Turner's syndrome, and may be caused by nondisjunction of the chromosomes during the second meiotic division of gametogenesis or by some error in chromosome distribution during cell division of the fertilized ovum.

sex-controlled. See **sex-influenced.**

sex determination, an examination of the cellular differences between male and female organisms, to find the XY chromosome combination in genetic male or the Barr body in genetic female chromosomes. Whole body differences include secondary sexual characteristics and skeletal variations.

sex factor. See **F factor.**

sex-influenced, of or pertaining to an autosomal genetic trait or condition, such as patterned baldness or gout, that in one sex is expressed phenotypically in both homozygotes and heterozygotes, whereas in the other sex a phenotypic effect is produced in homozygotes only.

sexism /sek'sizəm/, a belief that one sex is superior to the other and that the superior sex has endowments, rights, prerogatives, and status greater than those of the inferior sex. **−sexist,** *n.*

sex-limited, of or pertaining to an autosomal genetic trait or condition that is expressed phenotypically in only one sex, although the genes for them may be carried by both sexes.

sex-linked, pertaining to genes or to the normal or abnormal characteristics or conditions they transmit. The genes are carried on the sex chromosomes, particularly the X chromosome. **−sex-linkage,** *n.*

sex-linked disorder, any disease or abnormal condition that is determined by the sex chromosomes or a defective gene on a sex chromosome. These may involve a deviation in the number of either the X or Y chromosomes, as occurs in Turner's syndrome and Klinefelter's syndrome. Most occurrences are a result of nondisjunction during meiosis.

sex-linked ichthyosis, a congenital skin disorder characterized by large, thick, dry scales that are dark in color and that cover the neck, scalp, ears, face, trunk, and flexor surfaces of the body, such as the folds of the arms and the backs of the knees. It is transmitted by females as an X-linked recessive trait and appears only in males.

sex mosaic. See **sex chromosome mosaic.**

sex role, the expectations held by society regarding what behavior is appropriate or inappropriate for each sex.

sex surrogate [L *sexus, surrogare* substitute], (in sex therapy) a professional substitute trained to help the patient overcome inhibitions.

sextuplet /seks′tup′lit/ [L *sextus* six], one of six children born of a single pregnancy.

sexual /sek′shŏŏ·əl/, of or pertaining to sex.

sexual abuse, the sexual mistreatment of another person by fondling, rape, or forced participation in unnatural sex acts or other perverted behavior.

sexual assault, the forcible perpetration of an act of sexual contact on the body of another person, male or female, without his or her consent. Legal criteria vary among different communities.

sexual aversion disorder, a persistent or extreme aversion to or avoidance of all or nearly all genital sexual contact with a partner.

sexual dwarf, an adult dwarf whose genital organs are normally developed.

sexual dysfunction, a NANDA-accepted nursing diagnosis of a state in which an individual experiences a change in sexual function that is viewed as unsatisfying, unrewarding, or inadequate. Defining characteristics include a statement by the cli-

ent of the perceived dysfunction, a physical alteration or limitation imposed by disease or treatment, a reported inability to achieve sexual satisfaction, an alteration in the sexual relationship with the partner, and a change in interest in the self or in others.

sexual fantasy, mental images of an erotic nature that can lead to sexual arousal.

sexual generation, reproduction by the union of male and female gametes.

sexual harassment, an aggressive, sexually motivated act of physical or verbal violation of a person over whom the aggressor has some power. Sexual harassment may be heterosexual or, as is common in prison, homosexual.

sexual health, a condition, defined by the World Health Organization as freedom from sexual diseases or disorders and a capacity to enjoy and control sexual behavior without fear, shame, or guilt.

sexual history, (in a patient record) the portion of the patient's personal history concerned with sexual function and dysfunction. It may include age at onset of sexual intercourse, the kind and frequency of sexual activity, and the satisfaction derived from it.

sexual hormones, chemical substances produced in the body that cause specific regulatory effects on the activity of organs of the reproductive system.

sexual intercourse. See **coitus.**

sexuality /sek′shŏŏ·al′itē/, **1.** the sum of the physical, functional, and psychologic attributes that are expressed by one's gender identity and sexual behavior, whether or not related to the sex organs or to procreation. **2.** the genital characteristics that distinguish male from female.

sexuality patterns, altered, a NANDA-accepted nursing diagnosis of an individual's concern regarding his or her sexuality. Defining characteristics include reported difficulties, limitations, or changes in sexual behaviors or activities. Related factors include a knowledge or skill deficit about alternative responses to health-related transitions or altered body functions or structure (illness or medical).

sexually deviant personality /sek′shŏŏ·-əlē/, a sexual behavior that differs significantly from what is considered normal for a society.

sexually transmitted disease (STD), a contagious disease usually acquired by sexual intercourse or genital contact. Historically, the five venereal diseases were gonorrhea, syphilis, chancroid, granuloma inguinale, and lymphogranuloma venereum. To these have been added scabies,

S

herpes genitalis and anorectal herpes and warts, pediculosis, trichomoniasis, genital candidiasis, molluscum contagiosum, nonspecific urethritis, chlamydial infections, cytomegalovirus, and AIDS.

sexual mores, socially acceptable sexual behavior, usually based on fixed, morally binding customs governing sexual behaviors that are harmful to others or the group, such as rape, incest, and sexual abuse of children.

sexual orientation, the clear, persistent desire of a person for affiliation with one sex rather than the other.

sexual psychopath, an individual whose sexual behavior is openly perverted, antisocial, and criminal.

sexual reassignment, a change in the gender identity of a person by legal, surgical, hormonal, or social means.

sexual reflex, (in males) a reflex in which tactile or cerebral stimulation results in penile erection, priapism, or ejaculation.

sexual reproduction [L sexus male or female, re, producere to produce], replication of an organism by the formation of gametes. Generally, this requires the fusion of male spermatozoa and female ova, but parthenogenesis is an exception.

sexual response cycle, the four phases of biologic sexual response: excitement, plateau, orgasm, and resolution.

sexual sadism. See **sadism.**

sexual selection, the theory that mates are chosen according to the attraction of or preference for certain characteristics, such as coloration or behavior patterns, so that eventually only those particular traits appear in succeeding generations.

sexual tasks, specific skills learned in various phases of development in the life cycle continuum to allow an adult to function normally in the sexual realm.

sexual therapist, a health care professional with specialized knowledge, skill, and competence in assisting individuals who experience sexual difficulties.

sexual therapy, a type of counseling that aids in the resolution of pathologic conditions so that a healthy sexuality can be maintained.

sfc, abbreviation for *spinal fluid count.*

SFD, abbreviation for *small for dates.*

SGA, abbreviation for **small for gestational age.**

SGOT, abbreviation for **serum glutamic oxaloacetic transaminase.**

SGPT, abbreviation for **serum glutamic pyruvic transaminase.**

shadow /shad'ō/ [AS sceadu], (in psychology) an archetype that represents the unacceptable aspects and components of behavior.

shaken baby syndrome, a condition of whiplash-type injuries, ranging from bruises on the arms and trunk to retinal hemorrhages, coma, or convulsions, as observed in infants and children who have been violently shaken. Physicians are required by law to report suspected cases of child abuse.

shake test, a "foam" test for fetal lung maturity. It is more rapid than determination of the L/S ratio.

shaking palsy. See **parkinsonism.**

shallow breathing /shal'ō/ [ME schalowe little depth], a respiration pattern marked by slow, shallow, and generally ineffective inspirations and expirations. It is usually caused by drugs and indicates depression of the medullary respiratory centers.

shaping [AS scieppan to shape], a procedure used for conditioning a person undergoing behavior therapy to develop new behavioral responses.

shared governance, an organized, systematic approach to decision making that enables all levels of nurses to participate in the resolution of clinical, professional, and administrative practice issues.

shared paranoid disorder [AS scearan to shear], a psychopathologic condition characterized by identical manifestations of the same mental disorder, usually ideas, in two closely associated or related people.

shared services, administrative, clinical, or other service functions that are common to two or more hospitals or other health care facilities and which are used jointly or cooperatively by them.

Sharpey's fiber [William Sharpey, English anatomist, b. 1802], (in dentistry) any one of the many collagenous bundles of fibers of the periodontal ligament that have become embedded in the cementum during its formation.

sharps, any needles, scapels, or other articles that could cause wounds or punctures to personnel handling them.

shaving stroke [AS scafan to shave; strican to stroke], a phase of the working stroke of a periodontal curet, used for smoothing or planing a tooth or tooth root surface.

SHCC, abbreviation for **Statewide Health Coordinating Committee.**

shear /shir/ [AS scearan to cut], an applied force or pressure exerted against the surface and layers of the skin as tissues slide in opposite but parallel planes.

shearling /shir'ling/, a sheepskin placed on a bed to help prevent decubitus ulcers.

sheath [AS scaeth], a tubular structure that surrounds an organ or any other part of the body, such as the sheath of the rectus abdominis muscle.

sheath of Schwann [AS, *scaeth;* Friedrich Theodor Schwann, German anatomist, b. 1810], a neurilemma sheath of nucleated cells enclosing a nerve fiber.

Sheehan's syndrome [Harold L. Sheehan, English pathologist, b. 1900], a postpartum condition of pituitary necrosis and hypopituitarism after circulatory collapse resulting from uterine hemorrhaging.

sheep cell agglutination test (SCAT), a test for the presence of the rheumatoid factor in blood serum, using red blood cells of sheep that have been sensitized with rabbit antisheep erythrocyte immune globulin. The globulin will be agglutinated if the serum contains the rheumatoid factor.

sheep cell test [AS *sceap;* L *cella* storeroom; *testum* crucible], a method that mixes human blood cells with the red blood cells of sheep to determine the absence or the deficiency of human T-lymphocytes. When mixed with human blood cells, the red blood cells of sheep cluster around the human T-lymphocytes and form characteristic rosettes.

sheet bath [AS *scete, baeth*], the application of wet sheets to the body, used primarily as an antipyretic procedure.

sheet wadding, stretchable sheets of cotton padding used to cover the skin before a cast is applied. The stretching allows for some extremity edema without the cast becoming too tight.

shellfish poisoning [AS *scell, fisc*], a toxic, neurologic condition that results from eating clams, oysters, or mussels that have ingested the poisonous protozoa commonly called the "red tide." The characteristic symptoms appear within a few minutes and include nausea, lightheadedness, vomiting, and tingling or numbness around the mouth, followed by paralysis of the extremities and, possibly, respiratory paralysis. Saxitoxin, the causative agent, is not destroyed by cooking.

shell shock [AS *scell;* Fr *choc*], any of a number of mental disorders, ranging from extreme fear to dementia, resulting from a traumatic reaction to the stress of combat.

shell teeth, a type of dental dysplasia characterized by large pulp chambers, insufficient coronal dentin, and, usually, no roots.

sheltered workshop [ME *sheltrun* body of guards; AS *werc, sceoppa* stall], a facility or program, either for outpatients or for residents of an institution, that provides vocational experience in a controlled working environment.

shield [AS *scild*], (in radiation technology) a material for preventing or reducing the passage of charged particles or radiation. A shield may be designated by the ra-

diation it is intended to absorb, such as a gamma ray shield, or according to the kind of protection it is intended to give, such as a background, biological, or thermal shield.

shift [AS *sciftan* to divide], **1.** (in nursing) the particular hours of the day during which a nurse is scheduled to work. The evening shift is also called "relief," presumably because nurses originally worked 12-hour shifts and the evening and night shift was thought to be relief for the day nurse. **2.** an abrupt change in an analytic system that continues at the new level.

shift to the left, *informal;* a predominance of immature lymphocytes, noted in a differential white blood cell count. The term derives from a graph of blood components in which immature cell frequencies appear on the left side of the graph.

shift to the right, (in hematology) a preponderance of polymorphonuclear neutrophils having three or more lobes, indicating maturity of the cell. It indicates a relative lack of blood-forming activity.

Shigella /shigel′ə/ [Kiyoshi Shiga, Japanese bacteriologist, b. 1870], a genus of gram-negative pathogenic bacteria that causes gastroenteritis and bacterial dysentery, such as *Shigella dysenteriae.*

Shigella dysenteriae, a species of the bacterial family *Enterobacteriaceae* that causes a severe form of dysentery in humans. The *dysenteriae* subgroup of *Shigella* is most common in Asia and is particularly virulent.

shigellosis /shig′əlō′sis/ [Kiyoshi Shiga + Gk *osis* condition], an acute bacterial infection of the bowel, characterized by diarrhea, abdominal pain, and fever, that is transmitted by hand-to-mouth contact with the feces of individuals infected with bacteria of a pathogenic species of the genus *Shigella.* These organisms may be carried in the stools of asymptomatic people for up to several months and may be spread through contact with contaminated objects, food, or flies, especially in poor, crowded areas.

shin bone. See tibia.

shingles. See herpes zoster.

shin splints [AS *scinu* shin; ME *splinte*], a painful condition of the lower leg caused by strain of the long flexor muscle of the toes after strenuous athletic activity, such as running.

Shirodkar's operation /shir′odkärz′/, a surgical procedure called a cerclage in which the cervical canal is closed by a purse-string suture embedded in the uterine cervix encircling the canal. It is performed to correct an incompetent cervix that has failed to retain previous pregnancies. If labor begins with the suture in place, the suture is removed promptly or the infant is delivered by cesarean section, before rupture of the uterus occurs.

shock [Fr *choc*], an abnormal condition of inadequate blood flow to the body's peripheral tissues, with life-threatening cellular dysfunction, hypotension, and oliguria. The condition is usually associated with inadequate cardiac output, changes in peripheral blood flow resistance and distribution, and tissue damage. Causal factors include hemorrhage, vomiting, diarrhea, inadequate fluid intake, or excessive renal loss, resulting in hypovolemia. The signs and symptoms of different kinds of shock are similar and are related to the condition of hypovolemia. There is decreased blood flow with a resulting reduction in the delivery of oxygen, nutrients, hormones, and electrolytes to the body's tissues and a concomitant decreased removal of metabolic wastes. Pulse and respirations are increased. There may be tachycardia. Blood pressure may decline moderately at first. The patient often shows signs of restlessness and anxiety, an effect related to decreased blood flow to the brain. There may also be weakness, lethargy, pallor, and cool, moist skin. As shock progresses, the body temperature falls, respirations become rapid and shallow, and the pulse pressure (the difference between systolic and diastolic blood pressures) narrows. Urinary output is reduced. Hemorrhage may be apparent or concealed although other factors, such as vomiting or diarrhea, may account for the deficiency of body fluids. Kinds of shock include **anaphylactic, bacteremic, cardiogenic, diabetic, electric, hypovolemic,** and **neurogenic shock.**

shock lung. See **acute respiratory distress syndrome.**

shock therapy, a psychotherapeutic procedure for treating depression and other severe disorders by producing an epileptiform convulsion in the patient. The shock is induced by delivering an electric current through the brain.

shock treatment, See **shock therapy.**

shock trousers, pneumatic trousers designed to counteract hypotension, associated with internal or external bleeding, and hypovolemia. Shock trousers may be contraindicated in patients with pulmonary edema, cardiogenic shock, increased intracranial pressure, or eviscerations. The shock trousers are required when the patient loses consciousness, has a decreased or falling blood pressure, and shows signs of respiratory distress, such as dyspnea, rapid breathing, a cough, and pink, frothy

sputum. The leg pulses may be diminished or absent, and the feet may appear pale, mottled, and cold.

short-acting [AS *sceort;* L *agere* to do], pertaining to or characterizing a therapeutic agent, usually a drug, with a brief period of effectiveness, generally beginning soon after the substance or measure is administered.

short-acting insulin, an aqueous preparation of the antidiabetic principle of beef pancreas or pork pancreas that begins to act within 1 hour of injection and reaches a peak of action in 2 to 4 hours.

shortage area /shôr'tij/ [AS *sceort;* L *acticum* process], a geographic area, county as a census tract, or area designated by the federal government as being undersupplied with certain kinds of health care services, hence possibly eligible for aid under certain federal programs, including the National Health Service Corps or the Rural Clinics Assistance Act.

short-arm cast, an orthopedic cast applied to immobilize the hand or the wrist. It is used in treating fractures, for postoperative positioning, and for correction or maintenance of correction of deformities of the hand and the wrist.

short bones, bones that occur in clusters and usually permit movement of the extremities, such as the carpals and tarsals.

short-bowel syndrome, a loss of intestinal surface for absorption of nutrients caused by the surgical removal of a section of bowel.

short course tuberculosis chemotherapy, a 6-month treatment regimen for patients with tuberculosis who would otherwise continue medications for at least 18 to 24 months after sputum has become negative for tubercle bacilli. The short course requires a combination of four drugs, isoniazid (INH), rifampin (RMP), pyrazinamide (PZA), and either ethambutol (EMB), or streptomycin.

short-gut syndrome, a congenital disorder in which an infant's intestine is too short or underdeveloped to allow normal food digestion. The child is maintained on parenteral nutrition until the intestine grows or develops further or is replaced by surgical transplant.

shorting [AS *sceort*], the fraudulent practice of dispensing a quantity of drug less than that called for in the prescription and of charging for the quantity specified in the prescription.

short-leg cast, an orthopedic cast used for immobilizing fractures in the lower extremities from the toes to the knee.

short-leg cast with walker, an orthopedic cast with rubber walkers on the bottom. It immobilizes the leg from the toes to the knee and allows the patient to walk.

Short Portable Mental Status Questionnaire, a 10-item questionnaire used to screen older adults for cognitive impairment. It tests orientation, remote and recent memory, practical skills, and mathematical ability.

short-PR-normal-QRS syndrome. See **Lown-Ganong-Levine syndrome.**

short-sightedness. See **myopia, near-sightedness.**

short stature, a body height that is less than 70% of the average for a population of the same age, culture, gender, and other peer factors.

short-term memory, memory of recent events.

short-wave diathermy [AS, *sceort + wafian*; Gk, *dia, therme,* heat], a method of providing heat deep in the body by short-wave electrical currents. The high-frequency short-wave uses wavelengths of from 3 to 30 meters. It is used to treat chronic arthritis, bursitis, sinusitis, and other conditions.

shotgun therapy [AS *scot;* ME *gonne;* Gk *therapeia* treatment], *informal;* any treatment that has a wide range of effect and which therefore can be expected to correct the abnormal condition even though the particular cause is unknown.

shoulder [AS *sculder*], the junction of the clavicle and scapula at the point where the arm attaches to the trunk of the body.

shoulder blade. See **scapula.**

shoulder girdle, a partial arch at the top of the trunk formed by the scapula and clavicle.

shoulder-hand syndrome, a neuromuscular condition characterized by pain and stiffness in the shoulder and arm, limited joint motion, swelling of the hand, muscle atrophy, and decalcification of the underlying bones. The condition occurs most commonly after myocardial infarction but may be associated with other known or unknown causes.

shoulder joint, the ball and socket articulation of the humerus with the scapula. The joint includes eight bursae and five ligaments.

shoulder presentation, the part of the fetus that occupies the center of the birth canal when the presentation is associated with a transverse or oblique lie.

shoulder spica cast, an orthopedic cast applied to immobilize the trunk of the body to the hips, the wrist, and the hand. It is used in the treatment of shoulder dislocations and injuries or in the positioning and immobilization of the shoulder after surgery.

shoulder subluxation, the separation of the humeral head from the glenoid cavity, resulting in strain on the soft tissues surrounding the joint.

show. See **vaginal bleeding.**

shreds [AS *screade* piece cut off], glossy filaments of mucus in the urine, indicating inflammation in the urinary tract.

shunt [ME *shunten*], **1.** to redirect the flow of a body fluid from one cavity or vessel to another. **2.** a tube or device implanted in the body to redirect a body fluid from one cavity or vessel to another.

shunt, left to right, a diversion of blood from the left side of the heart to the right, as through a septal defect, or from the systemic to the pulmonary circulation, as from a patent ductus arteriosus.

Shy-Drager syndrome /shī'drā'gǝr/ [G. Milton Shy, American neurologist, b. 1919; Glenn A. Drager, American physician, b. 1917], a rare, progressive neurologic disorder characterized by orthostatic hypotension, bladder and bowel incontinence, atrophy of the iris, anhidrosis, tremor, rigidity, incoordination, ataxia, and muscle wasting.

Si, symbol for the element **silicon.**

SI, abbreviation for *Système International d'Unités,* the French name for the **International System of Units.**

SIADH, abbreviation for **syndrome of inappropriate antidiuretic hormone secretion.**

sialadenitis /sī'ǝlad'ǝni'tis/, any inflammation of one or more of the salivary glands.

sialogogue /sī·al'ǝgog'/ [Gk *sialon* saliva, *agogos* leading], anything that stimulates the secretion of saliva.

sialogram /sī·al'ǝgram'/, a radiographic image of the salivary glands and ducts.

sialography /sī·ȯlog'rǝfē/ [Gk *sialon + graphein* to record], a technique in radiology in which a salivary gland is filmed after an opaque substance is injected into its duct. **–sialogram** /sī·al'ǝgram'/, *n.,* **sialographic,** *adj.*

sialolith /sī·al'ǝlith/ [Gk *sialon + lithos* stone], a calculus formed in a salivary gland or duct.

sialolithiasis /-lithī'ǝsis/, a pathologic condition in which one or more calculi or stones are formed in a salivary gland.

sialorrhea /sī·al·ǝrē'ǝ/ [Gk *sialon + rhoia* flow], an excessive flow of saliva that may be associated with a variety of conditions, such as acute inflammation of the mouth, mental retardation, mercurialism, pregnancy, teething, alcoholism, or malnutrition.

Siamese twins /sī'ǝmēz/ [Chang and Eng, conjoined twins born in Siam (now Thailand) in 1811], conjoined, equally developed twin fetuses that were produced from the same ovum. The severity of the condition ranges from superficial fusion, as of the umbilical vessels, to that in which the heads or complete torsos are united and several internal organs are shared.

sib [AS *sibb*], pertaining to a close blood relationship.

Siberian tick typhus /sībir′ē·ən/ [Siberia, Russia], a mild, acute febrile illness seen in Asia, caused by *Rickettsia siberica*, transmitted by ticks, and characterized by a diffuse maculopapular rash, headache, conjunctival inflammation, and a small ulcer or eschar at the site of the tick bite.

sibilant /sib′ilənt/ [L *sibilare* to hiss], a hissing sound or one in which the predominant sound is that of "S".

sibilant rale [L *sibalare* to hiss], an abnormal whistling sound that may emanate from the lungs of an individual with a respiratory disorder or disease. It is caused by the passage of air through a lumen narrowed by the accumulation of mucus or other viscid fluid.

sibling /sib′ling/ [AS *sibb* kin], **1.** also called (informal) **sib.** one of two or more children who have both parents in common; a brother or sister. **2.** of or pertaining to a brother or sister.

sibship /sib′ship/ [AS *sibb* kin, *scieppan* to shape], **1.** the state of being related by blood. **2.** a group of people descended from a common ancestor who are used as a basis for genetic studies. **3.** brothers and sisters considered as a group.

sic [L], thus.

sickle cell [AS *sicol* crescent; L *cella* storeroom], an abnormal, crescent-shaped red blood cell containing hemoglobin S, an abnormal form of hemoglobin characteristic of sickle cell anemia.

sickle cell anemia, a severe, chronic, incurable, anemic condition that occurs in people homozygous for hemoglobin S (Hb S). The abnormal hemoglobin results in distortion and fragility of the erythrocytes. Sickle cell anemia is characterized by crises of joint pain, thrombosis, and fever and by chronic anemia, with splenomegaly, lethargy, and weakness.

sickle cell crisis, an acute, episodic condition that occurs in children with sickle cell anemia. The crisis may be vasoocclusive, resulting from the aggregation of misshapen erythrocytes, or anemic, resulting from bone marrow aplasia, increased hemolysis, folate deficiency, or splenic sequestration of erythrocytes. Painful vasoocclusive crisis is the most common of the sickle cell crises. It is usually preceded by an upper respiratory or GI infection

without an exacerbation of anemia. The clumps of sickled erythrocytes obstruct blood vessels, resulting in occlusion, ischemia, and infarction of adjacent tissue. Characteristic of this kind of crisis are leukocytosis, acute abdominal pain from visceral hypoxia, painful swelling of the soft tissue of the hands and feet (hand-foot syndrome), and migratory, recurrent, or constant joint pain, often so severe that movement of the joint is limited. Persistent headache, dizziness, convulsions, visual or auditory disturbances, facial nerve palsies, coughing, shortness of breath, and tachypnea may occur if the central nervous system or lungs are affected.

sickle cell dactylitis [AS *sicol*; L *cella*; Gk *daktylos* finger, *itis*], a painful inflammation of one or more fingers caused by an attack of sickle cell anemia.

sickle cell thalassemia, a heterozygous blood disorder in which the genes for sickle cell and for thalassemia are both inherited. A mild form and a severe form may be identified, depending on the degree of suppression of beta-chain synthesis by the thalassemia gene. The clinical course is relatively mild. When beta-chain synthesis is completely suppressed, as in the severe form, only hemoglobin S appears in the red cells, and the clinical course is generally as severe as in homozygous sickle cell anemia.

sickle cell trait, the heterozygous form of sickle cell anemia, characterized by the presence of both hemoglobin S and hemoglobin A in the red blood cells. Anemia and the other signs of sickle cell anemia do not occur. People who have the trait are informed and counseled regarding the possibility of having an infant with sickle cell disease if both parents have the trait.

sick role [AS *seoc*; Fr, character], a pattern of behavior in which a person adopts the symptoms of a physical or mental disorder to be cared for, sympathized with, and protected from the demands and stresses of life.

sick sinus syndrome [AS *seoc*; L *sinus* hollow], a complex of syndromes associated with sinus node dysfunction. The condition may result from a variety of cardiac diseases. It is characterized by severe sinus bradycardia alone, sinus bradycardia alternating with tachycardia, or sinus bradycardia with atrioventricular block. The most common symptoms are lethargy, weakness, light-headedness, dizziness, and episodes of near syncope to actual loss of consciousness.

SICU, abbreviation for *surgical intensive care unit.*

side effect [AS *side*; L *effectus*], any reaction or consequence that results from a medication or therapy. Usually, although not necessarily, the effect is undesirable, and may manifest itself as nausea, dry mouth, dizziness, blood dyscrasias, blurred vision, discolored urine, or tinnitus.

sideroblast /sid′ərōblast′/ [Gk *sideros* iron + *blastos* germ cell], an iron-rich, nucleated red blood cell in the bone marrow.

sideroblastic anemia /sid′ərōblas′tik/ [Gk *sideros* iron, *blastos* germ], a heterogenous group of chronic hematologic disorders characterized by normocytic or slightly macrocytic anemia, hypochromic and normochromic red blood cells, and decreased erythropoiesis and hemoglobin synthesis. The red blood cells contain a perinuclear ring of iron-stained granules. The condition may be acquired or hereditary, primary or secondary to another condition or situation.

siderocyte /sid′ərosīt′/ [Gk *sideros* iron, *kytos* cell], an abnormal erythrocyte in which particles of nonhemoglobin iron are visible.

sideropenic dysphagia. See **Plummer-Vinson syndrome.**

siderosis /sid′ərō′sis/ [Gk *sideros* + *osis* condition] 1. a variety of pneumoconiosis caused by the inhalation of iron dust or particles. 2. the introduction of color in any tissue caused by the presence of excess iron. 3. an increase in the amounts of iron in the blood.

siderotic granules /sid′ərot′ik/, inclusion bodies seen in the red blood cells of splenectomy patients and in cases of hemoglobin synthesis and hemolytic anemia. The granules contain iron.

SIDS, abbreviation for **sudden infant death syndrome.**

SIECUS /sē′kəs/, abbreviation for *Sex Information and Education Council of the United States.*

sievert (Sv) /sē′vərt/ [R. M. Sievert, twentieth-century Swedish physicist], a unit dose equivalent radiation. The sievert has identical units to the gray and is arrived at by multiplying the absorbed dose by the quality factor, a number that has been determined to accurately compare the health consequences of that type of radiation to x-rays.

sig., abbreviation for the Latin word, *signatura,* meaning "let it be labeled according to prescription."

sigh. a deep breath that may be 1.5 times the normal V_t. It plays a role in pulmonary hygiene.

sight /sīt/ [AS *gesiht*], 1. the special sense that enables the shape, size, position, and color of objects to be perceived; the faculty of vision. It is the principal function of the eye. 2. that which is seen.

sigma, Σ, **c,** the eighteenth letter of the Greek alphabet.

Sigma Theta Tau International /sig′mə thā′tə tou′/, an international honor society for nurses.

sigmoid /sig′moid/ [Gk *sigma* S-shaped, *eidos* form] 1. of or pertaining to an S shape. 2. the sigmoid colon.

sigmoid colon, the portion of the colon that extends from the end of the descending colon in the pelvis to the juncture of the rectum.

sigmoid flexure. See **sigmoid colon.**

sigmoid mesocolon /mez′ōkō′lən/ [Gk *sigma, eidos* + *mesos* middle, *kolon*], a fold of peritoneum that connects the sigmoid colon with the pelvic wall.

sigmoid notch, a concavity on the superior surface of the mandibular ramus between the coronoid and condyloid processes.

sigmoidectomy /sig′moidek′təmē/ [Gk *sigma, eidos* + *ektome* excision], excision of the sigmoid flexure of the colon, most commonly performed to remove a malignant tumor.

sigmoidoscope /sigmoi′dəskōp′/ [Gk *sigma, eidos* + *skopein* to look], an instrument used to examine the lumen of the sigmoid colon. It consists of a tube and a light, allowing direct visualization of the mucous membrane lining the colon.

sigmoidoscopy /sig′moidos′kəpē/, the inspection of the rectum and sigmoid colon by the aid of a sigmoidoscope.

sign /sīn/ [L *signum* mark], an objective finding as perceived by an examiner, such as a fever, a rash, the whisper heard over the chest in pleural effusion, or the light band of hair seen in children after recovery from kwashiorkor. Many signs accompany symptoms, as erythema and a maculopapular rash are often seen when a patient complains of pruritus.

signal molecule /sig′nəl/ [L *signum* mark], a hormone, neurotransmitter, or other agent that transfers information from one cell or organ to another. Examples include steroid hormones, insulin, and growth factors.

signal node. See **Virchow's node.**

signal symptom. See **symptom.**

signal-to-noise ratio (SNR), the number used to describe the relative contribution to a detected signal of the true signal and random superimposed signals or "noise."

signe de journal. See **thumb sign.**

significance /signif′ikəns/ [L *significare* to signify], 1. (in research) the statistical probability that a given finding is very unlikely to have occurred by chance alone.

S

2. the importance of a study in developing a practice or theory, as in nursing practice.

significant other /signif′ikənt/, a person who is considered by an individual as being special and as having an impact on that individual.

sign language [L *signum* + *lingua* tongue], a form of communication often used with and among deaf persons consisting of hand and body movements. Many variations exist, including American Sign Language, Signed English, and finger spelling.

silanization /sil′ənizā′shən/, (in chromatography) the chemical process of converting the SiOH moieties of a stationary form to the ester form.

silent disease /sī′ənt/, a disease or other disorder that produces no clinically obvious signs or symptoms.

silent ischemia [L *silere* to be silent], an asymptomatic form of myocardial ischemia that may result in severe damage (myocardial infarction) or sudden death. Ischemia is most likely to occur during the first 6 hours after awakening in the morning.

silent mutation, (in molecular genetics) an alteration in a sequence of nucleotides that does not result in an amino acid change.

silent peritonitis, a case of peritonitis that develops without clinical signs or symptoms.

silhouette sign /sil′ oo·et′/, an x-ray artifact caused by an infiltrate that obscures the demarcating line between lung segments.

silicate dental cement /sil′ikāt/ [L *silex* flint], a relatively hard, translucent material used primarily to restore anterior teeth.

silicon (Si) /sil′ikon/ [L *silex* flint], a nonmetallic element, second to oxygen as the most abundant of the elements. Its atomic number is 14; its atomic weight is 28. It occurs in nature as silicon dioxide and in silicates. The silicates are used as detergents, corrosion inhibitors, adhesives, and sealants.

silicone /sil′ikōn/ [L *silex* flint], any organic silicon polymer compound used in medicine, as an adhesive, a lubricant, or a substitute for rubber, especially in prosthetic devices.

silicone septum, a vascular access device used in intravenous therapy. It consists of a silicone partition that covers the port chamber housed in the metal or plastic body of an implanted infusion port.

silicosis /sil′ikō′sis/, a lung disorder caused by continued, long-term inhalation of the dust of an inorganic compound, silicon dioxide, which is found in sands, quartzes, flints, and in many other stones. Silicosis is characterized by the development of nodular fibrosis in the lungs. In advanced cases, severe dyspnea may develop.

silk suture [AS *seolc*; L *sutura* seam], a braided, fine, black suture material, usually used to close incisions, wounds, and cuts in the skin. It is not absorbed by the body.

silo filler's disease /sī′lō/ [Fr *ensilotage* ensilage; AS *fyllan* to fill], a rare, acute, respiratory condition seen in agricultural workers who have inhaled nitrogen oxide as they work with fermented fodder in closed, poorly ventilated areas such as silos. Characteristically, symptoms of respiratory distress and pulmonary edema occur several hours after exposure. Loss of consciousness may occur.

silver (Ag) [AS *seolfor*], a whitish precious metal occurring mainly as a sulfide. Its atomic number is 47; its atomic weight is 107.88. It is used extensively as a component of amalgams of dental fillings and many medications, especially antiseptics and astringents. Silver nitrate is used externally as an antiseptic and astringent, especially in the prevention of ophthalmia neonatorum.

silver amalgam, an alloy of silver, tin, copper, mercury, and zinc used in dentistry to fill prepared tooth cavities.

silver cone method, a technique for filling tooth root canals. A prefitted silver cone is sealed to the apex of a root canal, and any remaining canal space is filled with gutta-percha or sealer.

Silver dwarf [Henry K. Silver, American pediatrician, b. 1918], a person who has **Silver's syndrome,** a congenital disorder in which short stature is associated with lateral asymmetry, various anomalies of the head, face, and skeleton, and precocious puberty.

silver-fork fracture. See **Colles' fracture.**

silver nitrate, a topical antiinfective. A 1% solution is prescribed for the prevention of gonococcal ophthalmia in newborns and in stronger concentrations for use on wet dressings.

silver salts poisoning, a toxic condition caused by the ingestion of silver nitrate, characterized by discoloration of the lips, vomiting, abdominal pain, dizziness, and convulsions.

Silver's syndrome. See **Silver dwarf.**

silver sulfadiazine, a topical antimicrobial prescribed to prevent or treat infection in second- and third-degree burns.

Silverman-Anderson score, a system of

assessing the degree of respiratory distress.

simethicone /simeth′ikōn/, an antiflatulent prescribed to decrease excess gas in the GI tract.

simian crease /sim′ē-ən/ [L *simia* ape; ME *creste* crest], a single crease across the palm from the fusion of proximal and distal palmar creases, seen in congenital disorders, such as Down syndrome.

simian virus 40, a vacuolating virus isolated from the kidney tissue of rhesus monkeys.

Simmonds' disease. See **postpubertal panhypopituitarism.**

simplate bleeding time test /sim′plāt/, a blood test for determining how quickly platelets form a plug when exposed to air. Platelet plug formation is the first step in clotting.

simple angioma [L *simplex* not complicated], a tumor consisting of a network of small vessels or distended capillaries surrounded by connective tissue.

simple astigmatism, 1. simple myopic astigmatism in which one principal meridian is in focus on the retina and the other in front of it. **2.** simple hyperopic astigmatism in which one meridian is focused on the retina and the other behind it.

simple cavity, a cavity that involves only one surface of a tooth.

simple diarrhea, a form of diarrhea in which the loose stools contain normal feces.

simple dislocation, dislocation without a penetrating wound.

simple figure-of-eight roller arm sling, an open sling that fits under the arm and over the chest. The bandage is started with a single turn toward the uninjured side around the arm and chest, crossing the elbow above the external epicondyle. Finally, the bandage is brought down over the scapula and across the chest and arm, overlapping and continuing in a figure-of-eight pattern.

simple fission. See **binary fission.**

simple fracture, an uncomplicated, closed fracture in which the bone does not break the skin.

simple glaucoma, chronic open-angle glaucoma in which the angle is open when the intraocular fluid pressure is increased but with associated lowered outflow of fluid. There may be visual field loss and optic atrophy.

simple goiter, a goiter not accompanied by signs or symptoms of hyperthyroidism.

simple mastectomy, a surgical procedure in which a breast is completely removed and the underlying muscles and adjacent lymph nodes are left intact.

simple meningitis. See **sterile meningitis.**

simple periodontal pocket. See **periodontal pocket.**

simple phobia, an anxiety disorder characterized by a persistent, irrational fear of specific things, such as animals, dirt, light, or darkness.

simple protein, a protein that yields amino acids as the only or chief product on hydrolysis. The class includes albumins, globulins, glutelins, alcohol-soluble proteins, albuminoids, histones, and protamines.

simple reflex, a reflex with a motor nerve component that involves only one muscle.

simple stomatitis, a simple inflammation of the mucous membranes of the mouth with redness, swelling, and an excess of mucus.

simple sugar, a monosaccharide, such as glucose.

simple tubular gland, one of the many multicellular glands with only one tube-shaped duct, such as various glands within the epithelium of the intestine.

simple vulvectomy. See **vulvectomy.**

Simpson forceps. See **obstetric forceps.**

Sims' position [James M. Sims, American gynecologist, b. 1813], a position in which the patient lies on the left side with the right knee and thigh drawn upward toward the chest. The chest and abdomen are allowed to fall forward.

sinciput /sin′siput/ [L, half a head], the anterior or upper part of the head.

sinew /sin′yōō/ [ME *sinewe*], the tendon of a muscle, such as the thick, flattened tendon attached to the short head of the biceps brachii.

singer's nodule. See **vocal cord nodule.**

single-blind study [L *singulus* one alone; AS *blind*; L *studere* to be busy], an experiment in which the person collecting data knows whether the subject is in the control group or the experimental group, but the subject does not.

single component insulin, any highly purified insulin with less than 10 ppm of proinsulin.

single footling breech. See **footling breech.**

single monster, a fetus with a single body and head but severely malformed or duplicated parts or organs.

single-parent family, a family consisting of only the mother or the father and one or more dependent children.

single-photon emission computed tomography (SPECT), a variation of computed tomography (CT) scanning in which the ray sum is defined by the collimator holes on the gamma-ray detector rotating

single room occupant (SRO), a single person, usually an elderly individual, who lives alone in a single room of a low-cost hotel or apartment building.

singultus. See **hiccup.**

sinister /sin′istər/, the Latin for left, or the left hand.

sinistral /sinis′trəl, sin′istrəl/ [L *sinister* left], relating to the left side.

sinistrality. See **left-handedness.**

sinoatrial [L *sinus* + *atrium* hall], pertaining to the sinus node and atrium.

sinoatrial (SA) block /sī′nō·ā′trē·əl/ [L *sinus* hollow, *atrium* hall; Fr *bloc*], a conduction disturbance in the heart during which an impulse formed within the SA node is blocked from depolarizing the atrial myocardium. The condition is indicated on the electrocardiogram by the absence of some P waves. Causes include excessive vagal stimulation, acute infections, and atherosclerosis. SA block may also be an adverse reaction to quinidine or digitalis.

sinoatrial (SA) node, a cluster of hundreds of cells located in the right atrial wall of the heart, near the opening of the superior vena cava. It comprises a knot of modified heart muscle that generates impulses that travel swiftly throughout the muscle fibers of both atria, causing them to contract. Specialized pacemaker cells in the node have an intrinsic rhythm that is independent of any stimulation by nerve impulses from the brain and the spinal cord. The sinoatrial node will normally "fire" at a rhythmic rate of 70 to 75 beats per minute. If the node fails to generate an impulse, pacemaker function will shift to another excitable component of the cardiac conduction system, such as the atrioventricular node or Purkinje's fibers.

sinoauricular See **sinoatrial.**

sinus /sī′nəs/ [L, hollow], a cavity or channel, such as a cavity within a bone, a dilated channel for venous blood, or one permitting the escape of pus.

sinus bradycardia. See **bradycardia.**

sinus dysrhythmia, an irregular heart rhythm caused by interference in the impulses arising from the sinoatrial node.

sinusitis /sīnəsī′tis/ [L *sinus* + Gk *itis* inflammation], an inflammation of one or more paranasal sinuses. It may be a complication of an upper respiratory infection, dental infection, allergy, a change in atmosphere, as in air travel or underwater swimming, or a structural defect of the nose. With swelling of nasal mucous membranes, the openings from sinuses to the nose may be obstructed, resulting in an accumulation of sinus secretions, causing pressure, pain, headache, fever, and local tenderness. Complications include cavernous sinus thrombosis and spread of infection to bone, brain, or meninges.

sinus node, an area of specialized heart tissue near the entrance of the superior vena cava that generates the cardiac electric impulse and is in turn controlled by the autonomic nervous system.

sinusoid /sī′nəsoid/ [L *sinus* + Gk *eidos* form], an anastomosing blood vessel, somewhat larger than a capillary, lined with reticuloendothelial cells.

sinus pacemaker. See **sinus node.**

sinus rhythm, a cardiac rhythm stimulated by the sinus (sinoatrial) node.

sinus tachycardia [L *sinus*; Gk *tachys* fast + *kardia* heart], a rapid heartbeat generated by stimulation of the sinoatrial pacemaker. The rate is generally between 100 and 160 beats per minute.

sinus venosus defect. See **atrial septal defect.**

si op. sit [L, *si, opus, sit*], if necessary.

Sippy diet [Bertram W. Sippy, American physician, b. 1866], a severely restricted dietary regimen for peptic ulcer patients. It consists of hourly servings of milk and cream for several days, with the gradual addition of eggs, refined cereals, puréed vegetables, crackers, and other simple foods as tolerated until the regular bland diet is reached.

sireniform fetus. See **sirenomelus.**

sirenomelia /sī′rənəmē′lē·ə/ [Gk *seiren* mermaid, *melos* limb], a congenital anomaly in which there is complete fusion of the lower extremities and no feet.

sirenomelus /sī′rənom′ələs/, an infant who has sirenomelia.

siriasis /sirī′əsis/ [Gk *sieros* scorching], sunstroke.

Sister Kenny's treatment [Elizabeth Kenny, Australian nurse, b. 1886; Fr *traitment*], poliomyelitis therapy in which the patient's limbs and back are wrapped in warm, moist woolen cloths and, after the pain subsides, the patient is taught to exercise affected muscles, especially by swimming. Equally important is passive movement of affected limbs with simultaneous stimulation at the site of muscle origins, carried out after hot packs.

site [L *situs* location], **1.** location. **2.** a quantum of space occupied and defined by a cluster of people.

site visit, a visit made by designated officials to evaluate or to gather information about a department or institution. A site visit is a step in the accreditation of an institution.

sitosterol, a mixture of sterols derived from plants and used for treating hyperbetalipoproteinemia and hypercholesterolemia that are unresponsive to dietary measures. Its use is controversial.

situational anxiety /sich′o͞o·äshənəl/ [L *situs* location], a state of apprehension, discomfort, and anxiety precipitated by the experience of new or changed situations or events. Situational anxiety is not abnormal and requires no treatment; it usually disappears as the person adjusts to the new experiences.

situational crisis, (in psychiatry) a crisis that arises suddenly in response to an external event or a conflict concerning a specific circumstance.

situational depression, (in psychiatry) an episode of emotional and psychologic depression that occurs in response to a specific set of external conditions or circumstances.

situational loss, the loss of a person, thing, or quality, resulting from a change in a life situation, including changes related to illness, body image, environment, and death.

situational psychosis, (in psychiatry) a psychotic episode that results from a specific set of external circumstances.

situational supports, people who are available and can be depended on to help a patient solve problems.

situational theory, a leadership theory in which the manager chooses a leadership style to match the particular situation.

situational therapy, (in psychiatry) a kind of psychotherapy in which the milieu is part of the treatment program.

situation relating /sich′o͞o·ā′shən/ (in nursing research) a study design used to explain or predict phenomena in nursing practice in which a relationship is thought to exist among certain practices or characteristics of the population being studied.

situation therapy. See **milieu therapy.**

situs /sī′təs/ [L, location], the normal position or location of an organ or part of the body.

situs inversus viscerum, the transposition of the abdominal and thoracic organs to opposite sides of the body.

sitz bath /sits, zits/ [Ger *sitz* sitting; AS *baeth*], a bath in which only the hips and buttocks are immersed in water or saline solution. The procedure is used for patients who have had rectal or perineal surgery.

SI units, the international units of physical amounts. Examples of these units are the volume of a liter, the length of a meter, or the precise amount of time in a minute. A group of scientists (Comité International des Poids et Mesures) meets regularly to define the units.

sixth disease. See **roseola infantum.**

sixth cranial nerve. See **abducens nerve.**

Sjögren-Larsson syndrome /shō′gren-lär′sən/ [Torsten Sjögren, Swedish pediatrician, b. 1859; T. Larsson, twentieth-century Swedish pediatrician], a congenital condition inherited as an autosomal recessive trait characterized by ichthyosis, mental deficiency, and spastic paralysis.

Sjögren's syndrome [Henrik S. C. Sjögren, Swedish ophthalmologist, b. 1899], an immunologic disorder characterized by deficient moisture production of the lacrimal, salivary, and other glands and resulting in abnormal dryness of the mouth, eyes, and other mucous membranes. Atrophy of the lacrimal glands can lead to desiccation of the cornea and conjunctiva. When the lungs are affected, the dryness increases susceptibility to pneumonia and other respiratory infections. Treatment includes application of artificial tears.

SK, abbreviation for **streptokinase.**

skeletal enchondromatosis. See **enchondromatosis.**

skeletal fixation /skel′ətəl/ [Gk *skeletos* dried up; L *figere* to fasten], any method of holding together the fragments of a fractured bone by the attaching of wires, screws, pins, or nails.

skeletal muscle. See **striated muscle.**

skeletal system, all of the bones and cartilage of the body that collectively provide the supporting framework for the muscles and organs.

skeletal traction, one of the two basic kinds of traction used in orthopedics for the treatment of fractured bones and the correction of orthopedic abnormalities. Skeletal traction is applied to the affected structure by a metal pin or wire inserted in the tissue of the structure and attached to traction ropes. Skeletal traction is often used when continuous traction is desired to immobilize, position, and align a fractured bone properly during the healing process. Infection of the pin tract is one of the complications that may develop with skeletal traction.

skeleton /skel′ətən/ [Gk *skeletos* dried up], the supporting framework for the body, comprising 206 bones that protect delicate structures, provide attachments for muscles, allow body movement, serve as major reservoirs of blood, and produce red blood cells. The skeleton is divided into the axial skeleton, which has 74 bones, the

S

appendicular skeleton with 126 bones, and the 6 auditory ossicles. The skeleton is derived from the mesoderm that grows from the primitive streak as skeletal cells multiply, change, and migrate into various regions and form the membranous skeleton. Most of the membranous skeleton changes to cartilaginous skeleton in which ossification centers spread to form the bony skeleton. The four types of bones composing the skeleton are the long bones, including the humerus and the phalanges of the fingers; the short bones, including the carpals and the tarsals; the flat bones, including the frontal bone and the parietal bone of the cranium; and the irregular bones, including the vertebrae. **–skeletal,** *adj.*

Skene's duct. See **paraurethral duct.**

Skene's glands /skēnz/ [Alexander J. C. Skene, American gynecologist, b. 1838], the largest of the glands that open into the urethra of women.

skew /skyōō/ [ME *skewen* to escape], a deviation from a line or symmetric pattern, such as data in a research study that do not follow the expected statistical curve of distribution because of the unwitting introduction of another variable.

skilled nursing facility (SNF) [ME *skil* distinction], an institution or part of an institution that meets criteria for accreditation established by the sections of the Social Security Act that determine the basis for Medicaid and Medicare reimbursement for skilled nursing care, including rehabilitation and various medical and nursing procedures. Written policies and protocols are formulated with appropriate professional consultation.

Skillern's fracture /skil′ərnz/ [Penn G. Skillern, American surgeon, b. 1882], an open fracture of the distal radius associated with a greenstick fracture of the distal ulna.

skill play [ME *skil* + *plega* sport], a form of play in which a child persistently repeats an action or activity until it has been mastered, such as throwing or catching a ball.

skills training, the teaching of specific verbal and nonverbal behaviors and the practicing of these behaviors by the patient.

skimmed milk [Dan *skumme* scum removal; AS *meolc*], milk from which the fat has been removed. Most of the vitamin A is removed with the cream, although all other nutrients remain. It is available as fluid skimmed milk, fortified skimmed milk, nonfat dry milk, and a form of buttermilk.

skimming [Dan *skumme*], a practice, sometimes used by health programs that receive their income on a prepaid or capitation basis, of seeking to enroll only relatively healthy individuals as a means of increasing profits by decreasing costs.

skimping [Swed *skrympa* to shrink], a practice, sometimes used by health programs that receive their income on a prepaid or capitation basis, of delaying or denying services to enrolled members of the program as a means of increasing profits by decreasing costs.

skin [AS *scinn*], the tough, supple cutaneous membrane that covers the entire surface of the body. It is the largest organ of the body and is composed of five layers of cells. The deepest layer is the stratum basale. It anchors the more superficial layers to the underlying tissues, and it provides new cells to maintain the cells lost by abrasion from the outermost layer. The cells of each layer migrate upward as they mature. Above the stratum basale lies the stratum spinosum. The cells in this layer are polygonal with tiny spines on their surfaces. As the cells migrate to the next layer, the stratum granulosum, they become flat, lying parallel with the surface of the skin. Over this layer lies a clear, thin band of homogenous tissue called the stratum lucidum. The outermost layer, the stratum corneum, is composed of scaly, squamous plaques of dead cells that contain keratin. This horny layer is thick over areas of the body subject to abrasion, such as the palms of the hands. The color of the skin varies according to the amount of melanin in the epidermis. Genetic differences determine the amount of melanin.

skin barrier, an artificial layer of skin, usually made of plastic, applied to skin before the application of tape or ostomy drainage bags. It protects the real skin from chronic irritation.

skin button, a plastic and fabric device that covers the drivelines of an artificial heart at their exit point from the skin. Its purpose is to eliminate the transmission of pumping pressure to the surrounding tissues.

skin cancer, a cutaneous neoplasm caused by ionizing radiation, certain genetic defects, or chemical carcinogens, including arsenics, petroleum, tar products, and fumes from some molten metals, or by overexposure to the sun or other sources of ultraviolet light. Skin cancers, the most common and most curable malignancies, are also the most frequent secondary lesions in patients with cancer in other sites. Risk factors are a fair complexion, xeroderma pigmentosa, vitiligo, senile and seborrheic keratitis, Bowen's disease, radiation dermatitis, and hereditary basal cell nevus syndrome. The most common skin cancers are basal cell carcinomas and squamous cell carcinomas.

skin flap, a layer of skin, usually separated by dissection from deeper layers of tissue.

skinfold calipers, an instrument used to measure the breadth of a fold of skin, usually on the posterior aspect of the upper arm or over the lower ribs of the chest.

skinfold thickness, a measure of the amount of subcutaneous fat by inserting a fold of skin into the jaws of a caliper. The skinfolds are usually measured on the upper arm, thigh, or upper abdomen and the caliper measurements are later compared to precalibrated standard tables to indirectly assess the body fat content of an individual.

skin graft, a portion of skin implanted to cover areas where skin has been lost through burns or injury or by surgical removal of diseased tissue. To prevent tissue rejection of permanent grafts, the graft is taken from the patient's own body or from the body of an identical twin. Skin from another person or animal can be used as a temporary cover for large burned areas to decrease fluid loss. Various techniques are used including pinch, split-thickness, full-thickness, pedicle, and mesh grafts. In pinch grafting, 1-4 inch pieces of skin are placed as small islands on the recipient site that they will grow to cover. The split-thickness graft consists of sheets of superficial and some deep layers of skin. The grafts are sutured into place; compression dressings may be applied for firm contact, or the area may be left exposed to the air. A full-thickness graft contains all of the layers of skin and is more durable and effective for weight-bearing and friction-prone areas. A pedicle graft is one in which a portion remains attached to the donor site, whereas the remainder is transferred to the recipient site. Its own blood supply remains intact, and it is not detached until the new blood supply has fully developed. A mesh graft is composed of multiple slices of new skin. A successful new graft of any type is well established in about 72 hours.

skin integrity, impaired, a NANDA-accepted nursing diagnosis of a state in which an individual's skin is adversely altered. Defining characteristics include disruption of the surface of the skin, destruction of cell layers of the skin, and invasion of structures of the body through the skin.

skin integrity, impaired, high risk for, a NANDA-accepted nursing diagnosis of a state in which an individual's skin is at risk of being adversely altered. Defining characteristics include the environmental (external) or somatic (internal) risk factors that may contribute to the cause of the breakdown of the integument. Among the environmental factors are hypothermia or hyperthermia; presence of an injurious chemical substance; shearing force or pressure, restraint, or laceration; radiation; physical immobilization; presence on the skin of excretions or secretions; and an abnormally high humidity. Somatic factors include reaction to some medications; obesity or emaciation; an abnormal metabolic state; alteration in circulation, sensory function, or pigmentation; bony prominences; adverse developmental factors; decrease in normal skin turgor; and psychogenic or immunologic abnormalities.

Skinner box [Burrhus F. Skinner, American psychologist, b. 1904; L *buxus* boxwood], a boxlike laboratory apparatus used in operant conditioning in animals, usually containing a lever or other device that when pressed produces reinforcement by either giving a reward, such as food or an escape outlet, or avoiding a punishment, such as an electric shock.

skin pigment [AS *scinn;* L *pigmentum* paint], any skin coloring caused by melanin deposits in skin and hair. The coloring may be modified by substances in the blood, such as the several blood pigments, bile, or malarial parasites.

skin prep, a procedure for cleansing the skin with an antiseptic before surgery or venipuncture. Skin preps are performed to kill bacteria and pathologic organisms and to reduce the risk of infection. Various skin prep devices are available for this procedure. Such devices are commonly constructed of plastic, filled with a specific antiseptic, and equipped with an applicator. The antiseptic is applied by rubbing the device in a circular motion over the skin.

skin tag. See **cutaneous papilloma.**

skin test, a test to determine the reaction of the body to a substance by observing the results of injecting the substance intradermally or of applying it topically to the skin. Skin tests are used to detect allergens, to determine immunity, and to diagnose disease. Kinds of skin tests include **patch test, Schick test,** and **tuberculin test.**

skin traction, one of the two basic types of traction used in orthopedics for the treatment of fractured bones and the correction of orthopedic abnormalities. Skin traction applies pull to an affected body structure by straps attached to the skin surrounding the structure. Kinds of skin trac-

S

tion are **adhesive skin traction** and **non-adhesive skin traction.**

skin turgor [AS *scinn;* L *turgere* to swell], the resilience of the normal skin when subjected to physical distortion as by pinching or pressing. The relative speed with which the skin resumes its normal appearance after stretching or compression is an indicator of skin hydration. Turgor is slower in older persons.

skull [ME *skulle* shell], the bony structure of the head, consisting of the cranium and the skeleton of the face. The cranium, which contains and protects the brain, consists of eight bones. The skeleton of the face is composed of 14 bones.

SL, abbreviation for **soda lime.**

slander [Fr *esclandre* scandal], any words spoken with malice that are untrue and prejudicial to the reputation, professional practice, commercial trade, office, or business of another person.

slant of occlusal plane [ME *slenten* to slope], (in dentistry) the inclination measured by the angle between the extended occlusal plane and the axis-orbital plane.

SLE, abbreviation for **systemic lupus erythematosus.**

sleep [AS *slaepan* to sleep], a state marked by reduced consciousness, diminished activity of the skeletal muscles, and depressed metabolism. People normally experience sleep in patterns that follow four observable, progressive stages. During Stage 1, the brain waves are of the theta type, followed in Stage 2 by the appearance of distinctive sleep spindles; during Stages 3 and 4, the theta waves are replaced by delta waves. These four stages represent three fourths of a period of typical sleep and are called collectively, **non-rapid eye movement (NREM)** sleep. The remaining time is usually occupied with **rapid eye movement (REM)** sleep, which can be detected with electrodes placed on the skin around the eyes so that tiny electric discharges from contractions of the eye muscles are transmitted to recording equipment. The REM sleep periods, lasting from a few minutes to half an hour, alternate with the NREM periods. Dreaming occurs during REM time.

sleep apnea, a sleep disorder characterized by periods of an absence of attempts to breathe. The person is momentarily unable to move respiratory muscles or maintain airflow through the nose and mouth.

sleeping pill, 1. *informal;* a sedative taken for insomnia or for postoperative sedation. **2.** an over-the-counter pill, classified pharmaceutically as an aid to sleeping.

sleeping sickness. See **African trypanosomiasis.**

sleep pattern disturbance, NANDA-accepted nursing diagnosis of a disruption of the hours of sleep, causing discomfort or interference with normal daily activities. Defining characteristics include difficulty in falling asleep, wakening earlier than usual, interruption of the night's sleep by periods of wakefulness, or not feeling rested after sleep, and changes in behavior and performance, such as increased irritability, restlessness, disorientation, lack of energy, and fatigue.

sleep terror disorder [AS *slaepan;* L *terrere* to frighten], a condition occurring during stages 3 or 4 of nonrapid eye movement sleep that is characterized by repeated episodes of abrupt awakening, usually with a panicky scream, accompanied by intense anxiety, confusion, agitation, disorientation, unresponsiveness, marked motor movements, and total amnesia concerning the event. The disorder is seen usually in children.

sleepwalking. See **somnambulism.**

slide clamp [AS *slidan; clam* fastener], a device, usually constructed of plastic, used to regulate the flow of intravenous solution. The slide clamp has a graduated opening through which the intravenous tubing passes. Pushing the tube into the narrow end of the opening constricts the tube and reduces the flow rate.

sliding filaments [AS *slidan;* L *filamentum* thread], interdigitated thick and thin filaments of a sarcomere. In muscle contraction, they slide past each other so that the sarcomere becomes shorter, although the filament lengths do not change. The action of the sliding filaments contributes to the increased thickness of a muscle in contraction.

sliding transfer, the movement of a person in a sitting position from one site to another, as from a bed to a wheelchair, by sliding the person along a transfer board.

sling [ME *slingen* to hurl], a bandage or device used to support an injured part of the body.

sling restraint, a therapeutic device, usually constructed of felt, used to assist in the immobilization of patients, especially orthopedic patients in traction. The sling is placed over the pelvis to reduce pelvic motion with lower extremity traction or over the abdominal area as countertraction with Dunlop traction.

slip-on blood pump [ME *slippen* slippery; *on*], a plastic mesh device with an attached squeeze bulb, rubber tubing, and pressure gauge, used to help administer large amounts of blood quickly. The plastic mesh slips over the blood bag and applies pressure to the bag when the bulb is squeezed.

slipped disk. See **herniated intervertebral disk.**

slipped femoral epiphysis, a failure of the femoral epiphyseal plate that tends to occur primarily in overweight adolescents as a result of hormonal changes. Clinical features include hip stiffness and pain. There may also be knee pain and external rotation of the affected leg. The condition is treated by orthopedic surgery.

slipping patella [ME, *slippen;* L, *patella,* small disc], a patella that undergoes recurrent dislocation.

slipping rib, a chest pain caused by a loose ligament that allows slippage of one of the lower five ribs. One of the ribs may slip inside or outside an adjacent rib, causing pain or discomfort that may mimic a disorder of the pancreas, gallbladder, or other upper abdominal organ.

slit lamp [AS *slitan;* Gk *lampein* to shine], an instrument used in ophthalmology for examining the conjunctiva, lens, vitreous humor, iris, and cornea. A high-intensity beam of light is projected through a narrow slit, and a cross section of the illuminated part of the eye is examined through a magnifying lens.

slit lamp microscope, a microscope for ophthalmic examination. It permits the viewer to examine the endothelium of the posterior surface of the cornea in a projected band of light that is shaped like a slit.

slit scan radiography, a technique for producing x-rays of body structures without length distortion by scanning a fan-shaped beam through a narrow slit collimator. The beam divergence perpendicular to the scan results in some distortion of width.

slough /sluf/ [ME *sluh* husk], **1.** to shed or cast off dead tissue cells of the endometrium, which are shed during menstruation. **2.** the tissue that has been shed.

slow-acting insulin. See **long-acting insulin.**

slow diastolic depolarization [AS *slaw* dull], the slow loss of negativity that occurs during phase 4 of the action potential in cardiac cells having automaticity.

slow pulse, a pulse rate of less than 60 beats per minute. The rate is commonly found among older persons, conditioned athletes, and patients receiving beta-blocker medications.

slow-reacting substance of anaphylaxis (SRS-A), a group of active substances, including histamine and leukotrienes, that are released during an anaphylactic re-

action. They cause the smooth muscle contraction and vascular dilation that mark the signs and symptoms of anaphylaxis.

slow response action potential, (in cardiology) an action potential produced when none of the fast sodium channels is available for depolarization and the fiber is activated via slow calcium channels, producing an action potential with a slow upstroke velocity, low amplitude, and consequent slow conduction.

slow-twitch (ST) fiber, a muscle fiber that develops less tension more slowly than a fast-twitch fiber. The ST fiber is usually fatigue resistant and has adequate oxygen and enzyme activity.

slow virus, a virus that remains dormant in the body after initial infection. Years may elapse before symptoms occur.

slurred speech /slurd/ [D *sleuren* to drag; ME *speche*], abnormal speech in which words are not enunciated clearly or completely but are run together or partially eliminated. The condition may be caused by weakness of the muscles of articulation, damage to a motor neuron, cerebellar disease, drug usage, or carelessness.

Sm, symbol for the element **samarium.**

SMA, abbreviation for **sequential multiple analysis.**

SMA-6, SMA-12, SMA-18. See **sequential multiple analysis.**

small calorie. See **calorie.**

small cardiac vein [AS *smael*], one of the five tributaries of the coronary sinus that drains blood from the myocardium. It conveys blood from the back of the right atrium and the right ventricle and, in some individuals, is joined by the right marginal vein.

small cell carcinoma. See **oat cell carcinoma.**

smallest cardiac vein, one of the tiny vessels that drain deoxygenated blood from the myocardium into the atria. A few of these vessels end in the ventricles.

small for gestational age (SGA) infant, an infant whose weight and size at birth falls below the tenth percentile of appropriate for gestational age infants, whether delivered at term or earlier or later than term. Factors associated with smallness or retardation of intrauterine growth other than genetic influences include any disorder causing short stature, such as dwarfism; malnutrition caused by placental insufficiency; and certain infectious agents, including cytomegalovirus, rubella virus, and *Toxoplasma gondii.* Other factors associated with the smallness of an SGA infant include cigarette smoking by the mother during pregnancy, her addiction to alcohol or heroin, and her having received methadone treatment.

small intestine, the longest portion of the digestive tract, extending for about 7 m from the pylorus of the stomach to the iliocecal junction. It is divided into the duodenum, jejunum, and ileum.

small omentum. See **lesser omentum.**

smallpox /smôl′poks/ [AS *smael, pocc*], a highly contagious viral disease characterized by fever, prostration, and a vesicular, pustular rash. It is caused by one of two species of poxvirus, variola minor (alastrim) or variola major. Because human beings are the only reservoir for the virus, worldwide vaccination with vaccinia, a related poxvirus, has been effective in eradicating smallpox.

smallpox vaccine, a vaccine prepared from dried smallpox virus. It is indicated only for laboratory workers exposed to pox viruses.

small sciatic nerve [AS *smael*; Gk *ischiadikos* of the hip joint; L *nervus*], the posterior femoral cutaneous nerve, which pierces the fascia and subdivides into filaments, supplying the skin from the level of the greater trochanter to the middle of the thigh.

smear /smir/ [AS *smeoru* grease], a laboratory specimen for microscopic examination prepared by spreading a thin film of tissue on a glass slide. A dye, stain, reagent, diluent, or lysing agent may be applied to the specimen.

smegma /smeg′mə/ [Gk, soap], a secretion of sebaceous glands, especially the cheesy, foul-smelling secretion often found under the foreskin of the penis and at the base of the labia minora near the glans clitoris.

smell [ME *smellen* to detect odors], **1.** the special sense that enables odors to be perceived through the stimulation of the olfactory nerves; olfaction. **2.** any odor, pleasant or unpleasant.

smelling salt, aromatized ammonium carbonate to which may be added ammonia. It is used as a stimulant to arouse a person who has fainted.

Smith fracture [Robert W. Smith, Irish surgeon, b. 1807], a reverse Colles' fracture of the wrist, involving volar displacement and angulation of a distal bone fragment.

Smith-Hodge pessary. See **pessary.**

Smith-Petersen nail [Marius N. Smith-Petersen, American surgeon, b. 1886; AS *naegel* nail], a three-flanged stainless steel nail used in orthopedic surgery to anchor the fractured neck of the femur to its head. It is introduced below the prominence of the greater trochanter and passed through the fractured part into the head of the femur.

smog, a polluting combination of smoke and fog in the atmosphere.

smoke inhalation [AS *smoca*; L *in* within, *halare* to breathe], the inhalation of noxious fumes or irritating particulate matter that may cause severe pulmonary damage. Respiratory burns are difficult to distinguish from simple smoke inhalation. Chemical pneumonitis, asphyxiation, and physical trauma to the respiratory passages may occur. Characteristics include irritation of the upper respiratory tract, singed nasal hairs, dyspnea, hypoxia, dusty gray sputum, rhonchi, rales, restlessness, anxiety, cough, and hoarseness. Pulmonary edema may develop up to 48 hours after exposure.

smokeless tobacco, 1. chewing tobacco or tobacco powder that allows the stimulating components of tobacco to be absorbed through the digestive tract, or through the mucous membrane in the case of snuff. **2.** a transdermal nicotine patch that can be affixed to the upper part of the body to satisfy the patient's craving for nicotine.

smooth muscle [AS *smoth*], one of two kinds of muscle, composed of elongated, spindle-shaped cells in muscles not under voluntary control, such as the smooth muscle of the visceral organs. The heart muscle is an exception because it is a striated involuntary muscle. The nucleated cells of smooth muscle are arranged parallel to one another and to the long axis of the muscle they form. Smooth muscle fibers are shorter than striated muscle fibers and have only one nucleus per fiber.

smooth pursuit eye movement, the tracking of the eyes following a slowly moving object at a steady coordinated velocity, rather than in saccades.

smooth surface cavity, a cavity formed by decay that starts on surfaces of teeth without pits, fissures, or enamel faults.

SMR, abbreviation for **submucous resection.**

smudge cell /smuj/ [ME *sogen* to soil], a degenerated leukocyte as seen in blood smears from patients with chronic lymphatic leukemia.

Sn, symbol for the element **tin.**

SN, abbreviation for *student nurse,* used in signing nursing notes.

SNA, abbreviation for **State Nurses' Association.**

snail [AS *snagel* slug], an invertebrate of the order Gastropoda, several species of which are intermediate hosts of the blood flukes that cause schistosomiasis in humans.

snakebite [AS *snacan* to creep, *bitan*], a wound resulting from penetration of the flesh by the fangs of a snake. Bites by snakes known to be nonvenomous are treated as puncture wounds; those produced by an unidentified or poisonous snake require immediate attention.

snake venom [AS *snacan*; L *venenum*], a poison produced in glands of certain snakes and injected through fangs into a victim's flesh. The exact composition of snake venom varies with different species but generally are complex mixtures of neurotoxins, proteolytic enzymes, and phosphatases. About 20 of more than 100 North American species of snakes are venomous, accounting for around 8,000 snake venom poisonings a year. A venomous snake bite is considered a medical emergency.

snapping hip [ME *snappen*; AS *hype*], a condition in which a tendon slips over the greater trochanter when the hip is moved, possibly producing a loud snapping sound.

snare /sner/ [AS *sneare* noose], a device designed for holding a wire noose, used in removing small pedunculated growths. The operator tightens the wire around the peduncle, thus removing the growth.

sneeze [AS *snesen* to sneeze], a sudden, forceful, involuntary expulsion of air through the nose and mouth occurring as a result of irritation to the mucous membranes of the upper respiratory tract, as by dust, pollen, or viral inflammation.

Snellen chart [Hermann Snellen, Dutch ophthalmologist, b. 1834], one of several charts used in testing visual acuity. Letters, numbers, or symbols are arranged on the chart in decreasing size from top to bottom.

Snellen test, a test of visual acuity using a Snellen chart. The person being tested stands 20 feet from the chart and reads as many of the symbols as possible, reading each line and proceeding downward from the top. A score is assigned in the form of a ratio, comparing the subject's performance to that of a statistically normal subject's performance. A person who can read what the average person can read at 20 feet has 20/20 vision.

SNF, abbreviation for **skilled nursing facility.**

snout reflex [ME *snoute* muzzle], an abnormal sign elicited by tapping the nose, resulting in a marked facial grimace. It usually indicates bilateral corticopontine lesions.

snow blindness, a condition of photophobia, sometimes accompanied by conjunctivitis, as a result of overexposure of the eyes to the glare of sun on snow.

Snowden-Pencer scissors. See **scissors.**

SNP, abbreviation for **sodium nitroprusside.**

SNP, abbreviation for **school nurse practitioner.**

snuff dipping, the practice of extracting juices from chewing tobacco placed in the mucobuccal fold of the mouth. The practice has been associated with an increased incidence of leukoplakia, tooth and gum diseases, and possible oral cancer.

snuffles [D *snuffelen* to sniff], a nasal discharge in infancy characteristic of congenital syphilis.

soap [L *sapo*], **1.** a compound of fatty acids and an alkali. Soap cleanses because molecules of fat are attracted to molecules of soap in a water solution and are pulled off the dirty surface into the water. **2.** a metallic salt of any salt produced from an acid. Compare **detergent.**

SOAP /sōp, es'ō'ā'pē'/, (in a problem-oriented medical record) abbreviation for *subjective, objective, assessment, and plan,* the four parts of a written account of the health problem.

soapsuds enema, an evacuent enema made of one ounce of soft soap dissolved in two pints of hot water and administered at a temperature of 38° C or 100° F.

SOB, abbreviation for *short of breath.*

social adjustment rating scale. See **social readjustment rating scale.**

Social Behavior Assessment Scale /sō'shəl/, a semistructured interview guide that elicits information from significant others regarding a patient's functioning.

social breakdown syndrome [L *socius* partner; AS *brecan, dune*], the progressive deterioration of social and interpersonal skills in long-term psychiatric patients.

social class, a grouping of people with similar values, interests, income, education, and occupations.

social deviance, behavior that violates social standards, engendering anger, resentment, and a desire for punishment in a significant segment of the society.

social interaction, impaired, a NANDA-accepted nursing diagnosis of an insufficient or excessive quantity or ineffective quality of social exchange. Defining characteristics include verbalized or observed discomfort in social situations; verbalized or observed inability to receive or communicate a satisfying sense of belonging, caring, interest, or shared history; observed use of unsuccessful social interaction behaviors; and dysfunctional interaction with peers, family, and/or others.

S

social isolation, a NANDA-accepted nursing diagnosis of a condition in which a feeling of aloneness is experienced that the client acknowledges as a negative or threatening state imposed by others. Defining characteristics may be objective or subjective, or both. Objective characteristics include the absence of family and friends; the absence of a significant personal relationship with another person; the client's withdrawal and preoccupation with his or her own thoughts and interests; meaningless actions or interests and activities inappropriate to the client's developmental age; a physical or mental handicap or illness; or unacceptable social behavior. Subjective characteristics include the verbal expression of feeling different from and rejected by others, the acknowledgment of values unacceptable to the dominant cultural group, absence of a significant purpose in life, the inability to meet the expectations of others, and the expressed feeling of insecurity in social situations.

socialization /sō'shəlīzā'shən/, **1.** the process by which an individual learns to live in accordance with the expectations and standards of a group or society, acquiring the beliefs, habits, values, and accepted modes of behavior primarily through imitation, family interaction, and educational systems; the procedure by which society integrates the individual. **2.** (in psychoanalysis) the process of adjustment that begins in early childhood by which the individual becomes aware of the need to accommodate inner drives to the demands of external realty.

socialized medicine /sō'shəlīzd/, a system for the delivery of health care in which the expense of care is borne by a governmental agency supported by taxation rather than being paid for directly by the client on a fee-for-service or contract basis.

social learning theory, a concept that the impulse to behave aggressively is subject to the influence of learning, socialization, and experience.

social margin, the sum total of all resources (material, personal, and interpersonal) available to assist an individual in coping with stress.

social medicine, an approach to the prevention and treatment of disease that is based on the study of human heredity, environment, social structures, and cultural values.

social mobility, the process of moving upward or downward in the social hierarchy.

social motivation, an incentive or drive resulting from a sociocultural influence that initiates behavior toward a particular goal.

social network, an interconnected group of cooperating significant others, who may or may not be related, with whom a person interacts.

social network therapy, the gathering together of patient, family, and other social contacts into group sessions for the purpose of problem solving.

social order, the manner in which a society is organized and the rules and standards required to maintain that organization.

social phobia, an anxiety disorder characterized by a compelling desire for the avoidance of and a persistent, irrational fear of situations in which the individual may be exposed to scrutiny by others, such as speaking, eating, or performing in public, or using public lavatories or transportation.

social psychiatry, a branch of psychiatry based on the study of social influences on the development and course of mental diseases.

social psychology, the study of the effects of group membership on the behavior, attitudes, and beliefs of the individual.

social readjustment rating scale, a scale of 43 common life events associated with some degree of disruption of an individual's life. The scale was developed by psychologists T. J. Holmes and R. H. Rahe, who found that a number of serious physical disorders, such as myocardial infarction, peptic ulcer, and infections, and a variety of psychiatric disorders, were associated with an accumulation of 200 or more points on the rating scale within a period of 1 year. Most disruptive on one's life, according to the psychologists, was the death of a spouse, an event that warranted 100 points. The lowest rated event was a minor law violation, rated at 11 points.

social sanctions, the measures used by a society to enforce its rules of acceptable behavior.

Social Security Act, a U.S. federal statute that provides for a national system of old age assistance, survivors' and old age insurance benefits, unemployment insurance and compensation, and other public welfare programs, including Medicare and Medicaid.

social worker, a person with advanced education in dealing with social, emotional, and environmental problems associated with illness or disability. A **medical social worker** usually has completed a master's degree program that includes experience in counseling patients and their families in a hospital setting. A **psychiatric social worker** may specialize in counseling individuals and families in dealing with social, emotional, or environmental problems pertaining to mental illness.

society /səsī'ətē/, a nation, community, or broad group of people who establish particular aims, beliefs, or standards of living and conduct.

Society for Advancement in Nursing (SAIN), a group established for advancement of the profession of nursing through higher education.

sociobiology /sō'sē-ō'bī-ol'əjē/, the systematic study of biology as a basis for human behavior. Proponents contend that disease, stress, and aggression are natural pressures for maintaining an optimal level of population.

socioeconomic status /sō'sē-ō'ikənom'ik/ [L socius companion, oeconomicus methodical, status state], the position of an individual on a social-economic scale that measures such factors as education, income, type of occupation, place of residence, and in some populations, heritage and religion.

sociogenic /-jen'ik/ [L socius + Gk genesis origin], pertaining to personal or group activities that are motivated by social values and constraints.

sociolinguistics /-ling·gwis'tiks/, the study of the relationship between language and the social context in which it occurs.

sociology /sō'sē-ol'əjē/ [L socius + Gk logos science], the study of group behavior within a society.

sociopath. See psychopath.

sociopathic. See psychopathic.

sociopathic personality. See antisocial personality.

sociopathy /sō'sē-op'əthē/ [L socius + Gk pathos disease], a personality disorder characterized by a lack of social responsibility and failure to adapt to ethical and social standards of the community.

socket, the part of a prosthesis into which the stump of the remaining limb fits. Most modern prosthetic sockets are made of plastic materials, which are lighter, odorless, and easier to clean than traditional leather sockets.

soda [It sodo solid], a compound of sodium, particularly sodium bicarbonate, sodium carbonate, or sodium hydroxide.

soda lime (SL), a mixture of sodium and calcium hydroxides used to absorb exhaled carbon dioxide in an anesthesia rebreathing system.

sodium (Na) /sō'dē·əm/ [soda + L ium (coined by Sir Humphry Davy, English chemist, b. 1778)], a soft, grayish metal of the alkaline metals group. Its atomic number is 11; its atomic weight is 22.99. Sodium is one of the most important elements in the body. Sodium ions are involved in acid-base balance, water balance, the transmission of nerve impulses, and the contraction of muscles. Sodium is the chief electrolyte in interstitial fluid, and its interaction with potassium as the main intracellular electrolyte is critical to survival. A decrease in the sodium concentration of the interstitial fluid immediately decreases osmotic pressure, making it hypotonic to intracellular fluid osmotic pressure.

sodium acid glutamate. See sodium glutamate.

sodium arsenite poisoning, a toxic condition caused by the ingestion of sodium arsenite, an insecticide and weed-killer. The characteristic symptoms of arsenite poisoning are similar to those of arsenic poisoning.

sodium barbital, the sodium salt of 5,5-diethylbarbituric acid, a hypnotic and sedative drug.

sodium bicarbonate, an antacid, electrolyte, and urinary alkalinizing agent. It is prescribed in the treatment of acidosis, gastric acidity, peptic ulcer, and indigestion.

sodium chloride, common table salt (NaCl), used as a fluid and electrolyte replenisher, isotonic vehicle, irrigating solution, and enema.

sodium chloride and dextrose. See dextrose and sodium chloride injection.

sodium etidronate. See etidronate disodium.

sodium fluoride poisoning, a chronic condition of fluorine poisoning that occurs in some communities where the fluorine concentration in the water supply exceeds 1 ppm. Signs of the condition include mottling of tooth enamel and severe osteosclerosis.

sodium glutamate, a salt of glutamic acid used for the treatment of hepatic coma and the enhancement of the flavor of foods.

sodium hypochlorite solution, a 5% aqueous solution of NaOCl used as a disinfectant for utensils not harmed by its bleaching action.

sodium iodide, an iodine supplement prescribed in the treatment of thyrotoxic crisis, neonatal thyrotoxicosis, and in the management of hyperthyroidism before thyroidectomy.

sodium lactate injection, an electrolyte replenisher that has been prescribed for metabolic acidosis.

sodium nitroprusside (SNP), a vasodilator prescribed primarily in the emergency

S

treatment of hypertensive crises and in heart failure.

sodium perborate, an oxygen-liberating antiseptic ($NaBO_2.H_2O_2.3H_2O$) that may be used in the treatment of necrotizing ulcerative gingivitis and other kinds of gingival inflammation and for bleaching pulpless teeth.

sodium phenobarbital, the sodium salt of phenylethylbarbituric acid, a long-acting sedative and hypnotic. It can be administered orally or parenterally and is used in the therapeutic management of seizure disorders.

sodium phosphate, a saline cathartic prescribed to achieve prompt, thorough evacuation of the bowel and, in lower dosage, for laxative effect.

sodium phosphate P32, an antineoplastic, antipolycythemic, radioactive agent. It is prescribed for polycythemia vera and for neoplasms, including myelocytic leukemia, and for localizing tumors of the eye.

sodium pump, a mechanism for transporting sodium ions across cell membranes against an opposing concentration gradient. Energy for this transport system is obtained from the hydrolysis of adenosine triphosphate by special enzymes.

sodium-restricted diet. See **low-sodium diet.**

sodium salicylate, an analgesic, antipyretic, and antirheumatic prescribed to relieve pain and fever.

sodium stibocaptate, an investigational parasiticide for certain schistosomal infections. It is available from the Centers for Disease Control and Prevention.

sodium sulfate, a saline cathartic for habitual constipation caused by peristaltic disorders. It is prescribed to achieve prompt, thorough evacuation of the bowel and, in lower dosage, for laxative effect.

sodium sulfate anhydrous. See **salt cake.**

sodoku. See **rat-bite fever.**

sodomist /sod'əmist/ [Sodom, city cited in Bible], a person who practices sodomy.

sodomy /sod'əmē/ [Sodom, Biblical city in ancient Palestine], **1.** anal intercourse. **2.** intercourse with an animal. **3.** a vague term for "unnatural" sexual intercourse. –**sodomite,** *n.,* **sodomize,** *v.*

soft chancre, a usually painless local genital ulcer that follows an infection by *Haemophilus ducreyi* and is accompanied by suppuration of the inguinal lymphatic nodes, or inguinal buboes. Complications may include phimosis, urethral stricture or fistula, and marked tissue destruction.

soft contact lens, a contact lens made of a flexible plastic material that can be shaped more easily to fit the eyeball. Disadvantages are that soft lenses are more easily damaged, do not provide vision as sharp as alternative methods, and must be disinfected periodically because they tend to harbor bacteria.

soft data [AS *softe;* L *datum* something given], health information that is mainly subjective as provided by the patient and the patient's family, including pain or other sensations, life-style habits, and family health history.

soft diet, a diet that is soft in texture, low in residue, easily digested, and well tolerated. It provides the essential nutrients in the form of liquids and semisolid foods, such as milk, fruit juices, eggs, cheese, custards, tapioca and puddings, strained soups, and vegetables.

softening of bones /sô'fəning, sof'əning/, any disease that results in a loss of the mineral content of the bones.

soft fibroma, a fibroma that contains many cells.

soft money, *informal;* (in a university, school, or agency) income from unstable sources, such as grants or contracts.

soft neurologic sign, a mild or slight neurologic abnormality that is difficult to detect or interpret.

soft palate, the structure composed of mucous membrane, muscular fibers, and mucous glands, suspended from the posterior border of the hard palate forming the roof of the mouth. When the soft palate rises, as in swallowing and in sucking, it separates the nasal cavity and the nasopharynx from the posterior part of the oral cavity and the oral portion of the pharynx.

soft radiation, a relatively long wavelength with less penetrating radiation than short wavelength radiation.

soft tissue rheumatism. See **fibrositis.**

soft water, a water that does not contain salts of calcium or magnesium, which precipitate soap solutions.

sol, a colloidal state in which a solid is suspended throughout a liquid, such as a soap or starch in water. The fluidity of cytoplasm depends on its sol/gel balance.

sol., abbreviation for **solution.**

solar fever. See **dengue fever, sunstroke.**

solarium /sōler'ē·əm/ [L, terrace exposed to sun], a large, sunny room serving as a lounge for ambulatory patients in a hospital.

solar keratosis. See **actinic keratosis.**

solar plexus /sō'lər/ [L *sol* sun; *plexus* network], a dense network of nerve fibers and ganglia that surrounds the roots of the celiac and the superior mesenteric arteries at the level of the first lumbar vertebra. It is one of the great autonomic plexuses of the body in which the nerve fibers of the sympathetic system and the parasympathetic system combine.

solar radiation, the emission and diffusion of actinic rays from the sun. Overexposure may result in sunburn, keratosis, skin cancer, or lesions associated with photosensitivity.

solar sneeze reflex, a sneeze that may be caused by exposure to bright sunlight.

solar therapy [L *sol*; Gk *therapeia* treatment], the therapeutic use of sunlight.

sole [L *solea*], the plantar surface of the foot.

soleus /sō'lē-əs/ [L *solea* sole of foot], one of three superficial posterior muscles of the leg. It is a broad flat muscle lying just under the gastrocnemius. The soleus plantar flexes the foot.

solid /sol'id/ [L *solidus*], **1.** a dense body, figure, structure, or substance that has length, breadth, and thickness, is not a liquid or a gas, contains no significant cavity or hollowness, and has no breaks or openings on its surface. **2.** describing such a body, figure, structure, or substance.

solitary coin lesion /sol'īter'ē/ [L *solitarius* standing alone; *cuneus* wedge; *laesus* injury], a nodule identified on a chest x-ray film by clear normal lung tissue surrounding it. A coin lesion usually measures between 1 and 6 cm and is often malignant.

solitary play, a form of play among a group of children within the same room or area in which each child engages in an independent activity using toys that are different from the others' and showing no interest in joining in or interfering with the play of others.

solubility /sol'yəbil'itē/ [L *solubilis* able to dissolve], **1.** the maximum amount of a solute that can dissolve in a specific solvent under a given set of conditions. **2.** the concentration of a solute in a solvent at its saturation point.

solute /sol'yo͞ot, sō'lo͞ot/ [L *solutus* dissolved], a substance dissolved in a solution.

solution /səlo͞o'shən/ [L *solutus*], a mixture of one or more substances dissolved in another substance. The molecules of each of the substances disperse homogenously and do not change chemically. A solution may be a gas, a liquid, or a solid.

solvent /sol'vənt/ [L *solvere* to dissolve], **1.** any liquid in which another substance can be dissolved. **2.** *informal;* an organic liquid, such as benzene, carbon tetrachloride, and other volatile petroleum distillate, that when inhaled can cause intoxication, as well as damage to mucous membranes of the nose and throat and the tissues of the kidney, liver, and brain.

soma /sō'mə/, *pl.* **somas, somata** [Gk, body] **1.** the body as distinguished from the mind or psyche. **2.** the body, excluding germ cells. **3.** the body of a cell. **–somatic** /sōmat'ik/, **somal,** *adj.*

somatic. See **soma, psychosomatic.**

somatic cavity. See **coelom.**

somatic cell /sōmat'ik/, any of the cells of body tissue that have the diploid number of chromosomes as distinguished from germ cells, which contain the haploid number.

somatic chromosome, any chromosome in a diploid or somatic cell, as contrasted to those in a haploid or gametic cell; an autosome.

somatic delusion, a false notion or belief concerning body image or body function.

somatic mutation [Gk *soma*; L *mutare* to change], a sudden change in the chromosomal material in somatic cell nuclei affecting derived cells but not offspring.

somatic therapy, a form of treatment that affects one's physiologic functioning.

somatist /sō'mətist/, a psychotherapist or other health professional who believes that every neurosis and psychosis has an organic cause.

somatization /sō'mətīzā'shən/ [Gk *soma* body], a process whereby a mental event is expressed in a body disorder or physical symptom. Examples include peptic ulcers or asthma.

somatization disorder [Gk *soma* + *izein* to cause], a disorder characterized by recurrent, multiple, physical complaints and symptoms for which there is no organic cause. The symptoms vary according to the individual and the underlying emotional conflict. Some common symptoms are GI dysfunction, paralysis, temporary blindness, cardiopulmonary distress, painful or irregular menstruation, sexual indifference, and pain during intercourse.

somatoform   disorder /sōmat'əfôrm, sō'mətōfôrm'/ [Gk *soma* + L *forma* form], any of a group of neurotic disorders, characterized by symptoms suggesting physical illness or disease, for which there are no demonstrable organic causes or physiologic dysfunctions. Kinds of somatoform disorders are **conversion disorder, hypochondriasis, psychogenic pain disorder,** and **somatization disorder.**

somatogenesis /sō'mətəjen'əsis/ [Gk *soma* + *genein* to produce], **1.** (in embryology) the development of the body from the germ plasm. **2.** the development of a physical disease or of symptoms from an organic pathophysiologic cause. **–somatogenic, somatogenetic,** *adj.*

S

somatoliberin. See **growth hormone releasing factor.**

somatomedin. See **growth hormone.**

somatomegaly /sō'matōmeg'əlē/ [Gk *soma* + *megas* large], a condition in which the body is abnormally large because of an excessive secretion of somatotropin or an inadequate secretion of somatostatin.

somatoplasm /sō'mətōplaz'əm/ [Gk *soma* + *plasma* something formed], the nonreproductive protoplasmic material of the body cells as distinguished from the reproductive material of the germ cells.

somatopleure /sō'mətōploor'/ /sōmat'əploor/ [Gk *soma* + *pleura* side], the tissue layer that forms the body wall of the early developing embryo. **–somatopleural,** *adj.*

somatosensory evoked potential (SEP) /-sen'sərē/ [Gk *soma* + *sentire* to feel], evoked potential elicited by repeated stimulation of the pain and touch systems. It is the least reliable of the evoked potentials studied as monitors of neurologic function during surgery.

somatosplanchnic /sōmat'ōsplangk'nik/ [Gk *soma* + *splanchna* viscera], of or pertaining to the trunk of the body and the visceral organs.

somatostatin /sō'mətōstat'in/, a hormone produced in the hypothalamus that inhibits the factor that stimulates release of somatotropin from the anterior pituitary gland. It also inhibits the release of certain hormones, including thyrotropin, adrenocorticotropic hormone, glucagon, insulin, and cholecystokinin, and of some enzymes, including pepsin, renin, secretin, and gastrin.

somatotherapy /-ther'əpē/, the treatment of physical disorders, as distinguished from psychotherapy.

somatotropic /trop'ik/ [Gk *soma* + *trope* a turn], pertaining to an agent that influences the body or body cells.

somatotropic hormone, somatotropin. See **growth hormone.**

somatotype /sō'mətōtīp'/ [Gk *soma* + *typos* mark], **1.** body build or physique. **2.** the classification of individuals according to body build based on certain physical characteristics. The primary types are **ectomorph, endomorph,** and **mesomorph.**

somatrem /sō'mətrem/, a synthetic polypeptide growth hormone produced by recombinant DNA technology. It is prescribed for patients who fail to grow because of limited endogenous growth hormone secretion.

somite /sō'mīt/ [Gk *soma*], any of the paired, segmented masses of mesodermal tissue that form along the length of the neural tube during the early stage of embryonic development in vertebrates.

somite embryo, an embryo in any stage of development between the formation of the first and the last pairs of somites, which in humans occurs in the third and fourth weeks after fertilization of the ovum.

somnambulance /somnam'byələns/. See **somnambulism.**

somnambulism /somnam'byəliz'əm/ [L *somnus* sleep, *ambulare* to walk], **1.** a condition occurring during stages 3 or 4 of nonrapid eye movement sleep that is characterized by complex motor activity, usually culminating in leaving the bed and walking about, with no recall of the episode on awakening. The episodes usually last from several minutes to half an hour or longer. **2.** a hypnotic state in which the person has full possession of the senses but no recollection of the episode.

somnolent [L *somnolentia* sleepy], **1.** the condition of being sleepy or drowsy. **2.** tending to cause sleepiness. **–somnolence,** *n.*

somnolent detachment /som'nələnt/, (in psychology) a term introduced by Sullivan for a type of security operation in which a person falls asleep when confronted by a highly threatening, anxiety-producing experience.

Somogyi phenomenon [Michael Somogyi, American biochemist, b. 1883; Gk, *phainomenon*], a diabetes mellitus rebound effect in which an overdose of insulin induces hypoglycemia. This starts the release of hormones that stimulate lipolysis, gluconeogenesis, and glycogenolysis, leading to hyperglycemia and ketosis. Treatment involves gradually lowering the insulin dose to achieve an optimum level.

sonogram, sonography. See **ultrasonography.**

sonographer /sōnog'rəfər/, an allied health professional with special training in the use of ultrasound equipment for diagnostic and therapeutic purposes.

sonorous rale /sənō'əs/ [L *sonor* noise], a snoring sound that may be produced by the vibration of a mass of thick secretion lodged in a bronchus. This sound is associated with various lung or respiratory disorders.

soot wart. See **scrotal cancer.**

sopor /sō'pər/ [L, deep sleep], a sleep that is as deep or sound as the state of stupor.

soporiferous /sop'ərif'ərəs/ [L *sopor* + *ferre* to bear], tending to cause deep sleep, as an agent that induces deep sleep.

soporific /sop'ərif'ik/ [L *sopor* deep sleep, *facere* to make], **1.** of or pertaining to a substance, condition, or procedure that causes sleep. **2.** a soporific drug.

sorbent /sôr′bənt/ [L *sorbere* to swallow], the property of a substance that allows it to interact with another compound, usually to make it bind.

sorbic acid /sôr′bik/, a compound occurring naturally in berries of the mountain ash. Commercial sorbic acid derived from acetaldehyde is used in fungicides, food preservatives, lubricants, and plasticizers.

sordes /sôr′dēz/, *pl.* **sordes** [L *sordere* to be dirty], dirt or debris, especially the crusts consisting of food, microorganisms, and epithelial cells that accumulate on teeth and lips during a febrile illness. Sordes gastricae is undigested food and mucus in the stomach.

sore /sôr, sōr/ [AS *sar*], **1.** a wound, ulcer, or lesion. **2.** tender or painful.

sore throat, any inflammation of the larynx, pharynx, or tonsils.

Sorrin's operation, a surgical technique for treating a periodontal abscess, used especially when the marginal gingiva appears healthy and provides no access to the abscess. A semilunar incision is made below the abscess area in the attached gingiva, leaving the gingival margin undisturbed. The tissue flap produced by the incision is raised, accessing the abscessed area for curettage, after which the wound is sutured.

s.o.s., (in prescriptions) abbreviation for *si opus sit,* a Latin phrase meaning "if necessary."

souffle /sōo′fəl/ [Fr, breath], a soft murmur heard through a stethoscope. When detected over the uterus in a pregnant woman, it is coincident with the maternal pulse and is caused by blood circulating in the large uterine arteries.

soul food [AS *sawel, foda*], food linked with cultural or traditional origins, especially African-American, that contributes emotional significance and personal satisfaction to an individual.

sound [L *sonus*], an instrument used to locate the opening of a cavity or canal, to test the patency of a canal, to ascertain the depth of a cavity, or to reveal the contents of a canal or cavity.

source-image receptor distance /sôrs, sōrs/ [OFr *sourse* origin; L *imago* likeness], the distance between the focus of an x-ray beam and the x-ray film as measured along the beam.

South African genetic porphyria. See **variegate porphyria.**

South American blastomycosis. See **paracoccidioidomycosis.**

South American trypanosomiasis. See **Chagas' disease.**

Southern blot test /suth′ərn/, a gene analysis method used to identify specific DNA fragments and in the diagnosis of cancers and hemoglobinopathies.

sp. (*pl.* **sp., spp.**), abbreviation for **species.**

space [L *spatium*], an actual or a potential cavity of the body, such as the complemental spaces in the pleural cavity that are not occupied by lung tissue and the lymph spaces occupied by lymph.

space maintainer, a fixed or movable appliance for preserving the space created by the premature loss of one or more teeth.

space medicine, a branch of medicine concerned with the effects of travel in space, beyond the atmosphere and pull of gravity, including weightlessness, motion sickness, and restricted physical activity.

space obtainer, an appliance for increasing the space between adjoining teeth.

space regainer, a fixed or removable appliance for moving a displaced permanent tooth into its normal position in a dental arch.

space sickness, See **air sickness; motion sickness.**

Spanish fly. See **cantharis.**

sparganosis /spär′gənō′sis/ [Gk *sparganon* swaddling clothes, *osis* condition], an infection with larvae of the fish tapeworm of the pseudogenus Sparganum, characterized by painful subcutaneous swellings or swelling and destruction of the eye. It is acquired by ingesting larvae in contaminated water or in inadequately cooked, infected frog flesh.

sparteine sulfate, an alkaloid salt used to treat cardiac disorders and formerly used as an oxytocic to reduce uterine bleeding during the third stage of labor.

spasm /spaz′əm/ [Gk *spasmos*], **1.** an involuntary muscle contraction of sudden onset, such as habit spasms, hiccups, stuttering, or a tic. **2.** a convulsion or seizure. **3.** a sudden, transient constriction of a blood vessel, bronchus, esophagus, pylorus, ureter, or other hollow organ.

spasmatic asthma /spazmat′ik/, an airway obstruction characterized by paroxysms of wheezing and coughing caused by spasms of the bronchioles and inflammation of the bronchial mucosa.

spasmatic croup [Gk, *spasmos;* Scot, *kroak*], See **laryngismus.**

spasmodic croup, See **laryngismus.**

spasmodic dysphonia /spazmod′ik/ [Gk *spasmodes; dys* bad, *phone* voice], a speech disorder in which phonation is in-

S

termittently blocked by spasms of the larynx.

spasmodic stricture [Gk *spasmodes;* L *strictura* compression], a narrowing of a passage in which there is no organic change but merely muscle spasms.

spasmodic tic, any repetitive movement in which spasmodic muscle group contractions occur at variable intervals.

spasmodic torticollis, a form of torticollis characterized by episodes of spasms of the neck muscles. In some cases, severe stress and muscular spasm may be the cause.

spasmogen /spaz'məjən/, any substance that can produce smooth muscle contractions, as in the bronchioles, such as histamine, bradykinin, and serotonin.

spastic /spas'tik/ [Gk *spastikos* drawing in], of or pertaining to spasms or other uncontrolled contractions of the skeletal muscles. –**spasticity,** *n.*

spastic aphonia, a condition in which a person is unable to speak because of spasmodic contraction of the abductor muscles of the throat.

spastic bladder, a form of neurogenic bladder caused by a lesion of the spinal cord above the voiding reflex center. It is marked by loss of bladder control and bladder sensation, incontinence, and automatic, interrupted, incomplete voiding. It is often caused by trauma, a tumor, or multiple sclerosis.

spastic colon. See **irritable bowel syndrome.**

spastic constipation, a form of constipation associated with neurasthenia and constrictive spasms in part of the intestine. The condition may be a sign of lead poisoning.

spastic dysphonia. See **spasmodic dysphonia.**

spastic entropion. See **ectropion, entropion.**

spastic gait, a pattern of walking in which the legs are stiff, the feet plantar-flexed, and movements made by circumduction. The steps may also be accompanied by toe dragging.

spastic hemiplegia, paralysis of one side of the body with increased tendon reflexes and uncontrolled contraction occurring in the affected muscles.

spastic ileus, a form of intestinal obstruction caused by bowel spasms.

spasticity /spastis'itē/ [Gk *spastikos* drawing in], a form of muscular hypertonicity with increased resistance to stretch. It usually involves the flexors of the arms and the extensors of the legs. Moderate spasticity is characterized by movements that require great effort and lack of normal coordination. Slight spasticity may be marked by gross movements that are coordinated, but combined selective movement patterns are incoordinated.

spastic paralysis, an abnormal condition characterized by the involuntary contraction of one or more muscles with associated loss of muscular function.

spastic paraplegia, a form of partial paralysis affecting mainly older people. It is accompanied by irritability and spastic contractions of the leg muscles.

spastic pseudoparalysis. See **Creutzfeldt-Jakob disease.**

spastic strabismus, squint caused by spasmodic contractions of ocular muscles.

spatial dance /spā'shəl/ [L *spatium* space; ME *dauncen* to drag along], the body shifts or movements used by individuals as they try to adjust the distance between themselves and other individuals.

spatial relationships, 1. orientation in space; the ability to locate objects in the three-dimensional external world using visual or tactile recognition and make a spatial analysis of the observed information. 2. the relative locations of various personnel and equipment in an operating room with particular emphasis on what is sterile, clean, or contaminated.

spatial summation. See **summation.**

spatial zones, the areas of personal space in which most people interact. Four basic spatial zones are the intimate zone, in which distance between individuals is less than 18 inches; the personal zone, between 18 inches and 4 feet; the social zone, extending between 4 and 12 feet; and the public zone, beyond 12 feet.

SPE, abbreviation for **sucrose polyester.**

Spearman's rho /spir'mənz rō'/ [Charles E. Spearman, English psychologist, b. 1863; *rho,* seventeenth letter in Greek alphabet], a statistical test for correlation between two rank-ordered scales. It yields a statement of the degree of interdependence of the scores of the two scales.

special care unit /spesh'əl/ [L *specialis* individual], a hospital unit with the necessary specialized equipment and personnel for handling critically ill or injured patients, such as an intensive care unit, burn unit, or cardiac care unit.

special gene system, a plasmid, transposon, or other genetic fragment that is able to transfer genetic information from one cell to another.

specialing /spesh'əling/, *informal.* 1. (in psychiatric nursing) the constant attendance of a professional staff member on a disturbed patient to protect the patient from harming the self or others and to observe the patient's behavior. 2. (in nursing) the giving of nursing care to only one person, as when caring for a patient whose needs are so great that a nurse is required at all times.

specialist /spesh′əlist/, a health care professional who practices a specialty. A specialist usually has advanced clinical training and may have a postgraduate academic degree.

special sense, the sense of sight, smell, taste, touch, or hearing.

specialty /spesh′əltē/ [L *specialis*], a branch of medicine or nursing in which the professional is specially qualified to practice by having attended an advanced program of study, by having passed an examination given by an organization of the members of the specialty, or by having gained experience by extensive practice in the specialty.

specialty care, specialized medical services provided by a physician specialist.

species (sp) /spē′sēz, spē′shēz/, *pl.* **species (sp., spp.)** /spē′sēz, spē′shēz/ [L, form], the category of living things below genus in rank. A species includes individuals of the same genus who are similar in structure and chemical composition and who can interbreed.

species immunity, a form of natural immunity shared by all members of a species.

species-specific, 1. pertaining to the characteristics of a particular species. 2. having a characteristic effect on, or interaction with, cells, tissues, or membranes of a particular species; said of an antigen, drug, or infective agent.

specific absorption rate (SAR) /spisif′ik/ [L *species* form], (in hyperthermia treatment) the rate of absorption of heat energy (W) per unit mass of tissue in units of W/kg.

specific activity, 1. (in nuclear medicine) the radioactivity of a radioisotope per unit mass of the element or compound, expressed in microcuries per millimole or disintegrations per second per milligram. 2. the relative activity per unit mass, expressed as counts per minute per milligram.

specific gravity, the ratio of the density of a substance to the density of another substance accepted as a standard. The usual standard for liquids and solids is water. Thus, a liquid or solid with a specific gravity of 4 is four times as dense as water.

specific immune globulin, a special preparation obtained from human blood that is preselected for its high antibody count against a specific disease, such as varicella zoster immune globulin.

specific rates, statistical rates in which both the events in both the numerator and the denominator are restricted to a specific subgroup of a population.

specific treatment. See **treatment.**

specific ulcer, an ulcer associated with a specific disease, such as a syphilitic ulcer.

specific viscosity, the internal friction of a fluid, which may be measured by comparing the rate of flow of the fluid through a tube as compared with the rate of a standard liquid under standard conditions.

specificity /spes′əfis′itē/ [L *species* form, *facere* to make], the quality of being distinctive. Kinds of specificity may include: **group; species; type.**

specificity of association, the uniqueness of a relationship between a causal factor and the occurrence of a disease.

specimen /spes′imən/ [L *specere* to look], a small sample of something, intended to show the nature of the whole, such as a urine specimen.

SPECT, abbreviation for **single-photon emission computed tomography.**

spectator ions /spek′tātər/, ions that are not involved in proton transfer in a chemical reaction.

spectinomycin hydrochloride /spek′tinōmī′sin/, an antibiotic prescribed in the treatment of gonorrhea and certain infections in penicillin-allergic patients.

spectrometer /spektrom′ətər/ [L *spectrum* image; Gk *metron* measure], an instrument for measuring wavelengths of rays of the spectrum, the deviation of refracted rays, and the angles between faces of a prism. Kinds of spectrometer are **mass spectrometer** and **Mössbauer spectrometer.**

spectrometry /spektrom′ətrē/, the procedure of measuring wavelengths of light and other electromagnetic waves. **–spectrometric,** *adj.*

spectrophotometry /spek′trōfətom′ətrē/, the measurement of color in a solution by determining the amount of light absorbed in the ultraviolet, infrared, or visible spectrum, widely used in clinical chemistry to calculate the concentration of substances in solution. **–spectrophotometric,** *adj.*

spectrum /spek′trəm/, *pl.* **spectra** [L, image], 1. a range of phenomena or properties occurring in increasing or decreasing magnitude. Radiant or electromagnetic energy is arranged on the basis of wavelength and frequency. 2. the range of effectiveness of an antibiotic. A broad-spectrum antibiotic is effective against a wide range of microorganisms.

speculum /spek′yələm/ [L, mirror], a retractor used to separate the walls of a cavity to make examination possible, such as

S

an ear speculum, an eye speculum, or a vaginal speculum.

speech [ME *speche*], **1.** the utterance of articulate vocal sounds that form words to give expression to one's thoughts or ideas. **2.** communication by means of spoken words. **3.** the faculty of language production, which involves the complex coordination of the muscles and nerves of the organs of articulation.

speech audiometry. See **audiometry.**

speech center, a unilateral area in the posterior part of the inferior frontal gyrus and usually on the side contralateral to the dominant hand. Also associated with articulate speech are Brodmann's areas 44 and 45.

speech dysfunction, any defect or abnormality of speech, including aphasia, alexia, stammering, stuttering, aphonia, and slurring. Kinds of dysfunctions include **ataxic speech, explosive speech, mirror speech, scamping speech, scanning speech, slurred speech,** and **staccato speech.**

speech-language pathologist, an individual with graduate professional training in human communication, its development, and disorders. The person specializes in the measurement and evaluation of language abilities, auditory processes and speech production, clinical treatment of children and adults with speech, language, and hearing disorders, and research methods in the study of communication processes.

speech pathology, 1. the study of abnormalities of speech or of the organs of speech. **2.** the diagnosis and treatment of abnormalities of speech as practiced by a speech pathologist or a speech therapist.

speech reading, a method of verbal communication in which one utilizes the visual clues of the speaker's lip and facial movements, along with residual hearing. Gestures and "body language" are also observed.

speech synthesizer [AS *spaec;* Gk *synthesis* placing together], an electronic apparatus with a keyboard that produces sounds that imitate the human voice.

speech therapist, a person trained in speech pathology who treats people with disorders affecting normal oral communication.

speech therapy [AS *spaec;* Gk *therapeia* treatment], the application of treatments and counseling in the prevention or correction of speech and language disorders.

speed [AS *spedan* to hasten], **1.** the rate of change of position with time. **2.** *slang;* any stimulating drug, such as amphetamine. **3.** a reciprocal of the amount of ra-

diation used to produce an image with various components of an x-ray imaging system, such as screens, film, and image intensifiers. A system using little radiation is "fast," whereas one requiring more radiation is "slow." **4.** the amount of exposure of film to light or x-rays needed to produce a desired image.

speed shock, a sudden adverse physiologic reaction of a patient to intravenous medications or drugs that are administered too quickly. Some signs of speed shock are a flushed face, headache, a tight feeling in the chest, irregular pulse, loss of consciousness, and cardiac arrest.

sPEEP, abbreviation for **spontaneous PEEP.**

spell of illness [ME *spel, illr* bad], a period regarded by Medicare rules as the number of days between the admission of an insured patient to a hospital and the day that marks the end of a period during which the insured has not been an inpatient in a hospital or a skilled nursing facility.

sperm. See **semen, spermatozoon.**

spermatic cord /spərmat′ik/ [Gk *sperma* seed; *chorde* string], a structure extending from the deep inguinal ring in the abdomen to the testis, descending nearly vertically into the scrotum.

spermatic duct. See **vas deferens.**

spermatic fistula, an abnormal passage communicating with a testis or a seminal duct.

spermatid /spərmat′id/ [Gk *sperma* seed], a male germ cell that arises from a spermatocyte and that becomes a mature spermatozoon in the last phase of the continual process of spermatogenesis.

spermatocele /spərmat′əsēl′, spur′-/ [Gk *sperma* + *kele* tumor], a cystic swelling, either of the epididymis or of the rete testis, that contains spermatozoa.

spermatocide /spərmat′əsīd, spur′-/ [Gk *sperma* + L *caedere* to kill], a chemical substance that kills spermatozoa by reducing their surface tension, causing the cell wall to break down by a bactericidal effect or by creating a highly acidic environment.

spermatocyte /spur′mətōsīt′/ [Gk *sperma* + *kytos* cell], a male germ cell that arises from a spermatogonium.

spermatocytogenesis. See **spermatogenesis.**

spermatogenesis /spərmat′əjen′əsis, spur′-/ [Gk *sperma* + *genesis* origin], the process of development of spermatozoa, including the first stage, called spermatogenesis, in which spermatogonia become spermatocytes that develop into spermatids, and the second stage, called spermiogenesis, in which the spermatids become spermatozoa. **–spermatogenic, spermatogenous,** *adj.*

spermatogonium /spur′mətōgō′nē·əm/, *pl.* **spermatogonia** [Gk *sperma* + *gone* generation], a male germ cell that gives rise to a spermatocyte early in spermatogenesis.

spermatopathia /-path′ē-ə/ [Gk *sperma* + *pathos* disease], pertaining to diseased sperm or their associated organs.

spermatozoa. See **spermatozoon.**

spermatozoon /spur′mətəzō′an, spər-mat′-/, *pl.* **spermatozoa** /-zō′ə/ [Gk *sperma* + *zoon* animal], a mature male germ cell that develops in the seminiferous tubules of the testes. Resembling a tadpole, it is about 50 μm (1/500 inch) long and has a head with a nucleus, a neck, and a tail that provides propulsion.

sperm bank /spurm/, a facility for storage of semen to be used for artificial insemination.

spermicidal /spur′misī′dəl/, destructive to spermatozoa.

spermicide. See **spermatocide.**

spermiogenesis. See **spermatogenesis.**

sp.gr., abbreviation for **specific gravity.**

S-phase, the phase of a cell reproductive cycle in which DNA is synthesized before mitosis.

sphenoethmoid recess /sfē′nŏ·eth′moid/ [Gk *sphen* wedge, *eidos* form; L *recedere* to retreat], a narrow opening in the lateral wall of the nasal cavity bounded above by the cribriform plate of the ethmoid and the body of the sphenoid and below by the superior nasal concha. It opens into the sphenoidal sinus of the skull.

sphenoid /sfē′noid/ [Gk *sphen* + *eidos* form], an unpaired bone at the base of the skull, separating the maxilla, ethmoid and frontal bones from the temporal and occipital bones.

sphenoidal fissure /sfēnoi′dəl/ [Gk *sphen* wedge, *eidos* form], a cleft between the great and small wings of the sphenoid bone.

sphenoidal sinus, one of a pair of cavities in the sphenoid bone of the skull, lined with mucous membrane that is continuous with that of the nasal cavity.

sphenoid bone /sfē′noid/, the bone at the base of the skull, anterior to the temporal bones and the basilar part of the occipital bone.

sphenoid fontanel, an anterolateral fontanel that is usually not palpable.

sphenoiditis /sfē′noidī′tis/, an inflammation of the sphenoidal sinus.

sphenomandibular ligament /sfē′nōmandib′yələr/ [Gk *sphen, eidos* + L *mandere* to chew], one of a pair of flat, thin ligaments comprising part of the temporomandibular joint between the mandible of the jaw and the temporal bone of the skull.

sphere /sfir/ [Gk *sphaira* ball], a globe-shaped object, theoretically generated by a circle revolving on a diameter as its axis.

spherocyte /sfir′əsīt/ [Gk *sphaira* sphere, *kytos* cell], an abnormal spheric red blood cell that contains more than the normal amount of hemoglobin. **–spherocytic,** *adj.*

spherocytic anemia /sfir′əsit′ik/, a hematologic disorder characterized by hemolytic anemia caused by the presence of red blood cells that are spheric rather than round and biconcave. The cells are fragile and tend to hemolyze in the oxygen-poor peripheral circulatory system. Episodic crises of abdominal pain, fever, jaundice, and splenomegaly occur.

spherocytosis /sfir′ōsītō′sis/, the abnormal presence of spherocytes in the blood.

spheroidea. See **ball and socket joint.**

spherule /sfer′(y)ōōl/, a small ball.

sphincter /sfingk′tər/ [Gk *sphingein* to bind], a circular band of muscle fibers that constricts a passage or closes a natural opening in the body, such as the external anal sphincter, which closes the anus.

sphincter ani, a double set of circular muscles at the opening of the anus. One, the sphincter ani internus, consists of a thickened inner circular coat of the bowel; the other, the sphincter ani externus, is a flat sheet of muscle surrounding the anal orifice.

sphincter choledochus /kōled′əkəs/, a smooth muscle sphincter that encircles the lower end of the bile duct and is part of the sphincter of Oddi.

sphincter of Oddi [Ruggero Oddi, nineteenth-century Italian surgeon], a band of circular muscle fibers around the lower end of the common bile and pancreatic duct.

sphincter pupillae, a muscle that expands the iris, narrowing the diameter of the pupil of the eye. It is composed of circular fibers arranged in a narrow band about 1 mm wide, surrounding the margin of the pupil toward the posterior surface of the iris.

sphincter virginae. See **bulbocavernosus.**

sphingolipid /sfing′gōlip′id/ [Gk *sphingein* to bind, *lipos* fat], a compound that consists of a lipid and a sphingosine. It is found in high concentrations in the brain and other tissues of the nervous system.

sphingomyelin /sfing′gōmī′əlin/ [Gk *sphingein* + *myelos* marrow], any of a group of sphingolipids containing phosphorus. It occurs primarily in the tissue of the nervous system.

sphingomyelin lipidosis, any of a group of diseases characterized by an abnormality in the ability of the body to store sphingolipids. Kinds of sphingomyelin lipidosis include **Gaucher's disease, Niemann-Pick disease,** and **Tay-Sachs disease.**

sphingosine /sfing′gōsēn/, a long-chain unsaturated amino alcohol, a major constituent of sphingolipids and sphingomyelin.

sphygmogram /sfig′məgram/ [Gk *sphygmos* pulse, *gramma* record], a pulse tracing produced by a sphygmograph. Sphygmographic abnormalities of rate, rhythm, and form may be diagnostically useful in an assessment of cardiovascular function.

sphygmograph /sfig′məgraf/, an instrument that records the force of the arterial pulse on a tracing called a sphygmogram. **–sphygmographic,** *adj.*

sphygmomanometer /sfig′mōmənom′ətər/ [Gk *sphygmos* + *manos* thin, *metron* measure], an instrument for indirect measurement of blood pressure. It consists of an inflatable cuff that fits around the arm, a bulb for controlling air pressure within the cuff, and a mercury or aneroid manometer. Pressure in the brachial artery is estimated by the column of mercury it balances when the cuff is inflated.

sphygmoplethysmograph /-pləthis′məgraf′/ [Gk *sphygmos* + *plethysmos* increase, *graphein* to record], an instrument for measuring and recording the arterial pulse curve and blood flow in a limb.

spica [L, spike, or ear of wheat], a figure-of-eight bandage that, when applied to a joint, resembles the head of a stalk of wheat.

spica bandage /spī′kə/ [L *spica* spike of wheat; Fr *bande* strip], a figure-of-eight bandage in which each turn generally overlaps the previous to form a succession of V-like designs. It may be used to give support, to apply pressure, or to hold a dressing in place.

spica cast, an orthopedic cast applied to immobilize part or all of the trunk of the body and part or all of one or more extremities. Kinds of spica casts are **bilateral long-leg spica cast, one-and-a-half spica cast, shoulder spica cast,** and **unilateral long-leg spica cast.**

spicule /spik′yo̅o̅l/ [L *spiculus* sharp point], a sharp body with a needlelike point.

spider angioma [ME *spithre;* Gk *aggeion* vessel, *oma* tumor], a form of telangiectasis characterized by a central, elevated, red dot the size of a pinhead from which small blood vessels radiate.

spider antivenin. See **black widow spider antivenin.**

spider bite, a puncture wound produced by the bite by any of nearly 60 species of venomous spiders found in North America. Most spiders have fangs that are too short or fragile to penetrate the skin, but some are dangerous to humans.

spider nevus. See **spider angioma.**

spider telangiectasia, a branched group of dilated capillary blood vessels forming a spiderlike image on the skin.

spikeboard /spīk′bôrd/, a device that enables persons with upper extremity handicaps to stabilize foods when only one hand is available for meal preparation.

spillway [AS *spillan* to destroy, *weg* wagon track], a channel or passageway through which food normally escapes from the occlusal surfaces of the teeth during mastication.

spin [AS *spinnan* to draw threads], **1.** the intrinsic angular momentum of an elementary particle or a nucleus of an atom. **2.** intrinsic joint movements about an axis perpendicular to the articular surface.

spina /spī′nə/, *pl.* **spinae** [L, backbone], **1.** the spinal column. **2.** a spine or a thornlike projection, such as the bony projection on the anterior border of the ilium, forming the anterior end of the iliac crest.

spina bifida /spī′nə bif′ədə, bī′fədə/, congenital neural tube defect characterized by a developmental anomaly in the posterior vertebral arch. Spina bifida that does not involve herniation of the meninges or the contents of the spinal canal rarely requires treatment.

spina bifida anterior, incomplete closure along the anterior surface of the vertebral column.

spina bifida cystica, a developmental defect of the central nervous system in which a hernial cyst containing meninges (meningocele), spinal cord (myelocele), or both (myelomeningocele) protrudes through a congenital cleft in the vertebral column. The protruding sac is encased in a layer of skin or a fine membrane that can easily rupture, causing the leakage of cerebrospinal fluid and an increased risk of meningeal infection.

spina bifida occulta, defective closure of the laminae of the vertebral column in the lumbosacral region without hernial protrusion of the spinal cord or meninges. Because the neural tube has closed, there are usually no neurologic impairments associated with the defect. However, any abnormal adhesion of the spinal cord to the area of the malformation may lead to neuromuscular disturbances.

spinal /spī′nəl/ [L *spina*], **1.** of or pertaining to a spine, especially the spinal column. **2.** *informal;* spinal anesthesia, such as saddle block or caudal anesthesia.

spinal accessory nerve. See **accessory nerve.**

spinal anesthesia, a state of insensitivity to pain in the lower part of the body produced by injection of an analgesic drug or anesthetic drug into the subarachnoid space of the spinal cord.

spinal aperture, a large opening formed by the body of a vertebra and its arch.

spinal block, an obstruction of cerebrospinal fluid circulation.

spinal canal, the cavity within the vertebral column.

spinal caries. See **tuberculous spondylitis.**

spinal column. See **vertebral column.**

spinal cord, a long, nearly cylindric structure lodged in the vertebral canal and extending from the foramen magnum at the base of the skull to the upper part of the lumbar region. A major component of the central nervous system, the adult cord is approximately 1 cm in diameter with an average length of 42 to 45 cm and a weight of 30 g. The cord conducts sensory and motor impulses to and from the brain and controls many reflexes. Thirty-one spinal nerves originate from the cord: 8 cervical, 12 thoracic, 5 lumbar, 5 sacral, and 1 coccygeal. It has an inner core of gray material consisting mainly of nerve cells and is enclosed by three protective membranes (meninges): the dura mater, arachnoid, and pia mater. The cord is an extension of the medulla oblongata of the brain and ends near the third lumbar vertebra.

spinal cord compression, an abnormal and often serious condition resulting from pressure on the spinal cord. The symptoms range from temporary numbness of an extremity to permanent quadriplegia, depending on the cause, severity, and location of the pressure. Causes include spinal fracture, vertebral dislocation, tumor, hemorrhage, and edema associated with contusion.

spinal cord injury, any one of the traumatic disruptions of the spinal cord, often associated with extensive musculoskeletal involvement. Common spinal cord injuries are spinal fractures and dislocations, such as those commonly suffered by individuals involved in accidents. Such trauma may cause varying degrees of paraplegia and quadriplegia. Injuries to spinal structures below the first thoracic vertebra may produce paraplegia. Injuries to the spine above the first thoracic vertebra may cause quadriplegia. Injuries that completely transect the spinal cord cause permanent loss of motor and sensory functions activated by neurons below the level of the lesions involved. Spinal cord injuries produce a state of spinal shock, characterized by flaccid paralysis, and complete loss of skin sensation at the time of the injury. Musculoskeletal complications are associated with the neurologic involvement of spinal cord injuries.

spinal cord tumor, a neoplasm of the spinal cord of which more than 50% are extramedullary, about 25% are intramedullary, and the rest are extradural. Symptoms usually develop slowly and may progress from unilateral paresthesia and a dull ache to lancinating pain, weakness in one or both legs, abnormal deep tendon reflexes, and, in advanced cases, monoplegia, hemiplegia, or paraplegia. Function of the autonomic nervous system is sometimes disturbed, causing areas of dry, cold, bluish pink skin or profuse sweating of the lower extremities.

spinal curvature, any persistent, abnormal deviation of the vertebral column from its normal position. Kinds of spinal curvature are **kyphoscoliosis, kyphosis, lordosis,** and **scoliosis.**

spinal dysrhaphis. See **spina bifida.**

spinal fasciculi. See **spinal tract.**

spinal fluid. See **cerebrospinal fluid.**

spinal fusion, the fixation of an unstable segment of the spine, accomplished by skeletal traction or immobilization of the patient in a body cast but most frequently by a surgical procedure.

spinal headache, a headache occurring after spinal anesthesia or lumbar puncture, caused by a loss of cerebrospinal fluid (CSF) from the subarachnoid space, resulting in traction of the meninges on the pressure-sensitive intracranial structures. Severe spinal headache may be accompanied by diminished aural and visual acuity. Treatment usually includes keeping the patient flat in bed to relieve the meningeal irritation, encouraging an increased fluid intake to increase the production and volume of CSF, and administering analgesics to reduce pain.

spinal manipulation, the forced passive flexion, extension, and rotation of vertebral segments, carrying the elements of articulation beyond the usual range of movement to the limit of anatomic range.

spinal nerves, the 31 pairs of nerves without special names that are connected to the spinal cord and numbered according to the level of the cord at which they emerge. There are 8 cervical, 12 thoracic, 5 lumbar, and 5 sacral pairs, and 1 coccygeal pair. The first cervical pair of nerves

S

emerges from the spinal cord in the space between the first cervical vertebra and the occipital bone. The rest of the cervical pairs and all the thoracic pairs emerge horizontally through the intervertebral foramen of their respective vertebrae. The lumbar, the sacral, and the coccygeal nerve pairs descend from their points of origin at the lower end of the cord before reaching the intervertebral foramina of their respective vertebrae. Each spinal nerve attaches to the spinal cord by an anterior root and a posterior root. The posterior roots accompany a distended spinal ganglion within the vertebral foramina. Emerging from the cord, each spinal nerve divides into the anterior, the posterior, and the white rami, the anterior and the posterior rami serving the voluntary nervous system, the white rami serving the autonomic nervous system.

spinal puncture. See **lumbar puncture.**

spinal reflex, any reflex with a pathway through the spinal cord but not the brain.

spinal shock, a form of shock associated with acute injury to the spinal cord.

spinal tract, any one of the ascending and descending pathways for motor or sensory nerve impulses that is found in the white matter of the spinal cord. Twenty-one different tracts lie within the dorsal, the ventral, and the lateral funiculi of the white substance. Ascending tracts conduct impulses up the spinal cord to the brain; descending tracts conduct impulses down the cord from the brain. Touch, pressure, proprioception, temperature, and pain are sensory stimuli transmitted via the spinal tracts. Reflex and voluntary motor activity are regulated by motor nerve stimulation from the brain and brainstem to the motor neurons of the spinal cord.

spin density, (in nuclear magnetic resonance [NMR] imaging) a measure of the hydrogen concentration. It is a quantity proportional to the number of hydrogen nuclei precessing at the Larmor frequency and contributing to the NMR signal.

spindle [AS *spinel* to spin], **1.** the fusiform figure of achromatin in the cell nucleus during the late prophase and the metaphase of mitosis. **2.** a type of brain wave, consisting of a short series of changes in electric potential with a frequency of 14 per second. **3.** any one of the special receptor organs comprising the neurotendinous and the neuromuscular spindles distributed throughout the body.

spindle cell carcinoma, a rapidly growing neoplasm composed of fusiform squamous cells. It may be difficult to distinguish from a sarcoma.

spindle cell nevus. See **benign juvenile melanoma.**

spine, the vertebral column, or backbone.

spine of scapula, a sharp-edged plate of bone projecting backward from the flattened scapula base.

spin-lattice relaxation time. See **relaxation time.**

spinnbarkeit /spin′bärkīt, shpin′-/ [Ger, threadability], the clear, slippery, elastic consistency characteristic of cervical mucus during ovulation. It has the consistency of an uncooked egg white, and it is a valuable sign of the peak fertile period in a woman's menstrual cycle.

spinocerebellar /spī′nōser′əbel′ər/ [L *spina* + *cerebellum* small brain], of or pertaining to the spinal cord and the cerebellum.

spinocerebellar disorder, an inherited disorder characterized by a progressive degeneration of the spinal cord and cerebellum, often involving other parts of the nervous system as well. These disorders tend to occur within families and can be inherited as dominant or recessive traits. Some kinds of spinocerebellar degeneration are **ataxia telangiectasia, Charcot-Marie-Tooth atrophy, Dejerine-Sottas disease, Friedreich's ataxia, olivopontocerebellar atrophy,** and **Refsum's syndrome.**

spinofallopian tube shunt. See **ventriculofallopian tube shunt.**

spinous /spī′nəs/ [L, *spina* backbone], pertaining to an object that has the shape of a spine or thorn.

spinous process [L *spina* backbone, *processus*], a spinelike projection of bony tissue.

spinous process of vertebrae, the bony projection extending posteriorly from a vertebral arch.

spin-spin relaxation time. See **relaxation tme.**

spiral bandage /spī′rəl/ [Gk *speira* coil; Fr *bande* strip], any roller bandage applied around a limb that ascends the body part with each turn overlapping the previous one by half to two thirds of a bandage width.

spiral fracture [Gk *speira* coil], a bone break in which the disruption of bone tissue is spiral, oblique, or transverse to the long axis of the fractured bone.

spiral organ of Corti. See **organ of Corti.**

spiral reverse bandage, a spiral bandage that is turned and folded back on itself as necessary to make it fit the contour of the body more securely.

spirillary rat-bite fever, spirillum fever. See **rat-bite fever.**

spirit /spir′it/ [L *spiritus* breath], **1.** any

volatile liquid, particularly one that has been distilled. **2.** a volatile substance dissolved in alcohol.

spirit of ammonia [L *spiritus; Ammon* temple in Libya], a solution of 3% ammonium carbonate in alcohol with flavorings added. It is mixed with water for use as a stimulant and carminative.

spiritual distress (distress of the human spirit), NANDA-accepted nursing diagnosis of a disruption in the life principle that pervades a person's entire being and integrates and transcends biopsychosocial nature. Defining characteristics include stated anger against the deity or questions about the meaning of the suffering being experienced. The client may joke in a macabre fashion, regard the illness as punishment, have nightmares, cry, act in a hostile or apathetic manner, express self-blame or deny all responsibility for the problem, express anger or resentment against religious figures, and cease participation in religious practices.

spiritual therapy [L *spiritus;* Gk *therapeia* treatment], psychotherapy that involves moral and religious influences on behavior and physical health.

Spirochaeta pallida /spī'rəkē'təl/ [Gk *speira* coil, *chaite* hair; L *pallidus* pale], a species of flexible, spiral, motile microorganisms that is the cause of human syphilis.

spirochete /spī'rəkēt'/ [Gk *speira* coil, *chaite* hair], any bacterium of the genus *Spirochaeta* that is motile and spiral-shaped with flexible filaments. Kinds of spirochetes include the organisms responsible for leptospirosis, relapsing fever, syphilis, and yaws. **–spirochetal,** *adj.*

spirochetemia /spī'rōkətē'mē-ə/, the presence of spirochetal organisms in the blood.

spirogram /spī'rōgram/ [Gk *speira* + *gramma* record], a visual record of respiratory movements made by a spirometer, used in the assessment of pulmonary function and capacity.

spirograph /spī'rəgraf/ [Gk *speira* + *graphein* to record], a device for recording respiratory movements. **–spirographic,** *adj.*

spirometer /spīrom'ətər/ [Gk *speira* + *metron* measure], an instrument that measures and records the volume of inhaled and exhaled air, used to assess pulmonary function. **–spirometric,** *adj.*

spirometry /spīrom'ətrē/, laboratory evaluation of the air capacity of the lungs by means of a spirometer. **–spirometric,** *adj.*

spironolactone /spī'rənəlak'tōn/, an aldosterone antagonist prescribed in the treatment of primary hyperaldosteronism, edema of congestive heart failure, cirrhosis of the liver accompanied by edema, the nephrotic syndrome, essential hypertension, and hypokalemia.

spittle [AS *spittan* spew], saliva.

Spitz nevus. See **benign juvenile melanoma.**

splanchnic /splangk'nik/, of or pertaining to the internal organs; visceral.

splanchnic engorgement /splangk'nik/, the excessive filling or pooling of blood within the visceral vasculature following the removal of pressure from the abdomen, as in the excision of a large tumor, or birth of a child.

splanchnic nerves, a network of nerves, mainly preganglionic fibers, with filaments innervating the penis and clitoris, as well as the uterus, rectum, and other structures of the abdominal cavity.

splanchnocele [Gk *splanchna* viscera, *kele* hernia], hernial protrusion of any abdominal viscera.

splanchnocoele /splangk'nōsēl'/ [Gk *splanchna* viscera, *koilos* hollow], a part of the embryonic body cavity, or coelom, that gives rise to the abdominal, pericardial, and pleural cavities.

splanchnopleure /splangk'nōplŏŏr'/ [Gk *splanchna* + *pleura* side], a layer of tissue in the early developing embryo, formed by the union of endoderm and splanchnic mesoderm. **–splanchnopleural,** *adj.*

S-plasty /es'plas'tē/, a technique of plastic surgery in which an S-shaped instead of a straight line incision is made to reduce tension and improve healing in areas where the skin is loose.

splayfoot [ME *splaien;* AS *fot*], a foot that is flat and extremely everted, away from the midline.

spleen [Gk *splen*], a soft, highly vascular, roughly ovoid organ situated between the stomach and the diaphragm in the left hypochondriac region of the body. It is considered part of the lymphatic system because it contains lymphatic nodules. It has a dark purple color and varies in shape in different individuals. Macrophages lining the sinuses of the spleen destroy microorganisms by phagocytosis. The spleen also produces leukocytes, monocytes, lymphocytes, and plasma cells. If the body suffers severe hemorrhage, the spleen can increase the blood volume from 350 ml to 550 ml in less than 60 seconds. **–splenic** /splen'ik/, *adj.*

spleen scan, the scan of the spleen after the injection of radioactive red blood cells, performed to detect a tumor, damage, or other problem.

S

splenectomy /splənek'təmē/ [Gk *splen* + *ektome* excision], the surgical excision of the spleen.

splenic flexure /splen'ik/ [Gk *splen;* L *flectere* to bend], the left flexure of the colon, as it bends at the junction of the transverse and descending segments of the colon, near the spleen.

splenic flexure syndrome [Gk *splen* + L *flectere* to bend], a recurrent pain and abdominal distention in the left upper quadrant of the abdomen caused by a pocket of gas trapped in the large intestine below the spleen, at the flexure of the transverse and descending colon.

splenic gland. See **pancreaticolienal node.**

splenic vein. See **lienal vein.**

splenius capitis /splē'nē·əs/ [Gk *splenion* bandage; L *caput* head], one of a pair of deep muscles of the back. It acts to rotate, extend, and bend the head.

splenius cervicis, one of a pair of deep muscles of the back. The splenius cervicis acts to rotate, bend, and extend the head and neck.

splenohepatomegaly /splē'nōhep'ətō-meg'əlē/ [Gk *splen* + *hepar* liver, *megas* great], an abnormal simultaneous increase in the sizes of the liver and spleen.

splenomedullary leukemia. See **acute myelocytic leukemia, chronic myelocytic leukemia.**

splenomegaly /splē'nōmeg'əlē, splen'-/ [Gk *splen* + *megas* large], an abnormal enlargement of the spleen, as is associated with portal hypertension, hemolytic anemia, Niemann-Pick disease, or malaria.

splenomyelogenous leukemia. See **acute myelocytic leukemia, chronic myelocytic leukemia.**

splint [D *splinte* piece of wood], **1.** an orthopedic device for immobilization, restraint, or support of any part of the body. It may be rigid (of metal, plaster, or wood) or flexible (of felt or leather). **2.** (in dentistry) a device for anchoring the teeth or modifying the bite.

splinter [D *splinte*], a sharp pointed piece of bone or other substance.

splinter fracture [D *splinte*], a comminuted fracture with thin, sharp bone fragments.

splinter hemorrhage, linear bleeding under a fingernail or toenail, resembling a splinter.

splinting, the process of immobilizing, restraining, or supporting a body part.

split gene [D *splitten* to split], (in molecular genetics) a genetic unit whose continuity is interrupted.

split personality. See **multiple personality.**

split Russell traction, an orthopedic mechanism that combines suspension and traction to immobilize, position, and align the lower extremities in the treatment of congenital hip dislocation, hip and knee contractures, and in the correction of orthopedic deformities.

splitting, a primitive defense mechanism that when overused represents a developmental arrest. There is a failure to synthesize the experiences and ideas one has of oneself, other people, situations, and institutions.

spondylitic [Gk *sphondylos* vertebra], pertaining to a person afflicted with spondylitis.

spondylitis /spon'dəlī'tis/ [Gk *sphondylos* vertebra, *itis*], an inflammation of any of the spinal vertebrae, usually characterized by stiffness and pain. The condition may follow traumatic injury to the spine, or it may be the result of infection or rheumatoid disease.

spondylolisthesis /spon'dilōlisthē'sis/ [Gk *sphondylos* + *olisthanein* to slip], the partial forward dislocation of one vertebra over the one below it.

spondylosis /spon'dilō'sis/ [Gk *sphondylos* + *osis*], a condition of the spine characterized by fixation or stiffness of a vertebral joint.

spondylosyndesis. See **spinal fusion.**

spondylous /spon'diləs/ [Gk *sphondylos* vertebra], pertaining to a vertebra.

sponge /spunj/ [Gk *spongia*], **1.** a resilient, absorbent mass used to absorb fluids, to apply medication, or to cleanse. **2.** *informal;* a folded gauze square used in surgery.

sponge bath, the procedure of washing the patient with a damp washcloth or sponge, used when a full bath is not necessary or as a method of reducing body temperature.

sponge contraceptive. See **vaginal sponge.**

sponge gold. See **mat gold.**

spongioblastoma /spun'jē·ōblastō'mə/, *pl.* **spongioblastomas, spongioblastomata** [Gk *spongia* + *blastos* germ, *oma* tumor], a neoplasm composed of spongioblasts, embryonic epithelial cells that develop around the neural tube and transform into cells of the supporting connective tissue of nerve cells or cells of lining membranes of the ventricles and the spinal cord canal.

spongioblastoma multiforme. See **glioblastoma multiforme.**

spongioblastoma unipolare /yoo'ni-pōler'ē/, a rare neoplasm composed of approximately parallel spongioblasts. It may occur near the third ventricle, in the

spongiocytoma. See **spongioblastoma.**

spongy /spun'jē/ [Gk *spoggia*], pertaining to or resembling a sponge.

spongy bone, a latticelike arrangement of bony plates and trabeculae occurring at the ends of the long bones.

spontaneous /spontā'nē·əs/ [L *sponte* willingly], occurring naturally and without apparent cause, such as spontaneous remission.

spontaneous abortion, a termination of pregnancy before the twentieth week of gestation as a result of abnormalities of the conceptus or maternal environment.

spontaneous delivery, a vaginal birth occurring without the mechanical assistance of obstetric forceps or vacuum aspirator.

spontaneous evolution, the unassisted delivery of a fetus in the transverse position.

spontaneous fracture. See **neoplastic fracture.**

spontaneous generation, the theoretical origin of living organisms from inanimate matter; abiogenesis.

spontaneous labor, a labor beginning and progressing without mechanical or pharmacologic stimulation.

spontaneous PEEP (sPEEP), a spontaneous breathing system with end-expiratory pressure.

spontaneous phagocytosis [L *sponte*; Gk *phagein* to eat, *kytos* cell, *osis* condition], ingestion of antigenic particles by phagocytes of the reticuloendothelial system.

spontaneous pneumothorax [L *sponte*; Gk *pneuma* air, *thorax* chest], the presence of air or gas in the intrapleural space as a result of a rupture of the lung parenchyma and visceral pleura with no demonstrable cause.

spontaneous ventilation, normal breathing, unassisted, in which the patient creates the pressure gradient through muscle and chest wall movements that move the air into and out of the lungs.

spontaneous version [L *sponte, vertere* to turn], a change in the lie of a fetus that occurs without manipulation.

spoon nail [AS *spon, naegel*], a nail of the finger or toe that is thin and concave.

sporadic /spôrat'ik/ [Gk *sporaden* scattered], (of a number of events) occurring at scattered, intermittent, and apparently random intervals.

spore [Gk *sporos* seed], **1.** a reproductive unit of some genera of fungi or protozoa. **2.** a form assumed by some bacteria that is resistant to heat, drying, and chemicals. Diseases caused by spore-forming bacte-

ria include anthrax, botulism, gas gangrene, and tetanus.

sporicidal /spôrlisī'dəl/[Gk *sporos* seed; L *caedere* to kill], a chemical or other agent that kills spores.

sporicide /spôr'isīd/ [Gk *sporos* + L *caedere* to kill], any agent effective in destroying spores, such as compounds of chlorine and formaldehyde, and the gluteraldehydes.

sporiferous /spôrif'ərəs/, producing or bearing spores.

spork, a spoonlike food utensil with fork tines specially designed for persons with upper extremity disabilities.

sporoblast /spôr'əblast'/ [Gk *sporos* + *blastos* germ], any cell that gives rise to a sporozoite or spore during the sexual reproductive phase of the life cycle of a sporozoan, specifically the cells resulting from the multiple fission of the encysted zygote of the malarial parasite *Plasmodium* from which the sporozoites develop.

sporocyst /spôr'əsist'/ [Gk *sporos* + *kystis* bag], **1.** any structure containing spores or reproductive cells. **2.** a saclike structure, or oocyst, secreted by the zygote of certain protozoa before sporozoite formation. **3.** the second larval stage in the life cycle of parasitic flukes.

sporogenesis /spôr'ōjen'əsis/ [Gk *sporos* + *genesis* origin], **1.** the formation of spores. **2.** reproduction by means of spores. –**sporogenic,** *adj.*

sporogenous /spôroj'ənəs/ [Gk *sporos* + *genein* to produce], describing an animal or plant that reproduces by spores.

sporogeny. See **sporogenesis.**

sporogony /spôrog'ənē/ [Gk *sporos* + *genesis* origin], reproduction by means of spores, specifically the formation of sporozoites during the sexual stage of the life cycle of a sporozoan, primarily the malarial parasite *Plasmodium.*

sporont /spôr'ont/ [Gk *sporos* + *on* being], a mature protozoan parasite in the sexual reproductive stage of its life cycle.

sporonticide /spôron'tisīd/ [Gk *sporos, on* + L *caedere* to kill], any substance that destroys sporonts, such as chloroquine and other antimalarial drugs. –**sporonticidal,** *adj.*

sporophore /spôr'əfôr/ [Gk *sporos* + *pherein* to bear], the part of an organism or plant that produces spores.

sporophyte /spôr'əfīt/ [Gk *sporos* + *phyton* plant], the asexual, spore-bearing stage in plants that reproduce by alternation of generations.

sporotrichosis /spôr'ōtrikō'sis/ [Gk *sporos* + *thrix* hair, *osis* condition], a common, chronic fungal infection caused by the species *Sporothrix schenckii,* usually charac-

S

terized by skin ulcers and subcutaneous nodules along lymphatic channels. The fungus is found in soil and decaying vegetation and usually enters the skin by accidental injury.

Sporotrichum /spôrot′rikəm/ [Gk *sporos* + *thrix* hair], a genus of soil-inhabiting fungi formerly thought to cause sporotrichosis.

Sporozoa /spôr′əzō′ə/ [Gk *sporos* + *zoon* animal], a class of parasite in the phylum Protozoa that is characterized by the absence of any external organs of locomotion. Included in this class are the genera *Toxoplasma* and *Plasmodium.*

sporozoite /spôrəzō′it/ [Gk *sporos* + *zoon* animal], any of the cells resulting from the sexual union of spores during the life cycle of a sporozoan.

sport [ME *disporten* to amuse], 1. an individual or organism that differs drastically from its parents or others of its type because of genetic mutation; a mutant. 2. a genetic mutation.

sports medicine, a branch of medicine that specializes in the prevention and treatment of injuries resulting from training and participation in athletic events. Among the most common sports injuries are shin splints, runner's knee, pulled hamstring muscles, Achilles tendonitis, ankle sprain, tennis elbow, baseball finger, dislocations, muscle cramps, and bursitis.

sporulation /spôr′yəlā′shən/ [Gk *sporos* + L *atus* process], 1. a type of reproduction that occurs in lower plants and animals, such as fungi, algae, and protozoa, and involves the formation of spores by the spontaneous division of the cell into four or more daughter cells, each of which contains a portion of the original nucleus. 2. the formation of a refractile body, or resting spore, within certain bacteria that makes the cell resistant to unfavorable environmental conditions.

spot [ME, blot], (in psychotherapy) a small quantum of space that becomes the territorial object and extension of point behavior.

spot film, a radiograph made instantly during fluoroscopy.

spotted fever. See **Rocky Mountain spotted fever.**

spotting, the appearance of a blood-stained discharge from the vagina between menstrual periods, during pregnancy, or at the beginning of labor.

sprain [OFr *espeindre* to force out], a traumatic injury to the tendons, muscles, or ligaments around a joint, characterized by pain, swelling, and discoloration of the skin over the joint. The duration and se-

verity of the symptoms vary with the extent of damage to the supporting tissues.

sprain fracture, a fracture that results from the separation of a tendon or ligament at the point of insertion, associated with the separation of a bone at the same insertion site.

sprain of ankle or foot [OFr *espreindre;* AS *ancleow* + *fot*], sudden traction on a muscle, ligament, or capsule. The injury is not severe enough to cause a rupture of the tissue.

sprain of back [OFr *espreindre;* AS *baec*], a sudden traction injury to muscles and related tissues of the back. The tissues may have undergone traumatic strain without being ruptured.

spreader bar /spred′ər/, a metal bar with curved hoop areas for attaching hooks or pins for traction.

spring forceps [AS *springan* to jump], a kind of forceps that includes a spring mechanism, used for grasping an artery to arrest or prevent hemorrhage.

spring lancet, a lancet with a spring-triggered blade. It may be used for collecting small specimens of blood for laboratory tests.

sprinter's fracture [Swed *sprinta* to spurt; L *fractura* to break], a fracture of the anterior superior or the anterior inferior spine of the ilium, caused by a fragment of bone being forcibly pulled by a violent muscle spasm.

sprue /sprōō/ [D *sprouw* kind of tumor], a chronic disorder resulting from malabsorption of nutrients from the small intestine and characterized by diarrhea, weakness, weight loss, poor appetite, pallor, muscle cramps, bone pain, ulceration of the mucous membrane lining the digestive tract, and a smooth, shiny tongue. It occurs in both tropical and nontropical forms.

SPSS, (in statistics) abbreviation for **Statistical Package for the Social Sciences,** a computer program often used in research in clinical nursing for the analysis of complex data from large samples.

spur [AS *spura*], a projection of bone or metal from a body structure or appliance.

spurious pregnancy. See **pseudocyesis.**

sputum /spyōō′təm/ [L, spittle], material coughed up from the lungs and expectorated through the mouth. It contains mucus, cellular debris, or microorganisms, and it may also contain blood or pus. The amount, color, and constituents of the sputum are important in the diagnosis of many illnesses.

sputum specimen, a sample of material expelled from the respiratory passages taken for laboratory analysis to determine the presence of pathogens.

squama /skwā′mə/, *pl.* **squamae,** **1.** a flattened scale from the epidermis. **2.** the thin, expanded part of a bone, especially in the cranial wall. **–squamous,** *adj.*

squamous cell /skwā′məs/ [L *squama* scale; *cella* storeroom], a flat, scalelike epithelial cell.

squamous cell carcinoma, a slow-growing, malignant tumor of squamous epithelium, frequently found in the lungs and skin and occurring also in the anus, cervix, larynx, nose, bladder, and other sites. The typical skin lesion, a firm, red, horny, painless nodule is often the result of overexposure to the sun.

squamous epithelium [L *squama;* Gk *epi* above, *thele* nipple], a sheet of flattened scalelike cells, attached together at the edges.

square centimeter (cm²) /skwer/, a unit of area measurement equivalent to 1 centimeter long multiplied by 1 centimeter wide where 1 centimeter equals 0.3937 inch or 0.03281 foot.

square window [OFr *esquarre;* ME *windowe* wind-eye], an angle of the wrist between the hypothenar prominence and forearm. It is used as a reference point for estimating the gestational age of a newborn infant.

squeeze dynamometer /skwēz/ [AS *cwesan* to press tightly; Gk *dynamis* force, *metron* measure], a dynamometer for measuring the muscular strength of the grip of the hand.

squeeze-film lubrication, the exudation of fluid from the cartilage of joints, forming a film in the transient area of impending contact.

squint. See **strabismus.**

squinting eye /skwin′ting/ [D *schuinte* oblique; AS *eage*], the abnormal eye in a person with strabismus that cannot be focused with the fixated eye.

Sr, symbol for the element **strontium.**

SR, abbreviation for **sedimentation rate.**

sRNA, abbreviation for *soluble RNA.*

SRO, abbreviation for **single room occupant.**

SRS-A, abbreviation for **slow-reacting substance of anaphylaxis.**

SRY, symbol for a "maleness" gene found on the sex-determining region of the Y chromosome. The gene is believed to function as a master control switch with the ability to turn off or on other genes involved in sexual development.

ss, abbreviation for **steady state.**

SSE, abbreviation for **soapsuds enema.**

SSS, **1.** abbreviation for *sterile saline*

soak. **2.** abbreviation for **sick sinus syndrome.**

SSSS, abbreviation for **staphylococcal scalded skin syndrome.**

S's test. See **Sulkowitch's test.**

ST, abbreviation for *slow-twitch.*

stab [Swed *stabbe* thick stick], a nonsegmented neutrophil.

stab culture [ME *stabbe* piercing wound; L *colere* to cultivate], a culture made by dipping a needle into an inoculum and then into a transparent gelatin or agar medium.

stab form. See **band.**

stabile diabetes. See **non-insulin-dependent diabetes.**

stabilization /stab′ilīzā′shən/ [L *stabilis* firm, *atus* process], **1.** the physiologic and metabolic process of attaining homeostasis. **2.** the seating of a fixed or removable denture so that it will not tilt or be displaced under pressure. **3.** the control of induced stress loads and the development of measures to counteract such forces so that the movement of the teeth or of a prosthesis does not irritate surrounding tissues.

stable /stā′bəl/ [L *stabilis* stand], remaining unchanged.

stable condition, a state of health in which the prognosis indicates little if any immediate change.

stable element [L *stabilis* firm; *elementum*], a nonradioactive element, one not subject to spontaneous nuclear degeneration. Some kinds of stable elements are calcium, iron, lead, potassium, and sodium.

staccato speech /stəkä′tō/ [It, detached; ME *speche*], abnormal speech in which the person pauses between words, breaking the rhythm of the phrase or sentence. The condition is sometimes observed in association with multiple sclerosis.

stadium /stā′dē·əm/, *pl.* **stadia** [Gk *stadion* racetrack], a significant stage in a fever or illness, such as the fastigium of a febrile illness or the prodromal stage of a viral infection.

staff [AS *staef*], **1.** the people who work toward a common goal and are employed or supervised by someone of higher rank. **2.** a designation by which a staff nurse is distinguished from a head nurse or other nurse. **3.** (in nursing education) the nonprofessional employees of the institution, such as librarians, technicians, secretaries, and clerks. **4.** (in nursing service administration) the units of the organization that provide service to the "line," or administratively defined hierarchy.

staff development, (in nursing) a process

S

that assists individual nurses in an agency or organization in attaining new skills and knowledge, gaining increasing levels of competence, and growing professionally. The process may include such programs as orientation, in-service education, and continuing education.

staffing, the process of assigning people to fill the roles designed for an organizational structure through recruitment, selection, and placement.

staffing pattern, (in hospital or nursing administration) the number and kinds of staff assigned to the particular units and departments of a hospital. Staffing patterns vary with the unit, department, and shift.

staff of Æsculapius, a staff carried by Æsculapius, the Greek god of medicine. It is used as the traditional symbol of the physician. A single serpent entwines the staff of Æsculapius.

stage [OFr *estage*], 1. a platform. 2. a period or phase.

stages of anesthesia. See **Guedel's signs.**

stages of dying [OFr *estage* stage; ME *dyen* to lose life], the five emotional and behavioral stages that often occur after a person first learns of approaching death. The stages, identified and described by Elizabeth Kübler-Ross, are denial and shock, anger, bargaining, depression, and acceptance. The stages may occur in sequence or they may recur, as the person moves forward and backward—especially between denial, anger, and bargaining.

stagnant anoxia /stag′nənt/ [L *stagnum* standing water; Gk *a* without, *oxys* sharp, *genein* to produce], a condition in which there is inadequate blood flow in the capillaries causing low tissue oxygen tension and reduced oxygen exchange.

stain [OFr *desteindre* to dye], 1. a pigment, dye, or substance used to impart color to microscopic objects or tissues to facilitate their examination and identification. Kinds of stains include **acid-fast stain, Gram stain,** and **Wright's stain. 2.** to apply pigment to a substance or tissue to examine it under a microscope. 3. an area of discoloration.

stained film fault, a defect in a radiograph or developed photographic film that appears as a streaky discoloration or abnormal opacity.

stammering [AS *stamerian* to stutter], a speech dysfunction characterized by spasmodic pauses, hesitations, and faltering utterances, such as mispronunciation or the transposition of letters within a word.

stamp cusp [ME *stampen*; L *cuspis* point], a cusp that works in a fossa, such as any of the maxillary lingual cusps.

stance phase of gait [L *stare* to stand; Gk *phainein* to show; ME *gate* a way], the first phase of the normal gait cycle that begins with the strike of the heel on the ground and ends with the lift of the toe at the beginning of the swing phase of gait: the brief period in which both feet are on the ground.

standard [OFr *estandart*], 1. an evaluation that serves as a basis for comparison for evaluating similar phenomena or substances, such as a standard for the preparation of a pharmaceutical substance, or a standard for the practice of a profession. 2. a pharmaceutical preparation or a chemical substance of known quantity, ingredients, and strength that is used to determine the constituents or the strength of another preparation. 3. of known value, strength, quality, or ingredients. 4. predetermined criteria used to provide guidance in the operation of a health care or other facility to ensure quality performance by the personnel. **–standardize,** *v.,* **standardization,** *n.*

standard air chamber, a radiation measuring device used by national and international calibration laboratories to provide exposure calibrations of ion chambers for use in the diagnostic or orthovoltage energy range.

standard bicarbonate, the bicarbonate ion concentration of plasma separated anaerobically from whole blood that has been saturated with oxygen and equilibrated at carbon dioxide pressure of 40 torr at 38° C. It is a measure of the metabolic disturbance of acid-base balance in a sample of blood after any respiratory disturbance present has been corrected.

standard death certificate, a form for a death certificate that is commonly used throughout the United States.

standard deviation (SD), (in statistics) a mathematic statement of the dispersion of a set of values or scores from the mean. Each sample value is subtracted from the sample mean and squared, and the squares are summed. The square root of the summed squares gives a mathematically standardized value so that sample deviations can be compared.

standard environmental chamber. See **Skinner box.**

standard error, (in statistics) the variability in scores that can be expected if measurements are made on random samples of the same size from the same universe of population, phenomena, or observations. The standard error provides a framework within which a determination of the difference between groups may be made.

standardized death rate /stan′dərdīzd′/,

the number of deaths per 1,000 people of a specified population during 1 year. This rate is adjusted to avoid distortion by the age composition of the population.

standard of care, a written statement describing the rules, actions, or conditions that direct patient care. Standards of care guide practice and can be used to evaluate performance.

standards of nursing practice, a set of guidelines for providing quality nursing care and a criteria for evaluating care. Such guidelines help assure patients that they are receiving high-quality care. The standards are important if a legal dispute arises over the quality of care provided a patient.

standing orders [L *stare* to stand; *ordo* rank], a written document containing rules, policies, procedures, regulations, and orders for the conduct of patient care in various stipulated clinical situations. Standing orders usually name the condition and prescribe the action to be taken in caring for the patient, including the dosage and route of administration for a drug or the schedule for the administration of a therapeutic procedure.

stannous fluoride /stan′əs/ [L *stannum* tin, *fluere* to flow], a salt of fluorine and tin used in oral hygiene products to reduce caries activity.

stanozolol /stənō′zəlol, -ōl/, an androgenic anabolic steroid prescribed in the treatment of aplastic anemia and osteoporosis.

stapedectomy /stā′pədek′təmē/ [L *stapes* stirrup; Gk *ektome* excision], removal of the stapes of the middle ear and insertion of a graft and prosthesis, performed to restore hearing in the treatment of otosclerosis. The stapes that has become fixed is replaced so that vibrations again transmit sound waves through the oval window to the fluid of the inner ear.

stapedius /stəpē′dē·əs/, a small muscle on the wall of the tympanic cavity of the middle ear. It pulls the head of the stapes posteriorly, tilting the baseplate, and, with the tensor tympani, acts reflexively in response to loud sounds to reduce excessive vibrations that could injure the internal ear.

stapes /stā′pēz/ [L, stirrup], one of the three ossicles in the middle ear, resembling a tiny stirrup. It transmits sound vibrations from the incus to the internal ear.

staphylococcal infection /staf′ilōkok′əl/ [Gk *staphlye* bunch of grapes, *kokkos* berry; L *inficere* to taint], an infection caused by any one of several pathogenic species of *Staphylococcus,* commonly characterized by the formation of abscesses of the skin or other organs. Staphylococcal infections of the skin include carbuncles, folliculitis, furuncles, and hidradenitis suppurativa. Bacteremia is common and may result in endocarditis, meningitis, or osteomyelitis. Staphylococcal pneumonia often follows influenza or other viral disease and may be associated with chronic or debilitating illness. Acute gastroenteritis may result from an enterotoxin produced by certain species of staphylococci in contaminated food.

staphylococcal pneumonia, pneumonia caused by a staphylococcus infection.

staphylococcal scalded skin syndrome (SSSS), an abnormal skin condition characterized by epidermal erythema, peeling, and necrosis that gives the skin a scalded appearance. This disorder primarily affects infants 1 to 3 months of age and other children, but it may also affect adults. It is caused by strains of *Staphylococcus aureus,* especially group II phage types. Deficient immune functions and renal insufficiency. may predispose individuals to the disease. SSSS is more common in the newborn infant because of undeveloped immunity and renal systems.

Staphylococcus /staf′ilōkok′əs/ *pl.* **staphylococci** [Gk *staphlye* + *kokkos* berry], a genus of nonmotile, spheric, gram-positive bacteria. Some species are normally found on the skin and in the throat; certain species cause severe, purulent infections or produce an enterotoxin, which may cause nausea, vomiting, and diarrhea. *Staphylococcus aureus* is a species frequently responsible for abscesses, endocarditis, impetigo, osteomyelitis, pneumonia, and septicemia. **–staphylococcal,** *adj.*

Staphylococcus aureus [Gk *staphyle* + *kokkos*; L *aurum* gold], a species of *Staphylococcus* that produces a golden pigment with some color variations. It is also responsible for a number of pyogenic infections, such as boils, carbuncles, and abscesses.

staphylokinase /staf′ilōkī′nās/, an enzyme, produced by certain strains of staphylococci, that catalyzes the conversion of plasminogen to plasmin in various animal hosts of the microorganism.

staple /stā′pəl/, a piece of stainless steel wire used to close certain surgical wounds.

stapling [ME *stapel* stake], a method of fastening tissues together at the end of surgery by using a U-shaped piece of wire as a suture. The ends of the wire are bent toward the center close the staple.

starch [AS *stearc* strong], the principal molecule used for the storage of food in plants. Starch is a polysaccharide and is composed of long chains of glucose sub-

S

units. In animals, excess glucose is stored as glycogen.

Starling's law of the heart [Ernest H. Starling, English physiologist, b. 1866; AS *lagu* law, *heorte* heart], a rule that the force of the heartbeat is determined by the length of the fibers comprising the myocardial walls.

Starr-Edwards prosthesis [A. Starr, twentieth-century American physician; M. L. Edwards, twentieth-century American physician; Gk *prosthesis* attachment], an artificial cardiac valve. A caged-ball form of device, it obstructs the valve opening and prevents the backward flow of blood.

start codon. See **initiation codon.**

startle reflex /stä′təl/ [ME *stertlen* to rush; Gk *syn,* together, *dromos* course], a reflex response to a sudden, unexpected stimulus. The reaction may be accompanied by physiologic effects including increased heartbeat and respiration, closing the eyes. and flexion of trunk muscles. The reaction is rapid, pervasive, and uncontrollable, regardless of the unexpected stimulus, which may be as simple as a touch. However, premature and immature infants may not show the reaction.

start point [ME *sterte;* L *punctus* pricked], (in molecular genetics) the initial nucleotide transcribed from the DNA template in the formation of messenger RNA.

starvation /stärvā′shən/ [ME *sterven* to die], **1.** a condition resulting from the lack of essential nutrients over a long period of time and characterized by multiple physiologic and metabolic dysfunctions. **2.** the act or state of starving or being starved.

stasis /stā′sis, stas′is/ [Gk, standing], **1.** a disorder in which the normal flow of a fluid through a vessel of the body is slowed or halted. **2.** stillness.

stasis dermatitis, a common result of venous insufficiency of the legs beginning with ankle edema and progressing to tan pigmentation, patchy erythema, petechiae, and induration. Ultimately, there may be atrophy and fibrosis of the skin and subcutaneous tissue, with ulcerations that are slow to heal. The tan pigment is hemosiderin from blood leaking through capillary walls under elevated venous pressure. The involved skin is very easily irritated or sensitized to topical medications.

stasis ulcer, a necrotic craterlike lesion of the skin of the lower leg caused by chronic venous congestion. The ulcer is often associated with stasis dermatitis and varicose veins.

stat., abbreviation for the Latin word, *statim,* meaning "immediately."

state /stāt/ [L *status* condition], the circumstances or qualities that characterize a person, thing, or way of being at a particular time.

State Board Test Pool Examination (SBTPE), revised and retitled in 1982 as the NCLEX-RN, an examination prepared by the National Council of State Boards of Nursing for testing the competency of a person to perform safely as a newly licensed registered nurse. Each jurisdiction within the United States and its territories regulates entry into the practice of nursing; each requires the candidate to pass the examination. The content of the examination is planned to test the candidates' knowledge of the nursing process as applied to the broad areas of nursing practice, including maternal and child health, medical and surgical nursing, and psychiatric nursing.

state medicine. See **socialized medicine.**

State Nurses' Association (SNA), an association of nurses at the state level. The various State Nurses' Associations are constituent units of the American Nurses' Association.

Statewide Health Coordinating Committee (SHCC), a component of the national network of Health Systems Agencies.

static /stat′ik/ [Gk *statikos* causing to stand], without motion, at rest, in equilibrium.

static cardiac work, the energy transfer that occurs during the development and maintenance of ventricular pressure immediately before the opening of the aortic valve.

static electricity film fault, a defect in a radiograph or a developed photographic film, which appears as lightninglike streaks. It is caused by too rapid opening of the film packet or transfer of static electricity from the user to the film.

static equilibrium, the ability of an individual to adjust to displacements of his or her center of gravity while maintaining a constant base of support.

static imaging, (in nuclear medicine) a diagnostic procedure in which a radioactive substance is administered to a patient to visualize an internal organ or body compartment. An image or set of images is made of the fixed or slowly changing distribution of the radioactivity.

static pressure, a condition of equalized blood pressure throughout the body when the heart beat is stopped. A nonmoving fluid exerts a uniform pressure in all directions.

static reflex, a reflex that helps one maintain normal posture and muscle tone when the body is at rest.

static scoliosis, a form of scoliosis resulting from a difference in the length of the legs.

station /stā′shən/ [L *stare* to stand], the level of the biparietal plane of the fetal head relative to the level of the ischial spines of the maternal pelvis. An imaginary plane at the level of the spines is designated "zero station." Higher and lower stations are numbered at intervals of 1 cm and labeled as minus above and plus below.

stationary grid /stā′shənər′ē/ [L *stare* + ME *gridere* gridiron], (in radiography) an x-ray grid that does not move or oscillate during the exposure of a radiographic film.

stationary lingual arch, an orthodontic arch wire that is designed to fit the lingual surface of the teeth and is soldered to the associated anchor bands.

statistic /stətis′tik/ [L *status* condition], a number that describes a property of a set of data or other numbers.

Statistical Package for the Social Sciences. See SPSS.

statistical significance, an interpretation of statistical data that indicates an occurrence was probably due to a causative factor and not simply a chance result. Statistical significance at the 1% level indicates a 1 in 100 chance that a result can be ascribed to chance.

statistics /stətis′tiks/, a mathematical science concerned with measuring, classifying, and analyzing objective information.

statotonic reflex. See attitudinal reflex.

status /stā′təs, stat′əs/ [L, condition], **1.** a specified state or condition, such as emotional status. **2.** an unremitting state or condition, such as status asthmaticus.

status asthmaticus, an acute, severe, and prolonged asthma attack. Hypoxia, cyanosis, and unconsciousness may follow.

status dysraphicus. See dysraphia.

status epilepticus, a medical emergency characterized by continual seizures occurring without interruptions. Status epilepticus can be precipitated by the sudden withdrawal of anticonvulsant drugs, inadequate body levels of glucose, a brain tumor, a head injury, a high fever, or poisoning.

statute of limitations [L *statuere* to place; *limes* boundary], (in law) a statute that sets a limit of time during which a suit may be brought or criminal charges may be made.

statutory rape /stach′ətôr′ē/ [L *statuere* to place; *rapere* to seize], (in law) sexual intercourse with a female below the age of consent, which varies from state to state.

STD, abbreviation for **sexually transmitted disease.**

steady state (s, ss) /sted′ē/ [AS *stedefast* firm in its place; L *status* condition], a basic physiologic concept implying that the various forces and processes of life are in a state of homeostasis.

steam sterilization [ME *steme* vapor; L *sterilis* barren], the destruction of all forms of microbial life on an object by exposing the object to moist heat for 15 minutes at 121° C.

Stearns' alcoholic amentia /sturnz/ [A. Warren Stearns, American physician, b. 1885; Ar *alkohl* essence; L *ab* from, *mens* mind], a form of insanity brought on by alcohol, characterized by an emotional disturbance of a less severe nature than that of delirium tremens but of longer duration and with greater mental clouding and amnesia.

stearrhea [Gk *stear* fat, *rhoia* flow], excessive secretion of fat.

stearyl alcohol /stē′əril/, a solid substance, prepared by the catalytic hydrogenation of stearic acid, used in various ointments.

steatorrhea /stē′ətərē′ə/ [Gk *stear* fat, *rhoia* flow], greater than normal amounts of fat in the feces, characterized by frothy, foul-smelling fecal matter that floats, as in celiac disease, some malabsorption syndromes, and any condition in which fats are poorly absorbed by the small intestine.

steatorrhea simplex, See seborrhea.

Steele-Richardson-Olszewski syndrome [John C. Steele; J. Clifford Richardson; Jerzy Olszewski; twentieth-century Canadian neurologists], a rare, progressive, neurologic disorder of unknown cause, occurring in middle age, more often in men. It is characterized by paralysis of eye muscles, ataxia, neck and trunk rigidity, pseudobulbar palsy, and parkinsonian facies. Dementia and inappropriate emotional responses are also common.

steeple head. See oxycephaly.

Steinert's disease. See myotonic muscular dystrophy.

Stein-Leventhal syndrome. See polycystic ovary syndrome.

Steinmann pin /stīn′mən/ [Fritz Steinmann, Swiss surgeon, b. 1872; AS, *pinn*], a wide diameter pin used for heavy skeletal traction, as in the tibia or femur.

stellate /stel′it, -āt/ [L *stella* star], starshaped or arranged in the pattern of a star.

stellate fracture, a fracture that involves the central point of impact or injury and radiates numerous fissures throughout surrounding bone tissue.

stellate ganglion [L *stella*; Gk *gagglion*

S

knot], a large irregular ganglion on the lowest part of the cervical sympathetic trunk fused with the first thoracic ganglion. Its branches communicate with the seventh and eighth cervical nerves.

stem cell [AS *stemm* tree trunk; L *cella* storeroom], a formative cell; a cell whose daughter cells give rise to other cell types. A **pluripotential stem cell** is one that has the potential to develop into several different types of mature cells, including lymphocytes, granulocytes, thrombocytes, and erythrocytes.

stem cell leukemia, a neoplasm of blood-forming organs in which the predominant malignant cell is too immature to classify. The acute disease has a rapid, relentless course.

stem cell lymphoma. See **undifferentiated malignant lymphoma.**

stem pessary. See **pessary.**

stenosis /stinō′sis/ [Gk *stenos* narrow, *osis* condition], an abnormal condition characterized by the constriction or narrowing of an opening or passageway in a body structure. Kinds of stenosis include **aortic stenosis** and **pyloric stenosis. –stenotic,** *adj.*

Stensen's duct. See **parotid duct.**

stent [Charles R. Stent, nineteenth-century English dentist] **1.** a compound used in making dental impressions and medical molds. **2.** a mold or device made of stent, used in anchoring skin grafts and for supporting body openings and cavities during grafting or vessels and tubes of the body during surgical anastomosis.

step-care therapy, a therapeutic program that begins with a simple, conservative type of treatment but may advance to more complex stages as needed to achieve control of a disease or disorder.

steppage gait /step′ij/ [AS *staepe;* ONorse *gata* way], a gait in which the legs are raised abnormally high, as in cases of drop foot.

step reflex. See **dance reflex.**

stepwedge /step′wej/, an aluminum device that, when exposed to x-rays, displays a range of exposure intensities on a radiograph. These exposure "steps" are analyzed to determine the speed characteristics of the radiographic film.

stereognosis /ster′ōgnō′sis/ [Gk *stereos* solid, *gnosis* knowledge], **1.** the faculty of perceiving and understanding the form and nature of objects by the sense of touch. **2.** perception by the senses of the solidity of objects. **–stereognostic,** *adj.*

stereognostic perception /ster′ē-ōgnos′tik/ [Gk *stereos* solid, *gnosis* knowledge], the ability to recognize objects by the sense of touch.

stereoisomer /stir′ē-ō-ī′səmər/ [Gk *stereos* + *isos* equal, *meros* part], one of two or more chemical compounds that contain the same atoms linked in the same way but are organized differently in space. For example, one may be the mirror-image of the other.

stereoisomeric specificity /ī′səmer′ik/ [Gk *stereos* + *isos* equal, *meros* part], specificity of an enzyme for one enantiomer of a racemic mix.

stereo-ophthalmoscope /stir′ē-ō′ofthal′-məskōp′/, an ophthalmoscope fitted with two eyepieces so the examiner can view a three-dimensional interior of the eye.

stereopsis, the quality of visual fusion.

stereoradiography /-rā′dē-og′rəfē/ [Gk *stereos* + L *radiare* to shine; Gk *graphein* to record], a technique for producing radiograms that give a three-dimensional view of an internal body structure.

stereoscopic microscope /-skop′ik/ [Gk *stereos* + *skopein* to look], a microscope that produces three-dimensional images through the use of double eyepieces and double objectives.

stereoscopic parallax. See **binocular parallax.**

stereoscopic radiograph, a composite of two radiographs, made by shifting the position of the x-ray tube a few centimeters between each of two exposures. The result is a three-dimensional presentation of the radiograph when viewed through stereoscopic lenses.

stereotaxic neuroradiography /-tak′sik/ [Gk *stereos* + *taxis* arrangement; *neuron* nerve; L *radiare* to shine; Gk *graphein* to record], an x-ray procedure commonly performed during neurosurgery to guide the insertion of a needle into a specific area of the brain.

stereotype /stir′ē-ətīp/ [Gk *stereos* + *typos* mark], a generalization about a form of behavior, an individual, or a group.

stereotypic behavior /stir′ē-ōtip′ik/, a pattern of body movements that has autistic and symbolic meaning for an individual.

stereotypy /ster′ē-ətī′pē/ [Gk *stereos* + *typos* mark], the persistent, inappropriate, mechanical repetition of actions, body postures, or speech patterns, usually occurring with a lack of variation in thought processes or ideas. **–stereotypical,** *adj.*

sterile /ster′il/ [L *sterilis* barren], **1.** barren; unable to produce children because of a physical abnormality, often the absence of spermatogenesis in a man or blockage of the fallopian tubes in a woman. **2.** aseptic. **–sterility,** *n.*

sterile field, 1. a specified area that is considered free of microorganisms. **2.** an area immediately around a patient that has been prepared for a surgical procedure. The sterile field includes the scrubbed team members, and all furniture and fixtures in the area.

sterile meningitis, a form of meningitis, usually involving a viral infection, in which there is primarily a lymphocytic response in the cerebrospinal fluid.

sterility /stəril'itē/ [L *sterilis* barren], a condition of being unable to conceive or reproduce the species.

sterilization /ster'ilizā'shən/ [L *sterilis* + Gk *izein* to cause], **1.** a process or act that renders a person unable to produce children. **2.** a technique for destroying microorganisms using heat, water, chemicals, or gases. **–sterilize,** *v.*

sternal /stur'nəl/ [Gk *sternon* chest], pertaining to the sternum.

sternal node /stur'nəl/ [Gk *sternon* chest; L *nodus* knot], a node in one of the three groups of thoracic parietal lymph nodes.

sternal puncture, a diagnostic procedure in which a needle is inserted into the marrow of the sternum to remove blood samples for diagnosis.

Sternheimer-Malbin stain /sturn'hīmər-mal'bin/, a crystal violet and safranin stain used in urinalyses to provide additional contrast for certain casts and cells.

sternoclavicular /stur'noklavik'yələr/ [Gk *sternon* chest; L *clavicula* little key], pertaining to the sternum and clavicle.

sternoclavicular articulation, the double gliding joint between the sternum and the clavicle.

sternocleidomastoid /-klī'dōmas'toid/ [Gk *sternon* + *kleis* key, *mastos* breast, *eidos* form], a muscle of the neck that is attached to the mastoid process and superior nuchal line and by separate heads to the sternum and clavicle.

sternocostal articulation /-kos'təl/ [Gk *sternon* + L *costa* rib], the gliding articulation of the cartilage of each true rib and the sternum, except for the articulation of the first rib in which the cartilage is directly united with the sternum to form a synchondrosis.

sternohyoideus /stur'nōhī·oi'dē·əs/ [Gk *sternon* + *hyoeides* upsilon-shaped], one of the four infrahyoid muscles. It acts to depress the hyoid bone.

sternothyroideus /stur'nōthīroi'dē·əs/ [Gk *sternon* + *thyreos* shield, *eidos* form], one of the four infrahyoid muscles. It acts to depress the thyroid cartilage.

sternum /stur'nəm/ [Gk *sternon*], the elongated, flattened bone forming the middle portion of the thorax. It supports the clavicles, articulates with the first seven pairs of ribs, and comprises the ma-

nubrium, the gladiolus (body), and the xiphoid process.

sternutation. See **sneeze.**

steroid /stir'oid/ [Gk *stereos* solid, *eidos* form], any of a large number of hormonal substances with a similar basic chemical structure, produced mainly in the adrenal cortex and gonads.

steroid acne, a form of acne caused by the use of corticosteroids.

steroid hormones, any of the ductless gland secretions that contain the basic steroid nucleus in their chemical formulae. The natural steroid hormones include the androgens, estrogens, and adrenal cortex secretions.

steroid hormone therapy, treatment with any of the steroid hormones, such as in the use of estrogen to reduce symptoms of postmenopausal disorders.

sterol /stir'ôl/ [Gk *stereos* + Ar *alkohl* essence], a large subgroup of steroids containing an OH group at position 3 and a branched aliphatic side chain of eight or more carbon atoms at position 17. Kinds of sterols include **cholesterol** and **ergosterol.**

stertorous /stur'tərəs/ [L *stertere* to snore], pertaining to a respiratory effort that is strenuous or struggling; having a snoring sound.

stethomimetic /steth'ōmimet'ik/, pertaining to any condition causing or associated with a reduction of chest volume below its normal value.

stethoscope /steth'əskōp/ [Gk *stethos* chest, *skopein* to look], an instrument, used in mediate auscultation, consisting of two earpieces connected by means of flexible tubing to a diaphragm, which is placed against the skin of the patient's chest or back to hear heart and lung sounds.

Stevens-Johnson syndrome [Albert M. Stevens, American pediatrician, b. 1884; F. C. Johnson, American physician, b. 1894], a serious, sometimes fatal inflammatory disease affecting children and young adults. It is characterized by the acute onset of fever, bullae on the skin, and ulcers on the mucous membranes of the lips, eyes, mouth, nasal passage, and genitalia. Pneumonia, pain in the joints, and prostration are common. A complication may be perforation of the cornea. The syndrome may be an allergic reaction to certain drugs, or it may follow pregnancy, herpesvirus I, or other infection.

Stewart, Isabel Maitland (1878-1963), a Canadian-born American nursing educator and writer. The first nurse to receive a master's degree from Columbia University in New York, she was instrumental in upgrading the nursing curriculum and in di-

S

recting educational policies and became an important figure in international nursing affairs.

STH, abbreviation for **somatotropic hormone.**

sthenic fever /sthen′ik/ [Gk *sthenos* power; L *febris* fever], high body temperature associated with thirst, dry skin, and, often, delirium.

stibocaptate. See **sodium stibocaptate.**

stibogluconate sodium /stib′ōglōō′kənāt/, an antileishmanial available from the Centers for Disease Control. It is a drug of choice for the visceral form of leishmaniasis and has some effect on other forms.

stibophen /stib′əfin/, a schistosomicide prescribed in the treatment of infestations of *Schistosoma japonicum* or *S. haematobium.*

sticky ends. See **cohesive termini.**

Stieda's fracture /stē′dəz/ [Alfred Stieda, German surgeon, b. 1869], a fracture of the internal condyle of the femur.

stiff [OE *stif*], pertaining to a condition of rigidity or muscular inflexibility.

stiff joint [OE *stif*; L *jungere* to join], a rigid or inflexible joint, as may be due to arthritis or other rheumatic disorders.

stiff lung. See **ARDS.**

stigma /stig′mə/, *pl.* **stigmata, stigmas** [Gk, brand], **1.** a moral or physical blemish. **2.** a physical characteristic that serves to identify a disease or a condition.

stigmatism /stig′mətiz′əm/ [Gk *stigma* mark], **1.** normal visual accommodation and refraction whereby light rays fall onto the retina. **2.** a condition of abnormal skin markings.

stilbestrol. See **diethylstilbestrol.**

stilet, stilette. See **stylet.**

stillbirth [AS *stille;* ME *burth*], **1.** the birth of a fetus that died before or during delivery. **2.** a fetus, born dead, that weighs more than 1,000 g and would usually have been expected to live.

stillborn [AS *stille, boren*], **1.** an infant that was born dead. **2.** of or pertaining to an infant that was born dead.

Still's disease. See **juvenile rheumatoid arthritis.**

stimulant /stim′yələnt/ [L *stimulare* to incite], any agent that increases the rate of activity of a body system.

stimulant cathartic, a cathartic that acts by promoting the motility of the bowel, especially the longitudinal peristalsis of the colon. Kinds of stimulant cathartics are cascara and senna.

stimulating bath, a bath taken in water that contains an aromatic substance, an astringent, or a tonic.

stimulation /stim′yəlā′shən/ [L *stimulare*

to incite], the condition of being stimulated.

stimulus /stim′yələs/, *pl.* **stimuli** [L *stimulare* to incite], anything that excites or incites an organism or part to function, become active, or respond. **–stimulate,** *v.*

stimulus control, a strategy for self-modification that depends on manipulating the antecedents of behavior to increase goals or behaviors desired by a patient while decreasing those that are undesired.

stimulus duration, the length of time a stimulus must be applied for the resulting nerve impulse to produce excitation in the receptor tissue.

stimulus generalization, a type of conditioning in which the reaction to one stimulus is reinforced to allow transfer of the reaction to other occurrences.

sting [AS *stingan*], an injury caused by a sharp, painful penetration of the skin, often accompanied by exposure to an irritating chemical or the venom of an insect or other animal. Kinds of stings include bee, jellyfish, scorpion, sea urchin, and shellfish stings.

stingray /sting′rā/ [AS *stingan* + L *raia* ray-fish], a flat, long-tailed fish bearing barbed spines on its back that are connected to sacs of venom. Spasm of the skeletal muscles, severe local pain, seizures, and dyspnea may occur if the skin is broken by the spines.

stippling [D *stippen* to prick], the appearance of colored dots in some cells when stained. Red stippling in blood cells stained with eosin hematoxylin is a sign of malaria.

stitch [ME *stiche*], **1.** a suture. **2.** a sudden sharp pain.

stitch abscess, an abscess that develops around a suture.

St. Louis encephalitis /sāntlōō′is/ [St. Louis, Missouri; Gk *enkephalon* brain, *itis* inflammation], an arbovirus infection of the brain transmitted from birds to humans by the bite of an infected mosquito. It is characterized by headache, malaise, fever, stiff neck, delirium, and convulsions. Sequelae may include visual and speech disturbances, difficulty in walking, and personality changes. Convalescence may be prolonged, and death may result.

stocking aid, a device that enables a handicapped person to pull on a pair of stockings. One type consists of a dowel with a cuphook on the end.

stoker's cramp. See **heat cramp.**

Stokes-Adams syndrome. See **Adams-Stokes syndrome.**

stoma /stō′mə/, *pl.* **stomas, stomata** [Gk, mouth], **1.** a pore, orifice, or opening on a surface. **2.** an artificial opening of an internal organ on the surface of the body, created surgically, as for a colostomy, ileostomy, or tracheostomy. **3.** a new opening created surgically between two body structures, such as for a gastroenterostomy.

stomach /stum′ək/ [Gk *stomakhos* gullet], the major organ of digestion, located in the right upper quadrant of the abdomen and divided into a body and a pylorus. It receives and partially processes food and drink funneled from the mouth through the esophagus and moves nutritional bulk into the intestines. It is lined with a mucous coat, a submucous coat, a muscular coat, and a serous coat, all richly supplied with blood vessels and nerves, and contains fundic, cardiac, and pyloric gastric glands.

stomachache, pain in the stomach area.

stomach cancer [Gk *stomakhos, karkinos* crab], a malignant neoplasm of the stomach lining. Most stomach cancers are carcinomas, The remainder are classified as lymphomas and leiomyosarcomas. Commonly associated with gastritis and intestinal metaplasia, the etiology is unknown. The worldwide incidence varies: In Japan, stomach cancer is the most common malignancy while in the United States it ranks seventh as the most common cause of cancer deaths. No specific symptoms are present with early stages. Complaints such as anemia, fatigability, weight loss, and epigastric distress may suggest peptic ulcer, dysphagia, or other digestive disorders.

stomach pump, a pump for withdrawing the contents of the stomach through a tube passed through the mouth or nose into the stomach.

stomach tube, a tube used to introduce nutrients into the stomach, remove fluids and ingested poisons, or decompress the stomach.

stomadaeum, stomadeum. See **stomodeum.**

stomal /stō′məl/ [Gk, mouth], pertaining to one or more stomata or mouthlike openings.

stomal peptic ulcer, a marginal peptic ulcer.

stomatitis /stō′mətī′tis/ [Gk *stoma* + *itis* inflammation], any inflammatory condition of the mouth. It may result from infection by bacteria, viruses, or fungi, from exposure to certain chemicals or drugs, from vitamin deficiency, or from a systemic inflammatory disease. Kinds of stomatitis include **aphthous stomatitis, pseudomembranous stomatitis, thrush,** and **Vincent's infection.**

stomatitis parasitica [Gk *stoma* + *itis; parasitos* guest], an inflammation of the mucous membranes of the mouth by a yeast fungus, *Candida albicans,* typically expressed by a white coating on the tongue. It may affect infants or immunosuppressed persons with HIV or appear as an outgrowth secondary to antibiotic therapy.

stomatognathic system /stō′mətōnath′ik/ [Gk *stoma* + *gnathos* jaw; *systema*], the combination of organs, structures, and nerves involved in speech and reception, mastication, and deglutition of food. This system is composed of the teeth, jaws, masticatory muscles, tongue, lips, and surrounding tissues and the nerves that control these structures.

stomatology /stō′mətol′əjē/ [Gk *stoma* + *logos* science], the study of the morphology, structure, function, and diseases of the oral cavity. **–stomatologist,** *n.,* **stomatologic, stomatological,** *adj.*

stomion /stō′mē·on/ [Gk *stoma*], the median point of the oral slit when the mouth is closed.

stomodeum /stom′ədē′əm/, *pl.* **stomodeums, stomodea** [Gk *stoma* + *odaios* a way], an invagination in the ectoderm located in the foregut of the developing embryo that forms the mouth. **–stomodeal, stomodaeal, stomadeal,** *adj.*

stone. See **calculus.**

stool. See **feces.**

stool softener. See **fecal softener.**

stopcock, a valve that controls the flow of fluid or air through a tube.

stop needle [AS *stoppian* to stop; *naedel*], a needle with a shoulder flange that stops it from penetrating beyond a certain distance.

stored-energy foot, a lower-limb prosthesis designed to imitate the springlike action of a natural foot and leg. A device stores energy when weight is put on the artificial leg. When the weight is shifted to the other leg, the stored energy is released, returning the prosthesis to its original shape.

storing fermentation [L *staurare* to store; *fermentum* leaven], the rapid, gaseous clotting of milk caused by *Clostridium perfringens.*

stork bite. See **telangiectatic nevus.**

STP, *slang.* a psychedelic agent, dimethoxy-4-methylamphetamine (DOM). STP is an abbreviation for *serenity, tranquility, and peace.*

STPD, abbreviation for *standard temperature, standard pressure, dry.*

STPD conditions of a volume of gas, the conditions of a volume of gas at 0° C and

S

760 torr, and containing no water vapor. It should contain a calculable number of moles of a particular gas.

Str., abbreviation for *Streptococcus.*

strabismus /strəbiz′məs/ [Gk *strabismos* squinting], an abnormal ocular condition in which the eyes are crossed. There are two kinds of strabismus, paralytic and nonparalytic. Paralytic strabismus results from the inability of the ocular muscles to move the eye because of neurologic deficit or muscular dysfunction. The muscle that is dysfunctional may be identified by watching as the patient attempts to move the eyes to each of the cardinal positions of gaze. Nonparalytic strabismus is a defect in the position of the two eyes in relation to each other. The condition is inherited. The person cannot use the two eyes together but has to fix with one or the other. The eye that looks straight at a given time is the fixing eye. Some people have alternating strabismus, using one eye and then the other; some have monocular strabismus affecting only one eye. Visual acuity diminishes with diminished use of an eye, and suppression amblyopia may develop. **–strabismal, strabismic, strabismical,** *adj.*

straight line blood set /strāt/ [ME *streght*], a common device, composed of plastic components, for delivering blood infusions. It includes the plastic tubing, the clamp, the drip chamber, and the filter.

straight sinus [ME *streght* + L *sinus* hollow], one of the six posterosuperior venous channels of the dura mater, draining blood from the brain into the internal jugular vein. It has no valves and is located at the junction of the falx cerebri with the tentorium cerebelli.

straight wire fixed orthodontic appliance, an orthodontic appliance used for correcting and improving malocclusion. It is designed to decrease arch wire adjustments by reorienting arch wire slots.

strain [ME *streinen*], **1.** to exert physical force in a manner that may result in injury, usually muscular. **2.** to separate solids or particles from a liquid with a filter or sieve. **3.** damage, usually muscular, that results from excessive physical effort. **4.** a taxon that is a subgroup of a species. **5.** an emotional state reflecting mental pressure or fatigue.

straitjacket /strāt′jakit/[OFr *estreit* strict, *jaquette* short coat], a coatlike garment of canvas with long sleeves that can be tied behind the wearer's back to prevent movement of the arms. It is used for restraining violent or uncontrollable people.

strangle /strang′gəl/ [L *strangulare* to choke], an interruption of breathing caused by compression or constriction of the trachea.

strangulated hemorrhoids /strang′gyə-lā′tid/, prolapsed hemorrhoids that have become trapped by the anal sphincter, causing the blood supply to become occluded by the sphincter's constricting action.

strangulated hernia, a hernia in which the blood vessels have become constricted by the neck of the hernial sac, resulting in ischemia and possible gangrene if blood circulation is not quickly restored.

strangulation /strang′gyəlā′shən/ [L *strangulare* to choke], the constriction of a tubular structure of the body, such as the trachea, a segment of bowel, or the blood vessels of a limb, that prevents function or impedes circulation. **–strangulate,** *v.,* **strangulated,** *adj.*

strap [AS *stropp*], **1.** a band, such as that made of adhesive plaster, that is used to hold dressings in place or to attach one thing to another. **2.** to bind securely.

strapping, the application of overlapping strips of adhesive tape to an extremity or body area to exert pressure and hold a structure in place, performed in the treatment of strains, sprains, dislocations, and certain fractures.

stratified epithelium /strat′ifīd/, closely packed sheets of epithelial cells arranged in layers over the external surface of the body and lining most of the hollow structures. The layers may include stratified squamous, stratified columnar, or stratified columnar ciliated types of cells.

stratiform cartilage. See **fibrocartilage.**

stratiform fibrocartilage /strat′ifôrm/ [L *stratum* layer, *forma* form; *fibra* fiber, *cartilago* cartilage], a structure made of fibrocartilage that forms a thin coating of osseous grooves through which tendons of certain muscles glide.

stratum /strā′təm, strat′əm/, *pl.* **strata** [L, layer], a uniformly thick sheet or layer, usually associated with other layers, such as the stratum basale of the epidermis. **–stratified,** *adj.*

stratum basale, **1.** the deepest of the five layers of the skin, composed of tall cylindric cells. This layer provides new cells by mitotic cell division. **2.** the deepest layers of the uterine decidua, containing uterine gland terminals.

stratum corneum, the horny, outermost layer of the skin, composed of dead cells converted to keratin that continually flakes away. The stratum corneum is thick on the palms of the hands and the soles of the feet but thin over more protected areas.

stratum germinativum. See **stratum basale.**

stratum granulosum, one of the layers of the epidermis, situated just below the **stratum corneum** except in the palms of the hands and the soles of the feet, where it lies just under the **stratum lucidum.**

stratum lucidum, one of the layers of the epidermis, situated just beneath the **stratum corneum** and present only in the thick skin of the palms of the hands and the soles of the feet.

stratum spinosum, one of the layers of the epidermis, composed of several layers of polygonal cells. It lies on top of the **stratum basale** and beneath the **stratum granulosum** and contains tiny fibrils within its cellular cytoplasm.

stratum spongiosum, one of the three layers of the endometrium of the uterus, containing tortuous, dilated uterine glands and a small amount of interglandular tissue.

strawberry gallbladder /strô´berē/ [AS *streawberig*; ME *gal* gall; AS *blaedre*], a tiny, yellow gallbladder spotted with deposits on the red mucous membrane, characteristic of cholesterolosis.

strawberry hemangioma, strawberry mark. See **capillary hemangioma.**

strawberry tongue, a strawberry-like coloration of the inflamed tongue papillae. It is a clinical sign of scarlet fever and is also seen in Kawasaki syndrome.

stray light [OFr *estraier* to wander; AS *leoht* illumination], radiant energy that reaches a photodetector and which consists of wavelengths other than those defined by the filter or monochromator.

stray radiation. See **leakage radiation.**

streak [AS *strican* to stroke], a line or a stripe, such as the primitive streak at the caudal end of the embryonic disk.

strength [AS *strengou*], the ability of a muscle to produce or resist a physical force.

strength of association, the degree of relationship between a causal factor and the occurrence of a disease, usually expressed in terms of a relative risk ratio.

strep throat [*Streptococcus* + AS *throte*], *informal.* an infection of the oral pharynx and tonsils caused by a hemolytic species of *Streptococcus,* usually belonging to group A. The infection is characterized by sore throat, chills, fever, swollen lymph nodes in the neck, and, sometimes, nausea and vomiting. The symptoms usually begin abruptly a few days after exposure to the organism in airborne droplets or after direct contact with an infected person.

streptobacillary rat-bite fever. See **Haverhill fever.**

Streptobacillus moniliformis /strep´tō-bəsiləs/ [Gk *streptos* curved; L *bacillum*

small rod; *monile* necklace, *forma* form], a species of necklace-shaped bacteria that can cause rat-bite fever in humans.

streptococcal /-kok´əl/ [Gk *streptos* curved, *kokkos* berry], pertaining to any of the species of streptococcus.

streptococcal angina /strep´təkok´əl/ [Gk *streptos* + *kokkos* berry; L *angina* quinsy], a condition in which feelings of choking, suffocation, and pain occur as the result of a streptococcal infection.

streptococcal infection, an infection caused by pathogenic bacteria of one of several species of the genus *Streptococcus* or their toxins. The infections occur in many forms including cellulitis, endocarditis, erysipelas, impetigo, meningitis, pneumonia, scarlet fever, tonsillitis, and urinary tract infection.

streptococcal sore throat. See **strep throat.**

streptococcemia /-koksē´mē·ə/ [Gk *streptos* + *kokkos* berry], a condition of streptococci bacteria in the blood.

Streptococcus /strep´təkok´əs/ [Gk *streptos* + *kokkos* berry], a genus of nonmotile, gram-positive, cocci classified by serologic types (Lancefield groups A through T), by hemolytic action (alpha, beta, gamma) when grown on blood agar, and by reaction to bacterial viruses (phage types 1 to 86). Many species cause disease in humans. *Streptococcus viridans,* a member of the normal flora of the mouth, is the most common cause of bacterial endocarditis, especially when introduced into the bloodstream during dental procedures.

Streptococcus pneumoniae, any of 70 antigenic types of pneumococci that cause pneumonia and other diseases in humans.

Streptococcus pyogenes, a species of streptococcus with many strains that are pathogenic to humans, including the β-hemolytics in Lancefield Group A. It causes suppurative diseases such as scarlet fever and strep throat.

Streptococcus viridans, a species of streptococcus similar to *pyogens* strains. It produces α-hemolysis in cultures and is a common cause of subacute bacterial endocarditis and other infections in humans.

streptokinase /strep´təkī´nās/ [Gk *streptos* + *kinesis* motion; (ase) enzyme], a fibrinolytic activator that enhances the conversion of plasminogen to the fibrinolytic enzyme plasmin. It is used in the treatment of certain cases of pulmonary and coronary embolism.

streptokinase-streptodornase /-strep´tō-dôr´nās/, two enzymes derived from a strain of *Streptococcus hemolyticus.* It is prescribed for debridement of purulent exudates, clotted blood, radiation necrosis,

S

or fibrinous deposits resulting from trauma or infection.

streptolysin /streptol'isis/ [Gk *streptos* + *lysein* to loosen], a filterable substance, produced by various streptococci that liberates hemoglobin from red blood cells.

streptomycin sulfate /strep'təmī'sin/, an aminoglycoside antibiotic prescribed in the treatment of tuberculosis, endocarditis, and certain other infections.

streptozocin /strep'tōzō'sin/, an investigational antineoplastic used in the treatment of a variety of neoplasms, including metastatic islet cell tumors of the pancreas. It is an antibiotic substance from *Streptomyces acromogenes.*

stress [OFr *estrecier* to tighten], any emotional, physical, social, economic, or other factor that requires a response or change, such as dehydration, which can cause an increase in body temperature, or a separation from parents, which can cause a young child to cry.

stress-adaptation theory, a concept that stress depletes the reserve capacity of individuals, thereby increasing their vulnerability to health problems.

stress amenorrhea [OFr *estrecier;* GK *a, men,* month, *rhoia* to flow], a cessation in menstruation due to physical or mental stress.

stress behavior, a change from a person's normal behavior in response to a stressor.

stress fracture, a fracture, especially of one or more of the metatarsal bones, caused by repeated, prolonged, or abnormal stress.

stress inoculation, a procedure useful in helping patients control anxiety by substituting positive coping statements for statements that bring about anxiety.

stress kinesic, a type of behavioral characteristic of personal conversation, such as the use of body shifts or movements, that mark the flow of speech and generally coincide with linguistic stress patterns.

stress management, methods of controlling factors that require a response of change within a person by identifying the stressors, eliminating negative stressors, and developing effective coping mechanisms. Examples include progressive relaxation, guided imagery, biofeedback, and active problem solving.

stressor /stres'ər/ [OFr *estrecier* to tighten], anything that causes wear and tear on the body's physical or mental resources.

stress reaction. See **general adaptation syndrome, posttraumatic stress disorder.**

stress response syndrome. See **posttraumatic stress disorder.**

stress test, a test that measures the function of a system of the body when subjected to carefully controlled amounts of stress. The data produced allow the examiner to evaluate the condition of the system being tested.

stress ulcer, a gastric or duodenal ulcer that develops in previously unaffected individuals subjected to severe stress, as when severely burned.

stretching of contractures [AS *streccan;* L *contractura* drawing together], procedures for release of muscle that has been shortened due to paralysis, spasm, or fibrosis. The procedures may include tissue grafts, scar tissue removal, tendon transfer, and incision of a joint capsule.

stretch mark. See **stria.**

stretch receptors [AS *streccan;* L *recipere* to receive], specialized sensory nerve endings in muscle spindles or tendons that are stimulated by stretching movements.

stretch reflex [AS *streccan;* L *reflectere* to bend back], a reflex muscle contraction after it is stretched due to stimulation of proprioceptive receptors in the muscle. Tendon reflexes function in a similar manner.

stria /strī'ə/, *pl.* **striae** [L, furrow], a streak or a linear scar that often results from rapidly developing tension in the skin, as seen on the abdomen after pregnancy. Purplish striae are one of the classic findings in hyperadrenocorticism.

stria atrophica. See **linea albicantes.**

stria gravidarum, irregular depressions with red to purple colorations that appear in the skin of the abdomen, thighs, and buttocks of pregnant women.

striatal /strī·a'təl, strī'ətəl/ [L *striatus* striped], pertaining to the corpus striatum.

striate /strī'āt/ [L *striatus* striped], striped; marked by parallel lines; having structural lines.

striated muscle [L *stria* + *musculus* muscle], muscle tissue, including all the skeletal muscles, that appears microscopically to consist of striped myofibrils. Striated muscles are composed of bundles of parallel, striated fibers under voluntary control; the heart, a striated involuntary muscle, is an exception. Each myofibril comprises thick filaments that consist of molecules of myosin and of thin filaments that consist of actin and two other protein compounds. Muscle contraction occurs when an electrochemical impulse crosses the myoneural junction, causing the thin filaments to shorten.

stricture /strik'chər/ [L *stringere* to tighten], an abnormal temporary or permanent narrowing of the lumen of a hollow organ, such as the esophagus, pylorus of the stomach, ureter, or urethra because of inflammation, external pressure, or scarring. Treatment varies depending on the cause.

strict vegetarian [L *stringere* + *vegetare* to grow, *arius* believer], a vegetarian whose diet excludes the use of all foods of animal origin. Such diets may be deficient in many essential nutrients, particularly vitamin B$_{12}$.

stridor /strī'dôr/ [L, harsh sound], an abnormal, high-pitched, musical sound, caused by an obstruction in the trachea or larynx. It is usually heard during inspiration. Stridor may indicate several neoplastic or inflammatory conditions, including glottic edema, asthma, diphtheria, laryngospasm, or papilloma.

strike [AS *strican* to advance swiftly], an action taken by the employees of a company or institution in which they stop reporting for work in an effort to cause the employer to accede to certain demands.

string carcinoma [AS *strenge* cord; Gk *karkinos* cancer, *oma* tumor], a malignancy of the large intestine, usually of the ascending or transverse colon that, on radiologic visualization, causes the intestine to appear to be tied in segments like a string of large beads.

strip membranes [Ger *strippe* strap; L *membrana* thin skin], (in obstetrics) a procedure in which an examiner digitally frees the membranes of the amniotic sac from the wall of the lower segment of the uterus in the small area around the cervical os.

stripping, 1. *nontechnical;* a surgical procedure for the removal of the long and the short saphenous veins of the legs. 2. the mechanical removal of a very small amount of enamel from the mesial or distal surfaces of teeth to alleviate crowding.

stroboscopic illusion. See **phi phenomenon.**

stroke. See **cerebrovascular accident.**

stroke prone profile [AS *strac*], a predictive index using a complex of risk factors that indicate susceptibility of a person to cerebrovascular accident (CVA). The factors include advanced age, hypertension, a history of transient ischemic attacks, cigarette smoking, heart disorders, associated embolism, family history of CVA, use of oral contraceptives, diabetes mellitus, physical inactivity, obesity, hypercholesteremia, and hyperlipidemia.

stroke volume, the amount of blood ejected by the ventricle during a ventricle contraction.

stroke volume index, the stroke volume divided by the body surface area.

stroma /strō'mə/, *pl.* **stromata** [Gk, covering], the supporting tissue or the matrix of an organ as distinguished from its parenchyma. **–stromatic,** *adj.*

Strongyloides /stron'jiloi'dēz/ [Gk *strongylos* round, *eidos* form], a genus of parasitic intestinal nematode. A species of *Strongyloides, S. stercoralis,* causes strongyloidiasis.

strongyloidiasis /stron'jəloidī'əsis/, infection of the small intestine by the roundworm *Strongyloides stercoralis,* acquired when larvae from the soil penetrate intact skin, incidentally causing a pruritic rash. The larvae pass to the lungs via the bloodstream, sometimes causing pneumonia. Larvae then migrate up the air passages to the pharynx, are swallowed, and develop into adult worms in the small intestine. Bloody diarrhea and intestinal malabsorption may result. Wearing shoes prevents contagion from contaminated soil.

strontium (Sr) /stron'sh(ē)əm/ [Strontian, Scotland], a metallic element. Its atomic number is 38; its atomic weight is 87.62. Chemically similar to calcium, it is found in bone tissue. Isotopes of strontium are used in radioisotope scanning procedures of bone. Strontium 90, the longest lived, is the most dangerous constituent of fallout from atomic bomb tests. It can replace some of the calcium in food, become concentrated in teeth and bones, and continue to emit electrons that cause death in the host. Cows concentrate strontium 90 in their milk.

structural /struk'chərəl/ [L *structura* arrangement], pertaining to the arrangement or pattern of component parts of an object or organism.

structural chemistry [L *structura* arrangement], the science dealing with the molecular structure of chemical substances.

structural gene, (in molecular genetics) a unit of genetic information that specifies the amino acid sequence of a polypeptide.

structural integration, a technique of deep massage intended to help in the realignment of the body by altering the length and tone of myofascial tissues. The basis of the practice is the belief that misalignment of myofascial tissues may have an overall detrimental effect on a person's energy level, self-image, muscular efficiency, perceptions, and general health.

structural model, a model of family therapy that views the family as an open system and identifies subsystems within the family that carry out specific family functions.

structure /struk'chər/ [L *structura*], a part of the body, such as the heart, a bone, a gland, a cell, or a limb.

S

structure-activity relationship (SAR), the relationship between the chemical structure of a drug and its activity.

struma lymphomatosa. See **Hashimoto's disease.**

Strümpell-Marie disease /strim'pəlmärē'/ [Ernst Adolf Gustav Gottfried von Strümpell, German neurologist, b. 1853; Pierre Marie, French neurologist, b. 1853], ankylosing spondylitis.

strychnine /strik'nin, strik'nīn/ [Gr *strychnos* nightshade], a white crystalline alkaloid obtained from the leaves of the *Strychnos nux-vomica* plant. It is extremely toxic to the central nervous system, producing as a classic strychnine poisoning symptom an arched back.

strychnine poisoning, toxic effects of ingesting strychnine, a central nervous system stimulant. Symptoms include restlessness, hyperacuity of hearing and vision. Minor stimuli may produce convulsions, but there may be complete muscle relaxation between convulsions. One sign of strychnine poisoning is an arched back.

Stryker wedge frame /strī'kər/, an orthopedic bed that allows the patient to be rotated as required to either the supine or prone position. It is used in the immobilization of patients with unstable spines, postoperative management of multilevel spinal fusions, and management of severe burn patients.

S-T interval [L *intervallum* space between ramparts], the component of the cardiac cycle shown on an electrocardiogram as an isoelectric line following the QRS complex, before the ascent of the T wave. It represents phase 2 of the action potential. Elevation or depression of the S-T interval is the hallmark of myocardial ischemia or injury and coronary artery disease.

Stuart-Power factor. See **factor X.**

stump [ME *stumpe*], the part of a limb after amputation that is proximal to the portion amputated.

stump hallucination, the sensation of the continued presence of an amputated limb.

stunned myocardium, the presence of impaired myocardial contractile function, cellular biochemistry, and microvascular function in the absence of gross myocardial necrosis for minutes to days caused by ischemia of short duration.

stupefacient /st(y)o͞o'pəfā'shənt/ [L *stupere* to stun, *facere* to make], a narcotic or other agent that has the effect of making a person stuporous.

stupor /st(y)o͞o'pər/ [L, senselessness], a state of lethargy and unresponsiveness in which a person seems unaware of the surroundings. Kinds of stupor are **anergic,**

benign, delusion, and **epileptic stupor. –stuporous** /st(y)o͞o'pərəs/, *adj.*

Sturge-Weber syndrome /sturj'web'ər/ [William A. Sturge, English physician, b. 1850; Frederick P. Weber, English physician, b. 1863], a congenital neurocutaneous disease marked by a port-wine-colored capillary hemangioma over a sensory dermatome of a branch of the trigeminal nerve of the face. The cerebral cortex may atrophy, and generalized or focal seizures, angioma of the choroid, secondary glaucoma, optic atrophy, and new cutaneous hemangiomas may develop.

stuttering [D *stotteren*], a speech dysfunction characterized by spasmodic enunciation of words, involving excessive hesitations, stumbling, repetition of the same syllables, and prolongation of sounds. The condition may result from a cerebellar disease or a neuromuscular defect or injury of the organs of articulation, but in most cases the cause is emotional or psychologic.

sty [ME *styanye* eyelid tumor], a purulent infection of a meibomian or sebaceous gland of the eyelid, often caused by a staphylococcal organism.

stylet /stī'lət, stīlet'/ [It *stiletto* dagger], a thin metal probe for inserting into or passing through a needle, tube, or catheter to clean the hollow bore or for inserting in a soft, flexible catheter to make it shift as the catheter is placed in a vein or passed through an orifice of the body.

stylohyoideus /stī'lōhī·oi'dē·əs/ [Gk *stylos* pillar, *hyoeides* upsilon-shaped], one of four suprahyoid muscles, lying anterior and superior to the posterior belly of the digastricus. It serves to draw the hyoid bone up and back.

stylohyoid ligament /stī'lōhī'oid/, the ligament attached to the tip of the styloid process of the temporal bone and to the lesser cornu of the hyoid bone.

styloid /stī'loid/ [Gk *stylos* pillar, *eidos* form], long and tapered, like a pen or stylus.

styloid process, any of several projections of bone tissue, particularly a projection on the temporal bone.

stylomandibular ligament /stī'lōmandib'yələr/ [Gk *stylos* + L *mandere* to chew, *ligare* to bind], one of a pair of specialized bands of cervical fascia, forming an accessory part of the temporomandibular joint. It extends from the styloid process of the temporal bone to the ramus of the mandible between the masseter and pterygoideus muscles and separates the parotid gland from the submandibular gland.

styptic /stip'tik/ [Gk *styptikos* astringent],

1. a substance used as an astringent, often to control bleeding. A chemical styptic induces coagulation of blood. A cotton pledget used as a compress to control bleeding is a mechanical styptic. **2.** acting as an astringent or agent to control bleeding.

subacromial /-əkrō′mē·əl/ [L *sub* + Gk, *akron* extremity, *omos* shoulder], below the acromion.

subacromial bursa, the bursa separating the acromion and deltoid muscle from the insertion of the supraspinatus muscle and the greater tubercle of the humerus.

subacute /-əkyo̅o̅t′/ [L *sub* + *acutus* sharp], **1.** less than acute. **2.** of or pertaining to a disease or other abnormal condition present in a person who appears to be clinically well.

subacute bacterial endocarditis (SBE), a chronic bacterial infection of the valves of the heart, characterized by a slow, quiet onset with fever, heart murmur, splenomegaly, and the development of clumps of abnormal tissue, called vegetations, around an intracardiac prosthesis or on the cusps of a valve. Various species of *Streptococcus* or *Staphylococcus* are commonly the cause of SBE. Dental procedures are associated with infection by *Streptococcus viridans,* surgical procedures with *Streptococcus faecalis,* and self-infection (especially by drug abusers) with *Staphylococcus aureus.*

subacute glomerulonephritis, an uncommon noninfectious disease of the glomerulus of the kidney characterized by proteinuria, hematuria, decreased production of urine, and edema. Of unknown cause, the disease may progress rapidly, and renal failure may occur. Kidney transplantation and dialysis are the only treatments available.

subacute infection, a disease condition that is not chronic and which runs a rapid and severe, but less than acute, course.

subacute myeloptic neuropathy (SMON), a condition of muscular pain and weakness, usually below the T12 vertebra, painful dysesthesia of the limbs, and, in some cases, optic atrophy.

subacute sclerosing panencephalitis, an uncommon, slow virus infection caused by the measles virus and characterized by diffuse inflammation of brain tissue, personality change, seizures, blindness, dementia, fever, and death.

subacute thyroiditis. See **de Quervain's thyroiditis.**

subaortic /-ā-ôr′tik/ [L *sub* + Gk *aerein* to rise], pertaining to the area of the body below the aorta.

subaortic stenosis, a narrowing of the left ventricle outflow tract below the aortic valve.

subaponeurotic /-ap′ōn o̅o̅rot′ik/, beneath an aponeurosis.

subarachnoid /sub′arak′noid/ [L *sub* + Gk *arachne* spider, *eidos* form], situated under the arachnoid membrane and above the pia mater.

subarachnoid block anesthesia, a form of spinal anesthesia involving the injection of an anesthetic into the space between the arachnoidea and pia mater.

subarachnoid hemorrhage (SaH, SAH), an intracranial hemorrhage into the cerebrospinal fluid-filled space between the arachnoid and pial membranes on the surface of the brain. The hemorrhage may extend into the brain if the force of the bleeding from the broken vessel is sudden and severe. The cause may be trauma or rupture of a berry aneurysm or an arteriovenous anomaly. The first symptom of a subarachnoid hemorrhage is a sudden extremely severe headache that begins in one localized area and then spreads, becoming dull and throbbing. The localized pain results from vascular distortion and injury. The generalized ache is the result of meningeal irritation from blood in the subarachnoid space. Other characteristics of subarachnoid hemorrhage include dizziness, rigidity of the neck, pupillary inequality, vomiting, drowsiness, sweating and chills, stupor, and loss of consciousness. A brief period of unconsciousness immediately after the rupture is common; severe hemorrhage may result in continued unconsciousness, coma, and death. Delirium and confusion often persist through the first weeks of recovery, and permanent brain damage is common.

subarachnoid space, the space between the arachnoid and pia mater membranes.

subatomic /-ətom′ik/ [L *sub* + Gk, *atmos* indivisible], pertaining to the particles and phenomena that are within an atom.

subaxillary /-ak′siler′ē/ [L *sub* + *axilla* wing], beneath the axilla.

subcapital fracture /-kap′itəl/ [L *sub* + *caput* head], a fracture of tissue just below the head of a bone that pivots in a ball and socket joint, such as the head of the femur.

subcapsular /kap′s(y)ələr/ [L *sub* + *capsula* little box], below a capsule.

subcapsular cataract, a condition marked by opacity or cloudiness beneath the anterior or posterior capsule of the lens of the eye.

subclavian /səbklā′vē-ən/ [L *sub* + *clavicula* little key], situated under the clavicle, such as the subclavian vein.

subclavian artery, one of a pair of arteries that vary in origin, course, and the height to which they rise in the neck but having six similar main branches supplying the vertebral column, spinal cord, ear, and brain.

subclavian steal syndrome, a vascular syndrome caused by an occlusion in the subclavian artery proximal to the origin of the vertebral artery. The block results in a reversal of the normal blood pressure gradient in the vertebral artery and decreased blood flow distal to the occlusion. This condition is characterized by episodes of flaccid paralysis of the arm, pain in the mastoid and occipital areas, and a diminished or absent radial pulse on the involved side.

subclavian vein, the continuation of the axillary vein in the upper body, extending from the lateral border of the first rib to the sternal end of the clavicle, where it joins the internal jugular to form the brachiocephalic vein.

subclavius /səbklā′vē-əs/ [L *sub* + *clavicula*], a short muscle of the chest wall. It acts to draw the shoulder down and forward.

subclinical /-klin′ikəl/ [L *sub* + Gk *kline* bed], of or pertaining to a disease or abnormal condition that is so mild it produces no symptoms.

subclinical diabetes. See **impaired glucose tolerance.**

subcollateral gyrus /-kəlat′ərəl/, below the collateral fissure or sulcus of the cerebrum.

subconscious /-kon′shəs/ [L *sub* + *conscire* to be aware], imperfectly or partially conscious. –**subconsciousness,** *n.*

subconscious memory, a thought, sensation, or feeling that is not immediately available for recall to the conscious mind.

subcrepitant rale /-krep′itənt/, a rale that is only faintly crepitant.

subculture /sub′kulchər/ [L *sub* + *colere* to cultivate], an ethnic, regional, economic, or social group with characteristic patterns of behavior and ideals that distinguish it from the rest of a culture or society.

subcutaneous /sub′kyo͞otā′nē-əs/ [L *sub* + *cutis* skin], beneath the skin.

subcutaneous adipose tissue, fat deposits beneath the skin.

subcutaneous emphysema, the presence of free air or gas in the subcutaneous tissues. The air or gas may originate in the rupture of an airway or alveoli and migrate through the subpleural spaces to the mediastinum and neck. The face, neck, and chest may appear swollen. Skin tissues can be painful and may produce a "crackling" sound as air moves under them. The patient may experience dyspnea and appear cyanotic if the air leak is severe. Treatment may require an incision to release the trapped air.

subcutaneous fascia, a continuous layer of connective tissue over the entire body between the skin and the deep fascial investment of the specialized structures of the body, such as the muscles. It comprises an outer, normally fatty layer and an inner, thin elastic layer.

subcutaneous fat necrosis. See **adiponecrosis subcutanea neonatorum.**

subcutaneous infusion. See **hypodermoclysis.**

subcutaneous injection, the introduction of a hypodermic needle into the subcutaneous tissue beneath the skin, usually on the upper arm, thigh, or abdomen.

subcutaneous mastectomy, a surgical procedure in which all the breast tissue of one or both breasts is removed leaving the skin, areola, and nipple intact. The adjacent lymph nodes and the pectoralis major and pectoralis minor are not removed. It may be performed on women who are at great risk of developing breast cancer.

subcutaneous nodule, a small, solid boss, or node, beneath the skin that can be detected by touch.

subcutaneous test. See **intradermal test.**

subcutaneous tunnel, a tunnel under the skin between the exit site of an atrial catheter and the entrance into the vein.

subcutaneous wound, an injury to internal organs such as by crushing or other violence, without a break in the surface of the skin.

subcuticular suture /-kyo͞otik′yələr/ [L *sub* + *cutis* skin, *sutura*], a continuous suture placed so as to bring together the tissues immediately beneath the skin. It is frequently a suture of nonabsorbable material that can later be removed by pulling on one end.

subdural /-d(y)o͞o′rəl/ [L *sub* + *durus* hard], situated under the dura mater and above the arachnoid membrane.

subdural hygroma, a collection of fluid between the dura mater and arachnoid layers, resulting from a spinal fluid leak through a rupture in the arachnoid tissue.

subdural space, the potential space between the dura mater and the arachnoid membrane.

subendocardial infarction /-en′dōkär′dē-əl/, a myocardial infarction that involves only the innermost layer of the myocardium, and in some cases portions of the middle layer of tissue, but does not extend to the epicardial region.

subepidermal /-ep′idur′məl/, beneath the epidermis.

suberosis. See **cork worker's lung.**

subgerminal cavity. See **blastocoele.**

subgingival calculus /-jinjī′vəl/ [L *sub* + *gingiva* gum], a deposit of various mineral salts, such as calcium phosphate and calcium carbonate, which accumulates with organic matter and oral debris on the teeth or within the gingival crevice, the gingival pocket, or the periodontal pocket. It is usually darker, more pigmented, and denser than supragingival calculus.

subgingival curettage, the debridement of an ulcerated epithelial attachment and subjacent gingival corium to eliminate inflammation and shrink and restore gingival tissue.

subintentional suicide. See **benign suicide.**

subintimal /-in′timəl/ [L *sub* + *intimus* innermost], the area beneath the intima or membrane lining a blood vessel, usually a large artery.

subinvolution /-in′vəloo′shən/ [L *sub* + *involere* to roll up], delayed or absent involution of the uterus during the postpartum period. The causes of subinvolution include retained fragments of placenta, uterine fibromyomas, and infection. It is characterized by longer and heavier bleeding after childbirth and, on pelvic examination, a larger and softer uterus than would be expected at that time.

subjective /-jek′tiv/ [L *subjicere* to expose], **1.** pertaining to the essential nature of an object as perceived in the mind rather than to a thing in itself. **2.** existing only in the mind. **3.** that which arises within or is perceived by the individual, as contrasted with something that is modified by external circumstances or something that may be evaluated by objective standards. **4.** pertaining to a person who places excessive importance on his or her own moods, attitudes, or opinions; egocentric.

subjective data collection, the process in which data relating to the patient's problem are elicited from the patient. The interviewer encourages a full description of the onset, the course, and the character of the problem and any factors that aggravate or ameliorate it.

subjective sensation, a feeling or impression that is not associated with or does not directly result from any external stimulus.

subjective symptoms, symptoms that are observed only by the patient and cannot be objectively confirmed.

subjects /sub′jekts/, people, animals, or events selected for a study to examine a particular variable or condition, such as the effects of a new medication or therapy.

sublethal dose /-lē′thəl/, a dose of a potentially lethal substance that is not large enough to cause death.

sublethal gene [L *sub* + *lethum* death; Gk *genein* to produce], a gene whose presence causes abnormalities or impairs the functioning of an organism but does not cause its death.

subleukemic leukemia. See **aleukemic leukemia.**

sublimate /sub′limāt/ [L *sublimare* to lift up], to refine or divert instinctual impulses and energy from their immediate goal to one that can be expressed in a social, moral, or aesthetic manner acceptable to the person and to society.

sublimation /-limā′shən/ [L *sublimare*], **1.** a defense mechanism by which an unacceptable instinctive drive is unconsciously diverted to and expressed through a personally approved, socially accepted means. **2.** (in psychoanalysis) the process of diverting certain components of the sex drive to a socially acceptable, nonsexual goal.

subliminal /-lim′inəl/ [L *sub* + *limen* threshold], taking place below the threshold of sensory perception or outside the range of conscious awareness.

subliminal self, a level of mental activity at which an individual under normal waking conditions may function without consciousness.

sublingual /səbling′gwəl/ [L *sub* + *lingua* tongue], beneath the tongue.

sublingual administration of a medication, the administration of a drug, such as nitroglycerin, usually in tablet form, by placing it beneath the tongue until the tablet dissolves.

sublingual caruncle, a small fleshy growth under the tongue.

sublingual duct. See **Bartholin's duct, duct of Rivinus.**

sublingual gland, one of a pair of small salivary glands situated under the mucous membrane of the floor of the mouth, beneath the tongue. A narrow, almond-shaped structure, it secretes mucus produced by its alveoli.

subluxation. See **incomplete dislocation.**

submandibular /-məndib′yələr/ [L, *sub* + *mandible*], below the mandible, or lower jaw.

submandibular duct [L *sub* + *mandere* to chew], a duct through which a submandibular gland secretes saliva.

submandibular gland, one of a pair of round, walnut-sized salivary glands in the submandibular triangle. The gland secretes both mucus and a thinner serous fluid, which aid the digestive process.

submaxillary /-mak′sīler′ē/ [L *sub* + *maxilla*], below the maxilla, or upper jaw.

submaxillary duct. See **submandibular duct.**

S

submeatal /-mē-ā'təl/ [L *sub* + *meatus* passage], pertaining to tissues beneath a meatus, as the mastoid air cells under the acoustic meatus or the hard palate beneath the nasal meatus.

submental /-men'təl/ [L *sub* + *mentum* chin], beneath the chin.

submentovertex /-men'tōvur'teks/ [L *sub* + *mentum* chin, *vertex* peak], a reference point at the base of the skull used in preparing radiographic projections of the skull and its associated structures.

submetacentric /sub'metəsen'trik/ [L *sub* + Gk *meta* besides, *kentron* center], pertaining to a chromosome in which the centromere is located approximately equidistant between the center and one end so that the arms of the chromatids are not equal in length.

submucous /-m(y)o͞o'kəs/, beneath a mucous membrane.

submucous resection (SMR), a surgical procedure for correcting a deviated nasal septum, leaving the mucous membrane of the septum intact.

suboccipitobregmatic /-aksip'itō'bregmat'ik/ [L *sub* + *occiput* back of the head; Gk *bregma* front of the head], pertaining to the smallest anteroposterior diameter of an infant's head when it is well flexed during labor.

subperiosteal fracture /sub'perē·os'tē·əl/ [L *sub* + Gk *peri* around, *osteon* bone], a fracture in a bone beneath the periosteum that does not disrupt the periosteal covering.

subphrenic /-fren'ik/ [L *sub* + Gk *phren* diaphragm], beneath or under the diaphragm.

subphrenic abscess, an abscess that develops on or near the undersurface of the diaphragm, usually as a result of peritonitis or from another visceral site.

subpoena /-pē'nə/ [L *sub* + *poena* penalty], (in law) a document from a court commanding that a person appear at a certain time and place to testify on a specific matter.

subpoena duces tecum, (in law) a subpoena commanding a person to bring books, papers, records, or other items to the court.

subpubic dislocation. See **dislocation of hip.**

subscapularis /-skap'yələr'is/, the muscle arising from the subscapular fossa with insertion in the humerus.

subserous fascia /sir'əs/ [L *sub* + *serum* whey; *fascia* band], one of three kinds of fascia, lying between the internal layer of deep fascia and the serous membranes lining the body cavities in much the same manner as the subcutaneous fascia lies between the skin and the deep fascia. It is thin in some areas, such as between the pleura and the chest wall, and thick in other areas, where it forms a pad of adipose tissue.

subsistence /-sis'təns/ [L *subsistere* to stand still], to continue to be sustained or remain alive with a minimum of life essentials.

subspecialty /-spesh'əltē/ [L *sub* + *specialis* individual], (in nursing) a nurse's particular professional and highly specialized field of practice, such as nursing in dialysis, oncology, neurology, or newborn intensive care.

substance /sub'stəns/ [L *substantia* essence], **1.** any drug, chemical, or biological entity. **2.** any material capable of being self-administered or abused because of its physiologic or psychologic effects.

substance abuse, the overindulgence in and dependence on a stimulant, depressant, or other chemical substance, leading to effects that are detrimental to the individual's physical or mental health, or the welfare of others.

substance P, a polypeptide neurotransmitting substance that is synthesized by the body and acts to stimulate vasodilatation and contraction of intestinal and other smooth muscles. It also plays a part in salivary secretion, diuresis, and natriuresis, and it affects the function of the peripheral and central nervous systems.

substandard [L *sub* + OFr *estandart*], below the predetermined model or measure.

substantia alba /-stan'shə/, the portion of the central nervous system that is enclosed in myelin sheaths. The myelin contributes a white coloring to otherwise gray nerve tissue.

substantia nigra, a dark band of gray matter lying between the tegmentum of the midbrain and the crus cerebri.

substantive epidemiology [L *substantia* + Gk *epi* upon, *demos* people, *logos* science], the body of knowledge derived from epidemiologic studies, including for each disease the natural history of the disorder, patterns of occurrence, and risk factors for developing the disease.

substantivity, the property of continuing therapeutic action despite removal of the vehicle, such as applied to certain shampoos.

substernal /-stur'nəl/, beneath the sternum.

substernal goiter [L *sub* + Gk *sternon* chest; L *guttur* throat], an enlargement of the thyroid gland, a portion of which is beneath the sternum.

substitution, a mental defense mechanism, operating unconsciously, by which an unattainable or unacceptable goal, emotion, or object is replaced by one that is more attainable or acceptable.

substitutive therapy [L *substituere* to put in place of; Gk *therapeia* treatment], a treatment that effects a condition incompatible with or antagonistic to the condition being treated.

substrate /sub'strāt/ [L *sub* + *stratum* layer], a substance acted on and changed by an enzyme in any chemical reaction.

substrate depletion phase, a period during an enzyme assay when the concentration of substrate is falling and the assay is not following zero-order kinetics.

substratum /-strā'təm/ [L *sub* + *stratum* layer], any underlying layer; a foundation.

subsystem, a smaller component of a large system composed of individuals or dyads, formed by generation, gender, interest, or function.

subthalamus /-thal'əməs/ [L *sub* + Gk *thalamos* chamber], a portion of the diencephalon that serves as a correlations center for optic and vestibular impulses relayed to the globus pallidus. **–subthalamic,** *adj.*

subtle /sut'əl/ [L *subtilis* finely woven], having a low intensity; not severe and having no serious sequelae, such as a mild infection or inflammation.

subtotal [L *sub* beneath, *totus* whole], less than complete.

subtotal hysterectomy, the surgical removal of the body of the uterus without removing the cervix.

subtrochanteric osteotomy /-trō'kənter'ik/ [L, *sub*; Gk, *trochanter*, runner + *osteon*, bone + *temnein*, to cut], a surgical procedure that divides the shaft of the femur below the lesser trochanter to correct ankylosis of the hip joint.

subungual /səbung'gwəl/ [L *sub* + *unguis* nail], under a fingernail or toenail.

subungual hematoma, a collection of blood beneath a nail, usually resulting from trauma.

succinic acid /suksin'ik/, a compound found in certain hydatid cysts and in lichens, amber, and fossils.

succinylcholine chloride /suk'sinilkō'lēn/, a skeletal muscle relaxant prescribed as an adjunct to anesthesia or to reduce muscle contractions during surgery or mechanical ventilation and to facilitate endotracheal intubation.

succus /suk'əs/, *pl.* **succi** /suk'sī/ [L, juice], a juice or fluid, usually one secreted by an organ, such as succus prostaticus of the prostate.

succussion splash /səkush'ən/ [L *succutere*

to shake up; ME *plasche* puddle], the sound elicited by shaking the body of an individual who has free fluid and air or gas in a hollow organ or body cavity. This sound may be present over a normal stomach but may also be heard with hydropneumothorax, large hiatal hernia, or intestinal or pyloric obstruction.

suck [L *sugere* to suck], **1.** to draw a liquid or semiliquid into the mouth by creating a partial vacuum through motions of the lips and tongue. **2.** to hold on the tongue and dissolve by the movements of the mouth and action of the saliva. **3.** to draw fluid into the mouth, specifically to draw milk from the breast or nursing bottle.

sucking blisters, the pale, soft pads on the upper and lower lips of a baby that look like blisters but are not. They seem to augment the seal of the lips around the nipple or breast. Some babies are born with them, having sucked on their own fingers, hand, or arm before birth.

sucking reflex, involuntary sucking movements of the circumoral area in newborns in response to stimulation. The reflex continues throughout infancy and often occurs without stimulation, such as during sleep.

suckle [L *sugere*], **1.** to provide nourishment, specifically to breastfeed. **2.** to take in as nourishment, especially by feeding from the breast.

suckling, an infant that has not been weaned.

sucrose /sōō'krōs/ [Fr *sucre* sugar], sugar derived from sugar cane, sugar beets, and sorghum.

sucrose polyester (SPE), a synthetic, nonabsorbable fat that, when added to the diet, reduces plasma cholesterol levels by increasing the excretion of cholesterol in the feces.

suction [L *sugere* to suck], the aspiration of a gas or fluid by reducing air pressure over its surface, usually by mechanical means.

suction biopsy [L *sugere*; Gk, *bios* life, *opsis* view], a procedure for obtaining tissue or fluid samples from lymph nodes or a deep lesion by using suction and a trochar or cannula.

suction curettage, a method of curettage in which a specimen of the endometrium or the products of conception are removed by aspiration.

suction drainage. See **drainage.**

suction lipectomy. See **liposuction.**

sudden death, death that occurs unexpectedly and within 1 hour after the onset of symptoms, with or without known preexisting conditions.

sudden infant death syndrome (SIDS)
[ME *sodain* to come up; L *infans* unable
to speak; AS *death;* Gk *syn* together,
dromos course], the unexpected and sudden death of an apparently normal and
healthy infant that occurs during sleep and
with no physical or autopsic evidence of
disease. Multiple causes have been proposed, including lack of biotin in the diet,
abnormality of the endogenous-opioid system, mechanical suffocation, a defect in
respiratory mucosal defense, prolonged
apnea, an unknown virus, anatomic abnormality of the larynx, and immunoglobulin
abnormalities. It is seen more often among
babies who have recently had a minor illness such as upper respiratory infection.
The syndrome is neither contagious nor
hereditary, although there is a greater than
average risk of its occurrence within the
same family, which may indicate the influence of polygenic factors.

sudor /sōō′dôr/, perspiration.

sudoriferous duct /sōō′dərif′ərəs/ [L *sudor* sweat, *facere* to make], a duct leading from a sweat gland to the surface of
the skin.

sudoriferous gland, one of about 3 million tiny structures within the dermis that
produce sweat. The average quantity of
sweat secreted in 24 hours varies from 700
to 900 g. Most of these glands are eccrine
glands, producing sweat that carries away
sodium chloride, the waste products urea
and lactic acid, and the breakdown products from garlic, spices, and other substances. Each sudoriferous gland consists
of a single tube with a deeply coiled body
and a superficial duct.

sudorific /sōō′dərif′ik/ [L *sudor* sweat,
facere to make], **1.** of or pertaining to a
substance or condition, such as heat or
emotional tension, that promotes sweating.
2. a sudorific agent. Sweat glands are
stimulated by cholinergic drugs.

sufentanil citrate /sufen′tənil/, an intravenous analgesic and anesthetic used as an
adjunct to general anesthesia and as a primary anesthetic with 100% oxygen.

suffocation /suf′əkā′shən/ [L *suffocare* to
choke], an interruption in breathing with
oxygen deprivation, usually caused by an
obstruction in the airways. The condition
may be accidental, intentional, the result
of disease, or inadequate levels of respi-
rable gases in the atmosphere.

suffocation, high risk for, a NANDA-
accepted nursing diagnosis of the accentuated risk of accidental suffocation (inadequate air available for inhalation). The
risk factors may be internal (individual) or
external (environmental). Internal risk factors include reduced olfactory sensation,

reduced motor abilities, lack of safety education, lack of safety precautions, cognitive or emotional difficulties, and disease
or injury processes. External risk factors
include a pillow or a propped bottle placed
in an infant's crib, a vehicle warming in a
closed garage, children playing with plastic bags or inserting small objects into
their mouths or noses, discarded or unused
refrigerators or freezers without removed
doors, unattended children in bathtubs or
pools, household gas leaks, smoking in
bed, eating too large mouthfuls of food,
use of fuel-burning heaters not vented to
outside, low-strung clothesline, and a pacifier hung around infant's neck.

suffocative goiter [L *suffocare* to choke;
guttur throat], an enlargement of the thyroid gland causing a sensation of suffocation on pressure.

sugar [Gk *sakcharon*], any of several
water-soluble carbohydrates. The two
principal categories of sugars are
monosaccharides and disaccharides. A
monosaccharide is a single sugar, such as
glucose, fructose, or galactose. A disaccharide is a double sugar, such as sucrose
(table sugar) or lactose.

sugar alcohol, an alcohol produced by
the reduction of an aldehyde or ketone of
a sugar.

suggestibility, pertaining to a person's
susceptibility to having his or her ideas or
actions changed by the influence of others.

suggestion [L *suggerere* to propose], **1.**
the process by which one thought or idea
leads to another, as in the association of
ideas. **2.** the use of persuasion, exhorta-
tion, or another device to implant an idea,
thought, attitude, or belief in the mind of
another as a means of influencing or altering behavior or states of mind. **3.** an
idea, belief, or attitude implanted in the
mind of another.

suicidal /sōō′isī′dəl/ [L *sui* of oneself, *caedere* to kill], of, relating to, or tending
toward self-destruction.

suicide /sōō′isīd/ [L *sui* of oneself, *caedere*
to kill], **1.** the intentional taking of one's
own life. **2.** *informal;* the ruin or destruction of one's own interests. **3.** a person
who commits or attempts self-destruction.

suicide gesture, (in psychiatric nursing)
an apparent attempt by a patient to cause
self-injury without lethal consequences
and generally without actual intent to commit suicide.

suicide prevention center, a crisis-
intervention facility dealing primarily with
people preoccupied with suicidal thoughts.
Such facilities are usually operated by professional social workers with special train-

ing in counseling possible suicide victims in person or by telephone.

suicidology /sōō′isīdol′əjē/ [L *sui, caedere* + Gk *logos* science], the study of the prevention and the causes of suicide. **–suicidologist,** *n.*

sulculus /sul′kyələs/ [L *sulcus*], a small sulcus.

sulcus /sul′kəs/, *pl.* **sulci** /sul′sī/ [L, furrow], a shallow groove, a depression, or a furrow on the surface of an organ, such as a sulcus that separates the convolutions of the cerebral hemisphere. **–sulcate,** *adj.*

sulcus centralis cerebri. See **fissure of Rolando.**

sulcus pulmonalis, a depression on each side of the vertebral bodies that accommodates the posterior portion of the lung.

sulfacetamide /sul′faset′əmīd/, a topical antibacterial prescribed for the prophylaxis of infection after injury to the cornea and in the treatment of bacterial conjunctivitis and urinary tract infections.

sulfachlorpyridazine /sul′fəklôr′pirid′-əzēn/, a sulfonamide antibacterial prescribed in the treatment of infection, particularly of the urinary tract.

sulfacytine /sulfas′itēn/, a sulfonamide antibacterial prescribed in the treatment of infection, particularly primary pyelonephritis, and cystitis.

sulfadiazine /sul′fədī′əzēn/, a sulfonamide antibacterial prescribed in the treatment of infection, particularly of the urinary tract, and as a rheumatic fever prophylaxis.

sulfa drugs, a group of bacteriostatic agents that inhibit the biosynthesis of folic acid.

sulfamethizole /sulfəmeth′izōl/, a sulfonamide antibacterial prescribed in the treatment of infection, particularly pyelonephritis, pyelitis, and cystitis.

sulfamethoxazole /sul′fəmethok′səzōl/, a sulfonamide antibacterial prescribed in the treatment of otitis media, bronchitis, and certain urinary tract infections.

sulfamethoxazole and trimethoprim /trī-meth′əprim/, a fixed-combination antibacterial prescribed in the treatment of urinary tract infections, otitis media, and shigellosis.

sulfanilic acid /sul′fənil′ik/, a red-tinged, white crystalline compound used in the synthesis of sulfonamides and as a reagent in tests for phenol, fecal matter in water, albumin, aldehydes, and glucose.

sulfasalazine /sul′fəsalaz′ēn/, a sulfonamide; salicylazosulfapyridine prescribed in the treatment of mild to moderate ulcerative colitis and as adjunctive therapy in severe cases.

sulfate /sul′fāt/, a salt of sulfuric acid. Natural sulfates, such as sodium sulfate, calcium sulfate, and potassium sulfate, are plentiful in the body.

sulfathiazole /sul′fəthī′əzōl/, a sulfonamide antibacterial no longer commonly used.

sulfatide lipidosis /sul′fətīd/, an inherited lipid metabolism disorder of childhood caused by a deficiency of cerebroside sulfatase enzyme. It results in an accumulation of metachromatic lipids in tissues of the central nervous system, kidney, spleen, and other organs, leading to dementia, paralysis, and death by the age of 10 years.

sulfhemoglobin /sulfhem′əglō′bin/, a form of hemoglobin containing an irreversibly bound sulfur molecule that prevents normal oxygen binding. It is present in the blood in trace amounts.

sulfhemoglobinemia /-ē′mē·ə/, the presence of abnormal sulfur-containing hemoglobin circulating in the blood.

sulfinpyrazone /sul′finpir′əzōn/, a uricosuric prescribed in the treatment of chronic gout and intermittent gouty arthritis.

sulfisoxazole /sul′fisok′səzōl/, a sulfonamide antibacterial prescribed in the treatment of conjunctivitis and urinary tract infections, including vaginitis, cystitis, and pyelonephritis.

sulfiting agents, food preservatives composed of potassium or sodium bisulfite or potassium metabisulfite. Sulfiting agents are used in processing of beer, wine, baked goods, soup mixes, and some imported seafoods and by restaurants to impart a "fresh" appearance to salad fruits and vegetables. The chemicals can cause a severe allergic reaction in persons who are hypersensitive to sulfites. The reactions are marked by flushing, faintness, hives, headache, GI distress, breathing difficulty, and, in extreme cases, loss of consciousness and death.

sulfobromophthalein /sul′fəbrō′məfthal′-ēn, -ē·in/, a substance used in its disodium salt form for evaluating the function of the liver.

sulfonamide /səlfon′əmīd/, one of a large group of synthetic, bacteriostatic drugs that are effective in treating infections caused by many gram-negative and gram-positive microorganisms. The drugs act by preventing the normal growth, development, and multiplication of the bacteria but do not kill mature organisms. They are bacteriostatic rather than bactericidal.

sulfonates /sul′fənāts/, a class of anticholinesterase compounds used as insecticides.

sulfonylurea /sul′fənilyōōr′ē·ə/, an oral antidiabetic agent that stimulates the pan-

S

creatic production of insulin. Hypersensitivity to sulfonamides is a contraindication for using such agents, and ethanol consumption is incompatible with all sulfonylureas. Aspirin or other salicylates taken with any sulfonylurea intensifies the hypoglycemic effect.

sulfosalicylic acid /sul'fōsalisil'ik/, a white or faintly pink crystalline substance that is highly water-soluble, used as a reagent in tests for albumin and as an intermediate compound in the manufacture of dyes and surfactants.

sulfoxone sodium /sulfok'sōn/, a bacteriostatic sulfone derivative prescribed in the treatment of leprosy and dermatitis herpetiformis.

sulfur (S) [L], a nonmetallic, multivalent, tasteless, odorless chemical element that occurs abundantly in yellow crystalline form or in masses, especially in volcanic areas. Its atomic number is 16; its atomic weight is 32.06. Sulfur has been used in the treatment of gout, rheumatism, and bronchitis and as a mild laxative. The sulfonamides, or sulfa drugs, are used in the treatment of various bacterial infections.

sulfuric acid /sulf(y)o͞o'oik/, a clear, colorless, oily, highly corrosive liquid that generates great heat when mixed with water. An extremely toxic substance, sulfuric acid causes severe skin burns, blindness on contact with the eyes, serious lung damage if the vapors are inhaled, and death if it is ingested.

sulfurous acid /sul'f(y)o͞orəs/, a weak inorganic acid used as a chemical reducing and bleaching agent. It has been used in medicine in skin lotions and nasal and throat sprays. Sulfites formed by the acid may be used in antiseptics, antifermentatives, and antizymotics.

sulindac /sulin'dek/, an antiinflammatory agent prescribed in the treatment of osteoarthritis, rheumatoid arthritis, and ankylosing spondylitis.

Sulkowitch's test /sul'kəwichs/ [Hirsh W. Sulkowitch, American physician, b. 1906], an examination of the urine for the presence of calcium. A reagent, containing oxalic acid, ammonium oxalate, and glacial acetic acid, mixed with urine, causes calcium to precipitate out of the urine.

sulphur. See **sulfur.**

sumac /so͞o'mak, sho͞o'mak/ [Ar *summaq*], any of a number of species of trees and shrubs in the *Anacardiaceae* family, including the *Rhus* varieties, which have poisonous properties.

summary judgment [L *summa* total; *jus* law, *dicere* to state], (in law) a judgment requested by any party to a civil action to end the action when it is believed that there is no genuine issue or material fact in dispute.

summation [L *summa* total], 1. an accumulative effect or action; a total aggregate; totality. 2. (in neurology), the accumulation of the concentration of a neurotransmitter at a synapse, either by increasing the frequency of nerve impulses in each fiber (temporal summation) or by increasing the number of fibers stimulated (spatial summation), so that the threshold of the postsynaptic neuron is overcome and an impulse is transmitted.

summons [OFr *somondre* to remind secretly], (in law) a document issued by a clerk of the court on the filing of a complaint. A sheriff, marshal, or other appointed person serves the summons, notifying a person that an action has been begun against him or her.

sun bath [AS *sunne, baeth*], the exposure of the naked body to the sun.

sundowning [AS *sunne + ofdune* off the hill], a condition in which elderly patients tend to become confused or disoriented at the end of the day. With less light, they lose visual cues that help them to compensate for their sensory impairments.

sunrise syndrome, a condition of unstable cognitive ability on arising in the morning.

sunscreen protective factor index (SPF), a system of evaluating the effectiveness of various formulations for protecting the skin from actinic rays of the sun. Protective agents are rated from one to 50 by the FDA. Among the most highly rated sunscreen lotions are nonopaque combinations of PABA ester and benzophenone.

sunstroke [AS *sunne + strac* stroke], a morbid condition caused by overexposure to the sun and characterized by a high fever, convulsions, and coma.

superego [L *super* over; Gk *ego* I], (in psychoanalysis) that part of the psyche, functioning mostly in the unconscious, that develops when the standards of the parents and of society are incorporated into the ego. The superego has two parts, the conscience and the ego ideal.

superfecundation /so͞o'pərfekəndē'shən/ [L *super + fecundare* to be fruitful], the fertilization of two or more ova released during one menstrual cycle by spermatozoa from the same or different males during separate acts of sexual intercourse.

superfetation /-fētā'shən/ [L *super + fetus* pregnancy], the fertilization of a second ovum after the onset of pregnancy, resulting in the presence of two fetuses of different degrees of maturity developing within the uterus simultaneously.

superficial /-fish'əl/ [L *superficialis* surface], **1.** of or pertaining to the skin or another surface. **2.** not grave or dangerous.

superficial abscess, an abscess that develops above the fascia layer.

superficial fading infantile hemangioma, a superficial, transient, salmon-colored patch in the center of the forehead, face, or occiput of many newborns.

superficial implantation, (in embryology) the partial embedding of the blastocyst within the uterine wall so that it and, later, the chorionic sac protrude into the uterine cavity.

superficial inguinal node, a node in one of the two groups of inguinal lymph glands in the upper femoral triangle of the thigh.

superficial reflex, any neural reflex initiated by stimulation of the skin. Kinds of superficial reflexes are **abdominal reflex, anal reflex,** and **cremasteric reflex.**

superficial sensation, the awareness or perception of feelings in the superficial layers of the skin in response to touch, pressure, temperature, and pain.

superficial spreading melanoma, a melanoma that grows outward, spreading over the surface of the affected organ or tissue, most commonly on the lower legs of women and the torso of men.

superficial temporal artery, an artery at each side of the head that can be easily felt in front of the ear and is often used for taking the pulse. It is the smaller of the two terminal branches of the external carotid.

superficial vein, one of the many veins between the subcutaneous fascia just under the skin.

superimpregnation. See **superfetation.**

superinfection [L *super* + *inficere* to taint], an infection occurring during antimicrobial treatment for another infection.

superior /səpir'ē·ər/ [L, to go above], situated above or oriented toward a higher place, as the head is superior to the torso.

superior aperture of minor pelvis, an opening bounded by the crest and pecten of the pubic bones, the arch-shaped lines of the ilia, and the anterior margin of the base of the sacrum.

superior aperture of thorax, an elliptic opening at the summit of the thorax bounded by the first thoracic vertebra, the first ribs, and the upper margin of the sternum.

superior carotid triangle, a triangle bounded by the sternocleidomastoid muscle, in front and below by the omohyoid muscle, and above by the stylohyoid and digastric muscles.

superior conjunctival fornix, the space in the fold of the conjunctiva created by the reflection of the conjunctiva covering the eyeball and the lining of the upper lid.

superior costotransverse ligament, one of five ligaments associated with each costotransverse joint, except that of the first rib. It passes from the neck of each rib to the transverse process of the vertebra immediately above.

superior gastric node, a node in one of two sets of gastric lymph glands, accompanying the left gastric artery.

superior hemorrhagic polioencephalitis. See **Wernicke's encephalopathy.**

superior mediastinum, the cranial portion of the mediastinum in the middle of the thorax, containing the trachea, esophagus, aortic arch, and origins of the sternohyoidei and the sternothyroidei.

superior mesenteric artery, a visceral branch of the abdominal aorta, arising caudal to the celiac artery, dividing into five branches, and supplying most of the small intestine and parts of the colon.

superior mesenteric node, a node in one of the three groups of visceral lymph nodes that serve the viscera of the abdomen and the pelvis.

superior mesenteric vein, a tributary of the portal vein that drains the blood from the small intestine, cecum, and ascending and transverse colons.

superior olivary nucleus, a collection of nerve cells appearing as clumps of gray matter in the pons. It assists in the localization of sound by comparing the time difference between sound received by the left and right ears.

superior profunda artery. See **deep brachial artery.**

superior radioulnar joint. See **proximal radioulnar articulation.**

superior sagittal sinus, one of the six venous channels in the posterior of the dura mater, draining blood from the brain into the internal jugular vein.

superior subscapular nerve /səb-skap'yələr/, one of two small nerves on opposite sides of the body that supply the superior part of the subscapularis.

superior thyroid artery, one of a pair of arteries in the neck, usually rising from the external carotid artery, that supplies the thyroid gland and several muscles in the head.

superior ulnar collateral artery, a long, slender division of the brachial artery, arising just distal to the middle of the arm, descending to the elbow, and anastomosing with the posterior ulnar recurrent and inferior ulnar collateral arteries.

superior vena cava, the second largest vein of the body, returning deoxygenated blood from the upper half of the body to the right atrium. It is formed by the junction of the two brachiocephalic veins at the level of the first intercostal space behind the sternum on the right side. The section of the superior vena cava closest to the heart comprises about one half of the vessel's length and is within the pericardial sac, covered by the serous pericardium.

supernatant /-nā′tənt/ [L *super* + *natare* to swim], the clear upper portion of any mixture after it has been centrifuged.

supernormal excitability, the ability of the myocardium to respond to a stimulus that would be ineffective earlier or later in the cardiac cycle.

supernormal period, a period at the end of phase 3 of the cardiac cycle when activation can be initiated with less stimulus than is required at maximal repolarization.

supernumerary nipples /-nōō′mərer′ē/ [L *super* + *numerus* number; ME *neb* beak], an excessive number of nipples, which are usually not associated with underlying glandular tissue. They may vary in size from small pink dots to that of normal nipples.

supernumerary tooth, any tooth in addition to the normal 32 teeth in permanent dentition or the 29 teeth in deciduous dentition.

superoxide /-ok′sīd/, a common reactive form of oxygen that is formed when molecular oxygen gains a single electron. Superoxide radicals can attack susceptible biologic targets, including lipids, proteins, and nucleic acids.

superoxide dismutase (SOD), an enzyme composed of metal-containing proteins that converts superoxide radicals into less toxic agents. It is the main enzymatic mechanism for clearing superoxide radicals from the body.

supersaturate [L *super* + *saturare* to fill], a solution that contains solute above the saturation point at a given temperature.

supervision, (in psychology) a process whereby a therapist is helped to become a more effective clinician through the direction of a supervisor who provides theoretical knowledge and therapeutic techniques.

supervisor [L *super* + *videre* to see], (in hospital or public health nursing) the midlevel management position between the director of nursing and head nurses of a division or of several units. In many hospitals *clinical director* is the preferred term.

supervitaminosis /-vī′təminō′sis/, a condition of ingesting an excessive amount of vitamins. Signs and symptoms vary with specific vitamin excesses.

supinate /sōō′pənāt/, pertaining to a su-

pine position or turning the palm upward.

supination /sōō′pinā′shən/ [L *supinus* lying on the back], 1. one of the kinds of rotation allowed by certain skeletal joints, such as the elbow and the wrist joints, which allow the palm of the hand to turn up. 2. the position of lying on the back, face up. –**supinate,** *v.*

supinator longus. See **brachioradialis.**

supinator longus reflex /sōō′pinā·tər/, a contraction of the brachioradialis muscle, causing flexion at the elbow joint, on tapping the point of insertion of the supinator longus muscle at the lower end of the radius.

supine /səpīn′, sōō′pīn/ [L *supinus*], lying horizontally on the back.

supine hypotension, a fall in blood pressure that occurs when a pregnant woman is lying on her back. It is caused by impaired venous return that results from pressure of the gravid uterus on the vena cava.

supplemental inheritance [L *supplere* to complete; *in* in, *hereditare* hereditary], the acquisition or expression of a genetic trait or condition from the presence of two independent pairs of nonallelic genes that interact in such a way that one gene supplements the action of the other.

supplementary gene [L *supplere* + Gk *genein* to produce], one of two pairs of nonallelic genes that interact in such a way that one pair needs the presence of the other to be expressed, whereas the second pair can produce an effect independent of the first.

support [L *supportare* to bring up], 1. to sustain, hold up, or maintain in a desired position or condition, as in physically supporting the abdominal muscles with a scultetus binder or emotionally supporting a patient under stress. 2. the assistance given to this end, such as physical support, emotional support, or life support.

supporting area [L *supportare* + *area* space], any of the areas of maxillary or mandibular edentulous ridges that are considered best suited to bear the forces of mastication with functioning dentures.

supportive psychotherapy, a form of psychotherapy that concentrates on creating an effective means of communication with an emotionally disturbed person rather than on trying to produce psychologic insight into the underlying conflicts.

supportive treatment. See **treatment.**

suppository /səpoz′ətôr′ē/ [L *sub* under, *pornere* to place], an easily melted medicated mass for insertion in the rectum, urethra, or vagina. Theobroma oil, glycerinated gelatin, and high-molecular-weight polyethylene glycols are common vehicles for drugs in suppositories that are cone- or spindle-shaped for insertion in the rectum, globular or egg-shaped for use in the vagina, and pencil-shaped for insertion in the urethra.

suppressant /səpres'ənt/ [L *supprimere* to press down], an agent that suppresses or diminishes a physical or mental activity, such as a medication that reduces hyperkinetic behavior.

suppressed menstruation [L *supprimere* to press down, *menstruare*], a failure of menstruation to occur when expected, as in amenorrhea.

suppression [L *supprimere*], (in psychoanalysis) the conscious inhibition or effort to conceal unacceptable or painful thoughts, desires, impulses, feelings, or acts.

suppression amblyopia, a partial loss of vision, usually in one eye, caused by cortical suppression of central vision to avoid diplopia. It occurs commonly in strabismus in the eye that deviates and does not fixate.

suppressor gene, (in molecular genetics) a genetic unit that is able to reverse the effect of a specific kind of mutation in other genes.

suppressor mutation, (in molecular genetics) a mutation that partially or completely restores a function lost by a primary mutation occurring in a different genetic site.

suppressor T cell. See **T cell.**

suppurate /sup'yərāt/ [L *suppurare* to produce pus], to produce purulent matter. **–suppuration,** *n.,* **suppurative** /sup'yərā'tiv/, *adj.*

suppuration [L *suppurare* to form pus], the production and exudation of pus.

suppurative fever, a fever accompanied by pus formation.

suppurative pancreatitis, a form of pancreas inflammation accompanied by the appearance of small abscesses.

suppurative phlebitis, a vein inflammation as a result of septicemia or a nearby pyogenic infection.

supracallosus gyrus /soo'prəkalō'səs/ [L *supra* + *callosus* hard; Gk *gyros* turn], the gray matter covering the corpus callosum of the brain.

supracervical hysterectomy /-sur'vikəl/, a subtotal hysterectomy in which the body of the uterus is removed, leaving the cervix.

supraclavicular /-kləvik'yələr/ [L *supra* above, *clavicula* little key], the area of the body above the clavicle, or collar bone.

supraclavicular nerve, one of a pair of cutaneous branches of the cervical plexus, arising from the third and the fourth cer-

vical nerves, mostly from the fourth nerve.

supraclavicular triangle, the lower and anterior areas of the neck, bounded by the omohyoid muscle above, the sternocleidomastoid muscle in front, and the clavicle below. The first rib is in the base of the triangle.

supracondylar [L *supra* + Gk *kondylos* knuckle], above a condyle.

supracondylar fracture /-kon'dīlər /soo'prəkon'dilər/ [L *supra* + *kondylos* knuckle], a fracture involving the area between the condyles of the humerus or the femur.

supragingival calculus /-jinjī'vəl/ [L *supra* + *gingiva* gum], a deposit composed of various mineral salts, such as calcium phosphate and calcium carbonate, which accumulates with organic matter and oral debris on the teeth occlusal or coronal to the gingival crest.

suprainfection [L *supra* + *inficere* to taint], a secondary infection usually caused by an opportunistic pathogen, such as a fungal infection after the antibiotic treatment of another infection.

supraoptic nucleus /-op'tik/ [L *supra* + Gk *optikos*; L *nucleus* nut], a hypothalamic nucleus that lies in the optic chiasma with fibers extending to the posterior lobe of the pituitary.

suprapatellar, above the patella.

suprapubic [L *supra* + *pubes* signs of maturity], located above the symphysis pubis.

suprapubic catheter, a urinary bladder catheter that is inserted through the skin about 1 inch above the symphysis pubis.

suprarenal /-rē'nəl/ [L *supra* + *ren* kidney], above the kidney, such as the suprarenal gland.

suprascapular ligament /-skap'yələr/, a ligament that extends from the base of the coracoid process to the medial end of the suprascapular notch.

suprascapular nerve /soo'prəskap'yələr/ [L *supra* + *scapula* shoulderblade], one of a pair of branches from the cords of the brachial plexus.

suprasellar cyst. See **craniopharyngioma.**

supraspinal [L *supra* + *spina* backbone], pertaining to something above the spine.

supraspinal ligament, the ligament that connects the apices of the spinous processes from the seventh cervical vertebra to the sacrum. Between the spinous processes it is continuous with the interspinal ligaments.

supraspinous fossa /-spī'nəs/, a depressed area on the dorsal surface of the scapula, above the spine.

S

suprasternal /-stur′nəl/, above the sternum, adjacent to the neck.

supratentorial /-tentôr′ē·əl/, above a tentorium.

supravaginal hysterectomy /-vaj′inəl/ [L *supra* + *vagina* sheath; Gk *hystera* womb, *ektome* excision], a subtotal hysterectomy in which the body of the uterus is removed but the cervix remains.

supraventricular tachycardia (SVT) [L *supra* + *ventriculum* belly], any cardiac rhythm exceeding 100 beats per minute that originates above the ventricles, in the SA node, atria, or AV junction.

suprofen /səprō′fən/, an oral nonsteroidal antiinflammatory analgesic used in the treatment of mild to moderate pain and primary dysmenorrhea.

suramin sodium /sŌŌ′rəmin/, an antitrypanosomal and an antifilarial available from the Centers for Disease Control and Prevention.

surface anatomy [L *superficies* the top], the study of the structural relationships of the external features of the body to the internal organs and parts.

surface anesthesia. See **topical anesthesia.**

surface area (SA), the total area exposed to the outside environment. The surface area of an object increases with the square of the object's linear dimensions; volume increases as the cube of the object's linear dimensions.

surface biopsy, the removal of living tissue for microscopic examination by scraping the surface of a lesion.

surface tension, the tendency of the surface of a liquid to minimize the area of its surface by contracting. This property causes liquids to rise in a capillary tube, affects the exchange of gases in the pulmonary alveoli, and alters the ability of various liquids to wet another surface.

surface therapy, a form of radiotherapy administered by placing one or more radioactive sources on or near an area of body surface.

surface thermometer, a device that detects and indicates the temperature of the surface of any part of the body.

surfactant /sərfak′tənt/ [L *superficies*], 1. an agent, such as soap or detergent, dissolved in water to reduce its surface tension or the tension at the interface between the water and another liquid. 2. certain lipoproteins that reduce the surface tension of pulmonary fluids, allowing the exchange of gases in the alveoli of the lungs and contributing to the elasticity of pulmonary tissue.

surfer's nodules [ME *suffe* rush; L *nodus* knot], nodules on the skin of the knees, ankles, feet, or toes of a surfer caused by repeated contact of the skin with an abrasive, sandy surfboard.

surgeon's assistant (SA) [Gk *cheirourgos* surgeon; L *assistere* to cause to stand], a medical professional trained to assist in surgery and in the preoperative and postoperative periods under the supervision of a licensed physician qualified to practice surgery.

surgery [Gk *cheirourgos*], a branch of medicine concerned with diseases and trauma requiring operative procedures. –**surgical,** *adj.*

surgical abdomen. See **acute abdomen.**

surgical anatomy, (in applied anatomy) the study of the structure and morphology of the tissues and organs of the body as they relate to surgery.

surgical anesthesia, the third stage of general anesthesia.

surgical diathermy. See **electrocoagulation.**

surgical fever, a fever that develops after surgery. Under modern aseptic techniques, fever is unlikely to accompany an operation.

surgical induction of labor. See **induction of labor.**

surgical ligature, the exposure of an unerupted tooth by placing a metal ligature around its cervix.

surgical menopause, the creation of a menopausal state by surgical termination of menstrual function.

surgical microscope. See **operating microscope.**

surgical neck of humerus, the shaft of the humerus distal to the tuberosities. It is a region particularly vulnerable to fracture and surgical correction.

surgical pathology, the study of tissue specimens obtained during surgery. The surgical pathologist often examines specimens during surgery to determine how the operation should be modified or completed. Various techniques are used. The appearance of the specimen is first noted; then slices of the tissue are prepared and microscopically examined.

surgical scrub, 1. a bactericidal soap or solution used by surgeons and surgical nurses before performing or assisting in surgery. 2. the act of washing the fingernails, hands, and forearms with a bactericidal soap or solution before a surgical procedure.

surgical sectioning, an oral surgery procedure for dividing a tooth to facilitate its removal.

surgical shock, a condition of shock that may follow surgery, with signs of low blood volume, failure of peripheral circulation, sweating, thirst, restlessness, and cyanosis of the extremities.

surgical suite, a group of one or more operating rooms and adjunct facilities, such as sterile storage area, scrub room, and recovery room.

surgical technologist, an allied health professional who prepares the operating room. Surgical technologists have primary responsibility for maintaining the sterile field and being constantly vigilant that all members of the surgical team adhere to aseptic technique.

surgical treatment. See **treatment.**

surrogate /sur'əgāt/ [L *surrogare* to substitute], **1.** a substitute; a person or thing that replaces another. **2.** (in psychoanalysis) a substitute parental figure, a symbolic image or representation of another, as may occur in a dream.

surrogate parenting, a form of artificial insemination in which a fertile woman who is not the wife of the sperm donor agrees to be impregnated by the husband and to carry the child to term, at which time the offspring is surrendered to the care of the infertile wife. The surrogate mother usually receives a fee for bearing the child.

surveillance /sərvā'ləns/ [Fr *surveiller* to watch over], supervising or observing a patient or a health condition.

surveyed height of contour [OFr *surveir* to survey; AS *heah* high; It *contornare* to round off], a line, scribed or marked on a cast, that designates the greatest convexity relative to a selected path of denture placement and removal.

survival curve [Fr *survivre* to survive; L *curvus* bent], a curve obtained by plotting the number or percentage of organisms surviving at different intervals against doses of radiation.

survivor guilt, feelings of guilt for surviving a tragedy in which others died. In some cases, the person may believe the tragedy occurred because he or she "did something bad"; in others, the person may feel guilty for not taking proper steps to avert the tragedy.

susceptibility [L *suscipere* to undertake], the condition of being more than normally vulnerable to a disease or disorder. **–susceptible,** *adj.*

suspension [L *suspendere* to hang], **1.** a liquid in which small particles of a solid are dispersed, but not dissolved, and in which the dispersal is maintained by stirring or shaking the mixture. **2.** a treatment, used primarily in spinal disorders, consisting of suspending the patient by the chin and shoulders. **3.** a temporary cessation of pain or of a vital process.

suspension sling, a sling usually made of muslin or lightweight canvas and used primarily to provide support. An example is a common triangular sling.

suspensory ligament [L *suspendere* + *ligare* to bind], any of a number of ligaments that helps support an organ or body structure, such as the suspensory ligaments inside the eye that hold the lens in tension.

suspensory ligament of the lens. See **zonula ciliaris.**

sustained release. See **prolonged release.**

sustenance /sus'tənəns/ [L *sustenare* to sustain], **1.** the act or process of supporting or maintaining life or health. **2.** the food or nutrients essential for maintaining life.

susto /sōōs'tō/, a culture-bound syndrome found in Central American populations. It is related to stress engendered by a self-perceived failure to fulfill sex-role expectations.

sutilains /sōō'tilānz/, a proteolytic enzyme prescribed for debridement of certain wounds, ulcers, and second- and third-degree burns.

sutura /sōōchōō'ra/, *pl.* **suturae** [L, suture], an immovable, fibrous joint in which certain bones of the skull are connected by a thin layer of fibrous tissue.

sutura dentata, an immovable fibrous joint that is one kind of true suture in which toothlike processes interlock along the margins of connecting bones of the skull.

sutura limbosa, an immovable fibrous joint that is one kind of true suture in which beveled and serrated edges of certain connecting bones of the skull overlap and interlock.

sutura plana, a fibrous joint that is one kind of false suture in which rough, contiguous edges of certain bones of the skull, such as the maxillae, form a connection.

sutura serrata, an immovable fibrous joint that is one kind of true suture in which connecting bones interlock along serrated edges that resemble fine-toothed saws.

sutura squamosa, an immovable fibrous joint that is one kind of false suture in which overlapping, beveled edges unite certain bones of the skull.

suture /sōō'chər/ [L *sutura*], **1.** a border or a joint, as between the bones of the cranium. **2.** to stitch together cut or torn edges of tissue with suture material. **3.** a surgical stitch taken to repair an incision, tear, or wound. **4.** material used for surgical stitches, such as absorbable or nonabsorbable silk, catgut, wire, or synthetic material.

suture forceps. See **needle holder.**

Sv, abbreviation for **sievert.**

SV40, abbreviation for **simian virus 40.**

SvO₂, symbol for the percent of saturation of mixed venous blood.

swab [D *swabber* ship's drudge], a stick or clamp for holding absorbent gauze or cotton, used for washing, cleansing, or drying a body surface, for collecting a specimen for laboratory examinations, or for applying a topical medication.

swaddling [OE *swethel* swaddling band], **1.** long narrow bands of cloth once used to wrap a newborn. **2.** a method of wrapping a newborn, especially a premature or at risk newborn, that provides maximal comfort.

swallowing [AS *swelgan*], the process that usually involves movement of food from the mouth to the stomach via the esophagus. Coordination of muscles is needed from the tongue to the esophageal sphincter.

swallowing, impaired, a NANDA-accepted nursing diagnosis of decreased ability to voluntarily pass fluids and/or solids from the mouth to the stomach. Defining characteristics include observed evidence of difficulty in swallowing, such as stasis of food in the oral cavity, coughing, choking, and evidence of aspiration.

swallowing reflex [AS *swelgan;* L *reflectere* to bend back], a sequence of reflexes that begins when a bolus of food is manipulated by the tongue and other oral cavity muscles to the palate or the pharynx.

swamp fever. See **leptospirosis, malaria.**

Swan-Ganz catheter /swän′ganz′/ [Harold J. C. Swan, American physician, b. 1922; William Ganz, American cardiologist, b. 1919; Gk *kather* something lowered], a long, thin cardiac catheter with a tiny balloon at the tip.

swan neck deformity [D *zwaan;* AS *hnecca* neck; L *deformis* misshapen], **1.** an abnormal condition of the finger characterized by flexion of the distal interphalangeal joint and hyperextension of the proximal interphalangeal joint. The condition is seen most often in rheumatoid arthritis. **2.** a structural abnormality of the kidney tubules associated with rickets. The kidney tubule connecting the glomerulus with the convoluted portion of the tubule is narrowed into a configuration referred to as *swan neck.*

S wave, the component of the cardiac cycle shown on an electrocardiogram as a line slanting downward sharply from the peak of the R wave to the beginning of the upward curve of the T wave. It represents the final phase of the QRS complex.

sweat. See **perspiration.**

sweat bath, a bath given to induce sweating.

sweat duct [AS *swaetan* to sweat; L *ducere* to lead], any one of the tiny tubules conveying sweat to the surface of the skin from sweat glands throughout the body. Each sweat duct is the most superficial part of a coiled tube that forms the body of each sweat gland and opens onto the surface through a funnel-shaped opening. The sweat ducts in the armpits and in the groin are larger than in other parts of the body.

sweat gland. See **sudoriferous gland.**

sweating. See **diaphoresis.**

sweat test, a method for evaluating sodium and chloride excretion from the sweat glands, often the first test performed in the diagnosis of cystic fibrosis. The sweat glands are stimulated with a drug, such as pilocarpine, and the perspiration produced is analyzed. The eccrine glands of patients with cystic fibrosis produce sodium and chloride concentrations that are three to six times those of the normal.

Swedish massage [Fr *masser*], a regimen of massage combined with physical exercises.

Sweet localization method, a radiographic technique for locating a foreign body in the eye by making two x-ray films of the eye while the patient's head is immobilized. A small metal ball and a cone are placed at precise distances from the center of the cornea as register marks while lateral and perpendicular x-ray views of the eye are made. A three-dimensional view of the eye is constructed from the two x-ray films, and the location of the foreign body in the eye is plotted from the intersection of lines through the ball and cone.

Swift's disease. See **acrodynia.**

swimmer's ear [AS *swimman* to swim; *eare*], *informal;* otitis externa resulting from infection transmitted in the water of a swimming pool.

swimmer's itch, an allergic dermatitis caused by sensitivity to schistosome cercariae that die under the skin, leading to erythema, urticaria, and a papular rash lasting 1 or 2 days.

swing phase of gait [AS *swingan* + Gk *phasis* appearance; ME *gate* a way], one of the two phases in the rhythmic process of walking. The swing phase of gait follows the stance phase and is divided into the initial swing stage, the midswing stage, and the terminal swing stage.

swoon [OE *geswogen* unconscious], a fainting spell.

sycosis barbae /sikō′sis/ [Gk *sycon* fig, *osis* condition; L *barba* beard], an inflammation of hair follicles of skin that has been shaved.

Sydenham's chorea /sid′ənhamz/ [Thomas Sydenham, English physician, b. 1624; Gk *choreia* dance], a form of chorea associated with rheumatic fever, usually occurring during childhood. The cause is a streptococcal infection of the vascular and perivascular tissues of the brain. The choreic movements increase over the first 2 weeks, reach a plateau, and then diminish.

sylvatic plague /silvat′ik/ [L *sylva* woodland; *plaga* stroke], an endemic disease of wild rodents caused by *Yersinia pestis* and transmissible to humans by the bite of an infected flea. It is found on every continent except Australia.

sylvian aqueduct /sil′vē-ən/ [Franciscus Sylvius, Dutch anatomist, b. 1614; L *aqueductus* canal], a canal from the third to the fourth ventricle of the midbrain.

sylvian fissure [Franciscus Sylvius; L *fissura* cleft], the lateral sulcus of the cerebral hemisphere.

symbiosis /sim′bē-ō′sis/ [Gk *syn* together, *bios* life] **1.** (in biology) a mode of living characterized by close association between organisms of different species, usually in a mutually beneficial relationship. **2.** (in psychiatry) a state in which two mentally disturbed people are emotionally dependent on each other. **3.** pathologic inability of a child to separate from its mother emotionally and, sometimes, physically. –**symbiotic,** *adj.*

symbiotic phase /sim′bē-ot′ik/, in Mahler's system of preoedipal development, the stage between 1 and 5 months when the infant participates in a "symbiotic orbit" with the mother. All parts of the mother, including voice, gestures, clothing, and space in which she moves, are joined with the infant.

symbol [Gk *symbolon* sign], **1.** an image, object, action, or other stimulus that represents something else by reason of conscious association, convention, or other relationship. **2.** an object, mode of behavior, or feeling that disguises a repressed emotional conflict through an unconscious association rather than through an objective relationship, as in dreams and neuroses.

symbolism, 1. the representation or evocation of one idea, action, or object by the use of another, as in systems of writing, poetic language, or dream metaphor. **2.** (in psychiatry) an unconscious mental mechanism characteristic of all human thinking in which a mental image stands for but disguises some other object, person, or thought.

symelus. See **symmelus.**

symmelia /simē′lyə/ [Gk *syn* together,

melos limb], a fetal anomaly characterized by the fusion of the lower limbs with or without feet. Kinds of symmelia are **apodial, dipodial, monopodial,** and **tripodial symmelia.**

symmelus /sim′ələs/, a malformed fetus characterized by symmelia.

Symmer's disease. See **giant follicular lymphoma.**

symmetric, symmetrical [Gk *syn* + *metron* measure], (of the body or parts of the body) equal in size or shape; very similar in relative placement or arrangement about an axis. –**symmetry,** *n.*

symmetric lipomatosis. See **nodular circumscribed lipomatosis.**

symmetric tonic neck reflex, a normal response in infants to assume the crawl position by extending the arms and bending the knees when the head and neck are extended.

symmetry, (in anatomy) the correspondence of parts on opposite sides of the body, or equality of parts on both sides of a dividing line.

sympathectomize, to interrupt conduction of nerve impulses along part of the sympathetic trunk by surgery or drugs.

sympathectomy /sim′pathek′təmē/ [Gk *sympathein* to feel with, *ektome* excision], a surgical interruption of part of the sympathetic nerve pathways, performed for the relief of chronic pain or to promote vasodilation in vascular diseases, such as arteriosclerosis, claudication, Buerger's disease, and Raynaud's phenomenon. The sheath around an artery carries the sympathetic nerve fibers that control constriction of the vessel. Removal of the sheath causes the vessel to relax and expand and allows more blood to pass through it.

sympathetic [Gk *sympathein* to feel with], **1.** displaying of compassion for another's grief. **2.** pertaining to a division of the autonomic nervous system.

sympathetic amine, a drug that produces effects resembling those manifested by stimulation of the sympathetic nervous system.

sympathetic ganglion [Gk *sympathein, gagglion* knot], a collection of multipolar nerve cells along the course of the sympathetic trunk. Nearly two dozen of the ganglia serve as "cell stations" on efferent pathways between the cervical and sacral parts of the sympathetic trunk.

sympathetic imbalance, pertaining to vagotony or vagus nerve tension and hyperexcitability of the parasympathetic nervous system as opposed to the sympathetic nervous system.

sympathetic irritation [Gk *sypathein*; L *irritare* to tease], inflammation of one organ following inflammation of a related organ, as when trauma to an eye is followed by similar symptoms in the uninjured eye.

sympathetic nerve, any nerve of the sympathetic branch of the autonomic nervous system.

sympathetic nervous system. See **autonomic nervous system.**

sympathetic ophthalmia, a granulomatous inflammation of the uveal tract of both eyes occurring after an injury to the uveal tract of one eye.

sympathetic symptom, a symptom occurring in one body area when the causative lesion is actually in another area.

sympathetic trunk, one of a pair of chains of ganglia extending along the side of the vertebral column from the base of the skull to the coccyx. Each trunk is part of the sympathetic nervous system and consists of a series of ganglia connected by cords containing various types of fibers. Each sympathetic trunk distributes branches with postganglionic fibers to the autonomic plexuses, the cranial nerves, the individual organs, the nerves accompanying arteries, and the spinal nerves.

sympathizing eye, (in sympathetic ophthalmia) the uninfected eye that becomes infected by lymphatic or blood-borne metastasis of the microorganism.

sympatholytic, sympatholytic agent. See **antiadrenergic.**

sympathomimetic /sim′pəthōmimet′ik/ [Gk *sympathein* + *mimesis* imitation], denoting a pharmacologic agent that mimics the effects of stimulation of organs and structures by the sympathetic nervous system by occupying adrenergic receptor sites and acting as an agonist or by increasing the release of the neurotransmitter norepinephrine at postganglionic nerve endings. Various sympathomimetic agents are used as decongestants of nasal and ocular mucosa, as bronchodilators in the treatment of asthma, bronchitis, bronchiectasis, and emphysema, and as vasopressors and cardiac stimulants in the treatment of acute hypotension and shock.

sympathomimetic amine. See **adrenergic.**

sympathomimetic bronchodilator, a medication that reduces bronchial muscle spasm because of action that mimics the sympathetic nervous system in producing smooth muscle relaxation.

sympathy [Gk *sympathein*], **1.** an expressed interest or concern regarding the problems, emotions, or states of mind of another. **2.** the relation that exists between the mind and body causing the one to be affected by the other. **3.** mental contagion or the influence exerted by one individual or group on another and the effects produced, such as the spread of panic, uncontrollable laughter, or yawning. **4.** the physiologic or pathologic relationship between two organs, systems, or parts of the body. –**sympathetic,** adj., **sympathize,** v.

symphalangia /sim′fəlan′jē·ə/ [Gk *syn* together, *phalanx* finger], **1.** a condition, usually inherited, characterized by ankylosis of the fingers or toes. **2.** a congenital anomaly in which webbing of the fingers or toes occurs in varying degrees.

symphocephalus /sim′fōsef′ələs/ [Gk *symphes* growing together, *kephale* head], twin fetuses joined at the head. The term is often used as a general designation for fetuses with varying degrees of the anomaly.

symphyseal angle /simfiz′ē·əl/ [Gk *symphysis* growing together; L *angulus* corner], (in dentistry) the angle of the chin, which may be protruding, straight, or receding, according to type.

symphysic teratism /simfiz′ik/, a congenital anomaly in which there is a fusion of normally separated parts or organs, such as a horseshoe kidney.

symphysis /sim′fəsis/, pl. **symphyses** /-ēz/ [Gk, growing together], **1.** a line of union, especially a cartilaginous joint in which adjacent bony surfaces are firmly united by fibrocartilage. **2.** *informal;* symphysis pubis. –**symphysic,** adj.

symphysis pubis. See **pubic symphysis.**

sympodia /simpō′dē·ə/ [Gk *syn* together, *pous* foot], a congenital developmental anomaly characterized by fusion of the lower extremities.

symptom [Gk *symptoma* that which happens], a subjective indication of a disease or a change in condition as perceived by the patient. Many symptoms are accompanied by objective signs, such as pruritus. Some symptoms may be objectively confirmed, such as numbness of a body part, which may be confirmed by absence of response to a pin prick. **Primary symptoms** are symptoms that are intrinsically associated with the disease process. **Secondary symptoms** are a consequence of the disease process. –**symptomatic,** adj.

symptomatic esophageal peristalsis, a condition in which peristaltic progression in the body of the esophagus is normal but contractions in the distal esophagus are of increased amplitude and duration.

symptomatic impotence, impotence that is the result of poor health or the use of medications.

symptomatic nanism, dwarfism associated with defects in bone growth, tooth formation, and sexual development.

symptomatic neuralgia [Gk *symptoma, neuron* nerve, *algos* pain], nerve pain that is secondary to a disease condition.

symptomatic torticollis [Gk *symptoma;* L *tortus* twisted, *collum* neck], stiff neck caused by a disease in the neck, such as rheumatoid torticollis or myogenic torticollis.

symptomatic treatment. See **treatment.**

symptomatology /simp′təmətol′əjē/, the science of symptoms of disease in general or of the symptoms of a specific disease.

symptom-bearer, (in psychology) a family member frequently seen as the patient who is functioning poorly because family dynamics interfere with functioning at a higher level.

symptom complex. See **syndrome.**

symptothermal method of family planning [Gk *symptoma* + *therme* heat], a natural method of family planning that incorporates the ovulation and basal body temperature methods of family planning.

sympus /sim′pəs/ [Gk *syn* together, *pous* foot], a malformed fetus in which the lower extremities are completely fused or rotated and the pelvis and genitalia are defective. Kinds of sympuses are **sirenomelus, sympus dipus,** and **sympus monopus.**

sympus apus. See **sirenomelus.**

sympus dipus /dē′pəs/, a malformed fetus in which the lower extremities are fused and both feet are formed.

sympus monopus /mon′əpəs/, a malformed fetus in which the lower extremities are fused and one foot is formed.

synadelphus /sin′ədel′fəs/, *pl.* **synadelphi** [Gk *syn* + *adelphos* brother], a conjoined twin fetal monster with a single head and trunk and eight limbs.

Synanon, a residential center that provides a therapeutic community approach to rehabilitation for drug abusers.

synapse /sinaps′/ /sin′aps/ [Gk *synaptein* to join], **1.** the region surrounding the point of contact between two neurons or between a neuron and an effector organ, across which nerve impulses are transmitted through the action of a neurotransmitter, such as acetylcholine or norepinephrine. Synapses are polarized so that nerve impulses normally travel in only one direction; they are also subject to fatigue, oxygen deficiency, anesthetics, and other chemical agents. Kinds of synapses include **axoaxonic, axodendritic, axodendrosomatic, axosomatic,** and **dendrodendritic synapse. 2.** to form a synapse or connection between neurons. **3.** (in genetics) to form a synaptic fusion between ho-

mologous chromosomes during meiosis. **–synaptic,** *adj.*

synapsis /sinap′sis/, *pl.* **synapses,** the pairing of homologous chromosomes during the early meiotic prophase stage in gametogenesis to form double or bivalent chromosomes.

synaptic cleft, the microscopic, extracellular space at the synapse that separates the membrane of the terminal nerve endings of a presynaptic neuron and the membrane of a postsynaptic cell.

synaptic junction, the membranes of both the presynaptic neuron and the postsynaptic receptor cell together with the synaptic cleft.

synaptic transmission, the passage of a neural impulse across a synapse from one nerve fiber to another by means of a neurotransmitter.

synarthrosis. See **fibrous joint.**

syncephalus /sinsef′ələs/ [Gk *syn* + *kephale* head], a conjoined twin monster having a single head and two bodies.

synchilia /singkē′lyə/ [Gk *syn* + *cheilos* lip], a congenital anomaly in which there is complete or partial fusion of the lips; atresia of the mouth.

synchondrosis /sing′kondrō′sis/, *pl.* **synchondroses** [Gk *syn* + *chondros* cartilage], a cartilaginous joint between two immovable bones, such as the pubic symphysis.

synchorial /singkôr′ē·əl/ [Gk *syn* + *chorion* skin], pertaining to multiple fetuses that share a common placenta, as in monozygosity.

synchronized intermittent mandatory ventilation (SIMV), periodic assisted mechanical breaths occurring at preset intervals when the patient makes an inspiratory effort that is sensed by the ventilator. Spontaneous breathing by the patient occurs between the assisted mechanical breaths.

synchronous, occurring at the same time.

synclitism /sing′klitiz′əm/ [Gk *syn* + *klinein* to lean] **1.** (in obstetrics) a condition in which the sagittal suture of the fetal head is in line with the transverse diameter of the inlet, equidistant from the maternal symphysis pubis and sacrum. **2.** (in hematology) the normal condition in which the nucleus and the cytoplasm of the blood cells mature simultaneously and at the same rate.

syncope /sing′kəpē/ [Gk *synkoptein* to cut short], a brief lapse in consciousness caused by transient cerebral hypoxia. It is usually preceded by a sensation of lightheadedness and may often be prevented by lying down or by sitting with the head between the knees.

S

syncretic thinking [Gk *synkretismos* combined beliefs; AS *thencan* to think], a stage in the development of the cognitive thought processes of the child. During this phase thought is based purely on what is perceived and experienced. The child is incapable of making deductions or generalizations. In Piaget's classification, this stage occurs between 2 and 7 years of age. –**syncresis,** *n.*

syncytial /sinsish′əl/, pertaining to a syncytium.

syncytial virus a virus that induces the formation of syncytia, particularly in cell cultures. Syncytial viruses are members of the spumavirinae subfamily of retroviridae.

syncytiotrophoblast /sinsish′ē·ōtrof′əblast′/ [Gk *syn* + *kytos* cell, *trophe* nutrition, *blastos* germ], the outer syncytial layer of the trophoblast of the early mammalian embryo that erodes the uterine wall during implantation and gives rise to the villi of the placenta. –**syncytiotrophoblastic,** *adj.*

syncytium /sinsit′ē·əm/, *pl.* **syncytia** [Gk *syn* + *kytos* cell], a group of cells in which the protoplasm of one cell is continuous with that of adjoining cells.

syndactylism /sindak′tiliz′əm/ [Gk *syn* + *daktylos* finger or toe], a condition in which two or more fingers or toes are fused.

syndactylus /sindek′tiləs/, a person with webbed fingers or toes.

syndactyly /sindak′təlē/ [Gk *syn* + *daktylos* finger], a congenital anomaly characterized by the fusion of the fingers or toes. –**syndactyl, syndactylous,** *adj.*

syndelphus. See synadelphus.

syndesis /sin′dəsis/ [Gk *syn* + *dein* to bind], surgical fixation of a joint.

syndesmosis /sin′desmō′sis/, *pl.* **syndesmoses** [Gk *syndesmos* ligament], a fibrous articulation in which two bones are connected by interosseous ligaments, such as the anterior and posterior ligaments in the tibiofibular articulation.

syndrome [Gk *syn* together, *dromos* course], a complex of signs and symptoms resulting from a common cause or appearing, in combination, to present a clinical picture of a disease or inherited abnormality.

syndrome of inappropriate antidiuretic hormone secretion (SIADH), an abnormal condition characterized by the excessive release of antidiuretic hormone (ADH) that upsets the fluid and electrolytic balances of the body. It results from various malfunctions, such as the inability of the body to produce and secrete dilute urine, water retention, increased extracellular fluid volume, and hyponatremia. SIADH develops in association with diseases that affect the osmoreceptors of the hypothalamus. Oat cell carcinoma of the lung is the most common cause. Common signs and symptoms of SIADH are weight gain despite anorexia, vomiting, nausea, muscle weakness, and irritability. In some patients SIADH may produce coma and convulsions. Most of the free water associated with this syndrome is intracellular, and associated edema is rare unless excess water volume exceeds 4 mOsm.

synechia /sinek′ē·ə/, *pl.* **synechiae** [Gk, continuity], an adhesion, especially of the iris to the cornea or lens of the eye. It may develop from glaucoma, cataracts, uveitis, or keratitis or as a complication of surgery or trauma to the eye. Synechiae prevent or impede flow of aqueous fluid between the anterior and posterior chambers of the eye and may lead rapidly to blindness.

syneresis /siner′əsis/ [Gk *syn* + *hairein* to draw], the drawing together or coagulation of particles of a gel with separation from the medium in which the particles were suspended, as occurs in blood clot retraction.

synergism. See synergy.

synergist /sin′ərjist/ [Gk *syn* + *ergein* to work], an organ, agent, or substance that augments the activity of another organ, agent, or substance.

synergistic agent /sin′ərjis′tik/, a substance that augments or adds to the activity of another substance or agent.

synergistic muscles, groups of muscles that contract together to accomplish the same body movement.

synergy /sin′ərjē/ [Gk *syn* + *ergein* to work] **1.** the process in which two organs, substances, or agents work simultaneously to enhance the function and effect of one another. **2.** the coordinated action of a set of muscles that work together to produce a specific movement. **3.** a combined action of different parts of the autonomic nervous system, as in the sympathetic and parasympathetic innervation of secreting cells of the salivary glands. **4.** the interaction of two or more drugs to produce a certain effect. –**synergistic, synergetic,** *adj.*

syngeneic /sin′jənē′ik/ [Gk *syn* + *genesis* origin] **1.** (in genetics) denoting an individual or cell type that has the same genotype as another individual or cell. **2.** (in transplantation biology) denoting tissues that are antigenically similar.

synkinesis /sin′kinē′sis/ [Gk *syn* + *kinesis* movement], an involuntary movement by one part of the body when an intentional movement is made by another part. In imitative synkinesis, movement may be detected in paralyzed muscles when normal muscles are moved and vice versa.

synophthalmia. See **cyclopia.**

synopsis [Gk *syn* + *opsis* vision], a brief review, condensation, summary, or abridgement.

synostosis /sin'asto'sis/ [Gk *syn* + *osteon* bone], the joining of two bones by the ossification of connecting tissues. Synostosis occurs normally in the fusion of cranial bones to form the skull.

synostotic joint /sin'ostot'ik/ [Gk *syn* + *osteon* bone], a joint in which bones are joined to bones and there is no movement between them, as in the bones of the adult sacrum or skull.

synotia /sīnō'shə/ [Gk *syn* + *ous* ear], a congenital malformation characterized by the union or approximation of the ears in front of the neck, often accompanied by the absence or defective development of the lower jaw.

synotus /sīnō'təs/, a fetus with synotia.

synovectomy /sin'ōvek'təmē/ [Gk *syn* + L *ovum* egg; Gk *ektome* excision], the excision of a synovial membrane of a joint.

synovia /sinō'vē·ə/ [Gk *syn* + L *ovum*], a transparent, viscous fluid, resembling the white of an egg, secreted by synovial membranes and acting as a lubricant for many joints, bursae, and tendons. It contains mucin, albumin, fat, and mineral salts. –**synovial,** *adj.*

synovial bursa /sinō'vē·əl/, one of the many closed sacs filled with synovial fluid in the connective tissue between the muscles, tendons, ligaments, and bones.

synovial chondroma, a rare cartilaginous growth developing in the connective tissue below the synovial membrane of the joints, tendon sheaths, or bursa.

synovial crypt, a pouch in the synovial membrane of a joint.

synovial fluid. See **synovia.**

synovial joint, a freely movable joint in which contiguous bony surfaces are covered by articular cartilage and connected by ligaments lined with synovial membrane. Kinds of synovial joints are **ball and socket, condyloid, gliding, hinge, pivot, saddle,** and **uniaxial.**

synovial membrane, the inner layer of an articular capsule surrounding a freely movable joint. The synovial membrane is loosely attached to the external fibrous capsule. It secretes into the joint a thick fluid that normally lubricates the joint but that may accumulate in painful amounts when the joint is injured.

synovial sarcoma, a malignant tumor, composed of synovioblasts, that begins as a soft swelling and often metastasizes through the bloodstream to the lung before it is discovered.

synovial sheath, any one of the membranous sacs that enclose a tendon of a muscle and facilitate the gliding of a tendon through a fibrous or a bony tunnel, such as that under the flexor retinaculum of the wrist.

synovial tendon sheath, one of the many membranous sacs enclosing various tendons that glide through fibrous and bony tunnels in the body, such as those under the flexor retinaculum of the wrist. One layer of the synovial sheath lines the tunnel; the other covers the tendon.

synovitis /sin'əvī'tis/ [Gk *syn* + L *ovum;* Gk *itis*], an inflammatory condition of the synovial membrane of a joint as the result of an aseptic wound or a traumatic injury, such as a sprain or severe strain. The knee is most commonly affected. Fluid accumulates around the capsule, the joint is swollen, tender, and painful, and motion is restricted.

synovium [Gk *syn* + L *ovum*], a synovial membrane.

syntactic aphasia, an inability to arrange words in a logical sequence, with the result that what is spoken is not understood.

syntax [Gk *syn* + *taxis* arrangement], a property of language involving structural cues for the arrangement of words as elements in a phrase, clause, or sentence.

syntaxic mode, the ability to perceive whole, logical, coherent pictures as they occur in reality, according to the Sullivan theory of psychology.

synteny /sin'tənē/ [Gk *syn* + *taina* ribbon], (in genetics) the presence on the same chromosome of two or more genes that may or may not be transmitted as a linkage group but that appear to be able to undergo independent assortment during meiosis.

synthesis /sin'thəsis/ [Gk *synthenai* to put together], a level of cognitive learning in which the individual puts together the elements of previous learning levels to create a unified whole.

synthesize /sin'thəsīz/ [Gk *synthesis* putting together], to form by building, as in forming complex chemical compounds such as proteins from simpler units of amino acids.

synthetic, of or pertaining to a substance that is produced by an artificial rather than a natural process or material.

synthetic chemistry, the science dealing with the formation of chemical compounds from simpler substances.

synthetic human growth hormone, a synthetic form of somatotropin produced

S

by recombinant DNA techniques from a strain of *E. coli* bacteria. The polypeptide hormone consists of 191 amino acid residues in a sequence identical to that of natural human growth hormone.

synthetic insulin [Gk *synthesis* putting together; L *insula* island (of Langerhans)], a form of insulin synthesized in a nondisease-producing strain of *E. coli* bacteria or in yeast cells that has been genetically altered by the addition of the human gene for insulin production.

synthetic oleovitamin D.　See **viosterol.**

syntrophoblast.　See　**syncytiotrophoblast.**

syphilis /sif'ilis/ [Gk *syn* + *philein* to love], a sexually transmitted disease caused by the spirochete, *Treponema pallidum,* characterized by distinct stages of effects over a period of years. Any organ system may become involved. The spirochete is able to pass through the human placenta, producing congenital syphilis. The first stage **(primary syphilis)** is marked by the appearance of a small, painless, red pustule on the skin or mucous membrane between 10 and 90 days after exposure. The lesion may appear anywhere on the body where contact with a lesion on an infected person has occurred, but is seen most often in the anogenital region. It quickly erodes, forming a painless, bloodless ulcer, called a chancre, exuding a fluid that swarms with spirochetes. It heals spontaneously within 10 to 40 days, often creating the mistaken impression that the sore was not a serious event. The second stage **(secondary syphilis)** occurs about 2 months later, after the spirochetes have increased in number and spread throughout the body. This stage is characterized by general malaise, anorexia, nausea, fever, headache, alopecia, bone and joint pain, or the appearance of a morbilliform rash that does not itch, flat white sores in the mouth and throat, or condylomata lata papules on the moist areas of the skin. The disease remains highly contagious at this stage and can be spread by kissing. The third stage **(tertiary syphilis)** may not develop for 3 to 15 or more years. It is characterized by the appearance of soft, rubbery tumors, called gummas, which ulcerate and heal by scarring. Gummas may develop anywhere on the surface of the body and in the eye, liver, lungs, stomach, or reproductive organs. Tertiary syphilis may be painless, unnoticed except for gummas, or it may be accompanied by deep, burrowing pain. The ulceration of the gummas may result in punched-out areas of the palate, nasal septum, or larynx. Various tissues and structures of the body, including the central nervous system, myocardium, and the valves of the heart, may be damaged or destroyed, leading to mental or physical disability and premature death. **Congenital syphilis** resulting from prenatal infection may result in the birth of a deformed or blind infant. In some cases, the infant appears to be well until, at several weeks of age, snuffles, sometimes with a bloodstained or mucopurulent discharge, and skin lesions are observed, particularly on the palms and soles or in the genital region. Such children may also have visual or hearing defects, and progeria and poor health may develop. In many states, active, serologically documented cases of syphilis must, by law, be reported to the Department of Health.

syphilitic /sif'ilit'ik/ [Gk *syn* + *philein* to love], pertaining to, resembling, or infected with syphilis.

syphilitic aortitis, an inflammatory condition of the aorta, occurring in tertiary syphilis and characterized by diffuse dilatation with gray, wheal-like plaques containing calcium on the inner coat and scars and wrinkles on the outer coat. The middle layer of the vascular wall is usually infiltrated with plasma cells and contains fragments of damaged elastic tissue and many newly formed blood vessels. There may be damage to the aortic valves, narrowing of the mouths of the coronary arteries, and the formation of thrombi. Cerebral embolism may result. Signs of syphilitic aortitis are substernal pain, dyspnea, bounding pulse, and high systolic blood pressure.

syphilitic dementia, a general mental deterioration disorder resulting from a syphilis infection. Specific symptoms may vary from memory impairment to personality changes and are severe enough to interfere with social and occupational activities. If untreated, the disease may progress to dementia paralytica, paralysis, and death.

syphilitic endocarditis, a thickening and stretching of the cusps of the aortic valve, with aortic valve incompetence, caused by a syphilis infection of the aorta.

syphilitic fever, pyrexia that is due to a syphilis infection.

syphilitic meningoencephalitis. See **general paresis.**

syphilitic periarteritis, an inflammatory condition of the outer coat of one or more arteries occurring in tertiary syphilis and characterized by soft gummatous perivascular lesions infiltrated with lymphocytes and plasma cells.

syphilitic retinopathy, an invasion of the retina and optic nerve by a spreading syphilis infection. Primary retinal lesions are associated with the blood vessels and the choroid layer is often affected first. There may be occlusion of the retinal vessels.

syr. [L *syrupus*], Latin abbreviation for syrup.

syringe [Gk *syrinx* tube], a device for withdrawing, injecting, or instilling fluids. A syringe for the injection of medication usually consists of a calibrated glass or plastic cylindric barrel having a close-fitting plunger at one end and a small opening at the other to which the head of a hollow-bore needle is fitted. Medication of the desired amount may be pulled up into the barrel by suction as the plunger is withdrawn and injected by pushing the plunger back into the barrel, forcing the liquid out through the needle. Kinds of syringe include **Asepto, bulb, hypodermic, Luer-Lok,** and **tuberculin syringe.**

syringectomy /sir′injek′təmē/, a surgical procedure for excising the walls of a fistula.

syringomeningocele /siring′gōməning′gōsēl/, a meningocele that is connected to the central canal of the spinal cord.

syringomyelia /-mī-ē′lyə/, a chronic progressive disease of the spinal cord, marked by elongated central fluid-containing cavities, surrounded by gliosis, or a proliferation of neurologic tissue. Symptoms begin early in adulthood, usually involving the cervical region, with muscular wasting in the upper limbs.

syringomyelocele /siring′gōmī′əlosēl′/ [Gk *syrinx* + *myelos* marrow, *kele* hernia], a hernial protrusion of the spinal cord through a congenital defect in the vertebral column in which the cerebrospinal fluid within the central cavities of the cord is greatly increased so that the cord tissue forms a thin-walled sac that lies close to the membrane of the cavity.

syrup of ipecac, an emetic preparation of ipecac fluid extract, glycerin, and syrup used to treat certain types of poisonings and drug overdoses.

system [Gk *systema*], **1.** a collection or assemblage of parts that, unified, make a whole. Physiologic systems, such as the cardiovascular or reproductive systems, are made up of structures specifically able to engage in processes that are essential for a vital function in the body. **2.** a set of computer programs and hardware that work together for some specific purpose. –**systematic,** *adj.*

systematic error [Gk *systema*; L *errare* to wander], a nonrandom statistical error that affects the mean of a population of data and defines the bias between the means of two populations.

systematic heating, the elevation of the temperature of the whole body.

systematic tabulation, (in research) mechanical or manual techniques for recording and classifying data for statistical analysis.

systemic /sistem′ik/ [Gk *systema*], of or pertaining to the whole body rather than to a localized area or regional portion of the body.

systemic circulation, the general blood circulation of the body, not including the lungs.

systemic desensitization, a technique used in behavior therapy for eliminating maladaptive anxiety associated with phobias. The procedure involves the construction by the person of a hierarchy of anxiety-producing stimuli and the general presentation of these stimuli until they no longer elicit the initial response of fear.

systemic infection [Gk *systema*; L *inficere* to stain], an infection in which the pathogen is distributed throughout the body rather than concentrated in one area.

systemic lesion [Gk *systema*; L *laesio* lesion], a pathologic disturbance that involves a system of tissues with a common function.

systemic lupus erythematosus (SLE), a chronic inflammatory disease affecting many systems of the body. The pathophysiology of the disease includes severe vasculitis, renal involvement, and lesions of the skin and nervous system. The primary cause of the disease has not been determined; viral infection or dysfunction of the immune system has been suggested. Adverse reaction to certain drugs may also cause a lupuslike syndrome. Four times more women than men have SLE. The initial manifestation is often arthritis. An erythematous rash over the nose and malar eminences, weakness, fatigue, and weight loss are also frequently seen early in the disease. Photosensitivity, fever, skin lesions on the neck, and alopecia where the skin lesions extend beyond the hairline may occur. The skin lesions may spread to the mucous membranes and other tissues of the body. They do not ulcerate but cause degeneration of the tissues affected. Depending on the organs involved, the patient may also have glomerulonephritis, pleuritis, pericarditis, peritonitis, neuritis, or anemia. Renal failure and severe neurologic abnormalities are among the most serious manifestations of the disease.

systemic mycosis, a fungal infection that involves more than one body system or area.

systemic oxygen consumption, the amount of oxygen consumed by the body's tissues as measured during a period of 60 seconds.

systemic remedy, a medicinal substance that is given orally, parenterally, or rectally to be absorbed into the circulation for treatment of a health problem. Medication administered systemically may have various local effects, but the intent is to treat the whole body.

systemic vascular resistance (SVR), the resistance against which the left ventricle must eject to force out its stroke volume with each beat. As the peripheral vessels constrict, the SVR increases.

systemic vein, one of a number of veins that drain deoxygenated blood from most of the body. Systemic veins arise in tiny plexuses that receive blood from the billions of capillaries lacing the body tissues and converge into trunks that increase in size as they pass toward the heart. They are larger and more numerous than the arteries, have thinner walls, and collapse when they are empty. Kinds of systemic veins are identified according to location, such as deep veins, superficial veins, and venous sinuses.

system of care, a framework within which health care is provided, comprising health care professionals; recipients, consumers, or patients; energy resources or dynamics; organizational and political contexts or frameworks; and processes or procedures.

system overload, an inability to cope with messages and expectations from a number of sources within a given time limit.

systems theory, a holistic medical concept in which the human patient is viewed as an integrated complex of open systems rather than as semiindependent parts.

systole /sis'təlē/ [Gk, contraction], the contraction of the heart, driving blood into the aorta and pulmonary arteries. The occurrence of systole is indicated by the first heart sound heard on auscultation, by the palpable apex beat, and by the peripheral pulse. –systolic, adj.

systolic click /sistol'ik/ [Gk systole contraction; Fr cilqueter to click], an extra sound having a clicklike quality heard in mid- or late systole, and believed to originate from the abnormal motion of the mitral valve. The most frequent cause of systolic clicks is prolapse of a mitral valve leaflet.

systolic dysfunction a loss of cardiac muscle with volume overload and decreased contractility.

systolic ejection period, the amount of time spent in systole per minute.

systolic gradient, the difference in pressure in the left atrium and left ventricle during systole.

systolic murmur, cardiac murmur occurring during systole. Systolic murmurs are generally less significant than diastolic murmurs and occur in many people with no evidence of heart disease.

systolic pressure, the blood pressure measured during the period of ventricular contraction (systole). In blood pressure readings, it is normally the higher of the two measurements.

T, 1. symbol for **temperature.** 2. abbreviation for **tumor.**

T₁, T₂, See **relaxation time.**

T₃, symbol for **triiodothyronine.**

T₄, symbol for **thyroxine.**

Ta, symbol for the element **tantalum.**

TA, abbreviation for **transactional analysis.**

tabes /tā'bēz/ [L *tabes* wasting], a gradual, progressive wasting of the body in any chronic disease.

tabes dorsalis [L *tabes* wasting; *dorsum* the back], an abnormal condition characterized by the slow degeneration of all or part of the body and the progressive loss of peripheral reflexes. This disease involves the posterior columns and the posterior roots of the spinal cord and destroys the large joints of affected limbs in some individuals. It is often accompanied by incontinence and impotence and severe flashing pains in the abdomen and the extremities.

tabetic crisis /tābet'ik/[L *tabes;* Gk *krisis* turning point], an exacerbation of pain in tabes dorsalis due to syphilis.

tabetic gait [L *tabes;* ONorse *gata* a way], a high-steppage gait associated with the tertiary form of tabes. The condition results from degeneration of the dorsal columns of the spinal cord and of sensory nerve trunks.

tabetic neuritis, a form of neuritis that accompanies a syphilitic infection or tabes dorsalis, involving the dorsal posterior column spinal pathways.

tablet [Fr *tablette* lozenge], a small, solid dosage form of a medication. It may be of almost any size, shape, weight, and color. Most tablets are intended to be swallowed whole, but some may be dissolved in the mouth, chewed, or dissolved in liquid before swallowing; some may be placed in a body cavity.

taboo, something that is forbidden by a society as unacceptable or improper. Incest is a taboo common to many societies.

taboparesis /tā'bōpəre'sis/ [L *tabes;* Gk *paralyein* to be palsied], a form of paralysis associated with cerebral syphilis.

tabula rasa /tä'bŌŌlä rä'sä, tab'yəlä rä'sə/, a term used to describe a child's mind at birth as a receptive "blank slate."

tache laiteuse. See **macula albidae.**

tache noire /täshnô·är'/, a local ulcerous lesion marking the point of infection in certain rickettsial diseases, such as African tick typhus and scrub typhus.

tachycardia /tak'ikär'dē·ə/ [Gk *tachys* fast, *kardia* heart], an abnormal condition in which the myocardium contracts regularly but at a rate greater than 100 beats per minute. The heart rate normally accelerates in response to fever, exercise, or nervous excitement. Pathologic tachycardia accompanies anoxia, such as caused by anemia, congestive heart failure, hemorrhage, or shock. Tachycardia acts to increase the amount of oxygen delivered to the cells of the body by increasing the amount of blood circulated through the vessels.

tachycardiac, pertaining to or affected by tachycardia.

tachydysrythmia [Gk *tachys* + *a, rhythmos* rhythm], an abnormally rapid heart beat.

tachykinin. See **substance P.**

tachyphylaxis /tak'əfəlak'sis/ [Gk *tachys* + *phylax* guard], 1. (in pharmacology) a phenomenon in which the repeated administration of some drugs results in a marked decrease in effectiveness. 2. (in immunology) rapidly developing immunity to a toxin because of previous exposure, such as from previous injection of small amounts of the toxin.

tachypnea /tak'ipnē'ə/ [Gk *tachys* + *pnoia* breathing], an abnormally rapid rate of breathing, such as seen with hyperpyrexia.

tack, the degree of stickiness of an adhesive required to affix a therapeutic foreign substance, such as a transdermal delivery device, to the skin.

tactile /tak'təl/ [L *tactus* touch], of or pertaining to the sense of touch.

tactile amnesia [L *tactus;* Gk *amnesia* forgetfulness], a loss of the ability to determine the shape of objects through the sense of touch.

tactile anesthesia, the absence or lack of the sense of touch in the fingers, possibly resulting from injury or disease. This condition may cause the patient to incur severe burns, serious cuts, contusions, or abrasions.

tactile corpuscle, any one of many small,

oval end organs associated with the sense of touch, widely distributed throughout the body in peripheral areas, such as the skin of the lips, mucous membrane of the tongue, palpebral conjunctivae, and skin of the mammary papillae.

tactile corpuscle of Meissner. See **Wagner-Meissner corpuscle.**

tactile defensiveness, a sensory integrative dysfunction characterized by tactile sensations that cause excessive emotional reactions, hyperactivity, or other behavior problems.

tactile discrimination [L *tactus* + *discrimen* division], the ability to discriminate among objects by the sense of touch.

tactile fremitus, a tremulous vibration of the chest wall during respiration that is palpable on physical examination.

tactile hair, a hair shaft that is sensitive to the sensation of touch.

tactile hallucination, a subjective experience of touch in the absence of tactile stimulation.

tactile hyperesthesia [L *tactus;* Gk *hyper* excessive + *aesthesis* sensitivity], an abnormal increase in the sense of touch.

tactile image, a mental concept of an object as perceived through the sense of touch.

tactile localization [L *tactus, locus* place], the ability to identify, without looking, the exact point on the body that a tactile stimulus is applied. The localization test is applied in sensory evaluation tests.

tactile sensation [L *tactus, sentire* to feel], the sensation of touch.

tactile system, the part of the nervous system that is concerned with the sense of touch.

Taenia /tē'nē-ə/ [Gk *tainia* ribbon], a genus of large, parasitic, intestinal flatworm, having an armed scolex and a series of segments in a chain. Taeniae are among the most common parasites infecting humans and include **Taenia saginata,** the beef tapeworm, and **T. solium,** the pork tapeworm.

Taenia saginata, a species of tapeworm that inhabits the tissues of cattle during its larval stage and infects the intestine of humans in its adult form.

taeniasis /tēnī'əsis/ [Gk *tainia* + *osis* condition], an infection with a tapeworm of the genus *Taenia.*

Taenia solium, a species of tapeworm that most commonly inhabits the tissues of pigs during its larval stage and infects the intestine of humans in its adult form.

TAF, abbreviation for **tumor angiogenesis factor.**

TAG, abbreviation for 3,4,6-tri-O-acetyl-D-glucal.

tail bud. See **end bud.**

tail fold [AS *taegel; fealdan* to fold], a curved ridge formed at the caudal end of the early developing embryo.

tail of Spence, the upper outer tail of breast tissue that extends into the axilla.

tailor's bottom. See **weaver's bottom.**

tailor's bunion. See **bunionette.**

Takayasu's arteritis /tä'kəyä'sŏoz/ [Michishige Takayasu, Japanese physician, b. 1871], an inflammatory disorder characterized by progressive occlusion of the innominate and the left subclavian and left common carotid arteries above their origin in the aortic arch. Signs of the disorder are absence of a pulse in both arms and in the carotid arteries, transient paraplegia, transient blindness, and atrophy of facial muscles.

talbutal /tal'byŏŏtəl/, a barbiturate sedative-hypnotic prescribed as a hypnotic in the treatment of insomnia.

talipes /tal'ipēz/ [L *talus* ankle, *pes* foot], a deformity of the foot, usually congenital, in which the foot is twisted and relatively fixed in an abnormal position. Talipes refers to deformities that involve the foot and ankle.

talipes calcaneovalgus. See **clubfoot.**

talipes cavus. See **pes cavus.**

talipes equinovarus. See **clubfoot.**

talonavicular /tä'lōnəvik'yələr/ [L *talon* bird claw + *naviculus* scaphoid], pertaining to the talus and the navicular bones.

talus /tä'ləs/, *pl.* **tali** [L, ankle], the second largest tarsal bone. It supports the tibia, rests on the calcaneus, and articulates with the malleoli and with the navicular bones.

Tamm-Horsfall protein (THP), a mucoprotein found in the matrix of renal tubular casts. THP is secreted in the loop of Henle.

tamoxifen /təmok'səfin/, a nonsteroidal antiestrogen used in the palliative treatment of advanced breast cancer in premenopausal and postmenopausal women whose tumors are estrogen-dependent.

tampon [Fr, plug], a pack of cotton, a sponge, or other material for checking bleeding or absorbing secretions in cavities or canals or for holding displaced organs in position.

tamponade /tam'pənäd'/ [Fr *tamponner* to plug up], stoppage of the flow of blood to an organ or a part of the body by pressure, or by the compression of a part by an accumulation of fluid, such as in cardiac tamponade.

tangentiality /tanjen'chē·al'itē/ [L *tangere* to touch], expressions or responses characterized by a tendency to digress from an original topic of conversation. Tangentiality can destroy or seriously hamper the ability of people to communicate effectively.

tangible elements [L *tangere* + *elementum* first principle], objects that can be seen or touched, as distinguished from emotions, knowledge, or abstractions.

Tangier disease /tanjir'/ [Tangier Island, Virginia], a rare familial deficiency of high-density lipoproteins, characterized by low blood cholesterol and an abnormal orange or yellow discoloration of the tonsils and pharynx.

tannic acid [Celt *tann* oak; L *acidus* sour], a substance obtained from the bark and fruit of various trees and shrubs, particularly the nutgalls of oak trees. The acid is used as an astringent and protein precipitant.

tanning [Fr *tanner* to tan], a process in which the pigmentation of the skin deepens as a result of exposure to ultraviolet light. Skin cells containing melanin darken immediately.

tantalum (Ta) /tan'tələm/ [Gk *Tantalus* mythic king of Phrygia], a silvery metallic element. Its atomic number is 73; its atomic weight is 180.95. Relatively inert chemically, tantalum is used in prosthetic devices such as skull plates and wire sutures.

tantrum, a sudden outburst or violent display of rage, frustration, and bad temper, usually occurring in a maladjusted child and certain emotionally disturbed persons.

tapering arch [AS *tapor* slender; *arcus* bow], a dental arch that converges from the molars to the central incisors to such a degree that lines passing through the central grooves of the molars and premolars intersect within 1 inch (2.5 cm) anterior to the central incisors.

tapeworm [AS *taeppe, wyrm*], a parasitic, intestinal worm belonging to the class Cestoda and having a scolex and a ribbon-shaped body composed of segments in a chain. Humans usually acquire tapeworms by eating the undercooked meat of intermediate hosts contaminated by the cysticerus or larval form of the tapeworm.

tapeworm infection, an intestinal infection by one of several species of parasitic worms, caused by eating raw or undercooked meat infested with tapeworm or its larvae. Tapeworms live as larvae in one or more vertebrate intermediate hosts and grow to adulthood in the intestine of humans. Symptoms of intestinal infection with adult worms are usually mild or absent, but diarrhea, epigastric pain, and weight loss may occur.

tapotement /täpôtmäN'/ [Fr *tapoter* to pat], a type of massage in which the body is tapped in a rhythmic manner with the tips of the fingers or the sides of the hands, using short, rapid, repetitive movements.

tardive dyskinesia /tär'div/ [L *tardus* late; Gk *dys* difficult, *kinesis* movement], an abnormal condition characterized by involuntary, repetitious movements of the muscles of the face, the limbs, and the trunk. This disorder most commonly affects older people who have been treated for extended periods with phenothiazine drugs to alleviate the symptoms of parkinsonism.

tardy peroneal nerve palsy [L *tardus;* Gk *perone* brooch; L *nervus; paralyein* to lose control], a type of mononeuropathy in which the peroneal nerve is excessively compressed where it crosses the head of the fibula. Such compression may occur when an individual falls asleep with the legs crossed.

tardy ulnar nerve palsy, an abnormal condition characterized by atrophy of the first dorsal interosseous muscle and difficulty in the performance of fine manipulations. It may be caused by injury of the ulnar nerve at the elbow and commonly affects individuals with a shallow ulnar groove or those who persistently rest their weight on their elbows. Signs and symptoms of this disorder may include numbness of the small finger, of the contiguous half of the proximal and the middle phalanges of the ring finger, and of the ulnar border of the hand.

target [OFr *targuete* small shield], **1.** (in radiotherapy) any object area subjected to bombardment by radioactive particles or another form of diagnostic or therapeutic radiation. **2.** a device used to contain stable materials and subsequent radioactive materials during bombardment by high-energy nuclei from a cyclotron or other particle accelerator.

target cell, **1.** an abnormal red blood cell characterized, when stained and examined under a microscope, by a densely stained center surrounded by a pale unstained ring circled by a dark, irregular band. **2.** any cell having a specific receptor that reacts with a specific hormone, antigen, antibody, antibiotic, sensitized T cell, or other substance.

target organ, **1.** (in radiotherapy) an organ intended to receive a therapeutic dose of irradiation. **2.** (in nuclear medicine) an organ intended to receive the greatest concentration of a diagnostic radioactive tracer. **3.** (in endocrinology) an organ most affected by a specific hormone.

target symptoms, symptoms of an illness

T

that are most likely to respond to a specific treatment, such as a particular psychopharmacologic drug.

tarsal /tär′səl/ [L *tarsalis* eyelid or instep], of or pertaining to the tarsus, or ankle bone.

tarsal arches [Gk *tarsus;* L *arcus* bow], the superior and inferior branches of the palpebral artery supplying the eyelid.

tarsal bone, any one of seven bones comprising the tarsus of the foot, consisting of the talus, calcaneus, cuboid, navicular, and the three cuneiforms.

tarsal gland, one of numerous modified sebaceous glands on the inner surfaces of the eyelids.

tarsal plate. See **tarsus.**

tarsal tunnel syndrome, an abnormal condition and a kind of mononeuropathy, characterized by pain and numbness in the sole of the foot. This disorder may be caused by fractures of the ankle that compress the posterior tibial nerve.

tarsometatarsal /tär′sōmet′ətär′səl/ [Gk *tarsos* flat surface, *meta* beyond, *tarsos*], of or pertaining to the metatarsal bones and the tarsus of the foot.

tarsus, /tär′səs/ *pl.* **tarsi** [Gk *tarsos* flat surface], **1.** the area of articulation between the foot and the leg. **2.** any one of the plates of cartilage about 2.5 cm long forming the eyelids. One tarsal plate shapes each eyelid. The superior tarsal plates form the upper eyelids; the inferior tarsal plates form the lower eyelids.

tart, abbreviation for the *tartrate carboxylate anion.*

tartar /tär′tär/ [Fr *tartre*], **1.** a hard, gritty deposit composed of organic matter, phosphates, and carbonates that collects on the teeth and gums. **2.** any of several compounds containing tartrate, the salt of tartaric acid.

tartaric acid /tärter′ik/, a colorless or white powder found in various plants and prepared commercially from maleic anhydride and hydrogen peroxide. It is used in baking powder, certain beverages, and in tartar emetic.

Tarui's disease, a form of glycogen storage disease (type VII) in which abnormally large amounts of glycogen are deposited in the skeletal muscle. The disorder is characterized by cramping on exercise but no rise in blood lactate, and hemolysis.

task functions, behaviors that focus or direct activities toward movements with work or labor overtones.

task group, a group in which structured verbal or nonverbal exercises are used to help a person gain emotional, physical, and other personal awareness.

task-oriented behavior, actions involving a person's cognitive abilities in an attempt to solve problems and gratify the person's needs in order to reduce or avoid distress.

taste [ME *tasten*], the sense of perceiving different flavors in soluble substances that contact the tongue and trigger nerve impulses to special taste centers in the cortex and the thalamus of the brain. The four basic traditional tastes are sweet, salty, sour, and bitter. The front of the tongue is most sensitive to salty and sweet substances; the sides of the tongue are most sensitive to sour substances; and the back of the tongue is most sensitive to bitter substances. The middle of the tongue produces virtually no taste sensation. The sense of taste is intricately linked with the sense of smell.

taste bud, any one of many peripheral taste organs distributed over the tongue and the roof of the mouth. Each taste bud rests in a spheric pocket, which extends through the epithelium. Gustatory cells and supporting cells form each bud, which has a surface opening and an opening in the basement membrane.

taste papilla, small nipplelike elevations on the tongue. They contain sense organs that are sensitive to the chemicals identified with tastes, which vary with their location on the tongue.

TAT, abbreviation for **tetanus antitoxin.**

tattoo [Tahitian *tatau* marks], a permanent coloration of the skin by the introduction of foreign pigment. A tattoo may accidentally occur when a bit of graphite from a broken pencil point is embedded in the skin. **–tattoo,** *v.*

tau, τ, /tou/ the nineteenth letter of the Greek alphabet.

tautomer /tôtəmir/, structural isomers that differ only in the position of a hydrogen atom, or proton. Because tautomers can be rapidly interconverted by proton transfer in aqueous solutions, they are usually in equilibrium with one another. Keto and enol isomers are common examples of tautomers.

taxol, an anticancer drug derived from the bark of the rare, slow-growing Pacific yew tree. It is used in the treatment of ovarian cancer.

taxonomy /takson′əmē/ [Gk *taxis* arrangement, *nomos* rule], a system for classifying organisms on the basis of natural relationships and assigning them appropriate names. **–taxonomic,** *adj.*

Taylor, Effie J. (1874-1970), a Canadian-born American nurse who was graduated from Johns Hopkins School of Nursing. She served as president of the International Council of Nurses during World War II.

Taylor brace [Charles F. Taylor, American surgeon, b. 1827], a padded steel brace used to support the spine.

Tay-Sachs disease /tā'saks'/ [Warren Tay, English ophthalmologist, b. 1843; Bernard Sachs, American neurologist, b. 1858], an inherited, neurodegenerative disorder of lipid metabolism caused by a deficiency of the enzyme hexosaminidase A, which results in the accumulation of sphingolipids in the brain. The condition, which is transmitted as an autosomal recessive trait, occurs predominantly in families of Eastern European Jewish origin, specifically the Ashkenazic Jews, and is characterized by progressive mental and physical retardation and early death.

Tay's spot. See **cherry-red spot.**

Tb, symbol for the element **terbium.**

TB, 1. abbreviation for **tuberculosis.** 2. abbreviation for *tubercle bacillus.*

T bandage, a bandage in the shape of the letter T. It is used for the perineum and sometimes for the head.

TBP, 1. abbreviation for **bithionol.** 2. abbreviation for *total bypass.*

Tbs., tbsp., abbreviation for *tablespoon.*

TBT, abbreviation for **tracheobronchial tree.**

TBW, abbreviation for **total body water.**

TBZ, abbreviation for *tetrabenazine,* an anesthetic adjuvant.

t.c., abbreviation for *telephone call.*

Tc, symbol for the element **technetium.**

TC, abbreviation for **therapeutic community.**

T cell, a small circulating lymphocyte produced in the bone marrow that matures in the thymus or as a result of exposure to thymosin secreted by the thymus. T cells, which live for years, have several functions but primarily mediate cellular immune responses, such as graft rejection and delayed hypersensitivity. One kind of T cell, the **helper cell,** affects the production of antibodies by B cells; a **suppressor T cell** suppresses B cell activity.

T-4 cell, a thymus-derived lymphocyte of the body's immune system with a role of destroying or neutralizing cells or substances identified as "nonself." T-4 cells are "helper inducer" cells that secrete a substance, interleukin-2, which in turn stimulates the activity of natural killer cells, gamma interferon, and suppressor T-8 cells. The human immunodeficiency virus (HIV) commonly targets the T-4 cells, with the result that the body's immune defenses are severely damaged and opportunistic infections are allowed to flourish.

Td, abbreviation for **tetanus and diphtheria toxoids.**

TD, abbreviation for **toxic dose.**

TD50. See **median toxic dose.**

TDD, abbreviation for *transdermal drug delivery.*

tDNA, abbreviation for **transfer DNA.**

t.d.s. [L *ter die sumendum*], to be taken three times a day.

Te, symbol for the element **tellurium.**

tea. See **cannabis.**

teacher's nodule. See **vocal cord nodule.**

teaching hospital [AS *taecan* to show how], a hospital associated with a university that has accredited programs in various specialties of medical practice.

teaching rounds, informal conferences held regularly, often at the beginning of the day. Specific problems in the care of current patients are discussed.

team nursing [AS *team* family; L *nutrix* nourishment], a decentralized system in which the care of a patient is distributed among the members of a team. The charge nurse delegates authority to a team leader who must be a professional nurse. The team leader assigns tasks, schedules care, and instructs team members in details of care.

team practice, professional practice by a group of professionals that may include physicians, nurses, and others, such as a social worker, nutritionist, or physical therapist, who manage the care of a specified number of patients as a team, usually in an outpatient setting.

tear [ME *teren* to rend], to rip, rend, or pull apart by force.

teardrop fracture [AS *tear, dropa;* L *fractura* break], an avulsion fracture of one of the short bones, such as a vertebra, causing a tear-shaped disruption of bone tissue.

tear duct [AS *tear;* L *ducere* to lead], any duct that carries tears, including the lacrimal ducts, nasolacrimal ducts, and the excretory ducts of the lacrimal glands.

tearing /tir'ing/, watering of the eye usually caused by excessive tear production, such as by strong emotion, infection, or mechanical irritation by a foreign body. If the normal amount of fluid tears is produced but not drained into the lacrimal punctum at the nasal border of the eye, tearing will occur.

tears [ME *tere*], a watery saline or alkaline watery fluid secreted by the lacrimal glands to moisten the conjunctiva.

tears of the perineum [ME *teren;* Gk *perineos*], a rending of the tissues between the vulva and anus caused by overstretching of the vagina during child delivery. The damage is usually repaired by surgery.

tebutate, a contraction for tertiary butyl acetate.

technetium (Tc) [Gk *technectos* artificial], a radioactive, metallic element. Its atomic number is 43; its atomic weight is 99. Isotopes of technetium are used in radioisotope scanning procedures of internal organs.

technetium 99, the radionuclide most commonly used to image the body in nuclear medicine scans. It is preferred because of its short half-life and because the emitted photon has an appropriate energy for normal imaging techniques.

technician [Gk *technikos* skillful], a person with special training and experience in some form of technical procedures, usually those involving mechanical adjustments, such as maintaining and operating radiologic equipment.

technique [Gk *technikos* skillful], the method and details followed in performing a procedure, such as those used in conducting a laboratory test, a physical examination, a psychiatric interview, a surgical operation, or any process requiring certain skills or an ordered sequence of actions.

technologist, a person who studies the application of processes for making natural resources beneficial for humans. A medical technologist may work under the supervision of a physician in general clinical laboratory procedures.

teenager. See **adolescent.**

teether, an object, such as a teething ring, on which an infant can bite or chew during the teething process.

teething [AS *toth*], the physiologic process of the eruption of the deciduous teeth through the gums. It normally begins between the sixth and eighth months of life and occurs periodically until the complete set of 20 teeth has appeared at about 30 months. Discomfort and inflammation result from the pressure exerted against the periodontal tissue as the crown of the tooth breaks through the membranes. General signs of teething include excessive drooling, biting on hard objects, irritability, difficulty in sleeping, and refusal of food. –teethe, v.

teething ring, a circular device, usually made of plastic or rubber, on which an infant may chew or bite during the teething process.

TEIB, abbreviation for *triethylene-immunobenzoquinone.*

telangiectasia /təlan′jē·ektā′zhə/ [Gk *telos* end, *aggeion* vessel, *ektasis* dilatation], permanent dilatation of groups of superficial capillaries and venules. Common causes are actinic damage, atrophy-producing dermatoses, rosacea, elevated estrogen levels, and collagen vascular diseases.

telangiectasia lymphatica [Gk *telos* + *aggeion, ektasis* dilatation; L *lympha* water], a congenital or acquired condition of obstructed, dilated lymphatic vessels, resulting in lymphangiomata.

telangiectatic epulis /təlan′jē·ektat′ik/, a benign red tumor of the gingiva, containing prominent blood vessels. Low-grade or chronic irritation is a risk factor.

telangiectatic fibroma. See **angiofibroma.**

telangiectatic glioma, a tumor composed of glial cells and a network of blood vessels, which give the mass a vivid pink appearance.

telangiectatic granuloma. See **pyogenic granuloma.**

telangiectatic lipoma. See **angiolipoma.**

telangiectatic nevus, a common skin condition of neonates, characterized by flat, deep-pink localized areas of capillary dilatation that occur predominantly on the back of the neck, lower occiput, upper eyelids, upper lip, and bridge of the nose.

telangiectatic sarcoma, a malignant tumor of mesodermal cells with an unusually rich vascular network.

telediagnosis /tel′ədī′əgnō′sis/ [Gk, *tele,* far off + *dia,* through + *gnosis,* knowledge], a process whereby a disease diagnosis, or prognosis, is made by the electronic transmission of data between distant medical facilities.

telekinesis /tel′əkinē′sis/ [Gk *tele* + *kinesis* movement], a concept of parapsychology that one can control external events, such as the movement of a solid object, by the powers of the mind. For example, practitioners of telekinesis may believe it possible, by thought processes alone, to influence the roll of dice.

telemetry /telem′ətrē/ [Gk *tele* + *metron* measure], the electronic transmission of data between distant points.

telencephalon /tel′ensef′əlon/ [Gk *telos* end, *egkephalos* brain], the paired brain vesicles or endbrain from which the cerebral hemispheres are derived.

telepathist /təlep′əthist/, **1.** a person who believes in telepathy. **2.** a person who claims to have telepathic powers.

telepathy /təlep′əthē/ [Gk *tele* afar, *pathos* feeling], the alleged communication of thought from one person to another by means other than the physical senses. –telepathic, *adj.,* telepathize, *v.*

telereceptive /tel′ərisep′tiv/, pertaining to the exteroceptors of hearing, sight, and smell that detect stimuli distant from the body.

teletherapy [Gk *tele* + *therapeia* treatment], radiation therapy administered by a machine that is positioned at some distance from the patient.

tellurium (Te) /teloo̅'rē·əm/ [L *tellus* earth], an element exhibiting metallic and nonmetallic chemical properties. Its atomic number is 52; its atomic weight is 127.60.

telocentric /tel'əsen'trik/ [Gk *telos* end, *kentron* center], pertaining to a chromosome in which the centromere is located at the end, so that the chromatids appear as straight filaments.

telogen. See **hair.**

telophase /tel'əfāz/ [Gk *telos* + *phasis* appearance], the final of the four stages of nuclear division in mitosis and in each of the two divisions in meiosis.

temazepam /temaz'əpam/, a hypnotic agent prescribed for the relief of transient and intermittent insomnia.

temper [L *temperare* proper measure], **1.** to moderate or soften the effects. **2.** a state of mind regarding calmness or anger.

temperament [L *temperamentum* mixture in proper proportions], the features of a persona that reflect an individual's emotional disposition, the way he or she behaves, feels, and thinks.

temperate phage [L *temperare* to temper; Gk *phagein* to eat], a bacteriophage whose genome is incorporated into the host bacterium.

temperature [L *temperies* mildness], **1.** a relative measure of sensible heat or cold. **2.** (in physiology) a measure of sensible heat associated with the metabolism of the human body, normally maintained at a constant level of 98.6° F (37° C). **3.** *informal;* a fever.

temperature of infant, neonatal temperature that normally ranges from 35.5° to 37.5° C (96° F to 99.5° F). The temperature of an infant is unstable because of immature physiologic mechanisms.

temperature sense. See **thermic sense.**

temper tantrum. See **tantrum.**

template /tem'plit/ [L *templum* section], (in genetics) the strand of DNA that acts as a mold for the synthesis of messenger RNA.

temporal /tem'pərəl/ [L *tempus* temple], **1.** pertaining to a limited time. **2.** pertaining to the temporal bone of the skull.

temporal arteritis [L *temporalis* temporary, *arteria* air pipe, *itis* inflammation], a progressive inflammatory disorder of cranial blood vessels, principally the temporal artery. Symptoms are intractable headache, difficulty in chewing, weakness,

rheumatic pains, and loss of vision if the central retinal artery becomes occluded.

temporal artery, any one of three arteries on each side of the head: the superficial temporal artery, the middle temporal artery, and the deep temporal artery.

temporal bone, one of a pair of large bones forming part of the lower cranium and containing various cavities and recesses associated with the ear, such as the tympanic cavity and the auditory tube.

temporal bone fracture, a break of the temporal bone of the skull, sometimes characterized by bleeding from the ear.

temporal gyrus, any of three convolutions, inferior, middle, or superior, on the lateral surface of the temporal lobe of the brain.

temporalis /tem'pəral'is/ [L, temporary], one of the four muscles of mastication. It is a broad radiating muscle that arises from the whole of the temporal fossa and from the surface of the temporal fascia. The temporalis acts to close the jaws and retract the mandible.

temporal lobe, the lateral region of the cerebrum, below the lateral fissure.

temporal lobe epilepsy. See **psychomotor seizure.**

temporal muscle. See **temporalis.**

temporal subtraction, the subtraction of two or more digitized x-ray images that were acquired at different times. The subtraction process eliminates information in the image that was static.

temporal summation. See **summation.**

temporary pacemaker [L *temporarius* not permanent, *passus* step; ME *maken*], an artificial electronic heart pacemaker attached outside the patient's body and connected to a transvenous probe located within the heart. It is an interim procedure used when the heart rate is excessively slow.

temporary removable splint, any of a variety of dental appliances, including occlusal splints, used when limited stability of the teeth is required. It may be placed on or removed from teeth at will. Examples include *Hawley's orthodontic appliance* and *Elbrecht's cast metal splint.*

temporary stopping [L *temporalis* + AS *stoppian* to stop up], a mixture of gutta-percha, zinc oxide, white wax, and coloring, used for temporarily sealing dressings in tooth cavities.

temporary tooth. See **deciduous tooth.**

temporomandibular /tem'pərōmandib'yə-lər/ [L *temporalis* + *mandere* to chew], pertaining to the articulation between the temporal bone and the condyle of the mandible.

temporomandibular joint (TMJ) [L *tem-*

poralis + *mandere* to chew; *jungere* to join], one of two joints connecting the mandible of the jaw to the temporal bone of the skull. It is a combined hinge and gliding joint, formed by the anterior parts of the mandibular fossae of the temporal bone, the articular tubercles, the condyles of the mandible, and five ligaments.

temporomandibular joint pain dysfunction syndrome, an abnormal condition characterized by facial pain and by mandibular dysfunction, apparently caused by a defective or dislocated temporomandibular joint. Some common indications of this syndrome are the clicking of the joint when the jaws move, limitation of jaw movement, subluxation, and temporomandibular dislocation.

temporomandibular ligament, an oblique band of tissue that extends downward and backward from the zygomatic process to the neck of the mandible.

temporoparietal. See **parietotemporal.**

temporoparietalis /tem′pərōperī′ətal′is/ [L *temporalis* + *paries* wall], one of a pair of broad, thin muscles of the scalp that fans out over the temporal fascia. It acts in combination with the occipitofrontalis to wrinkle the forehead, to widen the eyes, and to raise the ears.

TEN, abbreviation for **toxic epidermal necrolysis.**

tenacious [L *tenax* holding fast], pertaining to secretions that are sticky or adhesive or otherwise tend to hold together, such as mucus and sputum.

tenacity [L *tenax* holding fast], the ability to be persistent or remain attached.

tenaculum /tənak′yələm/, *pl.* **tenacula** [L, holder], a clip or clamp with long handles used to grasp, immobilize, and hold an organ or a piece of tissue. Kinds of tenacula include the **abdominal tenaculum,** which has long arms and small hooks, the **forceps tenaculum,** which has long hooks and is used in gynecologic surgery, and the **uterine** or **cervical tenaculum,** which has short hooks or open, eye-shaped clamps used to hold the cervix.

tendinitis /ten′dənī′tis/ [L *tendo* tendon; Gk *itis* inflammation], an inflammatory condition of a tendon, usually resulting from strain.

tendinous /ten′dinəs/ [L *tendo*], pertaining to or resembling a tendon.

tendinous cords. See **chordae tendineae.**

tendo calcaneus. See **Achilles tendon.**

tendon [L *tendo*], one of many white, glistening fibrous bands of tissue that attach muscle to bone. Except at points of attachment, tendons are sheathed in delicate fibroelastic connective tissue. Ten-

dons are extremely strong and flexible, inelastic, and occur in various lengths and thicknesses. –**tendinous,** *adj.*

tendonitis. See **tendinitis.**

tendon of Achilles. See **Achilles tendon.**

tendon reflex. See **deep tendon reflex.**

tendosynovitis. See **tenosynovitis.**

tenesmus /tənez′məs/ [Gk *teinein* to stretch], persistent, ineffectual spasms of the rectum or bladder, accompanied by the desire to empty the bowel or bladder. –**tenesmic,** *adj.*

tennis elbow. See **lateral humeral epicondylitis.**

tenofibril. See **tonofibril.**

Tenon's capsule. See **fascia bulbi.**

tenosynovitis /ten′ōsin′əvī′tis/ [Gk *tenon* tendon, *syn* together; L *ovum* egg; L *itis*], inflammation of a tendon sheath caused by calcium deposits, repeated strain or trauma, high levels of blood cholesterol, rheumatoid arthritis, gout, or gonorrhea.

tenotomy /tənot′əmē/ [Gk *tenon* tendon, *temnein* to cut], the total or partial severing of a tendon, performed to correct a muscle imbalance, such as in the correction of strabismus of the eye or in clubfoot.

TENS, abbreviation for **transcutaneous electric nerve stimulation.**

tensiometer /ten′sē·om′ətər/ [L *tendere* to stretch; Gk *metron* measure], a device for measuring the surface tension of a liquid.

tension [L *tendere* to stretch], **1.** the act of pulling or straining until taut. **2.** the condition of being taut, tense, or under pressure. **3.** a state or condition resulting from the psychologic and physiologic reaction to a stressful situation, characterized physically by a general increase in muscle tonus, heart rate, respiration rate, and alertness and psychologically by feelings of strain, uneasiness, irritability, and anxiety.

tension headache, a pain that affects the head as the result of overwork or emotional strain, and involving tension in the muscles of the neck, face, and shoulder.

tension pneumothorax, a condition of air in the intrapleural space of the thorax caused by a rupture through the chest wall or lung parenchyma associated with the valvular opening. Air passes through the valve during coughing but cannot escape on exhalation.

tensor [L *tendere* to stretch], any one of the muscles of the body that tenses a structure, such as the tensor fasciae latae of the thigh.

tensor fasciae latae, one of the 10 muscles of the gluteal region. It functions to flex the thigh and to rotate it slightly medially.

tent [ME *tente*], **1.** a transparent cover, usually of plastic, supported over the upper part of a patient by a frame. Used in the treatment of respiratory conditions, it provides a controlled environment into which steam, oxygen, vaporized medication, or droplets of cool water may be sprayed, such as an oxygen tent. **2.** a cone made of various materials inserted into a cavity or orifice of the body to dilate its opening, such as a laminaria tent. **3.** a pack placed in a wound to hold it open to ensure that healing progresses from the base of the wound upward to the skin.

tentative [L *tentatare* to touch], not final or definite, such as an experimental finding that has not been validated.

tenth cranial nerve. See **vagus nerve.**

tenth-value layer (TVL) [ME *tenpe*; L *valere* to be worth; AS *lecgan* to lie], the thickness of material required to attentuate a beam of radiation to one tenth of its original intensity.

tentorial herniation /tentôr′ē·əl/ [L *tentorium* a tent; *hernia* rupture], the protrusion of brain tissue into the tentorial notch, caused by increased intracranial pressure resulting from edema, hemorrhage, or a tumor. Characteristic signs are severe headache, fever, flushing, sweating, abnormal pupillary reflex, drowsiness, hypotension, and loss of consciousness.

tentorial notch, an area occupied by the midbrain and enclosed by the free border of the tentorium cerebelli and the sphenoid bone.

tentorium /tentôr′ē·əm/, *pl.* **tentoria** [L, a tent], any part of the body that resembles a tent, such as the tentorium of the hypophysis that covers the hypophyseal fossa.

tentorium cerebelli, one of the three extensions of the dura mater that separates the cerebellum from the occipital lobe of the cerebrum.

tenure [L *tenere* to hold], (in a university) a faculty appointment with few limits on the number of years it may be held.

tepid, moderately warm to the touch.

teramorphous [Gk *teras* monster, *morphe* form], of the nature of or characteristic of a monster.

teras /ter′əs/, *pl.* **terata** [Gk, monster], a severely deformed fetus; a monster. –**teratic,** *adj.*

teratism /ter′ətiz′əm/, any congenital or developmental anomaly that is produced by inherited or environmental factors, or by a combination of the two; any condition in which a severely malformed fetus is produced. Kinds of teratism include atresic, ceasmic, ectopic, ectrogenic, hypergenetic, and symphysic teratism.

teratogen /ter′ətəjen′/ [Gk *teras* + *genein* to produce], any substance, agent, or process that interferes with normal prenatal development, causing the formation of one or more developmental abnormalities in the fetus. Teratogens act directly on the developing organism or indirectly, affecting such supplemental structures as the placenta or some maternal system. The period of highest vulnerability in the developing embryo is from about the third through the twelfth week of gestation, when differentiation of the major organs and systems occurs. –**teratogenic,** *adj.*

teratogenesis /ter′ətōjen′əsis/, the development of physical defects in the embryo. –**teratogenetic,** *adj.*

teratogenic agent. See **teratogen.**

teratogenous /ter′ətoj′ənəs/ [Gk *teras* monster, *genein* to produce], developed from fetal membranes.

teratogeny. See **teratogenesis.**

teratoid /ter′ətoid/ [Gk *teras* + *eidos* form], of or pertaining to abnormal physical development; resembling a monster.

teratoid tumor. See **dermoid cyst.**

teratologist, one who specializes in the science of teratology.

teratology /ter′ətol′əjē/ [Gk *teras* + *logos* science], the study of the causes and effects of congenital malformations and developmental abnormalities. –**teratologic, teratological,** *adj.*

teratoma /ter′ətō′mə/, *pl.* **teratomas, teratomata,** a tumor composed of different kinds of tissue, none of which normally occur together or at the site of the tumor.

terbium (Tr) /tur′bē·əm/ [Ytterby, Sweden], a rare earth metallic element. Its atomic number is 65; its atomic weight is 158.294.

terbutaline sulfate /terbyoo′təlēn/, a beta-adrenergic stimulant prescribed as a bronchodilator in the treatment of asthma, bronchitis, and emphysema and as a uterine relaxant to treat premature labor.

teres /tir′ēz, ter′ēz/, *pl.* **teretes** /ter′ətēz/ [L, rounded], a long, cylindric muscle, such as the teres minor or the teres major. –**teres,** *adj.*

teres major, a thick, flat muscle of the shoulder. It functions to adduct, extend, and rotate the arm medially.

teres minor, a cylindric, elongated muscle of the shoulder. The teres minor functions to rotate the arm laterally, weakly adduct the arm, and draw the humerus toward the glenoid fossa of the scapula, strengthening the shoulder joint.

terfenadine /terfen′ədēn/, a histamine

H₁-receptor antagonist used to relieve symptoms of seasonal allergic rhinitis.

terminal [L *terminus* end], (of a structure or process) near or approaching its end, such as a terminal bronchiole or a terminal disease. –**terminate**, *v.*, **terminus**, *n.*

terminal arteriole, an arteriole that divides into capillaries.

terminal bronchiole. See bronchiole.

terminal cancer, an advanced stage of a cancer with death as the inevitable prognosis.

terminal disinfection, the process of cleaning equipment and airing of a room after the release of a patient who has been treated for an infectious disease.

terminal drop, a rapid decline in cognitive function and coping ability that occurs 1 to 5 years before death.

terminal illness, an advanced stage of a disease with an unfavorable prognosis and no known cure.

terminal nerve, a small nerve originating in the cerebral hemisphere in the region of the olfactory trigone, classified by most anatomists as part of the olfactory, or first cranial, nerve.

terminal stance, one of the five stages in the stance phase of a walking gait, directly associated with the continuation of single limb support or the period during which the body moves forward on the supporting foot.

terminal sulcus of right atrium, a shallow channel on the external surface of the right atrium between the superior and inferior venae cavae.

termination codon, (in molecular genetics) a unit in the genetic code that specifies the end of the sequence of amino acids in a polypeptide.

termination phase, the last stage of a therapeutic relationship when attained goals are evaluated and outcomes achieved.

termination sequence, (in molecular genetics) a DNA segment at the end of a unit that is transcribed to messenger RNA from the DNA template.

term infant [Gk *terma* limit], any neonate, regardless of birth weight, born after the end of the thirty-seventh and before the beginning of the forty-third week of gestation.

terpin hydrate and codeine elixir /tur-'pin/, a preparation of the expectorant terpin hydrate, with sweet orange peel tincture, benzaldehyde, glycerin, alcohol, syrup, water, and the antitussive narcotic codeine.

territorial [L *territorium* district], a type of body movement that aids in communication. A territorial will frame an interaction and define an individual's "territory."

territoriality, an emotional attachment to and defense of certain areas related to one's existence.

tertian /tur'shən/ [L *tertianus* third], occurring every 48 hours or third day, including the first day of occurrence, such as vivax or tertian malaria, in which fever occurs every third day.

tertian malaria, a form of malaria, caused by the protozoan *Plasmodium vivax* or *Plasmodium ovale,* characterized by febrile paroxysms that occur every 48 hours. **Vivax malaria,** caused by *Plasmodium vivax,* is the most common form of malaria, and although it is rarely fatal, it is the most difficult form to cure. Relapses are common. **Ovale malaria,** caused by *Plasmodium ovale,* is usually milder and causes only a few short attacks.

tertiary /tur'shē·ərē, tursh'ərē/ [L *tertius* third], third in frequency or in order of use.

tertiary health care, a specialized, highly technical level of health care that includes diagnosis and treatment of disease and disability in sophisticated, large research and teaching hospitals. It offers a highly centralized care to the population of a large region, in some cases, to the world.

tertiary prevention, a level of preventive medicine that deals with the rehabilitation and return of a patient to a status of maximum usefulness with a minimum risk of recurrence of a physical or mental disorder.

tertiary syphilis, the most advanced stage of syphilis, resulting in infections of the cardiovascular and neurologic systems and marked by destructive lesions involving many tissues and organs. Late-stage syphilis is symptomatic but not contagious.

tesla /tes'lə/ [Nikola Tesla, American engineer, b. 1856], a unit of magnetic flux density, defined by the International System of Units as 1 weber per square meter, the equivalent of 1 volt/second per square meter.

test [L *testum* crucible], **1.** an examination or trial intended to establish a principle or determine a value. **2.** a chemical reaction or reagent that has clinical significance. **3.** to detect, identify, or conduct a trial.

testamentary capacity, a person's competency to make a will, including the requirement that he or she be aware that a will is being made, the nature and extent of the property covered by the will, and the identities of the beneficiaries.

testcross [L *testum* + *crux* cross], **1.** (in genetics) the cross of a dominant phenotype with a recessive phenotype to determine either the degree of genetic linkage or whether the dominant phenotype is homozygous or heterozygous. **2.** the subject undergoing such a test.

testes. See **testis.**

testes determining factor (TDF) /tes'tēz/, a Y-chromosome gene that is believed to determine male sexual development.

test for acetone in urine, a part of routine urinalysis. Normal findings are negative as acetone and other ketones are not normally present in urine. Exceptions include such cases as poorly controlled diabetic patients, alcoholics, and persons who may be fasting or on special high-protein diets.

test for lacrimation, a test for possible keratoconjunctivitis sicca conducted by placing a 35-mm long piece of filter paper in the lower fornix of the conjunctiva for five minutes. Failure of tears to wet as much as 10 mm of the strip indicates keratoconjunctivitis sicca.

testicle. See **testis.**

testicular /testik'yələr/ [L *testiculus* testicle], of or pertaining to the testicle.

testicular artery, one of a pair of long, slender branches of the abdominal aorta, arising caudal to the renal arteries and supplying the testis.

testicular cancer, a malignant neoplastic disease of the testis. An undescended testicle is often involved. In many cases the tumor is detected after an injury, but trauma is not considered a causative factor. Patients with early testicular cancer are often asymptomatic, and metastases may be seeded in lymph nodes, the lungs, and liver before the primary lesion is palpable. In the later stages there may be pulmonary symptoms, ureteral obstruction, gynecomastia, and an abdominal mass.

testicular duct. See **vas deferens.**

testicular feminization. See **feminization.**

testicular self-examination (TSE), a recommended (by the National Health Institute) procedure for detecting tumors or other abnormalities in the male testes. Each testicle is examined with both hands, placing the fingers under the testicle while the thumbs are placed on top. The testicle is then rolled gently between the thumbs and fingers.

testicular vein, one of a pair of veins that emerge from convoluted venous plexuses, forming the greater mass of the spermatic cords.

testimony [L *testimonium* evidence], the statement of a witness, usually made orally and given under oath, such as at a court trial.

testis /tes'tis/, *pl.* **testes** [L], one of the pair of male gonads that produce semen. The adult testes are suspended in the scrotum by the spermatic cords. Each testis is a laterally compressed oval body about 4 cm long, 2.5 cm wide, and weighs about 12 g. The convoluted epididymis lying on the posterior border of the testis is about 20 feet long and connects with the vas deferens through which spermatozoa pass during ejaculation. Each testis consists of several hundred conical lobules containing the tiny coiled seminiferous tubules in which spermatozoa develop.

test method, a method chosen for experimental testing or study by means of method evaluation.

test of patency of tear duct, a procedure in which drops of a weak sugar solution are placed in the eye. If the patient then detects a sweet taste the tear duct is assumed open.

testolactone /tes'tələk'tōn/, an antineoplastic androgen analog prescribed in the treatment of postmenopausal breast cancer and in premenopausal women whose ovarian function has been terminated.

testosterone /testos'tərōn/, a naturally occurring androgenic hormone prescribed for androgen deficiency, female breast cancer, and for stimulation of growth, weight gain, and red blood cell production.

testosterone cyclopentylpropionate. See **testosterone cypionate.**

testosterone cypionate, a long-acting form of testosterone.

testosterone derivative. See **anabolic steroid.**

testosterone enanthate, a long-acting form of testosterone.

testosterone propionate, an androgen given intramuscularly.

test tube, a tube made of transparent material having one open end. It is used in many common laboratory functions.

test tube baby, a popular term for an infant conceived through in vitro fertilization, using an ovum removed from the mother. After fertilization, the zygote is transplanted to the mother's uterus to develop normally.

tetanic contraction /tetan'ik/ [Gk *tetanos* convulsive tension; L *contractio* drawing together], a condition of continuous contraction in a voluntary muscle caused by a steady stream of efferent nerve impulses.

tetanic convulsion [Gk *tetanos*; L *convulsio* cramp], **1.** a generalized tonic muscular contraction. **2.** a prolonged violent involuntary muscular contraction.

tetanus /tet'ənəs/ [Gk *tetanos* extreme tension], an acute, potentially fatal infection of the central nervous system caused by an exotoxin, tetanospasmin, elaborated by an anaerobic bacillus, *Clostridium tetani.* The toxin is a neurotoxin and is one of the most lethal poisons known. *C. tetani* infects only wounds that contain dead tissue. The bacillus is a common resident of the superficial layers of the soil and a normal inhabitant of the intestinal tracts of cows and horses. The bacillus may enter the body through a puncture wound, abrasion, laceration, or burn. The infection occurs in two clinical forms: one with an abrupt onset, high mortality, and a short incubation period (3 to 21 days); the other with less severe symptoms, a lower mortality, and a longer incubation period (4 to 5 weeks). The disease is characterized by irritability, headache, fever, and painful spasms of the muscles resulting in lockjaw, risus sardonicus, opisthotonos, and laryngeal spasm; eventually, every muscle of the body is in tonic spasm. The motor nerves transmit the impulses from the infected central nervous system to the muscles. There is no lesion; even at autopsy no organic lesion is seen and the cerebrospinal fluid is clear and normal.

tetanus and diphtheria toxoids (Td), an active immunizing agent containing detoxified tetanus and diphtheria toxoids that slowly produce an antigenic response to the diseases. It is prescribed for immunization against tetanus and diphtheria in children under 7 years of age when pertussis vaccine present in the usual diphtheria, pertussis, and tetanus trivalent vaccine is contraindicated.

tetanus antitoxin (TAT), a tetanus immune serum that neutralizes exotoxins in tetanus infection. It is prescribed for short-term immunization against tetanus after possible exposure to the organism and in tetanus treatment.

tetanus immune globulin (TIG), an injectable solution prepared from the globulin of an immune human. It is effective and much safer than tetanus antitoxin. It is prescribed for short-term immunization against tetanus after possible exposure to the organism and tetanus treatment.

tetanus toxoid, an active immunizing agent prepared from detoxified tetanus toxin that produces an antigenic response in the body, conferring permanent immunity to tetanus infection. It is prescribed for primary active immunization against tetanus.

tetany /tet'ənē/ [Gk *tetanos* extreme tension], a condition characterized by cramps, convulsions, twitching of the muscles, and sharp flexion of the wrist and ankle joints. Tetany is a manifestation of an abnormality in calcium metabolism, which can occur in association with vitamin D deficiency, hypoparathyroidism, alkalosis, or the ingestion of alkaline salts. Kinds of tetany are **duration, grass, hyperventilation,** and **lactation tetany.**

tetrachlormethane. See **carbon tetrachloride.**

tetracycline /tet'rəsī'klēn/, a broad-spectrum antibiotic prescribed for the treatment of many bacterial and rickettsial infections.

tetracycline hydrochloride, a tetracycline antibiotic prescribed in the treatment of a variety of infections.

tetrad /tet'rad/ [Gk *tetras* quadrant], (in genetics) a group of four chromatids of a synapsed pair of homologous chromosomes during the first meiotic prophase stage of gametogenesis. **–tetradic,** *adj.*

tetradactyly /tet'rədak'tilē/ [Gk *tetra* + *dactylos*], the presence of only four fingers on each hand or four toes on each foot.

tetrahydrocannabinol (THC) /tet'rəhī'-drōkənab'inol/, the active principle, occurring as two psychomimetic isomers, in the hemp plant *Cannabis sativa,* used in the preparation of marijuana, hashish, bhang, and ganja. THC, a rapidly metabolized beta-adrenergic antagonist, increases pulse rate, causes conjunctival reddening, a feeling of euphoria, and has variable effects on blood pressure, respiratory rate, and pupil size. The drug affects memory, cognition, and the sensorium, decreases motor coordination, and increases appetite.

tetrahydrozoline hydrochloride /tet'rəhī-droz'əlēn/, an adrenergic vasoconstrictor prescribed for the treatment of nasal and nasopharyngeal congestion and as an ophthalmic vasoconstrictor.

tetraiodothyronine. See **thyroxine.**

tetralogy /tetrol'əjē/, any group of four writings, symptoms, or other related factors.

tetralogy of Fallot /falō'/ [Gk *tetra* four, *logos* word; Etienne-Louis A. Fallot, French physician, b. 1850], a congenital cardiac anomaly that consists of four defects: pulmonic stenosis, ventricular septal defect, malposition of the aorta so that it arises from the septal defect or the right ventricle, and right ventricular hypertrophy. The primary symptoms in the infant are cyanosis and hypoxia, usually during crying, difficulty in feeding, failure to gain weight, and poor development. In older children a typical squatting position and clubbing of the fingers and toes are evident.

tetramer /tet'rəmer/ [Gk *tetra* + *meros* part], something that is composed of four parts, such as a protein composed of four polypeptide subunits.

tetraplegia /tet'rəplē'jə/, paralysis of both arms and both legs.

tetraploid (4n) /tet'rəploid/ [Gk *tetraploos* fourfold, *eidos* form], **1.** of or pertaining to an individual, organism, strain, or cell that has four complete sets of chromosomes. **2.** such an individual, organism, strain, or cell.

tetraploidy /tet'rəploi'dē/, the state or condition of having four complete sets of chromosomes.

TFIIE, a general transcription factor involved in complementary DNA encoding. TFIIE consists of two subunits, TFIIE-alpha and TFIIE-beta.

T fracture, an intercondylar fracture in which the fracture lines are T-shaped.

TGF, abbreviation for **transforming growth factor.**

T group. See **sensitivity training group.**

Th, symbol for the element **thorium.**

thalamic peduncle /thalam'ik/ [Gk *thalamos* chamber; L *pes* foot], a group of fibers linking the thalamus with the hypothalamus.

thalamic syndrome, a vascular disorder involving the ventral and posterolateral nuclei of the thalamus and related nerve fibers causing disturbances of sensation and partial or complete paralysis of one side of the body. A major effect is an increased threshold to all stimuli on the opposite side of the body so that any stimuli may cause an exaggerated response.

thalamus /thal'əməs/, *pl.* **thalami** [Gk *thalamos* chamber], one of a pair of large oval organs forming most of the lateral walls of the third ventricle of the brain and part of the diencephalon. It relays sensory impulses to the cerebral cortex. It is composed mainly of gray substance and translates impulses from appropriate receptors into crude sensations of pain, temperature, and touch. It also participates in associating sensory impulses with pleasant and unpleasant feelings, in the arousal mechanisms of the body, and in the mechanisms that produce complex reflex movements. **–thalamic,** *adj.*

thalassemia /thal'əsē'mē·ə/ [Gk *thalassa* sea, *a, haima* not blood], hemolytic anemia characterized by microcytic, hypochromic, and short-lived red blood cells caused by deficient hemoglobin synthesis. It is genetically transmitted disease occurring in two forms. **Thalassemia major (Cooley's anemia),** the homozygous form, evident in infancy, is recognized by anemia, fever, failure to thrive, and splenomegaly and confirmed by characteristic changes in the red blood cells on microscopic examination. The spleen may become so enlarged that respiratory excursion is impeded, and the abdominal organs are crowded. Headache, abdominal pain, fatigue, and anorexia often occur. **Thalassemia minor,** the heterozygous form, is characterized only by a mild anemia and minimal red blood cell changes. Thalassemia minima is a form that lacks clinical symptoms, although patients show hematologic evidence of the disease.

thalidomide /thalid'əmīd/, a sedative-hypnotic, withdrawn from general use because of its potential for teratogenic effects, particularly phocomelia, when taken during pregnancy. It is sometimes prescribed for treatment of leprosy.

thallium (Tl) /thal'ē·əm/ [Gk *thallos* green line], a soft, bluish white metallic element that exhibits some nonmetallic chemical properties. Its atomic number is 81; its atomic weight is 204.37. Many of its compounds are highly toxic.

thallium poisoning, a toxic condition caused by the ingestion or the absorption through the skin of thallium salts, especially thallium sulfate. Characteristic of the condition are abdominal pain, vomiting, bloody diarrhea, tremor, delirium, and alopecia.

thanatology /than'ətol'əjē/ [Gk *thanatos* death, *logos* science], the study of death and dying. **–thanatologist,** *n.*

thanatophoric dwarf /than'ətōfôr'ik/ [Gk *thanatos* + *phoros* bearer; AS *dweorge*], an infant with severe micromelia, the limbs usually extending straight out from the trunk, an extremely narrow chest, and flattened vertebral bodies with wide intervertebral spaces.

thanotopsy. See **autopsy.**

Thanatos /than'ətəs/ [Gk, death], a freudian term for the death instinct.

THC, abbreviation for **tetrahydrocannabinol.**

the Blues, *informal.* a designation for Blue Cross (an insurance system that pays the costs of treatment by a hospital or clinic) and Blue Shield (an insurance system that pays the costs of treatment by a professional).

theca /thē'kə/, *pl.* **thecae** /thē'sē/, a sheath or capsule, such as the theca cordis or pericardium. **–thecal,** *adj.*

theca cell tumor [Gk *theke* sheath; L *cella* storeroom; *tumor* swelling], an uncommon benign fibroid tumor of the ovary, composed of theca cells and usually containing granulosa (follicular) cells.

thecocellulare xanthomatodes, thecoma. See **theca cell tumor.**

Theden's bandage /tā'dənz/ [Johann C. A. Theden, German surgeon, b. 1714], a roller bandage applied below the injury and continued upward over a compress; used to stop bleeding.

thelarche /thilär′kē/ [Gk *thele* nipple, *archaios* beginning], the beginning of female pubertal breast development that normally occurs before puberty at the beginning of the phase of rapid growth between 9 and 13 years of age. **Premature thelarche** is precocious breast development in a female without other evidence of sexual maturation.

thenar /thē′när/ [Gk, palm of hand], **1.** the ball of the thumb. **2.** of or pertaining to the thumb side of the palm.

thenar eminence, a raised rounded area on the palm of the hand near the base of the thumb.

theobromine /thē′əbrō′mīn/, a substance (methylxanthine) that is related chemically to caffeine and theophylline and differs from them by the number and distribution of methyl groups. Theobromine occurs naturally in cocoa, cola nuts, and tea. It acts as a diuretic, vasodilator, cardiac stimulant, and smooth muscle relaxant.

theophylline /thē·əfil′ēn/ [L *thea* tea; Gk *phyllon* leaf], a bronchodilator prescribed to relax the smooth muscle of the bronchial passages in the treatment of bronchospasm in bronchial asthma, bronchitis, and emphysema.

theorem [Gk *theorein* to look at], **1.** a proposition to be proved by a chain of reasoning and analysis. **2.** a rule expressed by symbols or formulae.

theoretic effectiveness [Gk *theorein* + L *efficere* to do], (of a contraceptive method) the effectiveness of a medication, device, or method in preventing pregnancy if used consistently and exactly as intended, without error.

theoretic plate number (N), a number defining the efficiency of a chromatographic column.

theory [Gk *theorein* to look at], an abstract statement formulated to predict, explain, or describe the relationships among concepts, constructs, or events.

theotherapy /thē′ōther′əpē/ [Gk *theos* god, *therapeia* treatment], a therapeutic approach to the prevention, diagnosis, and treatment of disease and dysfunction based on religious or spiritual beliefs.

therapeutic [Gk *therapeuein* to treat], **1.** beneficial. **2.** pertaining to a treatment.

therapeutic abortion, 1. a termination of early pregnancy deemed necessary by a physician. **2.** *informal;* any legal induced abortion.

therapeutic communication, (in psychiatric nursing) a process in which the nurse consciously influences a patient or helps the patient to a better understanding through verbal or nonverbal communication.

therapeutic community (TC), (in mental health) a treatment facility in which the entire milieu is part of the treatment. The physical environment, the other clients, the staff, and the policies of the facility influence the function of the individual.

therapeutic dose, the dose that may be required to produce a desired effect.

therapeutic equivalent, a drug that has essentially the same effect in the treatment of a disease or condition as one or more other drugs.

therapeutic exercise, any exercise planned and performed to attain a specific physical benefit, such as maintenance of the range of motion, strengthening of weakened muscles, increased flexibility of a joint, or improved cardiovascular and respiratory function.

therapeutic gain, the ratio of the biological effect of a therapy on a tumor compared with the effect on surrounding normal tissue.

therapeutic index, the difference between the minimum therapeutic and minimum toxic concentrations of a drug.

therapeutic pneumothorax, the intentional introduction of air in the intrapleural space, causing partial collapse of the lung. It was used in the 1940s for treatment of certain cases of tuberculosis.

therapeutic radiopharmaceutical, a radioactive drug administered to a patient to deliver radiation to body tissues internally, such as iodide 131, which is used to ablate thyroid tissue in hyperthyroid patients.

therapeutic recreation, an allied health category, staffed by persons with expertise in organizing and supervising recreational activities designed to accelerate recovery from mental or physical disorders.

therapeutic recreation specialist, a person who assists patients in their recovery or rehabilitation after physical or emotional illness or disability by planning and supervising recreation programs.

therapeutics [Gk *therapeia* treatment], a branch of health care that is concerned with the treatment of disease, seeking to relieve symptoms or to produce a cure.

therapeutic temperature, in hyperthermia treatment, temperatures between 42° C and 45° C (107° F and 113° F).

therapist, a person with special skills, obtained through education and experience, in one or more areas of health care.

therapy [Gk *therapeia*], the treatment of any disease or a pathologic condition, such as inhalation therapy, which administers various medicines for patients suffering from diseases of the respiratory tract.

thermal, thermic [Gk *therme* heat], of or pertaining to the production, application, or maintenance of heat.

thermal burn, tissue injury, usually of the skin, caused by exposure to extreme heat.

thermal dilution. See **thermodilution.**

thermal field size, the area over which therapeutic heating is likely to be produced.

thermalgesia /thur′məljē′zē·ə/ [Gk *therme* + *algos* pain], pain caused by exposure to high temperatures.

thermal radiation [Gk *therme*; L *radiare* to shine], the emission of energy in the form of heat.

thermic fever. See **heat hyperpyrexia.**

thermic sense, the network of sense organs and connecting pathways that allows an appreciation of temperature changes.

thermistor /thərmis′tər/ [Gk *therme* + L *resistere* to withstand], a kind of thermometer for measuring minute changes in temperature.

thermocautery /thur′mōkô′tərē/ [Gk *therme* + *kauterion* branding iron], the use of a needle or snare heated by direct flame, a heated hydrocarbon vapor, or an electric current in the destruction of tissue.

thermochemistry, a branch of chemistry that is concerned with the heat changes involved in chemical reactions.

thermocoagulation /thur′mōkō·ag′yəlā′shən/, the use of high-frequency electric currents to destroy tissue through heat coagulation.

thermocouple /thur′məkup′əl/ [Gk *therme* + Fr *couple* pair], a temperature-measuring device that relies on the production of a temperature-dependent voltage at the junction of two dissimilar metals.

thermodilution /thur′mōdilyōō′zhən/ [Gk *therme* + L *diluere* to wash], a method of cardiac output determination. A bolus of solution of known volume and temperature is added to the bloodstream, and the resultant cooling of blood temperature is detected by a thermistor previously placed in the pulmonary artery with a catheter.

thermodynamics, the science of the interconversion of heat and work.

thermogenesis /thur′mōjen′əsis/ [Gk *therme* + *genesis* origin], production of heat, especially by the cells of the body. **–thermogenetic,** *adj.*

thermograph [Gk, *therme* + *graphein,* to write], **1.** a photographic record of the amount of heat radiated from the surface of the body, revealing "hot spots" of potential tumors or other disorders. **2.** a device consisting of a thermometer, inked stylus, and chart for continuous recording of the ambient temperature.

thermography /thərmog′rəfē/, a technique for sensing and recording on film hot and cold areas of the body by means of an infrared detector that reacts to blood flow. **–thermographic,** *adj.*

thermoinhibitory center. See **thermoregulatory centers.**

thermolabile /thur′məlā′bəl/ [Gk *therme* + L *labilis* slipping], easily destroyed or altered by heat.

thermoluminescent dosimetry /thur′mōlōō′mines′ənt/ [Gk *therme* + L *lumen* light; Gk *dosis* giving something, *metron* measure], a method of measuring the ionizing radiation to which a person is exposed by a device that stores the radiant energy and releases it later as ultraviolet or visible light.

thermometer [Gk *therme* + *metron* measure], an instrument for measuring temperature. It usually consists of a sealed glass tube, marked in degrees of Celsius or Fahrenheit, containing liquid, such as mercury or alcohol. The liquid rises or falls as it expands or contracts according to changes in temperature. Some kinds of thermometers are **clinical, digital, electronic,** and **tympanic membrane thermometer.**

thermoneutral environment /thur′mōnōō′trəl/ [Gk *therme* + L *neutralis* neutral; ME *environ* around], **1.** an environment that keeps body temperature at an optimum point at which the least amount of oxygen is consumed for metabolism. **2.** an environment that enables a neonate to maintain a body temperature of 36.5° C (97.7° F) with a minimal requirement of energy and oxygen.

thermonuclear, pertaining to a reaction in which isotopes of hydrogen (protium, deuterium, or tritium) can be fused at temperatures of nearly 100,000,000° C into heavier nuclei of helium atoms. The process is the source of energy of the sun and is used in the explosion of thermonuclear weapons.

thermopenetration [Gk *therme* + L *penetrale* passing through], the use of diathermic techniques to produce warmth within the body tissues for therapeutic purposes.

thermophilic /thur′mōfil′ik/ [Gk *therme* + *philein* to love], pertaining to organisms that thrive in warmth of up to 70° C, well above normal human body temperature of 37° C.

thermoradiotherapy, a therapeutic process that applies ionizing radiation to any part of the body in which the temperature has been raised by artificial means.

T

thermoreceptor, nerve endings that are sensitive to heat or a rise in body temperature.

thermoregulation [Gk *therme* + L *regula* rule], the control of heat production and heat loss, specifically the maintenance of body temperature through physiologic mechanisms.

thermoregulation, ineffective, a NANDA-accepted nursing diagnosis of the state in which an individual's temperature fluctuates between hypothermia and hyperthermia. The critical defining characteristic is the fluctuation in body temperature above or below the normal range.

thermoregulatory centers, centers located in the hypothalamus concerned mainly with the regulation of heat production, heat inhibition, and heat conservation in order to maintain a normal body temperature. Kinds of thermoregulatory centers include **thermogenic, thermoinhibitory,** and **thermotaxic center.**

thermostable, unaffected by or resistant to change by an increase in temperature.

thermostat [Gk *therme* + *statos* standing], a device for the automatic control of a heating or cooling system. **–thermostatic,** *adj.*

thermotaxis /thur′mōtak′sis/ [Gk *therme* + taxis arrangement], **1.** the normal adjustment and regulation of body temperature. **2.** the movement of an organism in response to heat, either toward the stimulus (positive thermotaxis) or away from the stimulus (negative thermotaxis).

thermotaxic center. See **thermoregulatory centers.**

thermotherapeutic penetration, the depth to which heating to therapeutic temperatures is likely to extend.

thermotherapy [Gk *therme* + *therapeia* treatment], the treatment of disease by the application of heat. Thermotherapy may be administered as dry heat with heat lamps, diathermy machines, electric pads, or hot water bottles or as moist heat with warm compresses or immersion in warm water. **–thermotherapeutic,** *adj.*

thermotropism. See **thermotaxis.**

theta wave /thē′tə, thā′tə/ [Gk *theta* eighth letter of Greek alphabet; AS *wafian*], one of the several types of brain waves, characterized by a relatively low frequency of 4 to 7 Hz and a low amplitude of 10 μV. Theta waves are the "drowsy waves" of the temporal lobes of the brain.

thiabendazole /thī′əben′dazōl/, an anthelmintic prescribed in the treatment of a variety of worm infestations, including hookworms, roundworms, and pinworms.

thiamine /thī′əmin/ [Gk *theion* containing sulfur + *amine* ammonia], a water-soluble, crystalline compound of the B-complex vitamin group, essential for normal metabolism and for the health of the cardiovascular and nervous systems. Thiamine combines with pyruvic acid to form a coenzyme necessary for the breakdown of carbohydrates into glucose. A deficiency of thiamine affects chiefly the nervous system, the circulation, and the GI tract. Symptoms include irritability, emotional disturbances, loss of appetite, multiple neuritis, increased pulse rate, dyspnea, reduced intestinal motility, and heart irregularities. Severe deficiency causes beriberi. Also spelled **thiamin.**

thiazide diuretic. See **diuretic.**

thiethylperazine /thī′eth′ilper′əzēn/, a phenothiazine antiemetic prescribed to control nausea and vomiting.

thigh [AS *theoh*], the section of the lower limb between the hip and the knee.

thigh bone. See **femur.**

thinking [AS *thencan* to think], **1.** the cognitive process of forming mental images or concepts. **2.** the process of cognitive problem solving through the sorting, organizing, and classification of facts. Kinds of thinking include **abstract, concrete,** and **syncretic thinking.**

thin-layer chromatography (TLC), a method of separating two or more chemical compounds in a solution by their differential migrations over a thin layer of adsorbent spread over a glass or plastic plate.

thioamide derivative /thī′ō·am′īd/, one of a group of antithyroid drugs prescribed in the treatment of hyperthyroidism. Thioamide drugs act by inhibiting the synthesis of thyroid hormone.

thioctic acid /thī·ok′tik/, a pyruvate oxidation factor found in liver and yeast, used in bacterial culture media.

thioester /thī′ō·es′tər/, an important group of biologic chemicals formed by the hydrosulfides and carboxylic acids and identified by an ester bond involving the -SH radical. Examples include the coenzyme A thioesters.

thioguanine /thī′ōgwä′nēn/, an antineoplastic prescribed in the treatment of a variety of malignant neoplastic diseases, including the acute leukemias.

thiopental sodium /thī·əpen′təl/, a potent short-acting barbiturate, used as a general anesthetic for surgical procedures that are expected to require 15 minutes or less, as an induction agent for other general anesthetics, as a hypnotic component in balanced anesthesia, and as an adjunct to regional anesthesia.

thioridazine hydrochloride /thī·ôrid′əzēn/, a phenothiazine antipsychotic prescribed in the treatment of childhood behavioral disorders, geriatric mental disorders, depression, and alcohol withdrawal.

thiotepa /thī'ōtep'ə/, an antineoplastic alkylating agent prescribed in the treatment of a variety of malignant neoplastic diseases, including adenocarcinoma of the breast and ovary, and urinary bladder carcinomas.

thiothixene /thī·ōthī'ksēn/, a thioxanthene antipsychotic prescribed in the treatment of acute agitation and mild-to-severe psychotic disorders.

thiouracil /thī'ōyŏŏr'əsil/ [Gk *theion* sulfur, *ouron* urine], a chemical compound derived from thiourea that inhibits the formation of thyroxine in the thyroid gland and is used to treat hyperthyroidism.

thioxanthene derivative /thī·oksan'thēn/, any one of a group of antipsychotic drugs, each of which is similar to the phenothiazenes in indication, action, and adverse effects.

third cranial nerve. See **oculomotor nerve.**

third cuneiform bone. See **lateral cuneiform bone.**

third-party reimbursement, reimbursement for services rendered to a person in which an entity other than the giver or receiver of the service is responsible for the payment.

third stage of labor, the expulsion of the placenta, membranes, and a small amount of blood and amniotic fluid, occurring within 5 to 30 minutes after delivery of the fetus.

third ventricle [Gk *tritos* below second rank; L *ventriculum*], a cavity of the brain bounded on either side by a thalamus and the hypothalamus. It communicates anteriorly with the lateral ventricles and posteriorly with the aqueduct of the midbrain.

third ventriculostomy /ventrik'yəlos'təmē/ [L *tertius* three; *ventriculum* little belly; Gk *stoma* mouth], a surgical procedure for draining cerebrospinal fluid into the cisterna chiasmatis of the subarachnoid space in hydrocephalus, usually in the newborn.

thirst [AS *thurst*], a perceived desire for water or other fluid. The sensation of thirst is usually referred to the mouth and throat.

Thiry-Vella fistula /thī'rēvel'ə/ [Ludwig Thiry, Austrian physiologist, b. 1817; Luigi Vella, Italian physiologist, b. 1825], an artificial passage from the abdominal surface of an experimental animal to an isolated intestinal loop, created surgically for the study of intestinal secretions.

Thomas' splint [Hugh Owen Thomas, English surgeon, b. 1834] **1.** a rigid splint constructed of steel bars that are curved to fit the involved limb and held in place by a cast or a rigid bandage. **2.** a rigid metal splint that extends from a ring at the hip to beyond the foot.

Thompson scattering. See **scattering.**

Thomsen's disease. See **myotonia congenita.**

thoracentesis. See **thoracocentesis.**

thoracic /thôras'ik/, of or pertaining to the thorax.

thoracic actinomycocis. See **actinomycosis.**

thoracic aorta [Gk *thorax* chest; *aerein* to raise], the large upper portion of the descending aorta, starting at the caudal border of the fourth thoracic vertebra, dividing into seven branches, and supplying many parts of the body, such as the heart, ribs, chest muscles, and stomach.

thoracic cage, the bony framework that surrounds the organs and soft tissues of the chest. It consists of 12 thoracic vertebrae, 12 pairs of ribs, and the sternum.

thoracic cavity, the cavity enclosed by the ribs, the thoracic portion of the vertebral column, the sternum, the diaphragm, and associated muscles.

thoracic duct, the common trunk of all the lymphatic vessels in the body, except those on the right side of the head, the neck, and the thorax, the right upper limb, the right lung, the right side of the heart, and the diaphragmatic surface of the liver. The thoracic duct contains various valves, including two at this orifice that prevent venous blood from flowing into the lymphatic system.

thoracic fistula, an abnormal opening in the chest wall that ends blindly or that communicates with the thoracic cavity.

thoracic medicine, the branch of medicine concerned with the diagnosis and treatment of disorders of the structures and organs of the chest, especially the lungs.

thoracic nerves, the 12 spinal nerves on each side of the thorax, including 11 intercostal nerves and 1 subcostal nerve. They are distributed mainly to the walls of the thorax and the abdomen. The first 2 intercostal nerves innervate the upper limb and the thorax; the next 4 supply only the thorax; and the lower 5 supply the walls of the thorax and the abdomen.

thoracic outlet syndrome, an abnormal condition and a type of mononeuropathy characterized by paresthesia of the fingers. It may be caused by a nerve root compression by a cervical disk or by carpal tunnel syndrome.

thoracic parietal node, one of the lymph glands in the thorax, associated with various lymphatic vessels and divided into

T

sternal nodes, intercostal nodes, and diaphragmatic nodes.

thoracic surgery, a branch of medicine that deals with disease and injuries of the thoracic area by manipulative and operative methods.

thoracic vertebra, one of the 12 bony segments of the spinal column of the upper back, designated T1 to T12. T1 is just below the seventh cervical vertebra (C7) and T12 is just above the first lumbar vertebra (L1). The thoracic portion of the spine is flexible and has a concave ventral curvature.

thoracic visceral node, a node in the three groups of lymph nodes connected to the part of the lymphatic system that serves certain structures within the thorax, such as the thymus, pericardium, esophagus, trachea, lungs, and bronchi.

thoracocentesis /thôr′əkōsentē′sis/ [Gk *thorax* + *kentesis* puncture], the surgical perforation of the chest wall and pleural space with a needle for the aspiration of fluid for diagnostic or therapeutic purposes or for the removal of a specimen for biopsy.

thoracodorsal nerve /thôr′əkōdôr′səl/ [Gk *thorax* + L *dorsum* back], a branch of the brachial plexus, usually arising between the two subscapular nerves. It courses along the posterior wall of the axilla and terminates in branches that supply the latissimus dorsi.

thoracodynia /thôr′əkōdin′ē-ə/ [Gk *thorax* + *odyne* pain], chest pain.

thoracolumbar fascia /thôr′əkōkəlum′bər/, a noncontractile structure that functions in a manner similar to a ligament in the lumbar area. It extends from the iliac crest and sacrum to the thoracic cage and envelops the paravertebral musculature.

thoracostomy /thôr′əkos′təmē/ [Gk *thorax* + *stoma* mouth], an incision made into the chest wall to provide an opening for the purpose of drainage.

thoracotomy /thôr′əkot′əmē/ [Gk *thorax* + *temnein* to cut], a surgical opening into the thoracic cavity.

Thoraeus filters /thôrē′əs/, combinations of metals, usually tin, copper, and aluminum, used to modify the quality of orthovoltage x-ray beams to improve the penetrating ability.

thorax /thôr′aks/, *pl.* **thoraces, thoraxes** [Gk, chest], the cage of bone and cartilage containing the principal organs of respiration and circulation and covering part of the abdominal organs. It is formed ventrally by the sternum and costal cartilages and dorsally by the 12 thoracic vertebrae and the dorsal parts of the 12 ribs.

thorium (Th) /thôr′ē-əm/ [ONorse *Thor* god of thunder], a heavy, grayish, radioactive, metallic element. Its atomic number is 90; its atomic weight is 232.04. Thorium is used in radiographic procedures and in radiation therapy.

thought broadcasting [AS *thot*], a symptom of psychosis in which the patient believes that his or her thoughts are "broadcast" beyond the head so that other persons can hear them.

thought insertion, a belief by some mentally ill patients that thoughts of other persons can be inserted into their own minds.

thought processes, altered, a NANDA-accepted nursing diagnosis of a state in which an individual experiences disruption in cognitive operations and activities. Defining characteristics include distraction, egocentrism, abnormal cognitive function, abnormal interpretations of the environment; decreased ability to grasp ideas; impaired ability to reason, solve problems, calculate, conceptualize, or make decisions; disorientation; inappropriate social behavior; altered sleep patterns; delusions or hallucinations; and attention to environmental cues that is more or less acute than might normally be expected.

thought transference. See **telepathy.**

Thr, abbreviation for the amino acid **threonine.**

threadworm. See *Enterobius vermicularis.*

threadworm infection. See **strongyloidiasis.**

thready pulse [AS *thraed;* L *pulsare* to beat], an abnormal pulse that is weak and often fairly rapid; the artery does not feel full, and the rate may be difficult to count.

threatened abortion [AS *threat* coercion; L *ab* away, *oriri* to be born], a condition in pregnancy before the twentieth week of gestation characterized by uterine bleeding and cramping sufficient to suggest that miscarriage may result.

three-day fever. See **phlebotomus fever.**

three-day measles. See **rubella.**

3-methyl fentanyl, a potent heroin substitute and so-called designer drug. It is an analog of fentanyl.

three-point gait, a pattern of crutch walking in which the crutches and affected leg are advanced first with each step.

threonine (Thr), an essential amino acid needed for proper growth in infants and maintenance of nitrogen balance in adults.

threshold [AS *therscold*], the point at which a stimulus is great enough to produce an effect; for example, a pain threshold is the point at which a person becomes aware of pain.

threshold dose, a measure of a dose of radiation exposure defined in terms of conditions needed to produce a visible erythema in a given proportion of persons exposed.

threshold limit values, the maximum concentration of a chemical to which workers can be exposed for a fixed period, such as 8 hours per day, without developing a physical impairment.

threshold of consciousness, the lowest limit of perception of a stimulus.

threshold stimulus, a stimulus that is just sufficient to produce a response. Below that level, no action or response is likely without additional intensity of the stimulus.

thrill [AS *thyrlian* to pierce], a fine vibration, felt by an examiner's hand on the body of a patient over the site of an aneurysm or on the precordium, indicating the presence of an organic murmur.

throat. See **pharynx.**

throb [ME *throbben* to beat intensely], a deep, pulsating kind of discomfort or pain. **–throbbing,** *adj., n.*

thrombapheresis. See **plateletpheresis.**

thrombasthenia /throm′basthē′nē·ə/ [Gk *thrombos* lump, *a, sthenos* not strength], a rare hemorrhagic disease characterized by a defect in platelet-mediated hemostasis caused by an abnormality in the membrane surface of the platelet. The platelets do not aggregate, a clot does not form, and hemorrhage ensues, often from the mucous membrane.

thrombectomy /thrombek′təmē/ [Gk *thrombos* + *ektome* excision], the removal of a thrombus from a blood vessel, performed as emergency surgery to restore circulation to the affected part.

thrombi. See **thrombus.**

thrombin /throm′bin/, an enzyme formed in plasma during the clotting process from prothrombin, calcium, and thromboplastin.

thromboangiitis obliterans /throm′-bō·an′jē·ī′tis/ [Gk *thrombos* + *aggeion* vessel, *itis* inflammation; L *obliterare* to cancel], an occlusive vascular condition, usually of a leg or a foot, in which the small and medium-sized arteries become inflamed and thrombotic. Early signs of the condition are burning, numbness, and tingling of the foot or leg distal to the lesion. Phlebitis and gangrene may develop as the disease progresses. Pulsation in the limb below the damaged blood vessels is often absent.

thrombocytapheresis. See **plateletpheresis.**

thrombocyte. See **platelet.**

thrombocytopathy /throm′bōsītop′əthē/

[Gk *thrombos* + *kytos* cell, *pathos* disease], any disorder of the blood coagulation mechanism caused by an abnormality or dysfunction of platelets. Kinds of thrombocytopathies include **thrombocytopenia** and **thrombocytosis.** **–thrombocytopathic,** *adj.*

thrombocytopenia /throm′bōsī′təpē′nē·ə/ [Gk *thrombos, kytos* + *penia* poverty], an abnormal hematologic condition in which the number of platelets is reduced, usually by destruction of erythroid tissue in bone marrow associated with certain neoplastic diseases or an immune response to a drug. There may be decreased production of platelets, decreased survival of platelets, and increased consumption of platelets or splenomegaly. Thrombocytopenia is the most common cause of bleeding disorders.

thrombocytopenic purpura /throm′bō-sī′təpē′nik/, a bleeding disorder characterized by a marked decrease in the number of platelets, resulting in multiple bruises, petechiae, and hemorrhage into the tissues. Causes include infection and drug sensitivity and toxicity. It is considered to be a manifestation of an autoimmune response.

thrombocytosis /throm′bōsītō′sis/ [Gk *thrombos, kytos* + *osis* condition], an abnormal increase in the number of platelets in the blood. **Benign thrombocytosis,** or **secondary thrombocytosis,** is asymptomatic and usually occurs after splenectomy, inflammatory disease, hemolytic anemia, hemorrhage, or iron deficiency, as a response to exercise, or after treatment with vincristine. **Essential thrombocythemia** is characterized by episodes of spontaneous bleeding alternating with thrombotic episodes.

thromboembolism /throm′bō·em′-bəliz′əm/ [Gk *thrombos* + *embolos* plug], a condition in which a blood vessel is blocked by an embolus carried in the bloodstream from the site of formation of the clot. The area supplied by an obstructed artery may tingle and become cold, numb, and cyanotic. An embolus in the lungs causes a sudden, sharp thoracic or upper abdominal pain, dyspnea, a violent cough, fever, and hemoptysis. Obstruction of the pulmonary artery or one of its branches may be rapidly fatal.

thrombogenic /throm′bōjen′ik/ [Gk *thrombos* + *genein* to produce], pertaining to a thrombus or a factor causing a thrombus or clot.

thrombolytic /throm′bōlit′ik/ [Gk *thrombos* + *lysein* to loosen], pertaining to a drug or other agent that dissolves thrombi.

thrombophlebitis /throm′bōfləbī′tis/ [Gk

thrombos + *phleps* vein, *itis*], inflammation of a vein, often accompanied by formation of a clot. It occurs most commonly as the result of trauma to the vessel wall; hypercoagulability of the blood; infection; chemical irritation; postoperative venous stasis; prolonged sitting, standing, or immobilization; or a long period of intravenous catheterization. Thrombophlebitis of a superficial vein is generally evident; the vessel feels hard and thready or cordlike and is extremely sensitive to pressure; the surrounding area may be erythematous and warm to the touch, and the entire limb may be pale, cold, and swollen. Deep-vein thrombophlebitis is characterized by aching or cramping pain, especially in the calf when the patient walks or dorsiflexes the foot (Homan's sign).

thrombophlebitis migrans. See **migratory thrombophlebitis.**

thrombophlebitis purulenta, an inflammation of a vein associated with the formation of a soft purulent thrombus that infiltrates the wall of the vessel.

thromboplastin /throm′bōplas′tin/ [Gk *thrombos* + *plassein* to mold], a complex substance that initiates the clotting process by converting prothrombin to thrombin in the presence of calcium ion.

thrombosis /thrombō′sis/, *pl.* **thromboses,** an abnormal vascular condition in which thrombus develops within a blood vessel of the body.

thrombotic /thrombot′ik/, caused or characterized by thrombosis.

thrombotic phlegmasia. See **phlegmasia alba dolens.**

thrombotic thrombocytopenic purpura (TTP) [Gk *thrombos* lump; *thrombos, kytos* cell, *penia* poverty; L *purpura* purple], a disorder characterized by thrombocytopenia, hemolytic anemia, and neurologic abnormalities. It is accompanied by a generalized purpura together with the deposition of microthrombi within the capillaries and smaller arterioles.

thrombus /throm′bəs/, *pl.* **thrombi** [Gk *thrombos* lump], an aggregation of platelets, fibrin, clotting factors, and the cellular elements of the blood attached to the interior wall of a vein or artery, sometimes occluding the lumen of the vessel. Kinds of thrombi include **agonal, hyaline, laminated,** and **white thrombus.**

through-and-through drainage, a method of irrigating a body organ by inserting two tubes, one to introduce the fluid and another to drain the fluid that accumulates within the organ.

through transmission, (in ultrasonography) the process of imaging by transmitting the sound field through a specimen and picking up the transmitted energy on a far surface or a receiving transducer.

thrush [Dan *troeske* dryness], candidiasis of the tissues of the mouth.

thulium (Tm) /thōō′lē-əm/ [L *Thule* northern island], a rare earth metallic element. Its atomic number is 69; its atomic weight is 168.93.

thumb [AS *thuma*], the first and shortest digit of the hand, classified by some anatomists as one of the fingers because its metacarpal bone ossifies in the same manner as those of the phalanges. Other anatomists classify the thumb separately, regarding it as composed of one metacarpal bone and only two phalanges.

thumb forceps, a surgical instrument used to grasp soft tissue, especially while suturing.

thumb sign, the flexing of the terminal phalanx of the thumb against the flexed index finger, as in holding a piece of paper. It is observed in patients who are unable to adduct the thumb because of an ulnar lesion.

thumbsucking, the habit of sucking the thumb for oral gratification. It is normal in infants and young children as a pleasure-seeking or comforting device, especially when the child is hungry or tired. The habit reaches its peak when the child is between 18 and 20 months of age, and it normally disappears as the child develops and matures.

thymic /thī′mik/, of or pertaining to the thymus gland.

thymic hypoplasia, thymic parathyroid aplasia. See **DiGeorge's syndrome.**

thymine, a major pyrimidine base found in nucleotides and a fundamental constituent of DNA.

thymol /thī′mol/, a synthetic or natural thyme oil, used as an antibacterial and antifungal, that is an ingredient in some over-the-counter preparations for the treatment of hemorrhoids, acne, and tinea pedis.

thymoma /thīmō′mə/, *pl.* **thymomas, thymomata** [Gk *thymos* thyme flowers, *oma* tumor], a usually benign tumor of the thymus gland that may be associated with myasthenia gravis or an immune deficiency disorder.

thymosin /thī′məsin/, **1.** a naturally occurring immunologic hormone secreted by the thymus gland. It is present in greatest amounts in young children and decreases in amount throughout life. **2.** an investigational drug derived from bovine thymus extracts and prescribed as an immunomodulator.

thymus /thī′məs/, *pl.* **thymuses, thymi** [Gk *thymos* thyme flowers], a single unpaired gland that is located in the mediastinum, extending superiorly into the neck to the lower edge of the thyroid gland and inferiorly as far as the fourth costal cartilage. The thymus is the primary central gland of the lymphatic system. The T cells of the cell-mediated immune response develop in this gland before migrating to the lymph nodes and the spleen. The gland consists of two lateral lobes closely bound by connective tissue, which also encloses the entire organ in a capsule.

thyrocalcitonin. See calcitonin.

thyrocervical trunk /thī′rosur′vikəl/ [Gk *thyreos* shield, *eidos* form; L *cervix* neck; *truncus*], one of a pair of short, thick arterial branches, arising from the first portion of the subclavian arteries, close to the medial border of the scalenus anterior, supplying numerous muscles and bones in the head, neck, and back.

thyrocricotomy /thī′rokrīkot′əmē/ [Gk *thyreos* shield, *eidos* form, *krikos* ring, *temnein* to cut], a tracheotomy procedure in which the cricovocal membrane is divided.

thyrogenic /thī′rojen′ik/, **thyrogenous** /thīroj′ənəs/, pertaining to an origin in the thyroid gland.

thyroglobulin /thī′roglōb′yəlin/, a purified extract of porcine thyroid prescribed in the treatment of cretinism, myxedema, goiter, and other hypothyroid states.

thyroid. See thyroid gland, thyroid hormone.

thyroid acropathy /thī′roid/ [Gk *thyreos* shield, *eidos* form; *akron* extremity, *pathos* disease], swelling of subcutaneous tissue of the extremities and clubbing of the digits, occurring rarely in patients with thyroid disease and usually associated with pretibial myxedema or exophthalmos.

thyroid cancer, a neoplasm of the thyroid gland. The first sign of cancer may be an increase in size of the thyroid gland, a palpable nodule, hoarseness, dysphagia, dyspnea, or pain on pressure. Diagnostic measures include x-ray examination, transillumination of the gland, radioisotope scanning, needle biopsy, and ultrasonic examination. More than one half of thyroid malignancies are papillary carcinomas, about one third are follicular carcinomas, and the rest consist of rapidly growing invasive anaplastic carcinomas, medullary carcinomas that secrete calcitonin, and metastatic lesions from primary tumors in the breast, kidneys, or lungs.

thyroid cartilage, the largest cartilage of the larynx, consisting of two laminae fused together at an acute angle in the middle line of the neck to form the Adam's apple.

thyroid crisis, a sudden exacerbation of symptoms of thyrotoxicosis characterized by fever, sweating, tachycardia, extreme nervous excitability, and pulmonary edema. It usually occurs in a patient whose thyrotoxicosis treatment is inadequate and the paroxysm is triggered by a stressful infection or injury. If untreated, the crisis is often fatal.

thyroid dermoid cyst, a tumor derived from embryonal tissues that is believed to have developed in the thyroid gland or in the thyrolingual duct.

thyroidectomized, pertaining to a patient or condition in which the thyroid gland has been removed.

thyroidectomy /thī′roidek′təmē/ [Gk *thyreos* + *eidos* form, *ektome* excision], the surgical removal of the thyroid gland, performed for colloid goiter, tumors, or hyperthyroidism that does not respond to iodine therapy and antithyroid drugs. All but 5% to 10% of the gland is removed; regrowth usually begins shortly after surgery, and thyroid function may return to normal. For cancer of the thyroid, the entire gland is removed, along with surrounding structures from neck to collarbone, in a radical neck dissection.

thyroid function test, any of several laboratory tests performed to evaluate the function of the thyroid gland. Thyroid function tests include protein-bound iodine, butanol-extractable iodine, T3, T4, free thyroxine index, thyroxin-binding globulin, thyroid-stimulating hormone, long-acting thyroid stimulator, radioactive iodine uptake, and radioactive iodine excretion.

thyroid gland [Gk *thyreos* shield, *eidos* form], a highly vascular organ at the front of the neck, usually weighing about 30 g, consisting of bilateral lobes connected in the middle by a narrow isthmus. The thyroid gland secretes the hormone thyroxin directly into the blood and is part of the endocrine system of ductless glands. It is essential to normal body growth in infancy and childhood, and its removal greatly reduces the oxidative processes of the body, producing a lower metabolic rate characteristic of hypothyroidism.

thyroid hormone, an iodine-containing compound secreted by the thyroid gland, predominantly as thyroxine (T4) and in smaller amounts as four times more potent triiodothyronine (T3). These hormones increase the rate of metabolism, affect body temperature, regulate protein, fat, and carbohydrate catabolism in all cells, maintain growth hormone secretion, skeletal maturation, the cardiac rate, force, and output, promote central nervous system development, stimulate the synthesis of many enzymes, and are necessary for muscle tone

T

and vigor. Derivatives of thyronine, T4 and T3, are synthesized in the thyroid gland by a complex process involving the uptake, oxidation, and incorporation of iodide and the production of thyroglobulin; the form in which the hormones apparently are stored in thyroid follicular colloid.

thyroiditis /thī′roidī′tis/, inflammation of the thyroid gland. Acute thyroiditis, caused by staphylococcal, streptococcal, or other infections, is characterized by suppuration and abscess formation and may progress to subacute diffuse disease of the gland. Subacute thyroiditis is marked by fever, weakness, sore throat, and a painfully enlarged gland containing granulomas composed of colloid masses surrounded by giant cells and mononuclear cells. Chronic lymphocytic thyroiditis (Hashimoto's disease), characterized by lymphocyte and plasma cell infiltration of the gland and by diffuse enlargement, seems to be transmitted as a dominant trait and may be associated with various autoimmune disorders. Another chronic form of thyroiditis is Riedel's struma, a rare progressive fibrosis, usually of one lobe of the gland but sometimes involving both lobes, the trachea, and surrounding muscles, nerves, and blood vessels. Radiation thyroiditis occasionally occurs 7 to 10 days after the treatment of hyperthyroidism with radioactive iodine 131.

thyroid-releasing hormone. See **thyrotropin-releasing hormone.**

thyroid-stimulating hormone (TSH), a substance secreted by the anterior lobe of the pituitary gland that controls the release of thyroid hormone and is necessary for the growth and function of the thyroid gland. The secretion of TSH is regulated by thyrotropin-releasing factor, elaborated in the median eminence of the hypothalamus.

thyroid storm, a crisis in uncontrolled hyperthyroidism caused by the release into the bloodstream of increased amounts of thyroid hormones. The storm may occur spontaneously or be precipitated by infection, stress, or a thyroidectomy performed on a patient who had been inadequately prepared with antithyroid drugs. Characteristic signs are fever that may reach 106° F, a rapid pulse, acute respiratory distress, apprehension, restlessness, irritability, and prostration. The patient may become delirious, lapse into a coma, and die of heart failure.

thyromegaly /thī′romeg′əlē/ [Gk *thyreos* + *eidos* + *megas* large], enlargement of the thyroid gland.

thyrotonine (T3) triiodothyronine, See **thyroid hormone.**

thyrotoxic crisis. See **thyroid crisis.**

thyrotoxicosis. See **Graves' disease.**

thyrotrophic /thī′rotrof′ik/, **thyrotropic,** pertaining to something that influences the thyroid gland, such as the thyroid-stimulating hormone (TSH).

thyrotropic hormone. See **thyroid-stimulating hormone.**

thyrotropin. See **thyroid-stimulating hormone.**

thyrotropin (systemic) /thī′rotrō′pin/, a preparation of bovine thyroid-stimulating hormone that increases the uptake of radioactive iodine in the thyroid and the secretion of thyroxine by the thyroid. It is prescribed in diagnostic tests and to enhance uptake of ^{131} I in the treatment of thyroid cancer.

thyrotropin-releasing hormone, a substance elaborated in the median eminence of the hypothalamus that stimulates the release of thyrotropin (thyroid-stimulating hormone) from the anterior pituitary gland.

thyroxine (T4) /thīrok′sēn/, a hormone of the thyroid gland, derived from tyrosine, that influences metabolic rate.

thyroxine-binding globulin, a plasma protein that binds with and transports thyroxine in the blood.

Ti, symbol for the element **titanium.**

TI, abbreviation for **therapeutic index.**

TIA, abbreviation for **transient ischemic attack.**

tibia /tib′ē-ə/ [L, shin bone], the second longest bone of the skeleton, located at the medial side of the leg. It articulates with the fibula laterally, the talus distally, and the femur proximally, forming part of the knee joint. **–tibial,** *adj.*

tibialis anterior /tib′ē-ā′lis/ [L *tibia* + *anticus* in front], one of the anterior crural muscles of the leg, situated on the lateral side of the tibia. It dorsiflexes and supinates the foot.

tibial torsion [L *tibia* + *torquere* to twist], a lateral or a medial twisting rotation of the tibia on its longitudinal axis.

tibia valga, a bowed tibia with the convex surface toward the outside of the leg.

tic. See **mimic spasm.**

ticarcillin /tik′ärsil′in/, an antibiotic prescribed in the treatment of bacterial septicemia, and skin, soft tissue, and respiratory infections caused by both gram-negative and gram-positive organisms.

tic douloureux /tikdōōl′ōōrœ′/ [Fr, painful spasm], a brief extremely painful attack of trigeminal neuralgia. It is unilateral and limited to the distribution of the trigeminal, fifth cranial, nerve. An attack is easily and unexpectedly provoked by any stimulus of the facial muscles, from touching to speaking, and may occur repetitively.

tick bite [ME *tike;* AS *bitan* to bite], a puncture wound produced by the toothed beak of a bloodsucking tick, a small, tough-skinned, arachnid. Ticks transmit several diseases to humans, and a few species carry a neurotoxin in their saliva that may cause ascending paralysis beginning in the legs. Nervousness, loss of appetite, tingling, and headache, followed by muscle pain, and, in extreme cases, respiratory failure, may occur.

tick-borne rickettsiosis, any disease transmitted by Ixodid ticks carrying the *Rickettsia* pathogens, microorganisms smaller than bacteria but larger than viruses. A common infectious species in North America is *Rickettsia rickettsii,* the cause of Rocky Mountain spotted fever.

tick fever. See **relapsing fever.**

tick paralysis, a rare, progressive, reversible disorder caused by several species of ticks that release a neurotoxin that causes weakness, incoordination, and paralysis. The tick must feed on the host for several days before the symptoms appear.

t.i.d., (in prescriptions) abbreviation for *ter in die* /dē′ā/, a Latin phrase meaning "three times a day."

tidal [AS *tid* time] pertaining to an alternating process, such as a rise-and-fall, ebb-and-flow, or periodic lapse of time.

tidal drainage. See **drainage.**

tidal volume (TV) [AS *tid* time; L *volumen* paper roll], the amount of air inhaled and exhaled during normal ventilation. Inspiratory reserve volume, expiratory reserve volume, and tidal volume make up vital capacity.

tide [AS *tid*], a variation, increase or decrease, in the concentration of a particular component of body fluids, such as acid tide, fat tide. **–tidal,** *adj.*

tidemark, a transitional zone, appearing as a wavy line, that marks the junction between calcified and uncalcified cartilage.

Tietze's syndrome /tēt′sēz/, **1.** a disorder characterized by nonsuppurative swellings of one or more costal cartilages causing pain that may radiate to the neck, shoulder, or arm and mimic the pain of coronary artery disease. **2.** albinism, except for normal eye pigment, accompanied by deaf mutism and hypoplasia of the eyebrows.

TIG, abbreviation for **tetanus immune globulin.**

tight junction [ME *thight* strong; L *jungere* to join], the zonula occludens of the junctional complex between cells in which the plasma membranes of adjacent cells are in direct contact and there is no intercellular space.

tilt table, an examining table that can be rocked back and forth, seesaw fashion, during study of the response of a patient's circulatory system to gravitational forces.

timbre /tim′bər/ [Fr], **1.** a characteristic sound quality of a voice or musical instrument, as determined by harmonics of the sound and distinguished from intensity and pitch. **2.** a second metallic sound heard in aortic dilation.

timed collection, the collection of a specimen, such as a urine or stool sample, for a specific period of time.

timed release. See **prolonged release.**

timed vital capacity, a diagnostic test of certain lung disorders, determined by the percentage of predicted vital capacity that can be expired forcefully for at least 3 seconds in adults after a maximal inspiration.

timolol maleate /tim′ətōl/, a beta-adrenergic receptor blocking agent. It is prescribed for reducing intraocular pressure in chronic open-angle, aphakic, and secondary glaucoma.

tin (Sn) [AS], a whitish metallic element. Its atomic number is 50; its atomic weight is 118.69. Tin oxide is used in dentistry as a polishing agent for teeth and in some restorative procedures.

tincture, tinct., a substance in a solution that is diluted with alcohol.

tine, a sharp, projecting point such as a prong of a fork.

tinea /tin′ē·ə/ [L, worm], a group of fungal skin diseases caused by dermatophytes of several kinds, characterized by itching, scaling, and, sometimes, painful lesions. Tinea is a general term that refers to infections of various causes, which are seen on several sites; the specific type is usually designated by a modifying term.

tinea capitis, a superficial fungal infection of the scalp, most common in children. Most infections are caused by species of *Trichophyton*. The infection may lead to hair loss and may become secondarily infected with bacteria, causing a severe inflammation. Symptoms include severe itching and scaling of the scalp. Treatment with topical fungicidal agents is usually sufficient.

tinea corporis, a superficial fungal infection of the nonhairy skin of the body, most prevalent in hot, humid climates and usually caused by species of *Trichophyton* or *Microsporum*.

tinea cruris /kroo′ris/, a superficial fungal infection of the groin, caused by species of *Trichophyton* or *Epidermophyton floccosum*. It is most common in the tropics and among males.

tinea pedis, a chronic superficial fungal infection of the foot, especially of the skin between the toes and on the soles. It is common worldwide and is usually caused by *Trichophyton mentagrophytes, T. rubrum,* and *Epidermophyton floccosum.*

tinea unguium /tin'ē·ə un'gwē·əm/, a superficial fungal infection of the nails caused by various species of *Trichophyton* and, occasionally, by *Candida albicans.* It is more common on the toes than on the fingers and can cause complete crumbling and destruction of the nails.

tinea versicolor, a fungal infection of the skin caused by *Malassezia furfur* and characterized by finely desquamating, pale tan patches on the upper trunk and upper arms that may itch and do not tan. The fungus fluoresces under Wood's light and may be easily identified in scrapings viewed under a microscope.

Tinel's sign /tinelz'/ [Jules Tinel, French neurosurgeon, b. 1879], an indication of irritability of a nerve, resulting in a distal tingling sensation on percussion of a damaged nerve.

tine test /tīn/ [ME *tind* rake tooth; L *testum* crucible], a tuberculin skin test in which a small disposable disk with multiple tines bearing tuberculin antigen is used to puncture the skin. Induration around the puncture site indicates previous exposure or active disease, requiring further testing.

tingling [ME *tinklen* to tinkle], a prickly sensation in the skin or a part of the body, accompanied by diminished sensitivity to stimulation of the sensory nerves, felt by a person as the area is numbed by local anesthetic or by exposure to the cold, or as it "goes to sleep" from pressure on a nerve.

tinnitus /tinī'təs/ [L *tinnire* to tinkle], tinkling or ringing heard in one or both ears. It may be a sign of acoustic trauma, Ménière's disease, otosclerosis, presbycusis or an accumulation of cerumen impinging on the eardrum or occluding the external auditory canal.

tinnitus aurium. See **tinnitus.**

tinted denture base, a denture base that simulates the coloring of natural oral tissue.

tipped uterus, a uterus that is displaced from its normal position.

tip pinch, a grasp in which the tip of the thumb is pressed against any or each of the tips of the other fingers.

tip seal, the closure of an ampule accomplished by melting a bead of glass at the neck of the ampule.

tissue [Fr *tissu* fabric], a collection of similar cells that act together in the performance of a particular function.

tissue activator. See **fibrinokinase.**

tissue-base relationship, (in dentistry) the relationship of the base of a removable prosthesis to subjacent structures.

tissue committee, a group that evaluates all surgery performed in a hospital or other health care facility.

tissue culture, the maintenance of growth in vitro, under artificial conditions, of tissue or organ specimens.

tissue dextrin. See **glycogen.**

tissue dose, (in radiotherapy) the amount of radiation absorbed by tissue in the region of interest, expressed in rad.

tissue fixation, a process in which a tissue specimen is placed in a fluid that preserves the cells as nearly as is possible in their natural state.

tissue fixative, a fluid that preserves cells in their natural state, so that they may be identified and examined.

tissue integrity, impaired, a NANDA-accepted nursing diagnosis of a state in which an individual experiences damage to mucous membrane, corneal, integumentary, or subcutaneous tissue. The principal characteristic is damaged or destroyed tissue. Related factors are altered circulation, nutritional deficit or excess, knowledge deficit, and impaired physical mobility.

tissue kinase. See **fibrinokinase.**

tissue macrophage [OFr *tissu;* Gk *makros* large, *phagein* to eat], a large, mobile, highly phagocytic cell derived from monocytes. These cells become mobile when stimulated by inflammation, migrating to the affected area.

tissue perfusion, altered (renal, cerebral, cardiopulmonary, gastrointestinal, peripheral), a NANDA-accepted nursing diagnosis of a state in which an individual experiences a decrease in nutrition and oxygenation at the cellular level caused by a deficit in capillary blood supply. Defining characteristics include coldness of the affected extremity, paleness on elevation of the extremity, diminished arterial pulses, and changes in the arterial blood pressure when measured in the affected extremity. Claudication, gangrene, brittle nails, slowly healing ulcers or wounds, shiny skin, and lack of hair are also commonly seen.

tissue plasminogen activator (TPA), a clot-dissolving substance produced naturally by cells in the walls of blood vessels. TPA activates plasminogen to dissolve clots and has been used therapeutically to remove blood clots blocking coronary arteries.

tissue response, any reaction or change in living cellular tissue when it is acted on by disease, toxin, or other external stimulus. Some kinds of tissue responses are **immune response, inflammation,** and **necrosis.**

tissue review, a review of the surgery performed in a hospital or other health care facility. The evaluation is usually made on the basis of the extent of agreement of the preoperative, postoperative, and pathologic diagnoses and on the relevance and acceptability of the diagnostic procedures.

tissue typing, a systematized series of tests to evaluate the intraspecies compatibility of tissues of a donor and a recipient before transplantation.

titanium (Ti) [Gk *Titan* mythic giant], a grayish, brittle metallic element. Its atomic number is 22; its atomic weight is 47.9. An alloy of titanium is used in the manufacture of orthopedic prostheses.

titer /tī′tər/ [Fr *titre* to make a standard], **1.** the normality of a solution or substance, determined by titration to find the equivalence of two reactants. **2.** the extent to which an antibody can be diluted before losing its power to react with a specific antigen. **3.** the highest dilution of a serum that causes clumping of bacteria.

titillation, tickling.

Title [L *titulus* inscription], a section of the Social Security Act that provides for the establishment, funding, and regulation of a service to a specific segment of the population, such as Title XIX, which includes medical coverage under Medicaid.

titubation /tich′əbā′shən/ [L *titubare* to stagger], unsteady posture characterized by a staggering or stumbling gait and a swaying head or trunk while sitting. It may be a manifestation of cerebellar disease.

Tl, symbol for the element **thallium.**

TLC, 1. abbreviation for **total lung capacity. 2.** *informal;* abbreviation for *tender loving care.*

TLI, abbreviation for **total lymphoid irradiation.**

TLR, abbreviation for **tonic labyrinthine reflex.**

T lymphocyte. See **lymphocyte, T cell.**

Tm, symbol for the element **thulium.**

TMJ, abbreviation for **temporomandibular joint.**

TMP/SMX, abbreviation for *trimethoprim sulfamethoxazole.*

TNF, abbreviation for **tumor necrosis factor.**

TNM, a system for staging malignant neoplastic disease.

t.n.t.c., abbreviation for *too numerous to count,* usually applied to organisms or cells viewed on a slide under a microscope.

t.o., abbreviation for *telephone order.*

toadstool poisoning [AS *tadige, stol;* L *potio* drink], a toxic condition caused by ingestion of certain varieties of poisonous mushrooms.

tobacco [Sp *tabaco*], a plant whose leaves are dried and used for smoking and chewing, and in snuff.

tobacco withdrawal syndrome, a change in mood or performance associated with the cessation or reduction in exposure to nicotine. Symptoms may range from lack of concentration to anxiety and temper outbursts.

TOBEC, abbreviation for **total body electrical conductivity.**

tobramycin sulfate /tō′brəmī′sin/, an aminoglycoside antibiotic prescribed in the treatment of external ocular infection, septicemia, and lower respiratory tract and central nervous system infections.

Tobruk plaster /tō′brŏŏk/, a plaster cast splint with tapes for skin traction coming through openings in the plaster and connected with Thomas' splint. It covers and immobilizes the leg from foot to groin.

tocainide hydrochloride /tōkā′nīd/, an oral lidocaine-type antiarrhythmic drug prescribed for the suppression of symptomatic ventricular dysrhythmias.

tocodynamometer /tō′kōdī′nəmom′ətər/ [Gk *tokos* birth, *dynamis* force, *metron* measure], an electronic device for monitoring and recording uterine contractions in labor. It consists of a pressure transducer that is applied to the fundus of the uterus by means of a belt, which is connected to a machine that records the contractions on graph paper.

tocolytic drug /tō′kōlit′ik/, any drug used to suppress premature labor.

tocopherol. See **vitamin E.**

tocotransducer /tō′kōtransdl(y)ōō′sər/ [Gk *tokos* + L *trans* through, *ducer* to lead], an electronic device used to measure uterine contractions.

toddler [ME *toteren* to walk unsteadily], a child between 12 and 36 months of age. During this period of development the child acquires a sense of autonomy and independence through the mastery of various specialized tasks, such as control of bodily functions, refinement of motor and language skills, and acquisition of socially acceptable behavior.

toddlerhood, the state or condition of being a toddler.

Todd's paralysis [Robert Bentley Todd, English physician, b. 1809], a transient postepileptic paralysis of an arm or leg.

toe, any one of the digits of the feet.

toe clonus, an increased reflex activity in the large toe caused by a sudden extension of the first phalanx.

toe drop, a condition in which the toes droop and cannot be lifted because of paralysis of the tibial muscles.

toeing in. See **metatarsus varus.**

toeing out. See **metatarsus valgus.**

toenail [AS *ta, naegel*], one of the heavy ungual structures covering the terminal phalanges of the toes.

togaviruses /tō'gəvī'rəsəs/ [L *toga* cloak, *virus* poison], a family of arboviruses that includes the organisms causing encephalitis, dengue, yellow fever, and rubella.

toilet training, the process of teaching a child to control the functions of the bladder and bowel. Training often begins around 24 months of age, when voluntary control of the anal and urethral sphincters is achieved by most children. Nighttime bladder control may not be achieved until the child is 4 or 5 years of age or older.

token economy [AS *tacen* to show; Gk *oikonomia* household management], a technique of reinforcement used in behavior therapy in the management of a group of people, such as in hospitals, institutions, or classrooms. Individuals are rewarded for specific activities or behavior with tokens they can exchange for desired objects or privileges.

tokodynamometer. See **tocodynamometer.**

tolazamide /tolaz'əmīd/, an oral sulfonylurea antidiabetic prescribed in the treatment of stable or non-insulin-dependent diabetes mellitus and for some patients sensitive to other types of sulfonylureas or who have failed to respond to other similar drugs.

tolazoline hydrochloride /tolaz'əlēn/, a peripheral vasodilator prescribed in the treatment of spastic peripheral vascular disorders, including Buerger's disease, Raynaud's disease, and scleroderma.

tolbutamide /tolbo͞o'təmīd/, an oral sulfonylurea antidiabetic prescribed in the treatment of stable non-insulin-dependent diabetes mellitus uncontrolled by diet alone and for some patients changing from insulin to oral therapy.

tolerance [L *tolerare* to endure], the ability to endure hardship, pain, or ordinarily injurious substances, such as drugs, without apparent physiologic or psychologic injury. A kind of tolerance is **work tolerance.**

tolerance dose. See **maximum permissible dose.**

tolmetin sodium /tol'mətin/, a nonsteroi-

dal antiinflammatory agent prescribed primarily in the treatment of rheumatoid arthritis, juvenile rheumatoid arthritis, and osteoarthritis.

tolnaftate /tolnaf'tāt/, an antifungal prescribed in the treatment of superficial fungus infections of the skin, including tinea pedis, tinea cruris, and tinea versicolor.

tomogram /tō'məgram'/ [Gk *tome* section, *gramma* record], a radiograph produced by tomography.

tomographic DSA, the visualization of blood vessels in the body in three dimensions.

tomography /təmog'rəfē/ [Gk *tome* a slice, *graphein* to record], an x-ray technique that produces a film representing a detailed cross section of tissue structure at a predetermined depth. It is a valuable diagnostic tool for the discovery and identification of space-occupying lesions, such as might be found in the brain, liver, pancreas, and gallbladder.

tone. See **tonus.**

tone deafness [Gk *tonos* stretching; AS *déaf*], an inability to detect the pitch or changing pitch of a musical note or a voice change.

tongue [AS *tunge*], the principal organ of the sense of taste that also assists in the mastication and the deglutition of food. It is located in the floor of the mouth within the curve of the mandible. Its root is connected to the hyoid bone posteriorly by the hypoglossi and the genioglossi muscles. The use of the tongue as an organ of speech is not anatomic but a secondary acquired characteristic.

tongue-thrust swallow, an immature form of swallowing in which the tongue is projected forward instead of retracted during the act of swallowing. It may result in forward displacement of the maxilla with consequent malocclusion of the teeth.

tongue-tie. See **ankyloglossia.**

tonic, pertaining to a type of afferent or sensory nerve receptor that responds to length changes placed on the noncontractile portion of a muscle spindle. It may be triggered by a mechanical external force such as positioning, or from an internal stretch caused by intrafusal muscle contraction.

tonic convulsion, a prolonged generalized contraction of the skeletal muscles.

tonicity /tōnis'itē/ [Gk *tonikos* stretching], the quality of possessing tone, or tonus.

tonic labyrinthine reflex [Gk *tonikos* + *labyrinthos* maze; L *reflectere* to bend backward], a normal postural reflex in animals, abnormally accentuated in decerebrate humans, characterized by extension of all four limbs when the head is positioned in space at an angle above the horizontal in quadrupeds or in the neutral, erect position in humans.

tonic neck reflex, a normal response in newborns to extend the arm and the leg on the side of the body to which the head is quickly turned while the infant is supine and to flex the limbs of the opposite side.

tonic spasm, a sustained contraction of a muscle as distinguished from a transient clonic contraction.

tonoclonic /ton′əklon′ik/ [Gk *tonos* + *klonos* tumult], pertaining to muscular spasms that are tonic and then clonic.

tonofibril /ton′əfī′bril/ [Gk *tonos* + *fibrilla* small fiber], a bundle of fine filaments found in the cytoplasm of epithelial cells. The individual strands, or **tonofilaments,** spread throughout the cytoplasm and extend into the intercellular bridge to converge at the desmosome. In keratinizing epithelium, the strands are the main precursor of keratin.

tonometer /tōnom′ətər/ [Gk *tonos* + *metron* measure], an instrument used in measuring tension or pressure, especially intraocular pressure.

tonometry /tōnom′ətrē/, the measuring of intraocular pressure by determining the resistance of the eyeball to indentation by an applied force. The air-puff tonometer, which does not touch the eye, records deflections of the cornea from a puff of pressurized air. The Schiötz impression and the applanation tonometers record the pressure needed to indent or flatten the corneal surface.

tonsil [L *tonsilla*], a small rounded mass of tissue, especially lymphoid tissue, such as that comprising the palatine tonsils in the oropharynx.

tonsillar [L, *tonsilla*], pertaining to the palatine tonsil.

tonsillar crypt [L *tonsilla;* Gk *kryptos* hidden], a small tubular invagination on the surface of a palatine or pharyngeal tonsil.

tonsillar herniation, the herniation of tonsils of the cerebellum through the foramen magnum of the skull. It may occur as a result of intracranial pressure from an injury or tumor.

tonsillectomy /ton′silek′təmē/ [L *tonsilla* + Gk *ektome* excision], the surgical excision of the palatine tonsils, performed to prevent recurrent streptococcal tonsillitis. Tonsillectomy is often combined with adenoidectomy.

tonsillitis /ton′silī′tis/, an infection or inflammation of a tonsil. Acute tonsillitis, frequently caused by streptococcus infection, is characterized by severe sore throat, fever, headache, malaise, difficulty in swallowing, earache, and enlarged, tender lymph nodes in the neck. Acute tonsillitis may accompany scarlet fever.

tonsilloadenoidectomy /ton′silō·ad′-ənoidek′təmē/ [L *tonsilla* + Gk *aden* gland, *eidos* form, *ektome* excision], the surgical removal of tonsil and adenoid tissues.

tonus /tō′nəs/ [Gk *tonos* tension], **1.** the normal state of balanced tension in the tissues of the body, especially the muscles. Partial contraction or alternate contraction and relaxation of neighboring fibers of a group of muscles hold the organ or the part of the body in a neutral, functional position without fatigue. **2.** the state of the tissues of the body being strong and fit.

tooth, *pl.* **teeth** [AS *toth*], one of numerous dental structures that develop in the jaws as part of the digestive system and are used to cut, grind, and process food in the mouth for ingestion. Each tooth consists of a crown, which projects above the gum; two to four roots, embedded in the alveolus; and a neck, which stretches between the crown and the root. Each tooth also contains a cavity filled with pulp, richly supplied with blood vessels and nerves that enter the cavity through a small aperture at the base of each root. The solid portion of the tooth consists of dentin, enamel, and a thin layer of bone on the surface of the root. The dentin comprises the bulk of the tooth. The enamel covers the exposed portion of the crown. Two sets of teeth appear at different periods of life: the 20 deciduous teeth appear during infancy, the 32 permanent teeth during childhood and early adulthood.

tooth abscess, a collection of pus, usually close to the root of a tooth and often the result of an untreated cavity. If untreated, the pressure of the abscess may destroy the alveolar bone and adjoining soft tissues.

toothache, a pain in a tooth, usually caused by caries that have extended into the dentin or pulp, or by traumatic occlusion.

tooth alignment, the arrangement of the teeth in relation to their supporting bone or alveolar process, adjacent teeth, and opposing dentitions.

tooth-borne, describing a dental prosthesis or part of a prosthesis that depends entirely on abutment teeth for support.

tooth-borne base, a denture base restoring an edentulous area that has abutment teeth at each end for support.

toothbrush, an implement with bristles fixed to a head at the end of a handle, used for brushing and cleaning the teeth and

T

gingivae and for massaging the gingival tissues.

tooth form, the identifying curves, lines, angles, and contours of a tooth that differentiate it from other teeth.

tooth fulcrum, axis of movement of a tooth subjected to lateral forces, considered to be at the middle third of the portion of the tooth root embedded in the alveolus.

tooth germ, a primitive cell in the embryo that is the precursor of a tooth.

tooth inclination, the angle of slope of a tooth or teeth from the vertical plane, such as mesially, distally, lingually, buccally, or labially inclined.

tooth rotation, 1. the malposition of a tooth that has turned around its longitudinal axis, or that has been turned by orthdontic appliance to a normal position. **2.** the process by which the tooth is turned.

tophaceous /tōfā'shəs/, pertaining to the presence of tophi.

tophaceous gout [L *tufa*], a form of purine metabolism disorder characterized by formation of chalky deposits of sodium biurate under the skin and in the joints. If untreated, the deposits may eventually destroy the involved joints.

tophus /tō'fəs/, *pl.* **tophi** [L *tufa* porous rock], a calculus, containing sodium urate deposits, that develops in periarticular fibrous tissue, typically in patients with gout.

topical [Gk *topos* place], **1.** of or pertaining to the surface of a part of the body. **2.** of or pertaining to a drug or treatment applied topically.

topical anesthesia, surface analgesia produced by application of a topical anesthetic in the form of a solution, gel, or ointment to the skin, mucous membrane, or cornea.

topognosis /top'ognō'sis/ [Gk *topos* + *gnosis* recognition], the ability to recognize tactile stimuli.

topographic, pertaining to a freudian conceptualization of the layers of human consciousness.

topographic anatomy, the study of a specific region of a body structure, such as a lower leg, including all of the systems in the part and their relationship to each other.

topographic disorientation, a form of disorientation based on Freud's topographic model of the mental apparatus, consisting of conscious, preconscious, and unconscious sytems for interpreting perceptions of the outside world and internal perceptions.

topography /təpog'rəfē/ [Gk *topos* place,

graphein to write], (in medicine) the anatomic description of a body part in terms of the region in which it is located.

TOPV, abbreviation for *trivalent oral polio vaccine.*

TORCH /tôrch/, an abbreviation for *toxoplasmosis, other, rubella virus, cytomegalovirus, and herpes simplex viruses,* a group of agents that can infect the fetus or the newborn infant causing a constellation of morbid effects called the TORCH syndrome.

TORCH syndrome, infection of the fetus or newborn by one of the TORCH agents. The outcome of a pregnancy complicated by a TORCH agent may be abortion or stillbirth, intrauterine growth retardation, or premature delivery. At delivery and during the first days after birth an infant infected with any one of the organisms may demonstrate various clinical manifestations, such as fever, lethargy, poor feeding, petechiae on the skin, purpura, pneumonia, hepatosplenomegaly, jaundice, hemolytic and other anemias, encephalitis, microcephaly, hydrocephalus, intracranial calcifications, hearing deficits, chorioretinitis, and microophthalmia.

Torkildsen's procedure. See ventriculocisternostomy.

torque /tôrk/ [L *torquere* to twist], **1.** a twisting force produced by contraction of the medial femoral muscles that tend to rotate the thigh medially. **2.** (in dentistry) a force applied to a tooth to rotate it on a mesiodistal or buccolingual axis. **3.** a rotary force applied to a denture base.

torr /tôr/ [Evangelista Torricelli, Italian physicist, b. 1608], a unit of pressure equal to 1,333.22 dynes/cm^2, or 1.33322 millibars. One torr is the pressure required to support a column of mercury 1 mm high when the mercury is of standard density and subjected to standard acceleration.

torsades de pointes /tôrsäd' depô·äN', tôr'säd dəpoint'/ [Fr *torsader* to twist together, *pointes* tips], a type of ventricular tachycardia with a spiral-like appearance ("twisting of the points") and complexes that at first look positive and then negative on an electrocardiogram. It is precipitated by a long QT interval, which often is drug induced but which may be the result of hypokalemia or profound bradycardia.

torsion [L *torquere* to twist], **1.** the process of twisting in a positive (clockwise) or negative (counterclockwise) direction. **2.** the state of being turned. **3.** (in dentistry) the twisting of a tooth on its long axis.

torsion dystonia. See dystonia musculorum deformans.

torsion fracture, a spiral fracture, usually caused by a torsion injury.

torsion of the testis, the axial rotation of the spermatic cord that cuts off the blood supply to the testicle, epididymis, and other structures. Complete ischemia for 6 hours may result in gangrene of the testis. Partial loss of circulation may result in atrophy.

torsion spasm. See **dystonia musculorum deformans.**

torso [L *thrysus* stem], the body without the limbs.

tort [L *tortus* twisted], (in law) a civil wrong, other than a breach of contract. The elements of a tort are: a legal duty owed by the defendant to the plaintiff, a breach of duty, and damage from the breach of duty. **–tortious,** *adj.*

torticollis /tôr′tikol′is/ [L *tortus* twisted, *collum* neck], an abnormal condition in which the head is inclined to one side as a result of the contraction of the muscles on that side of the neck. It may be congenital or acquired.

tortipelvis /tôr′tipel′vis/ [L *tortus* + *pelvis* basin], a form of muscular dystonia resulting in a distortion of the pelvis, or spine and hips.

tortuous, having or making twists and turns.

Torula histolytica. See *Cryptococcus neoformans.*

torulopsosis /tôr′yəlopsō′sis/ [L *torulus* small swelling; Gk *opsis* appearance, *osis* condition], an infection with the yeast *Torulopsis glabrata,* a normal inhabitant of the oropharynx, GI tract, and skin, that causes disease in severely debilitated patients or in those with impaired immune function.

torulosis. See **cryptococcosis.**

torus fracture. See **lead pipe fracture.**

torus palatinus /tôr′əs/ [L *torus* swelling, *palatum* palate], a bony ridge along the hard palate at the line of fusion of the left and right jawbone segments. It is a hereditary feature.

total anomalous venous return [L *totus* whole; Gk *anomalos* uneven; L *vena* vein; ME *retournen* to turn back], a rare congenital cardiac anomaly in which the pulmonary veins attach directly to the right atrium or to various veins draining into the right atrium rather than directing flow to the left atrium. Clinical manifestations include cyanosis, pulmonary congestion, and heart failure.

total body electrical conductivity (TOBEC), a method of measuring body composition by the differences in electrical conductivity of fat, bone, and muscle. It is used in clinical studies of weight control in which physicians want to determine if weight loss results from fat, water, or other tissues.

total body radiation, radiation that exposes the entire body so that, theoretically, all cells in the body receive the same radiation.

total body water (TBW), all the water within the body, including intracellular and extracellular water plus the water in the GI and urinary tracts.

total cleavage, mitotic division of the fertilized ovum into blastomeres.

total communication, the combined use of oral language and manual communication by a person with hearing loss.

total hip replacement, a surgical procedure to correct a hip joint damaged by degenerative disease, often arthritis. The head of the femur and the acetabulum are replaced with metal components. The acetabulum is plastic coated to avoid metal-to-metal articulating surfaces.

total iron, the total iron concentration in the blood. The normal concentrations in serum are 50 to 150 μg/dl.

total joint replacement, a surgical procedure for the treatment of severe arthritis and other disorders in which the normal articulating surfaces are replaced by metal and plastic prostheses. The operation most commonly involves replacement of the hip joint with a metallic femur head and a plastic-coated metal acetabulum.

total lung capacity (TLC), the volume of gas in the lungs at the end of a maximum inspiration. It equals the vital capacity plus the residual capacity.

total lymphoid irradiation (TLI), a method of inducing a strong immunosuppresive effect in patients undergoing bone marrow transplants, treatment of certain lymphomas, or other therapies requiring immunosuppression. TLI involves exposing all lymph nodes, the thymus, and spleen to a total of 2,000 rad in 100-rad doses from a linear accelerator.

total macroglobulins, the heavy serum macroglobulins that are elevated in various diseases, such as cancer, and infections.

total nitrogen, the nitrogen content of the feces, measured to detect various disorders, such as pancreatic insufficiency and impaired protein digestion. The normal amount in a 24-hour fecal specimen is 10% of intake, or 1 to 2 g.

total parenteral nutrition (TPN), the administration of a nutritionally adequate hypertonic solution consisting of glucose, protein hydrolysates, minerals, and vitamins through an indwelling catheter into the superior vena cava. The procedure is used in prolonged coma, severe uncontrolled malabsorption, extensive burns, GI fistulas, and other conditions in which feeding by mouth cannot provide adequate amounts of the essential nutrients.

total peripheral resistance, the maximum degree of resistance to blood flow caused by constriction of the systemic blood vessels.

total renal blood flow (TRBF), the total volume of blood that flows into the renal arteries. The average TRBF in a normal adult is 1,200 ml per minute.

touch [Fr *toucher* to touch], **1.** the ability to feel objects and to distinguish their various characteristics; the tactile sense. **2.** the ability to perceive pressure when it is exerted on the skin or the mucosa of the body. **3.** to palpate or examine with the hand, such as the digital examination of the abdomen, rectum, or vagina.

touch deprivation, a lack of tactile stimulation, especially in early infancy, which if continued for a sufficient length of time may lead to serious developmental and emotional disturbances, such as stunted growth, personality disorders, and social regression.

touch receptors [Fr *toucher*; L *recipere* to receive], specialized sensory nerve endings that are sensitive to tactile stimuli.

Tourette's syndrome. See **Gilles de la Tourette's syndrome.**

tourniquet /tur′nikit, tŏŏr′-/ [Fr, turnstile], a device used in controlling hemorrhage, consisting of a wide constricting band applied to the limb proximal to the site of bleeding. The use of a tourniquet is a drastic measure and is to be employed only if the hemorrhage is life threatening and if other safer measures have proved ineffective.

tourniquet infusion method, a technique of intraarterial regional chemotherapy used in the treatment of osteogenic sarcoma. The technique uses one or two external tourniquets, depending on the location of the tumor, that slow or interrupt the blood flow to a limb temporarily while an anticancer drug, such as adriamycin, is infused into the area.

tourniquet test, a test of capillary fragility, in which a blood pressure cuff is applied for 5 minutes to a person's arm and is inflated to a pressure halfway between the diastolic and systolic blood pressure. The number of petechiae within a circumscribed area of the skin may be counted.

tower head, tower skull. See **oxycephaly.**

toxemia /toksē′mē·ə/ [Gk *toxikon* poison, *haima* blood], the presence of bacterial toxins in the bloodstream. **–toxemic,** *adj.*

toxemia of pregnancy. See **preeclampsia.**

toxic [Gk *toxikon*], **1.** of or pertaining to a poison. **2.** (of a disease or condition) severe and progressive.

toxic albuminuria [Gk *toxikon*; L *albus* white; Gk *ouron* urine], a condition of serum albumin in the urine caused by toxic substances in the body.

toxic allergic syndrome. See **Löffler syndrome; PIE**

toxic amblyopia, partial loss of vision because of retrooptic bulbar neuritis, caused by poisoning with quinine, lead, wood alcohol, nicotine, arsenic, or certain other poisons.

toxic delirium, a symptom of disordered mental status as a result of poisoning.

toxic dementia, dementia resulting from excessive use of or exposure to a poisonous substance.

toxic dilatation of colon, a condition of transverse colon dilatation as a complication of amebic colitis, ulcerative colitis, or other bowel disease. Symptoms may include cramping, fever, rapid heart beat, and mental confusion.

toxic dose (TD), (in toxicology) the amount of a substance that may be expected to produce a toxic effect.

toxic encephalitis, encephalitis caused by heavy metal poisoning. It is characterized by convulsions and cerebral edema.

toxic epidermal necrolysis (TEN), a rare skin disease, characterized by epidermal erythema, superficial necrosis, and skin erosions. This condition makes the skin appear scalded, often leaving scars. TEN may result from toxic or hypersensitive reactions. It is commonly associated with drug reactions and has also been associated with airborne toxins, such as carbon monoxide. TEN may also indicate an immune response, or it may be associated with severe physiologic stress. Early signs of the condition include inflammation of the mucous membranes, fever, malaise, a burning sensation in the conjunctivae, and pervasive tenderness of the skin. The first phase of TEN is manifested by diffuse erythema. The second phase involves vesiculation and blistering. The third phase is marked by extensive epidermal necrolysis and desquamation. As the disease progresses, large flaccid bullae develop and rupture, exposing wide expanses of denuded skin. Tissue fluids and electrolytes are consequently lost, resulting in extensive systemic complications, such as pulmonary edema, bronchopneumonia, GI and esophageal hemorrhage, sepsis, shock, renal failure, and disseminated intravascular coagulation. These extreme conditions contribute to the high mortality associated with TEN.

toxic erythema, an inexact term sometimes applied to reddish skin eruptions of undetermined origin.

toxic erythema of the newborn. See **erythema neonatorum.**

toxic gastritis. See **corrosive gastritis.**

toxic goiter, an enlargement of the thyroid gland associated with exophthalmia and systemic disease.

toxic hemoglobinuria. See **hemoglobinuria.**

toxicity /toksis′itē/ [Gk *toxikon*], **1.** the degree to which something is poisonous. **2.** a condition that results from exposure to a toxin or to toxic amounts of a substance that does not cause adverse effects in smaller amounts.

toxic neuritis, a painful nerve inflammation caused by a metallic, bacterial, or other poison.

toxic nodular goiter, an enlarged thyroid gland characterized by numerous discrete nodules and hypersecretion of thyroid hormones. Typical signs of thyrotoxicosis, such as nervousness, tremor, weakness, fatigue, weight loss, and irritability, are usually present, but exophthalmia is rare; anorexia is more common than hyperphagia, and cardiac arrhythmia or congestive heart failure may be a predominant manifestation.

toxicokinetics /tok′sikō′kinet′iks/, the passage through the body system of a toxic agent or its metabolites, usually in an action similar to that of pharmacokinetics.

toxicologist, a specialist in toxicology.

toxicology /tok′sikol′əjē/, the scientific study of poisons, their detection, their effects, and methods of treatment for conditions they produce. **–toxicologic, toxicological,** *adj.*

toxic or drug-induced hepatitis, hepatitis resulting from a chemical, parasitic, or metabolic poison.

toxicosis /tok′sikō′sis/, a disease condition caused by the absorption of metabolic or bacterial poisons.

toxic psychosis, psychosis that results from the effects of chemicals or drugs, including those produced by the body itself.

toxic shock syndrome (TSS), a severe acute disease caused by infection with strains of *Staphylococcus aureus*, phage group I, that produces a unique toxin, enterotoxin F. It is most common in menstruating women using high-absorbency tampons but has been seen in newborn infants, children, and men. The onset of the syndrome is characterized by sudden high fever, headache, sore throat with swelling of the mucous membranes, diarrhea, nausea,

and erythroderma. Acute renal failure, abnormal liver function, confusion, and refractory hypotension usually follow, and death may occur.

toxic substance, any poison.

toxin, a poison, usually one produced by or occurring in a plant or microorganism.

toxin-antitoxin [Gk *toxikon* poison; *anti* against, *toxikon*], a mixture of toxin and antitoxin. Diphtheria toxin-antitoxin was formerly used for active immunization.

toxocariasis /tok′sōkərī′əsis/ [Gk *toxo* bow, *kara* head, *osis* condition], infection with the larvae of *Toxocara canis*, the common roundworm of dogs and cats. Ingestion of viable eggs, commonly found in soil, leads to the spread of tiny larvae throughout the body, resulting in respiratory symptoms, enlarged liver, skin rashes, eosinophilia, and delayed ocular lesions. Children who eat dirt are particularly subject to this disease.

toxoid /tok′soid/ [Gk *toxikon* poison, *eidos* form], a toxin that has been treated with chemicals or with heat to decrease its toxic effect but that retains its antigenic power. It is given to produce immunity by stimulating the creation of antibodies.

Toxoplasma /tok′sōplaz′mə/ [Gk *toxikon* + *plasma* something formed], a genus of protozoa with only one known species, *Toxoplasma gondii*, an intracellular parasite of cats and other hosts that causes toxoplasmosis in humans.

toxoplasmosis /tok′sōplazmō′sis/ [Gk *toxikon, plasma* + *osis* condition], a common infection with the protozoan intracellular parasite *Toxoplasma gondii*, characterized in the congenital form by liver and brain involvement with cerebral calcification, convulsions, blindness, microcephaly or hydrocephaly, and mental retardation. The acquired form is characterized by rash, lymphadenopathy, fever, malaise, central nervous system disorders, myocarditis, and pneumonitis.

TPA, abbreviation for **tissue plasminogen activator.**

TPAL. See **parity.**

TPN, abbreviation for **total parenteral nutrition.**

TPR, abbreviation for *temperature, pulse, respiration.*

trabecula carnea /trəbek′yələ/, *pl.* **trabeculae carneae** [L, little beam; *carneus* flesh], any one of the irregular bands and bundles of muscle that project from the inner surfaces of the ventricles, except in the arterial cone of the right ventricle.

trabeculae, (in ophthalmology) the portion of the eye in front of the canal of Schlemm and within the angle created by the iris and the cornea.

trabecula septomarginalis. See **moderator band.**

trabeculectomy /trəbek´yəlek´təmē/ [L *trabecula* + Gk *ektome* excision], the surgical removal of a section of corneoscleral tissue to increase the outflow of aqueous humor in patients with severe glaucoma.

trabeculoplasty, a plastic surgery procedure used in the treatment of glaucoma. An argon laser beam is used to blanch the trabecular network of the eye, thereby permitting drainage of excess fluid causing increased pressure within the eyeball.

trabeculotomy, a surgical opening in an orbital trabecula to increase the outflow of aqueous humor.

trace element [L *trahere* to draw; *elementum* first principle], an element essential to nutrition or physiologic processes, found in such minute quantities that analysis yields a presence of virtually zero amounts.

trace gas, a gas or vapor that escapes into the atmosphere during an anesthetic procedure.

tracer [L *trahere* to draw], **1.** a radioactive isotope that is used in diagnostic x-ray techniques to allow a biological process to be seen. Kinds of tracers include **radioactive iodine (^{131}I)** and **radioactive carbon (^{14}C). 2.** a device that graphically records the outline or movements of an object or part of the body. **3.** a dissecting instrument that is used to isolate vessels and nerves. –**trace,** *v.*

tracer depot method, (in nuclear medicine) a technique used to determine local skin or muscle blood flow, based on the rate at which a radioactive tracer deposited in a tissue is removed by diffusion into the capillaries and washed out by the local blood supply.

trachea /trā´kē-ə/ [Gk *tracheia* rough artery], a nearly cylindric tube in the neck, composed of cartilage and membrane, that extends from the larynx at the level of the sixth cervical vertebra to the fifth thoracic vertebra, where it divides into two bronchi. The trachea conveys air to the lungs. –**tracheal,** *adj.*

tracheal breath sound /trā´kē-əl/, a normal breath sound heard in auscultation of the trachea. Inspiration and expiration are equally loud, the expiratory sound being heard during the greater part of expiration, whereas the inspiratory sound stops abruptly at the height of inspiration.

tracheal tugging [Gk, *tracheia,* rough artery; ME, *toggen*], an effect of an aortic aneurysm in which the trachea is tugged downward with each heart contraction.

tracheitis /trā´kē-ī´tis/, any inflammatory condition of the trachea. It may be acute or chronic, resulting from infection, allergy, or physical irritation.

trachelodynia. See **cervicodynia.**

tracheobronchial tree (TBT) /trā´kē-ō-brong´kē-əl/ [Gk *tracheia* + *bronchos* windpipe], an anatomic complex that includes the trachea, the bronchi, and the bronchial tubes. It conveys air to and from the lungs.

tracheobronchitis /trā´kē-ōbrongkī´tis/, inflammation of the trachea and bronchi, a common form of respiratory infection.

tracheobronchomegaly /trā´kē-ōbrong´-kōmeg´əlē/, an abnormally large upper airway, in which the trachea may be as wide as the spinal column.

tracheoesophageal fistula /trā´kē-ō-ē´-sofā´jēəl/, [Gk *tracheia* + *oisophagos* gullet], a congenital malformation in which there is an abnormal tubelike passage between the trachea and the esophagus.

tracheoesophageal shunt, a surgical procedure enabling a laryngectomee to speak by constructing a passageway between the trachea and the esophagus. The operation results in an ability to produce esophageal speech with normal respiration as a source of air and without the need to belch to produce voice sounds.

tracheomalacia /trā´kē-ōmolā´shə/, an eroding of the trachea, usually caused by excessive pressure from a cuffed endotracheal tube.

tracheostomy /trā´kē-os´təmē/ [Gk *tracheia* + *stoma* mouth], an opening through the neck into the trachea through which an indwelling tube may be inserted. After tracheostomy the patient's chest is auscultated for breath sounds indicative of pulmonary congestion, mucous membranes and fingertips are observed for cyanosis, and humidified oxygen is given via tent or directly into the tracheostomy tube. The patient is reassured that the tube is open and that air can pass through it. The tube is suctioned frequently to keep it free from tracheobronchial secretions using a suction catheter attached to a Y-connector. The patient is taught to cough to move secretions up and out of the bronchi. Pen and paper or a magic slate is kept available for communication because the patient cannot speak. If the procedure was done as an emergency, the tracheostomy is closed once normal breathing is restored. If the tracheostomy is permanent, such as with a laryngectomy, the patient is taught self-care.

tracheostomy care, care of the tracheostomy patient requires maintenance of a patent airway, adequate humidification, aseptic wound care, and sterile tracheal aspiration. Complications can include injury to the vocal cords, gastric distention and regurgitation, occlusion of the endotracheal tube, and an increased risk of infection.

tracheotomy /trā'kē·ot'əmē/ [Gk *tracheia* + *temnein* to cut], an incision made into the trachea through the neck below the larynx, performed to gain access to the airway below a blockage with a foreign body, tumor, or edema of the glottis. The opening may be made as an emergency measure at an accident site or at a hospitalized patient's bedside or in the operating room.

tracheotomy tube, a curved hollow tube of rubber, metal, or plastic, surgically inserted in the trachea to relieve a breathing obstruction.

trachoma /trəkō'mə/ [Gk, roughness], a chronic infectious disease of the eye caused by the bacterium *Chlamydia trachomatis,* characterized initially by inflammation, pain, photophobia, and lacrimation. If untreated, follicles form on the upper eyelids and grow larger until the granulations invade the cornea, eventually causing blindness.

tracing [L *trahere* to draw], a graphic record of a physical event, such as an electrocardiograph tracing made by pens on a moving sheet of paper while recording the electric impulses of heart muscle contractions.

tract [L *tractus* trail], **1.** an elongated group of tissues and structures that function together as a pathway, such as the digestive tract or the respiratory tract. **2.** (in neurology) the neuronal axons that are grouped together to form a pathway.

traction [L *trahere* to draw], **1.** (in orthopedics) the process of putting a limb, bone, or group of muscles under tension by means of weights and pulleys to align or to immobilize the part or to relieve pressure on it. **2.** the process of pulling a part of the body along, through, or out of its socket or cavity, such as axis traction with obstetric forceps in delivering an infant. Kinds of traction include **Bryant's traction, Buck's traction, Russell traction, skeletal traction, skin traction,** and **split Russell traction.**

traction frame, an orthopedic apparatus that supports the pulleys, the ropes, and the weights by which traction is applied to various parts of the body or by which various parts of the body are suspended. The main components of a traction frame are metal uprights that attach to the bed and support an overhead metal bar.

traction, 90-90, an orthopedic mechanism, used especially in pediatrics, that combines skeletal traction and suspension with a short-leg cast or a splint to immobilize and position the lower extremity in the treatment of a displaced fractured femur.

traction response, the response to traction applied to the spine. Alterations of certain signs and symptoms of a musculoskeletal disorder may be revealed by traction tests.

trademark, a word, symbol, or device assigned to a product by its manufacturer and registered as a part of its identity.

tragus /trā'gəs/, *pl.* **tragi** /trā'jī/ [Gk *tragos* goat], a small extension of the auricular cartilage of ear, anterior to the external meatus. **–tragal** /trā'gəl/, *adj.*

trainable [L *trahere* to draw], a term applied to a mentally retarded person who is capable of some degree of self-care and social adjustment in a supervised setting but would not benefit from formal education.

trained reflex. See **conditioned response.**

traineeship [L *trahere* to draw; AS *scieppan* to shape], a grant of money allocated to an individual for study in a given field.

training effect, a rehabilitation influence for heart patients that can be measured by changes in cardiac function.

training grant, a grant of money or other resources to provide training in a particular field.

trait [Fr, trace], **1.** a characteristic mode of behavior or any mannerism or physical feature that distinguishes one individual or culture from another. **2.** any characteristic quality or condition that is genetically determined and inherited as a specific genotype.

trance [L *transire* to be transformed], **1.** a sleeplike state characterized by the complete or partial suspension of consciousness and loss or diminution of motor activity. **2.** a dazed or bewildered condition; stupor. **3.** a state of detachment from one's immediate surroundings. Kinds of trances are **alcoholic trance, death trance, hypnotic trance, hysteric trance,** and **induced trance.**

tranquilizer [L *tranquillus* calm], a drug prescribed to calm anxious or agitated people, ideally without decreasing their consciousness. Major tranquilizers are generally used in the treatment of psychoses. Minor tranquilizers are usually prescribed for the treatment of anxiety, irritability, tension, or psychoneurosis. Tranquilizers tend to induce drowsiness and have the potential for causing physical and psychologic dependence.

T

transabdominal /trans'abdom'inəl/ [L *trans* across, *abdomen* belly], pertaining to a procedure through the abdominal wall.

transactional analysis (TA) [L *transigere* to drive through; Gk *analyein* to loosen], a form of psychotherapy based on a theory that three different, coherent, organized egos exist throughout life simultaneously in every person, representing the child, the adult, and the parent. Interactions between people are transactions, originating from a person in one of the ego states, received by another person who may be in a complementary or a crossed ego state.

transaminase /transam'inās/ [L *trans* through, *amine* ammonia; Fr *diastase* enzyme], an enzyme that catalyzes the transfer of an amino group from an alpha-amino acid to an alpha-keto acid, with pyridoxal phosphate and pyridoxamine phosphate acting as coenzymes.

transaortic /trans'ā·ôr'tik/ [L *trans* + Gk *aerein* to raise], pertaining to a procedure through the aorta.

transcellular water /trans'sel'yələr/ [L *trans* + *cella* storeroom], the portion of extracellular water that is enclosed by an epithelial membrane and whose volume and composition is determined by the cellular activity of that membrane.

transcendence [L *trans* + *scandere* to climb], the rising above one's previously perceived limits or restrictions.

transcervical fracture /transur'vikəl/ [L *trans* + *cervix* neck, *fractura*], a fracture through the neck of the femur.

transcondylar fracture /transkon'dilər/ [L *trans* + Gk *kondylos* condyle], a fracture that occurs transversally and distal to the epicondyles of any one of the long bones.

transconfiguration obL *trans* + *configuare* to form from], **1.** (in genetics) the presence of the dominant allele of one pair of genes and the recessive allele of another pair on the same chromosome. **2.** the presence of at least one mutant gene and one wild-type gene of a pair of pseudoalleles on each chromosome of a homologous pair.

transcortical apraxia. See **ideomotor apraxia.**

transcortin /trans'kôr'tin/, a diglobulin protein that binds a majority of cortisol in the plasma.

transcriptase /transkrip'tās/, an enzyme that induces transcription.

transcription [L *trans* + *scribere* to write], (in molecular genetics) the process by which RNA is formed from a DNA template in the process of manufacturing a protein.

transcultural nursing [L *trans* + *colere* to cultivate; *nutrix* nourishment], a field of nursing in which the nurse transcends ethnocentricity and practices nursing in other cultural environments.

transcutaneous /trans'k(y)ōōtā'nē·əs/ [L *trans* + *cutis* skin], pertaining to a procedure that is performed through the skin.

transcutaneous electric nerve stimulation (TENS), a method of pain control by the application of electric impulses to the nerve endings through electrodes placed on the skin. The electric impulses generated are similar to those of the body, but different enough to block transmission of pain signals to the brain.

transcutaneous oxygen/carbon dioxide monitoring, a method of measuring the oxygen or carbon dioxide in the blood by attaching electrodes to the skin. Oxygen is commonly measured through an oximeter, which contains heating coils to raise the skin temperature and increase blood flow at the surface. Transcutaneous carbon dioxide electrodes are similar to blood gas electrodes.

transdermal delivery system [L *trans* + Gk *derma* skin], a method of applying a drug to unbroken skin. The drug is absorbed continuously through the skin and enters the systemic system.

transducer [L *trans* + *ducer* to lead], a hand-held device that sends and receives a soundwave signal.

transduction, (in molecular genetics) a method of genetic recombination by which DNA is transferred from one cell to another by a viral vector.

transect [L *trans* + *secare* to cut], to sever or cut across, as in preparing a cross-section of tissue.

transfection [L *trans* + *inficere* to taint], (in molecular genetics) the process by which a cell is infected with DNA or RNA isolated from a virus or a viral vector.

transfer agreement [L *transferre* to carry over; *ad* toward, *gratus* pleasure], a written hospital agreement between two health care institutions for the transfer of patients from one to another and for the orderly exchange of pertinent clinical information on the patients transferred.

transferase /trans'fərās/ [L *transferre* + Fr *diastase* enzyme], any of a group of enzymes that catalyzes the transfer of a chemical group or radical, such as the phosphate, methyl, amine, or keto groups, from one molecule to another.

transfer DNA (tDNA), (in molecular genetics) DNA transferred from its original source and present in transformed cells.

transference [L *transferre*], **1.** the shifting of symptoms from one part of the body to another, such as occurs in conversion disorder. **2.** (in psychiatry) an unconscious defense mechanism whereby feelings and attitudes originally associated with important people and events in one's early life are attributed to others in current interpersonal situations. **3.** (in psychoanalysis and psychotherapy) the feelings of a patient for the analyst to whom the patient has attributed or assigned the qualities, attitudes, and feelings of a person or persons significant in his or her emotional development, usually a figure from childhood.

transfer factor, a leukocyte extract that transfers delayed hypersensitivity from one person to another.

transfer factor of lungs. See **diffusing capacity.**

transferrin /transfer′in/, a trace protein present in the blood that is essential in the transport of iron.

transferring [L *trans* + *ferre* to bring], relocating a person in need from one location to another.

transfer RNA (tRNA), (in molecular genetics) a kind of RNA that transfers the genetic code from messenger RNA for the production of a specific amino acid. There are at least 20 different kinds of tRNA, each of which is able to combine covalently with a specific amino acid.

transformation [L *transformare* to change shape], (in molecular genetics) the process in which exogenous genes are integrated into chromosomes in a form that is recognized by the replicative and transcriptional apparatus of the host cell.

transformer, an electrical apparatus that changes alternating current of one voltage into a different voltage of the same frequency.

transforming growth factor (TGF), a group of proteins produced by the cells of a tumor that, when inoculated into a normal cell culture, causes a disorderly and abnormal increase in the number of cells in the culture.

transfusion /trans′fyo͞o′zhən/ [L *trans* + *fundere* to pour], the introduction into the bloodstream of whole blood or blood components, such as plasma, platelets, or packed red cells. Whole blood may be infused into the recipient directly from a donor matched for the ABO blood group and antigenic subgroups, but more frequently the donor's blood is collected and stored by a blood bank.

transfusion reaction, a systemic response by the body to the administration of blood incompatible with that of the recipient. The causes include red cell incompatibility, allergic sensitivity to the leukocytes, the platelets, or the plasma protein components of the transfused blood or to

the potassium or citrate preservative in the banked blood. Fever is the most common transfusion reaction; urticaria is a relatively common allergic response. Asthma, vascular collapse, and renal failure occur less commonly. A hemolytic reaction from red cell incompatibility is serious and must be diagnosed and treated promptly. Symptoms develop shortly after beginning the transfusion, before 50 ml have been given, and include a throbbing headache, sudden, deep, and severe lumbar pain, precordial pain, dyspnea, and restlessness. Objective signs include ruddy facial flushing followed by cyanosis and distended neck veins, rapid, thready pulse, diaphoresis, and cold, clammy skin. Profound shock may occur within 1 hour.

transient /tran′shənt, tran′zē·ənt/ [L *transire* to go through], pertaining to a condition that is temporary, such as transient ischemic attack.

transient global amnesia (TGA), a temporary, short-term memory loss followed by full recovery. The disorder tends to affect middle-aged adults and may be attributed to cerebral ischemia. It is usually not accompanied by other mental deficiences.

transient ischemic attack (TIA), an episode of cerebrovascular insufficiency, usually associated with a partial occlusion of an artery by an atherosclerotic plaque or an embolism. Disturbance of normal vision in one or both eyes, dizziness, weakness, dysphasia, numbness, or unconsciousness may occur. The attack is usually brief, lasting a few minutes; rarely, symptoms continue for several hours.

transient myopia, a temporary change in visual accommodation secondary to trauma, high blood sugar level, sulfanilamide therapy, and other conditions.

transillumination /trans′ilo͞o′minā′shən/ [L *trans* through, *illuminare* to light up] **1.** the passage of light through a solid or liquid substance. **2.** the passage of light through body tissues for the purpose of examining a structure interposed between the observer and the light source.

transition [L *transire* to go through], the last phase of the first stage of labor, sometimes indicated by cervical dilation of 8 to 10 cm.

transitional, between a previous and a succeeding state, or in a state of becoming something else.

transitional cell carcinoma, a malignant, usually papillary tumor derived from transitional stratified epithelium, occurring most frequently in the bladder, ureter, urethra, or renal pelvis. The majority of tumors in the collecting system of the kidney are of this kind.

transitional dentition. See **mixed dentition.**

transitional object, an object used by a child to provide comfort and security while he or she is away from a secure base, such as mother or home.

transitional zone, a part of the crystalline lens of the eye where epithelial-capsule cells change into lens fibers.

transitory mania [L *transire* to go through; Gk *mania* madness], a mood disorder characterized by the sudden onset of manic reactions that are of short duration, usually lasting from 1 hour to a few days.

translation [L *translatio* handing over], (in molecular genetics) the process in which the genetic information carried by nucleotides in messenger RNA directs the amino acid sequence in the synthesis of a specific polypeptide.

translocation /trans′lōkā′shən/ [L *trans* + *locus* place], (in genetics) the rearrangement of genetic material within the same chromosome or the transfer of a segment of one chromosome to another nonhomologous one. Kinds of translocations are **balanced, reciprocal,** and **robertsonian.**

translucent [L *trans* + *lucens* shining], pertaining to a medium through which light can pass in a diffused manner so that a field is illuminated but objects cannot be seen distinctly.

transmigration [L *transmigrare* to migrate], a movement from one side to another, from inside to outside, or from outside to inside.

transmission [L *transmittere* to transmit], the transfer or conveyance of a thing or condition, such as a neural impulse, infectious or genetic disease, or a hereditary trait, from one person or place to another. –**transmissible,** *adj.*

transmission electron microscopy. See **electron microscopy.**

transmission scanning electron microscope, an instrument that transmits a highly magnified, well-resolved, three-dimensional image on a television screen, thus combining the advantages of the electron and the scanning electron microscopes.

transmission scanning electron microscopy (TSEM), a technique using a transmission scanning electron microscope in which the atomic number of the portion of the sample being scanned is determined and used to modulate a beam of electrons in a cathode-ray tube and in the beam scanning the sample.

transmitted light, light that has been transmitted through a transparent medium.

transmitter substance. See **neurotransmitter.**

transmural /trans′m(y)ŏŏ′rəl/ [L *trans* + *murus* wall], pertaining to the entire thickness of the wall of an organ, such as a transmural myocardial infarction.

transmural infarction, the death of myocardial tissue that extends from the endocardium to the epicardium as a result of a myocardial infarction.

transmutation /trans′m(y)ŏŏtā′shən/ [L *transmutare* to change], **1.** a mutation, as when a significant species change occurs during evolution. **2.** the conversion of one chemical element into another by radioactive bombardment.

transovarial transmission /trans′ōver′ē·əl/ [L *trans* + *ovum* egg], the transfer of pathogens to succeeding generations through invasion of the ovary and infection of the egg.

transparent [L *trans* + *parere* to appear], pertaining to a clear medium that allows for the transmission of light so that objects on the other side are distinguishable.

transplacental /trans′pləsen′təl/ [L *trans* + *placenta* cake], across or through the placenta, specifically in reference to the exchange of nutrients, waste products, and other material between the developing fetus and the mother.

transplant [L *transplantare*], **1.** to transfer an organ or tissue from one person to another or from one body part to another to replace a diseased structure, to restore function, or to change appearance. Skin and kidneys are the most frequently transplanted structures; others include cartilage, bone, corneal tissue, portions of blood vessels and tendons, and, recently but infrequently, hearts and livers. Preferred donors are identical twins or persons having the same blood type and immunologic characteristics. **2.** any tissue or organ that is transplanted. **3.** of or pertaining to a tissue or organ that is transplanted or to a recipient of a donated tissue or organ or to a phenomenon associated with the procedure.

transplantation, the transfer of tissue from one site to another or from one person or organism to another.

transplantation endometriosis, endometrial tissue that is accidentally transplanted to the incision wound during pelvic surgery.

transport [L *trans* + *portare* carry], the movement or transference of biochemical substances from one site to another. Active transport involves an expenditure of energy whereas passive transport allows movement down a gradient without an energy expenditure.

transposable element [L *transponere* to transpose; *elementum* first principle], (in molecular genetics) a DNA fragment or segment that can move or be moved from one site in the genome to another.

transposase /trans′pəzās/, (in molecular genetics) an enzyme involved in the movement of a DNA fragment or segment from one site in the genome to another.

transposition [L *transponere*], **1.** an abnormality occurring during embryonic development in which a part of the body normally on the left is found on the right or vice versa. **2.** the shifting of genetic material from one chromosome to another at some point in the reproductive process. –**transpose,** *v.*

transposition of the great vessels, a congenital cardiac anomaly in which the pulmonary artery arises from the left ventricle and the aorta from the right ventricle so that there is no communication between the systemic and pulmonary circulations. Life is impossible without associated cardiac defects, such as septal defects or a patent ductus arteriosus, that enable the mixing of oxygenated and unoxygenated blood.

transposon /transpō′son/ [L *transponere* + on], a gene or a group of genes that are mobile and, like plasmids, act to transfer genetic instructions from one place to another. Transposons travel piggyback from virus to virus on bacteriophages.

transpulmonary pressure /trans′pul′-mənər′ē/, the difference between alveolar and intrapleural pressure, or the pressure acting across the lung from the intrapleural space to the alveoli.

transsection /transek′shən/, a cross-section of a biological specimen or a cut across the long axis.

transseptal fiber /transep′təl/ [L *trans* + *saeptum* wall], (in dentistry) any one of the many fibers of the gingival fiber system that extends horizontally from the supraalveolar cementum of a tooth, through the interdental attached gingiva above the septum of the alveolar bone, to the cementum of an adjacent tooth.

transsexual /transek′cho͞o·əl/, a person whose gender identity is opposite his or her biologic sex.

transsexualism, a condition in which a person has an intense desire to discard his or her biological sex and live as a member of the opposite sex. It is considered a psychiatric disorder if the condition continues for more than 2 years. Some transsexual individuals cross-dress and seek medical or surgical help to change their physical sex characteristics.

transtentorial herniation /trans′ten-tôr′ē·əl/ [L *trans* + *tentorium* tent; *hernia* rupture], a bulge of brain tissue out of

the cranium through the tentorial notch, caused by increased intracranial pressure.

transthermia. See **thermopenetration.**

transthoracic pacemaker /trans′thôras′ik/ [L *trans* + Gk *thorax* chest; L *passus* step; ME *maken*], a permanent heart pacemaker with the pulse generator located in the abdominal wall and the pacing wires attached directly to the epicardium.

transtracheal oxygen [L *trans* + Gk *tracheia,*rough artery, *oxys* sharp, *genein* to produce], a method of administering oxygen to a patient requiring oxygen therapy by establishing a low-flow catheter route directly into the trachea. It is a sometimes preferred alternative to the administration of oxygen through a nasal canula.

transtrochanteric osteotomy /trans′trō′-kənter′ik/ [L *trans* + Gk *trochanter* runner], a surgical division of the upper end of the femur through the area of the trochanters.

transudate /trans′yədāt/ [L *trans* + *sudare* to sweat], a fluid passed through a membrane or squeezed through a tissue or into the space between the cells of a tissue.

transudation /trans′yədā′shən/, **1.** the passage of a substance through a membrane as a result of a difference in hydrostatic pressure. **2.** the passage of a fluid through a membrane with nearly all the solutes of the fluid remaining in solution or suspension.

transudative ascites /transy o͞o ′dətiv/, an abnormal accumulation in the peritoneal cavity of a fluid that characteristically contains scant amounts of protein and cells.

transurethral resection (TUR) /trans′y o͞o rē′thrəl/ [L *trans* + Gk *ourethra* urethra; L *re* again, *secare* to cut], a surgical procedure through the urethra, such as in transurethral prostatectomy.

transverse [L *transversus* oblique], at right angles to the long axis of any common part, such as the planes that cut the long axis of the body into upper and lower portions and are at right angles to the sagittal and frontal planes.

transverse colon, the segment of the colon that extends from the end of the ascending colon at the hepatic flexure on the right side across the midabdomen to the beginning of the descending colon at the splenic flexure on the left side.

transverse fissure, a fissure dividing the dorsal surface of the diencephalon and the ventral surface of the cerebral hemisphere.

transverse foramen, an opening through the transverse process of a cervical vertebra.

transverse fracture, a fracture that occurs at right angles to the longitudinal axis of the bone involved.

transverse lie, abnormal presentation of a fetus in which the long axis of the baby's body is across the long axis of the mother's body.

transverse ligament of the atlas, a thick, strong ligament stretched across the ring of the atlas, holding the dens against the anterior arch.

transverse mesocolon /mez′ōkō′lən/, a broad fold of the peritoneum connecting the transverse colon to the dorsal wall of the abdomen.

transverse myelitis, an acute attack of spinal cord inflammation involving both sides of the cord.

transverse palatine suture, the line of junction between the processes of the maxilla and the horizontal portions of the palatine bones that form the hard palate.

transverse plane, any one of the planes cutting across the body perpendicular to the sagittal and the frontal planes, dividing the body into caudal and cranial portions.

transverse presentation, a presentation of the fetal body in an oblique or transverse position across the birth canal.

transverse relaxation time. See **relaxation time.**

transverse sinus, one of a pair of large venous channels in the posterior superior group of sinuses serving the dura mater.

transversus abdominis /trans′vur′səs/, one of a pair of transverse abdominal muscles that are the anterolateral muscles of the abdomen, lying immediately under the obliquus internus abdominis. It serves to constrict the abdomen and by, compressing the contents, to assist in micturition, defecation, emesis, parturition, and forced expiration.

transvestism, a tendency to achieve psychic and sexual relief by dressing in the clothing of the opposite sex.

tranylcypromine sulfate /tran′əlsip′-rəmēn/, a monoamine oxidase inhibitor that acts as an antidepressant. It is prescribed in the treatment of severe reactive or endogenous mental depression.

trapezium /trəpē′zē·əm/, *pl.* **trapeziums, trapezia** [Gk *trapezion* small table], a carpal bone in the distal row of carpal bones. The trapezium articulates with the scaphoid proximally, the first metacarpal distally, and the trapezoideum and the second metacarpal medially.

trapezius /trəpē′zē·əs/ [Gk *trapezion* small table], a large, flat triangular muscle of the shoulder and upper back. It acts to rotate the scapula, raise the shoulder, and abduct and flex the arm.

trapezoid /trap′əzoid/, describing something in the shape of a trapeze, an irregular four-sided figure with one set of parallel sides.

trapezoidal arch [Gk *trapezion* + *eidos* form; L *arcus* bow], a dental arch that has slightly less convergence than that of a tapering arch.

trapezoid bone [Gk *trapezion, eidos* + AS *ban*], the smallest carpal bone, located in the distal row of carpal bones between the trapezium and the capitate.

trauma /trou′mə, trô′mə/ [Gk, wound], **1.** physical injury caused by violent or disruptive action, or by the introduction into the body of a toxic substance. **2.** psychic injury resulting from a severe emotional shock. **–traumatic,** *adj.,* **traumatize,** *v.*

trauma center, a service providing emergency and specialized intensive care to critically ill and injured patients.

trauma, high risk for, a NANDA-accepted nursing diagnosis of the accentuated risk of accidental tissue injury, such as a wound, burn, or fracture. The risk factors may be internal (individual) or external (environmental). Internal risk factors include weakness; poor vision; balancing difficulties; reduced temperature or tactile sensation; reduced muscle or eye-hand coordination; lack of safety education, precautions, or equipment; cognitive or emotional difficulties; and history of previous trauma. External risk factors include slippery floors, stairs, or walkways; a bathtub without antislip equipment; unsteady chairs or ladders; defective electric wires or appliances; obstructed passageway; potential igniting gas leaks; unscreened fires or heaters; inadequately stored combustibles or corrosives; contact with intense cold or heat (as very hot water); overexposure to sun, sunlamps, or radiotherapy; and exposure to dangerous machinery.

trauma registry, a repository of data on the incidence, diagnosis, and treatment of acute trauma victims treated by emergency service personnel.

Trauma Score, a system combining cardiopulmonary assessment with the Glasgow Coma Scale in estimating the degree of injury and the prognosis in a patient who has suffered a head injury. Cardiopulmonary factors include respiratory rate and chest expansion, systolic blood pressure, and capillary refill. The neurologic factors are eye opening, verbal response, and motor response.

traumatic anesthesia [Gk *trauma* + *anaisthesia* loss of feeling], a total lack of normal sensation in a part of the body, resulting from injury, destruction of nerves, or interruption of nerve pathways.

traumatic delirium, delirium after severe head injury, characterized by alertness and consciousness with disorientation, confabulation, and amnesia apparent.

traumatic dislocation, a dislocation caused by an injury.

traumatic epilepsy, a form of epilepsy caused by an injury.

traumatic fever, an elevation in body temperature secondary to mechanic trauma, particularly a crushing injury. The increased body temperature may help provide resistance to subsequent infection, and increased wound temperature may accelerate local healing.

traumatic gangrene, gangrene that follows a severe injury resulting in damage to blood vessels.

traumatic herpes, herpes that develops at the site of an injury.

traumatic meningitis, meningitis that develops as a result of injury to the skull or spinal column.

traumatic myelitis, a spinal cord inflammation resulting from an injury.

traumatic myositis, inflammation of the muscles resulting from a wound or other trauma.

traumatic neuritis, neuritis that is caused by injury to a nerve.

traumatic neuroma, a tangled mass of nerve elements and fibrous tissue produced by the proliferation of Schwann cells and fibroblasts after severe injury to a nerve. A kind of traumatic neuroma is **amputation neuroma.**

traumatic occlusion, a closure of the teeth that injures the teeth, the periodontal tissues, the residual ridge, or other oral structures.

traumatic psychosis, a form of psychosis that results from injury to the head, with symptoms usually indicating brain trauma. It is differentiated from psychic trauma in which personality damage can be traced to an unpleasant experience such as sexual assault.

traumatic shock, the emotional or psychologic state following trauma that may produce abnormal behavior. The most common types are hypovolemic shock from blood loss and neurogenic shock from a disruption of the integrity of the spinal cord.

traumatic thrombosis, intravascular coagulation of a vein or other blood vessel after injury or irritation. The condition may develop as an adverse effect of an intravenous injection that damages the wall of a vein.

traumatology /trô′mətol′əjē/ [Gk *trauma* + *logos* science], **1.** the study of wounds and injuries. **2.** a surgical specialty dealing with the treatment of wounds, injuries, and resulting disabilities. **–traumatologic, traumatological,** *adj.*

traumatopathy /trô′mətop′əthē/ [Gk *trauma* + *pathos* disease], a pathologic condition resulting from a wound or injury. **–traumatopathic,** *adj.*

traumatophilia /trô′mətōfil′ē·ə/ [Gk *trauma* + *philein* to love], a psychologic state in which the individual derives unconscious pleasure from injuries and surgical operations. **–traumatophiliac,** *n.,* **traumatophilic,** *adj.*

traumatopnea /trô′mətop′nē·ə/ [Gk *trauma* + *pnein* to breathe], partial asphyxia with collapse of the patient, caused by a penetrating thoracic wound permitting air to enter the pleural space and compress the lungs.

traumatopyra /trô′mətōpī′rə/ [Gk *trauma* + *pyr* fire], an elevated temperature resulting from a wound or injury.

traumatotherapy [Gk *trauma* + *therapeia* treatment], the medical, surgical, and psychologic treatment of wounds, injuries, and disabilities resulting from trauma. **–traumatotherapeutic,** *adj.*

traumatropism /trômat′rəpiz′əm/ [Gk *trauma* + *trepein* to turn], the tendency of damaged tissue to attract microorganisms and to promote their growth, frequently causing infections after injuries, especially burns.

travail /trəvāl′/ [Fr *travailler* to toil], **1.** physical or mental exertion, especially when distressful. **2.** (in obstetrics) the effort of labor and childbirth.

traveler's diarrhea [Fr *travailler* to toil; Gk *dia* through, *rhein* to flow], any of several diarrheal disorders commonly seen in people visiting regions of the world other than their own. Some strains of *Escherichia coli,* which produce a powerful exotoxin, are the common cause. Other causative organisms include *Giardia lamblia* and species of *Salmonella* and *Shigella.* Symptoms include abdominal cramps, nausea, vomiting, slight fever, and watery stools.

TRBF, abbreviation for **total renal blood flow.**

Treacher Collins' syndrome, an inherited disorder, characterized by mandibulofacial dysostosis.

treatment [Fr *traitement*], **1.** the care and management of a patient to combat, ameliorate, or prevent a disease, disorder, or injury. **2.** a method of combating, ameliorating, or preventing a disease, disorder, or injury. Active or curative treatment is designed to cure; palliative treatment is directed to relieve pain and distress; prophylactic treatment is for the prevention of a disease or disorder; causal treatment focuses on the cause of a disorder. Treatment may be pharmacologic, using drugs; surgical, involving operative procedures; or supportive, building the patient's strength.

treatment guardian, a person who is appointed by the court for the purpose of consenting to or refusing medical treatment for a patient.

treatment plan, a schedule of dental procedures and appointments designed to restore, step by step, the oral health of a patient. The plan contains the advantages, disadvantages, costs, alternatives, and sequelae of treatment. It must be presented to the patient for approval.

treatment room, a room in a patient care unit, usually in a hospital, in which various treatments or procedures requiring special equipment are performed, such as removing sutures.

Trechona /trikon'ə/, a genus of spiders, family Dipluridae, the bite of which is toxic and irritating to humans.

tree [AS *treow*], **1.** (in anatomy) an anatomic structure with branches that spread out like those of a tree, such as the bronchial tree. **2.** a pattern of searching for information in a computer data base, following a series of branching options from a general category.

trematode /trem'ətōd/ [Gk *trematodes* pierced], any species of flatworm of the class Trematoda, some of which are parasitic to humans, infecting the liver, the lungs, and the intestines. Kinds of trematodes include the organisms causing **clonorchiasis, fascioliasis, paragonimiasis,** and **schistosomiasis.**

tremor [L, shaking], rhythmic, purposeless, quivering movements resulting from the involuntary alternating contraction and relaxation of opposing groups of skeletal muscles, occurring in some elderly individuals, in certain families, and in patients with various neurodegenerative disorders. Kinds of tremors are **continuous tremor** and **intention tremor.**

tremulous [L *tremulare* to tremble], pertaining to tremors, or involuntary muscular contractions.

tremulous pulse, a feeble, fluttering pulse.

trench fever [OFr *trenchier* to carve; L *febris* fever], a self-limited infection, caused by *Rochalimaea quintana,* a rickettsial organism transmitted by body lice, characterized by weakness, fever, rash, and leg pains.

trench foot, a condition of moist gangrene of the foot caused by the freezing of wet skin.

trench mouth. See **acute necrotizing gingivitis.**

Trendelenburg gait /trendel'ənbərg, tren'd(e)lənburg'/ [Friederich Trendelenburg, German surgeon, b. 1844], an abnormal gait associated with a weakness of the gluteus medius. The Trendelenburg gait is characterized by the dropping of the pelvis on the unaffected side of the body at the moment of heelstrike on the affected side.

Trendelenburg's operation, the ligation of varicose veins whose valves are ineffective, performed to remove weakened portions of veins and pockets in which thrombi might lodge. The saphenous vein is ligated at the groin, where it joins the femoral vein. A wire device, called a stripper, is threaded through the lumen of the vein from groin to ankle; the wire and the vein are then pulled from the groin incision.

Trendelenburg's position, a position in which the head is low and the body and legs are on an inclined plane. It is sometimes used in pelvic surgery to displace the abdominal organs upward, out of the pelvis, or to increase the flow of blood to the brain in hypotension and shock.

Trendelenburg's test, a simple test for incompetent valves in a person who has varicose veins. The person lies down and elevates the leg to empty the vein, then stands, and the vein is observed as it fills. If the valves are incompetent, the vein fills from above; if the valves are normal, they do not allow backflow of blood, and the vein fills from below.

trephine /trifīn', trifēn'/ [Gk *trypan* to bore], a circular, sawlike instrument used in removing pieces of bone or tissue, usually from the skull.

trepidation [L *trepidare* to tremble], a state of anxiety.

Treponema /trep'ənē'mə/ [Gk *trepein* to turn, *nema* thread], a genus of spirochetes, including some pathogenic to humans, such as the organisms causing bejel, pinta, syphilis, and yaws.

Treponema pallidum, an actively motile, slender spirochetal organism that causes syphilis.

treponematosis /trep'ənē'mətō'sis/, *pl.* **treponematoses** [Gk *trepein, nema + osis* condition], any disease caused by spirochetes of the genus *Treponema.* All these infections are effectively treated with penicillin. Kinds of treponematoses are **bejel, pinta, syphilis,** and **yaws.**

tretinoin /tret'inō'in/, a keratolytic prescribed in the topical treatment of acne vulgaris.

TRF, abbreviation for *thyrotropin-releasing factor.*

TRH, abbreviation for **thyrotropin-releasing hormone.**

triacetin /trī·as'itin/, an antifungal prescribed in the treatment of superficial fungus infections of the skin, including athlete's foot.

triacetyloleandomycin. See **troleandomycin.**

triad [Gk *trias* three], a combination of three, such as two parents and a child.

triage /trē·äzh'/ [Fr *trier* to sort out], **1.** (in military medicine) a classification of casualties of war and other disasters according to the gravity of injuries, urgency of treatment, and place for treatment. **2.** a process in which a group of patients is sorted according to their need for care. **3.** (in disaster medicine) a process in which a large group of patients is sorted so that care can be concentrated on those who are likely to survive.

trial forceps [Fr *trier* to sort out], an obstetric operation consisting of an attempt to deliver an infant with obstetric forceps. The forceps are applied to the baby's head, and moderate traction is applied. The delivery is continued only if the trial indicates that delivery can be accomplished safely.

trial of labor, child delivery in which there is doubt as to whether the head of the fetus will pass through the pelvic brim and the situation must be monitored and assessed carefully to avoid fetal or maternal distress.

triamcinolone /trī'amsin'əlōn/, a glucocorticoid prescribed as an antiinflammatory agent in the treatment of dermatoses, stomatitis, and lichen planus lesions.

triamterene /trī·am'tərēn/, a potassium-sparing diuretic usually prescribed alone or with another diuretic in the treatment of edema, hypertension, and congestive heart failure.

triangle [L *triangulus* three-cornered], a predictable emotional process that takes place when there is difficulty in a relationship. The triangle can be composed of three people or two people and an object or group or issue.

triangular bandage, a square of cloth folded or cut into the shape of a triangle. It may be used as a sling, a cover, or a thick pad to control bleeding.

triangular bone, the pyramidal carpal bone in the proximal row on the ulnar side of the wrist.

triangular dullness. See **Koranyi's sign.**

triazolam /trī·az'əlam/, a benzodiazepine hypnotic agent prescribed in the short-term treatment of insomnia.

tribe [L *tribus*], a taxonomic division of organisms, subordinate to a family and superior to a genus, or subtribe.

tribology /tribol'əjē/ [Gk *tribo* to rub, *logos* science], the study of friction, wear, and lubrication of articulating surfaces.

TRIC /trik/, abbreviation for *trachoma inclusion conjunctivitis* agent, which refers to *Chlamydia trachomatis,* the organism that causes both inclusion conjunctivitis and trachoma.

tricarboxylic acid cycle. See **citric acid cycle, Krebs cycle.**

triceps brachii /trī'seps brak'ē·ī/ [L, three-headed; *brachium* arm], a large muscle that extends the entire length of the dorsal surface of the humerus. It functions to extend the forearm and to adduct the arm.

triceps reflex, a deep tendon reflex elicited by tapping sharply the triceps tendon proximal to the elbow with the forearm in a relaxed position.

triceps skinfold, the thickness of a fold of skin around the triceps muscle. It is measured primarily to estimate the amount of subcutaneous fat.

triceps surae limp, an abnormal action in the walking or gait cycle, associated with a deficiency in the elevating and the propulsive factors on the affected side of the body, especially a deficiency of the triceps surae. Such a deficiency prevents the triceps surae from raising the pelvis and carrying it forward during the walking cycle.

trichiasis /trikī'əsis/ [Gk *thrix* hair, *osis* condition], an abnormal inversion of the eyelashes that irritates the eyeball. It usually follows infection or inflammation.

trichinosis /trik'inō'sis/ [Gk *thrix* + *osis* condition], infestation with the parasitic roundworm *Trichinella spiralis,* transmitted by eating raw or undercooked pork or bear meat. Early symptoms of infection include abdominal pain, nausea, fever, and diarrhea; later, muscle pain, tenderness, fatigue, and eosinophilia are observed. Light infections may be asymptomatic.

trichlormethiazide /trī'klôrməthī'əzīd/, a thiazide diuretic and antihypertensive prescribed in the treatment of hypertension and edema.

trichloroethylene /trīklôr'ō·eth'ilēn/, a general anesthetic, administered by mask with N_2O, for dentistry, minor surgery, and the first stages of labor.

trichobasalioma hyalinicum. See **cylindroma.**

trichoepithelioma /trik'ō·ep'ithē'lē·ō'mə/,

pl. **trichoepitheliomas, trichoepitheliomata** [Gk *thrix + epi* above, *thele* nipple, *oma* tumor], a cutaneous tumor derived from the basal cells of the follicles of fine body hair.

trichoid /trik'oid/, resembling a hair.

trichologia /trik'əlō'jē·ə/ [Gk *thrix + legein* to pull], an abnormal condition in which a person pulls out his or her own hair, usually seen only in delirium.

trichomatous /trikom'ətəs/ [Gk *trichoma* hairy growth], **1.** pertaining to an introversion of the margin of the eyelid. **2.** pertaining to matted hair or ingrowing hair.

trichomonacide /trik'ōmon'əsīd/ [Gk *thrix + monas* unit; L *caedere* to kill], an agent destructive to *Trichomonas vaginalis*, a parasitic protozoan flagellate that causes a refractory type of vaginitis, cystitis, and urethritis. **–trichomonacidal**, *adj.*

Trichomonas vaginalis /trik'əmon'əs/ [Gk *thrix, monas* + L *vagina* sheath], a motile protozoan parasite that causes vaginitis with a copious malodorous discharge and pruritus.

trichomoniasis /trik'əmənī'əsis/ [Gk *thrix, monas + osis* condition], a vaginal infection caused by the protozoan *Trichomonas vaginalis*, characterized by itching, burning, and frothy, pale yellow to green, malodorous vaginal discharge. In men, infection is usually asymptomatic but may be evidenced by a persistent or recurrent urethritis.

tricopathy /trikop'əthē/ [Gk *thrix* hair, *pathos* disease], any disease condition involving the hair.

trichophytic   **granuloma.** See **Majocchi's granuloma.**

Trichophyton /trikof'iton/ [Gk *thrix + phyton* plant], a genus of fungi that infects skin, hair, and nails.

trichosis /trikō'sis/ [Gk *thrix + osis* condition], any abnormal condition of hair growth, including alopecia, excessive female hair growth, or abnormal hair color.

trichosporosis [Gk *thrix + spora* seed, *osis* condition], a fungus disease of the hair shaft, giving the hair a metallic appearance, and caused by *Trichosporon*.

trichostrongyliasis /trik'ōstron'jəlī'əsis/ [Gk *thrix + strongylos* round, *osis* condition], infestation with *Trichostrongylus*, a genus of nematode worm.

Trichostrongylus /trik'ōstron'jiləs/ [Gk *thrix + strongylos*], a genus of roundworm, some species of which are parasitic to humans, such as *Trichostrongylus orientalis*.

trichotillomania /trik'ōtil'ōmā'nē·ə/ [Gk *thrix + tillein* to pull, *mania* madness], a morbid impulse or desire to pull out one's hair, frequently seen in cases of severe mental retardation and delirium. **–trichotillomanic, trichomanic,** *adj.*

trichuriasis /trik'yŏŏrī'əsis/ [Gk *thrix + oura* tail, *osis* condition], infestation with the roundworm *Trichuris trichiura*. The condition is usually asymptomatic, but heavy infestation may cause nausea, abdominal pain, diarrhea, and, occasionally, anemia and rectal prolapse.

Trichuris /trikyŏŏr'is/ [Gk *thrix + oura*], a genus of parasitic roundworms of which the species *Trichuris trichiura* infects the intestinal tract.

trick knee. See **locked knee.**

tricrotic pulse /trīkrot'ik/, an abnormal pulse that has three peaks of elevation on a sphygmogram, representing the pressure wave from the heart in systole followed by two pressure waves in diastole.

tricuspal. See **tricuspid tooth.**

tricuspid /trīkus'pid/ [Gk *tri* three; L *cuspis* point] **1.** of or pertaining to three points or cusps. **2.** of or pertaining to the tricuspid valve of the heart.

tricuspid area, a region of the chest, near the left lower sternum and opposite the fourth and fifth costal cartilages, where sounds of the tricuspid heart valve are best heard by auscultation.

tricuspid atresia, a congenital cardiac anomaly characterized by the absence of the tricuspid valve so that there is no opening between the right atrium and right ventricle. Clinical manifestations include severe cyanosis, dyspnea, anoxia, and signs of right-sided heart failure. Definitive diagnosis is made by cardiac catheterization.

tricuspid murmur, one of the heart murmurs caused by a defective tricuspid valve. The tricuspid diastolic and systolic murmurs resemble mitral valve diastolic and systolic murmurs.

tricuspid stenosis, narrowing or stricture of the tricuspid value. It is relatively uncommon and usually associated with lesions of other values caused by rheumatic fever. Clinical characteristics include diastolic pressure gradient between the right atrium and ventricle, jugular vein distention, pulmonary congestion, and in severe cases, hepatic congestion and splenomegaly.

tricuspid tooth, a tooth with three cusps, rare in humans.

tricuspid valve, a valve with three main cusps situated between the right atrium and the right ventricle of the heart. As the right and the left ventricles relax during the diastole phase of the heartbeat, the tricuspid valve opens, allowing blood to flow into the ventricle. In the systole phase of the heartbeat both blood-filled ventricles contract, pumping out their contents, while the tricuspid and mitral valves close to prevent any backflow.

tricyclic antidepressant. See **antidepressant.**

tricyclic compound /trīsik′lik/ [Gk *tri* + *kyklos* circle; L *componere* to put together], a chemical substance containing three rings in the molecular structure, especially a tricyclic antidepressant drug used in the treatment of reactive or endogenous depression.

trident, a tooth with three points or cusps.

tridihexethyl chloride /trī′dīhek′səthil/, an anticholinergic prescribed in the treatment of GI muscle spasm and to reduce gastric secretion and GI motility.

trientine hydrochloride /trī·en′tēn/, an oral medication prescribed for the relief of symptoms of Wilson's disease, an inherited defect in copper metabolism.

triethanolamine polypeptide oleatecondensate /trī·eth′anol′əmēn/, a ceruminolytic agent prescribed to reduce excessive earwax, used as a solution in propylene glycol.

trifacial nerve. See **trigeminal nerve.**

trifluoperazine hydrochloride /trī′flōō·ōper′əzēn/, a phenothiazine tranquilizer prescribed in the treatment of anxiety, schizophrenia and other psychotic disorders, and as an antiemetic.

trifluorothymidine /trī′floōr′ōthī′mədēn/, an antiviral prescribed in the treatment of keratoconjunctivitis, herpetic keratitis, and other forms of keratitis caused by herpes simplex virus.

trifluopromazine hydrochloride /trī′fluprō′məzēn/, a phenothiazine tranquilizer prescribed in the treatment of severe agitation and other psychotic disorders and for the control of severe vomiting.

trifluridine. See **trifluorothymidine.**

trifocal lens, an eyeglass lens ground for viewing objects at three different distances—near, intermediate, and far.

trifurcation /trī′furkā′shən/, pertaining to a vessel or other structure with three branches.

trigeminal nerve /trījem′inəl/ [Gk *tri* + geminus twin], either of the largest pair of cranial nerves, essential for the act of chewing, general sensibility of the face, and muscular sensibility of the obliquus superior.

trigeminal neuralgia, a neurologic condition of the trigeminal facial nerve, characterized by paroxysms of flashing, stablike pain radiating along the course of a branch of the nerve from the angle of the jaw. It is caused by degeneration of the nerve or by pressure on it. Any of the three branches of the nerve may be affected.

Neuralgia of the first branch results in pain around the eyes and over the forehead; of the second branch, in pain in the upper lip, nose, and cheek; of the third branch, in pain on the side of the tongue and the lower lip. The momentary bursts of pain recur in clusters lasting many seconds; paroxysmal episodes of the pains may last for hours.

trigeminal pulse, an abnormal pulse in which every third beat is absent.

trigeminy /trījem′inē/ [Gk *tri* + L *geminus* twin] **1.** a grouping in threes. **2.** a cardiac arrhythmia characterized by the occurrence of three heartbeats, a normal beat followed by two ectopic beats in rapid succession. **–trigeminal,** *adj.*

trigger [D *trekker* that which pulls], a substance, object, or agent that initiates or stimulates an action.

triggered activity [D *trekker* that which pulls; L *activus*], rhythmic cardiac activity that results when a series of afterdepolarizations reach threshold potential.

trigger point, a point on the body that is particularly sensitive to touch and, when stimulated, becomes the site of a painful neuralgia.

triglyceride /trīglis′ərīd/, a compound consisting of a fatty acid (oleic, palmitic, or stearic) and glycerol. Triglycerides make up most animal and vegetable fats and are the principal lipids in the blood where they circulate, bound to a protein, forming high- and low-density lipoproteins.

trigone /trī′gōn/ [Gk *trigonos* three-cornered, **1.** a triangle. **2.** the first three dominant cusps, considered collectively, of an upper molar.

trigone of the bladder. See **trigonum vesicae.**

trigonitis /trī′gənī′tis/, inflammation of the trigone of the bladder, which often accompanies urethritis.

trigonum vesicae /trīsō′nəm/, a triangular area of the bladder between the opening of the ureters and the orifice of the urethra.

trihexyphenidyl hydrochloride /trīhex-′ifen′idil/, an anticholinergic agent prescribed in the treatment of Parkinson's disease and to control drug-induced extrapyramidal reactions.

trihybrid /trīhī′brid/ [Gk *tri* + *hybrida* mixed offspring], (in genetics) pertaining to or describing an individual, organism, or strain that is heterozygous for three specific traits, that is the offspring of parents differing in three specific gene pairs.

trihybrid cross, (in genetics) the mating of two individuals, organisms, or strains that have different gene pairs that determine three specific traits or in which three particular characteristics or gene loci are being followed.

trihydric alcohol /trīhīd′rik/, an alcohol containing three hydroxyl groups.

triiodothyronine (T₃) /trī′ī·ō′dōthī′rənēn/, a hormone that helps regulate growth and development, helps control metabolism and body temperature, and, by a negative feedback system, acts to inhibit the secretion of thyrotropin by the pituitary.

trilaminar blastoderm /trīlam′inər/ [Gk *tri* + L *lamina* plate; Gk *blastos* germ, *derma* skin], the stage of embryonic development in which all three of the primary germ layers, the ectoderm, mesoderm, and entoderm, have formed.

trill [It *trillare* to make a ringing sound], a vibratory, quavering, warbling sound, as produced by human voice, birds, insects, or musical instruments.

trilogy of Fallot /falō′/ [Gk *tri* + *logos* word; Etienne-Louis A. Fallot, French physician, b. 1850], a congenital cardiac anomaly consisting of the combination of pulmonic stenosis, interatrial septal defect, and right ventricular hypertrophy.

trilostane /tril′əstān/, a synthetic steroid that inhibits the synthesis of adrenal steroids. It is prescribed for the treatment of Cushing's syndrome.

trimalleolar fracture. See **Cotton's fracture.**

trimeprazine tartrate /trīmep′rəzēn/, an antipruritic prescribed in the treatment of pruritis and hypersensitivity reactions of the skin.

trimester /trīmes′tər, trī′-/ [L *trimestris* three months], one of the three periods of approximately 3 months into which pregnancy is divided. The first trimester includes the time from the first day of the last menstrual period to the end of 12 weeks. The second trimester extends from the twelfth to the twenty-eighth week of gestation. The third trimester begins at the twenty-eighth week and extends to the time of delivery.

trimethadione /trī′methədī′ōn/, an anticonvulsant prescribed to prevent seizures in petit mal epilepsy, particularly seizures that are resistant to other therapies.

trimethaphan camsylate /trīmeth′əfan/, a ganglionic blocking agent prescribed to produce controlled hypotension during surgery and to lower blood pressure in hypertensive emergencies.

trimethobenzamide hydrochloride /trī-meth′ōben′zəmīd/, an antiemetic prescribed for the relief of nausea and vomiting.

trimethoprim /trīmeth′əprim/, an antibacterial prescribed in the treatment of various infections, particularly of the urinary tract, middle ear, and bronchi.

trimethoprim and sulfamethoxazole. See **sulfamethoxazole and trimethoprim.**

trimethylene. See **cyclopropane.**

trimipramine maleate /trimip′rəmēn/, an antidepressant prescribed in the treatment of anxiety, depression, and insomnia.

trioxsalen /trī·ok′sələn/, a melanizing agent prescribed to enhance pigmentation, for repigmentation of the skin in idiopathic vitiligo, and to increase tolerance to sunlight.

tripelennamine citrate. See **tripelennamine hydrochloride.**

tripelennamine hydrochloride /trī′pel′-en′əmēn/, an antihistamine prescribed in the treatment of rhinitis and hypersensitivity reactions of the skin.

triphasic /trī-fā′zik/ [Gk *treis* three, *phasis* appearance], pertaining to something with three phases or stages.

triple-dye treatment, a therapy for burns in which three dyes, 6% gentian violet, 1% brilliant green, and 0.1% acriflavin base, are applied.

triplegia /trīplē′jə/ [Gk *treis* + *plege* stroke], a condition of paralysis on one side of the body plus paralysis of an arm or leg on the opposite side.

triple lumen catheter [Gk *triploos* triple; L *lumen* light; Gk *katheter* a thing lowered into], any catheter with three separate passages. In a triple-lumen urinary catheter one passage is for irrigation, one for drainage, and one for air.

triple point, a situation in which a given substance may exist in solid, liquid, and vapor forms at the same time. Every substance has a theoretical triple point, which depends on ideal conditions of temperature and pressure.

triple response, a triad of phenomena that occur in sequence after the intradermal injection of histamine. First, a red spot develops, spreading outward for a few millimeters, reaching its maximal size within 1 minute and then turning bluish. Next, a brighter red flush of color spreads slowly in an irregular flare around the original red spot. Finally, a wheal, filled with fluid, forms over the original spot.

triple sugar iron reaction, any one of several reactions seen in certain bacterial cultures growing on triple sugar iron agar, a culture medium used to aid in the identification of *Escherichia coli, Proteus, Salmonella, Shigella,* and other pathogenic enteric bacteria.

triple sulfonamides. See **trisulfapyrimidines.**

triplet [Gk *triploos*], **1.** any one of

three offspring born of the same gestation period during a single pregnancy. **2.** (in genetics) the unit of three consecutive bases in one polynucleotide chain of DNA or RNA that codes for a specific amino acid.

triple X syndrome. See **XXX syndrome.**

triploid (3n) /trip′loid/ [Gk *triploos* + *eidos*], **1.** of or pertaining to an individual, organism, strain, or cell that has three complete sets of chromosomes. In humans, the triploid number is 69, found in rare cases of aborted or stillborn fetuses. **2.** such an individual, organism, strain, or cell.

triploidy /trip′loidē/, the state or condition of having three complete sets of chromosomes.

tripod, any object with three legs or three feet.

tripodial symmelia /trīpō′de·əl/ [Gk *tri* three, *pous* foot; *syn* together, *melos* limb], a fetal anomaly characterized by the fusion of the lower extremities and the presence of three feet.

triprolidine hydrochloride /trī·prol′idēn/, an antihistamine prescribed in the treatment of a variety of hypersensitivity reactions, including rhinitis, skin rash, and pruritus.

tripsis /trip′sis/ [Gk, rubbing], **1.** massage. **2.** the process of reducing the particle size of a substance by grinding it with a mortar and pestle.

trisaccharide /trīsak′ərīd/ [Gk *treis* + *sakcharon* sugar], a carbohydrate composed of three monosaccharide units linked together.

trismus /triz′məs/ [Gk *trimos* gnashing], a prolonged tonic spasm of the muscles of the jaw.

trisomy /trī′səmē/ [Gk *tri* + *soma* body], a chromosomal aberration characterized by the presence of one more than the normal number of chromosomes in a diploid complement; in humans the trisomic cell contains 47 chromosomes and is designated $2n + 1$. **–trisomic,** *adj.*

trisomy C syndrome. See **trisomy 8.**
trisomy D syndrome. See **trisomy 13.**
trisomy E syndrome. See **trisomy 18.**
trisomy G syndrome. See **Down syndrome.**

trisomy 8, a congenital condition associated with the presence of an extra chromosome 8 within the C group. Those with the condition are slender and of normal height and have a large asymmetric head, prominent forehead, deep-set eyes, low-set prominent ears, and thick lips. There is mild to severe mental and motor retardation, often with delayed and poorly articulated speech. Skeletal anomalies and joint

limitation, especially camptodactyly, may occur, and there are unusually deep palmar and plantar creases, which are diagnostically significant. Most trisomy 8 individuals are mosaic.

trisomy 13, a congenital condition caused by the presence of an extra chromosome in the D group, predominantly chromosome 13, although in rare instances chromosome 14 or 15. It is characterized by multiple midline anomalies and central nervous system defects, including holoprosencephaly, microcephaly, myelomeningocele, microphthalmos, and cleft lip and palate. There are also severe mental retardation, polydactyly, deafness, convulsions, and abnormalities of the heart, viscera, and genitalia.

trisomy 18, a congenital condition caused by the presence of an extra chromosome 18, characterized by severe mental retardation and multiple deformities. Among the most common defects are scaphocephaly or other skull abnormalities, micrognathia, abnormal facies with low-set malformed ears and prominent occiput, cleft lip and palate, clenched fists with overlapping fingers, especially the index over the third finger, clubfeet, and syndactyly. Ventricular septal defect, patent ductus arteriosus, atrial septal defect, and renal anomalies are also common.

trisomy 21. See **Down syndrome.**

trisomy 22, a congenital condition caused by the presence of an extra chromosome 22 in the G group, characterized by psychomotor retardation and various developmental anomalies. Common defects include microcephaly, micrognathia, hypotonia, hypertelorism, abnormal ears with preauricular tags or fistulas, and congenital heart disease. In partial trisomy 22, the extra chromosome is much smaller than the normal pair and causes coloboma of the iris or anal atresia, or both, as well as various other defects.

trisomy syndrome, any condition caused by the addition of an extra member to a normal pair of homologous autosomes or to the sex chromosomes or by the translocation of a portion of one chromosome to another. Most trisomies occur as a result of complete or partial nondisjunction of the chromosomes during cell division.

tritium (3H) [Gk *tritos* third], a low-level radioactive isotope of the hydrogen atom, used as a tracer.

trivalence /trīvā′ləns/ [Gk *treis* + L *valere* to be worth], a triple state, usually a designation of three electrons in the outer orbit of an atom or an ability of a group of atoms to replace three monovalent elements in a compound.

T

trivalent, 1. pertaining to an atom or group of atoms with the capability of bonding with or replacing three monovalent elements. **2.** designating a vaccine that can prevent diseases or conditions.

tRNA, abbreviation for **transfer RNA.**

trocar /trō′kär/ [Fr *trois* three, *carres* sides], a sharp, pointed rod that fits inside a tube. It is used to pierce the skin and the wall of a cavity or canal in the body to aspirate fluids, to instill a medication or solution, or to guide the placement of a soft catheter.

trochanter /trōkan′tər/ [Gk, runner], one of the two bony projections on the proximal end of the femur that serve as the point of attachment of various muscles.

trochanter major, a large projection from the proximal end of the shaft of the femur. It is a point of attachment for the gluteus minimus and gluteus medius muscles.

trochanter minor, a bony prominence on the shaft of the femur, just below the neck. It is the site of insertion of the psoas major muscle.

troche /trō′kē/ [Gk *trochos* lozenge], a small oval, round, or oblong tablet containing a medicinal agent incorporated in a flavored, sweetened mucilage or fruit base that dissolves in the mouth, releasing the drug.

trochlea /trok′lē·ə/, a pulley-shaped part or structure. **–trochlear,** *adj.*

trochlear nerve /trok′lē·ər/ [L *trochlea* pulley; *nervus* nerve], either of the smallest pair of cranial nerves, essential for eye movement and eye muscle sensibility.

trochlear notch of ulna, a large depression in the ulna, formed by the olecranon and coronoid processes, that articulates with the trochlea of the humerus.

trochoid joint. See **pivot joint.**

trolamine /trol′əmēn/, a contraction for *triethanolamine.*

troleandomycin /trol′ē·an′dōmī′sin/, a macrolide antibiotic prescribed in the treatment of certain infections, including pneumococcal pneumonia and group A streptococcal infections of the upper respiratory tract.

trombiculosis /trombik′yəlō′sis/ [Gk *tromein* to tremble; *osis* condition], an infestation with mites of the genus *Trombicula,* some species of which carry scrub typhus.

trophectoderm. See **trophoblast.**

trophic /trof′ik/ [Gk *trophe* nutrition], pertaining to a nutritive effect on or quality of cellular activity.

trophic action [Gk *trophe* nutrition; L *agere* to do], the stimulation of cell reproduction and enlargement, by nurturing and causing growth.

trophic fracture, a fracture resulting from the weakening of bone tissue caused by nutritional disturbances.

trophic hormones, hormones secreted by the adenohypophysis that stimulate target organs.

trophic ulcer, a decubitus ulcer caused by external trauma to a part of the body that is in poor condition resulting from disease, vascular insufficiency, or loss of afferent nerve fibers.

trophism, the influence of nourishment.

trophoblast [Gk *trophe* + *blastos* germ], the layer of tissue that forms the wall of the blastocyst of placental mammals in the early stages of embryonic development. It functions in the implantation of the blastocyst in the uterine wall and in supplying nutrients to the embryo. **–trophoblastic,** *adj.*

trophoblastic cancer, a malignant neoplastic disease of the uterus derived from chorionic epithelium, characterized by the production of high levels of human chorionic gonadotropin (HCG). The tumor may be an invasive hydatid mole (chorioadenoma destruens) formed by grossly enlarged, vesicular chorionic villi or a malignant uterine choriocarcinoma that arises from nonvillous chorionic epithelium. Initial symptoms are vaginal bleeding and a profuse, foul-smelling discharge; a persistent cough or hemoptysis signals pulmonary involvement. As the disease progresses, there may be frequent hemorrhage, weakness, and emaciation.

trophotropic /trof′ətrop′ik/ [Gk *trophe* + *trepein* to turn], pertaining to a combination of parasympathetic nervous system activity, somatic muscle relaxation, and cortical beta rhythm synchronization, such as in a resting or sleep state.

trophozoite /trof′əzō′it/ [Gk *trophe* + *zoon* animal], an immature ameboid protozoon. When fully developed, a trophozoite may be identified as a schizont.

tropical acne, a form of acne that is caused or aggravated by high temperature and humidity. It is characterized by large nodules or pustules on the neck, back, upper arms, and buttocks.

tropical medicine [Gk *tropikos* of the solstice; L *medicina*], the branch of medicine concerned with the diagnosis and treatment of diseases commonly occurring in tropic and subtropic regions of the world, generally between 30 degrees north and south of the equator.

tropical sore. See **oriental sore.**

tropical sprue, a malabsorption syndrome of unknown cause that is endemic in the tropics and subtropics. It is characterized by abnormalities in the mucosa of the small intestine resulting in protein malnutrition and multiple nutritional deficiencies, often complicated by severe infection. Symptoms include diarrhea, anorexia, and weight loss. Megaloblastic anemia may result from folic acid and vitamin B_{12} deficiency.

tropical typhus. See **scrub typhus.**

tropocollagen /trop′əkol′əjən/ [Gk *trepein* to turn, *kolla* glue, *genein* to produce], fundamental units of collagen fibrils obtained by prolonged extraction of insoluble collagen with dilute acid.

tropomyosin /trop′əmī′əsin/ [Gk *trepein* + *mys* muscle], a protein component of sarcomere filaments, which, together with troponin, regulates interactions of actin and myosin in muscle contractions.

troponin /trō′pənin/ [Gk *trepein* to turn], a protein in the myocardial cell ultrastructure that modulates the interaction between actin and myosin molecules.

Trousseau's sign /trōōsōz′/ [Armand Trousseau, French physician, b. 1801; L *signum* mark], a test for latent tetany in which carpal spasm is induced by inflating a sphygmomanometer cuff on the upper arm to a pressure exceeding systolic blood pressure for 3 minutes.

Trp, abbreviation for the amino acid **tryptophan.**

true ankylosis, an abnormal fusion or union of the separate bones that usually form a joint.

true birth rate [AS *trywe;* ME *burthe;* L *reri* to calculate], the ratio of total births to the total female population of childbearing age, between 15 and 45 years of age.

true chondroma. See **enchondroma.**

true conjugate, a radiographic measurement of the distance from the upper margin of the symphysis pubis to the sacral promontory. It is usually 1.5 to 2 cm less than the diagonal conjugate.

true denticle, a calcified body, composed of irregular dentin, found in the pulp chamber of a tooth.

true diverticulum, diverticula that include all of the tissue layers as the organ from which it originates.

true dwarf. See **primordial dwarf.**

true glottis. See **glottis.**

true hermaphroditism, a condition in which an individual is born with both male and female gonads.

true labor, uterine contractions that result in a change in the cervix and in birth of an infant.

true neuroma, any neoplasm composed of nerve tissue.

true oxygen, the calculated concentration

as either a percentage or a fraction that when multiplied by the expiratory minute volume at STPD gives oxygen uptake.

true pelvis. See **pelvis.**

true hip. See **hip.**

true suture, an immovable fibrous joint of the skull in which the edges of bones interlock along a series of processes and indentations.

true twins. See **monozygotic twins.**

true value, (in statistics) a value that is closely approximated by the definitive value and somewhat less closely by the reference value.

true vocal cords, the vocal folds of the larynx, (plicae vocales), as distinguished from the vestibular folds (plicae vestibulares), called false vocal cords.

truncal /trung′kəl/ [L *truncus*], pertaining to the trunk of the body.

truncal ataxia, a loss of coordinated muscle movements for maintaining normal posture of the trunk.

truncal obesity, obesity that preferentially affects or is located in the trunk of the body, as opposed to the extremities.

truncus /trung′kəs/ [L, trunk], the main stem of an anatomic part from which branches may arise, as the sympathetic nerve chain or jugular lymph trunk.

truncus arteriosus [L, trunk; Gk *arteria* air pipe], the embryonic arterial trunk that initially opens from both ventricles of the heart and later divides into the aorta and the pulmonary trunk, the two portions separated by the bulbar septum.

truncus brachiocephalicus, a branch of the aorta that divides into the right common carotid and right subclavian arteries.

trunk balance, the ability to maintain postural control of the trunk, including the shifting and bearing of weight on each side so as to free an extremity for a particular function. Weight shifting can involve righting, equilibrium, and protective reactions. Head and neck control allows for dissociation of the shoulder and pelvic girdles from the trunk.

trunk incurvation reflex. See **Galant reflex.**

truss [Fr *trousser* to pack up], an apparatus worn to prevent or retard the herniation of the intestines or other organ through an opening in the abdominal wall.

trust [ME, protection], a risk-taking process whereby an individual's situation depends on the future behavior of another person.

truth [AS *treowo*], a rule or statement that conforms to fact or reality.

truth serum, a common name for any of several sedatives, such as the short-acting barbiturates, that have been administered

T

intravenously in subjects to elicit information that may have been repressed. It has been used successfully in helping to identify amnesia victims.

Trypanosoma /trip'ənōsō'mə/ [Gk *trypanon* borer, *soma* body], a genus of parasitic organisms, several species of which can cause significant diseases in humans. Most *Trypanosoma* organisms live part of their life cycle in insects and are transmitted to humans by insect bites.

Trypanosoma brucei gambiense. See **Gambian trypanosomiasis.**

Trypanosoma brucei rhodesiense. See **Rhodesian trypanosomiasis.**

Trypanosoma cruzi. See **Chagas' disease.**

trypanosomal infection. See **trypanosomiasis.**

trypanosome /trip'ənōsōm'/, tripan'-/, any organism of the genus *Trypanosoma.* –**trypanosomal,** *adj.*

trypanosomiasis /trip'ənōsōmī'əsis/ [Gk *trypanon, soma* + *osis* condition], an infection by an organism of the *Trypanosoma* genus. Kinds of trypanosomiasis are **African trypanosomiasis and Chagas' disease.**

trypanosomicide /trip'ənōsō'misīd/ [Gk *trypanon, soma* + L *caedere* to kill], a drug destructive to trypanosomes, especially the species of the protozoan parasite transmitted to humans by various insect vectors common in Africa and Central and South America. –**trypanosomicidal,** *adj.*

trypsin /trip'sin/ [Gk *tripsis* rubbing] a proteolytic digestive enzyme produced by the exocrine pancreas that catalyzes in the small intestine the breakdown of dietary proteins to peptones, peptides, and amino acids.

trypsin, crystallized, a proteolytic enzyme from the pancreas of the ox, *Bos taurus,* that has been used as a debriding agent for open wounds and ulcers.

trypsinogen /tripsin'əjən/ [Gk *tripsis* + *genein* to produce], the inactive precursor form of trypsin. Trypsinogen is secreted in pancreatic juice and converted to active trypsin through the action of enterokinase in the intestine.

tryptases. See **proteinase.**

tryptophan (Trp) /trip'təfan/, an amino acid essential for normal growth in infants and for nitrogen balance in adults. Tryptophan is the precursor of several substances, including serotonin and niacin.

TSEM, abbreviation for **transmission scanning electron microscopy.**

tsetse fly /tset'sē, tsē'tsē/ [Afr *tsetse;* AS *flyge*], a blood-sucking fly found in Africa. It is an insect of the genus *Glossina*

and a secondary host of trypanosomes, which cause African sleeping sickness.

TSH, abbreviation for **thyroid-stimulating hormone.**

TSH-releasing factor. See **thyrotropin-releasing hormone.**

tsp., abbreviation for *teaspoon.*

TSS, abbreviation for **toxic shock syndrome.**

TSTA, abbreviation for *tumor-specific transplantation antigen.*

tsutsugamushi disease. See **scrub typhus.**

t-**test,** a statistic test used to determine whether there are differences between two means or between a target value and a calculated mean.

TTP, abbreviation for **thrombotic thrombocytopenic purpura.**

T tube, 1. a tubular device in the shape of a T, inserted through the skin into a cavity or a wound, used for drainage. 2. an apparatus used to connect a source of humidified oxygen to the endotracheal tube so that a spirometer can be attached for the evaluation of tidal volume and appropriate removal of the endotracheal tube.

T tubule cholangiography, a type of biliary tract radiographic examination in which a water-soluble iodinated contrast medium is injected into the bile duct through an in-dwelling T-tube.

T tubule system, a system of invaginations along the surface of the myocardial cell membranes, providing an extension of the membrane into the cells. The system is believed to be a method of storing calcium ions and for the movement of substrates into the cells and the removal of metabolic end products from the cells.

TU, 1. abbreviation for *toxic unit.* 2. abbreviation for *toxin unit.* 3. abbreviation for *tuberculin unit.*

tuaminoheptane /tōō·am'inōhep'tān/, an adrenergic vasoconstrictor.

tubal abortion [L *tubus; ab* from, *oriri* to be born], a condition of pregnancy in which an embryo, ectopically implanted, is expelled from the uterine tube into the peritoneal cavity. Tubal abortion is often accompanied by significant internal bleeding, causing acute abdominal and pelvic pain.

tubal dermoid cyst, a tumor derived from embryonal tissues that develops in an oviduct.

tubal ligation, one of several sterilization procedures in which both fallopian tubes are blocked to prevent conception from occurring.

tubal pregnancy, an ectopic pregnancy in which the conceptus implants in the fallopian tube. The most important predisposing factor is prior tubal injury. Pelvic infection, scarring and adhesions from surgery, or IUD complications may result in damage that diminishes the motility of the tube. Transport of the ovum through the tube after fertilization is slowed, and implantation takes place before the conceptus reaches the uterine cavity.

tube [L *tubus*], a hollow, cylindric piece of equipment or structure of the body.

tube feeding, the administration of nutritionally balanced liquefied foods through a tube inserted into the stomach or duodenum. The procedure is used after mouth or gastric surgery, in severe burns, in paralysis or obstruction of the esophagus, in severe cases of anorexia nervosa, and for unconscious patients or those unable to chew or swallow.

tube feeding care, the nursing care and management of a patient receiving nourishment through a nasogastric tube.

tube gain, the overall electron gain of a photomultiplier tube, calculated as gn, where g is the dynode gain and n is the number of dynodes in the tube.

tubercle /t(y)ōō′bərkəl/ [L *tuber* swelling], **1.** a nodule or a small eminence, such as that on a bone. **2.** a nodule, especially an elevation of the skin that is larger than a papule, such as Morgagni's tubercles of the areolae of the breasts. **3.** a small rounded nodule produced by infection with *Mycobacterium tuberculosis,* consisting of a gray translucent mass of small spheric cells surrounded by connective cells.

tubercles of Montgomery [William Featherstone Montgomery, Irish gynecologist, b. 1797], small papillae on the surface of nipples and aerolas that secrete a fatty lubricating substance.

tubercular, pertaining to or resembling tuberculosis.

tuberculin. See **tuberculin test, tuberculosis.**

tuberculin purified protein derivative /tōōbur′kyōōlin/, a solution containing a purified protein fraction derived from isolated culture filtrates of strains of *Mycobacterium tuberculosis.* It is used as an aid in the diagnosis of tuberculosis, in the Mantoux test and, for the same purpose in a dried form, in multiple puncture devices.

tuberculin test [L *tuber* + *testum* crucible], a test to determine past or present tuberculosis infection based on a positive skin reaction, using one of several methods. A purified protein derivative (PPD) of tubercle bacilli, called **tuberculin,** is introduced into the skin by scratch, puncture, or intradermal injection. If a raised, red, or

hard zone forms surrounding the tuberculin test site, the person is said to be sensitive to tuberculin, and the test is read as positive. Kinds of tuberculin tests include **Heaf test, Mantoux test, Pirquet's test,** and **tine test.**

tuberculin tine test, a method of testing for the presence of tubercle bacilli by applying a device with multiple sharp prongs to the skin. The prongs penetrate the skin and inject tuberculin, a purified protein derivative (PPD) tubercle bacilli. A hardened raised area at the test site 48 to 72 hours later indicates the presence of the pathogens in the blood. Because of variations in sensitivity and strength of tuberculin units administered, a negative test result does not necessarily exclude a diagnosis of tuberculosis.

tuberculoid leprosy. See **leprosy.**

tuberculoma /t(y)ōōbur′kyəlō′mə/ [L *tuber* + Gk *oma* tumor], a rare tumorlike growth of tuberculous tissue in the central nervous system, characterized by symptoms of an expanding cerebral, cerebellar, or spinal mass.

tuberculosis (TB) /t(y)ōōbur′kyəlō′sis/ [L *tuber* + Gk *osis* condition], a chronic granulomatous infection caused by an acid-fast bacillus, *Mycobacterium tuberculosis,* generally transmitted by the inhalation or ingestion of infected droplets and usually affecting the lungs, although infection of other organ systems by other modes of transmission occurs. Listlessness, vague chest pain, pleurisy, anorexia, fever, and weight loss are early symptoms of pulmonary tuberculosis. Night sweats, pulmonary hemorrhage, expectoration of purulent sputum, and dyspnea develop as the disease progresses. The lung tissues react to the bacillus by producing protective cells that engulf the disease organism, forming tubercles. Untreated, the tubercles enlarge and merge to form larger tubercles that undergo caseation, eventually sloughing off into the cavities of the lungs. Hemoptysis occurs as a result of cavitary spread. Physical examination reveals apical rales, amphoric bronchial sounds, decreased respiratory excursion, and, in advanced cases, cyanosis.

tuberculosis vaccine. See **BCG vaccine.**

tuberculous /t(y)ōōbur′kyələs/ [L *tuberculum*], pertaining to tuberculosis.

tuberculous lymphadenitis, an inflammation of the lymph glands caused by the presence of *Mycobacterium tuberculosis.*

tuberculous peritonitis, an inflammation of the peritoneum that is secondary to a tuberculous infection in the viscera.

tuberculous pneumonia, a complication of tuberculosis in which caseous material

T

is inhaled into the bronchi, leading to bronchopneumonia or lobar pneumonia.

tuberculous spondylitis /tŏŏbur′kyələs/, a rare, grave form of tuberculosis caused by the invasion of *Mycobacterium tuberculosis* into the spinal vertebrae. The intervertebral disks may be destroyed, resulting in the collapse and wedging of affected vertebrae and the shortening and angulation of the spine.

tuberosity /t(y)ōŏ′bərəs′itē/ [L *tuber*], an elevation or protuberance, especially of a bone.

tuberosity of the tibia, a large oblong elevation at the proximal end of the tibia that attaches to the ligament of the patella.

tuberous carcinoma /t(y)ōŏ′bərəs/ [L *tuber;* Gk *karkinos* crab, *oma* tumor], a scirrhous carcinoma of the skin, characterized by nodular projections.

tuberous sclerosis, a familial, neurocutaneous disease characterized by epilepsy, mental deterioration, adenoma sebaceum, nodules and sclerotic patches on the cerebral cortex, retinal tumors, depigmented leaf-shaped macules on the skin, tumors of the heart or kidneys, and cerebral calcifications.

tuberous xanthoma. See **xanthoma tuberosum.**

tuboabdominal gestation /t(y)ōŏ′bō·abdom′inəl/ [L *tubus* + *abdomen* belly; L *gestare* to bear], an ectopic pregnancy in which the embryo develops while partly in the abdominal cavity and partly in the fallopian tube. The condition usually begins as a tubal pregnancy and extends into the abdomen as development continues.

tuboabdominal pregnancy. See **tuboabdominal gestation.**

tubo-ovarian /t(y)ōŏ′bō·ōver′ē·ən/ [L *tubus* + *ovum* egg], pertaining to the ovary and fallopian tube.

tubo-ovarian abscess, an abscess involving the ovary and fallopian tube. It is commonly associated with salpingitis.

tubo-ovarian cyst, a cyst that forms by adhesion of the ovary at the fimbriated end of the fallopian tube.

tubo-ovarian gestation, an ectopic pregnancy that develops partly in the fallopian tube and partly in the ovary.

tubo-ovarian pregnancy. See **tubo-ovarian gestation.**

tuboplasty /t(y)ōŏ′bōplas′tē/ [L *tubus* tube; Gk *plassein* to mold], a surgical procedure in which severed or damaged fallopian tubes are repaired.

tubular necrosis [L *tubulus* little tube; Gk *nekros* dead, *osis* condition], the death of cells in the small tubules of the kidneys as a result of disease or injury.

tubule /t(y)ōŏ′byōōl/ [L *tubulus*], a small

tube, such as one of the collecting tubules in the kidneys, the seminiferous tubules of the testes, or Henle's tubules between the distal and proximal convoluted tubules. **–tubular,** *adj.*

tuft [Fr *touffe* a helmet crest], an object resembling a tassle, such as a tuft of hair.

tuft fracture [Fr *touffe* + L *fractura* break], fracture of any one of the distal phalanges.

tularemia /tōŏ′lərē′mē·ə/ [Tulare, California; Gk *haima* blood], an infectious disease of animals caused by the bacillus *Francisella (Pasteurella) tularensis,* which may be transmitted by insect vectors or direct contact. It is characterized in humans by fever, headache, and an ulcerated skin lesion with localized lymph node enlargement, or by eye infection, GI ulcerations, or pneumonia, depending on the site of entry and the response of the host.

tumescence /t(y)ōōmes′əns/ [L *tumescere* to begin to swell], a state of swelling or edema.

tumor [L], **1.** a swelling or enlargement occurring in inflammatory conditions. **2.** a new growth of tissue characterized by progressive, uncontrolled proliferation of cells. The tumor may be localized or invasive, benign or malignant.

tumor albus, a white swelling occurring in a tuberculous bone or joint.

tumor angiogenesis factor (TAF), a protein that stimulates the formation of blood vessels in cancers.

tumoricide /t(y)ōōmôr′isīd/, a substance capable of destroying a tumor. **–tumoricidal,** *adj.*

tumorigenesis /t(y)ōŏ′mərijen′əsis/, the process of initiating and promoting the development of a tumor. **–tumorigenic,** *adj.*

tumor marker, a substance in the body that is associated with the presence of a cancer.

tumor necrosis factor (TNF), a natural body protein, also produced synthetically, with anticancer effects. It is produced in the body in response to the presence of toxic substances, such as bacterial toxins.

tumor registry, a repository of data on the incidence of cancers and personal characteristics, treatment, and treatment outcomes of patients diagnosed with cancer.

tumor viruses, viruses that are capable of directly or indirectly inducing tumor formation. Direct tumor formation may result from inoculation of living cells with tumorigenic viruses. Tumor formation may result from the influence of the virus on normal cells that are transformed into tumor cells.

tumor volume, a portion of an organ or

tissue that includes both the tumor and adjacent areas of invasion.

tungsten (W) [SW *tung* heavy, *sten* stone], a metallic element. Its atomic number is 74; its atomic weight is 183.85. It has the highest melting point of all metals.

tunica /t(y)ōō′nikə/ [L, tunic], an enveloping coat or covering membrane.

tunica adventitia, the outer layer or coat of an artery or other tubular structure.

tunica albugines [L *tunic* + *albus* white], a tissue covering of white collagenous fibers, such as the scleratic coat of the eyeball.

tunica intima, the membrane lining an artery.

tunica media, a muscular middle coat of an artery.

tunica vaginalis testis, the serous membrane surrounding the testis and epididymis.

tunica vasculosa bulbi. See **uvea.**

tuning fork [Gk *tonos* stretching; L *furca* fork], a small metal instrument consisting of a stem and two prongs that produces a constant pitch when either prong is struck. It is used in auditory tests of nerve function and of air and bone conduction.

tunnel [OFr *tonnel*], a canal or passage, such as the carpal tunnel.

tunnel vision [OFr *tonnel* fowl trap; L *videre* to see], a defect in sight in which there is a great reduction in the peripheral field of vision, as if looking through a hollow tube or tunnel. The condition occurs in advanced chronic glaucoma.

tunnel wound, a break in the surface of the body or an organ in which the entry and exit wounds are the same size.

TUR, abbreviation for **transurethral resection.**

turban tumor [Turk *tulbend* headdress; L *tumor* swelling], a benign neoplasm consisting of pink or maroon nodules that may cover the entire scalp, trunk, and extremities.

turbid /tur′bid/ [L *turbidus* confused], clouded or obscured, as in solids in suspension in a solution.

turbidimetry /tur′bidim′ətrē/ [L *turbidus* confused; Gk *metron* measure], measurement of the turbidity (cloudiness) of a solution or suspension in which the amount of transmitted light is quantified with a spectrophotometer or estimated by visual comparison with solutions of known turbidity.

turbidity /tərbid′itē/ [L *turbidus*], a condition of light scattering in a liquid resulting from the presence of suspended particles in the fluid.

turbinate /tur′binit/ [L *turbinum* top-

shaped], **1.** of or pertaining to a scroll shape. **2.** the concha nasalis.

turgid /tur′jid/ [L *turgidus*], swollen, hard, and congested, usually as a result of an accumulation of fluid. **–turgor,** *n.*

turgor /tur′gər/ [L *turgere* to swell], the normal resiliency of the skin caused by the outward pressure of the cells and interstitial fluid. An evaluation of the turgor of the skin is an essential part of physical assessment.

turista. See **traveler's diarrhea.**

turnbuckle cast [AS *tyrnan;* ME *bocle* small shield; ONorse *kasta*], an orthopedic device used to encase and immobilize the entire trunk, one arm to the elbow, and the opposite leg to the knee. It is constructed of plaster of paris or fiberglass and incorporates hinges as part of its design in the treatment of scoliosis. The hinges are placed at the level of the apex of the curvature.

Turner's sign. See **Grey Turner's sign.**

Turner's syndrome [Henry H. Turner, American physician, b. 1892], a chromosomal anomaly seen in about 1 in 3,000 live female births, characterized by the absence of one X chromosome, congenital ovarian failure, genital hypoplasia, cardiovascular anomalies, dwarfism, short metacarpals, "shield chest," extosis of tibia, and underdeveloped breasts, uterus, and vagina. Spatial disorientation and moderate degrees of learning disorders are common.

turricephaly. See **oxycephaly.**

tussis /tus′is/ [L *tussicula* a slight cough], a cough or pertussis.

tussive fremitus /tus′iv/ [L *tussis* + *fremitus* murmuring], a vibratory cough that can be felt by a hand over the chest of the patient.

TV, abbreviation for **tidal volume.**

TVL, abbreviation for **tenth-value layer.**

T wave, the component of the cardiac cycle shown on an electrocardiogram as a short, inverted, U-shaped curve following the ST segment.

Tweed triangle [Charles Tweed, American dentist, b. 1895; L *triangulus* three-cornered], a triangle used as a diagnostic aid, formed by the mandibular plane, the Frankfort plane, and the long axis of the lower central incisor.

twelfth cranial nerve. See **hypoglossal nerve.**

24-hour clock system, a method of designating time by using the numeric sequence from 00 to 23 for the hours and the numbers 00 to 59 for the minutes in a daily cycle beginning with 0000 (midnight) and ending with 2359 (1 minute before the following midnight).

twilight state [Ger *zweilicht* subdued light;

L *status*], an impaired state of consciousness in which the patient may experience visual or auditory hallucinations and responds to them with irrational behavior. The person may be unaware of the suroundings at the time of the experience and have no memory of it later, except perhaps to recall a related dream.

twin [AS *twinn* double], either of two offspring born of the same pregnancy and developed from either a single ovum or from two ova that were released from the ovary simultaneously and fertilized at the same time. The incidence of twin births is approximately 1 in 80 pregnancies. Kinds of twins include **conjoined, dizygotic, interlocked, monozygotic, Siamese,** and **unequal twins.**

twinge [ME *twengen* to pinch], a sudden, brief, darting pain.

twin monster. See **double monster.**

twinning [AS *twinn*], **1.** the development of two or more fetuses during the same pregnancy, either spontaneously or through external intervention for experimental purposes in animals. **2.** the duplication of like structures or parts by division.

twin-wire fixed orthodontic appliance, an orthodontic appliance employing a pair of 0.01 in (0.25 mm) wires to form the midsection of the arch wire. It is used to correct or improve malocclusion.

twitch [AS *twiccian*], **1.** the contraction of small muscle units, manifested as a quick, simple, spasmodic contraction of a muscle. **2.** to jerk convulsively.

twitching, a series of contractions by small muscle units. Twitching that involves large groups of muscle fibers is identified as **fascicular twitching.**

two-point discrimination test, a test of the ability of a person to differentiate touch stimuli at two nearby points on the body at the same time. It is used in studies of possible damage to the parietal regions of the brain.

two-point gait [OE *twa;* L *punctus* pricked; ONorse *gata* way], a pattern of crutchwalking with crutches in which the right foot and left crutch advance first, the step being completed by advancing the left foot and right crutch.

two-way catheter [AS *twa, weg;* Gk *katheter* something lowered], a catheter that has a double lumen, one channel for injection of medication or fluids and the other for removal of fluid or specimens.

tyloxapol /tīlok′səpôl/, a respiratory tract detergent prescribed for bronchitis, emphysema, pulmonary abscess, bronchiectasis, or atelectasis.

tympanectomy /tim′pənek′təmē/, the surgical removal of the tympanic membrane.

tympanic /timpan′ik/ [Gk *tympanum* drum], of or pertaining to a structure that resonates when struck; drumlike, such as a **tympanic abdomen** that resonates on percussion because the intestines are distended with gas. **–tympanum** /tim′-pənəm/ (*pl.* **tympana**), *n.*

tympanic antrum, a relatively large, irregular cavity in the superior anterior portion of the mastoid process of the temporal bone, communicating with the mastoid air cells and lined by the extension of the mucous membrane of the tympanic cavity.

tympanic cavity. See **middle ear.**

tympanic membrane, a thin semitransparent membrane in the middle ear that transmits sound vibrations to the internal ear by means of the auditory ossicles. It is nearly oval in form and separates the tympanic cavity from the bottom of the external acoustic meatus.

tympanic membrane thermometer, a device that measures the temperature of the tympanic membrane by detecting infrared radiation from the tissue. Results are obtained within 2 seconds and directly reflect the body's core temperature.

tympanic reflex, the reflection of a beam of light shining on the eardrum. In a normal ear a bright, wedge-shaped reflection is seen; its apex is at the end of the malleus, and its base is at the anterior inferior margin of the eardrum.

tympanic sulcus [Gk *tympanum;* L *sulcus* furrow], a narrow circular groove at the medial end of the osseous part of the external acoustic meatus that holds the tympanic membrane.

tympanic temperature, the body temperature as measured electronically at the tympanic membrane.

tympanitic resonance /tim′pənit′ik/, a drumlike or hollow sound heard over a large air space of the body, such as the pneumothorax.

tympanogram, a graphic representation of the acoustic impedance and air pressure of the middle ear and mobility of the tympanic membrane, measured as part of the audiologic test battery. Various middle ear pathologies, such as otitis media, otosclerosis, or tympanic membrane perforations, each yield distinctive tympanograms.

tympanoplasty /timpan′əplas′tē/ [Gk *tympanum* + *plassein* to mold], any of several operative procedures on the eardrum or ossicles of the middle ear, designed to restore or improve hearing in patients with conductive deafness. These operations may be used to repair a perforated eardrum, for otosclerosis, or dislocation or necrosis of one of the small bones of the middle ear.

tympanotomy. See **myringotomy.**

tympanum. See **tympanic.**

tympany /tim'pənē/, a low-pitched resonant sound heard on percussion over a pneumothorax or distended abdomen.

Type A personality [Gk *typos* mark], a behavior pattern associated with individuals who are highly competitive and work compulsively to meet deadlines. The behavior also is associated with a higher than usual incidence of coronary heart disease.

Type B personality, a form of behavior associated with persons who appear free of hostility and aggression and who lack a compulsion to meet deadlines, are not highly competitive at work and play, and have a lower risk of heart attack.

Type E personality, a term used to describe professional women who fit neither Type A nor Type B personality categories, but who have a marked sense of insecurity and strive to convince themselves that they are worthwhile.

type I diabetes mellitus. See **insulin-dependent diabetes mellitus.**

type II diabetes mellitus. See **non-insulin-dependent diabetes mellitus.**

type I hyperlipidemia. See **hyperlipidemia type I.**

type II hyperlipoproteinemia. See **familial hypercholesterolemia.**

type I hypersensitivity. See **anaphylactic hypersensitivity.**

type II hypersensitivity. See **cytotoxic hypersensitivity.**

type III hypersensitivity. See **immune complex hypersensitivity.**

type IV hypersensitivity. See **cell-mediated immune response.**

typhoid /tī'foid/ [Gk *typhos* fever, *eidos* form], pertaining to or resembling typhus.

typhoid carrier, a person without signs or symptoms of typhoid fever who carries on his or her body the bacteria that cause the disease and shed the pathogens in bodily excretions. The typical typhoid carrier is one who has recovered from an attack of the disease.

typhoid fever [Gk *typhos* typhus, *eidos* form; L *febris* fever], a bacterial infection usually caused by *Salmonella typhi,* transmitted by contaminated milk, water, or food and characterized by headache, delirium, cough, watery diarrhea, rash, and a high fever. Characteristic maculopapular rosy spots are scattered over the skin of the abdomen. Splenomegaly and leukopenia develop first. The disease is serious and may be fatal. Complications include intestinal hemorrhage or perforation and

thrombophlebitis. Some people who recover from the disease continue to be carriers and excrete the organism, spreading the disease.

typhoid nodules, a liver nodule consisting of a cluster of monocytes and lymphocytes surrounding the typhoid fever pathogen, *Salmonella typhi.*

typhoid pellagra, a form of pellagra in which the symptoms also include continued high temperatures.

typhoid vaccine, a bacterial vaccine prepared from an inactivated, dried strain of *Salmonella typhi.* It is prescribed for primary immunization against typhoid fever for adults and children.

typhous /tī'fəs/, pertaining to typhus fever.

typhus /tī'fəs/ [Gk *typhos* stupor], any of a group of acute infectious diseases caused by various species of *Rickettsia* and usually transmitted from infected rodents to humans by the bites of lice, fleas, mites, or ticks. These diseases are all characterized by headache, chills, fever, malaise, and a maculopapular rash. Kinds of typhus are **epidemic typhus, murine typhus,** and **scrub typhus.**

typhus vaccine, any one of three vaccines, each of which is prepared for the different rickettsial organisms that cause epidemic typhus, murine typhus, or Brill-Zinsser disease. Each of the vaccines is prescribed for immunization against a form of typhus.

typical, a representative example.

typing [Gk *typos* mark], the process of ascertaining the classification of a specimen of blood, tissue, or other substance.

Tyr, abbreviation for the amino acid tyrosine.

tyramine /tī'rəmēn/ [Gk *tyros* cheese, *amine* ammonia], an amino acid synthesized in the body from the essential acid tyrosine. Tyramine stimulates the release of the catecholamines epinephrine and norepinephrine. It is important that people taking monoamine oxidase inhibitors avoid the ingestion of foods and beverages containing tyramine.

tyroma /tīrō'mə/, *pl.* **tyromas, tyromata** [Gk *tyros* + *oma* tumor], a new growth or nodule with a caseous or cheesy consistency.

tyromatosis /tī'rōmətō'sis/ [Gk *tyros, oma* + *osis* condition], a process in which necrotic tissue is broken down and degenerates to a granular, amorphous, caseous mass.

tyrosine (Tyr) /tī'rəsēn/ [Gk *tyros*], an amino acid synthesized in the body from the essential amino acid phenylalanine. Tyrosine is found in most proteins and is

T

a precursor of melanin and several hormones, including epinephrine and thyroxin.

tyrosinemia /tī′rōsinē′mē·ə/ [Gk *tyros* + *haima* blood], **1.** a benign, transient condition of the newborn, especially premature infants, in which an excessive amount of the amino acid tyrosine is found in the blood and urine. The disorder is caused by an anomaly in amino acid metabolism, usually delayed development of the enzymes necessary to metabolize tyrosine. **2.** a hereditary disorder involving an inborn error of metabolism of the amino acid tyrosine. The condition is caused by an enzyme deficiency and results in liver failure or hepatic cirrhosis, renal tubular defects that can lead to renal rickets and renal glycosuria, generalized aminoaciduria, and mental retardation.

tyrosinosis /tī′rōsinō′sis/ [Gk *tyros* + *osis* condition], a rare condition resulting from a defect in amino acid metabolism and characterized by the excretion of an excessive amount of parahydroxyphenylpyruvic acid, an intermediate product of tyrosine, in the urine.

tyrosinurea /tī′rōsin ōōr′ē·ə/ [Gk *tyros* + *ouron* urine], the presence of tyrosine in the urine.

Tzanck test /tsangk/ [Arnault Tzanck, French dermatologist, b. 1886], a microscopic examination of cellular material from skin lesions to help diagnose certain vesicular diseases.

tzetze [Tswana dial]. See **tsetse fly.**

u, symbol sometimes used to stand for **micro-** (properly μ), as in "ul" or "um," representing μl or μm.

U, 1. abbreviation for **unit.** 2. symbol for the chemical element **uranium.**

UAO, abbreviation for **upper-airway obstruction.**

UGI, abbreviation for **upper GI.**

UICCC, abbreviation for *International Union Against Cancer, Union internacional contra el cancer, Union internationale contre le cancer, Unio internationalis contra cancrum,* or *Unione internazionale contro il cancro.*

ulcer /ul′sər/ [L *ulcus*], a circumscribed, craterlike lesion of the skin or mucous membrane resulting from necrosis that accompanies some inflammatory, infectious, or malignant processes. Some kinds of ulcer are **decubitus ulcer, peptic ulcer,** and **serpent ulcer. –ulcerate,** *v.,* **ulcerative** /ul′sərā′tiv/, *adj.*

ulceration, the process of ulcer formation.

ulcerative blepharitis /ul′sərā′tiv, ul′-sərətiv′/ [L *ulcus, atus* relating to; Gk *blepharon* eyelid, *itis* inflammation], a form of blepharitis in which a staphylococcal infection of the follicles of the eyelashes and glands of the eyelids results in sticky crusts forming on the lid margins. If the crusts are pulled off, the skin beneath bleeds. Tiny pustules develop in the follicles of the eyelashes and break down to form shallow ulcers.

ulcerative colitis, a chronic, episodic, inflammatory disease of the large intestine and rectum, characterized by profuse watery diarrhea containing varying amounts of blood, mucus, and pus. The attacks of diarrhea are accompanied by tenesmus, severe abdominal pain, fever, chills, anemia, and weight loss. Children with the disease may suffer retarded physical growth. The debilitating symptoms often prevent persons with ulcerative colitis from carrying on the normal activities of daily living.

ulcerative inflammation, the development of an ulcer over an area of inflammation.

ulcerative stomatitis [L *ulcus;* Gk *stoma* mouth, *itis* inflammation], an infectious disease of the mouth characterized by swollen, spongy gums, ulcers, and loose teeth.

ULD, abbreviation for **upper-level discriminator.**

ulna /ul′nə/ [L, elbow], the bone on the medial or little finger side of the forearm, lying parallel with the radius. The ulna articulates with the humerus and the radius. **–ulnar,** *adj.*

ulnar artery /ul′nər/, a large artery branching from the brachial artery, supplying muscles in the forearm, wrist, and hand; arising near the elbow, it passes obliquely in a distal direction to become the superficial palmar arch.

ulnar drift [L *ulna;* AS *drifan* to drive], a joint change in the metacarpophalangeal joints due to rheumatoid arthritis and chronic synovitis. The long axis of the fingers make an angle with the long axis of the wrist so that fingers are deviated to the ulnar side of the hand.

ulnar nerve, one of the terminal branches of the brachial plexus that arises on each side from the medial cord of the plexus. It receives fibers from both cervical and thoracic nerve roots and supplies the muscles and the skin on the ulnar side of the forearm and the hand. It can be easily palpated as the "funny bone" of the elbow.

ulocarcinoma /yo͞o′lōkär′sinō′mə/, *pl.* **ulocarcinomas, ulocarcinomata** [Gk *oule* scar, *karkinos* crab, *oma* tumor], any malignant neoplastic disease of the gums that is classified as a carcinoma.

ulterior transactions, (in psychiatry) transactions that are bilevel. The first level is usually of relevant verbal statements. The second level is usually nonverbal and has hidden psychologic meaning.

ultimate strain, the strain at the point of failure.

ultimate stress, the highest load that can be sustained by a material at the point of failure.

ultracentrifuge /ul′trəsen′trifyo͞oj/ [L *ultra* beyond; Gk *kentron* center; L *fugere* to flee], a high-speed centrifuge with a rotation rate fast enough to produce sedimentation of viruses, even in blood plasma.

ultradian /ul′trā′dē·ən/ [L *ultra + dies*

day], pertaining to a biorhythm that occurs in cycles of less than 24 hours.

ultrafiltrate /ul'trəfil'trāt/ [L *ultra* + Fr *filtre* filter], a solution that has passed through a special semipermeable ultrafilter membrane.

ultrafiltration, a type of filtration, sometimes conducted under pressure, through filters with very minute pores, as used by an artificial kidney. Ultrafiltration can separate large molecules from smaller molecules in body fluids.

ultra-high-speed handpiece, a device for holding rotary instruments, such as burs, that permits rotational speeds of 100,000 to 300,000 rpm. It is used primarily for tooth cavity preparation.

ultralente insulin. See **long-acting insulin.**

ultramicroscopy. See **darkfield microscopy.**

ultrasonic cardiography. See **echocardiography.**

ultrasonic [L *ultra* + *sonus* sound], pertaining to ultrasound, or sound frequencies so high (greater than 20 kilohertz) they cannot be perceived by the human ear.

ultrasonic nebulizer, a humidifier in which an electric current is used to produce high-frequency vibrations in a container of fluid. The vibrations break up the fluid into aerosol particles.

ultrasonic wave, a sound wave transmitted at a frequency greater than 20,000 per second, or beyond the normal hearing range of humans. The specific wavelength is equal to the velocity divided by the frequency.

ultrasonography [L *ultra* + *sonus* sound; Gk *graphein* to record], the process of imaging deep structures of the body by measuring and recording the reflection of pulsed or continuous high-frequency sound waves.

ultrasound [L *ultra* + *sonus*], sound waves at the very high frequency of over 20,000 vibrations per second. Ultrasound has many medical applications, including fetal monitoring, imaging of internal organs, and, at an extremely high frequency, the cleaning of dental and surgical instruments.

ultrasound imaging, the use of high-frequency sound to image internal structures by the differing reflection signals produced when a beam of sound waves is projected into the body and bounces back at interfaces between those structures.

ultraviolet (UV) [L *ultra* + Fr *violette*], light beyond the range of human vision, at the short end of the spectrum, or that portion of the electromagnetic spectrum with wavelengths between about 10 to 400 nm.

It occurs naturally in sunlight; it burns and tans the skin and converts precursors in the skin to vitamin D. Ultraviolet lamps are used in the control of infectious, airborne bacteria, and viruses and in the treatment of psoriasis and other skin conditions. Black light is ultraviolet light used in fluoroscopy.

ultraviolet microscopy. See **fluorescent microscopy.**

ultraviolet radiation, a range of electromagnetic waves extending from the violet or short-wavelength end of the spectrum to the beginning of the x-ray spectrum. Near-ultraviolet radiation covers a range of wavelengths from 380 to 320 mμ; middle-ultraviolet radiation covers a range from 320 to 280 mμ; and far-ultraviolet radiation extends from 280 to about 10 mμ. About 5% of the radiation from the sun is in the ultraviolet range, but little of this type of energy reaches the earth because much is absorbed by oxygen and ozone in the atmosphere. In medicine, ultraviolet radiation is used in the treatment of rickets and certain skin conditions. Milk and some other foods become activated with vitamin D when exposed to this type of energy.

ultraviolet rays. See **ultraviolet radiation.**

ultraviolet therapy, the application of electromagnetic radiations in the ultraviolet region of the spectrum to the body for therapeutic purposes. UV therapy is useful in the control of infectious, airborne bacteria and viruses and in the treatment of psoriasis and other skin conditions.

umbilical /umbil'ikəl/ [L *umbilicus* navel] **1.** of or pertaining to the umbilicus. **2.** of or pertaining to the umbilical cord.

umbilical artery catheter, a catheter inserted into the umbilical artery of a newborn.

umbilical catheterization, a procedure in which a radiopaque catheter is passed through an umbilical artery to provide a newborn infant with parenteral fluid, to obtain blood samples, or both, or through the umbilical vein for an exchange transfusion or the emergency administration of drugs, fluids, or volume expanders.

umbilical cord, a flexible structure connecting the umbilicus with the placenta in the gravid uterus and giving passage to the umbilical arteries and vein. In the newborn it is about 2 feet long and 1/2 inch in diameter.

umbilical duct. See **vitelline duct.**

umbilical fissure, a groove on the inferior surface of the liver that holds the ligamentum teres and separates the right and left lobes of the liver.

umbilical fistula, an abnormal passage from the umbilicus to the intestine or more frequently to the remnant of the canal in the median umbilical ligament that connects the fetal bladder with the allantois.

umbilical hernia, a soft, skin-covered protrusion of intestine and omentum through a weakness in the abdominal wall around the umbilicus.

umbilical region, the part of the abdomen surrounding the umbilicus, in the middle zone between the right and left lateral regions.

umbilical vasculitis, an inflammation of the umbilical cord and its blood vessels.

umbilical vein, one of a pair of embryonic vessels that return the blood from the placenta and fuse to form a single trunk in the body stalk.

umbilical vesicle, a pear-shaped structure formed from the yolk sac at about the fourth week of prenatal development that protrudes into the cavity of the chorion and connects to the developing embryo by the yolk stalk at the region of the future midgut.

umbilication /um'bilikā'shən/, becoming dimpled or pitted or acquiring a depressed area.

umbilicus /umbili'kəs, umbil'ikəs/ [L, navel], the point on the abdomen at which the umbilical cord joined the fetal abdomen. In most adults it is marked by a depression; in some it is marked by a small protrusion of skin.

umbo /um'bō/, *pl.* **umbones** /um'bōnēz/ [L *umbo* boss], a projection on the inner surface of the tympanic membrane where the malleus is attached.

umbrella filter, a small umbrella-shaped filter that can be inserted into the vena cava or other blood vessels to trap blood clots.

uncal herniation /ung'kəl/ [L *uncus* hook; *hernia* rupture], a condition in which the medial portion of the temporal lobe protrudes over the tentorial edge as a result of increased intracranial pressure. A dilated pupil on the side of the herniation is a diagnostic sign of the disorder.

unciform bone. See **hamate bone.**

Uncinaria /un'siner'ē·ə/ [L *uncinus* hook], a genus of nematode that causes hookworm in dogs, cats, and other carnivores.

uncompensated care [ME *un* against, not + L *compendere* to be equivalent], services provided by a hospital, a physician, or other health care professional for which no charge is made and for which no payment is expected.

uncompensated gluteal gait. See **Trendelenburg gait.**

uncompetitive inhibitor [ME *un* + L *com-**petere* to compete; *inhibere* to restrain], an enzymatic inhibitor that appears to bond only to the enzyme substrate complex and not to free enzyme molecules.

unconditioned response [ME *un* + L *conditio* condition; *respondere* to reply], a normal, instinctive, unlearned reaction to a stimulus; one that occurs naturally and is not acquired by association and training.

unconjugated monoclonal antibodies, hybrid antibodies of a single antigenic specificity used for highly selective targeting of tumor cells. These antibodies can destroy malignant cells by direct lysis, by binding to cell receptors, and by mobilization of effector cells.

unconscious [ME *un* + L *conscire* to be aware] **1.** unaware of the surrounding environment; insensible; incapable of responding to sensory stimuli. **2.** (in psychiatry) the part of the mental function in which thoughts, ideas, emotions, or memories are beyond awareness and not subject to ready recall.

unconsciousness, a state of complete or partial unawareness or lack of response to sensory stimuli as a result of hypoxia, resulting from respiratory insufficiency or shock; from metabolic or chemical brain depressants, such as drugs, poisons, ketones or electrolyte imbalance; or from a form of brain pathologic condition, such as trauma, seizures, cerebral vasular accident, or brain tumor or infection. Various degrees of unconsciousness can occur during stupor, fugue, catalepsy, and dream states.

unction. See **ointment.**

uncus /ung'kəs/ [L, hook], **1.** the hooklike anterior end of the hippocampal gyrus on the temporal lobe of the brain. **2.** a hook-shaped structure.

undecylenic acid /un'desilen'ik/, an antifungal agent prescribed in the treatment of athlete's foot and ringworm.

underdamping [AS *under* beneath, *dampen* to check], (in cardiology) the transmission of all frequency components without a reduction in amplitude.

underlying assumption, a set of rules one holds about oneself, others, and the world. These rules are regarded as unquestionably true.

underwater exercise [AS *under* + *woeter*], any physical activity performed in a pool or large tub where the buoyancy of the water facilitates the movement of weak or injured muscles.

underwater seal, a seal formed by water allowed to flow over a tube that exits from the chest cavity of a patient. The water acts as a one-way valve and permits the outflow of air but denies the ingress of air.

U

underweight [AS *under* + *wiht*], less than normal in body weight after adjustment for height, body build, and age.

undescended testis. See **cryptorchidism, monorchism.**

undifferentiated cell [AS *un* not + L *differentia* difference, *cella* storeroom], an embryonic-type cell that has not yet expressed signs of its future special type at maturity.

undifferentiated cell leukemia. See **stem cell leukemia.**

undifferentiated family ego mass, an emotional fusion in a family in which all members are similar in emotional expression.

undifferentiated malignant lymphoma [ME *un* + L *differe* to differ, *atus* process; *malignus* wicked; *lympha* water; Gk *oma* tumor], a lymphoid neoplasm containing many large stem cells that have large nuclei, a small amount of pale cytoplasm, and ill-defined borders.

undifferentiated schizophrenia. See **acute schizophrenia.**

undifferentiation, the lack or absence of normal cell differentiation into an identifiable cell type.

undisplaced fracture, a bone break in which cracks in the osseous tissue may radiate in several directions without the separation or displacement of fragmented sections.

undoing [ME *un* + AS *don*], the performance of a specific action that is intended to negate in part a previous action or communication. According to some psychologists, undoing is related to the magical thinking of childhood.

undulant /un′dyələnt/ [L *unda* wave], wavelike, such as a vibration, fluctuation, or oscillation.

undulant fever. See **brucellosis.**

unengaged head [ME *un* + Fr *engager* to involve; AS *heafod*], the head of a floating fetus.

unequal cleavage [ME *un* + L *aequare* to make equal; AS *cleofan* to split], mitotic division of the fertilized ovum into blastomeres that are larger near the yolk portion of protoplasm, or vegetal pole, and smaller near the nucleus, or animal pole.

unequal pulse, a pulse in which the beats vary in intensity.

unequal twins, two nonjoined fetuses born of the same pregnancy in which only one of the pair is fully formed, with the other showing various degrees of developmental defects.

unfinished business, the concerns of a dying patient that require resolution before death can be accepted by the patient.

ung., an abbreviation for the Latin word, *unguentum,* "unguenta, or ointment."

ungual phalanx. See **distal phalanx.**

unguent. See **ointment.**

unguis. See **nail.**

uniaxial joint /yōō′nē·ak′sē·əl/ [L *unus* one, *axis* axle; *jungere* to join], a synovial joint in which movement is only in one axis, such as a pivot or hinge joint.

UNICEF /yōō′nisef′/, abbreviation for **United Nations International Children's Emergency Fund.**

unicellular reproduction [L *unus* + *cella* storeroom; *re* again, *producere* to produce], the formation of a new organism from a female egg that has not been fertilized; parthenogenesis.

unicentric blastoma. See **blastoma.**

unidirectional block [L *unus* + *dirigere* to direct; Fr *bloc*], a pathologic failure of cardiac impulse conduction in one direction while conduction is possible in the other direction.

unidisciplinary health care team, a group of health care workers who are members of the same discipline.

unidose. See **unit dose.**

unification model /yōō′nifikā′shən/ [L *unus* + *ficare* to make whole, *atus* process; *modulus* small measure], a theoretic framework based on the close relationship of nursing education and clinical nursing service at the University of Rochester (New York). The faculty of the school of nursing holds joint appointments to the school and the hospital, teaching nursing students and providing clinical leadership in nursing service in the hospital.

uniform reporting, the reporting of service and financial data by a hospital in conformance with prescribed standard definitions to permit comparisons with other health facilities.

unilateral [L *unus* + *latus* side], involving only one side.

unilateral hypertrophy [L *unus* + *latus* side; Gk *hyper* above, *trophe* nourishment], enlargement of one side or a portion of one side of the body.

unilateral long-leg spica cast, an orthopedic cast applied to immobilize one leg and the trunk of the body cranially as far as the nipple line.

unilateral neglect, a NANDA-accepted nursing diagnosis of a state in which an individual is perceptually unaware of and inattentive to one side of the body. Defining characteristics include consistent inattention to stimuli on the affected side, inadequate self-care (as in positioning and/or safety precautions in regard to the affected side), lack of looking toward the affected side, and leaving food on the plate on the affected side.

unilateral paralysis. See **hemiplegia.**

uninterrupted suture, a continous suture running forward and backward without interruption.

uniocular diplopia, See **monocular diplopia.**

uniocular squint. See **monocular strabismus.**

uniocular vision. See **monocular vision.**

uniovular /yōō′nē-ov′yələr/ [L *unus* + *ovum* egg], developing from a single ovum as in monozygotic twins as contrasted with dizygotic twins.

uniovular twins. See **monozygotic twins.**

unipolar, pertaining to a nerve cell with only one pole, such as a nerve cell in which the cell body is connected to an axon but there is no dendrite.

unipolar depression a major disorder of mood that is characterized by symptoms of depression only.

unipolar lead [L *unus* + *polus* pole; AS *laedan* to lead] **1.** an electrocardiographic conductor in which the exploring electrode is placed on the precordium or a limb while the indifferent electrode is in the central terminal. **2.** *informal;* a tracing produced by such a lead on an electrocardiograph.

unique radiolytic product, a product, such as a food substance, that has undergone chemical changes as a result of exposure to ionizing radiation.

unisex, 1. concerning only one sex or having reproductive organs of only one sex. **2.** an interchange of sex roles in clothing and hairstyles, work assignments, shared restrooms, and other factors, such as encouraging boys to play with dolls.

unit (U) [L *unus*], **1.** a single item. **2.** a quantity designated as a standard of measurement. **3.** an area of a hospital that is staffed and equipped for treatment of patients with a specific condition or other common characteristics.

unitary human conceptual framework, a complex theory in nursing that emphasizes the importance of holistic health care and an understanding of the human being in relation to the universal environment.

unit clerk, a person who performs routine clerical and reception tasks in a hospital inpatient care unit.

unit dose, a method of preparing medications in which individual doses of patient medications are prepared by the pharmacy and delivered in individual labeled packets to the patient's unit to be administered by the nurses on the ordered schedule.

unit dose system, a system of drug distribution in which a portable cart containing a drawer for each patient's medications is prepared by the hospital pharmacy with a 24-hour supply of the medications.

United Nations International Children's Emergency Fund (UNICEF) /yōō′-nisef′/, a fund established by the General Assembly of the United Nations in 1946 to aid children in devastated areas of the world.

United Network for Organ Sharing (UNOS), a national organization for the collection and distribution of body organs that can be used in transplants. Hospitals advise relatives of newly deceased patients about the availability of UNOS service in arranging organ donations.

United States Pharmacopeia (USP), a compendium, recognized officially by the Federal Food, Drug, and Cosmetic Act, that contains descriptions, uses, strengths, and standards of purity for selected drugs and for all of their forms of dosage.

United States Public Health Service (USPHS), an agency of the federal government responsible for the control of the arrival from abroad of any people, goods, or substances that may affect the health of U.S. citizens. The agency sets standards for the domestic handling and processing of food and the manufacture of serums, vaccines, cosmetics, and drugs.

unit of service, any individual, family, aggregate, organization, or community given nursing care.

univalent /yōō′nivāl′ənt, yōōiv′ələnt/ [L *unus* + *valere* to be worth], referring to a chemical valency of one, or the capacity of one atom of a chemical element to attract one atom of hydrogen or to displace one atom of hydrogen.

univalent antiserum. See **antiserum.**

univalent reduction, a phenomenon during intracellular metabolism involving oxygen-reduction reactions in which superoxide radicals are produced.

universal, occurring everywhere and in all things.

universal antidote [L *universus* whole world; Gk *anti* against, *dotos* something given], a mixture of 50% activated charcoal, 25% magnesium oxide, and 25% tannic acid, formerly thought to be useful as an antidote for most types of acid, heavy metal, alkaloid, and glycoside poisons.

universal choking signal. See **Heimlich sign.**

universal cuff, an adaptive device worn on the hand to hold items such as utensils, shaver, or pencil, allowing a patient with a weak grasp to increase participation in self-care activities.

U

universal donor, a person with type O, Rh factor negative red blood cells. Packed red blood cells of this type may be used for emergency transfusion with minimal risk of incompatibility.

universalizability principle, a principle that an act is good if everyone should, in similar circumstances, do the same act without exception.

universal precautions an approach to infection control designed to prevent transmission of blood-borne diseases such as AIDS and hepatitis B in health care settings. The guidelines, initially developed in 1987 by the Centers for Disease Control in the United States and in 1989 by the Bureau of Communicable Disease Epidemiology in Canada, include specific recommendations for the use of gloves, masks, and protective eyewear.

universal qualifiers, (in neurolinguistic programming) the use of terms that give general impressions of limitations, such as all, common, every, only, and never.

universal recipient, a person with blood type AB, who can receive a transfusion of blood of any group type without agglutination or precipitation effects.

unmyelinated /unmī′əlinā′tid/ [AS *un* not + Gk *myelos* marrow], describing a nerve fiber that is not coated with a myelin sheath. An unmyelinated fiber, lacking the whitish sheath, appears as gray matter in the brain.

Unna paste boot /ōō′nəz/ [Paul G. Unna, German dermatologist, b. 1850; L *pasta* paste; ME *bote*], a dressing for varicose ulcers formed by applying a layer of a gelatin-glycerin-zinc oxide paste to the leg and then a spiral bandage that is covered with successive coats of paste to produce a rigid boot.

UNOS, abbreviation for **United Network for Organ Sharing.**

unresolved grief, a severe, chronic grief reaction in which a person does not complete the resolution stage of the grieving process within a reasonable time.

unsaturated [ME *un* + L *saturare* to fill], describing a solution that is capable of dissolving more of the solute; not saturated.

unsaturated alcohol, an alcohol derived from an unsaturated hydrocarbon, such as an alkene or olefin.

unsaturated compound [AS *un* + L *saturare* to fill, *componere* to put together], a chemical compound that contains double or triple bonds.

unsaturated fatty acid, any of a number of glyceryl esters of certain organic acids in which some of the atoms are joined by double or triple valence bonds. These bonds are easily split in chemical reactions, and other substances are joined to them. Monounsaturated fatty acids have only one double or triple bond per molecule. Polyunsaturated fatty acids have more than one double or triple bond per molecule.

unsaturated hydrocarbon, an organic compound in which two or more carbon atoms are united by double or triple valence bonds, such as in unsaturated fatty acids.

unscrubbed team members, the members of a surgical team, including the anesthetist and circulating nurse, who wear surgical attire but are not gowned or gloved and do not enter the sterile field.

unsocialized aggressive reaction [ME *un* + L *socialis* companion; *aggressio* an attack; *re, agere* again to act], a behavior disorder of childhood characterized by overt and covert hostility, disobedience, physical and verbal aggression, vengefulness, quarrelsome behavior, and destructiveness, often manifested in acts such as lying, stealing, temper tantrums, vandalism, and physical violence against others.

unstable, 1. in an excited or active state, such as an atom with a nucleus possessing excess energy. **2.** easily broken down.

unstable angina, a form of pain that is prodromal to acute myocardial infarction. It typically has a sudden onset, sudden worsening, and stuttering recurrence over days and weeks. It carries a more severe short-term prognosis than stable chronic angina. Nearly one third of unstable angina patients may experience myocardial infarction within 3 months.

unstriated muscle. See **smooth muscle.**

upper airway obstruction (UAO), any abnormal condition of the mouth, nose, or larynx that interferes with breathing when the rest of the respiratory system is functioning normally.

upper extremity suspension, an orthopedic procedure used in the treatment of bone fractures and the correction of orthopedic abnormalities of the upper limbs. The procedure uses traction equipment, including metal frames, ropes, and pulleys to relieve the weight of the upper limb involved rather than to exert traction.

upper GI (UGI), pertaining to the upper gastrointesinal tract, from the esophagus to and including the duodenum. The term is commonly applied to radiographic or fluoroscopic diagnostic views following ingestion of a barium sulfate "milkshake." Normal findings include normal size, contour, patency, filling, positioning, and transmission of barium through the lower esophagus, stomach, and duodenum.

upper level discriminator (ULD), an

electronic device used to discriminate against all pulses whose heights are above a given level.

upper motor neuron paralysis, an injury to or lesion in the brain or spinal cord that causes damage to the cell bodies, or axons, or both, of the upper motor neurons, which extend from the cerebral centers to the cells in the spinal column. Clinical manifestations include increased muscle tone and spasticity of the muscles involved with little or no atrophy, hyperactive deep tendon reflexes, diminished or absent superficial reflexes, the presence of pathologic reflexes, such as Babinski's and Hoffmann's reflexes, and no local twitching of muscle groups.

upper respiratory infection. See **respiratory tract infection.**

upper respiratory tract, one of the two divisions of the respiratory system. The upper respiratory tract consists of the nose, the nasal cavity, the ethmoidal air cells, the frontal sinuses, the sphenoidal sinuses, the maxillary sinus, the larynx, and the trachea. The upper respiratory tract conducts air to and from the lungs and filters and moistens and warms the air during each inspiration.

uptake [AS *uptacan*], the drawing up or absorption of a substance.

UR, abbreviation for **utilization review.**

urachus /yŏŏr′əkəs/ [Gk *ourachos* urinary tract], an epithelial tube connecting the apex of the urinary bladder with the allantois. Its connective tissue forms the median umbilical ligament.

uranium (U) [planet Uranus], a heavy, radioactive metallic element. Its atomic number is 92; its atomic weight is 238.03. Uranium is the heaviest of the natural elements.

urate /yŏŏr′āt/, any salt of uric acid, such as sodium urate. Urates are found in the urine, blood, and tophi or calcareous deposits in tissues. They may also be deposited as crystals in body joints.

urban typhus. See **murine typhus.**

urea /yŏŏrē′ə/ [Gk *ouron* urine], a systemic osmotic diuretic and topical keratolytic. It is prescribed to reduce cerebrospinal and intraocular fluid pressure and is used topically as a keratolytic agent.

urea cycle, a series of enzymatic reactions by which ammonia is detoxified in the liver. In the series of steps for disposing of the ammonia molecule, five enzymatic reactions occur as NH_2 radicals are combined with carbon and oxygen atoms from carbon dioxide to form urea, which is excreted. The amino acid arginine is synthesized during the same process.

urea nitrogen, See **blood urea nitrogen.**

Ureaplasma urealyticum /yŏŏrē′əplaz′-mə/, a sexually transmitted microorganism that is a common inhabitant of the urogenital systems of men and women in whom infection is asymptomatic. Neonatal death, prematurity, and perinatal morbidity are statistically associated with colonization of the chorionic surface of the placenta by *Ureaplasma urealyticum.*

uremia /yŏŏrē′mē·ə/ [Gk *ouron* + *haima* blood], the presence of excessive amounts of urea and other nitrogenous waste products in the blood, as occurs in renal failure. **−uremic,** *adj.*

uremic coma /yŏŏrē′mik/ [Gk *ouron* + *haima, koma* deep sleep], a stuporous condition resulting from acidosis and the the toxic effects of uremia with the retention in the blood of metabolic end products that would normally be excreted through the kidneys.

uremic frost, a pale, frostlike deposit of white crystals on the skin caused by kidney failure and uremia. Urea compounds and other waste products of metabolism that cannot be excreted by the kidneys into the urine are excreted through the small superficial capillaries into the skin, where they collect on the surface.

uremic gingivitis. See **nephritic gingivitis.**

ureter /yŏŏr′ətər, yŏŏrē′tər/ [Gk *oureter*], one of a pair of tubes, about 30 cm long, that carry the urine from the kidney into the bladder. The tubes are thick-walled, vary in diameter and are divided into an abdominal portion and a pelvic portion. The ureter enters the bladder through an oblique tunnel that functions as a valve to prevent backflow of urine into the ureter when the bladder contracts. Connecting with the kidneys, the ureters expand into funnel-shaped renal pelves that branch into calyces, each calyx containing a renal papilla. Urine draining through renal tubules drops into the papillae, passes through the calyces and the pelvis and down each ureter to the bladder. Urine is pumped through the ureters by peristaltic waves that occur an average of three times a minute. **−ureteral** /yŏŏrē′tərəl/, *adj.*

ureteral dysfunction [Gk *oureter* + *dys* bad; L *functio* performance], a disturbance of the normal peristaltic flow of urine through a ureter, resulting from dysfunction of ureteral motor nerves.

uretercystoscope /yŏŏr′ətərsis′təskōp′/ [Gk *oureter* + *kystis* bladder, *skopein* to view], a cystoscope equipped with ureteric catheters that can be inserted into either ureter.

U

ureteritis /yŏŏrē'tərī'tis/ [Gk *oureter* + *itis*], an inflammatory condition of a ureter caused by infection or by the mechanic irritation of a stone.

ureterocele /yŏŏrē'tərōsēl'/ [Gk *oureter* + *kele* hernia], a prolapse of the terminal portion of the ureter into the bladder. The condition may lead to obstruction of the flow of urine, hydronephrosis, and loss of renal function.

ureterodialysis /yŏŏrē'tərōdī·al'isis/ [Gk *oureter* + *dialysis* a breaking], the rupture of a ureter.

ureterography /yŏŏrē'tərog'rəfē/ [Gk *oureter* + *graphein* to record], the radiologic imaging of a ureter, usually conducted as part of an examination of the urinary tract. The examination may involve injection of a radiopaque medium through a urinary catheter.

ureterolysis. See **ureterodialysis.**

ureteroplasty /yŏŏrē'tərōplas'tē/ [Gk *oureter* + *plassein* to mold], a surgical procedure performed to restructure a ureter, as when a stricture blocks the normal flow of urine.

ureteropyelonephritis /yŏŏrē'tərōpī'-əlōəfrī'tis/ [Gk *oureter* + *pyelos* pelvis, *nephros* kidney, *itis*], an inflammation of the kidney, pelvis, and ureter.

ureterosigmoidostomy /yŏŏrē'tərōsig'-moidos'təmē/ [Gk *oureter* + *sigma* letter S, *eidos* form, *stoma* mouth], a surgical procedure in which a ureter is implanted in the sigmoid flexure of the intestinal tract.

ureterostomy /yŏŏrē'tərŏs'təmē/ [Gk *oureter* + *stoma* mouth], the surgical creation of a new opening from a ureter to the surface of the body or into another outlet, such as the rectum.

ureterotomy /yŏŏrē·ot'əmē/, an incision into a ureter.

urethra /yŏŏrē'thrə/ [Gk *ourethra*], a small tubular structure that drains urine from the bladder. In women, it is about 3 cm long and lies directly behind the symphysis pubis, anterior to the vagina. In men, it is about 20 cm long and begins at the bladder, passes through the center of the prostate gland, goes between two sheets of tissue connecting the pubic bones, and finally passes through the urinary meatus of the penis. In men the urethra serves as a passageway for semen during ejaculation, as well as a canal for urine during voiding.

urethral /yŏŏrē'thrəl/, of or pertaining to the urethra.

urethral caruncle [Gk *ourethra;* L *caruncula* small piece of flesh], a small painful growth in the mucous membrane of the female urethral meatus. It may be a source of bleeding.

urethral hematuria, blood in the urine as a result of a urethral lesion.

urethral papilla. See **papilla.**

urethral sphincter, the voluntary muscle at the neck of the bladder that relaxes to allow urination.

urethral swab, an absorbent pad on a slender rod used to treat lesions or to remove secretions.

urethritis /yŏŏr'ithrī'tis/, an inflammatory condition of the urethra that is characterized by dysuria, usually the result of an infection in the bladder or kidneys.

urethrocele /yŏŏrē'thrəsēl'/ [Gk *urethra* + *kele* hernia], (in women) a herniation of the urethra. It is characterized by a protrusion of a segment of the urethra and the connective tissue surrounding it into the anterior wall of the vagina.

urethrography yŏŏ'ethrog'rəfē/, the radiologic examination of the urethra after the injection of a radiopaque agent into the urethra, usually through a catheter.

urethroplasty /yŏŏrē'thrəplas'tē/, a surgical procedure for the repair of a urethra, as in the correction of hypospadias.

urethroscope /yŏŏrē'thrŏskŏp'/, an instrument used to examine the internal surfaces of the urethra.

urethrostenosis /yŏŏrē'thrōstənō'sis/, a stricture of the urethra.

urgency [L *urgere* to drive on], a feeling of the need to void urine immediately.

URI, abbreviation for **upper respiratory infection.**

uric acid /yŏŏr'ik/, a product of the metabolism of protein present in the blood and excreted in the urine.

uricaciduria /yŏŏr'ikas'idŏŏr'ē·ə/ [Gk *ouron* + L *acidus* sour; Gk *ouron*], a greater than normal amount of uric acid in the urine, often associated with urinary calculi or gout.

uricosuric drugs /yŏŏr'ikosŏŏr'ik/ [Gk *ouron* + L *acidus* sour; Gk *ouron;* Fr *drogue*], drugs administered to relieve the pain of gout or to increase the elimination of uric acid.

urinal, a plastic or metal receptacle for collecting urine.

urinalysis /yŏŏr'inal'isis/ [Gk *ouron* + *analysein* to loosen], a physical, microscopic, or chemical examination of urine. The specimen is physically examined for color, turbidity, specific gravity, and pH. Then it is spun in a centrifuge to allow collection of a small amount of sediment that is examined microscopically for blood cells, casts, crystals, pus, and bacteria. Chemical analysis may be performed for the identification and quantification of any of a large number of substances but most commonly for ketones, sugar, protein, and blood.

urinary, of or pertaining to urine or formation of urine.

urinary albumin [Gk *ouron;* L *albus* white], the presence of albumin, a protein, in the urine. Normally, protein is not found in the urine because the spaces in the glomerular membrane of the kidney are too small to allow escape of protein molecules. But if the membrane is damaged, as in some kidney diseases, albumin molecules can leak through into the urine. Normal findings: none or up to 8 mg/dl; 50-80 mg/24 hours at rest; less than 250 mg/24 hours after strenuous exercise.

urinary bladder [Gk *ouron* + AS *blaedre*], the muscular membranous sac in the pelvis that stores urine for discharge through the urethra.

urinary calculus, a calculus formed in any part of the urinary tract. Calculi may be large enough to cause an obstruction in the flow of urine or small enough to be passed with the urine. Kinds of urinary calculi are **renal calculus** and **vesicle calculus.**

urinary casts, cells or particles excreted in the urine having the shape of renal collecting tubules.

urinary elimination, altered, a NANDA-accepted nursing diagnosis of a state in which an individual experiences a disturbance in urine elimination. Defining characteristics include dysuria, urinary frequency, hesitancy, urinary incontinence, nocturia, urinary retention, and urinary urgency.

urinary frequency, a greater than normal frequency of the urge to void without an increase in the total daily volume of urine. The condition is characteristic of inflammation in the bladder or urethra or of diminished bladder capacity or other structural abnormalities.

urinary hesitancy, a decrease in the force of the stream of urine, often with difficulty in beginning the flow. Hesitancy is usually the result of an obstruction or stricture between the bladder and the urethral opening; in men it may indicate an enlargement of the prostate gland, in women, stenosis of the urethral opening.

urinary ileostomy [Gk *ouron;* L *ilia* intestines; Gk *stoma* mouth], the surgical creation of a passage between the urinary bladder and the ileum for the diversion of urinary flow from the ureters.

urinary incontinence, involuntary passage of urine, with the failure of voluntary control over bladder and urethral sphincters.

urinary infection. See **urinary tract infection.**

urinary meatus, the external opening of the urethra.

urinary output, the total volume of urine excreted daily, normally between 700 and 2,000 ml. Various metabolic and renal diseases may change the normal urinary output.

urinary retention, a NANDA-accepted nursing diagnosis of a state in which an individual experiences incomplete emptying of the bladder. Defining characteristics include bladder distention, small and infrequent voiding or absence of urine output, a sensation of bladder fullness, dribbling, residual urine, dysuria, and overflow incontinence.

urinary sediment [Gk *ouron;* L *sedimentum* a settling], solid matter that settles to the bottom of a urine sample that has been allowed to stand for several hours.

urinary system, all of the organs involved in the secretion and elimination of urine. These include the kidneys, ureters, bladder, and urethra.

urinary system assessment, an evaluation of the condition and functioning of the kidneys, bladder, ureters, and urethra and an investigation of concurrent and previous disorders that may be factors in abnormalities in the urinary system. The patient is asked if dysuria, frequency or burning on urination, dribbling, a decreased urinary stream, nocturia, stress incontinence, headache, back pain, or increased thirst has occurred. The color, odor, and amount of urine voided without a catheter and with one in place are determined. Diagnostic procedures may include cystoscopy, excretory and intravenous urography, renal angiography, retrograde studies, and x-ray film of the kidneys, ureters, and bladder.

urinary tract, all organs and ducts involved in the secretion and elimination of urine from the body.

urinary tract infection (UTI), an infection of one or more structures in the urinary tract. Most of these infections are caused by gram-negative bacteria, most commonly *Escherichia coli* or species of *Klebsiella, Proteus, Pseudomonas,* or *Enterobacter.* Urinary tract infection is usually characterized by urinary frequency, burning, pain with voiding, and, if the infection is severe, visible blood and pus in the urine. Kinds of urinary tract infections include **cystitis, pyelonephritis,** and **urethritis.**

urinate, to excrete urine from the bladder.

urination [Gk *ouron* + L *atus* process], the act of passing urine.

urine [Gk *ouron*], the fluid secreted by

U

the kidneys, transported by the ureters, stored in the bladder, and voided through the urethra. Normal urine is clear, straw-colored, slightly acid, and has the characteristic odor of urea. Its normal constituents include water, urea, sodium chloride and potassium chloride, phosphates, uric acid, organic salts, and the pigment urobilin.

urine osmolality, the osmotic pressure of urine. The normal values are 500 to 800 mOsm/L.

urine pH, the hydrogen ion concentration of the urine, or a measure of its acidity or alkalinity. The normal pH values for urine are 4.6 to 8.0.

urine specific gravity, a measure of the degree of concentration of a sample of urine. The normal range of urine specific gravity is 1.003 to 1.035, depending on the patient's previous fluid intake, renal perfusion, and renal function.

urinoma /yo͞or′ino͞o′mə/, pl. **urinoma, urinomatas,** a cyst filled with urine.

urinometer /yo͞or′inom′ətər/ [Gk *ouron* + *metron* measure], any device for determining the specific gravity of urine, including gravitometers and hydrometers.

urobilin /yo͞or′əbī′lin/, a brown pigment formed by the oxidation of urobilinogen, normally found in feces and, in small amounts, in urine.

urobilinogen /yo͞or′əbilin′əjən/, a colorless compound formed in the intestine after the breakdown of bilirubin by bacteria.

urodynamics /yo͞or′ōdīnam′iks/ [Gk *ouron* + *dynamis* force], the study of the hydrology and mechanics of urinary bladder filling and emptying.

urogenital /yo͞or′əjen′itəl/ [Gk *ouron* + L *genitalis* fruitful], of or pertaining to the urinary and the reproductive systems.

urogenital sinus, one of the elongated cavities, formed by the division of the cloaca in early embryonic development, into which open the ureter, mesonephric and paramesonephric ducts, and bladder.

urogenital system, the urinary and genital organs and the associated structures that develop in the fetus to form the kidneys, the ureters, the bladder, the urethra, and the genital structures of the male and female.

urogram /yo͞or′əgram′/, an x-ray film of the urinary tract, obtained by urography.

urography /yo͞oorog′rəfē/ [Gk *ouron* + *graphein* to record], any of a group of x-ray techniques used to examine the urinary system. A radiopaque substance is injected, and x-ray films are taken as the substance is passed through or excreted from the part of the system being studied. Some kinds of urography are **cystoscopic**

urography, intravenous pyelography, and **retrograde pyelography.**

urokinase /yo͞or′əkī′nās/, an enzyme, produced in the kidney and found in urine, that is a potent plasminogen activator of the fibrinolytic system.

urolagnia /yo͞or′əlag′nik/, sexual stimulation gained from acts involving urine, such as watching people urinate or being urinated on.

urolithiasis. See **urinary calculus.**

urologist /yo͞orol′əjist/, a licensed physician who has completed an approved residency program and who specializes in the practice of urology.

urology /yo͞orol′əjē/ [Gk *ouron* + *logos* science], the branch of medicine concerned with the study of the anatomy and physiology, the disorders, and the care of the urinary tract in men and women and of the male genital tract. **–urologic,** *adj.*

uromelus. See **sympus monopus.**

urometer, a type of hydrometer used to measure the specific gravity of a urine sample.

uropathy /yo͞oorop′əthē/ [Gk *ouron* + *pathos* disease], any disease or abnormal condition of any structure of the urinary tract. **–uropathic,** *adj.*

uroporphyria /yo͞or′ōpôrfir′ē·ə/ [Gk *ouron* + *porphyros* purple], a rare, genetic disease characterized by excessive secretion of uroporphyrin in the urine, blistering dermatitis, photosensitivity, splenomegaly, and hemolytic anemia.

uroporphyrin /yo͞or′ōpôr′firin/, a porphyrin normally excreted in the urine in small amounts.

uroradiology /yo͞or′ōrā′dē·ol′əjē/, the radiologic study of the urinary tract.

urorectal septum /yo͞or′ōrek′təl/ [Gk *ouron* + L *rectus* straight; *saeptum* wall], a ridge of mesoderm covered with endoderm that in the early developing embryo divides the endodermal cloaca into the urogenital sinus and the rectum.

uroscopy /yo͞oros′kəpē/ [Gk *ouron* + *skopein* to view], diagnostic examination of urine samples.

urostomy /yo͞oros′təmē/, the diversion of urine away from a diseased or defective bladder through a surgically created opening, or stoma, in the skin.

ursodeoxycholic acid /ur′sōdē·ok′sikol′ik/, a secondary bile salt. It is used in vivo to dissolve cholesterol gallstones.

urticaria /ur′tiker′ē·ə/ [L *urtica* nettle], a pruritic skin eruption characterized by transient wheals of varying shapes and sizes with well-defined erythematous margins and pale centers, caused by capillary dilatation in the dermis that results from the release of vasoactive mediators. **–ur-ticarial,** *adj.*

urticaria bullosa [L *urtica* + *bulla* bubble], a skin eruption in which the lesions are capped by blisters.

urticaria hemorrhagica. See **hemorrhagic urticaria.**

urticaria maculosa [L *urtica* + *macule* spot], a chronic skin eruption in which red lesions form with little or no edema present.

urticaria medicamentosa [L *urtica* + *medicina*], a form of skin eruption that follows the use of certain medications, including those containing quinine.

urticaria papulosa [L *urtica* + *papula* pimple], a form of skin eruption affecting mainly children and characterized by reddish macules upon which papules develop.

urticaria pigmentosa, an uncommon form of mastocytosis characterized by pigmented skin lesions that usually begin in infancy and become urticarial on mechanical or chemical irritation.

urushiol /ər oō′shē·ôl/, a toxic resin in the sap of certain plants of the genus *Rhus,* such as poison ivy, poison oak, and poison sumac, that produces allergic contact dermatitis in many people.

USAN /y oō′san, y oō′es′ā′en′/, for *United States Adopted Names,* a list of approved drugs compiled and published by U.S. Pharmacopeial Convention, Inc.

use effectiveness [L *usus* make use of; *efficere* to produce], (of a contraceptive method) the actual effectiveness of a medication, device, or method in preventing pregnancy.

useful radiation, the portion of direct radiation that is permitted to pass from an x-ray tube housing through the tube head port, aperture, or collimator.

use test, a procedure used to identify offending allergens in foods, cosmetics, or fabrics by the systematic elimination and addition of specific items associated with the life-style of the patient involved.

U-shaped arch, a dental arch in which there is little difference in width between the first premolars and the last molars and the curve from canine to canine is abrupt and U-shaped.

USP. See *United States Pharmacopeia.*

USP unit, a dose unit as recommended by the *United States Pharmacopeia,* the primary legally recognized national drug-standard compendium.

USPHS, abbreviation for **United States Public Health Service.**

uta /y oō′tə/ [Sp, facial ulcers], a mild cutaneous form of American leishmaniasis, occurring in the Andes of Peru and Argen-

tina, caused by *Leishmania peruana.* The lesions are small and usually occur on the exposed surfaces of the skin.

ut dict., an abbreviation for the Latin phrase, *ut dictum,* "as directed."

utend., an abbreviation for the Latin phrase, *utendus,* "to be used."

uterine /y oō′tərēn/ [L *uterus* womb], pertaining to the uterus.

uterine anteflexion [L *uterus* womb; *ante* before, *flectere* to bend], an abnormal position of the uterus in which the uterine body is bent forward on itself at the juncture of the isthmus of the uterine cervix and the lower uterine segment.

uterine anteversion, a position of the uterus in which the body of the uterus is directed ventrally. Mild degrees of anteversion are of no clinical significance.

uterine bleeding, any loss of blood from the uterus.

uterine bruit, a sound made by the passage of blood through the arteries of the pregnant uterus. The sounds are synchronized with the maternal heart rate.

uterine cancer, any malignancy of the uterus, including the cervix or endometrium.

uterine colic [L *uterus;* Gk *kolikos* pain in the colon], a spasmodic pain originating in the uterus, usually due to dysmenorrhea or extrusion of a fibroid polyp.

uterine fibroid [L *uterus, fibra* fiber; Gk *eidos* form], a growth of fibrous tissue in the uterus, usually a fibroma, fibromyoma, or leiomyofibroma.

uterine fibroma, a benign encapsulated uterine tumor that affects about 20% of women over the age of 30. Symptoms may include menstrual disorders, but are also likely to be related to the location of the tumor with respect to neighboring tissues. Uterine fibromas rarely spread or become life threatening.

uterine inertia, abnormal relaxation of the uterus during labor, causing a lack of obstetric progress, or after childbirth, causing uterine hemorrhage.

uterine ischemia, a decreasing or ineffective blood supply to the uterus.

uterine prolapse, the falling, sinking, or sliding of the uterus from its normal location in the body.

uterine retroflexion, a position of the uterus in which the body of the uterus is bent backward on itself at the isthmus of the cervix and the lower uterine segment. It has no clinical significance.

uterine retroversion, a position of the uterus in which the body of the uterus is directed away from the midline, toward the back. Mild degrees of retroversion are common and have no clinical significance.

U

uterine souffle, a soft, blowing sound made by the blood in the arteries of a pregnant uterus. It is synchronized with the maternal pulse.

uterine subinvolution [L *uterus, sub* under, *involere* to roll up], an incomplete involution of the uterus, such as after childbirth.

uterine swab, an absorbent material on a rod or flattened wire used to obtain specimens or to remove secretions from the uterus.

uterine tenaculum. See **tenaculum.**

uterine tetany, a condition characterized by uterine contractions that are extremely prolonged.

uterine tube. See **fallopian tube.**

uteritis. See **metritis.**

uteroabdominal pregnancy, a twin pregnancy in which one fetus develops in the uterus and the other develops in the abdomen.

uteroglobulin. See **blastokinin.**

uteroovarian varicocele /yōō′tərō-ōver′-ē-ən/ [L *uterus + ovum* egg; *varix* varicose vein; Gk *kele* tumor], a swelling of the veins of the pampiniform plexus of the female pelvis.

uteroplacental apoplexy. See **Couvelaire uterus.**

uterosalpingography /yōō′tərōsal′ping-gog′rəfē/ [L *uterus +* Gk *salpigx* tube, *graphein* to record], a radiographic examination of the uterus and fallopian tubes.

uterotomy /yōō′tərot′əmē/ [L *uterus +* Gk *temnein* to cut], a surgical incision into the uterus, such as in a cesarean section.

uterovesical. See **vesicouterine.**

uterus /yōō′tərəs/ [L, womb], the hollow, pear-shaped internal female organ of reproduction in which the fertilized ovum is implanted and the fetus develops, and from which the decidua of menses flows. Its anterior surface lies on the superior surface of the bladder. The uterus is composed of three layers: the endometrium, the myometrium, and the parametrium. The endometrium lines the uterus and becomes thicker and more vascular in pregnancy and during the second half of the menstrual cycle under the influence of the hormone progesterone. The myometrium is the muscular layer of the organ. The parametrium is the outermost layer of the uterus. It is composed of serous connective tissue and extends laterally into the broad ligament. During pregnancy it is able to grow to many times its usual size, almost entirely by cellular hypertrophy. The uterus has two parts: a body and a cervix. The body extends from the fundus to the cervix, just above the isthmus. The cavity within the body is only a potential space. The walls of the body touch, unless the woman is pregnant. The cervix has a vaginal portion, protruding into the vagina, and a supravaginal portion at the juncture of the lower uterine segment.

uterus bicornis, a uterus that is divided into two parts, usually separate at the upper end and joined at the lower end.

uterus masculinis. See **prostatic utricle.**

UTI, abbreviation for **urinary tract infection.**

utilitarianism [L *utilis* usefulness, *isma* practice], a doctrine that the purpose of all action should be to bring about the greatest happiness for the greatest number of people and that the value of anything is determined by its utility.

utilization review (UR) [L *utilis + atus* process], an assessment of the appropriateness and economy of an admission to a health care facility or a continued hospitalization.

utricle /yōō′trikəl/ [L *utriculus* small bag], larger of two membranous pouches in the vestibule of the membranous labyrinth of the ear. It is an oblong structure that communicates with the semicircular ducts by five openings and receives utricular filaments of the acoustic nerve.

utriculosaccular duct /yōōtrik′yəlōsak′-yələr/ [L *utriculus + sacculus* small sack; *ducere* to lead], a duct connecting the utricle with an endolymphatic duct of the membranous labyrinth.

UV, abbreviation for **ultraviolet.**

uvea /yōō′vē-ə/ [L *uva* grapes], the fibrous tunic beneath the sclera that includes the iris, the ciliary body, and the choroid of the eye. **–uveal,** *adj.*

uveitis /yōō′vē-ī′tis/ [L *uva +* Gk *itis*], inflammation of the uveal tract of the eye, including the iris, ciliary body, and choroid. It may be characterized by an irregularly shaped pupil, inflammation around the cornea, pus in the anterior chamber, opaque deposits on the cornea, pain, and lacrimation.

uvula /yōō′vyələ/, *pl.* **uvulae** [L *uva*], the small, cone-shaped process suspended in the mouth from the middle of the posterior border of the soft palate. **–uvular,** /yōō′vyələr/ *adj.*

uvulectomy /yōō′vyəlek′təmē/, the surgical removal of the uvula.

uvulitis /yōō′vyəlī′tis/, inflammation of the uvula. Common causes are allergy and infection.

U wave, (in electrocardiography) a small rounded positive wave that follows the T wave.

v, 1. abbreviation for *vein.* 2. abbreviation for *venous blood.*

V, 1. symbol for the element **vanadium.** 2. symbol for *ventilation capacity of the lung.*

V̇, symbol for *rate of gas flow.*

V̇max, the maximum rate of catalysis.

VAC, an anticancer drug combination of vincristine, dactinomycin, and cyclophosphamide.

vacc, abbreviation for **vaccination.**

vaccination [L *vaccinus* relating to a cow], any injection of attenuated microorganisms, such as bacteria, viruses, or rickettsiae, administered to induce immunity or to reduce the effects of associated infectious diseases. **–vaccinate,** *v.*

vaccine /vaksēn′, vak′sēn, -sin/ [L *vaccinus*], a suspension of attenuated or killed microorganisms administered intradermally, intramuscularly, orally, or subcutaneously to induce active immunity to infectious disease.

vaccinia /vaksin′ē·ə/ [L *vaccinus*], an infectious disease of cattle caused by a poxvirus that may be transmitted to humans by direct contact or by deliberate inoculation as a protection against smallpox. A pustule develops at the site of infection, usually followed by malaise and fever that last for several days. After 2 weeks the pustule becomes a crust that eventually drops off, leaving a scar.

vacuole /vak′yŏŏ·ōl/ [L *vacuus* empty] 1. a clear or fluid-filled space or cavity within a cell, such as occurs when a droplet of water is ingested by the cytoplasm. 2. a small space in the body enclosed by a membrane, usually containing fat, secretions, or cellular debris. **–vacuolar, vacuolated,** *adj.*

Vacu-tainer tube, a glass tube with a rubber stopper in which air can be removed to create a vacuum.

vacuum aspiration [L *vacuus* empty; *aspirare* to breathe], a method of removing tissues from the uterus by suction.

VAD, abbreviation for **vascular access device.**

vade mecum /vā′dē mē′kəm/ [L, go with me], something carried by a person for constant use.

vagal /vā′gəl/ [L *vagus* wandering], of or pertaining to the vagus nerve.

vagal tone, 1. pertaining to the hyperexcitability of the parasympathetic nervous system. 2. pertaining to the inhibitory control of the vagus nerve over heart rate and atrioventricular conduction.

vagina /vəji′nə/ [L, sheath], the part of the female genitalia that forms a canal from the orifice through the vestibule to the uterine cervix. It is behind the bladder and in front of the rectum. The canal is actually a potential space; the walls usually touch. The vagina widens from the vestibule upward and narrows toward the top, forming a curved vault around the protruding cervix. The vagina is lined with mucosa covering a layer of erectile tissue and muscle.

vaginal bleeding, an abnormal condition in which blood is passed from the vagina, other than during the menses. It may be caused by abnormalities of the uterus or cervix. The following terms are commonly used in describing the approximate amount of vaginal bleeding: **heavy vaginal bleeding,** which is greater than heaviest normal menstrual flow; **moderate vaginal bleeding,** which is equal to heaviest normal menstrual flow; **light vaginal bleeding,** which is less than heaviest normal menstrual flow; **vaginal staining,** which is a very light flow of blood barely requiring the use of a sanitary napkin or tampon; **vaginal spotting,** which is the passage vaginally of a few drops of blood; **bloody show,** which is an episode of light vaginal bleeding as often occurs in early labor, during labor, and, particularly, at the time of full dilation of the cervix at the end of the first stage of labor.

vaginal cancer, a malignancy of the vagina occurring rarely as a primary neoplasm and more often as a secondary lesion or extension of vulvar, cervical, endometrial, or ovarian cancer. Clear cell adenocarcinoma occurs in young women exposed in utero to diethylstilbestrol, given to their mothers to prevent abortion. A predisposing factor is cervical carcinoma. Vaginal leukoplakia, erythematosis, erosion, or granulation of the mucosa may prove to be carcinoma in situ. Symptoms of invasive lesions are postmenopausal bleeding, purulent discharge, pain, and dysuria.

vaginal cyst, an abnormal closed sac or pouch in the vaginal tissues.

vaginal discharge, any discharge from the vagina. A clear or pearly white discharge occurs normally. The discharge is largely composed of secretions of the endocervical glands. Inflammatory conditions of the vagina and cervix often cause an increase in the discharge, which may then have a foul odor and cause pruritus of the perineum and external genitalia.

vaginal fornix, a recess in the upper part of the vagina caused by the protrusion of the uterine cervix into the vagina.

vaginal hysterectomy [L *vagina*; Gk *hystera* womb, *ektome* excision], the surgical removal of the uterus through the vagina.

vaginal instillation of medication, the instillation of a medicated cream, a suppository, or a gel into the vagina, usually performed to treat a local infection of the vagina or uterine cervix.

vaginal jelly, a contraceptive product containing a spermicide in a jelly medium. It is usually used in conjunction with a contraceptive diaphragm or cervical cap. Some antimicrobial medications are also supplied in the form of a vaginal jelly.

vaginal speculum, a bivalved instrument, with two opening blades, used for inspection of the vaginal cavity.

vaginal sponge, a contraceptive sponge made of polyurethane and impregnated with the spermicide nonoxynol-9. The sponge is shaped like a mushroom and fits into the upper vagina. It is believed to work in three ways: by releasing spermicide, by absorbing semen, and by blocking the cervical opening.

vaginal spotting, vaginal staining. See vaginal bleeding.

vaginismus /vaj′iniz′məs/ [L *vagina* + *spasmus* spasm], a psychophysiologic genital reaction of women, characterized by intense contraction of the perineal and paravaginal musculature tightly closing the vaginal introitus. It occurs in response to fear of painful intromission before coitus or pelvic examination. Vaginismus is considered abnormal if it occurs in the absence of genital lesions and if it conflicts with a woman's desire to participate in coition or to permit examination, but it may be a normal or physiologic response if painful genital conditions exist or if forcible or premature intromission is anticipated.

vaginitis /vaj′inī′tis/, an inflammation of the vaginal tissues, such as trichomonas vaginitis.

vaginography /vaj′inog′rəfē/, the radiologic examination of the vagina after injection of a radiopaque contrast medium.

vagosympathetic /vā′gōsim′pəthet′ik/ [L *vagus* wandering; Gk *sympathein* to feel with] pertaining to the vagus nerve and the cervical portion of the sympathetic nervous system.

vagotomy /vāgot′əmē/ [L *vagus* wandering, *temnein* to cut], the cutting of certain branches of the vagus nerve, performed with gastric surgery, to reduce the amount of gastric acid secreted and lessen the chance of recurrence of a gastric ulcer. Because peristalsis will be diminished, a pyloroplasty or an anastomosis of the stomach to the jejunum may be done to ensure proper emptying of the stomach.

vagotonus /vā′gətō′nəs/ [L *vagus* + Gk *tonos* tension], an abnormal increase in parasympathetic activity caused by stimulation of the vagus nerve, especially bradycardia with decreased cardiac output, faintness, and syncope.

vagovagal reflex /vā′gōvā′gəl/ [L *vagus* + *vagus*; *reflectere* to bend backward], a stimulation of the vagus nerve by reflex in which irritation of the larynx or the trachea results in slowing of the pulse rate.

vagueness, a communication pattern involving the use of global pronouns and loose associations that lead to ambiguity and confusion in communication.

vagus nerve /vā′gəs/ [L *vagus* wandering, *nervus* nerve], either of the longest pair of cranial nerves essential for speech, swallowing, and the sensibilities and functions of many parts of the body. The vagus nerves communicate through 13 main branches, connecting to four areas in the brain.

vagus pulse, a slow, regular pulse caused by overactivity of the vagus nerve.

valence /vāl′əns/ [L *valere* to be strong] **1.** (in chemistry) a numeric expression of the capability of an element to combine chemically with atoms of hydrogen or their equivalent. A negative valence indicates the number of hydrogen atoms to which one atom of a chemical element can bond. A positive valence indicates the number of hydrogen atoms that one atom of a chemical element can displace. **2.** (in immunology) an expression of the number of antigen-binding sites for one molecule of any given antibody or the number of antibody-binding sites for any given antigen.

valence electron, any of the outermost orbiting electrons of an atom. They are responsible for the bonding of atoms into crystals, molecules, and compounds.

valeric acid /vəler'ik/, an organic acid with a penetrating odor found in the roots of *Valeriana officinalis.*

valgus /val'gəs/ [L, bowlegged], an abnormal position in which a part of a limb is bent or twisted outward, away from the midline, such as the heel of the foot in **talipes valgus.**

validation, an agreement of the listener with certain elements of the patient's communication.

validity, (in research) the extent to which a test measurement or other device measures what it is intended to measure. Kinds of validity include **content, current, construct, face,** and **predictive validity.**

valine (Val) /val'ēn/, an essential amino acid needed for optimal growth in infants and for nitrogen equilibrium in adults.

vallecula /vəlek'yələ/ [L, little valley], any groove or furrow on the surface of an organ or structure. **–vallecular,** *adj.*

vallecula epiglottica, a furrow between the glossoepiglottic folds of each side of the posterior oropharynx.

vallecular dysphagia /vəlek'yələr/, difficulty or pain on swallowing caused by inflammation of the vallecula epiglottica.

valley fever. See **coccidioidomycosis.**

valproic acid /valprō'ik/, an anticonvulsant prescribed to prevent certain types of seizure activity, particularly complex absence and petit mal seizures.

Valsalva maneuver /valsal'vəs/ [Antonio M. Valsalva, Italian surgeon, b. 1666; OFr *maneuvre* work done by hand], any forced expiratory effort against a closed airway, such as when an individual holds the breath and tightens the muscles in a concerted, strenuous effort to move a heavy object or to change position in bed. Most healthy individuals perform Valsalva maneuvers during normal daily activities without any injurious consequences.

Valsalva test [Antonio Valsalva; L *testum* crucible], a method for testing the patency of the eustachian tubes. With mouth and nose kept tightly closed, a forced expiratory effort is made; if the eustachian tubes are open, air will enter into the middle ear cavities.

value [L *valere* to be strong], a personal belief about the worth of a given idea or behavior.

value clarification, a method whereby a person can discover his or her own values by assessing and determining what those personal values are and how they affect personal decision making.

value system, the accepted mode of con-

duct and the set of norms, goals, and values binding any social group.

valve [L *valva* folding door], a natural structure or artificial device in a passage or vessel that prevents reflux of the fluid contents passing through it. **–valvular,** *adj.*

valve of Kerkring. See **circular fold.**

valve of lymphatics, one of the tiny semilunar structures in the vessels and trunks of the lymphatic system that helps regulate the flow of lymph and prevents venous blood from entering the system. There are no valves in the capillaries of the system, but there are many in the collecting vessels.

valvotomy /valvot'əmē/ [L *valva* + Gk *temnein* to cut], the incision into a valve, especially one in the heart, to correct a defect and allow proper opening and closure.

valvular endocarditis /val'vyələr/ [L *valva;* Gk *endon* within, *kardia* heart, *itis*], a form of chronic inflammation of the lining membrane of the heart in which the valves are stenotic or incompetent.

valvular heart disease [L *valva* + AS *hoert;* L *dis* opposite of; Fr *aise* ease], an acquired or congenital disorder of a cardiac valve, characterized by stenosis and obstructed blood flow or by valvular degeneration and regurgitation of blood. Diseases of aortic and mitral valves are most common and may be caused by congenital defects, bacterial endocarditis, syphilis, or, most frequently, rheumatic fever. Valvular dysfunction results in changes in intracardiac pressure and in pulmonary and peripheral circulation. It may lead to cardiac arrhythmia, heart failure, and cardiogenic shock.

valvular regurgitation [L *valva; re, gurgitare* to flow], a circulatory backflow that occurs when the heart contracts and the heart valves fail to close properly, allowing blood to be squeezed back into the atria from the ventricles.

valvular stenosis, a narrowing or constricture of any of the valves of the heart. The condition may result from a congenital defect, or it may be caused by some disease process.

valvulitis /val'vyəli'tis/, an inflammatory condition of a valve, especially a cardiac valve. Inflammatory changes in the aortic, mitral, and tricuspid valves of the heart are caused most commonly by rheumatic fever and less frequently by bacterial endocarditis and syphilis.

valvuloplasty /val'vyələplas'tē/, plastic surgery to repair a heart valve.

VAMP /vamp/, abbreviation for a combination drug regimen, used in the treatment of cancer, containing three antineoplastics (vincristine sulfate, methotrexate, and mercaptopurine) and a glucocorticoid (prednisone).

vanadium (V) /vənā'dē-əm/ [ONorse *Vanadis* (Freya) goddess of fertility], a grayish metallic element. Its atomic number is 23; its atomic weight is 50.942. Absorption of vanadium compounds results in a condition called **vanadiumism,** characterized by anemia, conjunctivitis, pneumonitis, and irritation of the respiratory tract.

van Bogaert's disease /vanbō'gərts/ [Ludo van Bogaert, twentieth-century Belgian physician], a rare familial disorder of lipid metabolism in which the substance cholestanol is deposited in the nervous system, blood, and connective tissue. Persons with the disease develop progressive ataxia and dementia, premature atherosclerosis, cataracts, and xanthomas of the tendons.

vancomycin /van'kōmī'sin/, an antibiotic prescribed in the treatment of infections, particularly staphylococcal infections resistant to other antibiotics.

Van Deemter's equation /vandēm'tərz/, an expression of a gas chromatography relationship between the height equivalent to the theoretic plate (HEPT) and the linear velocity of the carrier gas.

Van de Graaff generator /van'dəgräf'/ [Robert J. Van de Graaff, American physicist, b. 1901], an electrostatic machine in which electronically charged particles build up a high potential on an insulated terminal. The generator is often used to inject particles into a larger accelerator.

van den Bergh's test /van'dənburgs'/ [Albert A. H. van den Bergh, Dutch physician, b. 1869], a test for the presence of bilirubin in the blood serum. Blood is obtained from a patient who has fasted overnight, and the diluted serum is added to diazo reagent. A blue or violet color indicates the presence of bilirubin.

van der Waals forces /van'derwäls', fän-/, weak attractive forces between neutral atoms and molecules. It occurs because a fluctuating dipole moment in one molecule induces a dipole moment in another. The activity accounts for some deviation from Boyle's law at very low temperatures or very high pressures.

vanillylmandelic acid (VMA) /vanil'ilməndel'ik/, a urinary metabolite of epinephrine and norepinephrine. A greater than normal amount of VMA is characteristic of a pheochromocytoma and neuroblastomas.

Van Rensselaer, Euphenia /vanren'səlir/, (1840-1912), an American nurse who designed the first nurses' uniform, a blue and white seersucker dress with collar and cuffs, apron, and cap. She organized the Seton Hospital for Tuberculosis in New York.

vapor bath, the exposure of the body to vapor, such as steam.

vaporization [L *vapor* steam], the changing of a liquid or solid to a gaseous state.

vapor pressure depression, a phenomenon in which the addition of a solute molecule to a solvent will decrease the amount of solvent in equilibrium between the vapor phase and the liquid phase.

variability [L *variare* to diversify], the degree of divergence or ability of an object to vary from a given standard or average.

variable, a factor in an experiment or scientific test that tends to vary, or take on different values, while other elements remain constant.

variable behavior [L *variare* to vary; AS *bihabban* to behave], a response, activity, or action that may be modified by individual experience.

variable interval (VI) reinforcement, reinforcement that is offered after a specific lapse of time.

variable-performance oxygen delivery system. See **low-flow oxygen delivery system.**

variable ratio (VR) reinforcement, reinforcement that requires variable numbers of responses.

variable region, the N-terminal portion of an immunoglobulin polypeptide chain whose amino acid sequence can change. The region includes the antigen combining site.

variance [L *variare*], **1.** (in statistics) a numeric representation of the dispersion of data around the mean in a given sample. It is represented by the square of the standard deviation and is used principally in performing an analysis of variance. **2.** *nontechnical;* the general range of a group of findings.

variant [L *variare*], the differences between individuals of a species or between subpopulations of a species, as phenotypic or genotypic traits of mutants.

variant angina, a variation of angina pectoris, with symptoms of chest pain usually occurring during rest and at night. It is caused by focal spasm of proximal epicardial coronary arteries. An electrocardiogram shows an elevation of the ST segments, as opposed to the ST segment depression usually associated with angina pectoris.

varicella. See **chickenpox.**

varicella-zoster immune globulin (VZIG) /ver'isel'ə zos'tər/ [L *varius* spotted; Gk *zoster* girdle; L *immunis* free from, *globu-*

lus small globe], an immune globulin obtained from the blood of normal persons with high levels of varicella-zoster antibodies. The immune globulin can be administered to persons exposed to chicken pox to prevent or modify symptoms of the infection.

varicella zoster virus (VZV) [L *varius* diverse; Gk *zoster* girdle; L *virus* poison], a member of the herpesvirus family, which causes the diseases varicella (chickenpox) and herpes zoster (shingles). The virus has been isolated from vesicle fluid in chickenpox, is highly contagious, and may be spread by direct contact or droplets. Dried crusts of skin lesions do not contain active virus particles. Herpes zoster is produced by reactivation of latent varicella virus, usually several years after the initial infection.

varicelliform /ver′isel′ifôrm/, resembling the rash of chickenpox.

varices. See **varix.**

varicocele /ver′əkōsēl′/ [L *varix* varicose vein; Gk *kele* tumor], a dilatation of the pampiniform venous complex of the spermatic cord. The varicocele forms a soft, elastic swelling that can cause pain.

varicose /ver′əkōs/ [L *varix*], **1.** (of a vein) exhibiting varicosis, or a varicosity. **2.** abnormally and permanently distended, such as the bulging veins in some individuals.

varicose aneurysm, a blood-filled, saclike projection that connects an artery and one or several veins and that is formed from a localized dilatation of the adjoining vessels.

varicose ulcer. See **stasis ulcer.**

varicose vein, a tortuous, dilated vein with incompetent valves. Causes include congenitally defective valves, thrombophlebitis, pregnancy, and obesity. Varicose veins are common, especially in women. The saphenous veins of the legs are most often affected.

varicosis /ver′ikō′sis/ [L *varix* + Gk *osis* condition], a common condition characterized by one or more tortuous, abnormally dilated, or varicose veins, usually in the legs or the lower trunk. Varicosis may be caused by congenital defects of the valves or walls of the veins or by congestion and increased intraluminal pressure resulting from prolonged standing, poor posture, pregnancy, abdominal tumor, or chronic systemic disease. Symptoms include pain and muscle cramps with a feeling of fullness and heaviness in the legs. Dilatation of superficial veins is often evident before the condition produces discomfort.

varicosity /ver′ikōs′itē/, **1.** an abnormal condition, usually of a vein, characterized by swelling and tortuosity. **2.** a vein in this condition.

variegate /ver′ē·əgāt′/ [L *varius* diverse], having characteristics that vary, especially as to color.

variegate porphyria, an uncommon form of hepatic porphyria, characterized by skin lesions and photosensitivity. The condition may be congenital or acquired.

variola, variola major. See **smallpox.**

variola minor. See **alastrim.**

varioloid /ver′ē·əloid′/ [L *varius* + Gk *eidos* form], **1.** resembling smallpox. **2.** a mild form of smallpox in a vaccinated person or one who has previously had the disease.

varix /ver′iks/, *pl.* **varices** /ver′əsēz/ [L, varicose vein], **1.** a tortuous, dilated vein. **2.** an enlarged, tortuous artery or a distended, twisting lymphatic.

varus /ver′əs/ [L, bent], an abnormal position in which a part of a limb is turned inward toward the midline, such as the heel and foot in **talipes varus.**

vas /vas/, *pl.* **vasa** /vā′sə/ [L, vessel], any one of the many vessels of the body, especially those that convey blood, lymph, or spermatozoa.

vasa vasorum [L *vas* vessel], small blood vessels that supply the walls of the arteries and veins.

vascular /vas′kyələr/ [L *vasculum* little vessel], of or pertaining to a blood vessel.

vascular access device (VAD), an indwelling catheter, cannula, or other instrumentation used to obtain venous or arterial access.

vascular hemophilia. See **von Willebrand's disease.**

vascular insufficiency, inadequate peripheral blood flow caused by occlusion of vessels with atherosclerotic plaques, thrombi, or emboli, by damaged, diseased, or intrinsically weak vascular walls, arteriovenous fistulas, or hematologic hypercoagulability, or by heavy smoking. Signs of vascular insufficiency include pale, cyanotic, or mottled skin over the affected area, swelling of an extremity, absent or reduced tactile sensation, tingling, diminished sense of temperature, muscle pain, such as intermittent claudication in the calf, and, in advanced disease, atrophy of muscles of the involved extremity.

vascularity [L *vasculum*], the state of blood vessel development and functioning in an organ or tissue.

vascularization /vas′kyələr′īzā′shən/, the process by which body tissue becomes vascular and develops proliferating capillaries. It may be natural or may be induced by surgical techniques. **–vascularize,** *v.*

vascular leiomyoma, a neoplasm that is developed from smooth muscle fibers of a blood vessel.

vascular sclerosis [L *vasculum;* Gk *skerosis* hardening], a condition of hyaline degeneration of the blood vessels with hypertrophy of the media and subintimal fibrosis. Along with fibrosis and intimal thickening, there may be weakening and loss of elasticity in the artery walls.

vascular spider. See **spider angioma.**

vasculature /vas'kyələchər/, the distribution of blood vessels in an organ or tissue.

vasculitis /vas'kyəli'tis/, an inflammatory condition of the blood vessels that is characteristic of certain systemic diseases or that is caused by an allergic reaction. Kinds of vasculitis are **allergic vasculitis, necrotizing vasculitis,** and **segmented hyalinizing vasculitis.**

vasculogenic impotence /vas'kyəlōjen'ik/ [L *vasculum* + Gk *genein* to produce; L *in, potentia* power], an inability to perform the male sexual act because of an inadequate supply of arterial blood to the penis.

vasculomotor /vas'kyəlōmō'tər/ [L *vasculum* + *movere* to move], pertaining to the system of controlling constriction and dilatation of blood vessels.

vas deferens /def'ərənz/, *pl.* **vasa deferentia** /def'ərən'shē·ə/ [L *vas* + *deferens* carrying away], the extension of the epididymis of the testis that ascends from the scrotum and joins the seminal vesicle to form the ejaculatory duct.

vasectomy /vasek'təmē/ [L *vas* + Gk *ektome* excision], a procedure for male sterilization involving the bilateral surgical removal of a portion of the vas deferens. Vasectomy is most commonly performed at an outpatient surgery center using local anesthesia.

vasectomy reversal, a surgical procedure for rejoining the sections of the vas deferens previously severed in order to render the male infertile. Reanastomosis success varies from 45% to 60% and in some cases the severed ends of the vas deferens rejoin spontaneously.

vasoactive /vā'zō·ak'tiv/ [L *vas* + *activus* active], (of a drug) tending to cause vasodilation or vasoconstriction.

vasoactive intestinal polypeptide (VIP), a glucagon-secretin hormone found in the pancreas, intestine, and central nervous system. The hormone stimulates insulin and glucagon release. Gastric secretion, gastric motility, and peripheral vasodilation, as well as hyperglycemia by hepatic glycogenolysis are inhibited.

vasoconstriction /vas'ōkənstrik'shən/ [L *vas* + *constrigere* to tighten], narrowing of the lumen of any blood vessel, especially the arterioles and the veins in the blood reservoirs of the skin and the abdominal viscera. It is accomplished by various mechanisms that together control blood pressure and the distribution of blood throughout the body.

vasoconstrictive, able to cause a constriction of blood vessels.

vasoconstrictor [L *vas* + *constrigere*], **1.** of or pertaining to a process, condition, or substance that causes the constriction of blood vessels. **2.** an agent that promotes vasoconstriction. Cold, fear, stress, and nicotine are common exogenous vasoconstrictors. Internally secreted epinephrine and norepinephrine cause blood vessels to contract by stimulating adrenergic receptors of peripheral sympathetic nerves.

vasodepressor syncope. See **vasovagal syncope.**

vasodilation /vas'ōdīla'shən/, an increase in the diameter of a blood vessel caused by inhibition of its constrictor nerves or stimulation of dilator nerves.

vasodilator /vā'zōdī'lātər/ [L *vas* + *dilatare*], **1.** a nerve or agent that causes dilation of blood vessels. **2.** pertaining to the relaxation of the smooth muscle of the vascular system. **3.** producing dilation of blood vessels.

vasogenic shock /vas'ōjen'ik/ [L *vas* + *genein* to produce; Fr *choc*], shock resulting from peripheral vascular dilatation produced by factors, such as toxins, that directly affect the blood vessels.

vasomotor [L *vas* + *movere* to move], of or pertaining to the nerves and muscles that control the caliber of the lumen of the blood vessels. Circularly arranged fibers of the muscles of arteries can contract, causing vasoconstriction, or they can relax, causing vasodilatation.

vasomotor center, a collection of cell bodies in the medulla oblongata of the brain that regulates or modulates blood pressure and cardiac function primarily via the autonomic nervous system.

vasomotor reflex, any reflex response of the circulatory system due to stimulation of vasodilator or vasoconstrictive nerves.

vasomotor rhinitis, chronic rhinitis and nasal obstruction, without allergy or infection, characterized by sneezing, rhinorrhea, nasal obstruction, and vascular engorgement of the mucous membranes of the nose.

vasomotor spasm, an involuntary contraction of the muscles of the small arteries.

vasomotor system, the part of the nervous system that controls the constriction and dilatation of the blood vessels.

vasopressin. See **antidiuretic hormone.**

vasopressor. See **vasoconstrictor.**

vasospasm /vas'ōspaz'əm/, a spasm in a blood vessel.

vasospastic /vas'ōspas'tik/, 1. relating to a spasmodic constriction of a blood vessel. 2. any agent that produces spasms of the blood vessels.

vasospastic angina, an ischemic myocardial chest pain caused by spasms of the coronary arteries. It has features that differ from exertional angina.

vasostimulation /vas'ōstim'yəlā'shən/ [L vas + stimulare to incite], the promotion of vasomotor activity.

vasovagal attack. See **vasovagal syncope.**

vasovagal reflex /vas'ōvā'gəl/, a stimulation of the vagus nerve by reflex in which irritation of the larynx or the trachea results in slowing of the pulse rate.

vasovagal syncope, a sudden loss of consciousness, resulting from cerebral ischemia, secondary to decreased cardiac output, peripheral vasodilation, and bradycardia. The condition may be triggered by pain, fright, or trauma and be accompanied by symptoms of nausea, pallor, and perspiration.

vasovasostomy /vā'zōvəsos'təmē/ [L vas + vas; Gk stoma mouth], a surgical procedure in which the function of the vas deferens on each side of the testes is restored, having been cut and ligated in a preceding vasectomy. The procedure is performed if a man wants to regain his fertility.

vastus intermedius /vas'təs/ [L vastus enormous; inter between, mediare to divide], one of the four muscles of the quadriceps femoris, situated in the center of the thigh. It functions with the other three muscles of the quadriceps to extend the leg.

vastus internus. See **vastus medialis.**

vastus lateralis, the largest of the four muscles of the quadriceps femoris, situated on the lateral side of the thigh. It functions to help extend the leg.

vastus medialis, one of the four muscles of the quadriceps femoris, situated in the medial portion of the thigh. It functions in combination with other parts of the quadriceps femoris to extend the leg.

Vater-Pacini corpuscles /fä'tərpäsē'nē/ [Abraham Vater, German anatomist, b. 1684; Filippo Pacini, Italian anatomist, b. 1812], kinesioceptors located in joint capsules and ligaments.

Vater's ampulla /fä'tərz/ [Abraham Vater, German anatomist, b. 1684; L ampulla

jug], a flask-shaped dilatation at the end of the common bile duct where the duct joins with the duodenum.

VBP, an anticancer drug combination of vinblastine, bleomycin, and cisplatin.

VC, abbreviation for **vital capacity.**

Vco₂, symbol for carbon dioxide output per unit of time.

VD, abbreviation for **venereal disease.**

V deflection (HBE), a deflection on the HIS electrogram that represents ventricular activation.

VDRL, abbreviation for Venereal Disease Research Laboratories.

VDRL test, abbreviation for Venereal Disease Research Laboratory test, a serologic flocculation test for syphilis. It is also positive in other treponemal diseases, such as yaws.

VDT, abbreviation for video display terminal.

V̇e, symbol for expired volume.

VE, symbol for volume expired in 1 minute.

vector [L, carrier], 1. a quantity having direction and magnitude, usually depicted by a straight arrow whose length represents magnitude and whose head represents direction. 2. a carrier, especially one that transmits disease. A **biological vector** is usually an arthropod in which the infecting organism completes part of its life cycle. A **mechanical vector** transmits the infecting organism from one host to another but is not essential to the life cycle of the parasite. 3. a retrovirus that has been modified by alteration of its genetic component. Through recombinant DNA techniques, genes that cause harmful effects are removed and genes that mediate synthesis of essential enzymes are added. The vector can then be injected into a patient who suffers from an enzyme deficiency. –vector, v., vectorial, adj.

vectorcardiogram /vek'tərkär'dē·əgram'/, a tracing of the direction and magnitude of the electrical forces of a heart's activity during a cardiac cycle. It is produced by the simultaneous recording of three standard leads, using an oscilloscope.

vectorcardiography /vek'tərkär'dē·og'rəfē/, a method of recording the magnitude and direction of electrical forces acting on the heart as P-, QRS-, and T-wave vectors, using a continuous loop for each vector.

vecuronium bromide /vek'yərō'nē·əm/, an intravenous neuromuscular blocking drug used as an adjunct to general anesthesia, to facilitate endotracheal intubation, and to relax skeletal muscles during surgery or mechanical ventilation.

VEE, abbreviation for **Venezuelan**

equine encephalitis. See **equine encephalitis.**

vegan. See **strict vegetarian.**

veganism /vej′əniz′əm/ [L *vegetare* to grow, *ismus* practice], the adherence to a strict vegetable diet, with the exclusion of all protein of animal origin.

vegetable albumin, albumin produced in plants.

vegetal pole [L *vegetare* + *polus* pole], the relatively inactive part of the ovum protoplasm where the food yolk is situated, usually opposite the animal pole.

vegetarian /vej′əter′ē·ən/ [L *vegetare*], a person whose diet is restricted to foods of vegetable origin, including fruits, grains, and nuts. Many vegetarians eat eggs and milk products but avoid all animal flesh. Kinds of vegetarians are **lacto-ovo-vegetarian, lacto-vegetarian, ovo-vegetarian,** and *strict vegetarian.*

vegetarianism, the theory or practice of restricting the diet to food substances of vegetable origin.

vegetation, an abnormal growth of tissue around a valve, composed of fibrin, platelets, and bacteria.

vegetative /vej′ətā′tiv/ [L *vegerare*] **1.** of or pertaining to nutrition and growth. **2.** of or pertaining to the plant kingdom. **3.** denoting involuntary function, as produced by the parasympathetic nervous system. **4.** resting, not active; denoting the stage of the cell cycle in which the cell is not replicating. **5.** leading a secluded, dull existence without social or intellectual activity. **6.** (in psychiatry) emotionally withdrawn and passive, as may occur in the depressive phase of bipolar disorder. **–vegetate,** *v.*

vegetative endocarditis, a subacute form of bacterial endocarditis characterized by vegetation on the heart valves. The vegetation may cause ulceration and perforation of the heart valve cusps.

vegetative state, a physical condition in which a previously comatose patient appears to be awake but is unable to communicate or respond to stimuli. The eyes may be open but because of senile brain disease, cerebral arteriosclerosis, or injury to the cerebral cortex the patient remains immobile and must be fed and toileted.

vehicle [L *vehiculum* conveyance], **1.** an inert substance with which a medication is mixed to facilitate measurement and administration or application. **2.** any fluid or structure in the body that passively conveys a stimulus.

Veillonella /vā′yənel′ə/ [Adrien Veillon, French bacteriologist, b. 1864], a genus of gram-negative anaerobic bacteria. The species *Veillonella parvula* is normally present in the alimentary tract, especially in the mouth.

Veillon tube /vāyōn′/, a transparent tube whose ends are closed with removable stoppers, one cotton and one rubber. It is used for the laboratory growth of bacteriologic cultures.

vein [L *vena*], one of the many vessels that convey blood from the capillaries to the heart as part of the pulmonary venous system, the systemic venous network, or the portal venous complex. Most of the veins of the body are systemic veins that convey blood from the whole body (except the lungs) to the right atrium of the heart. Each vein is a macroscopic structure enclosed in three layers of different kinds of tissue homologous with the layers of the heart. Deep veins course through the more internal parts of the body, and superficial veins lie near the surface, where many of them can be seen through the skin. Veins have thinner coatings and are less elastic than arteries and collapse when cut. They also contain semilunar valves at various intervals.

vein ligation and stripping, a surgical procedure consisting of the ligation of the saphenous vein and its removal from groin to ankle.

vein lumen, the central opening through which blood flows in a vein.

vein of Thebesius. See **smallest cardiac vein.**

veins of the vertebral column, the veins that drain the blood from the vertebral column, the adjacent muscles, and the meninges of the spinal cord.

vellus hair. See **lanugo.**

velocity [L *velox* quick], the rate of change in the position of a body moving in a particular direction. Velocity along a straight line is linear velocity. Angular velocity is that of a body in circular motion.

velocity of growth, the rate of growth or change in growth measurements over a period of time.

velocity of ultrasound, the speed of ultrasound energy, measured in meters per second (m/sec), in a particular medium. The velocity varies from 331 m/sec in air to 1,450 m/sec in fat, 1570 m/sec in blood, and 4,080 m/sec in the skull.

velocity spectrum rehabilitation, a rehabilitation program that uses strength training at multiple speeds of movement, from slow to fast.

velopharyngeal insufficiency, an abnormal condition resulting from a congenital defect in the structure of the velopharyngeal sphincter. Closure of the oral cavity beneath the nasal passages is not complete.

Food may be regurgitated through the nose, and speech is impaired.

Velpeau's bandage /velpōz'/ [Alfred A. L. M. Velpeau, French surgeon, b. 1795], a roller bandage that immobilizes the elbow and shoulder by holding the brachium against the side and the flexed forearm on the chest.

vena cava /vē'nə kā'və/, *pl.* **venae cavae** [L *vena* vein; *cavum* cavity], one of two large veins returning blood from the peripheral circulation to the right atrium of the heart. **–vena caval,** *adj.*

vena caval syndrome. See **supine hypotension.**

vena comes /kō'mēz/, *pl.* **venae comites** /kom'itēz/, one of the deep paired veins that accompany the smaller arteries, one on each side of the artery. The three vessels are wrapped together in one sheath.

veneer /vənir'/ [Fr *fournir* to furnish], **1.** (in dentistry) a layer of tooth-colored material, usually porcelain or acrylic, attached to the surface of a crown or artificial tooth by direct fusion. **2.** a thin, tenacious film of calculus found subgingivally that is discolored blue-black.

venepuncture. See **venipuncture.**

venereal /vənir'ē·əl/ [L *Venus* goddess of love], pertaining to or caused by sexual intercourse or genital contact.

venereal bubo [L *Venus;* Gk, *boubon* groin], a swollen, inflamed lymph gland or node, usually in the groin and sometimes purulent. It is associated with a sexually transmitted disease.

venereal disease. See **sexually transmitted disease.**

venereal sore. See **chancre.**

venereal wart. See **condyloma acuminatum, genital wart.**

venereologist /vənir'ē·ol'əjist/ [L *Venus* + Gk *logos* science], a health professional who specializes in the study of the causes and treatments of venereal diseases.

venereology /vənir'ē·ol'əjē/, the study of the causes and treatments of venereal diseases. **–venereologic, venereological,** *adj.*

venerupin poisoning /ven'əroo'pin/, a potentially fatal form of shellfish poisoning that occurs from ingestion of oysters or clams contaminated with venerupin, a toxin that causes impaired liver functioning, GI distress, and leukocytosis. The shellfish toxin occurs in waters around Japan.

venesection. See **phlebotomy.**

Venezuelan equine encephalitis. See **equine encephalitis.**

venipuncture /ven'ipungk'chər/ [L *vena* + *pungere* to prick], a technique in which a vein is punctured transcutaneously by a sharp rigid stylet or cannula carrying a flexible plastic catheter or by a steel needle attached to a syringe or catheter. The purpose of the procedure is to withdraw a specimen of blood, to perform a phlebotomy, to instill a medication, to start an intravenous infusion, or to inject a radiopaque substance for radiologic examination of a part or system of the body.

venogram. See **phlebogram.**

venography. See **phlebography.**

venom [L *venenum* poison], a toxic fluid substance secreted by some snakes, arthropods, and other animals and transmitted by their stings or bites.

venom extract therapy, the administration of antivenin as prophylaxis against the toxic effects of the bite of a specific poisonous snake or spider, or other venomous animal.

venom immunotherapy, the reduction of sensitivity to the bite of a venomous insect or animal by the serial administration of gradually increasing amounts of the specific antigenic substance secreted by the insect or animal.

venospasm /ven'əspaz'əm/, a spasmodic contraction of a vein.

venotomy /vēnot'əmē/, the surgical opening of a vein.

venous /vē'nəs/, of or pertaining to a vein.

venous access device, a catheter designed for continuous access to the venous system. Such devices may be required for long-term parenteral feeding or the administration of IV fluids or medications for a period of several days.

venous blood, dark red blood that has been deoxygenated during passage from the left ventricle through the systemic circulation, en route to the right atrium.

venous blood gas [L *venosus* full of veins; AS *blod;* Gk *chaos* gas], the oxygen and carbon dioxide in venous blood measured by various methods to assess the adequacy of oxygenation and ventilation and to determine the acid-base status. The oxygen tension of venous blood normally averages 40 mm Hg; the dissolved oxygen averages 0.1% by volume, the total oxygen content 15.2%, and the oxygen saturation of venous hemoglobin 75%. The carbon dioxide tension normally averages 46 mm Hg, the dissolved carbon dioxide 2.9% by volume, and the total carbon dioxide content 50%. The normal average pH of venous plasma is 7.37.

venous capillaries [L *vena, capillaris* hairlike], capillaries that terminate in venules.

venous circulation [L *vena, circulare* to go around], the movement of blood from the venules, which drain deoxgenated blood from the cells, through the veins to the vena cava, and from there through the right atrium and ventricle to the pulmonary circulation of the lungs.

venous cutdown, a small surgical incision made in a vein of a patient who has suffered vascular collapse in order to permit the introduction of IV fluids or drugs. A cutdown also may be performed for the insertion of a cannula for the withdrawal of blood.

venous hum, a continuous murmur heard on auscultation over the major veins at the base of the neck, particularly when the patient is anemic, upright, and looking to the contralateral side.

venous insufficiency, an abnormal circulatory condition characterized by decreased return of the venous blood from the legs to the trunk of the body. Edema is usually the first sign of the condition; pain, varicosities, and ulceration may follow.

venous pressure, the stress exerted by circulating blood on the walls of veins; it is elevated in congestive heart failure, acute or chronic constrictive pericarditis, and in venous obstruction caused by a clot or external pressure against a vein. Indications of increased pressure are continued distention of veins on the back of the hand when it is raised above the sternal notch and distention of the neck veins when the individual is sitting with the head elevated 30 to 45 degrees.

venous pulse, the pulse of a vein usually palpated over the internal or external jugular veins in the neck. The pulse in the jugular vein is taken to evaluate the pressure of the pulse and the form of the pressure wave.

venous sinus, one of many sinuses that collect blood from the dura mater and drain it into the internal jugular vein. Each sinus is formed by the separation of the two layers of the dura mater.

venous stasis, a disorder in which the normal flow of blood through a vein is slowed or halted.

venous stasis dermatitis. See **stasis dermatitis.**

venous thrombosis, a condition characterized by the presence of a clot in a vein in which the wall of the vessel is not inflamed. Pain, swelling, and inflammation may follow if the vein is significantly occluded.

ventilate [L *ventilare* to wave], **1.** to provide with fresh air. **2.** to provide the lungs with air from the atmosphere and to aerate or oxygenate blood in the pulmonary capillaries. **3.** (in psychiatry) to open discussion of something, as to ventilate feelings.

ventilation [L *ventilare*], the process by which gases are moved into and out of the lungs. **–ventilatory,** *adj.*

ventilation, inability to sustain spontaneous, a NANDA-accepted diagnosis of a state in which the response pattern of decreased energy reserves results in an individual's inability to maintain breathing adequate to support life. Defining characteristics include dyspnea, increased metabolic and heart rates, increased restlessness and use of accessory muscles, decreased tidal volume, decreased P_{CO_2} level, and increased P_{CO_2} level.

ventilation lung scan, a radiographic examination of the lungs, performed while the patient inhales a radioactive gas as a contrast medium and the lungs are scanned to detect nonfunctional or impaired lung areas or other abnormalities.

ventilation perfusion defect, a disorder in which one or more areas of the lung receive oxygen but no blood, or blood but no oxygen.

ventilation/perfusion (V/Q) ratio, the ratio of pulmonary alveolar ventilation to pulmonary capillary perfusion, both measured quantities being expressed in the same units.

ventilator /ven'tilā'tər/, any of several devices used in respiratory therapy to provide assisted respiration and intensive positive pressure breathing. Kinds of ventilators are **pressure ventilator** and **volume ventilator.**

ventilatory rate /ven'tilətôr'ē/, the volume of air passing through the lungs per minute.

ventilatory standstill, the complete cessation of breathing activity.

ventilatory weaning process, dysfunctional (DVWR), a NANDA-accepted diagnosis of a state in which an individual cannot adjust to lowered levels of mechanical ventilatory support, which interrupts and prolongs the weaning process. DVWR may be classified as mild, moderate, or severe. For severe DVWR, the major defining characteristic is a response to lowered levels of mechanical ventilator support with agitation, deterioration in arterial blood gas levels from current baseline, increase from baseline blood pressure of greater than 20 mm Hg, an increase from baseline heart rate of greater than 20 beats/min, and a significant increase in respiratory rate. Related factors may be physical, such as ineffective airway clearance, or psychologic, such as decreased motivation, or situational, such as an adverse environment.

venting [Fr *vent* breath], (in intravenous therapy) a method for allowing air to enter the vacuum of the intravenous bottle and displace the intravenous solution as it flows out. Glass intravenous bottles are usually equipped with a venting tube attached to the primary IV tubing or to a vent port incorporated with the bottle stopper.

ventral [L *venter* belly], of or pertaining to a position toward the belly of the body; frontward; anterior.

ventral hernia. See **abdominal hernia.**

ventral horn, the anterior columns of the gray matter of the spinal cord.

ventral recumbent, a prone position of lying face down.

ventral root, the anterior or motor division of each spinal nerve.

ventricle /ven′trikəl/ [L *ventriculum* little belly], a small cavity, such as one of the cavities filled with cerebrospinal fluid in the brain, or the right and the left ventricles of the heart.

ventricular /ventrik′yələr/ [L *ventriculum* little belly], of or pertaining to a ventricle.

ventricular aneurysm, a localized dilatation or saccular protrusion in the wall of the left ventricle, occurring most often after a myocardial infarction. Scar tissue is formed in response to the inflammatory changes of the infarction. This tissue weakens the myocardium, allowing its walls to bulge outward when the ventricle contracts.

ventricular bigeminy, a dysrhythmia in which every other beat is caused by a premature ventricular beat.

ventricular block, an obstruction of the flow of cerebraospinal fluid. Causes usually are closure of the foramina of Magendie or Luschka. The condition results in a distention of the brain ventricles because of an increased accumulation of cerebrospinal fluid.

ventricular dysfunction, abnormalities in contraction and wall motion within the ventricles.

ventricular ejection, a forceful expulsion of blood from the ventricles to the main arteries.

ventricular escape, a release of the ventricles from inhibitory control of a sinus or junctional rhythm when the rate of discharges falls below the natural rate of impulse formation of the pacemaker cells in the bundle branches.

ventricular extrasystole, an extrasystole arising from the ventricle.

ventricular fibrillation, a cardiac arrhythmia marked by rapid, disorganized depolarizations of the ventricular myocardium. The condition is characterized by a complete lack of organized electric impulse, conduction, and ventricular contraction. Blood pressure falls to zero, resulting in unconsciousness. Death may occur within 4 minutes. Defibrillation and ventilation must be initiated immediately.

ventricular gallop, an abnormal cardiac rhythm in which a low-pitched extra heart sound (S_3) is heard early in diastole on auscultation of the heart. When it is heard in an older person with heart disease, it indicates myocardial failure.

ventricular gradient, the algebraic sum of the areas within the QRS complex and within the T wave in the electrocardiogram.

ventricular hemiblock, a failure to conduct an impulse down only one division of the left bundle branch, such as an anterior superior or posterior inferior hemiblock.

ventricular hypertrophy [L *ventriculum;* Gk *hyper* excessive, *trophe* nourishment], an abnormal enlargement of the heart ventricles, often caused by hypertension or a valvular disease.

ventricular pacing. See **pacing.**

ventricular remodeling, progressive myocardial ventricular dilation, eccentric hypertrophy, and distortion of left ventricular geometry that persist in the noninfarcted myocardium after a myocardial infarction has healed. It is associated with impaired functional capacity, congestive heart failure, and premature death.

ventricular rhythm, a cardiac dysrhythmia that results when the sinoatrial and the atrioventricular nodes are suppressed or discharge more slowly than the intrinsic rate of the ventricles.

ventricular septal defect (VSD), an abnormal opening in the septum separating the ventricles, permitting blood to flow from the left ventricle to the right ventricle and to recirculate through the pulmonary artery and lungs. It is the most common congenital heart defect.

ventricular septum. See **interventricular septum.**

ventricular systole [L *ventriculum;* Gk *systole* contraction], the contraction of the heart ventricles. It begins with the first heart sound.

ventricular tachycardia, tachycardia of at least three consecutive ventricular complexes with a rate of more than 100 beats/min that usually originates in the ventricular Purkinje system.

ventriculogram /ventrik′yələōgram′/, a radiographic examination of the ventricles of the heart in which contrast medium is injected during cardiac catheterization.

V

ventriculoatrial shunt /ventrik′ oōlō·ā′trē·əl/ [L *ventriculum* + *atrium* hall; ME *shunten*], a surgically created passageway, consisting of plastic tubing and one-way valves, implanted between a cerebral ventricle and the right atrium of the heart to drain excess cerebrospinal fluid from the brain in hydrocephalus.

ventriculocisternostomy /ventrik′ yəlōsis′-təros′təmē/ [L *ventriculum* + *cisterna* vessel; Gk *stoma* mouth], a surgical procedure performed to treat hydrocephalus. An opening is created that allows cerebrospinal fluid to drain through a shunt from the ventricles of the brain into the cisterna magna.

ventriculofallopian tube shunt /ventrik′-yəlōfəlō′pē·ən/, a surgical procedure with limited effectiveness for diverting cerebrospinal fluid into the peritoneal cavity. This procedure is used to correct both the obstructive and the communicating types of hydrocephalus.

ventriculography /ventrik′ yəlog′rəfē/ [L *ventriculum* + *graphein* to record], an x-ray examination of a ventricle of the heart, after injection of a radiopaque contrast medium.

ventriculoperitoneal shunt /ventrik′ yə-lōper′itənē′əl/ [L *ventriculum* + Gk *peri* around, *teinein* to stretch; ME *shunten*], a surgically created passageway, consisting of plastic tubing and one-way valves, between a cerebral ventricle and the peritoneum for the draining of excess cerebrospinal fluid from the brain in hydrocephalus.

ventriculoperitoneostomy /ventrik′ yoō-lōper′itōnēos′təmē/ [L *ventriculum* + Gk *peri* around, *teinein* to stretch, *stoma* mouth], a surgical procedure for temporarily diverting cerebrospinal fluid in hydrocephalus, usually in the newborn. In this procedure, a polyethylene tube is passed from the lateral ventricle subcutaneously down the dorsal spine and is re-inserted into the peritoneal cavity where the diverted fluid is absorbed.

ventriculopleural shunt /ventrik′yəlō-ploōr′əl/ [L *ventriculum* + Gk *pleura* rib; ME *shunten*], a surgical procedure for diverting cerebrospinal fluid from engorged ventricles in hydrocephalus, usually in the newborn. In this procedure, cerebrospinal fluid is diverted from the lateral ventricle into the pleural cavity.

ventriculostomy. See **ventriculocisternostomy.**

ventriculoureterostomy /ventrik′ yoō-dōlōy-ōōrē′təros′təmē/ [L *ventriculum* + Gk *oureter* ureter, *stoma* mouth], a surgical procedure for directing cerebrospinal fluid into the general circulation performed in

the treatment of hydrocephalus, usually in the newborn. In this procedure a polyethylene tube is passed from the lateral ventricle down the dorsal spine subcutaneously to the twelfth rib; the tube is inserted through the paraspinal muscles into a ureter.

Venturi effect /ventoō′rē/ [Giovanni B. Venturi, Italian physicist, b. 1746], a modification of the Bernoulli effect in which there is dilation of a gas passage just beyond an obstruction or restriction. The principle is used in respiratory therapy equipment for mixing medical gases.

Venturi mask, a respiratory therapy face mask designed to allow entrained air to mix with oxygen, which is supplied through a jet at a fixed concentration.

venule /ven′yoōl/ [L *venula* small vein], any one of the small blood vessels that gather blood from the capillary plexuses and anastomose to form the veins. **—venular,** *adj.*

VEP, abbreviation for **visual evoked potential.**

verapamil /verap′əmil/, a slow channel blocker or calcium ion antagonist. It is prescribed for the treatment of vasospastic and effort-associated angina, supraventricular tachycardia, atrial fibrillation, and atrial flutter.

Veratrum /vərā′trəm/ [L, hellebore], a genus of poisonous herbs of the lily family. The dried rhizomes of the British and American hellebore provide alkaloids that are used as antihypertensive agents.

verbal aphasia. See **motor aphasia.**

verbal language [L *verbum* a word; *lingua* tongue], a culturally organized system of vocal sounds that communicates meaning between individuals.

vergence /ver′jəns/, movement of the two eyes in opposite directions.

vermicide /vur′misīd/ [L *vermis* worm, *caedere* to kill], an agent that kills worms, particularly those in the intestine.

vermicular /vərmik′yələr/ [L *vermiculus* small worm], resembling a worm.

vermiform /vur′mifôrm/ [L *vermis* + *forma* form], resembling a worm.

vermiform appendix [L *vermis* + *forma* form; *appendix* appendage], a wormlike, blunt process extending from the cecum. Its length varies from 3 to 6 inches, and its diameter is about ⅓ inch.

vermifuge /vərmify oōj′/ [L *vermis* + *fugare* to chase away], an agent that causes the evacuation of parasitic worms.

vermilion border /vərmil′yən/ [L *vermillium* bright red; OFr *bordure* frame], the external pinkish to red area of the upper and lower lips, extending from the junction of the lips with the surrounding facial skin on the exterior to the labial mucosa within the mouth.

vermin [L *vermis* worm], any insects or small animals regarded as destructive or disease-carrying pests.

vermis /vur′mis/, *pl.* **vermes** [L], **1.** a worm. **2.** a structure resembling a worm, such as the median lobe of the cerebellum. –**vermiform,** *adj.*

vernal conjunctivitis /vur′nəl/ [L *vernare* springlike; *conjunctivus* connecting; Gk *itis* inflammation], a chronic, bilateral form of conjunctivitis, thought to be allergic in origin. Most common symptoms include intense itching and crusting discharge.

Vernet's syndrome /vernāz′/ [Maurice Vernet, French neurologist, b. 1887], a neurologic disorder caused by injury to the ninth, tenth, and eleventh cranial nerves as they pass through the jugular foramen when leaving the skull. The patient experiences dysphagia; the voice is nasal and hoarse; and there may be some loss of taste sensations.

Verneuil's neuroma. See **plexiform neuroma.**

vernix caseosa /vur′niks kas′ē·ō′sə/ [Gk, resin; L *caseus* cheese], a grayish white, cheeselike substance, consisting of sebaceous gland secretions, lanugo, and desquamated epithelial cells, that covers the skin of the fetus and newborn.

verruca /vərōō′kə/ [L, wart], a benign, viral, warty skin lesion with a rough, papillomatous surface. It is caused by a common, contagious papovavirus. –**verrucose, verrucous,** *adj.*

verruca acuminata. See **genital wart.**

verruca plana, a small, slightly elevated, smooth, tan or flesh-colored wart, sometimes occurring in large numbers on the face, neck, back of the hands, wrists, and knees, especially in children.

verruca vulgaris. See **verruca.**

verrucous carcinoma /vərōō′kəs/, a well-differentiated squamous cell neoplasm of soft tissue of the oral cavity, larynx, or genitalia. A slow-growing tumor, it tends to displace rather than invade surrounding tissue; it does not usually metastasize.

verrucous endocarditis [L *verruca;* Gk *endon* within, *kardia* heart, *itis*], a form of heart inflammation characterized by the development of wartlike growths on the heart valves.

verrucous dermatitis, any skin rash with wartlike lesions.

verruga peruana. See **bartonellosis.**

version [L *vertere* to turn], the changing of the position of the fetus in the uterus, usually done to facilitate delivery.

version and extraction, an obstetric operation in which a fetus presenting head first is turned and delivered feet first. It is performed by reaching deeply into the uterus, grasping the feet and pulling them down, and extracting the infant.

vertebra, *pl.* **vertebrae** [L, back joint], any one of the 33 bones of the spinal column, comprising the 7 cervical, 12 thoracic, 5 lumbar, 5 sacral, and 4 coccygeal vertebrae. The vertebrae, with the exception of the first and second cervical vertebrae, are much alike and are composed of a body, an arch, a spinous process for muscle attachment, and pairs of pedicles and processes. The first cervical vertebra is called the atlas and has no vertebral body. The second cervical vertebra is called the axis and forms the pivot on which the atlas rotates, permitting the head to turn. –**vertebral,** *adj.*

vertebral angiography, the diagnostic study of blood circulation in the spinal area after the injunction of radiopaque medium.

vertebral arch, the arch formed on the back of the vertebral body by the pedicles and laminae.

vertebral artery, each of two arteries branching from the subclavian arteries, arising deep in the neck from the cranial and dorsal subclavian surfaces. Each vertebral artery divides into two cervical and five cranial branches, supplying deep neck muscles, the spinal cord and spinal membranes, and the cerebellum.

vertebral body, the weight-supporting, solid central portion of a vertebra. The pedicles of the arch project from its dorsolateral surfaces.

vertebral canal, the passage formed anterior to the vertebral arches and posterior to the vertebral bodies and occupied by the spinal cord.

vertebral column, the flexible structure that forms the longitudinal axis of the skeleton. In the adult, it includes 26 vertebrae arranged in a straight line from the base of the skull to the coccyx. The vertebrae are separated by intervertebral disks. They provide attachment for various muscles, such as the iliocostalis thoracis and the longissimus thoracis, which give the column strength and flexibility. In the adult, the five sacral and four coccygeal vertebrae fuse to form the sacrum and the coccyx. The vertebral canal courses through the vertebral column and contains the spinal cord. The canal is formed by the posterior arches of the vertebrae.

vertebral foramen, the opening between

V

the neural arch and the body of a vertebra through which the spinal cord passes.

vertebral groove, a shallow depression on either side of the spinous processes of the vertebrae, occupied by the deep back muscles.

vertebral notch, either of the concavities on the lower or upper border of a vertebral pedicle.

vertebrate, pertaining to any animal possessing a backbone and thus a member of the subphylum *Vertebrata*. The group includes fish, birds, amphibians, reptiles, and mammals.

vertex [L, summit], **1.** the top of the head; crown. **2.** the apex or highest point of any structure.

vertex presentation, (in obstetrics) a fetal presentation in which the vertex of the fetus is the part nearest to the cervical os and can be expected to be born first.

vertical [L *vertex* summit], perpendicular or at a right angle to the plane of the horizon.

vertical angulation [L *vertex* + *angulus* corner], (in dentistry) the measured angle within the vertical plane at which the central beam of an x-ray is projected relative to a reference in the horizontal or occlusal plane.

vertical coordination, a system of community health nurses who serve as links between their level in the organization and those above and below their level.

vertical diplopia [L *vertex;* Gk *diploos* double, *opsis* vision], a form of double vision in which one image is displaced vertically above the other.

vertical-integrated health care, a health delivery system in which the complete spectrum of care, including financial services, is provided within a single organization, such as a health maintenance organization (HMO).

vertical plane. See **cardinal frontal plane.**

vertical resorption, a pattern of bone loss in which the alveolar bone adjacent to the affected tooth is destroyed without simultaneous crestal loss.

vertical strabismus, a deviation of one eye in a vertical direction from a point of fixation. A common cause is overaction by the inferior oblique muscles, resulting in a quick vertical movement of the eyeball on adduction.

vertical transmission, the transfer of a disease, condition, or trait from one generation to the next, either genetically or congenitally, such as the spread of an infection through breast milk or through the placenta.

verticosubmental /vur′tikō′submen′təl/ [L

vertex + *sub* below, *mentum* chin], a radiographic projection of the head in which the central ray passes from the vertex of the skull through its base.

vertigo. See **dizziness.**

very low-density lipoprotein (VLDL), a plasma protein that is composed chiefly of triglycerides with small amounts of cholesterol, phospholipid, and protein. It transports triglycerides primarily from the liver to peripheral sites in the tissues for use or storage.

vesical /ves′ikəl/ [L *vesica* bladder], pertaining to either the gall bladder or the urinary bladder.

vesical fistula [L *vesica* bladder; *fistula* pipe], an abnormal passage communicating with the urinary bladder.

vesical hematuria [L *vesica;* Gk *haima* blood, *ouron* urine], blood in the urine caused by bleeding in the bladder. The urine is bright red.

vesical sphincter, a circular muscle surrounding the opening of the urinary bladder.

vesicant /ves′ikənt/, a drug capable of causing tissue necrosis when extravasated.

vesicle /ves′ikəl/ [L *vesicula*], a small bladder or blister, such as a small, thin-walled, raised skin lesion containing clear fluid. **–vesicular,** *adj.*

vesicle calculus, a concretion occurring in the bladder.

vesicle reflex, the sensation of a need to urinate when the bladder is moderately distended.

vesicoureteral reflux /ves′ikōyŏŏrē′ərəl/ [L *vesica* + Gk *oureter* ureter; L *refluxus* backflow], an abnormal backflow of urine from the bladder to the ureter, resulting from a congenital defect, obstruction of the outlet of the bladder, or infection of the lower urinary tract. Reflux increases the hydrostatic pressure in the ureters and kidneys. The condition is characterized by abdominal or flank pain, enuresis, pyuria, hematuria, proteinuria, and bacteriuria accompanied by persistent or recurrent urinary tract infections.

vesicouterine /ves′ikōyŏŏ′tərin, -ēn/ [L *vesica* + *uterus* womb], of or pertaining to the bladder and uterus.

vesicula /vəsik′yələ/, a vesicle or small bladder.

vesicular /vesik′yələr/, pertaining to a blisterlike condition.

vesicular appendix, a cystic structure on the fimbriated end of each of the fallopian tubes. It represents a remnant of the mesonephric ducts.

vesicular breath sound, a normal sound of rustling or swishing heard with a stethoscope over the lung periphery, characteristically higher pitched during inspiration and fading rapidly during expiration.

vesicular mole. See **hydatid mole.**

vesicular rale, an abnormal breathing sound heard on auscultation of the chest during inspiration. Rales are discrete bubbling or crackling sounds often associated with pneumonia, pulmonary edema, and tuberculosis.

vesiculitis /vəsik′yəlī′tis/, inflammation of any vesicle, particularly the seminal vesicles.

vesiculography /vəsik′yəlog′rəfē/, the radiologic examination of the seminal vesicles and adjacent structures, usually conducted by injecting a radiopaque medium into the deferent ducts or by catheterization of the medium into the ejaculatory ducts.

vessel [L *vascellum* small vase], any one of the many tubules throughout the body that convey fluids, such as blood and lymph. The main kinds of vessels are the arteries, the veins, and the lymphatic vessels.

vestibular /vestib′yələr/ [L *vestibulum* courtyard], of or pertaining to a vestibule, such as the vestibular portion of the mouth, which lies between the cheeks and the teeth.

vestibular apparatus, the inner ear structures that are associated with balance and position sense. It includes the vestibule and semicircular canals.

vestibular extension. See **vestibuloplasty.**

vestibular function, the sense of balance.

vestibular gland, any one of four small glands, two on each side of the vaginal orifice. The vestibular glands secrete a lubricating substance.

vestibular nerve, a branch of the eighth cranial nerve associated with the sense of equilibrium. It arises in the vestibular ganglion (Scarpa's ganglion) of the ear.

vestibular toxicity, toxic effects (commonly of drugs) on the vestibule of the ear, resulting in dizziness, vertigo, and loss of balance.

vestibular window. See **oval window.**

vestibule /ves′tibyool/ [L *vestibulum* courtyard], a space or a cavity that serves as the entrance to a passageway, such as the vestibule of the vagina or the vestibule of the ear.

vestibule of the ear, the central portion of the inner ear, within the osseous labyrinth, involved with the sensation of position and movement.

vestibulocochlear nerve. See **auditory nerve.**

vestibulo-ocular reflex /vestib′yəlō·ok′-yələr/, a normal reflex in which eye po-

sition compensates for movement of the head. It is induced by excitation of the vestibular apparatus.

vestibuloplasty /vestib′yəlōplas′tē/, plastic surgery of the oral vestibule, particularly modification of the gingival tissues.

vestige /ves′tij/ [L *vestigium* track], an imperfectly developed, relatively useless organ or other structure of the body that had a vital function at an earlier stage of life or in a more primitive form of life. –**vestigial,** *adj.*

veterinarian [L *veterinarius* beasts of burden], a health professional who specializes in the causes and treatment of diseases and disorders of domestic and wild animals.

VF, 1. abbreviation for **ventricular fibrillation. 2.** abbreviation for **vocal fremitus.**

VH, abbreviation for **viral hepatitis.**

VI, abbreviation for *variable interval.* See **variable interval reinforcement.**

via [L, a way], any passage or course, such as the esophagus or trachea.

viable [Fr, likely to live], capable of developing, growing, and otherwise sustaining life, such as a normal human fetus at 24 weeks of gestation. –**viability,** *n.*

viable infant, an infant who at birth weighs at least 500 g or is 24 weeks or more of gestational age.

viability /vīabil′itē/ [L, *vita,* life], the ability to continue living.

vial /vī′əl/, a glass container with a metal-enclosed rubber seal.

vibrating. See **cupping and vibrating.**

vibration /vībrā′shən/ [L *vibrare* to vibrate], a type of massage administered by quick tapping with the fingertips, alternating the fingers in a rhythmic manner, or by a mechanical device.

vibratory, causing vibrations or a state of vibration.

vibratory sense, the ability to perceive vibratory sensations. Vibration receptors in the body are found in a variety of locations, from the skin surface to the membranes covering bones. Some respond only to certain vibration frequencies.

vibrio /vib′rē·ō/ [L *vibrare*], any bacterium that is curved and motile, such as those belonging to the genus *Vibrio.* Cholera and several other epidemic forms of gastroenteritis are caused by members of the genus.

Vibrio cholerae, the species of comma-shaped, motile bacillus that is the cause of cholera.

Vibrio fetus. See *Campylobacter.*

vibrio gastroenteritis, an infectious disease acquired from contaminated seafood

V

and characterized by nausea, vomiting, abdominal pain, and diarrhea, caused by *Vibrio parahaemolyticus.* Headache, mild fever, and bloody stools may also be present.

Vibrio parahaemolyticus /per'əhē'mōl-it'ikəs/, a species of microorganisms of the genus *Vibrio*, the causative agent in food poisoning associated with the ingestion of uncooked or undercooked shellfish, especially crabs and shrimp. Thorough cooking of seafood prevents the infection, which causes watery diarrhea, abdominal cramps, vomiting, headache, chills, and fever.

vicarious menstruation /vīker'ē·əs/ [L *vicarius* substituted; *menstruare* to menstruate], discharge of blood from a site other than the uterus at the time when the menstrual flow is normally expected. Such bleeding is usually caused by the increased capillary permeability that occurs during menstruation.

vidarabine /vider'əbēn/, an antiviral agent used systemically to treat herpes simplex encephalitis and locally to treat herpesvirus I keratoconjunctivitis and keratitis.

vigilance /vij'iləns/ [L *vigil* keep awake], a state of being attentive or alert.

vigil coma /vij'əl/, a semiconscious state of delirium in which the patient may appear awake, with eyes open and staring, and may make verbal sounds.

villi. See **villus.**

villoma /vilō'mə/, *pl.* **villomas, villomata** [L *villus* shaggy hair; Gk *oma* tumor], a villous neoplasm or papilloma, occurring chiefly in the bladder or rectum.

villous adenoma /vil'əs/ [L *villus*], a slow-growing, soft, spongy, potentially malignant papillary growth of the mucosa of the large intestine.

villous carcinoma, an epithelial tumor with many long, velvety papillary outgrowths.

villous papilloma, a benign tumor with long, slender processes, usually occurring in the bladder, breast, or a cerebral ventricle.

villus, *pl.* **villi** [L, shaggy hair], one of the many tiny projections, barely visible to the naked eye, clustered over the entire mucous surface of the small intestine. The villi diffuse and transport fluids and nutrients. Each villus has a core of delicate areolar and reticular connective tissue supporting the epithelium, various capillaries, and usually a single lymphatic lacteal that fills with milky white chyle during the digestion of a fatty meal. **–villous,** *adj.*

vinblastine sulfate /vinblas'tēn, -tin/, an antineoplastic prescribed in the treat-

ment of many neoplastic diseases, such as choriocarcinoma, testicular carcinoma, Hodgkin's disease, and non-Hodgkin's lymphoma.

Vincent's angina, Vincent's infection. See **acute necrotizing gingivitis.**

Vincent's stomatitis [Henri Vincent, French physician, b. 1862; Gk *stoma* mouth, *itis* inflammation], an infection of the mouth.

vincristine sulfate /vinkris'tēn, -tin/, an antineoplastic prescribed in the treatment of many neoplastic diseases, such as leukemia, neuroblastoma, lymphomas, and sarcomas.

vindesine sulfate /vin'dəsēn/, an antineoplastic agent prescribed in the treatment of acute lymphoblastic leukemia, breast cancer, malignant melanoma, lymphosarcoma, and non-small-cell lung carcinoma.

vinegar acid. See **glacial acetic acid.**

violence, high risk for: self-directed or directed at others, a NANDA-accepted nursing diagnosis of a state in which an individual exhibits behaviors that can be physically harmful either to the self or others. Risk factors are complex. Characteristics of clients who are potentially violent include anxiety, fear of the self or other people, lack of verbal ability, complaining or demanding vocalization, provocative, argumentative, or overreactive behavior, poor self-esteem, psychologic depression, a history of self-destructive behavior, pacing, excitement, agitation, or the possession of a weapon.

viosterol /vī·os'tərōl/, synthetic vitamin D_2 in an oil base.

VIP, 1. abbreviation for **vasoactive intestinal polypeptide 2.** abbreviation for *very important person.* A VIP suite in a hospital is one reserved for such persons.

vipoma /vipō'mə/, a type of pancreatic tumor that causes changes in secretion of vasoactive intestinal polypeptide (VIP). VIP causes dilation of blood vessels throughout the body and secretion of fluid and salt in the intestinal tract, resulting in diarrhea.

viral disease. See **viral infection.**

viral dysentery /vī'rəl/, a form of dysentery caused by a virus and usually characterized by an acute watery diarrhea.

viral gastroenteritis, an inflammation of the intestine caused by a virus. The symptoms usually include abdominal cramps, diarrhea, nausea, and vomiting.

viral hepatitis, a viral, inflammatory disease of the liver, caused by one of the hepatitis viruses, A, B, C, or delta. All have chronic forms except hepatitis A. The disease is transmitted sexually and through blood transfusions and is common among persons with behavior risks of HIV infection. Speed of onset, and probable course of the illness vary with the kind and strain of virus, but the characteristics of the disease and its treatment are the same.

viral infection, any of the diseases caused by one of approximately 200 viruses pathogenic to humans. Some are the most communicable and dangerous diseases known; some cause mild and transient conditions that pass virtually unnoticed. If cells are damaged by the viral attack, disease exists. The first step in the cycle, after entry into the body, is the attachment of the virus to a susceptible cell and the cell's adsorption of the virus. This is followed by penetration of the viral nucleic acid into the parasitized cell. The dissembled virus at this point causes no symptoms and cannot be recovered from the cells in infectious form. The virus begins to mature within the cell and, carrying its own genetic information, begins to replicate itself, using chemical building blocks and energy available in the parasitized cell. The virus has now taken over the cell. After a variable period of time, masses of fully grown viruses appear, each able to survive outside the cell until more susceptible cells are found. In many viral diseases, including mumps, smallpox, and measles, one attack confers permanent immunity. In others, immunity is short-lived. The incubation period for viral infection is short, the viruses do not circulate in the bloodstream, antibodies do not form, and, most often, immunity does not develop.

viral keratoconjunctivitis [L *virus;* Gk *keras* horn; L *conjunctivus* connecting; Gk *itis* inflammation], a combination of inflammation of the cornea and conjunctiva caused by a viral infection.

viral pneumonia, pulmonary infection caused by a virus.

Virchow-Robin space. See **perivascular space.**

Virchow's node /fĕr'shōz/ [Rudolf L. K. Virchow, German pathologist, b. 1821], a firm supraclavicular lymph node, particularly on the left side, that is so enlarged it is palpable.

viremia /vīrē'mē·ə/ [L *virus* + Gk *haima* blood], the presence of viruses in the blood.

virile /vir'əl/ [L *virilis* masculine], **1.** of, pertaining to, or characteristic of an adult male; masculine; manly. **2.** possessing or exhibiting masculine strength, vigor, force, or energy. **3.** of or pertaining to the male sexual functions; capable of procreatition. **–virility,** *n.*

virilism /vir'əliz'əm/ [L *virilis* + *ismus*

practice], **1.** pseudohermaphroditism in a female. **2.** premature development of masculine characteristics in the male. Kinds of virilism are **adrenal virilism** and **prosopopilary virilism.**

virilization [L *virilis* + *atus* process], a process in which secondary male sexual characteristics are acquired by a female, usually as the result of adrenal dysfunction or hormonal medication.

virion /vir'ē·on, vī'rē·on/ [L *virus* poison], a rudimentary virus particle with a central nucleoid surrounded by a protein sheath or capsid. The complete nucleocapsid with a nucleic acid core may constitute a complete virus, such as the adenoviruses and the picornaviruses, or it may be surrounded by an envelope, as in the herpesviruses and the myxoviruses.

virocytes /vī'rəsīts/ [L *virus* + Gk *kytos* cell], lymphocytes altered in appearance and in staining that are seen in blood smears from patients with certain viral diseases.

viroid /vī'roid/, a small infective segment of nucleic acid, usually RNA. It is not translated and is replicated by host cell enzymes. Viroids include segments that are complementary to introns and may bind to intron RNA.

virologist /vīrol'əjist, vir-/, a specialist who studies viruses and diseases caused by viruses.

virology /vīrol'əjē, vir-/ [L *virus* + Gk *logos* science], the study of viruses and viral diseases. **–virologic, virological,** *adj.*

virucidal /vī'rəsī'dəl/, pertaining to the destruction of viruses.

virucide [L *virus* + *caedere* to kill], any agent that destroys or inactivates a virus. **–virucidal,** *adj.*

virulence /vir'yŏŏləns/ [L *virulentus* poisonous], the power of a microorganism to produce disease.

virulent /vir'yŏŏlənt/ [L *virulentus*], of or pertaining to a very pathogenic or rapidly progressive condition.

virus [L, poison], a minute parasitic microorganism much smaller than a bacterium that, having no independent metabolic activity, may only replicate within a cell of a living plant or animal host. A virus consists of a core of nucleic acid (DNA or RNA) surrounded by a coat of antigenic protein sometimes surrounded by an envelope of lipoprotein. The virus provides the genetic code for replication, and the host cell provides the necessary energy and raw materials. More than 200 viruses have been identified as capable of causing disease in humans. Some kinds of viruses are **adenovirus, arenavirus, enterovirus,**

herpesvirus, and rhinovirus. –viral, adj.

virustatic /vī′rəstat′ik/, pertaining to the inhibition of the growth and development of viruses, as distinguished from their destruction.

vis [L, force], energy or power.

viscera /vis′ərə/, sing. viscus /vis′kəs/ [L, entrails], the internal organs enclosed within a body cavity, primarily the abdominal organs.

visceral /vis′ərəl/ [L viscus entrails], of or pertaining to the viscera, or internal organs in the abdominal cavity.

visceral afferent fibers, the nerve fibers of the visceral nervous system that receive stimuli and carry impulses toward the central nervous system and share the sensory ganglia of the cerebrospinal nerves with the somatic sensory fibers. Some of the parts of the body with visceral afferents are the face, scalp, nose, mouth, descending colon, lungs, abdomen, and rectum.

visceral cavity, 1. the abdominal cavity containing the viscera. 2. the cavity of any viscus, such as the stomach.

visceral efferent system [L viscus + effere to bear out; Gk systema], the part of the autonomic nervous system that supplies efferent nerve fibers from the central nervous system to the visceral organs.

visceral larva migrans, infestation with parasitic larvae or Toxocara or, occasionally, Ascaris, Strongyloides, or other nematodes.

visceral leishmaniasis. See kala-azar.

visceral lymph node, a small oval nodular gland that filters lymph circulating in the lymphatic vessels of the thoracic, abdominal, and pelvic viscera.

visceral nervous system, the visceral portion of the peripheral nervous system that comprises the whole complex of nerves, fibers, ganglia, and plexuses by which impulses travel from the central nervous system to the viscera and from the viscera to the central nervous system.

visceral pain, abdominal pain caused by any abnormal condition of the viscera. It is characteristically severe, diffuse, and difficult to localize.

visceral pericardium [L viscus; Gk peri around, kardia heart], the surface of the pericardial membrane that is in direct contact with the heart.

visceral peritoneum, one of two portions of the largest serous membrane in the body that invests the viscera. The free surface of the visceral peritoneum is a smooth layer of mesothelium exuding a serous fluid that lubricates the viscera and allows them to glide freely against the wall of the abdominal cavity or over each other.

visceral pleura, the inner layer of pleura that is adjacent to the external lung tissue.

visceral protein status, the amount of protein that is contained in the internal organs.

visceral reflex. See viscerosomatic reaction.

visceral skeleton, the portion of the skeleton, including sternum, ribs, pelvis, and vertebrae, that enclose the viscera.

viscerosomatic reaction /vis′ərō′sōmat′ik/ [L viscus; Gk soma body; L re, agere to act], a muscular response to stimulation of a nerve-receptor organ in a visceral organ.

viscid /vis′id/ [L viscidus sticky], sticky or glutinous. Also viscous /vis′kəs/.

viscosity [L viscosus sticky], a characteristic of a fluid solution relating to its ability to flow. A solution that has high viscosity is relatively thick and flows slowly because of the adhesive effect of adjacent molecules.

viscous /vis′kəs/ [L viscosus sticky], pertaining to something thick, viscid, sticky, or glutinous.

viscous fermentation [L viscosus], the formation of viscous material in milk, urine, and wine by the action of various bacilli.

viscus. See viscera.

visibility [L visibilitas being seen], a condition of being visible under the circumstances of light, distance, and other factors.

visible [L visibilis vision], pertaining to objects that are perceptible to the eye.

visible light [L visus sight; AS leoht], the radiant energy in the electromagnetic spectrum that is visible to the human eye. The wavelengths cover a range of approximately 390 to 780 nm.

visible radiation, electromagnetic radiation in the wavelengths between infrared and ultraviolet that can be perceived by most normal humans.

visible spectrum [L visibilis + spectrum image], the colors of the spectrum that can be observed by most people, from violet at about 4,000 Angstrom units through blue, green, yellow, and orange, to red, at about 6,500 Angstrom units.

vision [L visus], the capacity for sight.

visit [L visitare to see often], 1. a meeting between a practitioner and a client or patient. In the hospital and the home, the practitioner makes a visit to the patient; in the clinic or office the patient makes a visit to the practitioner. 2. (of a patient) to meet a practitioner to obtain professional services or (of a practitioner) to see a patient or client to render a professional service.

visual [L *visus* sight], pertaining to the sense of sight.

visual accommodation, a process by which the eye adjusts and is able to focus, producing a sharp image at various, changing distances from the object seen. The convexity of the anterior surface of the lens may be increased or decreased by contraction or relaxation of the ciliary muscle.

visual acuity [L *visus* + *acuitas* sharpness], **1.** a measure of the resolving power of the eye, particularly with its ability to distinguish letters and numbers at a given distance. **2.** pertaining to the sharpness or clearness of vision.

visual amnesia, an inability to recognize objects, including written words, previously seen.

visual angle, the angle between two lines passing from the extremities of an object looked at, through the nodal point of the eye.

visual aphasia, the inability to understand written language, caused by a lesion in the left visual cortex and the connections between the right visual cortex and the left hemisphere.

visual evoked potential (VEP), an evoked potential elicited by a repeatedly flashing light. High-risk infants are monitored with VEP to evaluate visual function.

visual field defect, one or more spots or defects in the vision that move with the eye, unlike a floater. This fixed defect is usually caused by damage to the retina or visual pathways, such as by chorioretinitis, traumatic injury, macular degeneration, glaucoma, or a vascular occlusion of the eye or the brain.

visual hallucinations, a subjective visual experience in the absence of objective evidence of a corresponding stimulus. Such hallucinations are most likely to be associated with acute organic disorders such as toxic confusional psychoses, delirium, focal brain diseases, and may occur with any stage of schizophrenia.

visualization, an effective means of deepening relaxation and desensitizing a real-life situation that is generally met with stress and tension. The imagery combines positive experiences with actual or perceived negative events or situations in an effort to desensitize the trauma.

visual memory, the ability to create an eidetic image of past visual experiences.

visual-motor coordination, the ability to coordinate vision with the movements of the body or parts of the body.

visual-motor function, the ability to draw or copy forms or to perform constructive tasks.

visual pathway, a pathway over which a visual sensation is transmitted from the retina to the brain. A pathway consists of an optic nerve, the fibers of an optic nerve traveling through or along the sides of the optic chiasm to the lateral geniculate body of the thalamus, and an optic tract terminating in an occipital lobe. Each optic nerve contains fibers from only one retina. The optic chiasm contains fibers from the nasal portions of the retinas of both eyes; these fibers cross to the opposite side of the brain at the optic chiasm.

visual purple. See **rhodopsin.**

vital [L *vita* life], pertaining to or contributing to life forces.

vital capacity (VC) [L *vita* life; *capacitas* breadth], a measurement of the amount of air that can be expelled slowly after a maximum inspiration, representing the greatest possible breathing capacity. The vital capacity equals the inspiratory reserve volume plus the tidal volume plus the expiratory reserve volume.

vital signs, the measurements of pulse rate, respiration rate, and body temperature. Although not strictly a vital sign, blood pressure is also customarily included.

vital stain [L *vita;* OFr *desteindre* to dye], any dye used to impart color to tissues or cells of living organisms.

vital statistics, data relating to births or natality, deaths or mortality, marriages, health, and disease or morbidity.

vitamin [L *vita* + *amine* ammonia], an organic compound essential in small quantities for normal physiologic and metabolic functioning of the body. With few exceptions, vitamins cannot be synthesized by the body and must be obtained from the diet or dietary supplements. No one food contains all the vitamins. Vitamin deficiency diseases produce specific symptoms usually alleviated by the administration of the appropriate vitamin. Vitamins are classified according to their fat or water solubility, their physiologic effects, or their chemical structures, and they are designated by alphabetic letters and chemical or other specific names. The fat-soluble vitamins are A, D, E, and K; the B complex and C vitamins are water soluble.

vitamin A, a fat-soluble, solid terpene alcohol essential for skeletal growth, maintenance of normal mucosal epithelium, and visual acuity. It is derived from various carotenoids, mainly carotene, and is present in leafy green vegetables, yellow fruits and vegetables, the liver oils of the cod and other fish, liver, milk, cheese, butter, and egg yolk. Deficiency leads to at-

V

rophy of epithelial tissue resulting in keratomalacia, xerophthalmia, night blindness, and lessened resistance to infection of mucous membranes.

vitamin A₁, one of the two forms of vitamin A that occur in nature. It is a fat-soluble unsaturated alcohol formed by hydrolysis of beta-carotene, one molecule of which yields two molecules of vitamin A₁. Natural sources include fish-liver oils, butterfat, and egg yolk. The vitamin is needed for healthy vision and skin epithelium. The RDA for adult men is 1,000 RE (retinol equivalents) and, because of average lower body weights, 800 RE for adult women.

vitamin A₂, an alternative form of vitamin A found in the tissues of freshwater fish but not in saltwater fish or mammals. Differences in ultraviolet light absorption spectra are used to distinguish the vitamin A forms.

vitamin B₁. See **thiamine.**

vitamin B₂. See **riboflavin.**

vitamin B₆. See **pyridoxine.**

vitamin B₁₂. See **cyanocobalamin.**

vitamin B₁₇. See **Laetrile.**

vitamin B complex, a group of water-soluble vitamins differing from each other structurally and in their biological effect. All of the B vitamins are found in large quantities in liver and yeast, and they are present separately or in combination in many foods.

vitamin C. See **ascorbic acid.**

vitamin D, a fat-soluble vitamin chemically related to the steroids and essential for the normal formation of bones and teeth and for the absorption of calcium and phosphorus from the GI tract. The natural foods containing vitamin D are of animal origin and include saltwater fish, especially salmon, sardines, and herring; organ meats; fish-liver oils; and egg yolk. Deficiency of the vitamin results in rickets in children, osteomalacia, osteoporosis, and osteodystrophy.

vitamin D₂. See **calciferol.**

vitamin D₃, an antirachitic, white, odorless, crystalline, unsaturated alcohol that is the predominant form of vitamin D of animal origin. It is found in most fish-liver oils, butter, brain, and egg yolk and is formed in the skin, fur, and feathers of animals and birds exposed to sunlight or ultraviolet rays.

vitamin deficiency, a state or condition resulting from the lack of or inability to use one or more vitamins. The symptoms and manifestations of each deficiency vary depending on the specific function of the vitamin in promoting growth and development and maintaining body health.

vitamin D resistant rickets, a disease clinically similar to rickets but resistant to treatment with large doses of vitamin D. It is caused by a congenital defect in renal tubular reabsorption of phosphate and is usually seen in men.

vitamin E, any of the group of fat-soluble vitamins that consist of the tocopherols and are essential for normal reproduction, muscle development, resistance of erythrocytes to hemolysis, and various other biochemical functions. It is an intracellular antioxidant and acts in maintaining the stability of polyunsaturated fatty acids and other fatlike substances, including vitamin A and hormones of the pituitary, adrenal, and sex glands. The richest dietary sources are wheat germ, soybean, cottonseed, peanut, and corn oils, margarine, whole raw seeds and nuts, soybeans, eggs, butter, liver, sweet potatoes, and the leaves of many vegetables.

vitamin H. See **biotin.**

vitamin K, a group of fat-soluble vitamins, known as *quinones,* that are essential for the synthesis of prothrombin in the liver and of several related proteins involved in the clotting of blood. The vitamin is widely distributed in foods, especially leafy green vegetables, pork liver, yogurt, egg yolk, kelp, alfalfa, fish-liver oils, and blackstrap molasses and is synthesized by the bacterial flora of the GI tract. Deficiency results in hypoprothrombinemia, characterized by poor coagulation of the blood and hemorrhage, and usually occurs from inadequate absorption of the vitamin from the GI tract or the inability to use it in the liver.

vitamin K₁, a yellow, viscous, fat-soluble vitamin, occurring naturally, especially in alfalfa, and produced synthetically. It is used as a prothrombinogenic agent.

vitamin K₂, a pale yellow, fat-soluble crystalline vitamin of the vitamin K group that is more unsaturated than vitamin K₁ and slightly less active biologically. It is isolated from putrefied fish meal and synthesized by various bacteria in the GI tract.

vitamin K₃. See **menadione.**

vitamin loss [L *vita + amine*], reduction in vitamin content of food resulting from the handling and preparation of fresh foods, during harvesting, heating, pickling, salting, milling, canning, and other food processing techniques. Further vitamin losses can occur because of digestive disorders that prevent absorption of nutrients and the use of drugs, such as isoniazid, that are vitamin antagonists.

vitaminology /vī'təminol'əjē/ [L *vita, amine* + Gk *logos* science], the study of vitamins, including their structures, modes of action, and function in maintaining the health of the body.

vitamin P. See **bioflavonoid.**

vitellin /vitel´in/ [L *vitellus* yolk], a phosphoprotein containing lecithin, found in the yolk of eggs. **–vitelline** /-ēn/, *adj.*

vitelline artery /vitel´in, vitel´ēn/ [L *vitellus* + Gk *arteria* air pipe], any of the embryonic arteries that circulate blood from the primitive aorta of the early developing embryo to the yolk sac.

vitelline circulation, the circulation of blood and nutrients between the developing embryo and the yolk sac by way of the vitelline arteries and veins.

vitelline duct, (in embryology) the narrow channel connecting the yolk sac with the intestine.

vitelline membrane, the delicate cytoplasmic membrane surrounding the ovum.

vitelline sac. See **yolk sac.**

vitelline sphere. See **morula.**

vitelline vein, any of the embryonic veins that return blood from the yolk sac to the primitive heart of the early developing embryo.

vitellogenesis /vitel´ōjen´əsis/ [L *vitellus* + Gk *genein* to produce], the formation or production of yolk. **–vitellogenetic,** *adj.*

vitellus /vitel´əs, vī-/ [L, yolk], the yolk of an ovum.

vitiligo /vit´ilē´gō/ [L *vitium* blemish], a benign, acquired skin disease of unknown cause, consisting of irregular patches of various sizes totally lacking in pigment and often having hyperpigmented borders. Exposed areas of skin are most often affected. **–vitiliginous,** *adj.*

vitrectomy /vitrek´təmē/ [L *vitreus* glassy; Gk *ektome* excision], a surgical procesure for replacing the contents of the vitreous chamber of the eye.

vitreous /vit´rē·əs/ [L *vitreus* glassy], pertaining to the vitreous body of the eye located in the posterior chamber of the eye.

vitreous body. See **vitreous humor.**

vitreous cavity [L *vitrum* glass; *cavum* cavity], the cavity posterior to the lens that contains the vitreous body and vitreous membrane and is transected by the vestigial remnants of the hyaloid canal.

vitreous degeneration [L *vitreus* glassy, *degenerare* to deviate from kind], a form of hyaline degeneration, the formation of glassy material in the connective tissue of blood vessels and other tissues.

vitreous hemorrhage, a hemorrhage into the vitreous humor of the eye.

vitreous humor, a transparent, semigelatinous substance contained in a thin hyoid membrane filling the cavity behind the crystalline lens of the eye.

vitreous membrane, a membrane that lines the posterior cavity of the eye and surrounds the vitreous body.

vitriol, oil of. See **sulfuric acid.**

vivax malaria. See **tertian malaria.**

viviparous /vivip´ərəs/ [L *vivus* alive, *parere* to bear], bearing living offspring rather than laying eggs, such as most mammals and some fishes and reptiles.

vivisection /viv´əsek´shən/ [L *vivus* + *secare* to cut out], the performance of surgical operations on living animals, particularly experimental surgery for the purpose of research.

VLDL, abbreviation for **very low-density lipoprotein.**

VMA, abbreviation for **vanillylmandelic acid.**

VNA, abbreviation for *Visiting Nurses Association.*

Vo₂, symbol for *oxygen uptake.*

vocal apparatus [L *vocalis* voice, *ad, parare* to prepare], the larynx, pharynx, and oral and nasal cavities involved in the production of sound.

vocal cord [L *vocalis* voice; Gk *chorde* string], either of two strong bands of yellow elastic tissue in the larynx enclosed by membranes called vocal folds and attached ventrally to the angle of the thyroid cartilage and dorsally to the vocal process of the arytenoid cartilage.

vocal cord nodule, a small, inflammatory or fibrous growth that develops on the vocal cords of people who constantly strain their voices.

vocal cues, a category of nonverbal communication that includes all the noises and sounds that are extra-speech sounds.

vocal folds, the true vocal cords.

vocal fremitus, the vibration of the chest wall as a person speaks or sings that allows the person's voice to be heard by the examiner during auscultation of the chest with a stethoscope. Vocal fremitus is decreased in emphysema, pleural effusion, pulmonary edema, or bronchial obstruction.

vocal resonance [L *vocalis; resonare* to sound again], **1.** auscultation. **2.** modification of the laryngeal tone as it passes through the throat and oral cavity so as to produce an increase in the intensity and quality of the sound.

voice, the acoustic component of speech that is normally produced by vibration of the vocal folds of the larynx.

voice box. See **larynx.**

void [ME *voide* empty], to empty, or evacuate, such as urine from the bladder.

voiding urethrography [ME, *voide;* Gk *ourethra, graphein* to record], radiography of the urethra during micturition after the introduction of a radiopaque fluid into the bladder.

vol., abbreviation for **volume.**

vol.%, symbol for *volume percent.*

volar /vō′lər/ [L *vola* palm, sole], of or pertaining to the palm of the hand or the sole of the foot.

volar ligament. See **retinaculum flexorum manus.**

volatile /vol′ətəl/ [L *volatilis* flying], (of a liquid) easily vaporized.

volatile solvent, an easily vaporized solvent.

volition /vōlish′ən/ [L *voluntas* inclination], **1.** the act, power, or state of willing or choosing. **2.** the conscious impulse to perform or to abstain from an act. **–volitional,** *adj.*

volitional tremor, a trembling that begins during voluntary effort, sometimes spreading throughout the body. It may occur in multiple sclerosis and cerebellar disorders.

Volkmann's canal /fōlk′munz/ [Alfred W. Volkmann, German physiologist, b. 1800], any one of the small blood vessel canals connecting haversian canals in bone tissue.

Volkmann's contracture [Richard von Volkmann, German surgeon, b. 1830], a serious, persistent flexion contraction of forearm and hand caused by ischemia. A pressure or crushing injury in the region of the elbow usually precedes this condition, and pressure from a cast or tight bandage about the elbow are common causes.

Volkmann's splint [Richard von Volkmann; AS *splinte* thin board], a splint that supports and immobilizes the lower leg. It has a footpiece attached to two sides that extends from the foot to the knee, allowing ambulation.

volsella forceps /volsel′ə/ [L *vosella* tweezers; *forceps* tongs], a kind of forceps having a small, sharp-pointed hook at the end of each blade.

volt (V) [Count Alessandro Volta, Italian physicist, b. 1745], the unit of electric potential. In an electric circuit a volt is the force required to send 1 ampere of current through 1 ohm of resistance, or the difference in potential between two points on a conductor carrying a charge of 1 ampere when there is a dissipation of 1 watt between them.

voltage [Alessandro Volta], an expression of electrical potential in terms of volts.

voltammetry /voltam′ətər/, the measurement of an electric current as a function of potential.

voltmeter, an instrument, such as a galvanometer, that measures in volts the differences in potential between different points of an electric circuit.

volume [L *volumen* paper roll], the amount of space occupied by a body, expressed in cubic units.

volume (ATPS), abbreviation for *ATPS (ambient temperature, ambient pressure, saturated with water vapor) conditions of a volume of gas.* The conditions exist in a water-sealed spirograph or gasometer when the water temperature equals ambient temperature.

volume (BTPS), abbreviation for *BTPS (body temperature, ambient pressure, saturated with water vapor) conditions of a volume of gas.* For humans, normal respiratory tract temperature is measured at 37° C, the pressure as ambient pressure, and the partial pressure of water vapor at 37° C as 47 torr.

volume control fluid chamber, any one of several types of transparent, plastic reservoirs with graduated volumetric markings, used to regulate the flow of intravenous solutions.

volume dose. See **integral dose.**

volume imaging, MR imaging techniques in which MR signals are gathered from the whole object volume to be imaged at once. Many sequential plane imaging techniques can be generalized to volume imaging, at least in principle.

volumetric analysis. See **quantitative analysis.**

volumetric flow rate, the rate at which a volume of fluid flows past a designated point, usually measured in liters per second.

volume ventilator, a ventilator that delivers a predetermined volume of gas with each cycle.

voluntary [L *voluntas* inclination], referring to an action or thought originated, undertaken, controlled, or accomplished as a result of a person's free will or choice.

voluntary abortion. See **elective abortion.**

voluntary agency, a service agency legally controlled by volunteers rather than by owners or a paid staff.

voluntary hospital system, a nationwide complex of autonomous, self-established, and self-supported private not for profit and investor owned hospitals in the United States.

voluntary muscle. See **striated muscle.**

volunteer [Fr *volontaire*], a person who serves a hospital without pay, augmenting but not replacing paid personnel and professional staff members.

volvulus /vol′vyələs/ [L *volvere* to turn], a twisting of the bowel on itself, causing intestinal obstruction. The condition is frequently the result of a prolapsed segment of mesentery and occurs most often in the ileum, the cecum, or the sigmoid portions of the bowel. If it is not corrected, the obstructed bowel becomes necrotic, and peritonitis and rupture of the bowel occur.

volvulus neonatorum, an intestinal obstruction in a newborn baby resulting from a twisting of the bowel caused by malrotation or nonfixation of the colon. Typical symptoms include abdominal distention, persistent regurgitation, often accompanied by fecal vomiting, and nonpassage of stools.

vomer /vō'mər/ [L, plowshare], the bone forming the posterior and inferior part of the nasal septum and having two surfaces and four borders.

vomit [L *vomere* to throw up], **1.** to expel the contents of the stomach through the esophagus and out of the mouth. **2.** the material expelled.

vomiting, the forcible voluntary or involuntary emptying of the stomach contents through the mouth.

vomiting of pregnancy, vomiting that occurs during the early months of pregnancy. Factors contributing to the condition include delayed stomach emptying during pregnancy, relaxation of the esophageal sphincter at the opening into the stomach, and relaxation of the diaphragmatic hiatus, which increase the risk of gastric reflux.

vomiting reflex. See **reflex emesis.**

vomitus /vom'itəs/ [L *vomere*], pertaining to the material expelled from the stomach during vomiting. Vomitus is sometimes clasified as to color or other appearances as an indicator of the cause of illness, such as a "coffee-ground" vomitus being a clinical sign of peptic ulcers.

VON, abbreviation for *Victorian Order of Nurses.*

von Economo's encephalitis. See **epidemic encephalitis.**

von Gierke's disease /fôngir'kəz/ [Edgar von Gierke, German pathologist, b. 1877], a form of glycogen storage disease in which abnormally large amounts of glycogen are deposited in the liver and kidneys. The disorder is characterized by hypoglycemia, ketoacidosis, and hyperlipemia.

von Hippel-Lindau disease. See **cerebroretinal angiomatosis.**

von Pirquet test. See **Pirquet test.**

von Recklinghausen's disease. See **neurofibromatosis.**

von Recklinghausen's tumor, See **Recklinghausen's tumor.**

von Willebrand's disease [Erick A. von Willebrand, Finnish physician, b. 1870], an inherited disorder characterized by abnormally slow coagulation of the blood and spontaneous epistaxis and gingival bleeding caused by a deficiency of factor VIII.

voracious [L *vorax* to devour], describing a greedy or gluttonous person or animal with an insatiable appetite.

vortex, *pl.* **vortexes, vortices** [L, whirl], a whirlpool effect produced by the whirling of a more or less cylindric mass of fluid (liquid or gas).

vox /voks'/ [L], voice, such as **vox cholerica,** the barely audible, hoarse voice of a patient in an advanced and severe case of cholera.

voxel /vok'səl/, abbreviation for *vo*lume *el*ement, the three-dimensional version of a pi*xel.*

voyeur /voiyur', vô·äyœr'/ [Fr *voir* to see], one whose sexual desire is gratified by the practice of voyeurism.

voyeurism /voi'yəriz'əm, voiyur'izəm/ [Fr *voyeur* + L *ismus* practice], a psychosexual disorder in which a person derives sexual excitement and gratification from looking at the naked bodies and genital organs or observing the sexual acts of others, especially from a secret vantage point.

VP-L-asparaginase, an anticancer drug combination of vincristine, prednisone, and L-asparaginase.

VS, 1. abbreviation for *vesicular sound.* **2.** abbreviation for *Veterinary Surgeon.* **3.** abbreviation for **vital signs. 4.** abbreviation for *volumetric solution.*

VSD, abbreviation for **ventricular septal defect.**

V$_t$, abbreviation for **tidal volume,** the amount of air in milliliters per breath.

vulgaris [L, common people], pertaining to something common or ordinary.

vulnerable [L *vulnus* wound], being in a dangerous position or condition and thereby susceptible to being infected or injured.

vulnerable period, a short period in the cardiac cycle during which activation may result in ectopy. The ventricular vulnerable period corresponds to the apex of the T wave toward its ascending side.

vulnerable population. See **population at risk.**

vulsella forceps. See **volsella forceps.**

vulva. See **pudendum.**

vulvar /vul'vər/, of or pertaining to the vulva.

vulvectomy /vulvek'təmē/ [L *vulva* wrapper; Gk *ektome* excision], the surgical removal of part or all of the tissues of the vulva, performed most frequently in the treatment of malignant or premalignant neoplastic disease. **Simple vulvectomy** includes the removal of the skin of the labia minora, the labia majora, and the clitoris. **Radical vulvectomy** involves excision of the labia majora, labia minora, clitoris, surrounding tissues, and pelvic lymph nodes.

vulvitis /vulvī'tis/, an inflammation of the vulva.

vulvocrural /vul'vōkr $\overline{oo}$'rəl/ [L *vulva* + *crus* leg], of or pertaining to the vulva and the thigh.

vulvovaginal /vul'vōvaj'inəl/ [L *vulva* + *vagina* sheath], of or pertaining to the vulva and the vagina.

vulvovaginitis /vul'vōvaj'inī'tis/, an inflammation of the vulva and vagina, or of the vulvovaginal glands.

vv, 1. abbreviation for *veins*. 2. abbreviation for *vice versa*.

v/v, 1. symbol for *volume of dissolved substance per volume of solvent*. 2. symbol for *volume per volume*.

v/w, symbol for *volume of substance per unit of weight of another component*.

VZIG, abbreviation for **varicella-zoster immune globulin.**

VZV, abbreviation for **varicella zoster virus.**

w, the amount of energy required to ionize a molecule of air, as expressed by w = 33.85 eV/ion pair. This is an important quantity for radiation dosimetry because it allows the extraction of dose from ionization measurements.

W, symbol for the element **tungsten.**

waddling gait [ME *waden* to wade; ONorse *gata* way], a gait observed in patients with progressive muscular dystrophy characterized by exaggerated lateral trunk movements and hip elevations.

Wagner-Meissner corpuscle /wag′nər-mīs′nər/ [Rudolf Wagner, German physiologist, b. 1805; Georg Meissner, German anatomist, b. 1829; L *corpusculum* little body], one of a number of small, special pressure-sensitive sensory end organs in the corium of the hand and foot, the front of the forearm, the skin of the lips, the mucous membrane of the tongue, the palpebral conjunctiva, and the skin of the mammary papilla.

Wagstaffe's fracture /wag′stafs/ [William Wagstaffe, English surgeon, b. 1834; L *fractura* break], a fracture characterized by separation of the internal malleolus.

waking imagined analgesia (WIA) [AS *wacian* to awaken; L *imaginari* to picture oneself; Gk *a, algos* without pain], the pain relief experienced by a patient who employs the psychologic technique, usually with the help of an attending nurse or a hospital aide, of concentrating on previous pleasant personal experiences that produced tranquility. This technique is often effective in reducing mild to moderate pain.

Wald /wôld/, **Lillian** (1867-1940), an American public health nurse, who was instrumental in establishing the school nursing system, the federal government's Children's Bureau, and the Nursing Service Division of the Metropolitan Life Insurance Company. She was the first nurse to be elected into the Hall of Fame for Great Americans.

Waldenström's disease. See **Perthes' disease.**

Waldenström's macroglobulinemia. See **macroglobulinemia.**

Waldeyer's throat ring /wäl′dī·ərz/ [Heinrich W. G. von Waldeyer-Hartz, German anatomist, b. 1836; AS *hring*], the palatine, pharyngeal, and lingual tonsils that encircle the pharynx.

walker [AS *wealcan* to roam], an extremely light, movable apparatus, about waist high, made of metal tubing, used to aid a patient in walking. It has four widely placed, sturdy legs. The patient holds onto the walker and takes a step, then moves the walker forward and takes another step.

walking belt, a leather or nylon device with handles that enables a health care provider to help a patient walk.

walking cast [AS *wealcan* to roam; ONorse *kasta*], a cast that permits a patient to walk. A short-leg walking cast has an attached rubber walker to accept a cast shoe for foot or ankle injuries. A long-leg walking cast covers the leg from the upper thigh to the toes, with an attached rubber sole device called a walker.

walking heel, a plastic or rubber heel placed in the sole of a leg cast to allow weight-bearing.

walking pneumonia. See **mycoplasma pneumonia.**

walking rounds [AS *wealcan* + Fr *rond*], rounds in which the clinician responsible leads a group of junior clinicians on a tour to visit the patients for whom they are collectively responsible.

walking typhoid [AS *wealcan* + Gk *typhos* stupor + *eidos* form], an ambulatory subclinical case of typhoid fever. The person may be infected with typhoid but with mild symptoms that do not interfere with the activities of daily living.

walking wounded [AS *wealcan* + *wund*], a military term for an injured person who is ambulatory.

wall [L *vallum* palisade], a limiting structure within the body, such as the wall of the abdominal, the thoracic, or the pelvic cavities, or the wall of a cell.

wallerian degeneration /waler′ē·ən/ [Augustus V. Waller, English physician, b. 1816; L *degenerare* to degenerate], the fatty degeneration of a nerve fiber after it has been severed from its cell body.

wander [AS *wandrian*], **1.** to move about purposelessly. **2.** to cause to move back and forth in an exploratory manner.

wandering abscess [AS *wandrian*; L *abscedere* to go away], an abscess that moves through tissues openings to a point some distance from its origin.

wandering atrial pacemaker [AS *wandrian*; L *passus;* ME *maken*], a heart arrhythmia caused by the shifting of a pacemaker stimulus site. The site usually moves throughout the atria. The arrhythmia is detected on an ECG as a varying P wave morphology and a P-R interval.

wandering goiter. See **diving goiter.**

wandering rash. See **geographic tongue.**

Wangensteen apparatus /wang′ənstēn/ [Owen H. Wagensteen, American surgeon, b. 1898; L *ad, parare* to prepare], a nasogastroduodenal catheter and a suction apparatus used for constant, gentle drainage and decompression of the stomach or duodenum.

Wangensteen tube [Owen H. Wagensteen], the catheter portion of a Wangensteen apparatus.

ward [AS *weard* guard], a hospital room designed and equipped to house more than four patients.

warfarin poisoning /wôr′fərin/ [Wisconsin Alumni Research Foundation + coumarin], a toxic condition caused by the ingestion of warfarin, accidentally in the form of a rodenticide or by overdose with the substance in its pharmacologic anticoagulant form. The poison accumulates in the body and results in nosebleed, bruising, hematuria, melena, and internal hemorrhage.

warfarin sodium, an anticoagulant prescribed for the prophylaxis and treatment of thrombosis and embolism.

warm-blooded [AS *wearm, blod*], having a relatively high and constant body temperature, such as the temperatures maintained by humans, other mammals, and birds, despite changes in environmental temperatures. Heat is produced in the warm-blooded human body by the catabolism of foods in proportion to the amount of work performed by the tissues in the body. Heat is lost from the body by evaporation, radiation, conduction, and convection. The average temperature of the healthy human is 98.6° F (37° C). The human body's tolerance for change in its temperature is very small, and significant changes can have drastic, even fatal consequences.

war neurosis. See **combat fatigue, shell shock.**

wart. See **verruca.**

Warthin's tumor. See **papillary adenocystoma lymphomatosum.**

washout [AS *wascan* to wash, ME *oute*], the elimination or expulsion of one gas or volatile anesthetic agent by the administration of another.

wasp [L *vespa*], a slender, narrow-waisted hymenopteran insect with two pairs of membranous wings that are folded lengthwise when at rest like parts of a fan. Many species of wasps may give painful stings that may have severe results in hypersensitive persons.

wasted ventilation, the volume of air that ventilates the physiologic dead space in a respiratory system.

waste products [L *vastare* to destroy + *producere*, to produce], the products of metabolic activity after oxygen and nutrients have been supplied to a cell. These include mainly carbon dioxide and water, along with sodium chloride, and soluble nitrogenous salts, which are excreted in feces, urine, and exhaled air.

wasting [L *vastare* to destroy], a process of deterioration marked by weight loss and decreased physical vigor, appetite, mental activity.

watchfulness, continuous supervision provided either openly or unobtrusively as the situation indicates.

water (H_2O) [AS *waeter*], a chemical compound, one molecule of which contains one atom of oxygen and two atoms of hydrogen. Almost three quarters of the earth's surface is covered by water. Essential to life as it exists on this planet, water comprises more than 70% of living things. Pure water freezes at 0° C (32° F) and boils at 100° C (212° F) at sea level.

waterborne, carried by water, such as a waterborne epidemic of typhoid fever.

water-hammer pulse [AS *waeter;* Gk *akme* point; L *pulsare* to beat], a pulse associated with aortic regurgitation. It is characterized by a full, forcible impulse and immediate collapse, causing a jerking sensation.

Waterhouse-Friderichsen syndrome /wô′tərhous′frid′ərik′sən/ [Rupert Waterhouse, English physician, b. 1873; Carl Friderichsen, Danish physician, b. 1886], overwhelming bacteremia, characterized by the sudden onset of fever, cyanosis, petechiae, and collapse from massive bilateral adrenal hemorrhage. The syndrome requires immediate emergency treatment, hospitalization, and intensive care.

water intoxication, an increase in the volume of free water in the body, resulting in dilutional hyponatremia.

water moccasin. See **cottonmouth.**

water pollution, the contamination of lakes, rivers, and streams by industrial or community sources of pollutants.

waters. See **amniotic fluid.**

water trap. See **underwater seal.**

Watson-Crick helix /wŏt′sənkrik′/ [John Dewey Watson, American biologist, b. 1928; Francis H. Crick, English biologist, b. 1916; Gk *helix* coil], a model of the DNA molecule proposed by Watson and Crick as two righthanded polynucleotide chains coiled around the same axis as a double helix. The purine and pyrimidine bases of each strand are on the inside of the double helix and paired according to a Watson-Crick base-pairing rule. Variations in the sequences of the bases determine the genetic information transmitted by the DNA molecule. Watson and Crick received the Nobel Prize in 1962.

watt [James Watt, Scottish engineer, b. 1736], the unit of electric power or work in the meter/kilogram/second system of notation. The watt is the product of the voltage and the amperage. One watt of power is dissipated when a current of 1 ampere flows across a difference in potential of 1 volt.

watt per square centimeter (W/cm²), a unit of power density or intensity used in ultrasonography.

wave [AS *wafian* to fluctuate], a periodic disturbance in which energy moves through a medium without permanently altering the constituents of the medium.

wavelength, the distance between a given point on one wave cycle and the corresponding point on the next successive wave cycle.

wax. See **cerumen.**

wax bath. See **paraffin bath.**

waxy flexibility. See **cerea flexibilitas.**

WBC, abbreviation for **white blood cell.**

wbt, abbreviation for *wet bulb thermometer.*

wc, abbreviation for **wheelchair.**

W chromosome and Z chromosome, the sex chromosomes of certain insects, birds, and fishes. Females of such species are heterogametic and have one W and one Z chromosome, whereas males are homogametic and have two Z chromosomes. The ZZ-ZW system of nomenclature was chosen to differentiate the chromosomes from the XX-XY type, which occurs in humans and various other animals and in which the female is homogametic and the male is heterogametic.

W/cm², abbreviation for **watt per square centimeter.**

W/D, abbreviation for *well developed,* often used in the initial identifying statement in a patient record.

wean [AS *wenian* to accustom], **1.** to induce a child to give up breast feeding and to accept other food in place of breast milk. Many children are ready for wean-

ing during the second half of the first year; some wean themselves. **2.** to withdraw a person from something on which he or she is dependent. **3.** to remove a patient gradually from dependency on mechanical ventilation.

weanling, a child who has recently been weaned.

wear-and-tear theory, a concept of the aging process in which structural and functional changes associated with growing old are accelerated by abuse of the body and retarded with health care.

weaver's bottom [AS *wefan* to weave; *botm* undersurface], a form of bursitis affecting the ischial bursae of the hips of people whose work requires prolonged sitting in one position.

web, a network of fibers forming a tissue or a membrane, such as the laryngeal web that spreads between the vocal cords.

webbed toes [AS *wefan* to weave + *tá*], an abnormality in which the toes are connected by webs of skin.

webbing, skinfolds connecting adjacent structures such as fingers or toes or the neck from the acromion to the mastoid, associated with genetic anomalies.

Weber (Wb), a unit of magnetic flux equal to m^2kg/s^2A.

Weber's tuning fork test, a method of determining if defective hearing in an ear is a conductive loss caused by a middle ear problem or a sensorineural loss. The test is performed by placing the stem of a vibrating tuning fork in the center of the person's forehead or on the maxillary incisors. The loudness of the sound is greater in an ear with a conductive hearing loss.

web of causation, an interrelationship of multiple factors that contribute to the occurrence of a disease.

Wechsler intelligence scales /weks′lər/ [David Wechsler, American psychologist, b. 1896], a series of standardized tests designed to measure the intelligence at several age levels, from preschool through adult, by means of questions that examine general information, arrangement of pictures and objects, vocabulary, memory, reasoning, and other abilities.

wedge fracture [AS *wecg* peg; L *fractura* break], a fracture of vertebral structures with anterior compression.

wedge pressure, the capillary pressure in the left atrium, determined by measuring the pressure in a cardiac catheter wedged in the most distal segment of the pulmonary artery.

wedge resection, the surgical excision of part of an organ, such as a part of an ovary containing a cyst. The segment excised may be wedge-shaped.

W

WEE, abbreviation for **western equine encephalitis.**

weed. See **cannabis.**

weeping [AS *wepan* to cry], **1.** crying, lacrimating. **2.** oozing or exuding fluid, such as a sore or rash.

weeping eczema [AS *wepan* + Gk *ekzein* to boil over], an inflammatory form of skin disease marked by a fluid exudate.

weeping lubrication, a form of hydrostatic lubrication in which the interstitial fluid of hydrated articular cartilage flows onto its surface when a load is applied.

Wegener's granulomatosis /wā'gənərz/ [F. Wegener, twentieth-century German pathologist; L *granulum* little grain; Gk *oma* tumor, *osis* condition], an uncommon, chronic inflammatory process leading to the formation of nodules or tumorlike masses in the air passages, necrotizing vasculitis, and glomerulonephritis. Symptoms, depending on the organs involved, may include sinus pain, a bloody, purulent nasal discharge, saddle-nose deformity, chest discomfort and cough, weakness, anorexia, weight loss, and skin lesions.

weight [AS *gewight*], the force exerted on a body by the gravity of the earth. Weight is sometimes measured in units of force, such as newtons or poundals, but it is usually expressed in pounds or kilograms, as is mass.

weight holder, a metal, T-shaped bar that holds weights for traction.

weightlessness [AS *gewiht;* ME *les*], a state of absence of apparent weight, as in being beyond the effects of gravitational force in space travel.

weight per volume (W/V) solution, the relationship of a solute to a solvent expressed as grams of solute per milliliter of the total solution. An example is 50 g of glucose in 1 L of water, considered a 5% W/V solution, even though it is not a true percent solution.

weights and measures, a system of establishing units or portions of quantities of substances, including standards of mass or volume.

weight traction [AS *gewiht;* L *trahere* to draw], traction applied to a limb or part of a limb by means of a suspended weight.

Weil's disease. See **leptospirosis.**

weismannism /vīs'muniz'əm/ [August F. L. Weismann, German biologist, b. 1834; L *ismus* practice], the basic concepts of heredity and development as proposed by A. Weismann. These state that the vehicle of inheritance is the germ plasm, which is distinct from the somatoplasm, and that acquired characteristics cannot be inherited. **–weismannian,** *adj., n.*

Weiss' sign. See **Chvostek's sign.**

well baby care [AS *wyllan* to wish; ME *babe;* L *garrire* to chatter], periodic health supervision for infants and children to promote optimal physical, emotional, and intellectual growth and development. Such health care measures include routine immunizations to prevent disease, screening procedures for early detection and treatment of illness, and parental guidance and instruction in proper nutrition, accident prevention, and specific care and rearing of the child at various stages of development.

well baby clinic, a clinic that specializes in medical supervision and services for healthy infants.

well-being [AS *wyllan* + *beon* to be], achievement of a good and satisfactory existence as defined by the individual.

well-differentiated lymphocytic malignant lymphoma, a lymphoid neoplasm characterized by the predominance of mature lymphocytes.

Wellen syndrome, in patients with unstable angina, the ECG signs of critical proximal left anterior descending coronary artery stenosis.

wellness, a dynamic state of health in which an individual progresses toward a higher level of functioning, achieving an optimum balance between internal and external environments.

welt [OE *wealtan* to roll], a raised ridge on the skin, usually caused by a blow.

wen. See **pilar cyst.**

Wenckebach heart block. See **Mobitz I heart block.**

Wenckebach periodicity /veng'kəbäk, veng'kəbäkh/ [Karel F. Wenckebach, Dutch-Austrian physician, b. 1864; Gk *peri* around, *hodos* way], a form of second-degree atrioventricular block with a progressive beat-to-beat prolongation of the PR interval, finally resulting in a nonconducting P wave.

Werdnig-Hoffmann disease /verd'nighôf'mun/ [Guido Werdnig, Austrian neurologist, b. 1862; Johann Hoffman, German neurologist, b. 1857], a genetic disorder beginning in infancy or young childhood, characterized by progressive atrophy of the skeletal muscle resulting from degeneration of the cells in the anterior horn of the spinal cord and the motor nuclei in the brainstem. Symptoms include congenital hypotonia, absence of stretch reflexes, flaccid paralysis, especially of the trunk and limbs, lack of sucking ability, fasciculations of the tongue and sometimes of other muscles, and, often, dysphagia.

Werlhof's disease. See **thrombocytopenic purpura.**

Wernicke's center [Karl Wernicke; Gk *kentron* center], a sensory speech center located in the posterior temporal gyrus and adjacent angular gyrus in the dominant hemisphere. Wernicke observed in 1874 that patients with brain damage in that area also suffered a loss of speech comprehension.

Wernicke's encephalopathy /ver'nikēz/ [Karl Wernicke, Polish neurologist, b. 1848], an inflammatory, hemorrhagic, degenerative condition of the brain. The condition is characterized by double vision, involuntary and rapid movements of the eyes, lack of muscular coordination, and decreased mental function, which may be mild or severe. Wernicke's encephalopathy is caused by a thiamine deficiency and is seen in association with chronic alcoholism.

Wernicke's syndrome. See **Wernicke's encephalopathy.**

West African sleeping sickness. See **Gambian trypanosomiasis.**

Westermark's sign, the absence of blood vessel markings beyond the location of a pulmonary embolism as seen on a radiograph.

Western blot test, a laboratory blood test to detect the presence of antibodies to specific antigens. It is regarded as more precise than the enzyme-linked immunosorbent assay (ELISA) and is sometimes used to check the validity of ELISA tests.

western equine encephalitis. See **equine encephalitis.**

West nomogram, a nomogram used in estimating the body surface area.

wet-and-dry-bulb thermometer, an instrument used to measure the relative humidity of the atmosphere. It consists of a thermometer with a bulb that is wet or moist and one that is kept dry. The relative humidity is calculated from difference in readings of the thermometers when water evaporates from the dry bulb, decreasing its temperature.

wet cough. See **productive cough.**

wet dream. See **nocturnal emission.**

wet dressing [AS *waet;* Ofr *dresser* to arrange], a moist dressing used to relieve symptoms of some skin diseases. As the moisture evaporates, it cools and dries the skin, softens dried blood and sera, and stimulates drainage.

wet lung, an abnormal condition of the lungs, characterized by a persistent cough and rales at the lung bases. It occurs in workers exposed to pulmonary irritants.

wet nurse, a woman who cares for and breast-feeds another's infant.

wet pack [AS *waet* moist; ME *pakke*], a therapy that involves wrapping the patient in wet sheets with a top covering of a dry blanket, usually to reduce fever.

wet pleurisy [AS *waet;* Gk *pleuritis*], pleurisy in which the inflammation has progressed to an effusive state, with the fluid having a high specific gravity because of the presence of blood clots and fibrin.

wetting agent, a detergent, such as tyloxapol, used as a mucolytic in respiratory therapy.

W/F, symbol for *white female,* often used in the initial identifying statement in a patient record.

Wharton's jelly /wôr'tanz/ [Thomas Wharton, English anatomist, b. 1614; L *gelare* to congeal], a gelatinous tissue that remains when the embryonic body stalk blends with the yolk sac within the umbilical cord.

wheal /wēl/ [AS *walu* pimple], an individual lesion of urticaria.

wheal and flare reaction [AS *walu* + *flare;* ME *fleare* to blaze up; L *re, agere* to act], a skin eruption that may follow injury or injection of an antigen. It is characterized by swelling and redness due to a release of histamine. The reaction usually occurs in three stages, beginning with appearance of an erythematous area at the site of injury followed by development of a flare surrounding the site, and finally, a wheal forms at the site as fluid leaks under the skin from surrounding capillaries.

wheat weevil disease, a hypersensitivity pneumonitis caused by allergy to weevil particles found in wheat flour.

wheelchair, a mobile chair equipped with large wheels and brakes.

wheeze [AS *hwesan* to hiss], **1.** a form of rhonchus, characterized by a high-pitched musical quality. It is caused by a high-velocity flow of air through a narrowed airway and is heard during both inspiration and expiration. **2.** to breathe with a wheeze.

whiplash injury [ME *whippen, lasshe;* L *ijuria*], *informal;* an injury to the cervical vertebrae or their supporting ligaments and muscles marked by pain and stiffness, usually resulting from sudden acceleration or deceleration, such as in a rear-end car collision that causes violent back and forth movement of the head and neck.

Whipple's disease [George Hoyt Whipple, American pathologist, b. 1878], a rare intestinal disease characterized by severe intestinal malabsorption, steatorrhea, anemia, weight loss, arthritis, and arthralgia. Persons with the disease are severely malnourished and have abdominal pain, chest pain, and a chronic nonproductive cough.

whipworm. See *Trichuris.*

W

whirlpool bath, the immersion of the body or a part of the body in a tank of hot water agitated by a jet of equally hot water and air.

whispered pectoriloquy, the transmission of a whisper through the pulmonary structures so that it is heard as normal audible speech on auscultation.

white blood cell. See leukocyte.

white cell, *informal;* white blood cell.

white corpuscle. See leukocyte.

white damp. See damp.

white fibrocartilage [AS *hwit;* L *fibra* fiber, *cartilago*], a mixture of tough, white fibrous tissue and flexible cartilaginous tissue.

white gold, a gold alloy with a high content of palladium or platinum used in some dental restorations, such as prepared tooth cavities and gold crowns.

whitehead. See milium.

white infarct [AS *hwit;* L *infarcire* to stuff], an infarct that is white because of an absence of blood.

white leg. See phlegmasia alba dolens.

white matter. See white substance.

white radiation, a form of radiation that results from the rapid deceleration of high-speed electrons striking a target, as when the electron beam of a tungsten cathode strikes the tungsten or molybdenum target of the anode in an x-ray tube.

white spots film fault, a defect in a radiograph or a developed photographic film, which appears as scattered white spots throughout the image area.

white substance, the tissue surrounding the gray substance of the spinal cord, consisting mainly of myelinated nerve fibers, but with some unmyelinated nerve fibers, embedded in a spongy network of neuroglia. It is subdivided in each half of the spinal cord into three funiculi: the anterior, the posterior, and the lateral white column. Each column subdivides into tracts that are closely associated in function.

white thrombus, 1. an aggregation of blood platelets, fibrin, clotting factors, and cellular elements containing few or no erythrocytes. 2. a thrombus comprised chiefly of white blood cells. 3. a thrombus composed primarily of blood platelets and fibrin.

whitlow /(h)wit′lō/ [Scan *whick* nail, *flaw* crack], an inflammation of the end of a finger or toe that results in suppuration.

WHO, abbreviation for World Health Organization.

whole blood [AS *hal, blod*], blood that is unmodified except for the presence of an anticoagulant. It is used for transfusion.

whole body hyperthermia. See systemic heating.

wholistic health /hōlis′tik/ [Gk *holos* whole + *ism;* AS *haelth*], a concept that concern for the health of an individual requires a perspective of the individual as an integrated system rather than one or more separate parts.

whoop, a noisy spasm of inspiration that terminates a coughing paroxysm in cases of pertussis. It is caused by a sudden, sharp increase in tension on the vocal cords.

whooping cough. See pertussis.

whorl /wurl, hwurl/ [ME *hwarwy*], a spiral turn, such as one of the turns of the cochlea or of the dermal ridges that form fingerprints.

WIA, abbreviation for waking imagined analgesia.

wick humidifier, a respiratory care device in which a material that absorbs water by capillary action is inserted in the path of the air flow. With the addition of heat, high levels of humidity can be achieved.

Widal's test /vēdäls′/ [Georges F. I. Widal, French physician, b. 1862], an agglutination test used to aid in the diagnosis of salmonella infections, such as typhoid fever.

wide-angle glaucoma. See glaucoma.

Wiedenbach /wē′dənbak/, **Ernestine** (b. 1900), an American nursing educator and writer. She was a leader in family-centered maternity nursing, and developed the full range of the art and science of obstetric nursing.

wild-type gene [AS *wilde* untamed; Gk *typos* mark, *genein* to produce], a normal or standard form of a gene, as contrasted with a mutant form.

will [AS *wyllan*], 1. the mental faculty that enables one consciously to choose or decide on a course of action. 2. the act or process of exercising the power of choice. 3. a wish, desire, or deliberate intention. 4. a disposition or attitude toward another or others. 5. determination or purpose; willfulness. 6. (in law) an expression or declaration of a person's wishes as to the disposition of property, to be performed or take effect after death.

Willis' circle. See circle of Willis.

willow fracture. See greenstick fracture.

Wilms' tumor /vilms/ [Max Wilms, German surgeon, b. 1867], a malignant neoplasm of the kidney, occurring in young children, before the fifth year in 75% of the cases. The most frequent early sign of this large malignant tumor of childhood is hypertension, followed by the appearance of a palpable mass, pain, and hematuria. The tumor, an embryonal adenomyosarcoma, is well encapsulated in the early stage, but it may later extend into lymph nodes and the renal vein or vena cava and metastasize to the lungs or other sites.

Wilson's disease [Samuel A. K. Wilson, English neurologist, b. 1877], a rare, inherited disorder of copper metabolism, in which copper accumulates slowly in the liver and is then released and taken up in other parts of the body. Hemolysis, then hemolytic anemia occur as the copper accumulates in the red blood cells. Accumulation in the brain destroys certain tissue and may cause tremors, muscle rigidity, dysarthria, and dementia. Kidney function is diminished; the liver becomes cirrhotic.

Winckel's disease. See **hemoglobinuria.**

windburn [AS *wind* + *baernan*], a skin disorder caused by exposure to winds.

wind chill /win′chil/, the loss of heat from the body when it is exposed to wind of a given speed at a given temperature and humidity.

wind chill factor [AS *wind* + *cele* cold], the amount of chilling of the body, beyond that due to a cold ambient temperature, because of exposure to cool air currents. The wind chill factor is expressed in degrees Celsius or Fahrenheit as the effective temperature felt by a person exposed to the weather. Because wind chill factors are based on exposure of dry skin to cool air currents, air blowing at the same speed over a wet skin surface would cause additional body heat loss and a greater wind chill.

wind chill index, a chart that compares temperatures of the atmosphere with various wind speeds, enabling one to calculate the windchill factor. The comparison is expressed in kilocalories per hour per square meter of skin surface.

winding sheet, a shroud for wrapping a dead body.

window [AS *wind* air, *owe* eye], a surgically created opening in the surface of a structure or an anatomically occurring opening in the surface or between the chambers of a structure. **2.** a specific time period during which a phenomenon can be observed, a reaction monitored, or a procedure initiated.

windowed, (of an orthopedic cast) having an opening, especially to relieve pressure that may irritate and inflame the skin.

winged scapula [ONorse *vaengr*; L *scapulae* shoulderblades], an abnormal prominence of the scapula caused by either projection of posterior angles of the ribs in a flat chest or paralysis of the serratus anterior muscle.

winter cough [AS *winter, cohhetan*], *nontechnical.* a chronic condition characterized by a persistent cough occasioned by cold weather.

wintergreen oil. See **methyl salicylate.**

winter itch, pruritus occurring in cold weather in people who have dry skin, particularly in those who have atopic dermatitis.

wire suture [AS *wir*; L *sutura*], a stainless steel or silver wire used for uniting bone fracture fragments or in dentistry.

wiry pulse [AS *wir*; L *pulsare* to beat], an abnormal pulse that is strong but small.

wisdom tooth [AS *wisdom, toth*], either of the last teeth on each side of the upper and lower jaw. These are third molars and are the last teeth to erupt, usually between 17 and 21 years of age, often causing considerable pain, dental problems, and the need for extraction.

wish fulfillment [AS *wiscan* to wish; *fullfyllan* to fill full] **1.** the gratification of a desire. **2.** (in psychology) the satisfaction of a desire or the release of emotional tension through such processes as dreams, daydreams, and neurotic symptoms. **3.** (in psychoanalysis) one of the primary motivations for dreams in which an unconscious desire or urge is given expression.

wishful thinking [AS *wiscan* + *thencan* to think], the interpretation of facts or situations according to one's desires or wishes rather than as they exist in reality, usually used as an unconscious device to avoid painful or unpleasant feelings.

Wiskott-Aldrich syndrome /wis′kotôl′-drich/ [Alfred Wiskott, German pediatrician, b. 1898; Robert Anderson Aldrich, American pediatrician, b. 1917], an immunodeficiency disorder inherited as a recessive, X-linked trait, characterized by thrombocytopenia, eczema, inadequate T- and B-cell function, and an increased susceptibility to viral, bacterial, and fungal infections and to cancer.

witch hazel [AS *wican* to bend; Ger *hasel*], **1.** a shrub, *Hamamelis virginiana,* indigenous to North America, from which an astringent extract is derived. **2.** a solution comprised of the extract, alcohol, and water, used as an astringent.

witch's milk, a milklike substance secreted from the breast of the newborn, caused by circulating maternal lactating hormone.

withdrawal [ME *with, drawen* to take away], a common response to physical danger or severe stress characterized by a state of apathy, lethargy, depression, retreat into oneself, and, in grave cases, catatonia and stupor.

withdrawal behavior, the physical or psychologic removal of oneself from a stressor.

withdrawal bleeding, the passage of blood from the uterus, associated with the

W

shedding of endometrium that has been stimulated and maintained by hormonal medication. It occurs when the medication is discontinued.

withdrawal method, a contraceptive technique in coitus wherein the penis is withdrawn from the vagina before ejaculation.

withdrawal reflex. See **flexor withdrawal reflex.**

withdrawal symptoms, the unpleasant, sometimes life-threatening physiologic changes that occur when some drugs are withdrawn after prolonged, regular use.

withdrawal syndrome [ME *withdrawen;* Gk *syn* together + *dromos* course], a physical reaction following cessation or severe reduction in intake of a substance, such as alcohol or opiates, that has been used regularly to induce euphoria, intoxication, or relief from pain or distress. The body tissues become dependent upon the regular reinforcing effect of the chemical so that interruption of the dosage induces an organic mental state characterized by anxiety, restlessness, insomnia, irritability, impaired attention, and, often, physical illness.

withdrawn behavior, a condition in which there is a blunting of the emotions and a lack of social responsiveness.

witness, a person who is present and can testify that he or she has personally observed an event, such as the signing of a will or consent form.

Wittmaack-Ekbom syndrome. See **restless legs syndrome.**

W/M, symbol for *white male,* often used in the initial identifying statement in a patient record.

W/N, symbol for *well nourished,* often used in the initial identifying statement in a patient record.

wobble, an eccentric rotation that permits increased resolution of tomographic imaging devices composed of discrete detector systems.

Wolff-Chaikoff effect /woolf′chīkəf/, the decreased formation and release of thyroid hormone in the presence of an excess of iodine.

wolffian body. See **mesonephros.**

wolffian cyst /wôl′fē-ən/ [Kaspar Friedrich Wolff, German anatomist, b. 1733; Gk *kystis* bag], **1.** a cyst of the wolffian duct. **2.** a cyst of a broad ligament of the uterus.

wolffian duct. See **mesonephric duct.**

Wolff-Parkinson-White syndrome /woolf′pär′kinsən(h)wīt′/ [Louis Wolff, American physician, b. 1898; Sir John Parkinson, English cardiologist, b. 1885; Paul Dudley White, American cardiologist, b.

1886], a disorder of atrioventricular conduction, characterized by two AV conduction pathways.

wolfram. See **tungsten.**

Wolman's disease. See **cholesteryl ester storage disease.**

woman-year [AS *wifman, gear*], (in statistics) 1 year in the reproductive life of a sexually active woman; a unit that represents 12 months of exposure to the risk of pregnancy.

womb. See **uterus.**

wood alcohol. See **methanol.**

Wood's glass [Robert Williams Wood, American physicist, b. 1868; AS *glaes*], a nickel oxide filter that holds back all light except for a few violet rays of the visible spectrum and ultraviolet wavelengths of about 365 nm. It is used extensively to help diagnose fungus infections of the scalp and erythrasma.

Wood's light [Robert Williams Wood; AS *leoht*], an ultraviolet light of about 365-nm wavelength used to diagnose certain scalp and skin diseases. The light causes hairs infected with a fungus, such as *tinea capitis,* to become brilliantly fluorescent.

wood tick [AS *wudu;* ME *tike*], a hard-shelled tick of the *Ioxidae* family and a natural reservoir of *Rickettsia rickettsii.* One species of wood tick, *Dermacentor andersoni,* is the principal vector in western North America of **Rocky Mountain spotted fever,** transmitted by *R. rickettsii.*

wool fat, a fatty substance obtained from sheep's wool and of which lanolin is a common chemical component.

woolsorter's disease [AS *wull;* Fr *sorte;* L *dis* opposite of; Fr *aise* ease], the pulmonary form of anthrax, so named because it is an occupational hazard to those who handle sheep's wool. Early symptoms mimic influenza, but the patient soon develops high fever, respiratory distress, and cyanosis.

word association. See **controlled association.**

word association test. See **association test.**

word blindness [AS *word* + *blind*], an inability to understand written language, a form of receptive aphasia caused by lesions in the parietal or parietal-occipital areas of the brain. The condition may be congenital or acquired as a result of disease or injury.

word salad, a jumble of words and phrases that lacks logical coherence and meaning, often characteristic of disoriented individuals and schizophrenics.

working occlusion [AS *weorc;* L *occludere* to shut], the occlusal contacts of teeth on the side of the jaw toward which the mandible is moved.

working phase, (in psychology) the second stage of the nurse-patient relationship. During this stage patients explore their experiences. Nurses assist patients by helping them to plan courses of action and try out the plans, and to begin to evaluate the effectiveness of their new behavior.

working pressure, (in respiratory therapy) a recommended beginning pressure of about 50 pounds per square inch, gauge (psig) for oxygen or compressed air leaving a cylinder for use in respiratory therapy.

working through, a process by which repressed feelings are released and reintegrated into the personality.

work of worrying, a coping strategy in which inner preparation through worrying increases the level of tolerance for subsequent threats.

work simplification, the utilization of special equipment, ergonomics, functional planning, and behavior modification to reduce the physical and psychologic stresses of home maintenance for disabled persons or their family members.

work therapy [AS *weorc;* Gk *therapeia* treatment], a therapeutic approach in which the client performs a useful activity or learns an occupation, as in occupational therapy.

work tolerance, the kind and amount of work that a physically or mentally ill person can or should perform.

workup, the process of performing a complete evaluation of a patient, including history, physical examination, laboratory tests, and x-ray or other diagnostic procedures to acquire an accurate data base on which a diagnosis and treatment plan may be established.

World Health Organization (WHO), an agency of the United Nations, affiliated with the Food and Agricultural Organization of the UN, the International Atomic Energy Agency, the International Labor Organization, the Pan American Health Organization, and UNESCO. The WHO is primarily concerned with worldwide or regional health problems, but in emergencies it is authorized to render local assistance on request. Its functions include furnishing technical assistance, stimulating and advancing epidemiologic investigation of diseases, recommending health regulations, promoting cooperation among scientific and professional health groups, and providing information and counsel relating to health matters. Its headquarters are in Geneva, Switzerland. Its French name is **Organisation Mondiale de la Santé** /ôr-gänizäsyôN′ môNdē·äl′ dǝlä säNtā′/ **(OMS).**

worm [AS *wyrm*], any of the soft-bodied, elongated invertebrates of the phyla Annelida, Nemathelminthes, or Platyhelminthes. Some kinds of worms parasitic for humans are **hookworm, pinworm,** and **tapeworm.**

wormian bone /vôr′mē·ǝn/ [Olaus Worm, Danish anatomist, b. 1588], any of several tiny, smooth, segmented bones that are soft, moist, and tepid to the touch, usually found as the serrated borders of the sutures between the cranial bones.

worthlessness, a component of low self-esteem, characterized by feelings of uselessness and inability to contribute meaningfully to the well-being of others or to one's environment.

wound [AS *wund*], **1.** any physical injury involving a break in the skin, usually caused by an act or accident rather than by a disease, such as a gunshot wound. **2.** to cause an injury, especially one that breaks the skin.

wound irrigation, the rinsing of a wound or the cavity formed by a wound using a medicated solution, water, or antimicrobial liquid preparation.

wound repair, restoration of the normal structure after an injury, especially of the skin.

Wright's stain [James H. Wright; American pathologist, b. 1869; Fr *teindre* to dye], a stain containing methylene blue and eosin, used to color blood specimens for microscopic examination, as for complete blood count and, particularly, for malarial parasites.

wrinkle test [AS *gewrinclian* to wind; L *testum* crucible], a test for nerve function in the hand by observing the presence of skin wrinkles after the hand has been placed in warm water for 20 to 30 minutes. Denervated skin does not wrinkle.

wrist. See **carpus.**

wrist drop [AS *wrist* + *dropa*], a condition caused by paralysis of the extensor muscles of the hand and fingers or by injury of the radial nerve that results in flexion of the wrist.

wrist joint. See **radiocarpal articulation.**

writer's cramp [AS *writan* to write; *crammian* to fill], a painful involuntary contraction of the muscles of the hand when attempting to write.

wrongful birth [OE *wrang* twisted; ME *burth*], a belief that a birth could have been avoided if the parents had been properly advised by a physician that a pregnancy could occur or that a fetus would be deformed.

wrongful death statute [AS *wrang, death;* L *statuere* to set up], (in law) a statute existing in all states that provides that the death of a person can give rise to a cause of legal action brought by the person's beneficiaries in a civil suit against the person whose willful or negligent acts caused the death.

wrongful life. See **wrongful birth.**

wrongful life action, (in law) a civil suit usually brought against a physician or health facility on the basis of negligence that resulted in the wrongful birth or life of an infant. The parents of the unwanted child seek to obtain payment from the defendant for the medical expenses of pregnancy and delivery, for pain and suffering, and for the education and upbringing of the child.

wryneck. See **torticollis.**

wt., abbreviation for **weight.**

Wuchereria /vōō′kərē′rē·ə/ [Otto Wucherer, German physician, b. 1820], a genus of filarial worms found in warm, humid climates. *Wuchereria bancrofti,* transmitted by mosquitoes, is the cause of elephantiasis.

w/v, abbreviation for **weight per volume.**

w/w, abbreviation for *weight per weight.*

xanthelasma, xanthelasma palpebrarum.
See **xanthoma palpebrarum.**

xanthelasmatosis /zan'thilaz'mətō'sis/ [Gk *xanthos* yellow, *elasma* plate, *osis* condition], a disseminated, generalized form of planar xanthoma frequently associated with reticuloendothelial disorders, especially multiple myeloma.

xanthemia. See **carotenemia.**

xanthene /zan'thēn/ [Gk *xanthos* yellow], a crystalline organic compound in which two benzene rings are fused to a central pyran ring. The pyran oxygen bridges the two benzene rings. It is a parent chemical structure of many medicinal elements.

xanthine /zan'thīn/ [Gk *xanthos* yellow], a nitrogenous byproduct of the metabolism of nucleoproteins. It is normally found in the muscles, liver, spleen, pancreas, and urine. –**xanthic,** *adj.*

xanthine base, a purine compound occurring in plants and animals as a metabolite of adenine and guanine. It is the parent structure of the methyl xanthine akaloids that include caffeine in coffee, theophylline in tea, and theobromine in cocoa.

xanthine derivative, any one of the closely related alkaloids caffeine, theobromine, or theophylline. They are found in plants widely distributed geographically and are variously ingested as components in different beverages, such as coffee, tea, cocoa, and cola drinks. The xanthine derivatives or methyl-xanthines have pharmacologic properties that stimulate the central nervous system, produce diuresis, and relax smooth muscles.

xanthinuria /zan'thinyŏŏr'ē·ə/ [Gk *xanthos* + *ouron* urine], **1.** the presence of excessive quantities of xanthine in the urine. **2.** a rare disorder of purine metabolism, resulting in the excretion of large amounts of xanthine in the urine because of the absence of an enzyme, xanthine oxidase, that is necessary in xanthine metabolism.

xanthochromia /zan'thəkrō'mē·ə/, a yellow or straw-colored substance in cerebrospinal fluid. It is caused by the presence of hemoglobin breakdown products.

xanthochromic /zan'thəkrō'mik/ [Gk *xanthos* + *chroma* color], having a yellowish color, such as cerebrospinal fluid that contains blood or bile.

xanthogranuloma /zan'thəgran'y ŏŏlō'mə/, *pl.* **xanthogranulomas, xanthogranulomata** [Gk *xanthos* + L *granulum* little grain; Gk *oma* tumor], a tumor or nodule of granulation tissue containing lipid deposits. A kind of xanthogranuloma is **juvenile xanthogranuloma.**

xanthoma /zanthō'mə/, *pl.* **xanthomas, xanthomata** [Gk *xanthos* + *oma* tumor], a benign, fatty, yellowish plaque, nodule, or tumor that develops in the subcutaneous layer of skin, often around tendons.

xanthoma disseminatum, a benign, chronic condition in which small orange or brown papules and nodules develop on many body surfaces.

xanthoma eruptivum. See **eruptive xanthoma.**

xanthoma multiplex. See **xanthoma disseminatum.**

xanthoma palpebrarum, a soft, yellow spot or plaque usually occurring in groups on the eyelids.

xanthoma planum. See **planar xanthoma.**

xanthomasarcoma /zan'thōməsärkō'mə/, *pl.* **xanthomasarcomas, xanthomasarcomata,** [Gk *xanthos, oma* + *sarx* flesh, *oma* tumor] a giant cell sarcoma of the tendon sheaths and aponeuroses that contains xanthoma cells.

xanthoma striatum palmare, a yellow or orange flat plaque or slightly raised nodule occurring in groups on the palms of the hands.

xanthoma tendinosum, a yellow or orange elevated or flat, round papule or nodule occurring in clusters on tendons, especially the extensor tendons of the hands and feet, of individuals with hereditary lipid storage disease.

xanthomatosis /zan'thōmətō'sis/ [Gk *xanthos, oma* + *osis* condition], an abnormal condition in which there are deposits of yellowish fatty material in the skin, internal organs, and reticuloendothelial system.

xanthoma tuberosum, a yellow or orange, flat or elevated, round papule occurring in clusters on the skin of joints, espe-

X

cially the elbows and knees, usually in people who have a hereditary lipid storage disease.

xanthopsia /zanthop′sē·ə/ [Gk *xanthos* + *opsis* sight], an abnormal visual condition in which everything appears to have a yellow hue.

xanthosis /zanthō′sis/ [Gk *xanthos* + *osis* condition] **1.** a yellowish discoloration sometimes seen in degenerating tissues of malignant diseases. **2.** a reversible yellow discoloration of the skin most commonly caused by the ingestion of large amounts of yellow vegetables containing carotene pigment.

xanthureic acid /zanth′yŏŏrē′ik/, a metabolite of tryptophan that occurs in normal urine and in elevated levels in patients with vitamin B_6 deficiency.

X chromosome, a sex chromosome that in humans and many other species is present in both sexes, appearing singly in the cells of normal males and in duplicate in the cells of normal females. The chromosome is carried as a sex determinant by all of the female gametes and one half of all male gametes.

Xe, symbol for the element **xenon.**

xenobiotic /zen′ōbī·ot′ik/ [Gk *xenos* stranger, *bios* life], pertaining to organic substances that are foreign to the body, such as drugs or organic poisons.

xenogeneic /zen′ōjənē′ik/ [Gk *xenos* + *genein* to produce], **1.** (in genetics) denoting individuals or cell types from different species and different genotypes. **2.** (in transplantation biology) denoting tissues from different species that are therefore antigenically dissimilar.

xenogenesis /zen′əjen′əsis/ **1.** alternation of traits in successive generations; heterogenesis. **2.** the theoretic production of offspring that are totally different from both of the parents. –**xenogenetic, xenogenic,** *adj.*

xenograft /zen′əgraft′/ [Gk *xenos* + *graphion* stylus], tissue from another species used as a temporary graft in certain cases, as in treating a severely burned patient when sufficient tissue from the patient or from a tissue bank is not available.

xenon (Xe) /zen′on, zē′non/ [Gk *xenos* stranger], an inert, gaseous, nonmetallic element. Its atomic number is 54; its atomic weight is 131.30.

xenon-133, a radioactive isotope of an inert colorless gas used in radiographic studies of the lung.

xenophobia /zen′əfō′bē·ə/ [Gk *xenos* + *phobos* fear], an anxiety disorder characterized by a pervasive, irrational fear or uneasiness in the presence of strangers, es-

pecially foreigners, or in new surroundings.

xeroderma /zir′ədur′mə/ [Gk *xeros* dry, *derma* skin], a chronic skin condition characterized by dryness and roughness.

xeroderma pigmentosum (XP), a rare, inherited skin disease characterized by extreme sensitivity to ultraviolet light, exposure to which results in freckles, telangiectases, keratoses, papillomas, carcinoma, and, possibly, melanoma. Keratitis and tumors developing on the eyelids and cornea may result in blindness.

xerogram /zir′əgram′/ [Gk *xeros* + *gramma* record], an x-ray image produced by xerography.

xerography /zirog′rəfē/ [Gk *xeros* + *graphein* to record], a dry radiologic process in which an image is made on a metal plate coated with powdered selenium.

xeromammogram, a type of breast radiograph.

xeromammography, the use of xerographic methods to produce radiographic images of the breasts.

xerophthalmia /zir′ofthal′mē·ə/ [Gk *xeros* + *ophthalmos* eye], a condition of dry and lusterless corneas and conjunctival areas, usually the result of vitamin A deficiency and associated with night blindness.

xeroradiography /zir′rā′dē·og′rəfē/ [Gk *xeros* + L *radiare* to shine; Gk *graphein* to record], a diagnostic x-ray technique in which an image is produced electrically rather than chemically, permitting lower exposure times and radiation of lower energy than that of ordinary x-rays. The latent image is made visible with a powder toner similar to that used in a copying machine. Xeroradiography is used primarily for mammography.

xerosis. See **dry skin.**

xerotic keratitis /zirot′ik/ [Gk *xeros* + *keras* horn, *itis*], an inflammation of the cornea caused by dryness of the conjunctiva. Underlying causes may be malnutrition, a deficiency of vitamin A, or autoimmune diseases.

xerostomia /zirostrō′mēə/ [Gk *xeros* + *stoma* mouth], dryness of the mouth caused by cessation of normal salivary secretion. The condition is a symptom of various diseases, such as diabetes, acute infections, hysteria, and Sjögren's syndrome, and can be caused by paralysis of facial nerves.

Xi /zi, si/, Ξ ξ, the fourteenth letter of the Greek alphabet.

X-inactivation theory. See **Lyon hypothesis.**

xiphisternal articulation /zif′istur′nəl/

[Gk *xiphos* sword, *sternon* chest; L *articularis* pertaining to joints], the cartilaginous connection between the xiphoid process and the body of the sternum.

xiphisternum. See **xiphoid process.**

xiphoid /zif′oid/ [Gk *xiphos* sword, *eidos* form], shaped like a sword; the xiphoid process of the sternum.

xiphoid process /zif′oid/ [Gk *xiphos* + *eidos* form; L *processus* going forth], the smallest of three parts of the sternum, articulating caudally with the body of the sternum and laterally with the seventh rib.

X-linked, pertaining to genes or to the characteristics or conditions they transmit that are carried on the X chromosome. Women may inherit the genes, but the recessive effects are usually masked by the normal dominant alleles carried on the second X chromosome. **–X-linkage,** *n.*

X-linked disorders, diseases and disorders associated with genetic abnormalities on the X chromosomes. Examples are the muscular dystrophies and hemophilias.

X-linked dominant inheritance, a pattern of inheritance in which the transmission of a dominant gene on the X chromosome causes a characteristic to be manifested. Affected individuals all have an affected parent. All of the daughters of an affected male are affected but none of the sons. One half of the sons and one half of the daughters of an affected female are affected.

X-linked ichthyosis. See **sex-linked ichthyosis.**

X-linked inheritance, a pattern of inheritance in which the transmission of traits varies according to the sex of the person, because the genes on the X chromosome have no counterparts on the Y chromosome. The inheritance pattern may be recessive or dominant. Kinds of X-linked inheritance are **X-linked dominant inheritance** and **X-linked recessive inheritance.**

X-linked mucopolysaccharidosis. See **Hunter's syndrome.**

X-linked recessive inheritance, a pattern of inheritance in which transmission of an abnormal recessive gene on the X chromosome results in a carrier state in females and characteristics of the condition in males.

XO, (in genetics) the designation for the presence of only one sex chromosome; either the X or Y chromosome is missing so that each cell is monosomic and contains a total of 45 chromosomes.

XP, abbreviation for **xeroderma pigmentosum.**

x radiation [*X*, an unknown quantity], radiation of electromagnetic energy in the wavelengths of 10^{-8} meters, longer than gamma rays but shorter than ultraviolet rays.

x-ray, 1. electromagnetic radiation of shorter wavelength than visible light. X-rays are produced when electrons, traveling at high speed, strike certain materials, such as tungsten. They can penetrate most substances and are used to investigate the integrity of certain structures, to therapeutically destroy diseased tissue, and to make photographic images for diagnostic purposes, as in radiography and fluoroscopy. **Discrete x-rays** are those with precisely fixed energies that are characteristic of differences between electron-binding energies of a particular element. **2.** a radiograph made by projecting x-rays through organs or structures of the body onto a photographic plate. **3.** to make a radiograph. **–x-ray,** *adj.*

x-ray dermatitis, a skin inflammation caused by exposure to x-rays. Excessive exposure to x-rays can lead to skin cancer.

x-ray fluoroscopy, real-time imaging using an x-ray source that projects through the patient onto a fluorescent screen or image intensifier.

x-ray microscope, a microscope that produces images by x-rays and records them on fine-grain film or projects them as enlargements.

x-ray pelvimetry, a radiographic examination used to determine the dimensions of the bony pelvis of a pregnant woman and, if possible, the biparietal diameter of her baby's head. It is performed when there is doubt that the head can pass safely through the pelvis in labor.

x-ray technician. See **radiologic technologist.**

x-ray tube, a large vacuum tube containing a tungsten filament cathode and an anode that often is a rotating tungsten disk. When heated to incandescence, the cathode emits a cloud of electrons that produce x-rays when they strike the surface of the anode at high speed. The anode is designed to deflect the x-rays toward a focal spot in the object being radiographed.

X-tra densities, images on x-ray film caused by the presence of foreign objects, such as bullets or surgical clips, in the patient's body.

XX /ekseks′/, (in genetics) the designation for the normal sex chromosome complement in the human female.

XXX syndrome /trip′əliks/, a human sex chromosomal aberration characterized by the presence of three X chromosomes and two Barr bodies instead of the normal XX complement, so that somatic cells contain a total of 47 chromosomes.

XXXX, XXXXX /fôreks', fīveks'/, (in genetics) the designation for an abnormal sex chromosome complement in the human female in which there are, respectively, four or five instead of the normal two X chromosomes so that each somatic cell contains a total of 48 or 49 chromosomes.

XXXY, XXXXY, XXYY /thrē'ekswī, fôr'-ekswī, dob'əleks'dob'əlwī'/, (in genetics) the designation for an abnormal sex chromosome complement in the human male in which there are more than the normal one X chromosome, resulting, respectively, in a total of 48, 49, or more chromosomes in each somatic cell.

XXY syndrome. See **Klinefelter's syndrome.**

XY, (in genetics) the designation for the normal sex chromosome complement in the human male.

xylitol /zī'litôl/, a sweet, crystalline pentahydroxy alcohol obtained by the reduction of xylose and used as an artificial sweetener.

xylometazoline hydrochloride /zī'-lōmetaz'əlēn/, an adrenergic vasoconstrictor prescribed in the treatment of nasal congestion in colds, hay fever, sinusitis, and other upper respiratory allergies.

xylose /zī'lōs/, an aldopentose sugar produced by hydrolyzing straw and corn cobs. It is incompletely absorbed when taken by mouth and is used in diagnostic studies of the digestive tract.

XYY syndrome /eks'dob'əlwī'/, the phenotypic manifestation of an extra Y chromosome, which tends to have a positive effect on height and may have a negative effect on mental and psychologic development. However, the anomaly also occurs in normal males.

Y, symbol for the element **yttrium.**

YACs, abbreviation for **yeast artificial chromosomes.**

yang, a polarized aspect of ch'i that is active or positive energy.

yaw /yô/ [Carib *ïaïa*], a lesion of the syphilis-like tropical disease of yaws. The initial lesion or primary sore is identified as the **mother yaw.**

yawn /yôn/ [AS *geonian*], an involuntary act of opening the mouth wide and taking a deep breath. It tends to occur when a person is bored, drowsy, or depressed and may be accompanied by upper body movements to aid chest expansion.

yaws /yôs/ [Afr *yaw* raspberry], a nonvenereal infection caused by the spirochete *Treponema pertenue,* transmitted by direct contact and characterized by chronic, ulcerating sores anywhere on the body with eventual tissue and bone destruction, leading to crippling if untreated. All serologic tests for syphilis may be positive in yaws.

Yb, symbol for the element **ytterbium.**

Y chromosome, a sex chromosome that in humans and many other species is present only in the male, appearing singly in the normal male. It is carried as a sex determinant by one half of the male gametes and none of the female gametes, is morphologically much smaller than the X chromosome, and has genes associated with triggering the development and differentiation of male characteristics. There are no known medically significant traits or conditions associated with the genes on the Y chromosome.

yeast /yēst/ [AS *gist*], any unicellular, usually oval, nucleated fungus that reproduces by budding. *Candida albicans* is a kind of pathogenic yeast.

yeast artificial chromosomes (YACs), yeast chromosomes used in recombinant DNA procedures. They carry large segments of foreign DNA in the sequencing of nucleic acids.

yellow cartilage [AS *geolu;* L *cartilago*], the most elastic of the three kinds of cartilage, consisting of elastic fibers in a flexible fibrous matrix. It is yellow and is located in various parts of the body, such as the external ear, the auditory tube, the epiglottis, and the larynx.

yellow fever, an acute arbovirus infection transmitted by mosquitoes, characterized by headache, fever, jaundice, vomiting, and bleeding. There is no specific treatment, and mortality is about 5%. Recovery is followed by lifelong immunity.

yellow fever vaccine, a vaccine produced from live, attenuated yellow fever virus grown in chick embryos. It is prescribed for immunization against yellow fever.

yellow marrow. See bone marrow.

Yersinia [Alexandre Emile Jean Yersin, French bacteriologist, b. 1863], a genus of nonmotile ovoid or rod-shaped gramnegative bacteria of the *Enterobacteriaceae* family. The genus includes *Y. pestis,* which causes plague in rats and humans, *Y. enterolitica,* a cause of enterocolitis and other diseases, and *Y. pseudotuberculosis,* a cause of pseudotuberculosis.

Yersinia arthritis /yursin'ē-ə/ [Alexandre E. J. Yersin, French bacteriologist, b. 1863], a polyarticular inflammation occurring a few days to 1 month after the onset of infection caused by *Yersinia enterocolitica* or *Y. pseudotuberculosis* and usually persisting longer than 1 month. Knees, ankles, toes, fingers, and wrists are most often affected. The clinical presentation may mimic juvenile rheumatoid arthritis, rheumatic fever, or Reiter's syndrome.

Yersinia pestis [Alexandre Yersin; L *pestis* plague], a small, gram-negative bacillus that causes plague. The primary host is the rat, but other small rodents also harbor the organism.

Y fracture, a Y-shaped intercondylar fracture.

yin, a polarized aspect of ch'i that is passive or negative energy.

Y-linked, pertaining to genes or to the characteristics or conditions they transmit that are carried on the Y chromosome.

yoga (hatha), a discipline that focuses on the body's musculature, posture, breathing mechanisms, and consciousness. The goal of yoga is attainment of physical and mental well-being.

yogurt [Turk *yoghurt*], a slightly acid, semisolid, curdled milk preparation made from either whole or skimmed cow's milk and milk solids by fermentation with organisms from the genus *Lactobacillus*.

yoke [L *jungere* to join], a connector used to link small cylinders of medical gases, such as portable oxygen tanks, to respiratory equipment.

yolk [AS *geolca*], the nutritive material, rich in fats and proteins, contained in the ovum to supply nourishment to the developing embryo. In humans and most mammals the yolk is absent or greatly diffused through the cell, because embryos absorb nutrients directly from the mother through the placenta.

yolk membrane. See **vitelline membrane.**

yolk sac, a structure that develops in the inner cell mass of the embryo and expands into a vesicle with a thick part that becomes the primitive gut and a thin part that grows into the cavity of the chorion. After supplying the nourishment for the embryo, the yolk sac usually disappears during the seventh week of pregnancy.

yolk sphere. See **morula.**

yolk stalk, the narrow duct connecting the yolk sac with the midgut of the embryo during the early stages of prenatal development.

young and middle adult, the stages of life from 22 to 65 years of age.

Young's rule [Thomas Young, English physician, b. 1773], a method for the calculation of the appropriate dose of a drug for a child 2 years of age or more using the formula (age in years) ÷ (age + 12) × adult dose.

Y-plasty, a method of surgical revision of a scar, using a Y-shaped incision to reduce scar contractures.

Y-set, a device composed of plastic components, used for delivering intravenous fluids through a primary intravenous line connected to a combination drip chamber filter section from which two separate plastic tubes lead to fluid sources. The Y-set also includes three clamps, one for the primary intravenous line and one for each of the two separate tubes. It is often used to transfuse packed blood cells that must be diluted with saline solution to decrease their viscosity.

ytterbium (Yb) /itur'bē·əm/ [Ytterby, Sweden], a rare earth metallic element. Its atomic number is 70; its atomic weight is 173.04.

yttrium (Y) /it'rē·əm/ [Ytterby, Sweden], a scaly, grayish metallic element. Its atomic number is 39; its atomic weight is 88.905. Radioactive isotopes of yttrium have been used in cancer therapy.

Zahorsky's disease. See **roseola infantum.**

Zakrzewski /zakshef'skē/, **Marie** (1829-1902), a Polish-German-American midwife who studied medicine, receiving her medical degree in Cleveland, and organized in 1872 the first successful American school of nursing at the New England Hospital for Women and Children.

zalcitabine the proposed generic name for the antiretroviral drug, **dideoxycytidine (DDC).**

Z chromosome. See **W chromosome and Z chromosome.**

Z disk, a thin membrane seen on longitudinal sections as a dark line in striated muscle. It occurs in the center of an I band, the distance between z bands serving to delimit the striated sarcomeres.

ZEEP, abbreviation for **zero end-expiratory pressure.**

Zenker's diverticulum /tseng'kərz/ [Friedrich A. Zenker, German pathologist, b. 1825; L *diverticulare* to turn aside], a circumscribed herniation of the mucous membrane of the pharynx as it joins the esophagus. Food may become trapped in the diverticulum and may be aspirated.

zeranol /zer'ənol/, an estrogenic substance used to fatten livestock. Consumption of beef from zeranol-treated cattle has been associated with precocious puberty in some boys and girls.

zero [Ar *sifr* cipher], **1.** a symbol for nothing. **2.** the point on most scales from which measurements begin. **3.** absolute zero, the temperature at which there is no molecular movement, corresponds to $-273.15°$ C on the Kelvin scale or $-459.67°$ F.

zero end-expiratory pressure (ZEEP) [Ar *zefiro;* ME *ende*], pressure that has returned to ambient or atmospheric at the end of exhalation.

zero fluid balance, a state in which the amount of fluid intake is equal to the amount of fluid output.

zero order kinetics, a state at which the rate of an enzyme reaction is independent of the concentration of the substrate.

zero population growth (ZPG), a situation in which there is no population increase during a given year because the total of live births is equal to the total of deaths.

zero-to-three infant stimulation groups, groups that provide therapeutic services for children from birth to 3 years of age.

zeta potential [Gk *zeta* sixth letter of Greek alphabet; L *potentia* power], the potential produced by the effective charge of a macromolecule, usually measured at the boundary between what is moving in a solution with the macromolecule and the rest of the solution.

zeugmatography /zoog'mətog'rəfē/ [Gk *zeugnynai* to join, *graphein* to record], another name for MR imaging, suggesting the role of the gradient magnetic field in joining the rf magnetic field to a desired local spatial region through nuclear magnetic resonance.

zidovudine /zīdov'ədēn/, an HIV virus inhibitor, formerly called azidothymidine (AZT), that interferes with DNA synthesis. Trade name is Retrovir.

Ziehl-Neelsen test /zēl'nēl'sən/ [Franz Ziehl, German physician, b. 1859; Friedrich K. A. Neelsen, German pathologist, b. 1854], one of the most widely used methods of acid-fast staining, commonly used in the microscopic examination of a smear of sputum suspected of containing *Mycobacterium tuberculosis.*

Ziehl's stain. See **carbol-fuchsin stain.**

ZIG, abbreviation for **zoster immune globulin.**

zinc (Zn) /zingk/ [Ger *zink*], a bluish white crystalline metal commonly associated with lead ores. Its atomic number is 30; its atomic weight is 65.38. Zinc is an essential nutrient in the body and is used in numerous pharmaceutics, such as zinc oxide.

zinc chill. See **metal fume fever.**

zinc deficiency, a condition resulting from insufficient amounts of zinc in the diet, characterized by abnormal fatigue, decreased alertness, a decrease in taste and odor sensitivity, poor appetite, retarded growth, delayed sexual maturity, prolonged healing of wounds, and susceptibility to infection and injury.

zinc finger, a loop or sequence of transcription factor subunits with a zinc atom linked to four carbon atoms at the base of

1139

a sequence. It is an important step in the cloning and sequencing of human general transcription factors.

zinc gelatin, a topical protectant for varicosities and other lesions of the lower limbs.

zinc ointment [Ger *zink;* OFr *oignement*], a preparation of 20% zinc oxide in mineral oil or a white petrolatum semisolid base, used as a local surface treatment for various skin disorders. Some preparations may also contain salicylic acid.

zinc oxide, a topical protectant prescribed for a wide range of minor skin irritations.

zinc oxide and eugenol (ZOE), a dental cement composed primarily of zinc salts, eugenol, and rosin, used chiefly in temporary tooth fillings. It has low relative strength and abrasion resistance, but its nearly neutral pH causes minimal irritation to dental pulp. It is intended as a sedative dressing until pain subsides and a more permanent filling can be inserted.

zinc oxide eugenol dental cement, a luting agent consisting of a powder that is essentially zinc oxide with strengtheners and accelerators, combined with a liquid that is basically eugenol.

zinc phosphate dental cement, a material for luting of dental inlays, crowns, bridges, and orthodontic appliances and for some temporary restorations of dentitions.

zinc salt poisoning, a toxic condition caused by the ingestion or inhalation of a zinc salt. Symptoms of ingestion include a burning sensation of the mouth and throat, vomiting, diarrhea, abdominal and chest pain, and, in severe cases, shock and coma.

zinc sulfate, an ophthalmic astringent given in drops for nasal congestion or irritation of the eye, applied topically in deodorants, and given orally in tablets to promote healing and as a dietary supplement.

ZIP, abbreviation for *zoster immune plasma.*

zirconium (Zr) /zərkō'nē·əm/ [Ar *zarqun* zircon], a steel-gray, tetravalent metallic element. Its atomic number is 40; its atomic weight is 91.22.

Z line. See Z disk.

Zn, symbol for the element zinc.

zoanthropy /zō·an'thrəpē/ [Gk *zoon* animal, *anthropos* human], the delusion that one has assumed the form and characteristics of an animal. **–zoanthropic,** *adj.*

ZOE, abbreviation for **zinc oxide and eugenol.**

Zollinger-Ellison syndrome /zol'injərel'-isən/ [Robert M. Zollinger, American surgeon, b. 1903; Edwin H. Ellison, American physician, b. 1918], a condition characterized by severe peptic ulceration, gastric hypersecretion, elevated serum gastrin, and gastrinoma of the pancreas or the duodenum.

zona /zō'nə/, *pl.* **zonae** [L; Gk *zone* belt], a zone, or girdlelike segment of a rounded or spheric structure.

zona ciliaris. See **ciliary zone.**

zona fasciculata, the middle portion of the adrenal cortex, which is the site of production of glucocorticoids and sex hormones.

zona glomerulosa, the outer portion of the adrenal cortex, where mineralocorticoids are produced.

zona pellucida /pəloo'sidə/, the thick, transparent, noncellular membrane that encloses the mammalian ovum. It is secreted by the ovum during its development in the ovary and is retained until near the time of implantation.

zona radiata, a zona pellucida that has a striated appearance caused by radiating canals within the membrane.

zona reticularis, the innermost portion of the adrenal cortex, which borders on the adrenal medulla portion of the gland. It acts in consort with the zona fasciculata in producing various sex hormones and glucocorticoids.

zona striata. See **zona radiata.**

Zondek-Aschheim test. See **Aschheim-Zondek test.**

zone [Gk, belt], an area with specific boundaries and characteristics, such as the epigastric, the mesogastric, or hypogastric zones of the abdomen.

zone of equivalence, a region of an antigen-antibody reaction in which concentrations of both reactants are equal.

zonesthesia /zō'nesthē'zhə/ [Gk *zone* + *aisthesis* feeling], a painful sensation of constriction, as of a bandage bound too tightly, especially experienced around the waist or abdomen.

zone therapy, the treatment of a disorder by mechanical stimulation and counterirritation of a body area in the same longitudinal zone as the affected organ or region.

zonifugal /zōnif'yəgəl/ [Gk *zone* + L *fugere* to flee], moving from within a zone or area outward.

zonography /zōnog'rəfē/ [Gk *zone* + *graphein* to record], an x-ray imaging technique used to produce films of body sections similar to those made by tomography.

zonula /zōn'yələ/, *pl.* **zonulae** [Gk *zonule* small belt], a small zone.

zonula adherens [L *zona* + *adhesio* sticking to], a continuous zone running around the outer surface of a cell in which there is an intercellular space of about 200 angstroms' width. A component of the junctional complex between cells, the zone contains dense filamentous material.

zonula ciliaris, a ligament composed of straight fibrils radiating from the ciliary body of the eye to the crystalline lens, holding the lens in place and relaxing by the contraction of the ciliary muscle. Relaxation of the ligament allows the lens to become more convex.

zonula occludens [L *zona* + *occludere* to close up], a component of the junctional complex between cells in which there is no intercellular space and the plasma membranes of adjacent cells are in direct contact.

zoobiology [Gk *zoon* animal, *bios* life, *logos* science], the biology of animals.

zoochemistry [Gk *zoon* + *chemeia* alchemy], the biochemistry of animals.

zooerastia. See **bestiality.**

zoogenous /zō·oj′ənəs/ [Gk *zoon* animal, *genein* to produce], acquired from or originating in animals.

zoograft /zō′əgraft/ [Gk *zoon* + *graphion* stylus], tissue of an animal transplanted to a human, such as a heart valve from a pig to replace a damaged heart valve in a human.

zoologist /zō·ol′əjist/ [Gk *zoon* + *logos* science], a person concerned with the scientific study of animals.

zoology /zō·ol′əjē/, the study of animal life.

zoomania /zō·əmā′nē·ə/ [Gk *zoon* + *mania* madness], a psychopathologic state characterized by an excessive fondness for and preoccupation with animals. **–zoomaniac,** *n.*

zoonosis /zō·on′əsis, zō′ənō′sis/ [Gk *zoon* + *nosis* disease], a disease of animals that is transmissible to humans from its primary animal host. Some kinds of zoonoses are **equine encephalitis, leptospirosis, rabies,** and **yellow fever.**

zooparasite /zō·əper′əsīt/ [Gk *zoon* + *parasitos* guest], any parasitic animal organism. Kinds of zooparasites are **arthropods, protozoa,** and **worms. –zooparasitic,** *adj.*

zoopathology, the study of the diseases of animals.

zoophilia /zō·əfil′ē·ə/ [Gk *zoon* + *philein* to love], **1.** an abnormal fondness for animals. **2.** (in psychiatry) a psychosexual disorder in which sexual excitement and gratification are derived from the fondling of animals or from the fantasy or act of engaging in sexual activity with animals. **–zoophile,** *n.,* **zoophilic, zoophilous,** *adj.*

zoophobia /zōfō′bē·ə/ [Gk *zoon* + *phobos*

fear], an anxiety disorder characterized by a persistent, irrational fear of animals, particularly dogs, snakes, insects, and mice.

zoopsia /zō·op′sē·ə/ [Gk *zoon* + *opsis* vision], a visual hallucination of animals or insects, often occurring in delirium tremens.

zootoxin /zō′ətok′sin/ [Gk *zoon* + *toxikon* poison], a poisonous substance from an animal, such as the venom of snakes, spiders, and scorpions. **–zootoxic,** *adj.*

zoster /zos′tər/. See **herpes zoster.**

zosteriform /zoster′ifôrm/ [Gk *zoster* girdle; L *forma* form], resembling the pocks seen in herpes zoster infection.

zoster immune globulin (ZIG) [Gk *zoster* + L *immunis* freedom; *globulus* small sphere], a passive immunizing agent currently in limited experimental use for preventing or attenuating herpes zoster virus infection in immunosuppressed individuals who are at great risk of severe herpes zoster virus infection.

zoster ophthalmicus [Gk *zoster* + *ophthalmos* eye], a herpes infection of the eye, particularly of the optic nerve. The infection frequently involves the cornea. There may be lid edema, ciliary and conjunctival involvement, and pain. Keratitis may be severe. Scarring and glaucoma are common sequelae. Topical corticosteroids are commonly prescribed and intraocular pressure is monitored.

ZPG, abbreviation for **zero population growth.**

Z-plasty /zē′plas′tē/, a method of surgical revision of a scar or closure of a wound using a Z-shaped incision to reduce contractures of the adjacent skin.

Zr, symbol for the element **zirconium.**

Z-track, a technique for injecting irritating preparations into muscle without tracking residual medication through sensitive tissues.

Zung Self-Rating Depression Scale, a "self-report test" of 20 negatively stated items administered to determine the presence of depression.

zwieback /zwī′bak, zwē′bak/ [Ger *zwie* twice, *backen* to bake], a sweetened bread that is enriched with eggs and baked, then sliced and toasted until dry and crisp. It is used as a snack food for children, especially teething infants.

zwitterion /tvit′əri′ən/, an ion that has regions of both negative and positive charge. Amino acids, such as glycine, may act as zwitterions when in a neutral solution.

zygocyte. See **zygote.**

zygogenesis /zī′gōjen′əsis/ [Gk *zygon* yoke, *genesis* origin], **1.** the formation of a zygote. **2.** reproduction by the union

Z

of gametes. **–zygogenetic, zygogenic,** *adj.*

zygoma /zīgō'mə, zig-/ [Gk *zygon* yoke] **1.** a long slender zygomatic process of the temporal bone, arising from the lower part of the squamous portion of the temporal bone, passing forward to join the zygomatic bone, and forming part of the zygomatic arch. **2.** the zygomatic bone that forms the prominence of the cheek.

zygomatic /zī'gōmat'ik/ [Gk *zygoma* bar], pertaining to the zygoma, or malar bone of the face.

zygomatic arch [Gk *zygoma;* L *arcus* bow], an arch formed by the temporal process of the zygomatic bone with the zygomatic process of the temporal bone. The tendon of the temporal muscle passes beneath it.

zygomatic bone [Gk *zygon; ban*], one of the pair of bones that forms the prominence of the cheek, the lower part of the orbit of the eye, and parts of the temporal and infratemporal fossae.

zygomatic head. See **zygomaticus minor.**

zygomatic process [Gk *zygoma;* L *processus*], **1.** a projection of the frontal bone forming the lateral boundary of the superciliary arch. **2.** a process of the maxilla. **3.** a process of the temporal bone.

zygomatic reflex [Gk *zygoma;* L *reflectere* to bend back], movement of the lower jaw toward the percussed side when the zygoma is tapped lightly but sharply.

zygomaticus major /zī'gōmat'ikəs/, one of the 12 muscles of the mouth. It acts to draw the angle of the mouth up and back to smile or laugh.

zygomaticus minor, one of the 12 muscles of the mouth. It acts to deepen the nasolabial furrow in a sad facial expression.

zygomaxillare. See **key ridge.**

zygomycosis /zī'gōmīkō'sis/ [Gk *zygon + mykes* fungus], an acute, often fulminant and sometimes fatal fungal infection caused by a class of Phycomycetal water molds, seen primarily in patients with chronic debilitating diseases. It begins with fever and with pain and discharge in the nose and paranasal sinuses that

progresses to invade the eye and lower respiratory tract. The fungus may enter blood vessels and spread to the brain and other organs.

zygonema /zī'gənē'mə/ [Gk *zygon + nema* thread], the synaptic chromosome formation that occurs in the zygotene stage of the first meiotic prophase of gametogenesis. **–zygonematic,** *adj.*

zygosis /zīgō'sis/, a form of sexual reproduction in unicellular organisms, consisting of the union of the two cells and fusion of the nuclei. **–zygotic** /zīgot'ik/, *adj.*

zygosity /zīgos'itē/, the characteristics or conditions of a zygote. The form occurs primarily as a suffix combining form to denote genetic makeup, referring specifically as to whether the paired alleles determining a particular trait are identical (homozygosity) or different (heterozygosity).

zygospore /zī'gōspôr'/ [Gk *zygon + sporos* seed], the spore resulting from the conjugation of two isogametes, as in certain fungi and algae.

zygote /zī'gōt/ [Gk *zygon* yoke], (in embryology) the developing ovum from the time it is fertilized until, as a blastocyst, it is implanted in the uterus.

zygotene /zī'gətēn/ [Gk *zygon + tainia* band], the second stage in the first meiotic prophase of gametogenesis in which synapsis of homologous chromosomes occurs.

zymogen granules /zī'məjən/ [Gk *zyme* ferment, *genein* to produce; L *granulum* little grain], granules found in some secretory exocrine cells. They contain the precursors of enzymes that become active after the granules leave the cell.

zymogenic cell. See **chief cell.**

zymoprotein /zīmoprō'ēn/ [Gk *zyme + proteios* first rank], **1.** a yeast protein. **2.** any protein that functions as an enzyme.

zymorphic, zymorphous /zīmôr'fik, zīmôr'fəs/ [Gk *zyme + morphe* form], pertaining to fermentation properties.

Z.Z.'Z'', symbol for increasing strength or intensity of contraction.